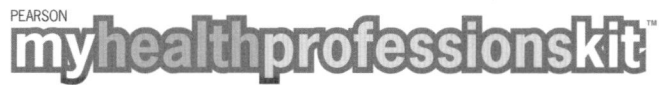

W9-CCN-239

Use the registration code below to gain 12-month access to the online study companion that supports this book. Simply go to this website and follow the registration instructions below. You will find a wealth of opportunities to further your understanding of your course material. Use this website in conjunction with your textbook for a multidimensional learning experience. Enjoy!

STEP 1: Student Registration

1. Go to **www.myhealthprofessionskit.com**.
2. Choose Medical Assisting from the **Select a Discipline** menu.
3. Find this book and click on the cover.
4. Click **Redeem Code**.
5. Using a coin scratch off the silver coating below to reveal your access code. Do not use a knife or other sharp object, which can damage the code.
6. Follow the on-screen instructions to complete registration. Be sure to enter your access code in lowercase or uppercase, without the dashes.

During registration, you will establish a personal login name and password to use for logging into the website. You will also be sent a registration confirmation email that contains your login name and password.

Your Access Code is:

Book cannot be returned once panel is scratched off.
Note: If there is no silver foil covering the access code, it may already have been redeemed, and therefore may no longer be valid. In that case, you can purchase access online using a major credit card. To do so, click **Purchase Code** and follow the on-screen instructions. Or you may order a Standalone Access Card at **www.MyPearsonStore.com** and enter ISBN: 0-13-507956-X.

STEP 2: Log in

Once your have a username and password:
1. Follow Steps 1-3 above under Student Registration and click **Student Login**.
2. Enter the username and password that you created during registration. If unsure of this information, refer to your registration confirmation email.

Instructor Access

1. Follow Steps 1-3 above and **Request Access** by clicking the button at the bottom of the screen.
2. Follow the on-screen instructions. If you already have a Pearson username and password you can link it to this book. If you do not already have a Pearson username and password, you can register here. For further assistance contact your local Pearson representative or call 800-852-4508.

Technical Support

Students: http://247pearsoned.custhelp.com to ask a question, post feedback, or search our knowledgebase for common solutions.
Faculty: 888-433-8435

PEARSON'S
COMPREHENSIVE
MEDICAL ASSISTING

SECOND EDITION

PEARSON'S
COMPREHENSIVE
MEDICAL ASSISTING

Administrative and Clinical Competencies

NINA BEAMAN, MS, RNC, CMA (AAMA)
Bryant and Stratton College
Richmond, VA

LORRAINE FLEMING-McPHILLIPS, MS, MT, CMA (AAMA)
Quinebaug Valley Community College
Danielson, CT

KRISTIANA SUE ROUTH, RMA, CHI
Allied Health Consulting Services
Girard, PA

ROBYN GOHSMAN, RMA, CMAS
Riverside Health System
Newport News, VA

STACIA REAGAN, CMA (AAMA), BA
Spokane Community College
Spokane, WA

Pearson

Boston   Columbus   Indianapolis   New York   San Francisco   Upper Saddle River
Amsterdam   Cape Town   Dubai   London   Madrid   Milan   Munich   Paris
Montreal   Toronto   Delhi   Mexico City   São Paulo   Sydney
Hong Kong   Seoul   Singapore   Taipei   Tokyo

Library of Congress Cataloging-in-Publication Data

Beaman, Nina.
    Pearson's comprehensive medical assisting: administrative and clinical competencies/Nina Beaman,
Lorraine Fleming-McPhillips.—2nd ed.
    p.; cm.
    Includes index.
    ISBN-13: 978-0-13-500883-6
    ISBN-10: 0-13-500883-2
  1. Medical assistants.   2. Medical secretaries.   3. Medical offices—Management.   I. Fleming-McPhillips, Lorraine.
II. Title.   III. Title: Comprehensive medical assisting.
    [DNLM: 1. Physician Assistants.   2. Medical Secretaries.   3. Practice Management, Medical.   W 21.5 B366p 2011]
    R728.8.B425 2011
    610.73'7—dc22

                                                                                                    2009040673

Publisher: Julie Levin Alexander
Publisher's Assistant: Regina Bruno
Editor-in-Chief: Mark Cohen
Executive Editor: Joan Gill
Associate Editor: Bronwen Glowacki
Editorial Assistant: Mary Ellen Ruitenberg
Development Editor: Teri Zak
Director of Marketing: Dave Gesell
Senior Marketing Manager: Harper Coles
Marketing Specialist: Michael Sirinides
Marketing Assistant: Judy Noh
Managing Production Editor: Patrick Walsh
Production Liaison: Julie Boddorf

Production Editor: Kelly Ricci
Manufacturing Manager: Ilene Sanford
Manufacturing Buyer: Pat Brown
Art Director: Miguel Ortiz
Interior Designer: Candace Rowley, cfishdesign
Cover Designer: Candace Rowley, cfishdesign
Director, Image Resource Center: Melinda Reo
Manager, Rights and Permissions: Zina Arabia
Manager, Visual Research: Beth Brenzel
Manager, Cover Visual Research and Permissions: Nancy Seise
Composition: Aptara®, Inc.
Printing and Binding: Courier Kendallville
Cover Printer: Lehigh-Phoenix Color

10 9 8 7 6 5 4 3

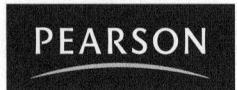
www.pearsonhighered.com

ISBN 13: 978-0-13-500883-6
ISBN 10:   0-13-500883-2

Brief Contents

Contents

UNIT ONE Introduction to Health Care 1

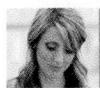

UNIT TWO   Administrative Medical Assisting   157

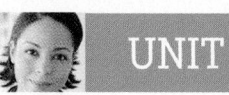

UNIT FOUR   Clinical Medical Assisting   651

CHAPTER 36

Assisting with Physical Examinations   730

CHAPTER 37

Assisting with Medical Specialties   762

CHAPTER 38

Assisting with Reproductive and Urinary Specialties   798

CHAPTER 39

Assisting with Eye and Ear Care   828

CHAPTER 40

Assisting with Life Span Specialties: Pediatrics 852

CHAPTER 41

Assisting with Life Span Specialties: Geriatrics 878

CHAPTER 42

Assisting with Minor Surgery 900

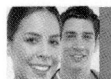

UNIT FIVE   Career Assistance   1329

Procedures

Supplements Package

Title	Student Ancillary	Instructor Ancillary	Product Type	What is it?
Medical Assisting Videos	✓	✓	DVD in the back of the book	Videos showing both psychomotor and affective skills
Workbook	✓		Printed book	Weighted Competency Checklists, note-taking activities, hands-on activities, quizzes, and critical thinking exercises
MyHealthProfessionsKit (for students) myhealthprofessionskit	✓		Web site (access code in front of book)	www.MyHealthProfessionsKit.com Charting and Scheduling activities, A & P activities, critical thinking activities, Games and Links and much, much, more
E-book	✓	✓	Web Access	Media-enriched e-text
Instructor's Resource Manual		✓	Printed book	Chapter objectives and outlines; general chapter information, answers to in-text exercises
Instructor's Resource CD-ROM		✓	CD in the back of the IRM	Lesson Plans PowerPoint Presentations Classroom Response PowerPoint Presentation Image Library TestGen Answers to Workbook Exercises
PowerPoint Slides		✓	On the CD in back of IRM; MyKit	Lecture Notes—coordinate with the lesson plans Classroom Response System Image Library
TestGen		✓	On the CD in back of IRM; MyKit	More than 5000 questions
Lesson Plans		✓	On the CD in back of IRM; MyKit	Detailed lesson outlines for each chapter.
Teacher's Wrap-Around Edition		✓	Printed book	The actual textbook with lecture notes and hints written on the pages
CourseConnect	✓	✓	Web Access	Sample of Textbook online
Electronic Gradebook		✓	Web Access	Electronic grader for weighted competency checklists
MyHealthProfessionsKit (for instructors) myhealthprofessionskit		✓	Web Access	One stop shopping for all your Pearson resources
Medical Assisting Interactive	✓	✓	Web Access or CD-ROM	A hands-on, virtual doctor's office with patient-driven medical assisting scenarios emphasizing the major skills and procedures required by all entry level Medical Assistants
Mock Clinic		✓	CD-ROM	Printable patient files and forms to create a "mock clinic" right in the classroom

Preface

Medical Assistants connect with people every hour of every day. They are the first line of medical care for many patients. Their clinical and administrative skills must be finely honed, and they must have thorough knowledge of both procedures and also every body system. But mainly, they must make every patient in a physician's office feel secure. They must comfort. They must explain. They must listen. They must demonstrate techniques. Medical Assistants help every patient feel like the only patient.

Pearson's Comprehensive Medical Assisting has set out on a journey to speak directly to the student, because, after all, it is the student who will need to effectively reach the patient.

Pearson's Comprehensive Medical Assisting, 2e is all about people, skills, and attitudes. This new edition of the successful text, carries even further the idea that the Medical Assistant is the vital link between people, their personal health and medical well-being. The concepts and ideas of the first edition have been finely tuned and expanded in this new second edition. The themes of professionalism and people skills run throughout the text and almost every special feature is designed and written to enhance the student's knowledge and demonstration of professionalism in the workplace. Skill building is also emphasized, with skills and procedures included in the text.

New to the Edition

In addition to enhancing the fundamental themes of professionalism and skill building, many changes and updates to the new text were also made. *Pearson's Comprehensive Medical Assisting, 2e* now covers over 175 key skills and procedures. Other updates and changes include:

New Chapters

- Chapter 4 Medical Terminology
- Chapter 14 Electronic Health Records
- Chapter 58 Professionalism
- Chapter 37 Assisting with Medical Specialties
- Chapter 38 Assisting with Reproductive and Urinary Specialties
- Chapter 40 Assisting with Life Span Specialties: Pediatrics
- Chapter 41 Assisting with Life Span Specialties: Geriatrics

- Chapter 49 Electrocardiography
- Chapter 50 Pulmonary Function

New Features

- Certification Link—chart of topics covered in the chapter that will be found on the CMA (AAMA), RMA, and CMAS examinations
- New Case Studies—placed at the beginning of each chapter
- Professionalism: The Workplace—provides short tips for the workplace
- Judgment Call—presents an ethical issue or dilemma and one critical thinking question

End-of-Chapter

- All new Preparing for the Certification Examination questions

Content Additions and Enhancements

- The new format for the Common Disorders sections of the anatomy and physiology and medical specialties chapters consists of a description of the condition followed by "Signs and Symptoms" and "Treatment" headings. More information related to pathology and pharmacology is also provided.
- Chapter 43 Assisting with Medical Emergencies and Emergency Preparedness includes a new Emergency Preparedness section on natural disasters such as earthquakes, tornados, fires, floods, hurricanes, and terrorism.
- Chapter 34 Infection Control and Asepsis includes new material on multidrug resistant organisms and bioterrorism.
- Additional HIPAA-related material has been provided when appropriate in each chapter.

Organization

The text is organized into 5 sections. **Introduction to Health Care** is the first section, covering information about the history of health care, the professional medical assistant, medical law and ethics, medical terminology, and communications. **Administrative Medical Assisting** addresses all the front office topics like medical billing and coding, reception, scheduling, electronic health records, and much, much more. **Anatomy and Physiology** covers the structure, function, and diseases of the human body systems. **Clinical Medical Assisting** deals with all those procedures and techniques that occur in the back office of the clinic, including examinations, vital signs, administering medications, phlebotomy, lab techniques, testing, and other medical procedures. **Career Assistance** focuses on professionalism and those skills the new medical assistant will need, to obtain a position in a medical office.

A Commitment to Accuracy

Finally, we were repeatedly reminded about the importance of ensuring complete accuracy in the content of the book and all ancillary resources. It was important to us to attain the highest level of accuracy possible throughout this educational program in order to match the requirement for precision in today's health care environment. To this end, our thorough manuscript review process charged members of our development team to read every page, every test question, and every vocabulary word. Content experts have read each chapter for accuracy and analyzed every bit of content that comprises the ancillary resources. While our intent and actions have been directed at creating an error-free text, it is still possible for some mistakes to occur. Pearson Education takes this issue seriously and therefore welcomes any and all feedback that you can provide along the lines of helping us enhance the accuracy of this text. If you identify any errors that need to be corrected in a subsequent printing, please send them to:

Pearson Health Science Editorial; Medical Assisting Corrections; 1 Lake St.; Upper Saddle River, NJ 07458.

Reviewers

The invaluable editorial advice and direction provided by the following educators and health care professionals is deeply appreciated:

Cindy Abel, BS, CMA (AAMA), Pbt
Program Chair
Ivy Tech Community College
Lafayette, IN

Kendra Allen, LPN
Program Manager Healthcare Office
   Technologies
Ohio Institute of Health Careers
Columbus, OH

Michaelann M. Allen, MA.Ed, CMA (AAMA)
Medical Assisting Program Director
North Seattle Community College
Seattle, WA

Peter F. Andrus, MD
Instructor
Bryant and Stratton College
Albany, NY

Yvonne Denise Arnold-Jenkins, NRCMA
Instructor
Remington College
Garland, TX

James Baird, MBA, CAHI
Medical Program Director
Computer Career Center
El Paso, TX

Jennifer Barr, MT, M.Ed., CMA (AAMA)
Chairperson, Medical Assisting Technology
Sinclair Community College
Dayton, OH

Sue Beaman, RN
Wayne Community College
Goldsboro, NC

Julie A. Benson, AAS, RMA. R. Phbt
Medical Assistant and Phlebotomy
   Program Chair
Oklahoma Health Academy
Tulsa, OK

Tricia Berry, MATL, OTR/L
Assistant Dean of Clinical Placement
Kaplan University
Ft. Lauderdale, FL

Suzanne Bitters, RMA-NCPT/NCICS
Program Manager
Harris School of Business
Wilmington, DE

Lou Brown, MT (ASCP), CMA (AAMA)
Medical Assisting Program Director
Wayne Community College
Goldsboro, NC

Minda Brown, RMA
Pima Medical Institute
Colorado Springs, CO

Beth A. Buchholz, CMA (AAMA), BS
Medical Assistant Program Director
Wichita Area Technical College
Wichita, KS

Caren Burford-Henry, NRCMA, CMBS, CCA
Medical Insurance and Coding Program
   Chair
Remington College
Garland, TX

Cara Carreon, BS, RRT, CMA (AAMA), CPC
Faculty
Ivy Tech Community College
Lafayette, IN

Denise Carsillo, MS, BS, RMA
Associate Dean
Lincoln College of Technology
West Palm Beach, FL

Lisa Cook, CMA (AAMA)
Medical Assisting Education Program
   Chair
Bryman College
Port Orchard, WA

Janie Corbitt, RN, BSL
Central Georgia Technical College
Milledgeville, GA

Bonnie J. Crist, BS, AAS, CMA (AAMA)
Medical Program Chair and Coordinator
Harrison College
Indianapolis, IN

Anita Denson, CMA (AAMA)
Director of Health Care Education
National College of Business & Technology
Danville, KY

Susan DeGirolamo, AAH, RMA, NCPT, NCICS, NCMHT
Instructor
Pennsylvania Institute of Technology
Media, PA

Hany Eissa, MD
Medical Assisting Program Director
South University
Savannah, GA

Cassandra R. Farris, BS, RMA
Former Director of Medical Programs
Vatterott College
Joplin, MO

George Fakhoury, MD, DORCP, CMA (AAMA)
Academic Program Manager Healthcare
Heald College's Central Administrative
   Office
San Francisco, CA

Suzanne Feathers, CMA (AAMA), EMT
Medical Program Coordinator
YTI Career Institute
Altoona, PA

Pamela Fleming, RN, CMA (AAMA), MPA
Professor
Quinsigamond Community College
Worcester, MA

Cheryl Garman, RN
Assistant Academic Dean
Berks Technical Institute
Wyomissing, PA

Beverley Giteles, CPC, CMM
Instructor
Gibbs College
Livingston, NJ

Wendy Hall-Campbell, ADN
Medical Assisting Program Director
Concorde Career Institute
Portland, OR

Carrie Hammond, CMA (AAMA)
Medical Assisting Program Director
Utah Career College
West Jordan, UT

Jessica Hart, CMA (AAMA)
Director of Healthcare Education
National College
Lexington, KY

Marsha Perkins Hemby, RN, CMA
(AAMA)
Medical Assisting Department Chair
Pitt Community College
Greenville, NC

Elizabeth Henisse, BAS, MA
Allied Health Program Director
Florida Metropolitan University
Orlando, FL

Jessica Holtsberry
HIT Program Instructor
Ohio Institute of Health Careers
Columbus, OH

Marsha M. Holtsberry, CMA (AAMA)
HOT Program Director
Ohio Institute of Health Careers
Columbus, OH

Susan Horn, AAS, CMA (AAMA)
Medical Program Coordinator
Harrison College
Lafayette, IN

Demetria Jackson
Former Program Director
Virginia College
Birmingham, AL

Shirley Jelmo, CMA (AAMA)
Faculty Coordinator
Pima Medical Institute
Colorado Springs, CO

Linda L. Kennedy, MBA, CMA
(AAMA)
Program Director Medical Assisting
Everest University
Largo, FL

Amy Knight, CMA (AAMA)
Allied Health Instructor
Remington College
Largo, FL

Holly A. Lincoln, BA
Academic Coordinator
St. Louis College of Health Careers
Fenton, MO

Marta Lopez, LM, CPM
Medical Assisting Program Coordinator
Miami Dade College
Miami, FL

Paul Lucas, CMA (AAMA), CPbt,
PN, AS
Program Director Medical Assisting
Brown Mackie College
Fort Wayne, IN

Tabitha Lyons, AS, NCMA
Corporate Medical Assistant Program
Manager
High-Tech Institute
Phoenix, AZ

Alice Macomber, RN, RMA, RPT,
BXP, AHI, CPI
Medical Assisting Program Coordinator
Keiser University
Port Saint Lucie, FL

Mary M. Marks, MSN, RN-BC,
Pbt (ASCP)
Program Coordinator
Mitchell Community College
Mooresville, NC

Natalie McBride, CMA (AAMA)
Instructor
ICM School of Business & Medical Careers
Pittsburgh, PA

DeLeesa G. Meashintubby, BS, CMA
(AAMA), RMA
MOA/HRT Program Coordinator
Lane Community College
Eugene, OR

Tanya Mercer, BS, RN, RMA
Curriculum Specialist
KAPLAN Higher Education
Rowell, GA

Kelly Miller, MPH, CHES, CST, RMA
Allied Health Department Chair
Remington College
Nashville, TN

Lisa Nagle, BS.Ed., CMA (AAMA)
Medical Assisting Program Director
Augusta Technical College
Augusta, GA

Kay Nave, CMA (AAMA), MRT
Medical Assisting Program Director
Kaplan University
Hagerstown, MD

Michelle Newman, LPN
Instructor
Florida Career College
Riverview, FL

Lisa K. Nicewarner
Program Director Medical Office
Administration
Vatterott College
O'Fallon, MO

Marion D. Odom, NCMA
Medical Assisting Department
Chairperson
Illinois School of Health Careers
Chicago, IL

Kathleen M. Olewinski, MS, RHIA,
NHA, FACHE
Medical Assisting Program Director
Bryant and Stratton College
East Milwaukee, WI

Everlee O'Nan, RMA
Director of Health Care Education
National College
Florence, KY

Karen Patrick, NCMA, CPI
Director
CAPPS College
Dothan, AL

Diane Peavy, RN, ASN, AHI
Director of Educational Services
Capps College
Foley, AL

Sonya Phipps, BA, MBA
Instructor
Everest College
Fort Worth, TX

Christina Rauberts-Conklin, AA, RMA
Medical Department Chair
Everest University
Tampa, FL

Deanna T. Rieke, BSRN, MSHA
Program Director
Montana State University—Billings
    College of Technology
Billings, MT

Jim Rocco, MS, CAHI, RMA, COLT,
    RPT, CPI, CEI, CPCI, CPhT
PCT Program Chair
Illinois School of Health Careers
Chicago, IL

Susan Saullo, RN, MS, MT (ASCP)
Medical Assisting Program Coordinator
Webster College
Ocala, FL

Wandagayle Sciambi, LPN, CMA
    (AAMA)
National Director of Medical Programs
Educational Affiliates
Baltimore, MD

Kristen Schoville, RN/BSN
Medical Assistant Instructor
Southwest Wisconsin Technical College
Fennimore, WI

Lory Lee Serrato, CCS-P
Everest College
Springfield, MO

Janet Sesser, RMA, CMA (AAMA), BS
    Ed.Admin.
Corporate Director of Education
Chubb Institute
Phoenix, AZ

Gary Shandrew, MSIA
Campus Director
Certified Careers Institute
Clearfield, UT

Maria L. Simard, LVN
Director of Allied Health Programs
Kaplan College
San Diego, CA

Lynn Slack, CMA (AAMA)
Medical Programs Director
Kaplan Career Institute
Pittsburgh, PA

Richard Snyder
Director of Medical Assisting Program
Kaplan University
Hagerstown, MD

Peggy Smith, MEd
Medical Assisting Program Director
Marion Technical College
Marion, OH

Sherry Stanfield, RN, BSN, MS
Assistant Program Director, Medical
    Assisting
Miller-Motte Technical College
North Charleston, SC

Lisa Stephens, CMA (AAMA), AAS
Medical Assisting Program Director
Kaplan College
Indianapolis, IN

Donna Lee Stevenson, LPN, BA
Allied Health Department Chair
Remington College
Largo, FL

Pollyanna Strunk, RN, BSN
Lead Medical Instructor
Daymar College
Louisville, KY

Deborah Sulkowski, CMA (AAMA)
Medical Department Chair
Pittsburgh Technical Institute
Oakdale, PA

Pamela H. Swann, RN
Assistant Program Director, Medical
    Assisting Department
Virginia College
Pensacola, FL

Dr. Ruth Torres, MD, MA
Medical Instructor
Harrison College
Terre Haute, IN

Drew D. Totten, BA, NRCMA
Director of Education
Charter College
Canyon Country, CA

Wendi Walker, RN, MSN
Medical Assisting Lead Instructor
Draughons Junior College
Murfreesboro, TN

Angela Woodson, RMA
Medical Assistant Program Director
Virginia College
Montgomery, AL

Lisa Wright, MS, CMA (AAMA), MT
    (ASCP), SH
Medical Assisting Program Coordinator
Bristol Community College
Fall River, MA

Carole A. Zeglin, MS, BS, RMA
Director of Medical Assisting Program
Westmoreland County Community
    College
Youngwood, PA

About the Authors

Nina Beaman, MS, RNC, CMA (AAMA)

Nina Beaman has been a Certified Medical Assistant since 1994 and has participated actively on the local, state, and national levels of the American Association of Medical Assistants. She is also a dually-certified Registered Nurse with certifications in Psychiatric/Mental Health and Ambulatory Women's Health. She is completing her doctoral dissertation at Walden University in using simulation for teaching disaster mitigation to medical assisting students. Nina has been Allied Health Program Director of Bryant & Stratton College's Richmond, Virginia campus since 1993. She recently was appointed Program Director for Nursing on the same campus. A popular speaker and author, she writes on her farm in the Shenandoah Valley of Virginia. In her spare time, she works as a forensic nurse consultant with the Nelson County Sheriff's department on violence and substance abuse prevention education and behavioral profiling.

Lorraine Fleming-McPhillips, MS, MT (ASCP), CMA (AAMA)

Lorrie, as she is known to family and friends, graduated with High Honors from the University of Connecticut with a BA in Medical Technology. She earned her registration from the American Society of Clinical Pathologists and maintains that registration currently. Lorrie worked at a number of hospitals and private clinical laboratories as a general medical technologist for 11 years before beginning as a medical assisting teacher. In 1995 she graduated from the University of Connecticut with a MS in Allied Health focusing on education and research and was elected to Phi Kappa Phi National Honor Society. She established a medical assisting program at Quinebaug Valley Community College in Connecticut, accredited by the CAAHEP. As program chair she created other allied health programs, namely phlebotomy, health information management, coding specialist, and an Allied Health Certificate program. Lorrie has been a member of AAMA since 1992 and has maintained active certifi-

cation since then. She served the organization on local and state levels in Connecticut, including state president. Currently Lorrie serves as a member of the Advisory Board for the Medical Assisting Program at Indian River State College, Fort Pierce, Florida. Lorrie is married and has four children, three step children and 17 grandchildren. She resides in Florida and spends summers in Connecticut at a small summer cottage with her husband Norman.

Kristiana Sue Routh, RMA, CHI

Kristiana Routh is a Registered Medical Assistant and a Certified Healthcare Instructor. She owns her own business, Allied Health Consulting Services, which specializes in consulting with allied health education programs and physician groups, as well as the general health care industry. Kristiana is very passionate about both her work and her faith. She is actively involved with children's ministry and outreach teams at her home church. Kristiana resides near Erie, PA with her husband and daughter.

Robyn Gohsman, RMA, CMAS

Robyn Gohsman graduated from Delta College in 1997 with a degree in medical assisting. Robyn started as a medical receptionist in an Ob/Gyn office, and within a year had moved into the Clinical Coordinator position. During that time, she worked closely with a local vocational medical assisting program's extern students. She found mentoring and teaching these students very rewarding and fulfilling. In 2002 Robyn accepted the position of Medical Assisting Program Director for that same vocational school. From 2002 through 2008 Robyn shared her love of the medical assisting profession with her students while at the same time emphasizing that we must treat our patients and their families as we, ourselves, would want to be treated. In 2008 Robyn accepted the position of Special Projects Coordinator with Riverside Health System, where she is currently helping lead Riverside toward CPOE (Computerized Physician Order Entry) and has been responsible for helping develop evidence-based physician orders. Robyn, her husband Terry, and their son Travis reside in Virginia.

Stacia Reagan, CMA (AAMA), BA

Stacia Marie Reagan serves as the program director for Spokane Community College and is a tenured instructor in Spokane, Washington. Before entering the education field, Stacia was the medical assistant for Dr. Richard Lambert and remains passionate about pulmonary medicine. Stacia is an active member of the Greater Spokane Chapter of the American Association of Medical Assistants. Raised in Craig, Alaska, Stacia was greatly inspired by her biology and chemistry instructor, Cheryl Fecko. Stacia is completing her final quarter for her Master's degree at Eastern Washington University.

Acknowledgments

Cover Photo Credits

Thomas Barwick/Getty Images Inc./Riser

Professionalism Features Credits

iStockphoto.com; Pawel Strykowski\Shutterstock; Image Source\Superstock Royalty Free

Interior Photo Credits

Allscripts LLC, 280; American Association of Medical Assistants, 5; © 1972–2004 American College of Rheumatology Clinical Slide Collection. Used with permission, 467; Bartee Photgraphy Inc./Pearson Education/PH College, 38 (BL); Thomas Barwick/Getty Images/Digital Vision, 1; © K. Beebe/Custom Medical Stock Photo, 425; Birn/Custom Medical Stock Photo, Inc., 1012 (BR); Dr. Klaus Boller/Photo Researchers, Inc., 1004 (TR); © R. Calentine/Visuals Unlimited, 1005 (BR); Cardiac Science, 1151 (BR); CNRI/Photo Researchers, Inc., 1093; Stewart Cohen/Getty Images Inc. - Stone Allstock, 31 (BR); Corbis RF, 38 (BR); JIM CUMMINS/Getty Images, Inc. - Taxi, 1315 (BR); Custom Medical Stock Photo, Inc., 1145 (MR); Custom Medical Stock Photo/Newscom, 1023; James Darell/Getty Images Inc. - Stone Allstock, 1323; George Dodson/Pearson Education/PH College, 1313; Michael Donne/Photo Researchers, Inc., 276; Elena Dorfman, 785; © Dorling Kindersley, 435, 530, 531, 982, 1005 (TR), 1087; George Draper/Pearson Education/PH College, 702, 705; Laura Dwight/Laura Dwight Photography, 1315 (BL); Laura Elliott/Jupiter Images Royalty Free, 1315 (TL); EMG Education Management Group, 23; Denis Finnin and Jackie Beckett © The American Museum of Natural History, 1002, 1005 (TL); Mike Gallitelli/Pearson Education/PH College, 951; Getty Images, Inc. - Photodisc./Royalty Free, 1281; © Eric Grave/Phototake, 1004 (TL); Will Hart, 1319 (BR); Michal Heron/Pearson Education/PH College, 6, 33, 34, 35, 53, 62, 66, 100, 108, 111, 125, 126, 127, 128, 132, 133, 139, 143, 144, 169, 171, 200, 218, 225, 238, 250, 258, 264, 289, 293, 300, 304, 361, 374, 378, 380, 399, 400, 403, 662, 663, 670, 672, 675, 692, 703, 704, 710, 722, 755, 840, 861, 891, 892, 941, 945, 946, 947, 948, 950, 960, 961, 967, 983, 984, 1013, 1017, 1024, 1037, 1039, 1045, 1046, 1070, 1136, 1149, 1151 (TR), 1183, 1209, 1233, 1235, 1239, 1241, 1280, 1318, 1324, 1334, 1335; Image Source/Getty Images Inc. - Image Source Royalty Free, 415; ImpactMD Document Scanner. Photo courtesy of Allscripts LLC, 278; IQmark™ Advanced Holter. Photo courtesy of Midmark Diagnostics Group, 277; IQMark™ Digital Spirometer. Photo Courtesy of Midmark Diagnostics Group, 281; iStockphoto.com, 157; Dennis Kunkel/Phototake NYC, 1003 (TL); Richard Lord/The Image Works, 1321; Dick Luria/Photo Researchers, Inc., 1145 (ML); David Mager/Pearson Learning Photo Studio, 31 (TL); Dylan Malone/Pearson Education/PH College; Dr. P. Marazzi/Photo Researchers, Inc., 542; David Matsumoto and Paul Ekman, www.PaulEkman.com, 1318; The Medical File, Inc., 32; Meridian Bioscience, Inc., 1022; Moredun Animal Health Ltd./Photo Researchers, Inc., 1003 (BR); National Library of Medicine, 21; Tony Neste/Anthony Neste, 725; Courtesy of Nonin Medical, Inc., 1152; Faye Norman/Photo Researchers, Inc.; Nova Biomedical, 240; Jim Olive/Peter Arnold, Inc., 26; Art Overlay/Pearson Education/PH College, 956, 999; Tom Pantages, 698; Pearson Education/PH College, 40, 151, 259, 1005 (BL); R. Spencer Phippen/Phototake NYC, 542; Chris Priest/Science Photo Library/Photo Researchers, Inc., 236; Peter_Purdy/Getty Images Inc. - Hulton Archive Photos, 25; Science Heritage/Custom Medical Stock Photo, Inc., 1012 (TR); Science Photo Library/Photo Researchers, Inc., 1137; A.M. Siegelman/Visuals Unlimited, 1000; Justin Slide © Dorling Kindersley, 1319 (BL); Jeffrey Smith/iStockphoto.com, 651; Verity Smith/Jupiter Images - PictureArts Corporation/Brand X Pictures Royalty Free, 1229; SUI/Photo Researchers, Inc., 766; William Taufic/CORBIS - NY, 314; Sheila Terry/Photo Researchers, Inc., 22; Courtesy of 3M Medical Division - 3M Health Care, 704; Jim Varney/Photo Researchers, Inc., 1010; Brian Warling/Pearson Education/PH College, 374; James Wilson/Woodfin Camp & Associates, Inc., 1314; John Woodcock © Dorling Kindersley, 517

Illustration Credits

All illustrations created by Imagineering for Prentice Hall unless listed. Berman, *Skills in Clinical Nursing,* 6/e, 664, 665, 705 (B), 718 (BR), 721, 773 (B), 791, 848, 1034, 1154; Ellis: *EKG Plain and Simple,* 2/e, 1127 (B), 1128, 1137 (T); Frazier, Malone: *Medical Assisting: Foundations and Practices,* 1/e, 109 (TL), 283, 342, 946, 947, 966 (L and R); Frazier, Morgan: *Clinical Medical Assisting: Foundations and Practice,* 1/e, 701, 733, 735, 864, 953, 957, 1118–1119, 1121; Fremgen & Frecht: *Medical Terminology: A Living Language,* 3/e, 428, 772, 780, 786; Garza, Becan-McBride: *Phlebotomy Handbook: Blood Specimen Collection from Basic to Advanced,* 8/e, 985, 988; Kozier & Erb: *Fundamentals of Nursing,* 8/e, 1113; Malone: *Administrative Medical Assisting: Foundations and Practices,* 1/e, 55, 56, 276, 278, 280, 281; Rice: *Medical Terminology: A Word-Building Approach,* 6/e, 87, 437, 455, 460 (T), 464, 478 (T), 479, 480, 490, 496, 500, 501, 502, 794, 811, 812, 815, 818, 822, 824, 1115; Turley: *Medical Language,* 1/e, 865, 1034; Vines: *Comprehensive Health Insurance: Billing, Coding and Reimbursement,* 1/e, 72, 168, 357, 358, 364; Walraven: *Basic Arrhythmias,* 6/e, 1114, 1116, 1117, 1124, 1125, 1127 (T), 1129, 1130–1132, 1137 (B), 1139; Wolgin: *Being a Nursing Assistant,* 9/e: 783 (R)

Successful Connections

Chapter Opener Features

The chapter opener highlights some of the most important aspects of the chapter.

LEARNING OBJECTIVES
focus students on what they should get out of the chapter.

CHAPTER OUTLINE
guides students through the topics of the chapter.

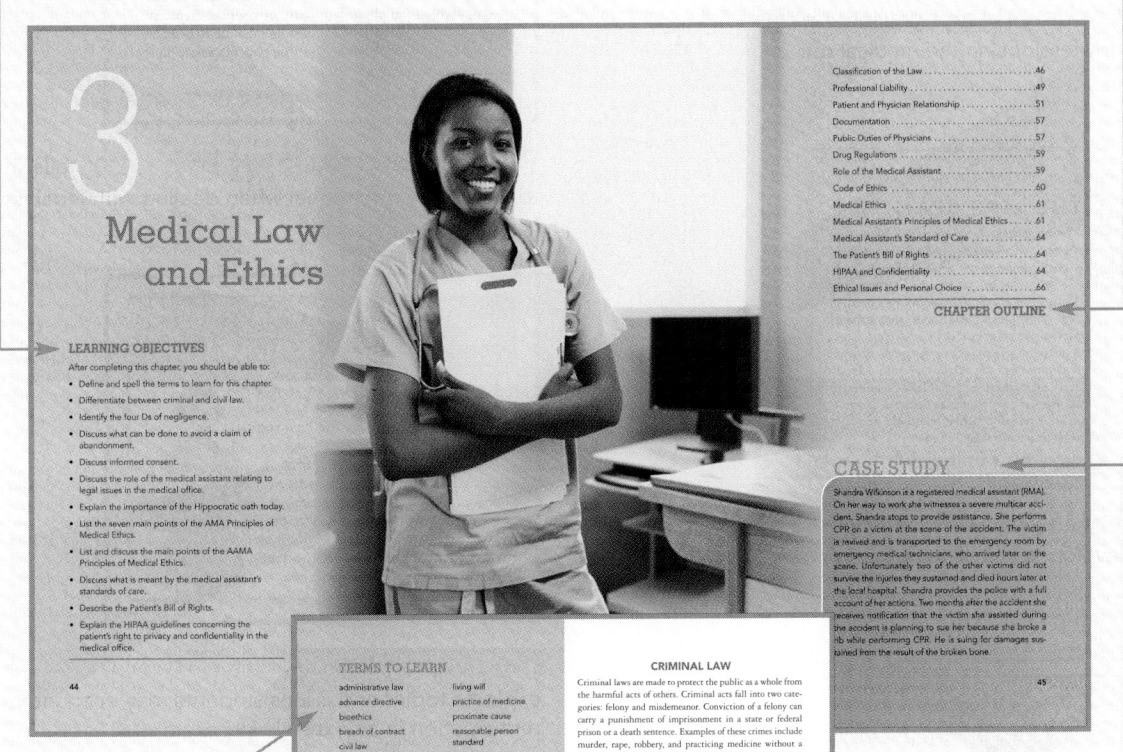

TERMS TO LEARN
present key words and concepts that are highlighted the first time they appear in the chapter.

CERTIFICATION LINK
connects chapter content to the CMA (AAMA), RMA, and CMAS (AMT) certification exams.

CASE STUDIES
give brief scenarios that help students understand how the chapter information relates to their careers. Questions at the end of the chapter refer back to the case study, providing a critical thinking opportunity.

Special Features

The features in this book focus on professionalism and highlight special topics for students. These help students connect the importance of adopting and maintaining a professional demeanor with success on the job.

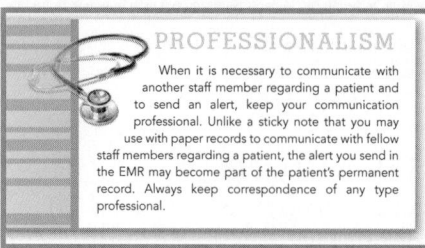

PROFESSIONALISM
When it is necessary to communicate with another staff member regarding a patient and to send an alert, keep your communication professional. Unlike a sticky note that you may use with paper records to communicate with fellow staff members regarding a patient, the alert you send in the EMR may become part of the patient's permanent record. Always keep correspondence of any type professional.

PROFESSIONALISM provides tips for how to be professional in the medical office.

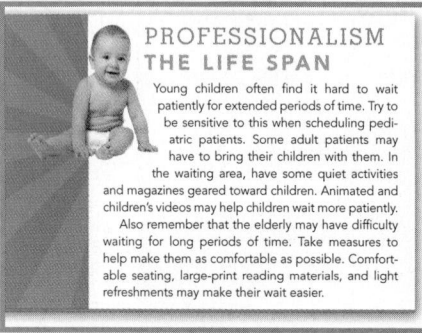

PROFESSIONALISM THE LIFE SPAN
Young children often find it hard to wait patiently for extended periods of time. Try to be sensitive to this when scheduling pediatric patients. Some adult patients may have to bring their children in with them. In the waiting area, have some quiet activities and magazines geared toward children. Animated and children's videos may help children wait more patiently. Also remember that the elderly may have difficulty waiting for long periods of time. Take measures to help make them as comfortable as possible. Comfortable seating, large-print reading materials, and light refreshments may make their wait easier.

PROFESSIONALISM: THE LIFESPAN helps students develop the skills to relate to patients of all ages.

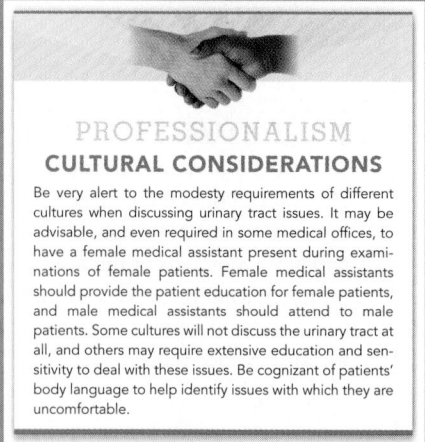

PROFESSIONALISM CULTURAL CONSIDERATIONS
Be very alert to the modesty requirements of different cultures when discussing urinary tract issues. It may be advisable, and even required in some medical offices, to have a female medical assistant present during examinations of female patients. Female medical assistants should provide the patient education for female patients, and male medical assistants should attend to male patients. Some cultures will not discuss the urinary tract at all, and others may require extensive education and sensitivity to deal with these issues. Be cognizant of patients' body language to help identify issues with which they are uncomfortable.

PROFESSIONALISM: CULTURAL CONSIDERATIONS give students the skills to connect with both patients and other health professionals from diverse backgrounds.

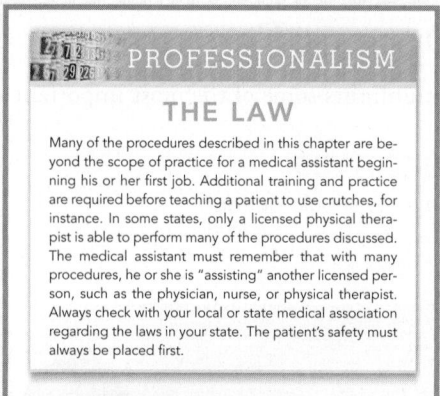

PROFESSIONALISM THE LAW
Many of the procedures described in this chapter are beyond the scope of practice for a medical assistant beginning his or her first job. Additional training and practice are required before teaching a patient to use crutches, for instance. In some states, only a licensed physical therapist is able to perform many of the procedures discussed. The medical assistant must remember that with many procedures, he or she is "assisting" another licensed person, such as the physician, nurse, or physical therapist. Always check with your local or state medical association regarding the laws in your state. The patient's safety must always be placed first.

PROFESSIONALISM: THE LAW tells students how to act like a professional when dealing with legal issues.

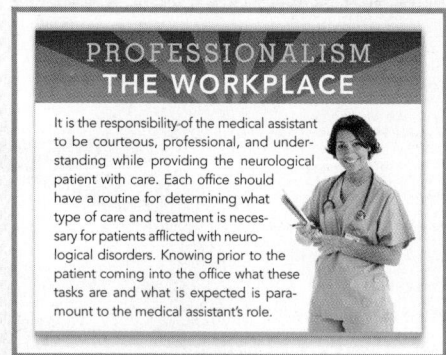

PROFESSIONALISM THE WORKPLACE
It is the responsibility of the medical assistant to be courteous, professional, and understanding while providing the neurological patient with care. Each office should have a routine for determining what type of care and treatment is necessary for patients afflicted with neurological disorders. Knowing prior to the patient coming into the office what these tasks are and what is expected is paramount to the medical assistant's role.

PROFESSIONALISM: THE WORKPLACE explores topics and issues students may encounter during participation in an externship program.

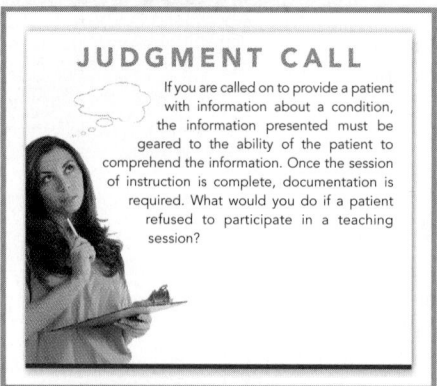

JUDGMENT CALL
If you are called on to provide a patient with information about a condition, the information presented must be geared to the ability of the patient to comprehend the information. Once the session of instruction is complete, documentation is required. What would you do if a patient refused to participate in a teaching session?

JUDGMENT CALL provides critical thinking opportunities for students throughout the chapters.

Visual Learning

The open design of this book is ideal for visual learners.

TABLES present topics in an at-a-glance format.

TABLE 5-3 Comparison of Assertive and Aggressive Behavior

Assertive Behavior	Aggressive Behavior
"This medication works best when it is taken on a regular daily basis."	"You know you can't expect this medication to work when you're not taking it every day."
"Let me find someone who can answer that question for you."	"That's not my job."
"Your behavior is inappropriate."	"Why did you do that? It was stupid."
Knocking on door and then coming into an exam to say "Excuse me, Dr. Thompson. You are needed on the telephone."	Rushing into an exam room to say "Doctor, you've got a telephone call."

- Describe the appropriate, reasonable, and enforceable consequences that will result if the person does not change his or her behavior.
- Follow through with consequences if the behavior does not change.
- Commend the individual for the behavioral change.
- Evaluate your confrontation.

Discussing Sensitive Issues

Numerous sensitive issues arise during contact with patients. Discussing issues involving money, such as the patient's bill and personal financial responsibility, can be very sensitive. Discussing issues involving money, such as the patient's bill and personal financial responsibility, can be very sensitive. Patients should be advised before the first visit of the physician's charges for specific services or treatment. Inquiries regarding the patient's medical insurance and procedures for payment of fees should also be reviewed prior to the first visit. Compliance with federal regulations regarding the patient's right to privacy for all health-related information should be addressed at the first visit. This includes reviewing the Health Insurance Portability and Accountability Act (HIPAA) and following its guidelines as discussed in Chapter 4. The medical assistant should have each patient sign a release of information form on his or her first visit stating that the medical information obtained from visits may be disclosed to insurance companies and others for payment purposes as designated.

A CUSTOMER-FRIENDLY ENVIRONMENT

Using good interpersonal skills to set a positive environment in the health care setting generates a customer-friendly atmosphere and comfortable workplace. A warm, friendly greeting, showing respect to the patient, being sincere and sensitive, and demonstrating empathy can help set a positive tone.

Greeting Patients

A patient should be greeted within one minute of entering the office. If you are speaking on the telephone when the patient comes in, be sure to acknowledge the patient's presence

with a smile and nod. Give your full attention to the patient as soon as you complete the telephone conversation.

Barriers to Communication

There are many barriers to communication. Identifying and overcoming these barriers is essential for effective communication. Some are obvious barriers, such as the distraction of loud background noise, and can be eliminated by the medical assistant. However, we may not be aware of other barriers that result in either no communication or a distorted message being received. To understand the patient, you must overcome the barriers to effective communication (Figure 5-5).

Giving the patient false reassurance by saying "Everything will be all right" can result in the patient's reluctance to talk to you about personal or health-related fears. Such comments can also lead to liability issues for the physician if the patient believes that a promise for recovery has been made.

The medical assistant also may put up barriers to communication unintentionally. To name a few, such obstacles include not looking at the patient when he or she is speaking,

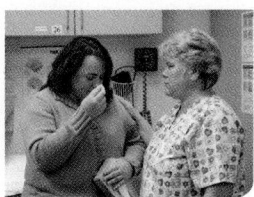

FIGURE 5-5 Effective listening skills demonstrate empathy to the patient and break down barriers to communication.

104   CHAPTER 5 Communication: Verbal and Nonverbal

Color **PHOTOGRAPHS** and **DRAWINGS** bring the world of medical assisting to life. They illustrate key procedures, important concepts, equipment, and interactions between MAs, patients and other staff.

BOXES separate and highlight special information.

Box 39-2 Other Professionals in Health CARE

Your occupation as a medical assistant often brings you into contact with other allied health professionals. To improve communication with other health care workers, it is important that you understand the duties and training of other members of the allied health team. Ophthalmic assistants work under the supervision of an ophthalmologist and work in offices or clinics. While some ophthalmologists hire medical assistants and train them on the job to perform the functions necessary in their office, others will only hire an ophthalmic assistant (OA). There are specific programs of training for the OA as there are for the medical assistant. The OA must have a high school diploma or equivalency and attend a clinical program approved by a review committee of ophthalmic medical personnel. An OA's duties include conducting acuity testing, tonometry, adjusting glasses, assisting during surgical procedures, and administering some eye medications. In addition, the OA may be trained

in the use and care of more highly technical instruments. OA students who pass a national certification examination earn the title of certified ophthalmic assistant (COA). For information on this field, contact the Joint Commission on Allied Health Personnel in Ophthalmology, 2025 Woodlane Drive, St. Paul, MN 55125-2995, (800) 232-3937.

Another health professional you may encounter is the audiologist. An audiologist is an allied health professional who performs diagnostic hearing tests, assesses patient's hearing, fits hearing aids, teaches proper use of the hearing aid, and rehabilitates clients with hearing loss. To become an audiologist, one must graduate from an accredited, five-year master's degree program and pass a national certification examination. Audiologists work in hospitals, schools, and private offices. For further information on this profession contact the American Academy of Audiology.

policies and procedures manual. See Box 39-2 for information about dealing with other allied health professionals.

The medical assistant may be asked to perform an audiometer test and may do so if he or she has undergone the proper training. The physician will interpret the results and inform the patient of the outcome. You are not permitted to release results to a patient unless you have been specifically instructed to do so by the physician. Procedure 39-8 describes the steps for performing an audiometric test on a

patient. Table 39-1 lists and explains some of the tests and procedures related to the ear.

ADDITIONAL DIAGNOSTIC TESTS

Tympanometry, a diagnostic test, is used to measure the ability of the myringa to move, thereby estimating the pressure in the middle ear. If the middle ear is filled with fluid, the tympanic membrane will be more rigid. A printout of the results is produced for the physician to evaluate.

procedure
39-8

ASSISTING WITH AUDIOMETRY
Objective: Perform audiometric test without error.

EQUIPMENT AND SUPPLIES
audiometer with headphones; quiet room or small, enclosed cubicle; patient's record; pen

METHOD
1. Check the physician's orders.
2. Perform hand hygiene.
3. Prepare the equipment.
4. Test the equipment and make sure the power is on.
5. Identify the patient, and explain the procedure.
6. Establish signal response that patient will give if no automatic button is available; nodding head or holding up a finger are acceptable signals (Figure 39-19).
7. Have the patient assume a comfortable position.
8. Place headphones over the patient's ears.

Procedures

More than 175 procedures give students all they need to know to perform medical assisting skills.

The **OBJECTIVE** helps students focus on the purpose of completing the procedure.

EQUIPMENT AND SUPPLIES lists what is needed for the procedure.

CHARTING EXAMPLE shows students how to document the procedure.

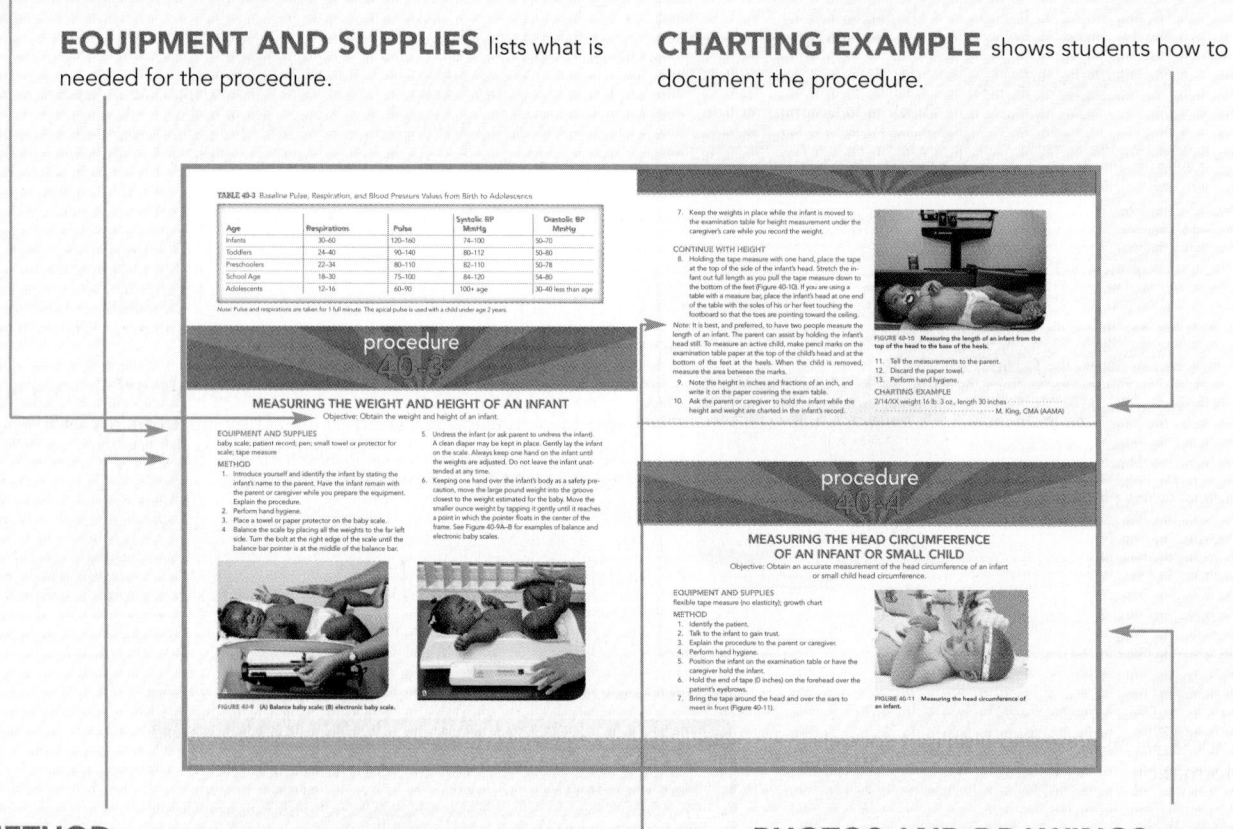

METHOD presents how-to in an easy to follow, step-by-step format.

PHOTOS AND DRAWINGS Illustrate the procedure where possible.

NOTES give tips or additional information to help students perform procedures.

End of Chapter

This section at the end of the chapter highlights the importance of the chapter using a variety of learning styles.

SUMMARY of the important topics from the chapter.

ON THE JOB help students increase retention and success by linking concepts to their job functions.

COMPETENCY REVIEW tests student retention of key concepts.

CRITICAL THINKING questions refer back to the case study at the beginning of the chapter.

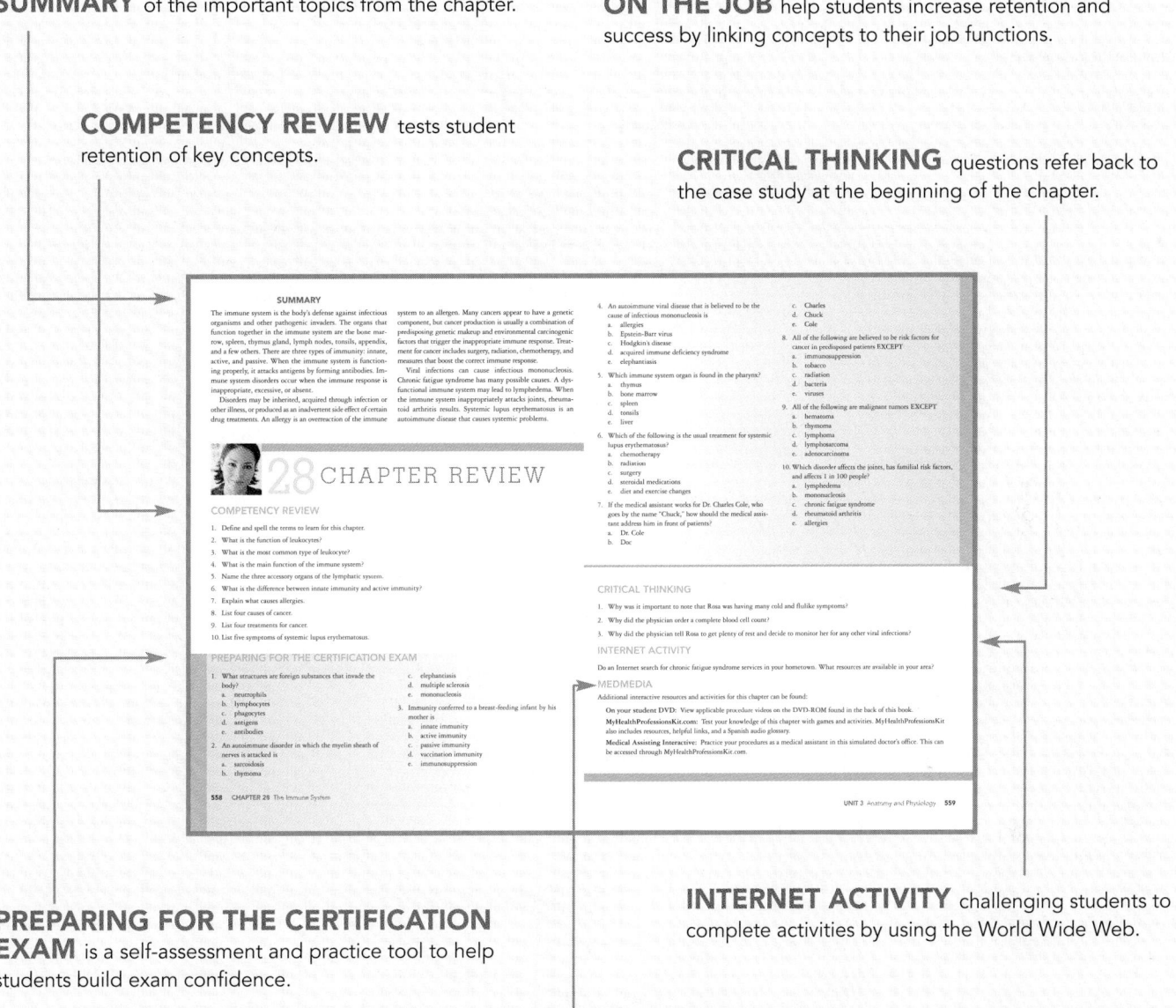

PREPARING FOR THE CERTIFICATION EXAM is a self-assessment and practice tool to help students build exam confidence.

INTERNET ACTIVITY challenging students to complete activities by using the World Wide Web.

MEDMEDIA points students to the media resources that are available at their fingertips, including the **DVD** of medical assisting skills videos found in the back of the book, **MYHEALTHPROFESSIONSKIT,** and **MEDICAL ASSISTING INTERACTIVE**.

Unit One

Introduction to Health Care

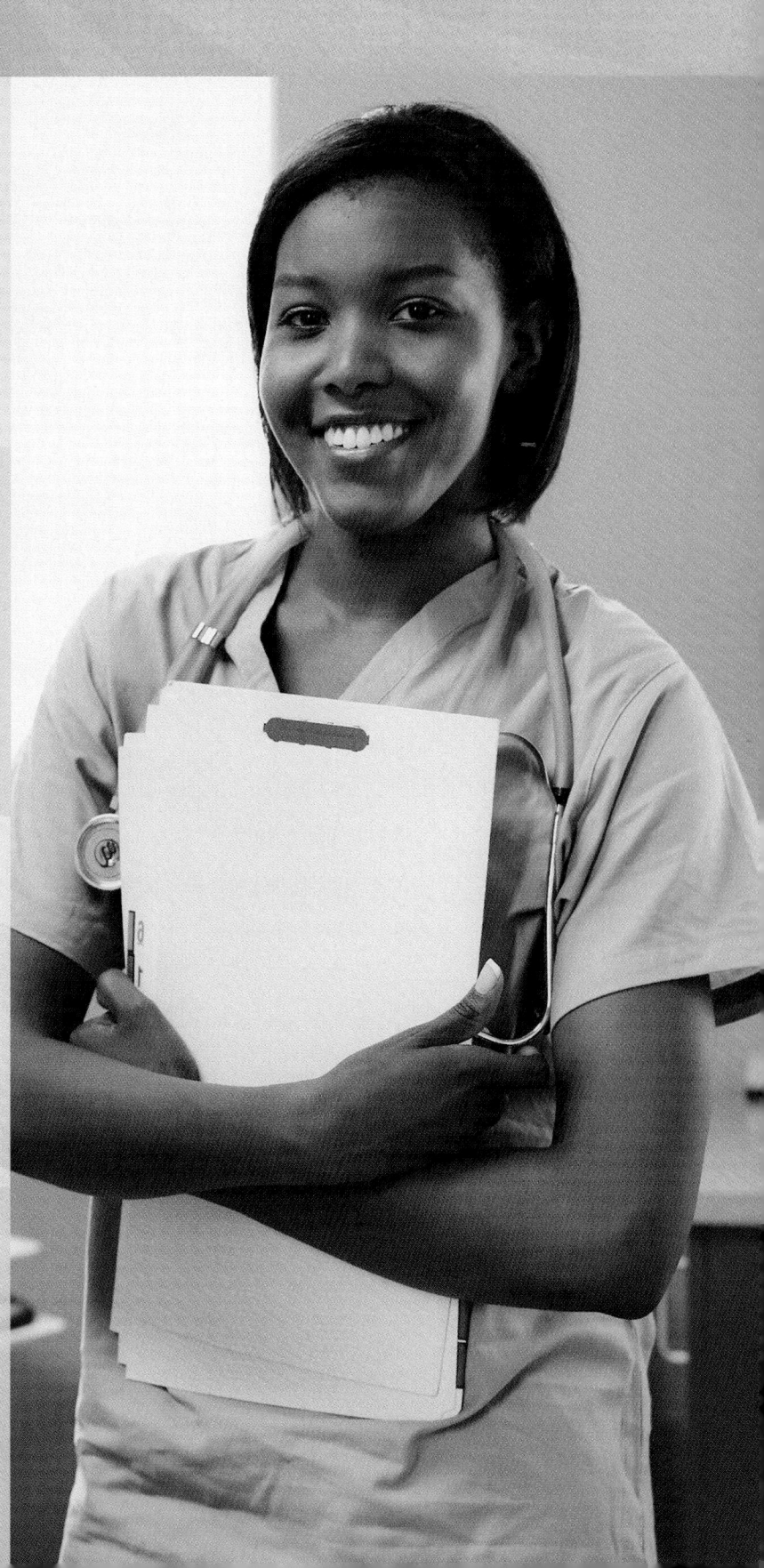

1

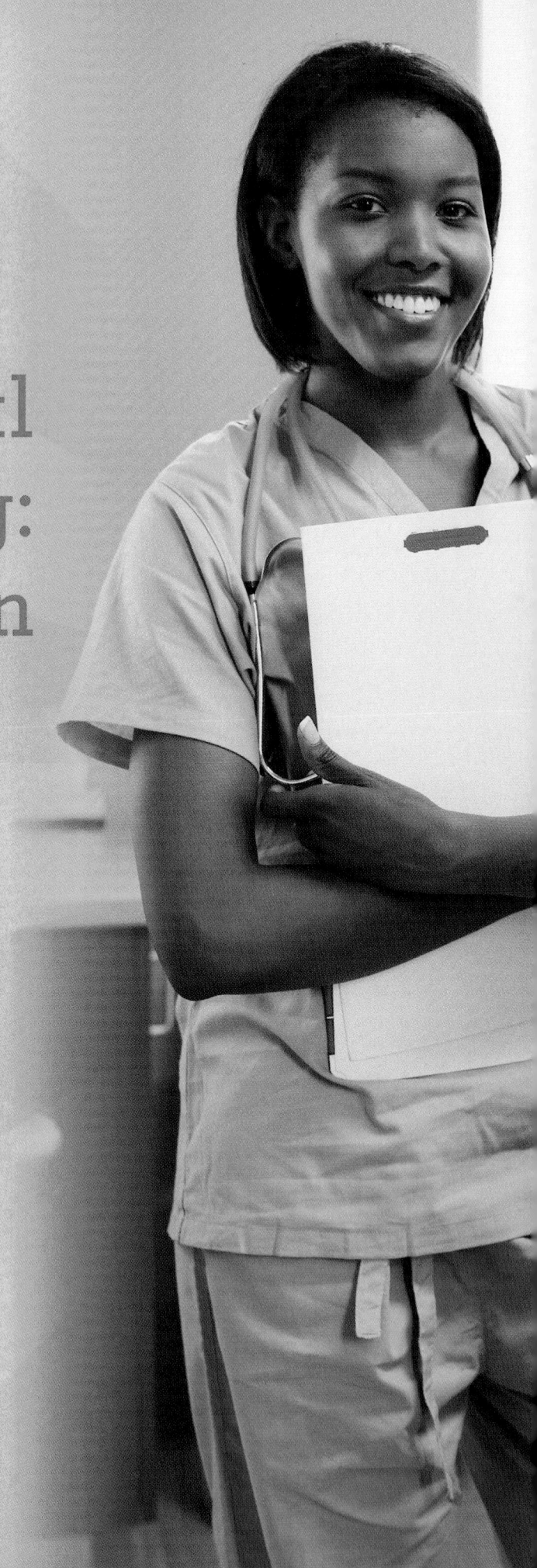

Medical Assisting: The Profession

LEARNING OBJECTIVES

After completing this chapter, you should be able to:

- Define and spell the terms to learn for this chapter.

- Discuss the history of medical assisting as a profession.

- Discuss educational opportunities available for medical assistants.

- Identify accrediting agencies for medical assisting programs.

- List ten administrative duties of the medical assistant.

- List ten clinical skills medical assistants need to know.

- List qualities usually found in a good medical assistant.

- Discuss the professional organizations that certify medical assistants.

- Identify career opportunities available to medical assistants, and give examples of areas in which you may choose to work.

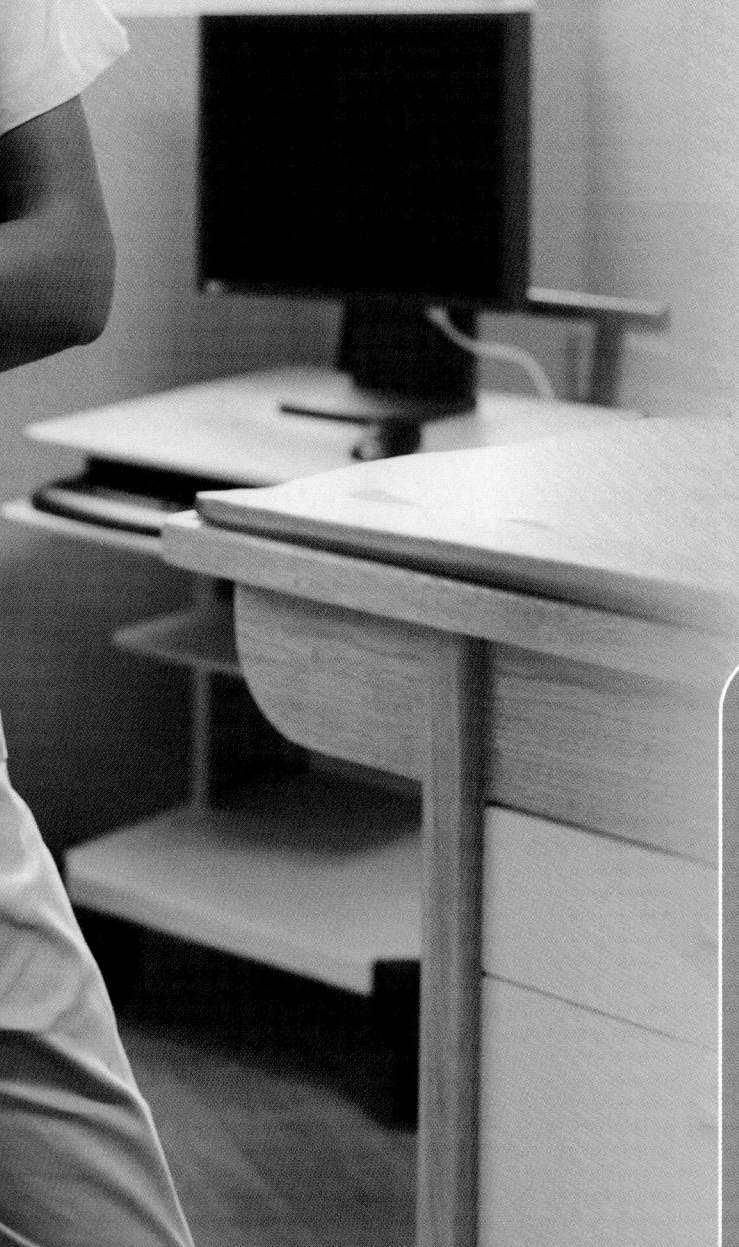

CHAPTER OUTLINE

CASE STUDY

Lucy Guttierez has been working a full-time job since graduating from high school three years ago. Lucy has always been interested in the health care field and wants to begin schooling for a health care profession. After weeks of research she has decided to enroll in a medical assistant program. Valley Heights Community College offers an associate degree for medical assisting, and Valley Heights Business School offers a 9-month certificate program. Lucy has not decided in which program she will enroll.

The rapidly changing health care environment has caused health care providers to rely more heavily on assistive personnel. As a result, medical assistants have become an important part of the health care team. No matter the setting, these multifunctional team members provide valuable services and support. Medical assistants can be found in a variety of settings from pediatric to chiropractic offices. No matter how varied the roles or duties of the medical assistant (MA), the essential skills and personal qualities required of all good medical assistants are quite similar.

As a well-trained, multiskilled health care professional, the medical assistant fulfills many roles in the allied health field where the everyday challenges are balanced by opportunities for advancement, personal growth, and satisfaction. Professional organizations that oversee or regulate the education, training, and certification of medical assistants are also discussed in this chapter, along with current career opportunities and the future of the medical assisting field.

History of Medical Assisting

Historically, medical assistants were trained on the job by a physician. They became skilled through the day-to-day education and training provided in the medical office. Due to the increasing responsibilities and liability issues, most clinics today staff their offices with individuals who have received some type of formal training. Many physicians had become familiar with the clinical skills of nurses while working closely with nurses in the hospital setting, so they chose to hire registered nurses to work in their offices. When a shortage of nursing personnel occurred, physicians had to look elsewhere for professionally trained office personnel who were specifically trained to handle both the administrative and clinical responsibilities of a medical office (Figure 1-1). Physicians began to hire credentialed medical assistants.

The **American Association of Medical Assistants (AAMA)** was adopted as a national professional organization in 1955 after previously being the Kansas Medical Assistant Society. In 1957 the first annual meeting of the AAMA was held, and Maxine Williams, who is considered the founder of the AAMA, was selected president. The AAMA was the first organization to place an emphasis on the educational objectives of medical assisting. Today the Commission on Accreditation of Allied Health Educational Programs (CAAHEP) offers the following definition of the medical assisting profession:

> Medical assistants are multiskilled health professionals specifically educated to work in ambulatory settings performing administrative and clinical duties. The practice of medical assisting directly influences the public's health and well-being, and requires mastery of a complex body of knowledge and specialized skills requiring both formal education and practical experience that serve as standards for entry into the profession.

Source: CAAHEP Standards and Guidelines for Medical Assistants, 2008.

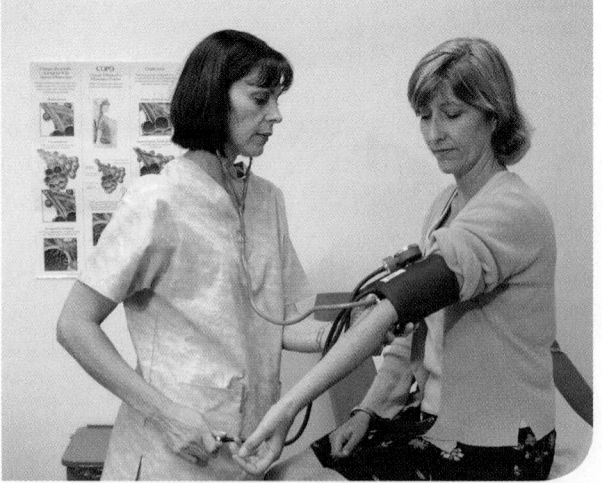

FIGURE 1-1 Medical assistants perform many functions in a physician's office or a clinic.

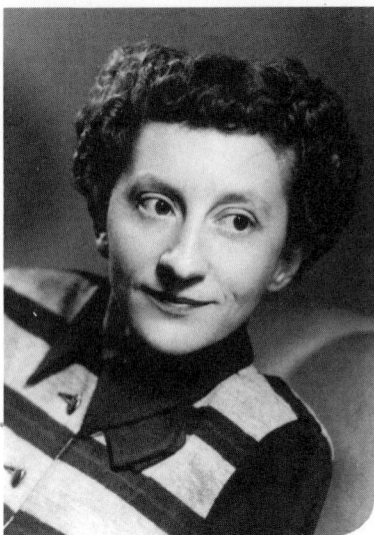

FIGURE 1-2 Maxine Williams was the founder and first president of the AAMA.
Source: American Association of Medical Assistants, Chicago, IL

Education and Training for the Medical Assistant

Over the years, education and training of medical assistants have undergone many changes. Today's medical assistants are well-trained and respected practitioners in the allied health field. Students may obtain a certificate, diploma, or associate degree in the field of medical assisting.

- **Certificate programs**—The length of the course of study varies from one institution to the next. Some programs are six weeks in length, while others may take up to a year to complete. These programs are usually offered in either vocational schools or career colleges. With certificate programs, the focus tends to be on the development of clinical skills. Students may choose the traditional classroom setting or may opt for distance learning (online). Most certificate programs require a hands-on externship to complete the program. Depending on the accreditation, graduates of certificate programs may be eligible to sit for a national certification examination. Students who choose this training option may be supplementing prior training or may simply want an introductory career in the health care field.

- **Diploma program**—These programs tend to be similar to certificate programs. Most programs are nine months to a year in length. Career and community colleges most often offer this course of study. Training focuses on developing clinical skills, as well as limited administrative skills. Students selecting this option may be interested in a career as a medical assistant while others may want to use this as a stepping stone to other health care careers.

- **Degree program**—This course of study can range from as brief as eight months to approximately two years in length. It is usually offered in a traditional classroom setting at a career or community college. Along with clinical and administrative courses, courses to assist in professional development and some general education courses may be offered as part of the curriculum. This option is usually chosen by those who know that they want a career as a medical assistant.

ACCREDITATION

Accreditation is the process in which an institution voluntarily completes a process of determining whether or not their school meets or exceeds standards set forth by an accrediting body. This detailed process ensures that a school meets an established list of criteria. It is important to understand that schools are accredited, people are not.

Schools may also seek programmatic accreditation for their medical assisting programs. The learning outcomes for these programs are competency based. The U.S. Department of Education recognizes two agencies that may accredit programs in medical assisting:

- **Commission on Accreditation of Allied Health Education Programs (CAAHEP)**

- **Accrediting Bureau of Health Education Schools (ABHES)**

The CAAHEP Standards and Guidelines state that to provide for student attainment of "Entry-Level Competencies for the Medical Assistant," the curriculum—"shall include, but is not limited to the following units, modules, and/or courses of instruction:"

Anatomy and Physiology

Applied Mathematics

Microbiology and Applied Infection Control

PROFESSIONALISM

Lifelong learning is an important professional responsibility. Even when schooling seems over after a certification exam is passed, professionals will continue to search for opportunities to keep their credentials current by continuing education. Since the health care industry undergoes constant change, it is important to stay current in medical assisting education.

Concepts of Effective Communication

Administrative Functions

Basic Practice Finances

Managed Care/Insurance

Legal Implications

Ethical Considerations

Protective Practices

An **externship** or **practicum** experience is a required component of the medical assistant's education. During a practicum, students work without payment in a physician's office, clinic, or hospital setting for 160 hours over a minimum of four weeks during the final stage of their training under the supervision of someone at the site.

Role of the Medical Assistant

The medical assistant's main responsibility is to assist the physician in providing patient care. Central to a medical assistant's responsibilities are sound clinical skills. He or she must be able to obtain vital signs, collect specimens, administer medication, and run basic laboratory tests. It is not unusual to find medical assistants who conduct cardiac stress tests and assist with minor office surgeries. Administrative duties may be part of the job description. In small clinics or physicians' offices, the medical assistant may function as the receptionist or insurance clerk.

The field of medical assisting is open to both men and women in a variety of work settings, such as physicians' offices, ambulatory care (outpatient) clinics, government agencies, urgent care facilities, and free-standing facilities (Figure 1-3). While traditionally medical assistants only worked in physician offices, increasingly they are being employed in urgent care facilities. These facilities are typically open beyond the traditional hours—at night and on weekends.

RESPONSIBILITIES OF THE MEDICAL ASSISTANT

The list of responsibilities that medical assistants perform is extensive. For this reason, the education and training for this field is carefully designed and must involve both theory and hands-on experience. The actual duties of the medical assistant vary from office to office. However, a good medical assistant, who has received a well-rounded education, will be able to adjust to different work environments. Never per-

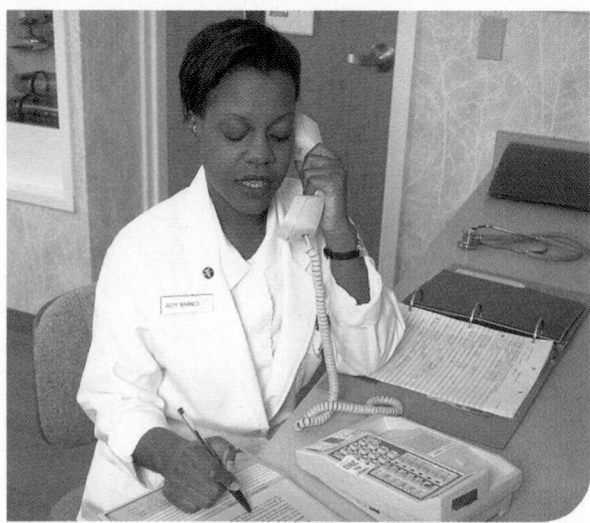

FIGURE 1-3   The medical assisting profession offers many settings in which to pursue your career. Good communication and social skills are required in each of them.
Source: Michal Heron/Pearson Education/PH College

form duties that are beyond your level of responsibility, education, and training.

Medical assistants' responsibilities will also vary according to the size and type of setting and state laws that apply. Always familiarize yourself with federal and state regulations and guidelines governing the procedures that medical assistants are allowed to perform in whatever environment you work. Generally, the medical assistants' duties are

PROFESSIONALISM

THE LAW

It is important to fully understand what your credentials allow you to do. The medical assistant is uniquely qualified to perform the administrative and clinical procedures associated with responsibilities assigned in the particular setting by the physician. In fulfilling these responsibilities, however, you must always be aware that the potential for psychological, financial, and physical injury to the patient exists. It is your ethical responsibility to patients and your employer that you do your utmost to maintain a high level of skill performance in all that you do. The medical assistant always works as an agent of the physician.

It is also very important that you only practice within the scope of practice for medical assisting. It is a crime to perform procedures that only nurses or physicians are licensed to do. Be sure to understand your role as a medical assistant and not deviate from it.

grouped into two categories—administrative and clinical—and include the following competencies:

Administrative Competencies: Business and Front Office

- Scheduling patients, including referrals to specialists
- Greeting and receiving patients
- Screening nonpatients and visitors
- Making arrangements for patient admissions to hospitals, patient tests, and procedures such as X-rays and laboratory tests
- Providing patient instruction regarding procedures and tests performed in the physician's office and hospitals
- Updating and filing patient medical records
- Coding diagnoses and procedures for insurance purposes
- Computer skills (Figure 1-4)
- Handling financial arrangements with patients
- Managing the telephone, reports, correspondence, and filing
- Handling mail, billing, insurance claims, credit, and collections
- Operating office equipment
- Preparing and maintaining employee records
- Handling petty cash
- Reconciling bank statements
- Maintaining records for license renewals, membership fees, and insurance premiums
- Handling the office in the physician's absence
- Assisting the physician with articles, lectures, and manuscripts

- Utilization review of necessary procedures and referrals
- Coordinating managed-care coverage for patients and physicians
- Ensure compliance with HIPAA guidelines

Clinical Competencies: Care and Treatment of Patients

- Assisting patients in preparation for physical examinations and procedures
- Obtaining a medical history (Figure 1-5)
- Performing routine clinical and laboratory procedures under the supervision of a physician
- Collecting, preparing, and transporting laboratory specimens
- Venipuncture, where permitted
- Assisting the physician with procedures
- Instructing and educating patients on treatments and procedures
- Cleaning and sterilizing equipment
- Obtaining patient's height, weight, and vital signs
- Preparing and maintaining examination and treatment rooms
- Inventory control—ordering and storing of supplies
- Disposing of hazardous waste and other materials
- Administering medications under the supervision and orders of the physician, where permitted
- Changing bandages and dressings, as well as suture removal where permitted
- Handling drug refills as directed by the physician
- Performing electrocardiograms (ECGs)

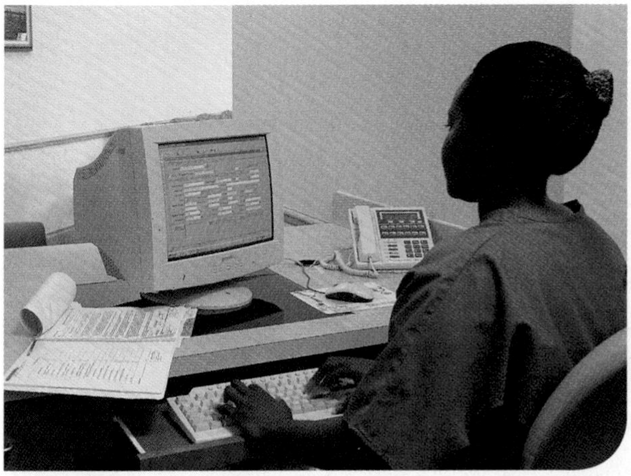

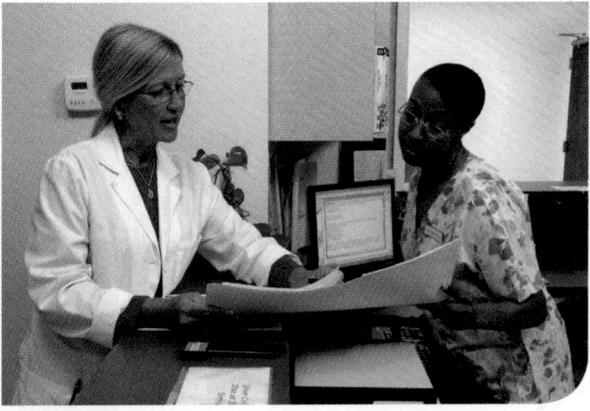

FIGURE 1-4 Good computer skills are now required to be a successful member of an office staff.

FIGURE 1-5 Helping maintain accurate patient records is a critical part of the medical assistant's work.

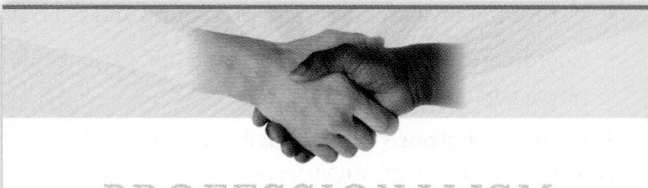

- Complying with Occupational Safety and Health Administration (OSHA) guidelines and employee instruction
- Performing skills relevant to a particular practice (for example, audiometry, spirometry, Holter monitor)
- Disposing of contaminated supplies
- Sterilizing medical instruments
- Preparing patients for X-rays

Medical assistants who work in specialty offices, such as pediatric or ophthalmic offices, will have additional duties for which they will be trained by appropriate personnel.

Occupational Analysis

From 1979 to 1996 the AAMA utilized a document called DACUM (Developing a Curriculum) to define specific areas of instruction and competencies for medical assisting. In 1997 the AAMA issued the Role Delineation Study, which was later revised in 2003 and again in 2007-2008, and is now known as the *Occupational Analysis of the CMA (AAMA)*. This study is the result of a composite of current competencies essential for medical assistants based upon the practice experience of an expert panel. The analysis identifies three major categories of competence-administrative, clinical, and general skills - for entry-level medical assistants. These areas are further expanded to include competencies that should be taught in medical assisting programs. (See General, Administrative, and Clinical Competencies of the CMA (AAMA) in Appendix I)

Characteristics of a Good Medical Assistant

In addition to having a general medical knowledge, including medical terminology, and being able to perform administrative and clinical responsibilities, medical assistants must genuinely care about others.

The nature of the patient and health care worker relationship demands that medical assistants be able to communicate effectively and get along with others. Qualities or characteristics regularly found in good medical assistants include integrity, empathy, discretion, the ability to safeguard the patient's right to confidentiality, thoroughness, punctuality, congeniality, proactivity, and competence (Figure 1-6).

- **Integrity**—A medical assistant with integrity will do what is expected, when it is expected, for the simple reason that it is expected. Someone with integrity is honest, dependable, dedicated to high standards, and adheres to a code of values.

- **Empathy**—The ability to work with the sick and the infirm depends on one's ability and willingness to show empathy. A medical assistant with empathy has the ability to be sensitive to or understand the feelings of another individual. An empathic person is able to stand in the shoes of another and identify with what he or she is experiencing. For example, when a medical assistant has some insight or understanding of the pain or distress a patient is feeling, he or she acts in a kindly way that expresses sensitivity to the patient's feelings.

- **Discretion**—A medical assistant who uses discretion is able to make decisions responsibly. Someone who uses

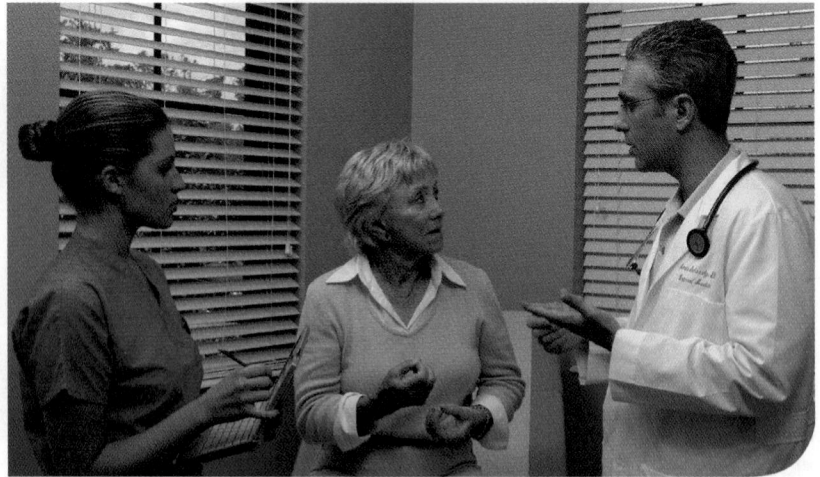

FIGURE 1-6 Medical assistants are often involved in confidential conversations between the physician and the patient.

discretion is tactful in communicating with others. It is important to be able to be fair and to be familiar with policies and regulations. Discretion is important in patient interaction, as well as interaction with coworkers.

- **Confidentiality**—The ability to safeguard patient confidences, particularly information in the medical record regarding family history, past or current diseases or illnesses, test results, and medications—is vital to the patient and health care professional relationship. No information about the patient is to be disclosed without the written permission of the patient. This is a legal and ethical issue with penalties for violating patient confidentiality. Without this trust, there can be no relationship. As the person with most frequent access to patient records and verbal confidences, the medical assistant has a serious professional responsibility to safeguard the patient's right to confidentiality.

- **Thoroughness**—The role of the medical assistant is varied, and often requires multitasking. However, a medical assistant should show pride in the work done by thoroughly completing every task the physician orders performed. If a medical assistant is not thorough, errors can jeopardize patient health.

- **Punctuality**—If a medical assistant is frequently absent, the office not only loses a valuable asset, but also the physician must pay extra for temporary help. It is a workplace expectation that medical assistants come to the office early and stay until the last patient leaves.

- **Congeniality**—A good medical assistant will get along with a diversity of people. The ability to get along with all patients is an asset for the medical assistant. Sometimes sick patients are hostile or aggressive, but a wise medical assistant will be friendly and helpful to all patients.

- **Proactivity**—The medical assistant must anticipate the needs of the physician and patients. Supplies should be laid out prior to procedures, charts should be pulled, and the physician should be briefed before the patient is even seen.

- **Competence**—As the practice of medical assisting changes, it is important for the medical assistant to keep competencies current. Continuing education should be an expectation of the lifelong learner.

In many cases, the medical assistant will be the first health professional with whom the patient interacts and on whom the patient bases his or her opinion of the physician.

PROFESSIONALISM THE LIFE SPAN

Some medical clinics and physicians' offices provide care to patients within a specific age range or stage of life. Pediatric offices treat young children and adolescents. A physician who specializes in gerontology or geriatrics provides care to an elderly population of patients. Each age group is unique in its stage of physical and emotional development. Therefore, each group has different needs and considerations. You cannot expect to communicate with a 5-year-old patient and a 45-year-old patient in the same manner. In your interactions with patients, you must consider their developmental stage and provide age-appropriate care and instruction.

It is important to present a confident, professional image that helps put the patient at ease. A calm, pleasant speaking voice conveys a professional attitude. Remember that eating, drinking, or chewing gum while working are not appropriate in areas open to the public. Along with a basic understanding of human behavior and good communication skills—written, spoken, and nonverbal—the medical assistant must be able to handle tasks requiring basic mathematics, grammar, and spelling skills.

Daily habits of good personal hygiene and grooming are expected from the medical assistant. The use of strong perfumes and showy jewelry is unprofessional and may even be harmful. For example, strong perfume may actually trigger allergies or headaches in some individuals and may be bothersome to a patient who is ill. Loose dangling jewelry may get in the way while treating a patient. Loose, long hair and extended nails should also be avoided.

Medical assistants provide the quality of care that they would wish to have given to themselves or to members of their own families. The medical assistant must have the ability to see beyond the gruff or complaining manner of the patient who is not feeling well and project a professional, pleasant, and caring attitude.

Certifying Professional Organizations

Several professional organizations train, certify, and represent medical assistants. It is a positive career move to align oneself with a professional organization. These organizations provide medical assistants with a network of career professionals who promote their profession as well as serve as a source of ongoing education. **Certification** is the issuance by an official body or professional organization of a certificate and credentials to one who has met the education and experience standards of the organization. It is voluntary and signifies that a medical assistant has met professional standards, usually by receiving professional training, passing a rigorous examination, and choosing to continue his or her education to retain currency at a high standard of professionalism.

AMERICAN ASSOCIATION OF MEDICAL ASSISTANTS

The American Association of Medical Assistants (AAMA) is a key association in the field of medical assisting. The national headquarters for the AAMA is located in Chicago, Illinois. This organization offers the **Certified Medical Assistant (CMA)** or **CMA (AAMA),** credential. Those who meet eligibility requirements for sitting for this examination must complete an application process. Computerized certification examinations are available throughout the year. Certification indicates that a candidate has met the education and experience standards of the AAMA and achieved a satisfactory test result. The first examination given to certify medical assistants was administered in 1963.

The certification examination is offered to graduates of programs accredited by the Commission on Accreditation of Allied Health Education Programs (CAAHEP) or by the Accrediting Bureau of Health Education Schools (ABHES). Upon successful completion of the certification examination, candidates receive a certificate, confirming them as certified medical assistants. To continue to be certified, a CMA (AAMA) must either show evidence of 60 hours of continuing education in five years or retake and pass the CMA (AAMA) exam every five years (Figure 1-7).

Membership in the AAMA is not necessary to take the certification examination. For the credential to remain

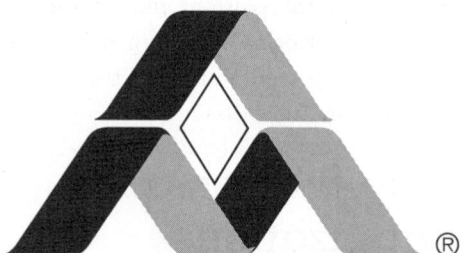

FIGURE 1-7 Becoming a Certified Medical Assistant may demonstrate your commitment to the profession and the continuing education required to maintain the CMA credential.
Source: American Association of Medical Assistants, Chicago, IL

current, it must be revalidated every five years, either by earning a designated number of **continuing education units (CEUs)** or through re-examination. The AAMA sponsors workshops, seminars, and county, state, and national conferences for medical assistants to remain current in their field and earn CEUs. The national office also offers online **monographs** (short books, each of which contains text and a test) for CEUs.

AMERICAN MEDICAL TECHNOLOGISTS

American Medical Technologists (AMT) provides oversight for the registration and testing of medical assistants, medical technologists, and phlebotomists. This association, in cooperation with the AMT Institute for Education (AMTIE), has developed a continuing education program and recording system.

The AMT, a nonprofit certifying body, provides a **Registered Medical Assistant (RMA)** certification examination for medical assistants who meet the eligibility requirements and can prove their competency to perform entry-level skills through written examination. The RMA is awarded to candidates who pass the AMT certification examination. The RMA certification examination is formed around the following parameters:

I. General Medical Assisting Knowledge
   a. Anatomy and Physiology
   b. Medical Terminology
   c. Medical Law
   d. Medical Ethics
   e. Human Rights
   f. Patient Education

II. Administrative Medical Assisting
   a. Insurance
   b. Financial Bookkeeping
   c. Medical Secretarial—Receptionist

III. Clinical Medical Assisting
   a. Asepsis
   b. Sterilization
   c. Instruments
   d. Vital Signs
   e. Physical Examinations
   f. Clinical Pharmacology
   g. Minor Surgery
   h. Therapeutic Modalities
   i. Laboratory Procedures
   j. Electrocardiography
   k. First Aid

Certification requirements include the applicant (1) being of good moral character and (2) being either a graduate of either a medical assistant program accredited by ABHES or CAAHEP, a graduate of a postsecondary school or college that is accredited by the Regional Accrediting Commission, or an accredited member of a national accrediting organization approved by the U.S. Department of Education, and (3) completing a minimum of 720 clock-hours or equivalent of training in medical assisting skills, including a clinical practicum or externship (supervised training in an actual medical setting) or a formal medical services training program (which the military refers to as an externship) of the United States Armed Forces.

The applicant also must have recent medical assisting experience. See Table 1-1 for further information. Qualified applicants can take a computerized exam at over 200 locations in the United States and Canada through Pearson VUE.

After becoming certified as an RMA and acquiring additional administrative experience, a medical assistant can apply for the **Certified Medical Administrative Specialist (CMAS)** credential. A qualified applicant also can take this computerized exam at over 200 locations in the United States and Canada through Pearson VUE. See Table 1-2 for qualifications for the CMAS exam.

TABLE 1-1 Qualifications of RMA Certification

Qualifications

To qualify for RMA Certification:

1. Applicant shall be of good moral character.

2. Applicant shall meet one of the following requirements

    A. Applicant shall be a recent graduate of, or scheduled to graduate from:

        1. A medical assistant program that holds programmatic accreditation by (or is in a post-secondary school or college that holds institutional accreditation by) the Accrediting Bureau of Health Education Schools (ABHES) or the Commission on Accreditation of Allied Health Education Programs (CAAHEP).

        2. A medical assistant program in a post-secondary school or college that has institutional accreditation by a Regional Accrediting Commission or by a national accrediting organization approved by the U.S. Department of Education, which program includes a minimum of 720 clock-hours (or equivalent) of training in Medical Assisting skills (including a clinical externship).

        3. A formal medical services training program of the United States Armed Forces.

    * If you graduated within the last three years proof of work experience is not required. If you graduated over three years ago, you will be required to show proof of current work experience.

    B. Applicant shall have been employed in the profession of Medical Assisting for a minimum of five (5) years, no more than two (2) years of which may have been as an instructor in the post-secondary medical assistant program (proof of current work experience and high school education or equivalent is needed). Employment dates must be within the last five (5) years.

    C. The AMT Board of Directors has further determined that applicants who have passed a generalist medical assistant certification examination offered by another medical assisting certification body (provided that exam has been approved for this purpose by the AMT Board of Directors) and who have been working in the medical assisting field for the past three out of five years and who have met all other AMT training and experience requirements, may be considered for RMA certification without further examination.

If you have any questions, please email AMT at: rma@amt1.com

Source: American Medical Technologists, Rosemont, IL

TABLE 1-2 Certified Medical Administrative Specialist AMT

Medical Administrative Specialist

A Medical Administrative Specialist serves a key role in medical office, clinic and hospital settings. This multi-skilled practitioner is competent in medical records management. Insurance processing, coding and billing, management of practice finances, information processing, and fundamental office management tasks. A Medical Administrative Specialist is very familiar with clinical and technical concepts required to coordinate administrative office functions in the health-care setting.

Nature of the Work

A Medical Administrative Specialist must have a sincere desire to help people and a willingness to learn the complexities of the health care industry. Medical Administrative Specialists work most of their time in the "front" office of a physician office, clinic or hospital. A medical administrative specialist must be outgoing, patient, and have an attention to detail. Also, this individual must be willing to learn new procedures, laws and insurance filing forms. Some of the duties performed by a Medical Administrative Specialist include:

- Set appointment times
- Greet patients
- File and pull charts
- Handle insurance information
- Assist new patients with paperwork
- Know word processing
- Know bookkeeping
- Type medical correspondence
- Transcribe medical dictation
- Understand and know insurance coding information
- Scheduling hospital admissions
- Types case histories
- Fill out and submit insurance medical forms
- Collects and records payments
- Must know medical terminology

Education and Training

A Medical Administrative Specialist must have a high school diploma or G.E.D. with acceptable training. Many colleges, career schools and technical schools offer Medical Administrative Assistant, Medical Office Assistant, or Medical Secretary programs. Graduates from these programs will receive either a certificate or diploma depending on the program. Graduation from a school that is accredited makes it easier to apply for certification.

Certification/Licensing: Each individual state decides the scope of practice for Medical Administrative Specialists. Most states do not have licensure laws, but many states do have a scope of practice for Medical Administrative Specialists or Medical Assistants.

Certification by a recognized organization enables Medical Administrative Specialists to be promoted faster, earn a higher pay and great respect. Employers prefer to hire experienced workers and many prefer certified applicants who have passed a national examination, indicating that the Medical Administrative Specialist meets certain standards of competence.

Employment

The job outlook for Medical Administrative Specialists is excellent. The field is expected to grow much faster than average, which means an increase in 36% or more between 2000 and 2010. The health services industry is expected to expand because of technological advances in medicine and the aging population.

Salary

Earnings vary depending on experience, education and skill level.

Profession Source: US Bureau of Labor statistics:

Source: American Medical Technologists, Rosemont, IL

NATIONAL CENTER FOR COMPETENCY TESTING

The **National Certified Medical Assistant (NCMA)** credential is issued by the National Center for Competency Testing. To qualify, a candidate must have a high school diploma and must have completed a medical assisting program. Those who are not graduates of a medical assisting program but are able to provide documentation of two years experience working as a medical assistant under the training and direction of a physician are also eligible to sit for the NCMA examination. To remain certified after passing the exam, 14 hours per year of continuing education are required.

The National Certified Medical Office Assistant (NCMOA) is also offered by the National Center for Competency Testing. To qualify to sit for this credential, medical assistants must provide documentation of least one year of experience as a medical office assistant or must be a graduate of an approved medical office assistant program of study.

NATIONAL HEALTHCAREER ASSOCIATION

The National Healthcareer Association (NHA) was founded in 1989 and has certified thousands of professional medical assistants. Two credentials, the Certified Clinical Medical Assistant (CCMA) and the Certified Medical Administrative Assistant (CMAA) are granted to certify medical assistants. To qualify, the applicant must be over 18 years of age, have a high school diploma, have two years of work in the field in which they certify, and pass a professional examination. Home study is available. Without home study, the applicant must have been graduated from an NHA-approved medical assisting program or had one year of experience in the field and a high school diploma.

Career Opportunities

According to the U.S. Department of Labor Statistics, "employment is expected to grow much faster than average, ranking medical assistants among the fastest growing occupations over the 2006–2016 decade. Job opportunities should be excellent, particularly for those with formal training or experience, and certification." In fact, the employment of medical assistants is projected by the U.S. Department of Labor to grow 35 percent in the decade following 2006. Technological advances in medicine and the growth in numbers of aging members of the U.S. population will necessitate more medical assistants. This boom in job growth is helped by the increasing number of medical settings where medical assistants work. Health care facilities will need support personnel, particularly medical assistants who can handle both administrative and clinical duties. Medical assistants work primarily in outpatient settings, a rapidly growing sector of the health care industry.

The anticipated need for more health professionals is based on the expected increase in the number of older adults who will require the care of a physician and the tremendous growth in the number of outpatient facilities. The wide range of health care settings presents many opportunities for the medical assistant who is trained in both clinical and administrative duties. Table 1-3 lists several inpatient and ambulatory care facilities or settings with descriptions of some possible job opportunities for medical assistants in each setting. Table 1-4 lists departments or specialties in which medical assistants may seek employment in either inpatient or ambulatory care settings. In some states and settings, additional education and training may be required for medical assistants to fulfill certain responsibilities. While the general category "medical assistant" may be used in some career ads, some of the job title opportunities may include the following:

- Patient technician
- Data processing clerk

PROFESSIONALISM THE WORKPLACE

Many of the jobs and careers discussed in this chapter require additional education, including passing a written certification examination. Be mindful that patients understand what your title—Certified Medical Assistant, or CMA (AAMA) or Registered Medical Assistant (RMA)—means. Never be afraid to say "I am not qualified to do that." Likewise, if you note a colleague misrepresenting qualifications, you must report this to your professional organization. Safety also is important on the job. Although you may have learned correct safety practices, you may observe others not practicing safe medical assisting. If you witness behaviors that are unsafe to patients, you must report that to your supervisor. If you witness behaviors that are unsafe to workers, you must notify OSHA.

TABLE 1-3 Job Opportunities for Medical Assistants in Inpatient and Ambulatory Care Settings

Ambulatory Care Setting	Description of Job
Clinic	Use clinical and administrative skills to schedule and assist with patients who require special medical attention (e.g., eye clinic, orthopedic clinic, mental health clinic).
Free-standing Facility	Care for patients who require immediate medical treatment.
Physician's Office	Use clinical and administrative skills in the private office setting for physicians of all specialties.
Rehabilitation Center	Provide care for patients recovering from illness or injury.

TABLE 1-4 Job Opportunities for Medical Assistants in Health Care Departments and Specialties

Department/Specialty	Description of Job
Admissions	Handle pre-admission interviews, schedule laboratory testing, and document insurance coverage.
Billing and Insurance	Work with patients, third-party payers, insurance companies to process insurance forms, claims forms, and DRG, ICD9, CPT, and HCPC coding.
ECG/EKG Technician	Perform electrocardiogram studies on patients.
Medical Records	Use administrative skills of transcription, medical terminology, and insurance coding. Requires use of the computer.
Phlebotomy	Use clinical skills to draw blood samples for testing and blood bank use.
Surgery	Use clinical skills to sterilize surgical instruments and set up surgical trays, assist when needed.
Treatment/Procedure/ Emergency Department	Assist with minor surgeries and procedures performed in physicians' offices, hospitals, rehabilitation centers, and emergency departments.

- Billing or collections assistant
- Insurance claims processor
- Clinic aide
- Unit clerk
- Patient care technician
- Insurance claims coder
- Medical records clerk
- Clinical assistant
- Medical receptionist
- Multifunctional technician

With additional education and credentials, you may even respond to ads for the following:

- Medical laboratory assistant
- Electrocardiography (ECG) technician
- Phlebotomist

Experienced medical assistants may find work as office managers, medical records managers, hospital unit secretaries, and instructors for medical assistant programs. With additional schooling, medical assistants can enter other health care occupations, such as nursing, occupational therapy, physical therapy, medical and x-ray technologists.

SUMMARY

The field of medical assisting is growing in response to increasing health care needs of consumers. The profession of medical assistant offers many opportunities, roles, responsibilities, and settings for employment. Most medical assistants work in ambulatory settings such as physicians' offices, where they fulfill the administrative and clinical responsibilities associated with running medical offices.

The size and nature of the medical office practice will determine the number of medical assistants and the actual work they will do.

Caring individuals, who are dedicated professionals with a commitment to maintain their skills through continuing education, make the best medical assistants. Qualities or characteristics regularly found in good medical assistants are integrity, discretion, empathy, the ability to safeguard the patient's right to confidentiality, thoroughness, punctuality, congeniality, proactivity, and competence.

It is most important to remember that the opportunities presented are many and the future of medical assisting looks promising. A career in medical assisting is emotionally and professionally challenging. Certification and alignment with a professional organization are essential for professional development, and lifelong learning is expected in the medical assisting profession.

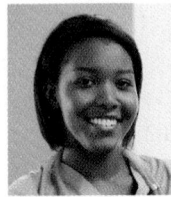

1 CHAPTER REVIEW

COMPETENCY REVIEW

1. Define and spell the terms to learn for this chapter.

2. List several health care facilities or specialties to work at as a medical assistant.

3. Explain the difference between the administrative and clinical functions of medical assisting.

4. Name a medical assistant's professional organization.

5. What qualities are regularly found in good medical assistants?

6. Explain what the curriculum in medical assisting should include.

7. List the job titles for which a medical assistant may qualify.

8. List the educational options available to one who is interested in medical assisting.

PREPARING FOR THE CERTIFICATION EXAM

1. What is the AAMA?
   a. American Medical Association
   b. American Allied Medical Association
   c. Administrative (division) of the American Medical Association
   d. American Association of Medical Assistants
   e. American Association of Medical Assistance

2. What are two general categories that BEST describe the responsibilities of a medical assistant?
   a. phlebotomy and laboratory
   b. secretarial and direct patient care
   c. assisting the physician and paperwork
   d. clinical and secretarial
   e. administrative and clinical

3. Which organization awards the Registered Medical Assistant?
   a. AAMA
   b. NCCT
   c. AMT
   d. AMA
   e. DOE

4. Which administrative tasks falls beyond the scope of practice for a medical assistant?
   a. coordinating managed care coverage
   b. handling petty cash
   c. assisting the physician with a journal article
   d. utilization review of necessary procedures
   e. signing prescriptions

5. Which of the following clinical tasks falls beyond the scope of practice for a medical assistant?
   a. vital signs
   b. suturing
   c. phlebotomy
   d. handling drug refills
   e. patient education

6. How many total CEUs over what period of time must a CMA (AAMA) obtain to remain certified?
   a. 10 CEUs over two years
   b. 30 CEUs over five years
   c. 60 CEUs over five years
   d. 45 CEUs over five years
   e. 50 CEUs over five years

7. Which of the following statements is TRUE?
   a. A medical assistant is equivalent to a nurse.
   b. A medical assistant is equivalent to a physician assistant.
   c. A medical assistant is equivalent to a pharmacy technician.
   d. It is acceptable for patients to refer to a medical assistant as a "nurse."
   e. An advertisement for a medical assistant might include "medical records clerk."

8. As per the CAAHEP Essentials, at a minimum, the curriculum of a medical assisting school does NOT include
   a. medical assistant administrative procedures.
   b. medical assistant clinical procedures.
   c. emergency medical technician training.
   d. medical law and ethics.
   e. externship of 160 to 190 hours.

9. Necessary characteristics of a good medical assistant should include all EXCEPT
   a. confidentiality.
   b. sympathy.
   c. thoroughness.
   d. integrity.
   e. discretion.

10. Which of the following statements is TRUE?
   a. Medical assistants work only in physicians' offices.
   b. All medical assistant programs are diploma programs.
   c. With additional training, medical assistants may work as ECG technicians.
   d. Medical assistants can perform minor surgeries without physicians present.
   e. Medical assistants do not need good communication skills.

CRITICAL THINKING

1. Lucy would like to have a career as a medical assistant, not simply a job. What decisions might Lucy make to support her goals?

2. Lucy is told that the medical assistant program at Valley Heights Community College is accredited by the Accrediting Bureau of Health Education Schools. What does this mean for Lucy?

3. Rosa, Lucy's mother, has asked Lucy what type of jobs would be available to Lucy after she graduates from a medical assistant program. What might Lucy tell her mother?

ON THE JOB

Kayla Christianson, a CMA, has been employed six years by the cardiology practice of three physicians. She is a graduate of a CAAHEP-accredited school. Furthermore, Kayla received extensive hands-on training performing ECGs while doing her required externship.

Kayla has completed an ECG ordered by Dr. Hsu for Mrs. Warner, a 76-year-old patient. Dr. Hsu, Kayla's boss, has telephoned her explaining that he was behind schedule doing rounds at the hospital. He asked her to do him a favor and interpret Mrs. Warner's ECG, sign his name, and fax the report to Mrs. Warner's referring internist who is expecting the results.

1. Given the scope of Kayla's education, training, and years of experience as a CMA, would this "favor" fall within the AAMA guidelines of her responsibilities?
2. Would any portion of Dr. Hsu's request fall within the guidelines? If so, which portion(s)? Is an exception to these guidelines ever allowed?
3. What, if anything, should Kayla say to Dr. Hsu?

INTERNET ACTIVITY

Conduct an Internet search for local medical assistant positions. How many positions require certification? What other job titles would a medical assistant be qualified to take?

MEDMEDIA

Additional interactive resources and activities for this chapter can be found:

On your student DVD: View applicable procedure videos on the DVD-ROM found in the back of this book.

MyHealthProfessionsKit.com: Test your knowledge of the chapter with games and activities. MyHealthProfessionsKit also includes resources, helpful links, and a Spanish audio glossary.

Medical Assisting Interactive: Practice your procedures as a medical assistant in this simulated doctor's office. This can be accessed through MyHealthProfessionsKit.com.

2

Medical Science: History and Practice

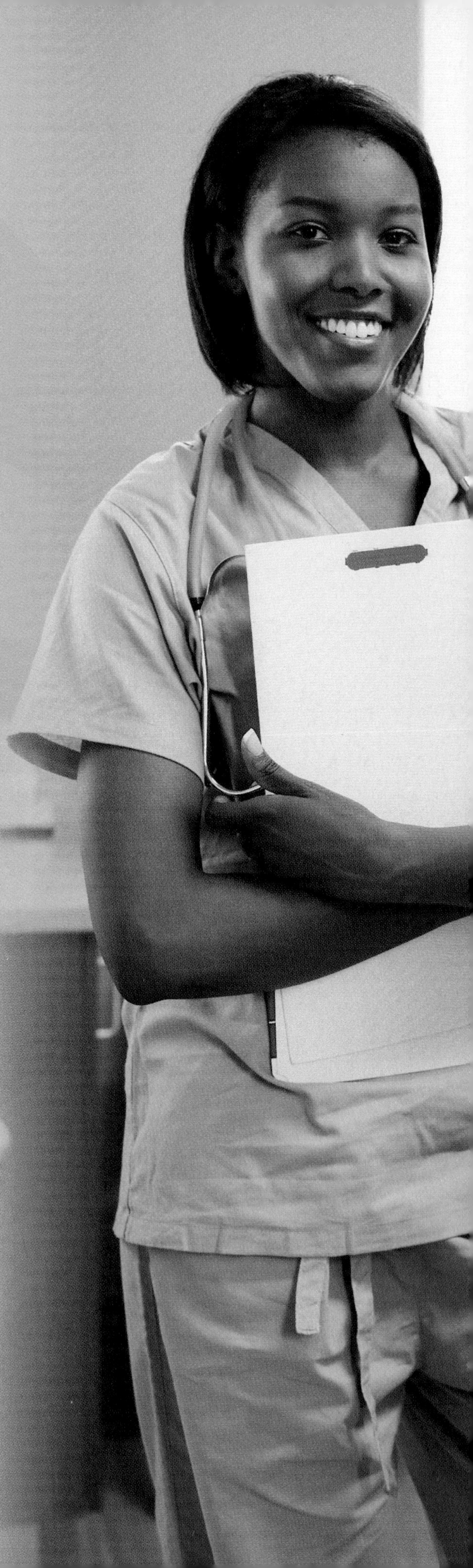

LEARNING OBJECTIVES

After completing this chapter, you should be able to:

- Define and spell the terms to learn for this chapter.

- Discuss the contributions of early medicine to health care.

- Discuss medical contributors of the eighteenth, nineteenth, and twentieth centuries.

- Identify and discuss the role women played in the history of medicine.

- Discuss modern medicine and the future of medicine.

- Describe the difference between an internship and a residency in the training of physicians.

- State which type of medical practice is addressed under the medical and surgical specialties.

- Discuss ten allied health fields and the educational requirements for each.

- Discuss the current trends in health care that are driving changes in medical practice.

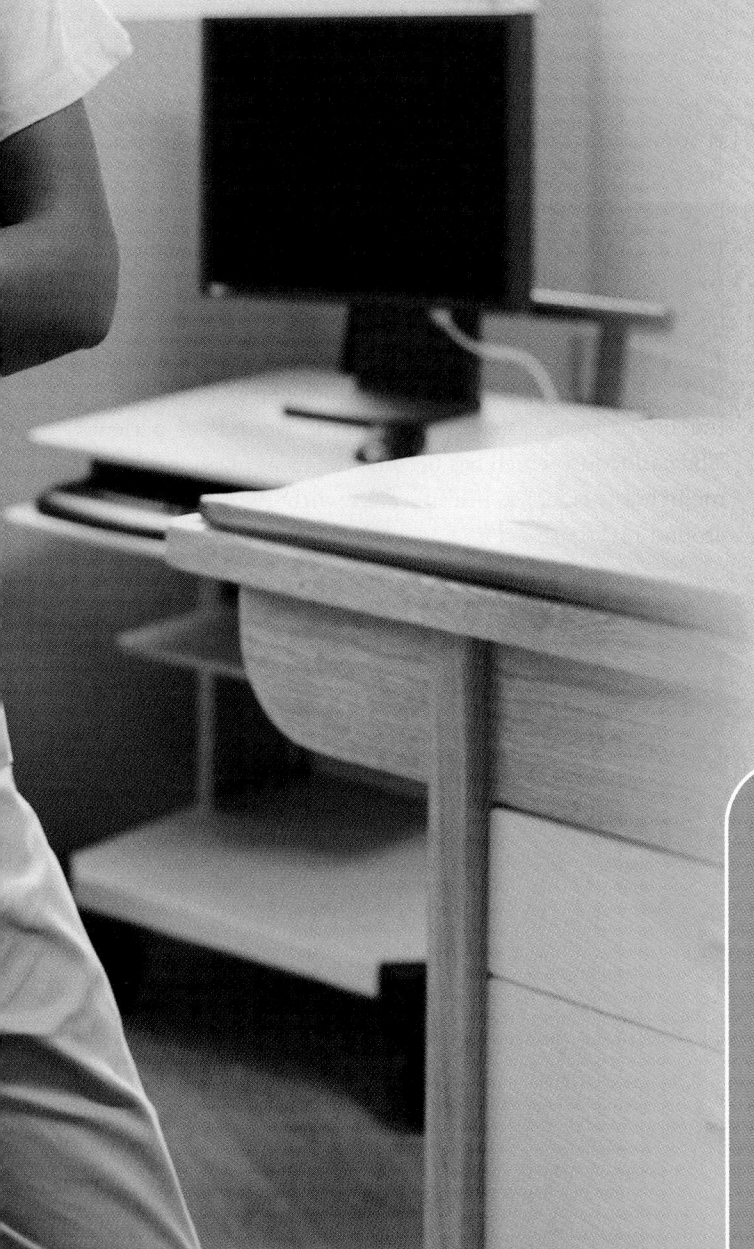

CHAPTER OUTLINE

CASE STUDY

Tania Washington has been an office manager for Pearson Physicians Group for the past eight years. During the past five years, the patient load has continued to grow. Dr. Bahjat, one of the managing partners of Pearson Physicians Group, has asked Tania to help the practice find a physician who will be added to the list of providers and help with the patient load.

The healing art of medicine was taught and practiced before written records were kept. This chapter describes the science and practice of medicine from the earliest evidence of healing, when disease was considered to be of supernatural origin, to the present—a time of astounding research, discovery, and healing. Contributions of many ancient peoples still influence medicine today. The discussion of present-day medical codes of ethics, rules pertaining to sanitization, personal hygiene, herbal cures, acupuncture, and other medical and surgical practices highlights the specific contributions of early medicine and those whose accomplishments catapulted the science of medicine into the amazing field that it is today.

This chapter provides a picture of today's medical practitioners—issues of licensure, including evaluations, credentials, reciprocity, renewals, suspensions, and doctor's titles. In addition, current trends in health care, health care costs, types of practices, medical and surgical specialties, and roles and educational requirements of a variety of health care team members are covered.

History of Medicine

Drawings, bony remains, and archaic surgical tools are evidence of early human attempts to practice medicine. Folk medicine, which incorporated plants, adopted a trial-and-error method to determine which were poisonous and which had medicinal value. Early humans attributed supernatural origins to some ailments. In early medicine, some diseases were considered the work of a demon, an evil spirit, or an offended god who had placed some object, such as a worm, into the body of the patient. Treatment consisted of trying to remove the evil intruder.

The first doctors—considered "medicine men" and "medicine women"—were shamans, witch doctors, or sorcerers. In 3000 BC, Babylonian physicians practiced medicine using the written Code of Hammurabi, named after an early king of Babylon. This code has laws relating to the practice of medicine, which included severe penalties for errors. For example, according to the code, a doctor who killed a patient while opening an abscess would have his hands cut off.

CONTRIBUTIONS OF ANCIENT CIVILIZATIONS

A study of medical practices in early Egypt offers greater insight into the basis of modern medicine. The Egyptians left behind lists of remedies, surgical treatments of wounds and injuries, and records for rules of sanitation. Personal hygiene, the sanitary preparation of food, and other matters of public health were pioneered by the practices of the Jewish religion and culture.

Some records of early Greek practitioners depict them using nonpoisonous snakes to treat the wounds of patients. The **caduceus**, which has become the recognized symbol for medicine, depicts a healing staff with two snakes coiled around it (Figure 2-1).

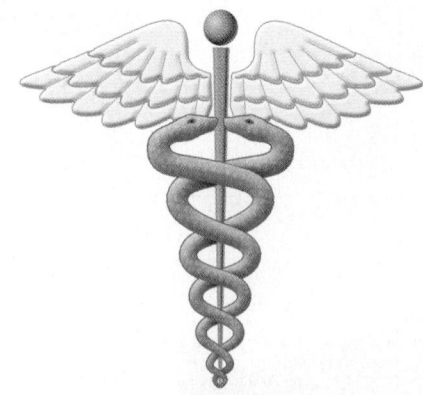

FIGURE 2-1 A caduceus, the emblem of the medical profession.

Herbal medical remedies originating from ancient India are recorded as early as 800 BC. The Chinese culture wrote about human blood pulses around the time of 250 BC. Both early Japanese and Chinese cultures practiced acupuncture successfully.

Ancient Cures Are Today's Legacy

Early medicine, while often based on superstition, actually provided medicinal remedies that are still in use today. The effects of opium, which is produced by the poppy plant, was known in ancient times to relieve severe pain. Today opium derivatives are used in the medication morphine. The following are early remedies still used today:

- Nitroglycerine to treat heart patients
- Digitalis from the foxglove plant to regulate and strengthen the heartbeat
- Sulfur and cayenne pepper to stop bleeding
- Chamomile and licorice to aid digestion
- Cranberry to treat urinary tract infections

EARLY MEDICINE

Early medicine began with Hippocrates and the shift from the belief in magical sources of illness and disease to more scientific study, which looked to physical causes of disease. The medieval period from the fifth century to the sixteenth century was a time of little or no progress in medical practices. Poor personal hygiene, poor nutrition, and the lack of sanitation led to many epidemics. (An epidemic is a disease that infects a large part of a population in one region or location at the same time.) The bubonic plague was a **pandemic** because it affected many people in different countries at the same time. It was known as the black plague or black death because the corpses appeared dark due to hemorrhage under the skin. Death from it also was extensive in China, India, Europe, Russia, Egypt, and North Africa. The cause of bubonic plague was not discovered until 1905. It was determined then that it was **bacteria** that grew in the fleas of infected rats. Bacteria are **microorganisms**, which are minute living organisms, some of which are capable of causing disease.

During the medieval period, medical teaching was mostly oral. Surgeons, at the time, only treated the wealthy. Other patients had to rely on the local barber to perform surgical procedures. The red-and-white striped pole we are familiar with today was the sign that barbers used—a white pole wrapped with bloody bandages to solicit business. This period concludes with the introduction of the microscope and the ability to see and measure bacteria previously not observed with the naked eye.

Hippocrates: Father of Medicine

Historically, the first scientific system of medicine is of Greek origin and is usually associated with Hippocrates (460–377 BC), who has become known as the Father of Medicine. Hippocrates shifted medicine from the realm of mysticism and into the area of scientific practice. He stressed the body's healing nature, clinical descriptions of diseases, and the ability to discover some diseases by listening to the chest. He practiced medicine at a time in history when little was known about anatomy and physiology. Nevertheless, his writings and descriptions of symptoms remain accurate today. See Figure 2-2 for a photo of Hippocrates.

The Hippocratic Oath (Box 2-1) is part of the writings of this fifth-century BC physician. The oath serves as a widely used ethical guide for physicians who pledge to work for the good of the patient, to do him or her no harm, to prescribe no deadly drugs, to give no advice that could cause death, and to keep confidential medical information regarding the patient. The oath is still often administered as part of graduation ceremonies in medical schools.

Galen

Galen (130–201 AD), a Greek physician who practiced in Rome (Figure 2-3), initially followed the Hippocratic method. He stressed the value of anatomy and founded experimental physiology. He stated that arteries contained blood and not air as previously believed. Since the dissection of humans was illegal during Galen's time, he based his theories on the examination of pigs and apes. While some of his work is inaccurate due to the lack of human **cadavers**, or dead bodies used to study human anatomy, he is still known as the Prince of Physicians.

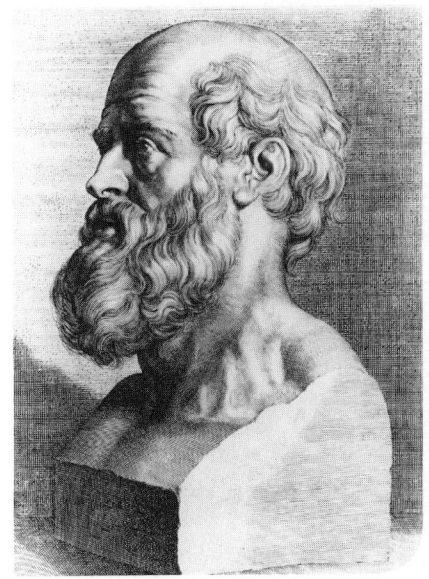

FIGURE 2-2 Hippocrates.
Source: National Library of Medicine

Box 2-1 The Hippocratic OATH

I swear by Apollo Physician, by Asclepias, by Health, by Heal All, and by all the gods and goddesses, that according to my ability and judgment, I will keep this oath and stipulation; to reckon him who taught me this art equally dear to me as my parents, and share my substance with him and relieve his necessities if required. To regard his offspring as on the same footing with my own brothers and to teach them this art if they should wish to learn it, without fee or stipulation; and that by precept, lecture, and every other mode of instruction I will impart a knowledge of my art to my own sons and to those of my teachers and to disciples bound by a stipulation and oath according to the law of medicine, but to none others.

I will follow that method of treatment which according to my ability and judgment, I consider for the benefit of my patients, and abstain from whatever is deleterious and mischievous. I will give not deadly medicine to anyone if asked, nor suggest any counsel.

Furthermore, I will not give to a woman an instrument to produce an abortion.

With Purity and with Holiness, I will pass my life and practice my art. I will not cut a person who is suffering with a stone, but will leave this to the practitioners of this work. Into whatever houses I enter I will go into them for the benefit of the sick and will abstain from every voluntary act of mischief and corruption; and further from the seduction of females or males, bond or free.

Whatever, in connection with my professional practice, or not in connection with it, I may see or hear in the lives of men which ought not to be spoken abroad, I will not divulge, as reckoning that all such should be kept secret.

While I continue to keep this oath inviolate, may it be granted to me to enjoy life and practice the art respected by all men, at all times, but should I trespass and violate this oath, may the reverse be my lot.

Galileo

Galileo (1564–1642) was the first to use a telescope to study the skies. Applications of the telescope lens led to the invention of the microscope.

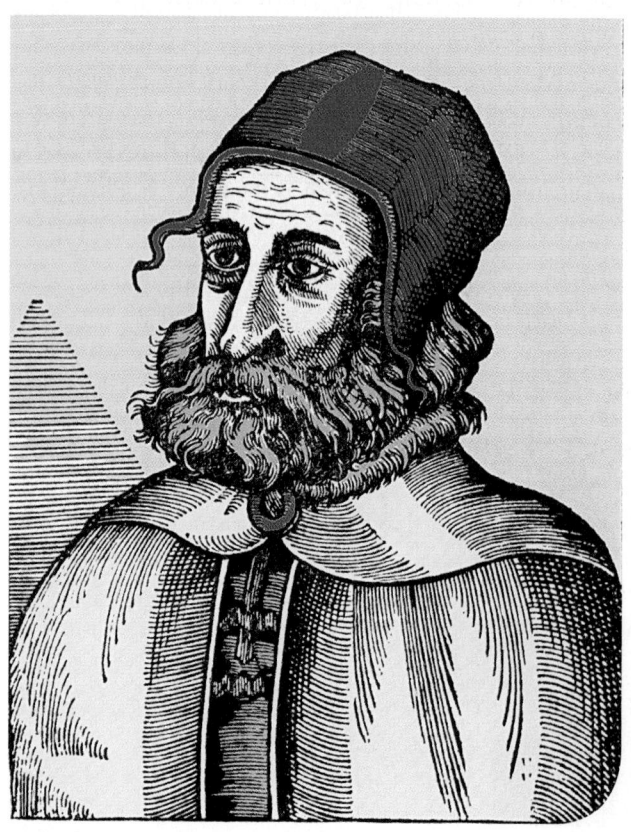

FIGURE 2-3   Galen.
Source: Photo Researchers Inc.

William Harvey

In England during the seventeenth century, William Harvey (1578–1657) began writing about blood circulation and using the experimental method in medicine. Unfortunately for Harvey, the microscope had not yet been invented, and he was never able to view capillaries.

Zacharias Jansen

Zacharias Janssen (1580–1638) was the Dutch eyeglass maker who invented the microscope.

Anton van Leeuwenhoek

Anton van Leeuwenhoek (1632–1723) of Holland devoted his life to microscopic studies. He is known as the first person to observe and describe bacteria, which he referred to as "tiny little beasties." He is also responsible for describing protozoa—the simplest forms, usually one cell, of animals—and spermatozoa (mature male sex cells).

MEDICINE DURING THE EIGHTEENTH CENTURY

In England, formal medical training began when it was required that anyone wishing to become a doctor must first become an apprentice. Medical schools in Scotland—Edinburgh and Glasgow—were developed during this era.

John Hunter

John Hunter (1728–1793) developed surgery and surgical pathology into a science. He is noted as the Founder of Scientific Surgery. Some of his contributions to medical science include the introduction of a flexible feeding tube into the stomach. The term *surgeon* comes from the Greek words *cheir,* which means "hand," and *ergeon,* which means "work."

Edward Jenner

Public health and hygiene began to attract attention during the eighteenth century. A country doctor, Edward Jenner (1749–1823), a pupil of John Hunter, observed that dairy maids who had become infected with the disease cowpox would not become infected with the deadly disease smallpox. Jenner overcame ridicule from the medical community and went on to perform the first vaccination using the smallpox vaccine.

The term *vaccination* comes from the Latin word *vacca,* meaning "cow." Cowpox was referred to as *vaccinia.* Today the term *vaccine* means "live or attenuated material given to a person to establish resistance to disease." Today's vaccines come from animals other than cows and from synthetic sources.

Rene Laennec

Another major advancement in medicine was made by Rene Laennec (1781–1826), who invented the stethoscope. His invention, the precursor of today's modern instrument, was based on the use of paper wrapped into a cone shape that was then placed over the patient's chest to listen to the heart.

Benjamin Franklin

The American statesman Benjamin Franklin (1706–1790) was an inventor. In addition to his invention of bifocals, his discovery that colds could be passed from one person to another was an important contribution to medical science.

MEDICINE DURING THE NINETEENTH CENTURY

During the nineteenth century, the practice of medicine advanced rapidly. The documentation of accurate anatomy and physiology allowed physicians to better understand the human body. The use of sophisticated microscopes, injection materials, and instruments such as the ophthalmoscope all moved the practice of medicine forward.

The discovery of the cell was one of the most enlightening discoveries of this era. Many believe that the greatest achievement of the nineteenth century was the knowledge that certain diseases, as well as surgical wound infections, were directly caused by microorganisms. The practice of surgery changed as a result of this knowledge, along with advances in the use of anesthetics.

Louis Pasteur

Louis Pasteur (1822–1895) (Figure 2-4) is credited for establishing the science of bacteriology. His experiments proved

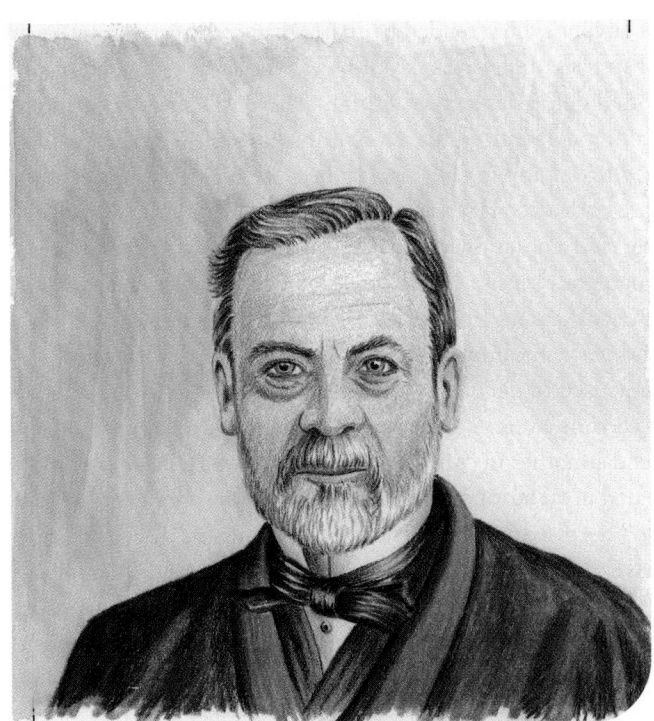

FIGURE 2-4 Louis Pasteur.
Source: Education Management Group (EMG)

that putrefaction or decay was caused by living organisms known as bacteria. His work solved many medical problems during his day, including rabies, anthrax in sheep and cattle, and chicken cholera.

Anthrax is a deadly infectious disease caused by *Bacillus anthracisis.* Humans can contract the disease from infected animal hair, hides, or waste. Cholera, an acute infection of the small bowel causing severe diarrhea, was determined to be a bacillus transmitted through water, milk, or food contaminated with excreta of carriers.

The process of **pasteurization** is named after Pasteur. It is the process during which substances, such as milk and cheese, are heated to a certain temperature to eliminate bacteria.

Joseph Lister

Joseph Lister (1827–1912) borrowed Pasteur's theories and eventually introduced the antiseptic system in surgery. Until that time, surgeons and obstetricians did not wash their hands between patients, so disease was being spread from one patient to another. Lister advised placing an antiseptic barrier between the wound and the germ-containing atmosphere. Present-day aseptic techniques can be attributed to Lister's work.

Ignaz Semmelweiss

Ignaz Semmelweiss (1818–1865), an obstetrician in Vienna, advised medical students to disinfect the hands and clothing of anyone who attended a birth. During the early practice of obstetrics, a physician would wear the same "butcher's coat" for all deliveries in the hospital. There was a high death rate from puerperal sepsis or childbed fever. Women avoided having a baby in the hospital because of the high mortality rate or death rate. Eventually, the use of contaminated clothing and contaminated hands were traced to the spread of puerperal sepsis thanks to Dr. Semmelweiss. The term *puerperal* comes from the Latin words *puer,* meaning "child," and *pario,* meaning "to bring forth." The term *puerperium* is now used to denote a period of time after a delivery.

Semmelweiss noted that the medical students would attend a mother in childbirth immediately after having participated in an **autopsy**, an examination of the organs and tissues of a deceased body to determine the cause of death. After he advised students to disinfect their hands before attending childbirth, the incidence of disease went down dramatically. In the 1800s, the men who advocated disinfection were ridiculed and in Semmelweiss's case were considered insane.

Robert Koch

Robert Koch (1843–1910) showed how bacteria could be cultivated and stained. He discovered the tubercle bacillus, the cause of tuberculosis. His investigation into the cause of cholera led to knowledge that contaminated food and water can cause disease.

Paul Ehrlich

Paul Ehrlich (1854–1915) was a pioneer in the study of microbiology. He was a pioneer in the fields of immunology, bacteriology, and the use of chemotherapy. **Immunology** is the study of immunity, the resistance to or protection from disease. **Chemotherapy** is the use of chemicals, including drugs, to treat or control infections and disease. He developed a method for staining bacteria and cells, which eventually led to a means for providing a differential diagnosis based on classifying organisms. He was one of the original "microbe hunters." **Microbes** are one-celled forms of life, such as bacteria. His greatest achievement was the discovery, on his 606th attempt, of the "magic bullet" to treat **syphilis**, an infectious and chronic venereal disease.

Other Major Advances During This Period

William Roentgen (1845–1923) discovered X-rays, Pierre Curie (1859–1906) and Marie Curie (1867–1934) discovered radium, and Sigmund Freud (1856–1939) worked in the field of psychiatry.

American Medicine During This Period

Significant contributions were made to medicine through the work of William Norton, Crawford Long, and Walter Reed. The specific work of each of these individuals is highlighted here.

William Morton and Crawford Long. An important American contribution to the practice of medicine during this period was the discovery of anesthesia. William Morton (1819–1868), a dentist at Massachusetts General Hospital, and Crawford Long (1815–1878), a Georgia physician, are generally credited with having first demonstrated the use of ether as a general anesthetic. **Anesthesia** refers to the partial or complete absence of sensation. An anesthetic is a substance used to produce anesthesia. Morton and Long worked independently of each other and made possible life-saving operations that previously could not be performed without anesthetics.

Walter Reed. Walter Reed (1851–1902) and others helped to conquer yellow fever, which allowed for completion of the construction of the Panama Canal by reducing the death rate for the workers. Dr. Reed gathered volunteers who allowed him to inject them with yellow fever in order to find a cure.

MEDICINE DURING THE TWENTIETH CENTURY

The first half of the twentieth century resulted in major medical advances. Death rates from diseases such as tuberculosis and diphtheria dropped dramatically. The overall mortality rates decreased due to improved medical care, and new emphasis was placed on **morbidity rates** (rates of disease and illness). Four major developments dominate this period:

- The development of chemotherapy and the specialty of oncology
- The development of immunology
- Progress in endocrinology
- Progress in nutrition

Alexander Fleming

One of the most dramatic episodes of the modern era was the discovery of antibiotics. Sir Alexander Fleming (1881–1955) (Figure 2-5) accidentally discovered that a stray mold on his culture plate of staphylococci would cause the bacteria to stop growing. He called this mold penicillium, and it has become known throughout the world as penicillin. Fleming's discovery took place in 1928.

Fleming and two other scientists won the Nobel Prize for their work with penicillin. It was one of the first chemicals used to treat infections. Today, the term *chemotherapy* generally refers to drugs used to treat forms of cancer.

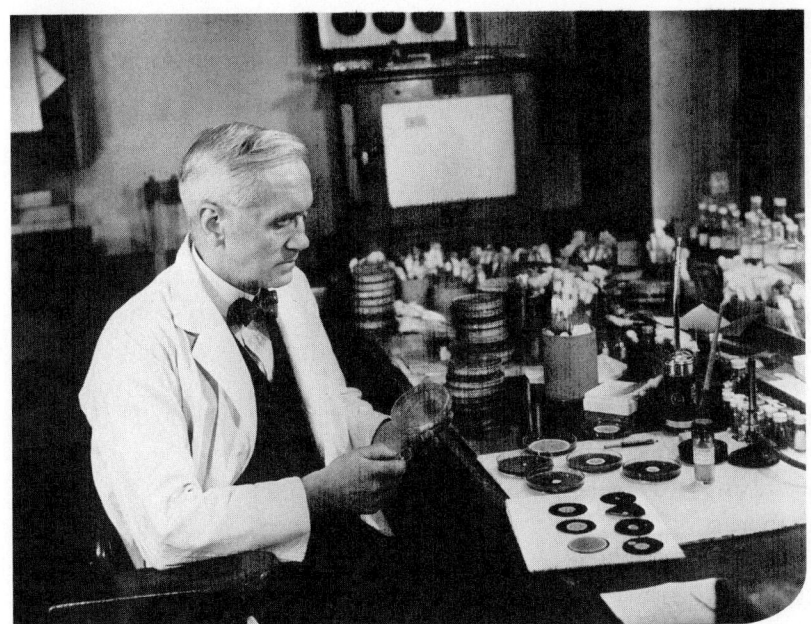

FIGURE 2-5 Alexander Fleming.
Source: Getty images - Hulton Archive photos

Jonas Salk and Albert Sabin

The study of immunology advanced with the discovery of vaccines against typhoid, tetanus, diphtheria, tuberculosis, yellow fever, influenza, and measles. During the 1950s, Doctors Jonas Salk (1914–1996) and Albert Sabin (1906–1993) developed vaccines that eradicated the crippling disease polio.

WOMEN IN MEDICINE

Few women were allowed to practice medicine in the early years. In part, this was due to social constraints on women appearing in public. However, many women did practice as midwives and became skilled at delivering babies. Some remarkable female physicians and nurses overcame great odds to practice in their profession.

Elizabeth Blackwell

Elizabeth Blackwell (1821–1910) was the first female physician in the United States. After being turned down by several medical schools, she was finally awarded a degree in 1849 in New York. She went on to open a medical college for women and her own dispensary.

Florence Nightingale

Florence Nightingale (1820–1910) is considered the founder of modern nursing. She studied nursing in Europe and cared for wounded soldiers during the Crimean War (1850–1853). Nightingale and her fellow nurses were treated poorly by the doctors at that time.

Nightingale's attention to detail, record keeping, and compassionate nursing care changed the way nursing was practiced. She advocated the use of the nursing process and elevated nursing to an honored profession. She is referred to as "The Lady with the Lamp" due to her tireless work night and day to supervise the nursing care of wounded soldiers. She started the first school of nursing in 1860 at St. Thomas Hospital in London.

Clara Barton

Clara Barton (1821–1912) was a contemporary of Florence Nightingale who nursed soldiers in a different war, the Civil War in the United States. She established the American Red Cross when she became aware of the need for support services for the soldiers. She also established the Federal Bureau of Records to help track injured and dead soldiers.

MODERN MEDICINE AND THE FUTURE

In the last 25 years, technological discoveries have permitted medical science to advance faster than in the previous one hundred years. The twenty-first century holds even more potential for greater advances. The average life span of ancient humans was 30 years. According to the U.S. Census Bureau in 2001, a person born in 1900 had the life expectancy of 47 years and someone born in 1991 had the life expectancy of 76 years. With rapid medical advancements, some estimate a life expectancy of 100 years will be possible.

Improved communication techniques now allow patients' results to be examined by physicians across the country. Robotics is being used in surgery. It is considered routine to successfully replace knees, hips, kidneys, and corneas. The future of medical science in the twenty-first century is vast.

Medical Firsts

In 1954, doctors at Brigham Hospital in Boston performed the first successful kidney transplant. In earlier attempts, patients died because physicians did not know that organs had to be compatible for a successful transplant. In this successful transplant, an organ was used from the patient's twin.

Dr. Michael DeBakey (Figure 2-6) invented the heart pump in 1960, which made open-heart surgery possible for millions. In 1962, doctors in Boston successfully reattached the severed arm on a young boy. In 1967, Dr. Christian Barnard completed the first heart transplant. A totally implantable heart was placed in the chest of several critically ill patients in 2001.

The discovery of the human immunodeficiency virus (HIV) as the cause of AIDS in 1984 was a major breakthrough in understanding **acquired immune deficiency**

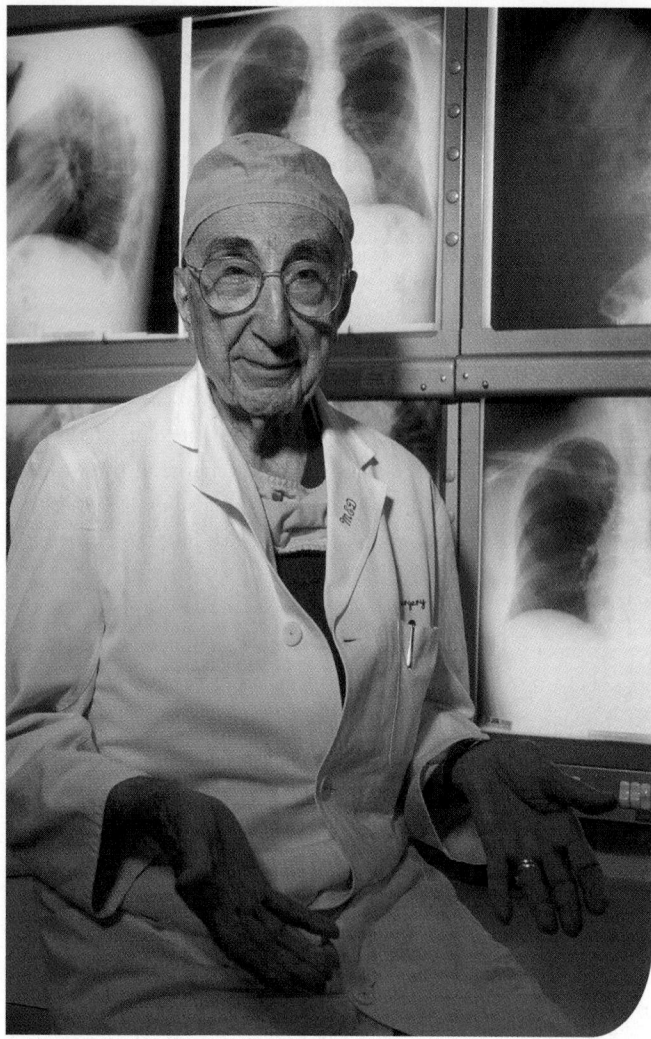

FIGURE 2-6 Dr. Michael DeBakey.
Source: Peter Arnold, Inc.

syndrome (AIDS). AIDS is a series of illnesses that occur as a result of infection by HIV, which causes the immune system to break down. Although there is as yet no cure for AIDS, a combination of drugs has stopped HIV replication to the extent that the virus is undetectable in some people. Treatment of pregnant woman with AZT and a combination of other drugs has greatly reduced the number of HIV-positive babies. Hopefully, a cure for HIV and better treatments for AIDS will be forthcoming.

Other breakthroughs include genetic engineering during the 1980s, which permitted greater production of vaccines, the birth of the first test-tube baby in England in 1978, and the cloning of the first sheep in 1997.

The Medical Frontier

The **human genome project**, a publicly funded international research project to sequence and identify human genes and record their positions on chromosomes, was completed in 2001. Information from the project enables doctors to routinely screen donor eggs for many inherited diseases. Mapping human genes has allowed for DNA testing to identify criminals, provide genetic counseling for prospective parents, and design treatments for diseases. With identification of the gene that causes Alzheimer's disease, certain types of breast cancer, and cystic fibrosis, better treatments and potential cures may be possible.

A **stem cell** is an undifferentiated cell that can give rise to other cells of the same type or from which specialized cells can develop. Stem cell research will play an important part in medical science over the next 20 years and beyond. It is already being used to induce cells in the diseased pancreas of a diabetic to produce insulin.

Hopes for the future include the following:

- A cure for AIDS
- A vaccine to prevent HIV
- Cloning organs to overcome the shortage of donors
- Better treatment and outcomes for mental illness
- Cures for heart disease, cancer, and obesity
- Methods to slow aging
- Regeneration of brain and nerve cells to overcome paralysis
- Development of antibiotics that do not allow bacteria to develop a resistant strain

Medical Practitioners

The medical assistance training and skills that you receive will enable you to work for physicians who practice in a variety of specializations. As a medical assistant, you will encounter many allied health professionals from a wide range of fields. It is important that you understand and respect the role and educational requirements of others.

In this section, we discuss the different types of credentials for those practicing medicine. Areas covered include fields of practice as well as educational requirements for medical doctors, osteopaths, and chiropractors. In addition, the Medical Practice Act and licensure issues, such as examination, reciprocity, and suspension are covered.

TITLE OF DOCTOR

The title of doctor designates a person who holds a doctoral degree. Commonly "doctor" refers to a medical doctor (an MD). The practice of medicine, which is the science of diagnosis, treatment, and prevention of disease, requires a minimum of 9 to 10 years of education and training, which generally includes a four-year college degree in premedical studies, four years of medical school, and a period of internship. During the first year of residency or internship, the medical student obtains vital practical experience under the supervision of a licensed physician. At the end of the residency or internship he or she takes a state medical board examination. If the candidate passes the state examination, he or she then becomes licensed to practice medicine in that state.

However, if the new physician wishes, he or she may seek graduate training in a specialty area or residency. This is a paid, on-the-job training position lasting anywhere from two to six years, depending on the specialty chosen. Then, the resident/doctor must sit for an American Board of Medical Specialties (ABMS) examination in his or her area of study. For example, a physician who specializes in obstetrics and passes the examination would be board certified by the American Board of Obstetrics and Gynecology. At this point, the new physician chooses how and where he or she would like to practice medicine. Types of medical practices are discussed later in this chapter.

OTHERS WITH TITLE OF DOCTOR

The designation "doctor" is also used as a proper way of addressing—verbally or in writing—someone who holds a doctoral degree of any kind. The abbreviation for doctor is "Dr." In the medical field, the title Doctor (Dr.) indicates that a person is qualified to practice medicine. In other fields, the title Doctor (Dr.) means that a person has attained the highest educational degree in his or her field. Several designations for doctor are listed in Table 2-1 with the corresponding initials.

A Doctor of Osteopathy (DO) degree has educational requirements similar to those for the medical doctor. Both MDs and DOs are licensed physicians. Both categories of

TABLE 2-1 Designations and Initials for Doctors

Term	Initials
Doctor of Chiropractic	DC
Doctor of Dental Medicine	DMD
Doctor of Dental Surgery	DDS
Doctor of Education	EdD
Doctor of Medicine	MD
Doctor of Optometry	OD
Doctor of Osteopathy	DO
Doctor of Philosophy	PhD
Doctor of Podiatric Medicine	DPM

physicians use similar approaches to medicine, including the use of drugs, therapy, and radiation. Both groups must pass state board examinations to become licensed in their states. Doctors of Osteopathy learn the skill of manipulation therapy in schools of osteopathy. The **osteopath** places great emphasis on the relationship between the musculoskeletal system and the organs of the body. In most states, the osteopath is able to perform the same procedures as a medical doctor.

A chiropractor (DC) is trained in manipulation of the spinal cord and other areas of the body. This field requires two years of premedical studies and four years of training in a licensed chiropractic school. Most states license chiropractors.

Medical Practice Acts

Each state has regulations that direct the practice of medicine within that state. While slight differences are found from state to state, in general, medical practice acts uphold who must be licensed to perform certain procedures. These acts also maintain the requirements for licensure (granting of a license), duties associated with that license, grounds on which the license can be revoked or taken away, and reports that must be made to the government. Medical practice acts also cover the penalties for practicing without a valid license.

If a physician moves to another state, he or she must obtain a license to practice in that state. This may require taking and passing another state medical examination. Some states allow reciprocity of physician licenses, which is discussed later in this chapter.

Generally, physicians in different states may consult with each other without being licensed in each other's states. Physicians who practice in governmental institutions, such as Department of Veterans Affairs hospitals or military service, may practice medicine without local licensure.

LICENSURE

The Board of Medical Examiners in each state grants a license to practice medicine. Licensure may be granted in any of three ways: examination, endorsement, or reciprocity.

Examination

Each state offers its own examination for licensure. This examination is usually taken before the end of medical school. Within the United States, the official medical licensing examination is called the Federation Licensing Examination (FLEX). The license is then issued after an internship is completed. Successful performance on this examination entitles one to set up private practice as a general practitioner. The United States Medical Licensing Examination (USMLE), which was first administered in 1992, provides a single three-step licensing examination for graduates from accredited medical schools that can facilitate the process of obtaining reciprocity.

Endorsement

Endorsement, meaning an approval or sanction, is granted to applicants who have successfully passed the National Board Medical Examiners (NBME). In fact, most physicians in the United States are licensed by endorsement. Any medical school graduate who is not licensed by endorsement is required to pass the state board examination (FLEX). Graduates of foreign medical schools must pass the same requirements as U.S. graduates.

Reciprocity

In some cases, the state to which the physician is applying for a license will accept the state license that the physician already holds so that the physician will not have to take another examination. This practice is known as reciprocity.

REGISTRATION

It is necessary for physicians to maintain their license by periodic re-registration either annually or biannually. The physician is notified by mail when to re-register and must submit the re-registration fee within a designated time period. In addition to payment of a fee to re-register, 75 hours of continuing medical education (CME) units in a three-year period are required to ensure that the physician remains current in the field of practice.

PROFESSIONALISM

Licensure and continuing medical education (CME) are two areas in which the medical assistant can assist the physician. The renewal of licenses is usually dependent on the completion of re-registration forms and filing these forms on time along with the necessary fees. Accurate records of continuing medical education units should always be maintained because CME is an important part of the licensing process. Be alert to this legal obligation for yourself, and remind your employing physician in advance of such renewals.

Medical assistants dedicate themselves to the care and well-being of all patients, according to the American Association of Medical Assistants code of ethics. In addition, medical assistants should take the Oath of Hippocrates, "Do no harm to the patient," as seriously as the physicians who state it at the time of their graduation from medical school. As a medical assistant, you will act as a representative of the physician and must be well versed on all legal issues that affect the physician's practice.

SUSPENSION AND REVOCATION

A physician's license may be revoked in cases of severe misconduct, which include unprofessional conduct, commission of a crime, or personal incapacity to perform one's duties. Unprofessional conduct relates to behavior that fails to meet the ethical standards of the profession, such as inappropriate use of drugs or alcohol. Crimes include rape, murder, larceny, and narcotics convictions. The physician, however, does not automatically lose the license in case of a felony or malpractice conviction. Due process requires a trial by the state board of medicine before a physician's license is revoked. Personal incapacity relates to the physician's inability to perform due to physical or mental incapacities.

Health Care Costs and Payments

Before discussing medical specialties, types of medical practices, health care facilities, and the role and education of allied health professions, it is important to look at some health care costs and trends. Comprehending these trends and their impact on health care makes you a more informed professional and will lead to a better understanding of problems that patients may have obtaining and paying for health care.

Health care has changed dramatically in the past 25 years. It has become the largest industry in the nation, providing 12.9 million jobs according to the Bureau of Labor Statistics. The costs of health care are increasing faster than the cost of living. It is estimated that more than 17 percent of the U.S. gross national product (GNP) is spent on health care, an average of $8,160 per person. According to the Kaiser Family Foundation, more than 45 million Americans were uninsured in 2007. The number of working Americans without health care is increasing because they cannot afford the premiums. According to the Kaiser Family Foundation, the annual premium for a family would be more than $12,000 a year for health care coverage. The United States is the only industrialized nation that does not provide some sort of basic health care for all citizens.

What are some of the factors that are driving the skyrocketing costs of health care delivery today?

- Technological advances are expensive.
- Knowledge growth and technology have led to physician specialization.
- Specialization has damaged the long-term doctor–patient relationship; patients do not feel close to the specialists and are more inclined to sue these doctors.

- Drug costs are skyrocketing.
- The population is aging, and the older segment of the population uses the most health care services.
- Longer life expectancy means greater need for care for a longer time.
- Patients are not passive; they are active, informed consumers who demand more tests and options.
- The uninsured rely on emergency room visits for primary care and do not seek medical care until absolutely necessary.
- The uninsured have less or no access to preventive care and often require treatment for more advanced illness or ailments.
- Social conditions—such as homelessness, substance abuse, poverty, child abuse, breakup of the family unit, and more people living alone—impact individual health, health care delivery systems, and health care costs.

These trends must be considered as we continue with our discussion of the types of practices, governmental regulations, and steps utilized to control the costs of health care. Insurance companies, managed care plans such as health maintenance organizations (HMOs), diagnosis related groups (DRGs), and government legislation have attempted to control costs and have had significant impact on the way health care services are delivered.

In 1983, Medicare instituted the **diagnosis related groups (DRGs)** hospital payment system, which classifies each Medicare patient according to his or her illness within 467 illness categories. Under this system, hospitals receive a preset sum for treatment, regardless of the actual number of bed days of care used by a patient. This method of payment provides further incentive to keep costs down. However, it has also led to early discharge of patients, has increased the number of readmissions, and has discouraged treatment of severely ill patients.

Types of Medical Practices

In the early part of the twentieth century, the main form of medical practice was the solo practice, in which a family practitioner set up a medical practice within a designated town or geographic area. Solo practices are becoming less and less popular due to the increased costs and changes associated with practicing medicine and the legal environment associated with it. Other forms of medical practice have become popular to meet patients' needs for around-the-clock medical coverage. Alternate types of medical practices also provide the opportunity for a group of physicians to share insurance premium costs, staff, and investments in facilities.

SOLO PRACTICE

In a solo practice, a physician practices alone and is responsible for all administrative decisions associated with his or her practice. Physicians generally enter into agreements with each other in order to establish coverage for patient care during off-duty times. It is also common for two solo practice physicians to work out of the same building or office in order to share office expenses.

SOLE PROPRIETORSHIP

In a sole proprietorship, one physician is still responsible for making all the administrative decisions. However, this physician may employ other physicians and pay them a salary. The physician-owner will pay all expenses and retain all assets. In the sole proprietorship form of practice, the owner is responsible and liable for the actions of all the employees.

PARTNERSHIP

A partnership is a legal agreement to share in the business operation of a medical practice. A partnership is between two or more physicians. In this legal arrangement, each of the partners becomes responsible for the actions of all the partners. This refers to debts and all legal actions, unless otherwise stipulated in the legal partnership agreement.

ASSOCIATE PRACTICE

The associate practice is a legal arrangement in which physicians agree to share a facility and staff. They do not, as a general rule, share responsibility for the legal actions of each other as in the partnership. The legal contract of agreement stipulates the responsibilities of each party. The physicians act as if each practice is a sole proprietorship.

The legal arrangement must be carefully described and discussed with patients. In some cases, patients have mistakenly believed that there was a shared responsibility by all the physicians in the practice.

GROUP PRACTICE

A group practice consists of three or more physicians who share the same facility (office or clinic) and practice medicine together. This is a legal form of practice in which the physicians share all expenses, income, personnel, equipment, and records. Some areas of medicine frequently found in group practice are anesthesiology, rehabilitative or obstetrical services, radiology, and pathology.

A group practice can also be designated as a health maintenance organization (HMO) or as an independent practice association (IPA). Group practices have grown rapidly during the last decade. Large group practices with over a hundred doctors are not uncommon. A large group practice will often form a legal corporation.

PROFESSIONAL CORPORATION

During the 1960s, state legislatures passed laws (statutes) allowing professionals (e.g., physicians, lawyers, and accountants) to incorporate. A corporation is managed by a board of directors. Both legal and financial benefits result from incorporating.

Professional corporation members are known as shareholders. Therefore, the physician-members become the shareholders in the corporation. Some of the benefits that can be offered to employees of a corporation include reimbursement for medical expense, profit sharing, pension plans, and disability insurance. These fringe benefits would not be taxable to the employee and are generally tax deductible to the employer. While a corporation can be sued, the individual assets of the members cannot be touched. This is not the case in solo practices or sole proprietorships. A corporation will remain intact after a member leaves or dies. Other forms of practice, such as the sole proprietorship, may end with the death of the owner.

Medical and Surgical Specialties

Due to the dramatic advances in medicine over the past two decades, physicians continue to be interested in specialization. In addition, transplant surgery, including the liver, kidneys, lungs, and pancreas, has expanded the need for medical and surgical specialties.

MEDICAL SPECIALTIES

Descriptions of some of the more common medical specialties follows.

Allergy and Immunology

An allergist treats abnormal responses or acquired hypersensitivity to substances with medical methods that include testing and desensitization. Pediatricians and internists may sit for the board examination in allergy and immunology after taking several years of additional training.

Anesthesiology

An anesthesiologist is trained to administer drugs both locally and generally to induce a partial or complete loss of feeling (anesthesia) during a surgical procedure. This specialist also provides respiratory and cardiovascular support during surgery. The anesthesiologist meets with the patient before the surgical procedure to explain the type of anesthetic that will be used. Certified registered nurse anesthesiologists (CRNA) also may administer anesthetics.

Bariatrics

This relatively new specialty was created in response to the obesity epidemic. Physicians specializing in **bariatrics** treat patients who are obese. Their offices usually have extra-large wheelchairs, doors, scales, and examining tables. Nutritional counseling and weight reduction therapy are key components of bariatric care.

Cardiology

A cardiologist is trained to treat cardiovascular disease. This physician has received special training in the diseases and disorders of the heart and blood vessels. A cardiologist specializing in the treatment of children's heart disease would receive special training as a pediatric cardiologist.

Dermatology

A dermatologist treats injuries, growths, and infections relating to the skin, hair, and nails, either medically or surgically. A dermatologist may remove growths such as warts, moles, benign cysts, birthmarks, and skin cancers.

Emergency Medicine

The physician who specializes in emergency medicine has received additional training as an emergency medicine resident. Emergency medicine specialists typically work in hospital emergency rooms and freestanding, walk-in emergency centers. They acquire the ability and skills to quickly recognize and prioritize (triage) acute injuries, trauma, and illnesses. They also supervise paramedic prehospital care. Figure 2-7 shows an emergency department physician at work.

Endocrinology

The endocrinologist ensures that the endocrine system communicates throughout body systems. When that system fails to work properly, an endocrinologist may be called upon to diagnose, treat, and coordinate the complex therapies necessary to help the patient. The patients most frequently treated by the endocrinologist are those with diabetes mellitus and thyroid disorders.

Family Practice (Primary Care Medicine)

Family practice physicians treat the entire family regardless of age and gender. In some cases, they will refer patients with specific medical conditions to specialists.

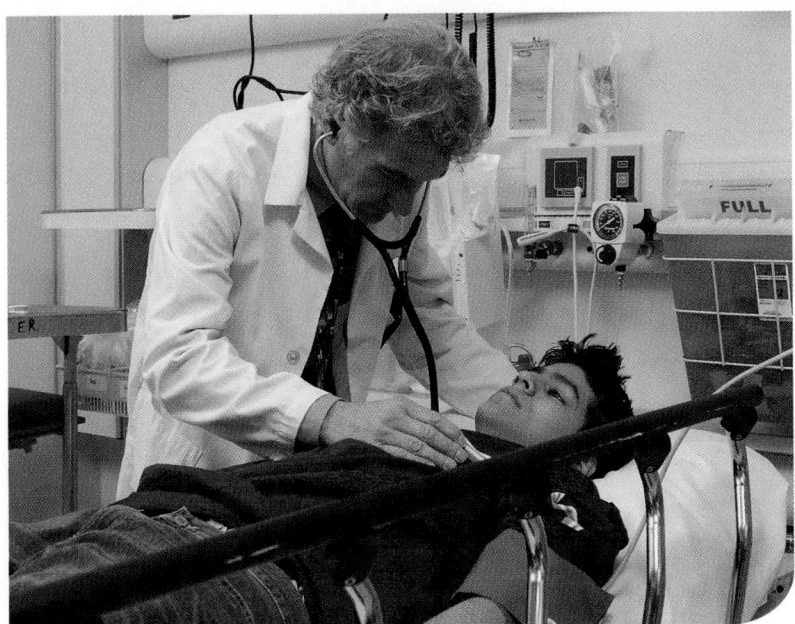

FIGURE 2-7 An emergency department physician at work.

Gastroenterology

The gastroenterologist diagnoses and treats illnesses of the gastrointestinal system. This specialty includes treatment of ulcers, digestive problems, and obesity. The gastroenterologist may need to work closely with the bariatric specialist when obesity leads to gastrointestinal diseases and disorders. Gastroenterologists perform examinations of the colon in outpatient settings.

Geriatric Medicine

The practice of geriatrics is focused on the care of diseases and disorders of the elderly. Gerontology is a relatively new field of medicine and is the direct result of the increase in the aging population.

Hematology

Hematology is the study of blood and blood-forming tissues. Hematologists specialize in laboratory research and in the care and treatment of patients with hematological diseases.

Nephrology

A nephrologist specializes in kidney pathology, including disorders and diseases. A nephrologist is skilled in both medical and surgical treatments, including kidney dialysis.

Neurology

The neurologist provides nonsurgical treatment of patients who have a disorder or disease of the nervous system.

Nuclear Medicine

The physician specializing in this field uses radioactive substances to diagnose and treat diseases such as cancer.

Obstetrics and Gynecology

An obstetrician treats the pregnant female from prenatal care through labor, delivery, and the postpartum period (Figure 2-8). A gynecologist provides both medical and surgical treatment of diseases and disorders of the female reproductive system. Gynecology is a subspecialty and also deals with infertility, which is the study of a diminished capacity or inability to produce offspring.

Oncology

Oncology is the study of cancer and cancer-related tumors, and oncologists diagnose and treat patients with such diseases.

Ophthalmology

An ophthalmologist treats disorders of the eye. The study of ophthalmology includes the diagnosis and treatment of vision problems using both medical and surgical procedures.

Orthopedics

An orthopedist, or orthopod, specializes in the branch of medicine that deals with the prevention and correction of disorders of the musculoskeletal system. An orthopedic surgeon specializes in surgical procedures relating to this specialty.

Otorhinolaryngology

Otorhinolaryngology includes the study of otology (ear), rhinology (nose), and laryngology (throat). Thus, the otorhinolaryngologist (ENT) specializes in the medical and surgical treatment of ear, nose, and throat disorders.

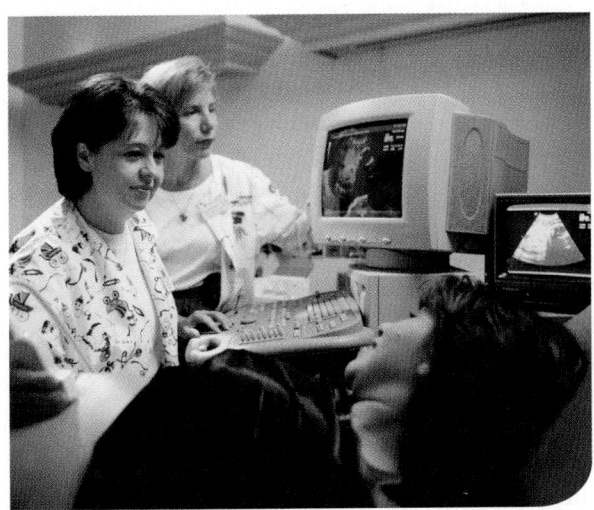

FIGURE 2-8 An obstetrician at work.

Pathology

A pathologist specializes in diagnosing abnormal changes in tissues that are removed during a surgical operation and in postmortem examinations. A forensic pathologist is an expert in determining the identity of a person based on such evidence as body parts, dental records, and tissue samples.

Pediatrics

The pediatrician specializes in the development and care of children from birth to maturity (Figure 2-9).

Physical Medicine and Rehabilitative Medicine

Physical medicine and rehabilitative medicine specialists (physiatrists) treat patients after they have suffered an injury or disability. The purpose of treatment is to return patients to their former state of physical health if possible. This rapidly growing field is closely associated with sports medicine in which the physician treats athletes using preventive and diagnostic medicine.

Primary Care (Internal Medicine)

The primary care specialist (internist) treats adult patients. This physician is skilled in diagnosis and treatment of nonsurgical problems. Subspecialties include cardiology, endocrinology, gastroenterology, hematology, immunology, nephrology, oncology, and pulmonary medicine, among others.

Psychiatry

The psychiatrist specializes in the diagnosis and treatment of patients with mental, behavioral, or emotional disorders and may also practice psychotherapy. A psychiatrist is qualified to prescribe and administer medications.

Pulmonology

This respiratory specialist treats lung problems. The pulmonologist works to ensure maximum oxygenation of patients who have respiratory disorders, such as pneumonia. The pulmonologist may work closely with respiratory therapists and internists.

Radiology

A radiologist specializes in X-ray visualization and study of tissues and organs. This physician has been tested and approved by the American Board of Radiology.

Rheumatology

A rheumatologist treats disorders and diseases characterized by inflammation of the joints such as arthritis.

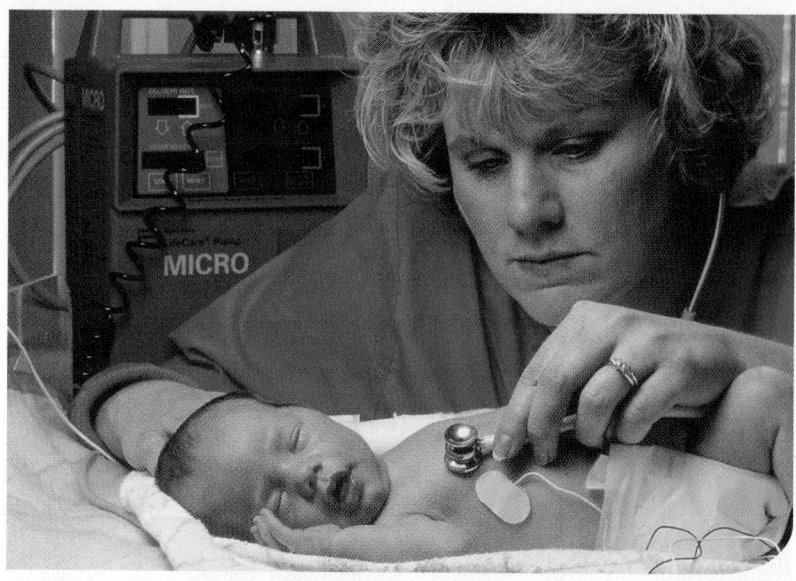

FIGURE 2-9 **A pediatrician with a baby.**

Urology

Urologists help patients with urinary system problems. Further, since the urological and reproductive systems are intimately entwined in the male, the urologist provides reproductive health initiatives for men. Urologists treat illnesses such as incontinence and erectile dysfunction.

SURGERY

Surgery is any invasive procedure that requires entering the body by making an incision or passing instruments through the skin and organs. Surgeons correct illness, trauma, and deformities using such procedures.

Surgical Specialties

General surgery includes all areas of surgery. General surgeons may restrict their practices to abdominal surgical procedures. However, many surgeons specialize in areas such as neurosurgery, cardiovascular surgery, and orthopedic surgery. Some of the more common surgical specialties are described in Table 2-2.

Health Care Institutions

Hospitals are the largest employers in the United States. In recent years, the public, government, and insurance companies have voiced increasing demand to curb hospital expenses. The length of stay in the hospital has been decreasing steadily over the past decade as a result of the DRGs system of payment and better medical and surgical procedures. The result has been an increased emphasis on outpatient rather than inpatient care, especially in the area of minor surgery. **Outpatient** care refers to services provided to patients on a walk-in basis where no overnight stay is required.

TABLE 2-2 Surgical Specialties and Their Descriptions

Surgical Specialty	Description
Cardiovascular	Cardiovascular surgery is the surgical treatment of the heart and blood vessels.
Colorectal	Colorectal surgery involves the surgical treatment of the lower intestinal tract (colon and rectum).
Cosmetic/Plastic	Cosmetic or plastic surgery involves the reconstruction of underlying tissues. This surgical intervention is used to correct structural defects or remove scars and signs of aging.
Hand	Hand surgery is orthopedic surgery that involves surgical treatment of defects, traumas, and disorders of the hand. Hand surgeons may employ a physical therapy staff and have x-ray equipment at their disposal.
Neurosurgery	Neurosurgery involves surgical intervention for diseases and disorders of the central nervous system.
Orthopedic	Orthopedic surgery treats musculoskeletal injuries and disorders, congenital deformities, and spinal curvatures through surgical means.
Oral (Periodontics, Orthodontics)	Oral surgery involves treatment of disorders of the jaws and teeth by means of incision and surgery as well as extraction of teeth.
Thoracic	Thoracic surgery involves treatment of disorders and diseases of the chest with surgical intervention.

Inpatient care refers to services provided to patients who are in a facility overnight or on a long-term basis.

Same-day surgery sites, home health agencies, and physical therapy/rehabilitative and sports medicine clinics are all multiplying rapidly. Also, care that can be provided to older adults in their own homes is encouraged.

HOSPITALS

The hospital is still considered the key resource for health care in the United States. While the patient's primary care is delivered in the physician's office, care for acute illnesses is delivered in hospitals, major surgical procedures are performed, health care professionals are trained and educated, research is conducted, and educational resources are provided to the public. Hospital sizes (measured by the number of patient beds) vary depending on the needs within the community where the hospital is located.

To ensure quality health care, many hospitals seek accreditation. The Joint Commission, formerly the Joint Commission on the Accreditation of Healthcare Organizations (JCAHO), is a private nonprofit organization that encourages high standards of medical care. Strict guidelines must be met by the institution seeking accreditation.

Hospitals are divided into four categories:

- General hospitals (Figure 2-10) provide both routine and specialized care, such as intensive care units and emergency rooms. They range in size from 50 to several hundred beds and are usually found in most towns and communities.

- Teaching hospitals provide the same type of care as in a general hospital. Generally, teaching hospitals are located near a university medical school and medical students, interns, and residents treat patients under the supervision of staff physicians. More specialists may be on staff to educate and train interns and residents.

- Research hospitals provide patient care and conduct research to combat disease. Examples include Department of Veterans Affairs hospitals throughout the United States and Shriners hospitals for crippled children.

- Specialty hospitals provide specialized care for certain types of patients, such as children, psychiatric patients, or burn victims.

Many larger hospitals provide all three services: general patient care, teaching, and research. The hospital organization contains many departments that interact to provide comprehensive health care for the patient. Hospital departments

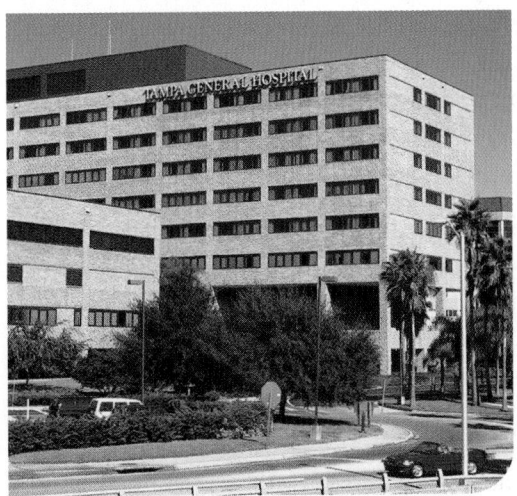

FIGURE 2-10 A general hospital.

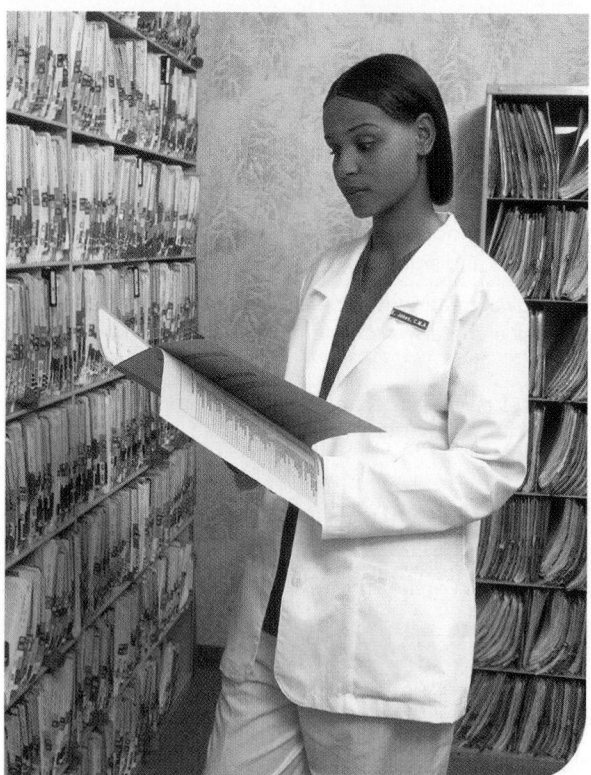

FIGURE 2-11 A medical records department.

include emergency services, laboratory, radiology, oncology, nuclear medicine, psychiatry, pathology, immunology, respiratory therapy, physical and occupational therapy, nursing, dietary services, pharmacy, central supply, housekeeping, engineering, health information, social services (to assist in locating medical care, treatment or placement for the patient after discharge from the hospital), and medical records (Figure 2-11).

Physicians generally serve on the staff of more than one hospital but seldom more than three. They refer their patients to one of the hospitals in which they have medical privileges. **Medical privilege** refers to the physician's right to practice medicine in a particular hospital or other health care facility. A physician may also have courtesy or visiting privileges at a hospital where he or she may be called to see a patient on a referral basis but does not have admitting privileges.

OUTPATIENT SURGICAL CENTERS

Although historically patients used to have all surgeries performed in hospitals, the modern trend is to have minor surgical procedures performed in freestanding or hospital-based outpatient surgical centers. Surgical procedures performed in outpatient centers generally require very little recovery time. In this setting the medical assistant can assist the patient with scheduling and preparing for surgery, receive and admit the patient, assist with some surgeries, and discharge the patient with postoperative instructions.

URGENT CARE CENTERS

Due to the need for quick care of nonemergent situations, a new variety of freestanding and hospital-based centers have emerged. The urgent care center has been created to treat nonemergent but urgent situations, such as performing sports physical examinations, setting fractures, drawing blood levels, treating infections, and providing care other than during the usual physician office hours. Some of these centers are also designated as primary care facilities in some managed care systems. Because of the quick assessment and treatment provided, these centers are popular for workers' compensation cases and occupational medicine coverage for many companies.

NURSING HOMES

Nursing homes were established in the nineteenth century to provide food, clothing, and shelter for the poor. Over the past century, the quality of care has improved in nursing homes, and most such homes care for the elderly. Many nursing homes are owned and operated by church groups, but the majority of homes are for-profit establishments run by nursing home corporations. Control over the quality of care is much tighter than in years past because of stricter regulations by state public health departments and Medicare. Due to the increased costs of nursing home care, some patients have to convert to Medicaid (the national health insurance for the poor) when their funds are depleted. The present-day nursing home is a long-term facility that cares for elderly persons who are sick, too feeble to care for themselves, and have no other source of care. According to the the U.S. Medicare, approximately nine million men and women over the age of 65 needed long-term care in 2009. Family and friends were caring for 70 percent. The remaining 30 percent or three million were resident in long-term care facilities.

Types of Long-Term Care Institutions

Long-term care institutions are classified by federal regulations either as skilled nursing facilities (SNF), intermediate care facilities (ICF), or extended care facilities (ECF). A description of these facilities and of assisted living follows.

- **Skilled nursing facility (SNF)** (Figure 2-12)— Intended for patients who require skilled nursing care around the clock. Patients must be recertified every 100 days to allow them to remain in an SNF.

- **Intermediate care facility (ICF)**—Intended for patients who are no longer able to live alone and care for themselves but do not require skilled nursing care on a 24-hour basis. Many ICFs also have occupational

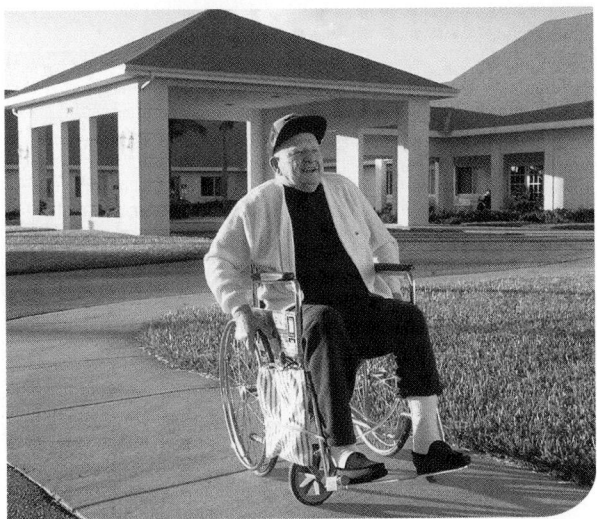

FIGURE 2-12 Skilled nursing facilities provide care for patients requiring longer stays than hospitals allow.

and rehabilitative therapists on their staff. ICFs must meet federal guidelines in order to receive federal funds for services provided to Medicare patients.

- **Extended care facility (ECF)**—Provides services to patients who no longer need the skilled nursing care of a hospital but are still too ill or incapacitated to return home. Many hospitals have opened extended care facilities for such patients (Figure 2-13). ECFs provide custodial care and thus do not employ skilled personnel.

- **Assisted-living facility**—Offers living arrangements for the older adult in which each resident or couple has a separate apartment and pays a fixed fee to have some meals and services provided. Older adults who are able to care for themselves and require a minimum of supervision are living in this relatively new environment.

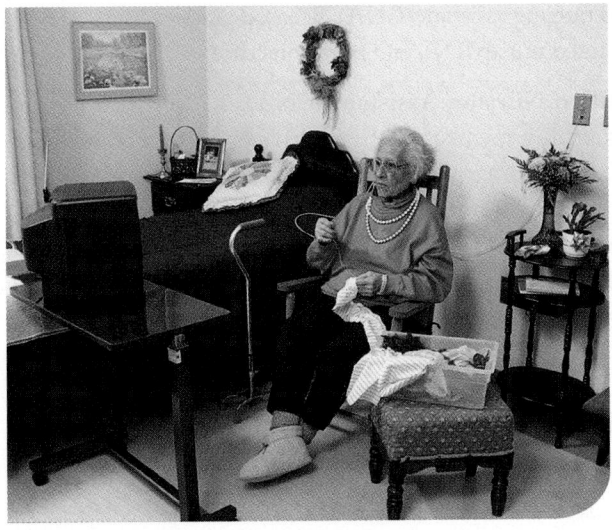

FIGURE 2-13 An extended care facility.

Hospice

Hospice is an interdisciplinary program of care and supportive services that facilitates the care of the patient by family members or significant others in the privacy of the patient's home or in a hospice facility. In the original hospice movement, which began in medieval England, the wounded, sick, and dying were cared for by religious communities of nuns. Today's modern hospice movement emphasizes improved quality of care for the dying. Most hospice care is provided at home, but some programs also provide care in homelike centers.

Hospice patients are suffering from the end stages of terminal illnesses, such as cancer, and Medicare currently covers part of end-stage care in a hospice setting. Medicare (Part B) will cover part of home care with a qualifying diagnosis. During home visits, hospice personnel provide nursing care for the special needs of the dying patient, including pain management but not necessarily treatment for the terminal illness. These visits often provide great emotional support to the patient and the patient's family. Often the visiting health care worker will offer suggestions to make the patient more comfortable.

Allied Health Professionals

It would be impossible in this single chapter to cover all of the many health care professions. Yet as a member of the health care team, it is essential that you understand others' roles and educational requirements. Before we consider some specific professions, you will need an understanding as they relate to allied health professionals of the terms *certification, licensure,* and *registration* as well as levels of education and degree titles.

Certification involves the issuing of a certificate and credentials by a professional organization to one who has met the educational and experience standards of that organization. Examples are certification as a medical assistant or CMA by the AAMA, or RMA certification by the AMT after a candidate has passed the national examination. **Registration** means that a professional organization in a specific health care field administers examinations, maintains a list of qualified individuals, or both. **Licensure** means that a government agency authorizes individuals to work in a given occupation, such as registered nurses (RN), licensed practical nurses (LPN), and physical therapists (PT).

Educational requirements for health careers vary from state to state. In all cases, a high school diploma or equivalency is necessary. Postsecondary education in a vocational/technical school, community college, or university may be required. Table 2-3 illustrates a career ladder in health care,

TABLE 2-3 Career Titles and Educational Levels

Professional	Educational Requirement	Diploma/Degree	Examples
Professional	4-year degree, advanced degree, and clinical training	Bachelor's (BA, BS), Master's, or Doctorate	Medical Doctor (MD), Pathologist
Technologist	4-year college program	Bachelor's (BA, BS)	Medical Technologist (MT)
Technician	2-year community college or vocational program	Associate's degree (AS)	Medical Laboratory Technician (MLT)
Assistant	Up to 1-year classroom and clinical preparation	Diploma	Laboratory Assistant
Aide	On-the-job training	High school diploma or GED	Laboratory Aide

educational requirements, degree designations, and some examples of professions in each category. Health care institutions may require the applicant to pass a national registration or certification examination in his or her field of study as a condition of hire.

PROFESSIONALISM

Physicians must obtain continuing education to retain their license. Medical assistants also need to keep abreast of new medical information. The AAMA requires Certified Medical Assistants (CMA) to earn 60 continuing education credits (CEUs) in five years to maintain their certification. Registered Medical Assistants (RMAs) who earn certification by passing the American Medical Technologists' examination are also encouraged to earn CEUs. Being a lifelong learner should be the goal of every medical assistant. The body of knowledge in health care is growing tremendously each year, and you will need to be vigilant about keeping up with new information. The following are a few ideas to help you become a well-informed, lifelong learner:

- Read *CMA Today,* the AAMA medical assisting journal, or *AMT Events,* the RMA professional publication, and complete the continuing education articles and tests provided in each publication.
- Select an interesting condition or disease each month to research on the Internet or at your local library. Keep this research information in a binder for future reference.
- Subscribe to other medical publications, or ask your physician employer if you may read some periodicals that he or she receives.
- Attend seminars provided by the local hospital, HMO, and state or local chapters of medical assisting groups.

Careers in the health care field involve many types of duties or responsibilities. An extensive list of possible career choices follows and are categorized into National Heath Care Skills Standards (NHCSS) career clusters. The NHCSS were developed to define the body of knowledge and specific skills health care workers are expected to possess for entry-level and technical-level positions. These core standards are used by schools, colleges, and health care facilities to establish curriculum and competencies for a wide variety of fields. The health care careers discussed are categorized according to NHCSS career clusters, and a few examples from each category are examined.

THERAPEUTIC CLUSTER CAREERS

Careers in this cluster include those that involve the health care status of the patient, including treatment, evaluation, collection of patient data, and evaluation of patient status.

Nurse

The term *nurse* refers to a diversified group of health care professionals with a range of qualifications. Descriptions of a certified nursing assistant (CNA), licensed practical nurse (LPN), registered nurse (RN), and nurse practitioner (NP) follow.

Certified Nursing Assistant (CNA). A certified nursing assistant is a member of the health care team who has completed a training program and taken a state examination to qualify to assist nurses in nursing homes, hospitals, and other health care facilities. The CNA provides such patient care as bed baths, vital signs, feeding, and ambulation. Cross-training of employees has led to positions such as patient care technician (PCT). The PCT may have a CNA or medical assisting background and perform more technical tasks, such as drawing blood and performing ECGs. The nursing assistant may also be referred to as a nurse's aide or orderly.

Licensed Practical Nurse (LPN). A licensed practical nurse performs some of the same, but not all, clinical nursing tasks as a registered nurse does. The LPN must have graduated from a recognized one-year program and become licensed by the National Federation of Licensed Practical Nurses. In some states, the LPN is known as a licensed vocational nurse (LVN).

Registered Nurse (RN). A nursing career is ideal for the person who wishes to provide hands-on patient care. Nurses work in hospitals, physicians' offices, industry, governmental agencies, ambulatory care units, emergency services, and schools. Their work ranges from managed care organizations providing direct patient care, to teaching and supervising other staff, performing research, and managing agencies. Nurses receive their education and training in either a two-year or four-year program. To become licensed as an RN requires successful completion of the National Council Licensure Examination (NCLEX), a national licensure examination. A nurse practitioner (NP) is a registered nurse who has a master's degree and has received additional training to provide basic patient care that includes diagnosing and prescribing medications and treatments for common illnesses.

Occupational Therapist (OT)

Occupational therapy provides treatment to people who are physically, mentally, developmentally, or emotionally disabled. Occupational therapists evaluate the patient's skills for self-care, work, and leisure. The goal of the occupational therapist is to develop programs that will help to restore the patient's ability to manage activities of daily living (ADL). Occupational therapists require a bachelor's degree from an approved program in occupational therapy, plus certification by the American Occupational Therapy Association (AOTA) and six months of on-the-job training.

An *occupational therapy assistant* must complete a two-year vocational training program and be certified by AOTA. This assistant works under the supervision of an OT and implements patient treatments designated by the OT.

Physical Therapist (PT)

Physical therapy is the treatment of diseases or disabilities of the joints, bones, and nerves by massage, therapeutic exercises, and heat and cold treatments. Examples of conditions treated by means of physical therapy include multiple sclerosis, cerebral palsy, arthritis, fractures, spinal cord injuries, and heart disease. Practitioners work in a variety of facilities including hospitals, ambulatory care centers, rehabilitation centers, private practice, and schools for the physically challenged. A PT is required to hold a four-year degree in physical therapy, participate in a four-month clinical internship, and successfully pass the state licensure examination. After obtaining a master's degree, some PTs set up private practices and provide services on a contract basis.

A *physical therapy assistant* may be required in some states to have a degree from an accredited two-year college and pass a written licensure examination. He or she works under the supervision of a physical therapist and implements treatments designated by the PT.

Physician Assistant (PA)

The field of physician assistant is relatively new, emerging since the 1970s. The goal of this profession is to assist the physician in the primary care of patients. The job description for a PA includes evaluation, monitoring, diagnosis, therapeutics, counseling, and referral skills. In nearly all states, the PA can prescribe medications. The profession has expanded to include surgeon's, pathologist's, anesthesiologist's, and radiologist's assistants, among others. The general educational program is similar to a master's-level program with two years education after a bachelor's degree. In most programs, the student must have some combination of work or internship experience and pass an accreditation examination.

Respiratory Therapist (RT)

A respiratory therapist evaluates, treats, and cares for patients with breathing problems. A respiratory therapist tests lung capacity, administers breathing treatments, teaches self-care to patients, and provides emergency care. An RT can be employed in hospitals, cardiopulmonary laboratories, nursing homes, health maintenance organizations (HMOs), and ambulatory care facilities. To become a certified respiratory therapy technician (CRTT), the candidate must complete a one-year internship and pass a written examination given by the National Board of Respiratory Therapy.

Becoming a registered respiratory therapist (RRT) requires completion of a college program, an approved training program, one year's experience in the field, and the successful completion of a written examination given by the National Board of Respiratory Therapy.

Dietician

Dietitians are skilled in applying the principles of good nutrition to food selection and meal preparation. They work closely with a patient's physician to coordinate the patient's diet with such other treatments as medications. Dietitians also provide consulting services, offer seminars, author books, counsel patients, plan food service systems, and design nutrition plans within fitness programs for athletes. A dietitian must have a bachelor's degree with a major in foods and nutrition. In addition, an internship in a dietary department is required. To become registered requires successful completion of an examination. Dietitians work in a variety of settings including hospitals, long-term care facilities, schools, and prisons. The employment opportunities for dietitians are currently excellent.

Dental Hygienist

A dental hygienist (Figure 2-14) works directly with the patient to clean teeth, take oral X-rays, and teach oral health and discusses results of dental examinations with the dentist. The dental hygienist must graduate from a two-year community college program or a four-year bachelor's program and pass both a state written and clinical examination.

Emergency Medical Technician (EMT) and Paramedics

Emergency medical technicians (EMTs) and paramedics are trained in providing emergency care and transporting injured patients to a medical facility. They are skilled in recognizing emergency conditions such as cardiac arrhythmias, airway obstruction, and psychological crisis. EMTs and paramedics always work under the direct supervision of a physician and follow a physician's orders.

There are different levels of EMTs:

- **Basic**—The beginner EMT performs basic life support.
- **Advanced**—The advanced EMT has more training and advanced skills beyond the basic level.
- **Paramedic**—As the highest level of EMT, a paramedic is able to treat cardiac arrest, perform defibrillation, and administer certain drugs.

EMTs receive certification after completion of an approved EMT program. They must be recertified every two years and receive ongoing education and training in their field.

Pharmacist

The field of pharmacy deals with the ordering, maintaining, preparing, and distributing of prescription medications. A pharmacist (Figure 2-15) must complete five years of education by an accredited pharmacy program. In addition, a pharmacy student must serve a one-year internship and become licensed in the state where he or she is employed. A registered pharmacist can work in a variety of institutions including hospitals, drug stores, and nursing homes. Some pharmacists may choose to open their own pharmacy.

Pharmacy technicians attend a community college or private vocational program. They are able to assist the pharmacist in preparing medications. In some states, they are issued a Pharmacy Technician Certificate upon completion of an examination. A *pharmacy clerk,* a position for which a high school degree is necessary, assists the pharmacist with typing prescription labels, assigning prescription numbers, and maintaining supplies and records.

Medical Social Worker

Social work involves programs and services that are developed to meet the special needs of the ill, the physically and mentally challenged, and the elderly. A medical social worker cares for the total person, including the emotional, cultural, social, and physical needs of the patient.

Medical social workers assist patients and their families in handling problems associated with a long-term illness or disability. Social workers need a thorough understanding

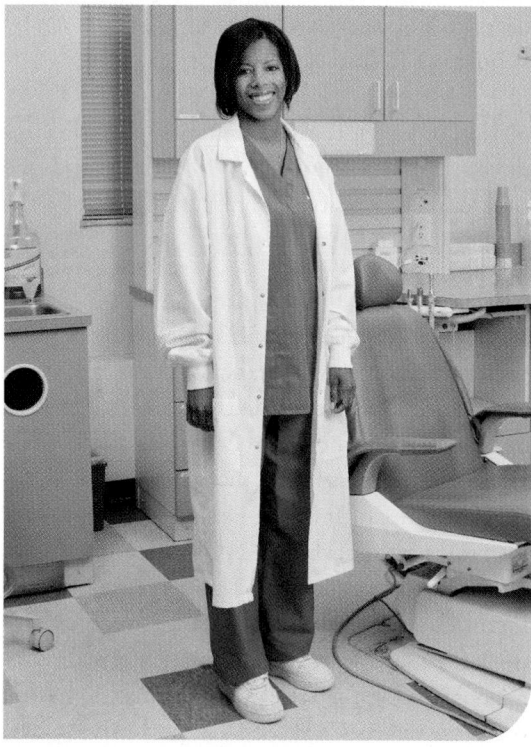

FIGURE 2-14 A dental hygienist.

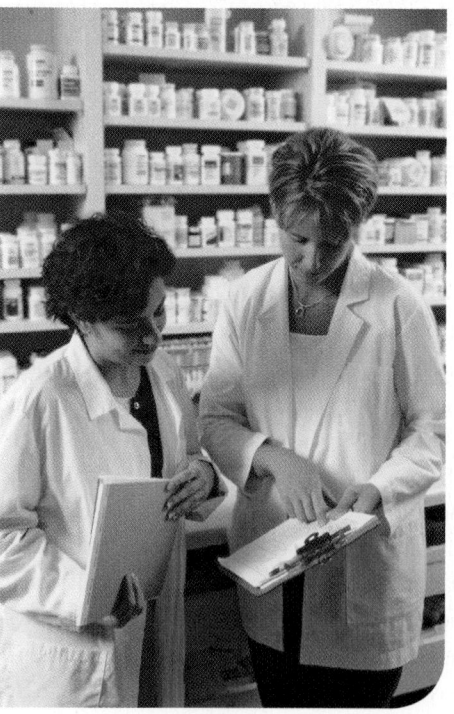

FIGURE 2-15 Two pharmacists consulting.
Source: Corbis - Brand X Pictures

of a community's resources for the disabled. A medical social worker requires a bachelor's degree. Many states require licensing or registration for social workers and a master's degree.

DIAGNOSTIC CLUSTER CAREERS

The careers in this cluster are involved with procedures that create a picture of the patient's health status at a specific point in time. These careers involve measuring, evaluating, and reporting patient information.

Ultrasound Technologist

An ultrasound technologist receives training in the use of ultrasound equipment, which uses inaudible sound waves to outline shapes of tissues and organs. Ultrasound equipment produces an image of the shapes. Ultrasound images of fetal development in the uterus are commonly used to assist with fetal monitoring.

X-ray Technologist (Radiologic Technologist)

An x-ray or radiologic technologist must hold a bachelor's degree in radiologic technology, have experience in two or more radiologic disciplines, such as nuclear medicine and radiation therapy, and be a registered radiologic technologist (ARRT).

Electroencephalograph Technician

Electroencephalography (EEG) is the field devoted to recording and studying the electrical activity of the brain. An EEG technician operates an electroencephalograph, which records the activity of the brain with a written tracing of the brain's electrical impulses. EEG technologists work primarily in hospitals.

Diagnostic Imaging Technician

Diagnostic imaging technicians are trained in the operation of x-ray equipment such as ultrasound, computerized tomography (CT), and magnetic resonance imaging (MRI) equipment. Radiology practitioners include darkroom attendants with a minimum of education or training; radiologic technicians who are graduates of an accredited program; radiologists, who are graduates of an accredited medical school; and licensed physicians with specialized training in radiology. Employment opportunities are available in physicians' offices, hospitals, trauma centers, and other ambulatory care facilities.

Medical Laboratory Careers

A medical laboratory is a facility that is equipped for testing, research, scientific experimentation, or clinical studies of materials, fluids, or tissues taken from patients. Independent laboratories provide routine analysis of patients' blood,

urine, tissue, and other materials. Hospital laboratories perform tests for both inpatients and outpatients. In some instances, a physician's office will contain a small laboratory (POL) where routine tests can be conducted.

Phlebotomist or Venipuncture Technician. A phlebotomist is skilled in drawing blood from patients. This requires the ability to maintain standard precautions, aseptic technique, excellent venipuncture technique, and good communication skills. Training in a vocational education program is required. Phlebotomy training courses at colleges or career schools vary in length but should prepare the student for certification. Every state decides licensing requirements, but most states do not require licensure for phlebotomists. California, on the other hand, requires both certification and licensure for phlebotomy technicians. Many employers prefer to hire workers with prior experience and may require certification through a national examination, indicating that the phlebotomy technician meets standards of competence.

The American Society for Clinical Pathology (ASCP) has a certification program for phlebotomy technicians (ASCP-PBT) that requires proof of phlebotomy skills and a rigorous examination. The route to certification includes high school graduation or equivalency and completion of a National Accrediting Agency for Clinical Laboratory Science (NAACLS)-approved phlebotomy program, one approved by the Joint Commission, one approved by the California Department of Health, or after experience of one year as a full-time phlebotomy technician in a laboratory that is accredited and regulated by the Clinical Laboratory Improvement Amendments (CLIA) within five years of application. Completion of an RN, LPN, or other acceptable accredited allied health professional or occupational education program can also qualify an applicant. The American Medical Technologists (AMT) organization has a certification program for AMT-RPT. Prior to taking the AMT's certification exam, an applicant for phlebotomy technician must have a high school diploma or GED and acceptable training. The American Society for Clinical Laboratory Sciences (ASCLS) also has a certification known as ASCLS-CLPlb.

Laboratory Technician (MLT and CLT). The medical laboratory technician (MLT) (Figure 2-16) is a certification obtained from the American Society of Clinical Pathology (ASCP). The American Society for Clinical Laboratory Sciences (ASCLS) is another highly regarded professional organization that promotes the Clinical Laboratory Technician (CLT) and Clinical Laboratory Scientist (CLS) certifications, which are administered through the National Credentialing Association. Both these highly regarded credentials are awarded to laboratory technicians skilled in testing blood, urine, lymph, and body tissues. This career requires two years of training in a vocational education program prior to certification. The AMT also certifies medical laboratory technicians.

Medical Technologist (MT) or Clinical Laboratory Scientist (CLS). A laboratory or medical technologist must complete a four-year medical technology program in a college or university to become a certified medical technologist (CMT) or certified laboratory scientist (CLS). This person directs the work of other laboratory staff, is responsible for maintaining quality assurance standards for all equipment, and performs laboratory analysis. The examination for this profession is prepared by the Board of Registry of the ASCP. The AMT also certifies medical technologists.

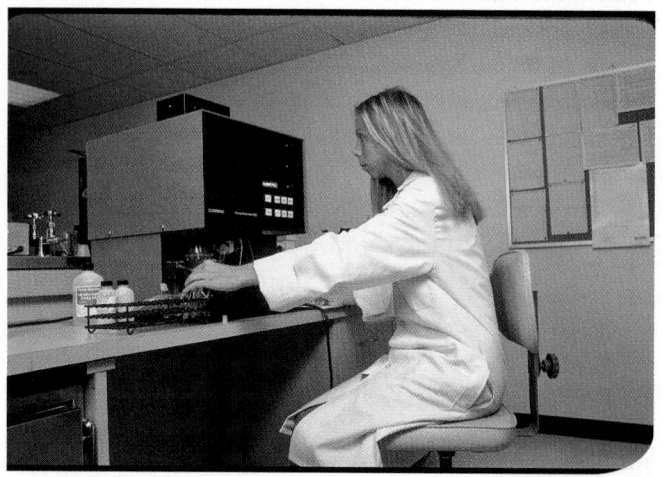

FIGURE 2-16 A medical lab technician.

INFORMATION SERVICES CLUSTER CAREERS

Careers in this cluster are involved with documenting client information, including managing, coding, analyzing, maintaining, and retrieving information.

Health Information Technology (Medical Records Technician)

Health information technology refers to the massive database known as medical records. Every person seen by a health care professional has a medical record. Medical records technicians, now more commonly referred to as health information technologists, maintain the permanent records relating to a patient's condition and treatment. The medical record is a legal document that can be used in a court of law.

A medical records technician must graduate from an accredited medical records program and must have a two-year associate's degree, several years of experience as a medical records clerk, and 30 credit hours from an accredited college. Successful completion of the accredited record technical examination offered by the American Medical record Association allows the technician to use the initials ART after his or her name. The American Health Information Management Association (AHIMA) offers the Registered Health Information Technician (RHIT) examination. A registered medical records administrator (RRA) requires a bachelor's degree in health information technology and the successful completion of an examination administered by the American Medical Record Association.

Medical Transcription

A medical transcriptionist types or enters into a computer dictation that is taken from a recording machine or an audio tape. This dictation consists of medical reports from physicians and surgeons. Skills required for this profession include typing ability, good spelling, understanding of medical terminology, and the ability to operate data processing equipment.

Office Management

The role of office manager is a choice open to some allied health professionals, including medical assistants and nurses. Office managers supervise the entire support staff. The position requires someone with a sound knowledge of the type of work performed in the office or institution, strong supervisory skills, and the ability to work closely with top management. Excellent time-management and communication skills are a must for office managers.

Unit Clerk/Communications Clerk

The unit clerk, or ward secretary, is responsible for clerical duties, reception work, and other communication duties in hospitals, long-term care facilities, and clinics. The unit clerk in a hospital performs varied tasks, for example, taking physicians' orders from charts and assisting the nursing staff. A knowledge of medical terminology is required.

ENVIRONMENTAL SERVICES CAREER CLUSTER

This career cluster includes careers involved with the patient's health care environment, such as aseptic procedures, resource management, maintaining equipment, and providing sterile supplies.

Biomedical Equipment Technician

A biomedical equipment technician maintains and repairs medical testing equipment either in a health care facility or for a private company. Educational requirements vary from an associate's to a bachelor's degree.

Other health care careers in this cluster that do not require postsecondary education, include central supply/sterile supply workers, housekeeping staff, and food-service aides.

SUMMARY

The medical profession contains a rich history of achievement and progress. The history of medicine can be broken into four categories: early medicine going back to 3000 BC, the eighteenth century, the nineteenth century, and the twentieth century. Major advancements include the eradication of many deadly diseases with the advent of vaccines, the decrease of infections due to the discovery of aseptic technique and antibiotics, the harnessing of radium to treat disease, the inventions of the microscope and surgical instruments, the discovery of anesthesia, and a better understanding of anatomy and physiology.

Today licensed physicians must maintain their knowledge base by completing 75 continuing medical education (CME) units over a period of three years. The medical assistant will have the opportunity to pursue a career working for physicians in all areas of specialization.

The health care environment can be confusing and intimidating to the patient. It is important to have an understanding of the health care system and the diversity of institutions that deliver health care services. The descriptions provided in this chapter of inpatient facilities, including hospitals, nursing homes, hospices, and ambulatory care settings and services, provide a basic explanation of a rather complex structure. Patients need to know the options that are available as they seek out services and follow up on the referrals made by their primary physician for treatment, procedures, or further diagnosis. The medical assistant's understanding of the system is key to providing clear explanations

Centers for Disease Control and Prevention (CDC)

The Centers for Disease Control and Prevention (CDC), a division of the U.S. Department of Health and Human Services (DHHS), was established in 1946. The CDC's main headquarters and laboratories are in Atlanta, Georgia. This is a governmental agency that employs more than 8,600 people.

The purpose of the CDC is to safeguard public health by preventing and controlling disease and to act as a resource for the medical profession. The CDC seeks information about causes of disease to find cures, alerts the medical profession to potential outbreaks of diseases such as influenza, describes those who will be at highest risk during an outbreak of disease such as the elderly, and recommends proper treatment. In addition, the CDC conducts disease research, prevention, control, and education programs nationally and in several other countries. These programs help to train doctors, provide public health information, develop immunization services with state and local agencies, and establish standards for healthful working conditions.

to the patient. Understanding managed care plans and using the proper insurance codes (see CPT and ICD-9 in Chapter 17) for services provided to patients are necessary to ensure proper insurance claims reimbursement.

There are numerous types of medical practices. The physician decides after rotations in medical school which area of medicine he or she prefers. After a residency in a specialty, a physician can practice in that specialty. Board certification in a specialty requires completing an approved residency, passing a challenging examination, and practicing in the field for years. New specialties, such as bariatrics, are created when a subspecialty is required. Physicians can take additional training and do another residency to change to a different area of medical interest after an initial residency. For example, a board-certified obstetrician may decide to become a pathologist or a surgeon. This would require another residency in that discipline.

Varied and numerous allied health professionals are enlisted to support physicians with patient care. Some of these professions include therapeutic cluster careers (such as nurses and dieticians), diagnostic cluster careers (such as x-ray and ultrasound technologists), laboratory cluster careers (such as phlebotomists and clinical laboratory scientists), information services cluster careers (such as unit clerks and office managers), and environmental cluster careers (such as biomedical equipment technicians). The medical assistant is a key part of the allied health team.

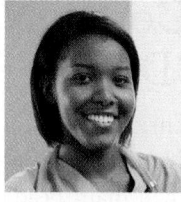

2 CHAPTER REVIEW

COMPETENCY REVIEW

1. Define and spell the terms to learn for this chapter.

2. State at least three of the major achievements in medicine during each of these periods: early medicine, eighteenth century, nineteenth century, and twentieth century (or modern medicine).

3. List the three methods by which a physician can become licensed.

4. Explain three circumstances that would justify the suspension or revocation of a physician's license.

5. Describe four types of medical practices.

6. Identify and explain issues in this chapter that might require patient education.

7. Find examples of four board-certified physicians in your local telephone directory.

8. Describe the role of the medical assistant as it relates to patient education concerning the physician's credentials.

9. Using the local telephone directory, find within your area examples of names and addresses of three hospitals, a hospice, an extended care facility, and a medical laboratory.

10. Discuss the role of the medical assistant in relationship to other health care providers.

PREPARING FOR THE CERTIFICATION EXAM

1. Which of the following is NOT an ancient remedy?
   a. digitalis
   b. ibuprofen
   c. chamomile
   d. nitroglycerine
   e. sulfur

2. Who is considered the Father of Medicine?
   a. Galen
   b. Galileo
   c. Hippocrates
   d. Socrates
   e. Curie

3. Who found the cure for smallpox?
   a. Harvey
   b. Hippocrates
   c. Galen
   d. Jenner
   e. Pasteur

4. Who established the science of bacteriology?
   a. Nightingale
   b. Pasteur
   c. Jenner
   d. Galileo
   e. Lister

5. The science of treating obese patients is:
   a. geriatrics
   b. gynecology
   c. dermatology
   d. bariatrics
   e. radiology

6. Which allied health professional performs phlebotomy as a career?
   a. unit clerk
   b. medical transcriptionist
   c. venipuncture technician
   d. dietician
   e. respiratory therapist

7. Which allied health professional would help a patient find an appropriate nursing home?
   a. clinical laboratory scientist
   b. certified nursing assistant
   c. physical therapist
   d. occupational therapist
   e. medical social worker

8. Which type of practice is managed by a board of directors?
   a. solo practice
   b. corporation
   c. group practice

d. sole proprietorship

e. partnership

9. Where should a patient go with a stomach infection?

a. urgent care facility

b. long-term care facility

c. hospice

d. nursing home

e. outpatient surgical center

10. Which of the following medical specialties would treat a patient with hearing loss?

a. bariatrics

b. ophthalmology

c. otorhinolaryngology

d. orthopedics

e. obstetrics

CRITICAL THINKING

1. During a meeting about finding a new physician, Dr. Bahjat informs Tania that the new physician will not be a partner in the practice. What will this mean for the new physician that the physicians group decides to hire?

2. Pearson Physicians Group decides to hire Dr. Shania McWalter. Dr. McWalter is a DO. Tania has been receiving many phone calls from patients inquiring about the difference between an MD and a DO. What should Tania tell these patients?

3. More than 30 percent of the patients seen by Pearson Physicians Group are between the ages of 68 and 93. Dr. Bahjat has asked that Tania create a brochure for patients and their family members regarding the differences between skilled nursing facilities and assisted living facilities. What information should Tania include in the brochure?

ON THE JOB

One of the important characteristics of a medical assistant is to have a concrete foundation in the practice of medicine. This would include a complete understanding of the many medical and surgical specialties and subspecialties in which a physician can be board certified.

An important responsibility for the medical assistant is to have the ability to convey this information about the treating physician to the anxious patient and the patient's family. This is part of patient education.

Bonnie is employed as a medical assistant for a physician who is a pediatric cardiovascular surgeon. She is taking a history on the patient, a newborn, by interviewing the parents, Mr. and Mrs. Appleby. They are extremely upset and anxious over the condition of their newborn who was diagnosed shortly after birth with a serious, yet quite treatable, heart defect. The prognosis, should the parents agree to the corrective surgery, is quite good. However, the parents are having a difficult time understanding how the physician could help their newborn. They are not even quite sure why they were referred to this specialist and why their pediatrician could not treat the infant.

1. How could Bonnie comfort and reassure these parents?

2. What could Bonnie possibly say about the physician that might help the parents to understand why they were referred and how their newborn could be helped?

INTERNET ACTIVITY

Research ethical arguments for and against the use of fetal stem cells for medical treatment.

MEDMEDIA

Additional interactive resources and activities for this chapter can be found:

On your student DVD: View applicable procedure videos on the DVD-ROM found in the back of this book.

MyHealthProfessionsKit.com: Test your knowledge of the chapter with games and activities. MyHealthProfessionsKit also includes resources, helpful links, and a Spanish audio glossary.

Medical Assisting Interactive: Practice your procedures as a medical assistant in this simulated doctor's office. This can be accessed through MyHealthProfessionsKit.com.

3

Medical Law and Ethics

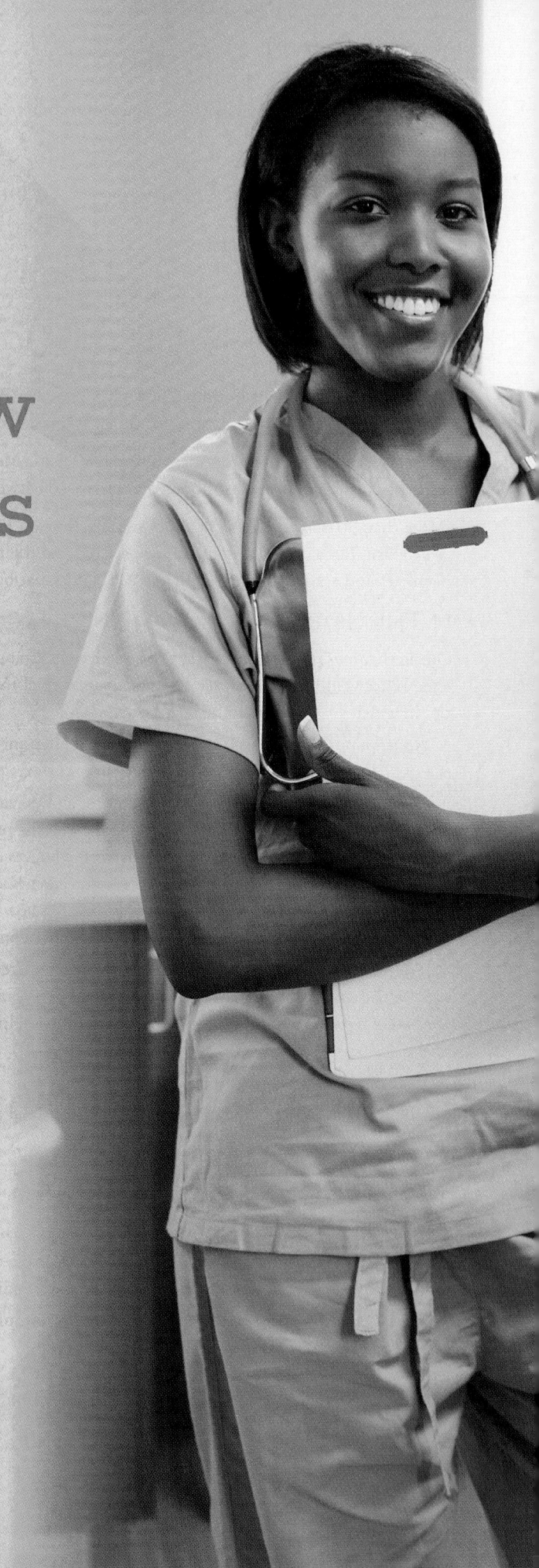

LEARNING OBJECTIVES

After completing this chapter, you should be able to:

- Define and spell the terms to learn for this chapter.

- Differentiate between criminal and civil law.

- Identify the four Ds of negligence.

- Discuss what can be done to avoid a claim of abandonment.

- Discuss informed consent.

- Discuss the role of the medical assistant relating to legal issues in the medical office.

- Explain the importance of the Hippocratic oath today.

- List the seven main points of the AMA Principles of Medical Ethics.

- List and discuss the main points of the AAMA Principles of Medical Ethics.

- Discuss what is meant by the medical assistant's standards of care.

- Describe the Patient's Bill of Rights.

- Explain the HIPAA guidelines concerning the patient's right to privacy and confidentiality in the medical office.

CHAPTER OUTLINE

CASE STUDY

Shandra Wilkinson is a registered medical assistant (RMA). On her way to work she witnesses a severe multicar accident. Shandra stops to provide assistance. She performs CPR on a victim at the scene of the accident. The victim is revived and is transported to the emergency room by emergency medical technicians, who arrived later on the scene. Unfortunately two of the other victims did not survive the injuries they sustained and died hours later at the local hospital. Shandra provides the police with a full account of her actions. Two months after the accident she receives notification that the victim she assisted during the accident is planning to sue her because she broke a rib while performing CPR. He is suing for damages sustained from the result of the broken bone.

TERMS TO LEARN

administrative law

advance directive

bioethics

breach of contract

civil law

contract law

contributory negligence

defamation of character

guardian ad litem

informed consent

living will

practice of medicine

proximate cause

reasonable person standard

res ipsa loquitur

respondeat superior

standard of care

statute of limitations

tort

CERTIFICATION LINK

CMA (AAMA)
Medicolegal guidelines and requirements
  Licenses
  Legislation

RMA
Medical law
Medical ethics

CMAS (AMT)
Medical office management
  Risk management and quality assurance

oday's health care consumer demands more of a partnership with the physician and the rest of the health care team. Patients should be part of the decision-making process regarding their care and treatment. This chapter discusses issues such as malpractice, abandonment, and litigation, as well as specific regulations and documents protecting the patient, the patient's family, physicians, and medical staff involved in care and treatment. Other topics presented include the public duties of the physician, documentation in medical records and electronic health records, regulations relating to controlled substances, and the medical assistant's role in preventing liability suits.

Classification of the Law

Laws are classified into four types:

- Criminal
- Civil
- International
- Military

Only criminal and civil law are discussed in this chapter.

CRIMINAL LAW

Criminal laws are made to protect the public as a whole from the harmful acts of others. Criminal acts fall into two categories: felony and misdemeanor. Conviction of a felony can carry a punishment of imprisonment in a state or federal prison or a death sentence. Examples of these crimes include murder, rape, robbery, and practicing medicine without a license. *Miranda laws* require that a defendant (the person being charged with the offense) be read his or her rights before being questioned. Among these rights are the right to remain silent, the right to have an attorney present at questioning, and the right to free court-appointed counsel if the defendant cannot afford a lawyer. Court cases have been dismissed on the grounds that the defendant did not know that his answers during questioning would be admissible in court.

Misdemeanors are less serious offenses and carry a punishment of fines or imprisonment in jail for up to a year. They include traffic violations, disturbing the peace, and theft.

A physician's license may be revoked or taken away if he or she is convicted of a crime. Criminal cases against physicians have included the revocation of a license for sexual misconduct, murder, violating narcotics laws, and practicing medicine without a license. The **practice of medicine** is defined as diagnosing and prescribing treatment or medication. The medical assistant must make sure that he or she always assists the physician and does not try to treat or diagnose a patient's condition.

CIVIL LAW

Civil law concerns relationships between individuals or between individuals and the government. Civil law includes contract law, tort law, and administrative law. **Contract law** includes enforceable promises and agreements between two or more persons to do or not do a particular action. Tort law covers acts that result in harm to another. **Administrative law** covers regulations that are set by governmental agencies. Health care employees are most frequently involved in cases of civil law, particularly tort and contract law.

Tort Law

A **tort** is a wrongful act, resulting in harm, that is committed against another person or property. Regarding medical laws, in order for a court case to meet the definition of a tort, there must be damage or injury to the patient that was caused by the physician or the physician's employee.

Intentional torts include assault, battery, false imprisonment, defamation of character, fraud, and invasion of privacy. Table 3-1 provides a description and example of intentional torts.

TABLE 3-1 Intentional Torts

Tort	Description	Example
Assault	The threat of bodily harm to another. Actual touching (battery) or injury does not have to occur for assault to take place.	Threatening to harm a patient or to perform a procedure for which he or she does not consent.
Battery	Actual bodily harm to another person without permission. This is also referred to as unlawful touching or touching without consent.	Performing surgery or a procedure without the informed consent (permission) of the patient.
False imprisonment	A violation of the personal liberty of another person through unlawful restraint.	Refusing to allow a patient to leave an office, hospital, or medical facility when he or she requests.
Defamation of character	Damage caused to a person's reputation through spoken or written word.	Making a negative statement about another physician's ability.
Fraud	Deceitful practice.	Promising a miracle cure.
Invasion of privacy	The unauthorized publicizing of information about a patient.	Allowing personal information, such as test results for HIV, to become public without the patient's permission.

Unintentional torts, such as negligence, occur when the patient is injured as a result of the health care professional not exercising the ordinary standard of care. The health care professional must exercise the type of care that a "reasonable" person would use in a similar circumstance. This is known as the reasonable person standard.

Negligence and malpractice have the same meaning when referring to medical lawsuits. Negligence is easier to prevent than it is to defend. Physicians can take steps to avoid negligence suits by:

- protecting the physician–client relationship, and
- being above reproach in the performance of their medical duties.

To obtain a judgment for negligence against a physician, the patient must be able to show proof of what is referred to as the "four Ds of negligence": duty, dereliction or neglect of duty, direct cause, and damages (Box 3-1).

In a case of negligence, the plaintiff (the person who files the lawsuit) must prove proximate cause. This means that the plaintiff must prove that the defendant's acts (or failure to act) directly caused the injury. For example, if a patient returns to his room after having prostate surgery and experiences severe headaches that were not present before having the surgery, the patient must prove that the physician's performance of the prostate surgery was the cause of the headaches. Contributory negligence relates to the patient's

Box 3-1 The Four Ds of NEGLIGENCE

- **Duty** refers to the physician–client relationship. The patient must prove that this relationship has been established. When the patient has made an appointment and been seen by the physician, a relationship has been established. Further office visits and treatment will establish that the physician had a duty or obligation to the patient. (Contract)
- **Dereliction or neglect of duty** refers to a physician's failure to act as any ordinary and prudent physician (a peer) within the same community would act in a similar circumstance when treating a patient. To prove dereliction

or neglect of duty, a patient would have to prove that the physician's performance or treatment did not comply with the acceptable standard of care based on the norm of the ordinary and prudent physician. (Standard of Care)
- **Direct cause** requires the patient to prove that the physician's dereliction or breach of duty was the direct cause for the injury that resulted.
- **Damages** refers to any injuries that were received by the patient. The court may award compensatory damages to pay for the patient's injuries.

TABLE 3-2 Penalties in Malpractice Suits

Type of Damages	Purpose	Example
Punitive Damages	Meant to punish the person for behavior.	A manufacturer dumps toxins into the water supply and might be given a high fine to prevent further occurrence.
Nominal Damages	A penalty that is not a high monetary value is given to punish.	A behavior leads to a loss of life. The defendant may be sentenced to write a letter weekly to the family to remind the person of the damage caused.
Compensatory Damages	A penalty, usually monetary, to compensate the person for damage.	A physician might be ordered to pay for the medical and rehabilitation bills of a patient he or she injured.

contribution to the injury. If it has been proven that the patient contributed to the deterioration of his or her medical status, the physician could be released of either a portion of or all of the negligent damages that are being sought by the patient (e.g., the patient did not keep an appointment causing an undetected infection to advance). Table 3-2 lists the various types of damages awarded to patients in medical malpractice suits.

Contract Law

The branch of law known as contract law is generally concerned with a breach or the neglect of an understanding between two parties.

A contract is a voluntary agreement that two parties enter into with the intent of mutual benefit for both parties. A contract between two parties is composed of four distinct parts:

- **Offer**—An individual makes the effort to provide services. For example, a physician offers dermatological services in a certain part of town. The physician is not compelled to offer all services in all places to all people.

- **Acceptance**—Another individual accepts the first person's offer. For example, the patient makes an appointment to see a physician. The patient agrees to see the physician in a certain office at a certain time.

- **Consideration**—This occurs when something of value is exchanged. A physician provides the service and the patient pays for the service.

- **Competence**—Both parties involved in the contract must be competent individuals. For example, minors or those with certain developmental delays may want to have services, but some parent or guardian who is deemed competent to act on their behalf signs the contract.

For a contract to be legal, several considerations are relevant. For one, the concerned party (the patient) must be mentally competent at the time the contract is made. For example, the patient must not be under the influence of drugs or alcohol at the time the contract is entered. A **breach of contract** occurs when either party fails to comply with the terms of the agreement. In the previous example, a breach of contract would occur if the patient failed to pay the agreed-upon fee.

Abandonment

Once a physician has agreed to take care of a patient that contract may not be terminated improperly. A physician may choose to end the physician–patient contract for reasons including failure to pay medical bills or failure to comply with a prescribed course of treatment. If a physician does not follow the proper steps to end the physician–patient contract, he or she may be charged with patient abandonment. A physician choosing to discontinue the treatment of a patient should notify the patient in writing. This is usually done by sending a certified letter with return receipt via the U.S. Postal Service. The letter should indicate that the physician is willing to continue treatment, generally for a period of 30 days, in order to allow the patient to seek the services of another physician. A copy of the certified letter and the return receipt should be placed in the patient's file.

Termination of Contract

The termination of the contract between a physician and a patient generally occurs when the treatment has ended and the fee has been paid. However, serious issues do arise causing premature termination of a contract between the physician and the patient. It should be noted that both physicians and patients have the right to terminate the contractual relationship. Letters from the physician should indicate the date the physician's services will be terminated. The medical

Box 3-2 Premature Termination of the Physician–Patient CONTRACT

A medical office should document any of the following incidents with a certified letter sent to the patient.

- Failure to pay for service.
- Missed appointments.
- Failure to follow instructions.

- The patient states (orally or in writing) that he or she is seeking the care of another physician. Reasons for seeking another physician are many. For example, the patient's insurance may have changed and the patient's physician may not be covered by the new insurance, or the patient may move.

---

assistant needs to understand these situations and handle them correctly (Box 3-2).

Collections

Several laws have been enacted to provide protection against unscrupulous collection practices that harm individuals. The medical assistant needs to be familiar with these laws since he or she is responsible for following the administrative procedures these laws require. The laws relating to the collection process are discussed in Table 3-3.

Professional Liability

Lawsuits related to health care have greatly increased during the past decade and the average liability award granted to plaintiffs in medical malpractice cases is now over $1 million. Professional liability is determined by the federal, state, and local laws governing the physician–patient relationship and relates to the standard of care, legal contracts, and informed consent. An important issue in the question of liability is the physician–employee relationship. Some factors impacting this relationship are discussed here. They include *respondeat superior,* standard of care, malpractice, *res ipsa loquitur,* statute of limitations, Good Samaritan laws, and defamation of character.

RESPONDEAT SUPERIOR

Physician-employers are especially concerned that their employees have a complete understanding of the law. The Latin term *respondeat superior* literally means "Let the master answer." What this means to your employer, the physician, is that he or she is liable for the negligent actions of anyone working for him or her. In some cases and in some states, both the physician and the employee may be held liable.

In effect, under *respondeat superior,* the physician delegates certain duties to you and, if you perform them incorrectly, the ultimate liability rests with the physician-employer. However, medical assistants and other health care workers can also be named in malpractice suits.

TABLE 3-3 Laws Governing Collection

Law	Description
Notice on "Use of Telephone for Debt Collection" from the Federal Communications Commission	Provides guidelines for the specific times that credit collection phone calls can be made. It prohibits using the telephone for harassment and threats. Telephone calls for the purposes of collections must be made between the hours of 8:00 A.M. and 9:00 P.M.
Fair Debt Collection Practices Act of 1978	Provides a guide for determining what are considered the fair collections practices for creditors.
Equal Credit Opportunity Act of 1975	Prohibits discrimination—unfair treatment—in the granting of credit. This law mandates that women and minorities must be issued credit if they qualify for it, based on the premise that if credit is given to one patient it should be given to all patients who request it.
Fair Credit Reporting Act of 1971	Provides guidelines for collecting an individual's credit information. Individuals are able to learn what credit information is available about them. Consumers can correct and update this credit information.
Truth in Lending Act of 1969	Requires a full, written disclosure concerning the payment of any fee that will be collected in more than four installments. Also referred to as Regulation Z of the Consumer Protection Act.

For example, if you are authorized by your employer to draw a sample of blood from a patient and you inadvertently enter a nerve causing permanent damage to the patient's arm, then you may also be liable for that patient's injury. Since the physician's medical license is in jeopardy when errors are made, it is vital that you have an understanding of the laws in your state.

STANDARD OF CARE

While a physician is under no obligation to treat everyone, once he or she does accept a patient for treatment, the physician has then entered into the physician–patient relationship and must provide a certain standard of care. This standard of care asserts that the physician must provide the same knowledge, care, and skill that a similarly trained physician would provide under the same circumstances in the same locality. The law requires only reasonable, ordinary care and skill.

The physician is expected to perform the same acts that a "reasonable and prudent" physician would. This standard also states that a physician will not perform any acts that a "reasonable and prudent" physician would not. Physicians are expected to exhaust all the resources available to them when they are treating a patient. These would include the following:

- Taking a thorough medical history
- Giving a complete physical examination
- Administering the necessary laboratory tests and X-rays

Physicians are not expected to expose their patients to undue risk. If the physician violates this standard of care, he or she is liable for negligence.

The medical assistant must also adhere to a standard of care. This standard will depend on training, skills, experience, education, and the responsibility assigned. Employees going outside of their competency risk being sued for negligence. Medical assistants should review applicable laws in their own states and regions to determine the standard of care.

MALPRACTICE

Professional misconduct or demonstration of an unreasonable lack of skill with the result of injury, loss, or damage to the patient is considered malpractice. It means the physician was negligent. Every mistake or error, however, is not considered malpractice. Therefore, when a treatment or diagnosis does not turn out well, the physician is not necessarily liable. The physician-employer and all staff must each act within the standard of care appropriate for the particular practice of medicine. All health care providers are held to this same standard.

Malpractice Insurance

In modern times, all physicians are expected to carry malpractice insurance. Rates are based on type of specialty and prior suits. Physicians can carry insurance that covers only claims made in that year, or they can carry occurrence coverage that covers occurrences in that year. To be sure that they are covered for occurrences before and after the insured years, complete coverage from beginning to end of career is also available. In most cases, employers carry insurance to cover acts of their employees while performing their duties. This is termed general liability coverage. Employees should request to see their employer's certificate of insurance to determine policy coverage.

To cover any negligence on the part of their clinical assistants, some physicians carry a rider, or addition, to their professional liability or malpractice policy. Once again, it is important for the medical assistant to determine the type of coverage their physician-employer carries and to clarify coverage. If the medical assistant is not covered by the employer's malpractice policy, then he or she may choose to purchase professional liability coverage from an insurance carrier who specializes in this type of coverage. By purchasing liability coverage, the medical assistant minimizes personal liability and risk. Ultimately, the employer is responsible for the actions of the employee (*respondeat superior*). However, both may be sued for the action of the employee.

RES IPSA LOQUITUR

The doctrine of res ipsa loquitur, which means "the thing speaks for itself," applies to the law of negligence. This doctrine tells us that the breach (neglect) of duty is so obvious that it does not need further explanation, or "it speaks for itself." For instance, leaving a sponge in the patient during abdominal surgery, dropping a surgical instrument causing injury to the patient, and operating on the wrong body part are all examples of *res ipsa loquitur*. None of these examples would have occurred without the negligence of someone involved in the procedure.

STATUTE OF LIMITATIONS

The statute of limitations refers to the period of time during which a patient may file a lawsuit. The court will not hear a case that is filed after the time limit has run out. Statutes of limitation vary from state to state; in some states, the time period is only one or two years.

The statute of limitations does not always start when the treatment is administered. It may begin when the problem is discovered, which may be some time after the actual treatment. This is known as the *rule of discovery*. For instance, a physician accidentally left a surgical sponge in a patient's body during an abdominal operation. After sixteen years of abdominal discomfort, the patient required more surgery, but the physician who had performed the original operation had died. So, another surgeon, who found the sponge and removed it, performed the second surgery. The patient then sued the estate of the original surgeon for malpractice and won because the statute of limitations, which was two years in that state, started when the sponge was discovered. The reverse of a statute being in effect is a situation in which the statute is prevented from coming into play. This occurs when the injury is to a minor child. Generally, the court will appoint a **guardian ad litem,** an adult who will act in court on behalf of the child. However, the child does not have to sue through a guardian ad litem as a minor but may wait until he or she reaches adulthood. In such a case, an obstetrician and his or her assistants can be sued twenty-one years and nine months (plus the statute of limitations period in that state) after a birth injury has occurred.

GOOD SAMARITAN LAWS

Good Samaritan laws are state laws that help to protect a health care professional from liability while giving emergency care to an accident victim. Such laws are in effect in all states to encourage physicians and other health care professionals to offer cardiopulmonary resuscitation (CPR) and first aid, as needed.

No one is required to provide aid in the event of an emergency, except in the state of Vermont. Someone responding in an emergency situation is only required to act within the limits of his or her skill and training. A medical assistant would neither be expected, nor advised, to perform emergency treatment that is within the area practiced by physicians and nurses.

DEFAMATION OF CHARACTER

Defamation of character is a scandalous statement about someone that can injure the person's reputation. Defamation can result even when the statement is true. *Slander* occurs when the defaming statement is spoken. *Libel* refers to written defamation.

As a medical assistant, you will have access to privileged information about patients that may seem harmless, but, in reality, the information could be very damaging to their reputations. For instance, a patient who undergoes a test for an infectious disease, such as hepatitis or AIDS, may not wish an employer to know the test took place even if the test result is negative. If you call the patient's place of employment and leave a message regarding a test result of this nature, the action could be considered a breach of confidentiality and defamation.

The fact that a physician saw a patient must be kept confidential. The medical assistant should not fax information or leave messages on answering machines unless specifically instructed to do so in writing by the patient. Such instructions should be documented in the patient's medical record.

To protect yourself and avoid involvement in lawsuits, you must practice your skills with care, be concerned about maintaining good public relations with patients and other staff members, and understand the law. Always ask your supervisor for guidance on the appropriate action to take.

WORKPLACE SEXUAL HARASSMENT

The employer must maintain a workplace where people are comfortable to work without being the target of unwanted sexual advances. Although employees are free to date each other outside the workplace, professional behavior is expected at all times in the medical office. It is inappropriate for supervisors to date direct subordinates. If two people meet at work and subsequently marry, it is best if one accepts a position that allows their relationship to flourish without needing to be concerned about workplace subordination.

It is against the law to create a hostile work environment in which employees must accept unwanted advances or listen to inappropriate talk. If sexual or romantic advances are made toward the medical assistant and are not appreciated, the medical assistant should make it clear that the advances must stop. If they do not stop, the medical assistant should report the incident(s) to a supervisor. Supervisors are held accountable under the law for maintaining a workplace that is free of sexual harassment. *Quid pro quo* is the Latin term for giving something for something else. It is usually used in reference to pressure for sexual behaviors forced on someone not wanting them in return for promotions or rewards. Any inference of sexual *quid pro quo* should be reported to supervisors.

Patient and Physician Relationship

Both the physician and the patient must agree to form a relationship if there is to be a contract for service and treatment. To receive proper treatment, the patient must confide truthfully in the physician regarding all aspects of his or her health. Failure to state all the facts may result in serious consequences for the patient. The physician is not liable if the patient has withheld critical information that directly affects his or her medical care.

PHYSICIAN RIGHTS

Physicians have the right to select the patients they wish to treat. They also have the right to refuse service to patients. From an ethical standpoint, most physicians do treat patients who need their skills. This is particularly true in cases of emergency.

Physicians may also state the type of services they will provide, the hours their offices will be open, and where the offices are located. The physician has the right to expect payment for treatment given.

Physicians have a right to take vacations and time off from their practices. Care must be taken to inform patients if their physician will be unavailable. In most cases, another physician will cover or take care of a colleague's patients while he or she is away.

PATIENT RIGHTS

The patient has the right to give consent, or permission, for all treatment. In giving consent for treatment, the patient reasonably expects that his or her physician will use the appropriate standard of care in providing care and treatment. Patients also expect that all information and records about their cases will be kept confidential by the physician and staff. The patient's right to privacy prohibits the presence of unauthorized persons during physical examinations or treatments.

In addition to these rights, the patient also has certain obligations. For example, the patient is expected to follow the instructions given by the physician. In addition, the patient is expected to pay the physician for medical services.

INFORMED CONSENT

The patient can expect to receive information concerning the advantages and potential risks of all treatments. Informed consent means that the patient is instructed about the possible consequences of both having and not having certain procedures and treatment. The physician must carefully explain that in some cases the treatment may even make the patient's condition worse.

The Doctrine of Informed Consent (Figure 3-1) includes the following:

- Explanation of advantages and risks to the treatment
- Alternatives available to the patient

PEARSON GENERAL HOSPITAL

COMPLETE ORIGINAL IN INK FOR HOSPITAL CHART
PATIENT MUST BE AWAKE, ALERT AND ORIENTED WHEN SIGNING

DATE: _____ TIME: _____ ☐ AM ☐ PM

I AUTHORIZE THE PERFORMANCE UPON _____
OF THE FOLLOWING OPERATION (state nature and extent):_____
_____
_____

TO BE PERFORMED UNDER THE DIRECTION OF DR. _____

1. I HAVE BEEN ADVISED THAT THERE IS A FAVORABLE LIKELIHOOD OF SUCCESS, BUT I UNDERSTAND THAT A COMPLETELY SUCCESSFUL OUTCOME MAY NOT BE ACHIEVABLE, AND THERE ARE NO GUARANTEES REGARDING THE OUTCOME. I ALSO UNDERSTAND THAT CERTAIN ADVERSE EVENTS COULD OCCUR AS A RESULT OF THE PERFORMANCE OF THE PROCEDURE OR TREATMENT, INCLUDING PAIN, INFECTION, LACERATION OR PUNCTURE OF INTERNAL ORGANS, BLEEDING, NERVE DAMAGE OR EVEN IN RARE CASES, DEATH. I UNDERSTAND THAT HOSPITALIZATION OR OTHER INSTITUTIONAL CARE, HOME CARE OR CARE BY HEALTH PROFESSIONALS MAY BE NEEDED FOLLOWING THE PROCEDURE OR TREATMENT, RELATED TO FULL RECOVERY, RECUPERATION OR CONVALESCENCE. I UNDERSTAND THE ALTERNATIVES TO THIS PROCEDURE, INCLUDING MY RIGHT TO REFUSE TO CONSENT TO IT, AND I NEVERTHELESS HAVE DECIDED TO CONSENT TO PERFORMANCE OF THE PROCEDURE OR TREATMENT.

2. I CONSENT TO THE PERFORMANCE OF OPERATIONS AND PROCEDURES IN ADDITION TO OR DIFFERENT FROM THOSE NOW CONTEMPLATED, WHETHER OR NOT ARISING FROM PRESENTLY UNFORESEEN CONDITIONS WHICH THE ABOVE NAMED DOCTOR OR HIS/HER ASSOCIATES OR ASSISTANTS MAY CONSIDER NECESSARY OR ADVISABLE IN THE COURSE OF THE OPERATION.

3. I CONSENT TO THE DISPOSAL BY HOSPITAL AUTHORITIES OF ANY TISSUES OR PARTS WHICH MAY BE REMOVED.

4. THE NATURE AND PURPOSE OF THE OPERATION/PROCEDURE, POSSIBLE ALTERNATIVE METHODS OF TREATMENT, THE RISK AND BENEFITS INVOLVED, AND THE COURSE OF RECUPERATION HAVE BEEN FULLY EXPLAINED TO ME. NO GUARANTEE OR ASSURANCE HAS BEEN GIVEN BY ANYONE AS TO THE RESULTS THAT MAY BE OBTAINED.

5. I UNDERSTAND AND AGREE WITH THE ABOVE INFORMATION. I HAVE NO QUESTIONS WHICH HAVE NOT BEEN ANSWERED TO MY FULL SATISFACTION. I UNDERSTAND THAT I HAVE THE RIGHT TO ASK FOR FURTHER INFORMATION BEFORE SIGNING THIS CONSENT.

I have crossed out any paragraph above which does not apply or to which I do not give consent.

PATIENT SIGNATURE: _____
(OR PARENT OR GUARDIAN IF PATIENT IS UNDER 18 YEARS OF AGE)

RELATIONSHIP: _____

WITNESS SIGNATURE: _____
(OF PATIENT, PARENT OR GUARDIAN SIGNATURE)

WITNESS SIGNATURE: _____
☐ **TELEPHONE CONSENT** (2ND WITNESS NEEDED FOR TELEPHONE CONSENT)

FIGURE 3-1 Sample of an informed consent to perform an operation, sedation, anesthesia, and other medical services.

- Potential outcomes to the treatment
- What might occur if there is no treatment
- The use of understandable language

Touching someone without the person's consent is referred to as battery. When a patient is seen for a routine examination for medical treatment, there is implied consent that the physician will touch the person during the examination. Therefore, the touching required for the examination would not be considered a crime of battery. However, if a physician brings a fellow colleague into the examination room to examine (which would require touching) a patient without asking the patient's consent, the patient could view this "touching without consent" as a form of battery.

It is very difficult to fully inform a patient about all the things that can go wrong with a treatment. In an emergency situation, during which the patient is not able to understand the explanation or sign a consent form, a physician is protected by law to provide care. A physician cannot delegate the duty of obtaining informed consent to another person except in emergency situations. Even then, after the emergency is under control, it is important to find a responsible party with whom to discuss patient issues if the patient is unable to give consent. Sometimes consent for procedures is given by relatives or those holding medical proxies, which allows the person to act in the best interests of the patient if the patient is unable to give an informed consent. (See Durable Power of Attorney later in this chapter for more information.) Frequently, patients are asked at office visits to declare names of relatives or friends with whom the physician can discuss patient care. This is an important document not only for determining with whom the physician can share information on an ongoing basis but also in an emergency situation (Figure 3-2).

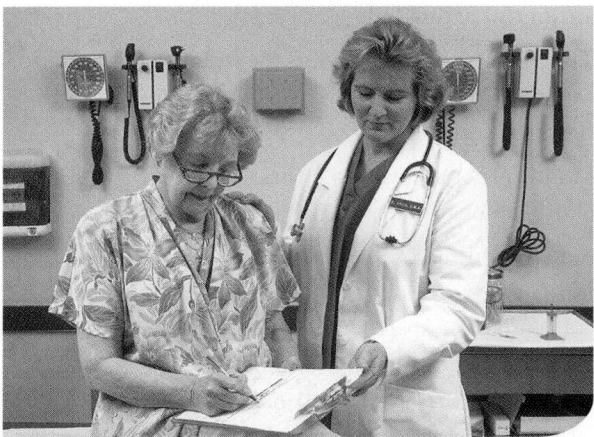

FIGURE 3-2 The patient's signature on the informed consent form indicates that the patient understands the limits and risks involved in the treatment or surgical procedure as explained by the physician.

Does a signed informed consent form protect both the physician and the staff from lawsuits? The answer generally is yes. As long as the physician has carefully explained the treatment or procedure and the patient acknowledges that he or she understands the risks involved by signing the consent form, some protection from lawsuits is usually in place. However, patients have sued and won cases in which they were presented the risks of a procedure, signed the form, and then proceeded to sue the physician when the treatment failed. Informed consent forms used in outpatient surgical and procedural facilities may be shorter in length and content than those used in physicians' offices. However, each state mandates unique exceptions to the informed consent doctrine. The following are the more general exceptions:

- A physician does not have to inform a patient about risks that are commonly known. For example, a patient could choke while swallowing a pill.
- If the physician feels the disclosure of risks may be detrimental to the patient, then he or she is not responsible for disclosing them. This might occur if a patient has a severe heart condition that may be worsened by an announcement of risks.
- If the patient requests the physician not to disclose the risks, then the physician is not responsible for failing to do so.

Patients have the right to refuse treatment. Different cultural and religious groups must be accommodated. Some members of religious groups, such as Jehovah's Witnesses and Christian Scientists, do not wish to receive blood transfusions or certain types of medical treatment. The adults would not receive the treatment against their wishes. In the case of a minor child, the court may appoint a guardian who can then give consent for the procedure.

RIGHTS OF MINORS

A minor is considered a person who has not reached the age of majority, which varies from state to state but usually is 18. In most states, minors are unable to give consent for treatment. Exceptions are special cases involving pregnancy, request for birth control information, abortion, testing and treatment for sexually transmitted diseases, problems with substance abuse, and a need for psychiatric care. Two types of minors can give consent for treatment:

A mature minor is a young person, generally under the age of 18, who possesses a maturity to understand the nature and consequences of the treatment. Emancipated minors actually have the same legal capacity as an adult under any of the following five conditions:

- They live on their own.
- They are married.
- They are self-supporting.
- They are in the armed forces.
- Any combination of the above conditions.

Since not all states recognize the categories of mature and emancipated minors, it is wise to handle consent on a case-by-case basis. The following are some legal implications to consider when treating a minor.

- **Right to confidentiality**—A 16-year-old who is seeking birth control information has a right to have her records remain confidential.
- **Financial responsibility**—The 16-year-old girl seeking birth control information may not be able to pay for the office visit. Contacting her parents for payment may breach confidentiality.
- **Minor's legal guardian**—This is sometimes difficult to determine if the child lives with the mother but the father is financially responsible for care and treatment, or vice versa. Always determine who is the legal guardian. In the case of divorce, the legal guardian will be the individual who a court has declared to be responsible. Sometimes, both parents share custody in a divorce. However, sometimes there is only one legal guardian. The other parent may be informed of some information regarding the patient and not others. The physician may choose to speak with his or her attorney about how to handle complex issues arising when one parent has custody and the other wants information.

PATIENT SELF-DETERMINATION ACT

Several documents executed by the patient provide protection for the patient and physician. Such documents also provide direction for the patient's caregiver, or proxy, to make health-care-related decisions according to the patient's wishes at a point in time when the patient is unable to do so. These documents include the living will, durable power of attorney, and Uniform Anatomical Gift Act card.

Living Will

The living will (Figure 3-3) allows patients to request that life-sustaining treatments and nutritional support not be used to prolong their life. This document gives patients the legal right to direct the type of care they wish to receive when their death is imminent. The document provides protection for physicians and hospitals when they follow the patient's wishes. This process is often discussed in the office with patients when they are capable of making the decision. Other family members or significant others can also be part of the discussion and decision. One copy of the living will should be kept with the patient's record. A living will is very similar to an advance directive, but the advanced directive generally includes not only the living will but also the durable power of attorney.

Durable Power of Attorney

The durable power of attorney (DPOA), when signed by the patient, allows an agent or representative to act on behalf of the patient. If the DPOA is for health care only, then the agent may only make health-care-related decisions on behalf of the patient. This agent may be a spouse, grown child, friend, or, in some cases, an attorney.

The DPOA is a safeguard that someone will be able to act on the patient's behalf if he or she becomes physically or mentally incapacitated. This document is in effect until the patient cancels it. A copy of the DPOA should be kept with the patient's record. The DPOA will act on behalf of the patient until the patient is again capable of making his or her own decisions. Figure 3-4 shows a durable power of attorney.

Uniform Anatomical Gift Act

The Uniform Anatomical Gift Act allows persons 18 years or older and of sound mind to make a gift of any or all parts of their body for purposes of organ transplantation or medical research at the time of death. Two regulations that are held within this act include:

- The physician performing the transplant operation cannot be the same physician to determine death or the time of death.
- Money is not allowed to change hands for the purpose of organ donation.

The donor will carry a card that has been signed in the presence of two witnesses (Figure 3-5). In some states the driver's license has a space to indicate the desire to be an organ donor with space for a signature.

In some cases, the family will make the decision for the donor if this was not done while the donor was alive. It is generally agreed that if a member of the family opposes the donation of organs, then the physician and hospital do not insist upon it.

LIVING WILL OF _____

I, _____, a resident of the City of _____,

_____ County, State of _____, being of sound and dispos-

ing mind, memory and understanding, do hereby willfully and voluntarily make, publish, and declare this to be my LIVING WILL, making known my desire that my life shall not be artificially prolonged under the circumstances set forth below, and do hereby declare:

1. This instrument is directed to my family, my physician(s), my attorney, my clergyman, any medical facility in whose care I happen to be, and to any individual who may become responsible for my health, welfare, or affairs.

2. Death is as much a reality as birth, growth, maturity, and old age. It is the one certainty of life. Let this statement stand as an expression of my wishes now that I am still of sound mind, for the time when I may no longer take part in decisions for my own future.

3. If at any time I should have a terminal condition and my attending physician has determined that there can be no recovery from such condition and my death is imminent, where the application of life-prolonging procedures and "heroic measures" would serve only to artificially prolong the dying process, I direct that such procedures be withheld or withdrawn, and that I be permitted to die naturally. I do not fear death itself as much as the indignities of deterioration, dependence, and hopeless pain. I therefore ask that medication be mercifully administered to me and that any medical procedures be performed on me which are deemed necessary to provide me with comfort or care or to alleviate pain.

4. In the absence of my ability to give directions regarding the use of such life-prolonging procedures, it is my intention that this declaration shall be honored by my family and physician as the final expression of my legal right to refuse medical or surgical treatment and accept the consequences for such refusal.

5. In the event that I am diagnosed as comatose, incompetent, or otherwise mentally or physically incapable of communication, I appoint _____ to make binding decisions concerning my medical treatment.

6. If I have been diagnosed as pregnant and my physician knows that diagnosis, this declaration shall have no force or effect during the course of my pregnancy.

7. I understand the full import of this declaration and I am emotionally and mentally competent to make this declaration. I hope you, who care for me, will feel morally bound to follow its mandate. I recognize that this appears to place a heavy responsibility on you, but it is with the intention of relieving you of such responsibility and of placing it on myself, in accordance with my strong convictions, that this statement is made.

IN WITNESS WHEREOF, I have hereunto subscribed my name and affixed my seal at _____,

_____, this _____ day of _____, 20 _____, in the presence of the subscribing witnesses whom I have requested to become attesting witnesses hereto. _____

Declarant

The declarant is known to me and I believe him/her to be of sound mind.

_____

_____Witness   Address

_____

_____Witness   Address

Subscribed and acknowledged, before me by _____, and subscribed and sworn to before the witnesses, on the _____ day of _____, 20_____.

_____

(SEAL)

NOTARY PUBLIC State of _____ My Commission

Expires:_____

Copies of this instrument have been given to:

Receipt and acknowledged & date:

FIGURE 3-3 Living will.

DURABLE POWER OF ATTORNEY FOR HEALTH CARE

I, _____,
(Printed or typed full name)
am of sound mind, and I voluntarily make this designation. I designate _____, (insert name of patient advocate) my _____, (Spouse, child, friend . . .) living at _____
(Address of patient advocate) as my patient advocate to make care, custody and medical treatment decisions for me in the event I become unable to participate in medical treatment decisions. If my first choice cannot serve, I designate
_____ (Name of successor) living at _____
_____
_____ (Address of successor) to serve as patient advocate.

The determination of when I am unable to participate in medical treatment decisions shall be made by my attending physician and another physician or licensed psychologist.

In making decisions for me, my patient advocate shall follow my wishes of which he or she is aware, whether expressed orally, in a living will, or in this designation.

My patient advocate has authority to consent to or refuse treatment on my behalf, to arrange medical services for me, including admission to a hospital or nursing care facility, and to pay for such services with my funds. My patient advocate shall have access to any of my medical records to which I have a right.

My specific wishes concerning health care are the following: (if none, write "none")

_____
_____
_____
_____
_____

I may change my mind at any time by communicating in any manner that this designation does not reflect my wishes.

It is my intent that my family, the medical facility, and any doctors, nurses and other medical personnel involved in my care shall have no civil or criminal liability for honoring my wishes as expressed in this designation or for implementing the decisions of my patient advocate.

Photostatic copies of this document, after it is signed and witnessed, shall have the same legal force as the original document.

I sign this document after careful consideration. I understand its meaning and I accept its consequences.

Signed: _____ Date: _____

Address: _____

NOTICE REGARDING WITNESSES

You must have two adult witnesses who will not receive your assets when you die (whether you die with or without a will), and who are not your spouse, child, grandchild, brother or sister, an employee of a company through which you have life or health insurance, or an employee at the health care facility where you are a patient.

STATEMENT OF WITNESSES

We sign below as witnesses. This declaration was signed in our presence.

The declarant appears to be of sound mind, and to be making this designation voluntarily, without duress, fraud or undue influence.

Signed by witness: _____
(Print or type full name)
Address: _____
Signed by witness: _____
(Print or type full name)
Address: _____

FIGURE 3-4 **Durable power of attorney.**

Uniform Donor Card

I,_____ , have spoken to my family about organ and tissue donation. The following people have witnessed my commitment to be a donor. I wish to donate the following:

◯ any needed organs and tissue

◯ only the following organs and tissue:_____
Donor Signature:_____ Date:_____
Witness:_____
Witness:_____
Next of Kin:_____
Telephone:(____)_____

FIGURE 3-5 Organ donor card.

Documentation

Carefully document all calls, visits, treatments, no-shows, appointment cancellations, medications, prescription refills, vital signs, and other pertinent information in the patient's chart. If an action is not recorded on the medical chart, then it is considered by most courts not to have been performed.

USE OF RECORDS IN LITIGATION

Litigation refers to a lawsuit tried in court. For this purpose, a court of law may subpoena a medical record. When this is done, only the parts of the record that are requested should be copied and sent to the requesting attorney. Unless the original record is subpoenaed, a certified photocopy may be sent. If the original record is subpoenaed, then make a copy and return the copy to the locked file. A receipt for the subpoenaed record should then be placed in the patient's file. The patient should also be notified that his or her record has been subpoenaed. Both the subpoenaed record and the notification to the patient should be sent by certified mail.

Be especially careful when using a fax transmission for medical records. The person receiving the fax should assure you that the receiving machine is located in a restricted area. Confidential material is not generally sent over a fax transmission. Of course, a fax is not usable when an original record is requested. A fax cover sheet compliant with the Health Insurance Portability and Accountability Act (HIPAA) should be used explaining that the records are confidential and should only be viewed by the intended recipient.

Should you or your employing physician receive a *subpoena ducestecum* (an order to appear in court and to bring along with you certain medical records or materials for trial), remember only the records specifically stated in the subpoena are required.

COURT TESTIMONY

Not everyone who has information relating to a case will be called into court to testify. An attorney may interrogate, or ask questions, of a witness. Another means of obtaining information from a witness to be used during a court case is to submit a deposition. In this case, a written statement is taken of oral testimony given in front of a court officer. The person who gives the oral testimony and then signs a deposition is not required to actually appear in court. An attorney submits the deposition during the court case. Arraignment occurs when a defendant is called before the court to answer a charge.

An expert witness is a person called upon to testify in court regarding the proper standard of care for a patient in a similar community. An expert witness in a medical malpractice suit is generally a physician.

In the event that you are called upon to appear in court, you will want to be as comfortable as you can when giving testimony. Remember the following pointers.

- **Be professional**—You will be judged by your appearance and behavior as well as by what you say. Your attorney can advise you on this more fully.

- **Remain calm, dignified, and serious at all times**—The opposing attorney may try to make you nervous.

- **Do not answer questions you do not understand**—Simply ask the attorney to repeat the question or state "I don't know."

- **Only present facts surrounding the case**—Do not give any additional information. Do not insert your opinion. Stating "He was angry" is stating your opinion. "The patient was shouting" is stating a fact.

- **Do not memorize your testimony ahead of time**—You will generally be allowed to take some notes with you to refresh your memory concerning dates.

- **Always tell the truth.**

Giving testimony in court is a crucial and sensitive matter. It is best to consult an attorney if you have any questions.

Public Duties of Physicians

Physicians have responsibilities to the general public. Some of these duties include reports of births, stillbirths, deaths, communicable illnesses or diseases, drug abuse, certain injuries

TABLE 3-4 Public Duties of the Physician

Duty	Description
Births	Issuing of a legal certificate, which will be maintained during a person's life as proof of age. Many benefits and documents, including Social Security, passport, and driver's license, depend on having a valid birth certificate.
Deaths	Physicians sign a certificate indicating the cause of a natural death. Check with your state public health department to determine specific requirements. For example, in the case of a stillbirth before the 20th week of gestation, the medical assistant will have to determine if both a birth and death certificate are required. A coroner or health official will have to sign a certificate in the following cases: • No physician present at the time of death • Violent death, unlawful death • Death as a result of criminal action • Death from an undetermined cause
Reportable communicable diseases	Physicians must report all diseases that can be transmitted from one person to another and are considered a general threat to the public. The list of reportable diseases differs from state to state. The report can be either by mail or phone. The following childhood vaccines and toxoids are required by law (National Childhood Vaccine Injury Act of 1986): • Diphtheria, tetanus toxoids, pertussis vaccine (DTP) • Pertussis vaccine (whooping cough) • Measles, mumps, rubella (MMR) • Poliovirus vaccine, live • Poliovirus vaccine, inactivated • Hepatitis B vaccine • Tuberculosis test
Reportable injuries	Certain injuries are reportable according to state requirements. These injuries include gun or knife wounds, rape and battered persons injuries, and spousal, child, and elder abuse.
Child abuse	Questionable injuries of children, including bruises, fractured bones, and burns, must be reported. Signs of neglect, such as malnutrition, poor growth, and lack of hygiene, are reportable in some states.
Elder abuse	Physical abuse, neglect, and abandonment of older adults is reportable in most states. The reporting agency varies by state but generally includes social service agencies.
Drug abuse	Abuse of prescription drugs is reportable according to the law. Such abuse can be difficult to determine since the abuser may seek prescriptions for the same drug from several different physicians. A physician will want to see a patient before prescribing a medication.

such as rape, abuse of children or older adults, gunshot and knife wounds, and animal bites.

Exact reporting requirements vary from state to state, so the medical assistant should be familiar with the requirements of his or her state. Office personnel, including the medical assistant, carry out many of the duties that relate to these responsibilities. Table 3-4 outlines the public duties of the physician.

Drug Regulations

The U.S. Food and Drug Administration (FDA) is the agency within the federal government that has jurisdiction over testing and approving drugs for public use. The Drug Enforcement Administration (DEA), a branch of the U.S. Justice Department, regulates the sale and use of schedule drugs.

The Controlled Substances Act of 1970 requires physicians to handle controlled drugs that are highly addictive in very specific ways. A physician who dispenses, purchases, administers, prescribes, or handles drugs is required to register with the DEA. The physician then receives a DEA registration number that must appear on all prescriptions for controlled substances. A DEA number is required for every location in which controlled drugs are stored. If a physician practices in two states, then two DEA numbers must be obtained. DEA registration numbers are generally printed on the physician's prescription blanks. See Chapter 53 for a sample prescription form.

Controlled drugs must be kept in a double-locked cabinet and any theft must be immediately reported to both the regional DEA office and the local police. In addition, the physician's black bag and prescription blanks should always be stored in a secure locked location.

Records must be kept to document the administering and dispensing of controlled drugs. In addition, federal regulations require that a written inventory in triplicate of drug supplies, based on daily use, be made every two years and kept for two more years.

Controlled drugs are classified into five schedules, or categories, that indicate levels of potential abuse. Schedule I drugs have the highest potential for addiction and abuse while Schedule V drugs have the least. In Chapter 53, a Schedule for Controlled Substances shows the meaning of each classification and examples of drugs for each category.

The physician's medical assistant may not dispense controlled substances; however, the medical assistant must be knowledgeable about the regulations governing the documentation and control of drugs. Only licensed personnel are permitted to dispense drugs. Be sure to report to the physician any unusual patient behavior indicating addictive drug use.

Role of the Medical Assistant

The role of the medical assistant in preventing liability suits is of paramount importance to both you and your employer. Remember that in many cases you are the only one in the office who will hear a patient's complaint. Your ability to handle the complaint professionally and efficiently may eliminate a potential lawsuit for the physician.

Acting under a code of ethics that compels you to safeguard any patient whose care and safety are affected by the negligent action of someone else, you must follow the chain of command and report to your immediate supervisor any negligent action you observe. It goes without saying that if you accidentally make an error, you will bring this to your supervisor's attention so that it can be corrected immediately.

You can help your employer and protect yourself by remembering the recommendations and cautions that follow. Though some of these recommendations have been discussed in previous parts of this chapter, it is important to understand how particular situations pertain directly to the role of the medical assistant.

OFFICE MANAGEMENT

- Treat all patients with the same courtesy and dignity you would expect to receive. Log and return telephone calls promptly. Explain any delays to patients who are waiting to see the physician. Offer to set up another appointment if the delay will be very long.

- Never make promises regarding what the physician can do for the patient.

- Carefully explain all fees and responsibilities for bills to the patient, relating any concerns the patient may have to the physician.

- Relay any dissatisfied patient's comments to the physician.

- If the physician will be out of town or absent from the office, post these dates. Include this announcement in the monthly billing envelopes. Also provide the name and telephone number of the physician available for patients who need care when their own physician is absent.

- If a physician is withdrawing from a case, then a certified letter must be sent to the patient declaring this. Send the letter certified mail with return receipt requested, and keep a copy of the letter and return receipt with the patient's record. The physician can be charged with abandonment if there is no documentation or evidence of formal withdrawal.

DOCUMENTATION

- Carefully sign or initial every note. *Remember:* Medical documents are considered legal documents and may be used in a court of law.

- If the patient did not keep an appointment, be sure to document the fact as a no-show. Document canceled appointments and follow-up attempts to determine why the patient missed the appointment.

- Document when a patient is referred to another physician, and follow up to make sure the patient did see the referral physician.

- Document all patient contacts, including telephone prescription refills and tests and procedures that have been ordered. Call all patients the day after surgery to check on their progress. Document this telephone call.

- Record all care and treatment given as soon as possible after the patient's visit. This will keep patient records current and ensure appropriate follow-up treatment if it is required.

- Be sure the physician sees and initials all diagnostic reports in a timely fashion before they are filed.

- Provide all instructions to patients in writing.

DRUG REGULATIONS

- A medical assistant may administer medication only under the direct supervision of a physician. This rule may vary from state to state. Follow the Controlled Substances Act by carefully adhering to designated procedures and documentation requirements.

- Secure the supply of prescription pads from theft at all times.

- When preparing medications for administration, check the medication three times. Remember the "three befores." Check the medication before removing it from the shelf; check the name and dosage again before preparing the dosage; and check the label again before returning the medication to the shelf.

CERTIFICATION AND LICENSING

- Have a thorough understanding of the limits of certification and standards of care for the medical assisting profession. Never perform any procedure for which you are not trained or qualified.

- Do not diagnose or prescribe over the telephone. This applies to all drugs even those that can be obtained over the counter. You could be charged with practicing medicine without a license.

- Do not call yourself a nurse or allow anyone else to refer to you as the nurse. You must be held to your own standard of care and not that of a nurse.

- Participate in continuing education and training programs to maintain your skill levels.

INFORMED CONSENT

- The physician must thoroughly explain all procedures to the patient. The medical assistant is responsible for making sure a signed consent form has been obtained and placed in the patient chart. Never have the patient sign a document that he or she does not understand.

PROFESSIONALISM THE WORKPLACE

It is important that every member of the office staff understand their respective roles. No one should pressure the medical assistant to practice outside his or her role. If a medical assistant is pressured to perform tasks that are outside the legal scope, according to state guidelines, or even the company policy, the medical assistant must notify a supervisor that he or she cannot practice outside the scope of responsibility and training.

- Obtain a parent or guardian's signature before any procedure is performed on a minor. The only exception is in a case of emergency, when the parent or guardian cannot be reached. File the signed consent form immediately.

SAFETY

- Maintain a safe environment in the office or work site for the patients and staff. Handle requests for maintenance repairs. Report any safety hazards at once. If you knowingly overlook a hazard that a reasonable person would report and eliminate, you can be guilty of negligence.

- Carefully check and document medical waste disposal. Be concerned about the safety of maintenance personnel who must handle the waste containers. Always correctly dispose of syringes and needles in designated hazardous waste containers.

- Maintain and document careful quality checks on laboratory testing equipment.

Code of Ethics

Ethics is the branch of philosophy relating to morals or moral principles. It involves the examination of human character and conduct, the distinction between right and wrong, and a person's moral duty and obligations to the community. Ethics has been part of the medical profession since the earliest days of the profession.

The earliest code of ethics, or principles to govern conduct, for those in medicine dates back to around 1800 B.C., to the Code of Hammurabi. In 400 B.C., Hippocrates, a Greek physician referred to as the "father of medicine," wrote a statement of principles for his medical students to follow. This statement of principles is known as the Hippocratic oath (Box 2-1 in Chapter 2) and remains important today. This oath reminds medical students of the importance of their profession, the need to teach others, and the obligation they have to act in such a way as to never knowingly harm a patient or divulge a confidence. The Hippocratic oath is still recited at medical school graduation ceremonies, and has been for centuries, as it carries an important ethical message for physicians. Modern codes of ethics have been developed as medical science has continued to advance.

Medical Ethics

Medical ethics refers to the moral conduct of people in medical professions. This moral conduct of medical professionals is governed by the high principles and standards that these professionals set for themselves and willingly choose to follow through personal dedication. Every medical profession has a code of ethics that sets the moral standards to which members of that profession are expected to adhere.

ETHICAL STANDARDS OF BEHAVIOR

Ethical standards are generally more severe than those standards that are required by law. In many cases, ethical standards are more demanding than the law. A violation of an ethical standard could mean the loss of the physician's reputation.

Ethical behavior, according to the American Medical Association (AMA), refers to moral principles or practices, the customs of the medical profession, and matters of medical policy. Unethical behavior would be any actions that do not follow these ethical standards. When a physician is accused of unethical behavior or conduct in violation of these standards, he or she can be issued a warning or censure (criticism) by the AMA. The AMA Board of Examiners may recommend the expulsion or suspension of a physician from membership in the association. Expulsion, or being forced out of the association, is a severe penalty for physicians because it limits the physician's ability to practice medicine. Not all physicians are members of the AMA, and the AMA does not have authority to bring legal action against nonmembers for unethical conduct. However, the state medical board that issued the physician his or her license may limit the physician's practice or revoke the license altogether for ethical misconduct. If it is alleged (asserted or declared without proof) that a physician has committed a criminal act, the medical society is required to report it to the state board or governmental agency. Violation of the law, which is followed by a conviction for the crime, may result in a fine, imprisonment, or both. The state medical board can then revoke (cancel) the physician's license to practice medicine.

AMA PRINCIPLES OF MEDICAL ETHICS

In the United States, the AMA has taken a leadership role in setting standards for the ethical behavior of physicians. The AMA was organized in New York City in 1846, and its first code of ethics was formed shortly after that in 1847.

The AMA Principles of Medical Ethics encompass human dignity, honesty, responsibility to society, confidentiality, the need for continued study, freedom of choice, and a responsibility of the physician to improve the community. Box 3-3 presents this statement of principles in its entirety.

Medical Assistant's Principles of Medical Ethics

Medical assistants may not be involved with the life-and-death ethical decisions that face the physician. However, they do face many dilemmas regarding right or wrong behavior on an almost daily basis. Examples include when a coworker violates patient confidentiality, use of foul language in front of a patient, or how the team treats a patient whose body may smell of urine or alcohol. Ethical issues involve doing the right thing at the right time.

AAMA CODE OF ETHICS

The Code of Ethics of the American Association of Medical Assistants (AAMA) is a standard that medical assistants are expected to follow. (Figure 3-6 shows a medical assistant assisting a physician with a patient.) The code, which describes ethical and moral conduct for the medical assistant, is similar to the AMA's Principles of Medical Ethics. Box 3-4 lists the code of ethics of the AAMA. Medical assistants assume a position of trust and must try to live up to the standards of the profession as stated in the code.

PROFESSIONALISM

THE LAW

As an agent, or representative of the physician, the medical assistant is responsible to understand ethical standards so that he or she can respond to questions related to any office issue. It is important to remember that the medical assistant cannot diagnose or treat illnesses, although educating the patient about information the physician has given is expected. Patient confidentiality cannot be breached for any reason. Staff members should not access or open any chart for which they do not have a specific work-related need.

Box 3-3 AMA Principles of Medical ETHICS

PREAMBLE

The medical profession has long subscribed to a body of ethical statements developed primarily for the benefit of the patient. As a member of this profession, a physician must recognize responsibility not only to patients, but also to society, to other health professionals, and to self. The following principles adopted by the American Medical Association are not law, but standards of conduct which define the essentials of honorable behavior for the physician.

Human Dignity

I. A physician shall be dedicated to providing competent medical service with compassion and respect for human dignity.

Honesty

II. A physician shall deal honestly with patients and colleagues, and strive to expose those physicians deficient in character or competence, or who engage in fraud or deception.

Responsibility to Society

III. A physician shall respect the law and recognize a responsibility to seek changes in those requirements which are contrary to the best interests of the patient.

Confidentiality

IV. A physician shall respect the rights of patients, of colleagues, and of other health professionals, and shall safeguard patient confidence within the constraints of the law.

Continued Study

V. A physician shall continue to study, apply and advance scientific knowledge, make relevant information available to patients, colleagues, and the public, obtain consultation, and use the talents of other health professionals where needed.

Freedom of Choice

VI. A physician shall, in the provision of appropriate patient care, except in emergencies, be free to choose whom to serve, with whom to associate, and the environment in which to provide service.

Responsibility to Improved Community

VII. A physician shall recognize a responsibility to participate in activities contributing to an improved community.

Copyright by the American Medical Association, Code of Medical Ethics. Reprinted by permission.

AAMA CREED

The Creed of the AAMA can be best followed by the medical assistant who spends time reading about and discussing ethical problems, such as transplants, artificial insemination, the right to die with dignity, and abortion. To be true to this creed, the medical assistant must know about the ethical issues the patient faces and be committed to treat the patient with respectful care regardless of the patient's religious beliefs or cultural practices.

Creed of the American Association of Medical Assistants

I believe in the principles and purposes of the profession of medical assisting.

I endeavor to be more effective.

I aspire to render greater service.

I protect the confidence entrusted to me.

I am dedicated to the care and well-being of all people.

I am loyal to my employer.

I am true to the ethics of my profession.

I am strengthened by compassion, courage, and faith.

Copyright by the American Association of Medical Assistants, Inc. Reprinted with permission.

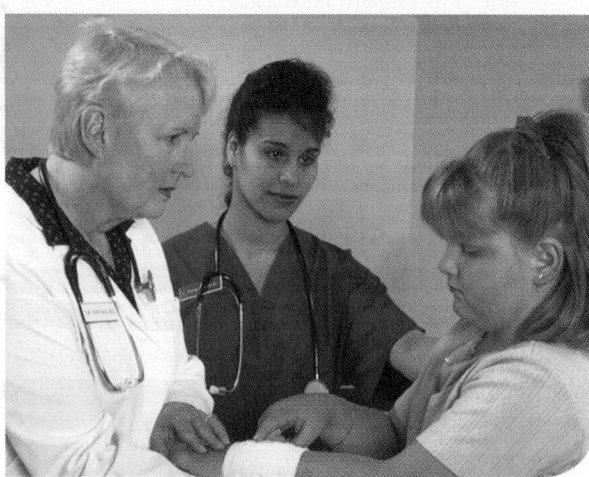

FIGURE 3-6 **A medical assistant helps the physician with a patient.**

Box 3-4 Code of Ethics of the American Association of Medical ASSISTANTS

PREAMBLE

The Code of Ethics of AAMA shall set forth principles of ethical and moral conduct as they relate to the medical profession and the particular practice of medical assisting.

Members of the AAMA dedicated to the conscientious pursuit of their profession, and thus desiring to merit the high regard of the entire medical profession and the respect of the general public which they serve, do hereby pledge themselves to strive always to:

Human Dignity

I. Render service with full respect for the dignity of humanity;

Confidentiality

II. Respect confidential information obtained through employment unless legally authorized or required by responsible performance of duty to divulge such information;

Honor

III. Uphold the honor and high principles of the profession and accept its disciplines;

Continued Study

IV. Seek to continually improve the knowledge and skills of medical assistants for the benefit of patients and professional colleagues;

Responsibility for Improved Community

V. Participate in additional service activities aimed toward improving the health and well-being of the community.

Copyright by the American Association of Medical Assistants, Inc. Reprinted with permission.

AMT STANDARDS OF PRACTICE

The American Medical Technologists (AMT) have standards of practice that reflect the ethical expectations for those with the Registered Medical Assistant (RMA) credential. Similar to the AAMA creed, the AMT Standards of Practice call for ethical behavior by medical assistants. AMT seeks to encourage, establish, and maintain the highest standards, traditions, and principles of the practices that constitute the profession of the registry. Members of the AMT Registry must recognize their responsibilities, not only to their patients but also to society, to other health care professionals, and to themselves. The following standards of practice are principles adopted by the AMT board of directors, which defines the essence of honorable and ethical behavior for a health care professional:

AMT STANDARDS OF PRACTICE

1. While engaged in the Arts and Sciences, which constitute the practice of their profession, AMT professionals shall be dedicated to the provision of competent service.
2. The AMT professional shall place the welfare of the patient above all else.
3. The AMT professional understands the importance of thoroughness in the performance of duty, compassion with patients, and the importance of the tasks which they may perform.
4. The AMT professional shall always seek to respect the rights of patients and of health care providers, and shall safeguard patient confidences.
5. The AMT professional will strive to increase his/her technical knowledge, shall continue to study, and apply scientific advances in his/her specialty.
6. The AMT professional shall respect the law and will pledge to avoid dishonest, unethical or illegal practices.
7. The AMT professional understands that he/she is not to make or offer a diagnosis or interpretation unless he/she is a duly licensed physician/dentist or unless asked by the attending physician/dentist.
8. The AMT professional shall protect and value the judgment of the attending physician or dentist, providing this does not conflict with the behavior necessary to carry out Standard Number 2 above.
9. The AMT professional recognizes that any personal wrongdoing is his/her responsibility. It is also the professional health care provider's obligation to report to the proper authorities any knowledge of professional abuse.
10. The AMT professional pledges personal honor and integrity to cooperate in the advancement and expansion, by every lawful means, of American Medical Technologists.

Copyright by the American Medical Technologists. Reprinted with permission.

Medical Assistant's Standard of Care

As a medical assistant, you must remember that your actions can have legal consequences for the physician who employs you. You are not held to the same standard of care as a physician due to differing credentials, licensure, and education. However, you will carry out your duties under the direction of a physician and, therefore, you must use the same approved methods that a physician would use. For example, you must uphold the same quality standard as any physician would use when taking an electrocardiogram, drawing blood, and collecting specimens.

A medical assistant is not expected to diagnose medical conditions, interpret electrocardiograms, or prescribe medications since these are all within the area of the physician's standard of care. In fact, a medical assistant must continually use caution and not take on any tasks or duties for which he or she is not trained within the scope of his or her practice.

The actions of medical assistants reflect upon their physician-employers. Many duties performed by medical assistants could result in harm to the patient if not done properly. In some lawsuits, the physician has been found guilty of negligence due to improper performance of his or her medical assistant.

The Patient's Bill of Rights

The American Hospital Association developed the "The Patient's Bill of Rights" (Box 3-5), which describes the patient–physician relationship. Medical assistants must also follow these guidelines when working with the physician's patients. Most offices have copies of this document available for patients to read.

HIPAA and Confidentiality

According to the Medical Patients Rights Act, all patients have the right to have their personal privacy respected and their medical records handled with confidentiality. No information—including test results, patient histories, and even the fact that the patient is a patient—can be told to another person without the patient's permission. Therefore it

Box 3-5 The Patient's Bill of RIGHTS

1. The patient has the right to considerate and respectful care.
2. The patient has the right to and is encouraged to obtain from physicians and other direct caregivers relevant, current, understandable information concerning diagnosis, treatment, and prognosis.
3. The patient has the right to make decisions about the plan of care prior to and during the course of treatment and to refuse a recommended treatment or plan of care to the extent permitted by law and hospital policy and to be informed of the consequences of this action.
4. The patient has the right to have an advance directive (such as a living will, health care proxy, or durable power of attorney for health care) concerning treatment or designating a surrogate decision maker with the expectation that the hospital will honor the intent of that directive to the extent permitted by law and hospital policy.
5. The patient has the right to every consideration of privacy.
6. The patient has the right to expect that all communications and records pertaining to his or her care will be treated as confidential by the hospital, except in cases such as suspected abuse and public health hazards when reporting is permitted or required by law.
7. The patient has the right to review the records pertaining to his or her medical care and to have the information explained or interpreted as necessary, except when restricted by law.
8. The patient has the right to expect that, within its capacity and policies, a hospital will make reasonable responses to the request of a patient for appropriate and medically indicated care and service.
9. The patient has the right to ask and be informed of the existence of business relationships among the hospital, educational institutions, other health care providers, or payers that may influence the patient's treatment or care.
10. The patient has the right to consent to or decline to participate in proposed research studies or human experimentation affecting care and treatment or requiring direct patient involvement, and to have those studies fully explained prior to consent.
11. The patient has the right to expect reasonable continuity of care when appropriate and to be informed by physicians and other caregivers of available and realistic patient care options when hospital care is no longer appropriate.
12. The patient has the right to be informed of hospital policies and practices that relate to patient care, treatment, and responsibilities.

Copyright by the American Hospital Association. Reprinted by permission.

important that a medical assistant adhere to the following guidelines:

- Never make any statements about your employing physician that could be interpreted as an admission of fault. On the other hand, as a medical assistant, you cannot remain silent if you are aware that your employing physician is doing something illegal. You can be held liable for remaining silent.
- Do not participate in negative or critical discussions of the physician(s) or other practitioners in your office with your patients. Do not comment on a patient's negative criticism of a current or former physician.
- Never discuss anything about a patient outside of the office.
- Make sure that a female medical assistant is present when the physician (male or female) examines a female patient.
- Treat all patients with dignity and respect.

This is not just a manner of ethics or professionalism; it is the law. After numerous complaints from patients about being unable to continue to pay premiums to the same insurance company when they changed jobs (portability), the United States Congress passed a law called the Health Insurance Portability and Accountability Act (HIPAA) of 1996. HIPAA, also known as Public Law 104-191, seeks to improve the efficiency and effectiveness of the health care system through insurance reform and administrative simplification. Many citizens feared that certain information about their health might prevent them from getting insurance coverage, and Congress responded by legislating rigorous standards of privacy for protected health information. The U.S. Department of Health and Human Services was charged with setting privacy and security standards for health information. Covered entities include health plans, health care clearinghouses, and providers who conduct certain health care transactions electronically. Medical practices are required to notify patients about the uses, disclosures, and rights of their protected information. These protocols, although sharing common concerns for the patient, are not standardized by the government. Each practice should have policies and procedures for handling confidential information, including privacy officers who guard the security of identifiable health information. All employees and business associates who will have access to identifiable health information must give written assurances that they will protect patient information before they may access it. Patients also must be informed about how their information might be shared with others. This act gives patients more control over their health information than they had before, sets boundaries and safeguards for release of information, and holds personnel accountable to protect the information. Patients can find out who had access to their private information and gives them the right to examine and copy their records. They also can request corrections to records. Penalties for the improper release of information are very expensive. There are few exceptions to this rule, such as government access, worker's compensation laws, research, and matters relating to public health and law enforcement. Medical assistants must always be vigilant about protecting patient information and following the safeguards established in their office. Complaints under HIPAA should be addressed to the U.S. Department of Health and Human Services.

All medical office employees must undergo HIPAA training during their orientation. HIPAA is organized into three parts: privacy regulations, transaction standards, and security regulations. To adhere to HIPAA regulations, the medical office must have an appointed privacy official, draft privacy policies and procedures, and implement a program to educate and train all employees and physicians on the mandates of HIPAA. These polices should be included in the office policy and procedures manual. Acknowledgement of receiving a copy of the privacy practices of the medical office should be signed by all new patients and clearly posted in the waiting area of the medical office. Patients should sign an authorization to release information to a spouse or adult children. Otherwise, the medical assistant should not share information with family members.

HIPAA extends its rules to making sure that computers with confidential patient information cannot be seen or accessed by individuals who are not authorized to see the information. All faxes and e-mails that contain private patient information must have a note stating that the information is confidential, and if the information is accidentally transmitted to someone without clearance to read the information, the recipient must immediately notify the office and destroy the information. Health care professionals should refrain from discussing patients' private information where other people without need for that information could overhear the discussion. The medical assistant should keep in mind that wireless telephones and cellular signals are not secure and should be cautious with the use of speakerphones because others may overhear. Even when the medical assistant reaches a patient's voice mail, it is important to leave only the minimal information that contains the name and telephone number of the person to call.

Although HIPAA is the law that protects the patient and promotes the portability of insurance, massive amounts of health care data must be controlled to ensure not only privacy but also efficiency. To simplify data use, the Centers for Medicare and Medicaid Services requires unique identification numbers for health care providers, individuals, health care plans, and employers. With these numbers, it is clear (even if names are similar) who the interested parties are in a transaction.

HIPAA further seeks to protect the transmission of data relating to health care. To improve the efficiency and effectiveness of the health care system, Congress, the public, and the health care industry have mutually agreed that standards are needed for the electronic exchange of administrative and financial health care transactions. The Secretary of Health and Human Services was designed by HIPAA to adopt protective and secure standards.

National standards for electronic health care transactions ultimately sought to simplify the processes involved in transmitting information required for quality patient care. Following these standards should promote savings resulting from the reduction in administrative burdens on health care providers and health plans. A standardized national claim form replaced over 400 different formats that existed before HIPAA. Health plans now use one standard form (CMS-1500) and standardize transactions such as remittance advices and referral authorizations to health care providers. These national standards also reduce paper usage.

The Secretary of Health and Human Services has adopted the standards for the following administrative and financial health care transactions:

1. Health claims and equivalent encounter information.
2. Enrollment and disenrollment in a health plan
3. Eligibility for a health plan
4. Health care payment and remittance advice
5. Health plan premium payments
6. Health claim status
7. Referral certification and authorization

The medical assistant must be sure to use the standardized forms for all these transactions.

The medical assistant's treatment of and concern for the patient reflects the physician's high standards of care. The human dignity of each patient must be preserved regardless of the patient's socioeconomic background, race, age, nationality, sexual orientation, or gender (Figure 3-7). Any promise or commitment that the medical assistant makes to a patient can be legally binding to his or her physician and employer. This means that the physician can be held responsible for something the staff has said or implied with regard to the physician improving the patient's condition.

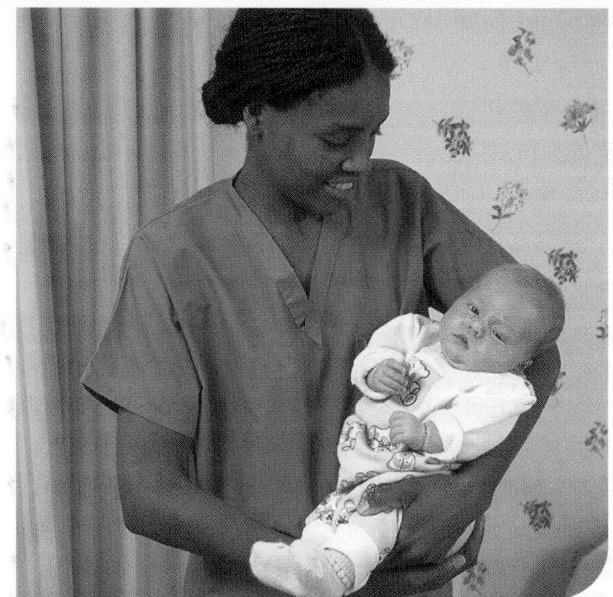

FIGURE 3-7 **Patients of all socioeconomic backgrounds should be given equal care.**

Any information that is given to a physician by a patient is considered confidential, and it may not be given to an unauthorized person. The physician's medical assistant is considered to be an authorized person with access to the patient's file and information. This information may not be divulged to anyone without permission of the doctor or patient. The physician must be notified of any information the patient gives the medical assistant, such as if the patient is not taking prescribed medications or complying with treatment (Figure 3-8).

Ethical Issues and Personal Choice

Ethics differ from laws in key ways. While laws are enforceable by governmental authorities with penalties such as fines and jail time, ethics are valued by professional organizations

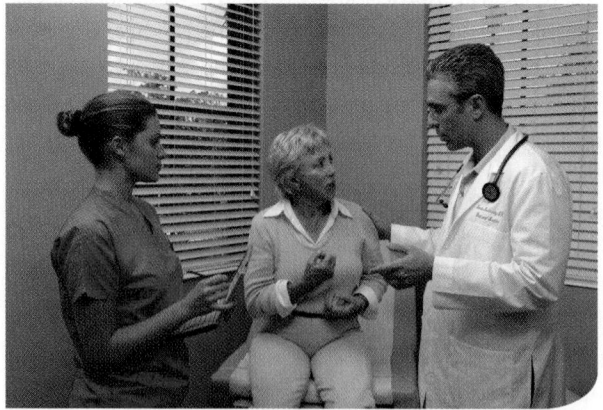

FIGURE 3-8 **A medical assistant listening to the patient and physician discuss the patient's care.**

but rarely are severe penalties attached to an ethical violation. If an ethical violation occurs, the guilty party may be shunned professionally or have a certification withheld, but no severe penalties exist for ethical violations. Ethical boards, such at that of the AMA, make ethical decisions (such as whether or not to perform certain procedures) for professional organizations. Bioethics refers to ethical decisions pertaining to life issues. For example, stem cell research, in vitro fertilization, and abortion rights are sometimes controversial issues about human life. Hospitals usually have ethics committees to assist in making ethical decisions about patient care.

Moral decisions are different from legal and ethical decisions. For example, a person might be legally able to have sex outside of marriage, but ethically this person should not have sex with a patient. However, morally, one might not believe that one can have sex outside of marriage at all. Moral decisions do not have a civil or professional penalty, but one might be socially shunned by a committee at a house of worship for making certain moral choices.

In some cases, the medical assistant may have a personal, religious, or ethical reason for wishing not to be involved in particular procedures, such as abortions or artificial insemination. These preferences should be stated to the employer prior to employment, allowing them to be considered when making a hiring decision. In the event that the situation arises after employment begins, all concerns should be communicated to the employer immediately. It is very important not to judge what the physician is doing since he or she is acting within ethical guidelines. An individual should request to be disallowed from participating in any procedures about which he or she has ethical doubts. If the medical assistant's choice to not assist the physician in a specific procedure jeopardizes the health and safety of a patient, or interferes with the physician's ability to do the procedures, it may be necessary for the medical assistant to seek other employment. The medical assistant must reflect on bioethical decisions but support the patient in the patient's own decision making.

SCIENTIFIC DISCOVERY AND ETHICAL ISSUES

Many areas of medical ethics—When should life support be withdrawn? When does a life begin? Is euthanasia ever permissible? Should the unborn baby's life be sacrificed to save the mother? and more—still encompass no conclusive answers. Scientific discoveries present new medical possibilities and choices every day. With these possibilities, more complicated ethical issues often need to be addressed before choices can be made. The medical assistant has a responsibility to keep current on medical advances and form opinions based on sound medical ethics and practice.

SUMMARY

In the United States, law is based on inalienable rights set forth in the U.S. Constitution. Laws are either criminal (against the state), civil (against people), military (involving military personnel), or international (between nations).

The medical and legal issues governing the medical profession and medical assistants are multifaceted. The medical assistant must be knowledgeable in many areas of the law. Laws governing medicine are different from those governing criminal behavior. Medicine is covered by civil law, often referred to as torts. It is the responsibility of both the physician and the medical assistant to be aware of these guidelines.

Medical ethics is based on the Hippocratic oath. Patients must be treated equally, using the best possible standards of care. Standard of care is determined to be what a reasonable person of the same education would probably have done. Both the American Medical Association (AMA) and the American Association of Medical Assistants (AAMA) have professional standards and values known as ethics.

Because health care providers can hurt the public, they can be held liable for damages done to patients. The physician–patient relationship is actually a contract, with rights granted to both parties. Care must be taken when terminating a relationship with a patient, or the physician can be charged with abandonment. The physician must obtain informed consent from the patient before performing invasive procedures on patients. A medical assistant can cause a physician to be held liable for the assistant's actions under the doctrine of *respondeat superior*. To prove malpractice the physician must have had duty to a patient, been derelict in the duty, and caused damages that were directly related to the dereliction of duty.

The Health Insurance Portability and Accountability Act (HIPAA) was enacted to encourage portability of insurance when citizens changed jobs, but it also includes strict provisions for maintaining confidentiality of patient information. Medical assistants have a professional duty to protect patient information.

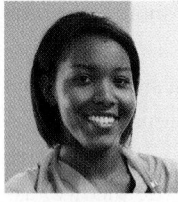

3 CHAPTER REVIEW

COMPETENCY REVIEW

1. Define and spell the key terms for this chapter.

2. What are the elements of a contract?

3. Compare the Code of Ethics of the AAMA with the AMT Standards of Practice.

4. What is informed consent?

5. Describe the medical assistant's responsibilities concerning medical ethics.

6. What is the difference between criminal and civil law?

7. List and describe the four Ds of negligence.

8. What are Good Samaritan laws, and how do they apply to you?

9. Why do you need thorough understanding of the law as it impacts your employer's practice?

10. State 10 steps that can be taken to help protect the physician and staff from liability.

PREPARING FOR THE CERTIFICATION EXAM

1. When a physician abandons a patient, it is an offense under which type of law?
   a. criminal
   b. civil
   c. military
   d. international
   e. corporate

2. Patients of which religious preference would probably refuse a blood transfusion?
   a. Catholic
   b. Christian Scientist
   c. Jewish
   d. Muslim
   e. Hindu

3. Which of the following lists the ethics of a medical assistant?
   a. Hippocratic oath
   b. AMA Code of Ethics
   c. state laws
   d. AAMA Code of Ethics
   e. The Patient's Bill of Rights

4. HIPAA protects which patient right?
   a. self-determination
   b. liberty
   c. beneficence
   d. confidentiality
   e. informed consent

5. Which expression describes that the physician is liable for the behavior of the medical assistant?

   a. *res ipsa loquitur*
   b. *respondeat superior*
   c. *quid pro quo*
   d. guardian ad litem
   e. rule of discovery

6. If a medical assistant is sued in court, the standards of care to which he or she would be compared would be that of a:
   a. medical student.
   b. prudent medical assistant.
   c. seasoned medical assistant.
   d. nurse.
   e. medical assisting student.

7. Which must be documented in writing before undergoing surgery?
   a. informed consent
   b. check for payment
   c. knowledge of The Patient's Bill of Rights
   d. AMA Code of Ethics
   e. collection notice

8. Which of the following does NOT emancipate minors?
   a. living on their own
   b. being married
   c. being self-supporting
   d. being in the armed forces
   e. having sexual relations

9. Which of the following is NOT one of the four Ds of negligence?
   a. direct cause   b. drug abuse
   c. damages   d. duty
   e. dereliction of duty

10. Injecting medication into someone without their consent is an example of:
   a. assault.   b. battery.   c. defamation.
   d. fraud.   e. abandonment.

CRITICAL THINKING

1. Does Shandra have protection from liability in this case?

2. One of the victims who did not survive the accident was an organ donor. What specific limitation has been placed on the physician who has declared this individual's time of death?

3. The organ donor had a signed organ donation card. If someone wishes to be an organ donor what else should be taken into consideration besides having an organ donor card?

ON THE JOB

Dr. Spring, a board-certified obstetrician and gynecologist, has been in practice for more than 10 years. He is licensed to practice medicine in both New York and Pennsylvania. Dr. Spring employs a staff that includes two medical assistants.

On Monday one of the medical assistants, Nancy Watts, took a history on a new patient who was referred to Dr. Spring by her internist. The 40-year-old, married patient had had vaginal spotting for more than six weeks.

As part of the history, Nancy learned that the patient has been under the care and supervision of a fertility specialist for more than two years. In fact, although not always compliant, the patient had been on a medication treatment regime for fertility problems.

After examining the patient, Dr. Spring ordered a uterine biopsy to be performed in the office. The patient returned the following week, underwent the biopsy, and was sent home. Soon after, the patient's husband had telephoned the office, requesting to speak to Dr. Spring immediately. His wife had just been admitted to the hospital because of intense vaginal bleeding.

1. Was there anything in the patient's history that should have caused Nancy to alert the physician about performing a uterine biopsy?
2. Should Nancy have given this patient special instructions prior to the biopsy because of her history?
3. How should Nancy have handled the husband's telephone call?
4. Would it violate patient confidentiality to fax the patient's records to the emergency room physician, if requested?
5. Is this a potential case of medical negligence and malpractice? Could Nancy, as the medical assistant, have complicity in this particular case?

INTERNET ACTIVITY

Do an Internet search for your local state health laws. Report back what you found to the class.

MEDMEDIA

Additional interactive resources and activities for this chapter can be found:

On your student DVD: View applicable procedure videos on the DVD-ROM found in the back of this book.

MyHealthProfessionsKit.com: Test your knowledge of the chapter with games and activities. MyHealthProfessionsKit also includes resources, helpful links, and a Spanish audio glossary.

Medical Assisting Interactive: Practice your procedures as a medical assistant in this simulated doctor's office. This can be accessed through MyHealthProfessionsKit.com.

4

Medical Terminology

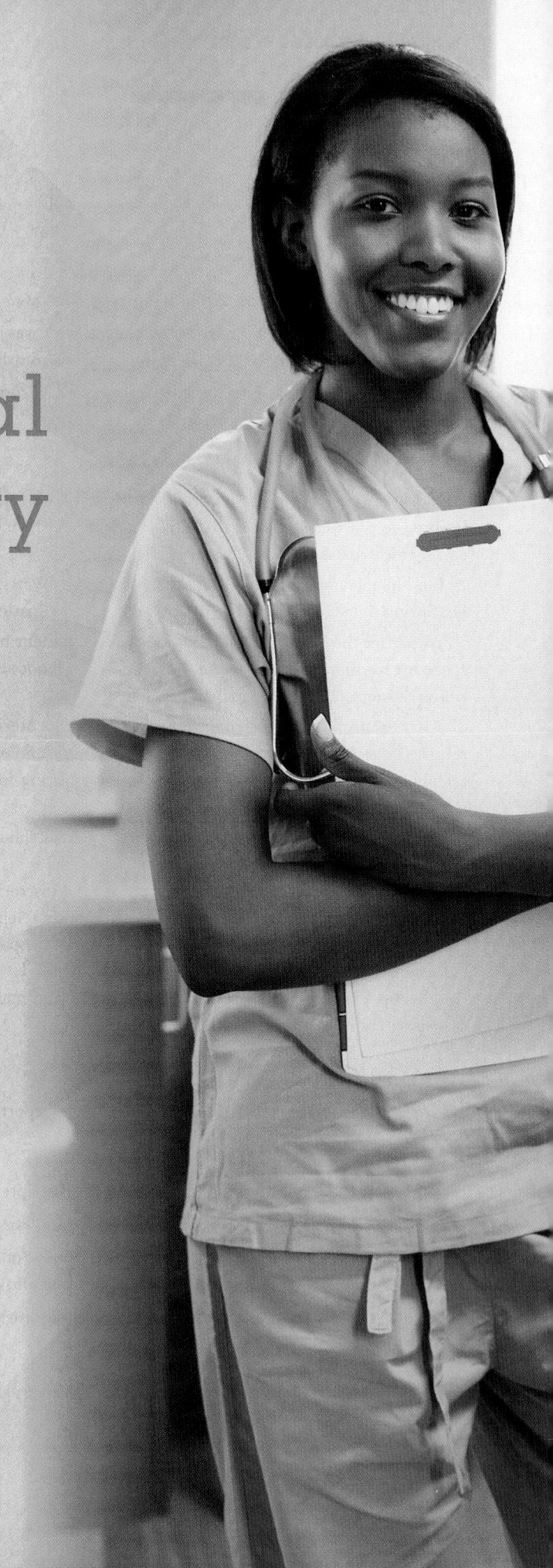

LEARNING OBJECTIVES

After completing this chapter, you should be able to:

- Define and spell the terms to learn for this chapter.
- Identify and discuss medical terminology word parts.
- Analyze, build, spell, and pronounce medical words.

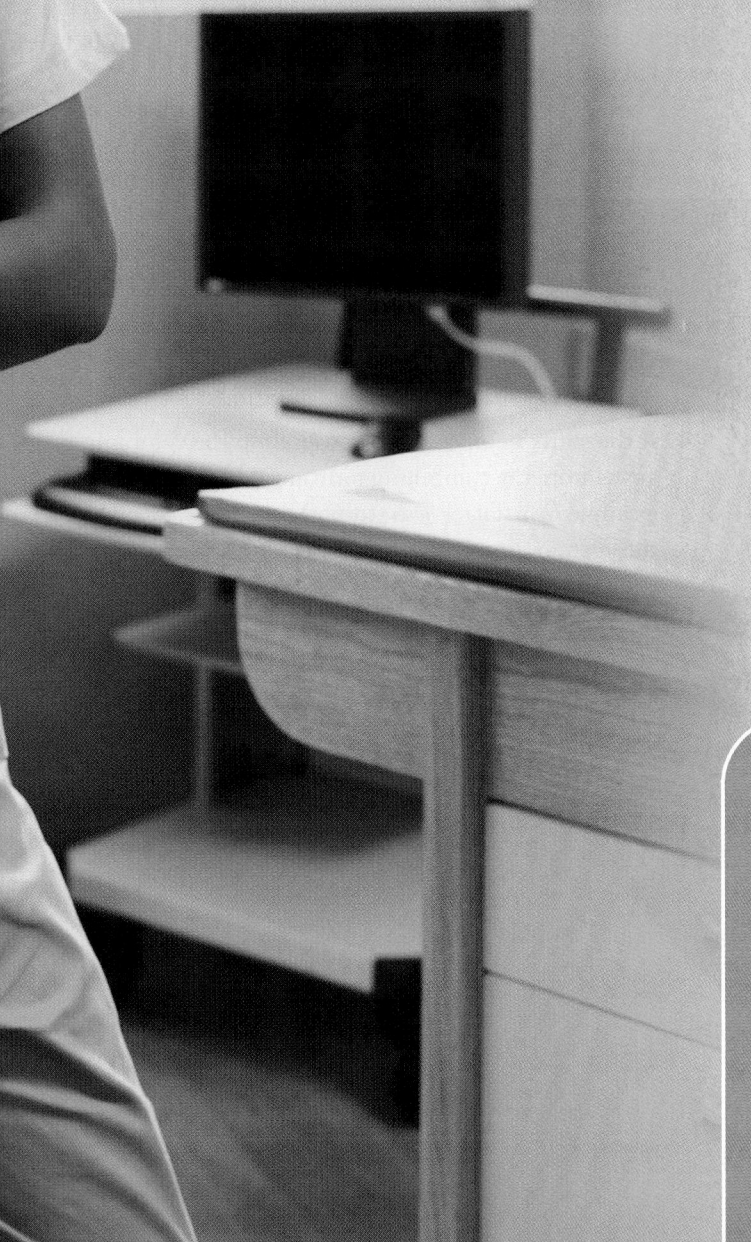

CHAPTER OUTLINE

CASE STUDY

Dr. McWalter saw Mickey Schultz in the office for abdominal pain. The pain was centered in the epigastric region, and Dr. McWalter needed to determine if the pain was cardiac or gastrointestinal in origin. She ordered a variety of tests to ensure that no chemical changes, musculoskeletal origins, or blockages in the soft tissue were causing the pain. Eventually, the pain was determined to be caused by a peptic ulcer.

The language of medicine is derived mostly from Latin and Greek words because the early fathers of the science of medicine spoke Latin and Greek. While these words may look unusual at first, once the medical assistant understands them and their meanings, communication becomes easier. Communication is very important in the medical office, and medical terminology is frequently used there. Therefore, it is important for medical assistants to have a solid, basic understanding of the structural components of medical terms. It is impossible for a medical assistant to know every possible medical term; therefore, it is helpful to become familiar with reputable Internet sites, medical dictionaries, and other sources of information.

Word Parts

Medical terms are frequently composed of word roots plus adjunctive parts; however, they can also be formed by adding together several word parts without a word root. If a word root is used, to prepare the word root for combining with another part, a **combining vowel** is sometimes added. This combining part is usually an "o" but is sometimes not used if a vowel is already present. Medical terms also will often contain prefixes and suffixes, both of which add further meaning to the given term (Figure 4-1). The medical assistant will dissect unknown words to determine their meanings and look up terms in reference resources.

WORD ROOTS AND COMBINING FORMS

A **word root** is a word or element from which other words are formed. Most medical terms have a word root on which other word parts are attached. For example, in Figure 4-2, the word root is *cardi*. The word root *cardi* means "heart," so the medical assistant knows that this word must have something to do with the heart. To fully understand the complete word, add to the central meaning of the word those parts that are attached to the front and back of the word part. To prepare a combining form for conjunction with a suffix or another word part, the medical assistant may need to add a combining vowel, usually an "o" or sometimes an "i." It is onto this combining form that a suffix or another word root or combining form can be added. Since it is difficult to say "electrcardiogram," the letter "o" is added to the word elements in Figure 4-1 to prepare the elements to be stuck together. When a word root has a vowel attached to it in order to add another element, it is termed a **combining form**. A combining form is a word root to which a vowel has been added. In the word shown in Figure 4-2, the combining forms are "electro" and "cardio." Since the suffix *gram* means "written record," the word *electrocardiogram* means a written record of the electrical activity of the heart.

Sometimes two combining forms are placed together to become a more complex word. An inflammation of the stomach is *gastritis,* and an inflammation of the intestines is *enteritis.* If both areas are inflamed, the term is *gastroenteritis.* Note that the letter "o" for the second combining form is not used because the suffix begins with a vowel. If a vowel follows the combining form, the combining letter (usually "o") is dropped. Combining letters are usually used when two consonants would otherwise be placed together. Here are some helpful guidelines:

1. If the suffix begins with a vowel, drop the combining vowel from the combining form and add the suffix. For example *lip/o* (fat) + *oma* (tumor) becomes *lipoma* when the *o* from *lipo* is deleted. Therefore, a lipoma is a tumor composed of fat.

Analyzing a Medical Term
You can often decipher the meaning of a medical term by breaking it down into its separate parts. Consider the following examples:

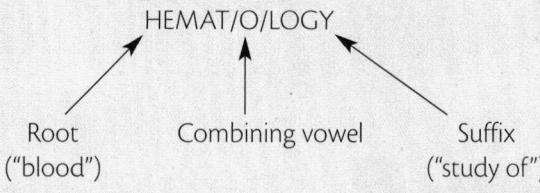

HEMAT/O/LOGY

Root
("blood")

Combining vowel

Suffix
("study of")

FIGURE 4-1 **Analyzing a medical term.**

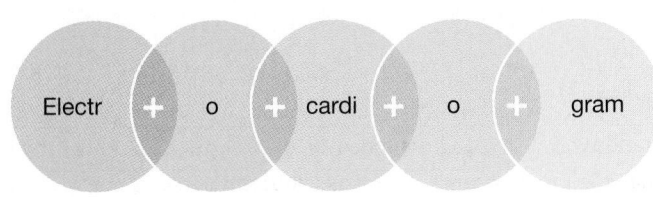

Electr + o + cardi + o + gram

FIGURE 4-2 Word building.

2. If the suffix begins with a consonant, keep the combining vowel and add the suffix to the combining form. For example *lip/o* (fat) + *lysis* (destruction) becomes *lipolysis,* and the *o* on that combining form

is retained. Therefore, lipolysis is the destruction of fat.

Table 4-1 shows common word roots in medical terminology. Table 4-2 shows common combining forms.

PREFIXES

A **prefix** is a word element that is placed before, or is affixed to the beginning of the word root. Prefixes are always placed at the beginning of words to alter or modify their meanings or to create new words. Table 4-3 shows some key prefixes.

TABLE 4-1 Selected Word Roots in Medical Terminology

Word Roots		cervic	neck; cervix
abdomin	abdomen	cheil	lip
aden	gland	chiro	hand
adren	adrenal gland	cholangi	bile duct
adrenal	adrenal gland	chole	gall; bile
aer	air; oxygen; gas	chondr	cartilage
alveol	alveolus	coccyg	coccyx; tailbone
angi	(blood) vessel; (lymph) vessel	col	colon; large intestine
ankyl	crooked; stiff; bent	conjunctiv	conjunctiva
appendic	appendix	corne	cornea
arteri, arter	artery	coron	heart; crown of the head
arteriol	arteriole (small artery)	cost	rib
arthr	joint	crani	cranium; skull
ather	yellowish; fatty plaque	cutane	skin
aur	ear	cyan	blue
aut	self	cyst	bladder; sac
bil	bile	cyt, cyte	cell
bio	life	dacry	tears; tear duct
blephar	eyelid	dactyl	fingers or toes
bronch	airway; bronchus	dent	tooth
bronchiol	bronchiole	derm	skin
burs	bursa	dermat	skin
carcin	cancer	dipl	two; double
cardi	heart	diverticul	diverticulum
caud	tail; toward lower part of the body	dors	back (of the body)
cephal	head	duoden	duodenum
cerebell	cerebellum	ectop	located away from usual place
cerebr	cerebrum; brain	edema	swelling

(continued)

TABLE 4-1 (*continued*)

electr	electricity; electrical activity		ili	ilium
encephal	brain		immun	immune
endocrin	endocrine		irid	iris
enter	intestines (usually small intestine)		kerat	horny tissue; hard
epiglott	epiglottis		kin	movement
epitheli	epithelium		kinesi	movement; motion
erythr	red		labi	lips
esophag	esophagus		lacrim	tear duct; tear
esthesi	sensation; feeling; sensitivity		lact	milk
eti	cause (of disease)		lapar	abdomen
exocrin	secrete out of		laryng	larynx
faci	face		later	side
fasci	fascia; fibrous band		lei	smooth
fract	break; broken		leuk	white
galact	milk		lingu	tongue
gastr	stomach		lip	fat
ger	old age; aged		lith	stone; calculus
geront	old age; aged		lob	lobe
gingiv	gums		lymph	lymph
glauc	gray		macr	abnormal largeness
gloss	tongue		mamm	breast
gluc	sweetness; sugar		mast	breast
glyc	sugar; glucose		meat	opening or passageway
glycos	sugar; glucose		melan	black
gnos	knowledge; a knowing		men	menstruation
gonad	gonad; sex glands		mening	meninges
gyn	woman		ment	mind
gynec	woman		mes, meso	middle
gyr	turning; folding		metr	uterus
hem	blood		mon	one
hemat	blood		morbid	disease; sickness
hepat	liver		muc	mucus
hidr	sweat		my, myos	muscle
hist	tissue		myc	fungus
hom	same		myel	bone marrow; spinal cord
home	sameness; unchanging		myelon	bone marrow
hydr	water		myring	eardrum
hyster	uterus		narc	stupor; numbness
ile	ileum		nas	nose

nat	birth
necr	death (cells; body)
nephr	kidney
neur	nerve
noct	night
nyct	night
nyctal	night
ocul	eye
onc	tumor
onych	nail
oophor	ovary
ophthalm	eye
or	mouth
orth	straight
oste	bone
ot	ear
ox	oxygen
palpat	touch; feel; stroke
pancreat	pancreas
par, part	bear; give birth to; labor
parathyroid	parathyroid
path	disease; suffering
pector	chest; muscle
ped	child; foot
pelv	pelvis; pelvic bone
pen	penis
perine	perineum
peritone	peritoneum
petr	stone; portion of temporal bone
phac, phak	lens of the eye
phag	eat; swallow
phalang	finger or toe bone
pharyng	pharynx, throat
phas	speech
phleb	vein
phot	light
phren	mind
physi	nature
pleur	pleura

pneum	lung; air
pneumat	lung; air
pneumon	lung; air
pod	foot
poli	gray matter
polyp	polyp; small growth
poster	back (of body)
prim	first
proct	rectum
pseud	fake; false
psych	mind
pulmon	lung
py	pus
pyel	renal pelvis
pylor	pylorus
pyr	fever; heat
quadr	four
rect	rectum
ren	kidney
retin	retina
rhin	nose
sacr	sacrum fallopian (uterine)
salping	tube
sanit	soundness; health
sarc	flesh; connective tissue
scler	sclera; white of eye; hard
scoli	crooked; curved
seb	sebum; oil
seps	infection
sept	infection; partition; septum
sial	saliva
sinus	inus
somat	body
somn	sleep
son	sound
sopor	sleep
sperm	sperm, spermatazoa; seed
spermat	sperm, spermatazoa; seed
spher	round; sphere; ball

(continued)

TABLE 4-1 (*continued*)

sphygm	pulse
spin	spine; backbone to
spir	breathe
splen	spleen
spondyl	vertebra; spinal or vertebral column
staphyl	grapelike clusters
stern	(breastbone)
steth	chest (muscles)
stoma	mouth; opening
stomat	mouth; opening
strab	squint; squint-eyed
synovi	synovia; synovial membrane
system	system
ten, tend	tendon
tendin	tendon
test	testis; testicle
therm	heat
thorac	thorax; chest
thromb	clot
thym	thymus gland; soul
thyr	thyroid gland
thyroid	thyroid gland
tom	cut; section
ton	tension; pressure
tone	to stretch
tonsill	tonsils
top	place; position; location
tox, toxic	poison; poisonous
trach, trache	trachea; windpipe
trachel	neck; necklike
trich	hair
tubercul	little knot; swelling
tympan	eardrum; middle ear
ulcer	sore; ulcer
ungu	nail

ur	urine; urinary tract
ureter	ureter
urethr	urethra
uria	urination; urine
urin	urine or urinary organs
uter	uterus
uvul	vula; little grape
vagin	vagina
valv	valve
valvul	valve
vas	vessel; duct
vascul	blood vessel; little vessel
ven	vein
versicul	seminal vesicles; blister
vertebr	vertebra; backbone
vesic	urinary bladder
vir	poison; virus
viril	masculine; manly
vis	seeing; sight
visc	sticky
viscer	viscera; internal organs sternum
viscos	sticky
vit	life
xanth	yellow
xen	strange; foreign
xer	dry
zygot	joined together

Additional Word Roots

caus	burning sensation; capable of burning
cusp	point; cusp
flexion	bending
genital	pertaining to birth
lumb	lumbar; loin region
mediastin	mediastinum
tens, tensi	pressure, force, stretching

TABLE 4-2 Selected Combining Forms in Medical Terminology

arter/o	artery	ophthalm/o	eye
arthr/o	joint	ot/o	ear
balan/o	penis	oste/o	bone
cardi/o	heart	pharyng/o	throat
cephal/o	head	phleb/o	vein
derm/o	skin	pulmon/o	lung
enter/o	intestines	ren/o	kidney
erythr/o	red	rhin/o	nose
gastr/o	stomach	stomat/o	mouth
hyster/o	uterus	thromb/o	clot
laryng/o	voice box	thyroid/o	thyroid
leuk/o	white	ureter/o	ureter
mamm/o, mast/o	breast	urethr/o	urethra
my/o	muscle	urin/o	urine
nas/o, rhin/o	nose	ven/o	vein

TABLE 4-3 Common Prefixes Used in Medical Terminology

Common Prefixes			
a	without or absence of	eso	inward
ab	from; away from	eu	normal; good
ad	to; toward	ex	outside; outward
an	without or absence of	exo	outside; outward
ante	before	extra	outside of; beyond
anti	against	hemi	half
bi	two	hyper	above; excessive
bin	two	hypo	below; incomplete; deficient
brady	slow	in	in; into; not
con	together	infra	under; below
contra	against	inter	between
de	from; down from; lack of	intra	within
dia	through; complete; between; apart	mal	bad
dis	to undo; free from	meso	middle
dys	difficult; labored; painful; abnormal	meta	after; beyond; change
ec	out	micro	small
ecto	outside	multi	many
endo	within	neo	new
epi	on; upon; over	nulli	none
		pan	all; total

(continued)

TABLE 4-3 *(continued)*

para	outside; beyond; around	sub	under; below
per	through	super	over; above
peri	surrounding (outer)	supra	above; beyond; on top
poly	many; much	sym	together; joined
post	after	syn	together; joined
pre	before; in front of	tachy	fast; rapid
pro	before	tetra	four
quadri	four	trans	through; across; beyond
re	back	tri	three
retro	back; behind	ultra	beyond; excess
semi	half	uni	one

Medical terminology must be learned carefully. Some prefixes, for example, may have several meanings. It is important to study the prefix in context to fully understand how it impacts the word meaning. In Figure 4-3, note how the use of the prefix *hypo* meaning "low," significantly changes the meaning of a word when replaced with the prefix *hyper* meaning "high." Table 4-4 lists some multiple meanings for the same prefix.

SUFFIXES

In medical terminology usage, a **suffix** is a word element that is affixed to the end of the word. A suffix could be a syllable or group of syllables attached to the end of a word to alter or modify its meaning or to create a new word. In the word in Figure 4-1, for example, the suffix *logy* means "the study of." Simply changing the suffix can alter the entire meaning of a word. If, as in Figure 4-1, the suffix was changed to *uria,* which means "urine," the word *hematuria* would mean "blood in the urine." Table 4-5 lists common suffixes used in medical terminology.

A medical assistant can utilize the same skills to learn medical terminology that are used to understand English. If the health care professional knew that a telegram was a written record from far away (*tele* means "far away"), the word can be taken apart to understand that *gram* is a written record—both in *telegram* and in *electrocardiogram.* For example, if the medical assistant knows that *appendicitis* means "inflammation of the appendix," then *tonsillitis* would mean "inflammation of the tonsils." Taking words apart can help the health care professional to understand the word-building patterns that form medical terminology.

Grammar and Medical Terms

SPELLING

Spelling is important in any language, but it is especially important in medical terminology. We have already noted how the simple changing of a prefix can cause a word to

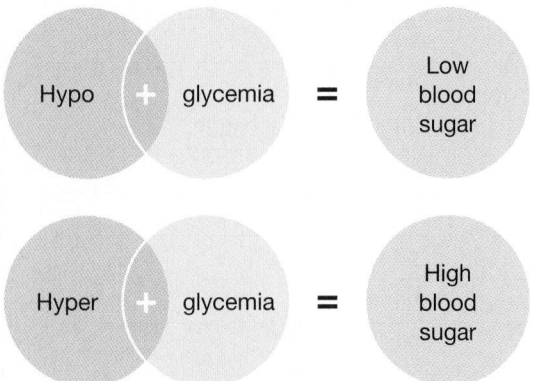

FIGURE 4-3 **Exchanging word parts to change meaning.**

TABLE 4-4 Selected Prefixes Used in Medical Terminology with More Than One Meaning

Prefix	Meanings	Prefix	Meanings
a-, an-	no, not, without, lack of, apart	extra-	outside, beyond
ad-	toward, near, to	hyper-	above, beyond, excessive
bi-	two, double	hypo-	below, under, deficient
de-	down, away from	in-	in, into, not
di-	two, double	mega-	large, great
dia-	through, between, complete	meta-	beyond, over, between, change
dif-, dis-	apart, free from, separate	para-	beside, alongside, abnormal
dys-	bad, difficult, painful, abnormal	poly-	many, much, excessive
ec-, ecto-	out, outside, outer	post-	after, behind
end-, endo-	within, inner	pre-	before, in front of
ep-, epi-	upon, over, above	pro-	before, in front of
eu-	good, normal	super-	upper, above
ex-, exo-	out, away from	supra-	above, beyond

mean its opposite. Some medical terms have various elements that cause them to be more difficult to spell. Table 4-6 lists common prefixes and suffixes that are frequently misspelled.

PLURALS

Not all medical terms are singular. Plurals can seem complicated if the health care professional has not studied the original Latin and Greek languages. Singular endings in Latin change considerably when in the plural form. Table 4-7 shows the patterns of forming plurals in Latin.

Gross Anatomy

Gross anatomy refers to the "big" picture of the body structure. To describe the gross anatomy of the patient, in terms of directions, body planes, positions, and cavities, certain terminology is used.

TABLE 4-5 Common Suffixes Used in Medical Terminology

algia	pain, suffering	crit	to separate
asthenia	weakness	cyte	cell
cele	hernia, protrusion	desis	fusion; to bind; tie together
centesis	surgical puncture to remove fluid	drome	run; running
cidal	killing	ductor	to lead or pull
clasia	break	dynia	pain
clasis	break	ectasis	stretching out; dilation; expansion
clast	break	ectomy	excision or surgical removal
clysis	irrigating; washing	ectopia	displacement
coccus	berry shaped (a form of bacterium)	emesis	vomiting
crine	separate; secrete	emia	blood; blood condition

(continued)

TABLE 4-5 (continued)

gen	producing; forming		physis	growth
genesis	producing; forming		plasia	formation; development; a growth
genic	producing; forming		plasm	growth; formation; substance
gnosis	a knowing		plasty	plastic or surgical repair
gram	record; x-ray		plegia	paralysis; stroke
graph	instrument used to record		pnea	breathing
graphy	process of recording; x-ray filming		porosis	lessening in density; porous condition
ictal	seizure; attack		praxia	in front of; before
ism	state of		ptosis	drooping; sagging; prolapse
itis	inflammation		ptysis	spitting
lepsy	seizure		rrhage	bursting forth, an abnormal excessive discharge or bleeding
logist	specialist		rrhagia	bursting forth, an abnormal excessive discharge or bleeding
logy	study of			
lysis	destruction; reduce; separation		rrhaphy	to suture or stitch
malacia	softening		rrhea	abnormal flow or discharge
mani	madness; insane desire		rrhexis	rupture
megaly	enlargement		schisis	split; fissure
meter	instrument used to measure		sclerosis	hardening
metry	measurement		scope	instrument used for visual exam
morph	form; shape		scopic	visual exam
oid, ode	resembling		scopy	visual exam with an instrument
oma	tumor; mass		sepsis	infection
opia	vision (condition)		sis	state of
opsy	to view		spasm	sudden involuntary muscle contraction
oxia	oxygen		stalsis	contraction; constriction
paresis	slight paralysis		stasis	control; stop; standing still
pathy	disease		stat	to stop
penia	abnormal reduction in number; lack of		stenosis	narrowing; constriction
peps, pepsia	digestion		stomy	new artificial opening
pexy	surgical fixation; suspension		therapy	treatment
phagia	eating; swallowing		tome	instrument used to cut
philia	love		tomy	cutting into; surgical incision
phily	love		tripsy	crushing
phobia	abnormal fear of or adversion to specific objects or things		trophy	nourishment
			ule	little
phonia	sound or voice		uria	urine; urination
phoria	feeling			

TABLE 4-6 Prefixes and Suffixes That Are Frequently Misspelled

Prefix	Meaning	Suffix	Meaning
ante-	before, forward	-poiesis	formation
anti-	against	-ptosis	prolapse, drooping, sagging, falling down
ecto-	out, outside, outer	-ptysis	spitting
endo-	within, inner	-rrhagia	to burst forth, bursting forth
hyper-	above, beyond, excessive	-rrhage	to burst forth, bursting forth
hypo-	below, under, deficient	-rrhaphy	suture
inter-	between	-rrhea	flow, discharge
intra-	within	-rrhexis	rupture
para-	beside, alongside, abnormal	-scope	instrument for examining
peri-	around	-scopy	visual examination, to view, examine
per-	through	-tome	instrument to cut
pre-	before, in front of	-tomy	incision
pro-	before	-tripsy	crushing
super-	above, beyond	-trophy	nourishment, development
supra-	above, beyond		

DIRECTIONS AND BODY PLANES

Terms that are used to indicate the body's direction are necessary when describing the location of a body part or organ. If the body were sliced down a *coronal* or *frontal plane*, the front would be referred to as the *anterior* or *ventral* side and the back would be referred to as *posterior* or *dorsal*. However, if a *transverse* or *horizontal* plane were used, the area above the plane would be referred to as either *superior*, *cranial*, or *cephalic*, and the area below the plane would be termed either *inferior* or *caudal*. Areas farther from the *medial* or *midsagittal* plane are *lateral*, those closer to the plane are *medial*. When referring to points relative to where the arms and legs attach to the body, those farther away are *distal*, those closer are *proximal*. Figure 4-4 illustrates the body planes. Table 4-8 summarizes the directional terms.

TABLE 4-7 Plurals in Medical Terminology

To change the following singular endings to plural endings, substitute the plural endings as illustrated:

Singular Ending	Plural Ending
a as in bursa	to ae as in bursae
ax as in thorax	to aces as in thoraces or es as in thoraxes
en as in foramen	to ina as in foramina
is as in crisis	to es as in crises
is as in iris	to ides as in irides
is as in femoris	to a as in femora
ix as in appendix	to ices as in appendices
nx as in phalanx	to ges as in phalanges
on as in spermatozoon	to a as in spermatozoa
um as in ovum	to a as in ova
us as in nucleus	to i as in nuclei
y as in artery	to i and add es as in arteries

POSITIONS

One of the main tasks of the medical assistant is to place the patient in the correct position for whatever procedure is to be performed. In some cases (such as for neck and back examinations), the patient should be lying on his or her abdomen. However, the vast majority of examinations require positioning patients on their backs. For a pelvic examination, the lithotomy position is used, with legs flexed in stirrups. For a proctological examination, the knee-chest position is favored. If a patient has low blood pressure, as is the case when a patient is in shock, the medical assistant should place the patient in the Trendelenburg position. It is important that the

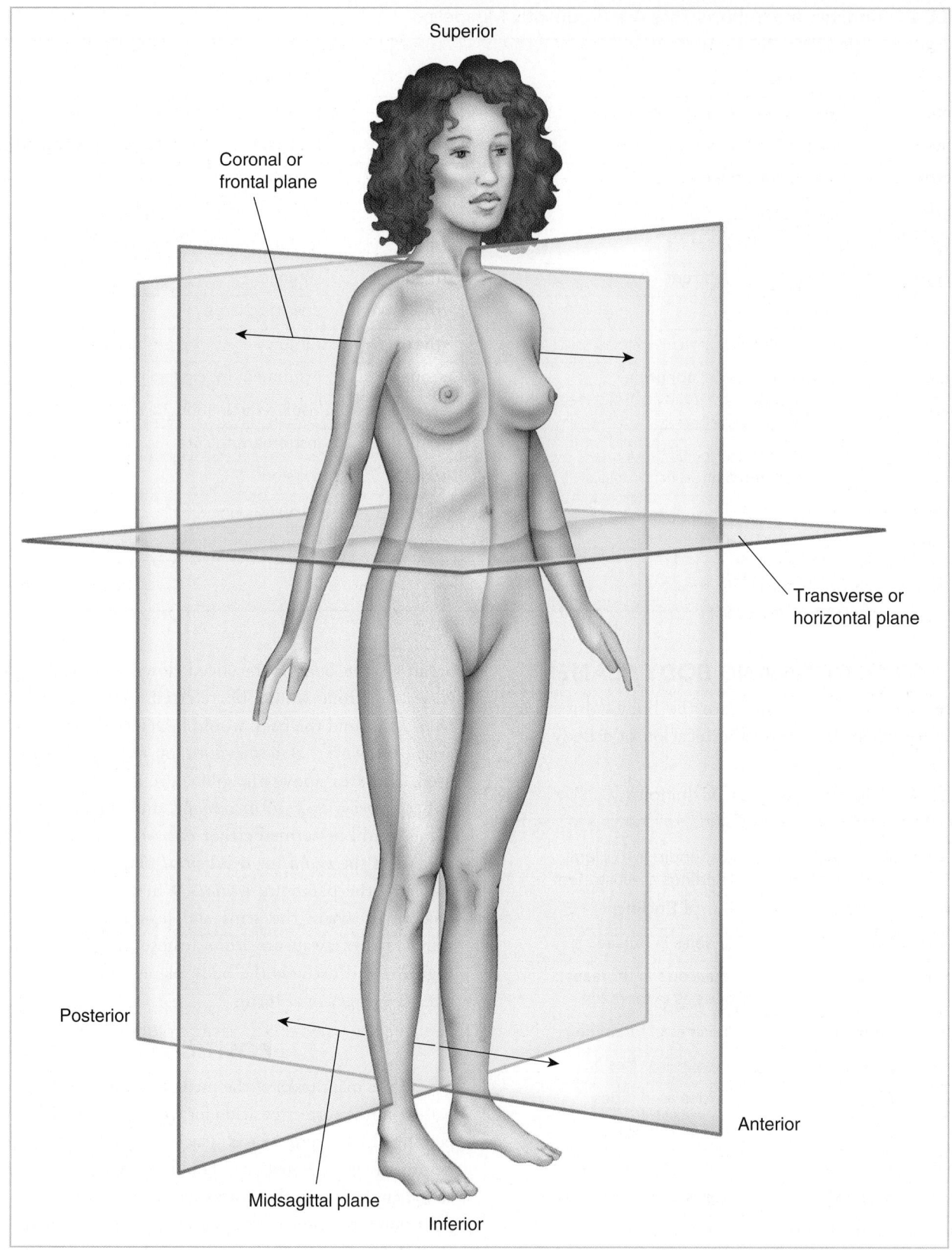

FIGURE 4-4   Planes of the body: coronal or frontal, transverse, and midsagittal.

TABLE 4-8 Directional Terms

Term	Description	Example
Superior	Above, in an upward direction, toward the head	The head is superior to the neck of the body.
Anterior (ventral)	In front of or before, the front side of the body	The breasts are located on the anterior side of the body.
Posterior (dorsal)	Toward the back, back side of the body	The nape is the back of the neck and is located on the posterior side of the body.
Cephalic	Pertaining to the head	A cephalic presentation is one in which any part of the head of the fetus is presented during delivery.
Medial	Nearest the midline or middle	The umbilicus is a depressed point in the medial area of the abdomen.
Lateral	To the side, away from the middle	In the anatomical position, the arm is located on the lateral side of the body.
Proximal	Nearest the point of attachment or near the beginning of a structure	The proximal end of the humerus (upper bone of the arm) joins with part of the shoulder bone.
Distal	Away from the point of attachment or far from the beginning of a structure	The distal end of the humerus joins with part of the elbow.

medical assistant understand in what position a patient must be placed. This way the physician does not have to wait for the patient to be positioned or repositioned, and the patient will be more comfortable because less movement is necessary. For more information about positions, see Table 4-9. The positions are discussed in depth in Chapter 36.

TABLE 4-9 Patient Positions

Position	Description
Anatomical	Body erect, head facing forward, arms by the sides with palms to the front; used as the position of reference in designating the site or direction of a body structure
Dorsal recumbent	On back with lower extremities flexed and rotated outward; used in application of obstetric forceps, vaginal and rectal examination, and bimanual palpation
Fowler's	Head of the bed or examining table is raised about 18 inches or 46 cm; patient sitting up with knees also elevated
Knee-chest	On knees, thighs upright, head and upper part of chest resting on bed or examining table, arms crossed and above head; used in sigmoidoscopy, displacement of prolapsed uterus, rectal exams, and flushing of intestinal canal
Lithotomy	On back with lower extremities flexed and feet placed in stirrups; used in vaginal examination, Pap smear, vaginal operations, and diagnosis and treatment of diseases of the urethra and bladder
Orthopneic	Sitting upright or erect; used for patients with dyspnea, shortness of breath (SOB)
Prone	Lying face downward; used in examination of the back, injections, and massage
Sims'	Lying on left side, right knee and thigh flexed well up above left leg that is slightly flexed, left arm behind the body, and right arm forward, flexed at elbow; used in examination of rectum, sigmoidoscopy, enema, and intrauterine irrigation after labor
Supine	Lying flat on back with face upward and arms at the sides; used in examining the head, neck, chest, abdomen, and extremities and in assessing vital signs
Trendelenburg	Body supine on a bed or examining table that is tilted at about 45° angle with the head lower than the feet; used to displace abdominal organs during surgery and in treating cardiovascular shock; also called the *shock position*

BODY CAVITIES

The body's vital organs are contained in cavities. The cranial cavity houses the brain. The spinal cord is located within the spinal cavity. The chest, or thoracic, cavity holds the lungs and heart. Under the diaphragm, the abdominopelvic cavity holds other vital organs including the intestines, stomach, reproductive organs, bladder, and liver. See Figure 4-5 to view the body cavities.

When referring to the abdominopelvic cavity, the medical assistant designates nine regions. The umbilical region describes the area where the umbilicus, or navel, is found. Above it is the epigastric region, and below it is the hypogastric region. To the left of these regions are the left hypochondriac, left lumbar, and left inguinal or iliac regions. To the right are the right hypochondriac, right lumbar, and right inguinal or iliac regions. These terms might be used when referring to where the medical assistant must prepare the patient's skin for a surgical procedure.

A patient may complain of pain coming from an organ that he or she feels may be injured; however, the pain may actually be coming from an entirely separate organ. For example, the patient might say "My stomach hurts." However the pain felt in that area might be from the spleen or

pancreas rather than the stomach. For that reason, the medical assistant refers to the four quadrants of the abdomen when describing this type of pain. These four quadrants are more generalized than the nine regions of the abdominopelvic cavity. In the preceding example, the medical assistant should document the pain as "left upper quadrant" pain. See Figure 4-6 for more information about the quadrants.

Body Structure and Function

When studying **anatomy**, which describes the structure of the body, and **physiology**, which describes the functions and processes of the body, it is important to understand that the body is divided into organ systems. Each organ system has a specific role in the body function but may interact with other systems to carry out the role. The anatomy and physiology of organ systems are further discussed in Chapters 21–33. Here, terminology related to those body systems is presented by body system. See Figure 4-7 for an illustration of the organs of the body and their functions.

INTEGUMENTARY SYSTEM

The integumentary system includes the largest organ of the body: the skin. The integument includes hair, oil, nails, sweat glands, fat cells, and other tissues that aid in protection, exchange of heat and fluids, and absorption. The combining forms for the skin are derm/o, dermat/o, and cutan/o. Thus, a physician who specializes in the skin is a dermatologist, who studied dermatology in depth. Placing medication into the layers of the skin is known as intradermal (ID), and placing medication under the skin is referred to as subcutaneous. Inflammation of the skin is known as dermatitis. See Table 4-10 for medical word parts related to the integumentary system.

SKELETAL SYSTEM

The skeletal system consists of bones that are used to store minerals, to give the body height and movement, and to protect and support the body organs. The combining form for bone is oste/o. A joint forms where two bones meet. Since the combining form for joint is arthr/o, inflammation of the bones and joints is called osteoarthritis. Orth/o is the combining form for straight. Ped/o is the combining form for foot. A physician specializing in (straightening) bones is an orthopedist. A specialist in arthritis, including rheumatoid arthritis, is a rheumatologist. A common abbreviation used in

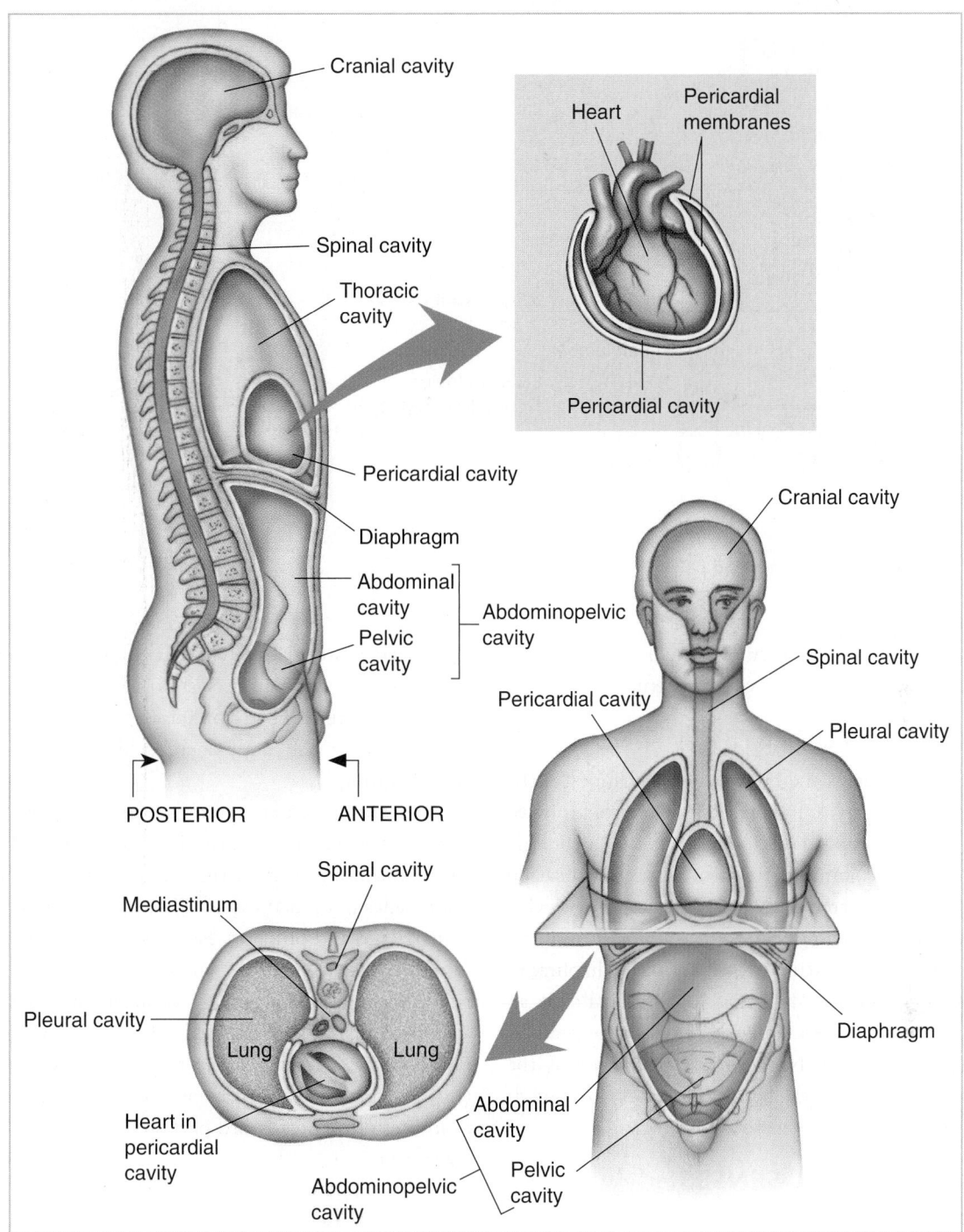

FIGURE 4-5 **Body cavities.**

relation to the skeletal system is *fx* for the word *fracture.* Table 4-11 lists medical word parts related to the skeletal system.

MUSCULAR SYSTEM

Muscles aid bones in movement. The combining forms for muscles are muscul/o and my/o. Thus, injecting medication into a muscle is known as an intramuscular (IM) injection. Fascia surrounds muscles. Inflammation of the fascia is termed fasciitis. The heart is also a muscle; thus, the death of a heart muscle is a myocardial infarction.

A medical assistant or physician may perform range-of-motion (ROM) activities to assess a muscle's ability to

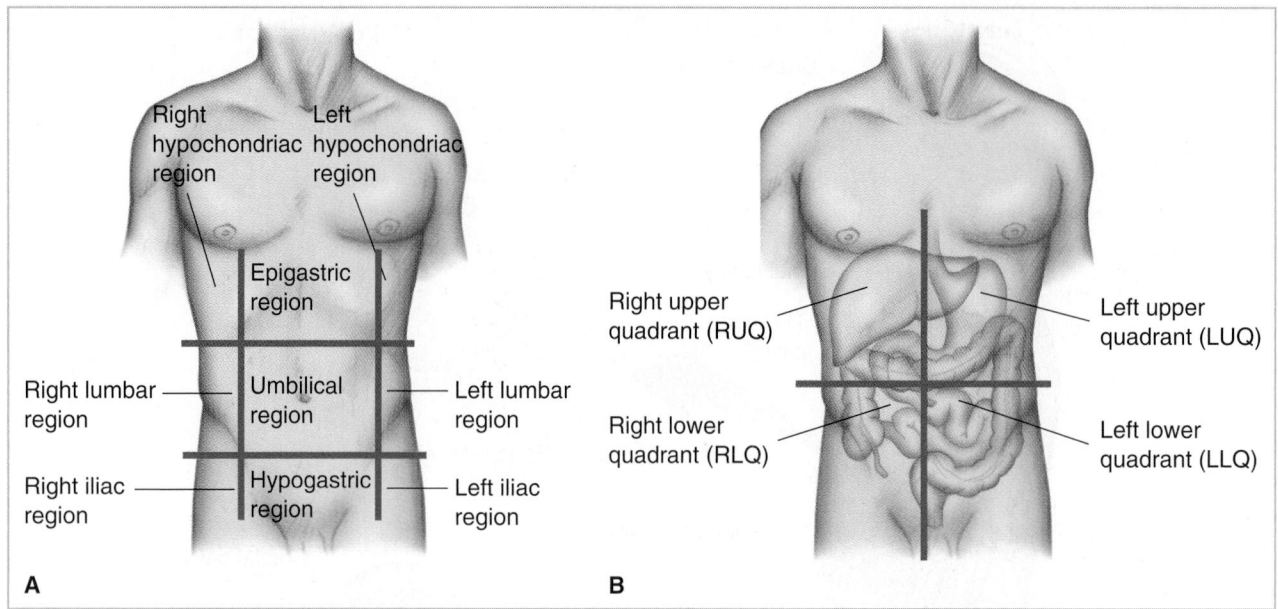

FIGURE 4-6 Regions of the abdomen and pelvis.

extend, flex, or rotate as necessary. See Table 4-12 for medical word parts related to the muscular system.

NERVOUS SYSTEM

The nervous system helps the body to sense changes in the external and internal environments. Pain is referred to with the suffixes –algia and –dynia. For example, arthralgia would be pain in the joint. A frequently used medication that reduces pain is referred to as an analgesic. This word is a combination of *a* (meaning "without") + *algia* (meaning "pain") + *ic* (meaning "relating to"). Pain in the diaphragm is known as phrenodynia. The brain, or encephal/o, is an organ of the nervous system. Inflammation of the brain is referred to as encephalitis. Notice how *cephal/o* means the "head," and *encephal/o* is "in the head." Table 4-13 lists medical word parts related to the nervous system.

SPECIAL SENSES

Special senses include vision, hearing, taste, touch, and smell. The combining forms for eye are ocul/o, ophthalm/o, and optic/o. Ophthalmologists and optometrists are health care providers who specialize in the care of the eye. The combining forms for the ear are ot/o and audi/o.

Audiometry measures the acuity of hearing. Gustatory means taste, and olfactory means smell. See Table 4-14 for medical word parts related to the special senses.

CIRCULATORY SYSTEM

The circulatory system consists of the heart, the blood vessels, the blood, and the structures that make up the lymphatic system. The lymphatic system, which is a subsystem of the circulatory system, acts as the body's transportation system. The lymphatic system is also responsible for defending the body against disease-causing agents, called pathogens.

The cardiovascular system is a subsystem of the circulatory system and is comprised of the heart and its vessels. The combining form for the heart is cardi/o. There are two main types of blood vessels. They are arteries (arteri/o) and veins (ven/o and phleb/o). Fatty plaque in the arteries is referred to as ather/o. A narrowing of an artery is arteriostenosis. The clogging of an artery by fatty plaques is atherosclerosis. The drawing of blood from the vein is phlebotomy. Entering a vein to place a catheter or medication is referred to as intravenous (IV). Table 4-15 provides examples of medical word parts related to the cardiovascular system.

IMMUNE SYSTEM

The immune system protects the body from disease. Cells in the immune system are sometimes named for their color or the color they become when stained. White blood cells (leukocytes) defend the body. The suffix –*phil* means "to love." Eosinophils "love" or turn pink when stained, whereas basophils "love" or turn blue. Neutrophils do not change color when stained; they might be said to be neutral in their "love" of colors. Macrophages (*phag/o* means "to eat") are cells that eat invader cells. Cells that are contained in the thymus are referred to as T-cells, and those defensive cells

Organ System	Major Functions

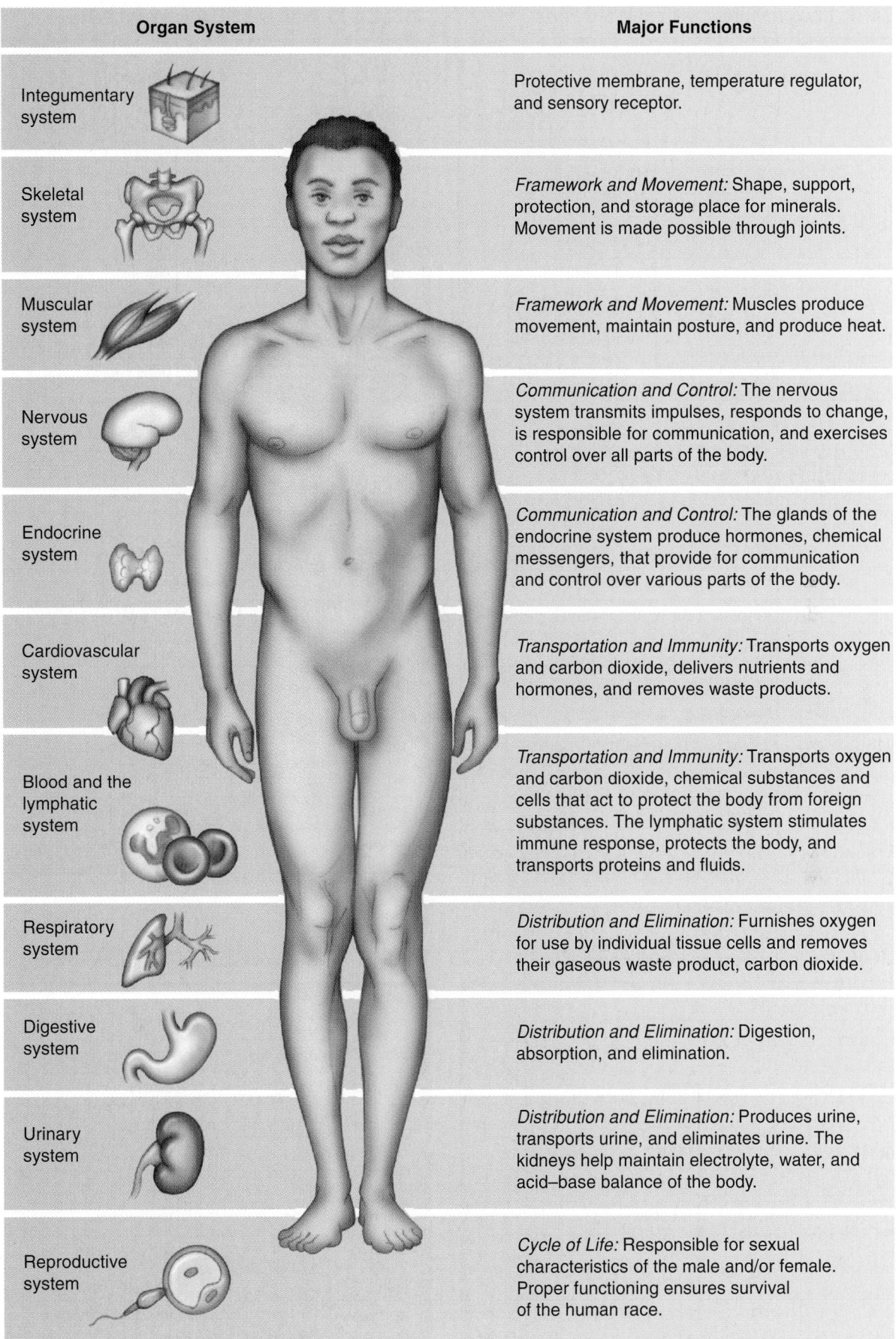

Integumentary system
Protective membrane, temperature regulator, and sensory receptor.

Skeletal system
Framework and Movement: Shape, support, protection, and storage place for minerals. Movement is made possible through joints.

Muscular system
Framework and Movement: Muscles produce movement, maintain posture, and produce heat.

Nervous system
Communication and Control: The nervous system transmits impulses, responds to change, is responsible for communication, and exercises control over all parts of the body.

Endocrine system
Communication and Control: The glands of the endocrine system produce hormones, chemical messengers, that provide for communication and control over various parts of the body.

Cardiovascular system
Transportation and Immunity: Transports oxygen and carbon dioxide, delivers nutrients and hormones, and removes waste products.

Blood and the lymphatic system
Transportation and Immunity: Transports oxygen and carbon dioxide, chemical substances and cells that act to protect the body from foreign substances. The lymphatic system stimulates immune response, protects the body, and transports proteins and fluids.

Respiratory system
Distribution and Elimination: Furnishes oxygen for use by individual tissue cells and removes their gaseous waste product, carbon dioxide.

Digestive system
Distribution and Elimination: Digestion, absorption, and elimination.

Urinary system
Distribution and Elimination: Produces urine, transports urine, and eliminates urine. The kidneys help maintain electrolyte, water, and acid–base balance of the body.

Reproductive system
Cycle of Life: Responsible for sexual characteristics of the male and/or female. Proper functioning ensures survival of the human race.

FIGURE 4-7 Organ systems of the body and their major functions.

TABLE 4-10 Integumentary System Word Parts

dermat/o, derm/o, cutane/o	skin
trich/o	hair
onycho/o	nail
adip/o	fatty deposits
seb/o	oily
epi-	upon, above
kerat/o	hard or horny
melan/o	black, extremely dark
-cyst	fluid-filled sac
ex-, ec-	out of

TABLE 4-13 Nervous System Word Parts

neur/o	nerve
-algia, -dynia	pain
-ethesia	feeling
mot/o	movement
astr/o	star
olig/o	scant
micr/o	small
-ase, -lysis	to break down
arachn/o	spider
dur/o	hard

TABLE 4-11 Skeletal System Word Parts

oste/o	bone
-clast	breaking
-blast	immature stage of cell development
arthr/o	joint
ab-	away from
ad-	toward
circum-	around
cost/o	ribs
-por/o	porous
-malacia	softening

TABLE 4-14 Special Senses Word Parts

ocul/o	eye
ophthalm/o	eye
opt/o	eye
ot/o	ear
gloss/o	tongue
gust/o	taste
olfact/o	smell
aqu/o	water
medi/o	middle
lingu/o	tongue

TABLE 4-12 Muscular System Word Parts

bi-	two
tri-	three
quad-	four
delt/o	triangular
maxim/o	large
vast/o	large
my/o	muscle
-trophy	growth
dys-	bad, painful
tax/o	coordination

TABLE 4-15 Cardiovascular System Word Parts

cardi/o	heart
vas/o	vessel
arteri/o	artery
ven/o	vein
phleb/o	vein
necr/o	death
-stenosis	narrowing
ather/o	fatty plaque
rhythm/o	heartbeat
congest/o	filled with fluid

TABLE 4-16 Immune System Word Parts

-cyte	cell
leuk/o	white
eosin/o	rosy pink
bas/o	blue
neutr/o	neutral, absorbs no color when stained
macro-	large
micro-	small
-phage	destroyer, eater
bacteri/o	bacteria
myc/o	fungus

TABLE 4-17 Respiratory System Word Parts

pulmon/o	lungs
pneum/o	air, lungs
pharyng/o	throat
oxyg/o, ox/o, ox/i	oxygen
capn/o	carbon dioxide
-pnea	breath
orth/o	straight
-thorax	chest
py/o	pus, infected material
spir/o	to breathe

that circulate are called CD cells. See Table 4-16 for more medical word parts related to the immune system.

RESPIRATORY SYSTEM

The respiratory system exchanges oxygen (O_2) in the environment for carbon dioxide (CO_2) in the body. The main organs of respiration are the lungs (pulmon/o). A specialist in the respiratory system is a pulmonologist. *Pneum/o* means "air" or "lungs" and is frequently used in referring to the respiratory system. *Pneumon/o* is a combining form that means "lung." For example, an infection of the lungs is pneumonia. Table 4-17 lists medical word parts related to the respiratory system.

DIGESTIVE SYSTEM

The digestive system either absorbs or rejects food and drugs for the body. It starts in the mouth (stom/o or stomat/o) and goes to the rectum (rect/o). The oral cavity is another term

for the mouth. Medically given through the mouth *per os* (po). Key organs of this system are stomach (gastr/o) and intestines (enter/o). Thus a physician with specialized training in the digestive system is a gastroenterologist. See Table 4-18 for medical word parts related to the digestive system.

URINARY SYSTEM

The urinary system rids the body of the toxic byproducts of metabolism. The combining form for the kidney is nephr/o, so a physician with specialized training related to the kidney is a nephrologist. Another combining form for kidney is ren/o, as in renal failure. Urine goes from the kidneys to the ureters, to the bladder, and out through the urethra. Careful attention must be paid to the spelling of two of the organs of this system. The ureters (uret/o) go toward the bladder (cyst/o), and the urethra (urethr/o) goes toward the outside of the body. A urologist is a physician with specialized training

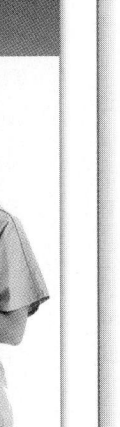

PROFESSIONALISM
THE WORKPLACE

Although abbreviations may save time in writing, they are frequently a source of misunderstandings in the workplace. Unless a list of approved abbreviations is established for the office, expand writing whenever possible.

TABLE 4-18 Digestive System Word Parts

stomat/o, stom/o, or/o	mouth
gastr/o	stomach
enter/o	intestines
col/o	colon
appendic/o, append/o	appendix
aliment/o	digestion
dent/o	teeth
retro-	behind
sigm/o	s-shaped
cholecyst/o	gallbladder

TABLE 4-19 Urinary System Word Parts

ur/o, urin/o	urinary
hemat/o	blood
poly-	many, much
oligo-	scanty amounts
protein-	protein
-dipsia	thirst
nephr/o	kidney
ren/o	kidney
cyst/o	bladder
ureter/o	ureter
urethr/o	urethra

TABLE 4-20 Endocrine System Word Parts

endo-	within
exo-	without
-crine	to secrete
somat/o	body
andr/o	man
estr/o	woman
gest/o	pregnancy
-stasis	stable
lact/o	milk
gonad/o	sexual organs

not only in the urinary system but also in the male reproductive system. A test used to analyze the content of urine to assess urinary function is urinalysis (U/A). Table 4-19 lists medical word parts related to the urinary system.

ENDOCRINE SYSTEM

The endocrine system is the ductless glandular system that controls other body systems by secreting hormones within the bloodstream. *Endo-* means "within" and *–crine* means "to secrete." Hormones used in the body are endocrine hormones. For example, follicle-stimulating hormone (FSH) stimulates ovaries to develop and release an ovum and the testes to develop sperm. Testosterone works in the testes of the male to create secondary sexual characteristics. The pituitary is the master gland of this system, and it gives its name to a synthetic form of oxytocin (pitocin), which is used to stimulate labor in women. See Table 4-20 for medical word parts related to the endocrine system.

REPRODUCTIVE SYSTEM

The reproductive system aids in reproducing offspring. The physician with specialized training in women's health is a gynecologist. The combining forms for the uterus are *metr/o* and *hyster/o*. The removal of a uterus is a hysterectomy. If it includes the ovaries, it is an oophorohysterectomy. The tying of fallopian tubes is a bilateral (two sides) tubal ligation (tying), or BTL. When the vessels (vas deferens) that conduct sperm through ejaculation are cut, it is referred to as a vasectomy. A common abbreviation related to the male reproductive system is benign (not cancerous) prostatic (pertaining to the prostate) hyperplasia (overgrowth of tissue),

or BPH. See Table 4-21 for some medical word parts relating to the reproductive system.

Surgical and Diagnostic Terms

Surgical terms are usually created by adding suffixes to a medical term to clearly define the surgery. For example, if a trachea is removed, it is a tracheotomy. If, instead, an opening (or mouth) is placed temporarily into the trachea, it is a tracheostomy. *Cis/o* is the combining form for "to cut." Thus, scissors cut. *Excision* means "to cut out or remove." *Incision* means to "cut into."

TABLE 4-21 Reproductive System Word Parts

gynec/o	female, woman
mamm/o	breast
mast/o	breast
oophor/o	ovary
metr/o	uterus
hyster/o	uterus
labi/o	lip
cervic/o	neck
balan/o	penis
orchid/o	testis
test/o	testis
testic/o	testis
crypt-	hidden

Diagnostic terms are used when a physician is trying to determine or diagnose what caused a disease. For example, an exploratory laparoscopy could be used to look into the abdomen to determine what might be wrong. A biopsy (the process of looking at life) is used to look at cells, perhaps to find if they are cancerous. Most surgical and diagnostic terms end with the letter y, which signifies a process.

An electrocardiogram is the written record of the electrical activity of the heart. However, the electrocardiograph is the instrument used to obtain the study. The process of recording the written record of the heart's electrical activity is electrocardiography. See Table 4-22 for medical word parts relating to surgical and diagnostic terms.

TABLE 4-22 Surgical and Diagnostic Word Parts

-graphy	to make a written record
-scopy	to observe
-analysis	to assess various parts
-tome	instrument to cut
-scope	instrument to view
-scopy	process of viewing
-stomy	to create an opening
-tomy	to cut into temporarily
-ectomy	to remove

SUMMARY

Words are made up of word elements. Word roots usually add a vowel before adding prefixes on the front and suffixes on the back of the word part, rendering a new word. Correct spelling is important in the practice of medical assisting because poor spelling reflects poor care and lack of professionalism. Wrong spelling also can infer a different word. Plurals are sometimes formed according to Latin rules, not always according to English rules, of grammar. To describe the body planes, directions, and positions, a medical vocabulary must be developed. The study of the structures and functions of the body is known as anatomy and physiology. The organs of the body are divided into body systems. Each system has its own organs and responsibilities, although they work together for the good of the body. Although medical terminology is often a challenge for the medical assistant, learning this language of medicine is crucial in this profession.

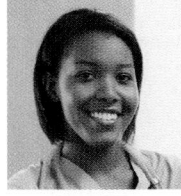

4 CHAPTER REVIEW

COMPETENCY REVIEW

1. Define and spell the terms to learn for this chapter.

2. Discuss how medical words are formed.

3. Label the word parts in *endoscopy*.

PREPARING FOR THE CERTIFICATION EXAM

1. Which of the following is a combining form?
   a. hyper-
   b. –emia
   c. glyc
   d. glyc/o
   e. lip

2. Which of the following is the combining form for the mouth?
   a. gastr/o
   b. enter/o
   c. stomat/o
   d. audi/o
   e. ot/o

3. Which of the following physicians specializes in male reproductive functions?
   a. gynecologist
   b. gastroenterologist
   c. dermatologist
   d. endocrinologist
   e. urologist

4. Which of the following is a combining form for bone?
   a. ophthalm/o
   b. ot/o
   c. oste/o
   d. arthr/o
   e. ather/o

5. Which of the following is the combining form for fatty plaque in blood vessels?
   a. phleb/o
   b. vas/o
   c. arthr/o
   d. arteri/o
   e. ather/o

6. In which position should a patient in cardiogenic shock be placed?
   a. lithotomy
   b. Trendelenburg
   c. Fowler's
   d. semi-Fowler's
   e. knee-chest

7. Which body system is responsible for using hormones for internal communication?
   a. reproductive
   b. cardiovascular
   c. gastrointestinal
   d. integumentary
   e. endocrine

8. Which word means "under the skin?"
   a. intravenous
   b. intradermal
   c. intramuscular
   d. subcutaneous
   e. oral

9. Which word means "in front of" or "before"?
   a. cephalic
   b. distal
   c. medial
   d. lateral
   e. anterior

10. The word part -algia means:
    a. enzyme.
    b. bacteria.
    c. hormone.
    d. pain.
    e. medication.

CRITICAL THINKING

1. Where is the epigastric region?

2. If Dr. McWalter ordered a test that required the patient to be supine, how would you position the patient?

3. Visualize the imaginary lines dividing the abdomen into quadrants. In which quadrant would Mr. Schultz's pain be localized?

ON THE JOB

George Tomlin RMA has been working for several years in a specialty practice. He applies for a position closer to his home with better hours and more pay. This office, however, sees patients with a variety of illnesses. For the first time since he graduated from college, he is encountering words and procedures with which he is not familiar.

1. What would be the best way for George to review his basic medical terminology?
2. What should George do when he encounters a new word?
3. What are some good ways for him to learn the new vocabulary for his new position?

INTERNET ACTIVITY

Conduct a search of medical terminology sites. Decide which ones you would go to if you needed to define words.

MEDMEDIA

Additional interactive resources and activities for this chapter can be found:

On your student DVD: View applicable procedure videos on the DVD-ROM found in the back of this book.

MyHealthProfessionsKit.com: Test your knowledge of the chapter with games and activities. MyHealthProfessionsKit also includes resources, helpful links, and a Spanish audio glossary.

Medical Assisting Interactive: Practice your procedures as a medical assistant in this simulated doctor's office. This can be accessed through MyHealthProfessionsKit.com.

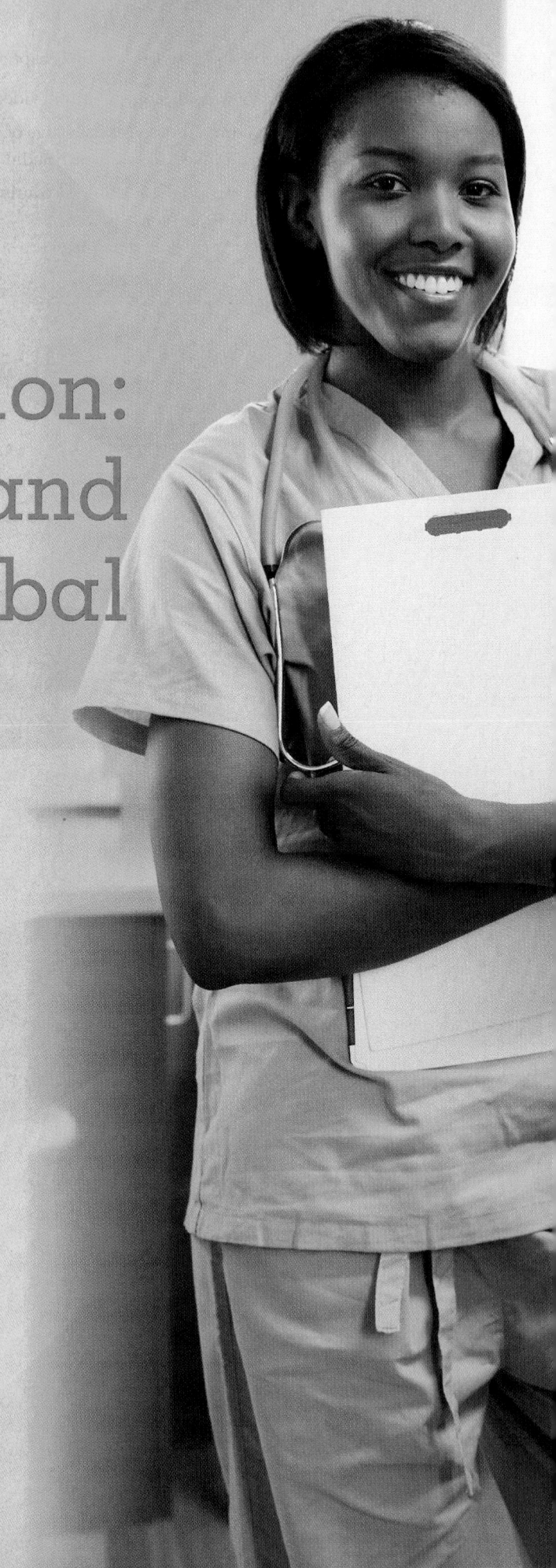

5

Communication: Verbal and Nonverbal

LEARNING OBJECTIVES

After reading this chapter, you should be able to:

- Define and spell the terms to learn for this chapter.

- Explain the importance of communication in health care today.

- Define the terms *values*, *attitudes*, and *behavior*, and explain their roles in self-awareness.

- Compare and contrast verbal and nonverbal communication.

- List five examples of nonverbal communication conveying impatience.

- List six guidelines for effective listening.

- Explain the importance of feedback in patient care.

- Describe the difference between assertive and aggressive behavior.

- List six types of defensive behavior, giving an example of each.

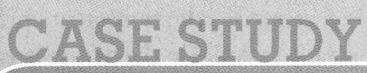

CHAPTER OUTLINE

CASE STUDY

Yun-qi Yeung, 65 years old, is returning to the medical office to receive the results of a biopsy for prostate cancer screening. Mr. Yeung speaks very little English and is usually accompanied by his son, Lou, for interpretation assistance. Today, Lou informs the front desk receptionist that his father is very apprehensive about receiving the results of the biopsy. Later, while in the physician's office, Mr. Yeung and his son find out that the biopsy was positive for the early stages of prostate cancer.

CERTIFICATION LINK

CMA (AAMA)
Communication
- Adapting communication according to an individual's needs
- Recognizing and responding to verbal and nonverbal communication
- Professional communication and behavior
- Patient interviewing techniques

RMA
Human relations
Patient education

CMAS (AMT)
Medical office
Clerical assisting
  Communication
  Patient information and community resources
Medical office management
Office communications

Communication is a necessary requirement in any field but is particularly essential in the health care field. As a medical assistant, you will relate to a variety of people, including sick and worried patients, your physician-employer, fellow staff members, vendors, and even some personal acquaintances of the physician. Some individuals you will interact with will be angry, frustrated, or simply ill and tired. Many patients who come into the physician's office or clinic will have physical or emotional problems that are not the main reason for their appointment. In addition, given the widely diverse population in the United States, you will encounter people from a variety of countries and cultures. The medical assistant must be able to care for the entire patient in a holistic fashion and treat everyone with respect and courtesy. **Holistic** medicine focuses on the whole patient and addresses the social, emotional, and spiritual needs, as well as the physical treatment of the patient.

It is not enough for the medical assistant to have excellent technical skills. Good interpersonal skills as well as good oral and written communication skills are needed to relate well to patients and fellow staff. In this chapter, you will learn about self-awareness and interpersonal dynamics. You will study the communication process, including directive techniques to improve effective communication, barriers to good communication, and defensive behaviors. Examining multicultural issues, communicating in special circumstances, and communicating with special needs patients will help you to be prepared for various situations you may encounter. Communication in the workplace, working as a member of a team, and understanding some conflict resolution strategies will help in your day-to-day work environment.

Interpersonal Dynamics

For the medical assistant to be able to provide effective communication in the delivery of health care, he or she must have a basic understanding of self. Why do you have the personality you exhibit? How do you communicate in everyday situations? Where do the impressions of others you hold originate? In other words, how did you get to be the person you are today? We will examine some concepts related to individuality and relationships with others.

SELF-AWARENESS

Understanding oneself and understanding the differences among others helps the medical assistant communicate more effectively. Personality is a sum of the traits, characteristics, and behaviors that make us individuals. We all recognize different personalities, even among close family members. **Character** is the sum of the values, attitudes, and behaviors a person exhibits. Psychologists tell us that **values** are a set of standards a person uses to measure the worth or importance of someone or something. **Attitudes** are opinions that develop from our value system. Values are acquired at home, in our family unit, in the culture we live in and often are difficult to change. **Prejudice** is a preformed and unfavorable belief or attitude toward a certain culture or group with little or no information about the culture or group. It is learned from experience and environment and impacts our actions towards and responses to others. An example of prejudice is viewing individuals with different skin color as inferior. **Behavior,** the actions others see, is based on our attitudes. To summarize, values form attitudes, and attitudes are reflected in behavior or actions that can be seen by others. Society prefers some behaviors and disapproves of others. For example, in the United States we are not permitted to have more than one spouse. In other cultures, this is perfectly acceptable.

To be an effective communicator in all areas of our lives, it is important to look at our attitudes and our prejudices. How do others see us? How do we see ourselves? Examining ourselves leads to greater self-awareness and can lead to better communication skills. Patients and coworkers expect certain attitudes and professional behaviors to be displayed in the health care setting.

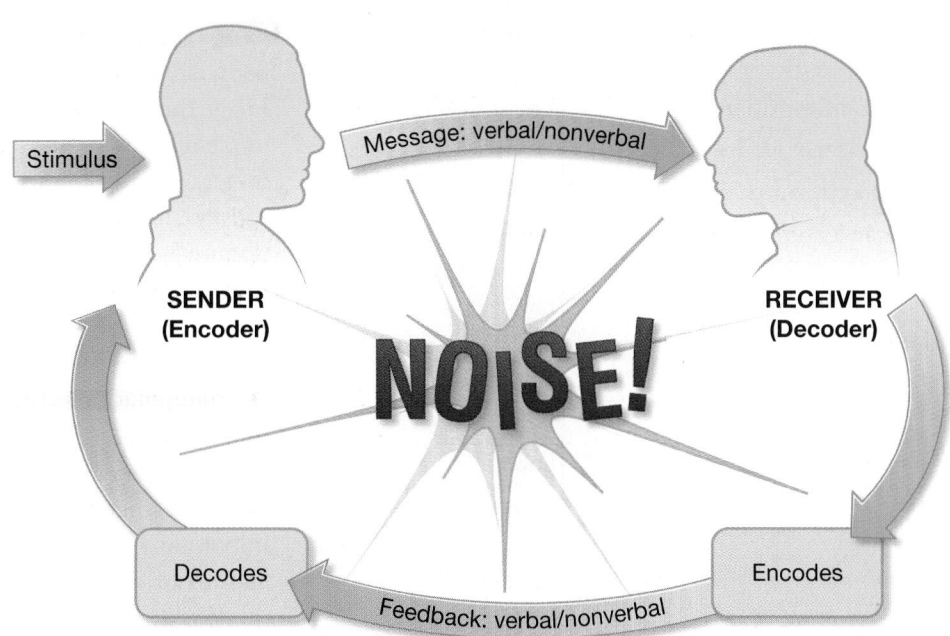

FIGURE 5-1 **After face-to-face discussion, telephone conversations are probably the most frequently used channel of communication.**

LEARNING STYLES

Examining the various styles of learning will increase our self-awareness. The three types of learning styles are auditory, visual, and kinesthetic. Most of us learn by using a combination of these styles, with one style tending to be more dominant. The auditory (by hearing) learner is one who retains information better by hearing lectures or listening to music and tapes. People who are auditory learners have difficulty retaining information presented in written format. The visual (by seeing) learner, as you would expect, learns better by seeing the information, by means of reading, drawings, diagrams, and films. Visual learners find it more difficult to follow lectures unless visual aids are used with the presentation. The kinesthetic (involving movement) learner assimilates knowledge better through hands-on activities, such as experiments, games, lab exercises, and movement. Such people have difficulty grasping a procedure until they have performed it themselves. Understanding these learning styles will help prepare you for your role as patient educator.

The Communication Process

The basic units of the communication process are the source, message, channel, and receiver. Think of this as the acronym SMCR:

S stands for the sender of the communication. Who is sending the message?

M represents the actual message. This could represent written or spoken words, as well as behavior.

C indicates the channel or channels through which the message moves from the source to the receiver. These channels include the senses: sight, smell, taste, hearing, and touch. Another set of channels consists of pathways such as the telephone or interoffice mail.

R stands for the receiver of the message.

For example, a physician (S) writes a prescription (M) that the medical assistant then reads over the telephone (C) to the pharmacist (R). If any link in this chain is broken, an incorrect message is relayed. The same holds true if you relay a message to a patient. If the medical assistant (S) explains a procedure (M) to a patient who has a hearing loss (C), then the patient (R) will not hear the message as it was intended.

The communication process, then, is a chain effect that requires a source (S) and a receiver (R). The source (S) acts on a stimulus to encode or transmit a message (M) in a particular form. The actual message can be transmitted in a variety of ways (C), including face to face, over the telephone, or in written form. The receiver (R) decodes or translates the message, based on his or her emotional state, perceptions, education, socioeconomic background, and many other factors.

CHANNELS OF COMMUNICATION

Channels of communication include the various means by which the spoken or written word is communicated from one person to another. Information is said to be "rich" if it conveys to the listener or reader the intent of the speaker. The "richest" information is gained from face-to-face discussion (Figure 5-1). The least amount of information is generally

TABLE 5-1 Information Richness Channels

Information Channel	Level of Richness
Face-to-face discussion	Highest
Telephone conversations	High
Written letter/memos (individually addressed)	Moderate
Formal written documents (general bulletins or reports)	Low
Fax (facsimile)	Low
E-mail	Low
Internet	Low
Formal numeric document (printouts, budget reports)	Lowest

gained from formal numeric documents, such as budget reports. When you wish to convey an important message to someone, it is better to do it face to face than to put the information into writing. This becomes important to remember when determining how to adequately educate patients regarding their medications. If you place all the important facts into a pamphlet, patients may never read it or might not understand your meaning. You must consider the learning styles discussed previously and the fact that using a variety of styles better reinforces the message. However, it is important to give written instructions in addition to any verbal explanation you give the patient. Table 5-1 illustrates the varying degrees of "richness" of various information channels.

Verbal and Nonverbal Communication

Virtually everything a person does from birth to death is a form of communication. Smiling is a form of nonverbal communication, whereas talking "with a smile in your voice" is verbal communication. **Nonverbal communica-** tion is the language of gestures and actions, which includes body language. In many cases, people are not aware of the image they are projecting with their bodies. The way a person holds his or her arms, makes eye contact, gestures, frowns, or turns toward or away from the speaker frequently conveys much more than just mere words could convey (Figure 5-2). Box 5-1 offers some examples of messages that convey impatience.

VERBAL COMMUNICATION

Verbal communication is based on words, sounds, and tone of voice. The sounds a person makes when speaking cover a wide range and can convey vastly different meanings. The tone in which you speak to a patient is vitally important in making a positive impression on the patient and his or her family. Generally, when someone is speaking, that person will raise his or her tone at the end of a statement when asking a question and drop the tone of voice when completing a sentence. When the speaker's tone drops, it is appropriate to begin your part of the conversation. Interrupting speakers is a negative behavior that creates a barrier to good communication.

The medical assistant should speak loudly enough to be heard but not so loudly that a patient's confidentiality is compromised. Speaking clearly and pronouncing your words properly is very important when conveying the message.

Word Selection

Choosing the right words to present a message is critical. We can all think of instances when we called a medical facility only to have been spoken to as though we were an annoyance to the person at the front desk. Other times, telephoning the medical assistant was a very pleasant experience, and when the conversation was completed, we had a positive feeling. Sarcasm and ridicule have no place in the professional setting. The goal of the medical assistant is to promote an open, comfortable environment for the patient while keeping in mind that the patient is the customer. Choose your words carefully, and take care not to be rude or impatient in your interpersonal relationships.

Box 5-1 Communication Messages Conveying IMPATIENCE

- Interrupting people when they are speaking
- Answering telephone calls curtly
- Finishing another person's sentence
- Rushing the patient
- Eating lunch at your desk
- Looking at your watch or the clock
- Doing two things at once
- Not looking up from your work when someone approaches
- Rushing around the office

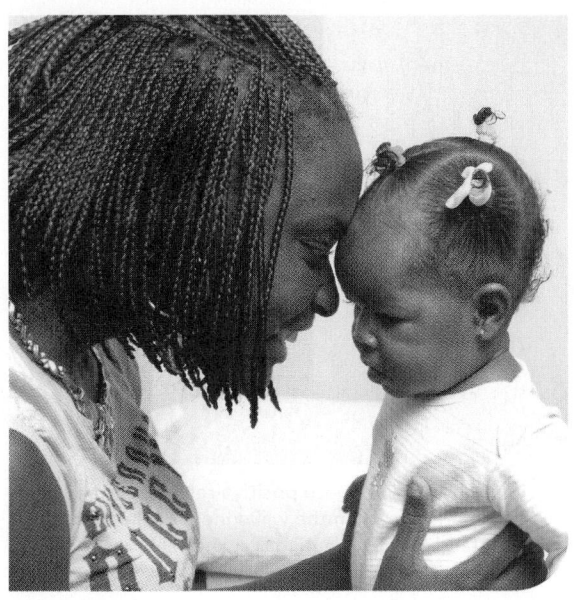
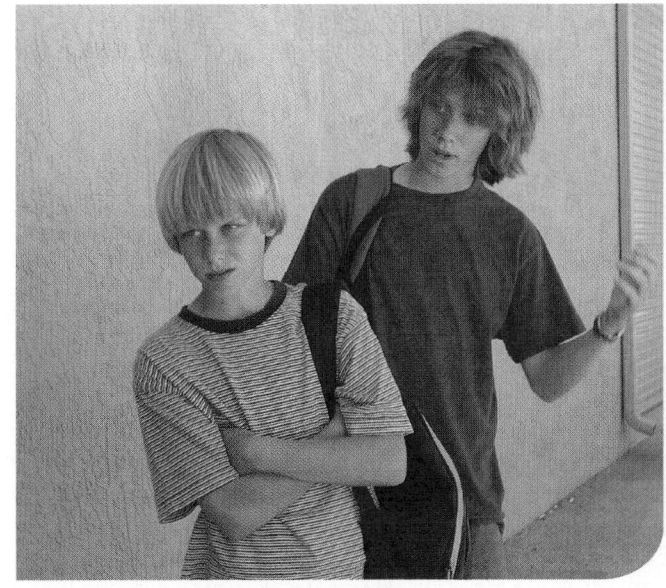
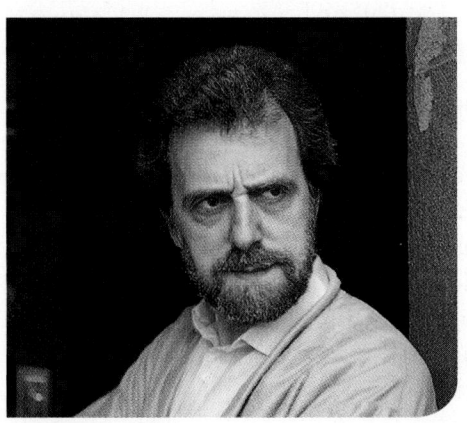
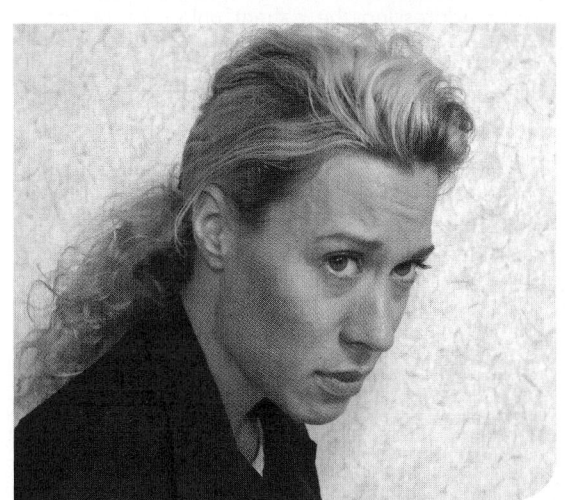

FIGURE 5-2 Nonverbal communications convey strong, powerful messages that may be negative or positive.

Positive Attitude

The ability to verbally convey a positive attitude is very important when working with people. When in the presence of a patient, always involve the patient in your conversation. Excluding the patient and talking in a manner incomprehensible to the patient "over his or her head" is disrespectful (Figure 5-3). If the conversation is of a business or confidential nature, it should be held elsewhere.

Effective medical assistants are able to demonstrate empathy but should be cautious about exhibiting sympathy for their patients. **Empathy** is the willingness or the ability to understand what the patient is feeling without necessarily experiencing the same thing. **Sympathy**, on the other hand, is feeling sorry for or pitying the patient. Patients react much better to an empathetic listener than to a sympathetic one. You can acquire the skill of empathetic listening by using some simple nonverbal techniques: nodding, leaning toward the patient, positioning yourself so you are at the patient's eye level, and indicating by your facial expression that you understand what he or she is saying (Figure 5-4).

Since we all share human emotions, at times you will become distressed over a patient's situation. It is not possible to be a concerned health care provider and remain totally unemotional at all times. If you become upset, you can excuse yourself for a few moments. Realize that your emotions and concerns are another indication that you have chosen the correct field.

NONVERBAL COMMUNICATION

Nonverbal communication involves facial expressions, gestures, body language, eye contact, good grooming, and mannerisms. It is important that verbal and nonverbal messages

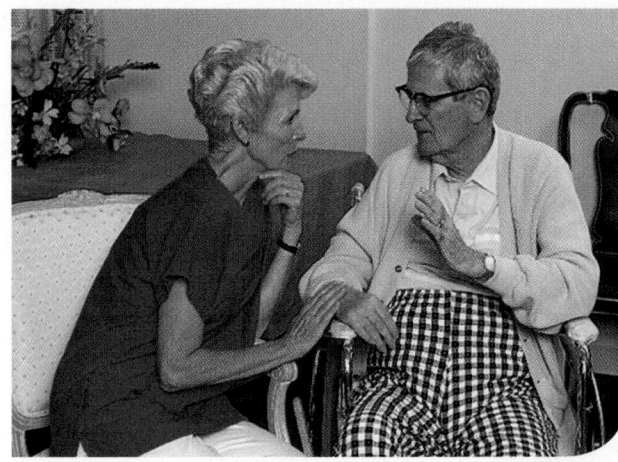
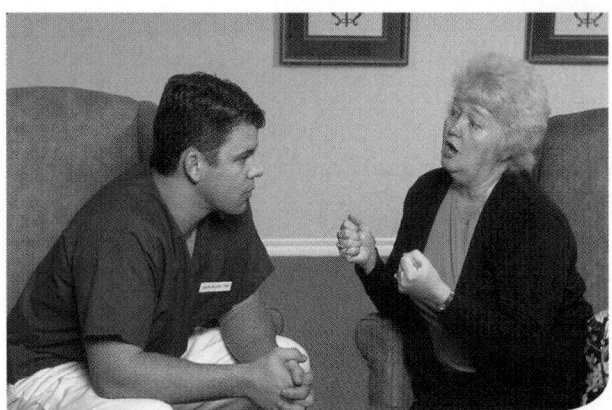

FIGURE 5-4 Empathy draws a more positive response from the patient because it is based on the willingness of the medical assistant to understand what the patient is experiencing.

match. Body language is learned through imitation, by being taught, and by instinct. Appearance is a nonverbal form of communication. Patients expect certain types of behaviors, attitudes, and appearance in the health care setting. Unprofessional attire, visible tattoos, and overpowering perfume can send a negative message.

The gesture of touch is considered a form of nonverbal communication and a form of body language. Gently touching a distraught patient's arm can provide reassurance and comfort. However, one must be cautious that the receiver does not misinterpret a touch. In some cultures, for instance, it is considered rude to touch a child's head without permission. At times, abused children can be fearful of even inno-

cent touching. Use caution when touching a patient unless you know him or her well.

Communication Techniques

The ability to encourage a patient to communicate effectively is critical when you wish to perform a patient assessment or evaluation to determine the patient's problems. For example, how can you stop a patient who is talking about seemingly irrelevant issues? Each communication experience has unique qualities and must be considered carefully. Before we discuss specific techniques, we need to consider several questions as we examine the overall communication process:

- What is the goal of your communication?
- What message do you want to give?
- Through what channel are you going to deliver (face to face, written, etc.)?
- How will you listen to the response (listening and observational skills)?
- How will you get clarification and feedback?
- Did you meet your goal, or do you need to revise the message (assess or evaluate)?

LISTENING SKILLS

Listening involves verbal and nonverbal cues. The medical assistant must pay attention to both. Listening is either active or passive. Active listening involves paying attention completely to the speaker, concentrating on the verbal message, watching for nonverbal cues, and offering a response. At times, it is difficult in a medical office to actively listen when so much is happening at once. One skill you will gain with experience is the

FIGURE 5-3 It is important to act concerned when a patient is upset.

ability to prioritize simultaneous events. **Passive listening** is listening to someone without having to reply, such as when you are listening as a member of an audience.

How we hear a message is often colored by the message being delivered. If it is criticism of your work and you disagree, you hear it one way. If it is praise for your work, you hear it another way. Sometimes we begin formulating a response before the speaker is finished with his or her message. In either circumstance, the listener's mind or thoughts may wander, the message may be delivered ineffectively, or it may be distorted. Part of effective listening is allowing enough time for the message to be completed and knowing when it is your turn to speak. With practice we can all become good listeners. Procedure 5-1 provides steps to practice effective listening skills with fellow students and to employ with patients. The following are some additional guidelines for good listening:

- Avoid distractions.
- Face the speaker.
- Give the person your full attention.
- Maintain the type of eye contact that is suitable for the culture of the patient.
- Do not be judgmental about what is said.
- Be aware of nonverbal cues.
- Note anything that seems unclear.
- Do not interrupt.

PROFESSIONALISM

As a health care representative, the medical assistant should set a good example. The medical assistant sets the first impression of the office and in many ways is the marketing representative of the practice. The medical assistant must always present a professional appearance. Good personal hygiene and grooming are musts. Nails should be kept according to office policy, and jewelry should be kept to a minimum.

- Maintain personal space.
- Ask questions if you do not understand.

DIRECTIVE COMMUNICATION TECHNIQUES

The medical assistant can often assist the communication process by directing the patient's comments, using specific communication techniques so that the sharing between the patient and the medical assistant is productive.

Types of Questions

Asking questions to deliver a message and to obtain information is a directive technique. The medical assistant will ask many questions of each patient. It is helpful to keep in mind the goal of your question before you choose the type of

procedure 5-1

EFFECTIVE LISTENING SKILLS

Objective: Use effective listening skills to obtain chief complaint from a patient.

EQUIPMENT AND SUPPLIES
Patient History Form

METHOD
1. Identify the patient.
2. Smile and establish eye contact.
3. Seat the patient in an appropriate area.
4. Focus full attention on the patient.
5. Ask the patient the reason for the current appointment.
6. Ask open-ended questions.
7. Do not interrupt the patient.
8. Provide feedback by paraphrasing what the patient says.
9. Observe the patient for signs of needing to give more information.
10. Restate the chief complaint before leaving the patient.
11. Conclude the patient interview in an appropriate manner.
12. Document the chief complaint.

CHARTING EXAMPLE
6/22/XX 4:30 P.M. *cc: gastrointestinal discomfort. Patient states,* "My belly hurts real bad." · · · · Nancy Beaumont CMA (AAMA)

question to ask. Four types of questions are discussed here: close-ended, open-ended, probing, and leading.

Close-ended questions can be answered with a yes or a no. Often these types of questions are appropriate to obtain background information, such as "Is your mother still living?" However, at times you may ask a patient "Do you understand what I mean?" and the patient will answer "Yes" even if he or she does not comprehend what you are saying. Usually this happens because the patient does not want to be bothersome or appear unintelligent. You need to consider the situation carefully when you use close-ended questions.

Open-ended questions are those that require more than yes or no responses. Such questions can be useful in gaining feedback or drawing out patient information. Using open-ended questions or directive methods, you will be able to obtain information that the physician will require to treat the patient. See Table 5-2 for a list of other directive communication techniques, including a description and an example of each technique.

Probing questions are used to ask the patient for further information to more fully discuss the subject. For example, if a patient says, "My head hurts," a probing question would ask, "Where does it hurt?" or "How long have you had this pain?" In this example, other probing questions would seek information about type of pain, when it started, and when it occurs. The medical assistant is often the person the patient feels more comfortable speaking to and questioning. It is important to be empathetic and endeavor to put the patient at ease.

Leading questions are those questions in which part of the answer is in the question. For example, when asked "Do you have to urinate two, three, or four times a night?" the patient then has to select one answer from your choices. This may be helpful in dealing with patients who do not understand English. However, the medical assistant must be careful not to ask a particular leading question in order to get the exact answer he or she desires.

FEEDBACK

Feedback, any response to a communication, is critically important when working with patients since you must determine if they truly understand what was said. Feedback can be either verbal or nonverbal. Sometimes the verbal message and the nonverbal message that patients send do not agree. For instance, as a medical assistant you may ask, "How are you feeling?" and the patient might state, "Fine." Since the patient is walking with a painful limp, you doubt the verbal statement. Always try to ask specific questions (e.g., "Do you have pain?" "Tell me about your medication." or "Tell me why you came in to see the doctor."). When documenting the information that the patient provides, write the patient's words in quotation marks.

TABLE 5-2 Directive Communication Techniques

Technique	Description	Example
Open-ended statement	Encourage the patient to discuss freely.	"Please describe your pain for me."
Closed-ended statement	Direct the patient to make a yes/no or simple response.	"Are you having pain?"
Reflecting	Direct the conversation back to the patient by repeating the patient's words.	Patient: "I'm afraid of what the doctor will find." MA: "You're afraid of what the doctor will find?"
Acknowledgment	Indicate understanding.	"I understand what you are saying."
Restating	State what the patient has said but in different terms.	Patient: "I can't sleep." MA: "You say you're having trouble getting to sleep at night?"
Add to an implied statement	Verbalize implied information.	Patient: "I'm usually relaxed." MA: "And today you're not relaxed?"
Seek clarification	Request more information to better understand.	Patient: "I don't feel good." MA: "Tell me what your symptoms are."
Silence	Remain silent, or make no gesture in response to a statement.	Patient: "I don't know what's wrong, but something is."

Reflecting

Reflecting is a directive technique in which you mirror the patient's message back to the individual to ensure that you have understood him or her correctly. For example, you may say in response to a patient who needs an appointment, "You say you can't come in on Wednesdays?" The reflecting technique is also helpful in resolving conflicts and clearing up confusing statements, and it requires more detail from the other person.

Restating

Restating or paraphrasing is repeating the patient's message to him or her in your own words. For example, "I heard you say that you will not be able to pay your bill this month. Is that correct?" This technique helps to confirm that both parties understand the message clearly.

Clarification

The ultimate goal in effective communication is to deliver the message so that it is understood clearly. Clarification is a directive technique in which the medical assistant requests more information in order to better understand what the patient has stated. Many times patients use words such as *a lot* or *much worse* in explaining their symptoms. It is important to ask them to be more specific in order to accurately diagnose or treat them. For example, the patient says, "My right arm hurts a lot." The medical assistant should employ the directive techniques mentioned to clarify this information. The following questions are examples of follow-up questions and statements useful in this situation:

- "You say that your right arm hurts. Is that correct? Where on your arm do you feel the pain?"
- "What kind of pain is it? When did it start? Does it hurt all the time?"
- "Are you able to sleep?"
- "Are you taking any medications for the pain?"

Assertive versus Aggressive Behavior

Most instances of communication within the work setting involve convincing someone else to cooperate with you. Whether patient or staff communication is your goal, the methods to achieve cooperation are the same. As a medical assistant, at times you will have to convince patients as well as staff members to listen to you. Using assertive behavior techniques can make this easier.

Being assertive means that you make a point in a positive manner by standing firm, making decisions based on your principles or values, and trusting your own ideas or instincts in the situation. On the other hand, being aggressive is trying to impose your point of view on others or trying to manipulate others. Aggressiveness is considered a negative behavior and indicates a type of pushiness when trying to convince others. In fact, it has been compared to making a verbal attack against another. Many people resort to aggressive behavior in order to impose their ideas on others or when they are angry or fearful. Aggressive people tend to be bossy and inconsiderate of the feelings of others.

ASSERTIVE BEHAVIOR TECHNIQUES

Acquiring the ability to use assertive behavior means that you will learn to offer new ideas or even unwanted ideas to people in such a manner that they will not feel threatened. Some assertive behaviors include being direct and honest, using positive body language, and using "I" statements such as "I feel." For instance, when calling a patient regarding non-payment of a bill, you will need to gain the patient's acceptance. The patient may become angry at the beginning of the conversation in response to an aggressive comment, such as "Are you aware that your bill is now two months overdue? When are you going to pay it?" He or she could become defensive and hang up. Since most patients know when they have not paid a bill, it is not necessary to use threatening language. A better approach would be to identify yourself and indicate that you are helping Dr. Thompson with his billings. In a calm but assertive manner, you would ask questions that would prompt a positive response from the patient. These questions might include "How can I help you in clearing up these payments? Perhaps we can discuss your making a small payment on your account twice a month. What would be an amount that you could afford?" Table 5-3 lists comparative examples of aggressive and assertive comments.

Assertive Behavior Guidelines

Assertiveness is a learned skill that helps one to maintain self-confidence under stressful conditions. The basis for assertiveness is that everyone has the right to express opinions or beliefs in an appropriate, respectful manner without fear of being humiliated or made to feel guilty. Aggressiveness results in violation of a person's rights during communication. The results of aggressive behavior are resentment and loss of respect. To practice assertive behavior, use the following steps:

- Take a few deep breaths to calm yourself.
- In unemotional tones, describe the behavior that you would like the other person to change.
- Describe how you feel when the behavior occurs.
- State the positive behavior you would like to see.

TABLE 5-3 Comparison of Assertive and Aggressive Behavior

Assertive Behavior	Aggressive Behavior
"This medication works best when it is taken on a regular daily basis."	"You know you can't expect this medication to work when you're not taking it every day."
"Let me find someone who can answer that question for you."	"That's not my job."
"Your behavior is inappropriate."	"Why did you do that? It was stupid."
Knocking on door and then coming into an exam to say "Excuse me, Dr. Thompson. You are needed on the telephone."	Rushing into an exam room to say "Doctor, you've got a telephone call."

- Describe the appropriate, reasonable, and enforceable consequences that will result if the person does not change his or her behavior.
- Follow through with consequences if the behavior does not change.
- Commend the individual for the behavioral change.
- Evaluate your confrontation.

Discussing Sensitive Issues

Numerous sensitive issues arise during contact with patients. Discussing issues involving money, such as the patient's bill and personal financial responsibility, can be very sensitive. Patients should be advised before the first visit of the physician's charges for specific services or treatment. Inquiries regarding the patient's medical insurance and procedures for payment of fees should also be reviewed prior to the first visit. Compliance with federal regulations regarding the patient's right to privacy for all health-related information should be addressed at the first visit. This includes reviewing the Health Insurance Portability and Accountability Act (HIPAA) and following its guidelines as discussed in Chapter 4. The medical assistant should have each patient sign a release of information form on his or her first visit stating that the medical information obtained from visits may be disclosed to insurance companies and others for payment purposes as designated.

A CUSTOMER-FRIENDLY ENVIRONMENT

Using good interpersonal skills to set a positive environment in the health care setting generates a customer-friendly atmosphere and comfortable workplace. A warm, friendly greeting, showing respect to the patient, being sincere and sensitive, and demonstrating empathy can help set a positive tone.

Greeting Patients

A patient should be greeted within one minute of entering the office. If you are speaking on the telephone when the patient comes in, be sure to acknowledge the patient's presence with a smile and nod. Give your full attention to the patient as soon as you complete the telephone conversation.

Barriers to Communication

There are many barriers to communication. Identifying and overcoming these barriers is essential for effective communication. Some are obvious barriers, such as the distraction of loud background noise, and can be eliminated by the medical assistant. However, we may not be aware of other barriers that result in either no communication or a distorted message being received. To understand the patient, you must overcome the barriers to effective communication (Figure 5-5).

Giving the patient false reassurance by saying "Everything will be all right" can result in the patient's reluctance to talk to you about personal or health-related fears. Such comments can also lead to liability issues for the physician if the patient believes that a promise for recovery has been made.

The medical assistant also may put up barriers to communication unintentionally. To name a few, such obstacles include not looking at the patient when he or she is speaking,

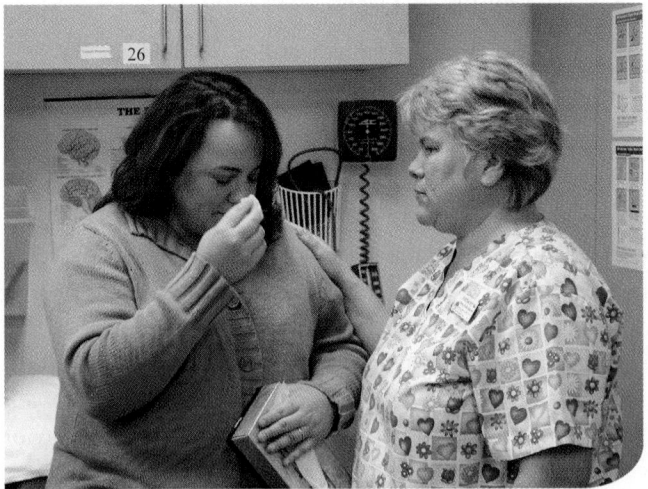

FIGURE 5-5 **Effective listening skills demonstrate empathy to the patient and break down barriers to communication.**

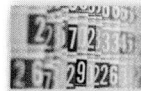
interrupting the patient, abruptly changing the subject, and using meaningless statements to soothe the patient. Medical assistants must remember that the patient is coming to see the physician because he or she has a problem. Patients should never be treated in a condescending manner.

DEFENSIVE BEHAVIORS

Patients also will put up barriers to effective communication when they are stressed by illness. These barriers are defensive behaviors. A **defensive behavior** is a reaction to a perceived threat that is usually unconscious in nature. Defensive behaviors are sometimes also referred to as *coping mechanisms*. Not all coping mechanisms are defensive or have a negative impact. For example, when trying to meet a deadline, you may have learned that using good time management skills and prioritizing tasks permits you to reach the deadline. Coping mechanisms are learned either consciously or unconsciously. As a member of the health care team, you must be aware of your defensive behaviors in the professional setting as well as at home. Some defensive behaviors are discussed in Table 5-4.

USE OF MEDICAL LANGUAGE

You will become adept at understanding the language of medicine. The abbreviations that are used in medicine are a form of communication for people working in the health care field. However, your patients have little understanding of medical terminology. You may wish to teach patients a few simple terms so that they can better understand the

physician's instructions about prescriptions. Otherwise, you must make an effort to avoid using medical terminology or abbreviations when speaking with patients. For example, abbreviations such as *NPO*, meaning "nothing by mouth," are not readily recognized or understood by patients. Always write out or state clear instructions regarding preparations for tests and taking medications. Patients may be reluctant to admit they do not understand, in which case you might assume that they have been properly instructed when they have not. Failure to inform patients in terms they are able to understand could be construed as negligence on the part of the health care provider and increase the risk of a lawsuit.

MULTICULTURAL ISSUES

As a medical assistant, you will come in contact with people from many different cultures. A **culture** consists of the values, beliefs, attitudes, and customs shared by a group of people and passed on through the generations. Behaviors exhibited by the members of a culture are based on their beliefs and values. Health care beliefs may differ widely from those to which you are accustomed. The medical assistant must be tolerant in attitude and treat each patient with respect, dignity, and empathy. The medical assistant will encounter cultural diversity when interacting with individuals from other cultures. Cultural diversity presents its own set of barriers to effective communication.

Language

A non–English-speaking patient is at a disadvantage when trying to obtain health care in the United States. Imagine, for a minute, how you would feel if you were traveling in a

TABLE 5-4 Defensive Behaviors

Behavior	Description	Example
Compensation	Substitution of an attitude, feeling, or behavior with its opposite	Mrs. Matthews believes the lump in her breast is cancer. However, she smiles and laughs whenever you talk to her about it.
Denial	Unconsciously avoiding an unwanted feeling or situation	Mr. Morgan cancels an appointment to have a PSA blood test for prostate cancer in spite of having symptoms associated with prostate trouble.
Displaced anger	Expressing angry feelings toward persons or objects that are unrelated to the problem	Mrs. Matthews is angry at being diagnosed with cancer. She takes this anger out on her family members.
Dissociation	Not connecting one event with another	Mary Sims is a nurse who works with alcoholic patients. In her free time, she drinks to excess.
Introjection	Adopting the feeling of someone else	Mr. Morgan's friends have said that the PSA test is reliable and could relieve his anxiety about having prostate cancer. He believes them and has the test.
Projection	Placing your own feelings on another person	Mr. Morgan becomes irritated when the medical assistant calls to remind him of his appointment. He wrongly decides that she is irritated with him or dislikes him. In reality, he is upset with himself.
Rationalization	Justifying thoughts or behavior to avoid the truth	Mary Sims believes that the appetite-suppressant benefit of smoking offsets the risk of developing cancer.
Regression	Turning back to former behavior patterns in times of stress	Jimmy, who is toilet trained, reverts to bed-wetting during hospitalization.
Repression	Keeping unpleasant thoughts or feelings out of one's mind	Mr. Morgan denies any urinary frequency when questioned by the physician.
Sublimation	Directing or changing unacceptable drives for security, affection, or power into socially or culturally acceptable channels	Mrs. Matthews is worried about having cancer and uses up energy cleaning her house.

foreign country and had an accident that required you to go to the hospital. Not only would you not understand anyone in the hospital, but the health care practices also might be very different from what you are accustomed to at home. The feelings of fear, frustration, and confusion you would feel would be increased if you had no one to act as an interpreter. It will help you to be more tolerant if you imagine yourself in the non–English-speaking patient's position.

You will encounter patients and other health care workers who speak a wide variety of languages. Hispanics make up the largest non–English-speaking group in the United States today. It would be helpful for you to learn a few phrases and some simple words in the Spanish language to help communicate with Hispanic patients and coworkers. The same is true for patients who speak other languages. If at all possible, you should get someone to interpret for the patient. Perhaps a fellow worker or family member could help. For patients with a limited ability to understand English, speak slowly and clearly, using simple words or phrases.

Smiling and other positive nonverbal cues are helpful. Use pictures if they are available.

Diverse Viewpoints

People from other cultures have different views and customs relating to health care delivery. Your views and customs are not better than theirs; they are just different. Patients may have different views about the causes of illness, the treatments, and the behavior expected of the health care provider. In some cultures, illness is thought to be caused by winds or other forces, blood being too thick or thin, or the ill will of others. The best way to learn about the views of someone from another culture is to ask them.

You may not always be successful in encouraging patients from a different culture to relate their symptoms and signs to you. Patients may feel that talking about physical pain is a sign of weakness, or they may be forbidden to mention psychological problems. One of the duties of the medical assistant is to help ensure that the patient complies with the

TABLE 5-5 Cultural Traditions in Health Care

Country	Sick Care Practices	Health Care Beliefs	Family Role in Care
China	Holistic and traditional includes acupuncture, herbal medicine	Upset in body energy causes disease. Stigma is attached to mental illness. Health promotion is important.	Family takes care of the sick, even in hospital.
Former Soviet Union	Holistic, folk, and Western medical practices	Health promotion is important. Acute sick care is practiced, rehabilitation is not stressed.	Family members provide care in hospital: bathing, feeding, changing linens.
Philippines	Health promotion is important. Mental illness is a disgrace. Evil cast from the eyes of another can cause illness.	Family may give hospital care.	Children feel obligated to care for elderly.
Vietnam	Health care practices contain magical and religious components. Eastern and herbal medicine are important. Self-care and self-medication are used to treat illness.	Only acute sick care is permitted. Health is believed to come from the restoration of yin and yang and hot and cold balance.	Patient care is a family responsibility.

treatment physicians prescribe, whether it is in the form of medication or therapy or diagnostic examinations. It may be necessary to ask for assistance from a family member who understands the issues and can communicate more easily. Table 5-5 lists some diverse cultural traditions.

Bias, Prejudice, and Stereotyping

Bias, prejudice, and stereotyping are barriers to effective communication that directly relate to cultural diversity. To understand these barriers, a few more definitions are in order. As discussed previously, culture is defined as the values, attitudes, and behaviors particular to a group of people. Ethnicity is a classification of people based on national origin. People from the same ethnic background share similar traditions, beliefs, and language.

Stereotyping results when negative generalities concerning specific characteristics of a group are applied unfairly to an entire population. Race is a classification of people based on their physical or biological characteristics, such as skin color, shape of eyes, hair type, bone structure, or facial features. Race is often used to classify people unfairly and unjustly in a negative way. Bias is an unfair preference or dislike of something. A bias prevents an impartial opinion of someone or something. People who are ethnocentric believe that their cultural background is better than any other. This leads to prejudice, prejudging, and stereotyping, which can negatively impact communication and the acceptance of others. To avoid these negative behaviors, the medical assistant should adhere to the following behaviors:

- Be aware of his or her own beliefs.
- Learn as much as possible about other cultures, races, and nationalities.
- Be sensitive to the feelings of others.
- Evaluate information before accepting it as a belief.
- Avoid ethnic jokes.
- Be open to differences.
- When unsure of a patient's cultural beliefs, ask the patient to help you understand.

Communication in Special Circumstances

The medical assistant will encounter special circumstances in the office when dealing with patients. It is likely that at some time you will encounter an angry patient, a patient who is terminally ill, or one who is anxious, visually or hearing impaired, or mentally or emotionally impaired. Regardless of the circumstances, all these patients must be treated with respect, empathy, and professionalism.

THE ANGRY PATIENT

One of the most difficult communication problems involves the angry patient. It can be a difficult task for the medical assistant to refrain from taking the patient's comments personally. People have different styles and coping behaviors when they are frightened (Figure 5-6). Many patients who enter the physician's office are fearful of the diagnosis they may hear. Some patients become frightened of the equipment in the office or have an unwarranted fear of pain. In addition to fear, another cause of anger is loss of control. If you have been hospitalized, you may be able to relate to this feeling.

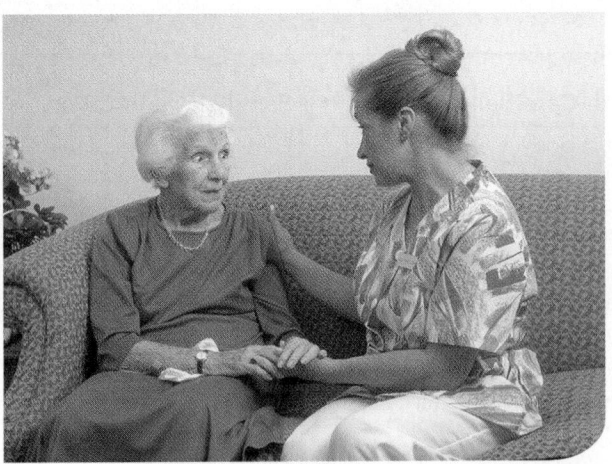

FIGURE 5-6 The medical assistant often has to reassure and comfort the patient before effective communication can take place.

The job of the medical assistant is to remain calm and use positive communication and professional techniques to direct the patient's anger into a positive channel. Try to defuse the patient's anger. For instance, many patients will gain control over their anger when the medical assistant offers a comment such as "I'm really sorry you feel this way. Let's see if we can solve the problem." You may have to take the patient into a private office if you cannot calm him or her immediately. Disruptive patients can upset others who are waiting to see the physician. Whereas it is not necessary to give in to the unreasonable demands of a patient, it is important to realize that an upset patient is often expressing the need for you to listen carefully, without judging, and to assist in solving the problem. Whenever possible, try to direct the patient's comments about a problem to a solution.

In the case of an angry caller, you must remember that no matter how angry a patient becomes, you cannot respond in anger. The role of the medical assistant is to assess or evaluate the situation. Remain calm and speak to the patient in a quiet, calm tone of voice, projecting your concern for the patient in the present situation. Often this will be enough to calm the patient. If that does not work, however, ask your supervisor or office manager for assistance. Alternatively, ask the patient if you may return the call after you have been able to gather more information that will enable you to be of help.

In the case of a patient who becomes abusive or violent, it is necessary to consider the safety of yourself, other staff members, and patients. Once the incident has been resolved, be sure to document it appropriately, according to office policies.

THE ANXIOUS PATIENT

Many patients exhibit what is known as *white coat syndrome*. This term was derived from the anxiety a patient feels when encountering medical staff, who would generally wear a white coat; however, attire is more varied in today's medical atmosphere. Some signs of anxiety are trembling, flushing, perspiring, fidgeting, talking excessively, and remaining unusually quiet. Hypertensive patients who suffer from white coat syndrome should have their blood pressure measured at the beginning and the end of the visit to get a more representative value. To deal with anxious patients, use the communication skills you have learned in this chapter: speak calmly, reassure patients, smile, touch them respectfully on the hand, and be empathetic.

PATIENTS WITH SPECIAL NEEDS

Meeting the needs of special needs patients requires extra sensitivity, patience, and empathy on the part of the medical assistant. Here we consider several types of patients individually, along with some procedural guidelines.

The Hearing-Impaired Patient

Hearing loss can vary from a slight loss to total deafness. Total hearing impairment is considered by many to be the most difficult of all handicaps because it can keep people isolated from communication and social interaction. If a child cannot hear, he or she will have difficulty speaking since learning speech involves imitating the speech of others. Many hearing-impaired individuals communicate by means of sign language. Figure 5-7 shows the alphabet in sign language. Basic sign language is not difficult to learn. Simple phrases in sign language should be a part of every medical professional's knowledge base. Hearing-impaired patients will often bring an interpreter to the medical office (Figure 5-8) shows a medical assistant with a hearing-impaired patient using an interpreter.

The manner in which you try to communicate will differ depending on whether the patient has a hearing aid, can lip-read, or has a family member or interpreter with him or her. Loss of hearing is a normal but frustrating sign of aging. The following are some guidelines to help the hearing impaired:

- Select a quiet environment to communicate with the patient.
- Reduce outside noise as much as possible.
- Never shout. Speak slowly and clearly.
- If the patient does not understand you the first time, rephrase the statement.
- Explain everything carefully before performing a procedure.
- Face the patient when speaking.
- Make sure light is on your mouth and not behind you. Light behind you may put shadows over the mouth and inhibit the patient's ability to lip-read.

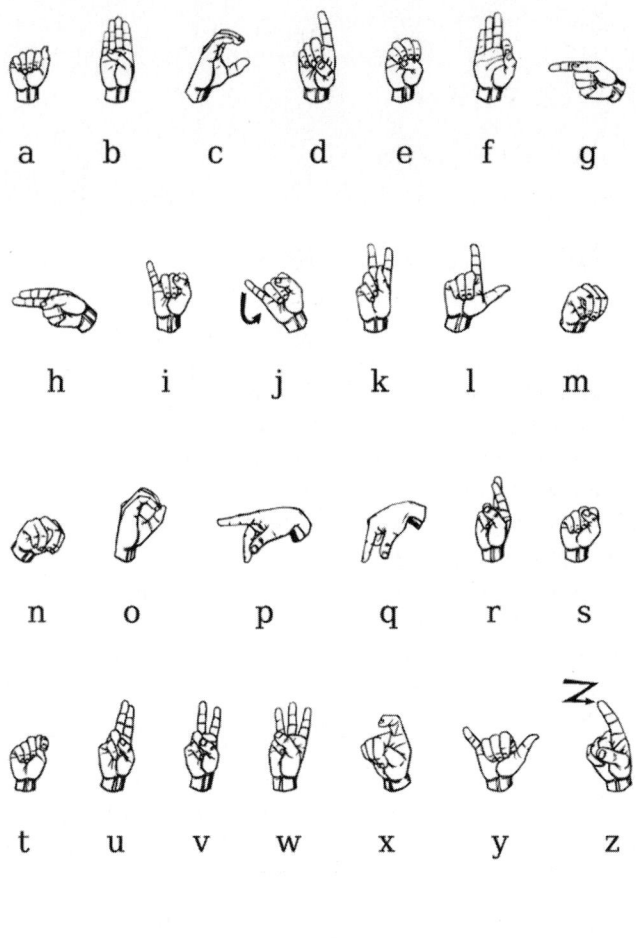

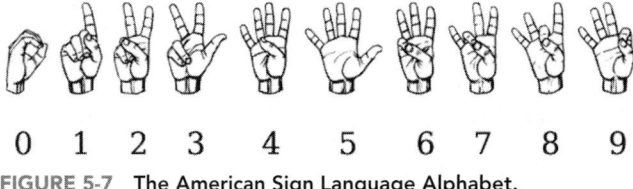

FIGURE 5-7 The American Sign Language Alphabet.

- Have a paper and pen available so that the patient can communicate in writing.
- Always provide written instructions or pamphlets for patient education purposes.

Basic hearing tests or screening tests are often performed by the medical assistant in the physician's office. An audiogram may be ordered by the physician when there is a suspicion of moderate to severe hearing loss. This test will determine the faintest sounds a patient can hear during audiometric testing. Audiometric testing, conducted by an audiologist, tests hearing ability by determining the lowest and highest intensities and frequencies that a person can distinguish. The patient may sit in a soundproof booth and receive sounds through earphones as the technician decreases the sounds or tones. Procedure 5-2 provides the steps to employ with the hearing impaired patient.

The Visually Impaired Patient

Blindness can be present at birth or may develop as a result of a disease, such as diabetes mellitus. Patients who are blind can remain independent. Specially trained service animals can help the visually impaired patient to be more independent. Figure 5-9 shows a patient with a service dog. The visually impaired patient cannot rely on nonverbal cues that make up much of the communication process for those with sight. The medical assistant can communicate and help the visually impaired patient by remembering to follow the following suggested guidelines:

- Always speak to announce your presence when you are near a blind person.
- Offer to guide the patient into the examination room by offering your arm. Do not grab the patient without offering your arm first.

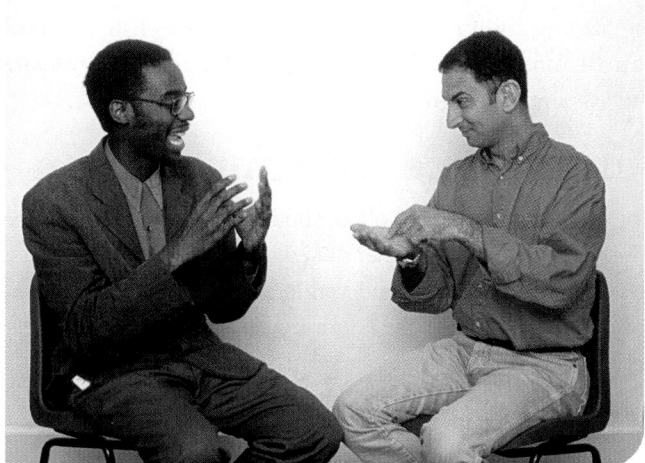

FIGURE 5-8 A hearing-impaired patient using an interpreter.

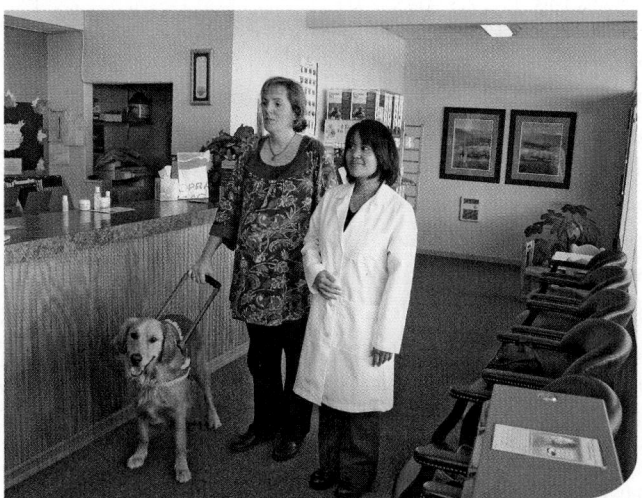

FIGURE 5-9 A visually impaired patient is assisted by a service dog.

ASSISTING THE HEARING-IMPAIRED PATIENT

Objective: Use effective communication skills to assist a hearing-impaired patient to prepare for a physical examination.

EQUIPMENT AND SUPPLIES

METHOD

1. Identify the patient.
2. Reduce external noise as much as possible.
3. Smile and establish eye contact and face the patient.
4. Speak slowly, and do not shout.
5. Provide careful explanation of the procedure.
6. Provide paper and pencil for the patient to use if desired.
7. Use written information to reinforce the message for the patient.
8. If possible, have the patient repeat your response to ensure that the message was received accurately.
9. Give directions using actions as well as words.
10. Be sensitive to the patient's needs.
11. Employ an empathetic, professional attitude.
12. Notify the physician of any patient concerns.

CHARTING EXAMPLE

6/24/XX 3:00 P.M. Patient is hearing impaired, so gave patient copy of attached handout on preparation for barium enema diagnostic testing. Patient was able to restate preparation steps.

. . . . Eric Williams RMA

- Face the patient, and speak clearly.
- Describe the patient's surroundings.
- Explain all procedures in detail before beginning.
- Try not to leave the patient alone for any length of time.
- Have available large-print educational materials for patients who might benefit from them.
- Do not be condescending toward the patient.

THE MENTALLY AND EMOTIONALLY IMPAIRED PATIENT

Psychology is the science of behavior and the human thought process. This behavioral science is primarily concerned with human beings acting alone or in groups. Normal and abnormal behavior are distinguished from each other in psychology. All social interactions, such as those that occur during the communication process, may pose a problem for some people. The medical assistant will encounter patients, family members, staff, and caregivers who exhibit a wide scope of behavioral patterns. These behavior patterns may be due to diseases, mental disorders, anxiety, drug abuse, trauma, the aging process, cultural customs, or a combination of several of these causes. The medical assistant must be tolerant and respectful of others in all circumstances.

When dealing with an emotionally or mentally impaired patient, it is important to determine, if possible, what level of communication the patient can understand. If a patient has a caregiver, he or she may be able to give you tips regarding how to communicate with the patient. In most cases, you should speak slowly and clearly, stay calm, and keep your messages short. If you have to touch the patient for a procedure, be sure first to explain what you are going to do. A caregiver may be able to give you assistance in calming the patient, if needed.

THE NON–ENGLISH-SPEAKING PATIENT

As mentioned in the previous discussion of cultural diversity, the non–English-speaking patient is at a disadvantage in the medical environment. You should employ the communication skills discussed previously and consider the following guidelines: Smile at the patient, determine if he or she has any ability to speak or understand English, speak in normal tones, use pantomime or pictures to demonstrate, and ask a family member for assistance.

Intraoffice Communication

The goal in the medical office should be to establish a sense of **rapport**—an environment of cooperation—with patients, coworkers, supervisors, and vendors. To create this cooperative environment, all the communication skills we have examined in this chapter must be utilized.

ESTABLISHING TRUST

To communicate effectively in the health care environment and in everyday life, we must establish trust in our relation-

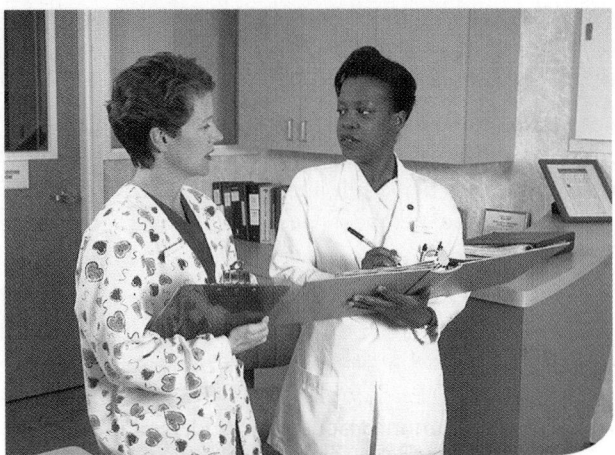

FIGURE 5-10 **Staff members often find it difficult to communicate with other coworkers.**

ships. Being open, honest, and firm in our convictions, presenting a professional image and using positive body language help create a positive environment. Some of the most difficult communication problems occur with other staff members (Figure 5-10). Good staff communication depends on positive respectful interactions. When thoughtless or condescending comments are made, permanent damage to relationships can occur. To be **condescending** is to adopt a superior attitude and act as though you are better than someone else. Withdrawing from the group, feeling angry and hurt, and discussing other staff members behind their backs causes office morale to suffer. Using assertive behavior with fellow staff means that you assert your own needs without threatening theirs. For instance, if it is your turn to have a holiday off and you have been scheduled to work, it is better to state "I'm sorry I can't work that day. Since I worked overtime on the last holiday, I have made plans for this one." An aggressive statement, such as "It's not fair; I always have to work on holidays and the others don't," would imply that favoritism or special treatment has been shown to some staff members and might cause the supervisor to become defensive.

RAPPORT AND TEAM BUILDING

A positive attitude can make the difference between keeping and losing a job. A positive attitude is easier to project if you are happy in your work. The work group you are part of is an important factor in your attitude. Work groups must become a cohesive team. To do this, some degree of socializing is beneficial. Discussions with other staff members about hobbies, travel, sports, family, and friends help to establish trust and understanding. However, the social aspect of staff communication should not interfere with work productivity.

Gossip is unnecessary and often results in a negative conversation, usually about someone who is not present. The medical assistant must learn to recognize gossip and not participate in it. Gossip can be extremely hurtful and is destructive to the cooperation needed in the medical facility.

THE PATIENT AS CONSUMER

The medical assistant should view the patient as a consumer of health care. Today, patients and family members are more knowledgeable about health care options because of the Internet and other media. They no longer place the physician on a pedestal as older patients may have done when physicians made house calls. In fact, many patients can experience a certain amount of alienation from their health care providers because most physicians are specialists. Specialization can lead to viewing the patient and his or her injury or procedure as one and the same—"a broken leg" or "an appendectomy"—a viewpoint that is degrading. Instead, the patient should be treated holistically and with dignity and respect.

Medical assistants are the first to encounter the patient in many instances. Therefore, they are responsible for the initial impression the patient has of the practice or facility. The concept of "The customer comes first" should be a primary goal for all health care providers and must be considered to sustain a satisfied client base. Communication with other physicians, hospitals, and clinics is vitally important to the economic stability of practices and facilities.

Staff Arrangements

Staffing arrangements are as varied as the types of medical practices. The solo practice with its staff of one, the multiphysician practice with a variety of staff, including an office manager, the clinic with many registered nurses (RNs) and other types of allied health care workers are only a few of the

Box 5-2 Steps for Problem SOLVING

- Recognize that a problem exists. Recognition may result from a feeling, observation, or conversation with others.
- Describe the problem and clarify what the basic issue or question is and the factors that affect it.
- Identify alternative methods of resolving the problem. Any alternative can be considered, even if is not immediately seen as practical.

- Choose the best method for resolving the problem, and implement it.
- As the plan is being put into affect, evaluate the results and adjust the method if necessary.

---

types of practices in which the medical assistant may work. Regardless of the type of practice, communication is vitally important to keep conflict to a minimum, establish a positive environment, and provide quality health care.

Whatever the staffing arrangements, the physician or office manager must be clear about the chain of command and convey that information to the employees. In the solo office with one medical assistant, problems rarely arise. However, in larger practices, the health care professional with most seniority is often the unofficial office manager. This person may not be the most qualified, the most multiskilled, or the most accomplished manager. Friction among coworkers is often a common problem in many of these larger practices. To avoid this problem, clearly defined areas of responsibility and authority should be established. The office policies and procedures manual can help resolve conflict about authority and responsibility.

CONFLICT RESOLUTION

Inevitably, coworkers will experience strife and conflict. The policies and procedures manual is a valuable tool when beginning to resolve issues. It should state clearly what standards are acceptable in all areas of the facility. Conflicts occur when miscommunication or misunderstanding of the message occurs. Conflict also can stem from prejudices or preconceived ideas. Conflict interferes with establishing rapport and cooperation, which are essential in the workplace. However, at times, conflict can be a positive experience if it resolves issues of disagreement in an appropriate manner.

PROBLEM SOLVING AND CRITICAL THINKING

Problem solving and critical thinking are necessary skills for health care workers. Problem solving is a way of looking at a problem and ultimately arriving at a decision. Box 5-2 lists the steps to evaluate the factors and risks involved in solving problems. Most problems have more than one solution. Weighing all the factors involved and evaluating the results will help later with other problems.

Critical thinking (Box 5-3) includes the ability to think imaginatively, solve problems, visualize situations, learn new information, and think logically. Both problem solving and critical thinking skills are important concepts to employ before trying to resolve any conflict. Box 5-4 illustrates the steps in conflict resolution.

Box 5-3 Elements of Critical THINKING

- Ask questions.
- Define a problem.
- Examine evidence.
- Avoid emotional reasoning.
- Analyze assumptions and bias.

- Avoid oversimplification.
- Consider other interpretations.
- Tolerate ambiguity.
- Think about one's own thinking.

Box 5-4 Steps in Conflict RESOLUTION

- Communicate your needs in simple terms.
- Know when to express your feelings.

- Do not assume you know the other person's feelings.
- Look at the issue from the other person's perspective.

SCOPE OF PRACTICE ISSUES

As a medical assistant, you are truly a multiskilled health care provider and are capable of functioning throughout a facility in many different areas. From the clinical area where you have direct patient contact, to working in the front office, and including your handling of administrative procedures, you are cross-trained to effectively perform all these duties. Other employees, like registered nurses (RNs) and licensed practical nurses (LPNs), who are working in the facility may only be able to handle the clinical areas. Medical secretaries, coding, and billing employees usually can only perform the administrative functions. Because of your multifunctional training, you may encounter some jealousy or resentment from other staff members. It is important to work within your own scope of practice and job description. In other words, do not perform skills that are beyond your training. On the other hand, do not be afraid to promote your profession and all for which it stands.

COMMUNICATING WITH SUPERIORS

In dealing with your superiors, as with your coworkers, communication should be kept positive. If conflicts do arise and you need to speak with your superior, choose an appropriate time or ask for an appointment to speak with him or her. Be direct and to the point, and do not promote any gossip you may have heard. If you have been given an order to do something and need clarification on how to complete it, ask for help. Most supervisors would rather be asked a question than to have you perform a function about which you are not clear. Show initiative in your daily work. If a task needs to be done, volunteer to do it without being asked, as long as it falls within your job description. Too often staff members are busy keeping score of which employees do more or less work as compared to others.

LOYALTY TO YOUR EMPLOYER

You represent your employer or physician every time you speak to a patient or caller. You must support the physician and his or her reputation in every instance. In your position, you may become privileged to personal information about your employer. Under no circumstances, whether inside or outside of the office, should you discuss that personal information. It is perfectly acceptable to state "I really can't answer that" or "I'm sorry, but I don't know" in response to a patient's or other staff member's questions.

A loyal employee protects and defends an employer when other employees engage in negative conversation. See Table 5-6 for examples of loyal responses to questions or comments about your employer's personal life.

Communication and Patients' Rights

Every patient has the right to privacy and confidentiality. Any information about a patient is considered privileged information.

CONFIDENTIALITY

All patients have the right to have their personal privacy respected and their medical records handled with confidentiality. Your treatment and concern for the patient reflect the physician's high standards of care. The human dignity of each patient must be preserved regardless of the patient's socioeconomic background, race, age, nationality, sexual orientation, or gender. The Health Insurance Portability and Accountability Act (HIPAA), as previously mentioned, was passed in 1996 by Congress. The HIPAA Privacy Rule, which is part of HIPAA, provides for the federal protection of health information. This rule, while protecting patients' privacy, also allows for patients to have better access to their medical records and to have more control about how and to whom the information can be released. HIPAA designates the following information as protected health information (PHI):

- Name
- Address

TABLE 5-6 Responses that Communicate Loyalty

Question/Comment	Sample Response
"I guess Dr. Thompson can't see me on Wednesday because he's playing golf."	"Dr. Thompson's day off is Wednesday, but he could see you on Saturday."
"I hear Dr. Thompson and his wife are divorcing."	"I really have no information about Dr. Thompson's personal life."
"I've been waiting one hour to see Dr. Thompson. Why is he so slow?"	"I'm sorry you've had a long wait. Dr. Thompson has had many very ill patients today. May I reschedule your appointment?"

- Phone numbers
- Fax numbers
- Dates (birth, death, admission, discharge, etc.)
- Social Security number
- E-mail address
- Medical record numbers
- Health plan beneficiary numbers
- Account numbers
- Certificate or license numbers
- Vehicle identifiers, serial numbers, and license plate numbers
- Device identifiers and serial numbers
- Web Universal Resource Locators (URLs)
- Internet Protocol (IP) address numbers

This means that none of this information can be given out by any means (electronic, paper, or orally) for any reason without the written authorization of the patient. The written authorization covers any information necessary for treatment, payment, and operations (TPO). If you are in doubt about whether to release personal patient information, do not do it. Always make sure that you have obtained the appropriate authorization.

Family members can pose special confidentiality problems. If a patient brings a family member into the examination room with them, you might presume that they are giving informed consent. However, it is prudent for the medical assistant to have the patient sign a form specifying with which family members or friends the office personnel may discuss the patient's case. Domestic violence victims may be intimidated into allowing their violent perpetrators to come to the office with them. A wise medical assistant may ask the significant other to leave the room for a few minutes so the assistant can assess whether the patient is safe at home. It is important to let patients know that they can exclude family members from the discussion of their health if they wish.

ADVISING PATIENTS

As a medical assistant, you are the physician's representative. Because you are part of the staff, wear a uniform, and assist with treatments, patients may view you as an authority figure. The physician advises the patient on a course of treatment or procedure based on his or her examination and diagnostic test results. You are not permitted to offer your opinion about the physician's diagnosis, discuss the course of action the physician has set forth, or tell the patient what you would do in his or her position. Those opinions are beyond your scope of practice and could put you and the physician at

risk of being sued. If asked by a patient "What would you do if you were me?" you must not offer advice. Explain to the patient that the physician will be pleased to review the course of action and answer any questions and that you will be happy to arrange for that meeting. A medical assistant giving advice to a patient could be construed as practicing medicine without a license and is a punishable offense in most states.

PATIENT DECISION MAKING

Patients who have received bad news from the physician or are faced with difficult choices do need help to come to a decision. Your role is to listen empathetically to the patient, ask him or her reflecting or clarifying questions, and make clear the information the physician has related to the patient to help him or her come to a decision on a course of treatment. For example, Mrs. Santos has been told by the physician that her breast biopsy was positive and a mastectomy is recommended as soon as possible. When the physician leaves the room, she asks you what she should do. Your response should be "Mrs. Santos, you seem upset about having to have a mastectomy. What concerns you about the procedure?" If she asks what you would do in her circumstances, suggest that she get a second opinion or offer to explain again in simple terms what the doctor has said. Sometimes patients are so nervous in the presence of a physician that they do not hear information correctly. It would be permissible to give Mrs. Santos written information about the procedure, offer to bring her concerns to the physician, and encourage her to call back once she is home if she has more questions.

RISK MANAGEMENT

The term **risk management** refers to planning and implementing strategies for reducing the physician's risk of a lawsuit in the medical setting. As a medical assistant, dealing so closely with patients, you are in a position to help reduce those risks. Communicating effectively with the patient is certainly one of the primary ways to reduce the risk of being sued. On the other hand, any promise or commitment that you make to a patient can be legally binding to the physician who employs you. This means that the physician can be held responsible for something you have said or implied to the patient with regard to how the physician might improve the patient's condition. Keep all matters relating to patients' personal health information confidential. If you believe that any health professional is acting in an unethical or unprofessional manner, discuss this with your employer or another physician. For example, a comment such as "Did Miss Jones come in for her pregnancy test?" can result in a breach of confidentiality lawsuit against the physician if it is overheard by others.

SUMMARY

Communication is a necessary requirement for everyday living. In the health care field, the ability to communicate effectively is essential for success, such as when calling and requesting a prescription be renewed, documenting the patient's symptoms and helping the patient be diagnosed properly, providing patient education, arranging travel plans for the physician, and so on. The concern you have for patients will show in your words, actions, gestures, and tone of voice. The values of the office personnel will reflect in their attitudes and behaviors. Effective listening is patient centered and requires practice to ensure that you understand the obvious and less obvious needs of the patients. The special needs of some patients may not be the presenting problems when they arrive in the physician's office; however, these special needs must be dealt with to accommodate the patients as much as possible. Special care must be taken with patients who are hearing impaired, do not speak English, cannot see, are angry or anxious, are terminally ill, or are mentally or emotionally impaired. The medical assistant must remain flexible and be able to handle all unusual situations professionally. Although medical assistants should advocate assertively for the patient, they should never become aggressive. They should understand that patients are vulnerable and may engage in defensive behaviors. Therefore, getting honest feedback from patients is vital.

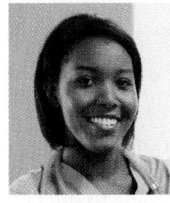 # 5 CHAPTER REVIEW

COMPETENCY REVIEW

1. Define and spell the terms to learn for this chapter.

2. What would you say to a patient who says that the medication Dr. Thompson gave her last week has made her sick?

3. What would you say to the patient who is angry at the delay in the waiting room?

4. What would you say to the patient who complains to you about Dr. Thompson?

5. What should you do if you are unfamiliar with the religious or cultural beliefs of a patient?.

6. Describe how to communicate to a profoundly deaf patient that he or she must remove all clothing and put on a gown.

7. Describe some cultural problems that can arise when treating patients from other cultures.

8. Discuss several defense mechanisms that you feel you sometimes exhibit. How do they impact negatively on your relationships with others?

9. Gladys Pierce's neighbor calls to see if she kept her appointment because she says Gladys is sometimes forgetful. What would you say?

PREPARING FOR THE CERTIFICATION EXAM

1. Which of the following is an open-ended question?
   a. Do you smoke?
   b. Have you ever had surgery?
   c. Do you take herbal supplements?
   d. Why are you here today?
   e. Are your parents still living?

2. If a patient is hearing impaired, which of the following would you do?
   a. Cover your mouth with your hand when talking.
   b. Stand with your back to the window.
   c. Give written instructions for surgical preparation.
   d. Speak more quickly than usual.
   e. Forgo getting informed consent.

3. Which of the following should you say to an angry patient?
   a. "Sit down and be quiet."
   b. "You need to calm down."
   c. "How may I help you resolve this problem?"
   d. "You should have been here on time."
   e. "I need to get the doctor first."

4. A 49-year-old patient has a developmental delay and is highly emotional. What would be the best course when approaching the patient in the reception area?
   a. Insist that he sit quietly in the reception area.
   b. Give him a toy truck to keep him occupied.
   c. Find a coloring book for him.
   d. Privately ask the caregiver how best to approach him.
   e. Offer him a cup of coffee.

5. Which of the following comprises the sum of all our values?
   a. behavior
   b. character
   c. beliefs
   d. attitudes
   e. prejudice

6. Which ethnic group comprises the largest number of non–English speakers in the United States?
   a. Hmong
   b. Hispanic
   c. Slavic
   d. Caucasian
   e. Persian

7. Which of the following is NOT a sign of impatience?
   a. tapping your finger
   b. interrupting conversation
   c. walking around the room
   d. sitting down
   e. checking your watch

8. Which of the following is assertive, not aggressive, behavior?
   a. demanding your way
   b. interrupting others
   c. telling others they are wrong
   d. advocating for patients
   e. shouting loudly

9. All of the following are protected under the Health Insurance Portability and Accountability Act (HIPAA) as protected health information (PHI) EXCEPT:
   a. vehicle license number.
   b. discharge date.
   c. age.
   d. gender.
   e. e-mail address.

10. Mrs. Hamsi has breast cancer. She does not want to offend her doctor, so she yells at her daughter as she leaves the office shouting. What defense mechanism is she exhibiting?
    a. denial
    b. depersonalization
    c. depression
    d. displacement
    e. dissociation

CRITICAL THINKING

1. The front desk receptionist informs the medical assistant that Mr. Yeung is very apprehensive. What are some things that the MA should or shouldn't do in this instance?

2. When working with a patient who has an interpreter, is it best to direct questions and comments to the interpreter or toward the patient? Explain your answer.

ON THE JOB

Amy Freeman is a new medical assistant who has recently passed the CMA examination. She has carefully studied the Health Insurance Portability and Accountability Act (HIPAA). When she is locking up the office at night, she notices that a patient's X-ray, bill, and driver's license photocopy have been left on a desk. Which documents, if any, must she put away under HIPAA regulations before leaving for the evening?

INTERNET ACTIVITY

Search using the term *deaf culture* for a chat room for the deaf. Communicate with people with hearing impairment about their culture.

MEDMEDIA

Additional interactive resources and activities for this chapter can be found:

On your student DVD: View applicable procedure videos on the DVD-ROM found in the back of this book.

MyHealthProfessionsKit.com: Test your knowledge of the chapter with games and activities. MyHealthProfessionsKit also includes resources, helpful links, and a Spanish audio glossary.

Medical Assisting Interactive: Practice your procedures as a medical assistant in this simulated doctor's office. This can be accessed through MyHealthProfessionsKit.com.

6

The Office Environment

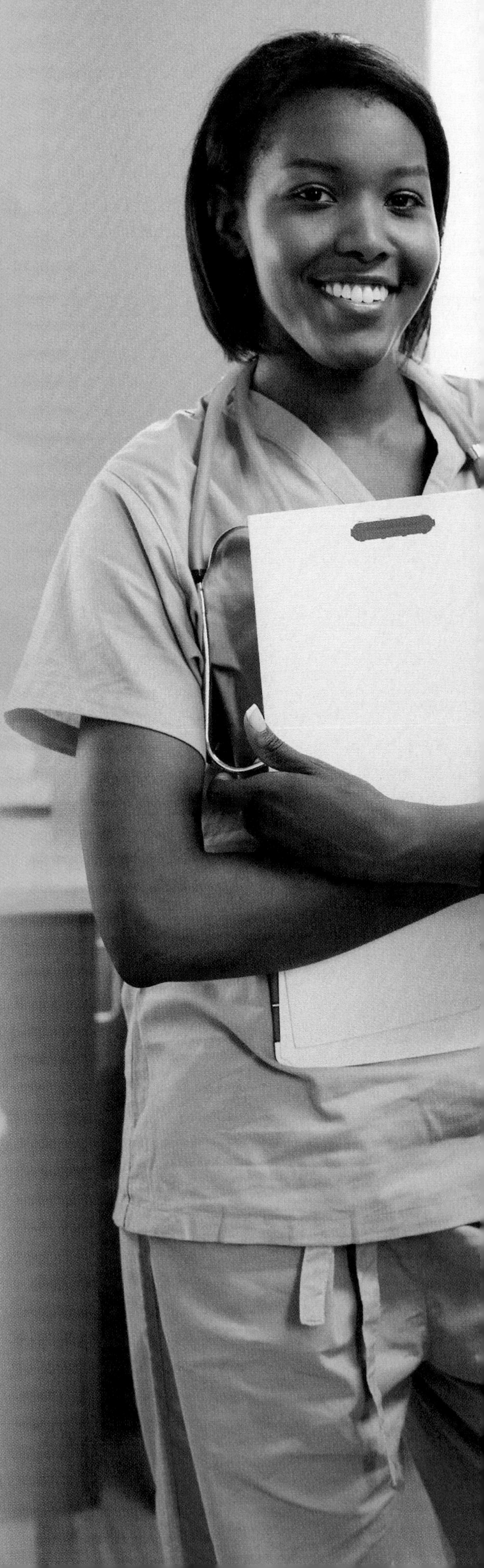

LEARNING OBJECTIVES

After completing this chapter, you should be able to:

- Define and spell the terms to learn for this chapter.

- Identify six general safety measures.

- Describe fire, electrical, mechanical, and chemical safety hazards.

- List and describe four types of medical waste.

- Define OSHA bloodborne pathogens standards.

- Describe the three points that must be included in an Exposure Control Plan.

- List and discuss five guidelines for using protective measures as indicated by OSHA.

- Discuss the importance of universal precautions for the medical assistant.

- List and describe six rules for proper body mechanics.

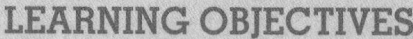

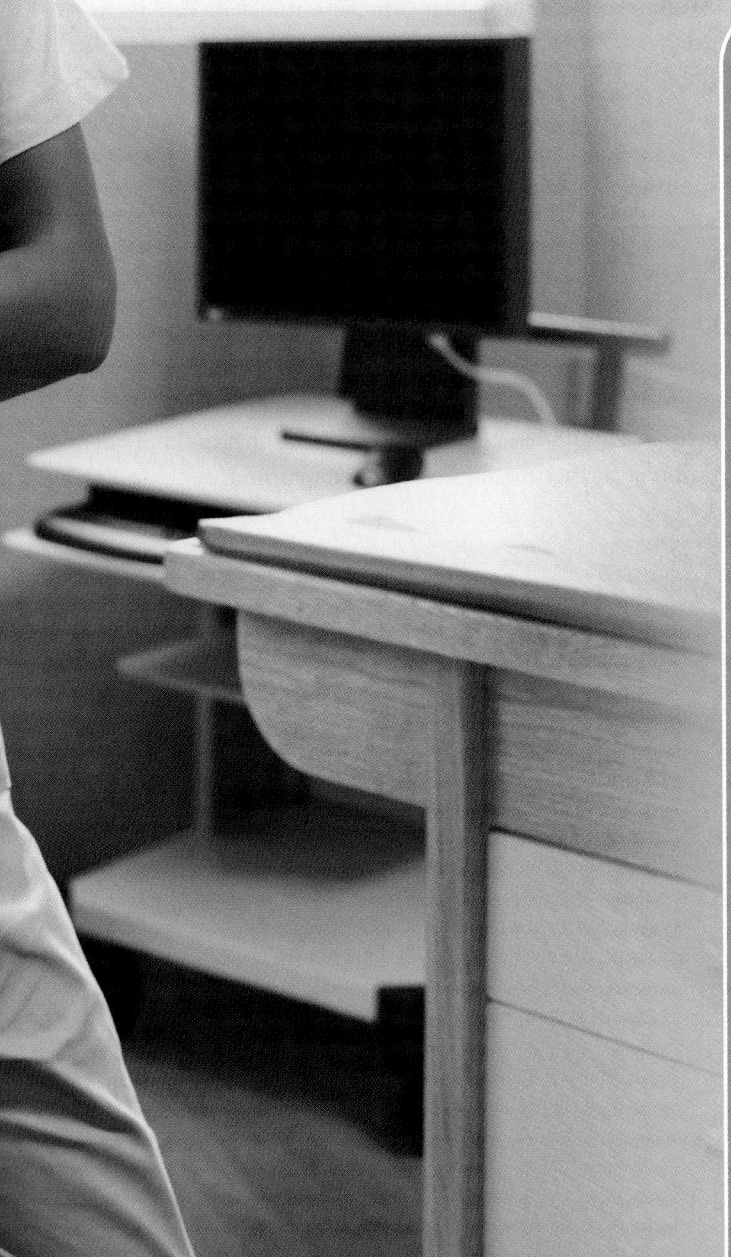

CHAPTER OUTLINE

CASE STUDY

Susan, a medical assistant, prepares a medication for Fei Yen Yeung that is to be given by an intramuscular injection technique. She has both safety needles and nonsafety needles at hand for use in this procedure. Since she has not been told to use only the safety needles and feels more comfortable with the old style because that is what she was taught in school, she chooses to use the nonsafety needle. After giving the injection, Susan proceeds to dispose of the needle and syringe in the sharps container. As she places the nonsafety needle on the flip-lid, it begins to slide off. Susan catches it, receiving a needlestick in the process. She continues to put the needle and syringe into the sharps container and finishes up with the patient.

After dismissing the patient, Susan reports the needlestick to her supervisor, Linda. Linda immediately asks Susan why she chose not to use a safety needle. Susan explains that she did not think she needed to and was not really trained to use them. Linda also asks if the patient is still in the office and how much time has elapsed since the needlestick occurred. Susan tells Linda the patient is no longer in the office and that the needlestick incident occurred approximately 10 minutes ago. Linda immediately asks Cindy, the phlebotomist, to draw several tubes of blood from Susan. Once Cindy is finished drawing Susan's lab specimens, Linda asks Susan to complete an incident report, describing the situation in full. Linda proceeds to call the patient and arrange for Mrs. Yeung to come into the office for lab draws.

J ust as in any workplace, general safety measures, employee safety, housekeeping, proper body mechanics, office security, and measures to ensure a clean, pleasant environment are critical to maintaining the safety and comfort of the medical assistant and the patient in the medical office. Additional safety issues may arise in a medical workplace, including biological hazards, bloodborne pathogens, and the handling of drug samples.

General Safety Measures

The **Occupational Safety and Health Administration (OSHA)** is a governmental agency responsible for the safety of all employees of companies operating in the United States. OSHA ensures the safety and health of America's workers by setting and enforcing standards; providing training, outreach, and education; establishing partnerships; and encouraging continual improvement in workplace safety and health. The agency has the authority to inspect a workplace without notification and to levy fines on any deficiencies relating to the health and safety of employees.

Many offices make the mistake of believing the only OSHA issues they need to be concerned with are the bloodborne pathogens standards. Whereas these regulations are important and will be covered later, many other safety factors fall under the regulations of OSHA.

OSHA is concerned with any workplace hazard that may impact the safety of an employee. Other governmental agencies may have standards regarding these factors as well, such as the local fire marshal or local law enforcement agencies. In addition, insurance companies with which the office may contract may have rules and regulations above and beyond these other agencies.

A workplace hazard can be defined as any issue that could affect the health or safety of an employee—either on immediate exposure or in the long term. Matters surrounding workplace hazards are discussed in the material that follows. See Guidelines 6-1 for some general safety measures to adhere to in the office.

PLANNING FOR OFFICE SAFETY

A disaster is anything that can cause injury or damage to a group of people. Disasters in a medical office include fire, flood, tornado, earthquake, hurricane, or explosions. Planning for natural and man-made disasters is discussed in Chapter 43. It is important for all employees to be aware of specific plans that have been put in place to protect the safety of the patients as well as the medical office staff. The safety measures discussed here address proper fire, electrical, mechanical, and chemical procedures. All new hires should be trained in all emergency steps within the first day of employment. This training should be documented in writing to ensure compliance with OSHA regulations. If a particular medical facility has radiation equipment on site, implementation of further regulations may be required.

PROFESSIONALISM
THE WORKPLACE

Safety precautions are the responsibility of all medical office personnel. It is especially important that medical assistants understand their role in an emergency because each employee may have a different responsibility. Regular disaster drills allow employees to act appropriately, carry out their assigned task, and ask questions if they are unsure of their role.

Fire Safety

Floor plans showing all exits, fire extinguishers, and stairwells should be placed in conspicuous areas all around the facility. These plans should clearly show the most direct route out of the building. They should be large enough to be easily read in dim light and from a reasonable distance. Prior to fire drills, it should be determined who will be designated for each area and responsible for ensuring all patients and staff are able to get out safely.

Portable fire extinguishers should be attached to walls in areas that are no more that 75 feet away from any employee area. Appropriate extinguishers for medical offices are the ABC types, which are capable of putting out many types of fires. Each employee should be instructed on the proper use of fire equipment.

Most of today's medical offices are located in buildings with smoke detectors and sprinkler systems. Smoke detectors and alarms should be tested regularly. Nothing should be placed within 18 inches of a sprinkler head.

Fire drills should be held at least once a year with all employees present. An ideal time to hold a fire drill is during a mandatory staff meeting. The drill should reinforce the location of fire exits, how to direct people to the fire exits, and how to act in a calm manner during such an emergency. Procedure 6-1 illustrates the proper procedure for handling a fire in the medical office and Figure 6-1 shows a basic plan for fire safety.

Many offices have adopted the acronym RACE to help employees remember what to do in the case of a fire. RACE stands for **R**escue, **A**lert, **C**onfine, and **E**xtinguish: Employees should rescue other employees and patients from the fire area, alert by calling 911, confine by closing doors and windows, and extinguish the fire.

Because of the widespread "No Smoking" policies now in place in medical facilities, cigarettes are not as much of a fire hazard inside the building as they used to be. However, safe disposal systems should be placed outside in designated areas to prevent people from throwing cigarettes into wastebaskets or other trash receptacles.

The following items should be in place in the event of a fire:

- Telephone numbers of fire and police departments should be attached to all telephones, including extensions.

- On fire extinguishers that have been properly maintained through monthly maintenance checks, the date and initials of the person responsible for testing the equipment should be legible.

- Exits and stairways should be clearly marked and free of debris, and a diagram of all exits should be posted near the fire extinguishers.

- File cabinets should be fireproof to protect vital records.

HANDLING A FIRE IN THE MEDICAL OFFICE

Objective: To respond to a fire in the medical office.

EQUIPMENT AND SUPPLIES

policy and procedures manual; evacuation maps of the office

Note: Planned fire drills should be executed at least annually and preferably more frequently so that all employees know their role and expectations in the event of a real disaster.

1. As soon as a fire is discovered, call 911 or the local fire department following the same procedure as practiced during fire drills.
2. Activate the established mechanism for signaling fire within the office. This may mean pulling the alarm, calling a code over the intercom, or taking other action.
3. All staff should calmly and quickly assist in getting all patients out of the office in an orderly manner, following the exit routes on the posted evacuation maps, and using the stairs, if applicable.
4. If the fire is contained, an attempt should be made to extinguish it using the fire extinguisher. However, if the fire is not contained, valuable time should not be spent in attempting to extinguish it.
5. The individual charged with ensuring that all rooms are cleared should quickly go through the office to ensure that no one is left behind.
6. After each room is evacuated, the door is to be closed.
7. Staff and patients should gather away from the building at the predetermined area.

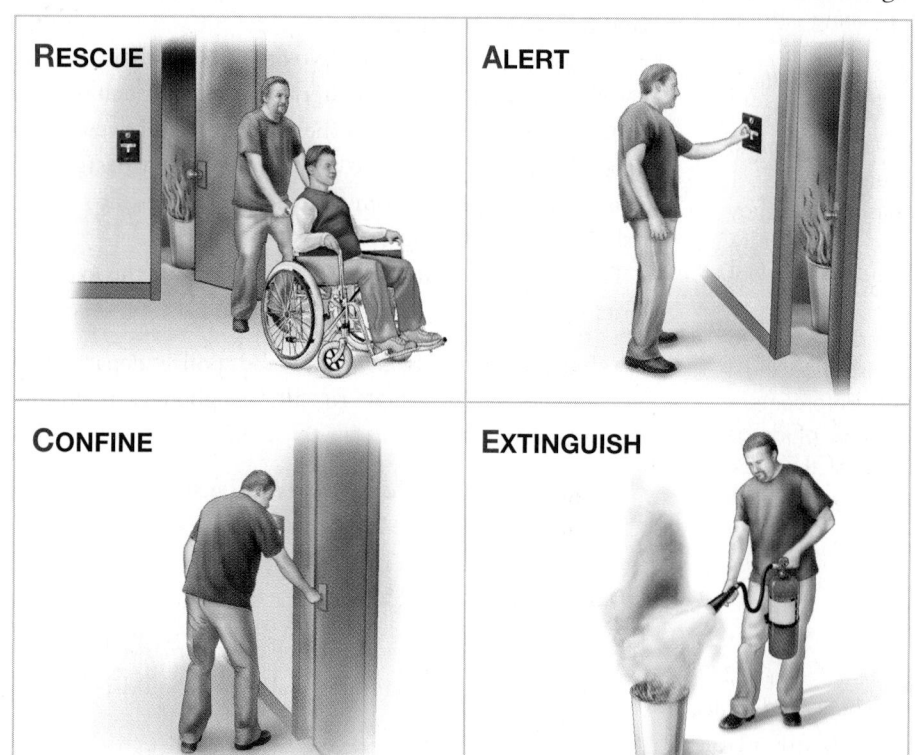

RESCUE

ALERT

CONFINE

EXTINGUISH

FIGURE 6-1 A fire safety plan like RACE saves lives.

Electrical Safety

Electrical shock is a hazard in the medical office. All equipment should be grounded according to the manufacturer's instructions. Never use extension cords because they are both an electrical and a trip-and-fall hazard. No circuit should be overloaded, and surge protectors should be used for all electronic equipment. If surge protectors are not used, a power surge can short-circuit or "fry" the sensitive components of electronic equipment, including computers. You should never plug a surge protector into another surge protector to double the number of outlets.

All electrical cords attached to equipment should be checked regularly for any cracks, loss of insulation, or other problems. In wet areas, such as near sinks, a **ground fault circuit interrupter (GFCI)** outlet must be used. GFCIs are designed to protect people from severe or fatal electric shocks. Because a GFCI detects ground faults, it can also prevent some electrical fires and reduce the severity of others by interrupting the flow of electric current. These outlets will break the circuit, or trip, if they become wet, protecting both the user and any plugged-in equipment.

Mechanical Safety

Many pieces of equipment in the medical office can cause harm if they are not used properly. Some of this equipment includes the centrifuge, autoclave, sterilizers, and oxygen equipment. Always read the entire instruction manual before installing or using any type of equipment. If you have any questions, ask your supervisor for clarification before continuing.

Chemical Hazards

Medical offices may contain chemicals that are hazardous to the human body. Materials may be considered harmful in several ways. **Biohazards** are biological substances, such as medical waste and samples of a virus or bacterium, that pose a threat to human beings and are potentially infectious. Corrosive materials cause burns, and flammable materials can burst into flames. Toxic materials can cause serious illness or death by exposure through skin contact, ingestion, or inhalation.

OSHA has very specific regulations regarding chemical hazards and hazardous communications. These are covered under the OSHA Hazardous Communications section of the regulations. Thee regulations are available from the U.S. Department fo Labor in Washington, DC. Each office should have an employee who is the designated OSHA compliance officer and is trained and aware of all the required controls for the use and storage of such materials. All employees must have documented annual training for hazardous communications.

Each manufacturer of a product is required to provide the consumer with a **Material Safety Data Sheet (MSDS)**, which contains printed material concerning a hazardous chemical. Each MSDS offers basic information needed to ensure the safety and health of the user at all stages of manufacture, storage, use, and disposal of a hazardous chemical product.

An MSDS will provide information regarding the hazards of using the product, how to protect oneself from injury by using the appropriate **personal protective equipment (PPE)**—such as gloves, fluid-resistant lab coats, safety glasses, and a surgical mask, shield, or respirator—and what actions to take if an accidental splash or exposure occurs. Each office must have an accessible hazardous communications (HAZCOM) binder where all MSDS information is filed, and all employees must know where the binder is kept. Figure 6-2 is an example of an MSDS label that should be attached to any product that does not already have such a label.

Employee Safety

Safety is the responsibility of every member of the staff. Whereas it is imperative that the medical office provides a safe working environment, the staff must also be constantly aware of their surroundings and any possible hazards. Employees must be willing to implement all safeguards to keep themselves and patients safe.

HAZARDOUS MEDICAL WASTE

Hospitals, dental practices, veterinary clinics, laboratories, nursing homes, medical offices, and other health care facilities generate 3.2 million tons of hazardous medical waste each year. Much of this waste is potentially infectious or radioactive. Following are the four major types of medical waste:

- **Solid**—generated in many areas of medicine, including patient rooms, and surgery suites. Solid waste is not always hazardous but can cause pollution of the environment. Mandatory recycling can reduce the amount of solid waste produced.

- **Chemical**—includes substances such as germicides, cleaning solvents, and pharmaceuticals. This waste material can be a causative factor in a fire or an explosion. The safe manner with which to handle and dispose of chemicals is included in the MSDS.

- **Radioactive**—any waste that contains or is contaminated with liquid or solid radioactive material, such as Iodine 123, Iodine 131, and Thallium 201. Radioactive waste must be clearly labeled as radioactive and must be removed by a licensed facility.

- **Infectious**—any waste material that has the potential to carry disease. This includes laboratory cultures, blood and blood products from blood banks, operating rooms, emergency rooms, doctor and dentist offices, autopsy suites, and patient rooms. Infectious waste must be separated from other solid and chemical waste at the point of origin. A licensed medical waste removal agency must dispose of these materials. This is covered in more detail in the following section.

OSHA BLOODBORNE PATHOGENS STANDARDS AND UNIVERSAL PRECAUTIONS

Medical offices must follow the OSHA regulations (available from the U.S. Department of Labor in Washington, DC) for handling contaminated materials. Offices may opt to contract with a private company to provide assistance in meeting OSHA regulations. OSHA rules and regulations govern all freestanding health care providers and ensure protection from contracting a contagious disease

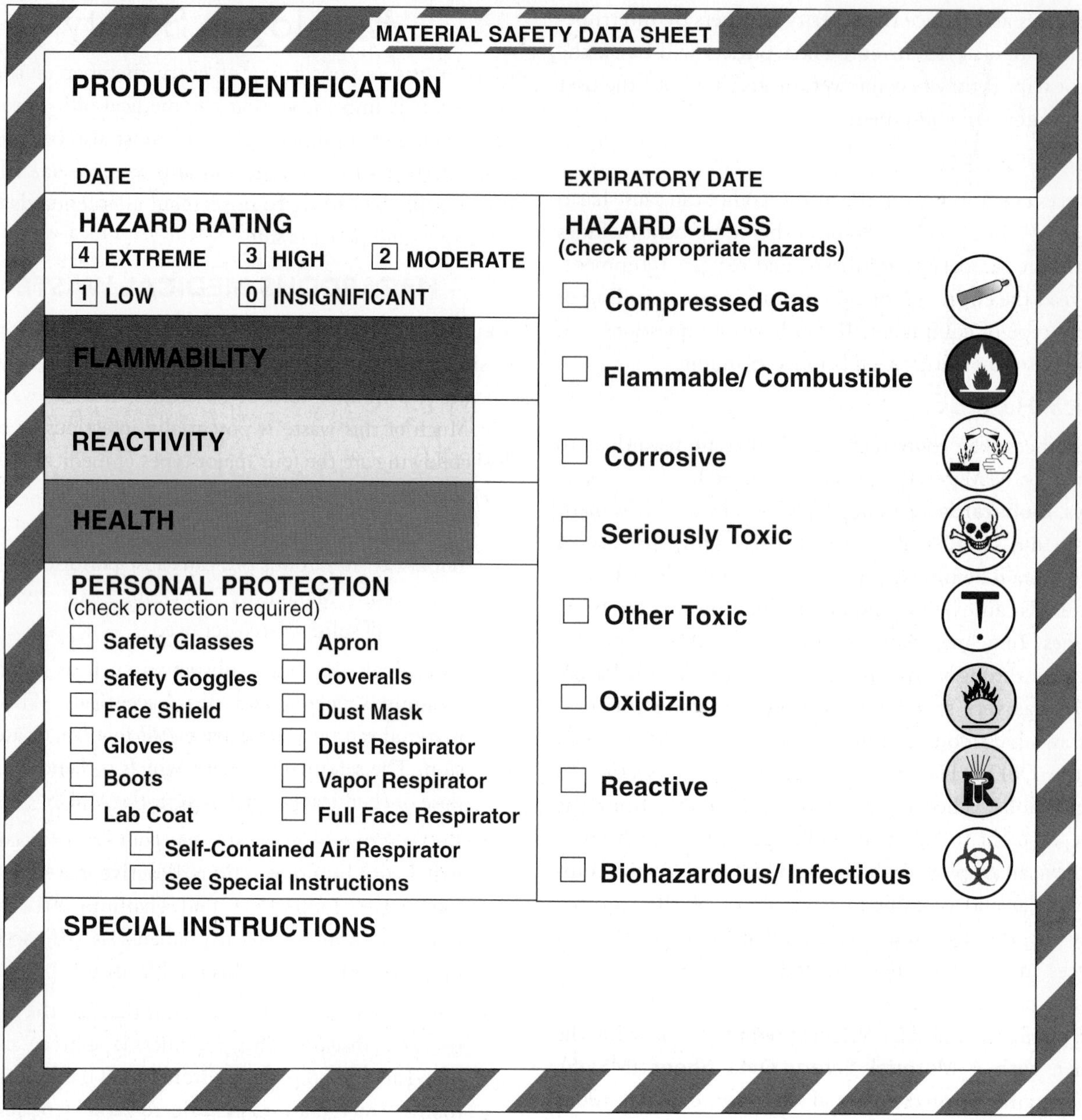
MATERIAL SAFETY DATA SHEET

PRODUCT IDENTIFICATION

DATE

EXPIRATORY DATE

HAZARD RATING

4 EXTREME 3 HIGH 2 MODERATE

1 LOW 0 INSIGNIFICANT

FLAMMABILITY

REACTIVITY

HEALTH

PERSONAL PROTECTION
(check protection required)

- ☐ Safety Glasses
- ☐ Apron
- ☐ Safety Goggles
- ☐ Coveralls
- ☐ Face Shield
- ☐ Dust Mask
- ☐ Gloves
- ☐ Dust Respirator
- ☐ Boots
- ☐ Vapor Respirator
- ☐ Lab Coat
- ☐ Full Face Respirator
- ☐ Self-Contained Air Respirator
- ☐ See Special Instructions

HAZARD CLASS
(check appropriate hazards)

- ☐ Compressed Gas
- ☐ Flammable/ Combustible
- ☐ Corrosive
- ☐ Seriously Toxic
- ☐ Other Toxic
- ☐ Oxidizing
- ☐ Reactive
- ☐ Biohazardous/ Infectious

SPECIAL INSTRUCTIONS

FIGURE 6-2 An example of a Material Safety Data Sheet (MSDS).

from any body fluids that may be handled by health care workers.

Occupational exposure is defined as a reasonable anticipation that the employee's duties may result in skin, mucous membrane, eye, or parenteral (for example, assisting with blood work) contact with infectious material. Every employee who has the possibility of occupational exposure to potentially infectious materials must adhere to the OSHA standards. Examples of employees at risk are physicians, nurses, laboratory workers, medical assistants, dental assistants, and, in some cases, housekeeping personnel. The OSHA standards mandate that each at-risk employee must be offered the hepatitis B (HBV) vaccine series within the first ten days of employment and at the expense of the employer. If an employee refuses the vaccine, he or she must sign a waiver. OSHA defines the following as body fluids:

- Blood
- Semen
- Amniotic fluid
- Cerebrospinal fluid
- Synovial fluid
- Vaginal secretions
- Pleural fluid
- Pericardial fluid

The best ways to prevent exposure to bloodborne pathogens are wearing PPE when applicable, and complying strictly with

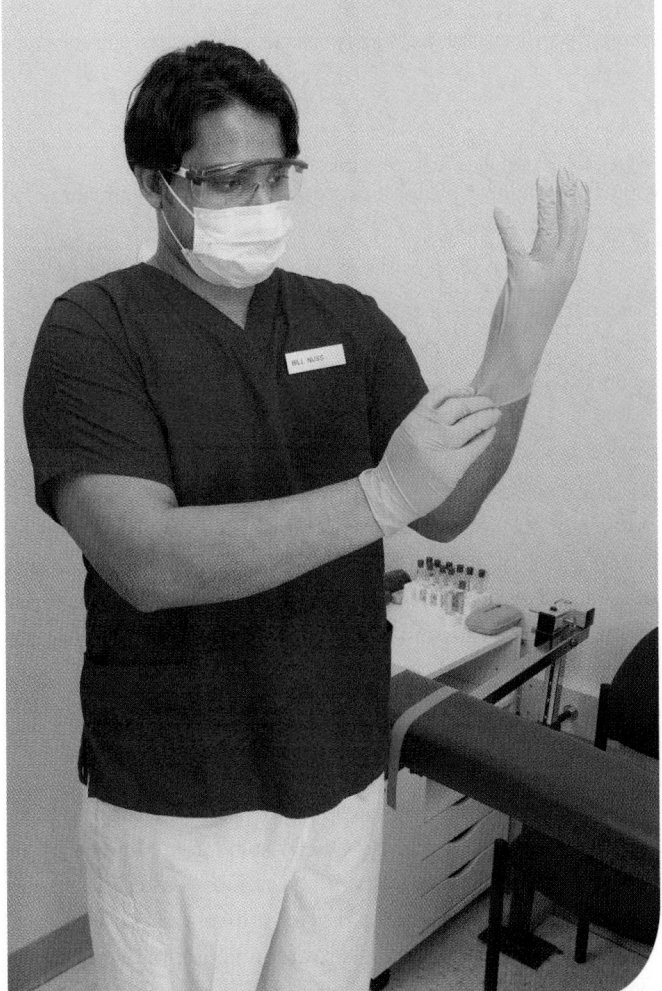

FIGURE 6-3 PPE used to prevent exposure to bloodborne pathogens.

THE LAW

The employer has the responsibility, according to OSHA guidelines, to protect each employee from infectious disease. The medical assistant has a responsibility to correctly follow OSHA guidelines for self-protection and to protect other employees and patients.

The medical assistant has a duty to report any incident, such as the accidental administration of medication to a patient, a patient fall or injury, or theft.

hepatitis B vaccine series or a waiver signed by the employee within ten days of initial employment, as well as a copy of any exposure incident reports. These records must be confidential and kept under lock and key.

Universal Precautions

The U.S. Centers for Disease Prevention and Control (CDC) in Atlanta issued recommendations for protection of health care workers. These became known as the universal precautions. According to universal precautions, all blood and body fluids should be treated as if they were contaminated with any bloodborne pathogen. The most commonly noted diseases related to bloodborne exposure are HIV and HBV. PPE used to fulfill the recommendations includes gloves, protective eyewear, masks, and fluid-resistant lab coats. Figure 6-3 shows a medical assistant applying PPE. Table 6-1 describes what protective clothing is appropriate, and Guidelines 6-2 lists details in the

hand hygiene protocol. All PPE must be provided by the employer and readily available for use. OSHA requires that each medical office have a written Exposure Control Plan to assist in minimizing employee exposure to infectious materials. This plan must be reviewed by all office staff and updated annually. An Exposure Control Plan must include the following:

- **Exposure Determination**—listing of job classifications within the office to determine at-risk employees (those with potential exposure to infectious materials).

- **Method of Compliance**—specific measures to reduce the risk of exposure.

- **Post-Exposure**—evaluation and follow-up, which specify the steps to follow when an exposure incident occurs.

A record for each employee must be kept on file for 30 years after the termination of employment. The record includes documentation of the employee's annual review of the Exposure Control Plan for the facility. In addition, the record must contain information regarding the administration of

GUIDELINES 6-2

OSHA GUIDELINES FOR USING PERSONAL PROTECTIVE EQUIPMENT AND CLOTHING

- The employer must supply the protective clothing and provide cleaning or disposal of it.
- The clothing or other equipment must be strong enough to act as a barrier to infectious materials that might reach the employee's street clothing, work clothing, eyes, mouth, or skin.
- Disposable gloves may not be reused.
- Protective eye equipment must have solid sides to prevent infectious material from entering the eye area from the side.
- All equipment and clothing must be removed and placed in a designated container before leaving the medical office.

TABLE 6-1 Personal Protective Equipment (PPE) and Clothing

Clothing and Equipment	When Used
Gloves	Anticipate contact with blood, infectious material, open wounds, or broken skin on hands. Examples: venipuncture, capillary stick, wound care, injections, minor surgery, cleaning contaminated equipment, such as contaminated surfaces of thermometers
Mask	Anticipate spray with blood or infectious materials. Often used with eye shields.
Eye/Face Shield	Anticipate spray with infectious materials, droplets of blood, or other infectious matter. Example: performing blood smear
Gowns, Lab Coats	Anticipate gross contamination of clothing during a procedure. Examples: minor surgery, laboratory procedures

use of PPE and clothing. In addition, the MSDS will contain information regarding PPE. In 1996, the CDC issued more complete guidelines known as standard precautions. These guidelines are discussed more fully in Chapter 34.

If infectious material has been spilled, proper procedures must be followed in the cleanup. A spill kit should be used. See Figure 6-4 for an example of a commercial spill kit. Commercial kits are available but a simple kit can be assembled with the following equipment:

- Plain clay kitty litter
- A small dust pan
- A biohazard bag

The kitty litter is used as a drying agent to allow sweep-up of the material without spreading it. The material should then be placed in a biohazard bag and disposed of properly with other biohazardous waste.

Most offices contract with outside vendors to pick up, transport, and dispose of biohazardous waste. Typically, the amount paid to the vendor is based on the total weight. From a cost perspective, this is one of the reasons why it is important for waste that is not considered biohazardous to be disposed of in regular trash receptacles. Placing items that have been used but are not soiled, such as used paper gowns or dry exam table paper, in the biohazardous waste container is frowned on.

HOUSEKEEPING SAFETY

All members of the housekeeping department must receive careful instruction regarding OSHA standards. Housekeeping personnel should not empty biohazardous waste and sharps containers. They only empty office trash containers. However, since housekeeping personnel are around potentially infectious materials, they must receive training. If the office contracts with an outside agency for housekeeping duties, the contract should state that all of the agency's employees should be trained in bloodborne pathogen standards and universal precautions. The medical office is then not required to train the personnel.

Proper storage of all chemical products is essential for the safety of employees and the patients. Figure 6-5 shows examples of waste and hazard containers that may be used, and

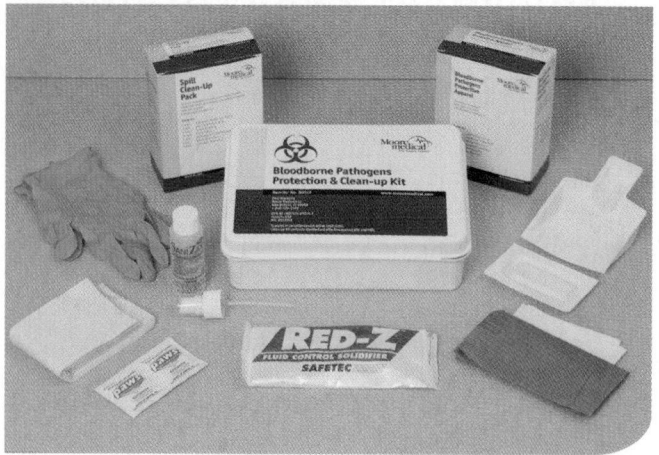

FIGURE 6-4 An example of a commercial spill kit.

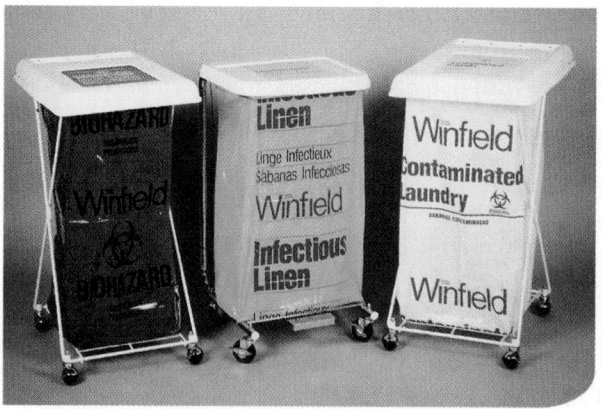

FIGURE 6-5 Examples of waste and hazard containers.

Procedure 6-2 provides information regarding housekeeping using OSHA guidelines.

Proper Body Mechanics

Ergonomics applies scientific information and data regarding human body mechanics to the design of objects and overall environments for human use. Whereas OSHA abandoned the ergonomic portion of regulations, proper **body mechanics**—coordination of body alignment, balance, and movement—should still be part of the medical assistant's training.

Medical assistants move, lift, and carry many things, including equipment, supplies, and even patients. Correct methods of standing and lifting objects will help prevent pain and injury. Table 6-2 describes the principles of proper body mechanics and provides a demonstration of proper lifting techniques.

procedure
6-2

HOUSEKEEPING USING OSHA GUIDELINES
Objective: Safely clean and disinfect contaminated surfaces

EQUIPMENT AND SUPPLIES
prepared spill kit; gloves; 1:10 bleach/water solution; dustpan; broom; sharps container; biohazard bag or container

1. Prior to performing any housekeeping procedures, the employee should ensure the appropriate PPE has been applied (Figure 6-6).
2. For any wet spills, use the prepared spill kit according to package directions.
3. Immediately after exposure to infectious materials, clean and disinfect contaminated surfaces with a 1:10 bleach/water solution. All surfaces must be decontaminated on a regular schedule. This schedule must be posted, signed by the person who performs the decontamination, and kept with OSHA records.
4. Properly bag contaminated clothing and laundry in leakproof labeled biohazard bags. Contaminated laundry should not be handled or washed at the medical office or with any uncontaminated clothing.
5. Replace a damaged biohazard bag by placing a second bag around the first. Do not remove infectious material from the damaged bag.
6. Biohazardous waste must be removed by a licensed waste disposal service and incinerated or autoclaved before it is placed in a designated landfill area.
7. Use puncture-proof, sealable, biohazard sharps containers for all needles and sharps, such as razors and glass pipettes.
8. Place each sharps container close to the work area, and ensure that each container remains upright.
9. Replace a sharps container when it is two-thirds full.
10. Seal and label each sharps container before placing it with the biohazardous waste for removal by the disposal service.
11. In the event of broken glass, use a dustpan or other mechanical device, such as a hemostat or another type of forceps, to pick it up. Never pick up broken glass with hands.
12. Properly dispose of any PPE used during housekeeping. Failure to do so may result in an OSHA citation.
13. Perform hand hygiene both before and after using gloves.

CHARTING EXAMPLE
6/23/XX 5:50 P.M. All examination room surfaces, including exam tables, chairs, writing surfaces, sink, countertop, and door handles, disinfected with 1:10 bleach/water solution. · · · · · · · · · · ·
· T Moreland, RMA
6/24/XX 6:10 P.M. All examination room surfaces, including exam tables, chairs, writing surfaces, sink, countertop, and door handles disinfected with 1:10 bleach/water solution. · · · · · · · · · · · · ·
· D Joyner, CMA (AAMA)

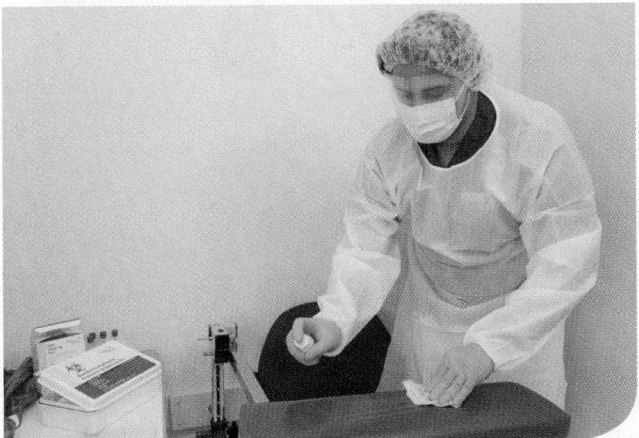

FIGURE 6-6   PPE used during spill clean-up.

TABLE 6-2 Principles of Proper Body Mechanics

Movement	Description
Stoop	• Do not bend from your back. • Stand close to the object you are moving. • Keep your feet 6 to 8 inches apart to create a base of support. • Place one foot slightly ahead of the other. • Bend at the hips and knees, keeping the back straight, and lower the body and hands down to the object (Figure 6-7). • Use the large leg muscles to assist in returning to a standing position (Figure 6-8).
Lift firmly and smoothly	• If you think you cannot move a heavy or awkward load, get help. • Grasp the load by using the large leg muscles. • Keep the load close to the body.
Use the center of gravity for carrying a load	• Keep your back as straight as possible. (Hint: You should not be able to feel your clothing touch your back if you are standing straight.) • Keep the weight of the load close to your body and centered over the hips. • Put the load down by bending at the hips and knees. • When two or more people carry the load, have one person give the commands to lift or move the object.
Pull or push (rather than lift or load)	• Remain close to the object you are moving. • Keep feet apart with one slightly forward. • Have a firm grasp on the object. • If the object is on the floor, crouch down with feet apart. • Bend your elbows, and place hands on the load at chest level. • Keep your back straight. • Push up with your legs in order to stand up with the load.
Avoid reaching	• Evaluate the distance before reaching too far for an object. • Stand close to the object. • Do not reach to the point of straining. • To change direction, point your feet in the direction you wish to go. • Keep the object close to your body as you lower it.
Avoid twisting	• Do not twist your body.

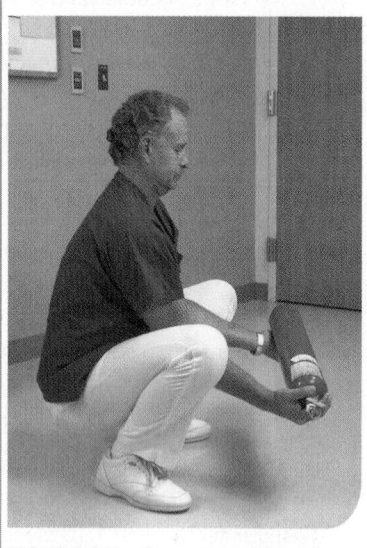

FIGURE 6-7 Correct position when lifting a heavy object off the floor.

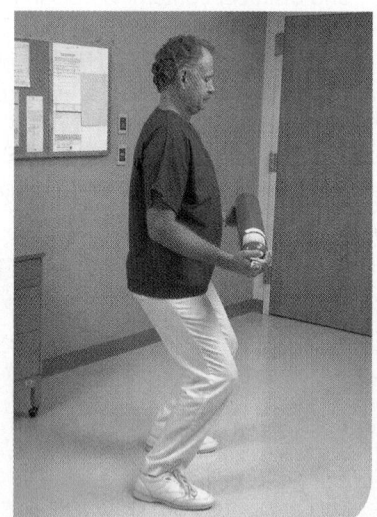

FIGURE 6-8 Use strong leg muscles, keeping back straight, when lifting.

ERGONOMICS

In the medical setting, ergonomics applies to all aspects of the facility. The most common area for problems is the computer workstation. The keyboard should be at elbow height, the monitor at eye level, and the chair adjustable, with a lumbar support. The operator's feet should rest on the floor comfortably, with no strain. A wrist rest and mouse wrist support should be used.

Lighting should be appropriate for the task. Overhead fluorescent lights should not reflect on the computer monitor screens, causing a glare. This can be prevented by adding an antiglare shield to the monitor or tilting the screen so that the light does not hit it directly. Clinical areas should be well lit. Repetitive motions should be limited, and the proper tools should be available for any procedure.

Office Security

Security issues in a physician's office are unique. Medical offices make an attractive target for a thief or addict looking for drugs. Doors and windows must be outfitted with secure locks. Depending on the opening and closing procedures of the office, every employee or only a few authorized personnel may have keys to the office. No matter how many keys have been authorized, when a key is reported as missing all locks must be changed.

Many offices have electronic security systems that are activated when the last person leaves the office and deactivated when the first person arrives at the office. To activate and deactivate the security system, a predetermined code must be entered into the system. When the first employee enters the building in the morning, an alarm will be activated at the security system company's office if the code is not properly entered within a specified number of seconds. The company will, in turn, alert the appropriate agency, such as fire or police. Depending on the system, an alarm may or may not sound within the building as well.

Security procedures should be implemented during the workday, too, taking into account the need to secure patients and staff, patient medical records, computer stations, medical supplies, and, particularly, prescription pads, from intruders and disorderly persons. Health Insurance Portability and Accountability Act (HIPAA) has raised awareness of many security issues regarding the privacy of each patient's personal medical history. It is every employee's responsibility to be vigilant when it comes to office safety.

If someone is acting suspiciously or demanding money or drugs, it is important to make mental note of such identifying characteristics as the individual's height, weight, facial hair, race, accent, tattoos, and scars. If possible, record this information so you will not be relying solely on memory if you are asked to describe the individual. Immediately report any suspicious concerns to the physician or office manager.

INCIDENT REPORTS

Any unusual occurrence or accident is referred to as an incident in the medical setting. Following are some examples of incidents:

- A patient falls on a wet floor.
- A housekeeping employee is stuck by a needle while emptying the trash.
- A prescription pad is missing.
- A patient receives the wrong medication.
- While in the office, a patient misplaces or loses personal property, such as a hearing aid or eyeglasses.
- Syringes or needles are found to be missing from the supply cupboard.
- A medical assistant receives a needlestick from a contaminated needle.
- An employee's purse is missing.
- A patient is abusive and uses vulgar language.

Whenever any accident, injury, or unusual occurrence takes place, the employee should immediately notify the supervisor. This is especially important if a needlestick accident is involved because time is of the essence when drawing appropriate baseline blood specimens. The supervisor also will require the employee to complete a written report immediately. This is called the **incident report** and should be completed in black ink. An incident report can protect both the employer and the medical assistant against possible lawsuits. Some incidents should also be reported to either the police or to the liability insurance carrier. For example, stolen property should be reported to the police, and a slip and fall should be reported to the insurance carrier. The incident should be described as simply as possible, stating only facts and not opinions. Keep in mind that the incident report may be used as a legal document; thus only objective information should be included, such as "Patient fell while getting onto exam table." Do not include subjective comments, such as "Patient was not paying attention to what he was doing."

Medical offices should have their own customized forms. However, most incident reports include the following information:

- Names of all persons involved
- Date and time of the incident

INCIDENT REPORT

Name of injured party ______________________ Date __________

Address ______________________ Telephone __________

____

The injured party was: ☐ Employee ☐ Patient ☐ Other __________

Date of accident/incident __________ Time of incident __________

Where did incident occur? ______________________

Names of witnesses (include titles):

______________________ ______________________

______________________ ______________________

What first aid/treatment was given at the time of the incident?

____

____

Who administered first aid? ______________________

Briefly describe the incident. ______________________

____

____

____

____

Names of employees present at time of incident/injury:

____

What, in your opinion, caused the accident? ______________________

____

Follow-up: What steps have been taken to prevent a similar accident? __________

____

____

__________ ______________________

Date Employee's signature

__________ ______________________

Date Supervisor's signature

FIGURE 6-9 An example of a typical incident report.

- Exact location of the incident (including the address of the medical facility and the location of the incident within the facility)
- Name of the person to whom the incident is reported
- Time of the report
- Brief description of what happened
- Names of all witnesses
- Name and description of any equipment involved in the incident
- Action taken at the time of the incident
- Action taken to prevent a recurrence
- Signature and title of the person completing the report

The incident report, like all other information relating to the patient, is subject to subpoena in litigation (lawsuits). A copy of the incident report should be placed in a master incident report file, the patient's file, and the employee's record. Figure 6-9 is an example of an incident report form.

Quality Medical Care

Quality medical care is an expectation of all patients and requires that the health care team use procedures and techniques that result in the best possible outcome for the patient. In addition, patients must be satisfied with the care and treatment they receive from everyone in the office.

The major parameters or attributes of health care that are regularly examined include treatment, outcome, cost/benefit, accessibility, and delivery location. The outcome factor actually requires a measurable change in the health status of the patient that is a direct result of the care received. Cost/benefit refers to the expenditure or cost in terms of time, money, and effort, along with the relationship of this cost to the actual benefit the patient receives. Accessibility to health care refers to the effort a patient must make to receive health care. The American Medical Association (AMA) has defined eight essential elements of quality care (Box 6-1).

What Is Quality Assurance?

In the early 1960s, the health care industry began to feel an increasing demand from the public for accountability regarding quality care. From that initial swell of public pressure developed a continuing effort on the part of health care providers to deliver satisfactory, achievable excellence in care. **Quality assurance (QA)** is the process of gathering and evaluating information about the services provided (as well as the results achieved) and comparing this information with an accepted standard typically referred to as a benchmark. Benchmarks may apply at a local, state, or national standard level.

Quality assessment measures consist of formal, systematic evaluations of overall patterns of care. The goal of the actual programs and activities of quality assurance have a

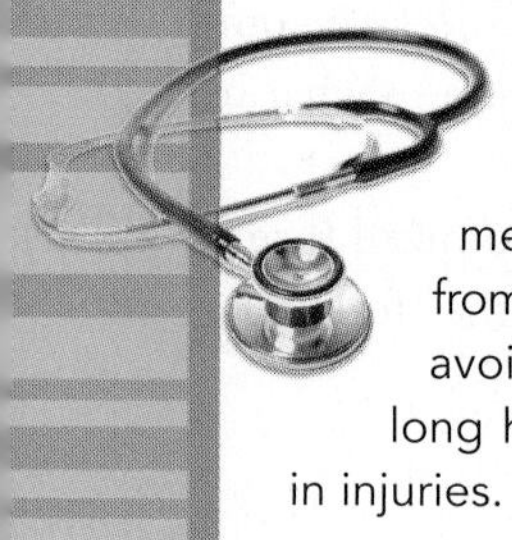

PROFESSIONALISM

Maintaining a professional demeanor in the medical office can prevent many incidents from occurring. Wearing the appropriate apparel, avoiding excessive jewelry, and pulling back long hair can eliminate hazards that might result in injuries.

desired degree of care in a health care setting. The results of the evaluations are then compared to standard results. As deficiencies are identified, recommendations for improvement in care are made. Quality improvement programs (QIPs) utilize the data gathered by quality assurance and assessment to make quality improvements in health care.

QUALITY ASSURANCE PROGRAM

A quality assurance program (QAP) in a hospital, ambulatory health care setting, long-term-care facility, or health maintenance organization (HMO) consists of a system for reviewing records maintained by staff. These records may consist of medical or nursing records, data regarding days of hospitalization or treatment, progress reports, and other statistics that provide a firm indication of the care received by patients. A quality assurance program must include evaluation and educational components to identify and correct problems. Quality assurance programs such as these are required in order for the facility to receive funding by the Public Health Service Act (which defines the requirements) as well as to achieve and maintain accreditation. The basic components of a quality assurance program include the following:

- Establish a QA committee. Representatives from the entire patient care team (such as physician, nurse, and medical assistant) should be part of a QA committee (Figure 6-10).
- Review all clinical and administrative services and procedures. Committee members or an assigned individual can conduct the review. All team members should have a role in the QA process, from designing the QA forms to selecting issues for review. Policies and procedures manuals are also subject to review during this process.

- Set up a structure for identifying items to review. Pay particular attention to problem issues.
- Quantify all issues, for example:
  - –average length of waiting time in minutes to see the physician
  - –number of errors in writing items on patient records
  - –number of insurance claims disallowed per 100 filed
  - –number of failed venipunctures per 50 attempts
- Limit the number of issues. Set a limit to the number of issues or problems reviewed at any one session. Place emphasis on taking corrective measures.
- Maintain careful records. Review all records, such as incident reports and committee records, and progress or improvement with the entire medical team.

Box 6-2 lists examples of issues that a QA committee might review in a physician's office.

IMPLEMENTING A QUALITY ASSURANCE PROGRAM

The ultimate goal of a formal QAP is to improve the quality of care so that there is no difference between what should be

Box 6-1 The AMA's Eight Essentials of Quality CARE

- Bring about the optimal in the patient's condition within the earliest time frame possible based on the patient's comfort and physical condition.
- Have an emphasis on early detection and treatment as well as health promotion and disease prevention.
- Receive treatment in a timely fashion without unnecessary delay, termination, interruption, or prolongation.
- Encourage the patient's participation in the decision process regarding his or her treatment.

- Base the treatment on skillful use of technology and the health professional's use of accepted principles of medical science.
- Demonstrate concern for the patient and the patient's family, with sensitivity to the stress caused by illness.
- Achieve the treatment goal through the wise use of technology and other resources.
- Provide adequate documentation in the patient's medical record to facilitate peer evaluation and continuity of care.

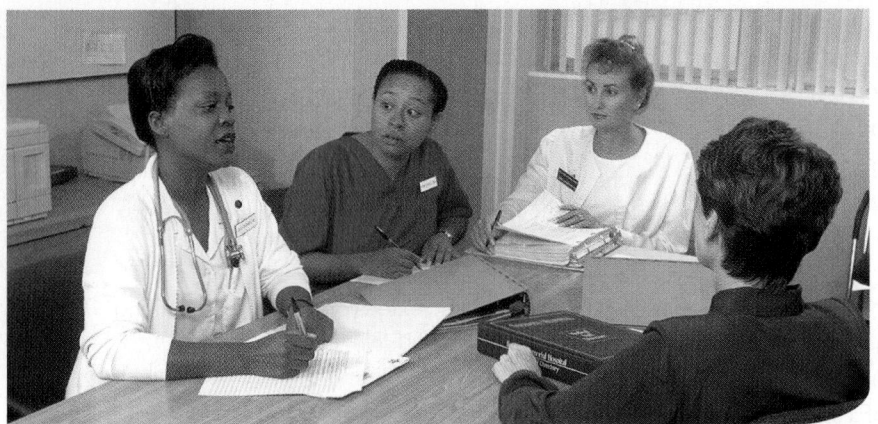

FIGURE 6-10 A quality assurance (QA) committee meeting.

process. If for some reason the discharge plan was overlooked and not provided for the patient, that particular patient would "fall out" in that performance measure and be counted against the facility in the overall percentage.

MEDICAL ASSISTANT'S ROLE IN A QAP

The medical assistant is trained in clinical and administrative skills with the expectation for the highest level of performance. To assist the physician/employer, the medical assistant should pay rigorous attention to the quality of care given to patients. Patient satisfaction is a key element in quality of care. The medical assistant may be the first and last person to respond to a patient's complaint or discomfort. Medical assistants have the opportunity to present patients' concerns or complaints at a team QA meeting so that corrective measures can be taken (Figure 6-11). Some of the areas in which the medical assistant may assist the physician with quality assurance are noted in Box 6-3.

done and what is being done. Professionals in the field who are experts in a particular health care area develop these norms or standards.

Putting a QAP into place requires the development of patient-centered criteria based on acceptable standards of care. Criteria are standards used to compare something in order to make a decision. For example, years ago some patients were discharged from a hospital without being given any formal information or education about what to do when they returned home. Now all hospitalized patients should receive instructions at discharge regarding medications, diet, activity, and follow-up appointments with the physician. This discharge plan is explained to the patient, who then signs the plan and keeps a copy. A copy of the signed plan is also put in the patient's chart, indicating that this instruction took place. A QAP would monitor the discharge planning

HEALTH PLAN EMPLOYER DATA AND INFORMATION SET

Under Health Plan Employer Data and Information Set (HEDIS), managed care plans that serve Medicare patients must collect data relating to eight categories of performance:

- Effectiveness of care
- Access to and availability of care

Box 6-2 Issues Reviewed by a Quality Assurance Committee in a Physician's OFFICE

- Disallowed insurance claims
- Errors in dispensing medications (use incident reports)
- Errors in labeling of laboratory specimens
- Incorrect coding of diagnosis for insurance claims
- Long waiting time for patients
- Adverse reactions to treatments and/or medications (use incident reports)
- Inability to obtain venous blood on the first attempt
- Patient satisfaction (from survey or questionnaire results)
- Patients who leave the office without seeing the physician
- Patient complaints relating to confidentiality
- Appearance of the office

- Handicapped parking availability
- Safety
- Provider availability
- Emergency preparations
- Treatment areas
- Safety and monitoring practices for radiology and laboratory
- Medications
- Infection control
- Patient education/rights
- Medical records
- Collection procedures
- Telephone and reception behaviors

- Member satisfaction
- Informed health care choices
- Health plan descriptive information
- Cost of care
- Health plan stability
- Use of service

Medicare, HMOs, and other plans seeking accreditation from the **National Committee for Quality Assurance (NCQA)**, must also report data. The NCQA evaluates the quality of health plans in order to help consumers and employers make more informed decisions about their health care. Eventually, most of the health plans (HMOs and preferred provider organizations [PPOs]) with which a physician contracts with will be collecting data for the medical practice.

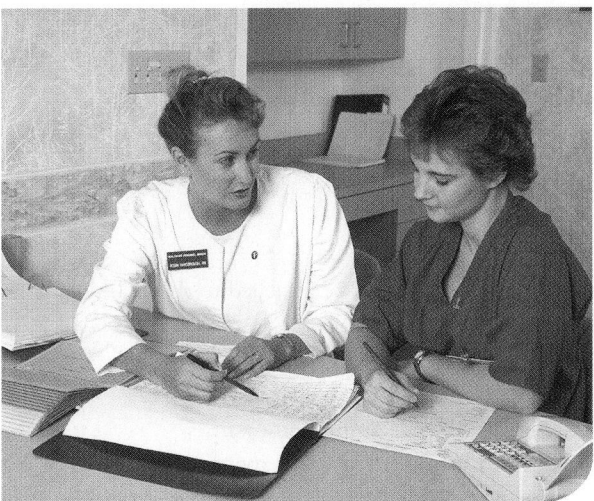

FIGURE 6-11 A medical assistant at a QA meeting.

CLINICAL LABORATORY IMPROVEMENT AMENDMENT

The federal government now requires that all clinical laboratories that test human specimens must be controlled. The Clinical Laboratories Improvement Amendment of 1988 (CLIA 1988) divides laboratories into three categories. These are described in Table 6-3. Refer to Chapter 44 for further discussion of the CLIA, which mandates quality control of laboratory tests by categories and documentation.

TABLE 6-3 Clinical Laboratory Improvement Amendment (CLIA)

Category	Explanation
Simple Testing	Incorrect test results pose little risk for the patient. Laboratory is subject to random inspectors only. Some physicians' laboratories fall in this category.
Intermediate-Level Testing (Level II)	Poses risk to patient if there is an incorrect test result. Must be certified by approved accrediting agency. Must be staffed by credentialed personnel. Must meet quality assurance standards.
Complex Testing (Level III)	Poses high risk to patient if there is an incorrect test result. Must be certified by approved accrediting agency. Must be staffed by credentialed personnel. Must meet quality assurance standards.

SUMMARY

Safety measures are an important aspect of the medical office for keeping patients and employees safe. These safety measures include general safety, employee safety, emergency plans (such as for fire, tornado, hurricane, etc.), and the handling of biological hazards and bloodborne pathogens.

Proper housekeeping procedures using OSHA guidelines, proper body mechanics, and office security are essential to maintaining a safe and pleasant workplace. The efforts of a medical assistant can be critical in ensuring that all these components are carefully regarded.

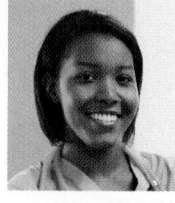

6 CHAPTER REVIEW

COMPETENCY REVIEW

1. Define and spell the terms to learn for this chapter.

2. List six safety rules to follow in medical offices.

3. You have been asked to draft the OSHA Exposure Control Plan for your office. What three points must you include in this plan?

PREPARING FOR THE CERTIFICATION EXAM

1. What acronym is frequently used in the event of a fire in the office?
   a. PASS
   b. RACE
   c. PPE
   d. GFCI
   e. HAZCOM

2. All of the following are safety measures except:
   a. always walk on the left side of the hallway.
   b. never carry uncapped syringes between exam rooms.
   c. open toe and open heel shoes are not recommended in the medical office.
   d. no eating or drinking in the medical office except in designated areas.
   e. floors should be clean but not highly polished.

3. Which of the following is typically used in wet areas such as near sinks?
   a. PASS
   b. RACE
   c. PPE
   d. GFCI
   e. HAZCOM

4. All of the following should be in place in the event of a fire except:
   a. fireproof file cabinets.
   b. exits clearly marked.

   c. diagram of all exits posted near fire extinguishers.
   d. fire extinguishers that have been maintained with annual maintenance checks.
   e. telephone numbers of fire and police departments.

5. All of the following are examples of PPE except:
   a. goggles.
   b. respirator.
   c. protective gloves.
   d. absorbent lab coat.
   e. surgical mask.

6. All of the following are major types of medical waste except:
   a. solid.
   b. infectious.
   c. chemical.
   d. radioactive.
   e. biohazardous.

7. Fire extinguishers should be attached to the wall no more than
   a. 70 feet from an employee area.
   b. 75 feet from an employee area.
   c. 70 feet from an examination room.
   d. 75 feet from an examination room.
   e. 75 feet from the reception area.

8. The governmental agency responsible for the safety of all employees operating in the United States is:
   a. PASS.
   b. CLIA.
   c. OSHA.
   d. HIPAA.
   e. OIG.

9. All of the following are considered sources of potential infectious material except:
   a. sweat.
   b. semen.

c. cerebrospinal fluid.
d. amniotic fluid.
e. pericardial fluid.

10. To help prevent an accidental needlestick, the sharps container should be replaced when it is:
    a. half full.
    b. two-thirds full.
    c. three-quarters full.
    d. three-fifths full.
    e. completely full.

CRITICAL THINKING

1. What errors did Susan make in preparing the injection?

2. What tests must be performed as a result of this needlestick?

3. Is Linda responsible for anything in this situation?

4. How would this pertain to OSHA's Bloodborne Pathogens Standards?

ON THE JOB

Bonnie feels that the office is always too cold, so she keeps a heater under her desk. To use the heater, she must run an extension cord across to another electrical outlet. Several times, the safety officer in the practice asks her to discontinue using the heater. Bonnie will put the heater away for a couple of days, then bring it back out when she feels it will not be noticed. The safety officer comes by one day and confiscates the heater and extension cord. Bonnie feels that this is unfair because she is cold during the day. She thinks she should be allowed to use the heater, which allows her to perform her duties in comfort and more efficiently.

1. What OSHA violations are of concern in this situation?
2. Did the safety officer handle the situation correctly the first few times?
3. Did the safety officer have the right to confiscate the heater and extension cord?
4. How might the situation be rectified to make Bonnie comfortable?

INTERNET ACTIVITY

Search the Internet to find private companies that are in business to provide services to help prepare an office to meet OSHA requirements.

MEDMEDIA

Additional interactive resources and activities for this chapter can be found:

On your student DVD: View applicable procedure videos on the DVD-ROM found in the back of this book.

MyHealthProfessionsKit.com: Test your knowledge of the chapter with games and activities. MyHealthProfessionsKit also includes resources, helpful links, and a Spanish audio glossary.

Medical Assisting Interactive: Practice your procedures as a medical assistant in this simulated doctor's office. This can be accessed through MyHealthProfessionsKit.com.

7

Telephone Techniques

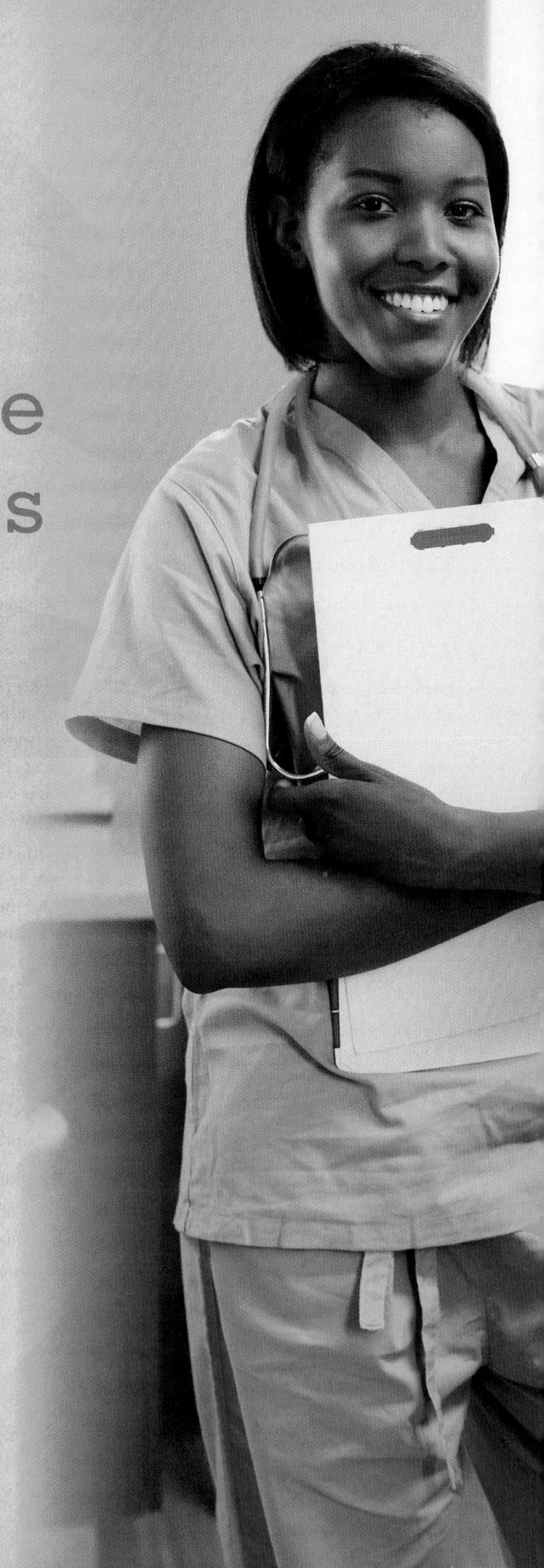

LEARNING OBJECTIVES

After completing this chapter, you should be able to:

- Define and spell the terms to learn for this chapter.

- Answer the telephone in a professional manner with a proper greeting and pleasant tone.

- Use the hold function effectively and professionally.

- Take detailed and efficient telephone messages.

- Adhere to HIPAA guidelines while placing telephone calls to patients.

- Describe telephone triage and how it is used in the medical office.

- Handle difficult callers.

- Place long distance calls and conference calls.

- Handle emergency phone calls.

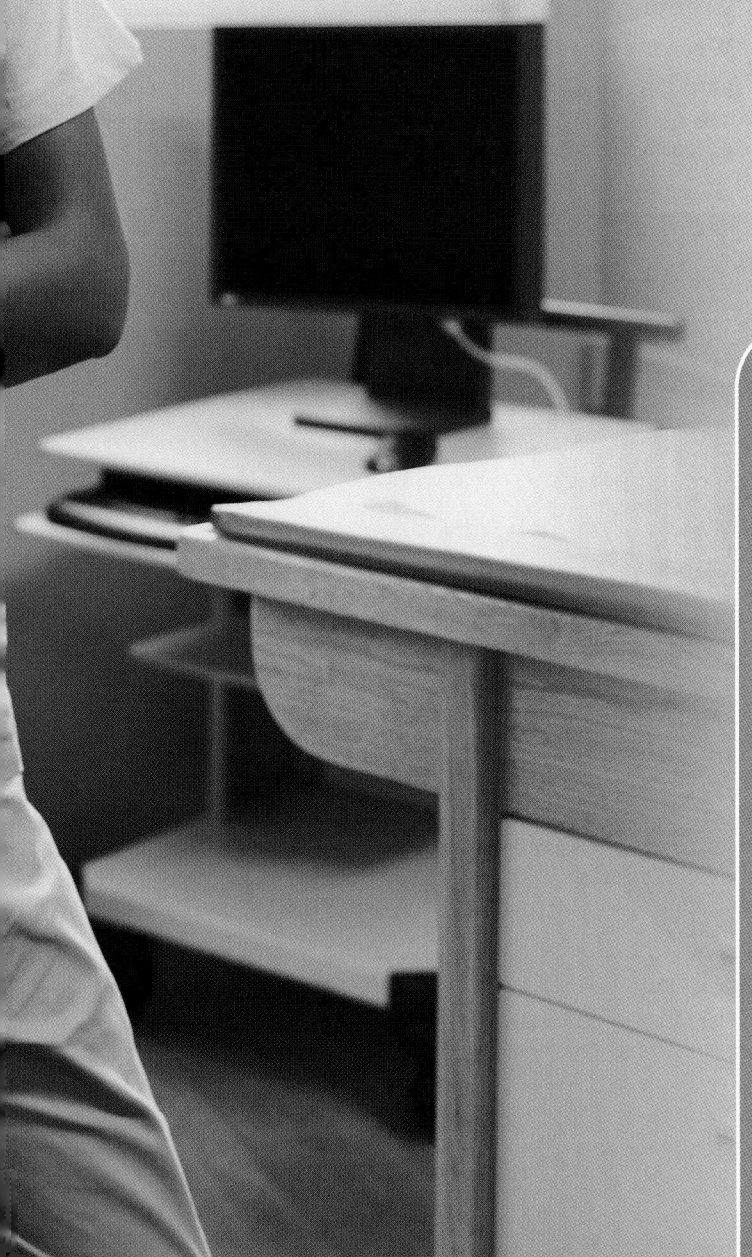

CHAPTER OUTLINE

CASE STUDY

Carmine DiStefano has been looking for a new physician. He has decided to try Pearson Physicians Group since the practice is near his office. When Carmine calls the office to set up an appointment, he is first greeted by an answering system. After he has been given many options, he decides to dial "2" to schedule an appointment. Carmine then waits as the system transfers him to the appropriate person. When the transfer is done, he is greeted by Tonya, a new medical assistant with the practice. Tonya greets Carmine by saying "Good afternoon. Pearson Physicians Group. This is Tonya. How may I help you?" Although Carmine is left with a cold feeling because he detects an insincere tone in Tonya's voice, he decides to go ahead and schedule an appointment. Tonya then tells Carmine to hold. When she finally returns after more than 2 minutes Tonya does not give Carmine a reason for the wait; nor does she offer an apology. Carmine is rather frustrated and informs Tonya that he will seek services from another physician.

The telephone is one the most vital tools used within the medical office. In addition, both the person answering the telephone and the communication used can "make or break" the practice. We have all been at the receiving end of poor telephone etiquette at one point or another. The key within the medical office is to ensure that every telephone encounter is efficient, accurate, and professional. Many times the patient's first impression of the office will be based on the initial interaction with the individual who answers the telephone. Attention to detail is required when answering the telephone, especially when taking messages or requests for prescription refills. Transposing one or two letters or numbers regarding a prescription can cause disastrous results.

Telephone Techniques

If you work in the front office area, much of your day will be spent on the telephone. A fundamental rule to remember when answering your medical office's telephone is that you are not answering a home telephone. The telephone techniques used when speaking on home telephones are generally more informal and chatty than the style of conversation that is expected in a medical office. It is inappropriate to answer the office line with personal greetings, such as

"Hello" or "Hi." Most offices will provide a script for you to follow when answering the telephone. A professional persona and voice must always be presented to your callers.

ANSWERING THE TELEPHONE

Your manner of answering the telephone frequently determines how the conversation will flow. It is also the first impression that callers, including potential new patients, receive of your office. The following are some important techniques that will assist you in answering your medical office's telephone in the most professional manner.

Smiling

Always answer the telephone with a smile. A human voice has so many nuances that most callers will often be able to sense the warmth or indifference in your voice. Until you can become comfortable with smiling when answering the telephone, you may want to look in a mirror as you answer. This will allow you to observe yourself and your facial expressions as you speak (see Figure 7-1).

Greetings

When the telephone rings in the medical office, it is important that it be answered quickly, generally by the third ring. The medical office supervisor will teach you the office's preferred method of answering the telephone. An appropriate greeting would include the following:

- The name of the office or the physician
- Your name
- Asking the caller how you can be of assistance

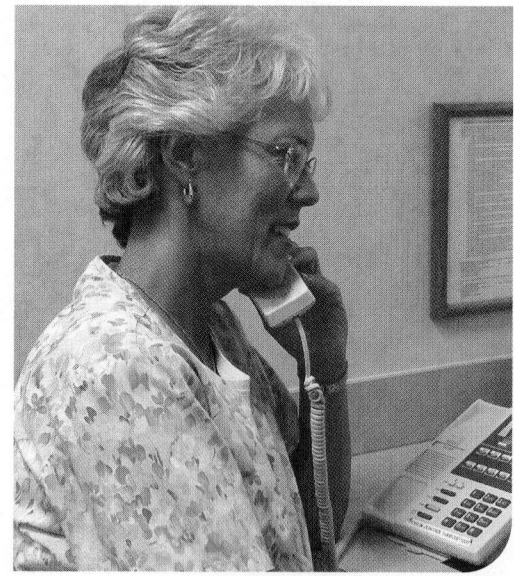

FIGURE 7-1 A pleasant smile can go a long way, even through telephone lines.

A greeting such as this will make the patient more comfortable in contacting your office. An example of a typical office greeting might be "Good morning. Main Street Physicians. This is Jessica. How may I help you?"

Speech

Many times we do not consider the importance of speaking clearly when on the telephone. However, speaking clearly is a key element in communicating effectively with patients. Four elements of speech are commonly evaluated: clarity, enunciation, inflection, and pitch.

Clarity refers to the quality or state of being understandable. How clear is your voice to the caller? Are you holding the telephone receiver 1 to 2 inches from your mouth so that the best sound gets through to the caller? Many people tend to drop the receiver so that it sits just below the chin. This does not produce clear sound for the person on the other end of the telephone. The telephone handset should be held in the middle, with the receiver to your ear and the mouthpiece 1 to 2 inches from your mouth. You also must have nothing in your mouth—no gum, candy, food, and so on—that could garble your words.

Enunciation refers to the clear articulation and pronouncement of words. Being careful not to speak too rapidly will help with word enunciation. Because you may use the same greeting and phrase repeatedly to answer the telephone, it is easy to fall into the habit of speaking too quickly. Slow down and pronounce your words slowly and properly. Correct pronunciation will help minimize confusion for the caller. See Table 7-1 for examples of words that are commonly misunderstood due to poor enunciation. Avoid using regional pronunciations in the office setting. Remember that your patients come from many different cultures and may not understand your particular pronunciation.

The sound of your voice ranges from high to low, depending on the context of your phrase. Have you ever noticed that when you ask a question your voice tends to rise at the end of

the phrase? This is an example of the **pitch** of your voice. You must be aware of pitch when speaking with patients.

Inflection refers to the changes in pitch and tone of your voice and the way you utter your words and phrases. Remember that speaking on the telephone is an opportunity to display excellent customer service. Try to avoid speaking in a monotone (one single tone). The caller may feel you are bored and not interested in helping.

Identify the Caller

Protection of a patient's information is vital in every medical office and health care facility. It is important to remember that some individuals may seek confidential information by unauthorized means, such as claiming to be the patient or even a specialist treating the patient. Therefore, steps must be taken to protect patient records. For example, each time a person phones and claims to be a patient, ask for some identifying information, including both first and last names, Social Security number, and date of birth. You can check this information against the patient's electronic or paper chart.

THE BUSINESS TELEPHONE SYSTEM

Many types of business telephone systems are in use today (Figure 7-2). Most medical offices will use some form of a multiline telephone. Some may have all separate lines, where

TABLE 7-1 Some Words Commonly Misunderstood Due to Poor Enunciation

Prostate	Prostrate
Ear	Air
Galactorrhea	Galacturia
Homeostasis	Hemostasis
Heart attack	Artifact
Palpation	Palpitation

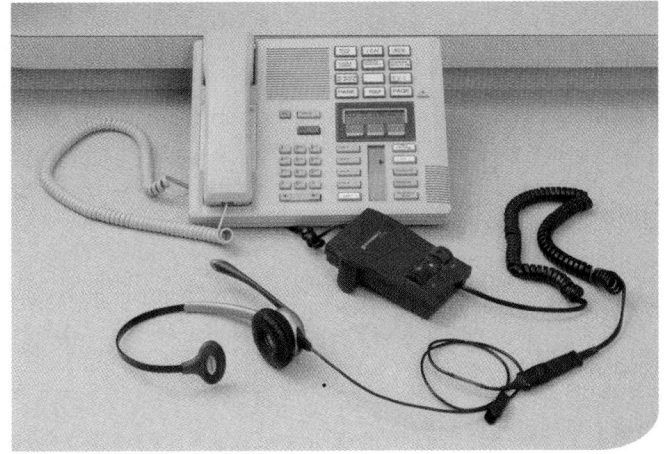

FIGURE 7-2 Choose the telephone unit that offers the features needed in your office.

procedure 7-1

ANSWERING THE TELEPHONE AND PLACING CALLS ON HOLD

Objective: Ensure that the telephone is answered in a professional manner and, if necessary, that patients are placed on hold appropriately.

EQUIPMENT AND SUPPLIES

telephone, message pad, pen, notepad

1. Answer the telephone by at least the third ring, with the mouthpiece 1 to 2 inches from your mouth.
2. Smile and speak clearly, using inflection, a pleasant tone, and a moderate rate of speech.
3. Answer using the greeting your office prefers (e.g., "Thank you for calling Dr. Smith's office. This is Carlos. How may I help you?").
4. At this point, callers will typically identify themselves. If not, ask callers to identify themselves and then verify the information against the patient's medical record.
5. Listen to the caller closely to verify the reason for the call, which may include, but it not limited to, the following:
   - a patient calling to schedule an appointment
   - a patient calling to request a prescription refill
   - another physician's office calling about a mutual patient
   - an insurance company calling regarding a patient's claim
6. Once you have determined the reason for the call, act accordingly while providing excellent customer service. The most common actions you will take during a telephone call are scheduling an appointment, taking a message, transferring the caller to a coworker, or requesting a prescription refill.
7. In busy offices, you may need to answer more than one incoming telephone line. When this occurs, you will combine the procedure just described with the following steps.
8. While speaking with one caller, another incoming line may ring. When this occurs, you must notify the current caller that another line is ringing and ask if the current caller can hold. Wait for the caller's response, then place the first call on hold.
9. Answer the second call following the procedures described, ask the second caller if he or she can hold, wait for a response, and then place the second call on hold. (If the second call is an emergency, you would not ask the person to hold and would assist the caller immediately.)
10. Return to the first call, thank the caller for holding, and continue assisting the person. When you return to that caller, do not ask "Who are you waiting for?" because it conveys the impression that you have forgotten about that person.
11. Once the first call is completed, return to the second call, thank the person for holding, and continue assisting that caller.
12. If the caller asks to speak with another employee who is not readily available and it is necessary to place the call on hold, be sure to check back with the caller about every 30 seconds. This lets the caller know you are actively working on their behalf, and it also provides an opportunity for the caller to leave a message instead of continuing to hold.

---

you must press a particular line's button to answer it, or a system that will feed calls to you from a **queue** or waiting line. More and more offices have systems that will answer the initial call with a recording and then feed the calls to the appropriate people.

Whether you answer initially (without an automated system) or an automated system answers (calls are queued), follow the rules of greeting callers.

Making Calls

You will have to make calls as often as you answer them. On most business telephones, you will be required to dial 9 to get an outside line, but some systems have an outside line button that you push in order to dial out. Depending on the office's location, you also may need to dial the area code with all calls. Large cities have begun to make this a common practice because of the existence of multiple area codes within a local calling zone.

The telephone calls that you make in the office should be limited to business calls. All offices have different policies on the use of the office telephone for personal calls. Some may prohibit them entirely, whereas others may allow them in limited number, or may ask that any personal calls be made on a private line, which may also be referred to as the back line. It is important to keep in mind that the office telephone is for patients and emergencies, so you must keep the lines open.

Using the Hold Function

One of the most sensitive issues relating to telephone courtesy is the use of the hold function, which refers to the ability to keep more than one call on the line at a time. Holding the call is permissible when you are speaking with a caller on one line and another call comes in, but you should never place a call on hold as you are placing it.

Be very mindful of how the hold function is used. Callers should never be left on hold for indefinite periods of time. If you anticipate that the call may need to be placed on hold for a long period of time, offer the patient the option of either continuing to hold or having their call returned.

If you are already speaking with a caller when a second call comes in, it is proper to ask the first caller if you may place him or her on hold for a moment in order to answer the second call (see Procedure 7-1). Once you have asked this question, be sure to listen for the caller's response before automatically placing the call on hold. It is possible the first caller has a billing question, in which case you may transfer the call instead of placing the caller on hold. It is discourteous to handle the second caller before returning to the first call. An example of a typical conversation follows:

FIRST CALLER:	"Mrs. Miller, may I place you on hold for a moment? I have another call."
MRS. MILLER:	"Yes, I can hold."
SECOND CALLER:	"Good afternoon. Doctors Garcia and Jensen. This is Tonya. How may I help you?"
MR. THOMPSON:	"This is Bobby Thompson, and I need to make an appointment to see the doctor."
TONYA:	"Mr. Thompson, can you please hold?"
MR. THOMPSON:	"Yes, I can."
TONYA:	"Mrs. Miller, thank you for holding." (Tonya continues with this first call as efficiently and expediently as possible without hurrying the caller.)

When you answer a second call and discover it is an emergency, you must take care of it before returning to the first call. If it is not an emergency, finish the first call before moving to the second. With all calls that you place on hold, try to keep the wait time to a minimum. Nobody likes to be on hold.

Other situations also may require you to place a caller on hold. For example, you may need to access a chart so you can answer a patient's question. When this happens, explain to the patient what you need to do and then ask if you may place him or her on hold. Always wait for a response, then retrieve the information in the timeliest manner possible. If you have trouble getting the information and need more time, let the caller know and offer the option of you calling back once you have found the needed information. If the patient agrees it would be best for you to call back, be sure you do just that.

Never leave callers on hold without checking back with them. Communication is key, and it is important that patients understand you are working to help them. To avoid forgetting about a caller on hold, be wary of distractions and do not complete any tasks that are unrelated to helping that caller.

Another situation that will require you to put a caller on hold is when a patient must speak with the doctor or another staff member who is not readily available. Verify and follow the protocol used in the office where you work. Many physicians will only accept calls from other physicians or family members while they are busy seeing patients. Physicians may choose to return patient phone calls during a specified time of day. If this is the policy in the office where you work, let the patient know the physician is seeing patients and when he or she generally returns calls. If the physician answers patient's calls while seeing patients, make sure the caller is aware that there will be a wait, and offer to take a message and a phone number for a return call. As much as possible, it is best to keep the telephone lines open. If the caller chooses to wait, you must check on him or her approximately every 30 seconds. Let the caller know that the person he or she is waiting on is still unavailable. Then check to see if the caller would like to leave a name and phone number so the call can be returned.

Transferring Calls

As you field calls in the medical office, you will find that it is often necessary to transfer or send them from one office telephone extension to another extension in the same office. Most business telephones will have a transfer feature. You should follow certain steps to make this a smooth transition for the caller:

1. Once you have identified the person to whom you will be transferring the call, tell the caller the name of this person. This lets the caller know who to expect on the other end of the line as well as who to call back in case of disconnection during the transfer. If you have an extension number available, it is also helpful to provide that number to the caller before transferring him or her.

2. When you start the transfer, make sure that the caller is aware of your actions. Do not transfer a patient without his or her prior knowledge and consent.

3. Most telephone systems allow you to announce a call that you are transferring. Let the person to whom you are transferring the call know the caller's name and the reason for the call. That person may tell you that he or she is unavailable to take the call.

4. Do not hang up before you know if the person was available to help the caller.

5. If you get a busy signal when you transfer the call, let the caller know that the line is busy and offer to take a message or let the caller leave a recorded message.

TAKING A MESSAGE

Medical offices are busy places. Medical assistants will often take messages from patients, other physicians, health care facilities, and businesses. Many medical offices have preprinted telephone message or note pads used for recording telephone messages. Most calls can be documented in the space provided on the pad. It is important to use the form as a guide for gathering all pertinent information. Occasionally, patients will provide much more information than necessary, and you may not know what is pertinent until you near the end of or have completed the call. Space on message pads is limited, and physicians want the facts conveyed in a concise bulleted list. To provide all the necessary information yet be brief, write down all information provided by the patient and transfer it (in bullet points) to the message form, then place that form in the chart for review by the physician. It is best to document as you go and not to trust your memory.

All messages should include the first and last name of the caller (with spelling verified), a telephone number including area code at which he or she can be reached for a callback, the reason for the call, and the name of the person he or she is trying to reach. If the patient is requesting a medication refill, it is important to also document the name, telephone number, and fax number of the appropriate pharmacy. If at any time you do not understand what a caller has stated, you must clarify the message with that caller. You may repeat to the caller what you believe you heard, or you may ask the caller to repeat back what was said to you. Always repeat the callback number and verify that the caller will be available at that number during normal business hours. If not, ask the patient for an alternate telephone number. If a callback doesn't occur because the phone number is incorrect, the caller may interpret it as a lack of concern or disrespect. All telephone messages regarding a patient should be placed in the patient's

chart as documentation of an interaction that occurred between the office and the patient.

It is very important to remember not to throw away but to shred anything that contains patient information. Even the written notes you use to take proper messages must be shredded if they contain patient information. It is a violation of the Health Insurance Portability and Accountability Act (HIPAA) privacy rule to throw patient information into the trash.

See Procedure 7-2 for instructions on how to take telephone messages.

The Voice Messaging System

In the medical office, you will deal with a **voice messaging system** for both incoming and outgoing calls. A voice messaging system allows messages (voice mail) to be left or recorded when the medical assistant is unavailable to answer the telephone. If your office uses such a system, inform callers in the initial greeting to hang up and dial 911 for a medical emergency.

For incoming calls, your office may have a voice messaging system to record messages for you when you are away from your desk. If you are using such a system, include your name and telephone number in your recorded greeting. Your voice messaging system should also allow for the caller to dial 0 for immediate assistance.

When calling patients, you will find that most of them will have some form of voice messaging system. This does present a problem in the context of patient privacy. Know both your office's policy regarding what kind of message should be left on a patient's voice messaging system and how to adhere to HIPAA guidelines when doing so. You must consider the patient's privacy, and if you were to leave a self-identifying message such as "This is Cathy from Carsonville OB/GYN," you may have disclosed patient confidential information. To leave a message, yet maintain patient

PROFESSIONALISM

THE LAW

Medical assistants must use a level of caution when speaking with patients over the telephone. Never diagnose a patient yourself—only the physician can diagnose. When handling calls, always follow your office's protocol manual. Document every call that you have with a patient. Document all details—even seemingly insignificant ones. Never discard any patient information in a trash can. When disposing of patient information, shred it.

procedure
7-2

TAKING A TELEPHONE MESSAGE

Objective: Ensure that correct and relevant information is retrieved when taking a telephone message.

EQUIPMENT AND SUPPLIES

message form or pad with carbon or carbonless for duplicates; pen; electronic medical record if available

1. Smile prior to answering the telephone and, in a warm voice, properly answer the telephone.
2. Use a message form to keep a record of the message, or document it directly into the electronic medical record (Figure 7-3).
3. Record the date and time of the call.
4. Record the caller's full name and a callback number with area code for use during office hours. (Always ask the caller to spell his or her name and provide another identifier, such as date of birth or Social Security number.) If recording the message in an electronic medical record, verify that you have the correct patient record.
5. Document for whom the message is intended.
6. Document the complete message. Avoid using abbreviations other than accepted medical abbreviations. Include symptoms (e.g., temperature, rash, emesis, duration of symptoms).
7. Thank the patient for calling and, prior to hanging up the telephone, ask if he or she has any other questions.
8. To indicate that you took a handwritten message, either write out your first and last name or record the initial of your first name and your last name spelled out. If using an electronic medical record, save the message and forward it to the intended recipient.

CHARTING EXAMPLE

Patient Name: Carl Toper   Date of Birth: 9/12/46
Date: 10/29/2010   Time: 9:15 am   Physician: Dr. Verde
Patient's Telephone Number (Home): 213-555-3424
                    (Other): 213-555-5946
Medical Record Number: 99574   Allergies: Penicillin
Pharmacy Name: Dispense for You
Pharmacy Telephone Number: 213-555-2359
Prescription Number:
Message Taken By: · Tonya Blue, RMA

MESSAGE

Patient called stating he has had nausea and diarrhea since he returned from seeing his grandkids in Seattle last week. On questioning, the patient stated his granddaughter had a fever the day he left to return home. Mr. Toper is wondering if the nausea and diarrhea will cause any problems with his insulin dosing. Per the patient, he will be home all day.

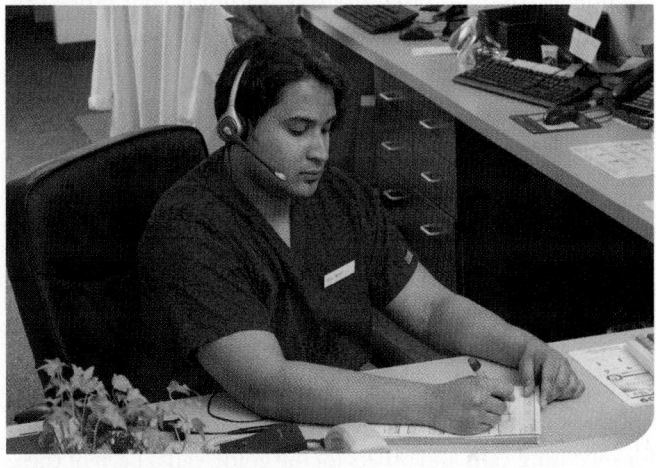

A

For _____ **Urgent** ☐
Date _____ **Time** _____
While You Were Out
M _____
Of _____
Phone _____
Area Code   Number   Extension

Telephoned ☐   Please Call ☐
Came To See You ☐   Will Call Again ☐
Returned Your Call ☐ Wants To See You ☐

Message _____
_____
_____
_____
_____
_____
Signed _____

B

FIGURE 7-3 (A) All messages must be documented and placed in the patient's chart. (B) A message pad.

privacy, it is best to leave a message such as "This is Cathy from Dr. Smith's office, and this message is for Charlene. Please return my call at your earliest convenience. You may reach me at 555-987-6543."

Call Forwarding

The call forwarding feature allows for a telephone user to forward calls to another telephone. For example, a physician may wish to forward his or her cell phone calls to a home telephone. You will often use this feature if your office utilizes an answering service. (Answering services are discussed later in this chapter.)

Caller ID

Caller ID is an increasingly popular telephone option. This function allows for telephone owners to know who is calling each time the telephone rings. In the office, it is unlikely that you will have caller ID, but many of your patients may have this telephone feature. It is important to understand that a medical office may need to block the office number from showing up on the patient's caller ID. This is because most offices often have multiple telephone lines, some designated for incoming calls and others for outgoing calls. Each of these lines may have a different telephone number. Back lines—those meant only for incoming calls from patients—should be left open at all times. If a patient has caller ID, he or she may get the number to one of your back lines. This can become very confusing to both the patient and the staff. Maintaining patient privacy is another reason commonly used to block the medical office's telephone number.

Privacy Manager

Privacy manager is a fairly recent addition to the variety of telephone options. It allows patients to block access to their home telephones. When you call a telephone number that has privacy manager attached, you will be asked to state from where you are calling. Once you have given this information, unless you are cleared, you'll be directed to a voice mail system, where you will leave a message.

Speakerphones and Headsets

At times you will need to free your hands for administrative duties, while still being available to answer the telephone. In such instances, you can use the speakerphone or the headset.

Most telephones have a built-in speakerphone or microphone and speaker. The speakerphone allows you to hear and speak without having to pick up the handset of the telephone. The speakerphone has a few drawbacks, however, such as others nearby may overhear your conversation or the caller on the other end will be able to hear background noise.

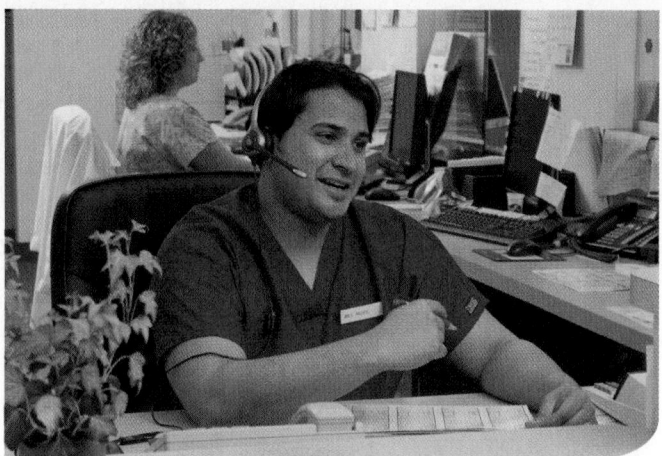

FIGURE 7-4 Headsets are ergonomically correct and allow the medical assistant or receptionist to use both hands for administrative duties, while still being available to answer the telephone.

Patient confidentiality should be a foremost concern when using the speakerphone.

Headsets are being used increasingly frequently in offices. They free your hands so you can document calls (Figure 7-4). They are ergonomically correct, as they help to prevent the neck and shoulder injuries that can result from cradling the receiver on the shoulder. Keep the headset microphone close to your mouth so the caller does not have difficulty hearing or understanding you.

PAGERS AND CELL PHONES

Many physicians carry pagers with them on a regular basis as it is the most expedient way of contacting him or her in an emergency. You must know if the physician(s) in your office carries one. You will find that most pager systems are user friendly. One simply has to call the pager number and, when instructed, enter in the callback telephone number. Some offices may use a coded message system. For example, certain numbers may be designated for different types of emergencies or situations. Using a specific number will give the physician a heads-up about the nature of the call. You must learn how your office uses its pager system.

Cell phones have become fundamental to business and social life. Most physicians and office managers now use cell phones to conduct day-to-day business (Figure 7-5). Some have even replaced their conventional pagers with cell phones because most cell phones also have a pager function. However, cell phones do have a disadvantage in that they can interfere with electronic monitors, and for that reason they are not allowed in parts of certain hospitals. Usually, signage clearly designates where cell phones are and are not allowed. In most cell-phone-free zones, pagers are allowed.

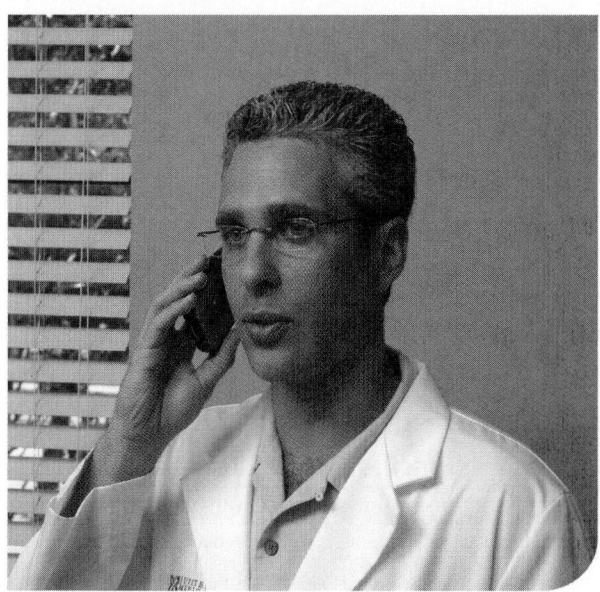

FIGURE 7-5 Many physicians use cell phones to stay in touch with their offices.

To understand and keep up to date with rules regarding cell phone and pager use, check frequently with those hospitals with which your office frequently communicates.

SCREENING TELEPHONE CALLS

One of the most important ways to keep the office running smoothly and one of the key functions of the front office is to screen telephone calls effectively. When answering the telephone, you must determine quickly what type of call you have received and the proper way to handle it. Whenever you answer the telephone, you should ask the person the reason for the call. From there, you will either transfer the call to the appropriate person, or you will handle the call yourself. (The different types of telephone calls you may receive are discussed later in this chapter.)

MAKING REMINDER CALLS AND CALLBACKS

Most offices require medical assistants to make calls to patients to remind them of upcoming appointments. Offices might do this a week before the appointment and then again the day before the appointment.

As a medical assistant, you also will be required to return calls to patients or other callers. For instance, messages left by patients may contain a question for the physician or deal with prescription refill

requests, and your callback will relay the physician's response. Sometimes the physician may have you call a patient to check on his or her status.

When making any calls to a patient's house or place of business, you must protect the patient's privacy. (Patient privacy is one of the most important matters for medical facilities.) The first thing to do when phoning any patient is to make sure that it is the patient to whom you are speaking. Start every patient callback by identifying yourself, then asking to speak to the patient. You should not indicate why you are calling until you have the patient on the phone. If the person who answers asks you why you are calling, explain that confidentiality laws prevent you from revealing that information.

Typical Incoming Calls

You will receive many types of calls in the medical office. The following are some types you will handle on a daily basis.

PATIENT CALLS

Most calls coming into the medical office will be from patients (Figure 7-6). They may be calling for an appointment, or about insurance, billing, fees, office hours and directions, laboratory results, or callbacks.

Appointment Requests

One of the most common types of calls you will receive in the medical office are appointment requests. These calls will often involve patients with health problems, so you

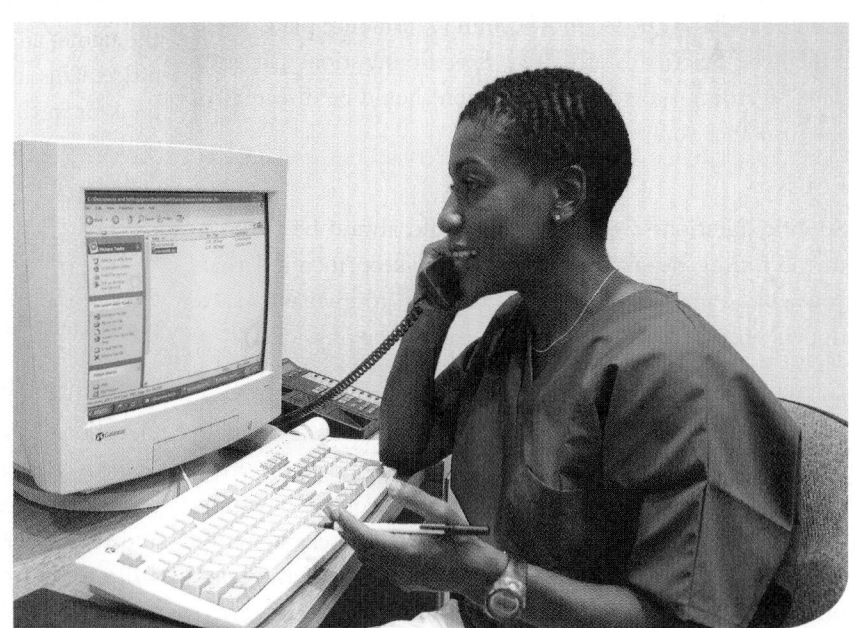

FIGURE 7-6 The medical assistant spends many hours on the telephone assisting patients.

need to follow telephone triage procedures (discussed later in this chapter) to schedule them appropriately. The caller may be a current patient or a new patient. For patients who need routine appointments, offer an appointment time that is convenient for both the patient and the medical office. (You will learn more about scheduling appointments in Chapter 9.)

Insurance and Billing Questions

It is a fact that most patients will not understand the way medical insurance works. You should anticipate receiving calls on a daily basis from patients with questions about their accounts and medical insurance. You may be able to answer some of these questions, but most will be directed to the billing department.

Patients will often call with questions regarding their bills. The most frequently asked question is "Why did I receive a bill?" Many patients have the misconception that their insurance company will pay the entire bill. You may have to explain to the patient the details of what was billed. In your explanation, you will need to include what steps the insurance company has taken in regard to covering the charges. This could include discussing deductibles, copayments, and coinsurance. You also may need to explain reasons for denial of certain charges. If you are unable to help with questions concerning insurance coverage, you may refer the patient to his or her insurance company or employer's human resources department.

New patients will often call prior to scheduling an appointment to inquire whether or not the provider participates with their insurance plan. The medical assistant should have a list of the most common insurance plans with which the practice is affiliated. Specific questions patients have regarding provider participation should be directed to the insurance company.

Fees

Specific questions regarding fees should always be referred to the billing department. You should keep in mind that you will be unable, more often than not, to give any exact figures until the patient has been seen by the physician.

Office Hours and Directions

Most offices now include the office hours and directions in the office's automated assistance systems. However, you may have to handle some of the calls yourself. You should have your office address and hours posted near your telephone. It is also a good idea to have directions posted near the telephone. The directions should include routes to the office from all directions—north, south, east, and west—when applicable.

Laboratory Test Results

Many patients will call the office to get the results of recent procedures and tests. Follow your office policy regarding disseminating results to patients. Certain tests may require follow-up testing or procedures. In that case, follow-up is necessary to ensure that the patient performed as instructed. Once the physician has reviewed the laboratory test results, he or she may ask the medical assistant to notify the patient of the results and to communicate any further instructions. Once the patient has been notified of the results and instructions, the medical assistant should document this in the patient's chart. If the patient has further questions, he or she will need to speak with the physician. It is important to understand that the medical assistant is not to read and interpret laboratory tests.

Follow-up Calls from Patients

It is common for a physician to have a patient call the office as a follow-up to certain procedures and to relate the status of certain problems. When these calls come into the office, the medical assistant must take a message and convey this information to the physician.

Referral Requests

Many insurance companies require that before patients see a specialist they must obtain a **referral** (which documents authorization) from their primary care physician by telephone or fax. Referrals are required for patients who have health management organizations (HMOs). Thus, patients may phone to request that the referral be prepared. You must get all the information necessary to place the referral, including the name, address, and telephone number of the specialist's office. This information may be found in the local telephone book or in the insurance company's provider book. You also will need to find out the reason the patient is seeing the specialist. You may obtain some of this information from the patient, and you also may need to check the patient's chart for the diagnosis that the referral references. All referrals need to be approved by the physician before being completed and released to the patient.

Patients Who Refuse to Identify Themselves

Occasionally, you will encounter patients who refuse to identify themselves to you. You must let the caller know that you will not be of assistance without his or her name and reason for calling. Inform the caller that the physician will not return calls to patients who refuse to identify themselves. If the caller continues to refuse to state his or her name, some offices will ask that the caller write a letter addressed to the physician.

The Persistent Talker

Every medical office has patients who call in and draw the staff into long conversations. Unfortunately, your time is limited. You must end such conversations kindly but promptly. You may simply state to the patient that you are busy helping another patient and apologize for the inconvenience.

NONPATIENT CALLS

Not all telephone calls to the office will be from patients. You will find that a large number of calls will come from salespeople, hospitals, physicians, and other health care facilities.

Sales Calls

Answering calls from sales representatives is part of the medical assistant's telephone responsibilities. You may have to become the wall between the sales calls and your physician and office manager. Most physicians will not take any type of sales calls while seeing patients. They may wish you to take messages or ask the sales representative to fax or email the information to them. The same will probably hold true with office managers. They will ask you to take messages for most sales calls so they can return the calls at a more convenient time.

Reports from Hospitals and Other Patient Care Facilities

If your physician has patients in a hospital or nursing facility, you will likely receive calls from those facilities. The facilities will often call with reports on the patients' status or changes in their conditions. In many cases, you will interrupt the physician for such calls. To do so, you should knock on the examination room door and let the physician know an important call is on hold.

Sometimes you will need only to take a message for the physician. The message may contain information to relay or may be a request that the physician return the call. In either case, you always should determine whether or not the call should be returned.

General Office Matters

Some calls received in the office deal with general office business, including telephone calls from accountants or calls regarding suppliers or rented office equipment. These calls should be handled on a case-by-case basis. It is important to carefully screen calls from the office's suppliers. Make sure the supplier gives you his or her name and the business's name, address, and telephone number. It is best that the office manager or person responsible handle calls regarding office equipment or supplies.

Physician's Personal Calls

The physician also will receive personal calls in the office. Physicians work long hours and often encourage family members to call them at the office. Most physicians will instruct you how they wish their personal calls to be handled. In some cases, they will want you to knock on the examination room door and simply state "Doctor, you are wanted on the telephone." In other cases, physicians may ask you to give them telephone messages as soon as they come out of the examination room. Generally, family members do not wish to interrupt the physician during a patient examination.

Calls from Other Physicians

The physician will let the office staff know how to handle calls from other physicians. He or she may wish to take such calls right away or when finished with an exam. Such calls may relate to a patient consultation and require an immediate answer. In certain circumstances, such as a consult on a patient, the physician receiving the call may want to have the patient's medical record available.

Obscene or Prank Calls

If you have a telephone, you are at risk for receiving obscene or prank calls. Hang up immediately if you receive such calls. You also may report the call to the telephone company, especially if it is an ongoing problem that seems to involve the same caller. Usually, the telephone company can trace the call.

Prescription Refill Requests

Phone requests for prescription refills are commonly received in medical offices. Because of the high volume of such calls, many offices have a voice mail system to answer most of these calls. The medical assistant is often responsible for taking messages off the voice mail system and responding to them at least twice each day, sometimes more frequently. The physician must sign off on all prescription refill requests. Some physicians will want to be given the patient's chart with the message before okaying the request, so be prepared to do so if necessary. See Procedure 7-3 for important information about taking a prescription refill message.

Telephone Triage

Triage is a process used to determine the order in which patients should be treated. The severity of the patient's illness or injury determines the order of treatment. **Telephone triage**—determining the order in which to take patient calls—is an issue for the telephone screening process. By asking specific questions, the medical assistant can determine how to handle a patient's problem. Each office should

procedure 7-3

TAKING A PRESCRIPTION REFILL MESSAGE

Objective: Ensure that correct information is acquired when refilling a patient's prescription.

EQUIPMENT AND SUPPLIES

message pad or paper; pen

1. Document the name of the patient. (This name may be different from the name of the caller.)
2. Document the patient's telephone number.
3. Document the name and dosage of the medication being requested. Ask the caller to spell the medication name if you do not understand what the caller is saying.
4. Document how long the patient has been on the medication.
5. Document the patient's symptoms and why the prescription is still needed.
6. Document the patient's age and (if a child) weight.
7. Ask for the name and telephone number (including area code) of the pharmacy and the prescription number if available.
8. Let the caller know you will forward the message to the physician.
9. Let the caller know you will call back if the prescription cannot be refilled or if the physician has any questions.

10. Attach the telephone message to the patient's medical record and give both to the physician to review.

CHARTING EXAMPLE

Patient Name: Lucy Coles   Date of Birth: 4/20/67

Date: 10/24/XX   Time: 10:05 am   Physician: Dr. Rudy

Patient's Telephone Number (Home): 213-555-1234
                              (Other): 213-555-3496

Medical Record Number: 89564   Allergies: NKDA

Pharmacy Name: Dispense for You

Pharmacy Telephone Number: 213-555-2359

Prescription Number: CC5679

Message Taken By: · · · · · · · · · · · · · · · · · · · Tonya Blue, RMA

MESSAGE

Patient called requesting refill on Celexa 20 mg. Patient stated she is doing well on the medication with no side effects. Patient scheduled for follow-up visit on 12/10/XX. Patient will be at home telephone number until 4:45 P.M.; after that, please call cell phone number above.

Box 7-1 Information to Request from CALLERS

- Patient's name
- The caller's name, if different from that of the patient
- Telephone number, including area code
- Date of the call
- Time of the call

- The patient's physician, if a multiphysician practice
- Any medications that the patient is taking
- Any allergies the patient may have
- The patient's insurance
- The patient's problem

have a policies and procedures manual that outlines the office's preferred method of screening telephone calls.

Most patients will be calling because they feel they need to see the physician. It will be one of your responsibilities to see that the patient is helped in the most appropriate manner. You will need to gather information from the patient. As with all telephone calls, the first thing you'll need to find

out is the patient's name and telephone number, in case you become disconnected. Have the patient spell out his or her name to avoid mistakes. During the course of your conversation, ask for some basic demographic information in addition to medical information. Box 7-1 lists information that you should request from the patient. When scheduling the patient, include the information you received from the patient, then place the information in the patient's chart so you or another medical assistant will know how to prepare for the appointment.

The medical assistant must be careful when screening patients on the telephone. You will be assessing a patient's symptoms. This, however, is very close to exceeding the medical assistant's scope of practice. Make sure that you are closely following the established telephone protocols that were agreed on by the physician. If ever a situation arises that is not covered in the policies and procedures manual, the medical assistant must ask the physician how to handle that particular problem. Physicians will often purchase one of many triage manuals that are available on the market. Follow only the protocols that the physician has approved.

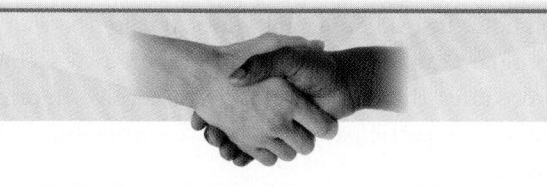

PROFESSIONALISM
CULTURAL CONSIDERATIONS

You will encounter an array of cultural differences when fielding calls in a medical office. When dealing with a patient, it is always best to speak directly with him or her to get the best information. However, some cultures may not allow direct contact with certain members of the family. Even though it is often difficult to obtain vital information by proxy (a third person), it is sometimes necessary to do so to avoid cultural clashes.

You also may deal with patients with very poor English skills. Sometimes a translator is necessary. If your office is affiliated with a hospital, the hospital has a list of available translators in your area. When the non–English-speaking patient schedules an appointment, the translator also should be scheduled. It is not advisable to have a patient's family member translate. Consider the effect of the family member's emotions if the physician has to ask the family member to translate and convey to the patient that he or she has a serious or terminal illness. If translators are not available in your area, contact the telephone company, which may be able to provide a dual phone system.

Your main goal when taking calls is to make the patient as comfortable as possible while providing appropriate assistance.

PROFESSIONALISM
THE LIFE SPAN

When handling pediatric cases, the information received about the patient will most likely be from a parent or guardian. You will find that first-time parents may call frequently. As the primary contact in the medical office, the medical assistant must always treat parents and guardians with respect and patience. Remember that what may be perceived as a minor health situation for most people can be perceived as a major health situation for first-time parents.

Handling Difficult Calls

You are likely to receive many types of problematic calls in a medical office, and the most important thing to remember when dealing with a difficult patient is not to lose your temper. Difficult patients can vary from those who are angry and yelling to those attempting to obtain confidential information. With any difficult caller, you must keep the situation as calm as possible. It is helpful to remember that the patient, more often than not, is displacing anger and is probably frustrated with some other situation, such as worry over an illness, having had a bad day, or even suffering from pain.

When you have a difficult patient on the phone, the best approach is to be empathetic while remaining in control of the situation. Take the time to listen and find out the exact problem. Once you determine the problem, you can begin to help. However, when patients use inappropriate language, you should state that you will not continue to speak with them if they continue to use foul language. Everyone is entitled to a certain level of respect and courtesy.

Using a Telephone Directory

When calling most insurance companies and hospitals, you encounter an automated telephone directory or **automated assistance program**—a telephone system that directs callers to the appropriate person through a series of questions.

After the call is answered automatically, the caller is presented with options so that the telephone system can direct the call to the proper person or department. Many large business systems will provide additional options. When using one of these systems, it is important to pay close attention to the options that are offered because it can be easy to miss your cue. When you hear an option, the system will instruct you either to press the appropriate button or to state the option verbally. In most systems, if you cannot find an option to fit your needs, you can dial 0 to have the operator of the system direct your call. Document the date, time, and name of the individual you speak with in case you need to follow up in the future. It is also advisable to document a telephone number or extension where you may contact the individual directly.

The term *telephone directory* can also pertain to the telephone book provided to you by your local telephone company. These directories have two main sections: white pages and yellow pages. The white pages list the names, addresses, and telephone numbers of telephone service customers; the yellow pages list the names, addresses, and telephone numbers of local businesses. In addition, you will find emergency numbers, local government numbers, national area codes, local zip codes, and directions on making long distance calls, including international calls. Telephone directories are also available on the Internet.

Telephones Used for Patient Education

The telephone system can be a great way of educating patients. The system can relay information to the patient in a number of ways.

If an automated assistance program is used, it is possible to program it to provide information to the patient. Most systems will provide the office's hours and directions. Emergency contact numbers are also provided. Some programs include an option that lets callers hear about new employees, such as a new physician or other practitioner.

Another opportunity to educate patients is while they are on hold. Instead of playing music during the wait time, the program can play a message explaining new techniques or procedures that the physician is offering. Information pertaining to participating insurance carriers may also be included.

Long Distance Calls

Occasionally, you will be asked to make long distance telephone calls for office business. For a time, a long distance call would be any call outside your area code. This is no longer true. Many larger cities have added area codes within local calling regions. Thus, you must know what is considered long distance in your area. Long distance calls can be very costly, so your office may limit how many are made. Some offices assign long distance codes to each employee and, prior to a call being placed, the employee is required to key in their long distance code. This measure can be used to track potential abuse of long distance calls.

TELEPHONE LOGS

Many offices maintain a telephone log to keep track of the long distance calls being made. When the telephone bill arrives, the log and the bill can be compared. This can help to identify any abuses of the business telephone with personal calls. Many logs will have you list the name of the person, the facility or company being called, the number being called, the name of the person placing the call, the date and time of the call, the city and state where the call is placed, the duration of the call, and the reason for it.

MAKING A LONG DISTANCE CALL

Direct Distance Dialing (DDD) is the most common way of making a long distance call. To place a long distance call using DDD, dial "1," then the area code followed by the number you are calling. If you need to find an area code, you will find the listing of area codes at the front of the telephone book. The telephone book also will give you instructions for making international calls, if you are required to make them.

Another way of calling long distance is to make a collect call—reversing the call charges to the person recieving the call. When collect calls are placed, the person being called is asked by the operator whether or not he or she will accept the charges. Your office should have a policy in place regarding accepting or denying collect calls.

CONFERENCE CALLS

A **conference call** is made when several people from different locations wish to have a joint discussion by phone. This means, for example, two physicians at a distance from each other may speak with a patient at a third location at the same time. These calls are more efficient and can save money in the long run because the participants do not have to make several separate long distance calls to relay the same information.

Most business telephone systems allow you to make conference calls without using the telephone operator. You will need to determine if your telephone system allows you to do so. If your system is not set up for making conference calls, you may use the operator to place the calls. See Procedure 7-4 for placing a conference call.

procedure
7-4

PLACING A CONFERENCE CALL

Objective: Allow for a discussion via the telephone between three or more parties from various locations.

EQUIPMENT AND SUPPLIES

telephone numbers of participating parties

1. Gather the telephone numbers of all participants before beginning the call.
2. Determine the time that everyone will be available for the conference call. You may have to call people in advance to determine a convenient time. Be aware of time zone differences when arranging conference calls.
3. Dial 0 for the operator and provide the name and telephone number (area code first) for each person to be called.
4. The operator will then place a call to each party. When all the participants are on the line, the operator will come back to the original caller (you) and the conversation can begin. If you are placing this call for your physician, he or she will pick up on your line (Figure 7-7).
5. If you are setting up the conference call ahead of time, tell the operator when you wish the conference call to begin.

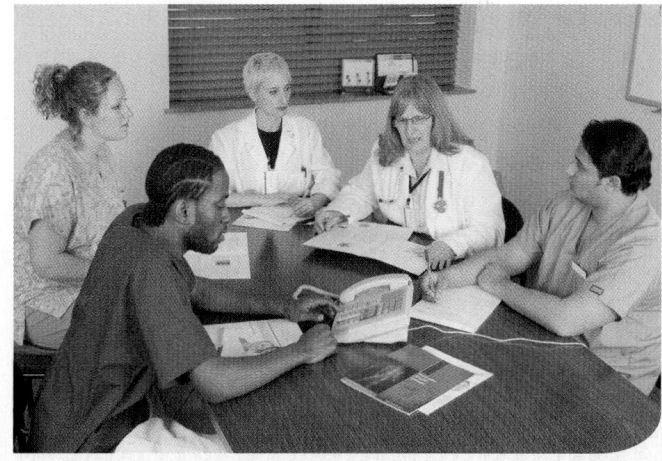

FIGURE 7-7 **Conference calling by telephone allows three or more persons in different locations to speak with each other at the same time.**

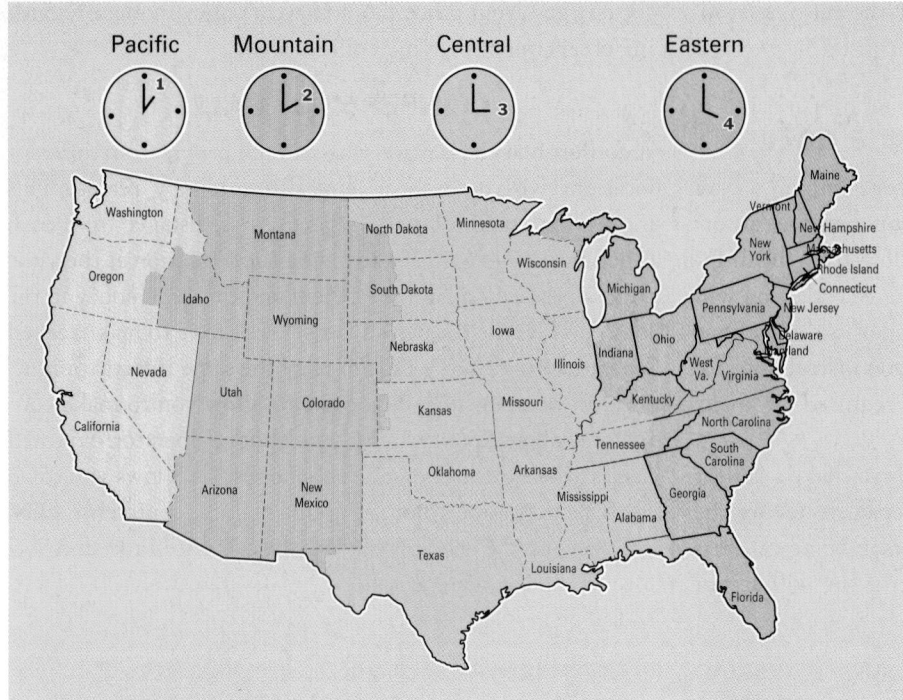

FIGURE 7-8 Having a time zone map located near the telephone will assist you when making long distance calls outside your time zone.

TIME ZONES

Time zones within the United States and foreign countries are important to consider when placing long distance telephone calls. The continental United States and parts of Canada are divided into four time zones based on their location in the country: Eastern, Central, Mountain, and Pacific. As you move from east to west across the United States, there is a 1-hour difference (earlier) in each time zone. For example, if it is 9:00 A.M. in Ohio (Eastern Time Zone), then it will be 8:00 A.M. in Illinois (Central Time Zone).

Keep a time zone map posted near your office telephone (Figure 7-8) so you can plan long distance calls based on office hours in each time zone. A call placed at 3:00 P.M. in California will be received in New York at 6:00 P.M., which is usually after offices close.

Using an Answering Service

Many offices use an **answering service** when no one is available in the office. This service can be in effect 24 hours a day or just at designated times such as during the night, during lunch, or during peak hours of the day to relieve office staff.

The system works by forwarding office calls to the service, which is at an off-site location. Answering service personnel answer the calls and inform the patients that the office is closed. They also will take some nonemergency messages, which will be delivered to the office when you return phone service to your care. When emergency calls come in, the answering service will contact the physician by pager or telephone. If a patient speaks with the answering service, it must be documented just as it would be if the call were answered by office staff. Most answering services will fax the calls received, and physicians in turn will document their responses and actions related to the call. Once the physician has completed the documentation, the information should be placed in the patient's record.

A fee is attached to answering services, but many offices consider this a necessary service. Offices have the option of using an answering machine or voice messaging system while the office is closed. This option is less expensive, but the patients' problems may not be addressed as quickly. If the office uses an answering machine or voice messaging system, you must ensure that the messages are retrieved in a timely manner and that the recorded office greeting provides a number to call in case of emergency.

Handling an Emergency Telephone Call

Every office should have a written protocol for handling emergency calls. Since you cannot see the telephone caller, it can be difficult to determine a true emergency when talking to someone over the telephone. It is critical to get the caller's name and telephone number immediately in case you are disconnected. You will then proceed by asking the patient specific questions. Examples of questions you may ask, depending on your office's procedure, are listed in Box 7-2. If an emergency is taking place during the telephone call, alert the physician immediately.

In some cases, the patient may be hysterical or crying. Your job, in a situation such as this, is to calm the patient. If your voice remains calm and reassuring, you may be able to soothe the patient. If the caller is extremely upset, ask if someone else can come to the telephone. Your role is to gain as much information from the caller as possible so that the emergency can be handled quickly. Following are some types of emergencies you may face:

- allergic reactions (anaphylactic shock)
- asthma
- broken bone
- drug overdose
- eye injury or foreign body in the eye
- gunshot or stabbing wound
- heart attack
- inability to breathe, or difficulty breathing
- loss of consciousness
- premature labor
- profuse bleeding
- severe pain, including chest pain
- severe vomiting or diarrhea
- suicide attempt or suicide threats
- high temperature

The office should have a policy in place for how to handle emergency calls when no physician is present. Many times, medical office policies and procedures will direct office staff to send the patient to a nearby emergency room. In this situation, *never* hang up the phone with the patient. Instead, while the patient is on the phone signal a coworker for help and have your coworker call 9-1-1 on behalf of the patient. It is important to remain on the line with the caller until emergency medical services arrive.

Never take an emergency call lightly. Emergencies can become life threatening if no treatment is provided. Even if you have questions about whether the call is actually an emergency, you must always assume it is and alert the physician. Malpractice suits have been brought against medical assistants who have failed to correctly handle an emergency.

SUMMARY

Working in a front desk position requires that the majority of the medical assistant's time is spent on the telephone. Most first impressions of the office will be generated based on the interaction on the telephone. Always greet the caller warmly and professionally. On a typical day, the medical assistant will field many different types of calls from patients, insurance companies, pharmacies, and others. Keep in mind that your ability to communicate and the telephone skills you have will greatly affect the way others perceive the office where you work. Attention to detail is required while taking telephone messages. You must understand what information is required in order to complete the message. You are representing your office every time you speak. Take each call one at a time, and use the techniques and procedures presented in this chapter to work more efficiently while maintaining patient confidentiality.

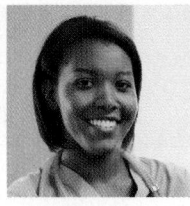

7 CHAPTER REVIEW

COMPETENCY REVIEW

1. Define and spell the terms to learn for this chapter

2. When it is 9:00 A.M. in New York, what time is it in (a) Pittsburgh, PA; (b) St. Paul, MN; (c) Los Angeles, CA; and (d) Denver, CO?

3. Write a telephone message for a patient who calls for a refill of Estrace 1 mg daily.

4. How might you handle receiving a prank telephone call?

5. Why should you smile when answering the telephone?

6. What do you do when you are helping a patient on one line and another line begins to ring?

PREPARING FOR THE CERTIFICATION EXAM

1. One of your patients is vacationing in San Diego, California, and calls your office located in Detroit, Michigan, at 5:15 P.M. What is the current time in San Diego?
   a. 5:15 P.M.
   b. 4:15 P.M.
   c. 3:15 P.M.
   d. 2:15 P.M.
   e. 1:15 P.M.

2. As the receptionist answering the telephone, you are required to triage incoming calls and determine those that are most urgent. From the following list, determine which call requires immediate attention:
   a. Patient is calling for laboratory results.
   b. Patient is calling to state her son is very groggy this morning and that he was tackled last night during a football game.
   c. Patient is calling to schedule an appointment for a school physical.
   d. Patient is calling to state she has developed hives since beginning a new medication last night.
   e. Patient is calling with a sliver in his knee.

3. If a second call is an emergency, which is the best behavior for handling the first call?
   a. Take care of the second caller before returning to the first.
   b. Put the second caller on hold and pick up the third call.

   c. Put the second caller on hold and go back to the first.
   d. Hand your phone to the physician to handle the second call.
   e. Tell the second caller to go immediately to the hospital.

4. If the medical assistant is on the telephone with one patient and the second line rings, which is the best way to handle the two calls?
   a. Hope that someone else picks up the second call.
   b. Ask the first caller if he or she can hold, place the call on hold, and then answer the second call. Ask the second caller if he or she can hold and return to the first call.
   c. Tell the first caller to hold, answer the second call, tell the second caller to hold, and return to the first call.
   d. Ask the first caller if he or she can hold, place the first caller on hold, and answer the second call.
   e. Tell the first caller to hold, answer the second call, ask the second caller to hold, and return to the first call.

5. When documenting a telephone message regarding an update on a patient's condition, all of the following must be recorded except the:
   a. name of the person taking the message.
   b. patient's telephone number.
   c. patient's medical insurance copayment.
   d. time of the call.
   e. date of the call.

6. When answering the telephone, the medical assistant or receptionist should always pay close attention to the following regarding his or her speaking voice except for:
   a. disinterest.
   b. enunciation.
   c. clarity.
   d. pitch.
   e. inflection.

7. Which of the following is an appropriate greeting for an incoming call?
   a. Thank you for calling. Dr. Smith's office. Please hold.
   b. Good morning. Dr. Smith's office.
   c. Good morning. Dr. Smith's office. This is Jenny. How may I help you?
   d. Good morning. Dr. Smith's office. This is Jenny. Hold, please.
   e. Dr. Smiths's office. This is Jenny

8. When transferring a call, the receptionist should do several things, except:
   a. notify the caller you are initating a transfer.
   b. provide the name of the person to whom the caller is being transferred.

c. stay on the line until the call has been transferred.
d. transfer directly to voice mail.
e. provide the extension number of the person to whom the caller is being transferred.

9. When taking a telephone message for a prescription refill, the following information must be obtained except for the:
   a. name of the patient.
   b. prescription number.
   c. pharmacy website address.
   d. pharmacy telephone number.
   e. name of the medication.

10. When working in a busy office, it is inevitable that you will need to place callers on hold. Once the caller is on hold, how often should you check back with them?
    a. every 3 minutes
    b. every 2 minutes
    c. every 1 minute
    d. every 30 seconds
    e. every 90 seconds

CRITICAL THINKING

1. What was wrong with the way Carmine was put on hold? How could this have been improved?

2. What should Tonya have done while Carmine was on hold for 2 minutes?

3. From the start of the conversation with Tonya, Carmine was displeased. What could Tonya have done differently?

ON THE JOB

For more than 2 years, medical assistant Linda Lewis has been employed by Drs. Norek and Klein, who are gerontologists. Also on staff are two registered nurses, a medical laboratory technician, and a medical social worker. The daughter of one of the doctor's patients has just called the office. She is very distraught at the seemingly diminished capacity of her mother and insists on speaking to the doctor.

Linda explains that both physicians only take emergency calls during patient appointment hours but that she will take a detailed message. The caller, however, suggests that not only should her call be considered an emergency but that she will sue the doctor if the call is not handled accordingly.

1. What should Linda do immediately to diffuse the situation?
2. Is this clearly a case where the call should be passed on to one of the registered nurses or the medical social worker?
3. Is this a case where, because of the threat of an impending suit, the physician should be called to the telephone?
4. How could Linda ascertain whether or not this is indeed an emergency? Is it up to her, as a medical assistant, to make such a determination?
5. Since this is the patient's daughter rather than the patient herself, does Linda have any reason to enter into a conversation with the caller? Could Linda be ethically bound by confidentiality not to admit the woman's mother is a patient?

INTERNET ACTIVITY

Use the Internet and research the ways HIPAA has affected the use of the telephone in the medical office.

MEDMEDIA

Additional interactive resources and activities for this chapter can be found:

On your student DVD: View applicable procedure videos on the DVD-ROM found in the back of this book.

MyHealthProfessionsKit.com: Test your knowledge of this chapter with games and activities. MyHealthProfessionsKit also includes resources, helpful links, and a Spanish audio glossary.

Medical Assisting Interactive: Practice your procedures as a medical assistant in this simulated doctor's office. This can be accessed through MyHealthProfessionsKit.com.

Unit One

Unit Two

Administrative
Medical
Assisting

Unit Three

Unit Four

Unit Five

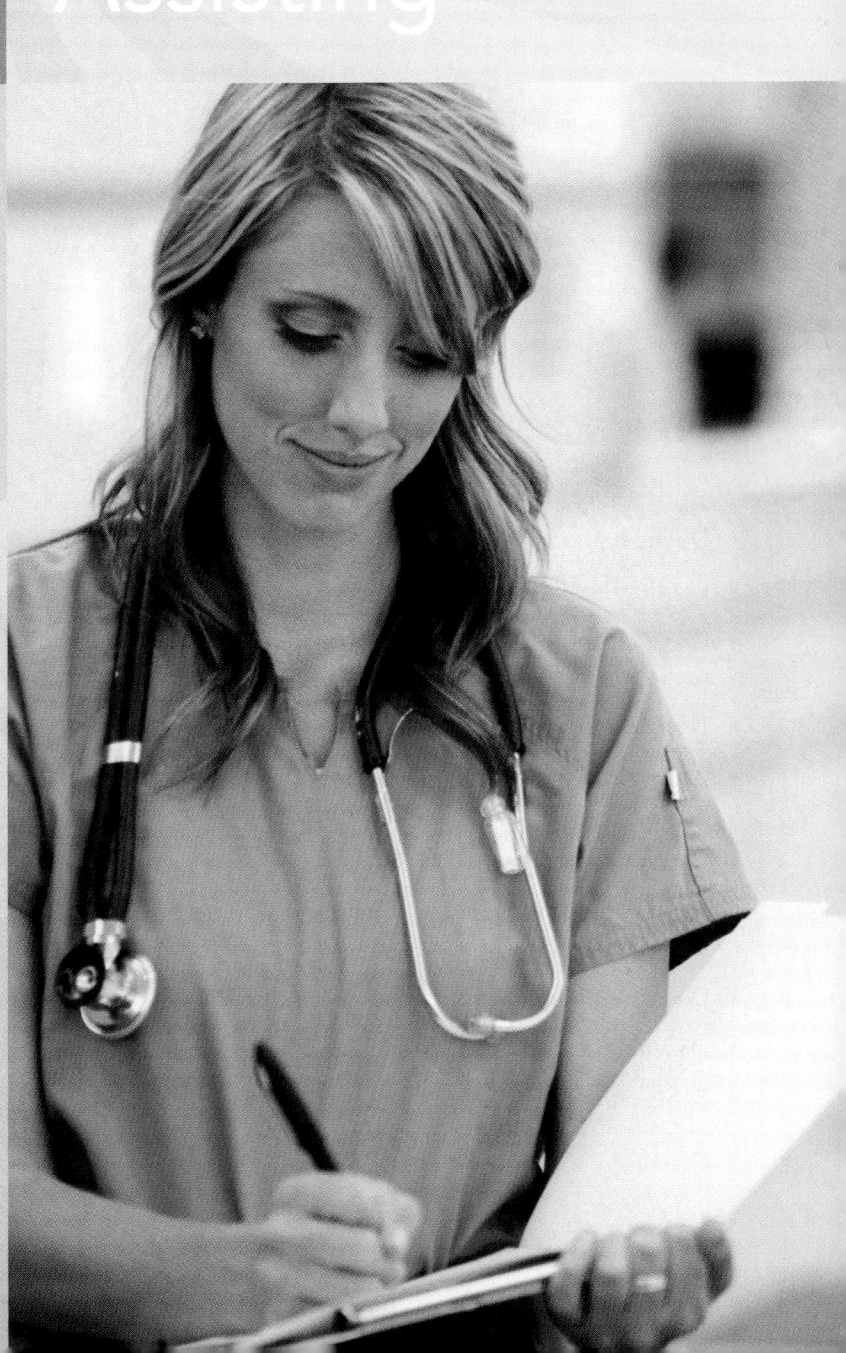

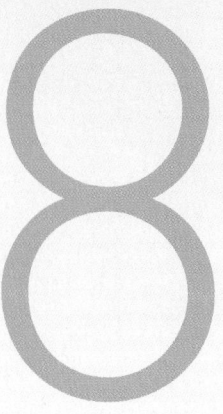

8

Patient Reception

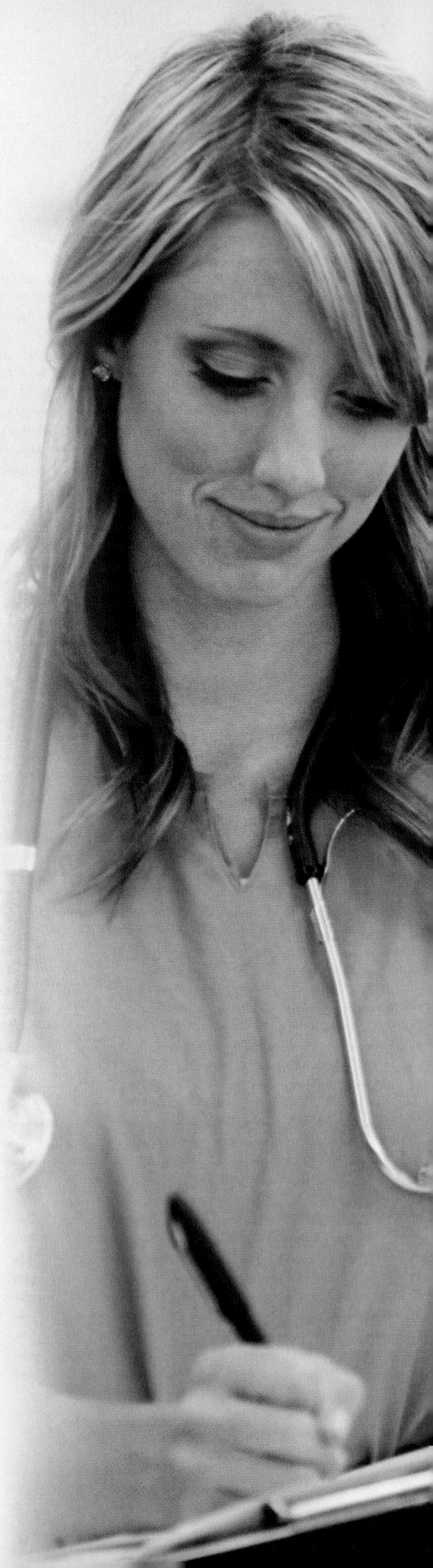

LEARNING OBJECTIVES

After completing this chapter, you should be able to:

- Define and spell the terms to learn for this chapter.

- List the receptionist's responsibilities.

- Describe the characteristics of an appropriate reception area.

- Describe the look of a professional medical assistant.

- Explain the procedure for opening the office.

- Explain the legal and ethical issues related to the duties of the receptionist.

- List the information to be obtained from the new patient.

- Describe how to handle the angry patient.

- Describe how to handle a waiting room emergency.

- Explain the procedure for closing the office.

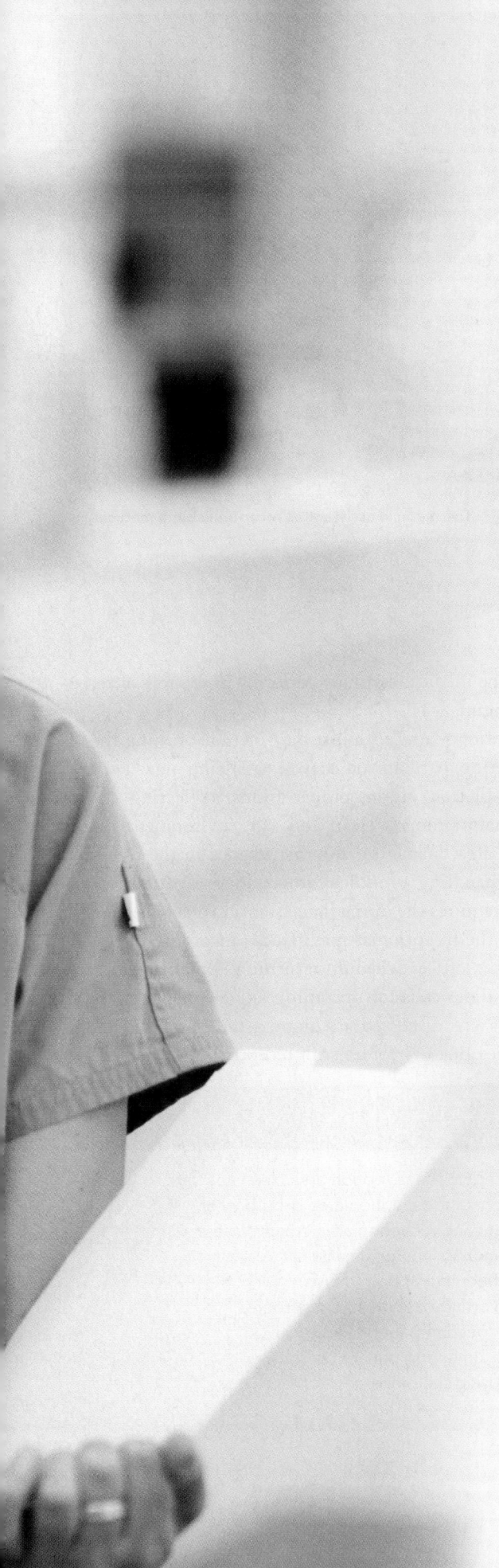

CHAPTER OUTLINE

CASE STUDY

Tania is responsible for opening Pearson Physicians Group on Tuesday and Thursday mornings. She arrives early and is the first employee at the office. There is a patient waiting at the front door to be let inside for his appointment that is scheduled for 45 minutes later, which is when the office is scheduled to open. When Tania opens the door to the office, she sees that the reception room has magazines strewn about, the children's books are not neatly piled, and the trash can was not emptied.

TERMS TO LEARN

collating

copayments

demographic

facsimile (fax)

medical emergency

no-show

overbooking

receptionist

CERTIFICATION LINK

CMA (AAMA)
Communication

Professionalism

Medicolegal guidelines and requirements

RMA
Human relations

Patient education

Medical receptionist/ Secretarial/Clerical

CMAS (AMT)
Medical office clerical assisting

Medical records management

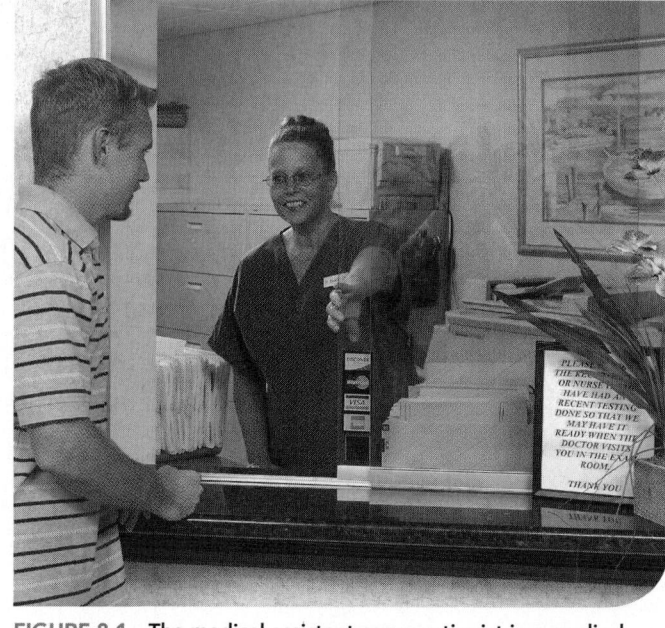

FIGURE 8-1 **The medical assistant as receptionist in a medical office.**

Patient reception requires a multiskilled individual who is able to multitask and whose manner, physical appearance, and tone of voice project a professional, confident, and caring persona. A small office will have fewer employees than one with several physicians; therefore, the medical assistant in a small office will perform many of the tasks described in this chapter. In the role of **receptionist**, the medical assistant greets and assists incoming patients and performs many important duties that make the office run smoothly and efficiently. Some of these duties are quiet and behind the scenes; others require constant interaction with patients. The medical assistant who functions as a receptionist must do everything possible to ensure patient safety and confidentiality at all times during the office visit.

Duties of a Receptionist

The number of patients as well as the nature of the medical practice—for example, whether it is a solo practice or a corporation of several physicians—will determine what duties or tasks the medical assistant performs in the role of receptionist (Figure 8-1).

The duties of a receptionist may include opening the office, greeting patients on arrival, assisting new patients with completion of the proper forms, collecting copayments, maintaining a clean and safe environment in the reception area, managing any disturbance in the reception area, and handling a **medical emergency** or patient condition that requires the immediate attention of a physician. In addition, the receptionist may handle incoming telephone calls for the office, schedule returning appointments, and make reminder calls for upcoming appointments. Many of these jobs are discussed in more detail throughout this chapter. See Box 8-1 for a list of reception duties.

Box 8-1 Duties of a Medical RECEPTIONIST

- Opening the office
- Pulling charts for the next day's appointments
- Collating patient records
- Checking in patients
- Greeting patients as they arrive
- Updating patient demographics
- Helping new patients fill out paperwork
- Collecting insurance copayments and patient balances due

- Keeping the reception area clean and safe
- Managing reception area disturbances
- Handling reception area emergencies
- Handling incoming calls
- Scheduling appointments
- Escorting patients to exam rooms
- Respecting patients' time
- Documenting patient no-shows
- Closing the office

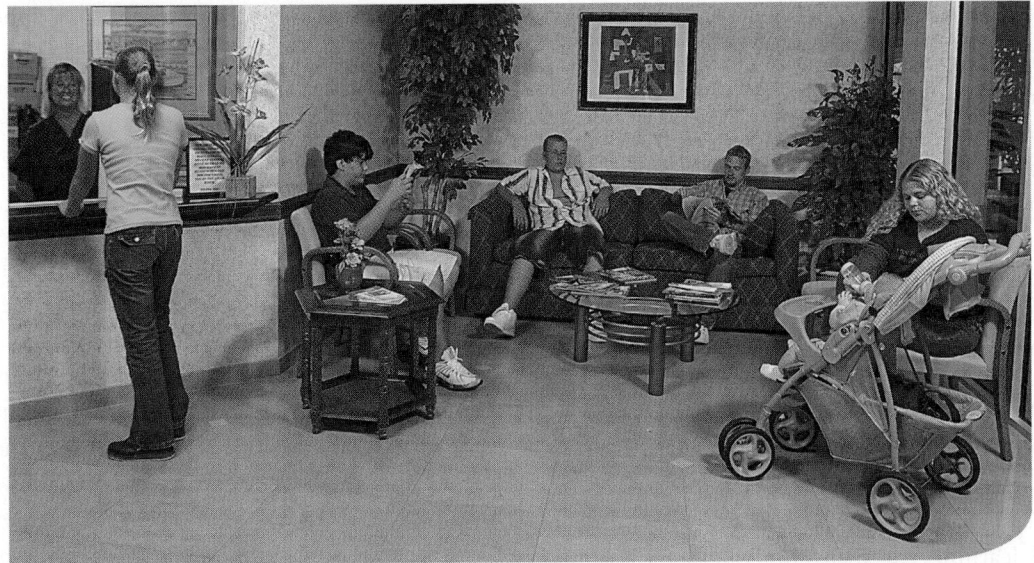

FIGURE 8-2 A typical reception area in a medical office.

RECEPTION ROOM

One of the most forgotten roles of the medical assistant is taking care of the reception area. Many offices still refer to this area as the waiting room; however, many now call it the reception area to avoid the term *waiting*. This area must be kept clean and free from any hazards that may injure a patient. It is often the reception area where the patient will develop his or her first impression of the office. Because first impressions are important, this area must be kept clean and organized (Figure 8-2). The receptionist must monitor the cleanliness of the room. If the room begins to get messy, the receptionist may need to take the time to straighten it up. Magazines, brochures, patient education documents, and toys should be arranged neatly. Any papers lying around must be thrown away or destroyed, depending on the information they contain.

In addition to keeping the reception room clean and organized, the receptionist may also be responsible for placement of furniture in that area. The path from the entrance to the receptionist's desk should be direct, with nothing in the way to trip the patient. Also, furniture should be placed to allow access and movement of wheelchairs. Most offices prefer placing furniture in conversational groups rather than around the perimeter of the reception area.

The type of furniture found in the office may be reflective of the patient population. For example, in addition to the traditional type of furniture found in the reception room of a pediatric office, you may find smaller chairs and couches for children. Low couches and chairs should be avoided in internal medicine and oncology practices as it is difficult for elderly and weak patients to rise from low furniture.

Many offices have a television patients can watch while they wait. Typically, educational health information is shown. Whatever the topic, it should always be appropriate for patients.

Lost and Found

It also may be the responsibility of the receptionist to take care of items mistakenly left in the office by patients. The office may have a lost-and-found box in which these items may be kept. Many offices will try to contact a patient if it is known that the item belongs to him or her. The office may have a policy as to how long unclaimed items are kept before they are thrown away or donated to a local charity.

PROFESSIONALISM

The receptionist is the first representative of the medical office that the patient is exposed to either by phone or in person. It is important that the patient's first impression inspires confidence in the office's ability to meet his or her needs. This means that receptionists must take great care in their appearance. Their clothes should be clean and pressed. The receptionist's hygiene influences the patient's perception of the cleanliness of the office. Receptionists must keep their office area neat and organized. If patients see a messy, disorganized area, they may wonder about how their information will be handled.

HANDLING INCOMING MONEY

The receptionist is often the person in charge of accepting office payments. They will often be responsible for collecting balances on accounts and copayments. **Copayments** are designated amounts that some medical insurance plans require patients to pay for medical services. Most medical offices expect to receive copayments at the time of service. It is important to keep excellent records of all incoming money so that balancing at the end of the day is easier. See Chapter 15 for more on the handling of money in the medical office.

CARE AND MAINTENANCE OF OFFICE EQUIPMENT

The receptionist is often responsible for taking care of certain equipment, such as copiers, computers, printers, and fax machines, and learning the many functions of these machines. Knowledge of how to repair small problems, such as paper jams, is also helpful. It is important that the receptionist troubleshoot the equipment prior to calling for service because solving issues through troubleshooting may save the office the cost of service calls. However, it is important to know what numbers to call for service if needed. The receptionist may also need to know how to replace printer toner and ink cartridges; it is very important that these machines remain filled with paper and operating correctly. See Chapter 12 for more information regarding the use of computers and troubleshooting.

Personal Characteristics and Physical Appearance

The receptionist is the first person a patient will see on entering the office. Presenting a positive public image is important because your appearance reflects on the entire staff.

PROFESSIONALISM THE LIFE SPAN

It is a fact that people of different generations feel differently about what constitutes appropriate personal appearance. For example, younger generations may not feel that multiple facial piercings or tattoos are offensive. However, older generations may feel these are inappropriate. As a medical assistant, you must achieve the highest level of professionalism so that you meet the highest standards of your patients. Even if you feel that a nose ring or tongue piercing is acceptable, remember that your patients may not agree.

Careful grooming, good hygiene, and appropriate dress must be observed. Office policy will dictate the preferred clothing. In most offices, the clinical staff members wear uniforms of the same type or color, which can consist of scrubs-type pants and top with a lab coat. The advantages of this type of uniform are that it can be worn by both male and female staff and is relatively inexpensive. Colors and patterns of uniforms are usually determined by the managers of the practice. Shoes must be closed-toe, and some offices ban wearing any shoes without a back, such as clogs. Whatever the type of shoe, it must be clean and skid resistant. Receptionists and other administrative personnel frequently wear the same style uniform as the clinical staff but without a lab coat, or they may be allowed to dress in business casual dress.

Hygiene, at a minimum, consists of daily bathing, use of a deodorant without a strong scent, good oral care, and clean, well-pressed clothing. Hairstyles and jewelry worn by male and female medical assistants should reflect professionalism, as should makeup. Accessories should be conservative and minimal—generally limited to one finger ring, a watch with a second hand, a name tag, and a professional association pin. Most offices will not tolerate any type of facial or tongue piercings, and tattoos may need to be covered. Long hair should be worn tied back and off the shoulders. Nails should be well trimmed, and only clear polish should be used. No perfumes should be worn as patients can be allergic to certain scents.

Name pins or tags should be visible at all times. Offices are increasingly requiring a picture ID for security reasons. These tags can serve dual purposes. With a magnetic strip, they can allow entrance into a secure area and can also be used to clock in and out for hours worked.

Opening the Office

The medical assistant whose responsibility it is to open the office should arrive 30 minutes prior to the start of office hours. In addition to the receptionist's friendly smile and welcoming greeting, a well-lighted, clean, and inviting environment does much to cheer patients. The receptionist should begin opening the office by checking the security alarm and disengaging it, turning on all lights, and checking the general status of the reception room, which should be tidy and clean. Any area used for children's toys should be neat and safe. Magazines and books should be stacked or placed in wall racks.

If the office uses paper charts, the medical assistant should check to make sure all charts are pulled and prepared for that day's patients; this task may often be performed

OPENING THE OFFICE

Objective: Prepare and set up the office to receive patients and operate efficiently.

EQUIPMENT AND SUPPLIES

Checklist of opening office procedures; office keys for rooms and files; message forms or pads; master lists of scheduled patients

1. Arrive at least 30 minutes prior to the first scheduled appointment.
2. Turn on the lights in the patient reception area before the first patient arrives.
3. Check that the heating or air conditioning and computers are working properly.
4. Check the reception room for safety hazards such as frayed electrical cords, a slippery floor, or torn carpeting. Place a warning sign near any safety hazard, and report it immediately to the office manager.
5. Check magazines, and recycle any that are torn, damaged, or outdated.
6. Check for cleanliness and report inadequate housekeeping services.
7. Unlock file rooms or cabinets where records are kept.
8. Take calls from the answering machine or faxes that may have come in from the answering service. Handle any that need immediate attention.
9. Unlock any money that may be used for the day. Count and balance the money to make sure that the amount is the same as it was when closing the office the day before.
10. Unlock the outer office door.
11. If you have not already done so the previous business day, compare the master list of all patients who will be seen during the day against the patient records that were pulled during previous office hours. If a patient has been added to the schedule after the records were pulled, pull, review, and add this patient's record to the other records.
12. Make phone calls to gather any laboratory test information that is missing from any patient's record. Provide the physician(s) and nurse(s) with a copy of the list of any laboratory test information that you have called for but have not yet received.
13. Print the day's patient schedule and place it on the physician's desk or other designated area.

the previous afternoon. Charge slips should be printed in advance for the day with any balances due highlighted. The previous day's receipts should have been taken to the bank, and the receptionist may have the responsibility of checking the cash box to see that the correct amount of change has been given. This will provide a way to double-check the balance at the end of the day.

For an efficient beginning to the day, all office machines should be turned on and made ready for use. Many copiers take several minutes to warm up. Any copiers, fax machines, and printers should be filled with paper. Nothing is more frustrating and time consuming than to find a fax machine without paper and a queue of faxes waiting to be printed.

A master list of patient appointments should be printed out, and copies of the master list should be placed on the desks of the clinical medical assistants and each of the doctors—but not in areas where patients may be able to see them. The final task prior to opening the office is to check the answering service and/or answering machine. If messages have come in, the receptionist should document all calls, place messages on charts, and distribute them to the appropriate individuals. Occasionally, messages may be left that will require immediate action. If such is the case, the receptionist should bring those messages to the attention of the appropriate individual. If additional appointments were made, the receptionist should pull the charts and print charge slips for these added patients. It may be the responsibility of the opening medical assistant to make sure that all examination rooms are prepared for use. See Procedure 8-1 for more about opening the office.

Collating Records

Collating refers to collecting all records, test results, and information pertaining to a patient who is scheduled to be seen by the physician. Collating also refers to organizing the subgroup information (for example, laboratory and X-ray results) in records for the day's appointments and for filing. This task should be part of pulling records, which may also be referred to as pulling charts. A record or chart is a medical record containing information such as laboratory and X-ray results. This is different from the patient's file. The file will refer to the financial record. It may contain billing, payment, and insurance information. The patient's file will most likely be an electronic record accessible on a computer, rather than a paper record.

Collating records is usually done the day before patients are seen. The records of patients scheduled for a Monday are typically pulled and collated on the previous Friday or Thursday. In some medical offices with several physicians, the number of patients seen may require collating records earlier than the day before the patient's visit. Always follow the policy of your office.

The physician's orders and notations from the previous visit must be reviewed to ensure that all necessary information has been received and is in the record. If information such as tests or lab results ordered at the last visit have not been received, the medical assistant will have to determine and phone whichever lab or facility was used and request either an oral, written, or electronic report. It is important that the information be available when the physician sees the patient. It is especially important if the patient's visit is solely to follow up on those results. When you are provided with an oral report,

the information should be documented on a message pad and flagged for the physician's review as the physician may request further reports depending on the findings. However, when the original report is received, it is also placed in the patient's record. This is done quite often by the clinical medical assistant. In some offices and laboratories, the facsimile (fax) machine can be used to send reports between facilities. A **facsimile (fax)** is an electronically transmitted document containing print and/or graphic information.

In some offices, the records are to be placed in the order in which the patients will be seen. A printed appointment list is placed on top of the collated records. This list serves as a checklist to keep track of patient arrivals and completed physician visits. As patients arrive you will verify their name on the schedule, and as they complete their visit and check out you will mark their names off the list. This system helps ensure that patients have checked in and checked out and that all encounter forms are accounted for. An encounter form, also called a charge slip or superbill, is a record of service for billing and for insurance processing. A copy of this same list is placed on the physician's desk on the morning of the patient's visit. A list may also be given to the person who will be rooming patients that day. Procedure 8-2 presents the steps in the process of collating records.

procedure 8-2

COLLATING RECORDS
Objective: Prepare medical records of scheduled patients for review by the physician.

EQUIPMENT AND SUPPLIES
Master list of scheduled patients; charts and records of scheduled patients

1. Print or copy the day's appointment schedule.
2. Pull all the medical records of patients scheduled to be seen.
3. In each record, review the patient's last appointment and make note of any results that should have been received, including laboratory tests, X-ray results, consultation notes, and other tests.
4. If any of the results are not in the patient's chart, call the appropriate facilities to retrieve the results. In the patient's chart, document the date, time, name of person with whom you spoke, and the expected action regarding the requested information. You may take oral results

and record them as a verbal report, but request that the hard copy results be faxed to the office as soon as possible.
5. Make a list of all results that have been received by phone and any that are outstanding. Let the physician know what remains outstanding.
6. Add all received information to each chart for the physician to review and sign off on.

CHARTING EXAMPLE
1/7/XX, 8:30 A.M. Spoke with Lisa at Saview Hospital lab, (555-1234). Requested Mr. Jones 12/20/XX CBC results. Lisa faxing results to office now. ········ K. Huerta, CMA (AAMA)

Greeting the Patient on Arrival

As stated previously in this chapter, the receptionist often provides patients with their first impressions of the medical office. The impression you make—good or bad—tends to flavor the patient's opinion of everyone related to the office. Therefore, that first impression is very, very important.

Emergency patients or those with a contagious disease should enter the office through a private office entrance (if there is one) and be escorted directly into an examination room. This is done to limit exposure to contagious germs and not to alarm the other patients.

In some offices, the receptionist sits behind a glass partition that slides open easily, allowing the receptionist to personally greet each patient entering the office (Figure 8-3). If the receptionist is on the telephone when a patient enters, looking up and smiling is a good way to acknowledge the patient's presence.

Patients must always take precedence over other visitors to the office (for example, a medical supplier or pharmaceutical representative). Scheduling such a visit when few or no patients are in the office might be a better solution. Nonemergency conversations with other staff persons should always be interrupted to respond to a patient.

Use caution and speak in a low voice when mentioning another patient's name over the telephone or to another staff member within hearing distance of any patients in the reception room. A violation of confidentiality can be grounds for a lawsuit. The reason for the glass partition is to protect the confidentiality of patients. Always close the partition when you are speaking on the telephone or to medical office staff members.

Quickly pick up ringing phones by the third ring, and always take a message if you are busy with another call or a patient in the office. It is better to call the patient back than to leave the patient on hold if you are unable to answer a question or have to look up information. Callers should not be left on hold for longer than 1 minute. See Chapter 7 for more information regarding use of the telephone.

It is important that special consideration and accommodation be provided for hearing and visually impaired, as well as physically challenged patients. The receptionist should ensure that these patients are treated the same as other patients, without overlooking their challenges. To communicate effectively with hearing and visually impaired as well as physically challenged patients, face the patient when you are speaking, speak slowly, do not raise your voice, offer a pen and piece of paper if the patient requests them, and provide any further assistance the patient requests. If the patient has a family member or companion accompanying them, do not communicate as if the patient is not there; communicate directly with the patient unless the patient instructs you otherwise.

SIGNING IN

A sign-in sheet or patient register is maintained at the reception desk. The sign-in sheet, which will differ from office to office, usually contains space for the patient's name, the time of arrival, and the name of the physician the patient will see. The sign-in sheet allows the receptionist to maintain a continuous record of all patients who come into the office. Be sure the sign-in sheet or patient register used in your office is Health Insurance Portability and Accountability Act (HIPAA) compliant. When patients arrive and sign in, they should not have access to the names of patients who have already signed in.

Several types of HIPAA compliant patient sign-in sheets are available. Some use a sticker with carbonless paper underneath. This type of system requires the patient to record their information on the sticker, peel off the sticker, and hand it to the receptionist. The information hidden under the carbonless paper is the information for office records, such as patient name, time of arrival, and reason for visit. A similar sign-in sheet uses shingled tickets, and instead of handing the receptionist the sticker, the patient hands the ticket to the receptionist and keeps the numbered stub. This method allows the office the option of calling patients back by either name or number. Calling patients back by numbers has received mixed

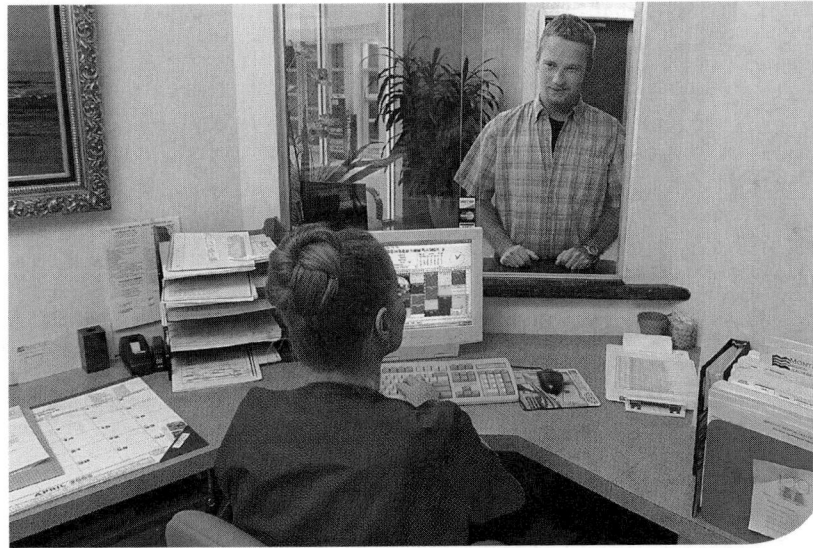

FIGURE 8-3 **Each patient is greeted by the receptionist.**

reviews. Some patients want to be called by name as going to the doctor is a very personal experience and using numbers is very impersonal. Others prefer not to have their name made known in the waiting room. This is a decision that must be made at the practice level, or even patient by patient. When registering the patient, the receptionist may want to ask whether the patient prefers to be called back by number or name. If it is determined patients will be called back by name, no other identifying marks are used to indicate the reason for their visit.

Many offices use a label system in which the patients sign in on a removable label. When the patient has signed the label, it is removed from the sheet and placed on a piece of paper behind the reception desk. In some offices, this piece of paper is maintained as a permanent record with all patient signatures from the day.

On signing in, it is important that the medical assistant ask patients to verbally confirm their current address and

telephone number without others hearing. HIPAA requires that every attempt be made to protect patient privacy. For example, in a quiet voice, the receptionist should ask the patient "Mr. Jones, will you please verify your address"? It is important that the office have current contact information for the patient. Confirming that all contact information is correct is critical for billing purposes. Current contact information is also vital for any follow-up that is required after the office visit.

In some offices, the sign-in sheet is filed in a designated folder at the end of the day to provide another record of the patients seen during that day. If the office policy is to destroy the sign-in sheet to maintain confidentiality, make sure these papers are shredded. (*Note:* Some offices are starting to move away from sign-in sheets due to confidentiality concerns. HIPAA does allow for the use of sign-in sheets, but you may not include the reason for the visit on the sign-in sheet. Only the patient's name, time of arrival, and the physician's name may be used.)

Registering New Patients

New patients must fill out a complete patient registration form requesting **demographic** information, such as age, gender, ethnic background, education, and Social Security number (Figure 8-4). Place the registration form on a clipboard with a pen attached and have the patient complete it while he or she is waiting to be seen by the physician.

PATIENT REGISTRATION FORM
(Please Print)

Date: _____

Patient's
Name: _____
    First   Middle   Last

DOB: _____ / _____ / _____
    Month   Day   Year

Address: _____
    Street   City   State   Zip

Phone: _____ / _____ - _____
    (Area code)

Patient's SS#: _____ - _____ - _____ Driver's License #: _____ Occupation: _____

Method of payment (circle): cash   check   credit card   insurance co-payment

Primary Insurance Co.: _____ Policy/Group #: _____

Medicare #: _____   Medicaid #: _____

Person
Responsible
For Payment: _____
    First   Middle   Last   Relationship

Address: _____
    Street   City   State   Zip

Phone: _____ / _____ - _____
    (Area code)

Employer Name: _____
    First   Middle   Last

Dept: _____

Address: _____
    Street   City   State   Zip

Phone: _____ / _____ - _____
    (Area code)

Spouse or
Nearest Relative: _____
    First   Middle   Last   Relationship

Address: _____
    Street   City   State   Zip

Phone: _____ / _____ - _____
    (Area code)

How were you referred to this office? _____

_____

Statement of Financial Responsibility: I, _____
do hereby agree to pay all medical charges incurred by the above listed patient. I further understand that these charges are my responsibility, regardless of insurance coverage.

Responsible Person's Signature: _____

FIGURE 8-4   **Patient registration form.**

Include the HIPAA privacy notification form, which is used to inform patients of their rights regarding HIPAA, with the registration form. Some offices mail these forms to patients to complete at home and submit at the first office visit; others ask new patients to arrive 15 to 30 minutes early to complete the necessary forms. Those offices using electronic medical records may have their patients supply the registration information online, or the office may have a computer in the reception area that allows the patient to complete registration electronically at the office (Figure 8-5).

No matter which registration method is used, provide the patient with precise instructions. Indicate the portions of the forms the patient must complete, if two sides are to be completed, and where the patient's signature is required. Assist patients who are unable to read and write due to illiteracy or a disability. Realize that many patients who cannot read or write may be embarrassed by this and do not readily admit they are unable to complete the forms. You may want to help them in a private area of the office.

You will need to explain to the patient your office's policies regarding billing and payment. Along with verbally explaining these policies, it is advisable to give each new patient informational brochures. The patient must also sign an assignment of benefits form so that the insurance company may send payments directly to the physician.

Make sure that all forms are completed correctly in their entirety and that all signatures are in place. With computer-assisted registration, you can input dictation directly onto the computer terminal. Refer to Chapters 12-14 for more information on computer-assisted office functions.

Request to see the patient's insurance card(s), and ask the patient politely if any insurance information has changed. This can decrease the chances of lapsed coverage. Photocopy both sides of the insurance card(s), and be sure that the copy is legible. Insurance billing cannot be processed without complete information. Check the insurance card to see if a patient copayment is required. Indicate the copayment in the appropriate place on the patient's file. (The copayment may be collected before or after the visit, depending upon office procedure.) Depending on the type of insurance the patient has, the receptionist may need to call and verify insurance coverage and the participation status of the physician with whom the visit is scheduled. See Procedure 8-3 for more information on how to register a new patient.

Charge Slips

The charge slip (also referred to as encounter form or superbill) used in most medical offices is a part of the billing process. The charge slip contains a list of the most common current procedural terminology (CPT) and International Classification of Diseases (ICD-9) codes, which correspond to the procedure- and diagnosis-related charges used by the office. Some offices use a charge plate system or computer program that will imprint the patient's name and identification number on all forms used in the medical office, including the charge slip. The appropriate charge slip is attached to the medical record of each patient who is to be seen by the physician on that day. At the end of the visit, the physician indicates what treatment was given, the supporting diagnosis and what the charge is. The charge slip is then given to

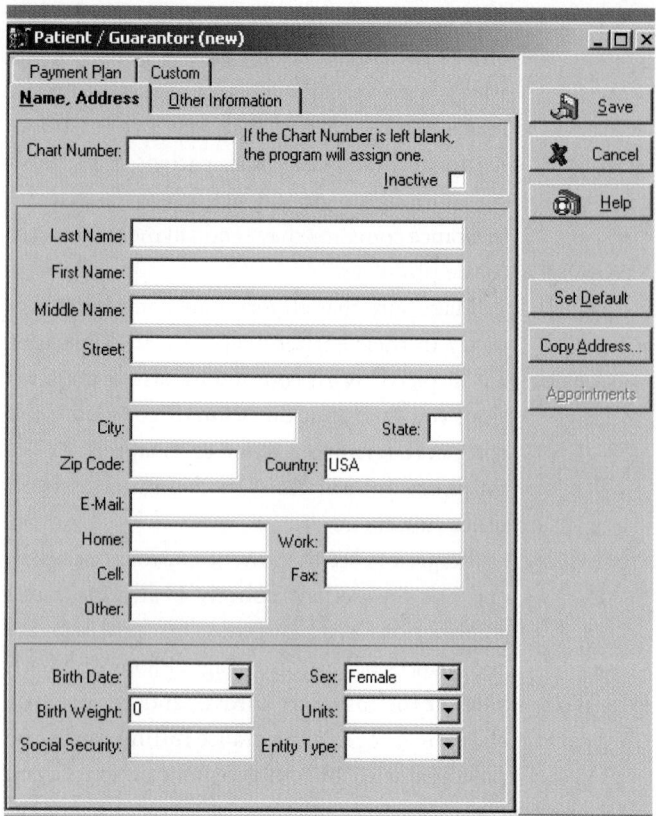

FIGURE 8-5 A patient registration form used in offices with electronic medical records. Many offices offer the convenience of completing the form online prior to the first visit or have computers set up in the reception area, which allows patients to complete the form once they are in the office.

the receptionist or the cashier. Payment or arrangements for payment are made before the patient leaves the office.

All patients are entitled to and should receive a copy of the charge slip before they leave the office. When there is no charge for the visit, as in a follow-up visit after surgery, the physician will write "no charge" or "N/C" on the slip. For accounting purposes, a charge slip number is assigned to each patient.

Consideration for the Patient's Time

One of the most common complaints expressed by patients is the excessive amount of time they have to spend in the reception room before being seen by a physician. Patients are generally understanding when they are told the physician has an emergency that has resulted in a schedule delay. However, in many cases, the physician is running behind schedule because of errors with the scheduling system, such as **overbooking**, when more than one patient is scheduled in the same time slot. Delays are also caused by not allowing enough time on the schedule for patient visits. This usually occurs because inaccurate information is obtained concerning the reason a patient wishes to see the doctor.

In general, a 20-minute wait is accepted by most patients. If the wait is going to be longer, then you should approach each patient and ask if the patient prefers to wait or wishes to reschedule the appointment. If the expected

procedure 8-3

REGISTERING A NEW PATIENT

Objective: Accurately complete a registration form for a new patient.

EQUIPMENT AND SUPPLIES

For paper-based charts: Registration form, pen, clipboard, private area

For electronic medical records: Computer and possibly online access

Note: If the patient has not completed a registration form prior to the appointment, the receptionist may need to assist the patient.

1. Gather the supplies.
2. Verify that the patient has not been seen in the office before.

3. Obtain and record the following information from the patient:
   - Full name spelled correctly
   - Date of birth
   - Home address, including zip code
   - Telephone number, including area code
   - Cell phone number, including area code
   - Marital status
   - Employer
   - Employer address
   - Employer telephone number
   - Social Security number

- Insurance information, including group number
- Insurance subscriber's name
- Insurance copayment amount (Photocopy both sides of the insurance card)
- Name of the guardian, if applicable
- Name of the person responsible for payment
- Address of the person responsible for payment
- Telephone number of person responsible for payment
- Photocopy of the patient's photo ID, such as a driver's license or military ID

4. Once the preceding information has been documented, review everything with the patient to ensure accuracy.
5. Ask the patient to read and sign the HIPAA privacy notification form. This form may vary from office to office, but the information it contains is the same.

6. For patients who are unable to complete the form themselves, document within the record that the patient verbally provided the documented demographic information, verify everything for accuracy, and have the patient sign in the appropriate area. The receptionist completing the form should also sign and date it.

CHARTING EXAMPLE

6/7/XX, 2:00 P.M. Information provided verbally by patient, Rena Jones. On completion of documentation, reviewed information with patient for accuracy. Patient confirmed information correct as noted. · L. Ritchie, RMA

wait time exceeds 20 minutes, the receptionist should inform the patient as soon as possible. This may mean notifying the patient of the delay either before or after they have checked in. For instance, if the physician is running 2 hours behind, the receptionist should attempt to contact the patient and let them know of the delay prior to the patient's arrival at the office. This affords the patient the opportunity to decide to wait or to reschedule.

Patients generally respond well to a quiet explanation from the receptionist regarding how long the wait will be. Unfortunately, after patients sign in they are sometimes forgotten by the receptionist. Since the patient's only contact in the office is the receptionist, it is critical that a concerned approach be used. Periodically check on your waiting patients. Know the office policy regarding which type of complaint is seen immediately by the physician.

When a patient complains of a long delay in seeing the physician, never express anger or say to the patient "It's not my fault." An empathetic medical assistant can imagine how nervous and ill the patient must feel. Make every effort to calm an angry patient so that he or she is no longer angry when going in to see the physician.

Escorting the Patient into the Examination Room

All patients should be personally escorted into the examination room (Figure 8-6). In most instances, this is done by a medical assistant assigned to patient care rather than by the receptionist. If, however, you are asked to help "room" patients, make sure you select the correct record and clearly call the patient by name (or number). To ensure that you have the correct patient and chart, ask the patient to state his

or her name and date of birth. Also make sure to ask the patient how he or she would like to be addressed. Never call a patient by his or her first name unless the patient has asked you to do so. Walk at the patient's speed, and offer special assistance to patients using a wheelchair, crutches, walker, or cane. You may wish to make pleasant conversation to make the patient feel at ease. If the patient is a small child or in a wheelchair, make sure you are at eye level when you speak with them.

Once the patient is in the exam room, clearly explain exactly what articles of clothing the patient should remove. It is important to be specific because it can extend a patient's appointment time if the physician is unable to perform an examination because the patient has not been correctly prepared. Point out the gown or sheet for the patient to use after undressing, and make sure the patient knows whether the gown is to open in the front or the back. If you suspect a

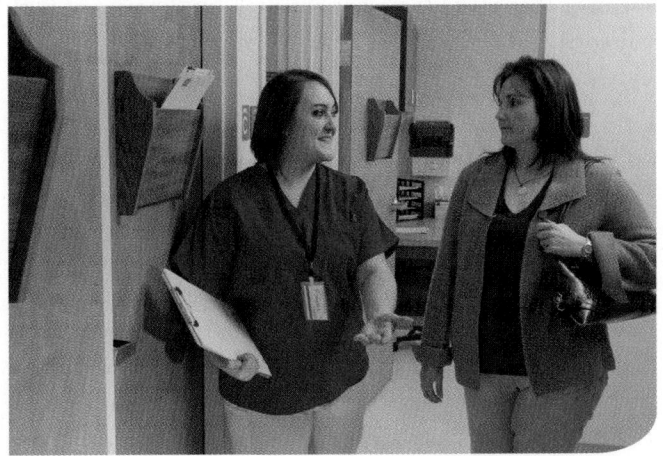

FIGURE 8-6 The medical assistant escorts the patient into the examination room.

patient will need assistance removing clothing, ask if he or she would like you to help. Always protect the patient's modesty; it will be appreciated by the patient.

Once the patient is situated, state approximately when the doctor will be in to see them. If the doctor is delayed, inform patients waiting in examination rooms that the doctor hasn't forgotten about them. If the patient has to wait in the exam room to see the doctor, make sure that appropriate reading material is available.

Never leave the patient alone with his or her chart. The patient might remove a page or pages, and if the patient were someday to bring legal charges against the physician, the chart would be incomplete and might not support the physician's case. Remember this "golden rule" of documentation: *If it is not documented, it didn't happen.*

The chart is often placed in a slot or box just outside the examination room. The patient's record should be placed in the proper location so that patient information is not visible to anyone walking by. This may require placing the chart in the box so the patient information faces the wall. Once the physician has completed the exam, return to the examination room and knock before entering. Give the patient instructions about what to do next. For example, you might say to the patient "You may dress now. The doctor will come back to talk to you shortly," or "Please stop at the reception desk (or other designated area) after you have dressed, and I'll explain the test the doctor has ordered."

Make it a point to speak with each patient before he or she leaves. In some cases, the patient may need to make a payment, talk to the cashier, make another appointment, or have a specific test or procedure explained. Always ask the patient if he or she has any additional questions. A simple "Good-bye" brings closure to each patient's office visit.

If discussion is needed, it should be done in a private area out of the hearing range and view of other patients. Remember that HIPAA regulations prohibit discussions with patients taking place in any area where another patient may overhear.

Patient Education

Patient education often begins when the patient calls for an appointment. Two other important sites for patient education are at the reception desk and in the reception room. For example, education regarding office hours, policies, insurance form submissions, and after-hours emergency telephone numbers can be handled at the reception desk. The receptionist may be responsible for providing and explaining instructions regarding tests and procedures such as fasting before a particular blood test. In smaller offices where the receptionist handles insurance processing, education can take place regarding the patient's responsibility in the insurance reimbursement process.

LEVEL OF UNDERSTANDING

Always ensure that patient education is provided at a level the patient understands. It is best to ask the patient to restate what they heard. This offers an opportunity to assess the patient's level of understanding. If it is apparent the patient didn't quite understand the first attempt, revise the information to an appropriate level and ask the patient to restate it again. If the educational information seems to confuse the patient or is extensive, it is best to provide written information for the patient. No matter the level of patient understanding, always stress the importance of calling the office if more instructions or clarification is needed. Many times patients feel more comfortable asking for clarification from the receptionist or medical assistant than from the physician. If the patient asks a question you cannot answer or are unsure how to answer, do not hesitate to ask the physician or another individual in the office who might be able to help.

ELECTRONIC PATIENT EDUCATION

Many of the offices that use electronic medical records are sending out targeted patient education information via e-mail. For instance, when an office uses electronic medical records, the patient's diagnosis and procedures are documented within the electronic record. The office is able to query its records and obtain diagnosis-specific information that can be e-mailed. For example, the system could search for all patients with a diabetes diagnosis. Once the patient data have been gathered, an e-mail can be sent out to all diabetic patients about coping with their diabetes during holidays. This type of system requires an authorization from the patient allowing the office to send such e-mails, but it is a very efficient and cost-effective means to deliver patient education.

Patient education also can be disseminated through descriptive informational office practice brochures; literature from established health care organizations such as the American Cancer Society, American Diabetic Association, and American Heart Association; and bulletin displays on various aspects of health. Some offices provide a brief video presentation about selected procedures or health concerns.

Managing Disturbances

If a patient becomes angry or starts speaking in a loud voice, try to handle the situation immediately. It is always advisable to ask the patient to come into a quiet office where the problem can be discussed and handled.

If a private office is not available, the problem must be handled quickly and quietly in another area. Generally, people will respond to a sincere statement, such as "I'm sorry there's a problem. Let's see how we can solve it." Never assume responsibility for an issue until all information has been acquired. Ask the patient to identify what he or she perceives the problem to be, and then discuss possible solutions. Frequently, the angry patient will respond well if the medical assistant uses a very quiet, calm manner. Keep your voice low to help calm the patient. With practice, a medical assistant can become adept at calming the angry patient. If the patient is drunk or disorderly, follow the office policy regarding when to call the police.

On occasion, the receptionist may need to interact with mentally challenged patients who may or may not require extra attention. If a mentally challenged patient becomes disruptive in the reception room, it is best to escort the patient to an exam room, if available, and allow the patient to wait there. This may alleviate anxiety for all involved.

CHILDREN

Children pose a special challenge. Usually, children go into the examination room with the adult patient and are removed only if private areas are to be examined on the parent. For several reasons, it is not advisable to have the medical assistant oversee the child in the reception area while the adult is being examined. It is advisable to explain to the parent during check-in that children cannot be left unattended.

On rare occasions, a physician treats a child without the parent being present. In such cases, a medical assistant or other staff person will stay with the child during the examination or procedure. Teenagers often have things to ask the doctor that they may not want their parents to hear.

MEDICAL EMERGENCIES IN THE RECEPTION ROOM

A medical emergency occurs occasionally in the physician's office (Figure 8-7). Ill patients may come directly to the physician's office instead of first calling the physician or 911. In such cases, you must stop whatever you are doing to give assistance immediately. Ask another staff member to alert the physician. Tell available staff to give you assistance or to call 911 if emergency transport to a hospital is necessary. If all the exam rooms are full, you may ask the other waiting patients to step into the hall to prevent them from becoming anxious during the emergency.

In certain emergency situations, the medical assistant may be required to start first aid procedures. It may be necessary to begin cardiopulmonary resuscitation (CPR) on the patient. Your office should have guidelines in place for proper handling of this form of in-office emergency.

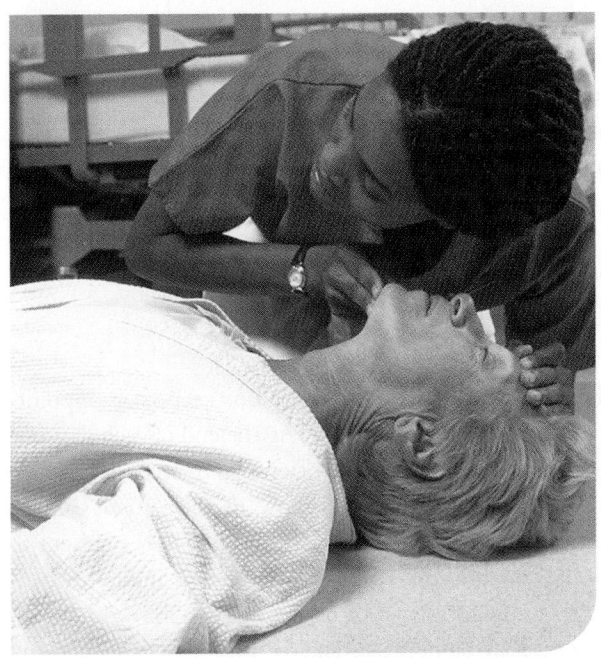

FIGURE 8-7 The medical assistant handles an emergency.

If a patient's condition requires emergency treatment and equipment, which the physician is able to provide in the office setting, then immediately take the patient into an examination room. Assist the patient onto an examination table if possible. Do not leave this patient unattended. Another staff member should alert the physician that the patient

PROFESSIONALISM

THE LAW

The receptionist must protect the safety of patients at all times during the office visit. Be sure to eliminate safety hazards, make sure exits are clearly marked, and place warning signs to identify wet floors. The receptionist must know how to evacuate the reception room in the event of fire. A map should be placed on the wall indicating where the patient reception area is in relation to the nearest exits.

In most offices, current CPR certification is required for all medical office staff, including the receptionist. The receptionist must be familiar with office policies regarding emergency treatment of patients and must respond quickly to reception room emergencies. Training in handling emergencies, including those initiated by phone, must be included in the receptionist's orientation to the job.

The receptionist also must always respect patient confidentiality. Be aware of what you are saying and whether or not you can be overheard by other people. Do not speak with patients about their care around other patients. Speak only in a private area where you cannot be overheard.

requires immediate attention. Many offices have an intercom system that allows communication from the reception area to all rooms in the office to quickly summon medical personnel.

If a family member who is present wishes to accompany the patient into the examination room, allow the person to do so unless prohibited by office policy. When treatment begins, a staff member should ask the family member to step out of the room.

No-Shows

No-show patients are those who do not keep their appointment and do not call to cancel it. At the end of each day, one of the responsibilities of the receptionist is to account for these patients and document the no-show in the patient's chart. Some offices have a standard practice to phone the patient to determine why the appointment was not kept and to reschedule another appointment. A policy to charge for no-show appointments may be in place. The receptionist must learn and use the procedure for no-shows as stated in the office's policies and procedures manual. Placing reminder calls to patients the day before their scheduled visit may lower the number of no-shows. One person, usually the office manager, is responsible for informing the physician of the patient no-shows.

Regardless of whether or not the patient was rescheduled, place a notation on the patient's record about the failed appointment, the date, any action taken and the result, and the initials of the person performing the documentation. This documentation is important in protecting the physician should there ever be a lawsuit.

If the patient fails to keep two or more appointments, the physician should definitely be informed. The physician may wish to send a letter declining to continue treating the patient. The letter should be sent both certified with return receipt requested and regular mail.

Closing the Office

Closing the office at the end of the day is a major function of the medical assistant. This function is key to operating a well-run office. A procedure for closing the office at the end of the day is presented in Procedure 8-4.

procedure 8-4

CLOSING THE OFFICE

Objective: Secure the office properly during nonoperating hours.

EQUIPMENT AND SUPPLIES

checklist of office closing procedures; bank deposit forms and envelope/pouch; office keys for rooms and files

1. Leave at least 15 to 30 minutes at the end of the day to close the office.
2. Check all records used during the day for any orders that may have been missed. In addition, make sure that every visit is posted to be billed.
3. Pull, review, and collate records for patients who will be seen the next day. Place the collated records with the charge slips attached and the master list of the next day's scheduled patients together in the appropriate place. Also, make a copy of this master list of patients for each physician.
4. Either deposit in a bank or lock in the office safe all money received from patient payments. It is wise to have the person designated to make the daily bank deposit vary the time of deposit. Many offices now use a courier for this task. For purposes of quality control, the person completing the bank deposit and the person making the deposit should not be the same. Both people should be bonded. Completing a bank deposit is discussed in Chapter 16.
5. Lock all files and file rooms, physician offices, and other individual offices within the medical practice.
6. Turn off electrical equipment and appliances. *Note:* Some equipment, such as incubators, fax machines, and computers, may require 24-hour operation. Check with your supervisor regarding the special requirements of your office.
7. Check all examination rooms to make sure they are clean and supplied for the next day. *Note:* This step may be done by the medical assistant who was in charge of rooming patients that day.
8. Straighten the reception room. Put away all magazines and pick up any toys.
9. Activate the answering service before leaving. Know the name of the physician who is accepting emergency calls or is on call until morning. Remind the physician who is on call.
10. Activate the security system if there is one.
11. Always double-check to make sure the door is locked.

SUMMARY

The receptionist's role can be one of the most demanding and most interesting positions in the medical office. While attending to the general running of the office, the medical assistant serving as receptionist must greet all patients, assist new patients in registering while obtaining updated health and insurance information, answer calls, schedule patients, open and close the office, contact and document no-shows, and more. All this requires a calm, caring, and organized individual who can keep patient information confidential and protect the safety of the patient during the office visit. The patient is most important.

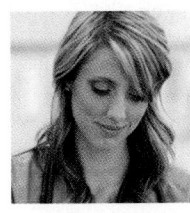

8 CHAPTER REVIEW

COMPETENCY REVIEW

1. Define and spell the terms to learn for this chapter.

2. Explain the steps to take if you are the first person to arrive and must open the medical office.

3. Describe how a professionally groomed receptionist would appear.

4. Explain what you would do if a patient suddenly collapsed in the reception room.

5. Discuss steps a medical assistant would take to assist in preventing a claim of abandonment against a physician.

6. Describe the important characteristics of a typical waiting area.

PREPARING FOR THE CERTIFICATION EXAM

1. Designated amounts that some medical insurance plans require patients to pay for medical services or medication, usually at the time of service, are known as:
   a. insurance premiums.
   b. deductibles.
   c. copayments.
   d. coinsurance.
   e. benefits.

2. The act of collecting all records, test results, and information pertaining to the patient is known as:
   a. filing.
   b. collating.
   c. tracking.
   d. sorting.
   e. indexing.

3. For hearing impaired patients to fully understand what is being said, it is best to:
   a. speak louder.
   b. write everything down.
   c. face the patient and speak slowly.
   d. try not to speak with them.
   e. talk to the accompanying family member.

4. When the patient is in a wheelchair, it is best to:
   a. make sure you are at eye level with the patient.
   b. speak to the person who brought the patient to the office.
   c. avoid using body language.
   d. speak louder.
   e. use paper and pencil.

5. If a patient doesn't show for their appointment, the receptionist should document:
   a. when the physician tells the receptionist to do so.
   b. only if the patient doesn't call to reschedule.
   c. at the end of the day when the appointment was missed.
   d. in the daily journal.
   e. when the office manager tells the receptionist to do so.

6. Typically, how long are most patients willing to wait in the office for their appointment before they become agitated?
   a. 50 minutes
   b. 40 minutes
   c. 30 minutes
   d. 20 minutes
   e. 1 hour

7. If it is apparent a new patient is unable to complete the registration form, the receptionist should:
   a. call the patient to the window and ask if he or she can read.
   b. call the patient to the window and ask them if he or she needs assistance.
   c. call the patient into an exam room and ask if he or she needs assistance.
   d. call across the reception room and ask if he or she needs assistance.
   e. ask the office manager to help the patient.

8. When calling a patient from the reception room to the exam room, it is proper to
   a. refer to the patient as Mrs. Smith.
   b. refer to the patient as Suzanne Smith.
   c. refer to the patient as "Honey."
   d. refer to the patient as Suzy.
   e. refer to the patient as Mrs. Robert Smith.

9. If a patient is a continual no-show for appointments, the physician has the option of:
   a. referring the patient to a physician partner.
   b. releasing the patient from his or her care.
   c. cancelling the patient's insurance.
   d. writing off the patient's balance.
   e. notifying the patient's insurance company.

10. Some offices use sign-in sheets that patients complete on arrival to the clinic. If using a sign-in sheet, what must not be included on the sheet?
    a. name
    b. time of arrival
    c. reason for visit
    d. physician's name
    e. date

CRITICAL THINKING

1. How should Tania handle the patient who is early for his appointment?

2. Tania checks the prior day's schedule and sees that Meghan closed the office on Monday night. How should Tania handle the disheveled reception room?

3. After other staff members have arrived for the day, Tania unlocks the office door. She sees the man from earlier in the morning exit his car and make his way to the door. When he arrives in the office, Tania notices that he has a bloody nose. What should she do with this patient?

ON THE JOB

Dr. Morrison, a child psychiatrist who is in solo practice, employs one medical assistant in her office. This medical assistant is multiskilled, like all medical assistants, and handles essentially all the administrative and clinical tasks in the office.

It is 3:00 P.M. and a parent has just arrived for a 3:30 P.M. appointment with her ten-year old daughter. The child is a new patient of Dr. Morrison and was referred by her attending physician. She has a relatively long history of combative and destructive behavior, and the referring pediatrician is seeking a psychological evaluation from Dr. Morrison. Psychotropic medication of some sort may be a viable treatment option. The medical assistant has politely asked the mother and daughter to be seated and to fill out some registration forms. The child is acting out—pulling cushions off the reception room couch, wildly ripping the pages of the magazines, whining, and kicking her mother. The behavior seems to be escalating as the mother tries to frantically control her child while, at the same time, follow the instructions of the medical assistant and fill out the registration forms.

1. What if anything, should the medical assistant do?
2. Would it be appropriate, for example, for the medical assistant to interrupt Dr. Morrison's current session?
3. Might this be considered a medical emergency?

INTERNET ACTIVITY

1. Find out how HIPAA has changed the way the medical office handles patient reception.

2. Look for companies that produce forms that can be used by a medical receptionist.

MEDMEDIA

Additional interactive resources and activities for this chapter can be found:

On your student DVD: View applicable procedure videos on the DVD-ROM found in the back of this book.

MyHealthProfessionsKit.com: Test your knowledge of the chapter with games and activities. MyHealthProfessionsKit also includes resources, helpful links, and a Spanish audio glossary.

Medical Assisting Interactive: Practice your procedures as a medical assistant in this simulated doctor's office. This can be accessed through MyHealthProfessionsKit.com.

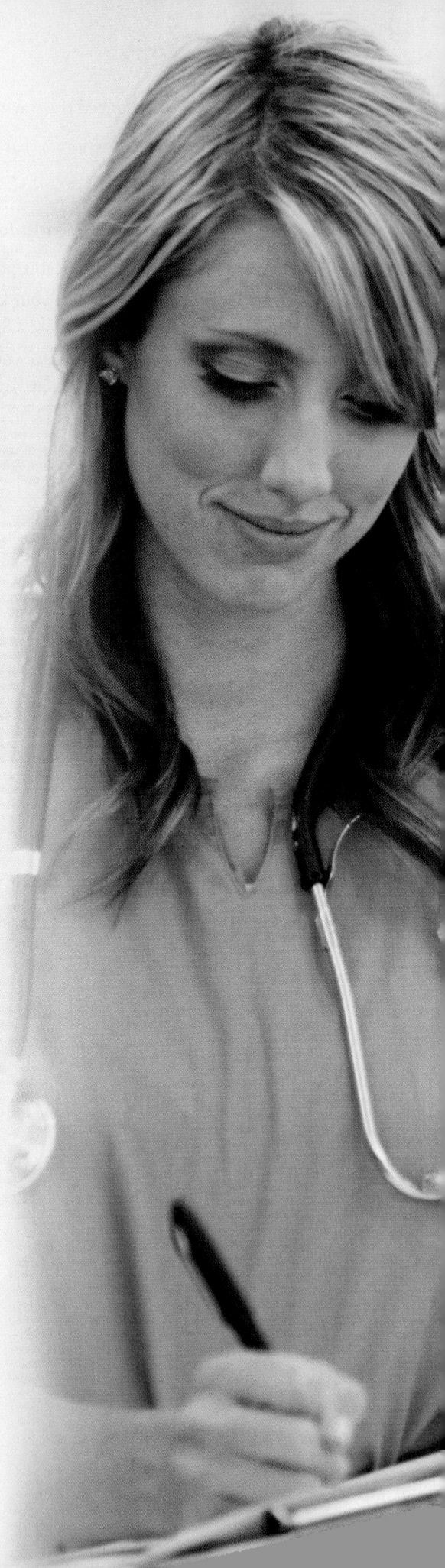

9

Appointment Scheduling

LEARNING OBJECTIVES

After completing this chapter, you should be able to:

- Define and spell the terms to learn for this chapter.

- Name and describe six scheduling systems.

- List and describe four pieces of equipment used in the scheduling process.

- Describe the appointment scheduling process.

- Explain the importance of correct documentation when a patient does not keep an appointment.

- Describe and arrange the process for scheduling a hospital admission and surgery.

- Summarize the ethical implications related to scheduling.

- Identify ten conditions that qualify as emergencies.

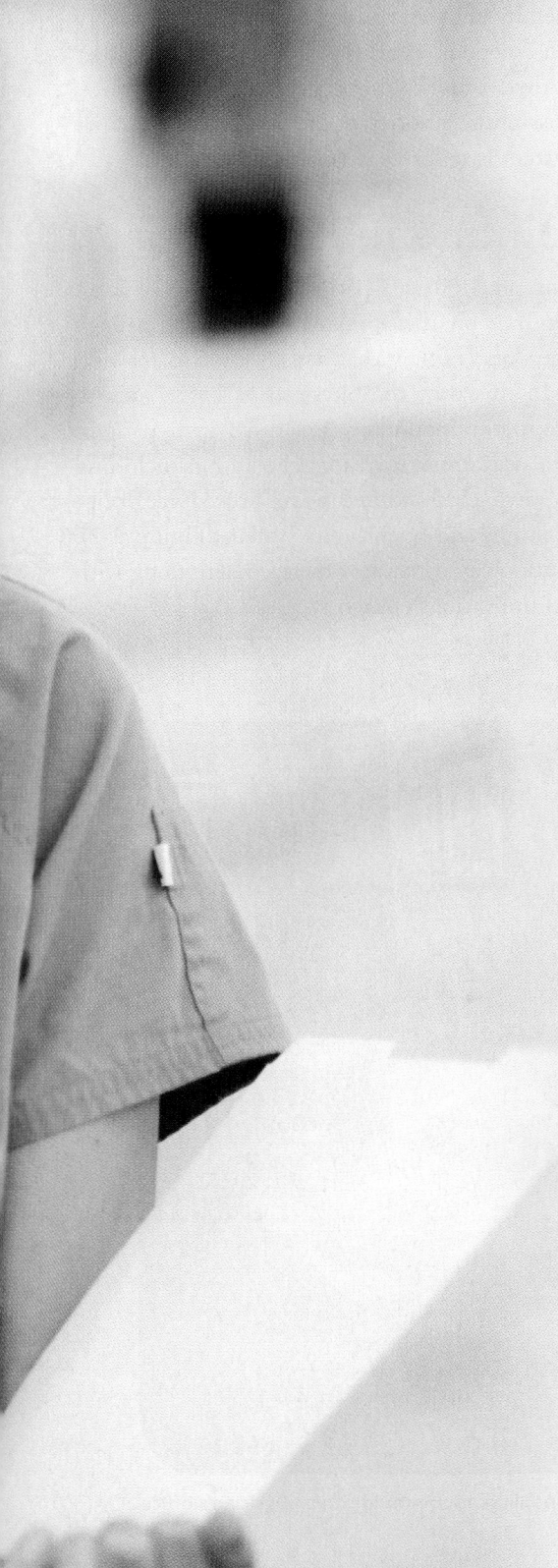

CHAPTER OUTLINE

CASE STUDY

Marc Rodgers, CMA (AAMA), is working the front desk today. He is looking ahead to tomorrow's (Friday) schedule. The office usually closes from noon until 1:00 P.M. for lunch. Marc takes note that tomorrow Dr. Miller is working a short day from 11:00 A.M. until 3:00 P.M. Marc sees that Dr. Miller has the following appointments scheduled:

11:00	Laura White	2:00	Rinna Brown
	Joe Tanner		Monica Floyd
	Lucy Smith		Peter Conner
1:00	Justin Ivy		
	Ramona Pierce		
	Lucas Abrams		

At 3:30 P.M., Rinna Brown calls to cancel her appointment for Friday. Shannon Reece wants to know if she can schedule a new patient appointment for tomorrow. Marcus Fowler, a familiar drug representative, wants to know if he can drop in briefly tomorrow.

TERMS TO LEARN

acute conditions	real time
advance booking	scheduling system
archived	screen saver
catch-up time	specific time
cycle time	subpoena
double booking	surgery scheduler
established patient	tickler file
matrix	time patterns
modified wave scheduling	triage
open-ended questions	wave scheduling
privacy screen	

CERTIFICATION LINK

CMA (AAMA)
General
Communication
Scheduling and monitoring appointments

RMA
General medical assisting knowledge
Administrative medical assisting

CMAS (AMT)
Basic clinical medical office assisting
Medical office clerical assisting

Office hours are usually determined by the physician or group of physicians in a practice. The scheduling system used in each office is dependent on a variety of factors, including the physician's preference, type and size of practice, equipment availability, staff availability, amount of flexibility required by the physician(s), insurance coverage issues, and patient needs (Figure 9-1). The two basic types of appointment scheduling systems are open office hours and scheduled appointments.

Some medical facilities, such as independent ambulatory urgent care clinics, offer extended evening hours and may be open 24 hours a day. Independent ambulatory urgent care clinics are facilities that are prepared to handle situations requiring immediate but not life-threatening medical care. These facilities are not always attached to a hospital or other large treatment center. The patients arrive without appointments and generally are seen in the order of arrival unless a patient with an emergent condition arrives, and then they would be seen first. This would occur as a result of triage, also known as assigning priority. A medical office or facility using such a system is said to have open office hours.

Appointment Schedules

Some physicians prefer to see patients according to a set schedule, depending on the specialty. As soon as a day's schedule of time slots is filled, that day is closed to any new appointments. In this way, the physician is better able to spend an appropriate amount of time with each patient. There are several variations used for scheduling, including specified time, wave and modified wave, procedure grouping, double booking, and open hours system (Figure 9-2). All these scheduling variations are described here along with the benefits and limitations of each type.

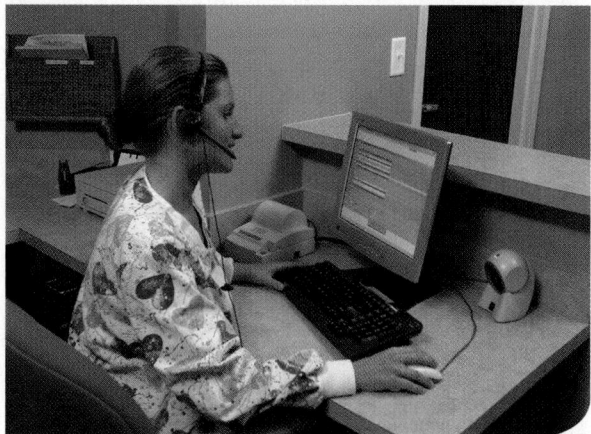

FIGURE 9-1 Scheduling patient appointments by telephone.

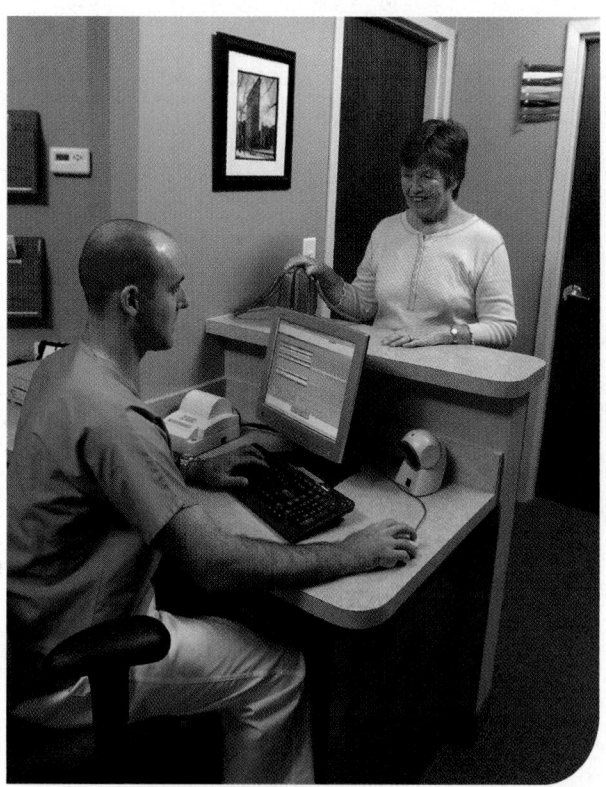

FIGURE 9-2 Scheduling appointments in a physician's office.

SPECIFIED TIME SCHEDULING

With specified time scheduling, each patient is given a **specific time** slot, which means the time allocated to each patient will depend on the reason for the office visit or the type of examination or testing that is to be done. For example, in some but not all offices, a complete physical examination may require one and one-half hours. In an office based on 15-minute increments, or time slots, this patient would be given six time slots in a row equaling the one and one-half hours needed. This method prevents a large backlog of waiting patients or **cycle time**—the length of time the average patient spends in the medical office. Each staff member has a chance to maintain the office flow by reducing patient cycle time.

The drawback to specified time scheduling is that some patients may not provide enough information about their medical problems at the time the appointment is scheduled, in spite of careful questioning by the medical assistant. For instance, consider the case of a patient who is given a 15-minute appointment when 45 minutes are needed for a thorough physical examination. Because not enough time was allocated for the visit, the schedule will back up.

Some patients will discuss topics that are unrelated to the complaint that brought them into the office. This can be time consuming, frustrating for the physician, and not beneficial to the patient. It is the receptionist's responsibility to get as much information as possible from the patient prior to scheduling an appointment. This allows the proper amount of time to be reserved for the patient. Occasionally, patients do not share all the information related to their condition, or they refuse to share any information with anyone other than the doctor. This creates special challenges for the receptionist. It is very helpful to establish rapport with the patients in order to make them feel comfortable enough discussing their symptoms, which at times can be very personal. If an appointment is scheduled and the patient ends up requiring more time than was originally scheduled, the physician might have to ask the patient to make another appointment. In an attempt to prevent this from happening, many offices will build in time—known as **catch-up time**—which is time built into the schedule, either in the morning or afternoon, for emergencies.

WAVE SCHEDULING

Wave scheduling provides built-in flexibility to accommodate unforeseen situations, such as patients who require more time with the physician, a late-arriving patient, or a patient who fails to keep an appointment (no-show). The purpose of wave scheduling is to begin and end each hour on time. Each hour is divided into equal segments of time, depending on how many patients can be seen within an hour.

For appointments averaging 20 minutes, three 20-minute appointments would be scheduled within each hour period, and for appointments averaging 15 minutes each, four appointments would be scheduled during the entire hour.

Using wave scheduling, all the patients are told to come in at the beginning of the hour in which they are to be seen. These patients are then seen in the order in which they arrive. Since some of the patients require more time, and others may be late, or some may not come in at all, wave scheduling allows for the actual time used by patient appointments to average out over the hour. This system tends to work very well in an office whose patients are often late. The disadvantage of wave scheduling is that all patients may arrive at nearly the same time; however, the last one signed in will have to wait the longest and may not be seen until 45 minutes after arrival. As discussed in Chapter 8, most patients consider 20 minutes as an acceptable wait time to be seen.

MODIFIED WAVE SCHEDULING

Wave scheduling can be modified to avoid the possibility that any patient would have to wait 45 minutes to be seen by the physician. **Modified wave scheduling** is also built on the hour as the base of each block of time.

There are many variations of this type of scheduling. One would be to have three patients scheduled at intervals during the first half hour with none scheduled for the second half hour. All three patients would be seen during the entire hour period, but the physician would not be waiting for a late arriving patient. With this system the physician can still spend 20 minutes with each patient without having to wait for any patients to arrive. Another form of modified wave scheduling is to have three patients arrive on the hour and to have them seen by the doctor within the first half of the hour in the order they arrived. During the second half of

TABLE 9-1 Comparison of Scheduling Methods

Specified Time		Wave		Modified Wave	
1:00	Ed Trombley—ear irrigation	1:00	Ed Trombley Jerry Richard Janet Orlando	1:00	Ed Trombley
1:20	Jerry Richard—well-baby checkup with vaccines			1:10	Jerry Richard
1:40	Janet Orlando—PAP smear			1:20	Janet Orlando
2:00	Lena Mezza—well-baby checkup with vaccines	2:00	Lena Mezza David Ingiolo Christina Soave	1:30	
2:20	David Ingiolo—BP check			1:40	
2:40	Christina Soave—skin rash (poss. contagious)			2:00	Lena Mezza
3:00		3:00		2:10	David Ingiolo
3:20				2:20	Christina Soave
3:40				2:30	
4:00		4:00		2:40	

the hour one patient would be scheduled, with another patient scheduled on the three-quarter hour. Table 9-1 is a comparison chart providing examples of specified time, wave, and modified wave scheduling.

SCHEDULING BY GROUPING PROCEDURES

Many physicians prefer to have similar procedures and examinations scheduled during a particular block of time. For example, an obstetrician may prefer to have all new patients scheduled together on two mornings a week because each will require a longer physical examination. An allergist may group all patients requiring skin testing together on three afternoons a week. A pediatrician may do well-baby checkups during particular hours each day. See Figure 9-3 for an example of scheduling by grouping procedures.

DOUBLE BOOKING PATIENTS

Double booking, which is the practice of scheduling two patients to be seen during the same time slot without allowing for any additional time in the schedule, is considered to be an ineffective but sometimes unavoidable method. If each patient needs a 20-minute appointment, and both are scheduled from 1:00 P.M. to 1:20 P.M., then the entire afternoon's schedule will be late by 20 minutes, at least. Using a modified form of wave scheduling will eliminate this problem since enough time is actually allowed in the schedule for all the patients.

OPEN OFFICE HOURS SYSTEM

An open office hours system is the least structured of all the systems. The hours in which the office is open are posted, and patients may arrive at any time during those hours. The patients are seen in the order of their arrival.

Some physicians prefer this method because the schedule is not disrupted by patients who miss appointments. The disadvantages to this method include having too many patients arrive at the same time, which frequently results in longer patient cycle time than necessary. The physician and staff can be overworked during peak times of the day while not having any patients during other times of the day.

Scheduling Systems

In most offices, one scheduling system will be used for all physicians within the practice; however, some multiphysician practices allow individual physicians to use the system they prefer. Scheduling systems as well as multiple scheduling systems can be very confusing for the staff until they learn each physician's preferences. No matter which system is used, appointment scheduling is key to the business aspects of the office process flow (Chapter 10), time management, increased efficiency, and quality patient care. A **scheduling system** facilitates the coordination of appropriate time segments for staff, patients, and the practice's available equipment. In order for a medical practice to coordinate time, an appointment scheduling system is applied, no matter what the practice size, specialty, and patient load. Scheduling systems establish the appropriate office process flow and coordination of time with the ability for flexibility as necessary. Appointment systems can be either computerized or manual; however the trend is leading toward computerized scheduling. Either system can accomplish coordination

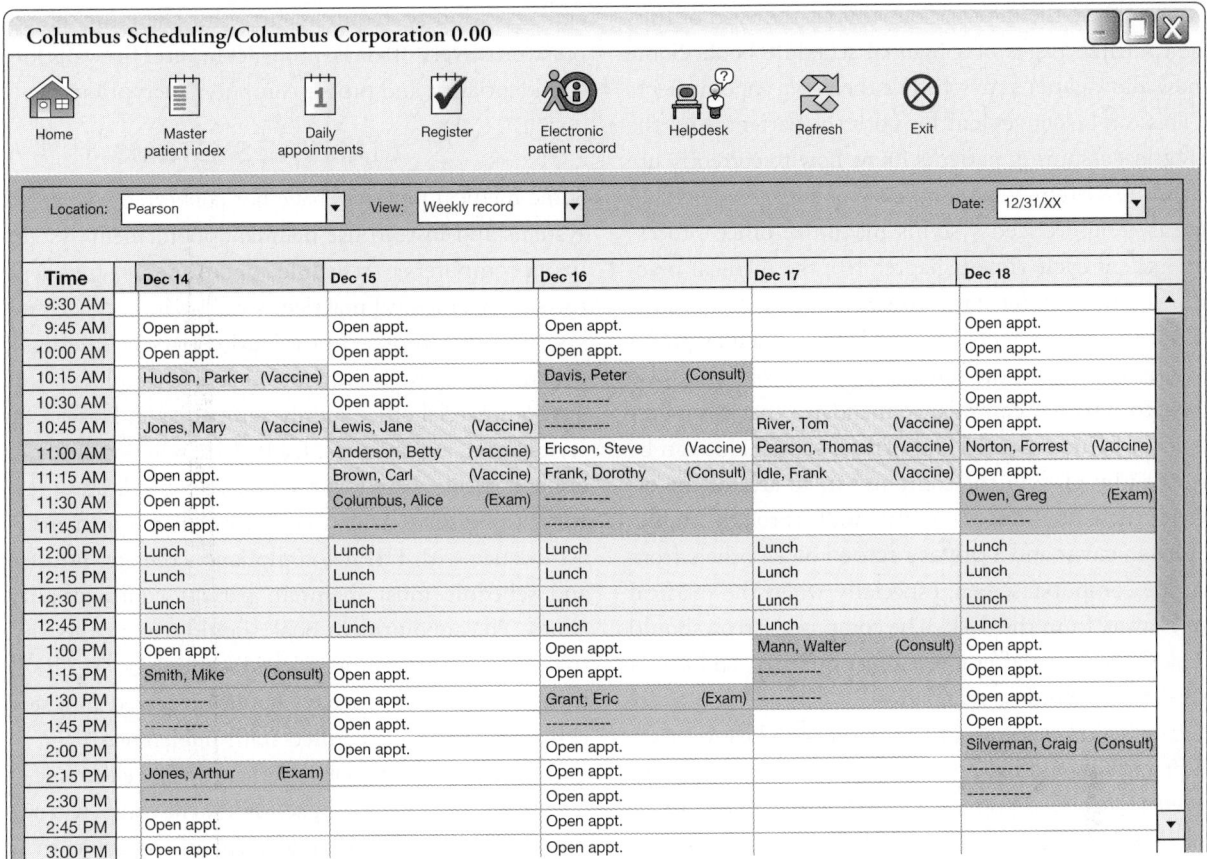

Time	Dec 14	Dec 15	Dec 16	Dec 17	Dec 18
9:30 AM					
9:45 AM	Open appt.	Open appt.	Open appt.		Open appt.
10:00 AM	Open appt.	Open appt.	Open appt.		Open appt.
10:15 AM	Hudson, Parker (Vaccine)	Open appt.	Davis, Peter (Consult)		Open appt.
10:30 AM		Open appt.	----------		Open appt.
10:45 AM	Jones, Mary (Vaccine)	Lewis, Jane (Vaccine)	----------	River, Tom (Vaccine)	Open appt.
11:00 AM		Anderson, Betty (Vaccine)	Ericson, Steve (Vaccine)	Pearson, Thomas (Vaccine)	Norton, Forrest (Vaccine)
11:15 AM	Open appt.	Brown, Carl (Vaccine)	Frank, Dorothy (Consult)	Idle, Frank (Vaccine)	Open appt.
11:30 AM	Open appt.	Columbus, Alice (Exam)	----------		Owen, Greg (Exam)
11:45 AM	Open appt.	----------	----------		
12:00 PM	Lunch	Lunch	Lunch	Lunch	Lunch
12:15 PM	Lunch	Lunch	Lunch	Lunch	Lunch
12:30 PM	Lunch	Lunch	Lunch	Lunch	Lunch
12:45 PM	Lunch	Lunch	Lunch	Lunch	Lunch
1:00 PM	Open appt.		Open appt.	Mann, Walter (Consult)	Open appt.
1:15 PM	Smith, Mike (Consult)	Open appt.	Open appt.	----------	Open appt.
1:30 PM	----------	Open appt.	Grant, Eric (Exam)	----------	Open appt.
1:45 PM	----------	Open appt.	----------		Open appt.
2:00 PM		Open appt.	Open appt.		Silverman, Craig (Consult)
2:15 PM	Jones, Arthur (Exam)		Open appt.		----------
2:30 PM	----------		Open appt.		----------
2:45 PM	Open appt.		Open appt.		
3:00 PM	Open appt.		Open appt.		

FIGURE 9-3 An example of scheduling by grouping. All immunizations are scheduled for morning appointments.

of scheduling time when managed appropriately for the medical practice while adhering to Health Insurance Portability and Accountability Act (HIPAA) compliance guidelines.

COMPUTERIZED SYSTEMS

Many medical practices of various sizes and specialties are utilizing computers to schedule appointments (Figure 9-4). Computerized systems may be purchased based on the medical practice's specific needs. Some practices will purchase a commercial software product, and others will contract a

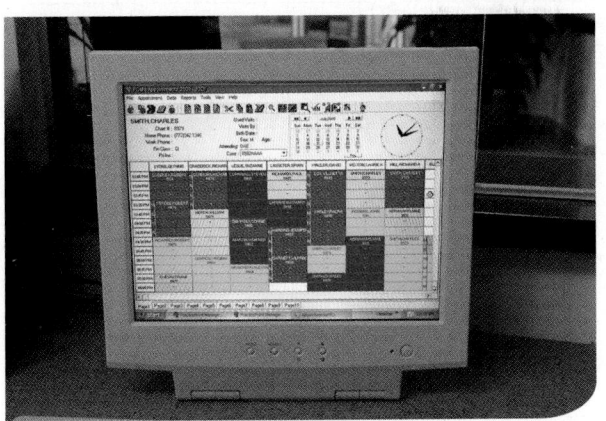

FIGURE 9-4 An example of a computerized scheduling format.

commercial appointment scheduling service. The responsibility of the medical assistant is to understand, demonstrate, and follow the computerized appointment system while adhering to HIPAA guidelines. No official government body or standards agency is established to certify a commercial computerized product or service as "HIPAA compliant." It is up to the health care providers to make sure the computerized product purchased for the medical practice will address the specific needs of the practice and its own HIPAA compliance issues, which will include patient safety, confidentiality, and security.

Computerized appointment systems are completed in a real-time environment. **Real time** refers to automatically placing the appointment, patient needs, and information within the appropriate areas of the computer program versus the manual systems. The medical professional can key in the information to maximize the efficiency of the workflow. In addition, a computerized system provides the medical assistant with the ability to search for and view times, dates, and open appointments with ease and consideration for the appointment criteria. Another advantage to computerized appointments is the ability to view and access patient appointments with a click or touch of a button. Whether a patient has a future appointment or a series of appointments, the computerized system can produce the information without the need of flipping the multiple pages of a manual schedule book. Some offices now allow patients to schedule their own appointments online. This can be convenient for both the patients and the medical office, assuming patients know how to correctly use the scheduling system.

Whereas computerized systems maximize office process flow and patient cycle time (Chapter 10), the medical practice will need to consider some disadvantages and concerns. In addition to privacy, technological factors, such as power outages, glitches within the software, and security, may also be of concern. HIPAA compliance mandates that computer systems must be in a secured and private space. This can be accomplished by placing the computer in an area of the office where there is limited public walk-through traffic. Both a **screen saver** and a **privacy screen** block others from viewing the computer screen, especially when the medical assistant is away from the desk. The computer screen should be set to a screen saver after a few short minutes, and use of a privacy screen should be mandatory.

For technological concerns, in accordance with HIPAA, each medical practice should have an action plan devised for emergency events, such as a power outage. The medical assistant must back up the computerized schedule frequently to prevent loss of important information. If a power outage were to occur, the emergency action plan should provide information that will ensure that the medical office can operate and function for 48 to 72 hours without power. Office policies and procedures would dictate how the scheduling would be handled during the power outages, such as printing a hard copy of the appointment schedule for the week rather than one day at a time.

Another advantage of computerized appointment scheduling includes the ability to track regular patterns within the medical practice. For example, the office could track the number of no-shows, or how many patients were scheduled for the same type of appointment (e.g., flu). These tracking features provide the medical practice with an additional tool and analytical report for audit and review of the best methods within the office. Time management could be modified as needed based on the reports.

Security concerns should be outlined in accordance with office policies and HIPAA compliance issues. Specified security guidelines are usually dictated by the medical office functions and flow. Security includes some of the following but is not limited to these: positioning and location of the computer monitor for visibility and confidentiality, employee computer authorization

and accessibility requirements, the changing of employee passwords every 30 days, proper computer firewalls for patient confidentiality, and proper computer encryption.

MANUAL SYSTEMS

Some medical practices have not converted to computerized systems and instead use manual appointment systems. Utilizing computers to schedule appointments often depends on the size of a medical practice as well as its specialties. Manual systems are comprised of a hard-copy schedule book and a pencil or pen. Appointment books are purchased from various commercial office supply companies and offer a variety of styles, sizes, and features. Each office will determine the type of book needed based on the practice's needs and preferences. Refer to Figure 9-5 for a sample of an appointment book. In accordance with HIPAA compliance, the appointment book and schedule must maintain patient confidentiality at all times. The appointment book should never be left in an area that is visible to visitors at the reception desk. The appointment schedule for the day should be placed in a secure and private location for required staff to reference.

The appointment book, whether paper or electronic, is a legal document that can be subpoenaed by the court. It is a record of the physician's day and time spent in contact with patients. Appointment books should be **archived** (stored) for future reference and kept for several years in the event of a court case that may **subpoena** information found in the appointment book. If subpoenaed, the office is required to present information such as the appointment book to the court. Files are archived by placing the appointment book or backup disks (in the case of electronic appointment scheduling) in a storage container or

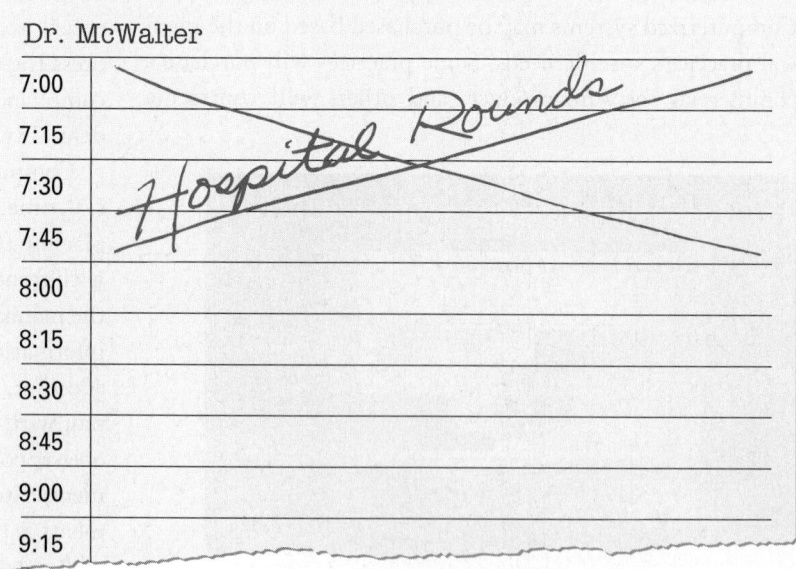

FIGURE 9-5 An example of a manual appointment book.

facility and keeping them for a predetermined number of years. If any changes are made to the schedule in the appointment book, such as a patient cancellation or no-show, these should be noted both in the appointment book and in the patient's medical record. If the appointment has been rescheduled, then this should be appropriately documented as well.

Patient Scheduling Process

Every office will utilize its own method for appointment scheduling in accordance with the needs of the practice. However, the scheduling process is generally the same for both the electronic and manual forms of appointment scheduling.

The first step in the patient scheduling process is to be organized and efficient. Gather all required equipment, including the patient chart, computer scheduling system, pencil, manual schedule book, and office criteria requirement checklist. The medical assistant should be sure the schedule depicts all unavailable times, which is known as forming a **matrix**—periods of time blocked out on the daily schedule when an appointment is unavailable (Figure 9-6). Some of

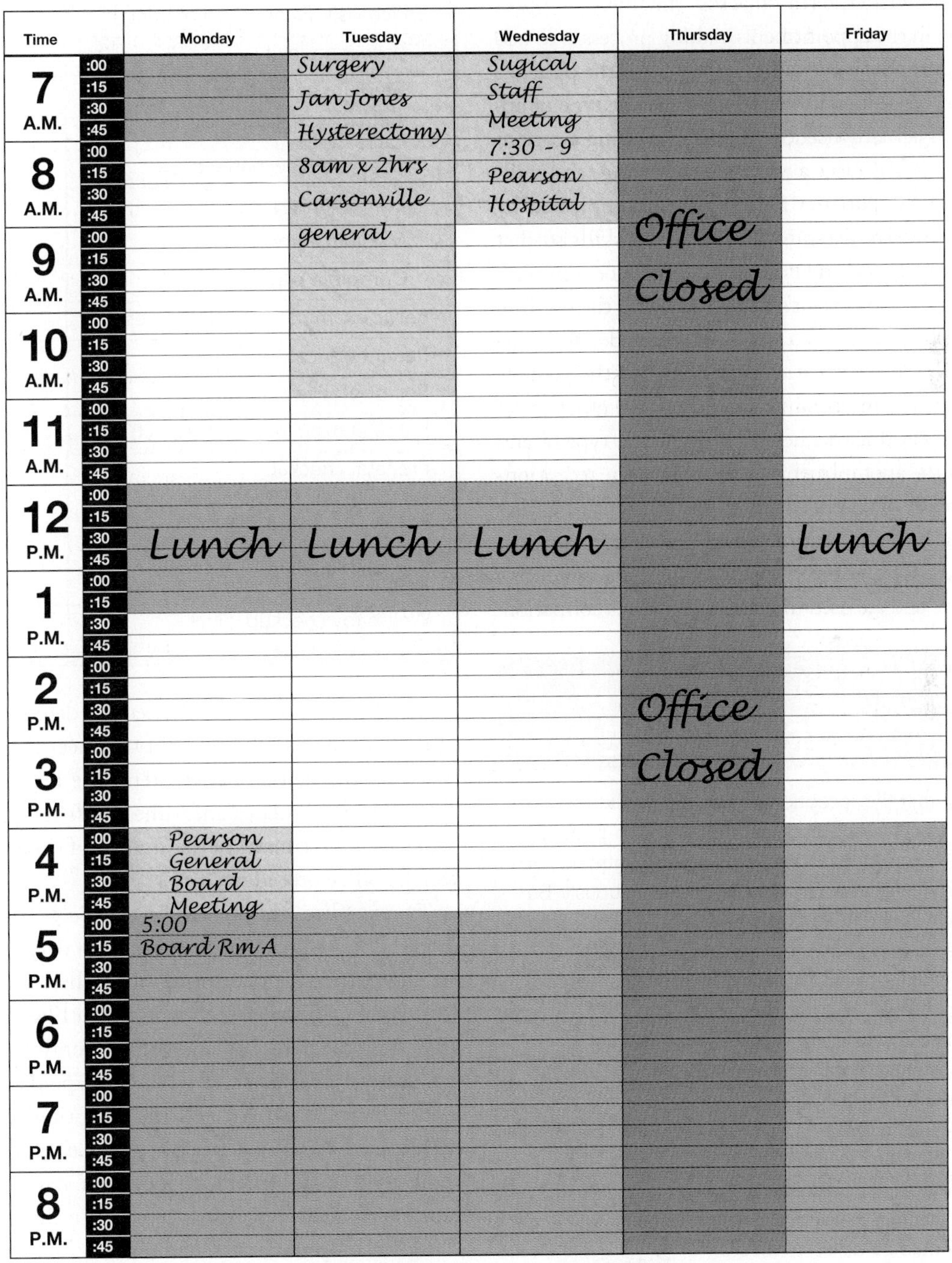

Time		Monday	Tuesday	Wednesday	Thursday	Friday
7 A.M.	:00 :15 :30 :45		Surgery Jan Jones Hysterectomy	Surgical Staff Meeting 7:30 - 9		
8 A.M.	:00 :15 :30 :45		8am x 2hrs Carsonville	Pearson Hospital		
9 A.M.	:00 :15 :30 :45		general		Office Closed	
10 A.M.	:00 :15 :30 :45					
11 A.M.	:00 :15 :30 :45					
12 P.M.	:00 :15 :30 :45	Lunch	Lunch	Lunch		Lunch
1 P.M.	:00 :15 :30 :45					
2 P.M.	:00 :15 :30 :45				Office Closed	
3 P.M.	:00 :15 :30 :45					
4 P.M.	:00 :15 :30 :45	Pearson General Board Meeting				
5 P.M.	:00 :15 :30 :45	5:00 Board Rm A				
6 P.M.	:00 :15 :30 :45					
7 P.M.	:00 :15 :30 :45					
8 P.M.	:00 :15 :30 :45					

FIGURE 9-6 An appointment schedule with a completed matrix.

these blocked-out segments include times when the physician is making hospital rounds or is in surgery, out to lunch, on break, returning telephone calls, in meetings, or out of town. Forming an appointment matrix is completed several weeks, if not even months, in advance. It is not good practice to block out the entire schedule for the year since there may be unexpected changes in either the physician's personal or professional schedule. When creating an appointment matrix for a manual appointment scheduling system, the blocking out and scheduling should be done in pencil. The medical assistant should cross out the blocks of time when the physician is unavailable and write the reason across the line.

The next step in the appointment-making process is to utilize effective communication skills. Listening to the patient's information and requests will help determine the type of appointment that is actually needed. When scheduling a patient appointment, always project a professional, caring, and willing demeanor to the patient. This can be accomplished by demonstrating effective listening and speaking skills so that the patient can understand and interpret the dialogue conveyed. Begin by asking for the patient's name (verifying the spelling if needed), telephone number including area code, and purpose for the visit. Once the patient has described the purpose of his or her visit, the receptionist should use the office criteria requirements checklist to help determine the type of and time needed for the appointment. Occasionally, the receptionist will need to ask open-ended questions in order to gather enough information to determine what type of appointment the patient needs. **Open-ended questions** require more than a yes or no answer and are used to gather pertinent information.

TABLE 9-2 Time Estimates for Specific Office Procedures

Procedure	Time in Minutes
Allergy testing	30–60
Cast check	10
Cast change	30
Complete physical with EKG	60
Blood pressure check	15
Dressing change	15
Minor surgery procedure	30–45
Office visit: Established patient	
Low complexity	5–10
Medium complexity	15–20
High complexity	20–30
Office visit: New patient	
Low complexity	10–15
Medium complexity	15–30
Complete physical	30–45
Pelvic examination with PAP test	30
Patient education	30–45
Postoperative checkup	15–20
Prenatal examination (first visit)	30–60
Prenatal checkup	15
Prostate examination	30
School physical	15–30
Suture removal	10
Well-baby checkup	15

PROFESSIONALISM
THE WORKPLACE

It is important that the receptionist is able to multitask and not become easily frustrated. While checking in patients, answering the telephone, and scheduling appointments, it is also important for the receptionist to continuously be aware of activity in the reception area. If a patient has an appointment with the physician because she is suffering from migraines and an exam room is available, it is best to offer the patient the opportunity to wait in the exam room instead of the reception area. This will allow the patient to lie down in a room away from the noise and lights of the reception room. If the receptionist is not able to periodically check on the patient, a member of the clinical staff should be asked to do so.

Next, the receptionist will need to determine the facility, equipment, and staff availability to meet the patient's needs. Based on the determination steps, the receptionist can then discuss available dates and times with the patient. Refer to Table 9-2 for estimates of the amount of time to be allotted for specific office procedures.

To expedite the scheduling process, the receptionist should offer only one or two choices of dates, days, and times for the patient to determine his or her availability. Avoid asking the patient "When would you like to come in?" Always state the date, day, and time to confirm that the patient has correctly understood when the appointment is scheduled. Once the patient and the receptionist have mutually determined the time, either key in the information into the computer or document the patient name and telephone number into the scheduled time slot in the schedule book. If using a computerized scheduling system, it is important that you click the save button once an appointment has been scheduled. Once the patient's name has been recorded on the schedule, repeat the date and time of the appointment again for the patient. This serves to verify that you have recorded the appointment correctly, and it offers the patient the opportunity to make any necessary corrections. If the patient is making the appointment in person, write the date, day, and time on an appointment card for the patient.

Established Patient Appointments

Any patient who has been previously seen by the physician within the past three years is considered an **established patient**. Established patients will have an existing medical record/chart that will need to be accessed each time the patient contacts the physician for an appointment. It is a good approach to verify the established patient's telephone number, address, and insurance information prior to scheduling an appointment. Maintaining good customer service with established patients includes appointment reminders and observing patient cycle time. Procedure 9-1 provides information on how to schedule established patients.

New Patient Appointments

Before scheduling someone as a new patient, be sure to verify that they truly are a new patient to the practice. Medical insurance companies have requirements that must be met in

procedure 9-1

SCHEDULING ESTABLISHED PATIENTS

Objective: Use an appointment scheduling system to schedule patients with efficiency.

EQUIPMENT AND SUPPLIES
Pencil or pen (if preferred by office management); appointment schedule book or computerized scheduling system

METHOD
1. Understand the scheduling system used in your office.
2. When scheduling manually, use a pencil so that appointments can be erased to make changes as needed. *Please note:* Some offices prefer the use of black or blue ink instead of pencil.
3. If using computerized scheduling, be sure the scheduling system is open.
4. Before scheduling patients, set up a matrix by blocking out all time periods when the physician is not available (hospital rounds, vacation, etc.) for appointments. Ideally, matrix setup or appointment blocking on the computer is done three months ahead of time.
5. Schedule appointments by beginning with the first empty appointment in the morning or early in the afternoon, and then fill in the day. Do not schedule appointments at the end of the day with large open gaps in between.
6. When scheduling manually, print the patient's full first and last name next to the appropriate time on the schedule. Add Jr. for *Junior* and Sr. for *Senior* if two patients in a family have the same name.
7. If using computerized scheduling, search for the correct patient. Some systems allow searching by the patient's

Social Security number or medical record number. This decreases the chances of pulling up the wrong patient if you have more than one patient with the same name.

8. When scheduling manually, ask the patient for a current work and home telephone number, including the area code. Write these numbers next to the patient's name. If using computerized scheduling, verify that the telephone numbers in the system are correct. If they are incorrect, take the time right then to update them. Correct contact information is necessary if the office needs to contact the patient prior to the appointment.
9. Record the reason for the visit on the schedule using accepted medical abbreviations only.
10. Allow the correct amount of time for the appointment. If an appointment will take more than the minimum time allotted on the schedule, then use an arrow to indicate that the patient will be using two or three blocks of time. In some offices, a line is drawn across the time blocks.
11. Once the appointment is recorded, repeat to the patient the date, time, and any special instructions.
12. If the patient is in the office while you are scheduling the appointment, record the appointment on a reminder card and hand it to the patient.

Note: In offices where scheduling is done by computer, follow any on-screen prompts in addition to the steps suggested above.

PROFESSIONALISM
THE LIFE SPAN

Young children often find it hard to wait patiently for extended periods of time. Try to be sensitive to this when scheduling pediatric patients. Some adult patients may have to bring their children with them. In the waiting area, have some quiet activities and magazines geared toward children. Animated and children's videos may help children wait more patiently.

Also remember that the elderly may have difficulty waiting for long periods of time. Take measures to help make them as comfortable as possible. Comfortable seating, large-print reading materials, and light refreshments may make their wait easier.

order to consider the patient as a truly "new" patient. This is because medical insurance companies compensate new patient visits at a higher level than established patient visits. Generally speaking, if it has been more than 3 years since a physician within the practice has seen the patient or the patient has never been seen by a physician in the practice, you may consider them a new patient.

Scheduling a new patient's appointment requires additional time, patience, and effective organizational skills. Always project a professional and positive image with the patient. Using effective communication skills will be most beneficial from a customer service perspective since managing this appointment will set the stage for the patient's actual in-office visit. Procedure 9-2 provides instruction on how to schedule new patients.

When scheduling pediatric and elderly patients, it is important to note that they may need specific times and may have other special needs.

procedure
9-2

SCHEDULING A NEW PATIENT APPOINTMENT
Objective: Schedule the first visit for a new patient.

EQUIPMENT AND SUPPLIES
Pencil or pen (if preferred by office management); appointment schedule book or computerized scheduling system

1. Assemble necessary appointment scheduling equipment.
2. Obtain the patient's full legal name and correct spelling, birth date, full address, telephone contacts (home, office, cell), and e-mail address.
3. Record the patient's chief complaint and symptoms.
4. Request the name of the patient's insurance carrier and policy number.
5. Ask how the patient was referred to the medical office (physician referral, friend, colleague, insurance company, etc.).
6. Ask the patient if he or she has a preference for morning or afternoon appointments.
7. Attempt to accommodate the new patient's request for a preferred appointment time.
8. Confirm the day, date, and time of the appointment and have the new patient repeat the information for verification and mutual understanding.
9. Many offices require new patients to arrive 15 to 30 minutes prior to their scheduled appointment time to provide

ample opportunity to enter the data provided on the initial history form.
10. Provide the new patient with directions to the office.
11. Inform the new patient of all materials to bring for the first visit (i.e., insurance verification, photo identification, list of current medications, past medical records, current lab, X-ray, and other medical reports, as available).
12. Welcome and thank the new patient by name for selecting your medical office.
13. Forward all information as discussed with the new patient via mail if there will be enough time between the day the appointment was made and the actual appointment date.
14. Document new patient information in a new medical record.

CHARTING EXAMPLE
1/05/XX 10:25 A.M. New patient appointment scheduled for patient John Samuel on 1/20/XX at 3:30 P.M. Patient requested new patient registration form and patient history form be forwarded to his home address at 1234 Carpenter Road, Smith Station, Chicago. Patient aware he needs to arrive 30 minutes prior to his appointment. Driving directions provided. · L. Battista, RMA

Maintaining the Schedule

Due to unforeseen circumstances, it is unlikely that a single day in a medical office will go by without some type of adjustment needing to be made to the schedule. Things such as missed appointments, delays, or cancellations will occur daily. It is important to remain positive when such variances occur.

MISSED APPOINTMENTS AND DELAYS

Appointments are cancelled for any number of reasons. Sometimes the patient experiences an unforeseen emergency, is too ill or too fatigued to get to the office, or actually forgets the appointment. Some medical practices charge patients for no-show appointments as well as rescheduled appointments. If the medical practice has a cancellation charge, the patients must be made aware of the policy prior to cancellation. Many offices place the cancellation policy in an office brochure that is given to all new patients and states the charge or fee for no-show appointments. Along with the office brochure, this information is often posted in the reception area near the front desk.

On the other hand, the physician may be delayed or need to cancel appointments due to an emergency at the hospital or even a patient emergency in the office. Also, the medical office may not have all the necessary physical equipment for certain procedures, or building issues may arise as well as other unforeseen circumstances. In all cases, the medical assistant should provide patients with an explanation and reschedule appointments. Missed appointments happen with no warning, so the medical assistant has less opportunity to make satisfactory adjustments. No matter what the reason for a missed appointment, the medical assistant must contact the patient, reschedule the appointment, and document it as a missed and rescheduled appointment in the patient medical record. Careful legible documentation is necessary for HIPAA compliance as well as to legally protect the physician from a claim of patient abandonment.

PATIENT NO-SHOWS

No-shows or failed appointments occur when a patient does not show up to keep an appointment. If a patient misses an appointment, write no-show (NS) or cancellation (cx) on both the appointment schedule sheet and in the patient chart. Make every attempt to fill up a void in the schedule caused by a patient cancellation. One method is to call the patient who has the last appointment for the day and ask the patient if it is possible to come in earlier. In the event that a long appointment, such as a 90-minute appointment for a complete physical, has been canceled, you will have to attempt to move up an entire group of patients. Many offices maintain a list of patients who wish to be called if an appointment becomes available at the last minute. This approach is beneficial to maintaining good customer service and is an effective use of time for the office schedule.

Future Appointments

Ideally, before leaving the office, the patient will schedule his or her next appointment. This is known as **advance booking**. Scheduling while the patient is in the office also reduces the number of incoming calls requesting appointments.

Advance booking allows patients to book their next appointment 3 to 6 months ahead of time. Advance booking is done for regularly scheduled checkups or required follow-up appointments, such as after blood pressure checks or completion of physical therapy treatments. The date and time of the next appointment can be written on appointment cards that also contain the name, address, and telephone number of the physician's practice, and such cards should be given to each patient at the time the next appointment is made (Figure 9-7).

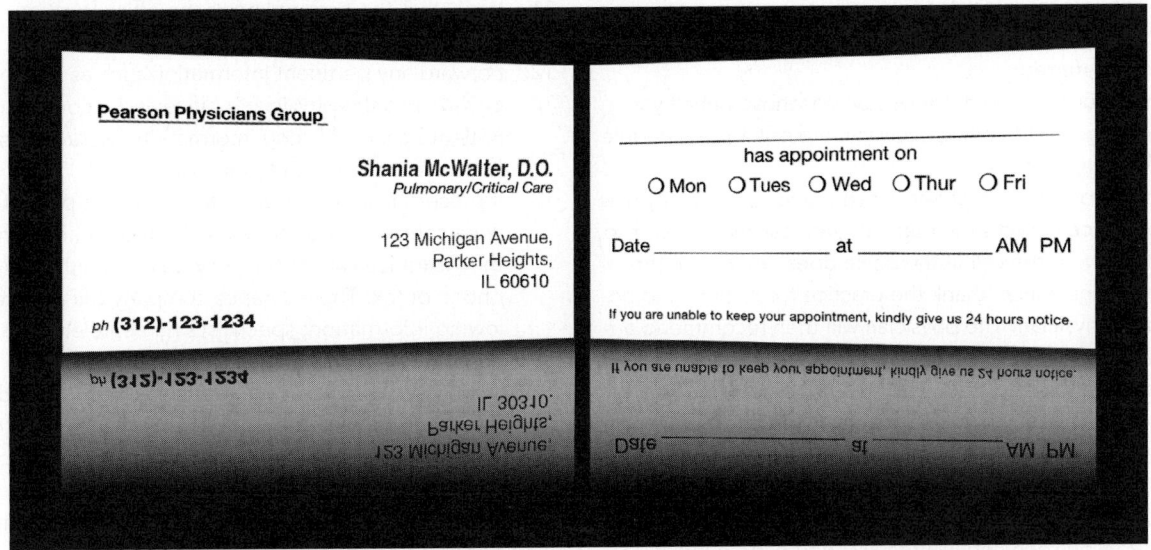

FIGURE 9-7 The reminder card should be completed and handed to the patient after the appointment is scheduled.

FOLLOW-UP

Some offices have the patient complete a self-addressed postcard, called a tickler card, to use in an appointment reminder system known as a **tickler file**. The tickler file is a small box in which the tickler card is filed under the date the postcard should be mailed. Such reminders are used for annual PAP tests, for example. The tickler file is very handy for any type of follow-up appointments. Follow-ups can be made in writing, by telephone, or by e-mail. All follow-up methods should include the day, date, and time of the next appointment. Some offices make personal telephone calls 1 to 2 days prior to the actual appointment. Either follow-up method is considered a good approach for maintaining customer service and smart office management to decrease the no-show rate. It is essential to comply with HIPAA confidentiality standards when sending reminder postcards or leaving appointment reminder messages on an answering machine or voice mail.

Patient Referrals

Physicians will often refer patients to another facility or physician when further treatment or testing is necessary. Ideally, the referral appointment is scheduled as soon as possible. Whether referring a patient to another location or receiving a referral from another physician, the receptionist or referral coordinator must exchange pertinent information regarding the patient's name, contact number, insurance, and referral needs, as well as the referral physician's name, address, and contact number. In some cases, depending on the insurance, precertification (approval) is necessary before scheduling the appointment. Procedure 9-3 reviews the steps to be taken when arranging for a referral appointment.

procedure 9-3

ARRANGING A REFERRAL APPOINTMENT

Objective: Schedule a referral appointment for the patient.

EQUIPMENT AND SUPPLIES
Patient chart; telephone; paper; pen; either Rolodex or physician directory; and physician request for referral information

METHOD
1. Gather supplies.
2. Open patient chart for insurance information and physician request for referral.
3. Place a call to the physician's office to whom the patient is being referred.
4. Identify yourself and the physician on whose behalf you are calling. Let the office know you are calling to schedule a referral appointment.
5. Before providing the patient's name and so on, verify that the practice accepts the patient's medical insurance. If so, continue with the call. If the office does not accept the patient's insurance, thank the practice for its time and notify the physician. The physician will then recommend another physician for the patient referral.
6. Once it has been determined that the office accepts the patient's insurance, provide the following information: patient's name, address, telephone number, and reason for referral.
7. The office may or may not ask how soon the patient needs to be seen and will then schedule the patient.

8. Record the referral appointment information in the patient's chart as well as on an appointment reminder card for the patient.
9. Be sure also to record the name of the individual with whom you spoke and the creation of the reminder card.
10. Notify the patient of the date and time of the appointment and provide the reminder card.
11. Verify that the patient knows the office location. If not, provide clearly written directions.
12. Forward any pertinent information such as laboratory tests or X-rays to the physician's office and record them in the patient's chart. If faxing information, be sure to place the fax confirmation in the patient's chart.
13. If precertification is required, contact the patient's insurance company and request authorization. Depending on the insurance carrier, this may be done either by telephone or fax. The insurance company will require the following information: specialist's name, telephone number, and reason for the visit or request.
14. If completing the precertification by telephone, document the precertification number and the name, and telephone number of the individual who provides the number.
15. Provide the precertification number and pertinent information to the physician's office where the patient is being referred.

10/9/XX, 2:15 P.M. Referral appointment scheduled for Patsy Smith. Patient scheduled to see Dr. Kendall on Friday, 10/16/XX, at 10:00 A.M. Verified Dr. Kendall's office participates with patient's insurance. Ms. Smith aware she is to arrive 30 minutes prior to appointment time to complete paperwork. Patient provided with written information regarding appointment, including driving directions to Dr. Kendall's office. 10/2/XX labs and ultrasound report faxed to Dr. Kendall's office. Confirmation received· D. Joyner, RMA
10/9/XX, 3:00 P.M. Contacted Humana, requested precertification for Ms. Smith's appointment with Dr. Kendall. Spoke with Jim Linday. Precertification authorized #JS123567 valid through 11/16/XX. J. Linday will fax confirmation. · · · · · D. Joyner, RMA

Hospital Admission Scheduling

The medical assistant may also be responsible for scheduling all patient admissions (admits) to the hospital. In a large medical practice, a scheduler may take care of all admissions. Patients do not schedule their own hospital admissions. When scheduling a direct admit to the hospital, be sure to contact the patient's insurance company for preadmission approval. Table 9-3 provides a description of the patient information supplied when scheduling hospital admissions. Procedure 9-4 provides instructions on scheduling inpatient surgical procedures.

Provide the patient with a detailed explanation of the day, date, time, and preparation needed for the admission. It is always better to place details in writing. Many offices distribute preprinted information to patients. Such information should, however, be personalized with the patient's name. Even when preprinted materials are used, the medical assistant should provide complete, concise, verbal explanations of important points pertaining to the admission/surgical procedure.

Scheduling Surgery and Outpatient Procedures

Scheduling an outpatient surgical procedure is based on the patient's need and diagnosis, type of surgery, insurance carrier, physician, anesthesia requirements (local or general), and facility availability. The medical assistant will contact the surgery scheduling department and make arrangements with the surgery scheduler. The surgery scheduler may request all patient information, including legal name, telephone contacts, insurance information (for example, prior authorization for some elective surgeries), advance directives, or other preadmittance information. Procedure 9-5 provides instructions on how to schedule an outpatient surgery.

TABLE 9-3 Patient Information Supplied When Scheduling Hospital Admissions

• Patient's full name	Verify spelling of first and last name.
• Address	Ask patient to state current address.
• Social Security number	May be taken from patient record.
• Age/date of birth	Verify birth date in patient record.
• Telephone number	Ask patient for current number and area code.
• Requirement	Type of room or special requirement.
• Admitting diagnosis	Give the physician's statement from the patient record.
• Recent prior admission	Ask the patient for last admission date in any hospital.
• Physician's name	Give physician's name.
• Insurance information	May fax copy of insurance card.
• Name of person at insurance company who gave preapproval.	Forms are also available from insurance company who gave preapproval.

SCHEDULING INPATIENT SURGICAL PROCEDURES

Objective: Perform proper procedure to schedule inpatient surgical procedures.

EQUIPMENT AND SUPPLIES

Patient's chart; patient's insurance card; notepad and pen; written instructions for patients (if required)

METHOD

1. Review the patient's chart for the most current information. Make sure the chart contains the physician's notes and orders regarding the surgical procedure.
2. Verify with the physician the type of procedure for which you are to schedule the patient, and gather the following information from the physician:
   - Category the surgical procedure falls under (routine, elective, urgent)
   - Name of the surgeon to perform the procedure
   - The surgeon's scheduling preference for this type of procedure
   - Estimated length of time for the procedure
   - Estimated length of stay
3. Gather the following information from the patient and patient's chart:
   - Patient's full name, age, sex, and any other pertinent identification or information
   - Physician's current diagnosis
   - Any allergies
   - Special preoperative orders and patient instructions
   - Patient's insurance information
4. Obtain preauthorization from the patient's insurance company, if required.
5. Contact the **surgery scheduler** and relay the requested surgery information. The surgery scheduler is the person in the surgery department who schedules the procedure, including the necessary preoperative appointments (i.e. blood work, chest X-ray, etc.), the actual surgery, and postoperative appointments, if necessary.
6. The surgery scheduler will confirm the date and time of surgery and any special instructions to be relayed to the patient.
7. Record the surgery scheduling information in the patient's chart.
8. Record the surgery information on the appropriate physician's schedule.
9. Follow office procedure and the surgeon's request for contacting other members of the surgical team.
10. Instruct the patient on special preparation and admission procedures. Provide written instructions, if available.

CHARTING EXAMPLE

6/5/XX, 9:15 A.M. Spoke with Jenny, surgery scheduler at Pearson General Hospital (PGH). Charles Wolf scheduled for total knee replacement surgery on 6/28/XX at PGH, Dr. Patel, surgeon. Patient aware he is to report to PGH on 6/15/XX at 8 A.M. for preoperative assessment and testing. Patient provided with written instructions and verbalized understanding he is not to eat or drink anything after midnight on 6/27/XX. He will call if he has any questions. · · · · · · · · · · · · · · · · · John Carter, RMA

SCHEDULING OUTPATIENT SURGICAL PROCEDURES

Objective: To demonstrate the ability to schedule outpatient procedures in the health care setting.

EQUIPMENT AND SUPPLIES

Telephone; patient's insurance card; notepad; pen; written instructions for patient

METHOD

1. Review the patient's chart for the most current information. Make sure the chart contains the physician's notes and orders regarding the surgical procedure.

2. Verify with the physician the type of procedure for which you are to schedule the patient and gather the following information from the physician:
   - Category under which the surgical procedure falls (i.e., routine, elective, urgent)
   - Name of the surgeon who will perform the procedure
   - The surgeon's scheduling preference for this type of procedure
   - Estimated length of time for the procedure
3. Gather the following information from the patient and the patient's chart:
   - Patient's full name, age, sex, and any other pertinent identification or information
   - Physician's current diagnosis for the patient
   - Any existing allergies
   - Special preoperative orders and patient instructions
   - Patient's insurance information
   - Days/times patient available for surgery
4. Obtain preauthorization from the patient's insurance company, if required.
5. According to the facility policy, contact the outpatient scheduler at the local hospital or clinic and identify yourself and your office.

6. Instruct the facility about the type of procedure and the amount of time the physician expects to need the operating room.
7. Determine available days at the facility.
8. If possible, offer options to the patient and have the patient choose the best option.
9. Notify the facility of the date and time chosen.
10. Create a patient instruction sheet to include date and time of procedure and necessary preoperative information.
11. Document the conversation in the patient chart.
12. Document the scheduled surgery on appropriate physician's schedule.

CHARTING EXAMPLE

10/20/XX, 10:30 A.M. Robin Jones scheduled for cervical conization at 12:30 P.M. on 11/9/XX. Patient instructed to arrive at hospital at 10:00 A.M. on day of surgery. Patient was given instruction sheet and stated she understood that she would have to go to the hospital for preoperative testing on 11/3 at 8 A.M. Ms. Jones is aware she is not to eat after midnight on the night prior to surgery—may take morning medications with small amount of water. Patient urged to call with any questions. · Celia Ruiz, CMAS (AMT)

Appointment Exceptions

On occasion, unscheduled patients will contact the office with a need for an immediate appointment. These include patient emergencies and patients with acute conditions. **Acute conditions** are illnesses or injuries that patients suddenly experience and that require treatment but may not be life threatening.

The medical assistant must listen carefully to all the patient's complaints and assess the seriousness of the patient's condition. It is important to ask the patient questions regarding where the pain is located, when it first appeared, the duration of strength or measure of the pain, and if the patient has experienced the same pain before. Also ask the patient for the telephone number from

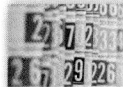

PROFESSIONALISM

THE LAW

There are many ethical concerns relating to the scheduling process. The appointment book is a legal document that records the physician's time spent with patients. This record can validate actual services provided and billed for Internal Revenue Service (IRS) verification. Documentation of canceled appointments and no-shows is critical. Keep in mind that a physician may be liable for a lawsuit on the grounds of abandonment and negligence if a patient who requests to see the physician is not seen by the physician through some fault of the physician or the physician's staff. The patient may claim that the physician did not offer treatment or provide follow-up care. If a patient cancels an appointment or does not show up for an appointment, the

physician is not at fault. This illustrates the need for correct documentation.

The medical assistant has a great responsibility to screen correctly and assess the patient's need for immediate treatment. The physician has a legal responsibility to see patients who are acutely ill or in need of emergency care. The severity of the patient's health problem should be related to the physician objectively. Subjective factors, such as like or dislike of a patient, are inappropriate and should never enter into the decision-making process. It is unethical for the medical assistant to decide that a patient is lying about his or her need to see the physician. All patients have the right to be seen by their physician.

where he or she is calling and determine if the patient is alone. It is best to follow office policies and procedures regarding handling emergency situations. The physician should always be informed immediately regarding a potential emergency.

The medical assistant will need to apply triage skills. **Triage** is the process of sorting or grouping patients according to the seriousness of their condition. Triage becomes necessary when more than one seriously ill patient is waiting to see the physician. In general, sudden onset of pain must be considered an emergency until otherwise determined.

If an emergency exists, such as in the case of severe chest pain, then the physician must be informed of the call immediately. If a physician is not available, then the medical assistant will follow office protocol, which may require referring the patient to the nearest emergency center. If the patient is not able to make his or her own arrangements for transportation, then the medical assistant will arrange for an ambulance and emergency medical personnel to transport the patient. Table 9-4 lists acute illnesses that require the patient to be seen by a physician as soon as possible. Table 9-5 lists emergency (life-threatening) conditions that require immediate physician assistance.

To eliminate the need to "squeeze in" an emergency or unscheduled appointment, the medical assistant should integrate **time patterns** into the office schedule, if office policy allows. Time patterns are similar to matrixing off time within the schedule to allow for catch-up time or unscheduled appointments. Ideally, a few minutes should be built into the schedule between the end of one patient visit and the beginning of another patient's visit. However, most scheduling systems do not allow for time between patients. Therefore, it is important to build small blocks of time into the schedule during the day when the physician can return

telephone calls, catch up on charting, read mail and journals, or rest. The best time for this is at the end of the morning's schedule and again at the end of the day. Some physicians prefer to return all morning telephone calls when they return from lunch, whereas others may work through lunch

TABLE 9-5 Examples of Emergency Conditions

Acute allergic reaction	Head injury
Allergic reaction with respiratory distress	Laceration
Chest pain	Loss of consciousness
Coma	Pain and/or numbness after the application of a cast for fracture
Convulsions	Poisoning
Diabetic reaction	Severe bleeding
Difficulty breathing	Severe dizziness
Drowning/ near-drowning	Severe nausea, vomiting, or diarrhea lasting more than 24 hours
Drug overdose	Severe pain
Foreign object in the eye	Sudden acute illness
Fracture	Sudden paralysis of part or all of the body
Gunshot wounds	Temperature over 104°F

TABLE 9-4 Examples of Acute Conditions

Earache	Eye infection
Fever lasting more than 24 hours	Infection that is visible to patient (e.g., a red, swollen area after an injury)
Pain or burning on urination	Pain in abdomen that is not severe
Skin rash	Unusually heavy uterine or vaginal bleeding
Unusual discharge (e.g., blood in urine)	Sore throat and/or swollen glands

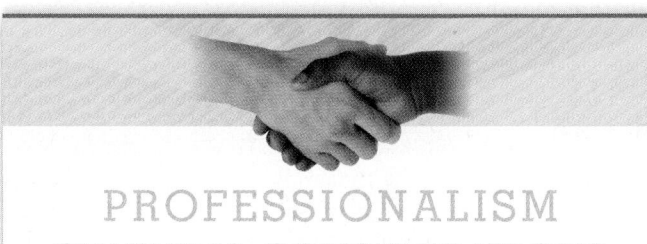

PROFESSIONALISM
CULTURAL CONSIDERATIONS

Scheduling appointments, particularly follow-up appointments, may sometimes be difficult due to a busy medical office and a patient's busy schedule. It is important not to try to convince a patient to make an unwanted appointment time. Some patients may adhere to strict religious conventions that are based on specific days of the week or times of the day, such as those who observe Islamic daily prayer schedules. Professional medical assistants must respect and facilitate any patient scheduling considerations.

and return all calls at the end of the day. It is important to inform patients when to expect the physician to return calls. This will help to reduce additional calls from patient(s) wondering when the physician will be calling.

Building this free time block into the daily office schedule at the same time each day is very important. Every effort should be made not to schedule last-minute appointments during this time. These "buffer" periods are excellent backup times for emergencies that may have to be seen that day.

Telephone and E-mail Scheduling

Many offices use the telephone and e-mail to schedule appointments. The medical assistant must apply professional, legal, and effective communication skills when using these forms of technology. Following are some professional considerations to include when communicating with the patient:

- Determine if you are speaking directly with the patient.
- Use the patient's name while addressing him or her on the telephone and in the e-mail.
- On the telephone, confirm the appointment by having the patient repeat the day, date, time, and location of the appointment.
- In an e-mail, be sure to use proper grammar and correct spelling and request that the patient provide a return communication for verification of received information.
- Communicate with the patient the desire to meet his or her requested appointment time; however, this is not always possible. An explanation may be necessary when offering an alternative time. If it is necessary to provide an explanation, be sure not to use any other patients' names.
- Be specific and inform the patient of the office policies for cancellations and missed appointments.
- Be sure to gather all pertinent information from the patient (i.e., name, telephone contacts, e-mail address, reason for visit, insurance carrier, and whether the patient needs directions to the office).
- As with any interaction with a patient, whether on the telephone, via e-mail, or in person, the medical assistant must always be aware of HIPAA regulations and take every measure possible to protect the patient's identity and verify that the individual the "patient" claims to be is indeed the patient. In addition to the common identifiers such as date of birth or address, many offices require PINs (personal identification numbers) or passwords, much like what is required for online banking. These provide another measure to prevent any information from being provided to someone other than the patient.

Scheduling Other Types of Appointments

Medical practices may have appointments to schedule for persons other than patients. These appointments may be for sales representatives from various companies—including office equipment, pharmaceuticals, and insurance—or community service leaders. Each visitor will need an appointment to update the staff and physician on the newest product, drug(s), equipment, or community issue(s). Most offices have a policy for working with nonpatient visitors and vendor representatives.

SUMMARY

An efficiently managed medical office requires careful attention to the scheduling function. The receptionist is responsible for carefully assessing the patient's need for an appointment. Providing the correct amount of time on the schedule for the patient visit works to ensure that the needs of patient and physician are met. However, the receptionist must remain flexible in scheduling since patients with emergencies and acute illnesses must be seen immediately. Keep in mind that flexibility is one key to being successful as a health care employee.

A professional and ethical manner is the best approach to handling a schedule that has fallen behind. Quick thinking and planning by rescheduling patients can alleviate stress for the physician who falls behind. Careful documentation and HIPAA compliance regarding all patients who fail to keep appointments, either through cancellation or no-show, can assist the physician in avoiding a lawsuit for abandonment of the patient.

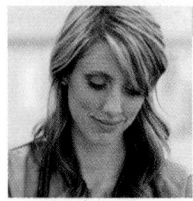

9 CHAPTER REVIEW

COMPETENCY REVIEW

1. Define and spell the terms to learn for this chapter.

2. Write an office policy for scheduling emergency appointments.

3. Role-play instructing a patient on admission to the hospital for a surgical procedure. Use another student as the patient.

4. Correctly document a patient appointment cancellation.

5. Use a computerized scheduling system to integrate patient information and appointment scheduling.

PREPARING FOR THE CERTIFICATION EXAM

1. The type of appointment scheduling where no appointments are made and first patient to sign in is the first patient seen is known as:
   a. wave.
   b. streaming.
   c. open hours.
   d. modified wave.
   e. double booking.

2. The type of appointment scheduling where patients are told to come in at the beginning of the hour in which they will be seen is known as:
   a. wave.
   b. streaming.
   c. open hours.
   d. modified wave.
   e. double booking.

3. When time is blocked off in the schedule for lunch this is known as establishing:
   a. a cluster.
   b. a schedule.
   c. a matrix.
   d. a calendar.
   e. an appointment.

4. Which of the following constitutes an emergency appointment?
   a. An 18-year-old college student leaving for school tomorrow needs a physical
   b. 58-year-old woman complaining of heavy vaginal bleeding
   c. 10-year-old child with a fever
   d. 34-year-old woman with sprained ankle
   e. 6-year-old with a 96°F fever

5. When scheduling an appointment for a patient over the telephone, it is most important to get what information?
   a. patient's date of birth
   b. patient's work telephone number
   c. patient's name, spelled correctly
   d. patient's home telephone number
   e. all of the above

6. Prior to calling the surgery scheduler for an inpatient surgery, the medical assistant should gather all of the following except:
   a. patient's medical insurance information.
   b. physician diagnosis.
   c. dietary preferences.
   d. known patient allergies.
   e. procedure to be performed.

7. If a patient is a no-show for an appointment, the receptionist should do all of the following except:
   a. record the no-show on the schedule.
   b. record the no-show in the patient's chart.
   c. refer the patient to a specialist.
   d. show the chart to the physician.
   e. if applicable, apply no-charge fee to patient's balance.

8. Appointment reminder cards should show all the following except:
   a. date of next appointment.
   b. time of next appointment.
   c. patient's name.
   d. patient's insurance information.
   e. name of physician patient is seeing.

9. Travis has an appointment at 10:00 A.M., and his roommate has an appointment the same day with the same

physician at 10:20 A.M. What type of appointment scheduling system is Travis's physician using?

a. double booking
b. specified time scheduling
c. wave scheduling
d. open office hours
e. modified wave

10. All of the following are examples of acute conditions except:

a. pain with urination.
b. earache.
c. abdominal pain.
d. laceration.
e. eye infection.

CRITICAL THINKING

1. Based on Dr. Miller's schedule, what scheduling variation is being used?

2. The office is usually closed from 12:00 P.M. to 1:00 P.M. for lunch. New patient visits usually last about 1 hour. Can Shannon Reece see Dr. Miller tomorrow?

3. How should Marc handle scheduling Marcus Fowler?

4. What needs to be done now that Rinna has cancelled her appointment?

ON THE JOB

A pharmaceutical representative has just arrived at the office of Dr. Joseph Henderson, a board-certified orthopedic surgeon. The waiting room is literally swarming with patients waiting to see Dr. Henderson because he was delayed with an unexpectedly complicated lumbar spinal fusion and laminectomy.

The representative is very insistent, almost belligerent, about seeing the physician immediately, even though she did not have an appointment to see him. In fact, the visit was totally unexpected as the representative had just been in 2 weeks ago. Last time the representative was in, she gave Dr. Henderson a variety of readily usable and dispensable medication. She has more of the same today—injectable cortisone with Novocain, muscle relaxants, NSAIDS, and even some Tylenol with codeine. Usually, Dr. Henderson is quite receptive to receiving these samples as they help ease the financial burden on his patients for whom he uses or to whom he dispenses the samples. The office is, in fact, running quite low on these particular medications because of Dr. Henderson's heavy patient load.

1. What is your response to the sales representative?
2. Should a representative ever take precedence over scheduled appointments?
3. Does the fact that Dr. Henderson is usually quite anxious to receive any and all samples for his patients enter in as a factor?
4. Does the diminished supply of these samples alter the situation?
5. Can the medical assistant ever accept delivery of any or all of these samples?

INTERNET ACTIVITY

Locate three different medical appointment-scheduling software programs on the Internet. Compare and contrast the products, services, features, and costs to fit the needs of a general practitioner's medical practice. Then locate the HIPAA compliance guidelines for appointment scheduling and develop a useful list for future reference.

MEDMEDIA

Additional interactive resources and activities for this chapter can be found:

On your student DVD: View applicable procedure videos on the DVD-ROM found in the back of this book.

MyHealthProfessionsKit.com: Test your knowledge of the chapter with games and activities. MyHealthProfessionsKit also includes resources, helpful links, and a Spanish audio glossary.

Medical Assisting Interactive: Practice your procedures as a medical assistant in this simulated doctor's office. This can be accessed through MyHealthProfessionsKit.com

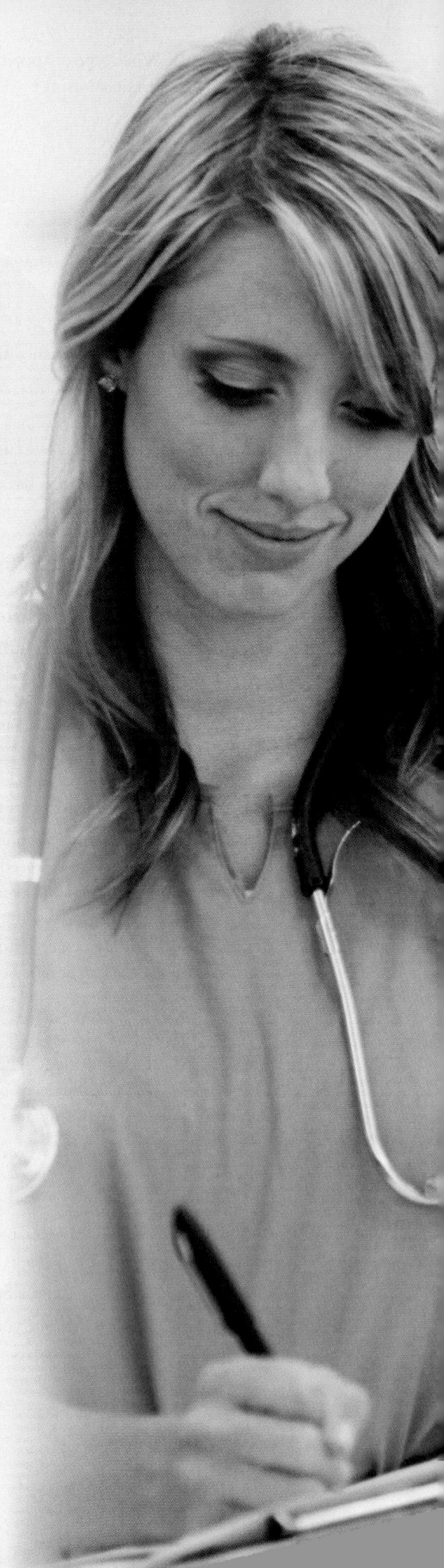

10

Office Facilities, Equipment, and Supplies

LEARNING OBJECTIVES

After completing this chapter, you should be able to:

- Define and spell the terms to learn for this chapter.

- Discuss the elements of office flow.

- Discuss HIPAA regulations as related to medical records.

- State the difference between capital equipment and expendable supplies.

- Discuss basic office equipment and the function of each.

- State the proper procedure for handling drug samples.

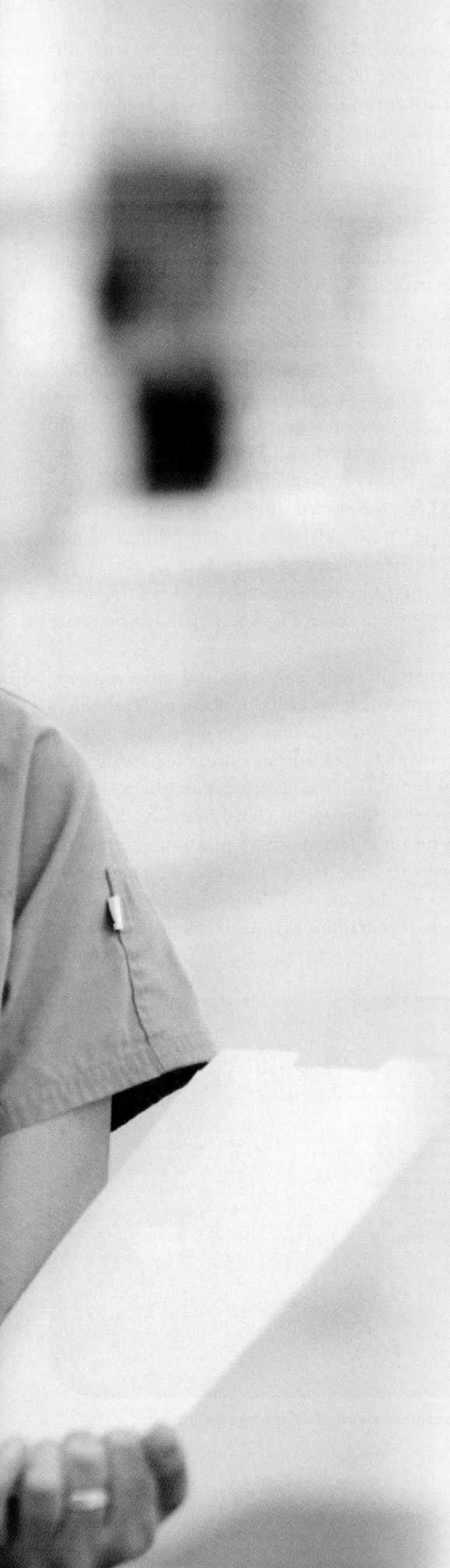

CHAPTER OUTLINE

CASE STUDY

Tanya Washington, a medical office manager, arrives at work to find the carpets have just been cleaned and all the patient waiting room furniture is stacked in the hallway. Several patients are starting to walk in the front door. The cleaning crew cleaned the office administration area, and most of the office equipment—including computers and the fax machine—have been moved or unplugged. Tanya finds an entire shelf of patient records on the floor and in her work area, and she also notices a few boxes in the hallway that contain patient supplies.

Americans with Disabilities
Act (ADA)

capital equipment

cycle time

depreciation

extended warranty

expendable supplies

financial life

inventory

life expectancy

morale

office flow

vendors

warranty

CERTIFICATION LINK

CMA (AAMA)
Professionalism
Communication
Medicolegal
guidelines and
requirements
Screening and
processing mail
Maintaining the
office environment

RMA
Medical law
Medical receptionist/
Secretarial/Clerical

CMAS (AMT)
Medical assisting
foundation
Medical office clerical
assisting
Medical office
management

Every medical workplace should be clean to ensure employee and patient safety and health, the traffic should flow smoothly, and it should adhere to federal, state, and local safety and health regulations. In recent years, changes have been made to many regulations that affect the medical office. As communication processes and technology become more sophisticated, it becomes necessary for the office personnel to stay informed and to adhere to the rules that make the medical office safe and protect everyone's right to privacy.

Medical Office Facility

The pleasant physical atmosphere created by a cheerful, clean office makes an immediate impression on patients. It also adds to the general positive morale of the employees. **Morale** refers to the positive or negative state of mind of employees (regarding a feeling of well-being) with relationship to their work or work environment. Things to be considered in setting up and maintaining a medical office include the office layout and design, which set the tone, attitude, climate, and culture of the office. Elements of the layout include the design of traffic flow, the color of the walls, room temperature, lighting, ventilation, furniture and placement of the furniture, equipment, supplies, and overall organization.

FACILITIES PLANNING

The medical assistant must view the medical office through the eyes of the patient. What does the patient see when he or she enters the doors and beyond?

One of the first considerations in planning a medical office facility is the **Americans with Disabilities Act (ADA)**. This legislation protects the rights of the disabled regarding access to employment, public buildings, transportation, housing, schools, and health care facilities. The law allows for every public facility to be easily accessible to the handicapped, including unrestricted hallways, elevators or ramps, and handicapped restroom facilities. Furnishings should be arranged to create an easy traffic pattern for patients to follow as they enter and leave the office. The waiting room should have adequate space for wheelchairs to be easily maneuvered.

All patients should walk into a medical office environment that is comfortable and bright. Some medical offices have patients walk into a reception room with a window that allows patients to look outside during their wait time. External light shines into the office, making the room well lit and comfortable. Reception rooms generally should be painted with bright colors and have pleasing and tasteful art on the walls (Figure 10-1). Fish tanks are common in medical offices as they are very inviting for children and adults to watch. If your office has a fish tank, it is important

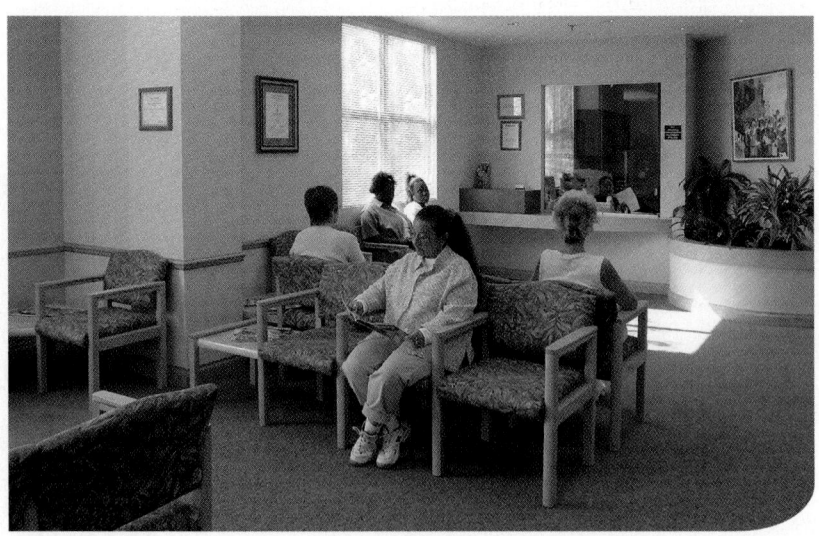

FIGURE 10-1 A reception area should be comfortable and bright.

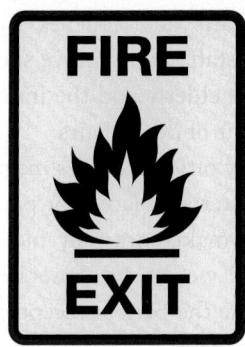

FIGURE 10-2 If a fire were to occur, follow the evacuation plan.

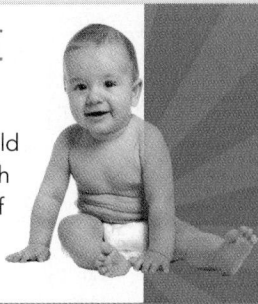

to regularly maintain the tank for patient safety and cleanliness. It is important to position the tank high enough so children cannot disturb the fish or push over the tank.

RECEPTION ROOM SAFETY

The medical assistant must monitor the office for safety hazards. Frayed cords, overloaded outlets, and extension cords can all pose safety risks. To identify potential safety hazards, the medical assistant must take a close look at the office with special concern for fire and fall hazards. If throw rugs are used, do they lie flat? Are any cords frayed? Are electrical outlets covered?

Fire Safety

To prevent fire, it is important to understand what it takes for a fire to start and continue burning. The three elements required for fire to occur are fuel, heat, and oxygen. If all three are not present, a fire will not ignite.

It is very important to act appropriately if a fire were to occur. To ensure safety not only for the patients but also for themselves, every staff member should know what their role is. An evacuation plan should be posted in a central location within every office, typically in the employee break area, and possibly other areas also. Fire safety and other emergencies in the medical office are discussed in Chapter 43. See Figure 10-2 for an example of the fire symbol that could be used in an evacuation plan.

Office Layout

Medical offices are generally divided into two areas: administrative and clinical. The administrative area may contain the reception area where patient processing and scheduling, file storage, payment collections, insurance, billing, and mail processing are performed. Office equipment such as computers, printers, scanners, fax machines, postage meters, calculators, telephone system, paper shredder, dictation and transcribing equipment, as well as all office supplies are also usually located in the administrative area. The reception area

may also include a children's play area. (See "Reception Area" for more detail.)

The clinical area contains the examination rooms, physician's office and consultation room, treatment room for office surgical procedures, supply room, clean and contaminated utility areas, restrooms, a laboratory that can house blood drawing, specimen analyzing, and electrocardiogram (ECG) equipment, and in some offices, a radiology room. Some medical facilities also have a small recovery room with a bed or cot for patients recovering from minor surgical procedures. Of course, not every office will have all these areas. Specialty practices may have other departments and equipment specific to the type of procedures performed.

OFFICE FLOW

The medical facility generally has a flow that lends itself easily to teamwork, time management, organized and efficient office equipment usage, and patient flow. This is known as **office flow**. The more organized the office area, the more effective the office flow will be managed by staff and patients. All staff members will be involved in the office flow process from the time the patients arrive to their departure time. Each staff member has a chance to maintain the office flow by reducing patient cycle time. **Cycle time** is the length of time the average patient spends in the medical office. With proper office layout, the cycle time can be managed more effectively for a smoother office flow (Figure 10-3).

The first element of the office flow is the patient entrance. The office entranceways should include handrails, elevators, ramps, wheelchair-accessible door frames, patient lifts if necessary, and well-lit walkways. High steps should be marked with reflector tape and should include slip-protection sheets. Doors and door handles should be marked with a push or pull indicator. Keeping doors clean and clear is vital to office aesthetics and patient safety.

RECEPTION AREA

The reception area consists of the waiting room and the reception desk. The desk should be enclosed with a glass partition that can be closed for privacy so that personal medical

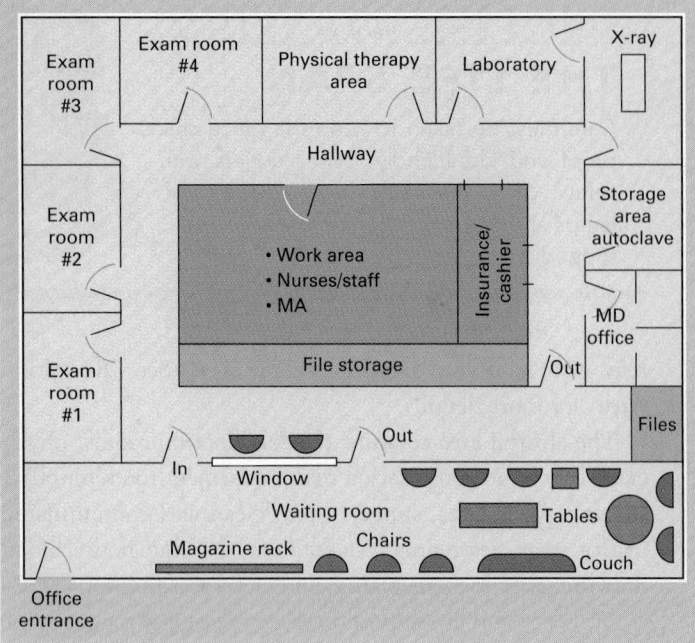

FIGURE 10-3   A typical office layout.

information cannot be overheard in the waiting room. The desk surface should be neat and not contain confidential patient information such as records, an open appointment book, or billing information.

The medical records area should be close to the receptionist's area for quick accessibility to charts for telephone calls. The Health Insurance Portability and Accountability Act (HIPAA) states that the medical records area should not be accessible to patients and that they should not be able to read the labels of the charts. Figure 10-4 shows a typical office file room.

Seating that provides good support and can be easily cleaned is most suitable for the patient reception area.

PROFESSIONALISM

Professional medical assistants must strive to keep their immediate work area neat, clean, and organized. This is especially important in the reception area of the office as a patient's first impression of the overall office, or you personally, may be formed based on the appearance of your work area. Be sure not to allow charts to stack up on the desk or have papers scattered. This may cause the patient to be concerned with how you may take care of their personal information, and this in turn may affect their confidence in the office.

Overstuffed chairs and couches should be avoided. Housekeeping staff cannot move such furniture easily. In addition, the elderly and the infirm find it difficult to get in and out of deep chairs.

Almost every office provides magazines for patients to read. All materials placed for patient reading must be screened to make sure they meet the standards of your office and would not upset any patients. Some offices opt to use the patient reception room to provide general patient education on topics such as healthy eating, exercise, and the adverse effects of smoking. Several types of media, such as DVDs, printed literature, and magazines, may be used to present this form of patient education. Magazines and materials should be organized neatly to show that the office is clean and well maintained. Typically, the receptionist or another staff member is assigned to straighten up the reception area and waiting room, especially magazines and brochures.

Children's toys and books should be washable and have no small or removable parts. Large building blocks, hardcover books, and appropriately sized plastic toys that can be sanitized may be placed on a small table for children. All toys should be disinfected daily with an appropriate cleaner to prevent the spread of infection.

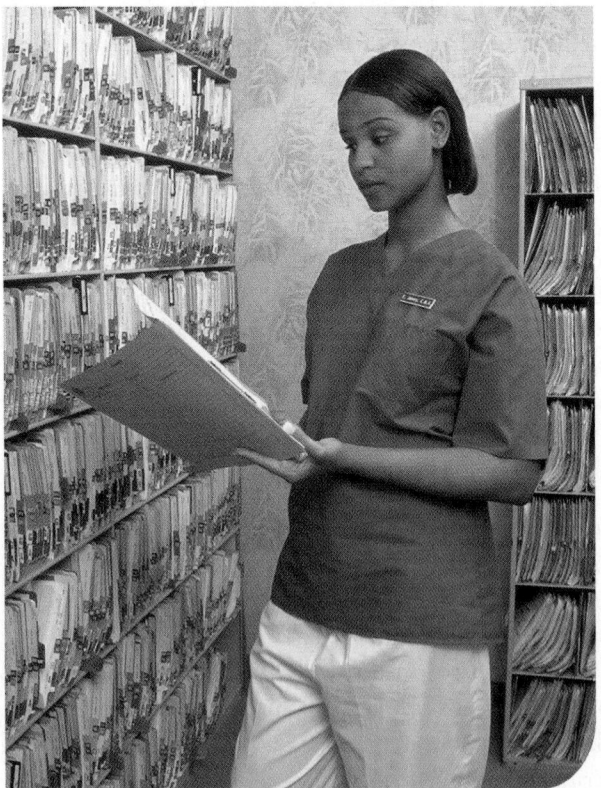

FIGURE 10-4   A typical office file room.

Smoking is not allowed in medical facilities. "No smoking" signs should be placed at the entrance of the building, and a container should be available for the disposal of cigarettes prior to entering the building.

If a person with a communicable disease visits the office, he or she should be placed in a designated area to minimize spreading the disease. After the visit is over, the office should be disinfected immediately.

Patient orientation begins when the patient arrives in the reception area. Clear markings and signs should indicate the location of the registration and check-in desk, office entrance and exits, where patients should sit if more than one doctor is in the office, and restroom locations. Hallways and walkways should be clear of any obstructions. In some offices, color-coded indicators on the floor or wall help to facilitate patient flow.

Proper signage helps patients get around the medical office. Clearly marked areas also assist patient exits. When a patient is ready to leave the office, it is important to confirm the route a patient needs to take to exit the office. For example, if a patient has just been seen by a physician and you are showing the patient out, it is best to lead the way. This will help prevent patients from accidentally walking into another examination room or into private areas of the office. Patients should have a direct, clearly marked route to the checkout desk.

EXAMINATION ROOMS

Examination rooms should contain only furnishings and equipment needed to examine a patient. Most examination rooms have only enough space for the necessities and little else. Figure 10-5 illustrates a typical patient examination room. A sufficient number of all instruments and supplies, such as disposable gowns, towels, tissues, and sheets, are kept

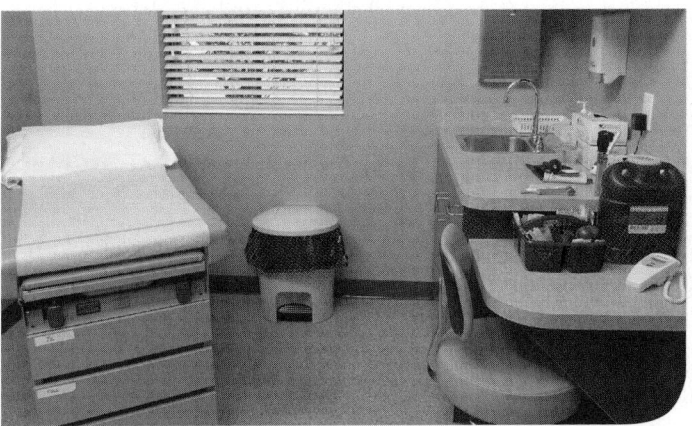

FIGURE 10-5 A patient examination room should be simple and efficiently designed.

in examination room supply cabinets. Most examination tables have drawers for the convenient storage of these items. A small sink for hand hygiene, an adjustable gooseneck lamp, chair, small writing desk, examination table, clothes hook, and physician's stool are the only furnishings necessary. Examination rooms should be painted in pleasant and comforting colors. Paintings or pictures can enhance the serenity of the room. Be sure no unpleasant odors are present in the examination rooms. If they are, you might need to close that room until the odor dissipates or the room is sanitized.

The temperature throughout the reception area and examination rooms should be maintained around 72°F. Patients in the examination rooms must frequently disrobe and may be chilled in just a disposable gown. If the examination room is too warm, patients will become drowsy. Controlling the room temperature so that all are comfortable is often one of the most difficult tasks to accomplish in the office.

At least one examination room should be configured for a wheelchair-bound patient. It should be larger than a normal-size examination room to allow both the patient and physician to maneuver comfortably.

Examination rooms should be soundproof so that conversations cannot be heard from one room to another. The examination table should be arranged so that the patient is not exposed when the door is opened. White noise, such as pleasant, soothing background music, can also filter sounds.

BATHROOMS

Bathrooms should be kept clean and odor free. Every bathroom should have hot and cold water, soap, paper towels or another drying system, a trash can, and toilet tissue. Since bathrooms in the medical office are multifunctional, they also should be large enough to accommodate a wheelchair, and at least one of the bathrooms should meet ADA guidelines for a handicapped restroom facility, such as handrails around the toilet. Although some offices have separate bathrooms for staff members, the same bathroom often is used by both staff and patients. Patient bathrooms should have a shelf or designated area to place urine specimens while the patient washes his or her hands after collecting the sample. This helps minimize the chance of specimens being spilled.

HOUSEKEEPING

Housekeeping or medical office cleaning services can be contracted to clean the front office area, clinical areas, and

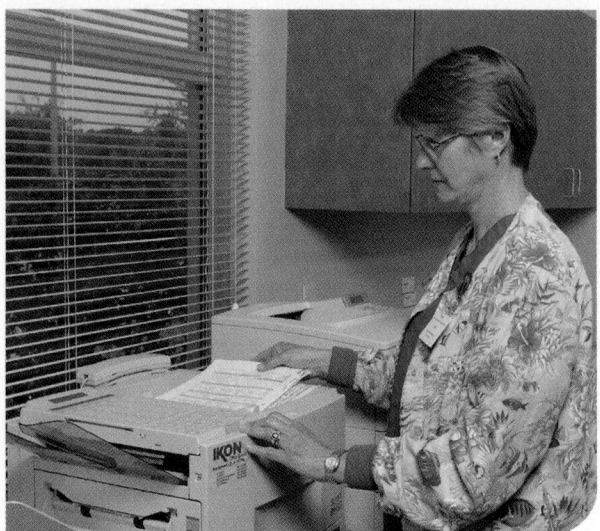

FIGURE 10-6   Fax machines are necessary in all medical offices.

examination rooms every night. Regular housekeeping services are usually not responsible for handling hazardous waste containers. Instead, hazardous waste, including sharps, should be disposed of in designated containers and removed from the office or facility properly. It is important if contracting an outside cleaning service that it operates in compliance with HIPAA standards. This often requires cleaning service personnel to sign forms stating they will adhere to HIPAA patient privacy laws.

Office Equipment

For a medical office to maintain effective office flow, certain office machines and equipment are most beneficial. As mentioned, a copier, computers, printers, scanners, fax machines (Figure 10-6), postage meters, calculators, telephone system, dictation and transcribing equipment, and paper shredder are considered essentials for the office. This and other equipment, such as examination tables, refrigerators, X-ray and EKG machines, office furnishings, and carpeting, are categorized as capital equipment.

CAPITAL EQUIPMENT

Capital equipment refers to items that require a large dollar amount to purchase (generally over $500) and have a relatively long life. The distinguishing factor between capital equipment and general office supplies is the **life expectancy** (functional life period) of the product.

Capital equipment also has a **financial life**, which is referred to as depreciation. **Depreciation** is a loss in value of the product resulting from normal aging, use, or deterioration. An allowance is made for this type of loss of value for tax purposes. Therefore, the office accountant will credit capital items differently than general office supplies. A master **inventory**, or list, should be detailed and maintained of all the physical assets, or capital equipment, in an office.

The needs of the office determine the equipment required. Obtaining the equipment requires research to gather equipment information, the actual purchase, delivery, setup, proper training, safe use, and general maintenance. Most medical offices have the following administrative capital equipment:

- **Computers**—Both laptops and desktops (see Chapter 12).
- **Color laser printer**—used in conjunction with a computer for letter-quality printing. Creates images with a laser beam and then transfers the color image to paper with pressure and heat.
- **Telephone system** (discussed in Chapter 7).
- **Scanners**—used to "read" text and graphic files.

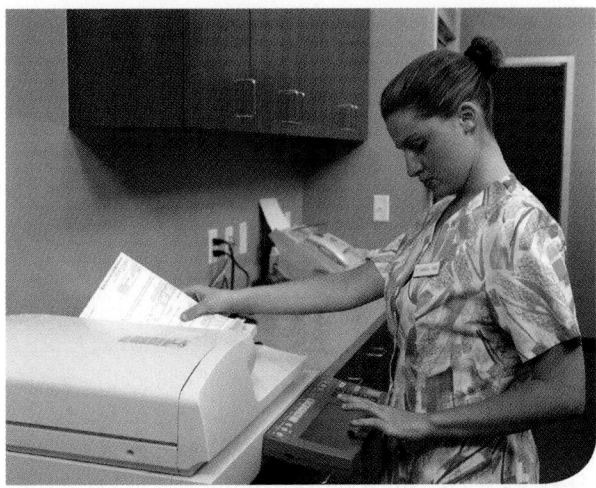

FIGURE 10-7 Copiers should meet the particular needs of the medical office.

- **Copy machine**—used to copy, reduce, enlarge, and collate documents in the medical office (Figure 10-7).
- **Postage meter**—used by offices with large mailings to stamp envelopes and packages.

WORD PROCESSING

Word processing has made creating and retrieving documents more efficient. The word processor has the ability to create and manipulate text without having to cut and paste a paper document. The word processor also allows the typist to work on a document, save it, retrieve it at a later time, and work on it again. Corrections during the typing process can easily be made, and word processors also have the ability to make multiple copies of a document.

VOICE RECOGNITION TECHNOLOGY

The latest voice recognition technology (VRT) allows the physician to speak into a microphone connected to a computer program that translates the physician's dictated office note into a typed report. VRT requires the physician to provide several samples of his or her speech by reading manufacturer-provided scripts to activate the program. Since this is a time-consuming process, relatively few physicians have adopted this system in their offices. However, it is used in some hospital medical records departments. As this equipment becomes more user friendly, it will become more accessible.

USING A POSTAGE METER

Many offices use a postage meter that includes a postage scale. The postage meter can automatically stamp large mailings. The postage can either be printed directly onto an envelope or onto an adhesive-backed strip that is placed directly on a package. A postage meter with a scale provides the option of weighing letters and packages, and the meter will then calculate the exact postage required and either print it directly onto the letter or print out a strip to be affixed to the package. This method can save significant amounts of money. Metered mail does not have to be stamped when it arrives at the post office. Postage is purchased for use with the machine, and as the machine applies postage to letters and packages, the monetary amount in the postage account decreases. When the amount of postage available begins to run low, the medical assistant may either take the meter to the post office or increase the available postage via the Internet if the office has established an account. The meter is occasionally taken into the post office for calibrating (Figure 10-8).

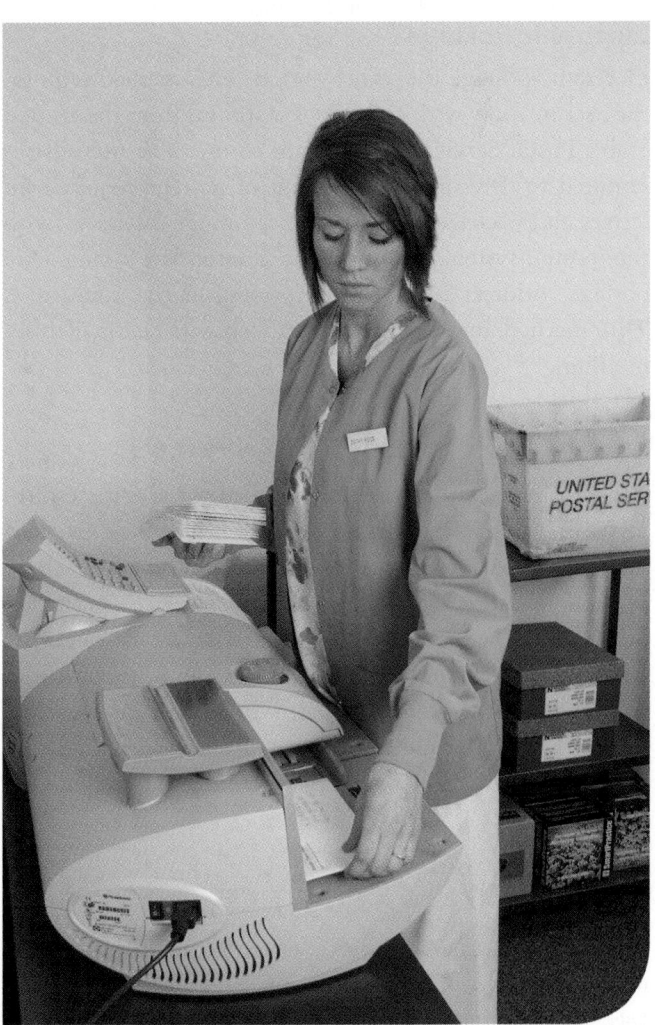

FIGURE 10-8 Postage meters are used for large mailings.

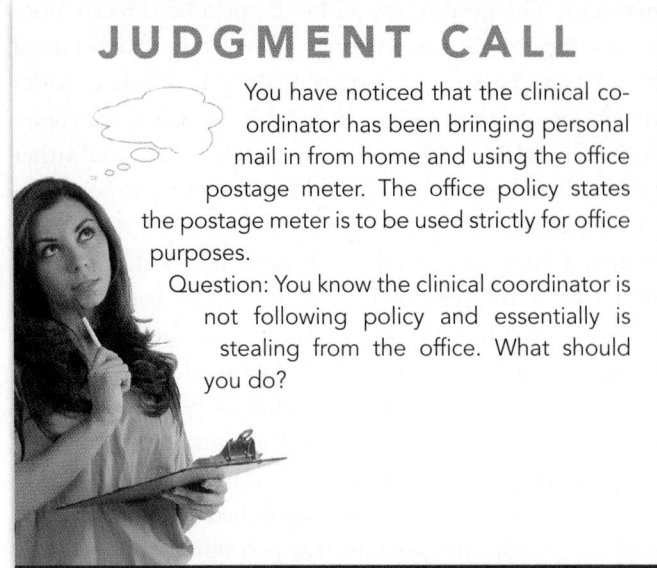
Electronic Postage

Electronic postage is another option. This method requires the user to apply with and receive approval from the United States Postal Service (USPS) prior to use. The user also is required to determine the amount of postage required for letters and packages, and then a computer interfaces with the postal system to print the appropriate amount of postage. Address labels can be printed at the same time. This method may be used in offices with a lot of bulk mailings.

PURCHASING EQUIPMENT

When a business determines the need for specific equipment, the purchase process begins. The medical assistant may be asked to research and compare equipment based on the manufacturer, quality, size, service, price, and other determining factors. The medical assistant can search the Internet and can contact local vendors and other offices as part of the fact-gathering quest. Collecting information, printed materials, and resources will enable the physician to make the right choice when actually purchasing the equipment.

WARRANTIES

A **warranty** is a manufacturer's guarantee in writing that its product will perform correctly under normal conditions of use. The warranty provides for a replacement of defective parts at no charge within a certain period of time. An **extended warranty** can be purchased to cover some period of time after the warranty has expired. For example, a copier may have a 1-year warranty, but an extended warranty can be purchased to cover parts replacement after that year has expired.

Some office equipment that is heavily used, such as a copy machine, has a service contract for preventive maintenance. To avoid a breakdown, a service contract provides maintenance and cleaning of equipment even when it is working properly. A service contract will state in detail what is actually covered by the contract. The dates and frequency of service should be noted carefully. Literature relating to warranties and preventive maintenance contracts should be kept in a designated location. Since office equipment is expensive, these contracts are important.

EQUIPMENT RECORDS

Records relating to office equipment must be maintained. Equipment records will include an office equipment maintenance log. This log is used to document the pieces of equipment that require regular maintenance, when the maintenance occurred, and which individual or company provided the service. A current maintenance log helps prove equipment has been well maintained. Depending on the type of practice, the maintenance log is a required document for insurance purposes and may be subpoenaed if a patient was injured due to equipment failure.

The medical assistant should record in writing any unusual occurrences of equipment. Memory of what actually happened may fail over time. A written record of exactly what happened and the corrective action that was taken can assist in determining cause as an accident or negligence.

Receipts for major purchases, operating manuals, instructions, warranties, and repair and maintenance instructions must be kept and filed appropriately. Lists of service people with contact information should be maintained. Many offices maintain a current file of business cards representing the companies from which equipment has been purchased. Ideally, the registration and ID number of each item is maintained in a separate file from the warranty.

An inventory list of items used for specific procedures may be found in the office's policies and procedures manual. This is especially helpful for new employees so they know what supplies are required for specific activities. The complete inventory record for the practice is typically also maintained in the computer and updated by the office manager or other individual responsible for ordering

TABLE 10-1 Equipment Inventory Record

Item	Serial #	Purchase Date	Location
Laptop	XX 12345	2/14/XX	Reception
IBM Selectric II Typewriter	XC54321	2/14/XX	Laboratory
IBM G40 Computer	4-190-L1001	9/19/XX	Reception
Hewlett-Packard Color LaserJet Printer	JPHAC15531	9/19/XX	Reception
Ricoh Copier	RC39C452	6/2/XX	Billing

supplies. Table 10-1 provides an example of an office inventory record.

EQUIPMENT LIFE AND SAFETY

All equipment is purchased with the accompanying manufacturer's training manual to maintain the life of the machine and the safety of the user. The medical assistant should read all manuals prior to use and have the vendor provide training for the office staff. Usually, the retailer's training and manual will suggest using the equipment defaults and turning the equipment off when not in use. Training and manuals provide cleaning, maintenance, and operation directions as well as other important information. The suggestions usually place safety of the user first, longevity of the equipment second, and reordering or service information third.

Supplies

Vendors, or suppliers, are selected based on several factors, including the quality, price, service, and availability that they provide. In general, it takes multiple vendors to provide all supplies for a medical practice. Catalog or online services can provide ease of availability, competitive pricing, and fast delivery. In preparation for negotiating a contract, a wise purchaser will develop a good working relationship with vendors, either in person, on the telephone, in writing, or online. Contracts or purchase agreements may include payment schedules, shipment times, product discounts, extended warranty, training sessions, and other incentives.

Many vendors will provide a discount on supplies when they are ordered in large quantities. This results in a unit cost savings. The drawback to this method is that many offices do not have enough storage space to handle a large inventory of supplies. Some suppliers will store excess inventory for you.

When ordering supplies, the person tasked with this responsibility should attempt to have an ample amount of supplies on hand without having too much or too little. Too much inventory costs money, not only from the paid goods perspective but also from an available space perspective. Most offices are switching to a just-in-time (JIT) method that requires more frequent ordering but has supplies arriving daily in some cases. Just-in-time ordering helps significantly with cash flow as well.

Several methods are used to determine when supplies should be ordered, and medical assistants should be familiar with the method used in the office where they work. Many offices use a card system where specific information regarding the product is recorded. The card may note the item name, name and address of the vendor, unit price, quantity typically ordered, date the order was placed, date the order was received, and any other information of note.

Supplies should be rotated on the shelves so that newer supplies are in the back of the shelf and older supplies are used first.

Expendable supplies and equipment include items that are used up quickly and have a relatively inexpensive unit cost. Examples of expendable office supplies are found in Table 10-2.

SUPPLY INVENTORY

Supply inventory control requires constant supervision since a medical office cannot afford to run out of supplies. As mentioned, many supplies are purchased in large quantities at lower cost. It can be costly to run out and have to suddenly purchase supplies at full price with additional shipping costs for faster service.

TABLE 10-2 Expendable Office Supplies

Paper Supplies	Examination table paper, disposable gowns, drapes, paper towels, sterilization bags and tapes, stationery, photocopy paper, insurance and chart forms, laboratory order forms, appointment books, ECG paper, receipt book, appointment cards, current CPT and ICD-9 coding books
Clinical Equipment	Disposable speculums, ear and nose speculum covers, catheters, tongue blades, thermometers, cotton-tipped applicators, lubricant, needles, syringes, suture material, dressings, tape, elastic bandages, gloves, goggles
Office Supplies	Pens, pencils, highlighters, copy paper, stapler(s), stapler removers, printer cartridge, CD-ROMs

Most offices maintain an ongoing inventory system that helps to determine when to reorder supplies. Whenever an item is removed from the supply cabinet, it should be marked on the inventory sheet. A staff member is assigned the responsibility of reordering all supplies when items get to a certain predetermined level so that the supply is never totally depleted. Along with the frequency in which supplies are used, the amount of time necessary to have the order processed and delivered should be factored in when reordering supplies. See Figure 10-9 for a sample inventory order form.

ORDER SYSTEM

It takes experience to be able to calculate how long inventory items will last. However, records can be reviewed to determine when half the supply has been used. Then, by calculating the amount of time it takes to receive a new order, an estimate can be made of when and how much to reorder. For example, if one printer cartridge is used in 1 month and the reorder period is 3 weeks, then a new order must be placed when half the supply has been used. Since print cartridges may be used more during a certain part of the billing period, or when the office is busier, it would be advisable to reorder cartridges in advance to prevent running out of the supply.

Many offices insert color-coded reorder reminder cards into the stack of inventory items. When the card comes to the top of the stack, it is time to reorder. Inventory reminder cards can be maintained with a date for reorder.

Some suppliers maintain their own records and will notify the medical office when it is time to reorder. Keep a list of inventory items in the procedure manual and maintain the inventory records on computer files. Some offices use an automated scanning system for inventory control and ordering system.

DRUG SAMPLES

The pharmaceutical representatives of drug companies will often supply medical offices with samples of medications. A drug sample is a small package of a medication for use by the physician or physician distribution to patients. An inventory list of all sample drugs must be maintained to adhere to Drug Enforcement Administration (DEA) and, in some cases, state regulations (check your local state requirements).

Even though these drug samples are small and "free," the medical office must secure and organize the samples in a supply cupboard

FIGURE 10-9 Sample inventory order form.

or drawer that is locked. It is advisable to keep all drugs together by category (e.g., sedatives, antibiotics, hypertensive drugs). The expiration dates on drug samples must be carefully monitored. All samples should be rotated like other supplies, with newer samples placed in the back behind samples of the same medication and strength with earlier expiration dates. Expired samples should be discarded following office policies and procedures and in accordance with federal, state, and DEA regulations.

SUMMARY

The office layout contributes to the physical atmosphere, organization, and impression that patients and employees will encounter. An organized office layout can affect the office flow, decrease patient cycle time, and positively impact employee morale and patients' attitudes.

The medical assistant must maintain an inventory list for all office equipment purchased, supplies, and drug samples. All staff members should be trained on the use and operational functions of the equipment.

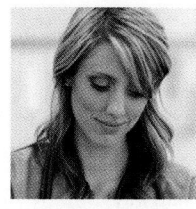

10 CHAPTER REVIEW

COMPETENCY REVIEW

1. Define and spell the terms to learn for this chapter.

2. Discuss how following the manufacturer's suggestions enhances equipment longevity.

3. Discuss the importance of patient flow.

4. Discuss how inventory control methods contribute to efficient office management.

5. Discuss the handling of pharmaceutical samples in the medical office.

PREPARING FOR THE CERTIFICATION EXAM

1. When asked to seek out a new vendor, the medical assistant should do all of the following except:
   a. gather information about available discounts.
   b. verify delivery procedures.
   c. speak with one vendor.
   d. verify payment policies.
   e. determine ease of availability.

2. When drug samples are left by the pharmaceutical representative, the samples should be kept in a locked cabinet and organized by:
   a. category.
   b. shipment date.
   c. alphabetical order.
   d. expiration date.
   e. cost.

3. An example of capital equipment found in the medical office would be:
   a. a computer.
   b. computer paper.
   c. a computer printer.
   d. a typewriter.
   e. computer ink cartridges.

4. What room temperature is most comfortable for the majority of patients?
   a. 70°F
   b. 71°F
   c. 72°F
   d. 73°F
   e. 74°F

5. What two distinct areas are typically found in a medical office?
   a. traffic flow and office areas
   b. administrative and clinical areas
   c. reception and staff areas
   d. staff and administrative areas
   e. reception and administrative areas

6. Once a vendor is chosen, the medical assistant should expect all of the following EXCEPT:
   a. quality assurance.
   b. fast delivery.
   c. unit pricing.
   d. inventory count.
   e. service.

7. Capital equipment includes all of the following EXCEPT:
   a. insurance forms.
   b. exam tables.
   c. EKG machine.
   d. microscope.
   e. copy machine.

8. Equipment purchase agreements may include the following EXCEPT:
   a. training.
   b. service.
   c. warranty.
   d. office flow.
   e. extended warranty.

9. Which supplies are NOT expendable clinical equipment supplies?
   a. disposable examination gowns
   b. paper towels
   c. syringes
   d. goggles
   e. disposable speculums

10. Office flow includes:
    a. lighting and ventilation.
    b. general eye appeal and traffic flow.
    c. current periodicals and furniture.
    d. ADA bathrooms and clearly marked hallways.
    e. exit signs.

CRITICAL THINKING

1. What is the first thing you would do to fix the situation after the office carpets were cleaned?

2. How do you function in the office? Based on your knowledge about physical hazards and office safety, what precautions should Tania take to resolve the problem?

3. What happens to patient flow in this situation?

ON THE JOB

Develop an inventory using an electronic spreadsheet of all equipment, machines, and supplies for the clinical and administrative areas. Include purchase date, maintenance schedule, and purchase price.

INTERNET ACTIVITY

Go to the Americans with Disabilities Act (ADA) website (www.ada.gov) and research the standards for bathrooms in public places that accommodate wheelchairs.

MEDMEDIA

Additional interactive resources and activities for this chapter can be found:

On your student DVD: View applicable procedure videos on the DVD-ROM found in the back of this book.

MyHealthProfessionsKit.com: Test your knowledge of the chapter with games and activities. MyHealthProfessionsKit also includes resources, helpful links, and a Spanish audio glossary.

Medical Assisting Interactive: Practice your procedures as a medical assistant in this simulated doctor's office. This can be accessed through MyHealthProfessionsKit.com.

11

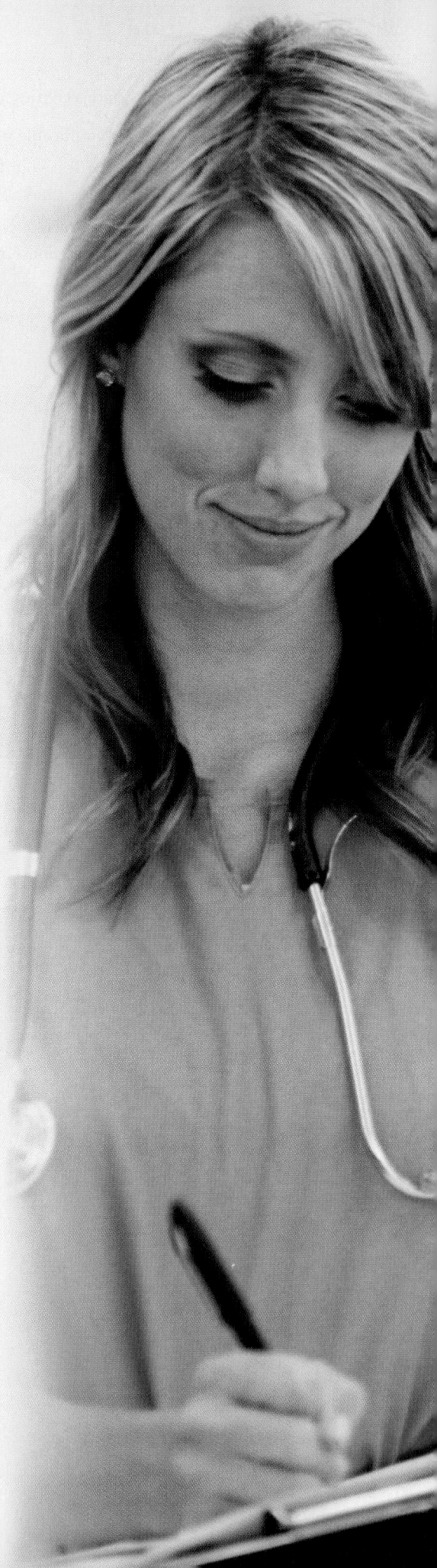

Written Communication

LEARNING OBJECTIVES

After completing this chapter, you should be able to:

- Define and spell the terms to learn for this chapter.

- Name and describe eight areas to consider when letter writing.

- Identify the eight parts of speech and use them correctly.

- Describe the process of drafting correspondence, using the four letter styles.

- Explain the process of proofreading and editing.

- List and describe how to prepare an envelope to meet the standards of the U.S. Postal Service.

- State the four classifications of mail service.

- List and describe six special services offered by the U.S. Postal Service.

- Define an instant message and identify its purpose.

CHAPTER OUTLINE

CASE STUDY

Lewis Jordan, RMA is working with a student in the Pearson Physicians Group externship program. The student has been asked by the physician to write a letter to refer a patient to another physician for a second opinion. The student writes the letter and asks Lewis to review it. Following is the letter written by the extern:

Dear Dr. Johnson

I am referring a patient to your office for further evaluation. I have been seeing this patient for several years now for right metatarsal injury. It is in my opinion that this patient should seek additional information on having the right metatarsal removed. This patient has been in my office on several occasions unable to walk with much swelling.

I trust your medical opinion and would appreciate you advising the proper action to take for this patient. For your review I have enclosed past X-rays, please feel free to contact my office as soon as possible.

Sincerely,
Dr. J. Ancella

211

TERMS TO LEARN

active voice

block

complimentary close

constant information

electronic mail (e-mail)

enclosure

gender bias

homophones

letterhead

memos

modified block

optical character recognition (OCR)

passive voice

proofreading

redundant

reference initials

salutation

signature line

thesaurus

variables

CERTIFICATION LINK

CMA (AAMA)
General
  Medical
  terminology
  Communication
Administrative
  Screening and
  processing mail

RMA
General medical
assisting knowledge
  Medical
  terminology
Administrative
medical assisting
  Medical
  receptionist/
  Secretarial/Clerical

CMAS (AMT)
Medical assisting
foundation
  Medical
  terminology
  Professionalism
Medical office clerical
assisting
  Communication
Medical office
management
  Office
  communications

Medical assistants draft many types of correspondence to be signed by the physician/employer. These letters must reflect the professionalism of the medical practice. Every piece of correspondence represents the medical office, and impressions of the office can be formed based on such correspondence. The physical appearance of letters depends on the quality of paper, letterhead design, and choice of formats used. However, even the most professional-looking correspondence is quickly and harshly judged when the letter is written in a negative or condescending tone or is filled with grammatical and spelling errors. Correspondence should be positive in tone and well written.

Handling incoming mail requires efficiency in sorting, dating, and reading all correspondence. Correct handling of the mail can save money and time for the medical practice. Initiative in handling mail quickly and accurately is paramount.

Letter Writing

Letters from a medical office must be professional, courteous, businesslike, positive in tone, and protective of the confidentiality of the physician and the patient. This requires some diplomacy. For example, when drafting a sensitive letter requesting payment for a long overdue bill or to advise a patient to seek the services of another physician, the writing should be clear and to the point. The situation should be explained and the expected outcome presented—"Please send a check for (amount due)" or "Please call to make payment arrangements." Threats or derogatory comments are never acceptable in professional correspondence and may have legal consequences for the sender. The following letters are examples of positive and negative tones in writing.

Negative Example:

Dear Mrs. Murray:

You have repeatedly failed to take medications as prescribed and follow my recommended treatment. Since you have again failed to keep an appointment, I am forced to withdraw as your physician, and I request that you find another physician immediately.

Positive Example:

Dear Mrs. Murray:

During your last visit, we discussed the necessity of continuing medical treatment for you to recover fully from your recent medical problems. Therefore, I am concerned that you failed to keep your appointment this week and have not called the office to schedule a new appointment. Your health continues to be important to me, so I am requesting that you call me as soon as possible to discuss future treatment.

If we are unable to reach a mutual understanding about your medical treatment and appointment schedule, I regret that I will not be able to continue as your physician. In that event, you will receive a letter indicating that you have a month's notice in which to secure the services of another physician.

Word Choice

The use of correct words when writing office correspondence includes avoidance of the use of technical terms, **gender bias** (indicating either male or female by the type of language used), long sentences and paragraphs, excessive use of the personal pronoun *I,* repetition, and passive voice.

TECHNICAL TERMINOLOGY

When writing a letter to medical professionals or institutions that employ medically trained staff, the correct use and

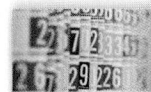

PROFESSIONALISM

THE LAW

The medical assistant must carefully monitor all dated material to ensure that replies are made on a timely basis. Confidential mail and correspondence, including checks and payments, are handled on a regular basis. This is an important responsibility that may be carried out by a medical assistant. Because the U.S. Postal Service is regulated by the federal government, any tampering or deliberate mishandling of mail is a federal offense.

A nonthreatening tone in correspondence can promote the medical profession to the reader. Any attempts to threaten a patient in writing can lead to charges of harassment. Courteous language, presented in a diplomatic manner, can result in compliance and prevent a lawsuit.

The medical assistant must carefully proofread all correspondence before it leaves the office to protect the physician from legal problems. An error in correspondence may not be caught by the physician before he or she signs the document. If you are unsure about proper grammar or spelling, ask someone else to read the document.

TABLE 11-1 Medical Terms and Corresponding Synonyms

Medical Term	Synonym
Carcinoma	Cancer
Cardiac	Heart
Dermatitis	Skin irritation
Diabetes mellitus	Diabetes
Gastric	Stomach
Gynecology	Study of female diseases
Hepatic disease	Liver disease
Hyperglycemic	Excessive blood sugar
Hypertension	High blood pressure
Larynx	Voice box
Leukocytes	White blood cells
MI	Myocardial infarction
Nephrosis	Kidney disease
NPO	Nothing by mouth
Otolaryngology	Study of ear, nose, and throat
Para I	First delivery
pc	After meals
Thrombus	Blood clot

spelling of medical terminology are essential. Medical terminology is easily understood by those trained in the profession. However, many patients are not familiar with medical terminology and, in fact, may not understand or may be intimidated by this style of writing. Table 11-1 lists selected medical terms with corresponding synonyms. The medical terms in the left column are appropriate for correspondence with medically trained personnel (physician to physician, physician to medical record, medical assistant to hospital); the terms in the right column are more easily understood by patients.

REMOVING GENDER BIAS

Unfortunately, it is quite common in the medical field to assume that every nurse is female and all physicians are male. Because this is no longer the case, gender-neutral terms are preferred. This means that any reference to a particular gender (male or female) should be eliminated. For example, a male orderly should be referred to as a medical attendant, and cleaning ladies are called housekeepers or cleaning personnel.

Written correspondence must also reflect this same neutral bias toward the genders. When writing, do not refer to physicians as males or to nurses and medical assistants as females. For example, "The patient was referred to a hospital dietitian for diabetic diet instruction. The patient was told to ask her about a food exchange list." This wording as-

sumes the dietitian is a female. A better statement would be "The patient was referred to a hospital dietitian for diabetic diet instruction. The patient was told to ask about a food exchange list." To write in a gender-neutral style, you may have to rewrite the sentence and choose alternate words or phrases.

SENTENCE AND PARAGRAPH LENGTH

Short, concise sentences and paragraphs are preferred in medical writing. Sentence length should never exceed 20 words. Eliminate all unnecessary words. Each paragraph should cover only one point. A good paragraph contains two to six sentences. Your reader may stop reading if the paragraph is too long.

PERSONAL PRONOUN

Whenever possible, it is preferable to avoid the use of the personal pronoun *I* in professional writing. It is better to use *you* or *we* since this involves the reader. For example, a message such as "I am asking that any overdue balance be cleared up immediately. I will have to take steps to send this account to a collection agency if it is not paid immediately" is negative in tone with personal implications. When requesting a patient to pay an overdue bill, it is better to write "We know that you will want to clear up any overdue account. This overdue balance may have been an oversight on your part. If that is the case, kindly remit your payment in the enclosed envelope."

REPETITION, REDUNDANCY, AND INFLATED PHRASES

Readers of your correspondence want to know in concise terms what you are telling them. Avoid being **redundant**—repeating the same word, expression, or statement. Redundant expressions include such phrases as *each and every, first and foremost,* and *physician's patient.* These examples can be simplified by stating *each, first,* or *the patient.*

Inflated phrases can usually be eliminated without any loss of meaning. Common examples are introductory word

TABLE 11-2 Inflated Phrases Compared to Concise Terms

Inflated	Concise
along the lines of	like
as a matter of fact	in fact
at all times	always
at the present time	now, currently
at this point in time	now, currently
because of the fact that	because
by means of	by
by virtue of the fact that	because
due to the fact that	because
for the purpose of	for
for the reason that	because
have the ability to	be able to
in light of the fact that	because
in the nature of	like
in order to	to
in spite of the fact that	although, though
in the event that	if
in the final analysis	finally
in the neighborhood of	about
until such time as	until

TABLE 11-3 Active Compared to Passive Voice

Active	Passive
The medical assistant took the patient's blood pressure measurement	The patient's blood pressure measurement was taken by the medical assistant.
The surgeon performed an appendectomy on the patient.	An appendectomy was performed on the patient by the surgeon.
The medical committee reached a decision.	A decision was reached by the medical committee.

groups such as *in my opinion, I think that, it seems that, one must,* and so on. Table 11-2 contains examples of inflated patterns of writing compared to concise terms.

ACTIVE VERSUS PASSIVE VOICE

Active verbs can make writing more interesting. In the **active voice**, the subject of the sentence performs the action; in the **passive voice**, the subject receives the action. Although both voices are grammatically correct, the active voice is considered more effective because it is simpler, more direct, and less wordy.

To transform a sentence from passive to active voice, make the actor the subject of the sentence. Table 11-3 contains examples of statements in both active and passive voice.

Composing Letters

Composing letters can be a simple process when using an organized approach. Prior to beginning the letter, think about the point(s) you are trying to make. If it is a long letter, you may want to write a bulleted list of the points you wish to cover. This approach ensures that you do not overlook any of the important points. Use the guidelines presented in this chapter. The most important element in writing an organized letter is to quickly make the point.

SPELLING

Several words in the English language have similar pronunciations but very different meanings and spellings. These words are **homophones**. They pose problems unless the writer is careful about their usage. Table 11-4 contains some of the most common homophones.

Computer software programs cannot be depended on to correct all word usage errors because they do not "understand" the data input or content of the correspondence. For

TABLE 11-4 Common Homophones

Word	Meaning	Word	Meaning
accept	to receive	loose	free; not secured
except	to take or leave out	lose	to be deprived of
advice	opinion about what to do for a problem	pair	set of two
advise	to offer advice	pare	to trim
affect	to exert an influence	pear	fruit
effect	result; accomplishment	patience	calm endurance
all ready	prepared	patients	a doctor's clients
already	by this time	personal	private; intimate
altar	a structure on which religious ceremonies are held	personnel	a group of employees
alter	to change	precede	to come before
always	every time; forever	proceed	to go forward
all ways	every way	quiet	silent; calm
bare	naked	quite	very
bear	to carry; to put up with	right	proper or just; correct
brake	something used to stop movement, to stop	rite	a ritual
break	to split or smash	write	to put words on paper
buy	to purchase	stationary	standing still
by	near	stationery	writing paper
choose	to select	taught	past tense of *teach*
chose	past tense of *choose*	taut	tight
cite	to quote	than	besides
sight	vision	then	at that time; next
site	position, place	their	belonging to them
complement	what makes a thing complete; to complete	they're	contraction of *they are*
compliment	an expression of admiration; to praise	there	that place or position
conscience	sense of right and wrong	through	by means of; finished
conscious	awake; aware	threw	past tense of *throw*
elicit	to draw or bring out	thorough	careful; complete
illicit	illegal	to	toward
fair	lovely; light-colored	too	also
fare	money for transportation, food, or drink	two	one or more in number
hear	to sense by the ear	waist	midsection
here	this place	waste	to squander
hole	hollow place	weak	feeble
whole	entire; unhurt	week	seven days
its	of or belonging to it	weather	state of the atmosphere
it's	contraction for *it is*	whether	indicating a choice between alternatives
know	to be aware of	who's	contraction of *who is*
no	opposite of yes	whose	possessive of *who*
lessen	to make less	your	possessive of *you*
lesson	something learned	you're	contraction of *you are*

TABLE 11-5 Commonly Misspelled Medical Terms

abscess	epistaxis	neuron	pneumonia
additive	eustachian	occlusion	polyp
aerosol	fissure	oscilloscope	prophylaxis
agglutination	glaucoma	osseous	prostate
albumin	gonorrhea	palliative	prosthesis
anastomosis	hemorrhage	parasite	pruritis
aneurysm	hemorrhoid	parenteral	psoriasis
anteflexion	homeostasis	parietal	pyrexia
arrhythmia	humerus	paroxysmal	respiratory
bilirubin	idiosyncrasy	pemphigus	roentgenology
bronchial	ileum	percussion	sagittal
calcaneus	ilium	perforation	sciatica
capillary	infarction	pericardium	serous
cervical	intussusception	perineum	sphincter
chromosome	ischemia	peristalsis	sphygmomanometer
cirrhosis	ischium	peritoneum	squamous
clavicle	larynx	petit mal	staphylococcus
curettage	leukemia	pharynx	suppuration
cyanosis	malaise	pituitary	trochanter
defibrillator	malleus	plantar	venous
ecchymosis	mellitus	pleura	wheal
effusion	menstruation	pleurisy	xiphoid
epididymis	metastasis		

example, use of the word *effect* or *affect* depends on the content and cannot be determined by the software program. Both spellings are correct, and only the individual using the word in the sentence can determine which word is the correct choice. Also, medical terms are not, generally, recognized by most spell-check software. Thus, it is always important to have a medical dictionary available when composing documents. See Table 11-5 for examples of the most commonly misspelled medical terms. General rules for capitalization are in Box 11-1.

Box 11-1 Rules for CAPITALIZATION

First word of:

- Sentences
- Expressions used as sentences
- Each item in a list or outline
- Salutation and closing of a letter

Proper name of person, place, or thing:

- John F. Kennedy
- New York City
- Sears Tower

Noun that is part of a proper name:

- Professor Mary King
- Dr. Shania McWalter
- Michigan Avenue

TABLE 11-6 Rules for Forming Plurals of Medical Terms (Nouns)

Ending	Rule	Example
a	ae	vertebra to vertebrae
ax	aces	thorax to thoraces
ex, ix	ices	apex to apices
is	es	metastasis to metastases
on	a	ganglion to ganglia
um	a	ovum to ova
us	i	nucleus to nuclei
y	ies	biopsy to biopsies
nx	ges	phalanx to phalanges

PLURALS

Following are some basic rules for forming plurals of words:

- Abbreviations are formed into plurals by adding an *s* (ECGs, DRGs).
- Plurals of nouns are formed by adding an *s* or an *es* (physicians, suffixes).

Basic rules for forming plurals of medical terms with specific endings are listed in Table 11-6 along with examples for each. More information relating to spelling and grammatical rules of medical terminology can be found in Chapter 4.

NUMBERS

In general, the numbers 1 to 10 are spelled out—one to ten—in correspondence. For numbers greater than ten, it is acceptable to use the number designation, as in 32, 128, and 1,020. The only exception to this rule is when the number is at the beginning of a sentence. It should then be spelled out. See Table 11-7 for a further description of the use of numbers in correspondence.

PARTS OF SPEECH

Traditional grammar recognizes eight parts of speech: noun, pronoun, verb, adjective, adverb, preposition, conjunction, and interjection. Many words function as more than one part of speech. For example, depending on its use in a sentence, the word *cut* can be a noun, as in "The *cut* is fresh," or a verb, as in "The surgeon *cut* into the organ." Table 11-8 provides a quick reference to parts of speech.

TABLE 11-7 Use of Numbers in Correspondence

Type	Explanation of When to Use
Decimals	Write using figure without commas (23.04).
Figures	Only numbers (including 1–10) are used in tables, statistical data, dates, money, percentages, and time.
Measurements	Write out in figures (23 inches).
Percentages	Write out in figures and spell out percent (20 percent).
Tables	When typing numbers or placing them in columns align as follows: • Arabic numerals (1, 2, 3) are aligned on the right. • Decimals (1.33) are aligned on the decimal. • Roman numerals (I, II, III) are aligned on the left.
Time	Do not use zeros when writing on-the-hour time. Use A.M. and P.M. with the time designation (10 A.M., not 10:00 A.M.).

TABLE 11-8 Eight Parts of Speech

Part of Speech	Definition
Noun	Names a person, place, or thing. *Examples:* medical assistant, office
Pronoun	Substitutes for a noun. *Examples:* I, me, you, he, him, she, her, it, we, us, they, them
Verb	Helping verb: comes before main verb. Main verb: asserts action, being, or state of being. *Examples:* operate, write, speak, obtain, is, are, am
Adjective	Modifies a noun or pronoun, usually answering the questions "Which one?" "What kind?" "How many?" *Example:* responsible medical assistant
Adverb	Modifies a verb, adjective, or adverb usually answering the questions "When?" "Where?" "Why?" "How?" "Under what conditions?" "To what degree?" *Examples:* gently, extremely, nicely, quietly
Preposition	Indicates the relationship between the noun and pronoun that follows it and another word in the sentence. *Examples:* about, above, after, for, in, on, over, through
Conjunction	Connects words or word groups. *Examples:* and, but, nor, or
Interjection	Word used to express strong feeling. *Examples:* oh, hooray, hurrah, ouch

ERROR CORRECTION IN OFFICE CORRECTION

Word processing has made correspondence correction much easier. Word processing allows the writer to display the document on the computer screen, enter the information, and make any necessary changes. This new document is then saved and printed or e-mailed.

Corrections made to letters typed on a typewriter require the use of correction ribbons, tapes, or fluids. Any corrections on correspondence should be inconspicuous. If more than a few words need correction, then the entire document should be retyped. It is considered unprofessional for a document to have correction fluid apparent on the document.

STANDARD COMPONENTS OF THE BUSINESS LETTER

All business letters contain the same basic components. These include the heading, date, inside address, salutation, body, closing, and reference initials. In some specialized cases, such as insurance correspondence, special components may be added for clarification, such as the insurer's identification number.

Heading

Medical office letters are usually typed on **letterhead**, which is stationery bearing the name of the physician (Shania McWalter, D.O.) or practice (Pearson Physicians Group), address, telephone number, and fax number. See Figure 11-1 for an illustration of letterhead. If the physician does not use letterhead, the letter should be typed or printed on good-quality bond paper with the return address typed above the date on the upper left side of the paper.

Date

Every correspondence must have a current date. The month must not be abbreviated and must be followed by the day and year (January 1, 2010). The date is usually placed three lines (spaces) below the letterhead or on line 15 if there is no letterhead. Four to six lines (spaces) are left after the date before the inside address.

Inside Address

The inside address contains the name, title, company name (if applicable), and address of the person who is to receive the correspondence. This is typed at the left margin and is single-spaced. If a company name is present (for example, Pearson Physicians Group, Pearson Clinic, or Pearson General Hospital), it must be typed exactly as shown on the company's own letterhead.

All words in the inside address (such as the street name) are spelled out fully. The name of the city is followed by a comma; the two-letter state abbreviation is followed by two spaces; then the ZIP code is added. If the inside address contains a long line, it may be divided into two lines so that the inside address is in balance. The second of these two lines would be indented two spaces. See the following example:

Marvin Hammer, MD
123 Bonneymeadow
   Plaza in the Park
Chicago, IL 60610

Business courtesy recommends always including a title with the receiver's name on the inside address.

Salutation

The **salutation**, a courteous greeting, is typed at the left margin and spaced two lines below the inside address. The name in the salutation must agree with the name in the inside address. If the letter is going to a physician named McWalter, the salutation would read "Dear Dr. McWalter" with a colon placed after the salutation ("Dear Dr. McWalter:"). If the person is well known to the writer, the first name is often used (e.g., "Dear Shania" followed by a comma, "Dear Shania,"). Guidelines 11-1 provides information on using courtesy titles in correspondence.

FIGURE 11-1 Different letterhead stationery and envelopes.

Body

The body contains the purpose of the letter. The body begins two spaces below the salutation and is single spaced, with a double space between each paragraph. The paragraphs of the body are either blocked or indented, depending on the style (format) of the letter. A letter may be any length; however, most letters bearing a single message are usually two to three paragraphs in length and confined to a single page.

Closing

The closing consists of a **complimentary close** containing a courtesy word(s), such as "Sincerely," "Sincerely yours," or "Yours truly." This appears two spaces below the end of the body of the letter.

The **signature line** is typed four spaces below the complimentary close and contains the name and title of the writer. If the name and title are on the same line, they are divided with a comma. The personal title of the writer (such as Mr. and Ms.) is not included in the signature line. The exception to this is when the writer may wish to indicate his or her gender to prevent the reader from being confused (for example, Ms. Leslie Lapointe or Mr. Pat Timmons). The handwritten signature of the writer must be placed directly above the typed signature line before the letter is sent.

Reference Initials

The medical professional uses **reference initials** to indicate who keyed the letter. Reference initials, when used, are placed at the lower left margin in lowercase. For example, if Brandy F. Forthing keyed a letter she would include the reference initials *bff*.

Enclosure Notation

When other documents are included along with the letter, a notation is made on the letter indicating the **enclosure**. Examples of enclosures are X-ray films, medical records, and brochures. The abbreviation *ENC.* is used or the word *Enclosure* can be spelled out.

For example:

> Enclosures (2)
> X-ray lumbar spine
> surgical report 12/10/20xx

Copy Notation

A copy of all correspondence is always filed in the office. In some cases, a copy of the letter is sent to someone other than the addressee. This is noted at the bottom left of the letter by typing the initial "c:" before the recipient's name. The title of the recipient is often added.

For example:

> c: Jane Paulson, Office Manager

Procedure 11-1 lists important guidelines for composing business letters.

TWO-PAGE LETTER

When the letter is too long to fit on one page, a second sheet of plain stationery is used. Letterhead stationery is used only for the top sheet. The plain-bond second sheet should be of the same quality and color as the letterhead stationery. A margin of 1 inch is left at the bottom of the first page. The second page and any pages following must begin with the date and subject line of the letter.

FORM LETTERS

Form letters can save time for the medical assistant. A form letter is developed when the same letter is sent once or

COMPOSING A BUSINESS LETTER

Objective: Compose a business letter using proper guidelines.

EQUIPMENT AND SUPPLIES

computer or typewriter; office stationery

METHOD

1. Gather all necessary information and supplies.
2. Determine the reason for the correspondence. Write down the main purpose of the letter.
3. Make a list of all the points you will cover in the letter. Prepare a rough draft.
4. Arrange the ideas in a logical manner. Make sure the letter has a beginning, middle, and end:
   - The beginning or introduction should be appropriate for the intended reader. Use appropriate greetings and titles.
   - The middle should contain all the supporting facts and details. Make sure the content relates to the purpose of the letter.
   - The end should be brief and pleasant and indicate any action that is to be taken by the reader or writer.
5. Use a natural style of writing. Avoid showy language, and avoid medical terms when writing to the layperson. Also avoid inflated phrases (refer to Table 11-2).
6. Use a positive tone. Negative writing should always be avoided.
7. Pay particular attention to spelling, punctuation, and grammar.
8. Once the rough draft is satisfactory, compose the final draft of the letter. Proofread for mistakes.
9. Obtain any necessary signatures. Include any enclosures as indicated.

CHARTING EXAMPLE

12/4/XX. Letter written and mailed to patient, Mrs. Ford, requesting that she contact the office to arrange payment for her outstanding balance. Return receipt requested. Copy of letter placed in chart. · B. Castle, CMAS

---

repeatedly to multiple recipients. Figure 11-2 contains an example of a form letter that can be used as a base when constructing a letter of withdrawal. Each letter would be personalized with the patient's name and the signature of the physician.

The use of a computer or a word processor with memory individualizes the form letter. The body of the letter, the **constant information**, is retained in the computer's memory or on a computer disk or CD. The areas of the letter that require personalization, such as the date, inside address, and salutation, are called the **variables**. The variables can be stored on a separate CD or database and then merged into the disk or main drive of the computer, which stores the constant information. In this manner, a set of data, such as names and addresses of patients for billing purposes, can be used with a form letter enclosed with the monthly bill. Chapter 12 contains more information regarding the use of computers in the medical office.

PEARSON PHYSICIANS GROUP
Shania McWalter, D.O.
123 Michigan Avenue
Parker Heights, IL 60610
(312) 123-1234

Date

Dear (Patient):

I find it necessary to inform you that I am withdrawing from providing you medical care for the following reason(s): _____

_____

_____

Since your condition requires medical attention, I suggest that you place yourself under the care of another physician. If you do not know of other physicians, you may wish to contact the county medical society for a referral.

I shall be available to attend to you for a reasonable time after you have received this letter, but in no event for more than 15 days.

When you have selected a new physician, I would be pleased to make available to him or her a copy of your medical chart or a summary of your treatment.

Sincerely yours,

Shania McWalter, D.O.

FIGURE 11-2 A form letter is used when the same letter is sent once or repeatedly to multiple recipients.

Letter Styles

Letter styles vary depending on the purpose. Letter styles include block, modified block (standard), modified block with indented paragraphs, and simplified. Block and modified block are used most often in the medical office.

The **block** letter style is spaced with all lines, from the date through the signature line, flush with the left margin. A space separates each paragraph as well as the inside address, salutation, body, and close. Since there are no indentations for paragraphs, this format saves typing time.

In the **modified block** (standard) style letter has the date, complimentary closing, and signature line begin at the center and continue toward the right margin. All other lines are flush with the left margin. This style is often preferred since it has a professional, neat appearance. It requires more time to type since the typist must set and use tabs. The modified block style with indented paragraphs is identical to the modified block except that the paragraphs are consistently indented a designated amount.

All lines in a simplified letter style are flush with the left margin. The salutation line is omitted. In its place is a subject line, which appears on the third line below the inside address. This subject line is in capital letters and draws the reader's attention to the purpose of the letter. A complimentary closing is also omitted. The signature is also typed in all capital letters on the fifth line below the body. This format is an abbreviated style of writing letters relating to patients. Figure 11-3 shows sample letter formats: block, modified block (standard), modified block with indented paragraphs, and simplified.

A semi-simplified letter style is spaced with all lines flush with the left margin except for the first line of each paragraph. The first line of each paragraph is indented. All other aspects of the simplified letter style apply to this format.

Interoffice Memoranda

Interoffice memoranda, also called **memos**, are written communications sent to people within the office or organization. They are used to inform personnel about meetings, general changes that affect all employees, special projects, or news items. The memo is an inexpensive means to communicate with others in the office setting. Memos do not require postage and are delivered through the interoffice mail route.

Memos are generally written on a short form developed for that purpose. They may contain a heading much like

letterhead stationery to indicate the office where they originated. They contain the word *Memorandum* at the top of the form. Also included are the typed words *DATE:*, *TO:*, *FROM:*, and *RE:* or *SUBJECT:*. The memo form is meant to be used within the office setting and should never be used to send information outside of the office. Figure 11-4 illustrates an example of a memo form.

Proofreading

Proofreading, or checking for errors in content and typing, is a critical activity. The professionalism of the office is judged, in part, by the appearance of correspondence and documents that come from that office. Proofreading cannot be overemphasized. Even small omissions, such as commas, are noticed by readers. Most computer programs contain spell-check and grammar-check components. These should always be used before printing the document. You may have to add frequently used medical terms to the program. After printing out any document, a careful reading should be done to catch any content or typing

PEARSON PHYSICIANS GROUP
Shania McWalter, D.O.
123 Michigan Avenue, Parker Heights, IL 60610
(312) 123-1234

August 1, 20xx

Thomas Moore
123 Lee Street
Louisville, KY 40223

Dear Mr. Moore:

With the season for colds and flu fast approaching, it is time once again for flu shots. Supplies have arrived and flu shots will be administered starting October 3. Please call the office to schedule a visit for your flu shot at your earliest convenience.

If you wish to wait to get your flu shot at the time of your next appointment, it is not necessary to call the office. An appointment card with the date and time of your next appointment is enclosed.

Sincerely,

Shania McWalter, D.O.

ENC: Appointment card
c: B. Reed, Office Manager

(A)

PEARSON PHYSICIANS GROUP
Shania McWalter, D.O.
123 Michigan Avenue, Parker Heights, IL 60610
(312) 123-1234

August 1, 20xx

Thomas Moore
123 Lee Street
Louisville, KY 40223

Dear Mr. Moore:

With the season for colds and flu fast approaching, it is time again for flu shots. Supplies have arrived and flu shots will be administered starting October 3. Please call the office to schedule a visit for your flu shot at your earliest convenience.

If you wish to wait to get your flu shot at the time of your next appointment, it is not necessary to call the office. An appointment card with the date and time of your next appointment is enclosed.

Sincerely,

Shania McWalter, D.O.

ENC: Appointment card
c: B. Reed, Office Manager

(B)

PEARSON PHYSICIANS GROUP
Shania McWalter, D.O.
123 Michigan Avenue, Parker Heights, IL 60610
(312) 123-1234

August 1, 20xx

Thomas Moore
123 Lee Street
Louisville, KY 40223

Dear Mr. Moore:

With the season for colds and flu fast approaching, it is time once again for flu shots. Supplies have arrived and flu shots will be administered starting October 3. Please call the office to schedule a visit for your flu shot at your earliest convenience.

If you wish to wait to get your flu shot at the time of your next appointment, it is not necessary to call the office. An appointment card with the date and time of your next appointment is enclosed.

Sincerely,

Shania McWalter, D.O.

ENC: Appointment card
c: B. Reed, Office Manager

(C)

PEARSON PHYSICIANS GROUP
Shania McWalter, D.O.
123 Michigan Avenue, Parker Heights, IL 60610
(312) 123-1234

August 1, 20xx

Thomas Moore
123 Lee Street
Louisville, KY 40223

RE: FLU SHOT

With the season for colds and flu fast approaching, it is time once again for flu shots. Supplies have arrived and flu shots will be administered starting October 3. Please call the office to schedule a visit for your flu shot at your earliest convenience.

If you wish to wait to get your flu shot at the time of your next appointment, it is not necessary to call the office. An appointment card with the date and time of your next appointment is enclosed.

Shania McWalter, D.O.

ENC: Appointment card
c: B. Reed, Office Manager

(D)

FIGURE 11-3 Examples of four letter formats: (A) block style; (B) modified block style; (C) modified block style with indented paragraphs; and (D) simplified letter style.

```
┌─────────────────────────────────────┐
│        PEARSON GENERAL HOSPITAL      │
│             MEMORANDUM               │
│  DATE:                               │
│    TO:                               │
│  FROM:                               │
│  SUBJECT:                            │
│                                      │
│  c:                                  │
└─────────────────────────────────────┘
```

FIGURE 11-4 An example of a memo form.

errors. Pay close attention to the spelling of names and procedures. When typing figures always double-check to make sure all decimal points are placed in the correct position. Look for sound-alike terms, such as *right* and *write* or *anti-* and *ante-*. Important points to remember when proofreading letters and other documents are listed in Procedure 11-2.

PROOFREADER'S MARKS

Specific marks are generally accepted for use when proofreading long documents. These are especially helpful when a second person is proofing the document, such as the physician. See Figure 11-5 for a list of proofreader's marks.

Editing

Editing is similar to proofreading in that you must read the final material to check for accuracy. Editing also involves reading the printed material to determine if it is clear. When editing medical reports, you cannot change the content of the report or alter the meaning in any way. If you believe the meaning is unclear, you must check with the writer of the report before making any content (editorial) changes.

When editing material you have composed, such as an informational form letter to be sent to all patients, changes can be made to increase clarity.

Abbreviations

Only accepted medical abbreviations can be used in medical reports and when filing insurance documents. The Joint Commission has released a list of unapproved abbreviations, and it is important that the abbreviations on that list are not used anywhere, including medical charts, reports and insurance documents. The Joint Commission's list was developed as a result of errors occurring because of abbreviations that

procedure
11-2

PROOFREADING WRITTEN DOCUMENTS
Objective: To draft grammatically correct correspondence with no spelling errors.

EQUIPMENT AND SUPPLIES
ruler; pencil; piece of paper; computer

1. Draft bulleted list of points to be made within the document.
2. Check the list to see if it flows in a logical order.
3. Key the document using proper grammar and correct spelling.
4. Review the document to ensure all points are covered.
5. Run the computer program spelling and grammar checks and consider the suggestions made.
6. Use a ruler, pencil, or edge of a piece of paper to follow each line as you proofread.
7. Check for missing and repeated words.
8. Verify the spelling of proper names and titles.
9. Check where the word breaks occur.
10. Verify numbers in dates, figures, and time (hours of the day).
11. Read the opening and closing carefully.
12. Proofread at least twice. If still unsure, ask a coworker to review the document.
13. Check the general appearance of the letter for spacing and format.
14. Print the document.

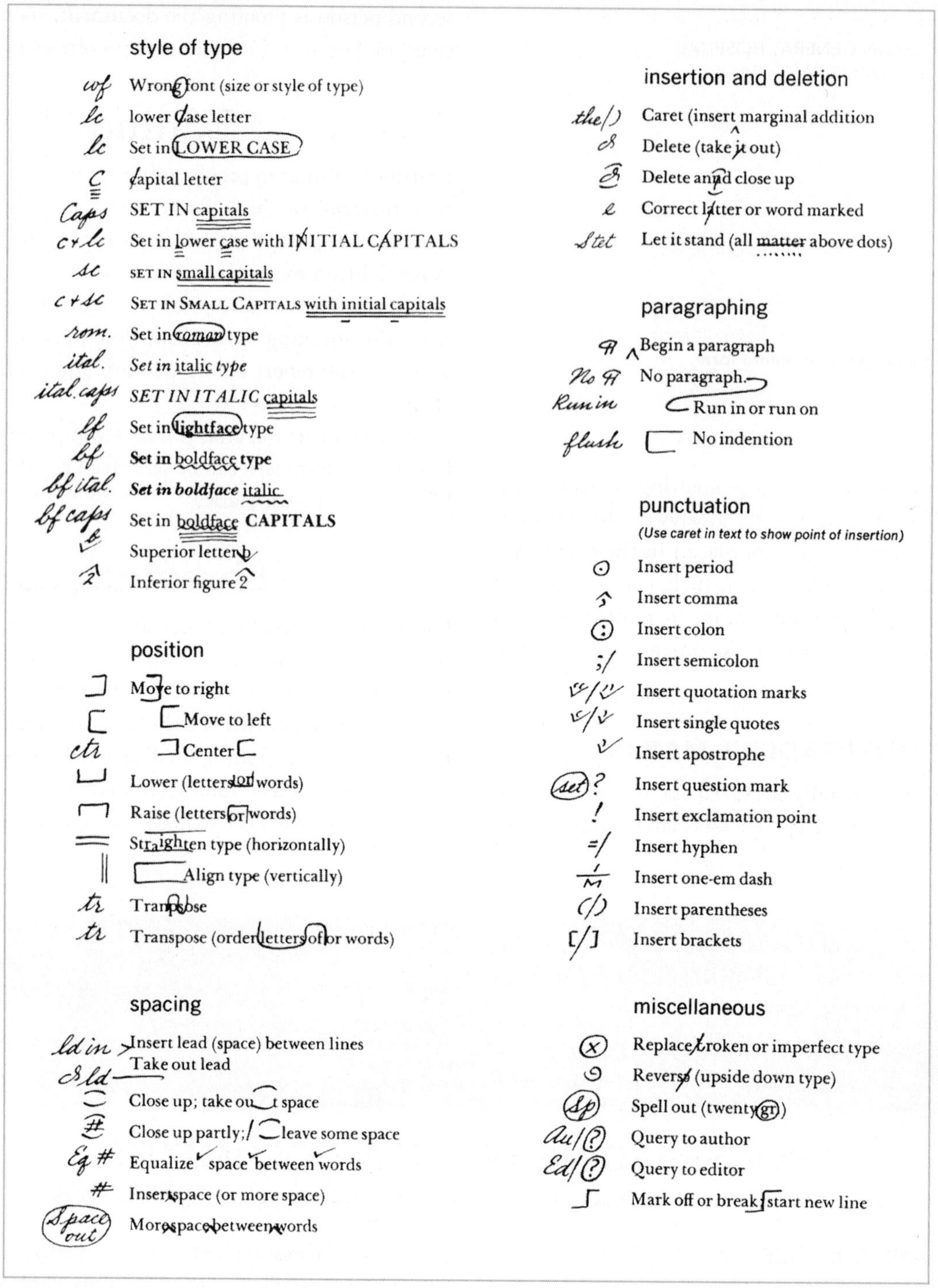

FIGURE 11-5 Proofreader's marks.

style of type

wf	Wrong font (size or style of type)
lc	lower case letter
lc	Set in LOWER CASE
C	capital letter
Caps	SET IN capitals
c + lc	Set in lower case with INITIAL CAPITALS
sc	SET IN small capitals
c + sc	SET IN SMALL CAPITALS with initial capitals
rom.	Set in roman type
ital.	Set in italic type
ital. caps	SET IN ITALIC capitals
lf	Set in lightface type
bf	Set in boldface type
bf ital.	Set in boldface italic
bf caps	Set in boldface CAPITALS
	Superior letter
	Inferior figure 2

position

]	Move to right
[	Move to left
ctr	Center
⊔	Lower (letters or words)
⊓	Raise (letters or words)
=	Straighten type (horizontally)
‖	Align type (vertically)
tr	Transpose
tr	Transpose (order letters of or words)

spacing

ld in	Insert lead (space) between lines
ld	Take out lead
⌣	Close up; take out space
#	Close up partly; leave some space
Eq #	Equalize space between words
#	Insert space (or more space)
Space out	More space between words

insertion and deletion

the/	Caret (insert marginal addition
♂	Delete (take it out)
♂	Delete and close up
e	Correct letter or word marked
Stet	Let it stand (all matter above dots)

paragraphing

¶	Begin a paragraph
No ¶	No paragraph.
Run in	Run in or run on
flush	No indention

punctuation

(Use caret in text to show point of insertion)

⊙	Insert period
⌃	Insert comma
⊙	Insert colon
;/	Insert semicolon
⸣/⸤	Insert quotation marks
⸣/⸤	Insert single quotes
⸌	Insert apostrophe
(set)?	Insert question mark
!	Insert exclamation point
=/	Insert hyphen
—/M	Insert one-em dash
(/)	Insert parentheses
[/]	Insert brackets

miscellaneous

⊗	Replace broken or imperfect type
⊙	Reverse (upside down type)
sp	Spell out (twenty gr)
Au/?	Query to author
Ed/?	Query to editor
	Mark off or break start new line

were too similar to other abbreviations. For instance, *qd* and *qod* are on The Joint Commission's "Official 'Do Not Use' List" because the two abbreviations look very similar yet have different meanings: *qd* indicates "every day," and *qod* indicates "every other day." A list of accepted medical abbreviations is included in Appendix IV.

Individual physician offices may use an abbreviation on progress notes that is related to that practice. For example, on progress notes a urologist may write "L," meaning leaking urine when coughing. Although this is not an acceptable abbreviation, it can be used to conserve space and simplify documentation within that particular office. So that all

TABLE 11-9 Stationery and Envelopes

Stationery	Dimensions	Envelope	Dimensions
Standard	8½" × 11"	No. 10	9½" × 4⅛"
Monarch	7¼" × 10½"	No. 7	7½" × 3⅞"
Baronial	5½" × 8½"	No. 6¾	6½" × 3⅝"

employees know the meaning of each abbreviation—and use all abbreviations correctly and consistently—each employee should have access to a list of abbreviations, and the list should be posted conveniently in the office.

Reference Materials

Every physician's office contains general reference books and medical dictionaries as well as textbooks related to the physician's specialization. A complete office library should include the following:

- A desk dictionary, and access to an online dictionary
- A medical dictionary, as well as access to an online medical dictionary, to assist with the correct spelling, pronunciation, acronyms, abbreviations, and meaning of medical terms and diagnoses
- A *Physician's Desk Reference (PDR)* to verify the correct spelling and use of drugs
- Current coding books, including CPT-4 (Current Procedural Terminology) and ICD-9-CM (International Classification of Diseases).
- A **thesaurus** (which provides synonyms or similar meanings for words), such as *Roget's International Thesaurus,* and access to an online thesaurus

Preparing Outgoing Mail

Letterhead stationery, which contains the name and address of the sender, comes in three commonly used sizes. These sizes are standard, monarch or executive, and baronial. The more common letter sizes with their matching envelope sizes are shown in Table 11-9.

Standard letterhead is used for most office correspondence. A smaller version of standard letterhead—monarch or executive style—is used by some physicians for their social correspondence. The baronial letterhead is half the size of a standard sheet and is used for brief letters and memoranda. Envelopes are sized to match different letter sizes. See Figure 11-6 for an illustration of different letter sizes.

FOLDING LETTERS AND INSERTING INTO ENVELOPES

Following are recommended methods for folding and inserting letters into envelopes so the contents can remain confidential and be easily removed. See Figure 11-7 for an illustration of folding a letter.

FIGURE 11-6 Letterhead stationery sizes are varied to suit the needs of the sender. Envelopes are sized to match different letter sizes.

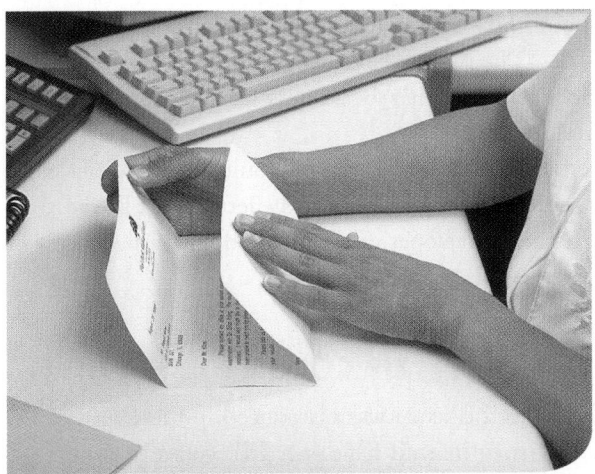

FIGURE 11-7 A well-folded letter fits easily into the envelope and is easily removed by the person who receives it.

Number 10 (Standard Business) Envelope

1. Bring up the bottom third of the letter and fold with a crease.

2. Fold the top of the letter down to ⅜ inch from the first creased edge.

3. Make a second crease at the fold, and place this edge into the envelope first.

Number 6¾ Envelope

1. Bring the bottom edge up to ⅜ inch from the top edge.

2. Make a crease at the fold.

3. Fold the right edge one-third of the width of the paper, and press a crease at this fold.

4. Fold the left edge to ⅜ inch from the previous crease, and insert this edge into the envelope first.

ENVELOPE FORMATS

The U.S. Postal Service (USPS) has recommended guidelines for addressing envelopes. This is meant to improve the handling and delivery of the mail. **Optical character recognition (OCR)** equipment used by the USPS scans, reads, and sorts envelopes. For optimal efficiency of OCR scanning, addresses must be typed, using single spacing and all capital letters with no punctuation. A more traditional style of typing envelopes with the initial letter of each word capitalized and remaining letters in each word lowercased is still accepted by the USPS.

The last line in the address must include the city, two-digit state abbreviation, and ZIP code. It cannot exceed 27 characters in length. See Figure 11-8 for a list of the two-digit state abbreviations.

The bottom margin of the No. 10 envelope (business size) should be ⅝ inch with 1-inch margins on the left and right sides. The No. 6¾ envelope should have a 2-inch margin on the left side with the address 12 lines from the top of the envelope.

A return address for the sender should always be placed in the upper left corner in the event the letter must be returned to the sender. Envelopes can be printed with the address of the sender in this position.

ZIP CODES

The five-digit ZIP code was introduced in the 1960s to increase efficiency in mail handling. ZIP codes begin on the East Coast with the number 0, eventually increasing to the number 9 on the West Coast and in Hawaii. The first three

TWO-LETTER ABBREVIATIONS

UNITED STATES and TERRITORIES

Alabama	AL	Montana	MT
Alaska	AK	Nebraska	NE
Arizona	AZ	Nevada	NV
Arkansas	AR	New Hampshire	NH
California	CA	New Jersey	NJ
Canal Zone	CZ	New Mexico	NM
Colorado	CO	New York	NY
Connecticut	CT	North Carolina	NC
Delaware	DE	North Dakota	ND
District of Columbia	DC	Ohio	OH
Florida	FL	Oklahoma	OK
Georgia	GA	Oregon	OR
Guam	GU	Pennsylvania	PA
Hawaii	HI	Puerto Rico	PR
Idaho	ID	Rhode Island	RI
Illinois	IL	South Carolina	SC
Indiana	IN	South Dakota	SD
Iowa	IA	Tennessee	TN
Kansas	KS	Texas	TX
Kentucky	KY	Utah	UT
Louisiana	LA	Vermont	VT
Maine	ME	Virgin Islands	VI
Maryland	MD	Virginia	VA
Massachusetts	MA	Washington	WA
Michigan	MI	West Virginia	WV
Minnesota	MN	Wisconsin	WI
Mississippi	MS	Wyoming	WY
Missouri	MO		

FIGURE 11-8 Every state has a two-digit letter abbreviation.

numbers of the ZIP code identify the city, and all five digits combine to identify the individual post office and zone within the city. Four more digits have been added to the ZIP code by the USPS. These four digits follow a hyphen placed after the first five digits and represent the addressee's street location. The 9-digit ZIP code has eliminated many handling steps at USPS collection and distribution centers and has improved service.

Classifications of Mail

The classifications of mail vary according to weight, type, and destination. Mail is weighed in ounces and pounds. The most common types of mail include first class, priority, second class, third class, fourth class, and express. Table 11-10 describes these classifications of mail.

SPECIAL POSTAL SERVICES

Specialized services include certified mail, certificate of mailing, special delivery, special handling, registered mail, insurance, postal money orders, forwarding of mail, mail recall, tracing lost mail, and returned mail.

TABLE 11-10 Classifications of Mail

Type	Description
First Class	Letters, postcards, business reply cards; letters weighing less than 11 ounces; sealed and unsealed, handwritten or typed material
Priority	First-class mail weighing more than 11 ounces; maximum weight of 70 pounds; postage calculated based on weight and destination
Second Class	Newspapers and periodicals that have received second-class mail authorization; not allowed for newspapers and periodicals mailed by the general public
Third Class	Catalogs, booklets, photographs, flyers, and other printed materials; must be marked "Third Class"; must be sealed; no size limitation; includes bulk mail
Fourth Class	Books, computer media, and merchandise not included in first and second class; must weigh between 16 ounces and 70 pounds; size limitations apply
Express Mail/ Next Day Service	Available 7 days a week; up to 70 pounds in weight and 108 inches around; expected delivery by noon; shipping containers are supplied; pickup service in some areas

Certified Mail

Mail that includes contracts, mortgages, birth certificates, deeds and checks, which are not valuable themselves but would be difficult to replace if lost, can be mailed as certified mail (Figure 11-9). Such items would need to be mailed at the first-class rate with a special fee added for certified mail. Certified mail assists in tracking and collecting this mail. A receipt verifying delivery can be requested for a fee. Certified mail can also be sent by special delivery if the extra fee is paid. Certified mail records are maintained at post office locations for 2 years.

If it is necessary to dismiss a patient from the practice, the patient must receive the notification in writing. Certified mail with a Return Receipt requested is used when documentation is needed that the patient did indeed receive the letter.

Certificate of Mailing

For a small fee, a Certificate of Mailing can be obtained at the post office. This document serves as proof that mail was posted. This is useful for mailing items such as tax returns, which need to be received by a certain date.

Special Delivery

When fast delivery of an item is needed, special delivery service can be requested from the USPS. Special delivery is useful for shipping perishables, such as specimens, since delivery of these items will be made after regular delivery service hours (for example, on Sundays and holidays). A fee is charged for this service.

Special Handling

Special handling can be requested for third- and fourth-class items. "Special Handling" is stamped across the package. The fee for this service is based on the weight of the item.

Registered Mail

Registered mail is the safest way to send first-class or priority mail. A fee is paid for this service, and a signed record is kept for each piece of registered mail. Registered mail is tracked as it moves throughout the mail system, which helps to reduce loss. Registered mail is insured for the value declared at the time of registration. For an additional fee, the sender can request a Return Receipt indicating the time, the place of delivery, and the receiver's signature.

Insurance

Insurance can be purchased for third-class, fourth-class, and priority mail. The sender will then be reimbursed for the content if this mail is lost or damaged. The sender receives a receipt at the time of purchasing the insurance. This receipt, along with the damaged goods, must be presented when reimbursement is necessary.

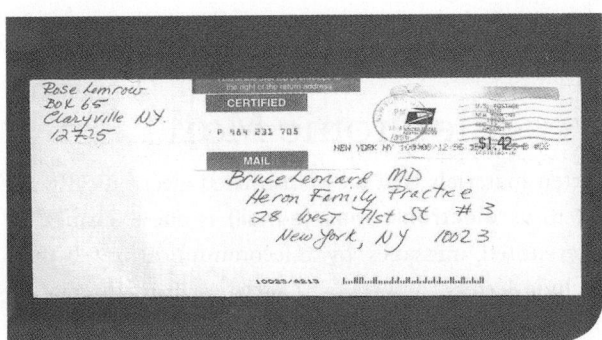

FIGURE 11-9 Items that would be difficult to replace bearing legal significance are sent by certified mail.

Postal Money Orders

A postal money order can be purchased at any post office. The money order can be mailed instead of actual cash and is replaceable if lost or stolen. It is available in several denominations. The fee varies according to the amount of the money order.

Forwarding Mail

First class is the only type of mail that can be forwarded to another address at no charge. To forward a piece of first-class mail, cross out the incorrect address, insert the new address, and return the item to the mail carrier or a post office. The post office will forward mail for up to 6 months.

Mail Recall

If mail has been placed in a mailbox or given to a postal carrier by mistake, it can be recalled by the sender. The sender can call the post office and request that the item be held for pickup. When the sender goes to the post office to reclaim the mail, he or she will be asked to complete a "Sender's Application for Recall of Mail." If the mail is still at the post office, it will be returned to the sender on completion of this form. If the mail has already left the post office, the postal clerk will call the post office where that mail has been sent and ask that the mail be returned. The sender must pay all the expenses incurred in an attempt to recall the mail, including any telephone calls placed by the postal service. If the mail has already been delivered to the addressee, the sender will be notified.

Tracing Lost Mail

All receipts for mailed goods should be retained until receipt of the mail has been acknowledged. If the mail has not arrived after a reasonable period of time, the post office will attempt to trace it upon request. First-class mail is not easy to trace since no receipt for it exists. A special form must be completed before the USPS will attempt to trace mail.

Returned Mail

When mail has been returned and marked "Undeliverable," it cannot be remailed until new postage is added. It is advisable to place the contents into a new envelope with the correct address, place the proper postage according to weight on the envelope, and remail it.

Size Requirements for Mail

The USPS standardizes envelope sizes for machine-sort mail. Minimum mail sizes have been established. Domestic mail must be at least 0.0007 inch thick. A further restriction on size requires that mail ¼ inch or less in thickness must be 3½ inches in height and at least 5 inches long. All mail not meeting this requirement is considered nonstandard.

Although postage is generally based on a package's weight, items that are bulky and lightweight are charged a 15-pound balloon rate surcharge. This balloon rate is applied to all Priority Mail and Parcel Post items that weigh less than 15 pounds and measure over 84 inches—but not more than 108 inches—in length and girth combined. Following are some general guidelines for preparing mail to be metered:

- Separate all international mail from domestic mail. Separate all mail to Canada or Mexico from other international mail.

- Face all letter-size envelopes in the same direction. Make sure none are upside down. When mailing letter-size envelopes, flaps must be sealed or tucked in.

- Try not to overstuff letter-size envelopes. If this is not possible, seal the envelopes with tape.

- All envelopes larger than a No. 10 must be sealed before being sent.

- Keep the top right corner of each mailing piece clear of all markings. This is where the postmark will appear.

The medical assistant should always consult the USPS for specific mailing, size, weight, and pricing requirements to ensure the outgoing mail is properly prepared. This may include either a visit to the nearest post office or browsing the USPS website.

Mail Handling Tips

To facilitate time management within the medical office, all mail should be handled only once. For ease and efficiency in handling large amounts of mail, follow the steps in Procedure 11-3.

Electronic Mail

All written materials that are transmitted electronically are referred to as **electronic mail (e-mail)** is the exchange of computer-stored messages by telecommunication. E-mail may include letters, reports, and pictures. E-mails may be sent over telephone lines, cables, computers, and satellites. E-mail allows the medical assistant to edit, correct, and transmit documents very quickly to another location. E-mail

OPENING AND SORTING THE DAILY MAIL

Objective: Sort and distribute the medical office's daily mail.

EQUIPMENT AND SUPPLIES

office stamps (one with date and one with the name of the medical office); ink pad; paper clips; pencil

METHOD

1. Have all supplies in one place when processing the mail.
2. Sort the mail before opening into first-class, personal or confidential, second-, third- and fourth class categories.
3. Discard and recycle all unwanted third-class mail.
4. Place a current date and time of arrival on each piece of mail. Purchase a rubber stamp and pad from an office supply store so that the date can be changed each day.
5. Stamp the name of the medical office across all periodicals and newspapers.
6. Lay all of the envelope flaps down to reduce the motions involved in opening a large amount of mail.
7. Do not open mail marked "Personal" or "Confidential." Place it unopened in the physician's inbox unless otherwise instructed.
8. Attach all enclosures in each envelope with a paper clip. Do not staple anything since staples would have to be removed later and could damage sensitive materials, such as X-rays. If an enclosure is noted in the correspondence but is not in the envelope, next to mention of the enclosure write "No" with your initials to indicate it was not included. Clip the opened envelope to the mail until the mail is completely processed. In some cases, a return address is only on the envelope and not on the inside correspondence.
9. Open all the mail, and clip together the inside contents before handling each piece of correspondence.
10. Annotate the mail as soon as possible after it is opened. An annotation consists of writing a short comment in pencil to indicate the purpose of the letter and underlining the critical portions of the letter. If another document is referred to in the letter, then take initiative by pulling it from the file and attaching it to this correspondence.
11. Route the mail immediately after opening it. Another department or physician may be waiting for the document.

---

cannot be used if the original signature on the document needs to be sent. When creating e-mail, remember that it is considered part of the patient's record and part of office management; therefore, all standard proofreading and confidentiality guidelines apply.

Like other correspondence, e-mail can take the form of a composed letter, form letter, or interoffice memorandum. Some offices use e-mail to confirm office visits. Every office has a particular format to utilize for this purpose.

Another form of e-mail is the instant message. Instant messages are a way to communicate via computer with another person in real time. The content of an instant message appears on the recipient's computer screen immediately after it is sent. Some offices allow users to instant message each other both internally (within the office) or externally. The internal instant message format is usually connected to the office computer server and allows messages to be sent quickly from person to person. External instant messages

PROFESSIONALISM
THE WORKPLACE

E-mail has become one of the most commonly used forms of written communication within the office. Most likely, you will find yourself receiving as well as composing e-mails to and from coworkers, patients, and other business associates. It is common courtesy to respond to any incoming e-mails as soon as possible. Set aside time each day to respond to your incoming e-mail. If it appears that you may not be able to respond within the same day, let the sender know you have received the e-mail and will respond either on a given day or when the information requested is available.

are generally linked to an account that is purchased from an Internet service provider. In such accounts, you would establish your own screen name and password so you can access and communicate with external users with instant messages.

It is important to remember that instant messages are not permanent documents and cannot be attached to a person's medical records or used in a court of law. You may be accustomed to abbreviating words when instant messaging at home; however, this is not acceptable for electronic messages sent from an office. The tone of the message should remain as professional as if you were keying in a letter to be sent through the USPS.

If e-mail is offered to patients as a mode of communication, it is imperative to check your e-mail inbox frequently in order to avoid liability. E-mail is not efficient for use in emergencies. As always, it is imperative to strictly adhere to all Health Insurance Portability and Accountability Act (HIPAA) confidentiality laws when using e-mail.

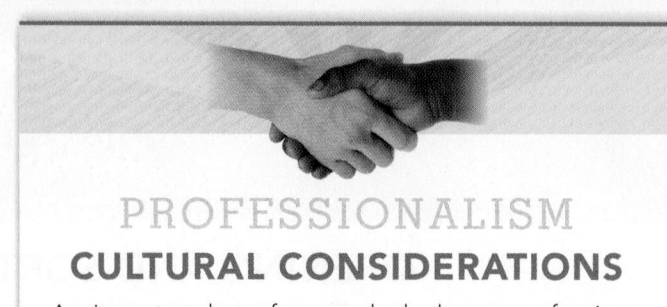

FACSIMILE (FAX)

The fax machine is another way to send a written communication electronically. The fax is an exact duplication of a document that is transmitted to another location via the facsimile (fax) machine. Telephone lines are used to transmit fax documents; thus, fax numbers look identical to telephone numbers. The original document is inserted into the fax machine, the receiver's fax phone number is dialed, and when the connection is made the document is transmitted over the telephone lines, resulting in a printed document at the receiver's fax machine. A cover sheet, which includes information about the sender (company, name, and telephone and fax numbers) telephone number of the receiver, date, and number of pages, should be the first page sent. It should contain a message that encourages the recipient to notify the sender if the fax has been received in error and also asks the recipient to destroy the document after notification. All fax cover letters must be HIPAA compliant.

Reflection on the Medical Practice

Medical assistants are often responsible for preparing interoffice memos and letters to patients. The letter you send is a direct reflection on the physician and the medical office as a whole. If the letter is filled with errors, contains an incorrect diagnosis, or is sent to the wrong patient, it reflects poorly on the medical office and can harm the physician's business. If your responsibilities as a medical assistant include letter writing, it is always a good idea to have someone in the office review your correspondence. To facilitate time management within the medical office, you can utilize a form letter that you or the physician has created. Proofread each document and check for any inappropriate content, misspellings, grammatical or punctuation errors, and margin restrictions.

SUMMARY

The responsibilities of the medical assistant relating to office correspondence are multifaceted. These include being able to draft correspondence using correct grammar and style and efficiently handling mail. Effective mail handling includes using the most efficient and cost-saving form of mail service. These responsibilities must be handled in a professional, courteous, and diplomatic manner. Correct handling of written communication allows the medical assistant to demonstrate competence.

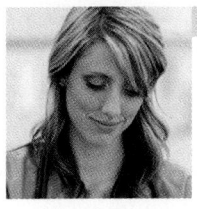

11 CHAPTER REVIEW

COMPETENCY REVIEW

1. Define and spell the terms to learn for this chapter.

2. How would you track a missing piece of mail?

3. Address an envelope using the method recommended by the USPS for use with optical character recognition (OCR) equipment.

4. Describe what types of material you would send by certified mail.

5. Type a short letter using both block and modified block with indented paragraph styles.

6. Why do you think companies (and medical offices) use letterhead stationery?

PREPARING FOR THE CERTIFICATION EXAM

1. When mailing a document that bears legal significance and would be difficult to replace, it should be mailed via:
   a. Insured Mail.
   b. Registered Mail.
   c. Special Delivery.
   d. Certified Mail.
   e. Special Handling.

2. Insurance can be purchased for all of the following types of mail EXCEPT:
   a. first class.
   b. third class.
   c. fourth class.
   d. Priority Mail.
   e. Special Handling.

3. A standard business envelope is:
   a. No. 6¾.
   b. No. 7.
   c. No. 9.
   d. No. 10.
   e. No. 11.

4. When composing a business letter, the date is usually placed how many lines (spaces) below the letterhead?
   a. 3
   b. 4
   c. 5
   d. 6
   e. 2

5. Catalogs, books, and photographs (also known as bulk mail) should be sent via which classification of mail?
   a. first class
   b. second class
   c. third class
   d. fourth class
   e. Special Delivery

6. A courteous greeting within a business letter is known as the:
   a. heading.
   b. salutation.
   c. body.
   d. closure.
   e. enclosure.

7. Which of the following is the two-letter abbreviation for Alabama?
   a. AB
   b. AK
   c. AL
   d. AM
   e. AA

8. When addressing an envelope, the last line in the address must contain the city, two-digit state code, and the ZIP code. This line cannot exceed how many characters in length?
   a. 25
   b. 26
   c. 27
   d. 28
   e. 24

9. The letter format in which all lines begin at the left margin, a salutation is used, and paragraphs are not indented is known as a:
   a. simplified letter.
   b. block letter.
   c. modified block letter.
   d. semi-simplified letter.
   e. semi-block letter.

10. Which of the following is the proofreader's mark that means "move left"?
    a. sp
    b. [
    c. //
    d. #
    e. ←

CRITICAL THINKING

1. According to the standard practices of written communication, is this letter okay? If not, explain why.

2. In what voice is this letter written?

3. If you were Lewis and you needed to rewrite the letter, what would you change about the letter? Why?

ON THE JOB

Diane Webb, a medical assistant in Pearson Physicians Group has been asked to proofread the following letter, which was prepared by a temporary assistant. Follow the rules for proofreading, grammar, capitalization, and spelling found in this chapter to correct the errors in this letter. Type this letter using the modified block style, and prepare it for Dr. Shania McWalter's signature.

Dear Docter Stacey:

I right this letter to inform you that I am pleased that you would chose me to present at your conference. Its a great complement.

Their are several cases which I can site. I would like you're recommendation since I no you will be frank with me. We must all ways be discrite and conscience of patience's rights when presenting cases relating to there conditions. We must remain mindful that patients have there legal rites.

I have the following x-ray studies which I can include: xyphoid process, greater trocanter, peretoneal abcess, left calcanus, fracture of right clavical, and a fractured ileum and ischeum. Let me know which of these rentgeneology studies you would prefer.

Please advise me on how to procede.

Sincerely yours,

Dr. Shania McWalter

INTERNET ACTIVITY

Access the Internet and locate information on how to write professional medical letters. Research other information you may need, such as your extended ZIP code, proofreader's marks you can use as a reference tool, an online dictionary, a medical dictionary, a thesaurus, and e-mail etiquette guidelines.

MEDMEDIA

Additional interactive resources and activities for this chapter can be found:

On your student DVD: View applicable procedure videos on the DVD-ROM found in the back of this book.

MyHealthProfessionsKit.com: Test your knowledge of the chapter with games and activities. MyHealthProfessionsKit also includes resources, helpful links, and a Spanish audio glossary.

Medical Assisting Interactive: Practice your procedures as a medical assistant in this simulated doctor's office. This can be accessed through MyHealthProfessionsKit.com.

12

Computers in the Medical Office

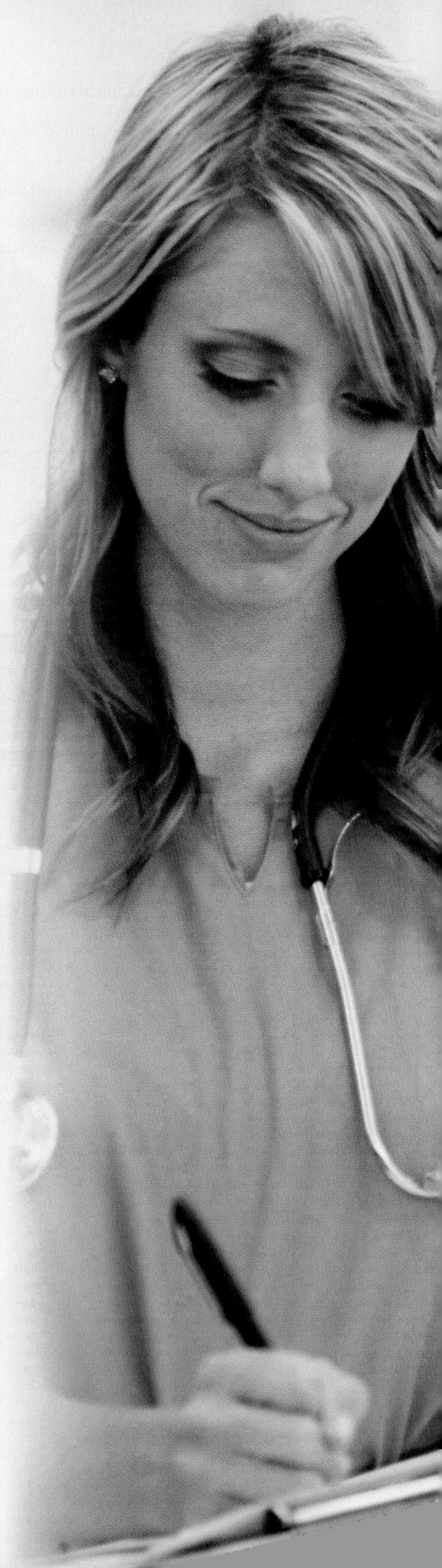

LEARNING OBJECTIVES

After completing this chapter, you should be able to:

- Define and spell the terms to learn for this chapter.

- Discuss the functions and applications of the computer.

- Explain the difference between hardware and software.

- Identify three methods to ensure confidentiality of medical records when using a computer.

- Describe computer security and maintenance.

- Distinguish the difference between the Internet and World Wide Web.

- List four methods to be ergonomically correct at your workstation.

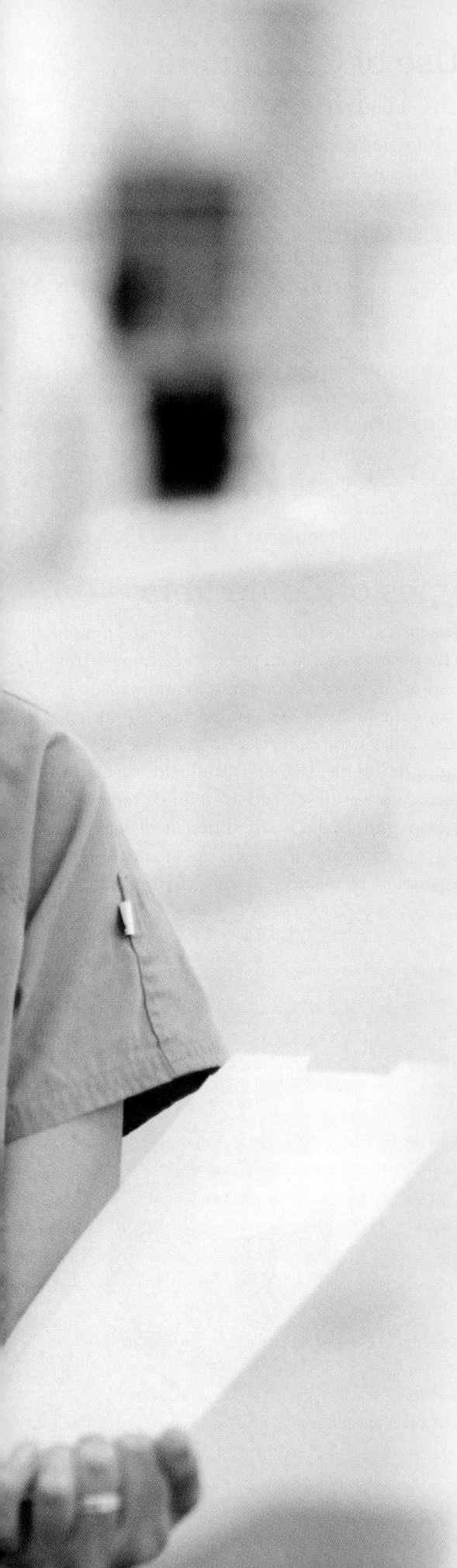

CHAPTER OUTLINE

CASE STUDY

Samra Belkovich is a medical assistant who works for Pearson Physicians Group. She has been asked to develop some continuing education materials for a community services project that the office will conduct at the local shopping mall. She is assigned to locate the most current information, design and develop the materials for distribution, and include marketing materials for the event and for the office.

Use of Computers in Medicine

Technology advancements have enabled medical offices to function with increased efficiency and speed using computers. Computers are considered a fundamental piece of operating equipment to perform and enhance quality patient care through data collection, eliminate duplication of work, and decrease errors. Figure 12-1 illustrates how computers have become invaluable in diagnosing, monitoring, and reporting the patient's progress. Medical assistants will be responsible for computer entries, electronic medical records, electronic bookkeeping, billing, insurance processing, appointment scheduling, inventory data, and many other functions. These responsibilities dictate the medical assistant's knowledge and application of computer literacy. Medical assistants must have competent computer skills and stay current as technology continues to advance.

Types of Computers

The computers used in medical offices today are microcomputers. This means that a small piece of electronic hardware, called a chip, allows the processing of information in a very small amount of space. The microchip revolutionized computers. Today computers can fit on a desk, in your lap, or even in a device the size of a handheld calculator. Before the microchip was developed, computers took up a great deal of room and used a vastly different technology. In the early days, a computer that took up an entire room had the same amount of memory as one that now fits on top of a desk.

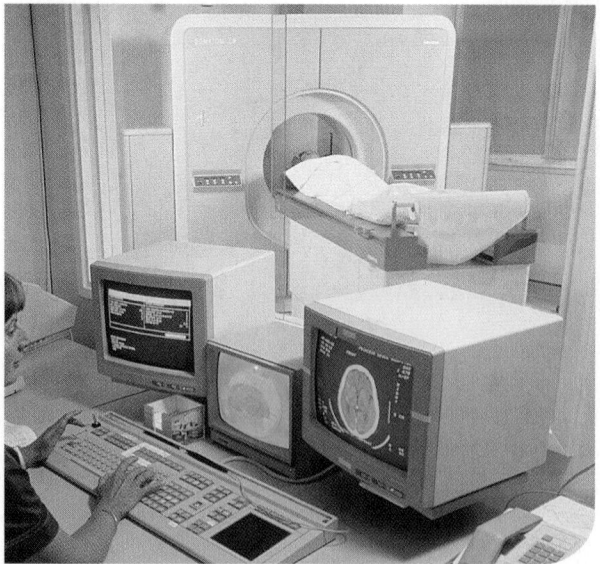

FIGURE 12-1 CT brain scanning.

The uses of computers in medicine are many and varied. Depending on the size of the medical practice, some or all of the functions normally performed in the front office may be done with computers and specialized programs. To be successful in both the administrative and clinical areas of a medical facility, the medical assistant must be familiar with computers and how they can be used.

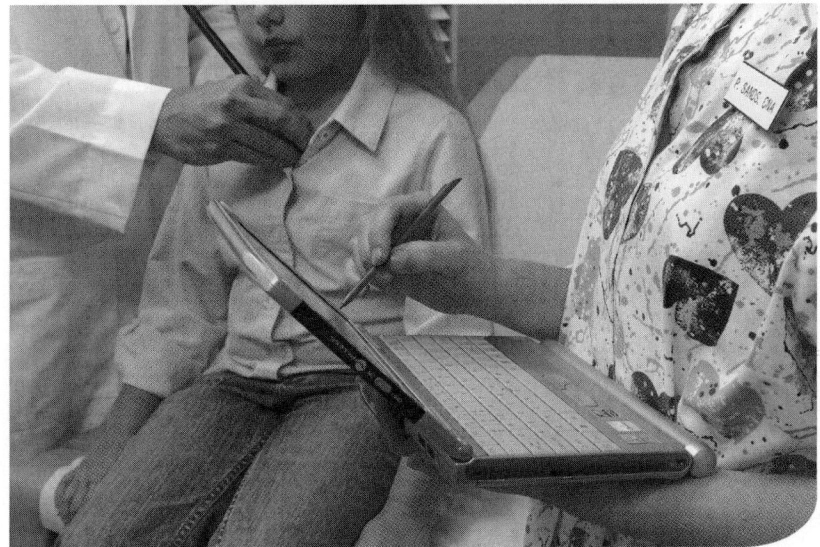

FIGURE 12-2 Medical assistant uses a laptop computer for bedside charting.

- **Input devices**, such as keyboards and scanners, feed data and instructions into a computer.

- **Output devices**, such as display screens, printers, and other devices, allow the user to see what the computer has accomplished.

- **Central processing unit (CPU)** is the brain of the computer that executes the specific set of instructions.

The CPU, or **main memory** of a computer, acts as a traffic controller, directing the computer's activities and sending electronic signals to the right place at the right time. The time it takes for the electronic signals to come and go is measured in **megahertz (MHz)**. One megahertz equals one million cycles per second. The higher the MHz, the faster the computer. At the heart of the CPU is the **microprocessor**, which has a number indicating its size. Microprocessors have three

As computers have evolved, two characteristics have changed: size and portability. For those offices using electronic medical records, it has become necessary for the physician to have computer access anywhere, including while away from the office. Laptop computers, also known as notebook computers, allow users to carry their work with them (Figure 12-2). A laptop computer can fit in a case about the size of a small briefcase. Laptop computers offer the same functionality as desktop computers, only in a smaller package. Palm Pilots and other personal digital assistants (PDAs) are other portable devices commonly used in the medical field. PDAs are small enough that they fit easily in the pocket of a lab coat. PDAs can store data (information) electronically, including an entire *Physicians' Desk Reference (PDR),* an annual compilation of manufacturers' prescribing information. The information in the PDA is, literally, at the physician's fingertips and can be recalled as needed.

Basic Computer Components

A **computer** is a programmable machine, or system of hardware (Figure 12-3) that responds to a specific set of instructions and performs a list of instructions in programmed language called **software**. Table 12-1 lists the different types of hardware, software, and storage components. Generally, computers require the following components to function:

- **Memory** makes it possible for a computer to temporarily store data and programs.

- **Mass storage device** makes it possible for a computer to permanently retain large amounts of data even when the computer is off. Common mass storage devices include disk drives or Zip drives.

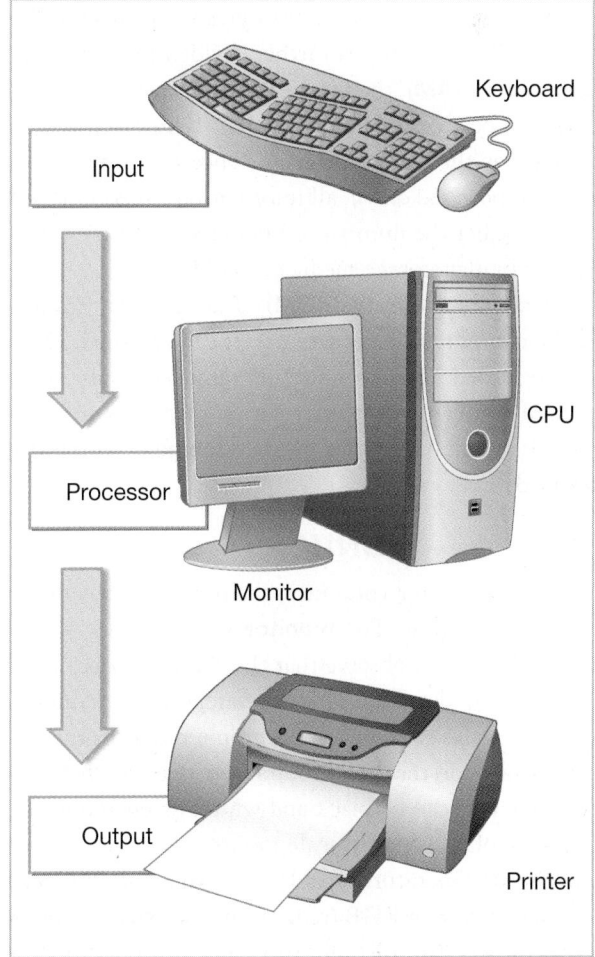

FIGURE 12-3 Components of a computer system.

TABLE 12-1 Hardware, Software, and Storage Components

Hardware	Software	Storage
Central processing unit (CPU)	Systems	Diskettes/floppy disks
Peripherals: monitor, printer, CD-ROM, modem, scanner, cables, and other equipment	Applications	Hard disks Magnetic tapes

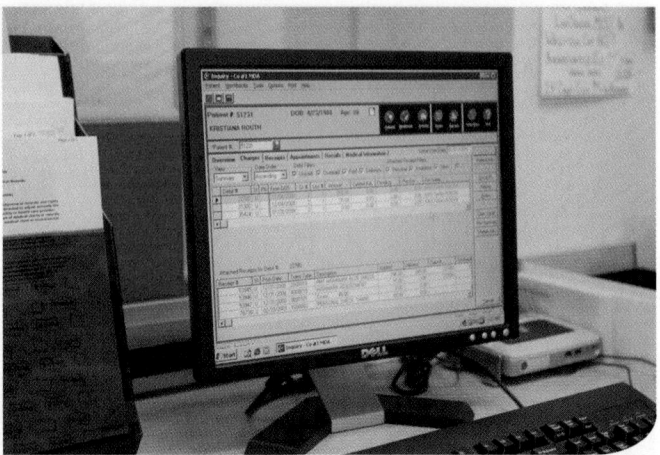

FIGURE 12-4 Color monitor for a computer system.

differentiated characteristics: instruction set; **bandwidth** (the amount of data that can be transmitted in a fixed amount of time); and **clock speed** (the speed at which the CPU can process instructions). The higher the numbers, the more power the CPU will have.

MEMORY

A computer's memory is measured and stored in **kilobytes (K or Kb)**. Each kilobyte is 1,000 bytes (or characters) of information. This memory is further divided into **random-access memory (RAM)**, the internal storage area in the computer that can be accessed randomly. RAM, however, is only good as long as the computer is on. Once the computer is turned off, or powered down, all information stored in RAM is lost. The higher the number of kilobytes, the more information a particular storage media can hold.

The **read-only memory (ROM)** is an internal storage area in the computer where data have been recorded. Once data are recorded, they cannot be removed, only read. Thus, ROM is used to store information that is not actively being used by the computer at that moment, primarily permanent data.

MONITORS

To communicate with a computer, the user must be able to see what is happening. The **monitor** is the display screen that allows the user to observe that the computer does what it is directed to do. Monitors are categorized as monochrome, gray scale, or color. Monochrome monitors display two colors: one for the background and one for the foreground; the colors can be black and white, green and black, or amber and black. A gray-scale monitor is a special type of monochrome monitor capable of displaying different shades of gray. Color or RGB (red, green, and blue) monitors display anywhere from 16 to over one million different colors (Figure 12-4). In addition to these monitor categories,

monitors are available in a variety of sizes and styles similar to television screens. The screen size is measured in diagonal inches, the distance from one corner to the opposite diagonal corner.

DRIVES

Computers are based on hard-disk drive technology. The hard-disk drive, a magnetic storage media inside the computer, is usually called the "C drive." This storage area is controlled by the CPU, and information written to the hard drive is accessed by the CPU when needed. Programs and information can be stored on a hard-disk drive. The more graphic elements produced by the software, the larger the amount of storage space required. Any of the several types of disk drives—hard-disk drive (HDD), floppy-disk drive (FDD), magnetic disk, and optical drive—can be either internal or external. Figure 12-5 shows a variety of storage devices.

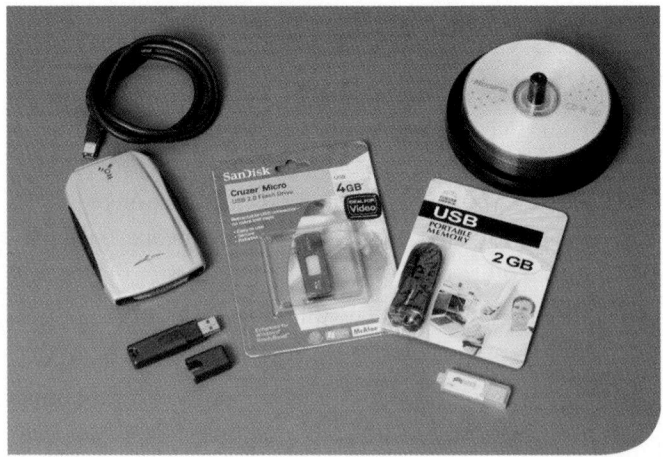

FIGURE 12-5 Information can be stored on a variety of storage devices: (A) hard disk drive, (B) flash drive, and (C) CD-ROMs.

CD-ROMs

CD-ROM stands for "compact disc read-only memory." It is a data storage system for computers that allows data to be stored on a compact disc. Computer programs, databases, and other large amounts of information on CD-ROM are digitally encoded and may not be changed by the user. Stored data may include simple text programs, entire encyclopedia programs, photo and sound libraries, and complex motion pictures or animations. The data are randomly accessed from the compact disc in the same manner as from a floppy disk, which is a small flexible, magnetic disk (in a rigid plastic case) on which data are stored and from which a computer can retrieve data. Floppy disks are now rarely used due to the increased use of CD-ROMs and DVD ROMs (digital videodisc or digital versatile disc). A CD-ROM can hold or store more information than 1,000 floppy disks.

Some computers have multimedia capabilities that allow the user to record and access a variety of sounds and music, photos, animations, and videos. Multimedia functions require the large storage capacity that a CD-ROM offers.

DVDs use a disc the same size as CD-ROMs; however, they can hold much more information and can be recorded on both sides. DVDs are used most often to record presentations that combine sound and graphics.

REMOVABLE DISK DRIVES

A removable external disk drive uses disks mounted in a disk enclosure similar to the hard disk drive in the computer. External disk drives come in a variety of sizes ranging from 1 to 500 gigabytes (GBs). Their advantage is that multiple disks can be used to increase the amount of stored material, and once removed, the disk can be stored away to prevent unauthorized use.

A portable **universal serial bus (USB)** drive, also known as a jump drive, thumb drive, or flash drive, is a small portable storage device that can hold up to 64 GB or more of data. USB hard-disk devices can be purchased in a variety of sizes, styles, and shapes depending on the overall need. As a courtesy to their patients, some medical facilities are storing the patient's medical record on a password-protected flash drive that allows the patient to essentially carry his or her record from office to office. This is especially helpful for patients with several physicians who are not all linked to the same electronic medical records system.

KEYBOARDS

The keyboard is a set of keys utilized to input data. The keyboard is designed with function keys, alphanumeric keys, punctuation keys, arrow keys, and conjunction keys. Function keys serve dual purposes, depending on the software program that is running. The F1-key and the F12-key execute specific word processing operations. Conjunction keys execute directions in conjunction with the program running and at least two other keys, for example the Control key + Alt key + Delete key (all pressed at the same time) will enable the user to access the Windows Task Manager.

MOUSE

Another device that gives the user control of the computer is a **mouse**. As the mouse rolls along a hard, flat surface, it controls the movement of the cursor, or pointer, on the monitor. The mouse contains at least one button, and up to three, each performing different functions depending on the program in use.

SCANNERS

Scanners are used for a variety of office tasks but most often to convert the patient's paper record or reports into an electronic record. This device "scans" printed paper records and converts them into a format the computer can read. Once the document has been converted into an appropriate format, it can be forwarded as an attachment in an e-mail.

DIGITAL CAMERAS

Digital cameras record pictures. Instead of the image being stored on film, it is stored digitally and can be downloaded to a computer system. Many offices using electronic medical records use digital cameras to take pictures of their patients and then download the pictures into the patient's record. This method helps the staff ensure they have the right patient and the right record.

PRINTERS

Printers are used to transfer information from the computer monitor onto paper or hard copy. The most popular printer options are inkjet and laser. Dot-matrix printers are also in use.

An inkjet printer works by forming dots when the ink is blown onto the paper. Inkjet printers can print graphics and in color if the proper ink cartridge and software have been installed.

Laser printers use lasers to burn the ink onto the paper. Although they are the most expensive of the three printer options, they are the most versatile printers available today. Laser printers are faster and quieter than either dot-matrix or inkjet printers, they can produce typewritten-quality work, and they can add color to documents with available options.

Some offices still use dot-matrix printers for multipage forms, such as carbonless NCR forms, which inkjet and laser printers are not able to print. Dot-matrix printers are noisier, have poor print quality, and are not as fast as inkjet and laser printers.

SOFTWARE

Software, or *program,* is the name given to the instructions that allow the computer to perform its functions. Every computer starts with an operating system. Computer programs that work with the operating system are called overlays. Overlays allow us to use menus instead of typing commands. The overlay programs that most users know are from Microsoft Windows, which lets the user choose a function from pictures or icons. Using a mouse, the user moves the cursor to the icon of the program and clicks the proper button on the mouse. The Windows program translates this command for the CPU, and the program is called to the screen.

Another layer of computer programs are application programs. These programs can perform special functions, such as word processing, data management, or spreadsheet formation.

Spreadsheet applications allow users to manipulate data by rows and by columns. Users input values into specific spreadsheet cells and with electronic formulas and labels define relationships between cells.

Word processing applications make it possible to create, edit, store, and print written documents such as letters, manuscripts, transmittals, and many other professional documents. Word processing programs can visually enhance a document's appearance with numerous features, such as boldface, italics, font choice, and color.

Data management applications are similar to electronic filing systems (Figure 12-6). Data are stored in collections of information that are organized within the software application and can be sorted for quick data selection of specific desired information pieces. For example, the user would select the field for creation of a directory of patient telephone numbers, diagnoses, or other needed information.

Several application programs may be used in the medical office; however, the most commonly used software is Microsoft Office. Within the Microsoft Office package. Microsoft Word is typically used to draft correspondence with patients, physicians, and insurance companies. Word also may be used in developing patient education materials, such as office brochures or handouts. Microsoft Excel is used to develop spreadsheets to track a variety of data, including income, expenses, insurance claims, and patient-specific data. Microsoft PowerPoint has a variety of uses but is used most often to develop presentations for patient education as a continuous loop on the waiting room monitor or for presentations the office manager or physician will deliver.

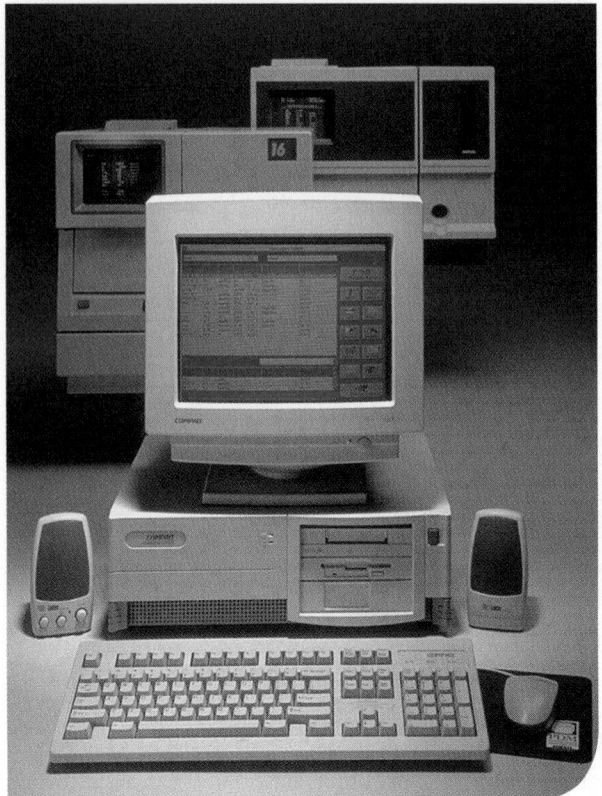

FIGURE 12-6 **Patient data management system.**

Advantages of medical management programs are many. After entering patient information into the program only once, the practice can schedule an appointment, record charges and payments, generate an insurance form, print a statement (including notices of delinquency accounts or aged accounts), track the number of days before payment is received from the insurance company, and write a reminder letter or postcard to the patient about an upcoming appointment.

Several medical management programs are available. The two programs most commonly used in the physician's office are Medical Manager and MediSoft. No matter which program is used, a few similarities exist. However, each program operates differently, including commands and required fields, so it is important that new employees understand the functions of the management program used in their office. Most offices will provide a one- or two-day training session for new users.

Security for the Computer System

The same legal standards of confidentiality and compliance with the Health Insurance Portability and Accountability Act (HIPAA) apply to all patient records, whether on paper or on the computer. It is important to reassure patients that their information will be used appropriately within the medical office. It is absolutely essential for the successful medical assistant to understand that other patients should not be able to see computerized records any more easily than paper records. This may require some thought and planning when a computer system is used for record keeping in the front office.

All computer screens should be positioned so they cannot be easily seen by patients. A privacy screen around key computer workstations may be necessary, depending on the office layout. Another available safeguard is a screen saver that uses an image or texture that covers up the screen at the touch of a key without removing any data, allowing no one but the user to see it.

It is imperative that patient records are accessible only to those who are authorized to use them. Keeping electronic patient records safe requires all users to have a unique password. Medical management programs often have several tiers of security, allowing one system administrator (the person in charge of the computer program) to limit access for patient records to those who need to see them. For example, the person who does appointment scheduling in a particular practice may not need to see a patient's financial records. The system administrator can lock the appointment scheduler out of financial records altogether or can assign limited access to the data.

Without a proper password, the user does not have access to data and must log in, or type in, his or her password, followed by an acceptance key (ENTER or RETURN), to use the program. It is important to guard a password carefully. It should not be shared with coworkers or written where someone else will see it. When choosing a password, avoid using the names of children or significant others (these would be too easy for someone else to guess). Use a word or a set of numbers that has significance to you but is also easily remembered. If you must write down your password, write it in a secure place and do not identify it as a system password. Change passwords on a regular basis. Many medical offices require you to change your password every 30 to 90 days for added security and HIPAA compliance measures. Once you have completed your task at the computer, log off or sign off your password before walking away. This prevents others from using your password inappropriately.

In addition to in-office security, a medical office must protect the computer from outside invaders. Outside invaders include hackers, crackers, viruses, and cyberbullies that access confidential information and commit identity theft. Computer security begins with protection of computer

systems with firewalls and antivirus programs. In addition, maintenance programs, such as defragmentation and deletion of temporary Internet files, cookies, and Internet history, should be scheduled automatically or manually and should be run often. In addition to internal maintenance, all equipment surfaces should be cleaned regularly with appropriate cleaning solution to maximize longevity and prevent users from spreading germs.

To avoid losing all data in the event of a system failure, fire, or equipment theft, it is also important to regularly back up files (copy files onto disks or CD-ROMs), and those backup files should be stored in a secure location outside the office. Again, confidentiality is of the utmost importance, and access to backup files should be carefully guarded.

Selecting a Computer System

Before beginning the search for a new computer system, it is important to establish the following:

- How will the computer be used?
- How many people will be using the computer system?
- How much storage space is needed now and for several years into the future?

Remember, the more graphic the computer program, the greater the amount of memory and storage required to run it. The greater the number of patients added to a particular database, the more storage space needed to keep pace with the size of the practice.

The second phase of selection of a computer system should focus on the software currently being used:

- Is it meeting the needs of the practice?
- Does everyone who uses it understand how to use it?
- Will the current programs transfer to a new system? Will it have the ability to interface with the hospitals in the area?
- If there are satellite offices, how do those offices exchange information with the "main" office?

The third critical element of selecting a computer system is the budget and costs related to the budget, such as monthly billing and insurance claim mailings. Changing programs adds to the cost of a new computer system and must be considered carefully in any system change.

Once the hardware and software analysis has been completed, it is time to look at the products on the market:

- Do some manufacturers have a better service record than others?
- What happens if the computer system malfunctions?
- Who pays to have the computer system fixed? Is a warranty provided?

Identify a support system of computer experts who can provide ongoing technical assistance and quick on-site service for computer software and hardware problems. Purchasing a service contract to take effect when the warranty covering parts, repair, and service expires is an option that you may wish to consider. Training contracts are available with firms that will provide employee training on new software and hardware.

Computer system selection is a large responsibility. Although the final decision usually rests with a financial manager, the system's users can make or break the success of any given installation. Users who are unhappy with the selection are not as apt to use the system to its fullest capability, and this will, in the end, cost the practice money. Therefore, to make sure that the money invested in a system is well spent, it is imperative that as many users as possible be involved in the selection process. Table 12-2 lists commonly used computer terms.

The Internet

The **Internet** is a computer network of thousands of interfacing networks worldwide. Millions of computers are connected to the Internet. There are organizations that develop technical aspects of this network and set standards for creating applications on it. However, no governing body is in control of the Internet. Access to the Internet is obtained through a commercial **Internet service provider (ISP)**. While using the ISP and a modem connection, you can browse the Internet for a wide variety of services: electronic mail, file transfer, vast information resources, interest group membership, interactive collaboration, multimedia displays, real-time broadcasting, shopping opportunities, breaking news, and much more.

With the advent of remote communications through electronic mail (e-mail) and modems, computers in one location can "talk" to computers across the street, across the state, across the country, and across the world.

JUDGMENT CALL

In the past, several medical office staff abused their Internet privilege and as a result the medical office where Janis, a medical assistant, works has developed a strict policy on using the Internet for personal business, especially any shopping sites. Prohibited sites are blocked, and when an employee accesses one of these sites, their computer screen immediately turns red and a report is filed with the information services (I/S) department at the main office.

Dr. Block has asked Janis to gather information about new computers for the office. While she is searching the Internet for information, her computer screen turns red and the message is as follows: "A report on Internet activity has been forwarded to the I/S supervisor." Janis is immediately concerned because she knows several people have been reprimanded as a result of such messages and one person was recently fired for visiting prohibited Internet sites. What should Janis do?

TABLE 12-2 Frequently Used Computer Terms

Term	Definition
Backup	A copy of work or software batch data stored for processing at periodic intervals.
Batch	Data stored for processing at periodic intervals.
Boot	To start up the computer.
Catalog	List of all files stored on a storage device.
Characters per second	Speed measurement for printers.
Cursor	Flashing bar, arrow, or symbol that indicates where the next character will be placed.
Daisy-wheel printer	An impact printer that "strikes" characters onto a page, much like a typewriter; unable to produce graphic images but does produce letter-quality output.
Database	Computer application that contains records or files.
Data debugging	Process of eliminating errors from input data.
Disk drive	A container that holds a read/write head, an access arm, and a magnetic disk for storage.
DOS	Disk operating system.
Downtime	Time a computer cannot be used because of maintenance or mechanical failure.
Electronic mail (e-mail)	Use of appropriate hardware and software (modem, computer, telephone, etc.) to allow transmission of data electronically from computer to computer.
File	A collection of related records.
File maintenance	Data entry operations including additions, deletions, and modifications.
Format	Methods for setting margins, tabs, line spacing, and other layout features.
GIGO	"Garbage in, garbage out," which means if you input incorrect information you will receive incorrect output.
Hard copy	A printed copy of data in a file.
Hardware	The actual physical equipment that is used by a computer to process data.
Input	To enter data into the computer system; data entered into the system.
Interface	Technology that allows two or more unconnected computers to exchange programs and data. Also referred to as a network.
Keyboard	An input device, similar to a typewriter keyboard.
Menu	A list of options available to the software user.
Modem	Hardware device that converts digital signals to analog signals for transfer over communication lines or links.
Output	To process data into final form; data produced by the computer system.
Peripheral	Device required for the input, output, processing, and storage of data; includes mouse, disk drives, keyboards, printers, and joysticks.
Scrolling	Feature that allows the computer operator to control the location of the cursor within a document.
Security code	A group of characters that allows an authorized computer operator access to certain programs or features; password.
Write-protect	Feature of storage devices that allows the data to be seen but not changed.

Internet technology has allowed many medical insurance companies to offer electronic claims services or ECT (electronic claims transmission). ECT service speeds up the insurance claim process and puts the payment for services rendered into the practice's bank account in as few as three working days. Such access can be obtained through a clearinghouse or remote computer with transfer to multiple insurance carriers.

Internet technology is also being used, though not commonly, to allow patients to store their medical records in one place on the Internet. When patients use this technology, they decide if they want to share their medical information, and if so, who may have access to it and, specifically, what can be shared. This creates a truly portable electronic medical record.

The **World Wide Web (WWW)**, or the Web, is a system of Internet servers. The initial purpose of the Web was to facilitate communication among its members, who were located in several countries. Rapid growth in the number of both developers and users ensued. In addition to hypertext (computer-based text), the Web began to incorporate graphics, video, and sound. The use of the Web has reached global

proportions and has become a defining aspect of human culture in an amazingly short time.

The World Wide Web provides almost instant access to information. Its convenient and user-friendly environment makes it easy for patients to research information about a new medication, for physicians to share test results with specialists assisting in diagnosing patients, or for use as a tool to further educate members of the health care team. Because of the Web's ability to work with multimedia and advanced programming languages, it is by far the most popular component of the Internet.

Electronic Signatures

The traditional signature on documents is becoming a thing of the past. The traditional signature can now be converted into a mathematical process (or a set of numbers) to create an electronic signature. This set of numbers (in computing terminology, it is a file), will be recorded temporarily in a computer's working memory or permanently on storage medium such as a disk. The file that constitutes the electronic document can be copied from place to place via telecommunication devices. An increasing proportion of both commercial and private communication takes place in purely electronic form. Some of those communications must be signed to achieve their intended legal status. Even when this is not strictly necessary, the parties involved in a transaction are likely to request that the transaction document or communication be signed.

HIPAA requires health care organizations to protect the privacy and security of confidential health information and requires standard formats for electronic transactions. These standardized national requirements apply to the electronic transmission of patient history and health records such as health insurance enrollment details and claims. The need to maintain confidentiality and privacy of medical information and rules for medical document security, including standards related to electronic signatures, is also outlined in HIPAA.

Computers and Ergonomics

If you are a longtime computer user, you might have noticed the occasional discomforts that accompany spending lengthy periods of time in front of the computer. After staring at a monitor for extended amounts of time, year after year, you may start to notice the discomfort increase in frequency and severity. As use and hours on the computer continue over the years, the discomfort could become part of the daily routine when you sit down to use a computer. To safely incorporate computer use in your daily routine and to work

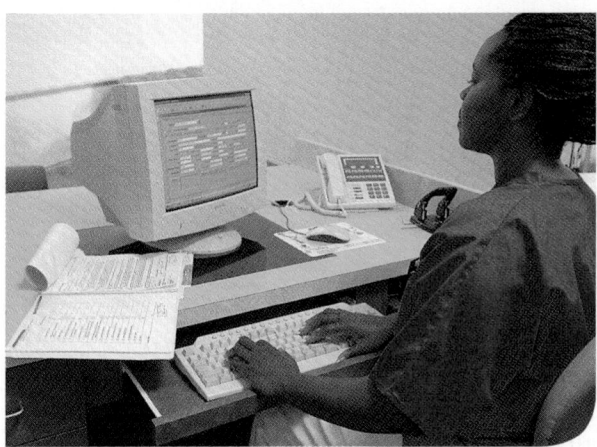

FIGURE 12-7 Ergonomically correct desk, chair, and keyboard.

effectively, you should be aware of some ergonomic tips, such as how to appropriately position computer equipment (Figure 12-7).

YOUR CHAIR

When sitting in your chair, make sure that you set your hips as far back as they can go in the chair. Adjust the seat height so your feet are flat on the floor and your knees are at the same level as, or slightly lower than, your hips. Adjust the back of the chair to a 100-degree to 110-degree reclined angle. Make sure your upper and lower back are supported. It may be necessary to use inflatable cushions or small pillows. If you have an active back mechanism on your chair, use it to make frequent position changes. For chairs with armrests, adjust them so that your shoulders are relaxed; remove the armrests if they are in the way.

YOUR KEYBOARD

An articulating keyboard tray allows you to adjust the angle and height of the keyboard and can provide optimal positioning of input devices. However, it should accommodate the mouse, provide leg clearance, and have an adjustable height and tilt mechanism. The tray should not push you too far away from other work materials, such as your telephone. It is helpful if you pull up close to your keyboard and position it directly in front of your body. If possible, adjust the keyboard height so that your shoulders are relaxed, your elbows are in a slightly open position, and your wrists and hands are straight. Wrist rests can help to maintain neutral postures and pad hard surfaces. However, the wrist rest should only be used to rest the palms of the hands between keystrokes.

YOUR MONITOR

Incorrect positioning of the monitor screen and source documents can result in awkward posture and muscle tension. Adjust the monitor and source documents so that your neck is in a neutral, relaxed position. Your monitor should be centered directly in front of you, above your keyboard. Position the top of the monitor approximately 2 to 3 inches above seated eye level. To reduce glare, it may be helpful to place the screen at right angles to windows and adjust curtains or blinds. Optical glass glare filters, light filters, or secondary task lights can also help reduce glare.

YOUR BODY

Once you have correctly set up your computer workstation, use good work habits. No matter how perfect the environment, prolonged, static postures will inhibit blood circulation and take a toll on your body. Take short 1- to 2-minute stretch breaks every 20 to 30 minutes. After each hour of work, take a break or change tasks for at least 5 to 10 minutes. Always try to get away from your computer during lunch breaks. Avoid eye fatigue by resting and refocusing your eyes periodically. Look away from the monitor and focus on something in the distance. Rest your eyes by covering them with your palms for 10 to 15 seconds. Use correct posture when working. Shift your position as much as possible.

SUMMARY

The use of computers is essential for medical offices to meet the process flow of business today. Computers enhance quality patient care through data collection, eliminate duplication of work, and decrease errors. Computers enable input, processing, output, and storage of medical data. In medical offices, computer use is especially valuable in eliminating some of the more time-consuming tasks associated with appointment scheduling, charting, billing, and insurance processing. Computers are composed of many parts, including the microprocessor, CPU, monitor, keyboard, and printer. Safety on the computer includes regular maintenance, passwords, antivirus protection, HIPAA compliance, and general cleaning. The successful medical assistant is a computer-literate professional who deals easily with the challenge of finding new and efficient ways to use available technology.

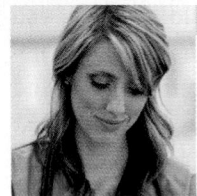

12 CHAPTER REVIEW

COMPETENCY REVIEW

1. Define and spell the terms to learn for this chapter.

2. Using a microcomputer, boot up the computer. Notice what information is displayed on the screen before the computer is "ready" to work. What disk operating system is being used? Does a menu or submenu appear when the computer has been booted, or is the computer using a version of Windows? Are any security codes required to use the programs listed? If so, what are they?

3. What type of printer is used by the computer system?

4. Print a list of all the files on the hard drive.

5. Select a word processing program and type a simple letter reminding a patient that he or she is due for a blood pressure check. Use the spell-check feature before printing the letter.

6. Enter a patient's information into a medical management software database. Use yourself and your own information as the data.

PREPARING FOR THE CERTIFICATION EXAM

1. What type of printer is fastest and most quiet?
   a. inkjet
   b. dot matrix
   c. laser
   d. word processor
   e. scanner

2. Which is considered a hardware element of computers?
   a. systems
   b. scanner
   c. diskettes
   d. central processing unit
   e. magnetic tapes

3. Which is NOT an advantage of a medical database management program?
   a. have to enter patient information only once
   b. can measure storage capacity
   c. can track days before payment is received from insurer
   d. can print delinquency notices
   e. can schedule appointments

4. Which is NOT recommended to establish computer security and protect patient information?
   a. screen saver to cover up the screen
   b. tiers of security that limit access to patient information to authorized employees
   c. password that is unknown to the patient but that you can remember easily

   d. screen positioned away from patients
   e. use of firewalls

5. Computer downtime is:
   a. data entry operations including additions, deletions, and modifications.
   b. a copy of work or software batch data stored for processing at periodic intervals.
   c. garbage in, garbage out.
   d. time of maintenance.
   e. processing of information in a very small amount of space.

6. A list of options available to the computer user is known as:
   a. password.
   b. menu.
   c. DOS.
   d. boot.
   e. a prompt.

7. The ergonomic concerns related to computing may be all of the following except:
   a. the document.
   b. keyboard.
   c. body.
   d. chair.
   e. monitor.

8. Which office function CANNOT be performed by word processing?
   a. User can correct errors on the screen before printing takes place.
   b. User can print X-ray films.
   c. User can input information using a typewriter-like keyboard.
   d. User can generate form letters.
   e. User can see the copy that will be printed before it is printed.

9. Which of the following is considered a software element of computers?
   a. peripherals
   b. mouse
   c. floppy disks
   d. medical billing programs
   e. monitor

10. The CPU is also known as:
    a. microprocessor.
    b. megahertz.
    c. main memory.
    d. bandwidth.
    e. kilobytes.

CRITICAL THINKING

1. Where should Samra begin?

2. Which software programs should she use to design and develop the educational materials and the marketing materials?

3. What should she do to become more familiar with the software features to design the materials?

ON THE JOB

Elizabeth Maxwell, a medical assistant for Dr. Casey, often works at the front desk. One of Dr. Casey's patients, Stephanie Cross, has arrived for a scheduled appointment. On her way in, Stephanie saw a neighbor leaving the office. She asks Elizabeth to look on the office system and tell her why her neighbor was in to see Dr. Casey.

Later the same day, Diana Mulderr, who sits at the desk next to Elizabeth, has forgotten her computer password. She asks to use Elizabeth's password "just for today."

1. What should Elizabeth tell Stephanie Cross?
2. Is it ever permissible to use the computer to look up information on patients for personal reasons?
3. What should Elizabeth tell Diana Mulderr?

INTERNET ACTIVITY

When researching information on the Internet, it is important that the websites used are reputable and provide accurate information. Perform a search using any of the search engines (a website that allows you to search the entire Web for related websites) available to you. Search for popular health-related websites. Make a list of ten websites and comment on each: ease of use, relevant information, easy to understand, and so on.

MEDMEDIA

Additional interactive resources and activities for this chapter can be found:

On your student DVD: View applicable procedure videos on the DVD-ROM found in the back of this book.

MyHealthProfessionsKit.com: Test your knowledge of the chapter with games and activities. MyHealthProfessionsKit also includes resources, helpful links, and a Spanish audio glossary.

Medical Assisting Interactive: Practice your procedures as a medical assistant in this simulated doctor's office. This can be accessed through MyHealthProfessionsKit.com.

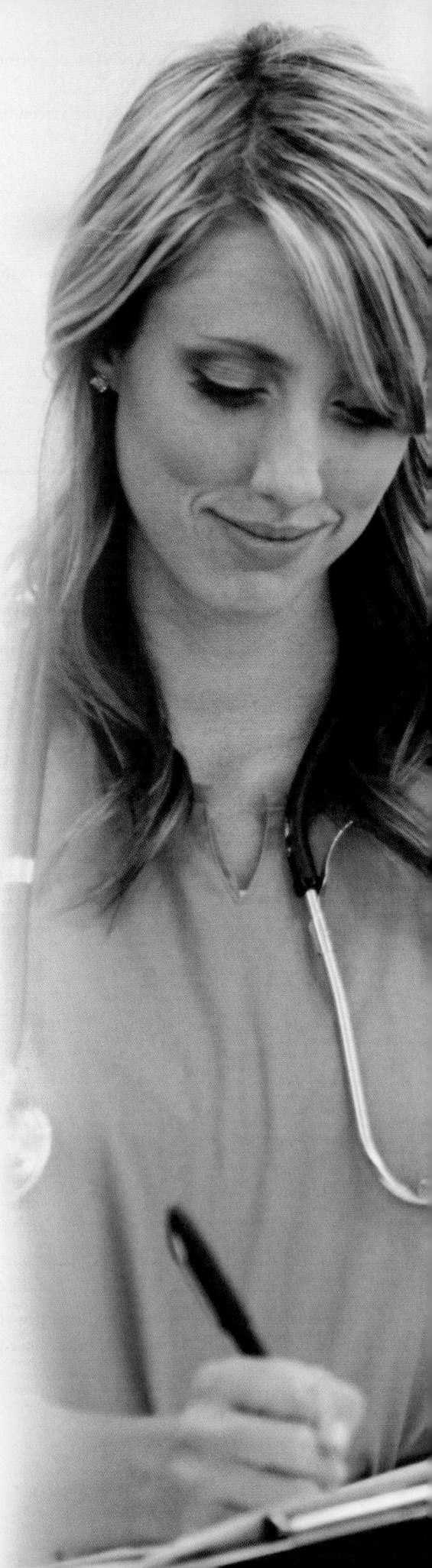

13

Managing Medical Records

LEARNING OBJECTIVES

After completing this chapter, you should be able to:

- Define and spell the terms to learn for this chapter.

- Discuss the problem-oriented medical record.

- Describe the four compontents of the SOAP charting method.

- Identify the three types of file storage units.

- Name the "Rules for Filing."

- Compare and contrast the alphabetic, numeric, and color-coded filing systems.

- List and discuss five types of numeric filing systems.

- State an effective system used for cross-referencing.

- Understand how to find a missing file.

- Describe a tickler file.

- Explain quality assurance.

- Discuss ownership of the medical record.

- Know the medical record's statute of limitations

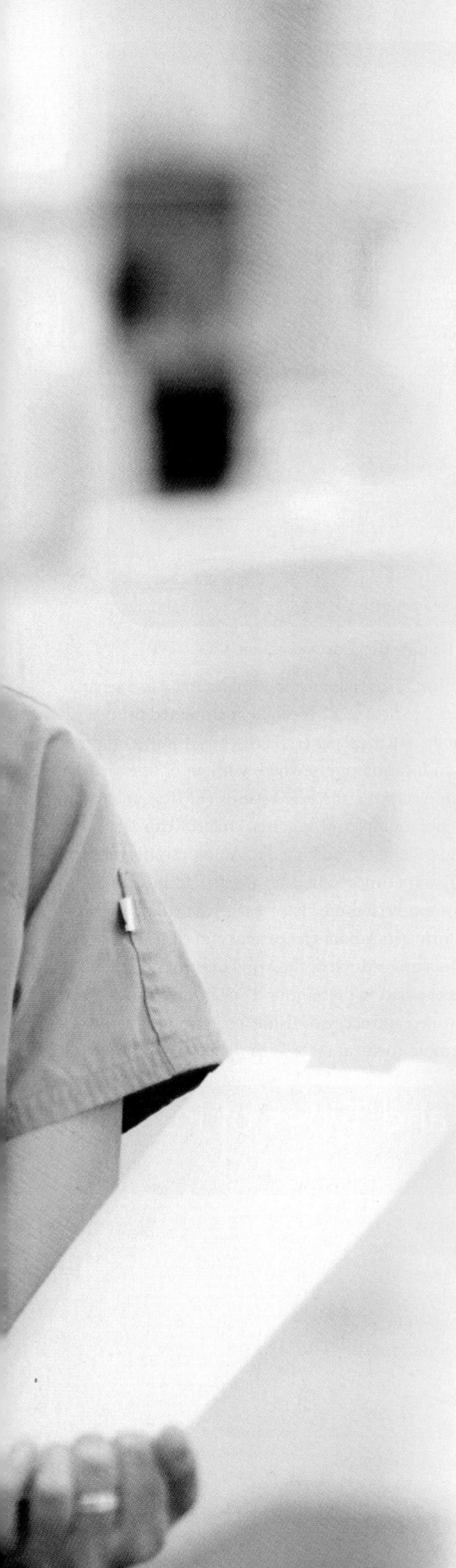

CHAPTER OUTLINE

CASE STUDY

Danita Coles has been a patient with Pearson Physicians Group for the past 10 years. Danita has recently gotten married to Richard Marley and now lives with her husband in a newly built home. She has legally changed her name to share the same last name as her husband. She is coming into the office today to see Dr. Miller. This is her first visit to the practice since she has been married.

249

active records

addendum

alphabetic filling

chronological medical record

closed records

electronic medical record (EMR)

inactive records

medical record

microfiche

microfilm

numeric filing

problem-oriented medical record (POMR)

source-oriented medical record (SOMR)

subjective, objective, assessment, and plan (SOAP)

terminal-digit filing

CERTIFICATION LINK

CMA (AAMA)

Medicolegal guidelines and requirements

  Legislation

Documentation/ Reporting

  Releasing medical information

  Physician-patient relationship

Records Management

  Needs, purposes and terminology of filing systems

  Filing guidelines

  Medical records (paper/electronic)

RMA

General medical assisting knowledge

  Medical law

  Medical ethics

Administrative medical assisting

  Medical receptionist/ Secretarial/ Clerical

CMAS (AMT)

Medical assisting foundation

  Legal and ethical considerations

  Professionalism

Medical records management

  Systems

  Procedures

  Confidentiality

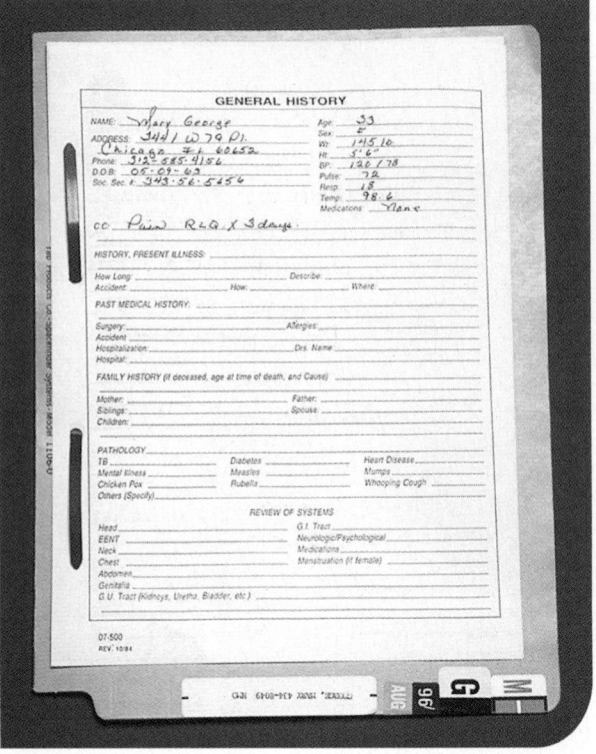

FIGURE 13-1 Handwritten documentation.

A medical record is the source of all documentation relating to the patient. The medical record contains past patient history, current diagnosis and treatment information, and correspondence relating to the patient. Billing materials are often maintained in a separate financial record. Medical records can be maintained using a variety of methods, such as paper (hard-copy files), computer database files on location or elsewhere with an online separate backup system, electronic medical records (EMRs), **microfilm** (miniaturized photographs of records), **microfiche** (sheets of microfilm), and other electronic media. An **electronic medical record (EMR)**, sometimes called an electronic health record (EHR), is a computerized means of gathering, documenting, and storing information about the patient and the care received in the medical setting. Much of the same information found in a patient's paper chart will be found in an electronic chart; however, it is stored and accessed using a computer. Chapter 14 discusses electronic medical records in detail. Medical records

Box 13-1 Standard Medical Record and Types of Reports Found in the RECORD

- Patient's past medical records
- History and physical
- Insurance information
- Office notes
- Progress notes
- Telephone messages
- Pathology results
- Nursing notes

- Medications
- Physician orders
- Radiology reports
- Laboratory reports
- Operative reports
- Consultation reports
- ECGs
- Miscellaneous

management requires careful attention to accuracy, confidentiality, and proper filing and storage.

The Medical Record

The medical record contains all the written documentation that relates to the patient's health care. Each patient's medical record will contain essentially the same categories of material but information unique to each patient. Information contained in a source-oriented medical record is filed within a section with tabs. Each medical record may or may not include all standard categories based on the patient's individual health care needs. For example, not every patient will have a consultation report from another physician, or a surgical report. See Box 13-1 for a summary list of standard categories and reports that are covered in more detail in this chapter. Figure 13-1 is an example of handwritten documentation in a medical chart. This demonstrates just one part of what is in the standard patient's chart.

Documentation of Patient Medical Information

Many different formats are used for recording medical information. Each practice will have its own format specific to its needs, but everyone in an office should chart with the same system.

CHRONOLOGICAL MEDICAL RECORD

The **chronological medical record** follows the patient over a period of time, with each visit consisting of a new entry by date, rather than by symptoms or diagnosis. Although this is one of the most common types of medical records, it does make some diagnoses, such as hypertension, more difficult to "catch." For such diagnoses, a problem-oriented medical record might be more appropriate.

PROBLEM-ORIENTED MEDICAL RECORD

The **problem-oriented medical record (POMR)** was developed by Dr. Lawrence Weed in 1970 and is used to identify patient problems and chart by those problems.

The functional aspect of this type of charting is the patient problem list found at the front of the chart (Figure 13-2). As new problems and diagnoses are identified, they are noted on the problem list, helping the health care provider to identify trends in the patient's medical history or emerging diagnoses. POMR also provides

NAME _____ AGE _____

OCCUPATION_____ SOC. SEC.# _____

	BLOOD PRESSURE	VISION Without Glasses		Diagnostic Tests	Results
Height ____	**Sitting**	Far R20/ L20/			
Weight ____		Near R / L /			
	R / :L /	**With Glasses**			
Build ____		Far R20/ L20/			
(Sm.Med.Lg.Obese.)	**Standing**	Near R / L /			
Pulse ____	R / :L /	**Tonometry** R ___ L ___			
Resp. ____		**Colorvision** ____			
	Lying	(Ishihara plates missed)			
Temp. ____	R / :L /	**Peripheral Fields** R ___ L ___			
AUDIOMETRIC TESTING	250 500 1000 2000 4000 8000 R ___ ___ ___ ___ ___ ___ L ___ ___ ___ ___ ___ ___				
	Gross Hearing _____				
PULMONARY FUNCTION					

Initial Problem List

_____
_____
_____
_____
_____
_____
_____
_____
_____
_____
_____
_____
_____
_____
_____
_____
_____
_____
_____
_____
_____

Employment status_____ Physician's signature _____
DATE _____

FIGURE 13-2   **An example of a medical history sheet to list patient problems.**

health care providers and physicians who do not already know a specific patient with an overview of previous visits and problems at a glance. A POMR has four parts:

- **Database**—Consists of the physical examination, the patient history, and the results of baseline laboratory or diagnostic procedures.
- **Problem list**—List of patient problems that is kept in the front of the chart much like a table of contents would be. The problem list assigns each problem a number with the date. The problem can be further explained by information in the database. Each problem the patient has experienced is titled and numbered in the problem list. Because each patient problem is numbered, that number can be referenced throughout the medical record when needed. Throughout the rest of the history, problems are referred to numerically. If one is resolved, the date of resolution is placed next to the problem listed. If a new problem arises, it is assigned a number and listed with the date.
- **Plan**—Indicates a written plan for each numbered problem identified on the problem list. The plan may include tests to be ordered, treatment plans, or plans for patient education about specific problems. The treatment plan is a very important part of the med-

ical record because it tells what is intended for the patient. Each treatment plan should have a title and should reference the problem number with which it is associated.

- **Progress notes**—Made up of several sections that follow a specific format; the first letter of each section title (Subjective, Objective, Assessment, and Plan) spells out the word SOAP. Thus, this portion of the POMR is known as SOAP notes. Sometimes E is added to SOAP if evaluation is completed. All progress notes should be maintained in chronological order. Each progress note also will reference the patient problem number.

SOAP Charting

The **SOAP** charting method is distinct because of the four parts of the approach. The subjective information gathered from the patient—the things that the patient believes he or she is seeing a physician for—are usually the same as a chief complaint (CC). The objective is comprised of the data gathered during the visit—such as vital signs, weight change, fevers, blood work, and other measurable data. The assessment is the physician's preliminary diagnosis. The plan section of the chart discusses the strategy for care of this patient (Figure 13-3). The SOAP method of documenting a medical record is described in Table 13-1.

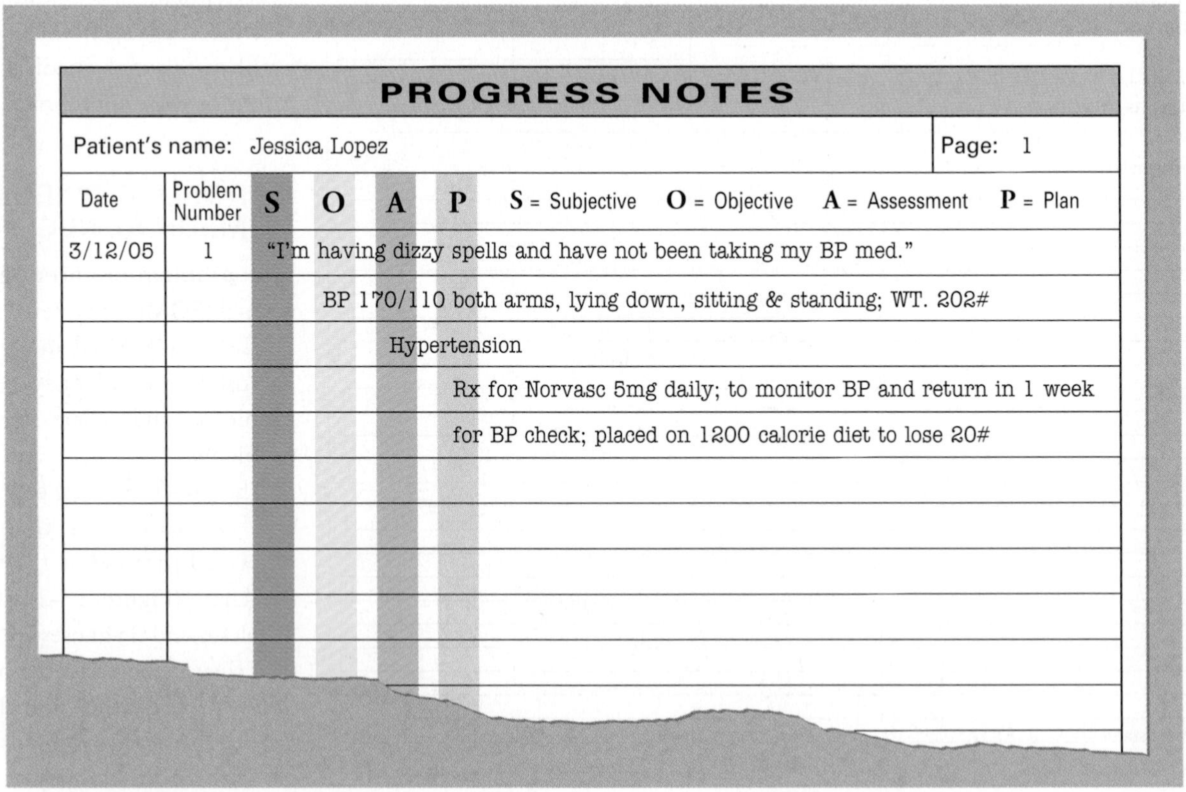

PROGRESS NOTES										
Patient's name: Jessica Lopez									Page: 1	
Date	Problem Number	**S**	**O**	**A**	**P**	**S** = Subjective	**O** = Objective	**A** = Assessment	**P** = Plan	
3/12/05	1	"I'm having dizzy spells and have not been taking my BP med."								
			BP 170/110 both arms, lying down, sitting & standing; WT. 202#							
				Hypertension						
					Rx for Norvasc 5mg daily; to monitor BP and return in 1 week					
					for BP check; placed on 1200 calorie diet to lose 20#					

FIGURE 13-3   **An example of SOAP charting.**

TABLE 13-1 SOAP Charting for 1/24/XX

S	Subjective symptoms provided by the patient and/or family. The actual patient's words are recorded	"I'm thirsty and eating all the time but I'm not gaining any weight. I feel tired all the time."
O	Objective findings from vital signs, physical examination, and laboratory and diagnostic tests	B/P: 158/96; T: 98°F; P: 76; R: 16 Skin turgor (resiliency) poor. Wt. 10# less than 6 weeks ago Urine 4 + sugar, FBS positive
A	Assessment, including the physician's diagnosis	Uncontrolled diabetes
P	Plan including recommended treatments, further tests, medications, consultation, surgery, physical therapy	Dx: Lab tests for diabetes Tx: Begin diabetic diet and insulin Instruct on diet and exercise follow-up

A problem list for the patient in the example given in Table 13-1 might appear as follows:

- *Problem List*
  2/14/XX
  Problem No. 1: Diabetes
  Problem No. 2: Hypertension, essential

- *Plan*
  2/14/XX
  Problem No. 1: Diabetic exchange diet
  Regular insulin, 20 units SC q AM
  Monitor blood sugar levels during day
  Problem No. 2: Norvasc 2.5 mg. daily
  Monitor blood pressure weekly

- *Progress Note*
  2/14/XX
  Problem No. 1: Diabetes
  S—Patient states thirst has diminished and hunger lessened
  O—Urine +2, FBS positive, gained 4 pounds in past 3 weeks, skin turgor good
  A—Diet and medication effective
  P—Continue medication, monitor blood sugar level daily, adjust insulin levels per instruction, return visit in 2 weeks
  Problem No. 2: Hypertension
  S—Patient states no complaints related to high blood pressure
  O—BP 138/86, down 10 points in past 3 weeks
  A—Medication effective
  P—Continue with medication and patient monitor of BP weekly; come in for check in 2 weeks

The POMR and SOAP methods can be combined in one chart, making for a very concise, clear set of information on any patient.

SOURCE-ORIENTED MEDICAL RECORD

The **source-oriented medical record (SOMR)** is commonly utilized in medical clinics. Patient information is placed in the medical record in reverse chronological order and organized in different sections. Each office determines which sections to be used and in what order they are to appear in the medical chart. The sections commonly used include history and physical, insurance, progress notes, medications, laboratory, and consultations. The most recent information is seen first in each section of the medical record. This method makes it complicated to identify and locate past medical problems, treatments, and results. Progress notes are included with each patient encounter whether it is an office visit, telephone call, or written communication.

THE MEDICAL RECORD: A LEGAL DOCUMENT

The medical record is a legal document, a permanent record, and a tool used by staff members to communicate not only in their office but also office to office regarding the services delivered to the patient. The patient's chart is not the place to document your opinion or internal office problems. Statements such as "Injection was not administered due to lack of staffing," or "Patient very angry with physician" are subjective comments (opinions). All documentation should be factual (objective).

Everything that is done during a patient's medical visit, ordered over the telephone, or discussed with a patient by telephone or e-mail must be documented in the medical record. Write legibly in black ink. If you make an error, do not erase or totally obliterate the original error with commercial products such as correcting fluid. Simply draw a single line through the error so the original entry can still be seen, initial above the single line, date and write "Error." Once this is complete, write in the correction. If an error is made while using a typewriter, it should be corrected as any other errors are corrected. However, if the error is noted later, then you must draw a line through the error, enter your initials and the date, and write in the correction. When documenting in an EMR, prior to saving the entry errors may be corrected by deleting as you would with any other type of computer program. However, if an error is discovered after the entry is saved, an **addendum** will be required. An addendum is an addition to the original document; in this case, the addendum should be titled "Correction." When using an EMR, the entry will be automatically dated and signed electroni-cally when saved. Procedure 13-1 lists steps the medical assistant should follow when changing or adding items to a patient's chart.

The following items cannot be overemphasized as part of the medical assistant's responsibility to ensure an efficiently run medical office.

- **Clear handwriting**—The medical records that are handwritten should be easily read by anyone. Pay particular attention to numbers and spelling.
- **Accurate records**—Keeping in mind that records are legal documents and can be used in a court of law, the physician must be able to trust the accuracy of the

procedure 13-1

ADDING OR CHANGING ITEMS ON A PATIENT'S RECORD
Objective: Add an item to a patient record and correctly change an error in documentation.

EQUIPMENT AND SUPPLIES
medical record to be added to or changed; black pen; correct information or documentation to be added or changed

METHOD
Adding items to a record:

1. An item is added to a patient record as soon as it is discovered that the item was omitted (Figure 13-4).
2. Locate the last entry in the medical record.
3. Using a pen with black ink, on the next line of the record, immediately after the last entry, place the current date.
4. On the same line, after the date, place the statement "Late entry."
5. Note the date on which the information to be added was gathered.
6. Enter the information that was originally omitted.

7. Sign the entry with your full name and credentials.

Changing items in a paper record:

1. If an incorrect entry was made in the medical record, or the entry was made in the wrong record, it must be corrected (Figure 13-5).
2. Locate the incorrect information.
3. Using a pen with black ink, draw one single line through the incorrect information so that the incorrect information is not obscured and can still be read.
4. Never erase entries in a medical record. Never use correction fluid in a medical record. NEVER mark through information so that it cannot be read.
5. Place the date of the correction, your initials, and "Error" above the incorrect information.
6. Enter the correct information.

Progress Notes
3-13-XX 10 $\frac{15}{aam}$ wt. 135, BP $^{130}/_{78}$ Temp 98.2°F
Patient presents for follow-up visit Re: B.P medication
Patient states he feels much better. Sam Smithick, CMA (AAMA)
3-14-XX Late entry, to be added to 3-13-XX entry. Fasting
lipid profile drawn and sent to HBC lab. Sam Smith CMA (AAMA)

FIGURE 13-4 An example of a late entry to the medical record.

Progress Notes
5-20-XX 2$\frac{30}{pm}$ Patient presents for staple removal
S/P hysterectomy on 5-10-XX. Patient states " I'm
improving, yet still tire easily." Explained to patient
she may feel this way for the next 2 ~~years~~.
months. Rita Gill, RMA

FIGURE 13-5 An example of a corrected chart notation.

data. As simple as it sounds, never guessing about information and double-checking your work each time will help ensure this is the case.

- **Records that are up to date and available**—Do not wait to update records; make it an office habit to update records either as they occur or daily. This updating must include telephone calls, lab reports, and office visits. Make sure that the files are easily accessible. If there is a patient emergency, for example, the medical history will be needed immediately.

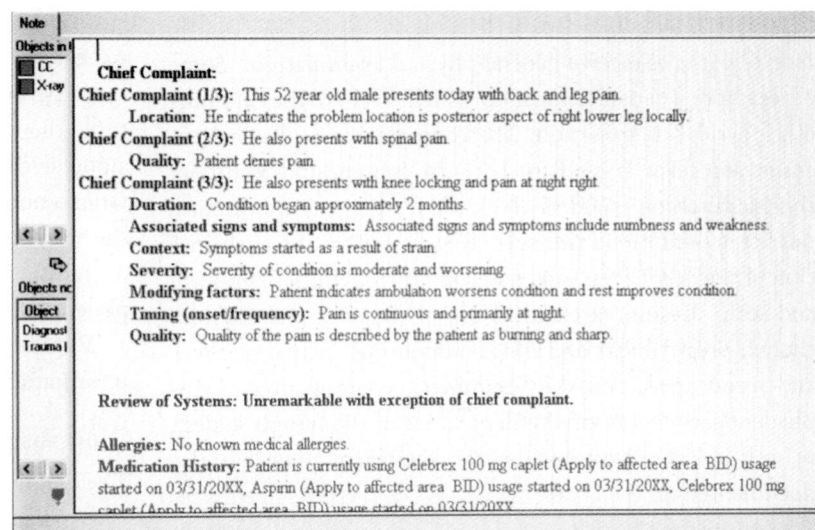

FIGURE 13-6 An example of a chief complaint chart notation in a computerized patient record.

Components of the Medical Record

Various medical reports are filed in the medical record with tabs that label the source, such as lab, X-ray, consultations, and special studies.

FORMS AND REPORTS

A standard medical record is one of the most important items in an office setting. It is imperative that you be familiar with all components of it, such as medical forms and reports, in order to maintain the integrity and accuracy of patient records.

Patient Registration

The patient registration form usually includes the patient's full name, address, contact information (including home phone, work phone, cell phone, and e-mail address if applicable), date of visit, age, date of birth (DOB), Social Security number, driver's license number (if applicable), medical insurance information, and person responsible for payment. The form should also request the patient's occupation, marital status, number of children (if applicable), and emergency contact information.

Family and Medical History

The patient's family and medical history is listed on a separate form. This information should include the patient's current medical problem with details of present illness (CC), as well as family medical history, patient's past medical history, past surgeries, allergies, and current prescription and over-the-counter medications. Figure 13-6 shows an example of a CC. The family and medical history form should request a list of herbal medications and recreational drugs used by the patient. It also should contain the patient's social and occupational history, including the amount of exercise done by the patient, whether the patient uses tobacco and the type of tobacco product, and alcohol use.

Managed care insurances often require that the patient's current chief complaint be entered into the medical record as a history against the diagnosis. Use of the patient's own words is often requested. When recording the patient's own words, be sure to use quotation marks. Relevant past family and social history is also vital, as well as the patient's medication history. Inventory of body systems also is usually included as part of the patient's history.

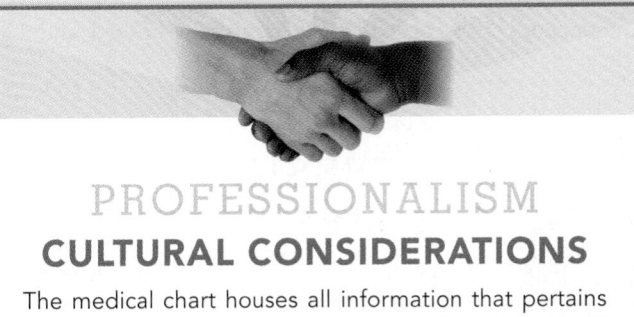

PROFESSIONALISM
CULTURAL CONSIDERATIONS

The medical chart houses all information that pertains to a patient. In addition to storing medical history and demographic and insurance information, the medical chart can be very useful regarding making notations regarding a patient's cultural background. Information relating to cultural background may include a patient's spoken language if it is not English, the need for an interpreter, and preferences regarding written, verbal, and nonverbal communication.

Physical Examination Results

Not all patients receive general physical examinations. Some offices have a separate form on which to chart the outcome of a physical examination. The comprehensive physical examination form is used to chart the content and results of the examination, such as the patient's general appearance, nutrition, and blood pressure (BP), as well as the examination of the head: eyes, ears, nose, and throat (EENT), mouth, and scalp. Results of examination of the neck and thyroid; thorax; breast; heart and lungs; abdominal, pelvic, genital, and rectal areas; and skin examinations are charted. Lymphadenopathy (abnormal enlargement of the lymph nodes), as well as overall impression and treatment plan, are also documented on the chart.

Results of All Tests

All results from tests performed on patients in the office, a laboratory, or a hospital should be tracked and filed in patients' records for easy accessibility should the physician need to consult them.

Records from Other Physicians and Hospital Visits

Records from other physicians and hospital visits should be obtained and placed in the record for all new and referred patients. The patient must make a request in writing for release and transfer of records from other offices. Relevant information and diagnoses from specialty physicians to whom the patient was referred for specific follow-up are also documented in the chart.

Informed Consent Forms

A signed informed consent form documents that a patient understands and consents to a treatment offered and has knowledge of the potential outcome and side effects of that treatment, including the expected outcome if the treatment is not performed. The form must contain the patient's signature, the physician's signature, and a witness's signature, along with the corresponding date. Moreover, it is important to note that the patient may withdraw consent if he or she so wishes. Should a patient choose to withdraw consent or refuse a procedure, it must be clearly noted in the patient's chart. Some medical offices require a patient to sign a "Refusal of Treatment" form. See Chapter 3 for more information on informed consent forms.

Diagnosis and Treatment Plan

The diagnosis and treatment plan should include the physician's diagnosis, the treatment plan, and all options and instructions presented to the patient.

Patient Correspondence and Follow-up Care

Any patient correspondence sent to the medical office, including procedures, follow-up visits, medical office care, and notations involving the patient, should be included in the patient's medical record. The date each piece of correspondence was forwarded should be noted in the chart, along with the initials of the individual who completed the action. Documentations of telephone calls—often a separate log—as well as correspondence with or about the patient from all sources, such as laboratories, health care agencies, and referred consultations, are also added to patient records.

Consultation Report

In many situations, a physician will ask another physician to provide a second opinion on a patient's case. Typically, the physician requesting the second opinion will forward a letter of introduction to the physician providing the second opinion. The letter of introduction includes a brief synopsis of the tests and results already performed. The second physician generally examines the patient and then dictates a report. The report is then sent to the attending physician (the requesting physician). The consultation report will include the following:

- Patient's name and medical record number
- Date of consultation
- Medical transcriptionist's initials
- Referring physician
- Reason for the consultation
- Physical and laboratory evaluations
- Consulting physician's impression and recommendations

PROFESSIONALISM
THE LIFE SPAN

For patients under the age of 18, it is especially important to document the name of the person responsible for any balances due the office. For children of divorced parents, it is possible that the parent bringing the child to the office for the visit is not the parent responsible for the copays or coinsurance. Depending on what is determined in the divorce decree, it is possible that one parent has primary custody and the other parent covers the child on his or her medical insurance.

It is appropriate to close this report, which is supplied in letter format, with a complimentary close, such as "Thank you for allowing me to participate in the care of this patient."

Operative Report

The operative report describes a surgical procedure. The surgeon is expected to dictate this report as soon as possible, preferably immediately after the procedure is completed. The surgeon's name, date of procedure, preoperative and postoperative diagnosis, and the actual findings during the procedure are contained in this report.

This report describes the actual procedure, including location and length of incisions, the layers of skin and tissue that were incised, the types of instruments used (in some cases), which tissues and organs (if any) were removed, all materials that were used in closing the wound, the estimated amount of blood loss, and a sponge count. The condition of the patient at the end of the procedure is stated, such as "Patient tolerated procedure well," "Patient awake and responding," or "Patient taken to recovery room."

Pathology Report

A pathology report focuses on microscopic (histology and cytology) findings, as well as gross (overall) description of tissues or organs. The pathology report is generated by the pathologist as the result of examining tissue and organs removed during a surgical procedure (such as a biopsy) or an autopsy. This report is related to disease findings and not laboratory findings, which are conducted on body fluids. An autopsy report is a pathology report generated after a patient's death to determine the cause of death.

Radiology Report

A radiology report, completed by a radiologist, documents results of diagnostic procedures, such as X-rays, CT (computerized tomography) scans, MRI (magnetic resonance imaging) scans, nuclear medicine procedures (scans of bone, thyroid, and other body parts), and other fluoroscopic examinations.

Discharge Summary

The discharge summary is completed on every hospitalized patient and summarizes the hospitalization. It explains why the patient was admitted, a summary of the patient's history, and a review of what occurred during the hospitalization. A discharge diagnosis is included in this report, and the patient's condition on leaving the hospital is noted.

Additional Reports

Other reports may be required concerning a patient, such as an emergency room report, a psychiatric note, and results of special procedures, such as a cardiac catheterization or an autopsy.

If information is not properly organized in the patient's medical record, errors can occur. It is very important that the medical assistant organize the patient's medical record according to facility policy. See Procedure 13-2 for instructions on how to organize a patient's medical record.

procedure 13-2

ORGANIZING A PATIENT'S MEDICAL RECORD

Objective: To update the patient's medical record, to verify that the correct record is in use, and to place the information in the correct place in the record.

EQUIPMENT AND SUPPLIES

patient medical record; assorted documents for filing in record

METHOD

1. Verify that you have the correct patient record for the patient documents you have been given.
2. File documents in chronological order in the correct areas of the file, according to your facility policy, for consistency. For example, file laboratory reports with other laboratory reports within the lab section, and with the most recent report on top.
3. Return the medical record to the correct place in alphabetic or numeric order with other patient files.

Filing

Choosing the type of file system for medical forms and reports, in accord with the file folder coding system used in the office, is an important decision since all files must be maintained within that system. Some large offices hire an office consultant to set up a filing system. Although office staff are generally consulted when setting up a new file system, the decision is made by the physician and the office manager. The three categories of files or records in a medical office are active, inactive, and closed:

- **Active records** are those of patients who have been seen within the past 3 years and are currently being treated. Each medical practice may have its own policy regarding what constitutes an active file, but the range is usually 3 to 5 years.

- **Inactive records** are those of patients who have not been seen within the past 3 years or another time period determined by office policy. These files are still maintained by the office but are generally kept in a separate storage file cabinet, which may be located off site. These patients have not received a formal notification that the physician has terminated caring for them. They may return when a medical problem develops.

- **Closed records** are those of patients who have actively terminated their contact with the physician. This occurs when they move away, ask to have their records sent to another physician, or death occurs. These files can be placed in storage boxes or converted and saved on a computer disk. These files are referred to as archives since they are no longer needed but must be kept for legal reasons.

Fireproof cabinets are used to file documents, such as patient records, tax records, insurance policies, and canceled checks.

FILE STORAGE

Three types of file storage commonly used in a physician's office are vertical, lateral, and movable:

- **Vertical files**—set up with two to four stacked pull-out drawers holding up to a hundred files per drawer. This type of file storage system is heavy and space consuming (Figure 13-7).

- **Lateral files**—set up with shelves that allow files to be easily pulled off them. A color-coded system for visual recognition of files if often used.

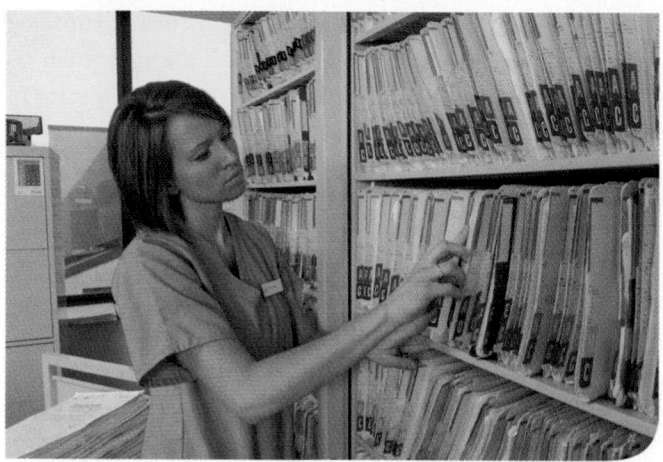

FIGURE 13-7 Vertical filing systems offer an alternative to traditional upright storage systems.

- **Movable files**—set up with electrically powered or manually controlled file units that move on stationary tracks in the floor. This type of open filing system saves space since the file units can be moved close together when they are not needed. This system is also useful for books and journals since the floor can be reinforced when the track is installed.

File Folders

File folders are also designed to meet special needs. The top or side edge contains tabs at spaced intervals. These tabs are marked with identification labels. If files are stored with alternating tab cuts, it is easier to read the labels in the file drawer. The identification label is attached to the top tab in a vertical file cabinet or to the side edge of the file in a lateral file cabinet.

The patient's record may be placed within a separate tabbed folder that remains in the filing cabinet. The file folders may be color coded to indicate the primary care physician. Each physician may be assigned a folder color and special indicators, such as for workers' compensation patients. These help keep files organized in large clinics.

Guides

Divider guides are used to separate files in drawers or on shelves. These guides are of heavy pressboard and should be placed every 1½ to 2 inches to separate the file folders. The divider guide separates the files into subsections using a letter (e.g., A, B, C, A–B, Invoices, etc.) or by patient number. An out guide is placed in the file when a file is removed to indicate where the file should be returned but can also be used to indicate who has removed the file and when it was removed. This is especially helpful in a

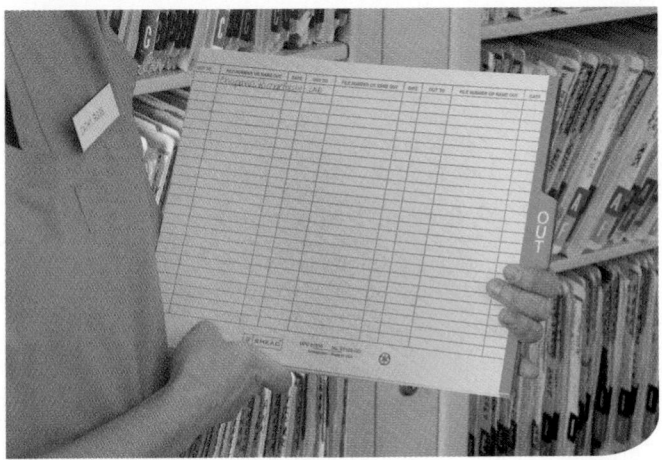

FIGURE 13-8 An example of an out guide.

large office when trying to locate charts. The out guide is usually a distinctive color, such as red, to indicate a file is missing (Figure 13-8).

Labels

The main purpose of the label on the file folder (such as the patient's name or medical record number) is to identify what is in the file. However, the label also can include a color-coded stripe that can be used for other purposes, such as identifying the primary care physician.

In addition to the labels identifying patient name or medical record number, offices also use special labels on charts to bring attention to patient allergies, required co-payments, and year of last visit. These special labels help the staff find pertinent information at a glance (Figure 13-9). For instance, a patient's allergy to penicillin is quickly identified

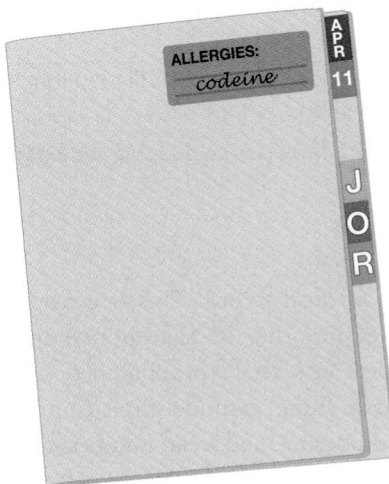

FIGURE 13-9 Using color coded labels enables the medical staff to quickly identify important information such as allergies.

if a bright allergy sticker that indicates the allergy is visible on the outside of the chart. It is important to update the information at every visit.

Rules for Filing

Three commonly used systems for filing are the alphabetic, numeric, and subject filing. Because the numeric system provides the most privacy, it is most commonly used in the office; however, alphabetizing is a component of all the methods and is explained in detail here. Color coding is used in all three systems to assist in locating files, refiling, and preventing misfiling.

Alphabetic System

In this system, Abbott would be filed before Bacon: A comes before B in the alphabet. If the first letter is the same, then move to the second letter in the name: Abbott is filed before Acker. This does not pose problems when filing a last name since everyone understands the alphabet. However, there could be confusion when filing Jacob James Jergens Jr. and Jacob James Jergens III, or determining how correspondence from 23rd Avenue Clinic should be filed.

The key to **alphabetic filing** is to divide the names and titles into units (first, second, and third). The unit is the portion of the name that is used for filing or indexing purposes. For example:

- Unit 1: Last name (Jergens)
- Unit 2: First name (Jacob)
- Unit 3: Middle name (James)

The first letter of each unit is then used to determine where the file is to be placed. When filing a large number of files, use the first letter of the first unit and place all the files from A to Z in order. Then take each group of A files and use the second letter and consecutive letters to place them in order. If the entire first unit is the same, as in Smith, then move onto the second unit and third unit. For example,

TABLE 13-2 Rules for Alphabetic Filing

Rules	Example
Names are filed: last name, first name, middle name (or middle initial). Each letter in the name is a separate unit.	Krause, Marvin K. is placed before Krause, Marvin L.
Initials come before a full name.	Brown, H. is placed before Brown, Henry.
Hyphenated names are treated as one unit. This applies to the names of individuals and businesses.	Amy Freeman-Smith is indexed under F for Freeman. It is considered Freemansmith for indexing purposes.
Titles (and initials) are disregarded for filing but placed in parentheses after the name.	Dr. Beth Ann Williams is indexed as Williams, Beth Ann (Dr).
Married women are indexed using their legal name. The husband's name can be used for cross-referencing.	Mrs. Mary Jane Smith is indexed as Smith, Mary Jane (Mrs. John).
Seniority units, such as Jr. and Sr., are filed in chronological (age) order from first to last.	Jacob James Jurgens, Sr. comes before Jacob James Jurgens, Jr.
Numeric seniority terms are filed before alphabetic terms.	Jurgens, Jacob James III is indexed before Jurgens, Jacob James, Jr.
Mac and Mc can be filed either alphabetically as they occur or grouped together depending on the preference of the office.	
Foreign language names are indexed as one unit.	Mary St. Claire is indexed as Stclaire, Mary. Carol van Damm is indexed as Vandamm, Carol.
If company names are identical, the address—by state, then city, then street—may be used in the index. The ZIP code is not used to index files.	ABC Drugs, 123 Michigan Blvd., Chicago, IL is indexed before ABC Drugs, 1450 N. Ash, Kalispell, MT.
If individual's names are identical, use the birth date or mother's maiden name. Avoid using an address since that can change.	Mark Richard Jones is indexed as Jones, Mark Richard (5/12/65) and Jones, Mark Richard (2/12/89).
Disregard apostrophes.	Megan O'Connor is indexed as OConnor, Megan.
Business organizations are indexed as they are written.	Lincoln Memorial Hospital is correct.
Disregard short terms, such as *a*, *and*, *the*, and *of*.	The Whitefish Drug Store is indexed as Whitefish Drug Store (The).
Numeric characters are indexed before alpha characters.	23rd Avenue Clinic would be indexed before the Nineteenth Street Medical Center. A separate file is set up for all numeric files.
Names with religious titles, such as Sister Mary Murphy, would be filed with the last name first, and then with the religious title.	Murphy, Sister Mary.
Compound words are filed as they are written.	South West Physician Service is filed before Southwest Physician Service.

Smith, Loren comes before Smith, Michael, which comes before Smith, Michelle. Table 13-2 describes basic rules for alphabetic filing. Procedure 13-3 lists steps to follow when using the alphabetic filing system.

Numeric Systems

A **numeric filing** or patient identification system is used in hospitals and many larger clinics. A number is assigned to each patient's medical record. This is generally a six-digit number divided into three sections of two digits each (e.g., 05-72-21). There are several types of numeric filing, including straight numeric filing, terminal-digit filing, middle-digit filing, unit numbering, and serial numbering.

Straight Numeric Filing. The simplest numeric method is the straight numeric filing system in which each record

procedure
13-3

FILING A RECORD ALPHABETICALLY

Objective: File a patient record in the correct order, using the alphabetic method for filing.

EQUIPMENT AND SUPPLIES

patient record; alphabetic files

METHOD

1. Locate medical record files or medical record room.
2. Observe the name on the record to be filed.
3. Records are filed in alphabetic order by last name first, then first name, then middle name or initial. Each letter in the name is a separate unit. Locate the set of records containing the same last name as the record to be filed.
4. Within the set of records containing the same last name as the record to be filed, locate the records with the same letter of the first name as the record to be filed.
5. Using the alphabet as a guide, place the record to be filed after the record that comes before it in the alphabet but before the record that comes after it in the alphabet.
6. A name with only an initial first name is filed before a full name. (Brown, H. is filed before Brown, Henry.) The filing rule "Nothing before something" is a useful tool here.

7. Hyphenated names are treated as one unit. (Mary Freeman-Smith is indexed as Freemansmith, Mary.)
8. Disregard apostrophes. (Megan O'Connor is indexed as Oconnor, Megan.)
9. Titles and initials are disregarded for filing, but placed in parentheses after the name. (Dr. Beth Ann Williams is indexed as Williams, Beth Ann, [Dr.].)
10. Married women are indexed using their legal name. The husband's name can be used for cross-referencing.
11. Seniority units, such as Jr. and Sr., are filed in numeric order from first to last.
12. Numeric seniority terms are filed before alphabetic terms.
13. After placing the file between the two records before and after it in the alphabet, check once more to be sure the file is properly placed.
14. If there is a marker or out guide in place of the removed record, then take out the marker when replacing the file.

---

is filed sequentially based on its assigned number. The numbers used in this system begin at 01 and continue upward.

Example:	01	101	886
	02	102	887
	03	103	888
	04	104	889

In this type of system, the file space is depleted rapidly as new files are added to one section. This requires constant reshifting of files to make room for new files.

Terminal-Digit Filing. **Terminal-digit filing**, based on the last digits of the ID number, evenly distributes the files within the entire filing system. This eliminates the need for frequent reshifting of files, providing enough space was

designated when the filing system was set up. Filing using terminal digits requires dividing the files into a hundred primary sections, starting with 00 and ending with 99. The three sections of numbers assigned to each file are designated as tertiary, secondary, and primary sections, respectively. To file a record using this system, find the file section matching the patient's primary digits (21). Within that section, match up the secondary digits (72) and file the record according to the tertiary digits (05).

Example:	05	72	21
	Tertiary	Secondary	Primary

Procedure 13-4 lists steps for using the terminal-digit filing system.

Middle-Digit Filing. Using the same six-digit numbering system as for the terminal-digit system, the middle-digit

FILING A RECORD NUMERICALLY USING THE TERMINAL-DIGIT FILING SYSTEM

Objective: File a patient record in the correct order, using the terminal-digit filing method for filing.

EQUIPMENT AND SUPPLIES

patient record; numeric files

METHOD

1. Locate medical record files or medical record room.
2. Observe the numbers on the record to be filed.
3. Locate the set of files with the same tertiary numbers as the record to be filed (these will be the first two numbers on the record).
4. Within the set of records with the same tertiary numbers, locate the row of records with the same secondary numbers as the record to be filed (the secondary numbers are the second two numbers on the record).
5. Within the set of records with the same tertiary and secondary numbers as the record to be filed, place the record to be filed in numeric order by primary numbers (last two numbers on the record).
6. After placing the file in numeric order by primary numbers, check once more to be sure the file is properly placed.
7. If there is a marker or out guide in place for the removed record, then take out the marker when replacing the file.

---

filing system places the middle digits as the primary numbers. In this example, find the section marked 72, within that section find the 05 area, then file the record according to the tertiary digit, 21.

Example:	05	72	21
	Secondary	Primary	Tertiary

Unit-Number Filing. A unit-number filing system assigns a number to patients the first time they are seen or admitted to a hospital. All other hospitalizations or hospital visits use the same number. This method requires that all records be kept at the same location.

Serial-Number Filing. With a serial-number filing system, the patient receives a different medical record number for each hospital visit. The patient acquires multiple records that are stored at different locations. For example, a hospitalization, laboratory work, and a mammogram will all receive different numbers and be filed within their own systems.

The assigned numbers are kept in an accession record in which numbers in sequential order (1, 2, 3, 4, 5, 6 . . .) have a name placed next to them as each new name is entered. This record can also be maintained on the computer.

SUBJECT MATTER

Filing by subject matter is used for general files, such as invoices, correspondence, résumés, and personnel records. This method is adequate as long as the files are relatively small. If these files become large, then another method, alphabetic or numeric, will have to be devised.

COLOR-CODING SYSTEMS

To decrease the number of misfiled charts and aid in file retrieval, many medical record departments will use a color-coded system on their file folders. This system assigns a color for each number from 0 to 9. Color bars on the edge of each file folder correspond to the medical record number. Usually only the three primary digits are color coded. When files are correctly placed, the color bands will all have the same pattern. In this manner, any misfiles are easily seen. Filing records is simplified since the correct color band can be located on the file shelf.

Color Bands

Two popular color-coding methods using a numeric system are the Ames Color File System and the Smead Manufacturing Company's method. Table 13-3 lists examples of the numeric color-coding systems used by these two systems.

Other color-coded methods use an alphabetic system. One example is the Alpha-Z system by the Smead Manufacturing Company. This system is based on 13 colors with

TABLE 13-3 Numeric Color-Coding Systems

Ames Color System	Smead Corporation File System
0–red	0–yellow
1–gray	1–blue
2–blue	2–pink
3–orange	3–purple
4–purple	4–orange
5–black	5–brown
6–yellow	6–green
7–brown	7–gray
8–pink	8–red
9–green	9–black

TABLE 13-4 The Alpha-Z Alphabetic Color-Coding System

Color	White Letter, No Stripe	White Letter, White Stripe
Red	A	N
Dark Blue	B	O
Dark Green	C	P
Light Blue	D	Q
Purple	E	R
Orange	F	S
Gray	G	T
Dark Brown	H	U
Pink	I	V
Yellow	J	W
Light Brown	K	X
Lavender	L	Y
Light Green	M	Z

white letters on a colored background (e.g., the white letter A is on a solid red background) for the first half of the alphabet, and a white stripe is added to the colored background for the second half of the alphabet (e.g., the letter N is on a red background with a white stripe).

The Alpha-Z system uses file labels to denote the patient's name and a color label with the letter of the alphabet to indicate the index unit. For example, Emily Jane Smith would be labeled Smith, Emily Jane with an orange color block containing a white stripe and the letter S. Two other color blocks would be added to the label for the secondary and tertiary letters of the index unit (in this example, E on a solid purple background and J on a solid yellow background).

This system is ideal for the large practice with many patients having the same surnames. It can be adapted to a particular office's needs. For example, only the last name is color coded (Joseph Evans has only one solid purple color label). After the files are color coded, they are then alphabetized within their particular color category.

In large practices with several physicians, a different color may be assigned to each physician (e.g., Dr. Williams's patients might all have medical file folders with a yellow label). This color-coding system is described in Table 13-4. Figure 13-10 shows a color-coded medical record.

In some medical practices, a color-coded "year" tab is placed on folders of patients who are seen once a year. This hastens the purging of "inactive" files.

CROSS-REFERENCING

Due to the large number of files processed in a busy office and the confusion over surnames—(e.g., how stepchildren's names are filed for easy access), cross-referencing of files is recommended. Cross-referencing refers to alerting the health worker that a file may be found under another name. For example, if Mrs. Henry Watts also uses her maiden name, Farideh Rahman, then a file insert into Henry Watts's file could state, "See Rahman, Farideh for Mrs. Henry Watts." Cross-referencing can be a simple but useful tool for finding and avoiding "lost" records.

LOCATING MISSING FILES

One of the most time-consuming and frustrating activities relating to medical records is locating a "missing" file. Ideally,

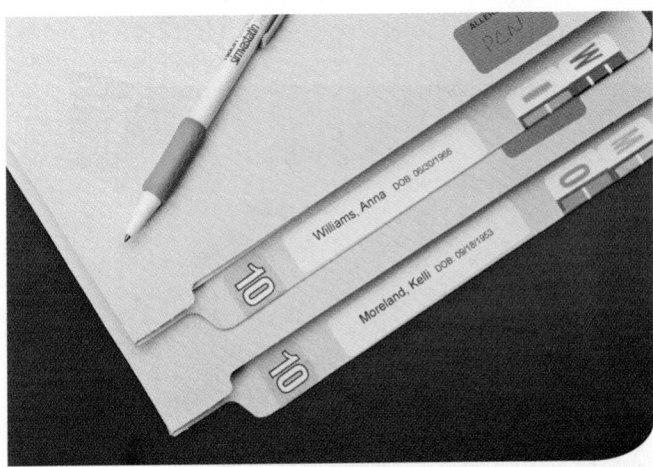

FIGURE 13-10 A color-coded record.
Source: Michal Heron/Pearson Education/PH College

procedure 13-5

LOCATING MISSING FILES

Objective: Locate misfiled records.

EQUIPMENT AND SUPPLIES

patient records

1. Begin by looking for a file with a sound-alike or look-alike name (e.g., Smith or Smits).
2. If the patient has a first name that might be considered as a last name (e.g., Samuel Jacob), look in the section where you would find Samuel.
3. If using a color-coded system, look for a folder that is out of place based on the color-coded label.
4. If using a numeric system, look for a transposition of numbers (e.g., 236984 for 263984).
5. Look for a transposing of letters.
6. Look for an alternative spelling (e.g., Keane for Kane).
7. Look at the folders that were filed before and after the missing record (e.g., pull out the schedule of all patients who were seen on the same day as the patient whose file is missing).
8. Look on the physician's desk and through in and out baskets. Also, ask other staff, such as the billing clerk, to examine his or her desk.
9. Ask others in the office to assist you. Many times a set of fresh eyes will spot the misfiled chart immediately.

everyone who takes a file from a cabinet should add that file name or number to a master file sheet. In addition, an out guide should be placed in the file indicating a record was removed.

If a systematic search takes place, the file can usually be located quickly. However, a single piece of paper that has been misfiled with other papers may not be located. In this case, the medical assistant will need to get another copy of the paper from the original source (e.g., a laboratory or radiology report).

The best way to avoid losing a file is to handle all records methodically and carefully. Procedure 13-5 provides steps you may take when looking for misplaced files.

TICKLER FILES

A tickler file is used to remind the medical assistant of an event or action that will take place at a future date. The tickler file contains patients' names and telephone numbers, dates when action or activities should occur, and actions to take. The tickler files should be reviewed daily so that actions are taken on time (e.g., tickler files can be used as reminders to call patients to set appointments, to pay certain invoices, or to send fees for the physician's license renewals). Figure 13-11 is an example of a tickler file, using a file drawer. Figure 13-12 illustrates an index card tickler file. See Chapter 9 for more on tickler files.

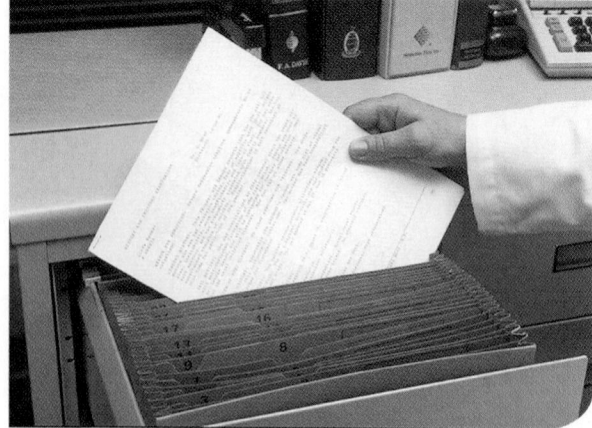

FIGURE 13-11 Tickler file using a file drawer.

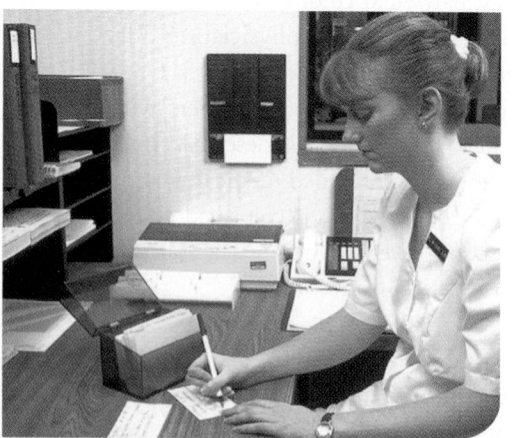

FIGURE 13-12 Index card tickler file.

Quality Assurance for Quality Medical Care

As discussed in Chapter 6, the primary goal of a formal quality assurance program (QAP) is to improve the quality of care so that there is no difference between what should be done and what actually is done. More physician offices and hospitals are moving toward standardization of care via evidence-based medicine and orders. This standardization helps to ensure that every patient receives the same care for a particular diagnosis.

Implementation of such a QAP requires the development of patient-centered criteria based on acceptable standards of care. An example of this is the formalization of discharge documents from hospitals: Every patient discharged from the hospital following an acute myocardial infarction (heart attack) should receive the same preprinted discharge instructions that should be documented as such in the patient's record; this helps prevent the possibility of something being overlooked, which may occur if the physician is writing individualized discharge instructions.

Maintaining a QAP will help significantly in the event of an audit or lawsuit. When documentation is consistent and complete with every patient encounter, it is less likely something will be overlooked, and it fares well with auditors.

INCIDENT REPORT

One means of documenting problem areas within the office or facility is through the incident report. (An example of a typical incident report appears in Chapter 6). This report should be completed for any unusual occurrence, such as a fall, error in medication dispensing, needlestick, fire, or patient complaint. The dual purpose is to document exactly what happened and to prevent another episode. Details on completing an incident report are usually included in every office's policies and procedures manual.

MEASURES TO ENSURE QUALITY ASSURANCE

Quality of patient care can be assessed from within the medical profession by organized groups of physicians. It is also monitored and assessed from outside the profession through governmental or insurance provider intervention.

The Joint Commission

The Joint Commission, formerly known as the Joint Commission on Accreditation of Health Organizations (JCAHO), headquartered in Chicago, Illinois, is a private, nongovernmental agency that establishes guidelines for hospitals and health care agencies to follow regarding quality of care. It is supported by representatives of the American Hospital Association (AHA), American College of Surgeons, American College of Physicians, and American Dental Association. In addition to forming guidelines for the operation of health care institutions, such as hospitals, ambulatory care facilities, and long-term care institutions, the Joint Commission conducts surveys and accreditation programs.

Joint Commission inspectors visit health care facilities and review patient medical records, medical staff organizations, and the general operations of the facility. Some survey and accreditation process indicators are mortality rate (the number of deaths in a given population), frequency of complication, nosocomial infection rate, and autopsy rate. Based on their assessment, the inspectors will issue either a full or a provisional accreditation report. The Joint Commission works with facilities to correct any deficiencies within a specified time frame.

The Joint Commission does not actually have authority or power to take punitive action against a physician or facility for poor treatment. However, the survey results of the Joint Commission are used by other agencies, that do have the authority to impose a sanction or penalty, such as the U.S. Department of Health and Human Services.

Occupational Safety and Health Administration

The Occupational Safety and Health Administration (OSHA) was established by the U.S. Congress in the Occupational Safety and Health Act of 1970 "to assure so far as possible every working man and woman in the nation safe and healthful working conditions." This act covers every employer whose business affects interstate commerce.

OSHA has the power to enforce federal regulations concerning the health and safety of employees. Every office and health care institution must be aware of OSHA recommendations and carefully monitor potential violations. For instance, the Centers for Disease Control and Prevention (CDC) has issued recommendations for a set of universal precautions that all health care workers must follow when dealing with hazardous materials. The CDC has authorized OSHA to enforce these precautions.

OSHA, in cooperation with other agencies, carries out research to establish basic safety standards. OSHA inspectors carry out frequent, surprise inspections of workplaces to see that standards are maintained. OSHA safety regulations include standards for exposure to noise, asbestos, toxic chemicals, lead, pesticides, and cotton dust. Violators of OSHA standards must correct the violations and pay fines if found guilty.

Since July 6, 1992, OSHA standards mandate that all health care employers must provide a means for protecting their employees from potential exposure to hepatitis B. In fact, every health care employee must be given the choice to elect or refuse the immunization series. If refused, the employee has the right to change his or her mind and receive the immunization series at no charge. All costs associated with this immunization series must be provided by the employer.

HIPAA and Confidentiality of Records

As the demand for both access and confidentiality of medical record information grows, how does the health care provider balance the competing, often clashing, interests? The laws relating to medical recordkeeping and access have been evolving in recent years.

The privacy provisions of the federal law, the Health Insurance Portability and Accountability Act of 1996 (HIPAA), apply to health information created or maintained by health care providers who engage in certain electronic transactions, health plans, and health care clearinghouses. The U.S. Department of Health and Human Services (HHS) has issued the regulation "Standards for Privacy of Individually Identifiable Health Information," applicable to entities covered by HIPAA. The Office for Civil Rights (OCR) is the departmental component responsible for implementing and enforcing the privacy regulation.

New rules require medical offices that maintain and transmit health information electronically to do the following:

- Provide reasonable and appropriate safeguards to protect the integrity and confidentiality of health care information.
- Train personnel to protect confidentiality of health care information.
- Provide policies and procedures on security and confidentiality protective measures within the medical office.

Medical information can be shared by a wide range of people, both inside and outside of the health care industry. Generally, access to medical records is obtained when the patient agrees to let others see them. Occasionally, patient medical information is used for health research and (in accordance with HIPAA) may be disclosed to public health agencies such as the CDC. Specific names are usually not given to researchers.

Releasing Medical Records

The physician owns the medical record, but the patient has the legal right of "privileged communication" and access to his or her records. Therefore, the patient must

PEARSON PHYSICIANS GROUP
Shania McWalter, D.O.
123 Michigan Avenue
Parker Heights, IL 60610
(312) 123-1234

RECORDS RELEASE   Date _____

To _____
                              Doctor

_____
                              Address

I hereby authorize and request you to release

to _____
                              Doctor

_____
                              Address

all medical records in your possession concerning any examination, diagnosis, and/or treatment rendered to me during the period from _____ to _____

_____
                    Signature of patient or closest relative

_____
                              Relationship

_____   _____
      Signature of witness   Address

FIGURE 13-13   A release form for medical records.

authorize release of his or her records and state in writing that the medical records may be released. An example of a release form is seen in Figure 13-13. Since the patient has access to his or her records, the patient may also request a copy of those records. Since some records are large and require excessive duplicating time and expense, the physician may charge a fee dictated by the state to provide this service.

Health care providers have specific procedures for handling and releasing medical records because of the confidential information contained in the records, as well as the federal and state laws concerning HIV, mental health, and substance abuse information.

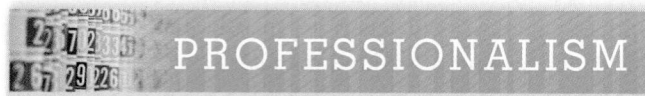

PROFESSIONALISM

THE LAW

Confidentiality of medical records must be maintained at all times. The medical record is the legal property of the physician. However, physicians and their staffs have a responsibility to treat the medical record with care because it contains documentation of the patient's medical history. Physicians must arrange for storage facilities to keep records of inactive or closed files since they could be needed at a future date for patient care or subpoenaed into court.

PERSONS AUTHORIZED TO RELEASE RECORDS

Generally, only a patient can authorize the release of his or her own medical records. However, there are some exceptions to the rule, and generally the following can sign a release:

- Parents of minor children
- Legal guardian
- Agent (someone you select to act on your behalf with a health care power of attorney)

Under some circumstances, a minor and not the parent must sign the release. If you have questions about who can authorize release of patient records, check with your office manager.

SPECIALLY PROTECTED MEDICAL INFORMATION

Federal law provides special protection for substance abuse treatment records. Some state laws also provide special protection for HIV/AIDS information and mental health records. These laws are meant to encourage people with these problems to obtain the medical treatment they need. To obtain a copy of the records or have them sent somewhere else, the patient may need to sign a form that specifically mentions this specially protected information.

DISCLOSURE WITHOUT CONSENT

Although medical records are confidential, at times they can be released without a patient's consent. In special cases, records are released to the following:

- Health care workers who have a need for the records to care for a patient

- Qualified people or organizations that perform services, such as data processing, medical record transcription, microfilming, administrative functions, or other such related services
- Qualified people or organizations for approved research and education functions
- Certain government authorities, as permitted or required by law, to investigate or regulate health-related issues such as child abuse, communicable diseases, and prescription drugs
- Certain lawyers and parties in a lawsuit if a patient's medical condition is an issue in the suit

Generally, strict rules apply to those who receive medical information. For example, they are often required to maintain procedures to protect the patient's confidentiality and prevent release of medical information and patient identity.

Storing Medical Records

Medical records may be stored in the medical office, if there is sufficient room, or in another office or building nearby. Medical record storage also may be outsourced to a business that specializes in managing and housing documents. Investigate the business to ensure that it is reputable and that the files will be safe and accessible. Either way, take steps to ensure that the files will be safe from fire, flood, or other damage.

Medical Transcription

Medical transcription involves translating dictated or written medical information and producing a permanent record into a typed format. The information can relate to a patient's office or hospital visit, a specific hospital report such as radiology, pathology or laboratory, or a manuscript for publication.

Absolute accuracy when transcribing is needed in order to ensure correct interpretation of the physician's dictation. And the same professional standard relating to confidentiality is necessary when handling transcription, even though the transcriptionist may never see the patient.

Medical records must be professionally prepared, following appropriate formats. They should be free of errors and correctly filed. Medical records are always subject to possible subpoena by a court of law.

MEDICAL TRANSCRIPTIONISTS

Transcriptionists are medical professionals who have excellent typing and grammar skills, knowledge of medical terminology, and a desire for accuracy and efficiency. The medical transcriptionist must understand words, know where and how to apply them, and have proper English grammar skills. This includes an understanding of etymology, phonetics, synonyms, acronyms, antonyms, homonyms, and eponyms.

Sound-Alike Words

Caution must be used when writing words that have the same or similar sound. When taking medical dictation off a recording device, such as a Dictaphone, it can be difficult to discern the term based on the physician's pronunciation. To compound the problem, many medical terms actually sound alike when spoken but have very different meanings.

Transcriptionists must take special precautions when transcribing tapes to ensure they have heard the correct terms. In many cases, the content of the material will determine which word is correct. For instance, *mastitis,* meaning an inflammation of a mammary gland, and *mastoiditis,* an inflammation of the mastoid bone in the middle ear, sound alike in pronunciation. However, the mammary gland in the female breast and the mastoid bone in the ear are located in different body systems and are not generally discussed in the same context.

Other terms, such as ureter and urethra, are organs located in close proximity to each other in a body system. Such terms must never be confused. When in doubt, always ask the dictating physician to clarify the term. You also may have to look up the exact definition of the word in a medical dictionary.

Ownership of the Medical Record

The medical assistant is frequently called on to explain the ownership of medical records and X-ray films. Although the patient has paid for the film, it is the property of the medical facility that performed the X-ray. Written reports prepared by the radiologist are sent to other physicians at the request of the patient, but the film generally remains in the original office. The reason for this is that if the film remains in one location it can always be accessed for future examination and comparison. Once it leaves the originating facility, it can be misplaced and lost.

Physicians can loan their films to referring physicians for further examination. The patient has to sign a release-of-records form for this to take place, but the film must then be returned to the original facility. Since films are a permanent record of the patient at a particular moment, they must be preserved carefully. It is possible, in some locations, for the patient to obtain a copy of a film. The patient might have to pay for the copy to be made.

As previously noted, patients may wish to view their medical records. If a patient makes such a request, you must allow them access unless the physician determines it may be detrimental, as may be the case in a mental health facility or with files related to the treatment of mental health disorders. Prior to allowing a patient to view his or her record, make sure either the physician or office manager has given approval. Never leave the patient alone with a record. The patient may write in the record, tear pages out, or become upset by information they see.

Retention and Destruction of Medical Records

From time to time in a practice, the question "How long should we keep medical records?" may arise. Although there are no definitive answers, the following can provide you with general guidelines:

- To be absolutely safe, all medical records should be retained forever. However, this is impractical in many circumstances. It is always a good idea to keep a patient's immunization records in case they need them in the future.

- The medical record is critical in a medical liability action, and its loss may considerably harm the physician in the defense of a claim.

- Each state varies somewhat on the legal time limits (statute of limitations) to keep records and documents.

In many cases, the statue of limitations is 2 years and begins at the point of discovery of damage and the connection between that damage and the treatment. In some circumstances, this could be many years later. Special rules apply when treating a child or an incompetent patient, in which case the time period is longer.

- Most states require that all patient records be retained for 2 to 7 years after the last treatment or 7 years after the patient reaches the age of majority (age 18 or 21 in most states), whichever comes last.

- The American Medical Association recommends keeping medical records for 10 years.

- In selected circumstances, you might consider saving the more complex records or those records with known serious patient problems for a longer period of time.

- The bottom line is there is no absolute answer. The medical assistant must be familiar with state laws.

If a physician cannot retain his or her patient records indefinitely, consideration must be given to the method of destruction. As with any office policy, a medical record destruction policy should follow a written procedure. The procedure should do the following:

- Outline the length of time records will be kept

- Define which records will be kept on site and which off site

- Designate a person to be responsible for deciding what to keep and what to purge

- Produce a log that details which patient records have been destroyed, as well as why, when, and how

- Provide a method of disposal (e.g., shred, pulp, or incinerate) that destroys all information in the record; (Patient confidentiality cannot be jeopardized because of an inadequate method of destruction. Many medical offices hire the services of a business that handles the destruction of medical records. That service must agree to abide by HIPAA guidelines.)

SUMMARY

Handling a patient's medical record requires an efficient system, which results in few missing or misfiled records. As a medical practice grows, it may be necessary to replace an alphabetic system with a numeric or even a color-coded system. Every medical practice needs a method for alerting staff when a file has been removed from the record area. A tickler system that is used faithfully can reduce the number of omissions, such as forgetting to remind the physician to renew a medical license. Medical transcription work can be a rewarding career for a skilled typist.

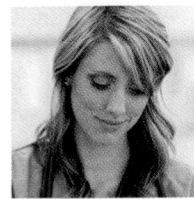

13 CHAPTER REVIEW

COMPETENCY REVIEW

1. Define and spell the terms to learn for this chapter.

2. Describe where you would find Emma Holmes' file. She has not been seen by Dr. Williams for two years and there has been no communication with her. Is this an active, inactive, or closed file?

3. Set up a tickler file system for your school assignments during this semester.

4. You are missing a file for Sean Roy. Discuss what process you would use to find it.

5. Mr. Crosby is angry and demanding that you give him his medical chart so that he can take it to another physician. How do you handle Mr. Crosby's anger and his request for his medical file?

PREPARING FOR THE CERTIFICATION EXAM

1. Which of the following would be first if filed alphabetically?
   a. Jacob James Jurgens III
   b. Jacob James Jurgens Jr
   c. Jacob James Jurgens Sr
   d. Jacob James Jurgens
   e. Jacob James Jurgens II

2. What is the second indexing unit in the following name: Mrs. Susan Donstead-Richards?
   a. Susan
   b. Richards
   c. Donstead
   d. Mrs.
   e. Donstead-Richards

3. To protect patient privacy, the most commonly used filing system is based on what method?
   a. alphabetic
   b. color coding
   c. numeric
   d. Social Security number
   e. tickler

4. South East Hospital Services would be filed as:
   a. Services South East Hospital.
   b. Southeast Hospital Services.
   c. South East Hospital Services.
   d. Services Southeast Hospital.
   e. Hospital South East Services.

5. Travis Willaims has been assigned the patient ID number 386492. To search for his file, you will look under 64, then 38, then 92. What system are you using?
   a. unit numbering
   b. straight numbering
   c. terminal-digit filing
   d. middle-digit filing
   e. service numbering

6. Which of the following would be indexed last?
   a. John Johnson
   b. John J Johnson
   c. Jon J Jonson
   d. John Jonson
   e. John Johnson II

7. If a patient has died, his or her medical record would be considered:
   a. dead.
   b. inactive.
   c. active.
   d. closed.
   e. terminated.

8. All of the following are sections in a POMR except:
   a. SOAP notes.
   b. progress notes.
   c. problem list.
   d. treatment plan.
   e. database.

9. All of the following would be found in the patient's medical record except:
   a. payment history.
   b. insurance information.
   c. date of birth.
   d. driver's license number.
   e. SOAP notes.

10. Which of the following agencies establishes guidelines for hospitals to follow regarding quality of care:
   a. OSHA
   b. Joint Commission
   c. HIPAA
   d. CDC
   e. HAS

CRITICAL THINKING

1. What type of updating would need to be done to Danita's medical record to reflect the recent changes since she has been married?

2. Danita would like to allow her husband Richard access to her medical information. Is this allowed? Explain why or why not.

3. Three months after their marriage, Richard is promoted to a new position within his company; however the position is out of state. Richard and Danita must move, causing Danita to find a new health care provider. How does this affect Danita's record status?

ON THE JOB

Marissa Lopez is asked to create a patient file and records for a new patient, Jonathan Schmidt. Please walk Marissa through each step of creating a new patient file, making sure that each component of the file is complete. Use the SOAP notes section of this chapter as part of your solution. Show how the patient's progress will be tracked by using POMR.

INTERNET ACTIVITY

Search the Internet for the newest legislation in your home state regarding the handling of medical records. Write a summary of the article, and discuss with your class whether the legislation adds to the efficiency of dealing with medical records or creates unnecessary obstacles.

MEDMEDIA

Additional interactive resources and activities for this chapter can be found:

On your student DVD: View applicable procedure videos on the DVD-ROM found in the back of this book.

MyHealthProfessionsKit.com: Test your knowledge of the chapter with games and activities. MyHealthProfessionsKit also includes resources, helpful links, and a Spanish audio glossary.

Medical Assisting Interactive: Practice your procedures as a medical assistant in this simulated doctor's office. This can be accessed through MyHealthProfessionsKit.com.

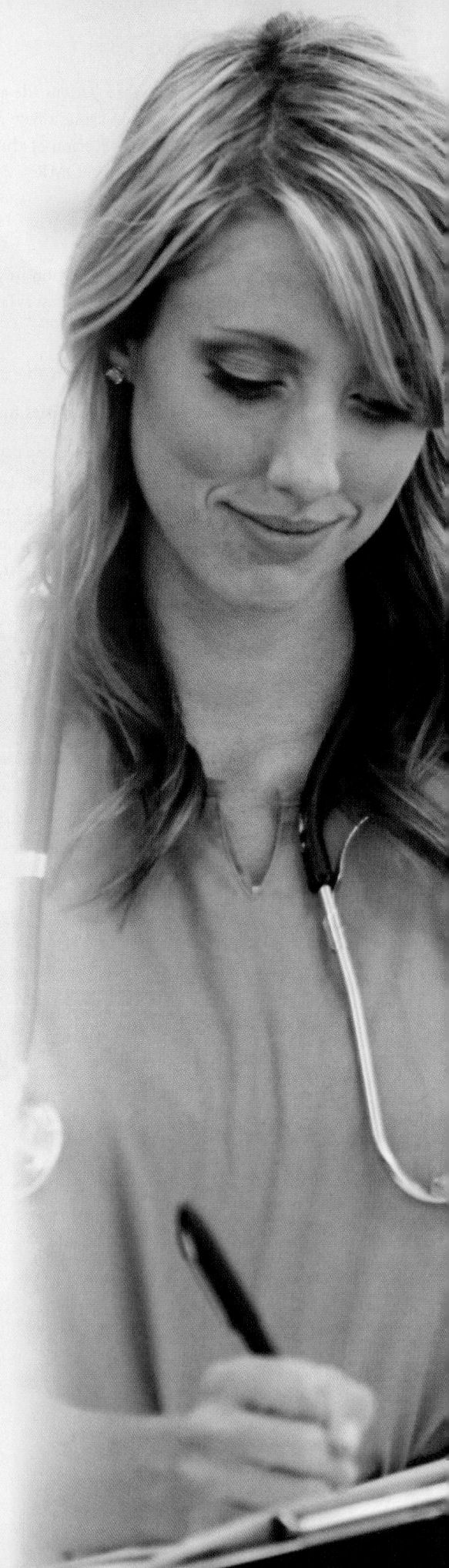

14

Electronic Medical Records

LEARNING OBJECTIVES

After completing this chapter, you should be able to:

- Define and spell the terms to learn for this chapter.

- Distinguish between the use of electronic medical records and paper medical records.

- Understand how to convert from paper to electronic medical records.

- Discuss the steps required to properly destroy a paper medical record after it has been converted to electronic format.

- Provide an example of HIPAA compliance with regard to the use of electronic medical records.

- Describe the use of personal digital assistants with electronic medical records.

- List the benefits of using electronic medical records.

- Explain the steps to correct a mistake in the electronic medical record.

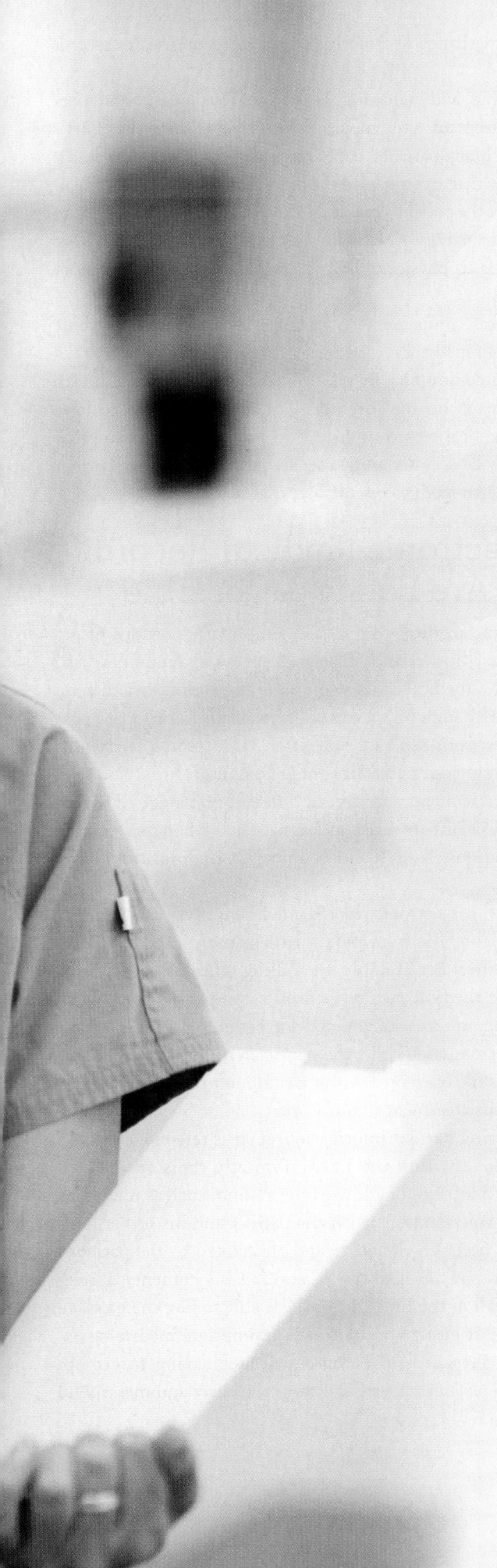

CHAPTER OUTLINE

CASE STUDY

Pearson Physicians Group is considering making the change from paper to electronic medical records. The physicians have assembled a team consisting of Lewis Jordan and Tania Washington to gather information relating to this possible change.

An **electronic medical record (EMR)**, sometimes called an **electronic health record (EHR)**, provides an electronic means of gathering, documenting, and storing information about the patient and the care received in the medical setting. Much of the same information found in a patient's paper chart is found in an electronic chart; however, electronic records are stored and accessed using a computer. The EMR/EHR are part of health care's future.

Although EMRs have been around since the Mayo Clinic began using them in the 1960s, ambulatory care has been slow to adopt the technology. However, with a greater understanding of technology, the EMR is gaining momentum. As today's health care providers strive to make health care safer and allow for efficient team communication, electronic records are playing a more prominent role.

In his 2004 State of the Union address, President George W. Bush stated, "By computerizing health records, we can avoid dangerous medical mistakes, reduce costs, and improve care." Shortly after this speech, President Bush outlined a plan to ensure that most Americans have electronic health records by 2014.

During and following Hurricane Katrina in September 2005, it became even more apparent how advantageous EMRs can be. Many patients' paper medical records were lost in the flooding that accompanied the hurricane. Inevitably, documentation of the patient's medical history was left for the patient to recall by memory. EMRs allow portability of information from physician to physician, hospital to hospital, and physician to hospital.

Several companies are working to make the electronic storage of medical records easier for the patient as well as the medical community by offering storage of electronic health information on the Internet. Patients may choose to have their medical records uploaded to a secure Internet site that can only be accessed with a secure password that the patient shares with medical doctors or hospitals.

Electronic Medical Records Are Easily Accessible

Electronic medical records are, simply, the portions of patients' medical records that are kept on a computer's hard drive or a medical office's computer network rather than on paper. Although physicians and their staffs must retrieve paper files from separate and often large rooms, electronic records are easily accessible on a computer. In large offices where patients may see several different providers, EMRs allow physicians to easily locate patients' laboratory results, consultations, X-rays, and examination findings from other providers.

By using electronic records, medical offices can access any one patient's file from more than one networked computer in the office. For example, the billing office might have the patient's medical record open on a computer screen while accessing information needed for coding a specific procedure. At the same time, the physician might have the same patient's file open on a separate computer screen while he or she inputs treatment notes.

Charting patient information, such as telephone calls, is easily done within the EMR. Typically the software will contain a section for adding information, such as telephone calls or conversations with the patient and his or her family that occur in the office and are related to the patient's medical care. When the receptionist documents a telephone call in the EMR, he or she is able to flag the message and send it electronically to the appropriate medical assistant or physician in the office without having to get up, pull the patient's chart, and carry the chart and message to the person.

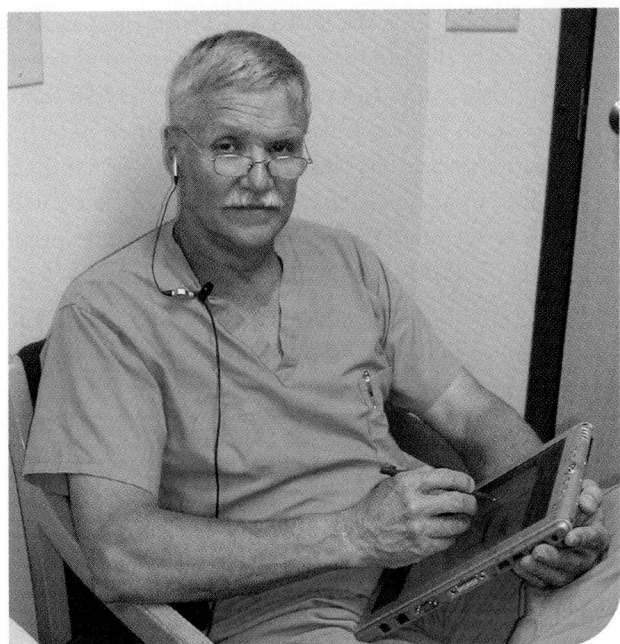

FIGURE 14-1 A physician uses a portable electronic tablet to enter patient data while in the examination room.

Many medical offices have computer terminals in each examination room, which allows medical personnel to add information to the patient's EMR, download test results, or research past medication records while the patient is in the room. In some offices, the physician or medical assistant uses a portable electronic tablet to enter patient data into the computer system (Figure 14-1).

How Does Paper Charting Differ from Electronic Charting?

With paper charting, the patient's chart is only available to one staff member at a time. The following example illustrates the steps an office using paper charting might take:

- The patient telephones the medical office and schedules an appointment to see the physician. The receptionist writes down the information the patient gives, such as name, address, telephone numbers, insurance information, and current complaint.

- Sometime before the patient's appointment, the receptionist or the billing office may call the patient's insurance carrier to verify the patient's benefits.

- The day before the patient's appointment, the receptionist may call the patient to remind him or her of the appointment scheduled for the next day.

- The day before the patient's appointment, the receptionist will prepare the new patient's chart. This is

typically done by gathering a paper file folder, color-coded labels to identify the patient's last name, and any other paper forms the patient and the medical staff will fill out on that first visit.

- If the patient is an established patient, the receptionist will locate the patient's paper chart and prepare it by adding the appropriate forms so it is ready for use the following day. It is possible the receptionist may not find the chart filed in the appropriate place. The chart may be in use by another staff member or physician, or it may be misfiled.

- When the patient arrives for his or her visit, the receptionist will give the patient the necessary papers to fill out.

- When the patient is taken back to the examination room, the clinical medical assistant will begin taking vital signs, such as blood pressure, pulse, and temperature, and begin noting this information by writing in the patient's paper medical chart.

- When the physician sees the patient, he or she will review the information the patient has filled out along with the information the medical assistant has filled out and will begin making notes of his or her own in the patient's paper chart. If the physician writes a

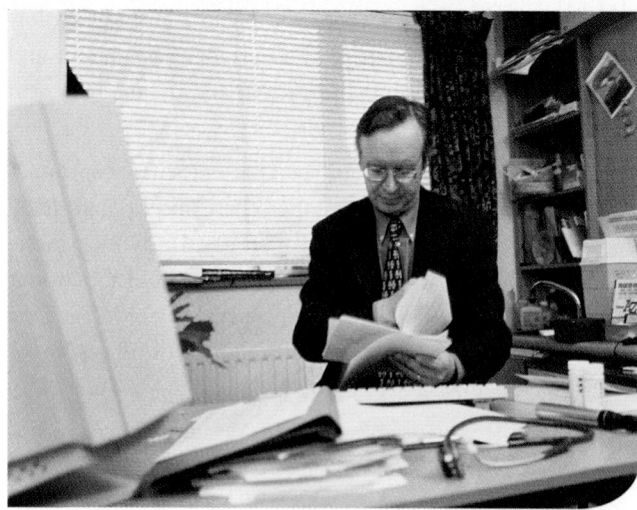

FIGURE 14-2 The physician will pull the patient's paper chart to review the results of tests alongside it.

prescription, he or she will note this in the patient's chart and will write the actual prescription on a paper form for the patient to take to the pharmacy. In some offices, the physician does not make written notes in the patient's chart and instead dictates his or her findings into some type of voice recorder. Those notes will be transcribed by a medical assistant or a transcription service, then added to the patient's paper chart.

• If the physician orders X-rays or laboratory tests, the patient's paper chart will be pulled once those reports are returned to the office so the physician can review the results along with the patient's chart (Figure 14-2). Figure 14-3 shows the workflow in a medical office using paper charts.

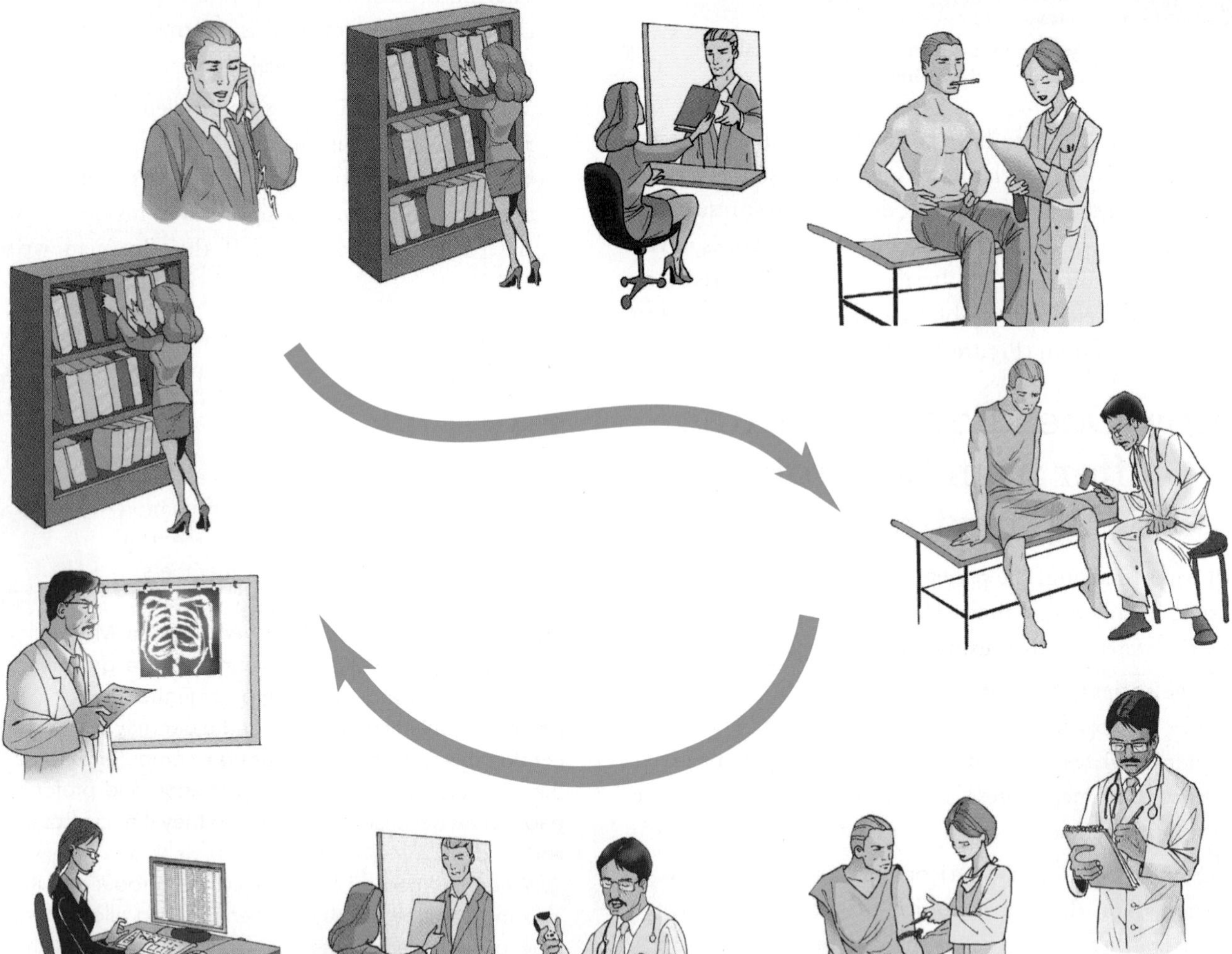

FIGURE 14-3 Workflow in a medical office using paper charts.

In contrast to the preceding approach to paper charting, the following example illustrates the steps an office using electronic charting might take:

- A patient calls the office to schedule a new patient appointment. The receptionist begins an electronic chart while she has the patient on the telephone, inserting information about the patient's telephone numbers, insurance information, and symptoms into the software program.

- Sometime before the patient's appointment, the software may be programmed to electronically confirm the patient's health insurance coverage. The software may also be programmed to call and remind the patient of his or her appointment the day before the appointment. Or, the software may set a reminder for office personnel to make this phone call.

- When the patient arrives in the office, he or she may be escorted to an examination room where a medical assistant will fill out the patient information form on the computer while the patient is present to answer any questions.

- The medical assistant will then take the patient's vital signs, entering all gathered information into the electronic medical record.

- When the physician comes into the room, he or she will review the patient's information in the EMR and make notes while interviewing and examining the patient. If a prescription is written, including faxing or e-mailing the prescription to the pharmacy the patient chooses, the physician will fill this information out in the electronic medical record. If any laboratory work or X-rays are ordered, the physician or medical assistant will fill this out within the EMR. If the physician wishes to give the patient any educational materials, such as information on reducing cholesterol, this information may be quickly printed from within the computer system, including making a notation within the patient's EMR that the information was given.

- If laboratory work or X-rays were ordered and completed, the physician will need only to review the results the patient's EMR on the computer, which may be done from any computer terminal within the facility (Figure 14-4). Figure 14-5 shows the workflow in a medical office using EMRs.

Making the Conversion from Paper to Electronic Medical Records

Although many health care providers and clinical support staff find that the process of changing from paper to EMRs format is time consuming, most would agree that once EMRs have been implemented, using the computer rather than writing in the patient's chart by hand saves a great deal of time.

The conversion from paper to EMR format is typically done over a period of time. Some clinics are able to use a scanner to scan documents from the patient's paper medical record to the electronic record. Other clinics may need to enter information from the paper chart to the electronic record manually. The process depends on the type of EMR software being used and the preferences of the medical staff (Figure 14-6).

PROFESSIONALISM

THE LAW

It is possible that the medical office where you work may be the only practice in the area that has converted to an EMR system. Other physicians in the area may have plans to convert to an EMR system but may still be using paper. When another physician forwards information such as a consult notice or laboratory results on a mutual patient, it will arrive in the typical form: on paper. To convert the information on paper into an electronic format to be used in your office, the paper must be scanned and entered into the EMR and flagged for the physician to review. Once the information is in the EMR, the original document may either be stored securely or shredded. Whether to store or shred is determined by the practice, and the associated policy will be in the office policies and procedures manual. If the policy states paper documents are to be destroyed, it is imperative that the document be shredded, either on site or by the company hired to accomplish this task.

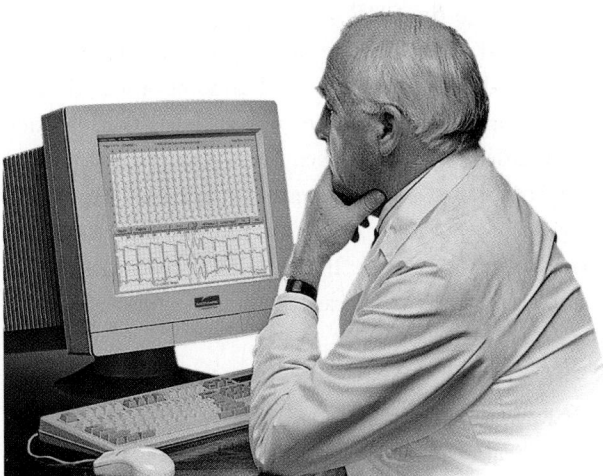

FIGURE 14-4 A physician uses a computer to access a patient's electronic medical record. *Courtesy of Midmark Diagnostic Group.*

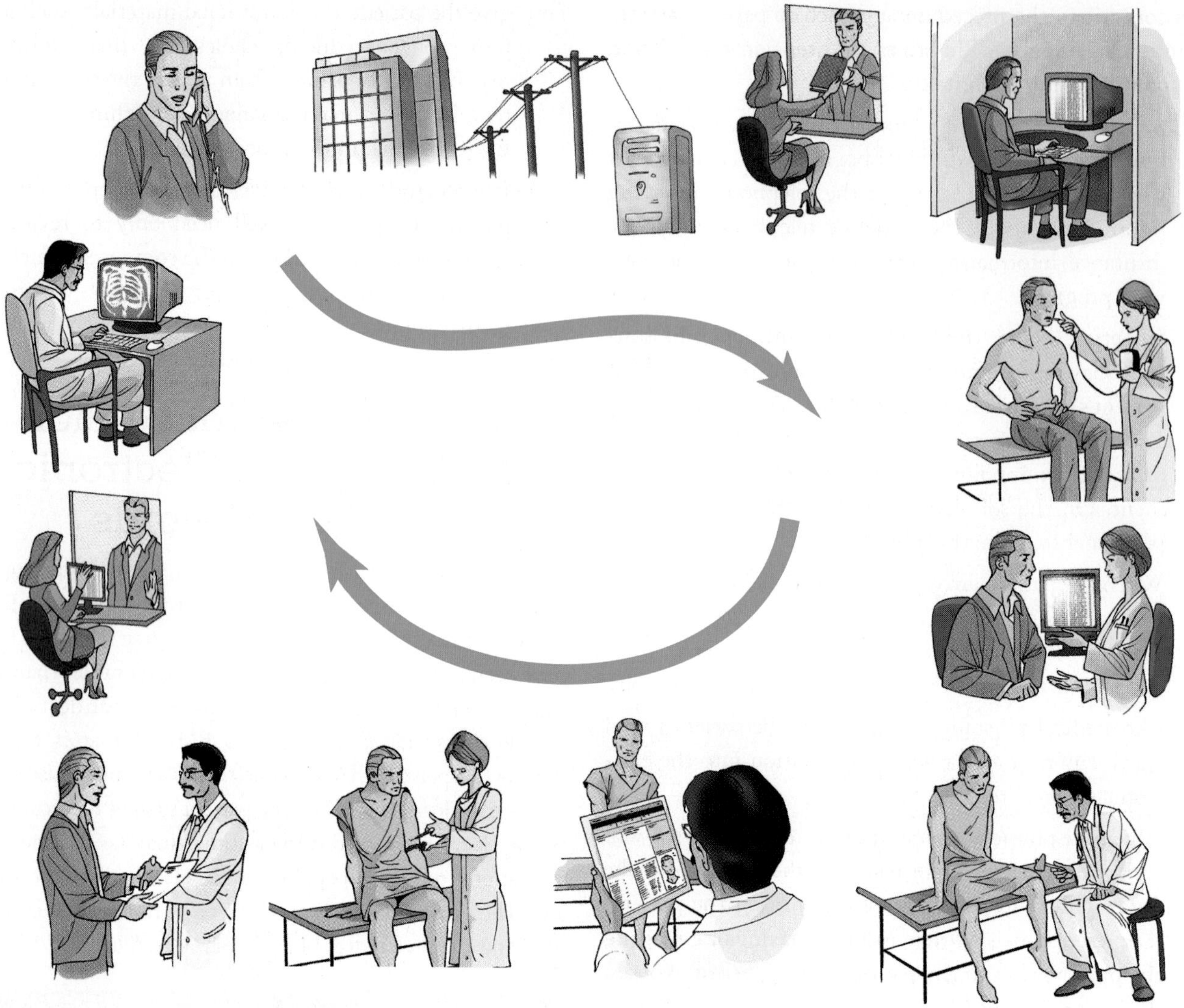

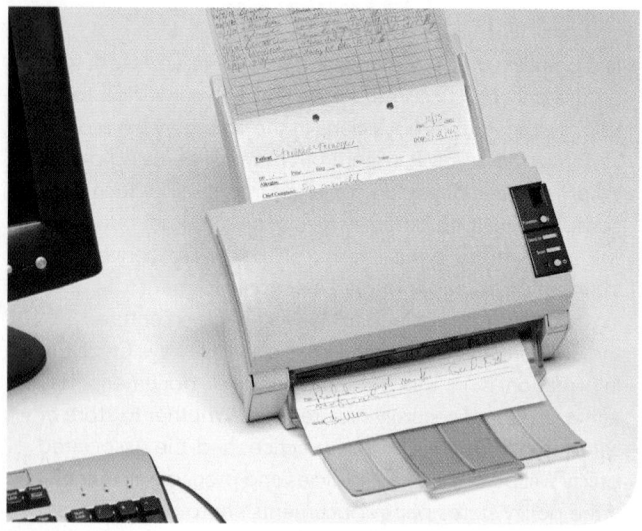

FIGURE 14-5 Workflow in a medical office using electronic medical records.

Once the information from the paper medical record has been transferred to the EMR, the staff may choose to destroy the paper record. This must be done by shredding the documents contained in the medical record. In some offices, the staff chooses to simply store the paper record in a secure location rather than destroy the file. When documents such as written reports or consultations from other facilities come into the office, these documents are typically added to the electronic medical record using a scanner. If the original document is no longer needed, it can be shredded to protect patient privacy.

TRAINING

Any software company that sells EMR software should supply the medical office with a certain amount of training for the staff to learn to use the equipment. This training should be attended by everyone within the office who will be using the software, including the physicians. In addition, a training

FIGURE 14-6 Some clinics are able to use a scanner to scan documents from the patient's paper medical record to the electronic medical record. *Courtesy of Allscripts LLC.*

manual should be supplied for use in training future staff members. Lastly, software companies that sell EMR software should supply the office with contact information to reach a technical support person in the event a question or concern with the new software should arise.

Electronic Medical Records and HIPAA Compliance

As with paper medical records, EMRs must be kept private. To ensure patient privacy and compliance with the **Health Information Portability and Accountability Act (HIPAA)** legislation, all computer users must have their own password to access the patient medical records. HIPAA is a legislative act that passed in 1996 and was fully enacted in 2003. Its purpose is to improve the access and portability of medical information and to decrease waste and abuse of health insurance. The overall goal of HIPAA is to simplify health insurance–related issues from an administrative point of view. With each person having login information, the software can track each entry or deletion and who made it. With paper records, it is not always obvious who last had a record and who made the latest changes if the user is not identified.

Each station must be logged off when the user is away from his or her desk, and computer screens must not be viewable by other patients while private patient information is displayed on the screen. Given the regulations in HIPAA legislation, computerized medical records are just as safe, if not more so, than paper medical records with regard to possible improper disclosure of information.

BACKING UP COMPUTERS AND ELECTRONIC MEDICAL RECORDS

To remain in compliance with HIPAA regulations, medical offices must use data backup systems to safeguard the information contained on office computer systems, including patient medical records. This is typically done on a daily basis, and in most offices the computer backup system is set to

work automatically. By having daily backup files, the medical office will not likely lose computer data, even if the entire computer system goes down.

Using Personal Digital Assistants with Electronic Medical Records

Depending on the software program being used, electronic records are available via a keyboard connected to a computer system, a stylus tapped on a notebook computer, or on a **personal digital assistant (PDA)**. A PDA is a lightweight, handheld, usually pen- or stylus-based computer used as a personal organizer. This device has many of the same functions as a full-size computer and has the added benefit of being small enough for physicians to carry with them from patient to patient. Most electronic medical records systems can be configured to work according to an office's specific needs. Box 14-1 lists the functions many of

Box 14-1 Functions of an EMR/EHR

The following can be documented in an EMR/EHR:

- Time-stamps on recordings
- Prescriptions printed or faxed to the pharmacy
- Patient education information given to the patient
- Digital photos of the patient and the patient's condition
- Electronically reported lab results, imaging studies, and other medical tests, as well as graphs of such data

- Graphs of height, weight, and blood pressure data
- Letters to or about patients
- Electronic data transmission to other health care providers

Capability to search electronically for patients with a certain condition or of a certain age or geographic location.

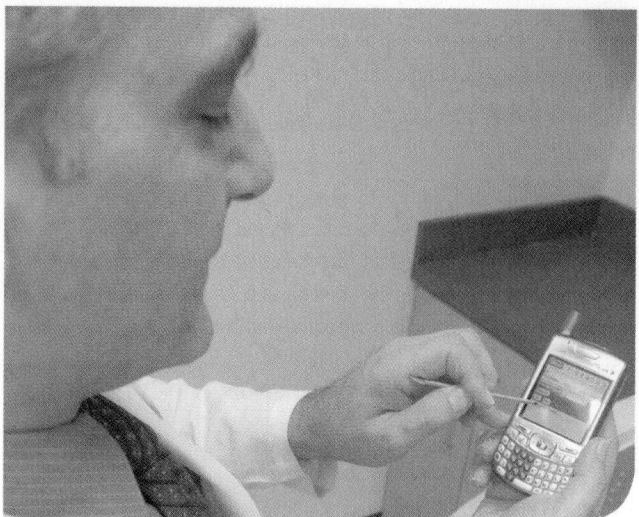

FIGURE 14-7 A handheld PDA.

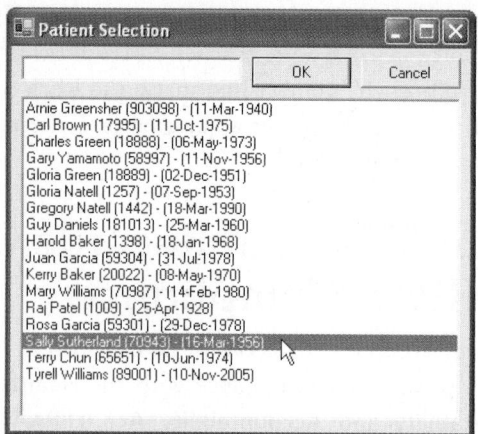

FIGURE 14-8 Selecting the right patient is easy with electronic medical records. *Courtesy of Medcin.*

these systems provide. One of the many benefits of such systems is the ability to access medical record information from many locations in the health care facility and to quickly search for and retrieve information in the patient's medical record (Figure 14-7).

Benefits of Electronic Medical Records

Using EMRs has additional benefits including electronic signatures, avoiding medical errors, saving time, facilitating patient health maintenance, immediate diagnostic test results, marketing, communicating, and online.

ELECTRONIC SIGNATURES

In offices where medical notes are dictated and printed for patient files, an **electronic signature** (an electronic version of a person's signature) or rubber-stamp signature may replace a handwritten signature. These offices must maintain on file a permanent record of the signer, as well as an original version of the signature.

Most EMRs will provide an electronic signature component that is based on the individual's login (user name and password). Once the entry is made in the patient's chart, the staff member or physician will click "Signature" and the entry will be electronically signed. Because the electronic signature is based on the computer login information, it is imperative that user names and passwords are not shared and are changed often.

AVOIDING MEDICAL ERRORS

Electronic medical records can be used to alert health care providers to possible medication reactions. This is especially helpful when treating patients who are being co-treated by several specialists. The software will typically have a built-in safeguard mechanism that alerts the prescribing physician to any contraindicated medications that a particular patient might be taking (Figure 14-8).

One of the most convincing arguments for converting paper medical records to an electronic format is based on patient safety. In 1999, the Institute of Medicine published a report called "To Err Is Human: Building a Safer Health System." This report stated, "At least 44,000 people, and perhaps as many as 98,000 people, die in hospitals every year as a result of medical errors that could have been prevented." One of the institute's recommendations was to move to EMRs. Their conclusions suggested that some medical errors are caused by **indecipherable**, or unreadable, handwriting, a problem that would be eliminated if health care providers made their entries electronically rather than in handwritten form.

Some states have enacted legislation to address the issue of bad handwriting and medical errors. In March 2006, Washington State passed a law that requires all prescriptions written by physicians to be electronically submitted to pharmacists or to be printed rather than written in cursive handwriting.

SAVING TIME

The time saved by EMRs may be better invested in patient care. Many health care providers believe they spend a great deal of time charting—far more time than they spend on actual patient care. With the cost of health care rising, it

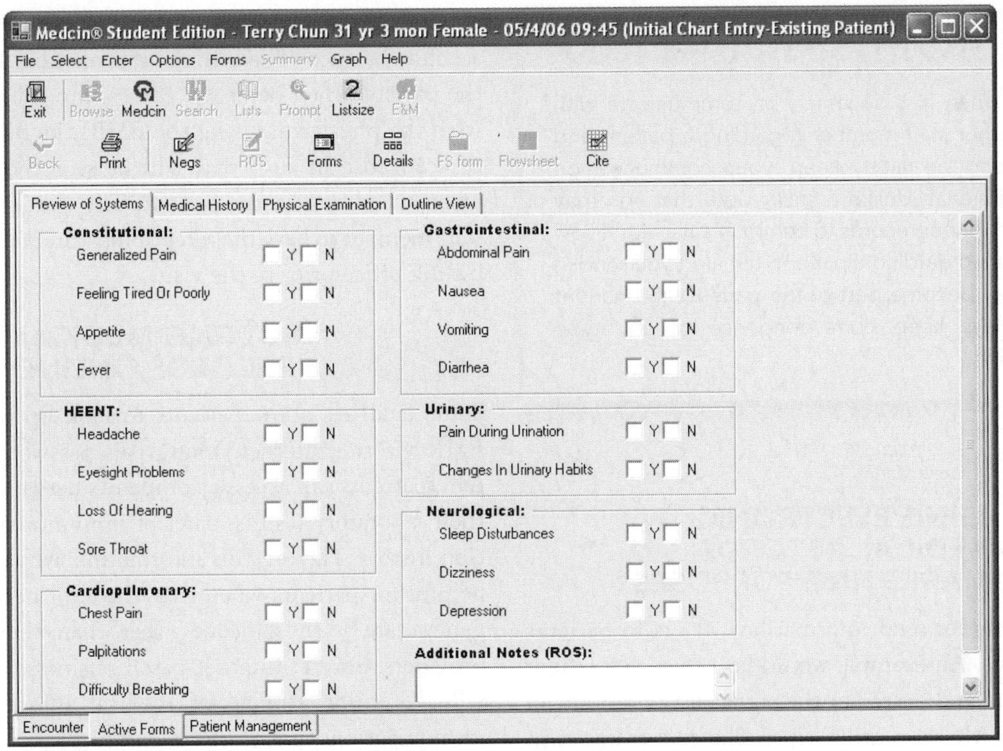

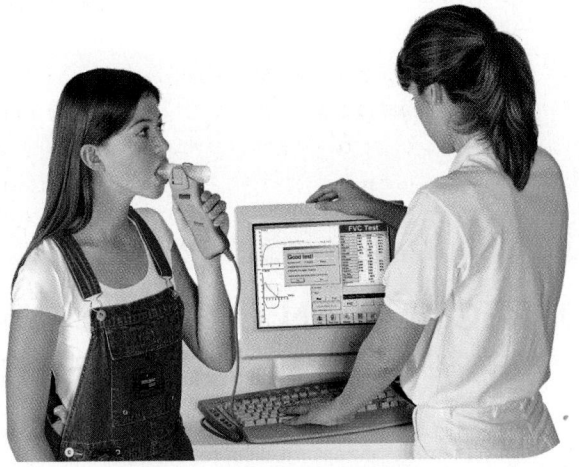

FIGURE 14-9 An example of an intake screen in an electronic medical record. *Courtesy of Medcin.*

makes sense to free up the health care provider's time while decreasing avoidable patient injuries (Figure 14-9).

Most EMR programs have drop-down menus that allow the user to choose information or symptoms from a preprogrammed list. For example, when the user inserts a diagnosis of "diabetes," the software may display a list of possible symptoms the patient may be having, such as excessive thirst or frequent urination. Many EMR programs also include lists of possible diagnoses for the physician to choose from based on the symptoms the patient lists; for example, if the patient complains of excessive thirst and frequent urination, the program may offer "diabetes" as a possible diagnosis for the physician to choose.

Electronic medical records allow medical staff to easily transmit patient information to patients' health insurance companies when requested, rather than having to photocopy the paper records and send them via the postal service. It is just as important to follow HIPAA guidelines for releasing medical records electronically as it is for releasing photocopies of the patient's paper medical record.

HEALTH MAINTENANCE

Many medical offices send reminder cards or letters to patients regarding the need for upcoming services. These are typically used to remind patients of the need for a colonoscopy, a mammogram, a yearly physical, immunizations, or well-child checkups. Using EMRs, the administra-

tive medical assistant can use the software program to print these reminders.

USING ELECTRONIC MEDICAL RECORDS WITH DIAGNOSTIC EQUIPMENT

With EMR software, the medical office can perform many tests in the office and have the results show immediately within the EMR. This can also be done with digital X-rays, Holter monitors, spirometers, and a number of laboratory tests on blood and urine samples (Figure 14-10).

FIGURE 14-10 A medical assistant performs a spirometry test using electronic medical record software. *Courtesy of Midmark Diagnostic Group.*

USING ELECTRONIC MEDICAL RECORDS FOR MARKETING PURPOSES

Many medical clinics send informational flyers to patients on a regular basis. An example would be a flyer that is sent during flu season and describes the signs and symptoms of the flu along with prevention tips. The prevention tips would be intended, in part, to encourage readers to come into the physician's office for a flu vaccine.

With EMRs, the medical assistant can create a list of patients according to specific parameters. For example, if the office has recently welcomed to the staff a physician who specializes in allergies, the medical assistant can create a list of patients who have been treated for allergies and can use that list to send a letter or an e-mail to patients to let them know of the availability of the new physician.

COMMUNICATING BETWEEN STAFF MEMBERS

At times one member of the medical office staff needs to communicate with another staff member about a particular patient. An example is a patient who has an outstanding account balance. The billing staff member may need to see the patient when he or she comes into the office for a visit with the physician. Using the EMR, the billing staff member can post an alert that will be seen by the receptionist when she checks in the patient. The alert allows the billing staff member to have the receptionist direct the patient to the billing office prior to the visit.

PUTTING MEDICAL RECORDS ONLINE

Some facilities allow patients to look up portions of their EMR via the Internet. Using this password-protected system, patients can access a company's network or intranet for their laboratory results, dates of immunizations, or medication history. Having this information available is especially helpful for patients when they travel or need to seek emergency care with someone other than their primary care providers. Several Internet-based businesses now offer individuals online storage of medical information, such as immunizations, medications, and surgeries.

Making Corrections in the Medical Record

As with paper medical records, medical staff entering data into the EMR may make errors in their entries. When this happens, the errors must be corrected as soon as possible. With EMRs, the steps to make the correction will depend on the software. Most often, the user will make the correction by crossing out the error and entering the correct information. The original entry will still be viewable, although it may show on a separate screen or with a line drawn through the entry. See Procedure 14-1 for correcting an entry in the EMR.

procedure 14-1

CORRECTING AN ENTRY IN THE ELECTRONIC MEDICAL RECORD

Objective: Appropriately correct an entry in the electronic medical record in an accurate manner following legal protocol.

MATERIALS
computer with electronic patient medical record software

METHOD

1. Identify the correct patient EMR where the error was made.

2. Locate the error within the record.

3. Using the rules associated with the software you are using, make the appropriate correction within the medical record.

4. Sign off on the changes as necessary, according to the steps required within the software program.
5. Verify that the change made is correct.
6. Save the changes made to the medical record before closing the patient's electronic medical record.

> Patient complains of ~~right~~ left leg pain.

FIGURE 14-11 Errors in the electronic medical record must be corrected as soon as possible. Most often, the user will cross out the error and enter the correct information, as shown in this example.

SUMMARY

Electronic medical records are gaining popularity over conventional paper files because they offer enhanced ease, efficiency, accessibility and portability. Once a paper medical record has been converted to an electronic version, the paper record may be kept in secure storage or may be shredded. Which action to take will be determined by the practice and outlined in the office policies and procedures manual. To avoid liability, medical offices must correct errors within the EMR using the accepted protocol. EMRs can save time by making such tasks as sending reminder postcards easier than performing these same tasks with paper medical records.

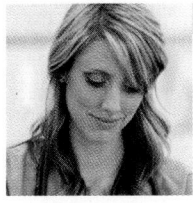

14 CHAPTER REVIEW

COMPETENCY REVIEW

1. Define and spell the terms to learn for this chapter.

2. Explain how the use of EMRs can help to avoid medication prescription errors.

3. Why would it be important for all staff members, even those with extensive computer experience, to attend a training session for new electronic medical records software?

4. Explain how a medical office might enter a letter from an outside medical facility into a patient's electronic medical record.

5. Explain how an electronic signature is used.

6. What is a drop-down menu?

7. How would using electronic medical records save time over using paper medical records?

8. Why should a medical office shred papers that contain patient information once those records have been entered?

PREPARING FOR THE CERTIFICATION EXAM

For the following questions, choose the best answer:

1. A PDA is often used in the medical office. What does *PDA* stand for?
   a. professional desk assistant
   b. personal digital assistant
   c. progressive digital assistant
   d. personal desk assistant
   e. professional digital assistant

2. Which of the following is an example of a reason the medical office would send post card reminders to patients?
   a. yearly physical examination
   b. mammogram
   c. immunizations
   d. 6-month follow-up exam
   e. All of the above

3. Using an electronic medical record system, the medical staff will typically be able to do which of the following?
   a. Locate possible contraindications with prescribed medications
   b. Allow two or more staff members to access the same patient file at the same time
   c. Save time looking for charts
   d. Fax medical records to other medical offices
   e. All of the above

4. Which of the following is a reason patients may want to access their own medical records online?
   a. View their current medications
   b. View the date of their vaccination
   c. Read their current lab report
   d. See when they are due for their annual exam
   e. All of the above

5. All of the following are means by which the physician can access the EMR except a:
   a. personal digital assistant.
   b. stylus tapped on a notebook computer.
   c. keyboard connected to a computer system.
   d. professional digital assistant.
   e. PDA.

6. All of the following are functions of an EMR/EHR except:
   a. electronic data transmission to other health care providers.
   b. search for certain types of conditions for a group of patients.
   c. ease of access by others.
   d. prescriptions printed.
   e. electronic graphs of lab results.

7. All of the following are benefits of using an EMR except:
   a. communicating between staff members.
   b. health maintenance.
   c. advertising purposes.
   d. putting records online.
   e. avoiding medical errors.

8. The most convincing argument for converting paper medical records to an electronic format is:
   a. easier for staff to use.
   b. patient safety.
   c. saves time.
   d. communication with staff.
   e. health maintenance.

9. How frequently should computers containing EMR information be backed up?
   a. every 1 hour
   b. every 4 hours
   c. every day
   d. every 2 days
   e. every week

10. Who said "By computerizing health records, we can avoid dangerous medical mistakes, reduce costs, and improve care"?
    a. Jimmy Carter
    b. George H.W. Bush
    c. Bill Clinton
    d. George W. Bush
    e. None of the above

CRITICAL THINKING

1. While gathering information, Lewis and Tania developed a list of pros and cons for converting to electronic medical records. What might have been included on their list?

2. The office has decided to make the conversion to EMRs. Once all records have been converted, what should be done with the original paper charts?

3. The office has recently received in the mail a typed consultation report from a local oncologist regarding a mutual patient, Yun-qi Yeung. What should be done with this report now that the office has converted to EMRs?

ON THE JOB

Dr. Jonas runs a private practice and admits patients and makes rounds in two local hospitals. He uses one type of EMR software in his private office and two other packages in the two hospitals. Not only must Dr. Jonas learn three software systems, but he also may at times be unable to move patient information between those systems due to incompatibility. What might Dr. Jonas do to address these issues?

INTERNET ACTIVITY

Using the Internet, research the different electronic medical records options available for the medical office.

MEDMEDIA

Additional interactive resources and activities for this chapter can be found:

On your student DVD: View applicable procedure videos on the DVD-ROM found in the back of this book.

MyHealthProfessionsKit.com: Test your knowledge of the chapter with games and activities. MyHealthProfessionsKit also includes resources, helpful links, and a Spanish audio glossary.

Medical Assisting Interactive: Practice your procedures as a medical assistant in this simulated doctor's office. This can be accessed through MyHealthProfessionsKit.com.

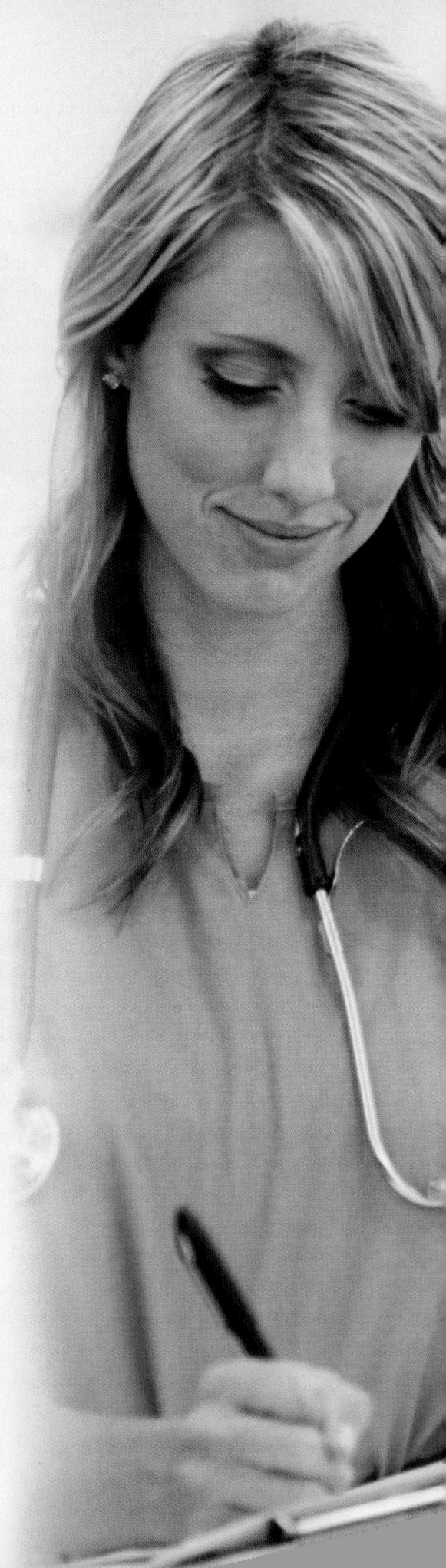

15

Fees, Billing, Collections, and Credit

LEARNING OBJECTIVES

After completing this chapter, you should be able to:

- Define and spell the terms to learn for this chapter.

- Discuss how fees are determined and be able to discuss this with patients.

- Describe the various billing methods and preparation of billing statements.

- Identify the patient information required at the time of registration and thereafter to maintain the records needed for billing.

- Explain credit policy.

- List the steps in the collection process and identify the legalities involved.

- Outline the procedures for aging accounts.

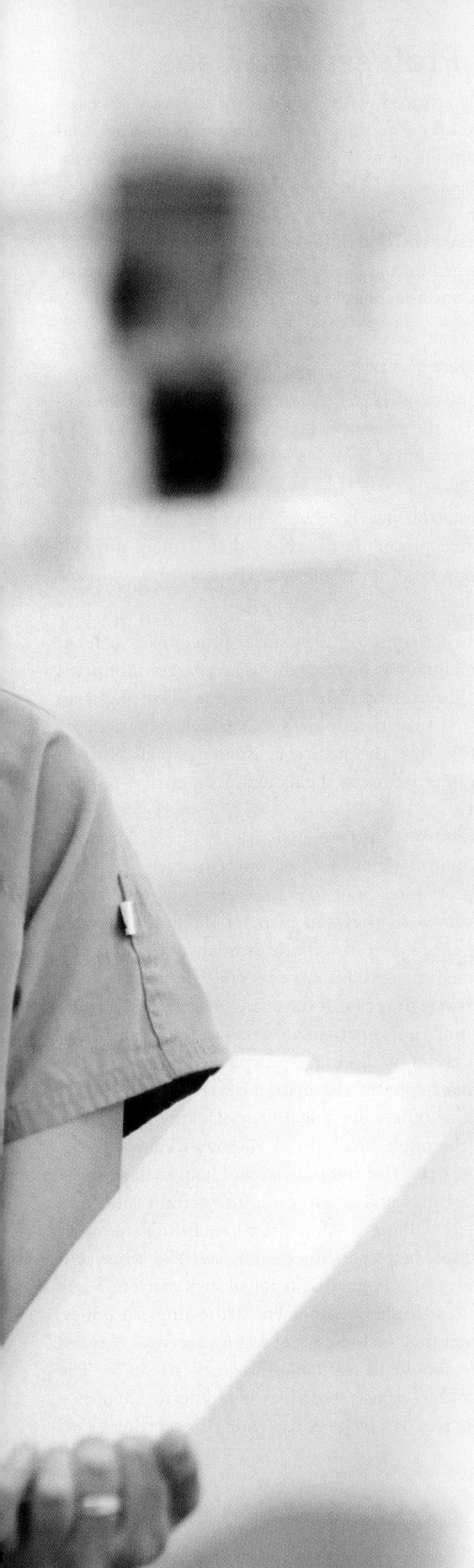

CHAPTER OUTLINE

CASE STUDY

Molly McConnley arrives at Pearson Physicians Group without an appointment at 3:45 P.M. She is complaining of radiating pain in her left leg and is visibly walking with a limp. Dr. Miller agrees to see Ms. McConnley because his last patient for the day has just checked out. While Dr. Miller is examining Mrs. McConnley, Samra, the medical assistant, begins to create a new superbill for her. Samra realizes that Ms. McConnley owes Pearson Physicians Group $328 for a procedure that was performed. No payment has been made to Ms. McConnley's account for the past 2 months.

Q uality service to the patient is the primary concern of any medical practice. However, revenue is also necessary to maintain a viable business. The process of setting up a fee schedule and extending credit, billing, and collection are important parts of any practice. To maintain a sound billing and collection system, the medical assistant must be aware of the importance that patients understand their financial responsibility to the doctor. The medical assistant should also offer assistance in setting up financial arrangements with patients.

Professional Fees

The fee is determined by the physician or the practice's partners as a result of taking into consideration the time and services involved, as well as the prevailing fee in the community. The economic level of the community, including whether the area is considered urban or rural, and the average fee charged will determine the prevailing rate fee.

Fees charged for medical services are referred to as **usual, customary, and reasonable (UCR)**:

- The usual fee is what a physician usually charges for a procedure or service.

- Customary refers to the fee charged for the same procedure by the majority of physicians with the same or similar training. This fee is also based on the socioeconomic and geographical area.

- A reasonable fee is what a physician charges for a modified procedure or service that is more difficult and requires more time and effort than a standard procedure.

Government-sponsored insurance programs, such as Medicare, maintain a record of the usual charges submitted for specific services by individual doctors. The physician will make the final determination as to what the fees for services will be. It is the medical assistant's responsibility to convey this information to the patient in a positive, responsible manner.

It is necessary to initiate a discussion of fees with patients and inform them of costs, office financial policies, and credit procedures prior to examinations and procedures being performed so they can plan for medical expenses. Patients are entitled to an accurate estimate of their obligations. The medical assistant must become comfortable with these discussions. It is best if the office financial policies are discussed prior to the patient's first visit. This can be accomplished through the initial telephone contact and by mailing a hard copy of the materials via the U.S. Postal Service. Many offices include financial expectations and policies in the office brochure. A thorough knowledge of the physician's practice and policies will help to handle any misunderstandings and would minimize certain collection problems later. Posted information regarding payment policies and fees helps patients become aware of office procedures. It also encourages discussion of such matters. Some medical offices display a statement addressing fee policy. The statement may include actual fees for services. A typed fee schedule should be available for quick reference. The medical assistant, if instructed by the physician, should be able to quote fees or a range of fees from this schedule. This

The patient must have a thorough understanding of office policy with regard to financial matters. The initial visit to the office should include information on fees, payment, and financial arrangements. This can be addressed in a patient information booklet or pamphlet given to the patient. Patients who will require surgical or other medical procedures should be made aware of fees, insurance allowances, and methods of payment. The patient must understand that he or she has the ultimate responsibility for all charges.

The informed patient will have a clear understanding of all obligations to the office and will be more likely to discuss financial arrangements. This mutual understanding helps to minimize the problems of collection for delinquent accounts.

schedule is approved by the physician and will be updated as needed. Medical offices should post in a prominent area for patients to view a notification that states, "Payment is due on the date of service."

Billing

Payment for medical services can be achieved in one of three ways. First is payment at the time of service, which is the preferred method (Figure 15-1). Recently, medical offices

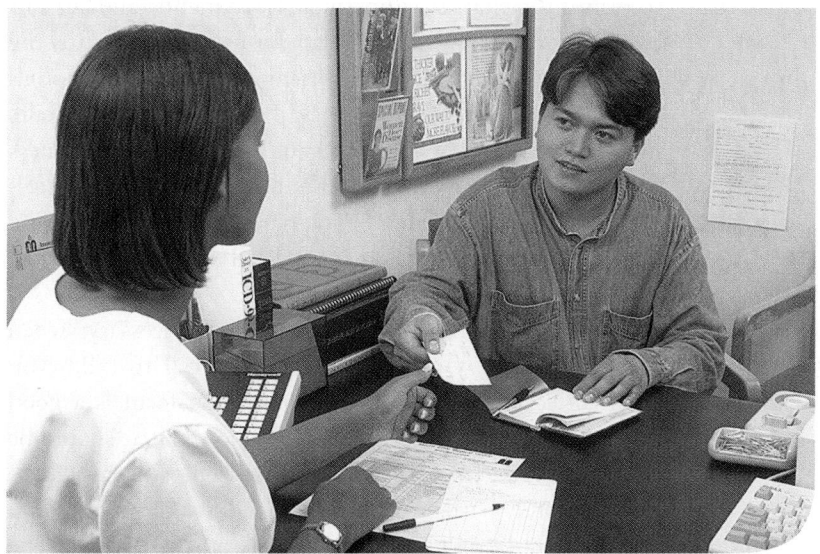

FIGURE 15-1 Payment at the time of medical service is the preferred method.

have begun to collect patient copayments prior to the patient being seen by the physician. A **copayment** is a predetermined amount of money the patient must pay for medical services at every visit, as determined by the insurance company. This helps to ensure that the medical office receives payment for services rendered. Payment at the time of services is the preferred method because it significantly reduces the costs of billing, including those related to the generation of bills, postage fees, and the use of human resources. The second payment method is billing the patient for services and extending credit. If credit is extended and it is determined that the patient will make set payments to the physician over four or more installments, the patient must sign a **Truth in Lending form** (Figure 15-2). This form must clearly state the amount financed, the finance charge, and the total of the payments. When no finance charges are to be assessed, that fact should be stated on the form. The original form is given to the patient, and a copy is retained by the doctor and must be kept on file for 2 years. The disclosure must be very specific, and the patient must sign it in the medical assistant's presence. The third type of payment, and usually the least desirable, is the use of an outside collection agency. Typically, this is used as a last resort because most collection agencies will keep a significant portion (sometimes up to 50 percent or more) of the amount actually collected. For example, the patient may have an outstanding balance of $1,000 that is sent to collections. The agency sends letters and makes telephone calls to the patient requesting payment. The patient forwards $500 to the collection agency, the agency will keep approximately half ($250) of the amount collected, and the remainder is forwarded to the office. The remaining $500 is written off as **bad debt**, an amount owed and not collectable.

The medical assistant must become familiar with health insurance coverage and the differences in the various plans. As health maintenance organizations (HMOs), individual practice associations (IPAs), and preferred provider organizations (PPOs) become a major influence in medical practices, the levels of benefits, copayments, and deductibles are important aspects of the fee and billing process. Patients can become easily confused about these matters; thus health care providers and their staff should be knowledgeable in these areas. See Chapter 17 for an explanation of HMOs, IPAs, and PPOs.

No matter which type of billing is used in the medical office, each patient must sign a

ANNUAL PERCENTAGE RATE The cost of your credit as a yearly rate.	FINANCE CHARGE The dollar amount the credit will cost you.	AMOUNT FINANCED The amount of credit provided to you or on your behalf.	TOTAL OF PAYMENTS The amount you will have paid after you have made all payments as scheduled.
%	$	$	$

Your Payment Schedule will be:

Number of Payments	Amount of Payments	When Payments are Due

Security: You will have a security interest in the following described property: (property description) _____

Late Charge: If any part of a payment is unpaid for 10 days after it is due, I may be charged 5% of the amount of payment.
Prepayment: (Scheduled Installment Earnings Method): If I pay off early, I may be entitled to a refund of part of the Finance Charge and I will not have to pay a penalty. **(True Daily Earnings Method):** If I pay off early, I will not have to pay a penalty.
Additional Information: See the contracts documents for any additional information about nonpayments, default, any required repayment in full before the scheduled date, and prepayment refunds and penalties.

Annual Percentage Rate	Finance Charge	Amount Financed	Total of Payments
The cost of your credit at a yearly rate.	The dollar amount your loan will cost you.	The amount of credit provided to you or on your behalf.	The amount you will have paid after you have made all scheduled payments.
10.16	71,855.17	71,600.00	151,455.017

FIGURE 15-2 Examples of Truth in Lending forms.

consent form that allows the medical office to bill the insurance carrier on behalf of the patient for services provided. Signing the form also grants the office permission to forward information regarding the patient's visit, including procedures and diagnoses to the insurance company if requested. This is a component of HIPAA regulations. The signed consent form should be placed on file and updated annually. Medicare requires specific wording on consent forms. For the most accurate wording, visit the MedLearn website. Each year the Center for Medicare and Medicaid Services (CMS) distributes a CD-ROM to health care providers that contains the updated fee schedule, general information on Medicare payment schedules, and payment policies. The CD also provides an immediate gateway to the MedLearn website.

BILLING METHODS

The faster you bill a patient or insurance company, the faster you will receive payment. Billing methods depend on the preferences and policies of the medical office. Billing may be performed internally, generated by the physician's office, or prepared externally by a billing service. External billing is used with large-volume billing. Internal billing can include the use of the superbill, ledger card, and follow-up mailed statements.

Superbill

The **superbill** also known as the **encounter form** or the **charge slip**, is the document generated by the medical office

that is a record of services for billing and for insurance processing (Figure 15-3). This document may be a two- or three-part carbonized form that performs several functions. It provides a comprehensive list of patient services, with respective diagnostic and procedural codes and fees, on which the physician indicates with a check mark the ser-vices that have been rendered. The superbill can be used to input computer information for billing, and it provides the patient with a record of the account activity (charges, payments, adjustments) for the day of service and, thus, can be used as a receipt. It also provides a record that can be used for insurance purposes. If the superbill is a triplicate form, the third copy can be kept in the patient's file. It is important that all superbills be accounted for at the end of each day as they are what the billing department will use to provide to the patient's insurance company all information and data regarding the patient's visit. When superbills are continuously lost or unaccounted for, it will have significant impact on the office's billing department and finances.

Ledger Card

Patients' monthly statements may be handwritten, computer generated, or photocopied. The **ledger card** is used to record the charges, adjustments, payments, and current balance for the patient and can be used to generate the monthly statement. The statement must be large enough to allow itemization of charges. Photocopied statements must be clear and legible and should be sent in a business envelope with a window through which the addressee's name is clearly visible. Envelopes should be imprinted with "Address Correction Requested" under the return address.

Accurate information is absolutely necessary when billing patients. Good records are essential to follow up with collections. The patient registration form is a good way to establish an information base; however, it should be updated every time the patient is seen. An inaccurate address for a patient will require additional work, and income may be lost while trying to find the patient. The

Pearson Physicians Group 312-123-1234

Patient Number	Ticket Number	Service Date	Prior Balance Pat
Patient Name		Gender	Ins
Address		Phone	Other
SSN	Referring Dr.		Total
Primary Insurance Co.	Policy/Group ID		Paymt
Secondary Insurance Co.	Policy/Group ID		Bal Due

Location

☐ ____________
☐ ____________
☐ ____________
☐ ____________
☐ ____________
☐ ____________
☐ ____________
☐ ____________
☐ ____________
☐ ____________
☐ ____________
☐ ____________

Cardiologist

☐ ____________
☐ ____________
☐ ____________
☐ ____________
☐ ____________
☐ ____________
☐ ____________
☐ ____________
☐ ____________
☐ ____________
☐ Other:

X	Code	Service	X	Code	Service	X	Code	Service
		New Patient			**Office Procedures**			**Diagnostic w/o Interp**
	99203	Limited/Simple (30m)		93000	EKG w/ Interp			**(Technical only)**
	99204	Comprehensive (45m)		93015	Stress Tread w/ Interp		93005	EKG
	99205	Complex (60m)		93040	Rhythm strip w/ Interp		93017	Stress Tread
				93307	2D Echo Compl.		93225	Holter Hookup
		New Patient Consult		93320	Doppler Compl.		93226	Holter Scan
		(Need Referring MD)		93325	Color Flow Compl.		93307-TC	2D Echo
	99243	Brief (40m)		93308	2D Echo F/U		93320-TC	Doppler Compl.
	99244	Full Consult (60m)		93321	Doppler F/U		93325-TC	Color Flow
	99245	Very Complex (80m)		ES	Stress Echo		93308-TC	2D Echo F/U
				BUB	Echo/Bubble/Doppler		93321-TC	Doppler F/U
		Established Patient					93880-TC	Carotid Doppler
	99211	Nurse Visit						
	99212	Very Brief FU (10m)			**Event Monitor**		**Phys**	**Interpretation**-Supervision,
	99213	Limited/Simple FU (15m)		93268	Loop- Non MC			Interpretation & Report Only
	99214	Comprehensive FU (25m)		G0005	Loop - Hookup - MC		93010	EKG Interp & Reortt only
	99215	Complex FU (40m)		G0007	Loop - Interp - MC		TR	Regular Stress Test--S, I & R
				93012	Chest Plate Tech - Non MC		NU	Nuclear Stress Test--S, I & R
		New Cons. 2nd Opin.		93014	Chest Pl - Interp Non MC		ES-26	Stress Echocardiogram--S, I & R
	99274	Moderate 2nd Opinion		G0016	Chest Pl - Interp MC		307	Echocardiogram 2-D
	99275	Complex 2nd Opinion					320-26	Doppler Echocardiogram
					Holter Monitor		325-26	Color Flow
		Home Health		93224	Holter w/ Interp Global		308	Echocardiogram 2-D F/U
	99375	Home Health 30 days					321-26	Doppler F/U
		Drugs:			**Other**		227	Holter Monitor - I & R only
	J3420	B-12 Injection		92960	Cardioversion		71250-26	UltraFast CT
	J1940	Lasix		93734	Pacer Eval - Single			
	90724	Flu (Dx V-04.8)		93735	Pacer Eval - Sngl w/ Prg		XXXXX	**LAB ORDERED**
	G0008	MC Flu Admin Fee		93731	Pacer Eval - Dual			(see attached sheet)
		Misc Rx ________		93732	Pacer Eval - Dual w/ Prg		36415	VeniPuncture (non MC)
	90782	IM Injections					99000	Specimen Collection (Lab)
	90784	IV Injections		99499	Review outside records			
	A4615	O2 Cannula		99080	Special Reports			

Next Appointment:
Return in: ___ (Wks) (Mo) (Yr)

Bl:

Before next appointment:
☐ Ekg ☐ Echo ☐ Doppler ☐ CXR ☐ Event Monitor
☐ TM ☐ Stress Echo ☐ CFD ☐ Holter ☐ Lab ________

Hospital Admission:
☐ Admit Cath
☐ Admit to ______________unit at:
☐ BAP ☐ WMC ☐CMC ☐ SHMC
☐ Other: ________________

Notes:

Cardiac Diagnoses

FIGURE 15-3 A superbill has multiple uses.

following information is needed to maintain a current billing file for each patient and should be included on the registration form:

Full name of patient (If the patient is a minor, then the full name and address of the parent or guardian who is responsible for the bill are also needed.)

Date of birth

Address (residence and mailing address, do not accept a post office box only)

Telephone number (home, work, and cell phone)

Occupation and employer (employer's address and telephone number)

Nearest relative (address and telephone number)

Insurance information (company name, address, and telephone number)

Copy of insurance card

Designated insurance identification number and group number

Copy of driver's license or other photo identification

If the patient and the **subscriber**, or the person who holds the insurance policy, are the same, this information only needs to be written once. If the patient is covered under a policy held by another family member (the subscriber), then the information regarding the subscriber must be obtained. It is possible that the patient may be the subscriber for his or her own policy (primary insurance) and also may have health insurance coverage under a spouse's insurance policy (secondary insurance). If this is the case, it is essential to verify primary and secondary insurance coverage at each patient visit. Once the patient's account has been established, the medical assistant must be made aware of any changes regarding patient information. A notice can be posted at the reception desk as a reminder to patients. The receptionist should also ask patients to state their name, address, and telephone number every time they are seen. If the receptionist asks the patient "Mrs. Smith, do you still live at 123 Fox Road?" the patient may not be listening and simply say "yes." Instead, if the patient is asked to state his or her address, you are more likely to consciously engage the patient and receive accurate information. This must be done out of the hearing range of other patients, as this information is considered confidential and is covered by Health Insurance Portability and Accountability Act (HIPAA) regulations. Procedure 15-1 describes how to complete a ledger card.

MANUAL BILLING

Manual billing was used by physician offices prior to the use of computerized billing. The entire bookkeeping system was completed by hand, and all billing was generated by the office. Most medical offices have converted to computerized billing because it is more cost effective and efficient.

and can be custom designed for the needs of the office (Figure 15-4). Database programs are used to collect and maintain patient information, procedure and diagnosis codes, and insurance company information. Software options make it possible to print statements, ledgers, and receipts. See Appendix VI regarding medical office software simulations.

THE BILLING PERIOD: FREQUENCY OF BILLING

Consistency in billing procedures is very important. The medical assistant must have a thorough understanding of office policy with regard to the timing of billing. When a billing date for an account has been established, it is extremely important not to vary the timing of the mailing statements.

There are two types of billing: once-a-month billing and cycle billing. Once-a-month billing requires that statements leave the office in time to reach the patient no later than the last day of the month. Cycle billing requires that certain portions of the **accounts receivable (AR)**, or money owed to the practice, are billed at given times during the month. For example, patients whose names begin with A through F would be billed on the first of the month, G through L on

However, some offices still use manual billing, so it is important that the concept be understood.

COMPUTERIZED BILLING

Computer software is available for internal billing purposes; however, many offices with regular, monthly, large-volume billing activity utilize outside computerized billing services. Many different computer programs exist

procedure
15-1

PREPARING A PATIENT LEDGER CARD
Objective: Prepare a patient ledger card with all pertinent information.

EQUIPMENT AND SUPPLIES
blank patient ledger card; black ink pen; completed patient demographic form; computer or typewriter

METHOD
If you are not using a computerized system, and instead use paper ledger cards, the same steps are followed as listed below; however, you will fill in the appropriate areas of the ledger card using a black ink pen instead of typing or keying into the computer.

1. Type or key into the computer the patient's name in the following format: last name first, first name, middle initial.
2. Type or key into the computer the patient's address, including zip code:

- If using copied paper ledger cards as patient bills, the patient name and address must be keyed as they would be for an addressed envelope.
3. Type or key into the computer the patient's telephone number, including area code. If applicable, document the patient's home, work, and cell phone numbers.
4. Type or key into the computer the patient's insurance information including name, address, and telephone number of the insurance company, subscriber name and ID, group number, and effective date.

If the previous ledger card has been filled to capacity, you will need to complete a new card following the preceding steps, but you must also forward the balance remaining from the previous card onto the new ledger card.

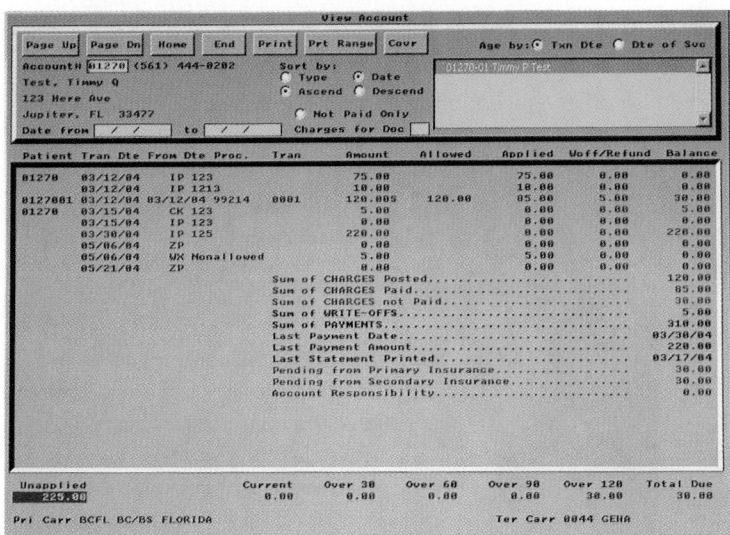

FIGURE 15-4 Computer programs can be customized to meet the medical office's billing needs.

the seventh, and so on. The advantages of cycle billing over once-a-month billing include the avoidance of once-a-month work overload and stabilization of cash flow. Thus, with cycle billing the medical assistant can handle routine duties including statements, rather than having to manage intensive billing responsibilities once a month. Also, by spacing the billing periods, more time can be given to each statement.

Patients must be made aware of the timing of billing statements. If a change is made, patients should be notified. This can be done by enclosing a notice of billing policy changes in each statement at least 2 months prior to the change.

PROFESSIONALISM

THE LAW

Financial information regarding the patient is confidential. All discussions, whether in person or on the telephone, should be conducted in an area that is out of view and hearing of other patients. Credit information about a patient is also confidential and may not be released without the patient's expressed permission. Statements outlining credit arrangements and interest charges must be in writing. If the responsibility for payment is to be handled by a person other than the patient, a signed statement by the third party is necessary to verify this obligation. In accordance with HIPAA, the physician is allowed to release a patient's outstanding balance to collection agencies.

BILLING THIRD-PARTY PAYERS AND MINORS

A **third-party payer** is a party or person other than the patient, such as an insurance company, responsible for paying the patient's bill. Patient registration must include information regarding all of the patient's medical insurance. Patients should be asked to provide all insurance identification cards, and copies should be made and kept in the patient's file. A signed **assignment of benefits** form, can be used by the office to ensure that insurance payments are made directly to the physician.

Bills for minors are addressed to parents or legal guardians (Figure 15-5). Minors, unless they are declared emancipated, are not responsible for bills; the subscriber to the primary insurance policy for the child is responsible for payment. The subscriber may not be the person who brings the child to the appointment, especially if the child has divorced parents. It is important to have accurate information in the child's chart regarding the financially responsible party.

Credit Policy

Payment at the time of service is the ideal method of collection. The medical assistants at the front desk must overcome any inhibitions regarding discussion of fees and payments. The final success of the practice may be due in part to the receptionist's ability to politely yet firmly ask for payment from patients. When patients call to schedule an appointment, inform them of office policies regarding payment. This is the first step in the collections process. Check with the office manager to verify the policy regarding patients who are not prepared to pay at the time of service. Depending on the type of practice and the reason for the

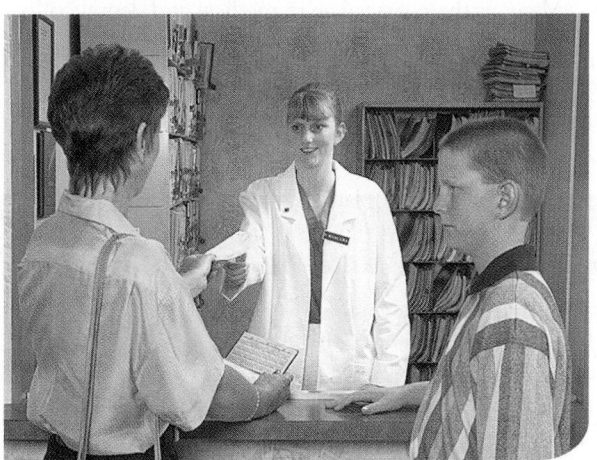

FIGURE 15-5 The subscriber to the primary insurance policy is responsible for paying a minor's medical bills.

appointment, if the patient is not prepared to make payment at the time of service he or she may be asked to reschedule the appointment. To avoid this practice, some offices will remind patients when they schedule an appointment that they will be expected to make their copayment prior to being seen by the physician, as discussed previously in this chapter. Other offices go as far as asking at the time reminder calls are made whether or not the patient will be paying by cash, check, or credit card.

Receptionists who do not feel comfortable asking for the patient's copayment at the time of service may think "What difference does a $20 or $30 copayment make?" But, if ten patients in 1 day were allowed to get by without making their copayments, it would have a significant impact on the AR balance and, potentially, the receptionist's future employment. If the office policy is to allow patients to still be seen without making their required payment, a billing statement should be prepared and mailed to the patient, requesting payment immediately.

The medical assistant must find out the policies the physician wants administered and consistently and fairly maintain them. A credit policy is an important part of any AR system.

Payment is often collected at the time of service, either before or immediately after the patient is seen by the physician. If it is anticipated that the patient will be responsible for a significant out-of-pocket amount, such as with surgery or similar procedures, credit arrangements often must be made. This is best done during the patient's initial visit prior to the time the surgery or procedure is scheduled. Never wait until after the procedure is completed to discuss payment arrangements. All necessary information should be gathered from the patient with regard to demographics, insurance, deductibles, employment, and signatures.

Credit bureaus operate as sources of credit data on individuals. Many of them specialize in medical and dental collections. They may supply data verifying a patient's employment, residence, and payment history. The medical office must be sure that it is working with a reputable credit bureau.

JUDGMENT CALL

Keri, the receptionist in Dr. David's office, is training a new employee to help out in the front office. Keri and the new employee will be responsible for making patient appointments and processing the monthly patient statements. Keri is aware that Mr. Wallace has a balance of $2,400, and after several attempts to communicate with him and his failure to respond to payment requests, his account is about to be turned over to collections. As Keri looks at the next day's schedule, she notices the new employee has scheduled Mr. Wallace for an annual physical. What should Keri do?

Collections

Every medical office should have a collection policy in place, as it is not advantageous to the office to have a haphazard method for collecting overdue accounts. The medical assistant must understand the collection policy of the medical practice and must administer it consistently and fairly according to the physician's directives. Most practices have a collection process in place that includes noting the patient's account status in his or her record. This is especially helpful if the patient calls the office to schedule an appointment or inquire about medication refills. Generally, once a patient's account is in the hands of a collection agency, most offices will terminate the physician–patient relationship using the proper notification procedure as determined in the office manual. Box 15-1 is useful in creating and maintaining positive collection procedures that will help deter many patients from going into collection status.

Box 15-1 COLLECTIONS

- Seek immediate payment.
- Use charge slips or superbills.
- Secure accurate patient information and update as needed.
- Inform the patient at the time of the appointment of possible fees and responsibility.
- Outline all fees and finance charges for the patient.
- Confirm third-party responsibility.
- Bill consistently following office policy.
- Institute collection procedures as needed with a personal interview, telephone calls, and letters.
- Follow up on all commitments made by the patient.

COLLECTION PROCESS

Accounts that are extremely overdue become very difficult and costly to collect. Patients must be educated on billing and collection procedures so that they have a clear understanding of what is expected of them financially. The patient information booklet given to new patients should have a section outlining office policy regarding billing and collection. This information also may be distributed in a formal financial policy document. Patients must be encouraged to openly discuss problems or questions they might have with respect to their bills.

The reasons why a bill is outstanding will vary. The following are some of the reasons:

- The patient does not feel that the bill is important.
- The patient believes that insurance will cover the bill.
- The patient is unable to pay (for various reasons).
- The patient has a misunderstanding about the fee.

The medical assistant must determine, in a timely manner, the reason that payments are overdue and then continue with the collection process. When all normal collection efforts have been exhausted and the account is slated for collection, the medical office can consider a "written off" policy for a designated predetermined amount that may be forgiven and becomes lost revenue. This is only considered when the cost of the collection efforts is greater than the designated predetermined amount. For example if the patient's bill is $80 and the cost of collection efforts exceeds $80, the billing office can refer to the office's policies and procedures manual to determine the specific threshold amount for collection services. Prior to any account being sent to a collection agency or writing off the amount, the physician must approve it.

DELINQUENT ACCOUNTS

Failure to collect delinquent accounts affects the medical practice in many ways. Patients who owe money may stay away from the office out of embarrassment due to their financial situation. Failure to collect delinquent accounts may imply guilt on the part of the physician as to the quality of care that the patient received. Ultimately, failure to collect delinquent accounts burdens the entire practice due to lost revenue.

AGING ACCOUNTS RECEIVABLE

It is extremely important to age all accounts receivable. **Age analysis** refers to the process of determining how long an account has been past due and then instituting the necessary collection procedures. Computerized systems will allow the medical assistant to print out an aging report with a 30-day, 60-day, 90-day, and longer analysis. This can be used to determine the next collection step. Manual systems may use a coding system to age accounts with various colors or flags to indicate the different ages. These may be attached directly to the patient's ledger card.

COLLECTION TECHNIQUES

The medical office may employ several methods of collection. Reminder notices, telephone calls, collection letters, and finally a collection agency may be used. The physician decides office policy regarding collection of overdue payments; the medical assistant has the responsibility to carry out the policy consistently and fairly.

A personal interview can be a very effective collection method. The patient who is seen in the office for an appointment and has an outstanding account is readily available for discussion with the office staff. This is the time to tactfully bring attention to the overdue account and to make arrangements with the patient for payment.

Reminder notices can be placed on bills when mailed to patients asking for their prompt attention to a past due bill. Other reminder notices may ask a patient to contact the office if there is a question about the past due bill. If no payment or contact is made, then a reminder letter is sent. It should not be a form letter but rather an individual letter that lets the patient know that his or her account is being reviewed and that there is concern about the unpaid debt. Tactful, professional telephone calls may also become part of the collection process and sometimes can be more effective than the letter. When these attempts have been exhausted, the account is often sent to the collection agency.

REGULATIONS

Some general rules should be followed when attempting to collect overdue accounts, and certain laws govern issues regarding collection, such as the **Fair Debt Collection Practices Act**. Office staff involved with billing and collections must be familiar with their particular state laws when applying collection techniques. Procedure 15-2 provides basic rules and guidelines to assist in the task of making collection calls. Violation of these rules could be an offense under the Fair Debt Collection Practices Act, which is a federal law that protects debtors from harassment.

TELEPHONE COLLECTIONS

A telephone call at the right time and in the right manner can be more effective than a letter. The medical assistant must be sure to make the call tactful, brief, and to the point. All conversation should be conducted only with the debtor.

procedure 15-2

MAKING COLLECTION CALLS

Objective: Place a call to a patient requesting payment.

EQUIPMENT AND SUPPLIES

patient's ledger card and/or financial record; demographic information; telephone; and black ink pen

1. Based on the collection policy of the office, determine how many days overdue the bill must be before the first call is made.
2. With the patient ledger card and/or financial record in front of you, review the account activity prior to placing the call.
3. Find a quiet area of the office in which to work while placing collection calls. Patients do not want their financial business shared, even unintentionally, with others, and background noise may be distracting.
4. Collection calls should only be made Monday through Saturday from 8:00 A.M. to 9:00 P.M. Do not call on Sundays or holidays.
5. Locate the patient's telephone number and place the call.
6. Once the call is answered, confidently ask to speak with the patient. Do not share information with anyone other than the patient or responsible party.
7. If the patient is unavailable, you may leave a message; however, the message should simply state the caller's name, who the message is for, and the telephone number where the caller may be reached.
8. When speaking with the patient, politely introduce yourself and ask if this is a good time to talk. If the patient

tells you it is not a good time, ask what time would be better, and make a note of that in the chart. Call back the patient at the stated time.
9. When speaking with the patient, be polite, project confidence, and state the facts and purpose of the call. Never threaten an action you do not intend to take.
10. Ask the patient if there is a reason for nonpayment. If the patient is able to provide a reason, document the response.
11. Ask the patient when you might expect payment and document that response as well.
12. Politely thank the patient for his or her time, and repeat the terms agreed upon.
13. Document the interaction in the patient's financial record.

CHARTING EXAMPLE

12/18/20XX. Spoke with Mrs. Ross regarding delinquent account. Patient stated she has recently lost her job and has been unable to keep up with her financial obligations. Mrs. Ross has agreed to make two payments of $20 each, due on the 1st of the month. Patient will contact the office if she is unable to make the payment. · · · · · · · · · · · · · · · · · ·
· C. Wood, CMA (AAMA)

A firm commitment to make payment should be obtained before ending the conversation. When you call and find the debtor is unavailable, leave only a message stating that the individual should contact the office.

COLLECTION LETTERS

The personalized letter has many advantages over the form letter. Patients who receive the personalized letter will feel that their account has been reviewed individually rather than that another form letter has been sent to every patient with an overdue balance. The letter may be inserted with the monthly statement. The letter should inquire why the bill has not been paid. There should be an offer to assist the patient with making payment arrangements. The letter must convey the message that action will be taken to resolve the payment obligation. Procedure 15-3 provides basic rules

and guidelines to assist in drafting a collection letter. Figure 15-6 shows an example of a reminder letter (see page 298).

SPECIAL PROBLEMS

Even with the best billing and collection system, problems may arise, thus making collection a challenge for even the most efficient medical offices. A *skip* is an individual who has a balance due and has moved without leaving a forwarding address. A skip is a collection problem that requires immediate action because the greater the amount of time it takes to locate the skip, the less likely it is that you will receive payment. Skips can be traced by checking the registration form to confirm addresses, calling all telephone numbers, and calling all references without divulging the nature of the call. "Address Correction Requested" on the statement's return envelope may help to get the patient's

WRITING A COLLECTION LETTER

Objective: Compose a collection letter requesting payment.

EQUIPMENT AND SUPPLIES

patient's ledger card and/or financial record; demographic information; computer; and black ink pen

METHOD

1. Based on the collection policy of the office, determine at what point the first letter is sent.
2. With the patient ledger card and/or financial record in front of you, review the account activity prior to drafting the letter.
3. Locate the patient's demographic information, including their address.
4. Using the computer, compose a rough draft of the letter, ensuring that proper formatting, grammar, and punctuation are used.
5. The first paragraph should summarize the reason for the letter and any payments the patient has made on the account.
6. The second paragraph should state the desired action of the patient. This may simply be to contact the office, or it may specifically state the expected payment amount and dates of the expected payment. Ensure that the letter is

written in a polite tone without any threats for lack of compliance.

7. The third paragraph, or closing paragraph, should thank the patient in advance for his or her prompt attention to the matter and should encourage the patient to contact the office.
8. Once the rough draft is complete, read through the document again, checking for spelling, grammar, and formatting errors.
9. Correct any errors, print, and sign the document.
10. Make a copy of the letter and place it in the patient's record.
11. Place the letter in an addressed envelope and mail it to the patient. In the patient's record, note the day the letter was mailed.

CHARTING EXAMPLE

3/29/XX. Letter mailed to Mr. Elders requesting payment by 4/29/XX. See copy of letter in patient record. · · · · · · · · · · ·
· J. Levy, RMA

---

statement delivered properly. The postal service may charge a fee for "Address Correction Requested," but it is a sound investment.

BANKRUPTCY

A patient who files for bankruptcy is protected by the court. When notice is received of a patient's bankruptcy, all collection attempts must cease and the medical office must file a claim for payment with the courts.

CLAIMS AGAINST ESTATES

When a patient dies, a bill should be sent to the estate of the deceased. Contacting next of kin will provide information regarding who is the administrator of the estate. It is important to follow-up on collection of bills to prevent any impression of physician's fault for medical care of the deceased patient.

STATUTE OF LIMITATIONS

Statute of limitations refers to the amount of time a legal collection suit may be brought against a debtor. This will vary from state to state and should be verified with state agencies. If you have aging accounts that are more than 2 or 3 years old, you should investigate the statute of limitations in your state before spending time, effort, and money to collect the debt.

USING A COLLECTION AGENCY

The collection agency used by the office should be chosen carefully. Reputable agencies will have references that can be checked and will readily discuss their collection methods. Further checks can be done with the Better Business Bureau and national credit agencies. If possible, interview the collection agency prior to choosing one and ask other medical offices which agency they use. The agency should

Pearson Physicians Group
Shania McWalter, D.O.
123 Michigan Avenue, Parker Heights, IL 60610
(312) 123-1234

Date

Patient Name
Street Address
City, State and ZIP Code

Dear Patient:

Your balance of $400.00 has been on our books for 18 months. Normally at this time, because your payment is long past due, your account would be handed over to our collection agency. However, we prefer to hear from you regarding your preference in this matter.

Please check one of the following options, and return this letter to our office:

☐ I would prefer to settle this account. Payment in full is enclosed.

☐ I would like to make regular weekly/monthly payments of $ _____ until this account is paid in full. My first payment is enclosed.

☐ I don't believe that I owe this amount for the following reasons(s):

_____

_____

_____

_____
patient's signature

Failure to return this letter will result in turning this account over to a collection agency.

Sincerely Yours,

Shania McWalter, D.O.

FIGURE 15-6   A reminder letter.

be professional and willing to discuss collection procedures with you.

Collection agencies charge for their services either by a flat fee per account or a percentage of the amount collected. In either case, the physician's office must be aware of the costs involved when using this method to collect past due accounts. Be certain not to include the patient's diagnosis when turning over an account for collection. This is a violation of the patient's privacy and HIPAA guidelines.

Once the patient is told his or her account is going to a collection agency, the account must, by law, be turned over to collection; otherwise notification could be considered an idle threat. After the account has been turned over, no further collection attempts can be made by the physician's office. The collection agency will need copies of patient information, such as itemized statements showing the dates and amounts of all transactions. (*Do not* include the patient diagnosis.) If the patient should contact the office after the account has been turned over for collection, the patient should be referred to the collection agency. Procedure 15-4 provides instructions on how to post a payment from a collection agency.

procedure 15-4

POSTING A PAYMENT FROM A COLLECTION AGENCY

EQUIPMENT AND SUPPLIES NEEDED FOR A MANUAL POSTING SYSTEM

Day sheet (a component of the pegboard system, used to list or post each day's financial transactions: charges, payments, adjustments, and credits); ledger card; pegboard; calculator; pen; collection agency payment

EQUIPMENT AND SUPPLIES NEEDED FOR A COMPUTERIZED POSTING SYSTEM

Calculator; computer; collection agency payment

STEPS FOR A MANUAL SYSTEM

1. After verifying the correct patient account to apply the payment to, align the patient's ledger card to the next line on the day sheet.
2. Enter the patient's name and previous balance into the appropriate column.
3. Enter the date of the payment, the name of the collection agency, and the amount of the payment in the appropriate columns.

4. Enter the amount of the payment on the deposit portion of the day sheet in the checks column.
5. Subtract the payment from the previous patient balance and record the new balance on the patient's ledger card.
6. If an adjustment is to be made to the account due to the collection agency fee, record the amount in brackets [ ] in the adjustment column of the ledger card. Enter it with the description "Collection agency fee."
7. Subtract the amount of the adjustment from the previous patient balance and record the new balance on the patient's ledger card.

STEPS FOR A COMPUTERIZED SYSTEM

1. Following instructions and training for the software program, locate the patient's account in the computer.
2. Verify that the patient account is correct and follow the steps appropriate for your software program to post the payment.
3. Choose "Collection Payment" to indicate the source of the payment.
4. Following the instructions and training you received for the software program, enter the amount of any fee due to the collection agency, if applicable.
5. Verify that the amount of the payment and the fee are correct, and save the changes in the program according to software specifications.

Accounting Systems

Accounting is the system of reporting the financial results of a business. The basis of accounting is the ability to make an analysis, statement, or summary about financial matters. Many physicians hire an accountant or accounting service to prepare tax returns and to prepare financial statements that are used to obtain bank financing. If the physician is in a partnership with other physicians, the accountant's financial statements will assist in dividing the earnings among the partners. Maintaining accurate financial records to be used by the accountant may be one of the medical assistant's responsibilities.

Bookkeeping is the process of managing the accounts for a business. Bookkeeping is a continual process and should be done on a daily basis. The medical assistant or office manager may assume this duty, or the medical practice could hire a bookkeeper. All receipts and charges should be entered immediately into a daily journal, day sheet, or record. Receipts, in duplicate, must be written for all money received. One copy is given to the patient, and one copy stays in the office file.

Bookkeeping is a precise skill requiring great attention to detail. Most offices use computer software for bookkeeping. However, the manual method is still used in some smaller offices and may also be used at times when the computer is down. See Box 15-2 for key points for accurate bookkeeping.

PATIENT ACCOUNTS

The medical office is unique as a business because its services are not always paid for at the time of delivery, as would be the case in some other businesses, such as retail. Patient accounts require careful bookkeeping. The bookkeeper or medical assistant must be sure that when insurance payments are received, they are correctly **posted**, or recorded, ensuring that patient's statements are accurate and that the physician receives payments for services rendered. Most medical offices are run on a cash basis, which means that the

Box 15-2 Key Points for Accurate BOOKKEEPING

- Use a black ink pen and clear penmanship. Do not use pencil.
- Keep the columns straight and decimal points lined up.
- Check all arithmetic carefully for errors, such as misplaced decimal points or errors in adding and subtracting.
- Do not erase, write over, or use opaque correction fluid. Make all corrections by drawing a straight line through the incorrect figure and writing the correct figure above it.
- Try to work in a quiet place each day without interruptions. Bookkeeping should not be done at the front desk while answering the telephone and greeting patients.
- Pay close attention to detail.
- Form all numbers carefully to avoid errors in calculations. Use care to avoid transposing numbers (e.g., 79 instead of 97).
- Always fix errors as soon as they appear. Do not carry the error forward in the account books.
- Double-check every entry.

charge for a medical service is entered in the financial records as income only when the payment is received. Many businesses, such as retailers and other merchants, use the accrual basis of accounting for income, which enters income when the service is rendered, even if a payment has not been received. For an example of the components of a manual patient billing system, see Figure 15-7.

The physician needs to be paid for the procedures done in the office. The medical assistant may need to ensure that patient accounts are in balance with financial obligations as described in Procedure 15-5.

ACCOUNTS RECEIVABLE

The AR ledger is a journal containing a record of all patients' accounts. Terms that relate to AR include the following:

- **Credit**—indicates that a payment has been received on an account. To credit an account means to subtract the payment from the account. A patient has a credit balance when an overpayment occurs. This may occur when either the patient or the insurance company pays more than is due. A credit balance may be noted on the patient's account either in red or by enclosing the amount in parentheses.

- **Debit**—indicates that a charge has been entered and added to the account balance. To debit an account means to add to that account's existing balance.

- **Adjustment**—indicates entering a change into the account record, such as a discount, write-off, or an amount not allowed by an insurance company (disallowance). A discount is entered as a credit since this amount will be subtracted from the total amount owed.

- **Balance**—indicates the difference between the debit (money owed) and the credit (money paid).

Accounts Receivable Insurance

Accounts receivable insurance may be purchased to protect against accounts receivable loss. The accounts receivable balance is reported each month, and ledgers are kept in a secure place within the office.

ACCOUNTS PAYABLE

Accounts payable (AP) are the amounts the physician owes to others for supplies, equipment, and services. The following are examples of AP expenditures in a medical office:

- Office supplies, such as paper goods, day sheets, appointment cards, scheduling books
- Medical supplies and equipment
- Equipment repair and maintenance, including housekeeping
- Utilities such as telephone and electric
- Taxes
- Payroll
- Rent

Typically, the largest AP account in the medical office is payroll.

Records relating to accounts payable include the purchase orders, the packing slips that come with the delivered goods, and the invoices requesting payment. The medical assistant, or bookkeeper, who is handling accounts payable payments must carefully document the payment made and place the check number and date paid on the retained invoice copy.

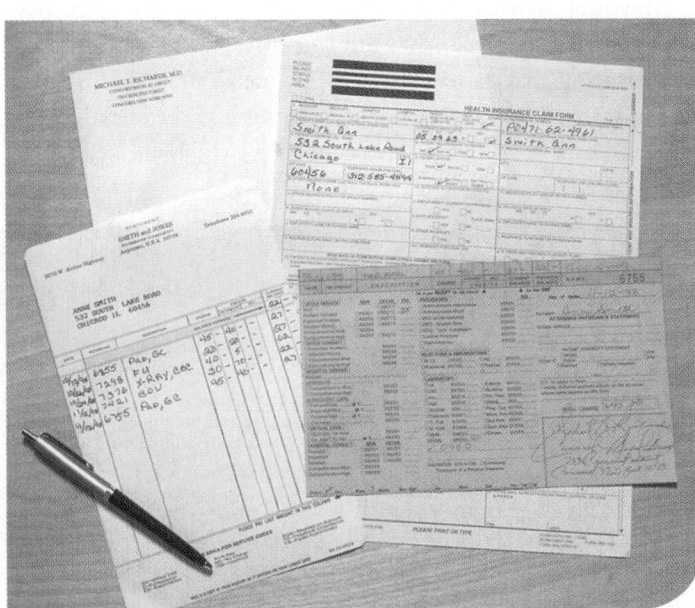

FIGURE 15-7 Components of the manual billing system.

PERFORM ACCOUNTS RECEIVABLE

Objective: Demonstrate skills to ensure that patient accounts are in balance and financial obligations are met in a timely manner.

EQUIPMENT AND SUPPLIES

data; computer or ledger; telephone

METHOD

1. Review the accounts receivable account aging.
2. Determine if third-party (insurance) payments have been received and posted to the patient accounts being reviewed.
3. Contact insurance carriers to resolve any outstanding payments, according to the facility policies.
4. Update the patient accounts with appropriate notes.

CHARTING EXAMPLE

12/18/XX. Contacted Marty Shapiro at United Healthcare. He stated that check in the amount of $169 for services rendered to patient was sent on December 12, 20XX. Have placed notice in tickler file to call again next week. · · · · · · · · · · R. Young, CMAS

Bookkeeping Systems

Most medical practices today use computerized rather than manual bookkeeping. Manual bookkeeping, however, is still used in many offices. Manual bookkeeping means that an item is entered by hand and is calculated using a handheld calculator. Computerized bookkeeping is most often utilized by medical practices for efficiency and accuracy. Many software programs are available for this purpose. Medical practices use two basic types of bookkeeping systems: single entry and double entry. The following are examples of manual bookkeeping.

SINGLE-ENTRY BOOKKEEPING

In a single-entry system, the bookkeeper or medical assistant records all financial transactions in the bookkeeping system just once. He or she makes a single entry. This is a simple, inexpensive system to learn and requires only three key records:

- Journal, or day sheet, which is also called the daily journal, or log
- Cash payment journal (See Figure 15-8 for an illustration of one type of cash payment record—a checkbook and stubs.)
- Accounts receivable ledger, containing a record of the money owed to the physician

Some offices also will have a journal for payroll records and petty cash (Figure 15-9). Petty cash vouchers are used to identify petty cash expenses (Figure 15-10).

DOUBLE-ENTRY BOOKKEEPING

In double-entry bookkeeping, a financial transaction is recorded in two different places. This system is inexpensive but requires a trained bookkeeper.

The double entry forces a balance since all accounting procedures require two entries to keep the accounting records in balance. For

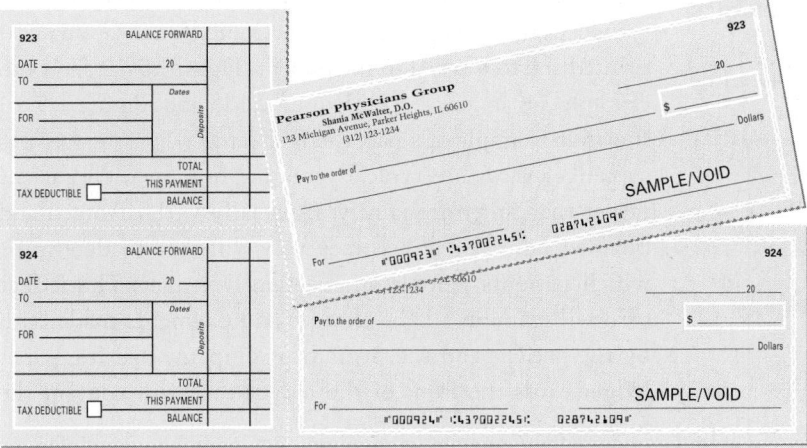

FIGURE 15-8 Cashbook and stubs are cash payment records.

Number	Date	Description	Amount	Office Expenses	Car	Misc.	Balance
	6-1	Fund established					75.00
1	6-2	Postage due	1.42	1.42			73.58
2	6-8	Taxi — (2)	8.00		8.00		65.58
3	6-10	Delivery charge	3.98			3.98	61.60
4	6-25	Supplies	11.62	11.62			49.98
		Total	25.02	13.04	8.00	3.98	
	7-1	Balance 49.98					
	ck #	790 25.02					
		75.00					

FIGURE 15-9 Petty cash record.

example, when a patient pays an outstanding bill, cash is recorded as an asset, and the receivable, which was the money owed or an asset, is eliminated.

Accounting is based on the premise that the assets of the business, less the liabilities of the business, equal the net worth of that business. This is expressed by the standard accounting formula:

$$\text{Assets} = \text{Liabilities} + \text{Net Worth}$$

The double-entry system ensures that the accounts are in balance.

Assets include everything owned by the medical practice, such as cash, bank accounts, money owed to the physician, equipment, and real estate. Liabilities are money the medical practice owes to its creditors, such as money owed for medical supplies to a vendor (supplier).

THE PEGBOARD SYSTEM

The pegboard, or write-it-once, system is not used as often as the computerized bookkeeping method. Computer software has replaced this style of bookkeeping in most physician offices, but a few offices may still utilize it.

The pegboard system is used to document patient bills and payments. The reason this system is sometimes called the write-it-once method is because a system of interrelated forms are placed onto the pegboard and used with the same master day sheet. It is an efficient system because the same

Amount $ 8.00   No. 2

RECEIVED OF PETTY CASH

June 8 20 XX

For Dr. McWalter — taxi
Charge to Medical Conference

Approved by   Received by
B.F.F.   Mary King

FIGURE 15-10 A petty cash voucher.

data are entered on all the forms at one time by using carbon receipts. The pegboard system is inexpensive as long as all employees are trained in its use. However, the forms manufactured by one company may not be compatible with forms from another company. See Figure 15-11 for an example of a pegboard system.

Required Pegboard System Forms

There are four components of the pegboard system:

- Day sheets
- Ledger cards
- Superbill
- Receipt forms

These forms have a carbon ribbon attached or are on special paper that will permit entering charges, payments, and adjustments onto the master day sheet, the superbill, and the patient's ledger card at the same time.

Day Sheets.   The day sheet, a component of the pegboard system, is used to list or post each day's financial transactions: charges, payments, adjustments, and credits. The day sheet, one for each day of the month, must be balanced at the end of each day. The balance from the previous day is carried over to the present day's day sheet as part of the balancing process. In a large or busy practice, more than one day sheet may be generated per day. The day sheet contains five basic sections that are described in Table 15-1.

Remember: The pegboard system, using the double-entry system based on the accounting equation, requires that each side of the equation must be balanced.

Ledger Cards.   Paper ledger cards are rarely used in modern office practice; however, computerized bookkeeping may use electronic ledger cards. An electronic ledger card may be printed and forwarded to the patient. Figure 15-12 shows an example of an electronic ledger card, and Figure 15-13 shows an example of a paper ledger card.

Ledger cards are typically maintained for each patient rather than an entire family. Especially with divorced and blended families, it becomes very difficult to determine which patients belong on the family ledger. The ledger card will contain all the charges and payments made both by the patient and the insurance company. If using paper ledger cards the front of the ledger card will contain the following:

Name of patient

Mailing address

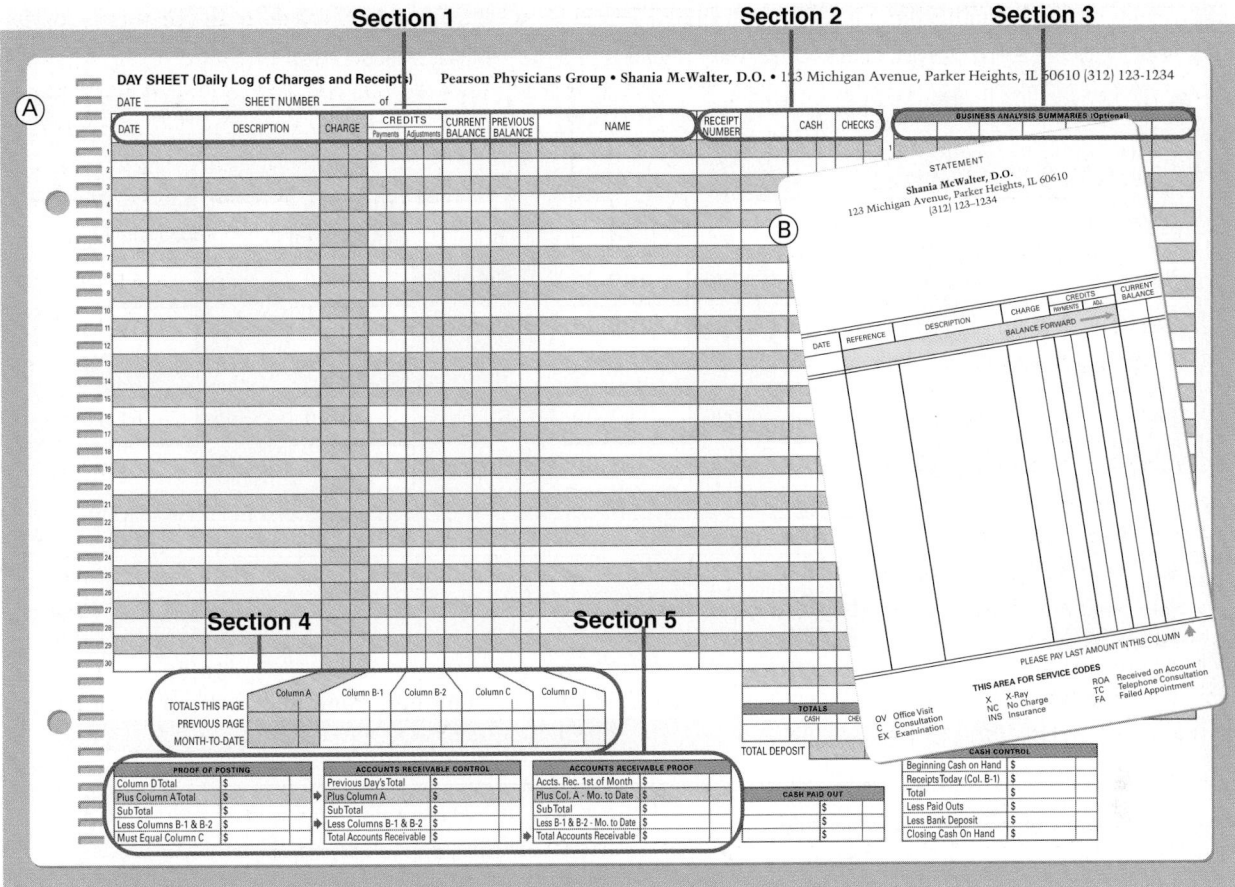

FIGURE 15-11 Example of a pegboard system.

Description of the activity (office visit, post-op visit, prenatal visit, injection, ECG)

Amount of the charge or payment

Adjustment(s), if any apply

Total balance due by that patient or by the patient's parent or guardian

TABLE 15-1 Day Sheet Sections

Section	Description
Section 1	The individual transaction, such as patient charges, are posted in this column. The ledger card, charge slip, and receipt forms are used when posting in this row and column. Included in this section are: • patient name. • description of transaction. • charges and credits. • previous and current balances.
Section 2	This is the deposit portion of the day sheet. Some forms actually include a detachable slip that can be used as a deposit slip for making a deposit in a bank account. A payment made by the patient would also be listed under the appropriate right-hand column (cash, check, insurance).
Section 3	This is an optional column and depends on the needs of the practice. For example, it can be used to specify the type of service that was provided (office visit, office surgery, hospital visit).
Section 4	This is the totals column/row. Each column feeding into the bottom section is totaled at the end of each day.
Section 5	This section is critical in checking that the accounts balance. It also keeps track of the cumulative accounts receivable figure owed by all the patients. This column is useful in determining, by looking at just one number, how much money is still owed to the physician.

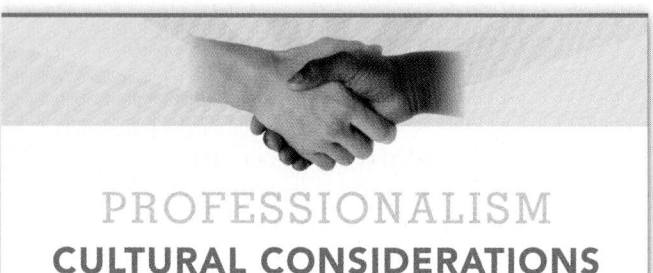

Columbus Scheduling/Columbus Corporation 0.00

File Edit Patient Billing Service Codes Clinic Daily Reports Forms Utilities Window Help

Ledger Card

Name	Mary A. Jones					Bill Type	1	Acct.	100	Doctor		10	Selected Ledger	Z

Curr	0.00	+60.	0.00	+120.	100.25	Surplus	0.00	Ins.	61.10
+30..	0.00	+90.	0.00	Total	100.25	End Bal	100.25	Pat.	39.15

Current Ledger

Curr	0.00	+60.	0.00	+120.	63.00	Surplus	0.00	Ins.	61.10
+30..	0.00	+90.	0.00	Total	63.00	End Bal	63.00	Pat.	1.90

Eff Date	#	Doc	CPT	Description	Bill	%	Ins. Bal.	Pat. Bal.	Amount	Total
01/30/20XX	2	1	67891	Balance Forward	P		000.00	000.00	000.00	375.00
01/30/20XX	3	1		Payment Check 00					66.00	309.00
01/30/20XX	1	1		Payment Check 01					198.00	111.00
01/30/20XX	2	1		Office Visit					50.00	161.00
02/07/20XX	1	1	45678	Cash Received	P		000.00	000.00	000.00	98.00
		***		END			***			63.00

FIGURE 15-12 Example of an electronic ledger card.

The back of the ledger card includes space for information regarding the collection process. This includes the name, address, and telephone number of the employer of the person responsible for the bill; the spouse's name, address, and telephone number; the name and address of the nearest relative; and insurance information. There is also a space for additional information, such as the name of a secondary insurer.

When using the pegboard system, the ledger card is placed under the superbill and directly over the day sheet, lining up the entry line on the ledger card with the next available space on the day sheet. It is important not to

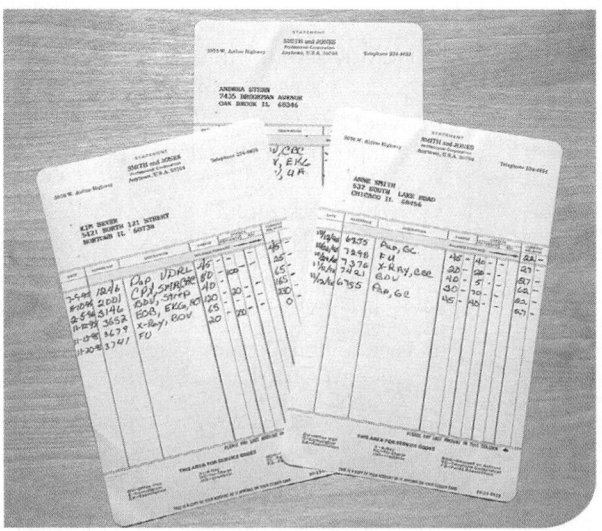

FIGURE 15-13 Examples of paper ledger cards.

miss any lines when entering information onto the day sheet.

Ledger cards can be copied and used as a statement that is sent to the patient. In offices using a computerized billing system, the bill is generated by the computer. Ledger cards are kept in a separate file container that is sized to fit them. This container is kept in an accessible spot close to the receptionist or person responsible for handling charges and billing.

Receipt Forms. A receipt form is used when a patient payment is made but no service is provided on that day. For example, a patient may come into the office or mail in a check to pay a bill. In some offices, this amount is entered onto the day sheet and ledger card, and at the same time the receipt form is completed for the patient. If the patient pays the bill with cash, a receipt is given. If the payment is made by check, the patient may use the canceled check as a receipt or may request a written receipt.

USING THE PEGBOARD SYSTEM

When using the pegboard system, every financial transaction, except the use of petty cash, is recorded on the day sheet. Each patient will have a ledger card on which individual financial activity is recorded. When the pegboard system is used, the patient's name, receipt number (the next chronological number on the day sheet), and previous balance are entered on the day sheet with a superbill attached when the patient arrives in the office. The superbill is then removed and attached to the patient's chart. After the patient is seen by the physician, the superbill is put back on the same line of the day sheet where it was originally written after placing the charge amounts next to the service rendered. Procedure 15-6 explains the pegboard system.

procedure 15-6

USING A PEGBOARD SYSTEM

Objective: Process patient accounts using the write-it-once system without error in posting or mathematics.

EQUIPMENT AND SUPPLIES

pegboard; superbills; new day sheet; ledger cards for each patient scheduled during the day; calculator

METHOD

1. Place a new day sheet and a strip of superbills on the pegboard, making sure they are fastened securely into the pegs.
2. Complete all the information required at the top of the day sheet (date and page number).
3. Carry balances forward from the previous day sheet and enter them in section 4. These include "Previous Page" columns A to D, "Previous Day's Total," and "Accounts Rec. 1st of the Month," which are entered into the "Accounts Receivable Control" and "Accounts Receivable Proof" boxes. Step 3 is necessary before the day sheet is ready to use.
4. Remove the superbill from the pegboard and clip it to the front of the patient's chart. The physician will enter the procedure performed that day on the appropriate line of the superbill, fill in the diagnosis, and sign the form after he or she sees the patient. The insurance code number is included on the superbill for ease of processing.

The superbill is then given to the receptionist by the medical assistant or the patient so that arrangements can be made for payment.

5. To record charges: Place the ledger card under the next superbill and turn back the top two pages of the superbill. Turn back these pages to correctly line up the space for the amount to be posted on the charge slip, and through to the ledger card and day sheet. Write the amount charged, pressing firmly and evenly to press through to the forms and day sheet.

6. To record payments: When the superbill is received at the front desk, the medical assistant or receptionist will enter the correct charge next to every procedure or service and place this total on the front of the superbill. The superbill is then again placed back on the pegboard, using care to line it up on top of the correct patient's name. The ledger card is then placed under the last page of the charge slip, aligning the first blank line of the ledger card with the carbonized entry strip on the superbill. On some types of superbills, you will turn back the first two pages of the superbill and enter the total charge and payment into the correct columns. Complete recording this transaction by

filling in all the information that the office requires in the far right-hand columns (e.g., method of payment such as cash or check).

7. To post adjustments: When an adjustment is made (e.g., a discount given to another health professional), the medical assistant or receptionist will enter the correct discounted amount into the computer system or subtract it from the balance due from the insurance company. If the adjustment is for nonsufficient funds, add the check amount and service fee charged by the bank to the patient balance. Always follow the facility's policy on adjustments.

8. To post collection agency payments: If the patient pays a collection agency and the collection agency forwards the money, credit that payment to the patient account and write "Collection agency payment of $ (amount received)" next to it.

9. If a credit balance then exists and the physician or office manager approves, issue a refund check to the patient.

If the patient makes a payment in person, then issue a receipt by placing a receipt form on the pegboard in place of the superbill. Place the patient's ledger card onto the day sheet. Enter the previous balance owed on the day sheet, credit the account and calculate the new balance after this payment. On the ledger card, post the date, patient's name, a description of the transaction (such as ROA, "received on account"), and the amount of the payment.

If a payment is made through the mail, a receipt is not sent. The amount credited to the account will appear on the next bill sent to the patient.

ADJUSTMENTS

Adjustments are any changes made that affect the patient's balance. They can occur when the physician reduces a fee or agrees to write off a portion of the charge and accept the insurance payment as full payment. For example, if the physician has charged $1,500 for a surgical procedure and agrees to accept the insurance payment of $1,200 as payment in full, then an adjustment is made for $300. The $300 appears in the adjustment column and is subtracted from the previous balance to indicate that $1,200 is now currently owed. If the $300 was not added to the adjustment column, the totals in section 4 on the balance sheet would not balance. An adjustment or correction also has to be made to correct an error in posting. See the following charting example:

11/12/20XX. Refunded $49 to patient for overpayment.
. . . . C. Baker, CMA (AAMA)

BALANCING THE DAY SHEETS

To ensure that the accounts and entries are correct, the day sheet(s) must be balanced at the end of the day. Use a calculator to balance day sheets, and always double-check each total. When balancing the day sheet, use a calculator with a paper tape, if possible. The tape can be used to search for calculation errors if the figures do not balance.

When errors in posting are corrected, the corrections should be made in the same column as the original posting (Table 15-2).

The steps for balancing the day sheets are presented in Table 15-3.

Accounts Receivable Control

It is important to keep a running record of all money owed to the physician (accounts receivable), and this is a figure most physicians are very interested in knowing. Some physicians will ask on a daily basis what the AR is. To make sure

TABLE 15-2 Correcting Posting Errors

Date	Description	Debit	Credit Payments	Adjustments	Balance
06/19/XX	OV	25.00			25.00
06/19/XX	Error in pstg	(25.00)			0

TABLE 15-3 Balancing the Day Sheets

1. Total columns A, B1, B2, C, and D and place the total for each column in the boxes marked "Totals This Page." These column totals then must be added to numbers brought forward and entered into the "Previous Page" column. This will provide the "Month to Date" total. "Month to Date" totals are important since they indicate all the credits, charges, and transactions that have occurred from the first day of the month to the present day.

2. The "Proof of Posting" box is used to ensure that all entries and the totals columns are correct. The numbers used to calculate this figure are taken from the "Totals This Page" column box.
   a. Enter the amount from today's column D total, which is the sum of the previous balances, in the appropriate box.
   b. Place the total for column A, which represents all the charges for this day, in the appropriate box ("Plus Column A Total"), and create a subtotal by adding column D and column A totals.
   c. Add columns B1 and B2, which are both credit columns (payments and adjustments), then enter this amount in the box "Less Columns B1 and B2." This amount will then be subtracted (minus) from the subtotal of column D and column A.
   d. If the calculations have been correct, this new subtotal obtained after subtracting columns B1 and B2 should be equal to column C, which is the current balance.

   Note: When doing a proof of posting, column D is added to column A minus the sum of columns B1 and B2, and this must equal column C. Therefore, a proof of posting formula is:

   $$D + A - (B1 + B2) = C$$

   This means the previous balance (D) plus the charge (A) minus the sum of the payments and adjustments (B1 and B2) is equal to the current balance (C).

this number is accurate, an "Accounts Receivable Control" column and an "Accounts Receivable Proof" column are maintained at the bottom of the day sheet.

On the first day of the month, the day sheet being used will have a zero placed in the box marked "Previous Page." If the day sheet page is for the second of the month through the end of the month, a "Previous Page" number is brought forward from the AR total on the previous page (day before).

The columns A and B totals are brought straight across from the "Proof of Posting" boxes into the correct spaces in the "Accounts Receivable Control" section. These two figures are added together for a subtotal, and then the sum of columns B1 and B2 are subtracted from this amount. This number is the new total accounts receivable figure.

The "Accounts Receivable Proof" is calculated in the same manner with the last box matching the last box on the "Accounts Receivable Control" for proof of posting. See Figure 15-14 for an illustration of accounts receivable control.

An AR ratio provides a measurement of how fast the outstanding accounts are being paid. The AR ratio equals the current AR balance divided by the average gross monthly charges.

For example, if the current AR balance is $20,000 and the annual gross charges are $120,000, then the average monthly charges are $10,000 ($120,000 ÷ 12). The AR ratio would equal $20,000 ÷ $10,000 = 2 months.

Since a desirable accounts receivable ratio, or the amount of time it takes to have the uncollected debts paid, is 2 months or less, this example is at the high end of the limit. The medical assistant will have to work hard to get collections under 2 months.

ACCOUNTS RECEIVABLE CONTROL

Month of ___March___ , 20__ __

Accounts receivable at end of preceding month: $22,500

	Services Rendered	Received from Patients	Adjustments Increase/ (Decrease)	Accounts Receivable Balance
1	$ 800	$ 1000		$22,300
2	$ 700	$ 400		$22,600
3	$ 900	$ 1100	($100)	$22,300
4	$ 1000	$ 700		$22,600

FIGURE 15-14 Accounts receivable control.

LOCATING ERRORS

The key to error control is to prevent errors in the first place. If there is a difference in the balances of the day sheet, there are several steps that can be taken to locate the error.

1. If the columns on the day sheet do not balance (using the "Proof of Posting" box at the bottom of the day sheet), check all calculations. Ideally you will have saved the calculator tape. Find the difference in the balances, and search for that identical amount on the ledger cards and superbill.

2. If an error is divisible by nine, it may be a transposition error. For example, if the difference in the balance is $63, you may find that you wrote $329 instead of $392.

3. Check all the columns, in particular the "Previous Balance" column to make sure you did not post the amount incorrectly when you carried it forward to the new day sheet.

4. Check the alignment of all digits to make sure a zero was not misaligned (e.g., in writing 200 instead of 20). One bookkeeping method for avoiding this type of error is to use a dash in the cents column instead of two zeros. Thus $45.00 would be written as $45.–.

Computerized Systems

Most offices perform the accounting function using a computer program. The computer system and program selected will depend on the needs of the office. Practice management software offers many services and can be modified to fit the needs of a particular office or specialty. When shopping for practice management software, offices often hire a consultant to evaluate the practice requirements. Specialized software is advertised in professional journals and is demonstrated at professional meetings for physicians and medical office personnel. Prior to making a final decision concerning office software, ask physicians' offices or practices with similar needs for their suggestions. Another concern in choosing new software is cost. New software may require an upgrade of the office hardware. A consultant will be able to advise the office concerning these needs. The new software must contain Current Procedural Terminology (CPT) and International Classification of Diseases (ICD) data. However, these data change yearly, and the system must be able to accommodate these updates.

When using a computerized system always back up data and information on a separate disk, such as a CD-ROM that is then stored separately in a fireproof box. Some systems also keep the information on the hard drive. Some offices keep one hard copy of printed material on file in the event the computer system goes down or there is a power failure.

HIPAA mandated use of the computer to submit bills to insurance companies electronically. Several comprehensive software systems are available that combine many office functions into one program. These software packages will make patient appointments, keep all patient records (including lab results and X-ray reports), maintain all insurance and billing information, and perform all bookkeeping functions, including insurance payments, patient payments, and accounts due. In addition, a function within these programs makes it possible to submit the bill electronically to an insurance clearinghouse for dissemination to the payment centers.

Most comprehensive software programs are quite expensive, so before deciding which one to buy, pay careful attention to the needs of the office, as well as which methods the office has chosen to follow to comply with HIPAA regulations.

To access the information in these programs, every employee must have his or her own unique login name and password. To be in compliance with HIPAA regulations, on leaving employment the employee's login name and password must be rendered unusable. Only those employees with a legitimate need to access the information may have login names and passwords. In addition, the person responsible for providing employees with access must keep records of who accesses the information, what information was accessed, and when (date and time) information is accessed. These logs must be kept for a designated period of time, usually at least 2 years.

A paper backup copy of the computer files is not necessary, but a disk backup file or an off-premises electronic backup file is necessary. The process by which the backup files can or should be accessed is written into the office's policies and procedures manual, along with the reasons and circumstances for granting access. One designated person has total access to the system and is responsible for the software, the passwords, and the backup files. This person is also documented in the office policies and procedures manual.

Professional Courtesy

Professional courtesy (PC) may be granted only by the physician and is not looked on kindly by the government. If the physician opts not to charge other physicians, staff, family members, or clergy, this is known as professional courtesy. When professional courtesy is granted it must meet insurance requirements and must be recorded in the patient's record. Some physician's offices will have the patient sign a letter stating that the patient was provided a service and was not charged out of professional courtesy. A copy of this letter should appear in the patient's medical record.

SUMMARY

The professional health care facility will have in place an office policy regarding fee setting, billing, and collection. The medical assistant has the responsibility to carry out the policy with a professional, courteous attitude. Informed patients will have a better understanding of office expectations. This helps to lessen the problems encountered with accounts receivable. When an account does become a collection dilemma, a series of steps can be instituted to quickly and efficiently address any problems. The goal of such policy is to protect the financial well-being and goodwill of the medical practice.

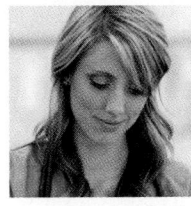

15 CHAPTER REVIEW

COMPETENCY REVIEW

1. Define and spell the terms to learn for this chapter.

2. With a fellow student, role-play a telephone conversation you would have with Samuel Jones, a patient who is unemployed, to collect a $225 bill overdue for 60 days.

3. Write a sample collection letter from Dr. Shania McWalter to Samuel Jones, based on the previous question.

4. What statements can you make to a patient to encourage payment at the time of service?

5. Discuss the ethical considerations involved when making collections.

PREPARING FOR THE CERTIFICATION EXAM

1. Petty cash is used to pay for:
   a. clinical supplies.
   b. administrative supplies.
   c. incidentals.
   d. annual parking fee.
   e. professional dues.

2. AR is money:
   a. owed to vendors for supplies received.
   b. owed to the practice.
   c. received by patients.
   d. owed to the insurance companies for overpayment.
   e. received by insurance companies from the patient.

3. When a patient leaves no forwarding address you should:
   a. close the patient's account.
   b. write off the patient's balance.
   c. consider the patient a skip.
   d. contact local law enforcement.
   e. consider the patient's account closed.

4. Which of the following individuals determine which accounts to turn over to collections?
   a. office manager
   b. physician
   c. administrative accounts representative

d. bookkeeper

e. billing manager

5. Which account is typically the largest AP account in the office?

a. rent

b. pending insurance payments

c. payroll

d. collection agency payments

e. medical malpractice premiums

6. UCR means:

a. usual customary receivable.

b. usual customary reasonable.

c. usual custom receivables.

d. usual customary responsibilities.

e. usual custom reasonable.

7. All of the following are components of the pegboard system EXCEPT:

a. encounter forms.

b. ledger cards.

c. checks.

d. day sheets.

e. superbills.

8. When the office is notified a patient has filed for bankruptcy, the office should:

a. attempt to contact the patient.

b. write off the balance.

c. send a reminder letter.

d. contact the patient's attorney.

e. file a claim with the courts.

9. A ledger card is used to record all of the following EXCEPT:

a. payments.

b. charges.

c. collection agency payments.

d. DRGs.

e. adjustments.

10. When a patient makes a payment, it would be recorded as what on the day sheet?

a. adjustment

b. debit

c. debit balance

d. credit

e. credit balance

CRITICAL THINKING

1. How should Samra handle the situation with Ms. McConnley?

2. When Ms. McConnley is ready to check out, she informs Samra that she does not have any cash to pay her $25 copayment. How should Samra respond?

3. Is it necessary for Samra to make any notations in the patient's chart?

ON THE JOB

Services were rendered to Jeffrey Boylan on October 1. It is now 45 days since Mr. Boylan received care, and he has not yet made a payment on his outstanding balance of $150. At this point, the office's policy requires that a reminder letter be sent. Compose a collection letter to Mr. Boylan, in accordance with HIPAA and office guidelines. Address: Mr. Jeffrey Boylan, 14 Meadow Road, Anytown, State 12345

INTERNET ACTIVITY

Your office is in the process of deciding between manual and computerized accounting systems. Search the Internet for the various accounting systems. Develop an Excel spreadsheet, and list the manual and computerized systems found online with all necessary equipment, components, warranties, and prices.

MEDMEDIA

Additional interactive resources and activities for this chapter can be found:

On your student DVD: View applicable procedure videos on the DVD-ROM found in the back of this book.

MyHealthProfessionsKit.com: Test your knowledge of the chapter with games and activities. MyHealthProfessionsKit also includes resources, helpful links, and a Spanish audio glossary.

Medical Assisting Interactive: Practice your procedures as a medical assistant in this simulated doctor's office. This can be accessed through MyHealthProfessionsKit.com.

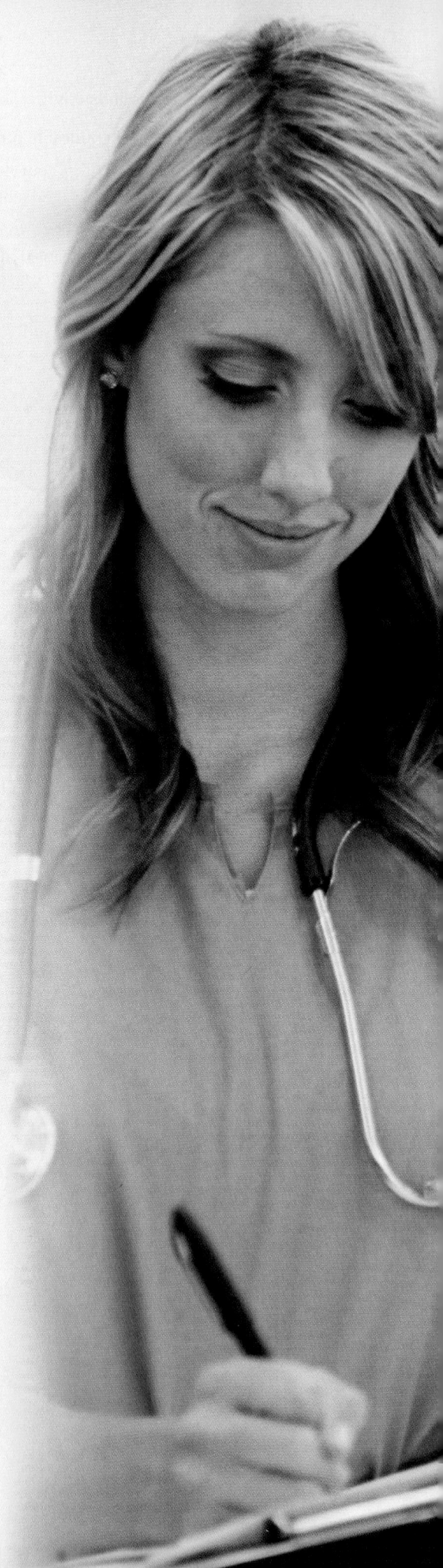

16 Financial Management

LEARNING OBJECTIVES

After completing this chapter, you should be able to:

- Define and spell the terms to learn for this chapter.

- List the criteria for a negotiable instrument.

- Differentiate between the ABA number and the MICR on a check.

- Describe the write-it-once check writing system.

- State the correct procedure for writing a check and check stub.

- State the risks associated with accepting a third-party check, cash, or check from an out-of-state bank.

- State the correct method for endorsing a check based on the guidelines issued by the federal government.

- State and describe three types of endorsements.

- List six recurring monthly expenses.

- Describe the five steps to follow when making a deposit.

- List and discuss nine steps for reconciling a bank statement.

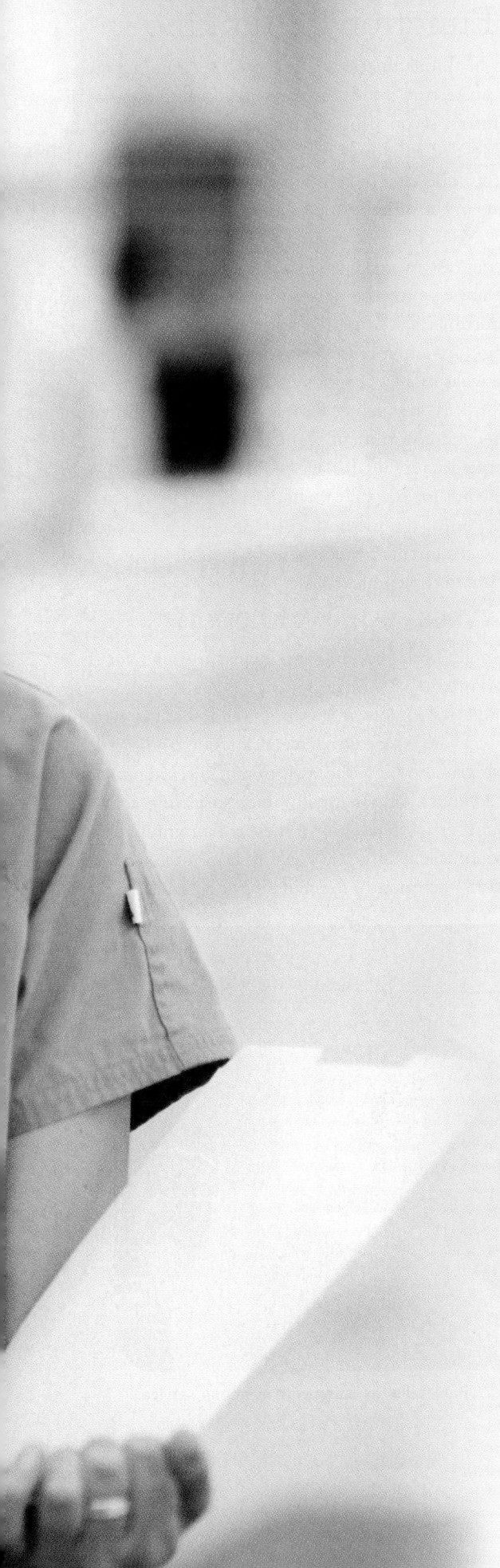

CHAPTER OUTLINE

CASE STUDY

Tania is a medical office co-manager for Pearson Physicians Group. She is in charge of managing the financial matters of the group practice. It is the end of the day, and Tania needs to collect the deposit slip, checks, and petty cash drawer from the front office. Susan hands Tania all the materials and leaves work for the day.

The medical assistant's responsibilities for maintaining control of the medical office's banking and accounting procedures are twofold. First, absolute accuracy is necessary when working with bank deposits, reconciliation of funds, and all related bookkeeping activities. The second responsibility relates to the trust that the physician has placed on the employee for handling cash, checks, and accounts. The medical assistant acts as the agent for the physician.

Function of Banking

The basic banking functions are depositing funds, writing checks, transferring funds between bank accounts, withdrawing funds, reconciling statements, and using banking services. Most of the funds that come into a medical office are from the collection of accounts receivable.

Someone in the office will have to use funds in a checking or savings account to pay business-related expenses. When funds (money) are moved from one account to another or used as cash, it always must be done in a systematic manner and carefully documented. Monthly statements for both checking and savings accounts must be reconciled or balanced to determine what money or funds are available for use.

Bank records are subject to government examination since the federal government regulates banking practices. In addition, the accountant for the medical practice will need accurate records for preparation of federal, and perhaps state, tax returns. Since the medical assistant will not be present when the accountant reviews the books, all information must be clear and accurate.

TYPES OF BANK ACCOUNTS

Banks maintain both checking and savings accounts for their customers (Figure 16-1). A checking account allows the owner of the account to withdraw money from the account by writing checks, which are used as payment for outstanding debts (bills). Cash can also be withdrawn from a checking account. Checking accounts are not usually interest-bearing accounts. Some accounts earn interest only if there is a minimum balance in the account. Generally, the bank charges a fee, or service charge (e.g., $5 per month) to maintain the account.

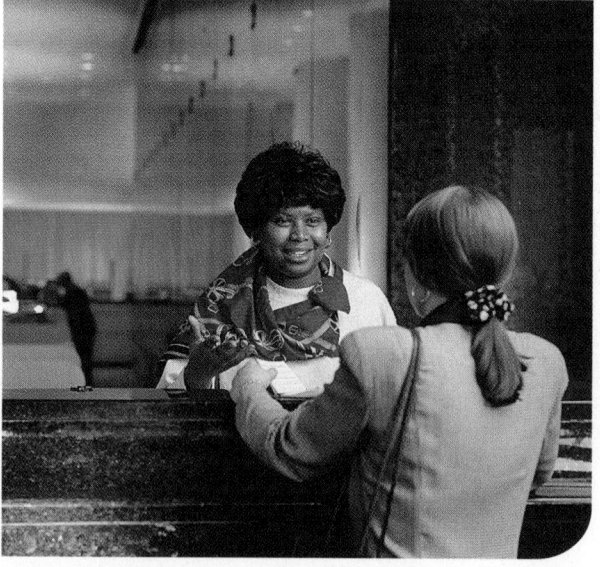

FIGURE 16-1 Bank teller assisting with customer service.

A savings account is an interest-bearing account in which funds not needed for daily expenses can be placed. Interest is earned monthly or quarterly. This means the bank will calculate a certain percentage (such as 3 percent) based on the average balance during a month and will pay that amount to the account. Cash can be withdrawn from a savings account or transferred into a checking account. There is usually a limit to the number of monthly withdrawals allowed before a fee is assessed.

A money market savings account is used more as an investment tool and usually pays a higher interest rate. It typically requires a minimum balance of $500 to $5,000, depending on the institution.

ONLINE BANKING

Most banks provide an online banking service to their customers. Online banking provides the customer access to his or her bank account 24 hours a day, 7 days a week. By using the computer to access the Internet, customers can enter the URL (Internet address) for their bank's home page. This address can be obtained from the bank. Once on the bank's home page, the customer chooses "Online Banking." A sign-in or log-in page will appear that asks for a username and password. The username and password are usually set by the customer and are unique to each customer. Some banks also require the account number to be entered.

Online banking allows customers to perform most transactions that previously required the account holder to physically go to the bank to complete the transaction. One of the benefits of using online banking is that you can perform transactions any time, day or night. If using online banking, you may perform all of the following: reconcile accounts on a daily basis if necessary, pay bills, view account activity including deposits and which checks have been processed, check the total amount of money in the account, and transfer money between accounts. Another advantage of online banking is the ability to download data from the bank website directly to the customer's money management software program.

Online banking is a paperless system, so it is important when using it that records be kept in the office. If a bill is paid, it must be noted in the accounts payable (AP) records. **Accounts payable** is money that is owed to vendors, suppliers, utility companies, and others for services rendered. It is important that notations are made in the AP record to ensure that the office's records always match the bank's records and that any money taken out of the account to pay a bill is posted in the office records.

Checks

A check is a written order to a bank to pay or transfer money to an individual, business, or entity. A check, which is payable on demand, is considered a negotiable instrument. A **negotiable instrument** is one that actualizes or permits the transfer of money to another person. In order to have a negotiable instrument, the check must:

- be written and signed by an authorized payer of the check.
- state a sum of money to be paid.
- be payable on demand or at a fixed date in the future.
- be payable to the holder (payee) of the check.

Checks are supplied, for a small fee, by the bank where the money is held or a company specializing in printing checks. These are referred to as blank checks since they contain only basic information, including the account number and name and address of the account owner.

Large medical offices that require a large supply of checks may request a business office checkbook that has several checks per page in a large bound checkbook. Each check has a stub on which to record the check information. Medical offices can also request a duplicate or write-it-once check system. A carbon strip on the back of the check allows a record of the check to be kept when written to ensure accountability for each check.

Standard information is included on all checks regardless of the bank that issues them. See Figure 16-2 for a labeled example of the standard parts of a check. This preprinted information includes the following:

- Name and address of the **payer** (person signing the check to release the money)

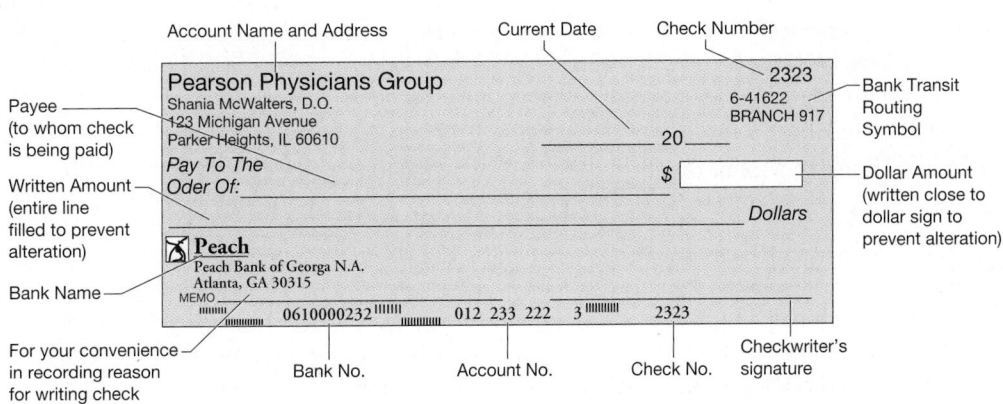

FIGURE 16-2 Labeled parts of a check.

- Preprinted sequential number on each check
- Space to enter the full date
- American Bank Association (ABA) number
- "Pay to the order of" space in which to enter the name of the **payee** (person or company to receive the money)
- Space in which to write the amount of the check
- Small box or space in which to enter the amount of the check in numbers
- Space for the signature of payer
- Preprinted name and address of bank
- Magnetic ink character recognition (MICR) figures used for bank processing of the check

The blank spaces must be completed before a bank will honor and cash the check.

ADVANTAGES OF CHECKS

Checks are recommended for a variety of reasons, including safety of funds, convenience, ease of maintaining a record or documentation of money transfer, reliability of records for tax purposes, summary of deposits from receipts, protection while money is in the bank account (banks carry insurance to cover loss), and stop-payment orders that can be issued by the payer to protect any lost or stolen checks.

TYPES OF CHECKS

The various types of checks include cashier's checks, certified checks, bank drafts, limited checks, money orders, traveler's checks, voucher checks, and warrants. Box 16-1 lists definitions of the different types of checks.

Box 16-1 Types of CHECKS

- *Cashier's checks* are written using the bank's own check or form and are issued by the bank. A cashier's check guarantees the money is available since the bank checks the payer's account before issuing the check. The purchaser can also pay cash to have a cashier's check issued. The funds to pay the check are debited against the payer's account when the check is issued by the bank. Cashier's checks can be requested of a bank by savings account holders who do not have a checking account. There is usually a charge for this service.
- *Certified checks* are similar to cashier's checks since the bank guarantees the money is available. A certified check is actually written on the payer's own check form. The teller will verify this check by placing an official stamp directly on the check. The bank actually withdraws the money from the payer's account when it certifies the check.
- *Bank drafts* are checks that are drawn up by a bank against funds (money) that are deposited to its account in another bank.
- *Limited checks* are issued on special check forms that contain a preprinted maximum dollar amount for which the check can be written. There may also be a time limit during which the check is valid or must be cashed. Limited checks are used for payroll checks and insurance payments.
- *Money orders* are purchased for the cash value typed on the check. Money orders can be purchased from banks, the United States Postal Service, and other authorized agents. International money orders can be purchased to be cashed in foreign countries. A money order is purchased with cash, and there is a charge for this service. Money orders are frequently used by individuals who do not have bank accounts since it is recommended that cash not be sent through the mail. Money orders are

considered safe to accept as payment since they are redeemable at the value typed on the check.
- *Traveler's checks* are familiar to most people who travel. These checks are preprinted in certain dollar amounts ($10, $20, $50, $100, $500 and $1,000) and are prepaid. Considered a safe means for carrying money when traveling, traveler's checks are also convenient since most places will accept a traveler's check and only the payer can cash it. There is a space for two signatures of the payer: one at the time of purchase and another when the check is cashed. The payee is able to check the two signatures, thus protecting the payer in the event the check is stolen or lost. People purchasing traveler's checks are advised to always sign the checks at the time of purchase before leaving the bank.
- *Voucher checks* contain three detachable sections for transaction information. This type of check is frequently used for payroll checks since additional information can be supplied to the payee. The upper portion of the check contains the actual check; the lower portion provides details about the transaction, such as any payroll deductions, account to which the check is to be credited, or reason for issuing the check; the third portion is a copy that remains with the payer as a record of the transaction. This copy can then be filed with any additional information that is available, such as invoices or receipts.
- *Warrants* are not actually negotiable checks. They are statements issued to indicate that debts should be paid. For example, an insurance adjuster may issue a warrant indicating that a fire insurance claim should be paid. This warrant then becomes authorization to the insurance company to issue a check as payment.

ABA NUMBER

The **American Banker's Association (ABA) number** is always located in the upper right corner of a printed check. It is printed as a fraction on a business check or as a straight series of numbers (1–109/210) on a personal check. The ABA originated this number to identify the area where the bank issuing the check is located, as well as to identify the individual bank.

MAGNETIC INK CHARACTER RECOGNITION

Magnetic ink character recognition (MICR) is a system of combining characters and numbers located at the bottom left side of checks and deposit slips. The MICR is read by high-speed machinery, increasing the speed and accuracy of processing bank statements and check sorting. It also facilitates the bookkeeping process within the bank. Printed on each check, the MICR is a form of identification for the bank and the account. The first series of numbers identifies the bank and its location. The second series of numbers identifies the individual account. When using a checking account in conjunction with online bill pay, it is necessary to be able to locate and identify these numbers. During bank processing, additional numbers are printed across the bottom of the check to indicate the amount of the check.

CHECK WRITING

The check writing process must be handled carefully to avoid errors. Methods for writing checks will vary from office to office depending on the preferences of the physician and the accountant. Your office may use a traditional checkbook with individual checks on each page, a business office checkbook, a write-it-once system, or a computer-generated check processing system. Procedure 16-1 provides instruction for the proper procedure to follow when writing checks.

Checks must be handwritten in ink or typewritten so they cannot be altered. Pencil is not used for check writing. The signature cannot be typewritten. Correctly written checks require legible handwriting. No blank space should be left before the name of the payee, the written dollar amount, and the numbered dollar amount. This is to prevent another

procedure 16-1

PREPARE A CHECK

Objective: Correctly prepare a check.

EQUIPMENT AND SUPPLIES

blank checks with stub or record; black ink pen

METHOD

1. Move all the checks in the pad to the left so that the lowest-numbered check will lay across the check register.
2. Fill in the check stub or check record before writing the check.
3. Use a black ink pen to complete check and stub.
4. Write the name of the payee on the "Pay to the order of" line.
5. Write out the full amount of the check on the "Pay" line.
6. Write the full date and check number in the designated boxes.
7. Write the amount of the check, using numbers in the designated area.
8. Fill in all blank spaces, and leave no room for anyone to add anything. Always begin writing or figures at the extreme left of the space.
9. Date the check on the day it is written. Never postdate a check. (Postdating a check means writing a future date on a check.)
10. Use care when spelling the name of the payee. Do not use abbreviations or titles, such as MD. Leave no space either before or after the payee's name. If space remains after the name, draw a straight line from the name to the end of the space.
11. Make sure the dollar amount written on the second line agrees with the numeric dollar amount entered in the space on the first line.
12. It is not advisable to write checks for less than one dollar. In addition to the time spent on bookkeeping such a small amount, many banks place a service charge for each check written. This can be costly. However, when you must write a check for less than one dollar, use care. Write out the amount with the word "only" indicating to the reader that the amount should be noted as less than one dollar. Do not cross out the word *dollars*.

13. Record what the check was written for (example: "Office Supplies") on the memo line at the bottom left of the check.
14. Make sure the check is signed. The signature is placed on the line found at the bottom right of the check. The individual signing checks should be the owner of the bank account or his or her authorized agent. In some offices, the office manager is designated to sign checks for the physician.
15. Look over the check carefully to ensure all spaces have been filled in.
16. Finally, subtract the amount of this check from the "Balance Brought Forward" line. Write this amount as the new balance brought forward.

person from altering any of these items. See Figure 16-3 for an example of correctly written checks.

In some cases, the net amount of the check is imprinted by machine. All the other information is entered by hand. Checks with stubs will have to be detached from the stub for typing. However, the stub must be completed immediately. Checks can be prepared ahead of time by the medical assistant or office manager and given to the physician to sign. Attach all materials, such as invoices and statements, to the check for the physician to sign. Writing a check payable to "Cash" ("cash" checks) is not advised. These checks are easily cashed since they have no payee designated and have been signed by the payer. Banks will usually require that the person cashing this type of check endorse the check while in front of the teller. Procedure 16-1 describes the check writing process using a write-it-once system.

WRITE-IT-ONCE SYSTEM

The write-it-once system is based on the use of a check with a carbon strip on the back that allows a record to be kept of the date, check number, payee, and net amount of the check. A pegboard system (see Chapter 15), check register sheet, and checks with a carbonized writing strip on the back are used for this method. The check register sheet is placed over the pegs of a pegboard. Checks with the carbonized strip on the back edge are then placed on top of the check register, lining up the first line of the check register with the writing line of the first check. Any information that is written on the check (e.g., payee or dollar amount) will then appear on the check register sheet as a permanent record.

Checks must be handwritten when using the write-it-once method. The user must press hard when writing on this type of check so that the impression will go through to the check register underneath. The check register has space for 25 checks to be recorded on one page.

ERRORS IN WRITING CHECKS

Banks are very suspicious of any alterations on a check. If when you are writing a check a mistake is made, such as writing out a different dollar amount than appears in the boxed space for the numeric amount, or the payee name is written in the space meant for the handwritten dollar amount, the check is not valid. In this case, draw a line through the check and write VOID, in ink, in large letters on the face of the check. Keep the voided check so that it is not considered missing when the bank statement is reconciled. If the check has already been signed, many people will tear off and discard just the signature and keep the remainder of the check for a record.

ACCEPTING CHECKS

An office policy should be in place to guide staff regarding accepting checks from patients as payment for services. Most of the time it is acceptable for patients to pay for services with a personal check. Most of the **accounts receivable (AR)**, the money owed to the physician or medical practice, are paid by checks written

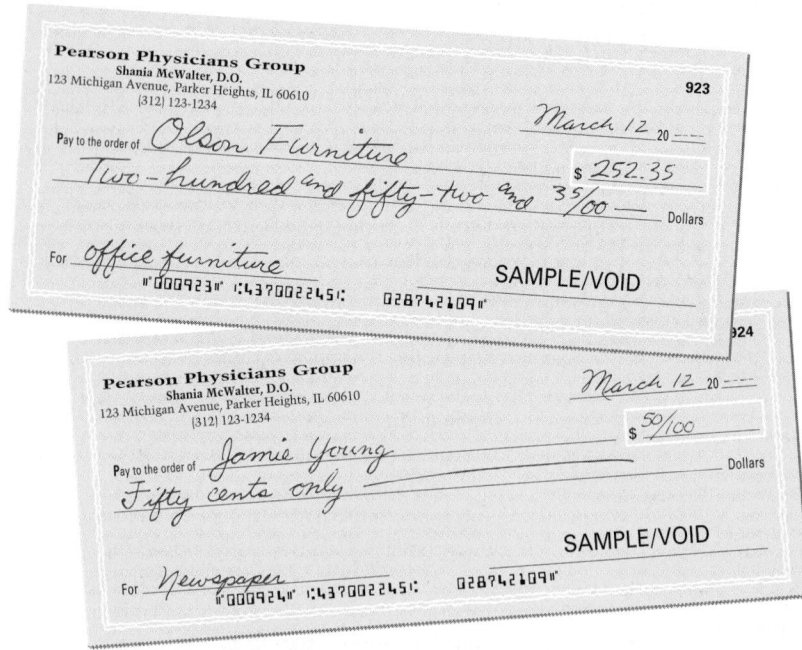

FIGURE 16-3 Correctly written checks.

against the bank accounts of patients. For a variety of reasons, there may be patients who have an agent delegated to sign his or her checks. If this is the case, a notation should be made in the financial section of the patient's medical record.

Third-Party Checks

Most medical offices consider certain checks risky and may not accept them. These include third-party checks, checks drawn on an out-of-town bank, overpayment of account checks, and "paid in full" checks.

A **third-party check** refers to a check written by a party unknown to you. You are considered the third party in this process. The patient (the second party), the payee, has received a check from another person to pay his or her medical bill. The person who wrote the check is considered the first party. You are at risk in accepting this check since you do not know the payer who has signed the check and have no contact information on the payer. You may encounter some trouble collecting the money for which the check is issued.

In many cases, these checks will be for an amount greater than the amount of the bill, and you would have to issue a refund in cash. This would require maintaining extra cash in the office and performing additional staff work, and it might result in financial loss if the check turns out to be invalid. Therefore, most offices do not accept third-party checks of any kind.

Out-of-Town Banks

Checks drawn on out-of-town banks are generally not accepted for payment unless identification is sought from the payee. It is difficult to collect payment if a check is not good, and it may not be easy to reach an out-of-town bank, concerning the validity of a check, prior to accepting it.

Overpayment

Occasionally, a patient writes a check for an overpayment of an account. This can happen accidentally if a patient has not maintained adequate records or if the patient's insurance company has also made a payment to the patient's account in the medical office. In this case, a refund must be made to the patient. This can be handled by issuing a refund check for the amount of overpayment or returning the incorrect check to the patient if it has not been deposited.

"Paid in Full"

Checks written with the statement added "Paid in Full" are to be avoided. Patients sometimes write this on their check when they believe they no longer owe any money to the physician. If you deposit the check you acknowledge that this is correct. Therefore, if the patient still owes money on the bill and you deposit the check, you may have difficulty collecting any further payments.

PROFESSIONALISM THE LIFE SPAN

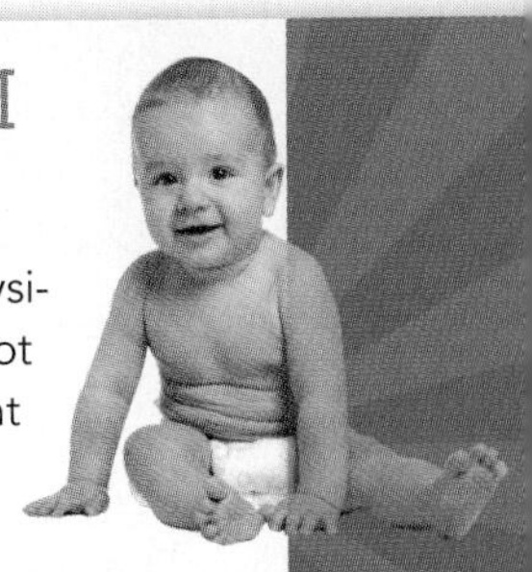

Sometimes an elderly person who is physically unable to write a check, or who cannot see to write a check, will designate an agent to write and sign checks for him or her. Most often it is a family member. This is an arrangement the person has made with the bank, and it is a perfectly legitimate and legal way to handle finances. When money is owed to the doctor's office, it is usually the agent who will write the check for the patient, but it will be credited to the patient's account.

COMPLETING THE CHECK STUB

A check stub can be used as a permanent record of the date, amount, payee, and purpose of the check. The check stub has room to place the new balance, which is obtained by subtracting the current check from the previous balance. See Figure 16-4 for an illustration of a correctly completed check stub.

ENDORSEMENT OF CHECKS

To transfer money from one person to another, the check must be endorsed. According to federal banking regulations, an endorsement is placed on the back of the check within the top 1.5 inches on the left side of the check as it is turned over. This upper-left corner is referred to as the "trailing edge" of a check. If the endorsement is not placed within this designated area or extends beyond the 1.5-inch mark, it can be refused by a bank.

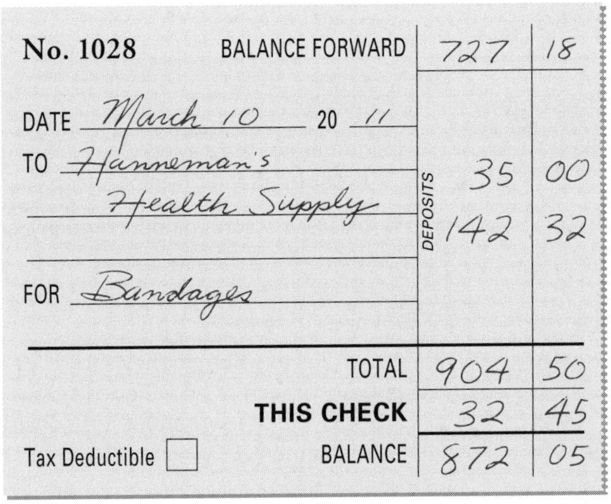

No. 1028 BALANCE FORWARD 727 | 18

DATE March 10 20 11

TO Hanneman's Health Supply

DEPOSITS 35 | 00
142 | 32

FOR Bandages

TOTAL 904 | 50
THIS CHECK 32 | 45
Tax Deductible ☐ BALANCE 872 | 05

FIGURE 16-4 Correctly completed check stub.

MAILING CHECKS

Care should be used when mailing checks so that the check is not visible through the envelope. Special security (non-transparent) envelopes can be purchased. Other methods include placing the check in a piece of folded paper or actually folding the check in half. When mailing a payment to a vendor for an item or a service received, a stub from the invoice being paid is usually mailed along with the check. It is important not to staple the check to the invoice as it could cause the check to tear, making it unacceptable for deposit.

RETURNED CHECKS

A check may be returned by the bank for a variety of reasons. When this occurs, a returned item notice detailing the reason for the return is also included with the check. Checks are returned, for example, when the payee name, date, or signature of payer is missing. If a check is returned with the payee's name or date missing, it is acceptable for the medical assistant to fill in the date and physician's name. If the payer's signature is missing, then the check will have to be returned to the payer. It is always wise to place a telephone call to a patient with the reasons for returning his or her check. All checks should be reviewed prior to adding a written or stamped endorsement for deposit.

Nonsufficient funds (NSF) (in the payer's account) and the stop-payment order (issued by the payer) are two of the more serious reasons for the return of a check. In the case of NSF, the payer's account does not have enough money to cover the amount of the check. Someone in the medical office, perhaps the medical assistant, will have to contact the writer of the check and ask how he or she wishes to make the payment. If funds have been added to the account, the patient (payer) may ask that the check be resubmitted. To resubmit a check, call the payer's bank to determine if

An endorsement can either be a payee's written or rubber-stamped signature. To prevent theft, checks should be endorsed "For Deposit Only" as soon as they arrive in the mail.

It is common procedure in a medical office to endorse checks as soon as they are received. This is often done with an endorsement stamp that contains the doctor's name, the account number, and the name of the bank. Some checks may specify that the check must be cashed within a set period of time, such as 90 or 180 days. If the check has not been presented for payment within the time suggested on the check, it would be considered a **stale check**.

Endorsements are regulated by the Uniform Negotiable Instrument Act. A check that has been transferred to more than one person (third-party payer) would have more than one endorsement on the back. Types of endorsements are discussed in Table 16-1.

TABLE 16-1 Endorsements

Endorsement	Description	Example
Blank	Signature of the payee. Check can be cashed by anyone. This is not used in the business office.	Shania McWalter
Full	Indicates person's name, company, account number, bank name, and payee's name.	Pay to the order of First Town Bank Shania McWalter, D.O. 123-123456
Restrictive	Specifies to whom money should be paid and the money's purpose, such as "For Deposit Only." You can rubber-stamp the physician's signature. It is considered the safest endorsement.	Pay to the order of First Town Bank For Deposit Only Shania McWalter, D.O. 123-123456

POST NONSUFFICIENT FUNDS (NSF) CHECKS

Objective: Demonstrate the process for posting nonsufficient funds (NSF) checks.

EQUIPMENT AND SUPPLIES

data; computer or ledger card; pen

METHOD

1. Record the amount of the NSF check and the service fee in the adjustment column on the day sheet and ledger card or in the appropriate field of an accounting computer software program.
2. Accurately record the NSF check to show that the amount is added to the balance, instead of subtracted from it.
3. Note the reason for the adjustment to the patient account.

CHARTING EXAMPLE

12/8/XX. $68 charge plus $20 NSF check fee = $88 was added to the patient balance. · · · · · · · · · · · · K. Taylor, CMAS

---

the account has sufficient funds, write the word *Resubmit* on both the face and the back of the check, make out another deposit slip, and resubmit it. Many banks charge the account a fee if a deposited check is NSF. Offices will then charge the patient, in addition to the amount of the NSF check, the fee charged to them by the bank and a handling charge. See Procedure 16-2 on posting nonsufficient funds checks.

Some medical offices have a policy that if a check is returned for NSF, they will not resubmit the check. They request the payment be made immediately, with either cash, money order, or a cashier's check. A **cashier's check** guarantees payment because it is written on a check drafted by a bank. Offices may also accept payment in the form of a **certified check**, which is a check written on the patient's check but is guaranteed by the bank because money has been set aside in the patient's account. Some medical offices now offer patients the opportunity to pay for services with a credit card. The returned check should be held until payment in one of these forms has been made. If the patient has not taken care of the bill after notification and a sufficient time has elapsed, then advise the physician of the patient's lack of response and follow the physician's suggestion. This may mean turning the bill over to a collection agency, which is discussed in Chapter 15. If this is the case, the patient must be notified in writing that the bill will be turned over to collections.

If a **stop-payment order** has been issued by the payer, then the bank will not allow the funds to be disbursed. The

bank will indicate that you should contact the payer with the terms "Refer to Maker" on the item notice. This procedure is used when a check has been lost or stolen.

Paying Bills

All bills should be paid by check for documentation and control purposes. The only exception to this policy would be very small payments, such as daily newspaper delivery and public transportation costs. In these instances, the payments could be made from petty cash. However, it is advisable that all payments, even the daily newspaper, be paid from accounts established with appropriate vendors.

An office policy must be established regarding how often checks are written. This may be weekly, biweekly, semimonthly, or monthly. This bill-paying schedule must match a schedule of when funds are available for payment of

PROFESSIONALISM

For many patients, money owed is a touchy and uncomfortable subject. Always address this topic in a calm, nonjudgmental way. If a patient requests to make payment arrangements, comply only if the office has a policy about payment arrangements. Always follow the office policy, and never veer from it. In this way, your honesty in dealing with money issues will never be questioned.

office expenses. For instance, your office policy may be to send all invoices to patients at the end of the month for payments that are due on the first of the next month. In this case, you would not want to write checks against your account to pay office expenses during the last week of the month since the payments from patients will not have arrived to cover your check writing.

The office banking policy should indicate who is responsible for writing and signing all checks. A smart policy is to separate the responsibilities; one person (the medical assistant) should write the checks and another person should be authorized to sign them (office manager or physician). In some medical offices, two authorized signatures are required to transfer funds from one account to another or to write checks over a certain dollar amount, such as $1,000.

It is not recommended to pay bills on the day they arrive since they are generally not due for 30 days. During that 30-day period, the money that is used to pay bills can remain in an interest-bearing account. The incentive for paying bills as they arrive occurs when a supplier (vendor) offers a discount if payment is included with the order or paid within a certain number of days, such as payment within 10 days. Since this discount could be as much as 10 to 20 percent, it is wise to take advantage of it.

A schedule for paying recurring monthly expenses should be kept on a master calendar or in a tickler (reminder) file. Examples of recurring monthly expenses may include the following:

- Insurance premium(s)
- Rent or mortgage
- Waste removal
- Utilities, including telephone charges
- Housekeeping and maintenance expenses
- Laundry
- Equipment rental, such as a copy machine
- Taxes
- Maintenance contracts for equipment
- Medical and office supplies
- Postage

If all checks for expenses are written on a particular day of the month, a planned transfer of funds can be made from a savings account to a checking account to cover these checks.

Some offices use a tickler file to remind the bookkeeper when each bill is due. The office will have some recurrent bills that are the same amount and paid at the same time each month. One example of a recurrent bill is the office rent. The rent for the office is typically the same amount

each month and is due on the same day of each month. For some offices, there may be an annual, bimonthly, or quarterly lease arrangement. In this case, the lease money may be paid up to 1 year in advance. The bills for the electricity, the water, the telephone, and the gas will vary in amount from month to month but will still be due on the same day each month. These bills should be paid early enough in the month to ensure that the payment for the service reaches the company to which it is owed before the actual due date listed on the bill. It is a good idea to file these bills for payment days earlier than the actual due date so the checks or payment for them will be sent several days in advance, allowing adequate time for delivery by the due date.

HIRING AN ACCOUNTANT OR BOOKKEEPING FIRM

Larger medical practices may hire an accountant or bookkeeping firm to process all checks. This is an accurate means of handling banking procedures. However, these services can be too costly for smaller medical offices. In some firms, a computerized check-writing service system is used.

Deposits

Deposits, which refer to money (cash, checks, and money orders) placed into a bank account, can be made to either checking or savings accounts. Offices will vary somewhat on specific methods of handling deposits, but the following procedures are usually followed:

- Prepare and make deposits daily.
- Maintain all records of daily receipts (for checks, cash, money orders, and credit card transactions) together in a safe location.
- Compare the total on the deposit slip against the total on the day sheet.
- Keep a duplicate copy of all deposits on file in the office. Photocopy the deposit slip before submitting it to the bank. Some offices copy checks for later reference.
- Keep bank receipts of all deposits on file in the office.
- Immediately note all deposits in the checkbook.

The frequency of making deposits may depend on several factors. If there is a significant distance between the office and the bank, deposits may not be made as frequently as if the bank were closer to the office. Also, depending on the volume of payments received, some offices may make several deposits per day. More frequent deposits may help reduce the possibility of losing money. It is important to remember that the sooner money is deposited, the sooner it will be available to pay bills. Until cash and checks can be deposited, they should be stored in a safe or other secure location that is not accessible to patients.

Always compare the total credited to the AR with the total on the deposit slip. Occasionally, a check is omitted from the AR record. Numbers may be transposed when completing the deposit slip or the AR total. Using the pegboard or write-it-once system results in a duplicate deposit slip. Maintain an accurate balance of all accounts on a daily basis.

COMPLETING THE DEPOSIT SLIP

A deposit slip is completed every time a deposit is made into a bank account. The slip indicates the total dollar amounts of cash and checks being deposited. Entries on the slip should be printed in black ink. Currency (coins and bills) is totaled separately from checks. The currency bills should be organized in descending order by face value, and all bills should be facing the same way. This helps reduce the likelihood for error. For instance, all $100 bills would be facing the same way, next all $50 bills would be facing the same way, and so on.

Each check must be entered on a different line, noting either the payer's name, the check number, or ABA number depending on the bank's preferred method. If more checks than lines are provided, the excessive checks can be entered on the back of the deposit slip. The currency and coin totals and check totals are added together. Then this amount, the total for the deposit, is entered on the bottom line of the deposit slip. Procedure 16-3 lists steps for preparing deposit slips. See Figure 16-5 for an example of a deposit slip.

Check all deposits on the deposit slip against the day sheet totals. If the two figures do not match, check for the error in several ways:

- Recheck addition.
- Check each item on the deposit slip.
- Check for transposed numbers.
- If the error is still not found, subtract the difference between the deposit slip and the day sheet, then search for an item with that number.
- Check for errors of omission.

The correct order for listing money on a bank deposit is as follows: currency, coins, checks, and money orders.

procedure 16-3

PREPARE A DEPOSIT SLIP

Objective: Complete a bank deposit slip.

EQUIPMENT AND SUPPLIES

pen; deposit slip; checks and currency to be deposited; endorsing stamp; calculator

METHOD

1. Using the endorsing stamp, endorse all checks to be deposited.
2. Complete the information on the front of the deposit slip:
   - Account name
   - Account number
   - Date of the deposit
3. If there is cash to be deposited, enter the total amount of the cash in the upper-right box of the deposit slip beside the CASH indicator. In the CURRENCY box, list the total amount of all cash paper money to be deposited. In the COIN box, list the total of all the cash coin money to be deposited.

4. List each check to be deposited on a different line. If you have more checks than will fit on the front, list each additional check on the reverse side of the deposit slip.
5. Beside the numbers, list who wrote the check. In the box beside the numbered box, list the amount of the check.
6. List each check in a different numbered box.
7. Use a calculator to add all the checks entered on the reverse side of the deposit slip, and enter the total of the checks in the space at the bottom of the deposit slip that reads TOTAL. This amount is also placed on the front of the deposit slip in the space that reads TOTAL FROM REVERSE SIDE.
8. Use the calculator to add the total amount of the cash and the checks being deposited. List this amount in the space labeled TOTAL and in the space labeled NET DEPOSIT on the front of the deposit slip.
9. Place the deposit slip and the cash and checks listed on the slip in an envelope for deposit to the bank.

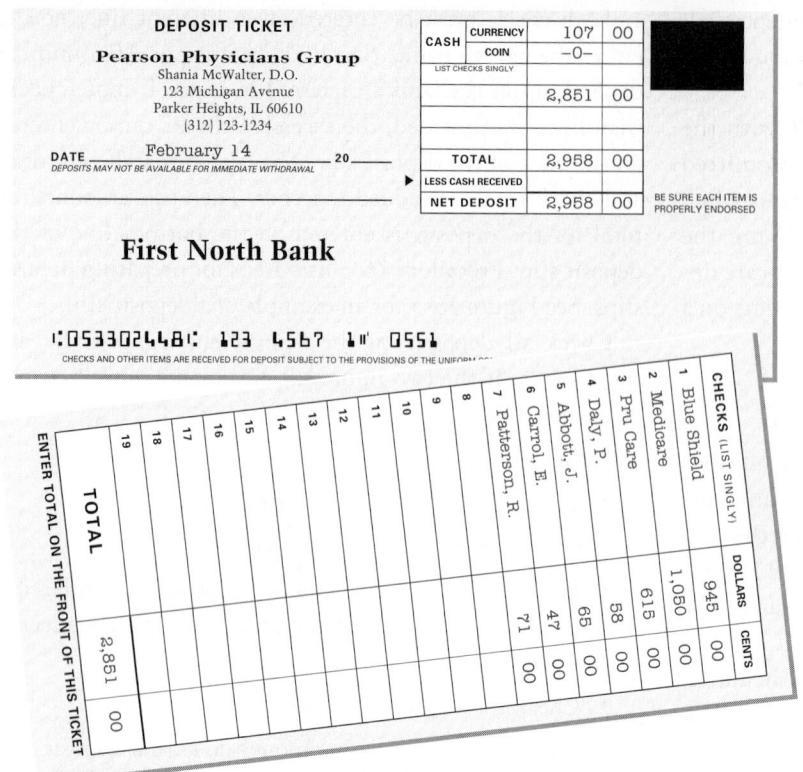

FIGURE 16-5 An example of the front and back sides of a deposit slip.

DEPOSIT TO SAVINGS ACCOUNTS

Cash and checks can also be deposited into a savings account. When the amount in a checking account becomes greater than the amount needed to cover the checks written on the account, deposits can be made into a savings account, which will have a greater interest return on the money than a checking account. When transferring funds from a checking account to a savings account, it is advisable to do so by check. This provides a record of the transaction.

A savings account is set up using a statement or a passbook, which is utilized for maintaining a record of deposits, withdrawals, interest earned, and account balance. The passbook should be kept in a safe place designated for banking materials in the office. Statement savings accounts are sent monthly or quarterly.

MAKING THE DEPOSIT

Deposits can be made to both the checking and savings accounts in person, by mail, or by night depository. If a deposit is made in person, there will be an immediate receipt of deposit. A deposit by mail will result in a receipt by mail. However, cash should not be sent in the mail.

The night depository method can be set up for a business by obtaining a night depository key and depository bags with security locks. The deposit slip, cash, and checks are placed in the bag and then dropped off at the end of the day when the bank may be closed. For security purposes, the office may require that two people take the deposit to the bank together.

It is preferable that one designated person be responsible for the deposits and another for the receivable records. This separation of responsibilities is a critical method of fiscal or financial control.

Accepting Cash

Cash can be accepted as a form of payment; however, most patients will pay either with check or credit card. Receipts must be given for all cash payments. Having large amounts of cash in an office poses a security risk and also holds the potential for the embezzlement of funds. **Embezzlement** is the unauthorized taking of funds and involves a breach of trust. Large cash amounts may necessitate making bank deposits more than once a day in order to minimize cash on hand.

Cash Disbursement

Cash disbursement refers to a payment made to creditors. The term *cash* is misleading since, in most cases, the disbursement is made by check, not cash. Payment by check provides a permanent document for proof of payment and tax purposes.

Bank Hold on Accounts

Occasionally, a bank will place a *hold* on funds in a checking account. Before allowing anyone to draw on those funds, an *Uncollected Funds Hold (UCF or UFH)* may be attached to the deposited funds that must "clear" before the bank knows the funds are present. This typically occurs with checks written for large sums. The bank will not actually credit the account in which the money was deposited until the check has been processed and the funds paid to the payer's bank. These funds cannot be used by the depositor until the check or funds have cleared and the hold is removed. The bank will notify the depositor of the length of time for the hold.

Bank Statement

The purpose of a statement from the bank is to confirm the amount of funds that are in each account. The bank statement can uncover errors that have been made in either the office bookkeeping system or the bank bookkeeping system.

A monthly bank statement includes all debits and credits that have been processed. **Debits** are charges against an account; **credits** are additions to an account. The statement will include **canceled checks**—checks that have been processed and paid out to the medical practice's creditors by the bank; deposits; and fees charged by the bank against the account. Many banks no longer return canceled checks, which indicates a further need to maintain excellent record keeping on the check stub when the check is written. Figure 16-6 is an example of a typical bank statement.

RECONCILIATION OF BANK STATEMENTS

Reconciliation refers to the comparison of the figures on the bank statements with the records maintained in the medical office and the adjustment of banking records so that both are in agreement. The purpose of this reconciliation is to match the account activity and totals against the medical office records. Bank statements include the following information:

- Account number
- Average collected balance
- Minimum balance
- Tax ID number (usually the Social Security number of the physician)
- Beginning balance
- Deposit history, including credit card transaction deposits
- Interest/credits
- Checks and debits
- Service charges
- Ending balance

Bank statements should be reconciled as soon as they are received, and errors that are found should be corrected immediately. Office policy may indicate an exact date when reconciliation should take place. For better fiscal control, the person reconciling the bank statement should be someone other than the person who prepares the checks and makes the deposits. This is another measure that can prevent embezzlement of funds.

For interest-bearing accounts, the interest earned will be based on the average collected balance (the average amount of money in that account during the period covered by the statement). Any interest credited to the account or any service fees charged to the account, as shown on the bank statement, should be recorded in the checking account records before beginning the reconciliation.

The processed checks will be listed by number. Any checks that are listed in nonconsecutive order may be indicated with an asterisk (*). For instance, you may have check numbers 1301 and 1303 showing as processed, with an asterisk beside the check numbers. This should prompt you to look in the check register for check 1302, which may be a voided check or a check that has not yet been cashed.

The reverse side of the bank statement includes information on how to handle errors or questions about the statement, along with a form to assist in reconciling the bank statement. Procedure 16-4 lists step-by-step instructions for reconciling a bank statement.

STATEMENT OF ACCOUNT

FIRST NORTH
BANK OF CHIGAGO
123 East Pearson, Chicago, IL 60611
(312) 321-1000

144808

┌ Pearson Physicians Group
  Shania McWalter, D.O.
  123 Michigan Avenue,
  Parker Heights, IL 60610

PAGE   1 OF   1
STATEMENT PERIOD
FROM   08/01/11
THRU   08/31/11
CUST #   300-30-3000

```
---------------- ADVANTAGE CHECKING ACCOUNT ----------------
ACCOUNT NBR DD          12345   BEGINNING BALANCE      $2,646.63
AVG COLL BAL       $4,732.52    DEPOSITS/CREDITS       $8,000.00
MINIMUM BAL        $2,502.88    INTEREST PAID              $.00
TAX ID NUMBER    300-30-3000    CHECKS/DEBITS         $7,871.32 -
                                SERVICE CHARGES           $5.00 -
                                ENDING BALANCE        $2,770.31
                                # DEPOSITS/CREDITS            1
                                #CHECKS/DEBITS               11

                                                       BALANCE
DATE      DESCRIPTION              AMOUNT              $2,646.63
08/01  BEGINNING BALANCE                               2,621.68
08/01  CK#        872              24.95-              2,618.68
08/06  CK#        879               3.00-              2,543.68
08/08  CK#        883              75.00-              2,527.88
08/14  CK#        885              15.80-              2,502.88
08/15  CK#        886              25.00-             10,502.88
08/19  DEPOSIT                   8,000.00             10,470.88
08/26  CK#        887              32.00-              7,970.88
08/26  CK#        888           2,500.00-              7,900.88
08/28  CK#        890              70.00-              7,775.31
08/28  CK#        889             125.57-              2,775.31
08/28  CK#        884           5,000.00-              2,770.31
08/31  MONTHLY MAINTENANCE FEE       5.00-            $2,770.31
08/31  ENDING BALANCE
                          CHECK REGISTER
   CHECK#    DATE     AMOUNT      CHECK#    DATE      AMOUNT
    872     08/01      24.95       886     08/15       25.00
    879*    08/06       3.00       887     08/26       32.00
    883*    08/08      75.00       888     08/26    2,500.00
    884     08/28   5,000.00       889     08/28      125.57
    885     08/14      15.80       890     08/28       70.00
 * INDICATES NON-CONSECUTIVE CHECK NUMBER(S)
```

FIGURE 16-6 A typical bank statement.

RECONCILING A BANK STATEMENT

Objective: Reconcile a bank statement for a checking account.

EQUIPMENT AND SUPPLIES

current and previous bank statements; cancelled checks (if returned by the bank); checkbook stubs

METHOD

1. Compare the beginning balance of the current statement with the ending balance of the previous statement. These should be the same.
2. Write the current ending balance in the appropriate space on the reverse side of the bank statement.
3. Compare deposits noted on the statement against your records or receipts by making a check mark next to each correct number.
4. List separately all outstanding deposits. These are deposits made toward the end of the month that have not been included in the current statement. Add these together and place the total on the reverse side of the statement in the space provided.
5. Add the ending balance to the total of deposits not already included and write this amount on the TOTAL line.
6. Compare the value of the checks listed on the statement with the value listed in the checkbook or check stubs, and place a check mark next to each correct number.
7. Note all numbers missing from the sequential list of check numbers; these are checks that have not yet cleared

your bank (outstanding checks). List all outstanding checks. Add the total for outstanding checks, and place that figure on the line indicated on the back of the statement.

8. Subtract the total figure for checks outstanding from the previous total on the back of the statement to determine the current balance. This amount should agree with the amount in your checkbook or stub balance.

EXAMPLE

1. Bank balance shown on this
   statement: $ _____
   ADD (+)
2. Deposits not credited in this statement,
   (if any) $ _____
3. TOTAL $ _____
   SUBTRACT (−)
4. Checks outstanding $ _____
5. BALANCE $ _____

SUMMARY OF RULES

#1 Note ending statement balance.
#2 Add all deposits not yet credited.
#3 Determine subtotal of step #1 and #2.
#4 Subtract total outstanding checks.
#5 Determine balance or final total.

Saving Documentation

Documents relating to banking procedures should be saved in an organized manner. In addition to banking documents, such as copies of deposit slips and check stubs, your records must include the following for verification of business expenses:

- Receipts
- Vouchers for expenses and salaries
- Invoices
- Statements from suppliers
- Proof of payments

These supporting documents should be saved in a file with check numbers of payments written on the document. After the bank statement has been reconciled each month, it

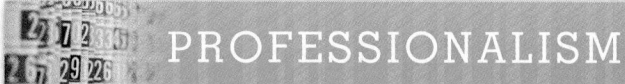

PROFESSIONALISM

THE LAW

The medical assistant acts as the physician's agent when performing the banking procedures for the medical office. In this capacity, the medical assistant must exercise great care and integrity to protect all cash and check receipts that come into the office. Similarly, all disbursements made by the medical assistant on behalf of the physician and the medical office must be handled responsibly. Information relating to the banking practices or the total assets of the physician or the medical practice is confidential and should never be discussed outside of the office.

should be stored with the canceled checks as further documentation of business activity. Remember that business expenses are subject to auditing by the Internal Revenue Service (IRS). Good recordkeeping is essential when providing documentation to the IRS.

Petty Cash

Petty cash is available for incidentals such as small purchases, reimbursements, postage due or other miscellaneous expenses within the medical office. For example, petty cash is used for postage due on certified mail or other letters received in the office. Petty cash must be tracked and recorded in a daily financial log. To replenish petty cash, a check is written for the predetermined amount. A designated amount of cash is usually placed in a drawer or box at the beginning of each month for this purpose. This amount will vary from office to office, depending on the needs of the office, and usually ranges from $50 to $100. At the end of a designated period (usually a week or a month), all the receipts for money taken out of the petty cash drawer are totaled and added to the money remaining in the drawer. This total should match the amount placed in the drawer at the beginning of the period. The cash used during the period will then be replaced to make the total cash available in the drawer equal to the beginning amount.

Petty cash is usually handled by one responsible office person and by a substitute in his or her absence. The petty cash drawer should be kept in a secret place under lock and key.

Payroll

Payroll responsibilities include calculating payroll checks for the entire staff. Some medical offices contract an independent payroll service. This may or may not include the physician, depending on how the office structure and payment system are set up. Payroll checks are generally issued weekly, biweekly, or monthly. These result in the following pay periods for a year:

Weekly—52 pay periods a year (Employees are paid every week on the same day of the week.)

Biweekly—26 pay periods a year (Employees are paid every 2 weeks.)

Semi-Monthly—24 pay periods a year (Employees are paid on predetermined dates during the month, for example, on the 15th and 30th of every month.)

NAME Tania Walker
SOCIAL SECURITY NO. 123-12-1234
ADDRESS 22 W. Elm Avenue, Apt 3C
DATE OF EMPLOYMENT 6-30-11
Goram City, MI 55555
TELEPHONE (010)123-4567
EXEMPTIONS 1
HOURLY RATE $10.00

HOURS		GROSS SALARY	DEDUCTIONS					NET SALARY	DATE	CHECK NO.
REG.	O.T.		FWT	SWT	FICA					
80		800 —	72 —	14 —	61⁶⁰			652⁴⁰	7/14	276
80		800 —	72 —	14 —	61⁶⁰			652⁴⁰	7/28	414
72		720 —	64⁸⁰	12⁶⁰	55⁴⁵			587¹⁵	8/11	565
80	4	860 —	77¹⁰	15⁰⁵	66²⁰			701³⁵	8/25	697
QUARTERLY TOTAL										
YEAR TO DATE										

FIGURE 16-7   **An example of a paper employee payroll record.**

Monthly—12 pay periods a year (Employees are paid on the same date every month.)

The physician determines the type of pay period the office will use. All employees will then be paid at the same time. Figure 16-7 is an example of a paper employee payroll record. Figure 16-8 is an example of a computerized employee payroll record.

HOURLY EMPLOYEES

The employee's payroll check is determined by first calculating the **gross annual wage** before taxes and any withholding amounts that are taken out. For hourly employees, use this formula:

(Hourly wage × Number of hours worked per week) × 52 Weeks in a year = Gross pay (or Hourly wage × 2080 Full-time hours in a year = Annual pay)

The following would be the annual gross wage for an employee earning $12.00 per hour working a 40-hour week:

$$\$12.00 \times 40 \times 52 = \$24,960$$

annual gross wage

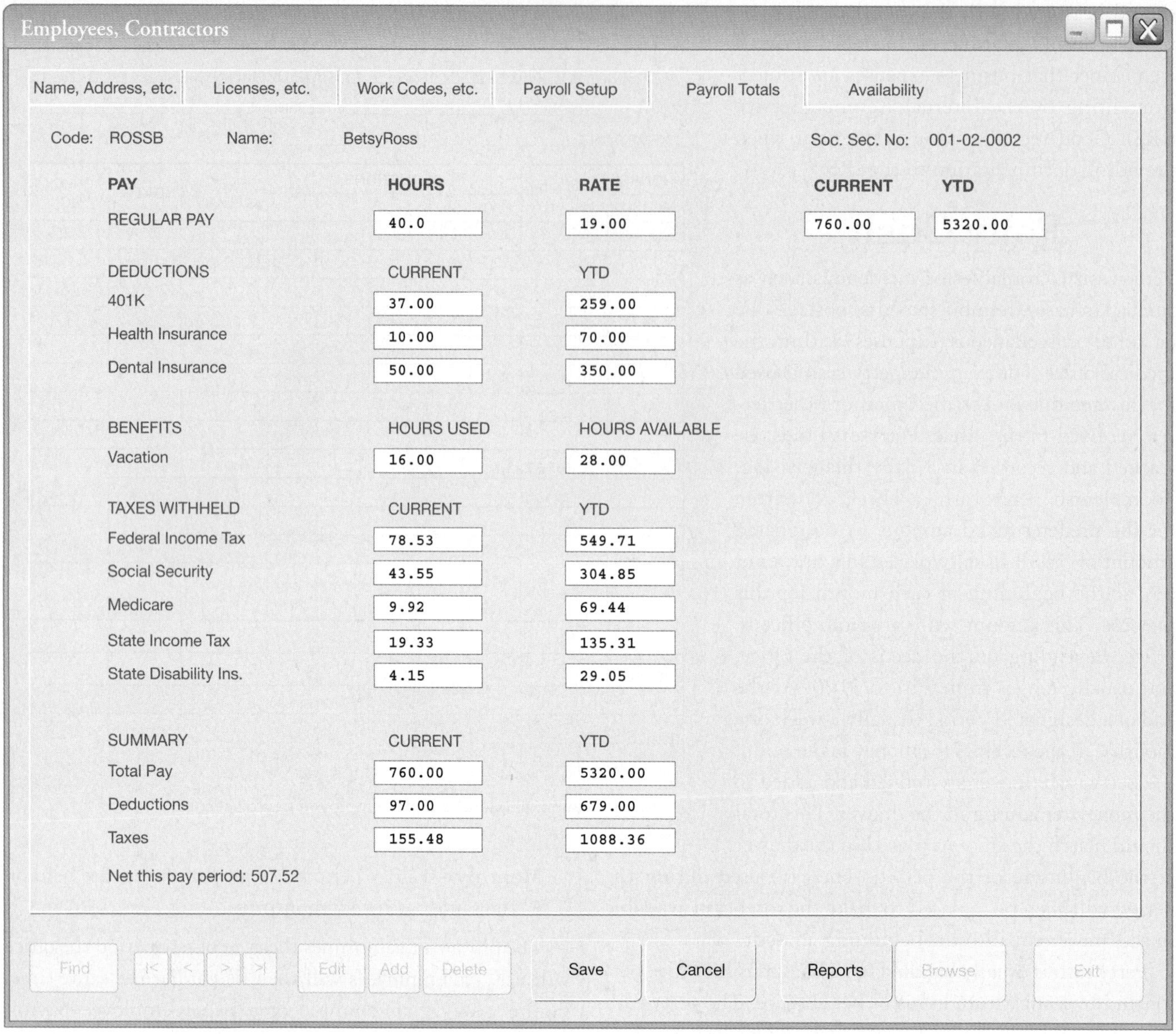

FIGURE 16-8 Example of a computerized employee payroll record.

To determine the amount the employee earns per day, use the following formula:

(Annual gross pay ÷ 52) ÷ 5 = Day's pay

For the example above:

($24,960 ÷ 52) = $480

$480 ÷ 5 = $96 pay per day

Therefore, if this employee missed a day of work, $96 would be deducted to arrive at the adjusted gross pay ($480 − $96 = $384). Occasionally, an employee will work overtime or more hours than normal (a 40-hour week at 8 hours a day for 5 days per week) for that pay period. To calculate the overtime pay of time and a half (1 hour of pay plus ½ hour of pay) for an employee who worked 1 day of over-

time at the hourly wage of $12.00, simply divide $12 in half ($6) and add that amount to the regular $12 hourly wage ($12 + $6 = $18). The payment for 1 hour of overtime for this employee would be $18 instead of the regular $12 payment.

SALARIED EMPLOYEES

Salaried employees receive a predetermined amount of money every pay period that is not dependent on the number of hours worked within the pay period. Unless the salaried employee is considered exempt, he or she is not entitled to overtime. No matter whether the employee works 40 hours or 50 hours in a week, the pay will remain the same; however, the salary is based on a 40-hour work week.

DEDUCTIONS

Money is withheld from the employee's paycheck, depending on the taxes, health and life insurance premiums, and any other deductions taken out of the employee's wages. Some deductions must be paid by the employee and the employer. This is referred to as **tax withholding**. For example, if the withholding tax is 4 percent, then this amount is calculated based on the employee's gross pay. The taxes are then subtracted from the gross or adjusted gross pay. The amount after subtracting the withholdings is what appears on the employee's paycheck. Figure 16-9 provides an example of computerized payroll processing and the deductions that may be taken.

Government regulations require that records must be maintained for each employee relating to the following payroll items:

- Amount of gross pay

- Social Security number of the employee
- Number of exemptions of each employee (taken from W-4 form completed by the employee at the time of hire)
- Deductions for federal, state, and city taxes and Social Security
- State disability insurance and unemployment tax, where applicable
- Any pretax deductions, such as 401K contributions

METHODS FOR CALCULATING PAYROLL CHECKS

Several systems may be used for calculating and issuing payroll checks. They include manual, pegboard, and computer.

Manual Method

Meticulous recordkeeping is necessary when performing any payroll function. Separate records are needed for

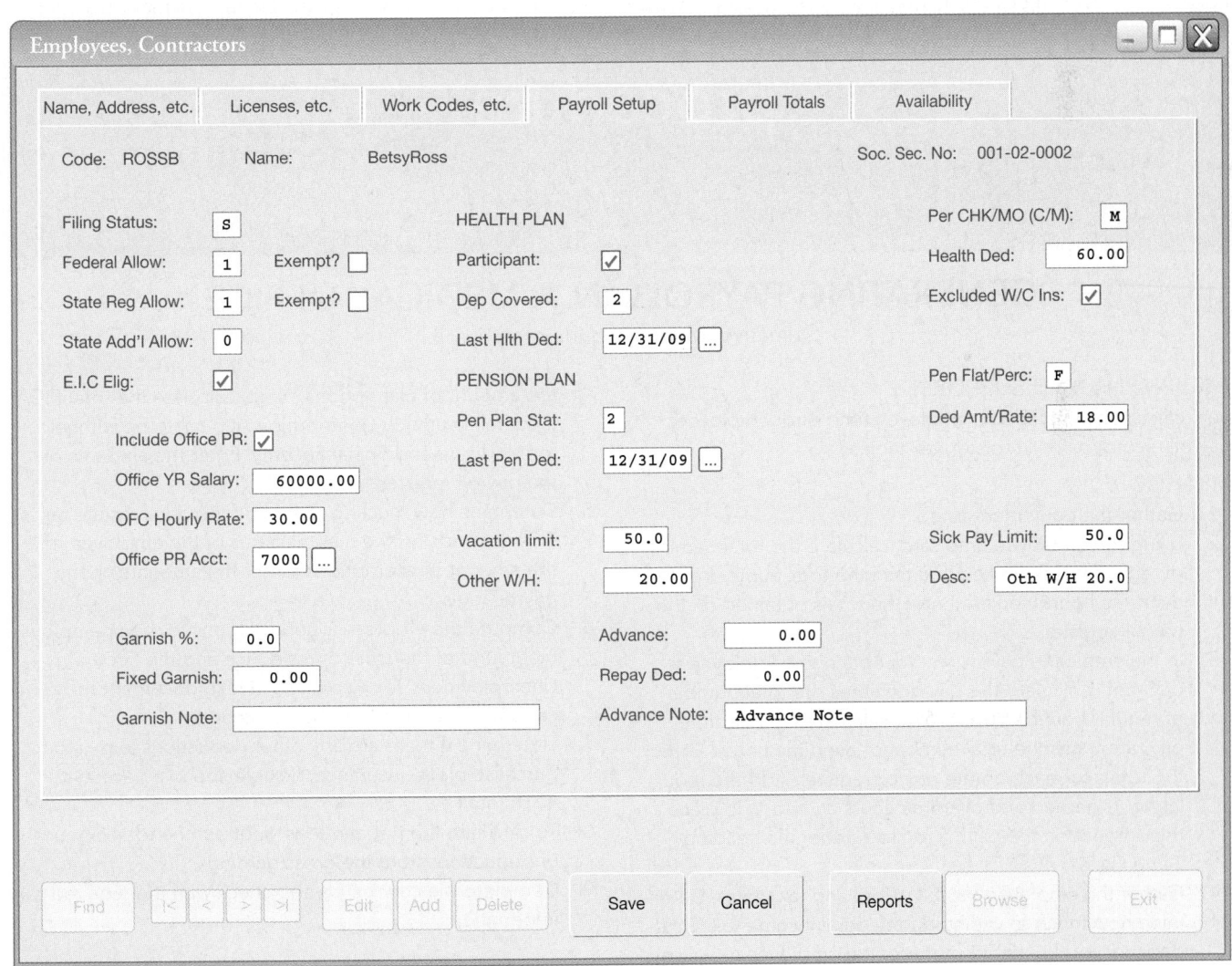

FIGURE 16-9 Example of a computerized payroll showing possible deductions.

documentation of gross income, tax withholding, and each check issued for all employees. This can mean that the records for payroll are kept in more than one record book or logbook. For example, the check stub will indicate the name, date, and amount of the payroll check, whereas a logbook is needed to track the gross income and withholding, which are totaled monthly, quarterly, and annually. Procedure 16-5 lists steps for manually generating a payroll in a medical office.

Pegboard Method

The advantage of using a pegboard (write-it-once) method is that all or most of the payroll record is in one record.

Computer Method

Several software packages are available that are used to calculate payroll and tax withholdings and print payroll checks. Such software programs can save time for office staff over the traditional manual method. In addition, the amounts calculated for withholding can be performed more accurately with the computer than with the manual method. In some offices, an outside payroll service is hired to process all payroll checks, calculate withholding payments, and keep records.

INCOME TAX WITHHOLDING

Federal, state, and city taxes are withheld from the paycheck of the employee. These tax payments are made directly to the government. Employers have an obligation by law to withhold a portion of each employee's earnings for tax purposes and to report and forward this amount to the government. To determine the amount of money to be withheld from each paycheck, each employee must complete a W-4 form when he or she is hired (Figure 16-10). The W-4 form must include the following:

- Employee's name and current address
- Social Security number
- Marital status
- The number of exemptions the employee claims should be used when calculating withheld tax money

procedure 16-5

GENERATING PAYROLL IN A MEDICAL OFFICE
Objective: Manually generate payroll.

EQUIPMENT AND SUPPLIES
pen; calculator; checkbook; employee time card; employee payroll record; payroll register; tax tables

METHOD
1. Gather the equipment listed.
2. Using the employee time card, calculate the total number of regular hours worked and then the total number of overtime hours worked. Enter the totals obtained on the payroll register.
3. In the employee payroll record, obtain the employee's pay rate. Calculate the pay rate times the total number of regular hours worked. Next, calculate the overtime pay rate times the total number of overtime hours. Enter the totals for each on the payroll register. Add the regular hours earned and overtime hours earned, and place this amount on the payroll register under the heading TOTAL GROSS.
4. Gather the employee payroll record and tax tables. Determine how much to withhold for federal income tax. This depends on the marital status of the employee as well as

the amount of exemptions. Next, calculate the total FICA (Federal Insurance Contribution Act) tax to be withheld for Medicare and Social Security. Enter the amounts on the payroll register.
5. Determine how much to withhold for local and state taxes. This depends on the marital status of the employee and the amount of exemptions. Enter the amounts on the payroll register.
6. Compute the employer's contributions to the unemployment fund of the state of residence and the Federal Unemployment Tax Act (FUTA). Next, document these calculations on the employer's account.
7. Determine if there are any other deductions (e.g., stock purchase plans, insurance, flexible spending account, 401K, etc.).
8. To calculate the net earnings, subtract the total amount of deductions from the gross earnings.
9. Complete the check stub and check with the required information.

Form W-4 (20XX)

Purpose. Complete Form W-4 so that your employer can withhold the correct federal income tax from your pay. Because your tax situation may change, you may want to refigure your withholding each year.

Exemption from withholding. If you are exempt, complete only lines 1, 2, 3, 4, and 7 and sign the form to validate it. Your exemption for 20XX expires February 16, 20XX. See Pub. 505, Tax Withholding and Estimated Tax.

Note. You cannot claim exemption from withholding if (a) your income exceeds $800 and includes more than $250 of unearned income (for example, interest and dividends) and (b) another person can claim you as a dependent on their tax return.

Basic instructions. If you are not exempt, complete the **Personal Allowances Worksheet** below. The worksheets on page 2 adjust your withholding allowances based on itemized deductions, certain credits, adjustments to income, or two-earner/two-job situations. Complete all worksheets that apply. However, you may claim fewer (or zero) allowances.

Head of household. Generally, you may claim head of household filing status on your tax return only if you are unmarried and pay more than 50% of the costs of keeping up a home for yourself and your dependent(s) or other qualifying individuals. See line **E** below.

Tax credits. You can take projected tax credits into account in figuring your allowable number of withholding allowances. Credits for child or dependent care expenses and the child tax credit may be claimed using the **Personal Allowances Worksheet** below. See Pub. 919, How Do I Adjust My Tax Withholding? for information on converting your other credits into withholding allowances.

Nonwage income. If you have a large amount of nonwage income, such as interest or dividends, consider making estimated tax payments using Form 1040-ES, Estimated Tax for Individuals. Otherwise, you may owe additional tax.

Two earners/two jobs. If you have a working spouse or more than one job, figure the total number of allowances you are entitled to claim on all jobs using worksheets from only one Form W-4. Your withholding usually will be most accurate when all allowances are claimed on the Form W-4 for the highest paying job and zero allowances are claimed on the others.

Nonresident alien. If you are a nonresident alien, see the Instructions for Form 8233 before completing this Form W-4.

Check your withholding. After your Form W-4 takes effect, use Pub. 919 to see how the dollar amount you are having withheld compares to your projected total tax for 20XX. See Pub. 919, especially if your earnings exceed $125,000 (Single) or $175,000 (Married).

Recent name change? If your name on line 1 differs from that shown on your social security card, call 1-800-772-1213 to initiate a name change and obtain a social security card showing your correct name.

Personal Allowances Worksheet (Keep for your records.)

A Enter "1" for **yourself** if no one else can claim you as a dependent . . . . **A** _____

B Enter "1" if:
- You are single and have only one job; or
- You are married, have only one job, and your spouse does not work; or
- Your wages from a second job or your spouse's wages (or the total of both) are $1,000 or less.

. . **B** _____

C Enter "1" for your **spouse**. But, you may choose to enter "-0-" if you are married and have either a working spouse or more than one job. (Entering "-0-" may help you avoid having too little tax withheld.) . . . . **C** _____

D Enter number of **dependents** (other than your spouse or yourself) you will claim on your tax return . . . . . . **D** _____

E Enter "1" if you will file as **head of household** on your tax return (see conditions under **Head of household** above) . **E** _____

F Enter "1" if you have at least $1,500 of **child or dependent care expenses** for which you plan to claim a credit . . **F** _____
(**Note.** Do **not** include child support payments. See **Pub. 503,** Child and Dependent Care Expenses, for details.)

G **Child Tax Credit** (including additional child tax credit):
- If your total income will be less than $54,000 ($79,000 if married), enter "2" for each eligible child.
- If your total income will be between $54,000 and $84,000 ($79,000 and $119,000 if married), enter "1" for each eligible child plus "1" **additional** if you have four or more eligible children. . . . . **G** _____

H Add lines A through G and enter total here. (**Note.** This may be different from the number of exemptions you claim on your tax return.) ▶ **H** _____

For accuracy, complete all worksheets that apply.
- If you plan to **itemize or claim adjustments to income** and want to reduce your withholding, see the **Deductions and Adjustments Worksheet** on page 2.
- If you have **more than one job** or are **married and you and your spouse both work** and the combined earnings from all jobs exceed $35,000 ($25,000 if married) see the **Two-Earner/Two-Job Worksheet** on page 2 to avoid having too little tax withheld.
- If **neither** of the above situations applies, **stop here** and enter the number from line H on line 5 of Form W-4 below.

------- Cut here and give Form W-4 to your employer. Keep the top part for your records. -------

Form W-4

Department of the Treasury
Internal Revenue Service

Employee's Withholding Allowance Certificate

OMB No. 1545-0010

20XX

▶ Whether you are entitled to claim a certain number of allowances or exemption from withholding is subject to review by the IRS. Your employer may be required to send a copy of this form to the IRS.

1 Type or print your first name and middle initial	Last name	2 Your social security number

Home address (number and street or rural route)	3 ☐ Single ☐ Married ☐ Married, but withhold at higher Single rate.
City or town, state, and ZIP code	**Note.** If married, but legally separated, or spouse is a nonresident alien, check the "Single" box.
	4 If your last name differs from that shown on your social security card, check here. You must call 1-800-772-1213 for a new card. ▶ ☐

5	Total number of allowances you are claiming (from line **H** above **or** from the applicable worksheet on page 2)	**5**	
6	Additional amount, if any, you want withheld from each paycheck	**6**	$
7	I claim exemption from withholding for 20XX, and I certify that I meet **both** of the following conditions for exemption.		

- Last year I had a right to a refund of **all** federal income tax withheld because I had **no** tax liability **and**
- This year I expect a refund of **all** federal income tax withheld because I expect to have **no** tax liability.

If you meet both conditions, write "Exempt" here . . . . ▶ **7** |

Under penalties of perjury, I declare that I have examined this certificate and to the best of my knowledge and belief, it is true, correct, and complete.

Employee's signature
(Form is not valid unless you sign it.) ▶   Date ▶

8 Employer's name and address (Employer: Complete lines 8 and 10 only if sending to the IRS.)	9 Office code (optional)	10 Employer identification number (EIN)

For Privacy Act and Paperwork Reduction Act Notice, see page 2.   Cat. No. 10220Q   Form **W-4** (20XX)

FIGURE 16-10 An example of a W-4 required by the IRS.

MARRIED Persons—**WEEKLY** Payroll Period
(For Wages Paid Through December 2009)

If the wages are—		And the number of withholding allowances claimed is—										
At least	But less than	0	1	2	3	4	5	6	7	8	9	10
		The amount of income tax to be withheld is—										
$0	$310	$0	$0	$0	$0	$0	$0	$0	$0	$0	$0	$0
310	320	1	0	0	0	0	0	0	0	0	0	0
320	330	2	0	0	0	0	0	0	0	0	0	0
330	340	3	0	0	0	0	0	0	0	0	0	0
340	350	4	0	0	0	0	0	0	0	0	0	0
350	360	5	0	0	0	0	0	0	0	0	0	0
360	370	6	0	0	0	0	0	0	0	0	0	0
370	380	7	0	0	0	0	0	0	0	0	0	0
380	390	8	1	0	0	0	0	0	0	0	0	0
390	400	9	2	0	0	0	0	0	0	0	0	0
400	410	10	3	0	0	0	0	0	0	0	0	0
410	420	11	4	0	0	0	0	0	0	0	0	0
420	430	12	5	0	0	0	0	0	0	0	0	0
430	440	13	6	0	0	0	0	0	0	0	0	0
440	450	14	7	0	0	0	0	0	0	0	0	0
450	460	15	8	1	0	0	0	0	0	0	0	0
460	470	16	9	2	0	0	0	0	0	0	0	0
470	480	17	10	3	0	0	0	0	0	0	0	0
480	490	19	11	4	0	0	0	0	0	0	0	0
490	500	20	12	5	0	0	0	0	0	0	0	0
500	510	22	13	6	0	0	0	0	0	0	0	0
510	520	23	14	7	0	0	0	0	0	0	0	0
520	530	25	15	8	1	0	0	0	0	0	0	0
530	540	26	16	9	2	0	0	0	0	0	0	0
540	550	28	17	10	3	0	0	0	0	0	0	0
550	560	29	19	11	4	0	0	0	0	0	0	0
560	570	31	20	12	5	0	0	0	0	0	0	0
570	580	32	22	13	6	0	0	0	0	0	0	0
580	590	34	23	14	7	0	0	0	0	0	0	0
590	600	35	25	15	8	1	0	0	0	0	0	0
600	610	37	26	16	9	2	0	0	0	0	0	0
610	620	38	28	17	10	3	0	0	0	0	0	0
620	630	40	29	19	11	4	0	0	0	0	0	0
630	640	41	31	20	12	5	0	0	0	0	0	0
640	650	43	32	22	13	6	0	0	0	0	0	0
650	660	44	34	23	14	7	0	0	0	0	0	0
660	670	46	35	25	15	8	1	0	0	0	0	0
670	680	47	37	26	16	9	2	0	0	0	0	0
680	690	49	38	28	17	10	3	0	0	0	0	0
690	700	50	40	29	19	11	4	0	0	0	0	0
700	710	52	41	31	20	12	5	0	0	0	0	0
710	720	53	43	32	22	13	6	0	0	0	0	0
720	730	55	44	34	23	14	7	0	0	0	0	0
730	740	56	46	35	25	15	8	1	0	0	0	0
740	750	58	47	37	26	16	9	2	0	0	0	0
750	760	59	49	38	28	17	10	3	0	0	0	0
760	770	61	50	40	29	19	11	4	0	0	0	0
770	780	62	52	41	31	20	12	5	0	0	0	0
780	790	64	53	43	32	22	13	6	0	0	0	0
790	800	65	55	44	34	23	14	7	0	0	0	0
800	810	67	56	46	35	25	15	8	1	0	0	0
810	820	68	58	47	37	26	16	9	2	0	0	0
820	830	70	59	49	38	28	17	10	3	0	0	0
830	840	71	61	50	40	29	19	11	4	0	0	0
840	850	73	62	52	41	31	20	12	5	0	0	0
850	860	74	64	53	43	32	22	13	6	0	0	0
860	870	76	65	55	44	34	23	14	7	0	0	0
870	880	77	67	56	46	35	25	15	8	1	0	0
880	890	79	68	58	47	37	26	16	9	2	0	0
890	900	80	70	59	49	38	28	17	10	3	0	0
900	910	82	71	61	50	40	29	19	11	4	0	0
910	920	83	73	62	52	41	31	20	12	5	0	0
920	930	85	74	64	53	43	32	22	13	6	0	0
930	940	86	76	65	55	44	34	23	14	7	0	0
940	950	88	77	67	56	46	35	25	15	8	1	0
950	960	89	79	68	58	47	37	26	16	9	2	0
960	970	91	80	70	59	49	38	28	17	10	3	0
970	980	92	82	71	61	50	40	29	19	11	4	0
980	990	94	83	73	62	52	41	31	20	12	5	0
990	1,000	95	85	74	64	53	43	32	22	13	6	0

FIGURE 16-11 An example of a federal tax withholding table for married couples.

total gross income (see "Hourly Employees" for method of calculating gross income). The number of exemptions claimed on the W-4 form and the marital status of the employee are taken into account when calculating the tax. The employer has an obligation to match the employee's payment for Social Security and Medicare. This means that if the employee has $100 withheld for Social Security and Medicare, the employer must match the $100 and make a total payment to the government for that employee of $200. The employer does not have to match the federal, state, and local taxes.

DEPOSIT REQUIREMENTS

The federal tax money withheld and the FICA payment are placed into a federal deposit account in a Federal Reserve Bank or into an authorized banking institution, either at the end of each period or at the end of the month. The Internal Revenue Service (IRS) has a severe penalty for failure to deposit this money.

Employers must file a quarterly report (Form 941: Employer's Quarterly Federal Tax Return) before the last day of the first month after the end of the quarter. These dates are April 30, July 31, October 31, and January 31.

Tables used to determine the amount of withholding are provided in the Federal Employer's Tax Guide. See Figure 16-11 for a sample federal tax withholding table. Tables are available for married persons, single persons, and unmarried heads of households and cover weekly, biweekly, monthly, semimonthly, and daily periods.

SOCIAL SECURITY, MEDICARE, AND INCOME TAX WITHHOLDING

The federal government mandates, or requires, that the following taxes be paid: Social Security (Federal Insurance Contribution Act or FICA), Medicare, and federal income tax. These taxes are based on a percentage of the employee's

FEDERAL UNEMPLOYMENT TAX

Every employer must contribute to the unemployment tax act as mandated under the Federal Unemployment Tax Act (FUTA). If the employer is making payments into a state unemployment fund, this can generally be applied as credit against the FUTA tax amount.

FUTA is the sole responsibility of the employer. It is based on the employee's gross income but must not be deducted from the employee's wage.

FUTA deposits are calculated quarterly, and the amount due must be paid by the last day of the first month after the quarter ends. Therefore, for the first quarter of the year ending on March 31, the payment must be made by April 30. An annual FUTA report must be filed to the federal government using Form 940 each year.

Control number: B1-049097-0	Company # 007252	ERU 000	State Form		

Employer's name, address, and ZIP code **Pearson Physicians Group** **123 Machigan Avenue** **Parker Heights, IL 60610**	1 Wages, tips, other compensation 32094.40	2 Federal income tax withheld 5559.06
	3 Social Security wages 32094.40	4 Social Security tax withheld 1989.85
	5 Medicare wages and tips 32094.40	6 Medicare tax withheld 465.37
Employer's identification number	7 Social Security tips	8 Allocated tips
Employee's social security number	9 Advance EIC payment	10 Dependent care benefits
Employee's name, address, and ZIP code	11 Nonqualified plans	12 Benefits included in Box 1
	13 See instr. for Box 13	14 Other

15 Statutory emp.	Deceased	Pension plan X	Legal rep.	942 emp.	Deferred comp.	Void

18 State and Employer's state ID number	17 State wages, tips, etc. 32094.40	18 State income tax 1305.46	19 Locality Name CASDI	20 Local wages, tips, etc.	21 Local income tax 412.97

1995 Wage and Tax Statement — For Employee's Records — Department of the Treasury – Internal Revenue Service

FORM W2 COPY C

FIGURE 16-12 An example of a W-2 form required by the IRS.

STATE UNEMPLOYMENT TAX

All states have unemployment compensation laws. Most states require only the employer to make payments toward this fund. However, a few states require both the employer and employee to make a payment. In this case, the employer would withhold a certain calculated amount from the employee's paycheck.

In some states, the employer does not have to make a payment to unemployment compensation if there are very few employees (four or fewer). Each state's regulation concerning tax requirements should be checked carefully before preparing the payroll.

STATE DISABILITY INSURANCE

Some states require a certain amount of money be withheld from the employee's check to cover a disability insurance plan. This insurance coverage assists employees in the event they become injured or disabled rendering them unable to work. Money may also be withheld, as requested by the employee, for health, life, and disability insurances, and pension plan contributions.

ANNUAL TAX RETURNS

W-2 forms must be completed at the end of each year and are provided to each employee. By law, employers must mail or hand deliver W-2 forms by January 31 of the year immediately following the upcoming tax reporting season. For instance, W-2 forms indicating wages earned in the year 2009 must be mailed to employees by January 31, 2010. The amount of wages that were taxable under Social Security and Medicare must be listed separately on the W-2 form. The employer must provide three copies of the W-2 form to each employee from whom these taxes were withheld (one each for federal and state filing and one for the employee's file). The W-2 form (Figure 16-12) lists the total gross income; total federal, state, and local taxes that were withheld; taxable fringe benefits, such as tips; and the employee's total net income for the year.

The preparation of reports to the federal government and the W-2 forms for the employees can be time consuming and requires some training. Many offices that do not have a bookkeeper or medical assistant assigned to perform this duty use the services of an accountant. The records and reports the accountant will use must be prepared ahead of time. The pegboard system, if used, can provide summaries of the income, expenses, and payroll for the office. If a manual system is used, the totals for all the tax payment periods should be calculated for the accountant. The accountant will then **audit** or reexamine all the financial statements for accuracy.

SUMMARY

Banking is one of the critical office procedures since it requires careful handling of money and records. A thorough understanding of banking procedures and terminology is vital to running an efficient medical office. Great trust is placed in the medical assistant by the physician to handle his or her banking needs with accuracy.

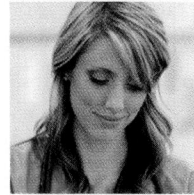# 16 CHAPTER REVIEW

COMPETENCY REVIEW

1. Define and spell the terms to learn for the chapter.

2. Using your own bank statement, reconcile it to your checkbook records.

3. Create and complete a check and check stub in the amount of 65 cents drafted to Bill Jay.

4. Call a local bank and request information regarding the various options for checking and savings accounts.

5. Create a bank deposit slip for $23.10 in cash and checks for $54.00, $21.25, $110.00, $29.00, and $9.25.

PREPARING FOR THE CERTIFICATION EXAM

1. A check that will become void if not cashed within the time stated on the check is a
   a. certified check.
   b. limited check.
   c. cashier's check.
   d. stale check.
   e. old check.

2. The person the check is made out to is the
   a. maker.
   b. payee.
   c. payer.
   d. teller.
   e. recipient.

3. The code number found in the lower-left corner of a printed check is the
   a. MICR.
   b. withdrawal number.
   c. registration number.
   d. ABA number.
   e. OCR.

4. A check written on the payer's own check yet guarantees payment is considered a
   a. cashier's check.
   b. voucher check.
   c. certified check.

   d. limited check.
   e. paycheck.

5. If an employee is paid on two set dates every month, he or she is paid
   a. bi-monthly.
   b. semi-monthly.
   c. bi-weekly.
   d. semi-weekly.
   e. bi-annually.

6. Gross annual wage is the
   a. amount of money the employee takes home in a year.
   b. amount of money the employee takes home each pay period.
   c. amount of money the employee earns in a year before deductions.
   d. amount of money the employee earns in a pay period before deductions.
   e. amount of money the employee pays into a fund every year.

7. Which of the following is purchased for the cash value typed on the check?
   a. cashier's check.
   b. certified check.
   c. voucher check.

d.   money order.

e.   payroll check.

8. Which of the following types of endorsement is not used in the business office?

a.   restrictive.

b.   full.

c.   blank.

d.   limited.

e.   exclusive.

9. An employer must provide how many copies of the employee's W-2 by January 31?

a.   1

b.   2

c.   3

d.   4

e.   none, unless the employee asks.

10. Which of the following types of checks are frequently used for payroll checks?

a.   cashier's check.

b.   certified check.

c.   voucher check.

d.   money order.

e.   traveler's check.

CRITICAL THINKING

1. As Tania reviews the checks for deposit, she realizes that one of the checks collected for a patient's copayment is postdated 2 days in advance. The office has a clear policy regarding not accepting postdated checks. The deposit slip, which today lists 18 checks, already includes the postdated check. What should Tania do?

2. While reviewing the petty cash drawer, Tania realizes that $5 is missing and unaccounted for. How should Tania handle this situation?

ON THE JOB

Your office has decided that all payroll should be handled through direct deposit into employee bank accounts. Call your bank and ask how that procedure would be handled for a medical office. There are forms to complete and information on other bank account numbers and ABA numbers that you will need to collect and complete, according to the bank's procedures.

INTERNET ACTIVITY

Call your bank and get its online address. Then go to the Internet and access the bank's home page. If you do not have a bank account, call several local banks and go to their home pages. List the steps in setting up an online banking account.

MEDMEDIA

Additional interactive resources and activities for this chapter can be found:

On your student DVD: View applicable procedure videos on the DVD-ROM found in the back of this book.

MyHealthProfessionsKit.com: Test your knowledge of the chapter with games and activities. MyHealthProfessionsKit also includes resources, helpful links, and a Spanish audio glossary.

Medical Assisting Interactive: Practice your procedures as a medical assistant in this simulated doctor's office. This can be accessed through MyHealthProfessionsKit.com.

17

Medical Insurance

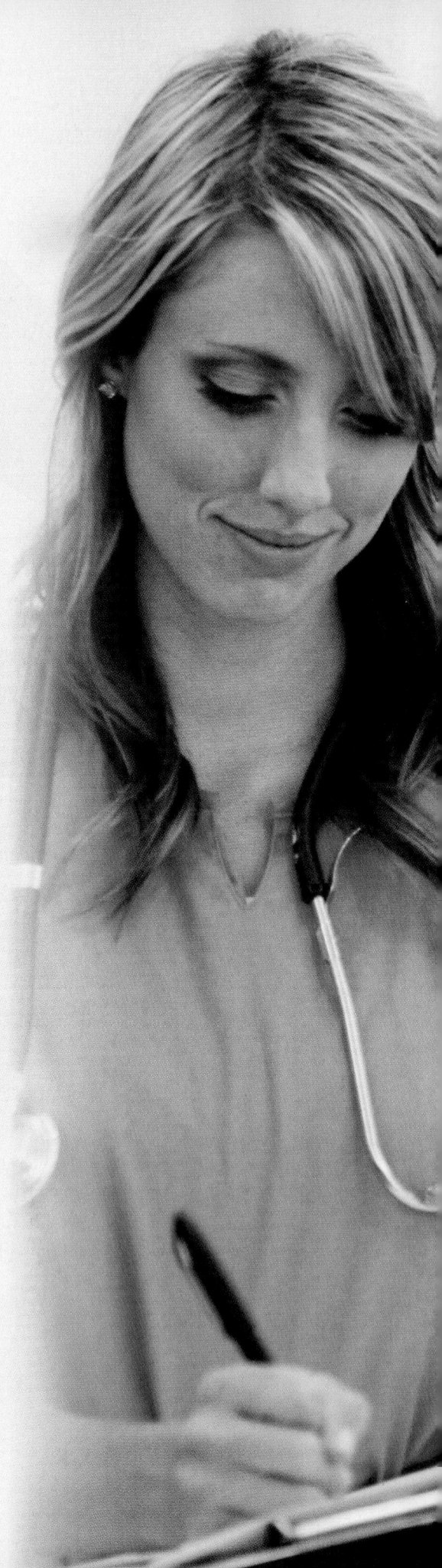

LEARNING OBJECTIVES

After completing this chapter, you should be able to:

- Define and spell the terms to learn for this chapter.

- Explain the differences among health maintenance organizations (HMOs), preferred provider organizations (PPOs), and traditional insurance programs.

- Describe group, individual, and government-sponsored (public) health benefits and explain the differences among them.

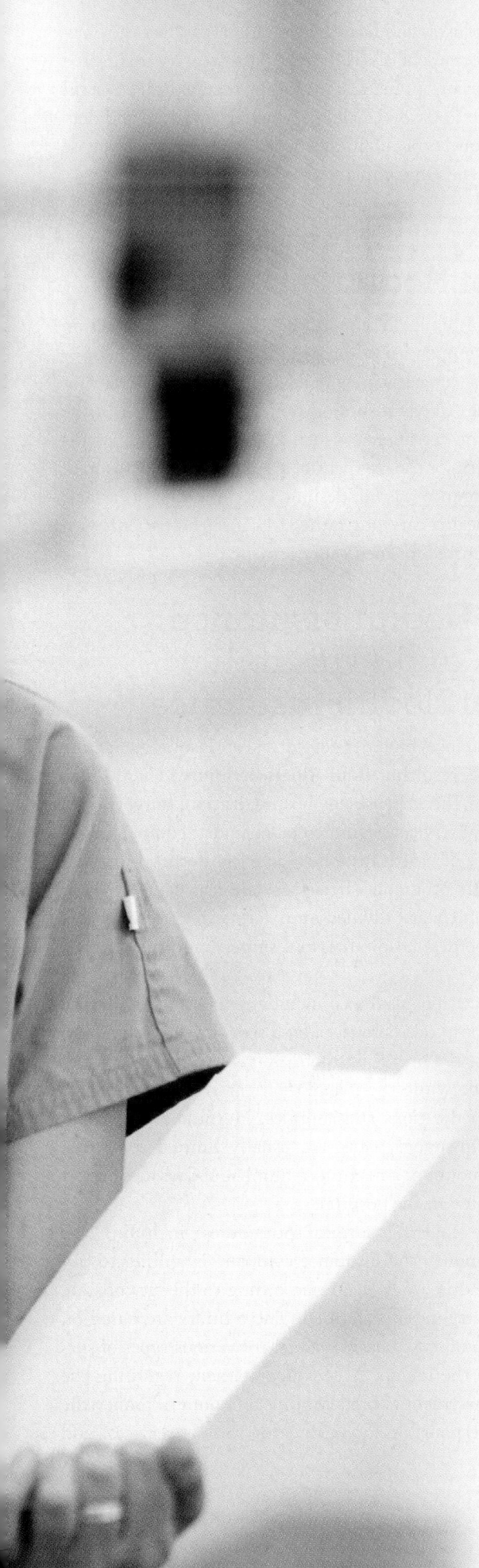

CHAPTER OUTLINE

CASE STUDY

Miriam Jones is the CMA (AAMA) working at the front desk today at Pearson Physicians Group. Shelly Flannery presents to the office today as a new patient. She is about to turn 65 years old. Shelly informs Miriam that she is a retired nurse from the United States Navy and is wondering how her upcoming birthday may affect her health care coverage.

benefit period

capitation rate

claim

closed-panel HMO

coordination of benefits (COB)

crossover claim

deductible

exclusive provider organizations (EPOs)

fee-for-service

fee schedule

formulary

gatekeeper

health maintenance organization (HMO)

integrated delivery system (IDS)

medical foundation

open-panel HMO

point-of-service plan (POS)

preauthorization

preferred provider organization (PPO)

premium

prepaid plan

primary care provider (PCP)

referral

self-referral

CERTIFICATION LINK

CMA (AAMA)
Practice finances
    Third-party billing

RMA
Administrative medical assisting
    Insurance
    Medical receptionist/ Secretarial/ Clerical

CMAS (AMT)
Medical office clerical assisting
    Communication
    Health care insurance processing, coding, and billing
        Insurance processing
        Insurance billing and finances

Health insurance was originally designed to help patients with catastrophic medical expenses that occurred as a result of an unexpected illness or injury. Health benefits were set up as a contract between the subscriber (insured) and the carrier (insurance company or third-party payer). The first medical or health insurance plans were not intended to cover all costs associated with health care. Over the years, insurance plans for medical and health care have expanded. As the cost of medical care has escalated, new and different types of health care plans and many regulations have come into being. In today's medical practices, as much as 85 percent of a physician's income is paid by some form of medical insurance.

The successful medical assistant understands the importance of insurance to both the patient and the practice. He or she keeps current with regulations governing the health insurance industry and how these regulations affect the practice's reimbursements as well as the patients who are insured under the various policies. This means the medical assistant must be able to process a **claim**, which is a written and documented request for reimbursement, for an eligible expense in a correct and timely manner.

The Purpose of Health Insurance

Generally, insurance is something that provides protection against or compensation for specific types of risk, loss, or ruin. It is a contract in which an insurance company or agency agrees to pay a sum of money to the insured in the event of some contingency, such as death, accident, or illness, in return for the payment of a premium by the insured. Medical insurance was not designed to cover all costs associated with health care but rather to assist the patient with expenses incurred for medical treatment.

Health Insurance and Availability of Health Insurance

Health insurance includes all forms of insurance against financial loss resulting from illness or injury. These losses may include the expenses of hospitalization, surgery, and other medical services. Commercial insurance companies sell various types of health insurance policies. Both commercial and nonprofit programs offer essentially the same types of coverage, which are divided into four categories: regular medical expenses, hospitalization, surgery, and major medical expenses.

Hospitalization insurance includes expenses such as the cost of the hospital room (usually a semi-private room) and meals, use of the operating room, X-ray and laboratory fees for tests done while the insured patient is in the hospital, and some medications and supplies. Hospitalization benefits, under insurance plans, are usually limited to a total monetary amount or a maximum number of days a patient is allowed to stay in the hospital.

Insurance covering surgical procedures, including the amount of money the insurance company is willing to pay for the procedure, may change according to the city or state where the surgery is performed. These limits are based on "reasonable and customary" charges for various types of surgery within the region. A general statement regarding the insured's copayment (a predetermined amount of money the patient is responsible for paying for various services) and

deductible (a predetermined amount of money the patient must pay prior to the insurance company beginning to cover services) may be required of the patient as designated by the insurance carrier.

Relatively new types of insurance are the fixed payment plans. These are offered by organizations that operate their own health care facilities or that have made arrangements with a specific hospital or health care provider within a city or region. The fixed-payment plan offers subscribers, or members, complete medical care in return for a fixed monthly fee or semimonthly fee. This fee is called a **premium**. When the premium is paid, reimbursement for certain benefits becomes available. Some contracts specify a maximum lifetime benefit.

Health care insurance today is available in three common options:

- **Managed Care**—fixed, prepaid-fee plans with contracted health care providers obtained either independently or as a group.

- **Group-Sponsored or Individual Policies**—purchased through commercial insurance companies.

- **Government-Sponsored Programs**—financed and regulated by federal or state governments for specific groups of people. Some examples of government-sponsored insurance include Medicare, Medicaid, workers' compensation, and military plans such as TRICARE and CHAMPVA.

Any of these plans will help with the cost of health care; however, they do not cover all expenses. For any of the insurance options, the insured pays a premium for specific coverage and usually has a deductible as well.

Managed Care Organizations

Managed care organizations (MCOs) offer options that are available through private insurance carriers and through some government programs. This type of plan is referred to as a **prepaid plan** because a group of providers will have a contractual agreement to provide services to subscribers on a negotiated fee-for-service basis. **Fee-for-service** is a set of fees for services established by a health care provider and paid for by the patient. A **fee schedule** lists the amount to be paid by the insurance company for each procedure or ser-vice subject to the managed care contract.

In some managed care situations, the patient is assigned a **primary care provider (PCP)**, also known as a primary care physician, who is responsible for the overall management of the patient's health. This PCP acts as a **gatekeeper** and will determine the medical necessity of specialist providers' services and will refer the patient to specialists if necessary. At the same time, the MCO stresses the concept of wellness, often paying higher benefits for health maintenance, such as physical examinations and routine immunizations. In this manner, the MCO tries to decrease the number of visits a patient makes each calendar year for health care services of an acute nature.

HISTORY OF MANAGED CARE SYSTEMS

The first privately owned, prepaid medical group in the United States was founded in 1929 in Southern California. The Ross-Loos Medical Group was composed of several medical group locations and provided services to Los Angeles Department of Water and Power employees. In the 1970s, Ross-Loos merged with a health plan group in Philadelphia to become CIGNA Healthplans of California. The federal Health Maintenance Organization Act of 1973 allowed this to occur. The act did the following:

- Provided funds (loans and grants) to assist in the development of new federally qualified HMOs

- Required most employers with more than 25 employees to offer HMO benefits as an alternative to traditional health insurance plans

- Established federal standards for HMOs

In 1985, the Preferred Provider Health Care Act impacted the **preferred provider organizations (PPOs)**.

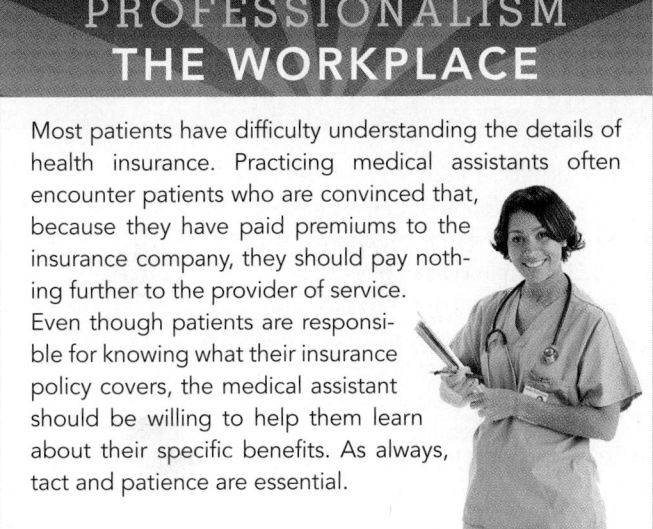

PROFESSIONALISM
THE WORKPLACE

Most patients have difficulty understanding the details of health insurance. Practicing medical assistants often encounter patients who are convinced that, because they have paid premiums to the insurance company, they should pay nothing further to the provider of service. Even though patients are responsible for knowing what their insurance policy covers, the medical assistant should be willing to help them learn about their specific benefits. As always, tact and patience are essential.

PPOs require the patient to use a provider under contract with the insurance company and reimburse the provider at a discounted rate. This act allows subscribers to utilize providers outside the defined network. A 1988 amendment to the HMO Act of 1973 made similar changes to the HMO system.

ADVANTAGES AND DISADVANTAGES OF MANAGED CARE

How has managed care impacted the cost of health care? Costs have been contained by controlling who provides the services (PCP or specialist), what services are provided (covered or noncovered), and where the services are provided (inpatient or outpatient). This means the MCO has a limited number of providers and facilities from which the patient may receive covered services. The MCO also determines the types of covered services the patient can or will receive. Box 17-1 lists advantages and disadvantages of managed care.

HEALTH MAINTENANCE ORGANIZATIONS

A **health maintenance organization (HMO)** is a type of managed care plan in which a range of health care services by a limited group of providers (such as physicians and hospitals) are made available to plan members for a predetermined fee called the **capitation rate**. The HMO concept was started to control the cost explosion in health care as a result of overutilization of services. Before HMOs became so widespread, insurance companies reimbursed providers for all their charges without questioning whether the services were medically necessary. Providers had little incentive to control costs. HMOs operate on a budget that is the total of their member patients' fees. For this reason, HMOs attempt to control the length of hospital stays or unnecessary surgery for their members. The following are two important components of an HMO:

- All medical services are provided based on a predetermined (per capita) fee and not on a fee-for-service basis. If the actual cost of services exceeds the predetermined (or capitation) amount, then the provider must absorb the excess in costs. This provides the incentive for the provider to control costs.

- A member patient must use the providers and hospitals that are identified by the HMO. The HMO will pay for any covered services that are provided by designated providers, hospitals, durable medical equipment, and pharmacies. Therefore preapproval must be granted through the PCP when and if a patient has to seek consultation or medical services out of the network. The exception to this is in the case of recognized emergency services.

As mentioned, HMOs place an emphasis on maintaining health. Regular physical examinations and patient education are strongly encouraged. The advantage of HMOs is the control of health costs that results from instructing providers to limit unnecessary tests and procedures. Premiums, therefore, are lower. The disadvantage is that providers may decide to cut costs by not providing services patients need.

A member patient who joins an HMO may either choose a personal provider from a list of provider physicians, nurse practitioners, and physician assistants or be assigned a PCP who is generally an internist, family practitioner, OB/GYN, or pediatrician. The PCP must provide all pri-

Box 17-1 Advantages and Disadvantages of Managed CARE

Advantages

- Smaller out-of-pocket expenses for the patient
- Nominal copayment
- No deductible for some plans
- Contains health care costs
- Pays for authorized services
- Fee schedules established
- Preventive medical treatment usually covered

Disadvantages

- Increased amount of paperwork
- Preauthorization requirements
- Lower reimbursement rates
- Limited provider choices
- Renewal of coverage not guaranteed
- Specialized care limited at times
- Referrals limited at times
- Limited flexibility
- Unapproved or unauthorized treatments not covered

mary care services since the HMO will not pay for the costs of a nonmember provider, except in the case of an emergency. HMOs are required to tell members, in the documents regarding their coverage, of the patient's right to ask for an investigation of any problems concerning care or coverage under the HMO.

HMO Models

There are two categories of HMO models: closed-panel HMO and open-panel HMO. In the **closed-panel HMO**, the clinic is owned by the HMO and the providers are employees of the HMO. There are two types of closed-panel models: the group model HMO and the staff model HMO. In the *group model,* the HMO may contract with providers who are part of an independent group practice. The HMO reimburses the group for providing care to subscribers. The group is responsible for reimbursing the treating provider. In the *staff model,* the providers are employees of the HMO. All premiums are paid to the HMO.

In the **open-panel HMO**, the health care providers are not employees of the HMO and do not belong to a medical group owned or managed by the HMO. There are three models under this category: direct contract model, individual practice association (IPA) model, and the network model. Individual physicians in the community provide contracted health care services to subscribers in the *direct contract model.* The *IPA model* is similar to the direct contract model in that the providers are not employees of the HMO. The difference is that the IPA can negotiate contracts and manage the capitation payment from the HMO. With the *network model* HMO, contracted services are provided by multiple provider group practices.

PREFERRED PROVIDER ORGANIZATIONS

Preferred provider organizations (PPOs) require the patient to use a medical provider or hospital) under contract with the insurer for an agreed-on fee. A PPO is similar to an HMO but differs in two main areas:

- The PPO is a fee-for-service program and is not based on a prepayment (also known as prospective payment) or capitation program, as is the case for the HMO. Thus the providers and hospitals, designated as PPOs, are reimbursed for each medical service they provide.

- The PPO members or enrollees are not restricted to certain designated providers or hospitals. The PPO member may receive care from a non-PPO provider; however, they will generally have to pay more out-of-pocket expenses when they do this.

PPOs manage cost containment in the following ways:

- They negotiate fees with providers that are less than the current market fees.

- They offer financial incentives for PPO members to use a PPO provider.

- They carefully monitor the quality and type of services offered by PPO providers.

Point-of-Service Plan

To allow for more flexibility, some HMOs and PPOs have created a **point-of-service plan (POS)**. Within such plans, patients may choose to use the panel of providers within the HMO network or to utilize the services of non-HMO providers. If the enrollee chooses to use a provider within the network, the enrollee is responsible only for the regular copayment and deductible amounts do not apply. The same benefits apply if the patient is referred by a provider to a specialist outside the network (with authorization from the HMO). If an enrollee chooses to see an out-of-network provider without authorization, it is known as **self-referral**. The enrollee may be responsible for greater out-of-pocket expenses, including larger deductible and coinsurance charges.

EXCLUSIVE PROVIDER ORGANIZATIONS

Exclusive provider organizations (EPOs) combine concepts developed by HMOs and PPOs. The EPO, a managed care system, allows the patient to select only from a defined panel of providers. This system reimburses these providers on a modified fee-for-service basis, not on the basis of capitation, as in an HMO. The EPO differs from a PPO since no insurance reimbursement is made if there is a nonemergency service provided by a non-EPO provider.

Integrated Delivery System

An organization of provider sites (e.g., ambulatory centers, clinics, or hospitals) with a contracted relationship that offer services to subscribers is known as an **integrated delivery system (IDS)**. One such organization is a physician-hospital organization (PHO). PHOs are composed of hospital(s) and physician groups, or clinics. The PHO obtains managed care plan contracts. In this organization, the physicians are able to maintain their own practices while providing care to contracted plan members. A nonprofit IDS is a **medical foundation**. This type of organization contracts and acquires assets of physician practices. The medical foundation manages the business and clinical aspects of the practice. Other examples of IDS organizations are management service organization (MSO), group practice without

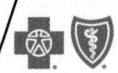

BlueCross BlueShield Of the National Capital Area	Capital Care
ADM. CERT **BC PLAN DBC**	**PRE-CERT**

9999999
Identification No.

DC000
Group

JOHN BROWN
Member Name

A1234567
Physician Number

01/11/61
Member Date of Birth

MARION WELBY, M.D.
Physician Name

PS $10 ER $25 UC $10 IPO Di
Copay Rider Information

FIGURE 17-1 Sample of an insurance card.

walls (GPWW), and integrated provider organization (IPO).

Group-Sponsored or Individual Policies

Group-sponsored or individual policies can be purchased through commercial insurance companies. Commercial health insurance carriers are usually for-profit organizations. These companies may offer traditional fee-for-service insurance as well as a managed care option. Generally, the insured pays a premium and receives coverage for specific services. Figure 17-1 shows a member insurance card, listing the name of the insured, the effective date of the coverage, and other information of importance such as the patient's copayment for various types of facilities. This is where the medical assistant will find the information regarding the copayment

the office should receive and, in turn, should be requesting as payment from the patient.

Always ask to see the patient's insurance card at every office visit. Just because a patient had a particular type of insurance one month does not mean they have the same insurance or policy the next month. Make a copy of both sides of the card and return it immediately to the patient. In addition to placing a copy of the card in the patient's chart, you also may wish to write the insurance plan number on the patient's chart. Verify the patient's name with a form of photo identification. Compare the name on the insurance card with the name on the photo ID.

It is also a good idea to become familiar with the insurance representatives who serve your area. The representatives are knowledgeable, conduct office seminars, and can answer many questions over the telephone.

BLUE CROSS/BLUE SHIELD

Perhaps the most well-known insurance plans are Blue Cross and Blue Shield plans that operate in all states and have become the largest prepayment medical insurance system in the country. These Blue plans date back to the 1930s when Blue Cross was introduced to provide coverage for hospital costs to teachers in Texas. This simple agreement between Baylor Hospital and a group of school teachers launched the programs that are known today as Blue Cross and Blue Shield. By 1939, Blue Shield was sponsored by state medical societies in Texas, Michigan, and California to provide both medical and surgical coverage. Both plans cover all services now and offer various types of health care plans similar to other commercial carriers. Blue Cross and Blue Shield plans exist in every state and operate locally under each individual state's laws.

Government Programs

Federal and state governments provide health care benefits for specific groups of people through various programs, such as Medicare, Medicaid, workers' compensation, and military plans.

MEDICARE

Perhaps the best-known government plan is Medicare. Medicare is health insurance for the elderly that is provided by the United States government. The Medicare system is operated by the Social Security Administration and paid for largely through Social Security funds. It is designed for

PROFESSIONALISM

A professional medical assistant will make every effort to stay current with health insurance procedures. Many sources from which you can obtain the most up-to-date information are available. Seminars and other professional development events may address changes in insurance plans. Another source is a representative from the actual health care plan. Establish a relationship with someone at each major insurance company so that you always can get accurate information.

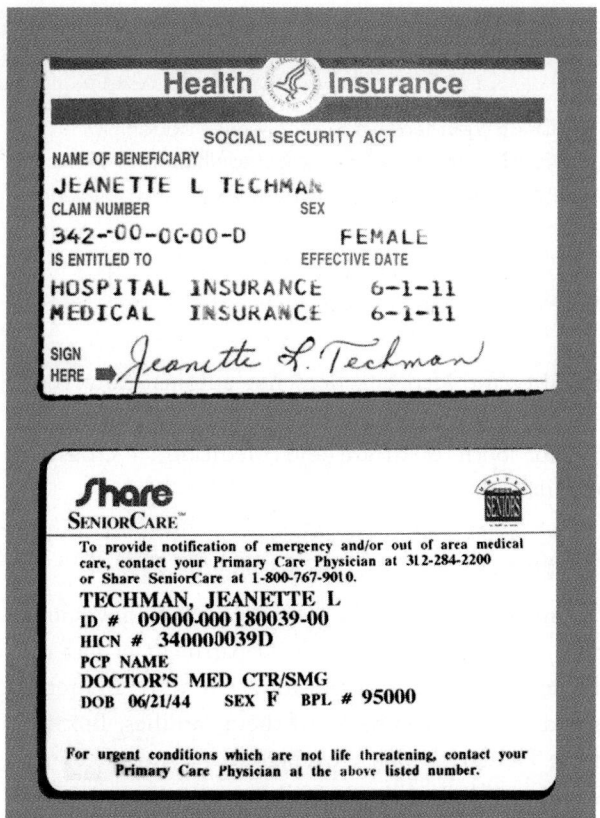

FIGURE 17-2 Medicare and supplemental private insurance cards.

persons 65 years old and older and for the severely disabled. Medicare covers approximately 32 million elderly citizens as well as 2 million permanently disabled persons. Eligible patients are issued a Medicare card (Figure 17-2) after applying for services.

Medicare is actually a two-part health care benefit system: Part A and Part B.

Part A, which covers hospital expenses, provides coverage when an insured becomes eligible for Social Security benefits. The patient must apply to receive Part A benefits from the Social Security Administration.

Part B covers medical expenses for doctors, medical services, outpatient hospital care, durable medical equipment, and some medical services not covered by Part A. To qualify for Part B Medicare coverage, the insured must pay a monthly premium. This coverage is not automatic, nor does the coverage pay for all services. The patient pays a yearly deductible. After this deductible is met, Medicare will pay for 80 percent of the approved amount of covered services and the insured is liable for the 20 percent coinsurance. Often, this is referred to as 80/20. The 80 percent reimbursement rate of Medicare is based on the program's resource-based relative value scale (RBRVS), which was developed using

values for procedures performed and based on what Medicare believes is the cost to provide the service.

Medicare covers all expenses for the first 60 days of hospitalization, except for an initial amount, or deductible, that is paid by the patient. Medicare also will pay for a portion of hospital costs for an additional 30 days. Medicare does not cover extended nursing-home care, or the costs of lengthy or chronic illnesses.

Prescription drugs are covered under a separate medical policy known as Medicare Part D. Medicare Part D was implemented in 2006 and is offered as a supplemental plan that Medicare recipients may purchase. Medicare Part D covers a predetermined list of prescription drugs at participating pharmacies. For those Medicare recipients who opt to participate in Medicare Part D, annual deductibles, applicable copayments or coinsurance, and maximum benefits apply.

Medicare supplement policies pay benefits related to the copayments and deductibles required of patients and not paid by Medicare. These amounts can be as little as $10. Some policies require special forms to be filed before benefits can be paid to the insured. It is important for the medical assistant to check coverage with the individual carrier of the supplement policy, as the coverage provided varies widely from carrier to carrier.

Medicare deductibles, covered services, and copayments change, so it is important to understand which services are covered under Medicare and which are not. Medical assistants should maintain their knowledge of Medicare coverage and be knowledgeable regarding the **benefit period**, or period of time that payments for Medicare hospital benefits are available.

- **TRICARE Prime**—a managed care option similar to a civilian health maintenance organization
- **TRICARE Extra**—a preferred provider option in which beneficiaries choose a doctor, hospital, or other medical provider within the TRICARE provider network

- **TRICARE Standard**—a fee-for-service option
- **TRICARE for Life**—an option available to Medicare-eligible beneficiaries age 65 and over

Information is courtesy of www.tricare.mil.

MEDICAID

Although not directly a federal program, Medicaid also qualifies as government insurance. Some of the cost of the Medicaid program, designed for the medically indigent, or persons without funds, comes from state funds, with some federal money to offset costs. Federal funds may supply 50 percent to 80 percent of the cost of the state's Medicaid program. Since Medicaid is administered by individual states, the rules for eligibility and for payment vary from state to state. In most instances, however, the patient must qualify for benefits on a monthly basis. Some services require **preauthorization** (prior approval from the insurance company administrator, including Medicaid); in such cases, the cost of services will not be paid without it. When dealing with Medicaid patients, the medical assistant should verify coverage at each and every visit and become familiar with the policies and procedures covering Medicaid in his or her individual state.

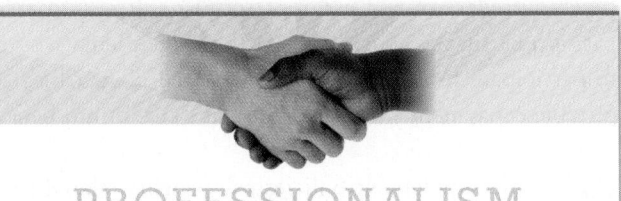

PROFESSIONALISM
CULTURAL CONSIDERATIONS

In this day and age, many individuals have intense and varying opinions regarding recent and past wars in foreign countries, as well as military involvement in other matters. It will be obvious when a patient presents to the office with a TRICARE or CHAMPVA insurance card that he or she is either involved with or related to someone who is a member of the armed services. Regardless of your opinion of the United States government and its decisions regarding military issues, remember that the medical office is never a place to promote a cause. All patients must be treated with respect and honor.

Eligibility for Medicare does not automatically confer Medicaid eligibility. In some cases in which a person is eligible for both Medicare and Medicaid, a **crossover claim** is filed.

MILITARY MEDICAL BENEFITS

Military medical benefits are also part of U.S. government programs. TRICARE is the U.S. Department of Defense's worldwide health care program for active duty and retired uniformed services members and theirs families. Box 17-2 shows the TRICARE plan's coverage.

A spouse, widow, widower, children of veterans with total or permanent service-connected disabilities, and surviving spouse or dependents of veterans who have died as a result of service-connected disabilities are covered under a program called CHAMPVA (Civilian Health and Medical Program of the Veterans Administration).

Providers of service must be approved in order for the patient to receive benefits for services. Special forms are required for claim filing. Certain services require approval from the government agency responsible for administering these programs before payment can be made.

WORKERS' COMPENSATION

Another type of government-mandated insurance is workers' compensation. This particular insurance is for injuries directly related to work. Payment of premiums is the employer's responsibility; the employee pays nothing. In workers' compensation cases, the provider of services must complete a Doctor's First Report form and must submit further reports at predetermined intervals. In addition, if the patient receives regular care in the same practice that treats the work injury, any information connected to the injury or illness being treated under workers' compensation must be kept separate from all other patient information. Billing is to be done separately, and the patient will not be billed for services. Billing statements are sent instead to the employer or insurer. Because of the special type of documentation required for workers' compensation claims, some providers of service will not see workers' compensation patients. In some states, the patient must see physicians who specialize in workers' comp cases.

DISABILITY INSURANCE

Disability insurance is a particular type of insurance that usually begins paying the patient (not the doctor or the hospital) after the insured has been disabled (unable to work) for a specific period of time. A waiting period of weeks or months before benefits are paid is not uncommon with these policies. The benefit period is the amount of time the insured will receive a monthly check after the policy begins to pay. This can be from 6 months to life. The payment is paid directly to the insured. This type of insurance coverage is not used to pay medical bills. Rather, it is to be used for the income that patient has lost due to his or her disability. Most disability insurance also requires completion and submission of special forms by the attending physician before benefits can be paid to the insured. Before the medical assistant has the physician sign the disability insurance form, he or she needs to proofread it very carefully. After the physician has signed the disability insurance form, the medical assistant will make a copy of it and place it in the patient's medical record.

Types of Health Insurance Benefits

Many patients (and medical assistants) find the proliferation of health care policies confusing. It is important to understand what type of insurance coverage the patient has and what types of services this insurance covers. Remember, insurance is considered a three-party contract between the insured (the patient or the patient's family), the insurance company, and the provider. Questions about specific coverage should be directed to the insurance carrier, as policies vary widely, even with the same carrier.

The most basic insurance policies cover doctor office visits, hospitalization, emergency room visits, surgical procedures, and wellness examinations. Some insurance policies may require an annual deductible, which is the portion the patient must pay before the insurance company will pay any benefits. Typically, the higher the deductible, the more inexpensive the monthly premium is. In addition, a fixed percentage of covered charges beyond the deductible, called

coinsurance, may be required. To reduce unnecessary patient visits to the provider's office, insurance companies frequently require a copayment.

Major medical insurance covers expenses related to catastrophic illnesses or injuries. It also covers prolonged illnesses. Major medical is usually a supplemental policy to basic insurance policies. Adding this type of policy increases the premium rate the insured will pay. There are other types of riders that may be available for an additional fee. The following is a list of possible riders:

- *Surgical insurance* is just what its name implies—an insurance policy covering surgical services. These policies are not as common today as they once were; most surgical services are now covered under basic medical coverage.

- *Long-term care* is an insurance policy designed to cover nursing home care costs. Other insurance policies have very limited coverage if any for long-term care.

- *Dental insurance* covers the dental examination, cleaning, polishing, fillings, and certain extractions, and selected other procedures. Most insurance carriers require a deductible. Depending on the insurance carrier, most procedures are covered from 50 percent to 100 percent.

- *Vision insurance* covers the cost of an eye examination, contact lens or prescription frames and lenses. Some vision insurance policies also covers laser corrective eye surgery. The percentage covered by the insurance carrier depends on the insured's policy.

- *International health and medical insurance* covers the insured while outside of the United States in countries where the policy applies.

PROFESSIONALISM

THE LAW

When dealing with insurance, confidentiality and honesty are major issues. The patient's right to confidentiality with regard to sensitive medical information must be scrupulously respected. Insurance reimbursement, as it is currently structured, provides a constant temptation to do what is necessary to recover the full amount of charges. As a successful medical assistant, be careful to release only information authorized by the patient and avoid becoming involved with insurance fraud in any manner.

- *Student health insurance* is important when a parent's insurance policy no longer covers a child or children who are attending school. Basic insurance, major medical, or both are available. This type of coverage is usually available at a rate that is affordable for the student.

Payment of Benefits

When a covered service has been rendered, the insurance carrier is obligated to pay its portion of the cost. How is this portion calculated? Many insurance carriers use the UCR (usual, customary, reasonable) method (also see Chapter 15). The UCR method allows the carrier to establish a payment base for allowed or covered services. In this model, payment is set by determining the following:

- The usual fee a provider charges the majority of patients for a particular service

- The geographic location of the practice and the provider's specialty

- Any complications or unusual services or procedures

Indemnity schedules—another means of determining the amount of payment made by an insurance carrier—are based on a maximum amount for a specific service. Payment to the provider of a service is based on the lower of either the provider's submitted charge or the provider's fee schedule. This method of payment is very common in managed care situations.

To communicate effectively and efficiently with providers of medical care, insurance companies have adopted several methods of standardizing information received. Many insurance companies, working together and separately, have developed a means of calculating pricing factors in reimbursement. The results of these efforts are called relative value studies (RVS). In each instance, the system takes into account the time, skill, and overhead expense of the provider as required for each service. These factors are then turned into unit counts applied to a specific service, allowing for the most efficient and effective method of calculating payment.

Since 1992, Medicare has established payment on a resource-based relative value scale (RBRVS), which incorporates the RVS but also allows for increases in charges tied to economic changes and other factors.

Each insurance carrier has a certain deadline for submitting insurance claims. Claims must be submitted in a timely manner in order to be processed, and if the deadline for filing has passed, no money can be recovered from the insurance carrier. It is extremely important to become familiar with these filing deadlines that vary from carrier to carrier and also to submit correct claims known as "clean claims" on the first attempt. If a carrier finds errors in the claim, it will send the claim back to the provider for correction. When this occurs, the deadline is not extended and the provider has fewer days to submit for reimbursement.

It is also important that the appropriate form be used for filing charges. Most carriers require claims to be submitted on the CMS-1500 (see Chapter 18); a few carriers may require forms specific to that carrier. Some carriers require supporting documentation (such as reports) that must be submitted in a timely manner. It is important that the medical assistant be familiar with the claim submission requirements of each carrier.

If a patient has more than one insurance carrier, it is crucial that the primary carrier be determined for proper billing to occur. Insurance carriers have procedures in place to prevent duplication of payment by more than one carrier. This is known as **coordination of benefits (COB)**. The claim must be submitted first to the primary carrier for processing. The claim must then be processed and a statement of remittance completed before the information can be sent to any secondary carrier.

Coverage for some expenses, such as cosmetic surgery, are excluded from policies and are called exclusions. Payments for some medications are excluded if they are not on an approved medication list, called a **formulary**, that is specific to each insurance carrier.

As with all aspects of insurance processing, accuracy and attention to detail are the primary concerns. The successful medical assistant keeps abreast of rules, regulations, and changes about insurance claims processing to prompt insurance reimbursement for the practice that is as high as is allowed for services rendered. The medical assistant may need to bill the third-party payer for the patient and collect the fees owed to the provider. See Procedure 17-1 for performing billing and collection procedures.

PREAUTHORIZATION OR PRECERTIFICATION

It may be necessary to seek preauthorization (also known as precertification) from the health insurance provider for certain services. Remember that part of the patient registration process is gathering all pertinent information, including the insurance plan requirements. The medical assistant must obtain any required preauthorization or precertification.

procedure

17-1

PERFORMING BILLING AND COLLECTION PROCEDURES

Objective: Demonstrate the ability to record payments received from a patient, to record patient information using a patient ledger card and day sheet, and to generate an insurance bill using a charge slip. Demonstrate the ability to then record a payment and provide receipt to the patient.

EQUIPMENT AND SUPPLIES

day sheet; ledger card; copayment check; receipt book; pen; calculator

METHOD

1. Pull the appropriate ledger card and place it directly on the day sheet.
2. Temporarily remove the strip of charge slips from the pegboard.
3. Enter the patient's previous balance on the day sheet. The ledger card does not extend to this column.
4. Post the date, patient's name, descriptions, and copayment amount.
5. Calculate the new balance by subtracting the payment from the previous balance.
6. Generate an insurance bill for the remaining balance.
7. Create a receipt for the patient.

CHARTING EXAMPLE

3/12/20XX. $20 copay paid by pt. at time of office visit on 3/11/20XX. Allied insurance billed for balance of $79 on 3/12/20XX. · J. Cleary, CMAS

Preauthorization consists of obtaining permission from the insurance plan before performing a procedure or providing certain services to subscribers. It is important to find out if preauthorization is necessary prior to the patient's scheduled appointment. Involve the patient in this process; he or she may not be aware that preauthorization is necessary for the particular plan. Failure to have this permission may delay treatment or require the patient to pay out of pocket. The insurance carrier may only pay for part of the procedure or may pay nothing at all if preauthorization is not granted beforehand. Preauthorization is usually obtained a minimum of 24 hours before a patient arrives for an office visit, hospitalization, certain procedures and treatments, and referrals to a specialist.

To acquire preauthorization, the medical assistant will contact the insurance carrier and provide all patient information and details regarding the procedure. The medical assistant should have the following information before contacting the insurance carrier:

- Patient's medical record with insurance information
- Preauthorization form
- Specific procedure or service requested, number of treatments, and period of time necessary for the treatments

- Specific documentation by the provider in the patient's medical record supporting the need for the requested procedure or service
- Name, address, telephone number, and fax number of the provider who will perform the procedure or service that has been requested

The insurance carrier will provide preauthorization information (usually a number) that will be have to be included on the insurance claim. The medical assistant should make a copy of the completed preauthorization form and place it in the patient's medical record.

In case an insurance plan rejects a preauthorization request, it may be necessary for the provider to write a letter to the carrier. With the consent of the patient, the provider should state the patient's diagnosis and professional rationale for prescribing a particular treatment. It may be helpful to recommend that the subscriber send a letter of appeal as well. A copy of the provider's letter to the carrier must be kept in the patient's medical record. If possible, obtain a copy of the patient's letter of appeal for placement in the patient's medical record. Third-party payers, usually insurance companies, expect medical assistants to follow their guidelines for preauthorization.

procedure

APPLYING THIRD-PARTY GUIDELINES

Objective: To apply knowledge of third-party guidelines to obtain prior approval for a procedure.

EQUIPMENT AND SUPPLIES

provider's report recommending procedure; telephone; notepad; pen

METHOD

1. Gather information about the patient.
2. Locate the insurance carrier's number.
3. Call the carrier and introduce yourself, indicating your office.
4. Instruct the carrier that the provider recommends the procedure but that the third-party carrier requires preauthorization.
5. Give the carrier the necessary information, as requested.
6. Document in the patient chart the preauthorization number for the procedure.

CHARTING EXAMPLE

9/15/20XX. Michelle Kimenhour at Allied Health Insurance preauthorized hysterectomy scheduled for 9/26/20XX for patient, Mary Mahoney. Preauthorization number GAQ3498.
.... M. Johns, CMA (AAMA)

See Procedure 17-2 for how to apply third-party payer guidelines.

REFERRALS AND AUTHORIZATION

When a patient needs more specialized care than the family physician can provide, the patient will be referred to another physician or facility.

A **referral** is used to send a patient for treatment to another facility or physician. There are three types of referrals: regular, urgent, and STAT. *Regular referrals* are requested when the PCP has determined the need for a specialist to continue quality care. A week may be needed to obtain the authorization from the insurance plan for a regular referral. An *urgent referral* is granted for a non–life-threatening need for quality of care, and preauthorization may take up to 48 hours. A *STAT referral* is approved for a life-threatening need for quality of care. Whether the referral is regular, urgent, or STAT, it will require preauthorization directly from the insurance carrier. Preauthorization may be obtained by telephone, fax, e-mail, or in writing on specific insurance carrier forms (Figure 17-3). A medical assistant must always have the referral authorization prior to patient treatment and must maintain all information for insurance billing and utilization review purposes.

When a provider requests that a patient be referred to a specialist, it is important to document this in the patient's medical record. The appropriate paperwork must be sent to the referred provider. Referral recommendations should be in writing. When submitting the request to the health insurance plan, be sure to follow the appropriate procedures for that plan. The medical assistant should have the following information before contacting the insurance carrier:

- Patient's medical record with insurance information
- Referral form

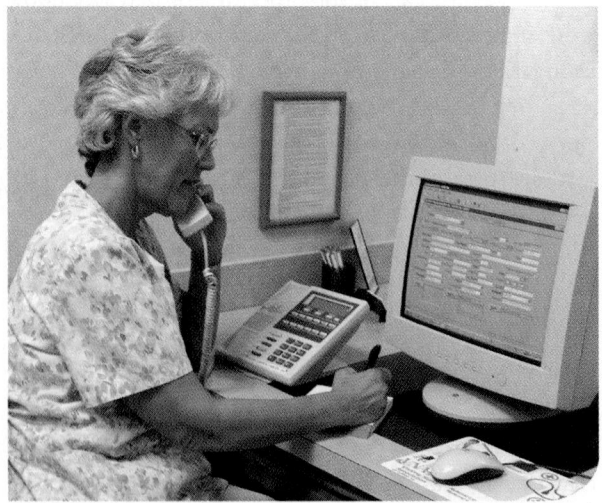

FIGURE 17-3 A medical assistant may obtain a referral over the telephone.

APPLYING MANAGED CARE POLICIES AND PROCEDURES
Objective: Demonstrate knowledge of managed care policies.

EQUIPMENT AND SUPPLIES
insurance card; patient record
METHOD
1. Greet patient and request insurance card.
2. Check the patient's insurance card to see if coverage is current. For some insurances, this may require calling an automated telephone system through which you will determine whether or not the patient has coverage on a particular date.
3. Correctly enter the insurance card information into the office database.
4. Photocopy the insurance card.
5. Return the card to the patient.

- Specific procedure or service requested, number of treatments, and period of time necessary for the treatments
- Specific documentation by the provider in the patient's medical record supporting the reason for the referral
- Name, address, telephone number, and fax number of the provider who will be providing the procedure or service
- Appointment date, time, and location
- Diagnostic and procedure codes

If certain forms are required, make sure that you have the current form and that it is filled out properly. Some requests are rejected due to incorrect or incomplete paperwork. The medical assistant should forward a copy to the provider to whom the patient is being referred, make a copy of the completed referral form, note to whom the referral was forwarded, and place the copy and note in the patient's medical record.

Verification of Insurance Benefits

A medical assistant must always confirm or verify the patient's eligibility for insurance benefits prior to the office visit. Verification may take time but, by performing the following guidelines, will be more effective for the insurance process.

Guidelines for insurance verification:

- In the initial contact with the patient, obtain all insurance information (i.e., insurer name, guarantor name, insurance identification number, patient's address, telephone number, and birth date).

- Obtain insurance company name, address, telephone number, fax number, copayment fees, deductibles, and preauthorizations.
- Provide the patient with written information regarding medical office policies and procedures for dealing with his or her insurance carrier.
- Discuss insurance benefits with the patient prior to services rendered.

As a medical assistant, you must apply managed care policies and procedures in the office as presented in Procedure 17-3.

JUDGMENT CALL

It is the second day of the month, and Johanna Sparks has arrived for a follow-up appointment regarding her blood pressure. When Miriam, the receptionist, asks for a copy of Johanna's insurance card, the patient states she does not have it with her. The patient was seen last week for her 6-week postpartum visit and had presented her Medicaid card at that time. Ms. Sparks asks why Keri cannot just use the copy of the card from last week. What should Keri do?

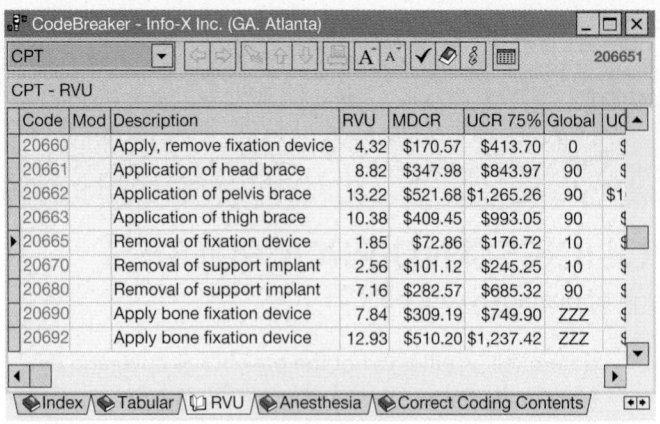

Code	Mod	Description	RVU	MDCR	UCR 75%	Global	UC
20660		Apply, remove fixation device	4.32	$170.57	$413.70	0	$
20661		Application of head brace	8.82	$347.98	$843.97	90	$
20662		Application of pelvis brace	13.22	$521.68	$1,265.26	90	$1
20663		Application of thigh brace	10.38	$409.45	$993.05	90	$
20665		Removal of fixation device	1.85	$72.86	$176.72	10	$
20670		Removal of support implant	2.56	$101.12	$245.25	10	$
20680		Removal of support implant	7.16	$282.57	$685.32	90	$
20690		Apply bone fixation device	7.84	$309.19	$749.90	ZZZ	$
20692		Apply bone fixation device	12.93	$510.20	$1,237.42	ZZZ	$

◇Index / ◇Tabular / ◇RVU / ◇Anesthesia / ◇Correct Coding Contents

FIGURE 17-4   Example of a computerized fee schedule.

Fee Schedules

Health care insurance providers determine fees based on several components. Determining factors include time, location of practice, type of practice, value of services, and allowable charge. Allowable charge is the highest amount that third-party payers will make for services rendered. Figure 17-4 is an example of a computerized fee schedule.

Health Care Cost Containment

Over time the cost of medicine has risen steadily. As new advances are discovered to treat and cure disease, heal injuries, and prolong life, the costs are passed on to the consumer or patient. Traditionally, medical care has been rendered on a fee-for-service basis, which was a separate charge or fee set up by individual physicians for every service. Insurance carriers initially set up their policies on this basis, as well. However, as medical care costs rose, the insurers and medical community began to offer cost-saving alternatives to higher medical costs and the escalating costs of medical insurance premiums.

The first cost-containment measure was initiated when Congress amended the Social Security Act of 1972 and established the Professional Standards Review Organization (PSRO). This was a voluntary group of physicians who monitored the necessity of hospital admissions and reviewed the treatment costs and medical records of hospitals. Unfortunately, the cost of operating this system was greater than the savings that the program could generate each year. To establish stricter controls over Medicare reimbursement for inpatient costs, Congress created control peer review organizations (PROs). These PROs were intended to determine whether proposed services were reasonable and medically necessary and whether or not the services provided on an inpatient basis could be provided more efficiently on an outpatient basis.

As part of the cost-containment process, a patient classification system was developed, which provides a means of relating the type of patients a hospital treats to the costs incurred by the hospital. Yale University developed the design of diagnosis-related groups (DRGs) in the late 1960s. The initial idea was to provide a means of monitoring the quality of care and the utilization of services in a hospital setting. Payment rates based on DRGs have now been established as the basis for a hospital's Medicare reimbursements. Although DRGs have an effect on hospital reimbursements, they are not used to calculate payments made to outpatient providers. Physicians now have contracts with managed care companies and insurance companies.

The *Federal Register*

The *Federal Register* is a daily legal publication of the National Archives and Records Administration (NARA). The medical assistant uses this register when seeking information on federal rules, regulations, notices, executive orders, proclamations, and presidential documents. The *Federal Register* may be accessed through the World Wide Web, microfiche, or as a daily newspaper.

SUMMARY

Most patients coming into the medical office have some form of health care insurance. These include commercial insurers, as well as government plans such as Medicare, Medicaid, workers' compensation, and military insurance (TRICARE and CHAMPVA). Many patients are members of health care plans, such as health maintenance organizations (HMOs) and preferred provider organizations (PPOs). The medical assistant should have a working knowledge of each type of insurance in order to be able to quickly and accurately process insurance forms.

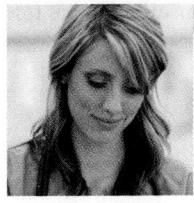

17 CHAPTER REVIEW

COMPETENCY REVIEW

1. Define and spell the terms to learn for this chapter.

2. List the three insurance options currently available.

3. What are the two important components of an HMO?

4. How does a PPO differ from an HMO?

5. What is the purpose of the peer review organization (PRO)?

PREPARING FOR THE CERTIFICATION EXAM

1. When the patient has a primary and secondary insurance carrier, which of the following is required to determine the amount payable by each carrier?
   a. explanation of benefits.
   b. assignment of benefits.
   c. coordination of benefits.
   d. acceptance of benefits.
   e. acceptance of care.

2. A government-sponsored insurance program that covers those 65 and older is
   a. Medicaid.
   b. Medicare.
   c. Part C supplemental insurance.
   d. BCBS.
   e. TRICARE.

3. The PCP is also known as the
   a. cardiologist.
   b. internist.
   c. primary consulting provider.
   d. gatekeeper.
   e. on-call physician.

4. When the insurance carrier makes payments to the PCP every month, regardless of whether the patient is seen, it is known as

   a. fee-for-service.
   b. prospective payment.
   c. POS.
   d. HMO fee payment.
   e. PPO.

5. Which part of Medicare covers doctor visits?
   a. Medicare Part A.
   b. Medicare Part B.
   c. Medicare Part C.
   d. Medicare Parts A and C.
   e. Medicare Part D.

6. When hospitals are paid based on the diagnosis and treatment, this is known as
   a. DRG.
   b. DTG.
   c. RPG.
   d. RDG.
   e. TDG.

7. The lump-sum money that must be paid by the patient before the insurance carrier begins to pay is known as the
   a. deductible.
   b. capitation.
   c. indemnity.

d. premium.

e. fee-for-service.

8. Health insurance contracts are considered which of the following?

   a. two-party contracts.

   b. third-party contracts.

   c. fourth-party contracts.

   d. elective-party contracts.

   e. none of the above.

9. The type of HMO insurance available to military personnel is which of the following?

   a. CHAMPVA.

   b. TRICARE Prime.

   c. TRICARE Extra.

   d. TRICARE Standard.

   e. TRICARE Basic.

10. All of the following are considered determining factors for fee schedules EXCEPT

   a. allowable charge.

   b. location of office.

   c. time.

   d. size of office.

   e. office overhead.

CRITICAL THINKING

1. Based on Shelly's status, what is likely to be her current form of health insurance?

2. With Shelly's 65th birthday approaching, how should Miriam handle the question regarding Shelly's health insurance coverage?

3. Shelly asks Miriam for any useful websites that she could use to explore her options. What websites might Miriam suggest?

ON THE JOB

Lisa Medina, CMA, processes insurance claims for a large internal medicine practice. You have recently been hired as Lisa's assistant, and she has asked you to verify insurance coverage for the patients who have appointments to see Dr. Williams in the next 2 days. Lisa "advises" you to be careful when obtaining preauthorizations. She hands you a list of "approved" services and tells you to use this information when calling the insurance companies.

1. Name some of the options that are possible for handling this situation.
2. For what types of services might you have to obtain preauthorizations?
3. Would Lisa's "advice" be considered fraud? Explain your response.
4. What is the proper procedure for obtaining preauthorizations?

INTERNET ACTIVITY

Most health insurance providers have websites to provide information to their members and the public. Because changes occur so quickly, important information regarding health plans is posted to keep those who are interested up to date. Conduct a search to find the websites for Medicaid, a commercial insurance company, and CHAMPVA. List the website addresses and list the different plans offered by each.

MEDMEDIA

Additional interactive resources and activities for this chapter can be found:

On your student DVD: View applicable procedure videos on the DVD-ROM found in the back of this book.

MyHealthProfessionsKit.com: Test your knowledge of this chapter with games and activities. MyHealthProfessionsKit also includes resources, helpful links, and a Spanish audio glossary.

Medical Assisting Interactive: Practice your procedures as a medical assistant in this simulated doctor's office. This can be accessed through MyHealthProfessionsKit.com.

18

Medical Insurance Claims

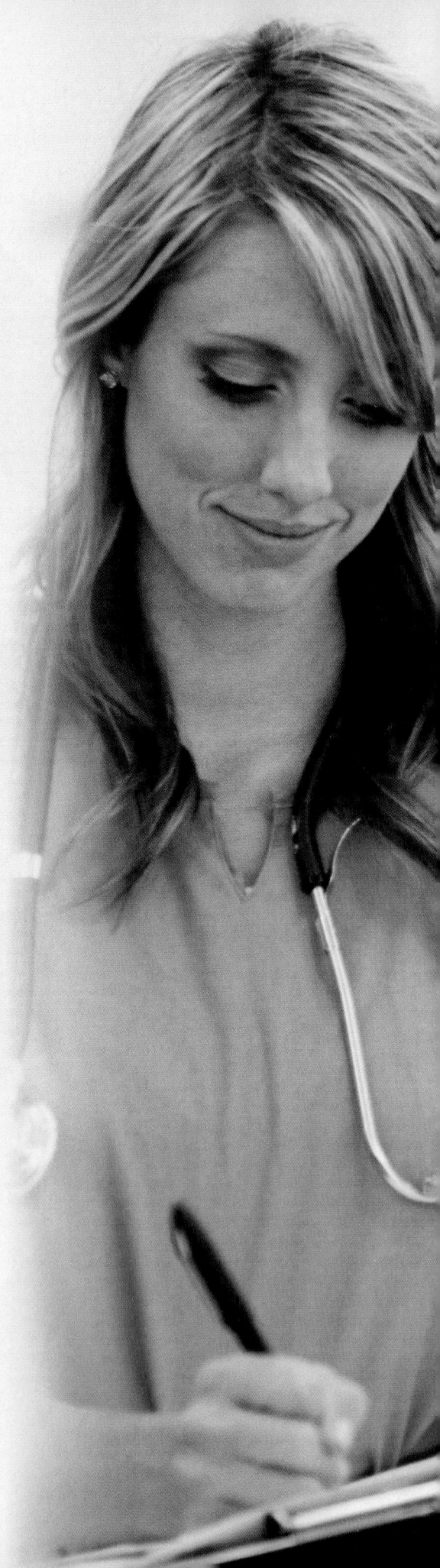

LEARNING OBJECTIVES

After completing this chapter, you should be able to:

- Define and spell the terms to learn for this chapter.

- Define and discuss various health insurance forms.

- Explain the differences among the discussed insurance policies.

- List the information required on a medical claim form and explain why each piece of information is needed.

- Discuss legal issues affecting medical claims submission.

- Discuss insurance claims processing.

- Explain why insurance claim security is so important.

- Discuss tracking insurance claims.

- List the reasons for insurance claims being rejected.

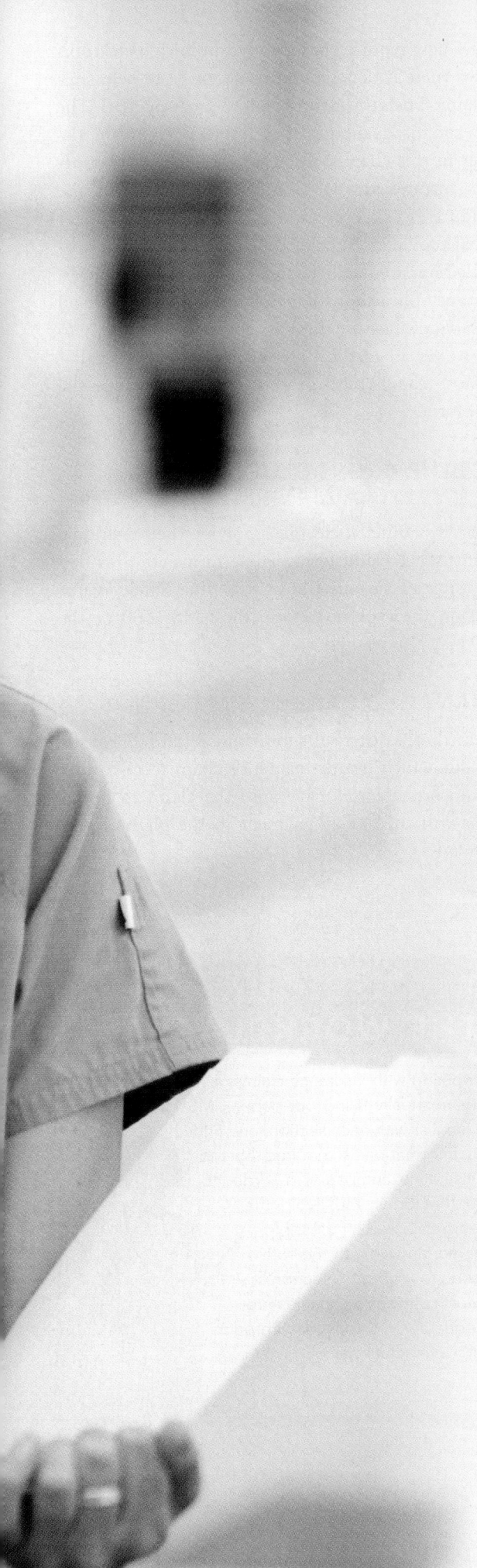

CHAPTER OUTLINE

CASE STUDY

Lewis Jordan, RMA, works at Pearson Physicians Group as a medical billing and insurance clerk. His duties include verifying insurance and processing claims. Sylvia Baker is a new patient and has an appointment to see Dr. Miller next week. She has Blue Cross/Blue Shield insurance. Mark Flannery is also a patient. He was in to see Dr. Miller last month, and the claim for his care was rejected. The codes, quantities, and modifiers were all correct on the CMS-1500. Lewis receives a call from Mr. Flannery, who is angry, because he has been billed for his last visit and has already paid his copayment.

assignment of benefits

birthday rule

breach of confidentiality

clean claim

clearinghouse

CMS-1500

denied claim

dirty claim

invalid claim

nonparticipating provider

participating provider

primary insurance

secondary insurance

write off

CERTIFICATION LINK

CMA (AAMA)
Medicolegal guidelines and requirements
  Legislation
  Documentation/ Reporting
  Releasing medical information
Practice finances
  Third-party billing

RMA
Administrative medical assisting
  Insurance
  Financial and bookkeeping
  Medical receptionist/ Secretarial/Clerical

CMAS (AMT)
Medical office clerical assisting
  Reception
Health care insurance processing, coding, and billing
  Insurance processing
  Insurance coding
  Insurance billing and finances
Medical office financial management
  Patient accounts

The health insurance claim form provides communication between the insurance company and the physician for the services the patient has received. Three main points to this communication process are critical in order to receive proper reimbursement from the insurance carrier.

First, the correct health insurance claim form must be used. Second, the information provided in the health insurance claim form must be accurate. One minor mistake can cause the claim to be rejected. The medical assistant must always proofread the claim form before submitting it. Third, the health insurance claim form must be submitted to the correct insurance carrier.

Types of Health Insurance Claim Forms

The **CMS-1500** (previously known as the HCFA 1500) is the most common health insurance claim form. This form is used to file claims for physicians' services. Most insur-

ance carriers now require claims to be submitted electronically unless there is documentation required to help support the claim. Then the claim would be sent by mail. The advantages and disadvantages of each type of claim are discussed later in this chapter. Another type of health insurance claim form is the CMS-1450, also known as the UB-04 (Figure 18-1). This form is used to file claims for institutional providers, such as those who practice in hospitals, skilled nursing facilities, and home health agencies. Since this type of health insurance claim form is used in an inpatient setting, most medical assistants are less likely to encounter it, yet all medical assistants should be familiar with it. Most commercial insurance carriers utilize the CMS-1500 form.

BLUE CROSS/BLUE SHIELD CLAIM FORM

Many Blue Cross/Blue Shield plans provide their own type of health insurance claim form. These forms are provided on the websites of various Blue Cross/Blue Shield plans. Depending on the type of service, the CMS-1500 or the CMS-1450 may also be used.

MANAGED CARE CLAIM FORM

When the medical assistant is submitting a claim, he or she must find out which health insurance claim form to use. Using the incorrect form may cause the claim to be rejected. This will then delay payment to the physician for services rendered.

PROFESSIONALISM
THE WORKPLACE

Prior to working with insurance claims, it may be helpful to practice manually filling out paper CMS-1500 forms. Become familiar with each section, and find out what information is required by the various insurance companies in order to complete the forms and avoid the claim being rejected. If possible, also become familiar with the software used to submit electronic claims. Most software companies provide a tutorial for you to work with prior to working with actual claims.

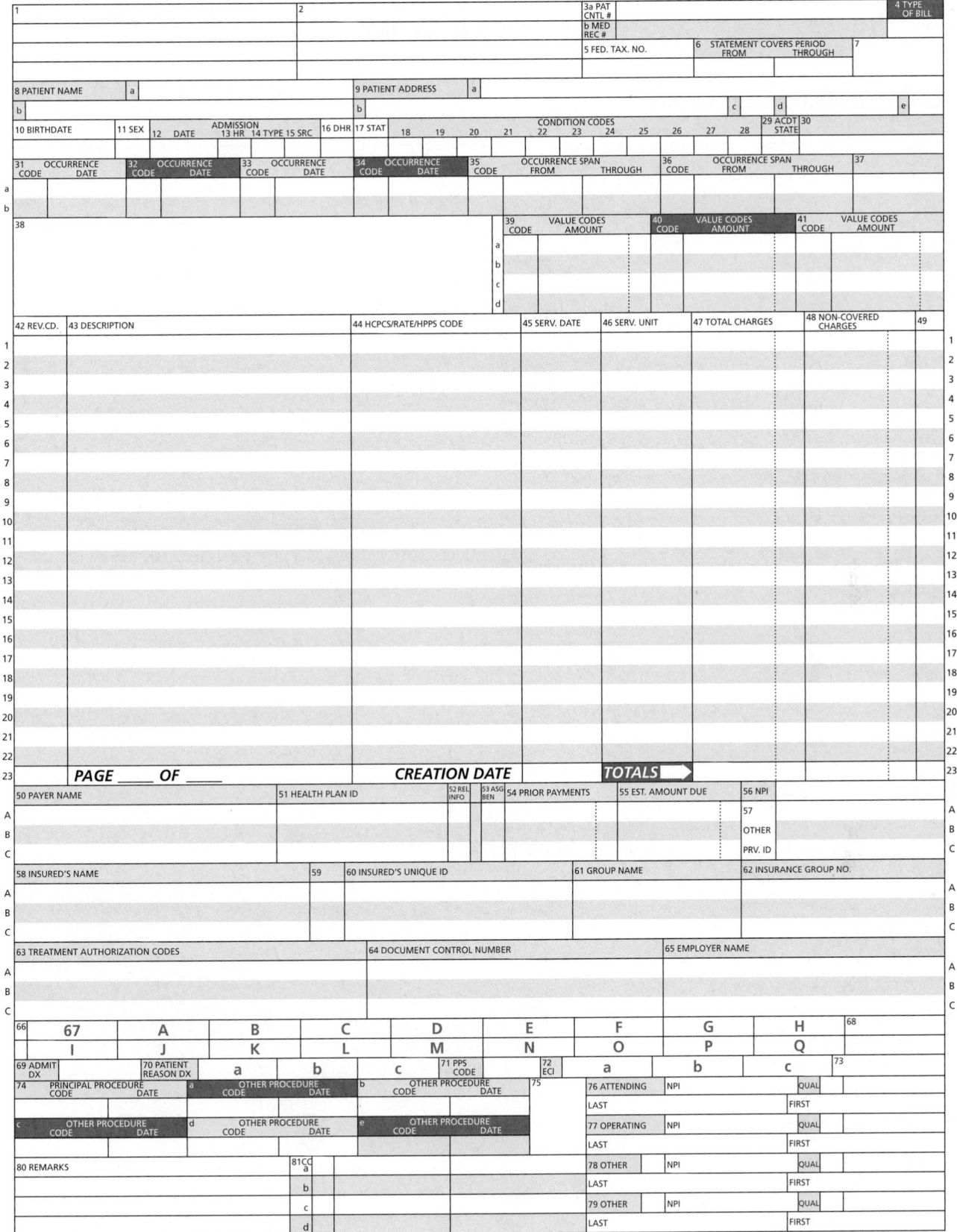

FIGURE 18-1 CMS-1500 (UB-04) paper claim form.

CMS-1500 CLAIM FORM

FIGURE 18-2 A blank paper CMS-1500 form.

MEDICARE CLAIM FORM

Medicare deductibles, covered services, and copayments change frequently, so it is important to understand which services are covered under Medicare and which are not at any given time. Many elderly patients may not fully understand what services Medicare does and does not cover, and it may be up to the administrative medical assistant to help the patient understand the coverage. Medical assistants must stay current with their knowledge regarding Medicare policies, coverage, and the benefit period, which is the period of time for which payments of Medicare hospital benefits are available.

The medical assistant working in a medical office also must be familiar with the CMS-1500 claim form and the requirements for completing it accurately. All Medicare claims must be submitted on the CMS-1500 (Figure 18-2) claim form. If the CMS-1500 claim form is not used, Medicare will reject the claim. Remember, when a claim is rejected, payment is delayed, and if enough claims have been rejected, it can have a significant impact on the office's cash flow.

MEDICAID CLAIM FORM

Medicaid is a governmental insurance program for those individuals who are considered medically indigent. To qualify, typically an individual's assets must not exceed set levels. Medicaid is funded in part by the federal government; however, it is administered by individual states, so the rules for eligibility and for payment vary from state to state. In most instances, however, the patient must qualify for benefits on a monthly basis. Some services and procedures require preauthorization (prior approval from the Medicaid administrator), also known as precertification, or the cost of services and procedures will not be paid. When working with Medicaid patients, the medical assistant must verify coverage prior to each and every visit and become familiar with the policies and procedures covering Medicaid in his or her individual state. It is very possible that the patient may have Medicaid coverage one month and no longer have the coverage the following month.

As noted in Chapter 17, eligibility for Medicare does not automatically confer Medicaid eligibility. In cases where a person is eligible for both Medicare and Medicaid (Medi/Medi), a crossover claim is filed.

After the patient has checked out of the office, the medical assistant will complete a CMS-1500 form and forward it to the appropriate address.

MILITARY CLAIM FORM

Military medical benefits are also part of federal government programs. Three types of health insurance claim

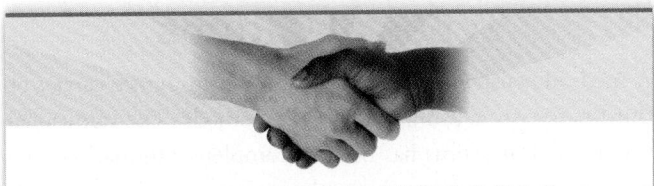

forms are used to submit services to TRICARE and CHAMPVA:

- DD *Form 2642,* Patient's Request for Medical Payment, is completed and sent by the patient or a family member. This form is completed when the patient or family member is requesting payment for medical services already provided. Payment will be sent directly to the patient or family member as reimbursement for the payment the patient or family member has already paid.

- *CMS-1500* is completed and sent by the physician's office. Payment will be sent to the physician's office to cover services already provided to the patient.

- *UB-04* is completed and sent by the hospital for services provided to the patient in a hospital setting. Payment will be sent directly to the hospital.

WORKERS' COMPENSATION CLAIM FORM

The most frequently used claim form for workers' compensation is the CMS-1500, but some states or insurance carriers require completion of specifically designed forms. Before the medical assistant completes a claim form, he or she must investigate which claim form to use. This can be accomplished by calling the insurance carrier or checking the insurance carrier's website.

Types of Claims

A medical assistant submits claims to an insurance carrier or third-party payer using one of two methods. The traditional way to submit claims has been to complete information on a paper claim form and mail it to the insurance carrier. The more current and faster way to submit insurance claims is done by using a computer to complete an electronic claim form and sending the claim electronically. The same information is provided when submitting either a paper or electronic claim.

PAPER CLAIMS

Only small providers (those institutional organizations with fewer than 25 full-time employees or physicians with fewer than 10 full-time employees) may file paper claims. Paper claims are completed manually by the medical assistant or person responsible for billing and are more likely to have errors. This means that the likelihood of the insurance carrier rejecting the claim is greater. Common errors include omissions of data, transpositions of numbers, and typographical and mathematical errors. When a claim form contains an error and is rejected by the insurance carrier, the claim form must be corrected and resubmitted for payment. This increases the time it takes for the medical office to receive payment and results in delayed cash flow. This also means that more personnel time is used to resubmit the claim, which is not efficient in a medical office. The patient may also be concerned when the insurance carrier takes a long time to make a payment because of delays in processing a claim. Many patients, especially the elderly, keep close track of outstanding balances, including outstanding insurance balances.

Advantages and Disadvantages of Paper Claims

The start-up costs involved with using paper claims are minimal. The equipment and supplies needed to complete the claim forms include the claim forms and current coding books. As long as the office has a sufficient amount of forms, they can be accessed at any time.

The disadvantages are found in the cost to complete a paper claim process that includes storage space, postage, mailing, resubmission, follow-up, and copies of claim forms that are submitted and resubmitted. When the medical assistant completes a claim form manually, it must be on an original claim form. It must be legible, completed in dark ink, and printed in capital letters. This can be very time consuming.

Preparing Paper Claim Forms

Never use punctuation, decimals, dollar signs, or correction aids on a paper claim form. If a mistake is made, you must begin again with a new claim form. Do not tape, staple, or clip items to the claim form. Always place the required documentation with the completed claim form in an envelope to be mailed and make sure the insurance address is correct. Never fold the claim forms.

ELECTRONIC CLAIMS

The Health Insurance Portability and Accountability Act (HIPAA) required that claims be transmitted electronically in the HIPAA format by providers who were not considered small by October 16, 2003. Electronic claims are sent to an insurance carrier or a **clearinghouse** via dial-up modem, direct data entry, or over the Internet rather than on paper. A clearinghouse is an independent entity that reviews claims, requests clarification from the provider, "cleans" claims ensuring accurate information is documented, and then submits them to insurance companies in the proper format.

Advantages of Electronic Claims

The electronic process of filing claims speeds processing time on both the provider's end and at the insurance carrier's end. Many plans make direct electronic deposits of insurance-claim payments into the provider's bank account. Processing claims electronically decreases payment turnaround time. It also shortens the payment cycle, thereby increasing cash flow into the medical office. Sending claim forms electronically instead of by mail saves postage and labor costs for the medical office. Even though it is less likely than with paper claims, errors may still occur with electronic filing. It is very important for the medical assistant to proofread all claims before submitting them.

When submitting claims directly to the insurance carrier, electronic claims submission requires the same information as on the CMS-1500 form, but instead of mailing the claim form, all information is sent directly from the medical office to the insurance carrier's computer server. This type of submission is referred to as a paperless claim. To send a claim electronically, the medical assistant must do the following:

- Collect all information needed about the patient, including diagnostic and procedure codes, as though you were completing a manual CMS-1500 form. The claim form on the screen may not be identical to a hard copy of the CMS form.

- Connect your computer to the insurance company's computer server, using instructions provided by the insurance company. Type in your identification number and password and follow the instructions and prompts on the screen.

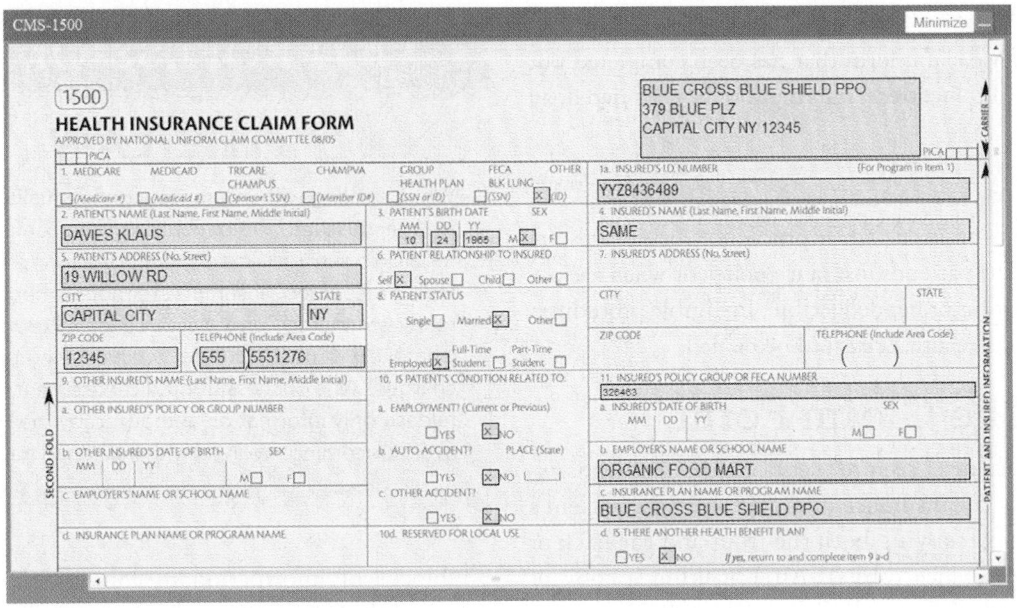

CMS-1500 Minimize

1500

HEALTH INSURANCE CLAIM FORM

APPROVED BY NATIONAL UNIFORM CLAIM COMMITTEE 08/05

BLUE CROSS BLUE SHIELD PPO
379 BLUE PLZ
CAPITAL CITY NY 12345

PICA

1. MEDICARE MEDICAID TRICARE CHAMPUS CHAMPVA GROUP HEALTH PLAN FECA BLK LUNG OTHER

(Medicare #) (Medicaid #) (Sponsor's SSN) (Member ID#) (SSN or ID) (SSN) [X] (ID)

1a. INSURED'S I.D. NUMBER (For Program in Item 1): YYZ8436489

2. PATIENT'S NAME (Last Name, First Name, Middle Initial): DAVIES KLAUS

3. PATIENT'S BIRTH DATE MM DD YY: 10 24 1965 SEX M [X] F

4. INSURED'S NAME (Last Name, First Name, Middle Initial): SAME

5. PATIENT'S ADDRESS (No. Street): 19 WILLOW RD

6. PATIENT RELATIONSHIP TO INSURED: Self [X] Spouse Child Other

7. INSURED'S ADDRESS (No. Street)

CITY: CAPITAL CITY STATE: NY

8. PATIENT STATUS: Single Married [X] Other

CITY STATE

ZIP CODE: 12345 TELEPHONE (Include Area Code): (555) 5551276

Employed [X] Full-Time Student Part-Time Student

ZIP CODE TELEPHONE (Include Area Code) ( )

9. OTHER INSURED'S NAME (Last Name, First Name, Middle Initial)

10. IS PATIENT'S CONDITION RELATED TO:

11. INSURED'S POLICY GROUP OR FECA NUMBER: 326463

a. OTHER INSURED'S POLICY OR GROUP NUMBER

a. EMPLOYMENT? (Current or Previous) YES [X] NO

a. INSURED'S DATE OF BIRTH MM DD YY SEX M F

b. OTHER INSURED'S DATE OF BIRTH MM DD YY SEX M F

b. AUTO ACCIDENT? PLACE (State) YES [X] NO

b. EMPLOYER'S NAME OR SCHOOL NAME: ORGANIC FOOD MART

c. EMPLOYER'S NAME OR SCHOOL NAME

c. OTHER ACCIDENT? YES [X] NO

c. INSURANCE PLAN NAME OR PROGRAM NAME: BLUE CROSS BLUE SHIELD PPO

d. INSURANCE PLAN NAME OR PROGRAM NAME

10d. RESERVED FOR LOCAL USE

d. IS THERE ANOTHER HEALTH BENEFIT PLAN? YES [X] NO *If yes, return to and complete item 9 a-d.*

SECOND FOLD

CARRIER

PATIENT AND INSURED INFORMATION

FIGURE 18-3 Sample of CMS-1500 in electronic format.

- Fill out the claim form as you would the CMS-1500. When the insurance carrier recognizes the physician's identification number, it will automatically assign a processing number to the claim. Keep track of this number for future reference; it is your confirmation that the claim has been received. The best place to document this information is in the insurance claims log.

Software programs are available that allow claims processing without the need to reenter some of the data more than once. To prevent delay of payment, it is important to be familiar with the procedures and software. Figure 18-3 provides an example of a CMS-1500 electronic claim submission.

Disadvantages of Electronic Claims

One of the disadvantages of submitting claims electronically is the initial start-up expense. The medical office requires an Internet service provider, computer, software, appropriate training for those using the system, printer, and backup or storage devices. In addition, glitches may occur with the computer that can delay processing time, transmission, and payments.

Transmitting Claims Electronically

Claims can be transmitted electronically in three ways. The first method is to send the transmission directly to the payer. To communicate electronically between the payer and the medical office, an electronic data interchange (EDI) information system must be utilized.

The second method is transmitting claims through a clearinghouse. The clearinghouse does not modify any of the data. Rather, the clearinghouse is responsible for putting the data in a format appropriate for EDI use. Clearinghouses charge for the services provided, yet they eliminate the need for medical offices to have specific software that may be required by different carriers. The clearinghouse also checks each claim form for accuracy and returns it to the medical office for correction, thereby reducing the incidence of claim rejection.

The last method is direct data entry (DDE), which is an online service provided by some carriers. The data from the claim is keyed in a specific format and then transmitted directly to the carrier.

STATUS OF INSURANCE CLAIMS

The status of insurance claims is a concern of every medical office. Lost, incomplete, or rejected claims cause delays in reimbursement to the practice. Over time, this is costly to any medical office.

Clean Claims

A health insurance claim form that has been completed correctly without any errors or omissions is called a **clean claim**. Clean claims are also submitted on time to the insurance carrier. The first time such a claim is submitted to the insurance carrier, it is processed and payment is sent to the provider.

Dirty Claims

When a health insurance claim form is incorrect because it has missing data or errors, it is considered to be incomplete and a **dirty claim**. This will cause the claim to be rejected.

Invalid Claims

A health insurance claim form that has been completed but has some type of incorrect information is considered an **invalid claim**.

Denied Claims

A **denied claim** can occur when procedures or services are not covered by the patient's insurance policy or when the patient has not met his or her deductible. Ineligible procedures or services can also cause a claim to be denied.

The Claim Form

Each time a patient is seen for services, the medial assistant must verify the insurance information in the patient's medical record by copying both the front and the back of the patient's insurance card(s). After making a copy of each insurance card, the medical assistant will file it with the patient's medical record. Then, the medical assistant will verify that the patient has signed the **assignment of benefits** form, which allows the insurance carrier to pay the physician directly for billed charges. After the patient has been seen by the physician, the medical assistant can complete the CMS-1500 form. The CMS-1500 contains

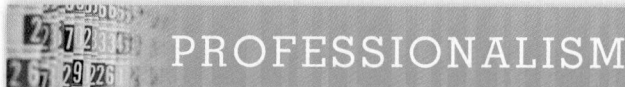
33 blocks of information to complete. Blocks 1 to 13 request information about the patient's demographics and insurance carrier. Blocks 14 to 33 request information about the patient's diagnosis, procedure(s) performed, dollar amount of each procedure, and total charge. The form also requires information about the physician. Procedure 18-1 reviews each step for correctly completing the CMS-1500 form.

procedure
18-1

COMPLETING THE CMS-1500 FORM
Objective: Correctly complete a CMS-1500 form.

EQUIPMENT AND SUPPLIES
patient's medical record; patient's insurance information; patient's ledger card; superbill; CMS-1500 form; black ink pen; computer and printer (or typewriter)

METHOD

1. Box 1 refers to government medical plans. Place an "X" in the appropriate box to indicate the type of insurance plan or program.
   a. Enter the identification number listed on the insurance card.
2. Enter the patient's name in the order requested on the form.
3. Enter the patient's 8-digit birth date. Place an "X" in the box that indicates the patient's gender.
4. Enter the insured's name in the order requested on the form. Enter the word "SAME" if the patient and insured are the same.
5. Enter the patient's complete address and telephone number.
6. Place an "X" in the box that indicates the patient's relationship to the insured.
7. Enter the insured's complete address and telephone number.
8. Place an "X" in the box that indicates the patient's marital status. Place an "X" in the box to indicate if the patient is employed or a full-time or part-time student.
9. If the patient has secondary insurance, enter the other insured's name in the order requested on the form; otherwise, leave blank.
   a. Enter the other insured's policy or group number.
   b. Enter the other insured's 8-digit birth date. Place an "X" in the box that indicates the other insured's gender.

c. Enter the other insured's employer name or school name.

d. Enter the other insured's insurance plan name or program name.

10. Place an "X" in either the YES or NO box to indicate if the patient's condition is related to:

a. employment,

b. auto accident, or

c. other accident.

d. Reserved for local use. Leave blank.

11. Leave blank if there is no private secondary insurance. If there is secondary insurance, see Blocks 9 through 9d.

a. Leave blank.

b. When submitting to a secondary insurance carrier, enter the name of the employer or school if the primary insurance is a group plan; otherwise, leave blank. The **primary insurance** is the coverage provided by the patient's employer. If the patient is not employed, the spouse's insurance is primary. **Secondary insurance** applies if the patient has primary insurance and also has coverage available through the spouse's employer.

c. When submitting to a secondary insurance carrier, enter the name of the primary insurance; otherwise, leave blank.

d. Place an "X" in either the YES or NO box to indicate the availability of another health benefit plan. If YES, complete 9a to 9d.

12. To release and use the patient's medical information to process the claim, have the patient or authorized person sign and date in the appropriate area, or if applicable, note SIGNATURE ON FILE. Some insurance carriers accept the acronym SOF.

13. To authorize payment for the claim dispersed to the provider, have the insured or authorized person sign in the appropriate area or, if applicable, note SIGNATURE ON FILE or SOF.

14. Enter the 8-digit date of current illness, injury, or pregnancy.

15. Enter dates if patient has had same or similar condition.

16. Enter the 8-digit from and to dates for which the patient is unable to work in his or her current occupation.

17. Enter the name of the referring physician or other source.

a. Enter the National Provider identifier (NPI) number of the referring or ordering physician.

18. Enter the 8-digit from and to hospitalization dates related to the current services.

19. This block may be completed in a number of different ways depending on the insurance carrier. Check with the insurance carrier for guidelines.

20. Place an "X" in either the YES or NO box to indicate if an outside laboratory was used. Enter the amount of the charges.

21. Enter the correct ICD-9-CM code (see Chapter 19) related to the diagnosis or nature of the illness or injury. Each ICD-9-CM code must be entered in priority order. Each form can only contain four ICD-9-CM codes.

22. Enter the Medicaid resubmission code and original reference number; otherwise, leave blank.

23. Enter the prior authorization number, if applicable.

24. Enter information into columns A through J.

a. Enter the 8-digit from and to dates the patient had services.

b. Enter the 2-digit code for place of service.

c. Leave blank.

d. Enter the correct CPT/HCPCS code and modifier for procedures, services, or supplies.

e. Enter the correct diagnosis code (1, 2, 3, or 4) that corresponds to the service that was rendered.

f. Enter the charges for the service rendered.

g. Enter the number of days or units of service.

h. Leave blank.

i. If the provider does not have an NPI number, enter the ID qualifier "1C" in the shaded portion of the block. This indicates the non-NPI number being reported; otherwise, leave blank.

j. Enter the rendering provider's NPI number in the lower portion.

25. Enter the federal tax ID number or Social Security Number.

26. Enter the patient's account number. When Medicare is billed electronically, this block must be completed.

27. Place an "X" in either the YES or NO box to indicate if assignment will be accepted.

28. Enter total charges.

29. Enter amount paid.

30. Enter balance due.

31. Enter signature of physician or supplier, including degrees or credentials.

32. Enter the complete name and address of the facility where the services were rendered.

33. Enter the physician or supplier's name, billing address, zip code, and telephone number.

a. Enter the NPI number of the billing provider or group.

b. Leave blank.

34. Proofread the CMS-1500 form for accuracy.

35. Make a copy of the CMS-1500 form to keep in the patient's financial record—for paper claim submissions only.

36. Enter required data into the insurance claims log.

37. Send the completed CMS-1500 form (Figure 18-4) and required documentation to the insurance carrier.

HEALTH INSURANCE CLAIM FORM
APPROVED BY NATIONAL UNIFORM CLAIM COMMITTEE 08/05

☐☐ PICA

1. MEDICARE MEDICAID TRICARE CHAMPVA GROUP FECA OTHER	1a. INSURED'S I.D. NUMBER (For Program in Item 1)
CHAMPUS HEALTH PLAN BLK LUNG	
☐(Medicare #) ☐(Medicaid #) ☐(Sponsor's SSN) ☐(Member ID#) ☒(SSN or ID) ☐(SSN) ☐(ID)	514258522

2. PATIENT'S NAME (Last Name, First Name, Middle Initial)
BLAKE NORBERT

3. PATIENT'S BIRTH DATE   SEX
MM 05 DD 07 YY 1984   M☒   F☐

4. INSURED'S NAME (Last Name, First Name, Middle Initial)
SAME

5. PATIENT'S ADDRESS (No, Street)
1721 ELM STREET

6. PATIENT RELATIONSHIP TO INSURED
Self☒ Spouse☐ Child☐ Other☐

7. INSURED'S ADDRESS (No, Street)

CITY RICHARDSON   STATE TX

8. PATIENT STATUS
Single☒ Married☐ Other☐

Full-Time Part-Time
Employed☒ Student☐ Student☐

CITY   STATE

ZIP CODE 12345
TELEPHONE (Include Area Code)
(912) 4148544

ZIP CODE
TELEPHONE (Include Area Code)
( )

9. OTHER INSURED'S NAME (Last Name, First Name, Middle Initial)

10. IS PATIENT'S CONDITION RELATED TO:

11. INSURED'S POLICY GROUP OR FECA NUMBER
58999

a. OTHER INSURED'S POLICY OR GROUP NUMBER

a. EMPLOYMENT? (Current or Previous)
☐YES ☒NO

a. INSURED'S DATE OF BIRTH   SEX
MM DD YY   M☐ F☐

b. OTHER INSURED'S DATE OF BIRTH   SEX
MM DD YY   M☐ F☐

b. AUTO ACCIDENT?   PLACE (State)
☐YES ☒NO

b. EMPLOYER'S NAME OR SCHOOL NAME
LIZIS CHICKEN

c. EMPLOYER'S NAME OR SCHOOL NAME

c. OTHER ACCIDENT?
☐YES ☒NO

c. INSURANCE PLAN NAME OR PROGRAM NAME
CIGNA HEALTH CARE

d. INSURANCE PLAN NAME OR PROGRAM NAME

10d. RESERVED FOR LOCAL USE

d. IS THERE ANOTHER HEALTH BENEFIT PLAN?
☐YES ☒NO   If yes, return to and complete item 9 a-d

READ BACK OF FORM BEFORE COMPLETING & SIGNING THIS FORM.

12. PATIENT'S OR AUTHORIZED PERSON'S SIGNATURE I authorize the release of any medical or other information necessary to process this claim. I also request payment of government benefits either to myself or to the party who accepts assignment below.

SIGNED SIGNATURE ON FILE   DATE XX XX XXXX

13. INSURED'S OR AUTHORIZED PERSON'S SIGNATURE I authorize payment of medical benefits to the undersigned physician or supplier for services described below.

SIGNED SIGNATURE ON FILE

14. DATE OF CURRENT   ILLNESS (First symptom) OR
MM DD YY   INJURY (Accident) OR
XX XX XXXX   PREGNANCY (LMP)

15. IF PATIENT HAS HAD SAME OR SIMILAR ILLNESS.
GIVE FIRST DATE MM DD YY

16. DATES PATIENT UNABLE TO WORK IN CURRENT OCCUPATION
MM DD YY   MM DD YY
FROM   TO

17. NAME OF REFERRING PHYSICIAN OR OTHER SOURCE
17a.
17b. NPI

18. HOSPITALIZATION DATES RELATED TO CURRENT SERVICES
MM DD YY   MM DD YY
FROM   TO

19. RESERVED FOR LOCAL USE

20. OUTSIDE LAB? $ CHARGES
☐YES ☒NO

21. DIAGNOSIS OR NATURE OF ILLNESS OR INJURY (Relate Items 1,2,3 or 4 to Item 24E by Line)

1. 959 . 4   3.
2.   4.

22. MEDICAID RESUBMISSION
CODE   ORIGINAL REF. NO.

23. PRIOR AUTHORIZATION NUMBER

24. A. DATE(S) OF SERVICE						B. PLACE OF SERVICE	C. EMG	D. PROCEDURES, SERVICES, OR SUPPLIES (Explain Unusual Circumstances)		E. DIAGNOSIS POINTER	F. $ CHARGES	G. DAYS OR UNITS	H. EPSDT Family Plan	I. ID. QUAL.	J. RENDERING PROVIDER ID. #
From			To					CPT/HCPCS	MODIFIER						
MM	DD	YY	MM	DD	YY										
														1G	234665212
XX	XX	XX	XX	XX	XX	11		99213		1	60 00	1		NPI	8888877777
														1G	234665212
XX	XX	XX	XX	XX	XX	11		73130		1	45 00	1		NPI	8888877777
														NPI	
														NPI	
														NPI	
														NPI	

25. FEDERAL TAX ID NUMBER   SSN EIN
725727222   ☐☒

26. PATIENT'S ACCOUNT NO.
BLANO

27. ACCEPT ASSIGNMENT? (For govt. claims, see back)
☒YES ☐NO

28. TOTAL CHARGE
$ 105 00

29. AMOUNT PAID
$

30. BALANCE DUE
$

31. SIGNATURE OF PHYSICIAN OR SUPPLIER INCLUDING DEGREES OR CREDENTIALS
(I certify that the statements on the reverse apply to this bill and are made a part thereof)

SIGNED SIGNATURE ON FILE   DATE XXXXXX

32. SERVICE FACILITY LOCATION INFORMATION
MALLARD & ASSOCIATES PA
19333 FORREST HAVEN
DALLAS TX 12345

a. 7777788888   b. 1GM 23548711

33. BILLING PROVIDER INFO & PH. #   (215) 5555040
MALLARD & ASSOCIATES PA
19333 FORREST HAVEN
DALLAS TX 12345

a. 7777788888   b. 1GM23548711

NUCC Instruction Manual available at: www.nucc.org
WCMS-1500CS

APPROVED OMB 0938-0999 FORM CMS-1500 (08/05)

FIGURE 18-4 A completed CMS-1500 form.

Assignment of Lifetime Medicare Benefits

Name of Beneficiary ____________________

Medicare Number ____________________

I, the undersigned, request that all authorized Medicare benefits be paid to me or on my behalf to ____________________ (Name of Physician or Supplier) for all services rendered to me by the aforementioned provider. I hereby authorize any holder of my medical records to release to the Health Care Financing Administration and its agents any information necessary to determine and secure the payment of all benefits.*

Signed ____________________ (Signature of Beneficiary) Date ____________

* If you are a patient in a hospital or skilled nursing home, this authorization is in effect for the period of your confinement. Otherwise, this authorization is in effect until you choose to revoke it.

FIGURE 18-5 **An Assignment of Lifetime Medicare Benefits form.**

Claims Processing

Claims are processed at insurance companies by a claims administrator. The claim form is a critical item in claims processing. Although several forms are used for claims processing, the most commonly used form (as noted previously) is the CMS-1500 designed by the Health Care Financing Administration (HCFA). For a claim to be processed, this form must be filled out completely and correctly. In addition to information about the patient, the diagnosis, and the services received, the following information regarding the insured, also known as the policyholder, is required for all claims:

- The name of the insured's insurance company
- The name of the insured
- The insured's identification number
- The address of the insured
- The telephone number of the insured

In general, the upper portion of the form describes the patient and the insured (which may or may not be the same individual) and the lower half of the form (separated by a heavy line) refers to the provider of services, the services provided to the patient, and the medical necessity of those services.

As with all patient information, all rules of confidentiality apply. Therefore, the patient must sign a release of information for a claim form to be completed. To make this process simpler, many offices have a standard release form for this purpose. Once the form has been signed and is on file in the patient's record, a notation of SIGNATURE ON FILE (or SOF) may be written or typed in box 12 of the CMS-1500 form. Box 13 deals with payment of benefits. If this box is signed, payment will frequently be made directly to the provider of services. If the box is not signed, or the insurance contract specifies that benefits cannot be assigned, payment is made to the insured. Many insurance carriers, including Medicare, allow for lifetime assignment of benefits (Figure 18-5). With a signature on one form, the notation SIGNATURE ON FILE (or SOF) can also be made in box 13. This saves the medical assistant the time required for a patient to sign an insurance claim form for each office visit. The forms, however, must be kept in the patient record and must be available at all times. If the insurance carrier were to request the signed form, the medical office must be able to produce a current, signed form to avoid penalty.

A confusing element in insurance processing is the concept of participating and nonparticipating providers, also known as par and nonpar. Most insurance companies will make special incentives available to those who choose to become participating providers. A **participating provider** has a contractual agreement with an insurance plan to render care to eligible beneficiaries and then bill the insurance carrier directly. Such providers may be physicians or medical facilities that agree to accept the insurance company's allowed amount as payment in full (less the patient's copayment).

PROFESSIONALISM THE LIFE SPAN

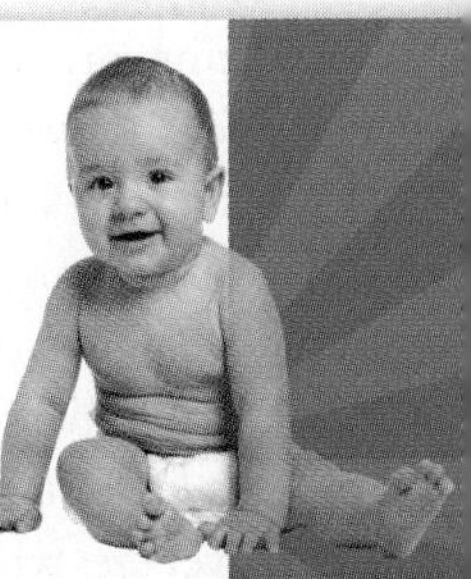

Some insurance plans require that the subscriber fill out the claim forms. To someone, especially an older patient, who has never worked with filing claims, this can be very confusing. Because the physician cannot receive payment for services until claims are filed, it can be helpful to assist the patient in filling out the appropriate forms. Some offices do this for a small fee, whereas others do it at no charge. In any case, have the patient sign an authorization to release medical information before submitting any claim.

A participating provider may not bill the patient for the difference between the amount billed the insurance company and the amount allowed by the insurance company. To become a participating provider, the physician must complete a form and sign a contract with the insurance carrier.

With most insurance plans, payment is made directly to participating providers, although payment is made directly to the patient for claims regarding care received by a nonparticipating provider. A **nonparticipating provider** bills the patient, and the patient is expected to pay the charges and then submit the claim to the insurance company. If and when payment is made by the insurance company, it is made directly to the patient.

Often, insurance companies reimburse at a lower rate than the physician bills. In this case, the physician must **write off** or agree to forfeit the amount the insurance company does not authorize. It is an expense to any practice when administrative staff (medical assistant or insurance claims processing clerk, for example) on the payroll must spend time submitting and tracking insurance claims. On the other hand, payment is made directly to the physician's practice, often within a few days (especially with electronic claim submission), ensuring that large charges do not accumulate on the physician's accounts receivable. Each practice must weigh the advantages and disadvantages carefully before making a decision to become either a participating or nonparticipating practice.

Many medical offices now use a single sheet to speed the process of reimbursement. This form is called a superbill. A superbill also known as an an encounter form or charge slip, includes the patient's name, diagnoses, treatments, and additional space to fill in claim information. Some insurance carriers will accept a superbill in lieu of a claim form, although this depends on the specific carrier. Originally, superbills were created to allow patients to file their own claims; however, as insurance rules and regulations have become more complex and coding and documentation requirements more stringent, most medical practices file insurance claims for their patients as a courtesy. It is important for the medical assistant to verify if a patient has primary and secondary medical insurance coverage. A patient who has health insurance coverage with more than one medical insurance plan will designate one plan as the primary insurance coverage and the other insurance plan as secondary coverage. If the patient has coverage with his or her employer as well as his or her spouse's employer, then the patient's medical insurance plan through his or her employer would be the primary insurance, and the spouse's medical insurance plan would be the secondary insurance. This prevents a patient from profiting on his or her medical insurance. It also prevents double payment on services provided.

The **birthday rule** is used by insurance claims administrators to determine which parent's benefit plan will be the primary insurance plan of a dependent child who is covered by employer-sponsored insurance plans of both parents. The plan of the parent whose birthday falls earliest in the year (not the oldest parent) will be the primary plan. For example if one parent's birthday is March 30 and the other parent's birthday is September 24, the parent with the March birthday would cover the child on his or her insurance plan, although the other parent's plan would be considered secondary insurance for the dependent child. If it happens that both parents have the same birth date, the parent who has had the coverage the longest is primary. This rule only applies to parents who are legally married.

If the parents are divorced, the court will determine which parent's medical insurance will be primary. Just because a parent has legal custody does not mean that his or her medical insurance will be the primary coverage plan.

Claims Security

Confidentiality is an important issue in regard to the sensitive information that is found in a patient's medical record. Care must be taken when processing insurance claims that only the appropriate information is released to the appropriate person. Security involves protection of patient information. Security is the responsibility of all who have access to patients' records. Care must be taken in the work area not to leave records unattended. When discussing patient information with insurance carriers over the telephone, it is best to be in an area where you cannot be easily overheard. It is considered to be a **breach of confidentiality**, or failure to keep something confidential, when patient information is released to others without authorization from the patient.

Before releasing patient information to anyone, you must obtain a signed Authorization for Release of Medical Information statement from the patient. Authorization can be given by having the patient sign block 12, Patient's or Authorized Person's Signature, on the CMS-1500. A practice can also create its own release form. It is good practice to have the patient renew this authorization annually.

Another element of claims security is making sure electronic data containing health information about a patient are secure when stored on a computer network. A firewall is used to prevent unauthorized access from another computer system to the data stored on the computer network.

Tracking Claim Forms

When a medical assistant is submitting paper claims, he or she must have a tracking system in place to follow up on claims that have been submitted. An insurance claims log is used for this purpose. An insurance claims log can be documented manually or kept on a computerized spreadsheet. Provided the claim log is continuously updated, it can quickly provide the status of a claim. After the medical assistant completes a claim form, he or she then enters data into the insurance claims log. The data entered at this time include the patient's name, date of service, insurance carrier, date of claim submission, and amount of the claim. When the medical assistant follows up on the claim, the date must be documented on the insurance claims log. Once the medical assistant receives payment on the claim, this date must also be documented on the insurance claims log. The difference between the submitted and paid amounts is also documented on the insurance claims log. After the claim is paid in full, the medical assistant can highlight that section of the insurance claims log to indicate that the claim is completely processed.

CLAIM FORM REJECTION

As mentioned elsewhere in this chapter, if a claim contains missing or incorrect information, the insurance company will reject the claim. Some of the most common reasons for claim rejection include the following:

- Incorrect or missing patient registration information (name, address, insurance number)
- Incorrect or missing name of a referring physician
- Incorrect or missing diagnosis code
- Overlapping, incorrect, or duplicate dates of service
- Incorrect place of service
- Invalid, incorrect, or missing procedure code
- Incorrect or missing number of days or units
- Incorrect or missing modifier

If a claim is rejected for any reason, it must be corrected and resubmitted to the insurance carrier. Time limits for re-filing rejected claims usually apply, so the medical assistant must be very aware of these deadlines and resubmit the claims before the time has expired. Expired claims will not be processed by the insurance carrier and will ultimately cost the practice money.

To minimize the number of rejected claims, the medical assistant must review every claim for accuracy prior to submitting it. Although no one process or procedure can guar-

antee that a claim will never be rejected or reviewed by the insurance carrier, a careful, studious approach to the claims process can ensure greater accuracy. Review by the insurance carrier is a random audit during which claims are pulled and reviewed for accuracy and compliance.

PREVENTING CLAIM FORM REJECTION

Some simple steps can be taken to minimize the possibility of having claims rejected. The following is a list of suggested steps:

- Pay close attention to detail.
- Keep current reference materials, books, and equipment readily available and use them.
- Limit distractions in the medical office to help ensure the claim form is completed correctly and completely.
- Since time to focus on claims processing is not always easy to come by, have the office team work together to provide it.
- Set aside a certain time each day for working only on claims. This can help the medical assistant complete the forms correctly and, most of the time, more quickly.
- Have another medical office staff member review each insurance claim form before it is submitted. A second set of eyes may notice errors or omissions not detected by the person processing the forms.

SUMMARY

The health insurance claim form provides communication between the insurance company and physician for the patient. When the medical assistant is submitting a claim, he or she must make sure the correct health insurance claim form is used. The most commonly used claim form is the CMS-1500.

Medical assistants must be familiar with the requirements for submitting clean claims. Diligent and concentrated work can help to produce claims that are clean and less likely to be denied. Claims are most often submitted electronically; however, they may also be submitted in paper form.

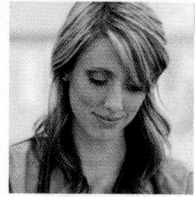

18 CHAPTER REVIEW

COMPETENCY REVIEW

1. Define and spell the terms to learn for this chapter.

2. Explain the birthday rule.

3. What is the name of the standardized form used to submit insurance claims? What information must be included on this form?

4. List the reasons a claim may be rejected.

5. Use the health insurance claim forms shown in Figures 18-4 and 18-5 to complete the forms for Jane Doe, address 123 Main Street, Anytown, ST 60000, U.S.A., telephone 444-555-1234, S/S# 123-45-6789, DOB 1/15/1973. She is single and self-insured. Jane Doe's insurance number is the same as her Social Security number. Jane saw Dr. Brent Smith for the first time on May 27, 2005, and he diagnosed her with primary hypertension. Jane paid $40 for the office visit. Jane's account number is 00321. Dr. Smith is located at 555 Frances Street, Anytown, ST 60000, U.S.A., telephone 444-555-1111, federal tax ID# 000000000.

PREPARING FOR THE CERTIFICATION EXAM

1. Once a patient has signed a release of information statement, what may be written in box 12 of the CMS-1500?
   a. Benefits Assigned.
   b. Confidential.
   c. NPI.
   d. Participating Provider.
   e. Signature on File.

2. All of the following are required for completing the CMS-1500 EXCEPT
   a. the insured's name.
   b. the patient's name.
   c. the patient's relationship to the insured.
   d. the number of people in the household.
   e. the patient's marital status.

3. Which of the following forms is used to submit claims for patients seen in the physician's office?
   a. CMS-1450
   b. CMS-1500
   c. CMS-1540
   d. UB-04
   e. UB-92

4. The upper portion of the CMS-1500 contains information regarding
   a. the patient's diagnosis.
   b. the referring physician.

   c. place of service.
   d. the insured.
   e. the balance due.

5. The CMS-1450 claim form
   a. is rarely used.
   b. must be filled out by the patient.
   c. must be filled out by the provider.
   d. is the claim form used for institutional providers.
   e. is accepted by every insurance company.

6. When a claim is rejected due to missing data this is known as a (an)
   a. invalid claim.
   b. dirty claim.
   c. crossover claim.
   d. clean claim.
   e. none of the above.

7. HIPAA requires that physician offices with this number or more full-time employees submit claims electronically:
   a. 10
   b. 15
   c. 20
   d. 25
   e. 30

8. When submitting paper claims, all of the following applies EXCEPT
   a. must be printed in all capital letters.
   b. must be on original form.
   c. must use dark ink.
   d. must staple supporting documents to form.
   e. must be legible.

9. All of the following is true regarding Medicaid EXCEPT
   a. eligibility is determined on a month-to-month basis.
   b. payment is the same across the nation.
   c. it is funded in part by the federal government.
   d. It is intended for those considered medically indigent.
   e. it is administered by individual states.

10. All of the following are advantages for submitting claims electronically EXCEPT
   a. payments made via direct deposit.
   b. increases cash flow.
   c. saves labor cost.
   d. decreases the time it takes to pay a claim.
   e. typically have more errors than paper claims.

CRITICAL THINKING

1. What steps should Lewis take to verify Sylvia Baker's insurance?

2. List some reasons the claim for Mark's care could have been rejected.

3. How should Lewis handle Mr. Flannery's angry call?

ON THE JOB

Drake Scott, CMA (AAMA), is responsible for processing insurance claims for a large medical clinic. You have just hired Anne Obermark, CMA (AAMA), to work with Drake in processing insurance claims. You determined that Anne will be responsible for tracking claims.

1. Why is it important for Anne to track insurance claims processed through the clinic?
2. What kind of information should the insurance claim log contain?
3. When Anne checks the insurance claim log, she finds five claims that have not been paid in the past 3 months. What should Anne do?

INTERNET ACTIVITY

There are many software packages available to help complete and submit insurance claims. Conduct a search to find five such packages. List the unique features, similar features, and cost.

MEDMEDIA

Additional interactive resources and activities for this chapter can be found:

On your student DVD: View applicable procedure videos on the DVD-ROM found in the back of this book.

MyHealthProfessionsKit.com: Test your knowledge of the chapter with games and activities. MyHealthProfessionsKit also includes resources, helpful links, and a Spanish audio glossary.

Medical Assisting Interactive: Practice your procedures as a medical assistant in this simulated doctor's office. This can be accessed through MyHealthProfessionsKit.com.

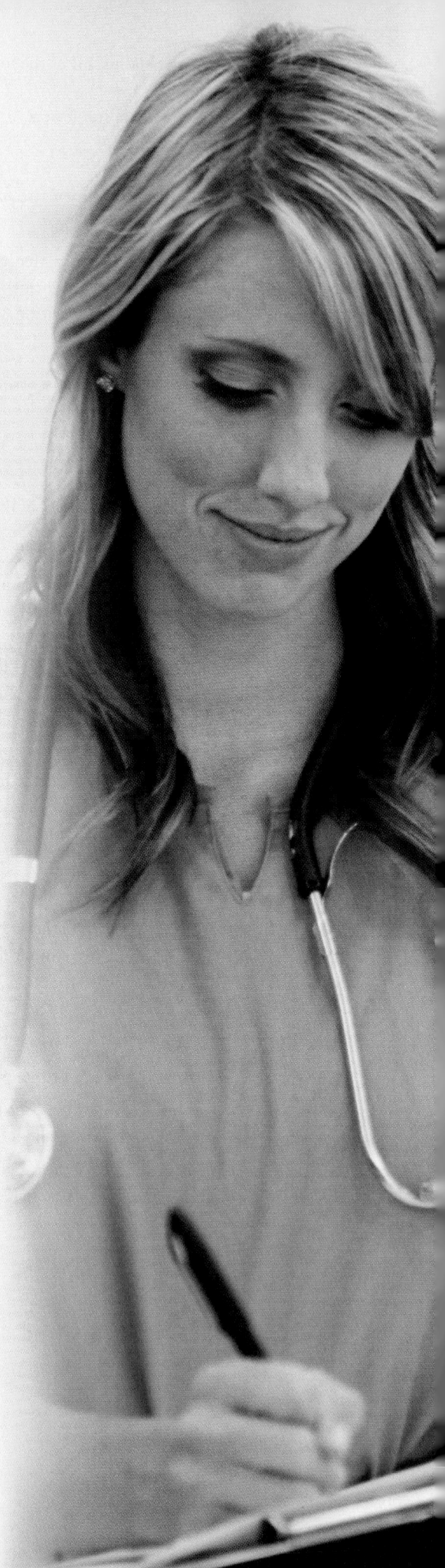

19

Medical Coding

LEARNING OBJECTIVES

After completing this chapter, you should be able to:

- Define and spell the terms to learn for this chapter.

- Describe the purpose of diagnostic coding.

- Correctly apply the principles of ICD-9-CM coding.

- Describe the purpose of CPT coding.

- Discuss basic coding rules for CPT.

- Correctly apply the principles of CPT coding.

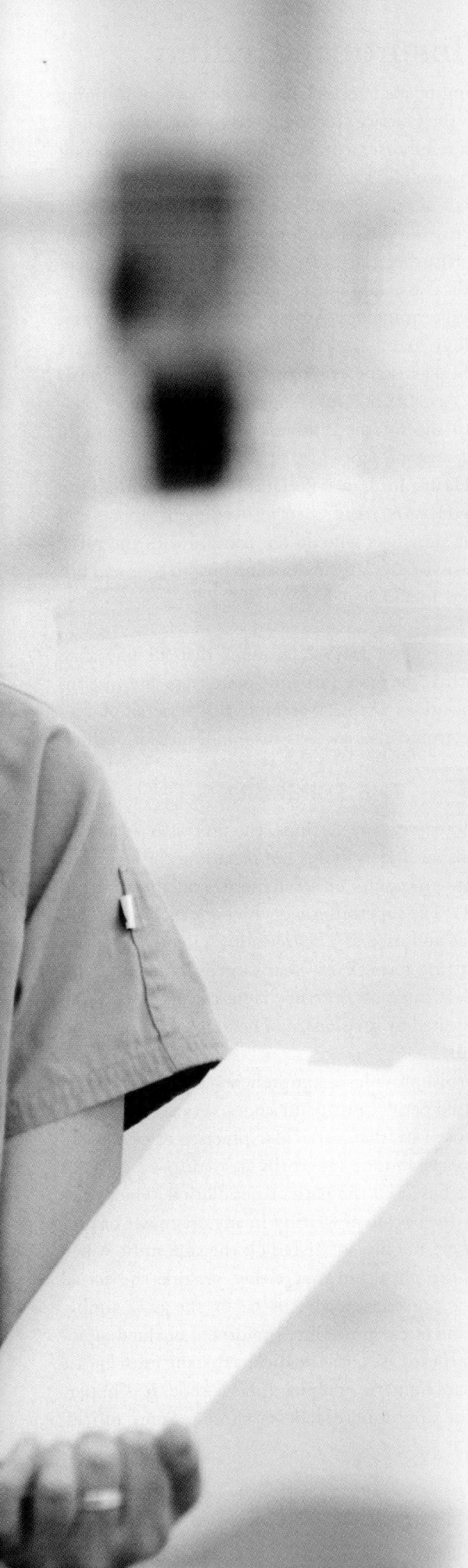

CHAPTER OUTLINE

CASE STUDY

Sophia DiStefano, a five-year-old female, was seen by Dr. Salpega. He diagnosed Sophia with chronic otitis media because this visit was the third bout of otits media she has had within the past 7 months. Dr. Salpega asked that David, a registered medical assistant, conduct an audiometry screening on Sophia. He also suggested that Edvige, Sophia's mother, consider having Sophia undergo bilateral myringotomies and tube placement for a more permanent treatment of the chronic otitis media.

Current Procedural
Terminology (CPT)

established patient

Evaluation and
Management (E/M)

International Classification
of Diseases, Ninth Revision,
Clinical Modification
(ICD-9-CM)

International Classification
of Diseases, Tenth Revision
(ICD-10)

kickback

modifier

new patient

principal diagnosis

procedural coding

symbols

upcoding

World Health Organization
(WHO)

CERTIFICATION LINK

CMA (AAMA)
Medical
terminology
  Uses of
  terminology
Medicolegal
guidelines and
requirements
  Legislation
  Physician–
  patient
  relationship
Practice finances
  Coding systems

RMA
Administrative
medical assisting
  Insurance
  Medical
  receptionist/
  Secretarial/Clerical

CMAS (AMT)
Medical assisting
foundation
  Legal and ethical
  considerations
Health care insurance
processing, coding,
and billing
  Insurance coding

The process of insurance billing includes the accurate identification of the diagnostic, procedure, and service codes on the medical insurance claim form discussed in Chapter 18. Diagnostic codes are located in the International Classification of Diseases, Ninth Revision, Clinical Modification (ICD-9-CM) listing. The procedure and service codes are located in the Current Procedural Terminology (CPT) listing. Each individual code specifically represents a numeric or alphanumeric identification for insurance carriers and aids in obtaining the maximum reimbursement. The medical assistant will need to identify the appropriate codes to reflect the correct diagnosis to support the procedure or service performed. This will help to maintain sound billing practices. Transposing any of the numbers will cause the claim to be rejected, so it is key to pay close attention to detail.

Insurance Coding

Proper coding of insurance claims is the basis of bringing income into the practice. Incorrect coding will cause delays or denials in reimbursement. Anytime the medical assistant does not observe clear and concise documentation in the patient's medical record to support the ICD-9-CM or CPT code (see "Procedural Coding"), he or she must consult the physician for further clarification. To be proficient in coding, the medical assistant must also have a good understanding of medical terminology, pathology, procedures, anatomy, and physiology. A medical dictionary is a handy resource for any medical assistant who has the responsibility of medical coding. Another helpful resource is the Internet. Having access to the Internet allows the medical assistant to research a disease or procedure he or she does not understand. The Health Insurance Portability and Accountability Act of 1996 (HIPAA) requires correct coding of services and may sanction providers who do not comply with the rules. The medical assistant must understand how to code and bill with accuracy. In addition, HIPAA requires electronic submission of the CMS-1500 form for Medicare billing and reimbursement. Also, HIPAA requires that all physician practices with 10 or more full-time employees and institutional organizations with 25 or more full-time employees complete electronic insurance claims for all medical billing.

THE SUPERBILL

In many ambulatory care settings, the process of insurance coding begins with identifying and recording the appropriate diagnosis, procedure, or service codes on the superbill (Figure 19-1). The superbill is a document generated by the medical office and used as a charge slip, statement, and insurance reporting form. Every year, superbills must be updated to reflect the most current diagnostic and procedural codes, as indicated by revisions, and new codes that are published annually.

The superbill provides a comprehensive list of the most frequently used patient procedure codes, services, and diagnosis codes used by that particular practice or physician. Most offices have unique superbills created specifically for each practice based on the patient population. The physician also has the option of writing in any diagnoses or procedures that are not already listed on the superbill. When this occurs, the physician may either provide the actual diagnostic or procedure code, or he or she may simply write the name of the procedure preformed or the diagnosis given. In these cases, the medical assistant must locate the appropriate numeric or alphanumeric code. It is imperative that the appropriate code is chosen. Some offices'

Pearson Physicians Group
Shania McWalter, D.O.
123 Michigan Avenue, Parker Heights, IL 60610
(312) 123-1234

ID.# 20-1342846
No. 4815

PATIENT INFORMATION

PATIENT'S LAST NAME	FIRST	INITIAL	BIRTHDATE	SEX ☐ MALE ☐ FEMALE	TODAY'S DATE /
ADDRESS	CITY	STATE	ZIP	RELATION TO SUBSCRIBER	REFERRING PHYSICIAN
SUBSCRIBER or POLICY HOLDER				INSURANCE	
ADDRESS	CITY	STATE	ZIP	INSURANCE ID.#	COVERAGE CODE	GROUP

OTHER HEALTH COVERAGE?
☐ NO
☐ YES   IDENTIFY

DISABILITY RELATED TO:
☐ ACCIDENT ☐ PREGNANCY
☐ INDEPENDENT ☐ OTHER

DATE SYMPTOMS APPEARED, INCEPTION OF PREGNANCY, OR ACCIDENT OCCURED: / /

ASSIGNMENT and RELEASE: *I hereby assign my insurance benefits to be paid directly to the undersigned physician. I am financially responsible for noncovered services. I also authorize the physician to release any information required to process this claim.*

SIGNATURE OF PATIENT (or Parent, if Minor) _____   DATE / /

PROCEDURES	CPT-Mod	AMOUNT	PROCEDURES	CPT-Mod	AMOUNT	PROCEDURES	CPT-Mod	AMOUNT
A. OFFICE VISITS			31 Post-Partum Only	59430		60 PG Test, Urine	81025	
1 New GYN, Prob Focused	99201		**F. GYN PROCEDURES**			61 PG test, hCG	84702	
2 New GYN, Exp Prob Focused	99202		32 Irrigation of Vagina	57150		62 Cytopathology Smear	88147	
3 New GYN, Detailed	99203		33 Insert Pessary	57160		63 Specimen Handling	99000	
4 New GYN, Comprehensive	99204		34 Pessary Supplies	99070		**I. MISCELLANEOUS**		
5 New GYN, High Complexity	99205		35 Colposcopy	57452		64 Surgical Tray	99070	
6 Return GYN, Nurse visit	99211		36 Biopsy, Cervix	57500		65 Therapeutic Injection	96372	
7 Return GYN, Prob Focused	99212		37 Biopsy, Vagina	57100		66 Injection, Kenalog	J3301	
8 Return GYN, Expanded Prob Foc	99213		38 Biopsy, Vulva	56605		67 Injection, Xylocaine	J2001	
9 Return GYN, Detailed	99214		39 Biopsy, Endometrium	58100		68 Injection, Estrogen	J1410	
10 Return GYN, Comprehensive	99215		40 Biopsy, Skin			69 Injection, Progesterone	J2675	
11 Return GYN, Post-Operative	99024		0.5 cm.	11420		70 Injection, Vitamin B12	J3420	
B. CONSULTATION			0.6 to 1.0 cm.	11421		71 Special Reports	99080	
12 GYN Consultation, Prob Focused	99241		1.1 to 2.0 cm.	11423				
13 GYN Consultation, Exp Prob	99242		41 Cryotherapy, Cervix	57511				
14 GYN Consultation, Detailed	99423		42 Destruct. Condyloma	56501				
15 GYN Consultation, Compreh.	99244		43 Diaphragm Fitting	57170				
16 GYN Consultation, Complex	99245		44 Diaphragm Supplies	99070				
C. TELEPHONE CONSULTATION			45 IUD Insertion	58300				
17 Telephone Consult., 5–10 min	99441		46 IUD Supplies	99070				
18 Telephone Consult., 11–20 min	99442		47 IUD Removal	58301				
19 Telephone Consult., 21–30 min	99443		**G. UROLOGIC PROCEDURES**					
D. SPECIAL SERVICES			48 Urethral Dilation	53660				
20 ER Service Out of Office	99060		49 Urethral Dilation, Repeat	53661				
21 Service out of Off. req by pt	99056		50 Bladder Instillation	51700				
22 Scheduled evening visit	99051		51 Periurethral Injection	53665				
23 Night Call after 10 pm	99053		52 Simple Catheterization	51702				
24 Sunday or Holiday Service	99050		53 Manual Electric Stimulation	97032				
25 Office Emergency	99058		**H. LAB**					
E. OB CARE			54 Urine Analysis	81000				
26 Antepartum only 4–6 visits	59425		55 Urine Culture	87088				
27 Routine OB, pre & post, Normal	59400		56 Hematocrit	85014				
28 Routine OB, pre & post, H.R.	59400.22		57 Hemogram	85027				
29 C-section pre & post care	59510		58 OB Panel	80055		TODAY'S TOTAL FEE	$	
30 C-section only	59514		59 Wet Mount	87210				

DIAGNOSIS	CODE	DIAGNOSIS	CODE	DIAGNOSIS	CODE	DIAGNOSIS	CODE
Abortion:		Breasts	216.5	Galactorrhea	676.6_	Pregnancy Postpartum	V24.2
Threatened	640.0_	Vulva	221.2	Hemorrhoids	455.0	Rectocele	618.04
Incomplete	637.91	Breast Disorder (Mass)	611.72	Hypertension	401.9	Retention of Urine	788.20
Habitual	646.3_	Bronchitis	491.0	Incontinence of Urine	788.3_	Stress Incontinence	625.6
Abnormal Urination	788.6_	Carcinoma In Situ:		Interstitial Cystitis	595.1	Urethral Stricture	598._
Abnormal PAP Smear	795.0_	Cervix	233.1	Irritable Colon	564.1	Urethral Syndrome	597.81
Adenomyosis	617.0	Uterus	233.2	Irregular Menstrual Cycle	626.4	Uterine Leiomyoma	218._
Adnexal Mass	625.8	Female Genital Organs	233.3	Malignant Neoplasm:		Uterine Prolapse:	
Amenorrhea	626.0	Cervical Dysplasia	622.1	Cervix	180.9	Incomplete	618.2
Anemia	285.9	Cervicitis	616.0	Uterus	182.0	Complete	618.3
Arthritis	716.9_	Contraceptive Management	V25.0_	Ovary	183.0	Vaginal Discharge-Non Specific	623.5
Artificial Menopause	627.4	Cystocele	618.0	Vagina	184.0	Vaginal Enterocele	618.6
Asthma-Hayfever	493.00	Cystourethritis	595.0	Vulva	184.4	Vaginal Prolapse	618.09
Atrophic Vaginitis	627.3	Diabetes Mellitus	250.0_	Menopausal Syndrome	627.2	Vaginal Vault Prolapse Post	
Bartholin Abscess	616.3	Thyroid Disorder	246.9	Menometrorrhagia	626.2	Hysterectomy	618.5
Benign Neoplasm:		Dysmenorrhea	625.3	Oligomenorrhea	626.1	Vulvovaginitis:	
Cervix	219.0	Dyspareunia	625.0	Obesity	278.0_	Non Specific	616.10
Uterus	219.1	Dysuria	788.1	Ovarian Cyst	620.2	Candida	112.1
Ovary	220	Ectopic Pregnancy	633.90	Pelvic Inflammatory Disease	614.9	Trichomonas	131.01
Vagina	221.1	Endometriosis	617.9	Pelvic Peritoneal Adhesions	614.6		
Vulva	221.2	Enuresis-Unstable Bladder	788.3	Polycystic Ovaries	256.4		
Benign Neoplasm of Skin:		Frequency of Urination	788.4_	Postmenopausal Bleeding	627.1		
Buttocks	216.5	Functional Disorder:		Post-Op Wound Infection	998.59		
Abdomen	216.5	Bladder Instability	596.52	Pregnancy Prenatal	V22_		

MISCELLANEOUS DIAGNOSIS

DOCTOR'S SIGNATURE _____   DATE / /

SERVICES PERFORMED AT: ☐ Office ☐ Emergency Room
☐ PEARSON PHYSICIANS GROUP   ADMITTED / /
  123 Michigan Avenue, Chicago, IL 60610
  (312) 123-1234
☐ Hospital Calls at $_____ per Visit   DISCHARGED / /

RETURN VISIT INFORMATION
15 · 30 · 45 · 60
___DAYS ___WEEKS ___MONTHS ☐ WILL CALL
Procedure: _____

ACCEPT ASSIGNMENT
☐ YES
☐ NO

INSTRUCTIONS TO PATIENT FOR FILING INSURANCE CLAIMS
1. Complete patient information portion of this form.
2. Sign and date.
3. Mail this form directly to your insurance company with your own insurance company's form.
4. Patients with health care insurance please remember:
   A. Professional services are charged to the patient, and not to the insurance company.
   B. Insured patients are expected to take care of their fees as services are rendered.
   C. This office cannot accept responsibility for collecting your insurance claim or for negotiating a settlement on a disputed claim.
   D. You are responsible for payment of your account.

TODAY'S FEE	$
OLD BALANCE	$
ADJUSTMENTS	$
TOTAL DUE	$
AMOUNT RECEIVED TODAY	$
☐ CASH ☐ CHECK ☐ C.C.	
NEW BALANCE	$

FIGURE 19-1 An example of a superbill.

superbills also include the fees associated with the services rendered. The superbill is used as a point of reference for traditional paper insurance forms and electronic claims (Figure 19-2).

History of Coding

In 1937, the International List of Causes of Death was introduced. In 1948, the World Health Organization (WHO) published the International Classification of Diseases. This provided a revised list of the first classification system. In 1979 the United States, the Department of Health and Human Services published the International Classification of Diseases, Ninth Revision, Clinical Modification (ICD-9-CM). By 1988, the Medicare Catastrophic Coverage Act had been passed. This law made it a requirement for physicians to use diagnosis codes to receive Medicare reimbursement.

Coding has gradually grown from an office task to a career that requires extensive training and knowledge of both the medical and insurance professions. Many medical practices will offer monetary bonuses to insurance billers and coders who are able to identify that their coding skills result in increased revenue and more accurate collections for the physician's practice. For information about becoming a certified medical coding specialist, contact the American Academy of Professional Coders (AAPC) or the American Health Information Management Association (AHIMA).

Understanding the ICD-9-CM

On the physician evaluation, each patient will be diagnosed in medical terms. These medical terms are converted into numeric and alphanumeric diagnosis codes. The diagnosis codes are systematically classified in the **International Classification of Diseases, Ninth Revision, Clinical Modification (ICD-9-CM)**, which is published by the **World Health Organization (WHO)**, a specialized agency of the United Nations.

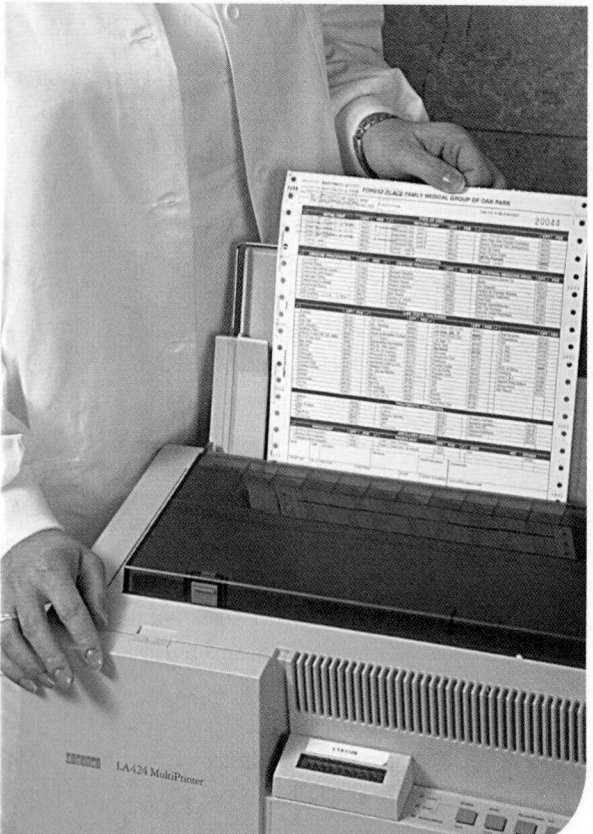

FIGURE 19-2   A computer-generated superbill.

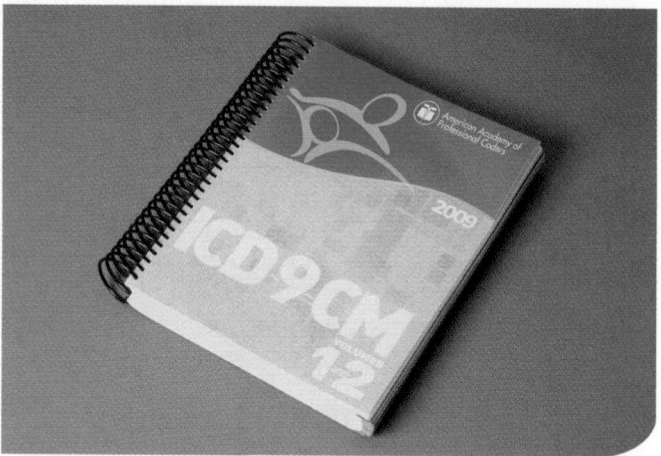

FIGURE 19-3   ICD-9-CM code book.

WHO accumulates all the diagnoses reported on claim forms and places the diagnostic codes into a computerized database. This database tracks statistical information, such as morbidity data throughout the world.

Every year the ICD-9-CM codes are updated. The newly published codes are available to the public on or before October 1. Every medical office should use the newest published revision (Figure 19-3) to perform coding. Failure to use the newest published copy of the codes could cause the claim to be rejected because of incorrect coding.

FORMATS AND CONVENTIONS OF THE ICD-9-CM

The ICD-9-CM provides three- to five-digit numeric and alphanumeric codes for patient diagnoses. For an insurance payment to be processed appropriately, the diagnosis code must appear on a claim form and must support the medical necessity of the procedure code (service rendered).

The ICD-9-CM coding manual contains three volumes of information. Volume III deals with inpatient treatment, which is used to code inpatient hospital-billed procedures. This volume is not used in most ambulatory care settings, such as physician offices. Therefore, we will concentrate on Volumes I: Tabular List and Volume II: Alphabetic Index.

Volume I: Tabular List contains 17 chapters of disease and injury codes, as well as supplementary classifications for V and E codes (see "Special Codes"). It also contains five appendices. In the Tabular List, codes are arranged in numeric order.

Volume II: Alphabetic Index lists the diseases and injuries found in the Tabular List in alphabetic order. In addition, Volume II contains an index of poisoning and adverse effects of chemicals and drugs and an index of injuries caused by external events, such as accidents.

STEPS IN ICD CODING

To understand how to code diagnoses, it is important that the medical assistant understand the organization of the ICD-9-CM. Diagnoses are given a three-digit main code. Fourth and fifth digits are required for certain conditions that define the code to the highest level of specificity.

To code properly, it is necessary to begin with Volume II: Alphabetic Index. Diagnoses and conditions are located

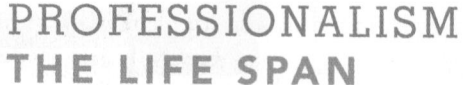

PROFESSIONALISM
THE LIFE SPAN

Elderly patients and caregivers of patients may not understand the diagnosis stated on the superbill. The medical assistant can help the patient or patient's parent or guardian with any questions he or she may have concerning the superbill.

alphabetically by condition, not body system. Therefore, when trying to find a code for a closed fracture of the right arm, the coder would begin by looking for the key word *fracture*. This term is listed in bold type. The coder would next locate the word *arm*. A code number of 818.0 is given. Next, the coder would turn to the numeric index (Volume I: Tabular List) and find the code number 818.0. After reading the description, the code 818.0 is determined to be the correct one. However, the diagnosis needs greater specification that requires an additional fifth digit to designate the specific bone of the arm that contains the fracture. Also, it may be possible that a different code would be used for a *closed fracture* than for an *open fracture*. The medical assistant must read all the information associated with that particular diagnosis to ensure that the correct diagnosis has been chosen. Special notes and symbols used in ICD-9-CM coding, such as "not otherwise specified" (NOS), are listed as reference material in the code books and should be used only when a higher level of specificity is not available.

PRINCIPAL DIAGNOSIS

When coding for claim reimbursement, the medical assistant must also understand the significance of a principal diagnosis. The **principal diagnosis** is used in the inpatient hospital setting to describe the condition chiefly responsible for hospitalization, based on the tests and procedures performed. The primary or first-listed diagnosis is used in the outpatient setting to describe the patient's major health problem for that particular visit. Asking "Why was the patient seen today?" will help determine the primary diagnosis for that particular visit. This is important when you file a claim for a patient who has more than one diagnosis (e.g., cancer and a urinary tract infection). If the urinary tract infection (UTI) is unrelated to the cancer and the cancer will not affect the treatment or recovery from the UTI, then the code used for that claim would be UTI by itself. Any other diagnoses treated at that time (up to four) must also be listed. For example, if a patient who has diabetes and hypertension is seen for an ear infection, the ear infection is the primary diagnosis, whereas diabetes and hypertension would be listed as secondary diagnoses because there would be consideration of the diabetes and hypertension when medication is prescribed. So when the claim was submitted, the diagnosis code for ear infection will be listed as the primary diagnosis, but codes for hypertension and diabetes also will be included on the claim form as secondary codes.

SPECIAL CODES

The ICD-9-CM coding system also allows for visits (V codes) not directly related to illness or injury. These codes could also add supportive information about the patient or family's personal history. The V codes are used to describe a person who may not have a current illness but uses the health care system for some specific purpose, such as well-baby care, birth control advice, pregnancy test, or immunizations. The codes are also used as supportive information when some current circumstance or problem may influence the patient's health but is not, in itself, a current illness or problem, such as an allergy to penicillin.

The ICD-9-CM manual also uses tables for certain diseases and conditions. A diagnosis of hypertension, for example, must be coded from the hypertension table. A neoplasm, whether benign or malignant, must be coded from the neoplasm table. In addition, adverse reactions or poisoning are included in a section listing various drugs and other agents. Again, the medical assistant must become familiar with the organization of the ICD-9-CM manual in order to code diagnoses correctly. Procedure 19-1 describes how to assign the correct ICD-9-CM codes.

E codes (Figure 19-4) are used to describe external causes of injury and poisoning or adverse effects. These codes should not be used as primary or principal diagnoses (they do not stand alone). E codes are used as additional information to help support a particular diagnosis and to further define the cause of a poisoning or adverse effect, such as therapeutic use, attempted suicide, or an accident (e.g., a drug overdose can be either an accident or a suicide attempt). The use of E codes (E930–E949) is mandatory when coding injury or illness due to the use of drugs.

ABBREVIATIONS AND SYMBOLS

Instructional notes are included in the listings to guide the user on how to accurately and precisely code. Following are some examples:

NEC—not elsewhere classifiable

NOS—not otherwise specified

[]—Brackets enclose synonyms, alternative terminology, or explanatory phrases.

()—Parentheses enclose supplementary words (nonessential modifiers) that may be present in the narrative description of a disease without affecting the code assignment.

}—The brace encloses a series of terms, each of which is modified by the statement appearing to the right of the brace.

•—The bullet indicates a new code.

procedure
19-1

ICD-9-CM CODING
Objective: Accurately assign an ICD-9-CM code.

EQUIPMENT AND SUPPLIES
patient's medical record; patient's insurance card; computer with printer or typewriter; medical billing software; current ICD-9-CM coding book; medical reference material; superbill with the doctor's diagnosis

METHOD
1. Locate the condition or diagnosis on the superbill or in the patient's medical record.
2. In Volume II: Alphabetic Index of the ICD-9-CM book, locate the condition or diagnosis. A condition may be expressed as a noun, an adjective, or an eponym (named after an individual).
3. Examine the diagnostic statement to determine if the main term specifically describes that disease. If it does not, then look at the modifiers listed under that main term to find a more specific code. Also read any notes or cross references that may apply.
4. Then, locate the code in Volume I: Tabular Index.
5. Match the code description in the Tabular Index with the diagnosis in the patient's medical record.
6. Any of the codes from 0021.0 through V82.9 in the ICD-9-CM can be used to describe the main reason for the patient's office visit.
7. First list the ICD-9-CM code for the condition, problem, or diagnosis that is the main reason for the visit. Then, list coexisting conditions under additional codes.

8. Use codes at their highest level of specificity—5th digit codes first, then 4th digit, 3rd digit, and so on.
9. Do not code questionable, probable, or rule-out (R/O) diagnoses. One of the signs or symptoms of the R/O diagnosis will have to be identified by the physician as the reason for the office visit. For example, in R/O cystic fibrosis, the symptom of dyspnea would be coded until a definitive diagnosis of cystic fibrosis is made.
10. V codes describe factors that influence the health status of the patient, such as pregnancy test or vaccination, and are not used to code current illnesses. V codes are located in Volume II.
11. E codes are used for identifying external environmental events or conditions as the cause of injury, some adverse effect, or poisoning (e.g., a drug overdose, either accidental or taken as a suicide attempt). The use of E codes (E930–E949) is mandatory when coding the use of drugs.
12. M codes, in Appendix A of Volume I, relate to the morphology of neoplasms. Morphology codes are used only by tumor registries for reporting purposes. Each M code begins with the letter M. The M codes cannot be used on claims for patient billing.
13. List all diagnosis codes (up to four) on the insurance claim form with the primary diagnosis listed first.
14. Always double-check your coding and ensure proper use of abbreviations and symbols prior to assigning the final code.

◆—The diamond indicates a revision in the Tabular List and a code change in the Alphabetic Index.

➤ ◄—Arrow brackets indicate revised text.

Boldface type is used for all codes and titles in the Tabular List.

Italicized type is used for all exclusion notes and to identify codes that should not be used for describing the primary diagnosis.

ICD-10

The diagnosis codes in the **International Classification of Diseases, Tenth Revision (ICD-10)** contain increased specificity and include recently discovered or diagnosed diseases. The ICD-10 has more codes, as well as organizational and

content modifications, and new features. One significant change will be the identification of left versus right. Currently, with the ICD-9, there is no differentiation between the two. The following shortcomings of the ICD-9 and expected benefits of the ICD-10 are found on the Centers for Medicare and Medicaid website:

Shortcomings of the ICD-9

- ICD-9 is outdated, with only a limited ability to accommodate new procedures and diagnoses;

- ICD-9 lacks the precision needed for a number of emerging uses such as pay-for-performance and bio-surveillance. Bio-surveillance is the automated monitoring of information sources that may help in detecting

SUPPLEMENTARY CLASSIFICATION OF EXTERNAL CAUSES OF INJURY AND POISONING (E000-E999)

This section is provided to permit the classification of environmental events, circumstances, and conditions as the cause of injury, poisoning, and other adverse effects. Where a code from this section is applicable, it is intended that it shall be used in addition to a code from one of the main chapters of *ICD-9-CM*, indicating the nature of the condition. Certain other conditions which may be stated to be due to external causes are classified in Chapters 1 to 16 of *ICD-9-CM*. For these, the "E" code classification should be used for more detailed analysis.

Machinery accidents [other than those connected with transport] are classifiable to category E919, in which the fourth-digit allows a broad classification of the type of machinery involved.

Categories for "late effects" of accidents and other external causes are to be found at E929, E959, E969, E977, E989, and E999.

EXTERNAL CAUSE STATUS (E000)

> Note: A code from category E000 should be used in conjunction with the external cause code(s) assigned to a record to indicate the status of the person at the time the event occurred. A single code from category E000 should be assigned for an encounter.

- ▪ **E000** **External cause status**
  - ● **E000.0** **Civilian activity done for income or pay**
    Civilian activity done for financial or other compensation
    Excludes: *military activity (E000.1)*

  - ● **E000.1** **Military activity**
    Excludes: *activity of off duty military personnel (E000.8)*

  - ▪ **E000.8** **Other external cause status**
    Activity NEC
    Hobby not done for income
    Leisure activity
    Off-duty activity of military personnel
    Recreation or sport not for income or while a student
    Student activity
    Volunteer activity
    Excludes: *civilian activity done for income or compensation (E000.0)*
    military activity (E000.1)

  - ● **E000.9** **Unspecified external cause status**

ACTIVITY (E001-E030)

> Note: Categories E001 to E030 are provided for use to indicate the activity of the person seeking healthcare for an injury or health condition, such as a heart attack while shoveling snow, which resulted from, or was contributed to, by the activity. These codes are appropriate for use for both acute injuries, such as those from chapter 17, and conditions that are due to the long-term, cumulative effects of an activity, such as those from chapter 13. They are also appropriate for use with external cause codes for cause and intent if identifying the activity provides additional information on the event.

> These codes should be used in conjunction with other external cause codes for external cause status (E000) and place of occurrence (E849).

> This section contains the following broad activity categories:
> E001 Activities involving walking and running
> E002 Activities involving water and water craft
> E003 Activities involving ice and snow
> E004 Activities involving climbing, rappelling, and jumping off
> E005 Activities involving dancing and other rhythmic movement
> E006 Activities involving other sports and athletics played individually
> E007 Activities involving other sports and athletics played as a team or group
> E008 Activities involving other specified sports and athletics
> E009 Activity involving other cardiorespiratory exercise
> E010 Activity involving other muscle strengthening exercises
> E011 Activities involving computer technology and electronic devices
> E012 Activities involving arts and handcrafts
> E013 Activities involving personal hygiene and household maintenance
> E014 Activities involving person providing caregiving
> E015 Activities involving food preparation, cooking and grilling

▪	Add 4th or 5th digit	▪	Nonspecific code	▪	Unspecified code	▪	Manifestation code

707

FIGURE 19-4 An E-code section of the ICD-9-CM 2010. *Copyright 2009 Practice Management Information Corporation (PMIC). Reprinted with permission.*

an emerging epidemic, whether naturally occurring or as the result of bioterrorism;

- ICD-9 limits the precision of diagnosis-related groups (DRGs) as a result of very different procedures being grouped together in one code;

- ICD-9 lacks specificity and detail, uses terminology inconsistently, cannot capture new technology, and lacks codes for preventive services; and

- ICD-9 will eventually run out of space, particularly for procedure codes.

Expected Benefits of the ICD-10

- Support value-based purchasing and Medicare's anti-fraud and anti-abuse activities by accurately defining services and providing specific diagnosis and treatment information;

- Support comprehensive reporting of quality data;

- Ensure more accurate payments for new procedures, fewer rejected claims, improved disease management, and harmonization of disease monitoring and reporting worldwide; and

- Allow the United States to compare its data with international data to track the incidence and spread of disease and treatment outcomes because the United States is one of the few developed countries not using ICD-10.

In August 2008, the U.S. Department of Health and Human Services established a deadline of October 2011 for the conversion to using ICD-10; however, that date has since been pushed back to 2013.

Procedural Coding

Required elements for reimbursement from insurance carriers are based on a coding system that converts uniform descriptions of medical, surgical, and diagnostic services into numbers. This system, developed by the American Medical Association (AMA) in 1966, allows providers to communicate the procedures and services provided to the patient with increased accuracy. Reimbursement is based on codes submitted for services rendered. The process of transferring a narrative description of procedures into numbers is referred to as **procedural coding**.

HEALTHCARE COMMON PROCEDURE CODING SYSTEM SECTIONS

To report services and procedures for Medicaid and Medicare patients, the Healthcare Common Procedure Coding System (HCPCS) is used. There are two coding levels (Level I and

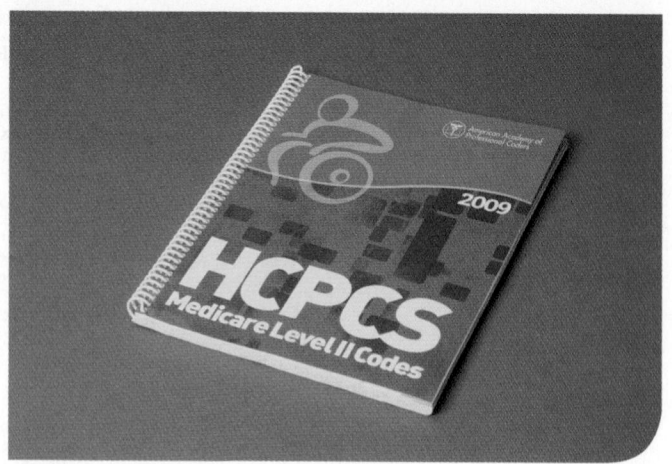

FIGURE 19-5 HCPCS Level II coding book.

Level II) available in HCPCS. See Figure 19-5 for an example of a HCPCS Level II Coding Book. Level I is the same as the **Current Procedural Terminology (CPT)** manual, which provides a comprehensive list of procedure and service codes. Level II has codes that are not available in the CPT. This part has 22 sections that contain five-digit alphanumeric codes (Figure 19-6). These codes are for items that Medicare covers, such as DME (durable medical equipment), materials, supplies, and injections. Each Level II code begins with a letter and is followed by four numbers (e.g., E1280 is a Level II HCPCS code). HCPCS also has modifiers. Each modifier consists of two letters. These can also be used in addition to the modifiers from the CPT manual.

Getting to Know the CPT

To code and receive maximum reimbursements for a particular practice, the medical assistant must be familiar with CPT codes and how they are used. Codes are reviewed and updated on a yearly basis by the American Medical Association (AMA). Utilizing codes from the most current edition of the CPT manual is essential (Figure 19-7). The CPT manual is available for purchase from the AMA as well as from bookstores and online venues.

The CPT manual is organized numerically or alphanumerically in sections according to classified types of service. The most commonly used codes are **Evaluation and Management (E/M)** services (office visits, consultations, the physician's component for emergency services, and inpatient hospital care) and are located in the front of the book. Codes for anesthesia, surgery, radiology, pathology and laboratory, and miscellaneous medical services follow. Several appendices

A4212 Non-coring needle or stylet with or without catheter

A4213 Syringe, sterile, 20cc or greater, each

A4215 Needle, sterile, any size, each

A4216 Sterile water, saline and/or dextrose (diluent/flush), 10 ml
MCM: 2049

A4217 Sterile water/saline, 500 ml
MCM: 2049

A4218 Sterile saline or water, metered dose dispenser, 10 ml

A4220 Refill kit for implantable infusion pump
CIM: 60-14

A4221 Supplies for maintenance of drug infusion catheter, per week (list drug separately)

A4222 Infusion supplies for external drug infusion pump, per cassette or bag (list drugs separately)

A4223 Infusion supplies not used with external infusion pump, per cassette or bag (list drugs separately)

A4230 Infusion set for external insulin pump, non needle cannula type
CIM: 60-14

A4231 Infusion set for external insulin pump, needle type
CIM: 60-14

A4232 Syringe with needle for external insulin pump, sterile, 3cc
CIM: 60-14

A4233 Replacement battery, alkaline (other than j cell), for use with medically necessary home blood glucose monitor owned by patient, each

A4234 Replacement battery, alkaline, j cell, for use with medically necessary home blood glucose monitor owned by patient, each

A4235 Replacement battery, lithium, for use with medically necessary home blood glucose monitor owned by patient, each

---

| | Not valid for Medicare | | Non-covered by Medicare | | Special coverage instructions | | Carrier discretion | 19 |

FIGURE 19-6 HCPCS 2010 Level II page. *Copyright 2009 Practice Management Information Corporation (PMIC). Reprinted with permission.*

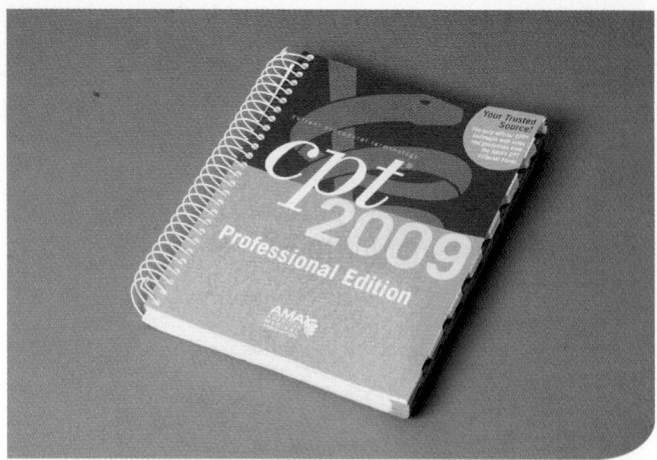

FIGURE 19-7 CPT coding book.

follow the numeric and alphabetic listings, including a complete list and descriptions of all modifiers used in procedural coding, as well as a quick reference summary of codes that have been added, deleted, or revised. See Table 19-1 for examples of CPT sections and codes.

UNDERSTANDING EVALUATION AND MANAGEMENT

For a beginning coder, the most complex section of the CPT coding system is assigning Evaluation and Management Services codes. E/M (E and M), as it is referred to, is based on the following criteria: history of the patient, complexity of the examination, and the degree of difficulty in medical decision making. Of these three factors, the medical decision-making factor can be the most complex.

Levels of Evaluation and Management

The four levels of decision-making are *straightforward, low complex, moderate complex,* and *high complex.* The E/M codes are ser-

TABLE 19-1 CPT Manual: Examples of Sections and Codes

CPT Section	CPT Code
Evaluation and Management	99201–99499
Anesthesia	00100–01999 99100–99140
Surgery	10021–69990
Radiology	70010–79999
Pathology and Laboratory	80048–89356
Medicine	90281–99199 99500–99602

vice oriented and were designed to link the procedure or diagnosis with the amount of time it takes the physician to diagnose and treat the patient. However, the decision-making component will not automatically be bumped up to the next level simply because a physician spent more time with the patient.

For coding purposes, all patients are either an established patient or a new patient. A **new patient** has never been seen by anyone in the practice or has not been seen by anyone of the same specialty in the practice for more than 3 years. An **established patient** is one who has been seen within the past 3 years by any practitioner of the same specialty in the practice. It is important to understand the difference between a new and established patient, the difference between a consultation and a referral, and how to code properly for the place of service (office, hospital, skilled nursing facility, emergency department).

Take a few moments to look through the CPT manual to become familiar with its structure and how codes are presented. Commonly accepted descriptions of services or procedures are presented after the code number. Two types of codes are listed. One type stands alone; the other is indented. Only the codes that stand alone have full descriptions. Indented codes include only that portion of the stand-alone code before the semicolon. (This is an extremely important concept to remember.)

Procedures and services are listed by name of service or procedure, anatomic site, condition or disease, synonym, eponym, or abbreviation. To code services correctly, locate the desired procedure in the index at the back of the CPT manual. Often a single code is given, although ranges of possible codes (joined with a hyphen) are presented and should be utilized, if necessary.

MODIFIERS

At times it is necessary to report a service not contained in the CPT manual. These procedures may be reported using the *unlisted procedure* code for that particular section or using a **modifier**—a two-digit code preceded by a hyphen that clarifies the procedure. This is used in circumstances in which the procedure code does not accurately describe the procedure. The two-digit modifier provides additional information about services provided to a patient. For example, the most common modifier is -50, which indicates the procedure was bilateral and done at the same time, such as bilateral myringotomies and tube insertion. The five-digit code for this procedure would be listed followed by a hyphen and the number 50. When using multiple modifiers always list the modifier -99 first. This indicates to the person checking the claim that multiple modifiers are being used (Figure 19-8).

Symbols

▲   Revised code

●   New code

►◄   New or revised text

⮂   Reference to *CPT Assistant, Clinical Examples in Radiology,* and *CPT Changes*

✚   Add-on code

⊘   Exemptions to modifier 51

⊙   Moderate sedation

⯁   Product pending FDA approval

○   Reinstated or recycled code

\#   Out-of-numerical sequence code

Modifiers (See Appendix A for Definitions)

22   Increased procedural services

23   Unusual anesthesia

24   Unrelated evaluation and management service by the same physician during a postoperative period

25   Significant, separately identifiable evaluation and management service by the same physician on the same day of the procedure or other service

26   Professional component

32   Mandated services

47   Anesthesia by surgeon

50   Bilateral procedure

51   Multiple procedures

52   Reduced services

53   Discontinued procedure

54   Surgical care only

55   Postoperative management only

56   Preoperative management only

57   Decision for surgery

58   Staged or related procedure or service by the same physician during the postoperative period

59   Distinct procedural service

62   Two surgeons

63   Procedure performed on infants less than 4 kgs

66   Surgical team

76   Repeat procedure or service by same physician

77   Repeat procedure or service by another physician

78   Unplanned return to the operating/procedure room by the same physician following initial procedure for a related procedure during the postoperative period

79   Unrelated procedure or service by the same physician during the postoperative period

80   Assistant surgeon

81   Minimum assistant surgeon

82   Assistant surgeon (when qualified resident surgeon not available)

90   Reference (outside) laboratory

91   Repeat clinical diagnostic laboratory test

92   Alternative laboratory platform testing

99   Multiple modifiers

Anesthesia Physical Status Modifiers

P1   A normal healthy patient

P2   A patient with mild systemic disease

P3   A patient with severe systemic disease

P4   A patient with severe systemic disease that is a constant threat to life

P5   A moribund patient who is not expected to survive without the operation

P6   A declared brain-dead patient whose organs are being removed for donor purposes

Modifiers Approved for Hospital Outpatient Use Level I (CPT)

25   Significant, separately identifiable evaluation and management service by the same physician on the same day of the procedure or other service

27   Multiple outpatient hospital E/M encounters on the same date

50   Bilateral procedure

52   Reduced services

58   Staged or related procedure or service by the same physician during the postoperative period

59   Distinct procedural service

73   Discontinued outpatient hospital/ambulatory surgical center (ASC) procedure prior to the administration of anesthesia

74   Discontinued outpatient hospital/ambulatory surgical center (ASC) procedure after the administration of anesthesia

76   Repeat procedure or service by same physician

77   Repeat procedure by another physician

78   Unplanned return to the operating/procedure room for a related procedure during the postoperative period

79   Unrelated procedure or service by the same physician during the postoperative period

91   Repeat clinical diagnostic laboratory test

Level II (HCPCS/National)

LT   Left side (used to identify procedures performed on the left side of the body)

RT   Right side (used to identify procedures performed on the right side of the body)

BL   Special acquisition of blood and blood products

CA   Procedure payable only in the inpatient setting when performed emergently on an outpatient who expires prior to admission

CR   Catastrophe/disaster related

E1   Upper left, eyelid

E2   Lower left, eyelid

E3   Upper right, eyelid

E4   Lower right, eyelid

FA   Left hand, thumb

F1   Left hand, second digit

F2   Left hand, third digit

F3   Left hand, fourth digit

F4   Left hand, fifth digit

F5   Right hand, thumb

F6   Right hand, second digit

F7   Right hand, third digit

F8   Right hand, fourth digit

F9   Right hand, fifth digit

FB   Item provided without cost to provider, supplier or practitioner, or full credit received for replaced device (examples, but not limited to covered under warranty, replaced due to defect, free samples)

FC   Partial credit received for replaced device

GA   Waiver of liability statement on file

GG   Performance and payment of a screening mammogram and diagnostic mammogram on the same patient, same day

GH   Diagnostic mammogram converted from screening mammogram on same day

LC   Left circumflex, coronary artery

LD   Left anterior descending coronary artery

RC   Right coronary artery

Q0   Investigational clinical service provided in a clinical research study that is in an approved clinical research study

Q1   Routine clinical service provided in a clinical research study that is in an approved clinical research study

QM   Ambulance service provided under arrangement by a provider of services

QN   Ambulance service furnished directly by a provider of services

TA   Left foot, great toe

T1   Left foot, second digit

T2   Left foot, third digit

T3   Left foot, fourth digit

T4   Left foot, fifth digit

T5   Right foot, great toe

T6   Right foot, second digit

T7   Right foot, third digit

T8   Right foot, fourth digit

T9   Right foot, fifth digit

FIGURE 19-8   Modifier page from the CPT. *Printed with permission by the American Medical Association. Copyright © 2009.*

MEDICAL CODING

The medicine section of the CPT manual is organized according to body system, not disease. This section of the manual also includes codes for noninvasive procedures and treatment procedures. Included in this section are many diagnostic tests, such as an ECG, and many noninvasive (does not enter the skin) procedures performed in a physician's office. If the procedure is invasive (enters the skin, other than by injection, or enters a body cavity), it is found in the surgical section of the manual. Procedure 19-2 reviews examples for assigning CPT codes.

SYMBOLS

Symbols are used in the CPT manual to distinguish changes or give instructions to be used when coding. These symbols add additional information or instructions for proper coding of certain procedures. To accurately code procedures, it is imperative that the coder be familiar with the symbols and their meanings.

Insurance Fraud

Unfortunately, insurance fraud and attempts at insurance fraud occur on a regular basis. The Centers for Medicare & Medicaid Services (CMS) website provides information to help you better understand insurance fraud. Even though this information comes from the CMS, the principles apply to anyone who has medical insurance coverage through other carriers.

PROFESSIONALISM
THE WORKPLACE

The medical assistant must have a thorough understanding of how to properly use the ICD-9-CM, CPT, and HCPCS Level II coding books as this is required for billing purposes and physician orders of extended services. The diagnosis code reflects detailed information about the illness or injury converted to numeric form.
The procedure code reflects detailed information about the service provided utilizing levels of care. Because diagnoses are not written out when submitted to insurance companies for reimbursement, the patient may question what "all those numbers" mean. It may be up to the medical assistant to explain the numbers, what they mean, and how they are used for billing purposes.

The Centers for Medicare & Medicaid Services (CMS) offers the following tips for preventing fraud and abuse:

- Look at your Medicaid bill carefully to make sure that Medicaid has been billed for medical services or goods that you really received. Check to see that the date of service is correct.
- DO NOT give your Medicaid card number to anyone except your doctor, clinic, hospital, or other health care provider.
- DO NOT let anyone borrow your Medicaid card. Treat your card the way you treat your credit card.
- DO NOT ask your doctor or other health care provider for medical care that you do not need.
- DO NOT sign your name to a blank form.
- Ask for a copy of everything you sign. Keep the copy for your records.
- DO NOT share your Medicaid records or other medical information with anyone except your doctor, clinic, hospital, or other health care provider.
- If you are offered free tests or screenings in exchange for your Medicaid card number, be suspicious. Be careful about accepting Medicaid services when you are told they will be free of charge.
- DO NOT give your Medicaid card number to anyone or do business with door-to-door or telephone salespeople who tell you that services of medical equipment are free.
- Give your Medicaid identification card only to those who have provided you with medical services.
- Never allow a medical provider to bill for services rendered without contacting you first.
- If anyone claims to know how to make Medicaid pay for health care services or goods that Medicaid usually does not pay for, you should avoid them.

FRAUDULENT BILLING AND CODING PRACTICES

As a medical assistant, it is important to understand insurance fraud as it relates to medical billing and coding. Insurance fraud is often committed within the Medicare system. Fraud is an intentional representation that an individual makes but knows to be false or does not believe to be true, knowing that the representation could result in some unauthorized benefit to himself or herself or some other person.

The most frequent kind of fraud arises from false statements or misrepresentations that claim to provide proof to

procedure

ASSIGNING A CPT CODE
Objective: Accurately assign a CPT code.

EQUIPMENT AND SUPPLIES
patient's medical record; computer; medical billing software; current CPT coding book; superbill with procedure marked

METHOD
1. Locate the completed procedure on the superbill.
2. If the only procedure was a physician visit, locate the E/M code 99200–99499 in the front of the CPT coding book.
3. Following the guidelines, determine by the patient's medical record whether this office visit was a first-time or a follow-up visit.
4. Also determine by the patient's medical record whether this visit was with the patient's attending physician or a consulting physician.
5. Note where the visit took place (nursing home, hospital, emergency room, office, etc.).
6. After locating the place of service in the CPT index, locate the level of the visit within the place-of-service codes. To determine the correct level of service and how many tests were done, it may be necessary to study the patient's personal, family, and social history, as well as the results of the physical examination. This is one of the most important codes you can list because improper level of service billing can result in nonpayment of the bill and very large monetary fines.
7. If a surgical procedure was performed, locate the CPT code in the index by using the procedure name or anatomical site, then look up the suggested codes, which will be between 10021 and 69990. For such codes, read the surgeon's operative report. For some situations, the anesthetic for the surgery is included in the surgery code. In other cases, the anesthesia must be billed as a separate code. In addition, some surgical procedure groups are billed under one code, whereas others are billed as separate procedures. It will usually be necessary to read the operative report to determine which situation applies.
8. Some equipment used in surgery is billable under the 10021 to 69990 codes, whereas other equipment is billed separately.
9. All radiological procedures are billed under the codes 70010 to 79999, including X-rays, diagnostic ultrasound, angiography, and computerized tomography.
10. Locate the radiological procedure codes in the index, using the procedure name or anatomical site.
11. In the section 70010 through 79999, read the description of the code(s) listed in the index.
12. Locate the correct radiological procedure, being careful to note if the test was bilateral or unilateral and if multiple different images were made.
13. If a laboratory test was run or a specimen was sent to the laboratory for pathology inspection, the code will be between 80048 and 89356. Look first in the index under the name of the test.
14. If the test was a laboratory test, it will be in the first part of this section. It is necessary to know what test was done and whether the test is a panel (many tests within one ordered block) or if the test is organ specific or disease specific.
15. In addition, if the test was performed by an outside laboratory, then the test itself cannot be billed. However, the cost of the venipuncture to obtain the specimen and the cost of transporting the specimen to the laboratory, if it was transported by the physician's staff, may be billed.
16. In some cases, some medicines can be billed to insurance. Some general rules apply to most billable medicines.
17. Usually billed medicines must be injected, not administered orally.
18. Many specialized procedures, such as ophthalmology services and pulmonary tests and services, can be billed under the CPT codes.
19. Before finalizing the bill, always compare the final CPT codes with the ICD codes to ensure that the diagnosis supports the procedure or service. There must be a logical match. For example, if the patient was seen in the physician's office for removal of a foreign body in the ear, the visit can be billed, but the blood sugar done at the same time cannot be billed under a diagnosis of foreign body in the ear. If a blood sugar test was done at the same time, an additional diagnosis code that justifies the need for the test is required.

entitlement or payment under the Medicare program. The violator may be a physician or other practitioner, a hospital or other institutional provider, a clinical laboratory or other supplier, an employee of any provider, a billing service, a beneficiary, a Medicare employee, or any person in a position to file a claim for Medicare benefits. Other violations fit within the broad definition of fraud, including the offering or acceptance of kickbacks and the routine waiver of copayments. A **kickback** is an incentive provided by another physician, laboratory, hospital, or pharmaceutical representative for using their services.

Fraud schemes range from those perpetrated by individuals acting alone to broad-based activities by institutions or groups of individuals, sometimes employing sophisticated telemarketing and other promotional techniques to lure consumers into serving as the unwitting tools in the schemes. Seldom do perpetrators exclusively target only one insurer or either the public or the private sector. Rather, most attempt to simultaneously defraud several private and public sector victims.

In Medicare, the most common forms of fraud include the following:

- Billing insurance companies for services not furnished
- Misrepresenting the diagnosis to justify payment
- Soliciting, offering, or receiving a kickback
- Unbundling (billing for separate services that are usually bundled in a single procedure code)
- Falsifying certificates of medical necessity, plans of treatment, and medical records to justify payment
- **Upcoding** (billing for a service at a higher level than was actually provided)

PROFESSIONALISM

The medical record must reflect all services and care for which the insurance company is billed. If a health care provider is found to have billed for services not received, or if a health care provider is found to have billed for a more complicated or expensive service than was actually received, the penalty will be denial of the claim or, worse, monetary sanctions and even prison. If the medical assistant believes that such a bill is being submitted, he or she should discuss the situation with the physician in order to be assured that the care being delivered is, in fact, the service being billed.

FRAUD TIPS

The Centers for Medicare & Medicaid Services website also offers consumers and patients information to help them identify fraud. The medical assistant can also watch for the following items, whether the health care provider gives the patient this information or you are asked by the health care provider to relay it:

- The test is free; the doctor only needs your Medicare number for his records.
- Medicare wants you to have the item or service.
- The medical office knows how to get Medicare to pay for it.
- The more tests the patient takes, the cheaper they are.
- The equipment or service is free; it will not cost the patient anything.

Consumers should also be suspicious of medical offices or employers who do the following:

- Routinely waive copayments without checking on ability to pay
- Advertise "free" consultations to Medicare beneficiaries
- Claim they represent Medicare
- Use pressure or scare tactics to sell high-priced medical services or diagnostic tests
- Bill Medicare for services the patient does not recall receiving
- Use telemarketing and door-to-door selling as marketing tools

Box 19-1 lists information on how to report suspected fraud.

Compliance Plan

Each medical office should have a compliance plan. A medical office without a compliance plan may be at risk for liability issues. It also demonstrates to the physician, fraud investigators, or insurance carriers that the medical office is attempting to locate and correct errors. Having a compliance plan gives the medical office staff a process for locating, correcting, and preventing practices that are illegal. The Office of Inspector General in the U.S. Department of Health & Human Services provides compliance guidance for fraud prevention and detection. The following are basic components for an effective compliance plan:

- Conducting periodic audits of billing and coding practices
- Developing written standards and procedures for compliance

Box 19-1 How to Report Suspected FRAUD

Before you get in touch with your state Medicaid contact or call the National Fraud Hotline, please be ready to provide as much information as possible, including the following:

- The name of the Medicaid client
- The client's Medicaid card number
- The name of the doctor, hospital, or other health care provider
- The date of service
- The amount of money that Medicaid approved or paid
- A description of the acts that you suspect involve fraud or abuse relating to your allegation

Who to Contact

Contact Your State Directly.   Medicaid is a joint federal- and state-funded program. Although the federal government deter-

mines who is eligible for Medicaid benefits and sets standards for quality of care, the states carry out most of the day-to-day business of Medicaid. If you suspect that fraud is being committed against Medicaid, your first contact should be the Program Integrity contact in the agency that oversees your state's Medicaid program, which is usually called the State Medicaid Agency.

Call the OIG National Fraud Hotline.   A second way to report suspected fraud in Medicaid is to call the National Fraud Hotline (1-800-HHS-TIPS) in the Office of Inspector General (OIG). This hotline handles calls about both Medicaid and Medicare, but it is not as direct as calling your state contact.

Source: Centers for Medicare & Medicaid website (www.cms.hhs.gov).

- Training and educating staff members on procedures
- Investigating violations and disclosing incidents to appropriate government agencies
- Discussing in staff meetings how to avoid erroneous or fraudulent conduct

As a medical assistant, it is important to research and understand practice standards so that the medical office is in compliance with various regulations.

CODING COMPLIANCE

Responsibility for accurate documentation, completion of health insurance claim forms, and regulation compliance falls ultimately on the physician. It is the medical assistant's responsibility to make certain these duties are followed.

CODE LINKAGE

When the medical assistant is completing the health insurance claim form, it is critical that the diagnosis be related to the procedure. An example of valid code linkage is a diagnosis

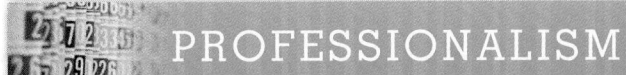

PROFESSIONALISM

THE LAW

Federal regulations on coding are specific and require full compliance. Coding of procedures and diagnoses must be supported by the documentation in the patient record. Providers as well as medical staff may be sanctioned with fines or prison terms if improper coding is discovered to increase reimbursement.

of diabetes mellitus and a glucose tolerance test. However, a diagnosis of hypertension and a procedure to remove five skin tags cannot be linked in a health insurance claim form because no connection can be made between the patient's diagnosis and the procedure the physician performed. Coding inaccuracies such as this can result in minor to severe penalties.

SUMMARY

Most patients coming into the medical office have some form of health care insurance, and the medical assistant should be familiar with the carriers in their particular geographic area. In addition to familiarity with the health insurance carriers, the medical assistant should also have a

general overview of the coding process, using the procedure coding process (CPT codes) and diagnostic coding (ICD-9-CM) to better serve patients and also to be able to assist the medical coder if necessary.

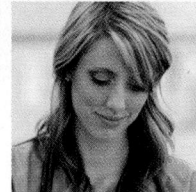

19 CHAPTER REVIEW

COMPETENCY REVIEW

1. Define and spell the terms to learn for this chapter.

2. Describe what steps you would take to determine if a patient has insurance coverage.

3. What code book is used to code a diagnosis?

4. What code book is used to code an office visit and procedure?

5. Explain the difference between a primary and secondary diagnosis, using the example of stroke and hypertension.

PREPARING FOR THE CERTIFICATION EXAM

For the following questions choose the best answer

1. HCPCS Level II codes are used to code
   a. modifiers.
   b. DME.
   c. procedures.
   d. morphology.
   e. diagnoses.

2. In ICD-9-CM coding conventions, V codes
   a. cannot stand alone.
   b. are required for all diagnoses.
   c. give external causes or factors for illness or injury.
   d. can be used when the family history includes a particular condition.
   e. are the same as CPT codes.

3. CPT stands for
   a. current physician's terminology.
   b. current procedure terminology.
   c. current procedural terminology.
   d. current procedural term.
   e. current procedural timetable.

4. The most commonly used codes in the CPT are:
   a. DCME.
   b. Medicine.
   c. Morphology.
   d. E/M.
   e. E Codes.

5. Modifiers consist of how many digits?
   a. 2
   b. 3
   c. 4
   d. 5
   e. 6

6. Which of the following indicates a new code in the ICD-9-CM?
   a. NEC
   b. NC
   c. ▲
   d. ●
   e. ►◄

7. The superbill may be used as all of the following EXCEPT
   a. charge slip.
   b. insurance reporting form.
   c. preauthorization.
   d. statement.
   e. encounter form.

8. Regarding diagnostic coding, all of the following statements are true EXCEPT
   a. Volume II is the numeric index.
   b. always code to the highest level of specificity.
   c. diagnoses will be three, four, or five digits.
   d. to code properly, start with Volume II.
   e. the medical assistant needs to understand the ICD-9-CM.

9. Levels of E/M decision making may be all of the following EXCEPT
   a. straightforward.
   b. low.
   c. low complex.

d. moderate complex.

e. high complex.

10. When coding illness or injury due to the use of drugs, which of the following codes is mandatory?

a. M codes.

b. V codes.

c. E codes.

d. D codes.

e. C codes.

CRITICAL THINKING

1. What CPT code would be assigned for audiometry (pure tone, air only) that was performed in the office by David?

2. What would the principal diagnosis be for Sophia's visit? How can the medical assistant responsible for billing and coding ensure that the diagnosis is correct?

3. What procedural code would be assigned if Sophia underwent bilateral myringotomies and tube insertion with local anesthesia? Would a modifier be necessary?

ON THE JOB

Lisa Medina, certified medical coding specialist, processes insurance claims for a large internal medicine practice. You have recently been hired as Lisa's assistant, and she has asked you to verify the accuracy of a group of claim forms. As you review the forms, you notice that one of the doctors regularly checks the superbill used in the office at one E/M code level higher than the actual level of service provided.

1. Name some of the options for handling this situation.

2. Tell which option you would select.

3. Give three reasons for your selection of this particular option.

4. Whose advice might you seek before acting on your choice?

INTERNET ACTIVITY

There are many places to purchase ICD-9-CM and CPT coding books. Search the Internet to find the cost of the ICD-9-CM and CPT coding books and coding software. What month are the new editions of the ICD-9-CM and CPT coding books available?

MEDMEDIA

Additional interactive resources and activities for this chapter can be found:

On your student DVD: View applicable procedure videos on the DVD-ROM found in the back of this book.

MyHealthProfessionsKit.com: Test your knowledge of this chapter with games and activities. MyHealthProfessionsKit also includes resources, helpful links, and a Spanish audio glossary.

Medical Assisting Interactive: Practice your procedures as a medical assistant in this simulated doctor's office. This can be accessed through MyHealthProfessionsKit.com.

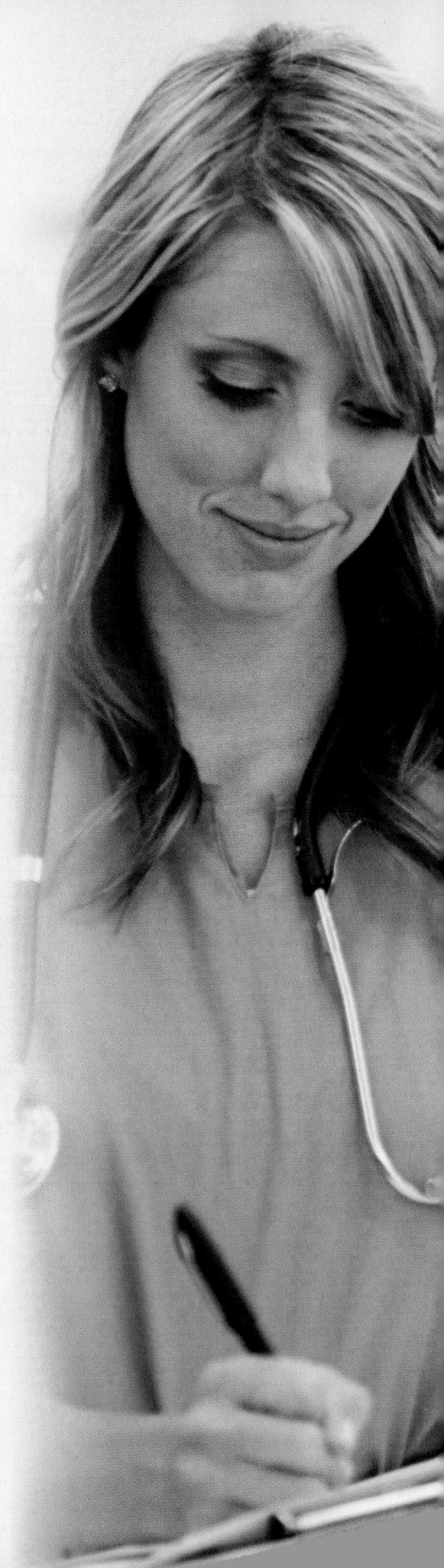

20

Medical Office Management

LEARNING OBJECTIVES

After reading this chapter, you should be able to:

- Define and spell the terms to learn for this chapter.

- Define the systems approach to management.

- List and discuss the personnel management duties as they relate to the medical office.

- Discuss the elements of monthly planning including holding staff meetings.

- Describe time management principles and how a To Do list would enhance office organization.

- Differentiate between the personnel policy manual and the office policies and procedures manual.

- Describe ten responsibilities in assisting the physician to prepare for a medical meeting.

- Discuss how to assist the physician when preparing to make a presentation at a medical meeting.

- List five items that belong in a patient information booklet.

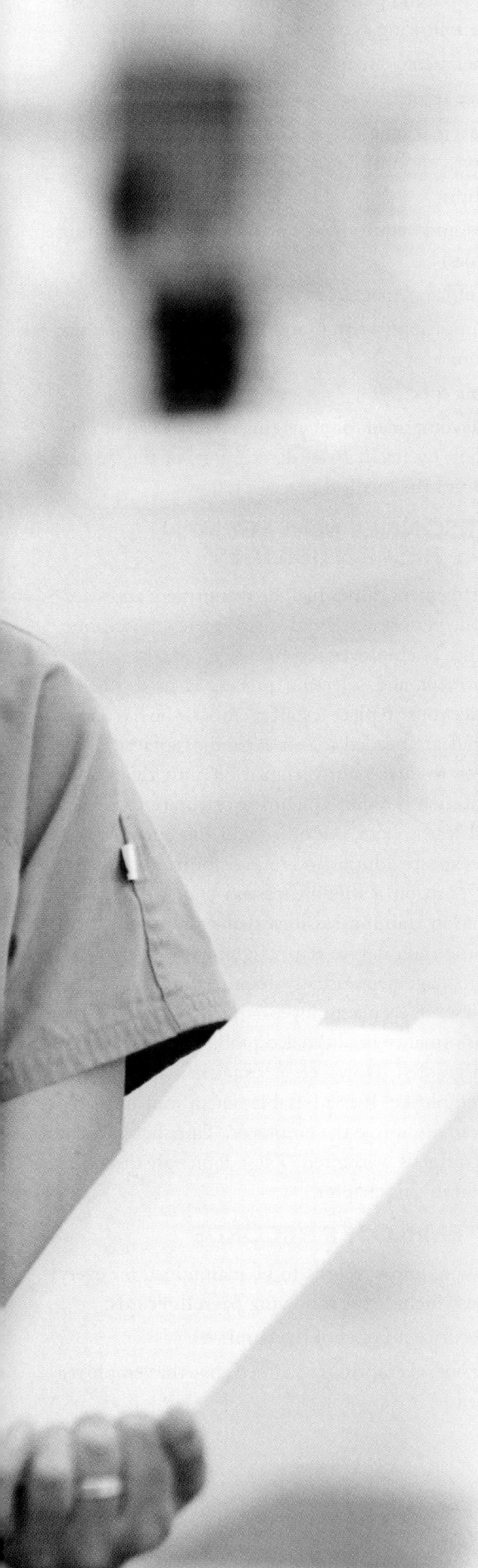

CHAPTER OUTLINE

CASE STUDY

Tania Washington is an office manager at Pearson Physicians Group. The group's business has been growing steadily, and the office is in need of a new certified medical assistant. Tania decided to put an advertisement in the local newspaper and on the newspaper's employment website. She received many résumés in response to the posted position. She took a couple of days to sort through the résumés and the accompanying cover letters, removing all that did not meet the minimum qualifications, as well as those with spelling and grammatical errors. On Monday, she contacted several individuals who had the best résumés and set up interviews for the week.

Prior to speaking with any of the candidates, Tania drafted a set of questions she would use for all candidates. She also made notes of specific questions she wanted to ask each applicant pertaining to the information found on his or her résumé or cover letter.

Tania's first interview went very well, but it was difficult to read the application form that the applicant completed. The second applicant had recently had her tongue pierced, and at times it was very difficult to understand her speech. The third applicant had the least experience but looked very professional, wrote neatly, and spoke well.

Office management requires special administrative and communication skills. Office management cannot be discussed without discussing time management. Careful planning of activities, delegation of tasks, and effective use of all personnel involve careful attention to how time is managed. Several documents are important for a medical office to run smoothly. These include the personnel policy manual, the office policies and procedures manual, and patient information booklets.

Systems Approach to Office Management

Current management philosophy recommends a systematic approach when managing a medical office. Under this approach, the functions of an office are categorized into systems that must function simultaneously and be integrated into a whole system: the medical office. For example, the administrative component of a medical office can be divided into the following systems:

- Personnel management
- Employee records
- Financial management (including banking, billing, collections, and insurance)
- Scheduling
- Facility and equipment management (including computers)
- Clnical office management
- Communication (written and oral, including patient education)
- Legal concepts

The clinical component of managing an office can be considered a system by itself. Brief descriptions of the various systems that form the medical practice follow.

PERSONNEL MANAGEMENT RESPONSIBILITIES

Personnel management duties include recruitment and selection, probation, performance and salary review, discipline, and maintenance of employee records.

The recruitment and selection process is used when a medical practice must replace a staff member who has left or when more staff are needed for an expanding practice. For new employees to successfully transition into their positions, an orientation is required. During orientation the new employee will learn about the office and the new position and about the expected duties and responsibilities associated with the new position. Large offices and clinics often have formal orientation training sessions that employees attend before beginning their day-to-day assignments.

Personnel management usually requires an annual performance review of each employee at which time, if the employee's performance has been acceptable, a merit raise in salary is often granted. However, at times it is necessary to discipline an employee. It is advisable not to wait until the annual review to discipline the employee. This should occur as soon as discipline is warranted. These topics are discussed in greater detail in this chapter.

EMPLOYEE RECORDS

The federal law requires records to be maintained for every employee. These include the following payroll records:

- Social Security number of the employee
- Number of exemptions claimed by the employee (W-4 form)

- Gross salary amount (salary before taxes are removed)
- Deductions for Social Security taxes, federal, state, and city withholding taxes, state disability tax, and state unemployment tax, if applicable.

Payroll is discussed further in Chapter 16.

FINANCIAL MANAGEMENT

Financial management includes banking, billing, collections, and insurance collections. This critical area is responsible for tracking the income necessary to keep the practice **solvent** or capable of paying its bills and salaries. Fees, billings, collections, and credit are discussed in Chapter 15. Financial management, including employee record keeping, is discussed in Chapter 16.

SCHEDULING

Typically, when scheduling is mentioned, most people automatically think about patient scheduling. However, effective and efficient scheduling of staff can contribute significantly to the satisfaction level of the practice at several levels. If the office staff is continuously scheduled inappropriately, it affects employee morale and may cause discontent among the physicians and patients. Yet there must be some flexibility with the staff schedule to allow for unanticipated occurrences, such as sick days and business appointments.

A successful patient scheduling process involves using a systematic method for patient appointments. This process is discussed in Chapter 9.

FACILITY AND EQUIPMENT MANAGEMENT

Facility and equipment management includes facility layout and planning, inventory, maintaining safety and Occupational Safety and Health Administration (OSHA) standards, and equipment replacement. This is discussed in Chapters 6 and 10. Computer use in the medical office is presented in Chapter 12.

CLINICAL OFFICE MANAGEMENT

The clinical aspects of office management are separate from the administrative aspects. Managing the clinical aspects of a medical office requires a wide variety of duties, including the training of any new clinical personnel, keeping track of medical supplies and purchasing supplies when the stock is low, and making sure that the physician's requests are met and that proper procedures are followed. As part of the clinical office duties, the office manager often will have to handle safety issues (such as employee hepatitis B injections) and OSHA regulations. Because of the many duties

required in managing the clinical aspects of the office, it is not uncommon to find that an office has a separate supervisor such as a clinical coordinator or nurse manager who will take on those duties to reduce the workload of the general office manager.

COMMUNICATION

An office manager's ability to effectively communicate at all levels is very important and will contribute significantly to the cohesiveness of the staff. Written communication skills are presented in Chapter 11, oral communication, including verbal and nonverbal, in Chapter 5, and patient education in Chapter 55.

LEGAL CONCEPTS

Physicians typically use attorneys to assist with handling legal documents and issues. However, medical assistants must have an understanding of legal terminology. Medical legal and ethical issues are discussed fully in Chapter 3.

The Office Manager

The office manager acts as the coordinator for business activities conducted in the office. Each office varies somewhat; however, the general duties include the following:

- Acting as liaison between staff and the physician-employer
- Conducting performance and salary reviews
- Delegating responsibilities to staff
- Orienting, developing, and training staff
- Improving office efficiency
- Maintaining the office policies and procedures manual
- Overseeing Health Insurances Portability and Accountability Act (HIPAA) compliance
- Planning and conducting staff meetings
- Preparing patient education materials
- Providing guidelines for patient education
- Recruiting, hiring, and firing
- Supervising cash, banking, and payroll operations
- Supervising employees on a day-to-day basis
- Supervising the purchase and storage of equipment and supplies

Along with the knowledge needed to run an efficient medical office, an office manager needs effective administrative and communication skills. Medical assistants who have demonstrated these skills may seek to be promoted into this

TABLE 20-1 Manager's Responsibilities to Employee and Physician-Employer

To Employee	To Physician-Employer
Interview	Increase efficiency of office
Hire/terminate	Meet with physician to discuss problems/plans
Orientate/train	Manage calendar for physician
Arrange work schedules	Assist with meetings
Arrange vacation coverage	Update physician on insurance changes related to Medicare fee schedules
Conduct performance evaluations	Order CPT and ICD code books and current pharmacology books annually
Consult with physician regarding salary increases	Renew insurance policies and pay premiums

position. The following are other qualities or skills observed in good managers:

- Ability to organize
- Ability to communicate effectively at all levels
- Ability to enforce policy, when necessary
- Ability to resolve conflicts
- Creativity
- Diplomacy
- Excellent judgment
- Flexibility
- Leadership and take-charge initiative
- Objectivity
- Sense of fairness
- Willingness to continue to learn and promote the same behavior in staff members

The office manager's time is generally spent on employee and administrative issues. The employees, on the other hand, spend most of their time working with patients. A good office manager does not strive to become "the boss" but, rather, to establish and implement a team approach to management by including all staff in the decision-making process. Ultimately, the manager must make the final decision in conjunction with the physician-employer, but compliance with decisions is much greater when employees have had the opportunity to participate and contribute to the process. Table 20-1 describes responsibilities the office manager has to the employees and also to the physician-employer.

Many office managers are promoted based on **seniority**—a status gained by being the individual who has worked for the physician the longest. This is not always a wise practice since not everyone is a skilled manager, and even individuals who have experience or have completed management classes are not always the best candidates. When no internal candidate with the necessary skills for, or interest in, the office manager position is available, the physician-employer will have to seek an outside candidate. This is usually handled by posting an advertisement under the medical heading of the employment section of the local newspaper and relevant websites. In some cases, the physicians' **colleagues** (fellow members of the profession) will recommend a qualified candidate for the position.

MONTHLY PLANNING

The office manager may wish to develop a system in which the schedule for the entire month is laid out on a calendar. All physicians' conferences, staff meetings, vacations, accountant meetings, and other vendor visits should be noted. One of the office manager's tasks is to approve and decline vacation requests from staff members. It is important to list staff vacations on a calendar because it helps to prevent overlapping of vacations, which can leave an office short staffed. This calendar should be placed in an accessible location. It may be helpful to purchase an erasable-style wall calendar so that corrections and changes can be made easily.

The manager will create and update the physician's own calendar. It is not necessary to include staff vacations on the physician's calendar. However, the office manager's own vacation schedule and days off should be included in both the physician's calendar and the staff calendar.

Many physicians carry a pocket-size electronic calendar in which they enter all hospital rounds, meetings, conferences, and time away from the office. It is wise to compare the office calendar with the physician's calendar on a periodic basis and to update the office's master calendar as necessary.

STAFF MEETINGS

Lack of communication between staff and management is a common complaint in the medical office. Staff members wish to have direct communication with the physician, but this is often not possible in a large practice. The office manager can help to resolve this problem by asking the physician(s) to attend all or part of regularly scheduled staff meetings, if this is not already being done. Many of the best ideas for office improvement are a result of suggestions made at staff meetings (Figure 20-1).

Staff meetings should be held on a regular basis. If it is necessary to hold weekly meetings because of the nature of the practice, then the physician(s) should be invited monthly to accommodate his or her busy schedule.

Meetings may need to be scheduled for when the staff members' work schedules overlap, either due to shift changes or staggered hours, or before or after regular office hours. For instance, if the practice is open from 9:00 A.M. to 9:00 P.M. on Thursdays, the meetings could be scheduled for 4:30 P.M. or 5:00 P.M. when all the staff would be present. Or the meetings may be scheduled at 8:00 A.M. prior to the office opening. If attendance at staff meetings is mandatory, then

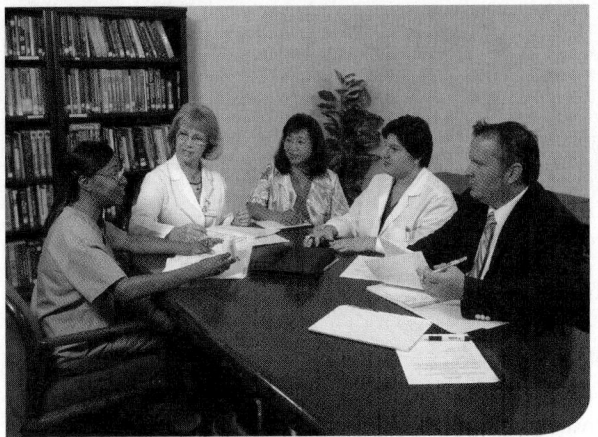

FIGURE 20-1 Regular staff meetings will increase the efficiency of the medical office staff.

staff members must be compensated for any meeting that is outside of their normal work schedule.

The office manager usually conducts staff meetings and facilitates team interaction. The office manager determines the time and date for the meeting and also prepares the agenda, frequently with input from the physician and other staff. The key to a good meeting is a concise agenda that identifies items for discussion, such as staff responsibilities, and limits the time allotted. Focusing staff meetings and discussions in this way limits the amount of time wasted. Generally, the minutes, including names of the individuals attending the meeting, are recorded for future reference and distributed for review prior to the next meeting. See Box 20-1 for an example of an office staff meeting

Box 20-1 Example of a Staff Meeting AGENDA

Pearson Physicians Group
Staff Meeting Agenda

Date: December 19, 20XX
Time: 4:30–5:30 P.M.
Place: Staff Conference Room

Time	Agenda	Person Responsible
4:30	Introduction of new staff Review of last meeting's minutes	T. Washington, Office Manager
4:35	New policies	
4:45	Problems with insurance	L. Turner/Insurance Coding Clerk
4:55	OSHA protocol for needlesticks	K. Wall/Lab Tech
5:05	Vacation schedules	T. Washington
5:10	New office location	Dr. McWalter
5:20	New business	Tania Washington
5:30	Meeting adjourned	

procedure 20-1

STAFF MEETING PROCEDURES

Objective: Explain and present the necessary steps to preparing and running a staff meeting.

EQUIPMENT AND SUPPLIES
agenda items received from staff; meeting agenda; means of keeping time (watch, clock, stopwatch, etc.); room for the meeting; any audio or video equipment that may be needed

METHOD
1. One week before the meeting, request agenda items from the staff.
2. Before the meeting, create a meeting agenda with all topics to be discussed. On the agenda include the date, time, and place of the meeting. List who will be running (facilitating) the meeting (most often, the office manager).

Assign a length of time to each topic and a person who will be responsible for that topic.
3. Start the meeting on time.
4. Begin by briefly covering the previous meeting.
5. Try to stay on schedule as much as possible.
6. Allow for time at the end of the meeting to have open discussion of any new business.
7. Adjourn the meeting.
8. After the meeting, have the minutes of the meeting typed and distributed to all involved.

---

agenda. Procedure 20-1 shows how to prepare and hold a staff meeting.

MOTIVATING EMPLOYEES

Motivating employees is vital to maintaining a positive working environment and an efficiently run medical office. Respect, ownership of personal space or environment, a sense of affiliation with the practice, fair compensation, acknowledgment, recognition, emotional rewards, communication, honesty, visibility of the management, empathy, trust, and equal treatment of all staff are a few items that employees expect from management.

Respect from management is a basic need of all employees. The office manager should greet employees in a pleasant manner, always acknowledge their hard work, and never reprimand them in front of their peers. The manager should be accessible and listen to employees when they need to talk and should consider their suggestions seriously. Satisfied employees are one of the best resources that the office manager has in running an efficient medical office.

In the medical office, many people often share one space. If possible, each employee should have some personal space. Preferably this would be a desk, but it may just be a small table or a locker located somewhere in the office. Allowing employees to place pictures in the area in which they work most often makes the employee feel settled, and in turn, tends to produce a greater level of productivity.

Creating a sense of affiliation to the medical office is often achieved by making simple considerations. Sharing in the highlights of staff member's lives, such as throwing a small birthday celebration or recognizing a special event (marriage or birth of a child), helps employees feel part of the office community or "family." Bringing the staff together outside of the office with special events, such as a company picnic, can also increase the sense of affiliation.

Generally, employees want to feel that they are being fairly compensated for the amount of work they produce. If an employee feels that he or she is producing the quality and quantity of work that is required but that it is not reflected in his or her pay, the employee will most likely seek a position elsewhere. One of the office manager's responsibilities is to make sure that all staff are appropriately compensated.

There are other rewards beyond pay. Employees need encouragement, recognition, and acknowledgement of their work, such as awards for meeting or exceeding set goals. Praise should be given to employees using a method that does not make them feel awkward. Some employees prefer public recognition, and other employees prefer private recognition. The employee who prefers private recognition will appreciate receiving a card from the office manager recognizing the achievement, more than a sign at the entrance to the workplace. Many offices now incorporate a questionnaire at the time of new employee orientation that asks how the employee prefers to be recognized.

Communication is essential to managing an efficient office and maintaining a cohesive work atmosphere. Employees like honest, straight talk from their employers. It is important to realize that secrets in an office breed distrust. It is always best for employees to receive news directly from their manager rather than through rumors. The office manager should always inform staff of both the positive and the negative issues affecting the practice.

It is essential for the office manager to be available to the employees. Being visible to employees creates a positive rapport, and any problems that may arise can often be dealt with swiftly and efficiently. A manager should not hide in an office, staying busy with business affairs. Employees are very aware of their manager's behavior, especially during the time spent in the office. For example, the office manager should be mindful of their own arrival and departure times to the office. It is difficult for the office manager to maintain credibility when counseling an employee regarding tardiness when he or she is late several times per week. The office manager needs to lead by example.

An office manager can often gain a great deal of loyalty from his or her employees through empathy. Though the office manager is a figure of authority to the employee, honest communication and a sincere regard for the employee's well-being go a long way in creating a comfortable and productive workplace.

Leadership Styles

The ability to make appropriate calls of judgment, the willingness to learn new ideas, staying calm during stressful situations, always maintaining a professional attitude, and good listening skills are all attributes of good leaders. As an office manager, you will be the team leader of the medical office. Think back to good managers that you have had in the past. What attributes made them good managers? Was it their knowledge, or was it that they were easy to approach, or both? If you think back, you may find traits in former managers that you can incorporate into your own behavior to create your version of an office manager.

The four standard types of leaders are authoritarian, democratic, permissive, and bureaucratic. Each type of leader is distinct and responds to different motivators. Knowledge of different management styles may help you fine-tune your own management style and give you ideas on how to benefit your employees.

Each leadership style has benefits and downfalls. Most managers find they exercise one particular style the majority of the time; however, they may shift to a different management style if the situation calls for it. For example, an office manager might be a democratic leader the majority of the time, but if a fire breaks out in the office, the manager may switch to an authoritarian style.

Authoritarian leaders tend to be very direct. They make most decisions on their own without the input of others. They probably will not be team players as much as solid leaders. Authoritarian leaders tend to want respect and obedience from their staff members and may even use fear to achieve staff obedience. The need for power and absolute authority often motivates this type of leader. Authoritarian leaders work best in times of great stress and crisis situations.

A *democratic leader* will concentrate more on the relations among staff members and will emphasize teamwork within the office. He or she tends to be motivated from within to provide a comfortable work environment for all. With a leader of this style, you will often find very open communication. Democratic leaders are more receptive to new ideas from staff members, which helps to create an atmosphere of cooperation among the staff, instituting greater participation in the decision-making process. This style of leadership often leads to a contented staff.

Permissive leaders are very open with the staff. They are not strict with rules and policies. Like the democratic leader, the permissive leader is self motivated. In many situations, he or she will let staff members make their own decisions and will not interfere with staff processes. However, medical offices must keep an ordered environment, and at times permissive leadership can lead to disorganization and even hazardous conditions.

Bureaucratic leaders are very strong at enforcing rules. Their motivation comes from external means. They prefer to rely on established management methods for office matters. Bureaucratic leaders tend to be rigid and set in their ways. Bureaucratic leaders are somewhat insecure, as witnessed in the fact that they do not trust themselves in making decisions that will affect the office. The staff often will find the bureaucratic leader to be very distant and formal.

For any manager to enact and enforce the rules that are necessary to run an efficient medical office, he or she must establish a level of power. A manager may establish several types of authoritative power. One type uses the power of rewards. This type of power incorporates rewards or some type of enticement in exchange for better job performance and teamwork. When managers use rewards to exact greater productivity from their employees, they are exercising a form of power over their employees. The degree to which this works will depend on the level of reward that the employee wants and receives.

Legitimate authority and responsibility are given to people based on their title. The president of a company will hold legitimate authority: the power of the title of president. *Expert authority* is given to those who have a great deal of knowledge. This is earned through experience and education. *Referent power* is given out of high regard and respect. It comes with a person's likability and even his or her success in the field. At some point in their lives most individuals have experienced *informative power*—the power wielded by those with information that others want or need. *Connective power*—the idea that if you know the right people you can get what you need—is one reason to network at local organizations. As a student, it is never too early to start making connections.

With all authority comes the ability to abuse or overuse it. The effects of overuse of authority will depend on the type of power wielded by the individual. With reward power, one downfall is that the employees can become reliant on rewards. Once this happens, the power becomes coercive, which is a negative power because it uses fear to motivate employees. The employee may be afraid of punishment or that the manager may withhold certain rewards to gain cooperation. Also there is the possibility of jealousy among employees. They may have the perception that someone is getting more attention or rewards than someone else, and thus the idea of favorites emerges. With coercive power, a misuse can lead to distrust and fear of the manager and of other employees. Misused legitimate power leads to fear of the person with the title or even the title itself. In the misuse of informative power, you will often see avoidance, a sense of unfairness, and a bit of hostility. Expert, referent, and connective powers all tend to lead to the same effects when misused: a perceived level of manipulation and intrusion among those affected.

Creating a Team Atmosphere

For a medical office to run at its most efficient level, the staff must work as a team. This can be difficult for the office manager to manage. Still, the office manager is in charge of strengthening and enhancing the team atmosphere. The following are some factors that must come together to create a successful office team:

- **Size**—The smaller a team, the better it will work together.
- **Team personalities**—It is inadvisable to put together a team made of the same personalities and similar mindsets.
- **Responsible team members**—All members of the team must be accountable for their actions.
- **Unified team approach**—Team members must come together to face the project with the same purpose and goals.

Every team must have its leader, and the office manager must realize that he or she is the team leader. Yet other team leaders may emerge from the team itself.

Managers should treat all members of a team equally. Showing favoritism, perceived or real, to one or two employees can easily break down any team atmosphere.

Managers also must show that they are an integral part of the team. It will make employees more confident and content in their jobs to know that their manager is willing to help out with employee duties when assistance is needed. Most successful managers adopt the attitude "I would not ask the employee to do anything I haven't already done myself or would be willing to do." For instance, if two members of the office team are both out sick, a manager who answers the telephone or files medical records in their place will show his or her team members a vital component to teamwork.

In some medical offices, it may also be necessary to have several levels of leaders among the office team. For example, one team leader may work at the front desk, and another may have clinical duties. To keep the team unified and productive, all team leaders must be highly organized, have a good deal of energy, and support the other team leaders.

TEAM SIZE

The size of a group can greatly affect the dynamics of how it will work. Small groups often will be very intimate. Close bonds may form, but because of the small group dynamics they also tend to be very unstable. As groups grow larger, they tend to become more stable but experience a loss of group intimacy. This information is important to know when assembling a team. You will find that the smaller a group, the more relaxed the atmosphere will be, whereas a larger group will have a more rigid structure. In similar fashion, the smaller the office, the easier going it may be. Larger multiphysician offices tend to be much more formal and systematic as a whole, but employees may be very close within their own small groups, such as a group of receptionists or clinical medical assistants.

TEAM PERSONALITY AND SKILLS

Staff members who feel they have no say in the people being hired tend to have a harder time adjusting to the presence of a new staff member. Thus, creating a team atmosphere begins during the hiring process by, for example, allowing some staff members to help in the hiring process, provided that all are aware of the legality of the questions to be asked. It is important that the staff understand what the office manager is looking for in potential employees. Staff members may be able to provide some insight into the personality of the job candidate, which would be helpful in maintaining a cohesive team atmosphere. Ultimately, the office manager and physician will have the final say in the

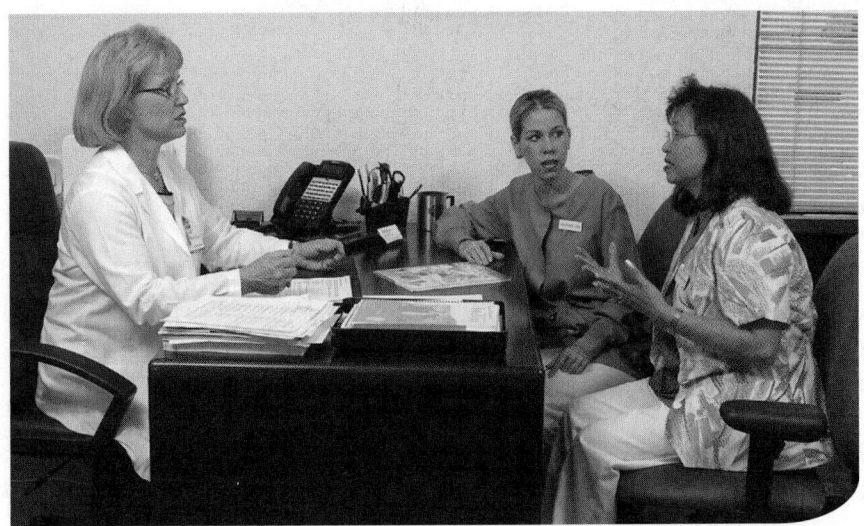

FIGURE 20-2 A medical office requires teamwork.

hiring of the candidate, but this process lets the staff know that their opinions also matter.

It takes the right mix of people to create a strong team. It is never a good idea to fill an office with people who are similar in personality and leadership style. Often, similar weaknesses will manifest in the day-to-day business of the office, which defeats the goal of efficiency and teamwork. A manager should look for staff members who complement each other's talents and traits. For example, one member of the staff who is really good with computers but is weak in filing will be complemented by a staff member who is weak in computers but an excellent filer. Creating this mix will give you the foundation for a strong team (Figure 20-2).

You will find that within any given team, the different team members will take on various roles. These roles can be task oriented in nature or more nurturing. Some of the task-oriented roles include the information seeker, the information giver, the coordinator, the energizer, the evaluator or critic, and the recorder. These roles all focus on the goal toward which the team is working. The nurturing roles may include the encourager, the harmonizer, the compromiser, and the follower. A team member may take on one or many roles within the team.

TEAM ACCOUNTABILITY

As a team, members must hold each other accountable for their actions. If something goes wrong, the team must come together to locate and fix the problem. This means that the team should not attack or try to blame a problem on any one member but that they must find where, as a team, they lost track and how they can prevent a similar problem from reoccurring.

TEAM PURPOSE AND GOALS

The team must find a way to work together. Ensuring that you have the correct personalities and talents is a good starting point. Encourage team members to concentrate on a single goal. Successful teams work with the same purpose in mind and approach a problem or task using similar means. That way there is little conflict among the team members as they work out problems that may get in the way of achieving their goal.

Any team will have some weaknesses, so it is important for the office manager to monitor the progress of the team. In a medical office that has employees who are strictly clinical and employees who are strictly administrative, you may find that the two types tend to divide themselves into separate teams. The employees may feel comfortable with this type of division, but it usually puts strains on running the practice. The office manager must prevent this from happening. When possible, it is good practice to have staff members switch places occasionally (e.g., have those who are strictly front-office employees trade with those who are accustomed only to back-office duties). This will help team members to experience the duties and responsibilities of the office as a whole. When employees are not working toward the goal of a cohesive team, the manager may wish to use team-building exercises. Many companies specialize in helping office managers pull their team together.

Hiring Procedures: Selecting the Right Staff Members

The office manager will need to hire new staff from time to time. It may be that someone has left the office or that a new position has been created. Recruitment can begin in house, with the job vacancy posted within the medical office so existing employees may apply for the vacant positions before the position is advertised elsewhere. If no internal candidates are interested or qualified, several methods may be used to seek applicants.

ADVERTISING THE POSITION

There are many ways of advertising for open positions. These include placement of job advertisements in newspaper and trade journals, professional organizations, the Internet, formal training programs, and employment agencies, which charge a fee to be paid by the employer to the agency if an agency's candidate is hired. Local training programs in colleges are also excellent resources.

In most cases, the newspaper or Internet will often be the best way to reach your local population. Many online providers offer options for job advertisements. Advertisements should describe the position and the required qualifications accurately. This will prevent the office from receiving too many résumés that do not pertain to the advertised position. If you are too general in your description, you may receive an excess of applicants. However, being too specific can cause the opposite problem: you may receive a very limited number of individuals applying for the position.

Once you have advertised and received résumés, you will begin the task of sorting through each applicant's résumé. Each office manager has his or her own way of doing this, but some of the most commonly used sorting methods include first removing any résumés that have obvious errors, such as poor grammar and spelling errors. Next, many office managers will remove all résumés that do not show the appropriate educational requirements, certifications, licensure, or work experience for the position that has been advertised. Once those résumés have been weeded out, office managers are usually left with the candidates they believe show the most promise for the position. At this point, the interview process begins.

THE INTERVIEW

Before each interview, it is good practice to have all applicants complete a job application either online or in paper format (Figure 20-3). You may choose to send this to applicants by mail and have them bring it with them to their interview or provide the link for them to access the online version (Figure 20-4). However, there are benefits to having the applicant fill out the form at the time of the interview. You will be able to see how the applicant handles filling out forms under a time constraint. You also will get to see the applicant's handwriting. Legible handwriting is important to have since most office employees will be writing directly in charts. The last thing you will learn from this process is how adept the applicants are at completing a requested task. Do they follow directions and complete every line, or do they take shortcuts? Their actions can indicate how they will handle on-the-spot tasks that may need to be resolved quickly and efficiently.

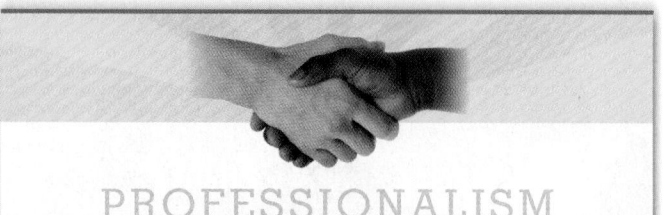

PROFESSIONALISM
CULTURAL CONSIDERATIONS

Many medical office managers seek to hire applicants who are multilingual, particularly if a medical office is situated in a region that is highly populated with a specific ethnic group. For instance, states in the southern part of the United States may be more populated with Spanish-speaking individuals because Texas borders Mexico and Florida is in close proximity to Cuba and Puerto Rico. Thus, a medical assistant who is bilingual in both Spanish and English would be very desirable in those states. Being multilingual is often a deciding factor between two candidates who are both equally qualified for a position in a medical office. Medical assistants should include all fluent languages on their résumés.

EMPLOYMENT APPLICATION FORM

Directions: Answer all questions using black ink (print).

PERSONAL NAME

(LAST)	(FIRST)	(MI)

ADDRESS-STREET	CITY	STATE	ZIP

PHONE NUMBER: SOCIAL SECURITY NUMBER:

POSITION DESIRED:

EXPECTED SALARY OR HOURLY WAGE:

EDUCATION

NAME OF SCHOOL	ADDRESS	DATE(S)	DEGREE/CERTIFICATE
HIGH SCHOOL			
VOCATIONAL/TECHNICAL			
COLLEGE			
OTHER			

WORK EXPERIENCE – Give present position (or last position held first).

JOB TITLE:	EMPLOYER	ADDRESS	DATES
DUTIES PERFORMED:			
JOB TITLE:	EMPLOYER	ADDRESS	DATES
DUTIES PERFORMED:			
JOB TITLE:	EMPLOYER	ADDRESS	DATES
DUTIES PERFORMED:			

REFERENCES – List three persons (other than relatives) who have known you for at least 2 years

NAME/TITLE	ADDRESS	TELEPHONE NUMBER

APPLICANT'S SIGNATURE _____

Date

FIGURE 20-3   A standard employment application form may be used.

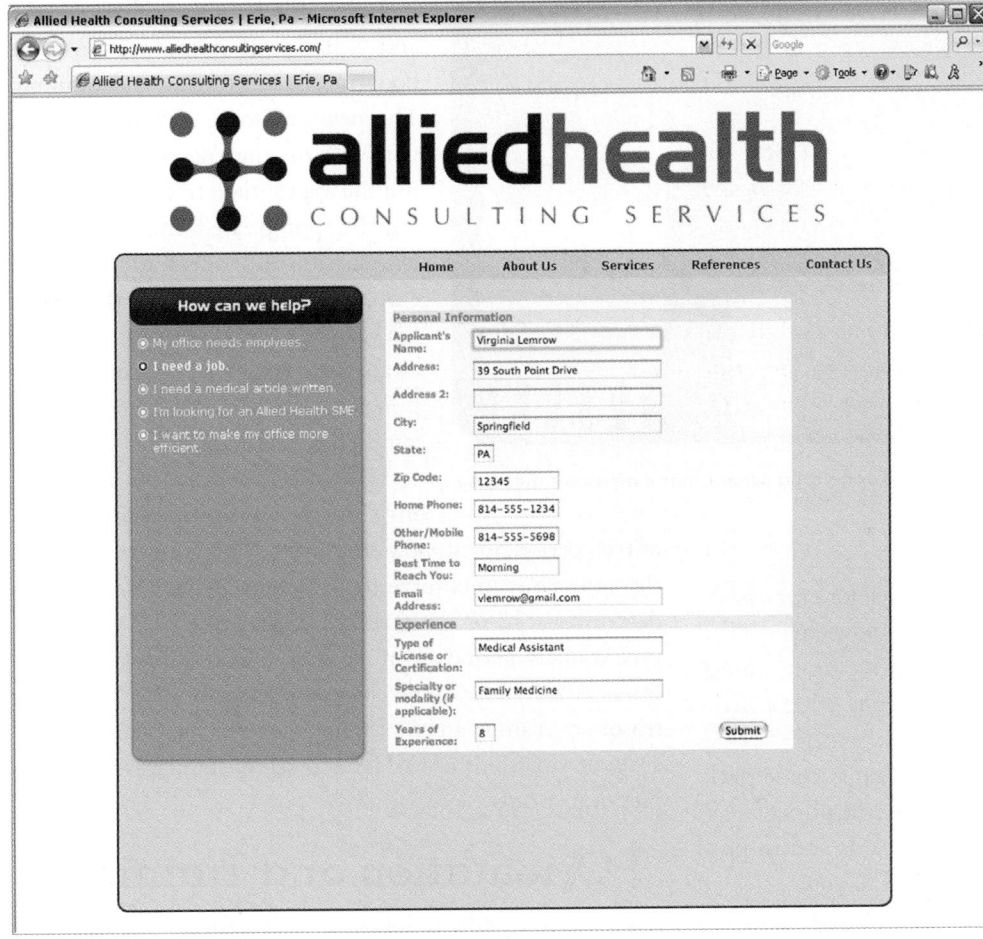

FIGURE 20-4 Example of an online employment application and posting of a résumé.

Learning important information about applicants is key to making sure that they would be a good fit for your practice. You may want to ask them about past office experience and what types of physicians they have worked with before.

Another good idea is to test applicants' ability to think on their feet. It has been an increasing practice to give applicants off-the-cuff questions to see how they respond. You are not looking for a correct answer but wish only to see how they reason through the question. Do they give up and guess, or do they try to make a logical guess by thinking through the possibilities? Many managers also will give applicants situational questions. For example, you may wish to ask how they would handle a patient who is upset about a test result.

As discussed in the sections on creating a team atmosphere, it is sometimes a good idea to allow certain staff members to ask questions of the applicant. Again, staff members can give input on whether or not the applicant will fit with the other staff.

While interviewing, applicants are also interviewing the interviewer and forming opinions regarding whether or not they want to work for the practice. Important aspects of the applicant should be assessed. Is the applicant dressed appropriately? Does he or she reflect a professional appearance? Is the résumé neatly prepared? The answers to these questions will give you insight into the type of employee the applicant will make and whether or not he or she will fit into your current team.

Many questions may be asked, but others are not allowed by law. You must keep in mind the fair-employment practice (FEP) laws that affect hiring. Title VII of the Civil Rights Act of 1964, later amended as the Equal Employment Opportunity Act of 1972 (and further amended in 1990), prohibits asking applicants questions about their race, color, religion, sex, or national origin both during the interview and on the application. For example, asking a female applicant questions such as "Did you have difficulty finding a baby-sitter today?" or "Do you plan to have children?" is considered **discriminatory**, or prejudicial treatment, and is therefore against the law.

PROFESSIONALISM
THE LIFE SPAN

When interviewing candidates for vacant positions in the medical office, it is important that stereotyping does not occur. This is especially important when interviewing older candidates and very young candidates.

All too often, older individuals may be typecast as not being computer literate, tiring easily, and having health issues. Younger individuals may be typecast as not being reliable, not serious about their work, and requiring additional supervision. Do not allow yourself to fall into this mindset. Some of the most productive and reliable employees may be the older or younger candidates.

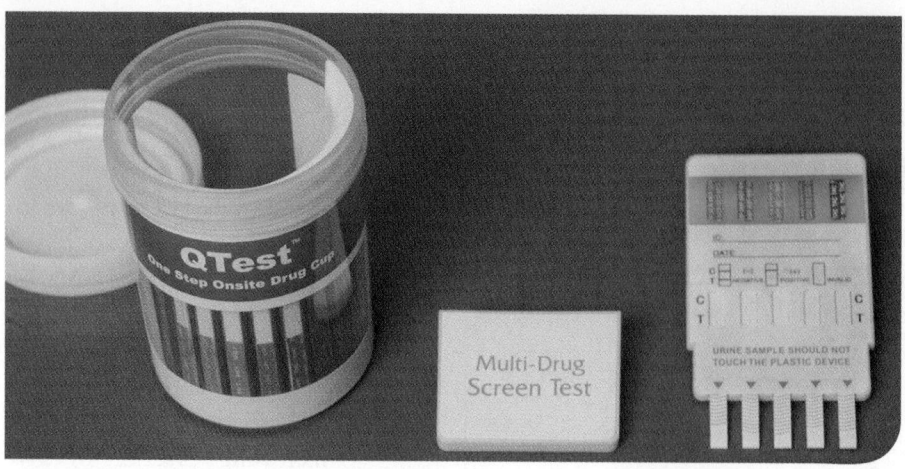

FIGURE 20-5 Example of equipment used for a urine drug screen that a medical office may require prior to employment.

It is important to find the right employee for every position. Always look beyond experience and knowledge to the applicant's personality. To maintain a positive team atmosphere, sometimes it is better to hire someone with a little less experience.

You may choose to have your top applicants come back for second interviews. You may wish to have the physician or other staff members interview these applicants and to provide time for the candidate to ask questions of you.

References

The next step in the selection process is to check the references of the applicants. This is done by conducting a brief telephone interview with the person(s) referenced by the applicant. After interviewing all the applicants of interest and checking their references, it will be time to decide whom to hire.

HIRING

Once you have verified the references of your applicants, you can begin the process of selecting your top choices for the position and making an offer. It may happen that you call your top choice and offer the position but he or she declines your offer. In such a case, you would then offer the position to your next choice.

After an applicant has accepted the position, all other applicants should be notified, either by telephone or in writing, that the position is filled. The new employee should receive a job description and written confirmation of the job offer that includes the salary and benefits offered. The office manager will usually sign this letter.

Some medical offices will require a post-offer drug screen (Figure 20-5), acceptable credit report, acceptable criminal background check, preemployment physical (which may include tuberculosis [TB] testing and hepatitis B immunization), and body mechanics testing and training. The new employee will be provided with information regarding scheduling the appropriate tests and completing the appropriate forms required for the position either prior to the offer of employment or at the time the offer is made. The candidate must be made aware that the official offer of the position is not valid until all screenings are completed satisfactorily.

The first 3 months (90 days) usually constitute a **probationary period**, or trial period, for all new employees. This time frame allows the supervisor to observe the new employee at work and to determine if he or she is suited to the position. During this probationary period an employee can be terminated without cause. After 90 days, the employer must show just cause, or reason, to dismiss an employee. Absenteeism, poor performance, or violations of OSHA and safety standards are examples of just cause.

Orientation and Training

If you were to take a poll of new employees and ask what was most frustrating about their first days on the job, they would reply "lack of orientation." An effective manager will have an organized, efficient method of orientation and training for all new hires. The time and effort will pay off in the long run as all employees will have received the same information. Many offices have an orientation checklist, which helps ensure all employees have received the proper orientation.

The following list presents the basic subjects that should be covered for all new hires at orientation:

- Work hours and schedule, including overtime approval procedures
- Office layout (locations of the restroom, break room, employee parking, employee entrances, etc.)
- Dress code
- Smoking policy (many offices have adopted a smoke-free environment policy)
- Lunch and break times and location
- Job description
- All employment records—including I-9s (Figure 20-6), emergency contact information, affidavit of citizenship, insurance enrollment, and so on

Department of Homeland Security
U.S. Citizenship and Immigration Services

Form I-9, Employment
Eligibility Verification

Read instructions carefully before completing this form. The instructions must be available during completion of this form.

ANTI-DISCRIMINATION NOTICE: It is illegal to discriminate against work-authorized individuals. Employers CANNOT specify which document(s) they will accept from an employee. The refusal to hire an individual because the documents have a future expiration date may also constitute illegal discrimination.

Section 1. Employee Information and Verification *(To be completed and signed by employee at the time employment begins.)*

Print Name: Last	First	Middle Initial	Maiden Name

Address *(Street Name and Number)*	Apt. #	Date of Birth *(month/day/year)*

City	State	Zip Code	Social Security #

I am aware that federal law provides for imprisonment and/or fines for false statements or use of false documents in connection with the completion of this form.

I attest, under penalty of perjury, that I am (check one of the following):

☐ A citizen of the United States

☐ A noncitizen national of the United States (see instructions)

☐ A lawful permanent resident (Alien #) _____

☐ An alien authorized to work (Alien # or Admission #) _____
until (expiration date, if applicable - *month/day/year*) _____

Employee's Signature	Date *(month/day/year)*

Preparer and/or Translator Certification *(To be completed and signed if Section 1 is prepared by a person other than the employee.)* I attest, under penalty of perjury, that I have assisted in the completion of this form and that to the best of my knowledge the information is true and correct.

Preparer's/Translator's Signature	Print Name

Address *(Street Name and Number, City, State, Zip Code)*	Date *(month/day/year)*

Section 2. Employer Review and Verification *(To be completed and signed by employer. Examine one document from List A OR examine one document from List B and one from List C, as listed on the reverse of this form, and record the title, number, and expiration date, if any, of the document(s).)*

List A	OR	List B	AND	List C
Document title:				
Issuing authority:				
Document #:				
Expiration Date *(if any):*				
Document #:				
Expiration Date *(if any):*				

CERTIFICATION: I attest, under penalty of perjury, that I have examined the document(s) presented by the above-named employee, that the above-listed document(s) appear to be genuine and to relate to the employee named, that the employee began employment on *(month/day/year)* _____ **and that to the best of my knowledge the employee is authorized to work in the United States. (State employment agencies may omit the date the employee began employment.)**

Signature of Employer or Authorized Representative	Print Name	Title

Business or Organization Name and Address *(Street Name and Number, City, State, Zip Code)*	Date *(month/day/year)*

Section 3. Updating and Reverification *(To be completed and signed by employer.)*

A. New Name *(if applicable)*	B. Date of Rehire *(month/day/year)* *(if applicable)*

C. If employee's previous grant of work authorization has expired, provide the information below for the document that establishes current employment authorization.

Document Title:	Document #:	Expiration Date *(if any):*

I attest, under penalty of perjury, that to the best of my knowledge, this employee is authorized to work in the United States, and if the employee presented document(s), the document(s) I have examined appear to be genuine and to relate to the individual.

Signature of Employer or Authorized Representative	Date *(month/day/year)*

Form I-9 (Rev. 02/02/09) N Page 4

FIGURE 20-6 A standard I-9 form.

LISTS OF ACCEPTABLE DOCUMENTS
All documents must be unexpired

LIST A	LIST B	LIST C
Documents that Establish Both Identity and Employment Authorization	Documents that Establish Identity	Documents that Establish Employment Authorization
	OR	AND
1. U.S. Passport or U.S. Passport Card	1. Driver's license or ID card issued by a State or outlying possession of the United States provided it contains a photograph or information such as name, date of birth, gender, height, eye color, and address	1. Social Security Account Number card other than one that specifies on the face that the issuance of the card does not authorize employment in the United States
2. Permanent Resident Card or Alien Registration Receipt Card (Form I-551)		
3. Foreign passport that contains a temporary I-551 stamp or temporary I-551 printed notation on a machine-readable immigrant visa	2. ID card issued by federal, state or local government agencies or entities, provided it contains a photograph or information such as name, date of birth, gender, height, eye color, and address	2. Certification of Birth Abroad issued by the Department of State (Form FS-545)
		3. Certification of Report of Birth issued by the Department of State (Form DS-1350)
4. Employment Authorization Document that contains a photograph (Form I-766)	3. School ID card with a photograph	
	4. Voter's registration card	4. Original or certified copy of birth certificate issued by a State, county, municipal authority, or territory of the United States bearing an official seal
5. In the case of a nonimmigrant alien authorized to work for a specific employer incident to status, a foreign passport with Form I-94 or Form I-94A bearing the same name as the passport and containing an endorsement of the alien's nonimmigrant status, as long as the period of endorsement has not yet expired and the proposed employment is not in conflict with any restrictions or limitations identified on the form	5. U.S. Military card or draft record	
	6. Military dependent's ID card	
	7. U.S. Coast Guard Merchant Mariner Card	5. Native American tribal document
	8. Native American tribal document	
	9. Driver's license issued by a Canadian government authority	6. U.S. Citizen ID Card (Form I-197)
	For persons under age 18 who are unable to present a document listed above:	7. Identification Card for Use of Resident Citizen in the United States (Form I-179)
6. Passport from the Federated States of Micronesia (FSM) or the Republic of the Marshall Islands (RMI) with Form I-94 or Form I-94A indicating nonimmigrant admission under the Compact of Free Association Between the United States and the FSM or RMI	10. School record or report card	8. Employment authorization document issued by the Department of Homeland Security
	11. Clinic, doctor, or hospital record	
	12. Day-care or nursery school record	

Illustrations of many of these documents appear in Part 8 of the Handbook for Employers (M-274)

Form I-9 (Rev. 02/02/09) N Page 5

FIGURE 20-6 (Continued)

- OSHA Bloodborne Pathogens Standards and universal precautions—including request for a waiver form for hepatitis B vaccine
- Health Insurance Portability and Accountability Act (HIPAA) training
- Fire safety—locations of fire extinguishers (Figure 20-7), exit procedures, stairwell locations (Figure 20-8)

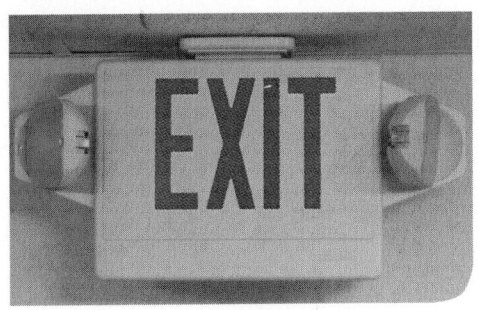

FIGURE 20-8 New employees should be shown all exits in case of an emergency.

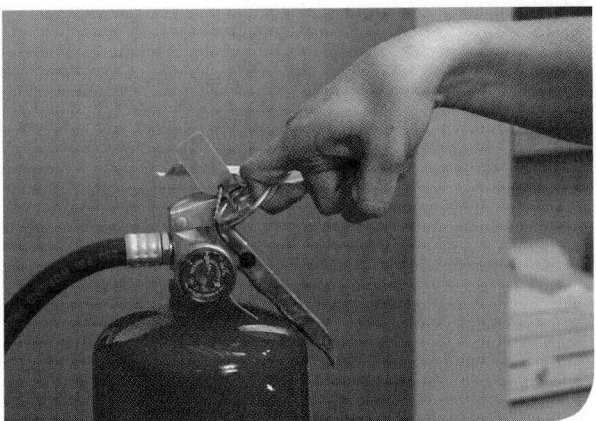

(A) Pull the pin on the upper handle of the fire extinguisher.

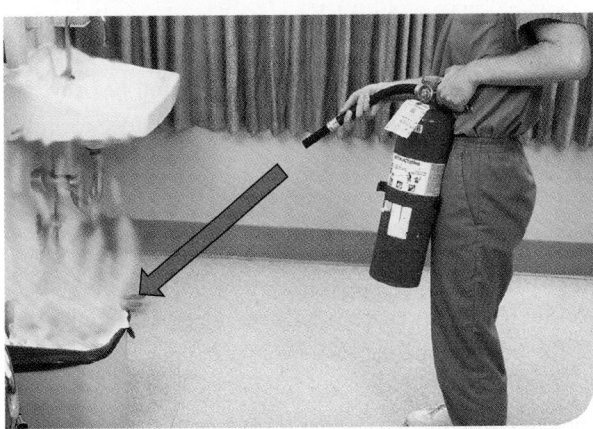

(B) Aim low toward the base of the fire.

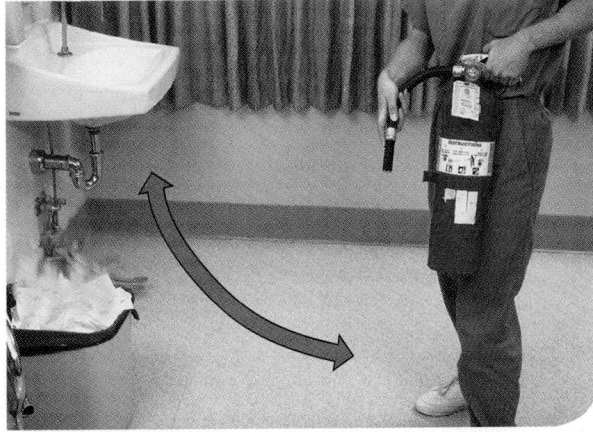

(C) Sweep the area from side to side.

FIGURE 20-7 It is important for new employees to know the location of all fire extinguishers.

- Confidentiality (obtain signature on confidentiality statement)
- Policies and procedures manual (Employee should read and sign a statement that the document has been read and understood.)
- Physician's work preferences—how the physician and the team prefer to work, including examples to help the medical assistant understand his or her role

Smaller offices with fewer employees may conduct orientation sessions on the job as the new employee begins working. This is not ideal but is often necessary. Orientation materials and a schedule can be developed to assist in this training process.

While some of these issues should have been covered during the interview process, many new employees need to be reminded. The pressure of the interview often causes applicants to forget important issues. Reiterating these issues during orientation can prevent confusion and errors. A confident employee is an efficient employee.

PROFESSIONALISM

THE LAW

Confidentiality, as both a legal and ethical concern, is a part of almost every function in the medical office. A good office manager will see that all employees put the patient's needs and confidentiality first. Special care must be taken that only selected office personnel have access to patient records.

The office manager must also protect the confidentiality of all employees by keeping employee records under lock and key. There should never be discussions about one employee's behavior with another employee present.

Using Performance Evaluation Effectively

All employees need feedback on how well they are performing in their assigned positions. In addition, management needs opportunities to introduce new goals for staff. The employee, in return, should be allowed to voice concerns and make suggestions for increasing the morale and productivity of the staff. Regular evaluations offer the chance for a productive give-and-take beyond the day-to-day interactions.

When it comes to any evaluation, preparation is the key. The office manager should never go into an evaluation unprepared. This will only cause problems. The appraisal should be given in a nonjudgmental manner and should focus on the entire review period, not just recent events. The manager should not take the stance of "the boss" versus "the employee" but, rather, should be open to understanding any problems the employee may be experiencing. Discussion of the job description and required duties should allow the employee to voice any frustration. At the same time, the manager should reinforce what is expected of the staff member. Teamwork should be emphasized.

The manager must look at the employee's performance as a whole. The employee's job description should be reexamined and the most important aspects of the position identified. Then the manager can rate the employee on those points. Is the employee's performance outstanding, good, average, poor, or unacceptable? Prior to assigning a rating, each rating must first be defined: What factors determine outstanding performance? What determines a good versus a poor performance? Next, the employee's social interaction skills, many times referred to as their "soft skills," should be examined: How does the employee get along with the other members of the office team? How does he or she interact with the patients? Depending on the employee's position within the office, it may be more important for the employee to excel in one set of skills than another.

In this general evaluation of the employee, it is also important to give him or her new goals to strive to meet before the next scheduled evaluation. The employee should be told about areas in which he or she might improve work performance and ways to help achieve the suggested goals, such as educational seminars and conferences. If possible, the evaluation meeting should end on a good note. Ideally, the employee should leave the meeting with the feeling that something valuable was gained from the review.

In situations in which employees are not performing up to the standard set for them, the performance evaluation may satisfy the legal requirements for documentation of rightful termination. If you are giving an employee a poor evaluation, it is a good idea to warn the employee at the start of the meeting. This will prevent the employee from being surprised when you begin to explain the problems with his or her performance.

Most employees look at an evaluation as the chance to be given or ask for a raise in pay. The office personnel manual should clearly delineate the types of performance reviews and the time intervals at which they will be given. Following is a list of different types of reviews.

- **Orientation or training**—Observe the new employee, and every few days ask the employee how the training is going. Make sure he or she has the materials, equipment, and supplies needed to perform the job. Ask the employee if he or she has any questions regarding policy and if supervision is being provided, and continue to reinforce the idea that you are available to address questions or concerns.

- **Routine performance review**—Reviews are normally performed at 90-day, 6-month and yearly intervals. Approximately 1 hour should be devoted to this meeting. These reviews should not come as a surprise to the employee. They should be stated in the policies and procedures manual. Many offices offer the staff member the opportunity to do a self-evaluation prior to the meeting. This allows the employee the chance to think about his or her performance to date.

  Figure 20-9 is an example of a form that may be used in a routine evaluation.

- **Poor performance reviews**—This type of review is conducted when there have been obvious deficiencies in the performance of the employee. They offer the opportunity to help the employee improve. Conversely, they document the poor performance and set the stage for dismissal.

- **Salary reviews**—A review of the employee's salary when a shift in job responsibility occurs.

Should salary reviews be tied to the performance evaluation? Several schools of thought address this issue. Whatever the policy of the office, fair and equal standards should be set.

What should the manager hope to accomplish with the meeting? It is important to target specific areas of performance. Following are some questions to ask to achieve effective management goals:

- How can improvement be achieved?

- How can you, as the manager, help the improvement?

- How can you remain fair and even in your opinion?

- How will you handle the possibility of a negative response from the employee?

PERFORMANCE EVALUATION AND DEVELOPMENT PLAN
(OFFICE AND CLERICAL)

NAME: _____ DATE OF EVALUATION: _____
DATE OF HIRE: _____ DEPARTMENT: _____
JOB TITLE: _____ SUPERVISOR: _____
DATE APPOINTED THIS JOB: _____ MANAGER: _____
LAST REVIEW DATE: _____ LAST REVIEW RATING: _____
NEXT REVIEW DATE: _____ CURRENT REVIEW RATING: _____

PURPOSE

The purpose of this evaluation is to:
1. SET GOALS WITHIN SCOPE OF PRESENT JOB.
2. COMMUNICATE OPENLY ABOUT PERFORMANCE.
3. EVALUATE PAST PERFORMANCE.
4. DISCUSS FUTURE DEVELOPMENT PLANS FOR GROWTH.

INSTRUCTIONS

1. Supervisor to review form prior to completion. If specific items are not applic[able] they should be left blank.
2. Supervisor and employee to review job description prior to review.
3. In "COMMENTS" section supervisor may indicate which factors should be more heavily weighted in this particular evaluation.
4. Comments should be specific and job-related. All appropriate evaluation fac[tors] should be commented on to some degree.

I. POSITION OBJECTIVES AND MAJOR RESPONSIBILITIES: Summarize specific respo[nsibilities]

II. ACCOMPLISHMENTS AND/OR IMPROVEMENTS: What specific accomplishments a[nd/or improvements] has employee made since last review with respect to set goals?

PLEASE CONSIDER THE EMPLOYEE'S DEMONSTRATED PERFORMANCE AND MARK THE C[ATEGORY THAT MOST] CLOSELY DESCRIBES THAT PERFORMANCE.

4 - Performance consistently far exceeds expectations and requirements.
3 - Performance consistently exceeds normal expectations and job requirements.
2 - Performance consistently meets expectations and job requirements.
1 - Performance usually meets expectations and minimum job requirements.
0 - Performance does not meet job requirements.

– CONTINUED, NEXT PAGE –

ORDER # 72-119 • PERSONNEL RECORDS SYSTEM • © 1987 BIBBERO SYSTEMS, INC., PETALUMA, CA • TO REORDER CALL TOLL FREE: (800) BIBBERO (800 242-2376) OR FA[X]

FIGURE 20-9 Standard employee performance evaluation forms are available for use.

7. DEPENDABILITY: Consider attendance, punctuality, idle time and reliance which can be placed on employee to persevere and carry through to completion all assigned tasks.

○ 0   ○ 1   ○ 2   ○ 3   ○ 4

8. COMPLIANCE WITH COMPANY POLICIES: Does the employee comply with rules and regulations which apply to safety, fair employment practices and general administrative procedure?

○ 0   ○ 1   ○ 2   ○ 3   ○ 4

9. SPECIFIC PERFORMANCE

	0	1	2	3	4	COMMENTS
A. Ability to handle scheduling:						
B. Willingness to work OT when necessary:						
C. Handling of calls and follow-up:						
D. Maintenance of equipment:						
E. Ability to handle patient complaints:						
F. Tact in dealing with patients:						
G. Speed (in specific technical procedures):						
H. Secretarial accuracy:						
I. Professional terminology:						
J. Assisting procedures:						
K. Laboratory techniques:						
L. X-ray techniques:						
M. Physical therapy:						
N. Collections:						
O. Medical Insurace:						
P. Bookkeeping:						

10. PERSONAL

	0	1	2	3	4	COMMENTS
A. Grooming:						
B. Professional conduct:						
C. Energy, enthusiasm:						
D. Ability to handle stress:						

ADDITIONAL COMMENTS:

– CONTINUED, NEXT PAGE –

ORDER # 72-119 • PERSONNEL RECORDS SYSTEM • © 1987 BIBBERO SYSTEMS, INC., PETALUMA, CA • TO REORDER CALL TOLL FREE: (800) BIBBERO (800 242-2376) OR FAX (800) 242-9330

Box 20-2 lists possible topics to cover during the review of front-office personnel. Typically, clinical staff will be evaluated either by the clinical coordinator or physician as they are the persons primarily working with the clinical employee. Finally, as in all aspects of medical office management, everything said during the evaluation should be documented objectively, leaving personal opinions aside.

DISCIPLINE AND PROBATION

Occasionally it is necessary to discipline an employee. Due to the sensitive nature of medical work, certain situations can result in immediate discharge. These include intoxication, drug use, breach of patient or office confidentiality, and sleeping on the job. The employee must be sent home on suspension while the incident is investigated. If the facts prove to be true, then the employee is dismissed. It is best to have a witness present when dismissing an employee.

For frequent tardiness or absenteeism, an employee may be placed on probation and told that if the situation occurs again within a set period of time (e.g., 30 days or 3 months), the employee will be discharged. In some facilities, both verbal and written warnings are issued before corrective action is taken. Investigating every employee incident prevents someone from being falsely fired. For instance, diabetic employees may appear to be on drugs when they are, in fact, having a diabetic reaction.

Box 20-2 Topics of Review for Front-Office PERSONNEL

Telephone technique
Daily balance of cash box
Accurate filing
Appointment scheduling
Communication and interaction with others
Treating patients with respect
Prioritizing tasks
Manging time effectively
Working neatly
Following directions
Cheerfulness and interest in the patient's comfort

Punctuality and attendance record
Grammar and spelling
Appropriate appearance and hygiene
Performance as a team member

Additional Topics for a Clinical Medical Assistant's Review

Accurate and concise charting
Ability to anticipate the needs of the doctor
Knowledge of procedures
Willingness to help fellow team members
Continuing education

Any employee incident must be carefully documented and include the time, date, and an objective statement regarding what happened. This is then placed in the employee's file. Document the incident immediately after it has occurred.

Time Management

One of the greatest attributes of an effective office manager is the ability to successfully manage time. If the manager is organized, the office is usually organized. Time management requires the ability to multitask and prioritize important tasks to complete them on schedule. This is quite different from doing every task as it comes along. The office manager generally has little control over the tasks presented. The control lies in how the tasks are handled and delegated.

One of the main responsibilities of the office manager and medical assistant is to manage all peripheral office functions so the physician is free to concentrate on practicing medicine. It is possible for the physician to gain an hour each day to devote to administrative and patient-related tasks that only he or she can do because tasks, such as opening the daily mail, searching for a drug sample to give to a patient, and dealing with pharmaceutical and other sales representatives, are handled by the office manager.

Before establishing a time management system, it is important to define the office goals with the physician. Physicians' goals vary from simple to complex and from long term to short term. These goals may include collecting all payments at the time of delivery of services, reorganizing or computerizing billing, limiting the practice, adding a partner or new service, writing a textbook, or planning for early retirement.

One of the dangers of strictly adhering to time management and goal-setting practices is that the patient may be forgotten in the process. The main concern always should be to take care of patients first. For example, it is more important to take care of a patient who is waiting at the reception desk than it is to straighten up the work area.

After goals have been established, priorities can be set. The office manager and medical assistant can establish a priority list of the goals. A priority list is a composite of all the tasks that must be accomplished to actualize each goal. These can be placed on a To Do list as they come to the office manager's attention. Each item is assigned a priority designation of 1, 2, or 3, depending on how critical the item is to completion of the task. For example, ordering supplies that are running out is a number 1, whereas rearranging a linen cupboard or a file drawer might be a number 3. Number 1 priority items must be done first and number 3 last. It is often tempting to do the easier tasks first since they take less time and show an immediate accomplishment. Good use of time management would determine that the inventory order should be placed immediately and the number 3 priority items should be delegated to someone else or completed later, if necessary. It is a good idea to date a To Do list and to cross off or check items as they are accomplished. Box 20-3 shows an example of one type of To Do list.

Make every attempt to complete each task, such as handling mail, only once. Mail should be handled immediately, if possible. As mail is opened, it must be quickly sorted according to importance, handled, and processed.

When leaving a telephone message, it is advisable to leave detailed voice mail messages, whenever possible, since it can actually save time. Leaving a detailed message during the first call can prevent having to make another telephone call. An exception would be when calling a patient. The patient's confidentiality should be protected. See Chapter 7 for more information regarding voice messaging.

Never trust anything to memory in the medical office. Always write down complete instructions from the physician

Box 20-3 Medical Office To Do LIST

Priority	To Do _____ Date: _____
2	Order paper supplies
1	Arrange Dr. Williams's air transportation to medical convention next week
2	Prepare performance appraisal for J. Jones
3	Reorganize storeroom
1	Type convention speech
1	Place ad for new medical assistant
3	Ask Janet to remove old magazines from reception room
1	Call for pap test report for Ms. Kohut
2	Block out schedule book for next quarter
1	Prepare agenda for Thursday's staff meeting

as well as information from the patient, another employee, or a supplier. It is better to maintain one small record book and keep all notations in that book rather than have several pieces of paper with information that can be misplaced. Many medical assistants carry a small notepad and pen in their pocket at all times.

Some offices require that the in basket of the day's mail and incoming laboratory reports be emptied before the end of the day. This is a good time management technique to develop.

Personnel Policy Manual

The personnel policy manual, also known as the employee handbook, contains information for the employee about the employer–employee relationship, the work environment, and the expectations of the particular medical facility. This manual contains general information about office policies relating to dress and behavior codes, punctuality, office safety, and the role of the employee in an emergency, such as a fire. It usually describes the circumstances or grounds for dismissal, such as sleeping or drinking while on the job, as well as breach of confidentiality on or off the job. OSHA guidelines and standard precautions may be included in the personnel policy manual or may be found in a separate OSHA handbook.

Employees should be provided with specific information about the following issues or benefits:

- Compensation and reimbursement for work-related activities, such as attending conventions and continuing education or degree courses, and parking fees

- Emergency leave
- **Grievance** (complaint) process
- Health benefits
- Holidays
- Jury duty
- Overtime policy
- Pension plan
- Performance review and evaluation
- Probationary period
- Sick leave
- Termination of employment
- Vacation
- Work hours, including flex time

An office manager will find that an updated personnel policy manual can be a useful tool when providing employee counseling. A well-designed personnel policy manual remains flexible enough in its design to allow for revisions, if and when policies change. Manuals for small offices consist of several pages that are copied on site. In large practices, the manual may be bound and copied at a printing service.

The personnel policy manual (sometimes referred to as the employee handbook) is often the first piece of office literature that the employee is asked to read. Employees should be asked to sign a statement indicating they have read and understood the information it contains. The signed statement should be placed in the employee's personnel file.

Office Policies and Procedures Manual

All offices should have a policies and procedures manual describing how to carry out tasks within a particular medical practice. This manual varies in content from the personnel policy manual. Detailed descriptions of the standard operating procedure (SOP) and how to perform both administrative and clinical tasks are included in this manual.

Policy refers to a plan of action, such as "It is office policy that all employees receive hepatitis B (HBV) vaccination." The procedure will describe the steps to be performed to carry out the policy. For example, "A series of three injections of HBV will be administered over a 7-month period of time, free of charge, to the employee." The terms *policy* and *procedure* are used interchangeably in many offices.

The primary functions of a policies and procedures manual are (1) list the tasks to be performed within the office, including equipment needed to complete the procedure; (2) standardize the procedure for each task; and (3) describe job responsibilities and titles. The policies and procedures manual, when properly updated, is an excellent reference tool for the new employee since it provides guidelines for performing specific tasks. Temporary or substitute employees also find it valuable.

Ideally, the policies and procedures manual is contained in a loose-leaf binder that allows the addition of new pages for ease of updating. Each policy is numbered and dated. As the policy is updated, the number remains the same, but the date changes to indicate the revision. The manual should be clearly labeled and available for employees to read.

New policies and procedures are usually distributed or posted for employees in addition to being added to the policies and procedures manual. In some offices, the staff is asked to initial the corner of the policy to indicate they have read it.

Table 20-2 contains a list of information that should be included in a policies and procedures manual. Writing and updating this manual is often a job function of the medical assistant or the office manager. Whereas one person may have responsibility for development of the manual, the best manuals are the result of input from a variety of personnel. The physician should always provide the final review of all written policies and procedures.

Medical Meetings and Speaking Engagements

The medical assistant may be asked to assist the physician in making travel arrangements for medical meetings or in preparing for medical speaking engagements. Travel arrangements may include making hotel, flight, and car rental reservations, and sometimes typing a travel itinerary for the trip.

When making the travel arrangements, the physician may wish to use a local travel agent or one of the many Internet sites available for booking flights and hotels. It is important to find out what the physician's preferences are before making any plans. The physician may prefer a nonsmoking hotel room and only business-class flight tickets. Make sure the reservations are in line with the wishes of the physician.

When putting together the travel **itinerary**, which is the travel plan, obtain all of the flight, hotel, car rental, and meeting or engagement information. Flight information includes travel dates, airline name, flight number, confirmation number or E-ticket number, and departure and arrival times. The hotel information includes the hotel name, address, telephone number, reservation dates, and confirmation number. Also assemble car rental reservations and any information pertinent to the meeting that the physician is attending. Keep a copy of the itinerary at the office and give a copy to the physician.

TABLE 20-2 Contents of an Office Policies and Procedures Manual

Content	Description
Routine Office Tasks	Clinical tasks such as venipuncture, taking vital signs, ECGs, assisting with physical examinations, assisting with pap test and other laboratory tests
Special Procedures	Surgical tray setup for individual physicians, assisting with special exams such as proctological exams, using specialized equipment such as ultrasound
Emergency Procedures	Protocol for handling telephone and office emergencies, description of equipment used for emergency care such as mouth shield for CPR, proper sequence for alerting physician, and 911 emergencies
Quality Assurance	Procedures for maintaining quality control over all laboratory testing and procedures
OSHA Compliance	Compliance regarding needles, other sharps, specimens, personal protective equipment, regulated waste control, hepatitis B vaccine, laundry disposal, and contaminated equipment

When helping a physician to prepare for a speaking engagement, you can help in a variety of capacities. It may include doing research. Be sure to provide all source material with any research that you reference and cite. The physician may ask you to create handouts for his or her presentation. When doing so, ensure that impeccable spelling and grammar are used. Always obtain the physician's approval on the handout prior to making an numerous copies. The physician may also ask you to create a computer presentation. Different software programs can assist you in creating a presentation.

Patient Information Booklet

Many medical practices use a professional advertising service to develop informational brochures as marketing tools. However, a patient information booklet or a variety of patient teaching materials can be developed in house. These materials should provide patient information regarding office hours, payment guidelines, appointment and cancellation policy, the telephone answering service, information about the physician(s), after-hours availability, directions to the facility, and parking information. A good patient information booklet can reduce the number of questions received by telephone from patients, enhance the office's image, and reduce the number of patients who fail to remember instructions.

Instruction booklets can be used either for patients with special needs or to teach methods of disease prevention. Developing and using a format and design is described in Procedure 20-2. A patient information booklet containing vital office information should be handed to each new patient at the time of registration or mailed prior to the first appointment. Patient information materials never diminish the need to give personal instructions to the patient. They simply augment, or reinforce, patient teaching.

procedure 20-2

DEVELOPING A PATIENT INFORMATION BOOKLET
Objective: Develop a booklet to inform patients about services provided by your medical office.

EQUIPMENT AND SUPPLIES
computer; design software (if including images); high-quality paper; printer (or an independent printing service)

METHOD
1. Make the booklet as appealing as possible. Leave a white border around all page edges. Use large print for the elderly reader's benefit. The booklet should be small enough that it will fit easily into a pocket or purse.
2. Write the booklet with the reader in mind and at a reading level appropriate for the target audience. Avoid the use of technical medical terms. Never use medical abbreviations in patient literature.
3. Avoid long paragraphs of explanation. Keep the sentences short and concise, and use as many bulleted points as possible.
4. Provide a list of the regular office hours.
5. List any special services offered by the practice or clinic, such as patient education classes or blood pressure testing programs.
6. Explain the procedure for having a prescription refilled.
7. Explain the procedure for processing medical insurance forms.
8. Include a general statement about payment of fees, especially if payment is expected at the time of delivery of services. Do not discuss specific fees in patient brochures.
9. Provide information about the physician and the staff. For example, "Dr. McWalter is in general practice specializing in family practice. Our pediatrician is Dr. Conway. Our physicians are on staff at two hospitals: Northwestern Memorial Hospital and Children's Memorial Hospital." Include the name and telephone number of the office manager, the personnel responsible for insurance processing and the patient educator.
10. State what procedure to follow in case of an emergency. For example, instruct the patients to call 911 if the emergency is life threatening. Also provide a 24-hour emergency telephone number. Ask the patient to keep this number near his or her telephone.
11. Include a telephone number at the end of the brochure where additional information may be obtained.
12. End the brochure by thanking the patient for taking the time to read the literature.

Patients need an introduction to all the caregivers with whom they come into contact in the office. Employees should always identify themselves to patients. Many patients need further education about the functions that individual employees are able to perform.

Patient information booklets are one of the best ways to educate the patient about the functions of the staff and medical office. Whereas verbal instructions are still necessary, the booklets can enhance learning. Medical assistants need to involve the entire staff in the production of patient literature.

Medical Practice Marketing and Customer Service

Marketing is a subject that most office managers do not think much about when running a medical office. Marketing a medical practice involves various activities to promote the services of a physician or group of physicians to a population of patients. Marketing can promote a new office and improve the image of an established office to compete with the new offices and to retain patients. Marketing can impact a medical office in many ways. Always remember that outstanding customer service can be a valuable marketing tool.

TARGET MARKET

In marketing a medical office or facility, one of the first things to look at is the target market of the physician(s). What kinds of services are being offered? This can affect the physician's office location. A new geriatric medical practice has a better chance of doing well if it is located near retirement communities rather than within communities comprised mostly of young families. Simply put, the services of the office should match the area in which it is located.

After assessing the target market and the needs of the target group, types of services the practice could offer can be determined and tailored to meet the expectations and needs of the target market. Services may include new procedures that could benefit patients' needs.

Once you have determined your services, a plan must be developed and put into place. The first step will be to look for any problems or opportunities that may come about in the execution of the plan. The plan should describe specific steps that need to be implemented, who is responsible for these steps, and a reasonable time frame. A plan must be thought through and in place before you begin to follow and execute it. Many ventures have failed due to poor planning. When the plan has been executed, it is a good idea to review the plan to determine if it has or has not met expectations. Make note of any particular problems that may have arisen and the positive lessons that may have been learned in the process.

MARKETING THE PRACTICE

A medical practice may be promoted in many ways. Some marketing plans may require large expense budgets to implement the plan. However, some marketing tools are available free or at low cost.

Free Marketing and Public Relations

One of the best ways of promoting a practice is by word of mouth, which is completely free. Many patients choose their physician based on friends and family recommending their own physician. Word of mouth is built on a base of good customer service (see "Customer Service").

Another method of promoting a practice is through public relations activities, such as local charities and events. Involvement in the community will spread the office's name and show that it is a participating member of the community. Goodwill in the community can translate into growing the practice.

Websites

Building a practice website is a relatively new marketing tool for medical professionals. This can be done using simple website building software or hiring a website firm. It is important to plan what should be included on the website. The main objective of the site must be determined. What is the site's function? Is it simply providing one-way information to the patient regarding the practice? Or is the website intended to provide interactive communication and allow the patient to ask questions, complete forms, and so on and have the physician or medical office staff member respond? Would the patient be able to access different forms and procedure instructions? Will patients be able to request appointments online? It is important to always consider HIPAA laws and confidentiality requirements if interactive communication is

Box 20-4 Phrases That Decrease Customer Service LEVEL

"It's not my job."
"I don't know."
"It's not my fault."
"What do you want?"

"I can't."
"You're wrong."
"It's not my problem."

---

the goal of your office's website. Keep the site easy to use. Graphics should be simple, and colors should be pleasing to the eye.

You will then have to choose a Web server to support your site. Many options are available and will need to be researched. Some are free, but they will add advertisements to your site. Others will require a fee.

CUSTOMER SERVICE

One of your most potent marketing tools will depend entirely on the level of customer service delivered to the patient. Just as word of mouth can bring you many customers, it can also drive them away if poor services are provided.

The patient, like a customer, will respond positively or negatively to his or her experience at the medical office. What impression does the patient have? Is the staff helpful and empathetic? Is the staff attentive and considerate of the patient's time and condition? It is important that all patients are treated with respect and concern. Box 20-4 includes spoken phrases that will leave the patient with a poor view of a medical office's customer service abilities. The most successful practices provide excellent customer service for their patients, which in turn usually means increased profits due to increased patient volume.

SUMMARY

A smooth-running office requires attention to many factors, including staff training, effective time management skills, up-to-date policies and procedures manuals, and careful attention to detail. A medical office requires the same management skills that any business organization uses. Maintaining good customer service is key to keeping a contented patient base while enhancing the possibility of growing the practice.

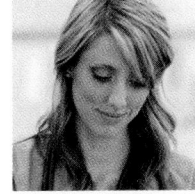

20 CHAPTER REVIEW

COMPETENCY REVIEW

1. Define and spell the terms to learn for this chapter.

2. Prepare an office procedure for any one of the following tasks: appointment scheduling, patient reception process, taking vital signs, OSHA guidelines.

3. Prepare a monthly calendar for the month of December, showing staff vacations and office coverage.

4. Develop a patient information booklet for your own physician's practice.

5. Prepare an employee policy for taking vacation days.

For the following questions choose the best answer:

1. For completion of the I-9 form, the employee must present an acceptable document from which of the following?
   a. List A only
   b. List B only
   c. List C only
   d. List A and B
   e. List A and C

2. All of the following should be found in an office procedure manual EXCEPT
   a. OSHA compliance
   b. routine office tasks
   c. special procedures
   d. termination
   e. emergency procedures

3. Which of the following laws affect the hiring of a new employee?
   a. EEOC
   b. AMA
   c. Title IV of the Civil Rights Act
   d. OSHA
   e. EEOA of 1972

4. During new employee orientation, all of the following should be covered EXCEPT
   a. personalities of coworkers
   b. personnel policy manual
   c. policies and procedures manual
   d. HIPAA training
   e. work hours

5. All of the following records are required for employee payroll EXCEPT
   a. gross salary
   b. 1-9
   c. W-4
   d. 1099
   e. Social Security number

6. All of the following are factors that contribute to a successful office team EXCEPT
   a. unified approach
   b. responsible members
   c. size
   d. job duties
   e. personalities

7. All of the following are qualities or skills found in good office managers EXCEPT
   a. organization skills
   b. effective communication skills
   c. subjectivity
   d. flexibility
   e. creativity

8. Patient instruction booklets should be
   a. used in place of individual instructions
   b. used to standardize instructions
   c. used to prevent lawsuits
   d. used for vision-impaired patients
   e. used only with hearing-impaired patients

9. Routine performance reviews are normally performed at all of the following intervals EXCEPT
   a. 30 days
   b. 2 months
   c. 3 months
   d. 6 months
   e. 1 year

10. Which of the following leadership styles is motivated by external means?
    a. bureaucratic
    b. permissive
    c. democratic
    d. authoritarian
    e. none of the above

CRITICAL THINKING

1. Where else could Tania have advertised the job opening?

2. Why is it important for Tania to have her applicants fill out paperwork by hand?

3. Which applicant do you think Tania should hire? Consider if personal appearance should outweigh professionalism. Explain your answer.

ON THE JOB

Sarah Egan is the office manager in Dr. Williams's practice. Nell Jacobs, who has worked as a CMA (AAMA) in the office for 1 year, has frequently been absent or tardy on Mondays. Sarah suspects that Nell has a drinking problem. However, Nell has never arrived at the office intoxicated—until today. Sarah has just observed Nell stumbling in the parking lot when getting out of her car. Her speech is slurred, and her breath has a fruity odor that Sarah thinks could be alcohol. Nell does not appear to understand anything that Sarah is saying to her.

1. Given the situation, as the office manager, what should Sarah do immediately regarding Nell?
2. If Sarah decides to send Nell home, should she call Nell's husband to come and get her, or, perhaps, insist that Nell go home in a cab?
3. Does Sarah have an obligation to tell Dr. Williams about her suspicions regarding Nell?
4. Should this incident become part of Nell's employment record?
5. Is this incident grounds for firing an employee?
6. Because Nell is a CMA (AAMA) and works with patients, is it within Sarah's rights to demand a blood and urine screening for alcohol and drugs?
7. Should the police be notified of the incident?
8. If Nell is indeed intoxicated or under the influence of alcohol or drugs, is Sarah obligated to refer Nell to counseling at an alcohol and drug rehabilitation facility?

INTERNET ACTIVITY

Research the different methods that the Internet provides for advertising job opportunities available at your medical office.

MEDMEDIA

Additional interactive resources and activities for this chapter can be found:

On your student DVD: View applicable procedure videos on the DVD-ROM found in the back of this book.

MyHealthProfessionsKit.com: Test your knowledge of the chapter with games and activities. MyHealthProfessionsKit also includes resources, helpful links, and a Spanish audio glossary.

Medical Assisting Interactive: Practice your procedures as a medical assistant in this simulated doctor's office. This can be accessed through MyHealthProfessionsKit.com.

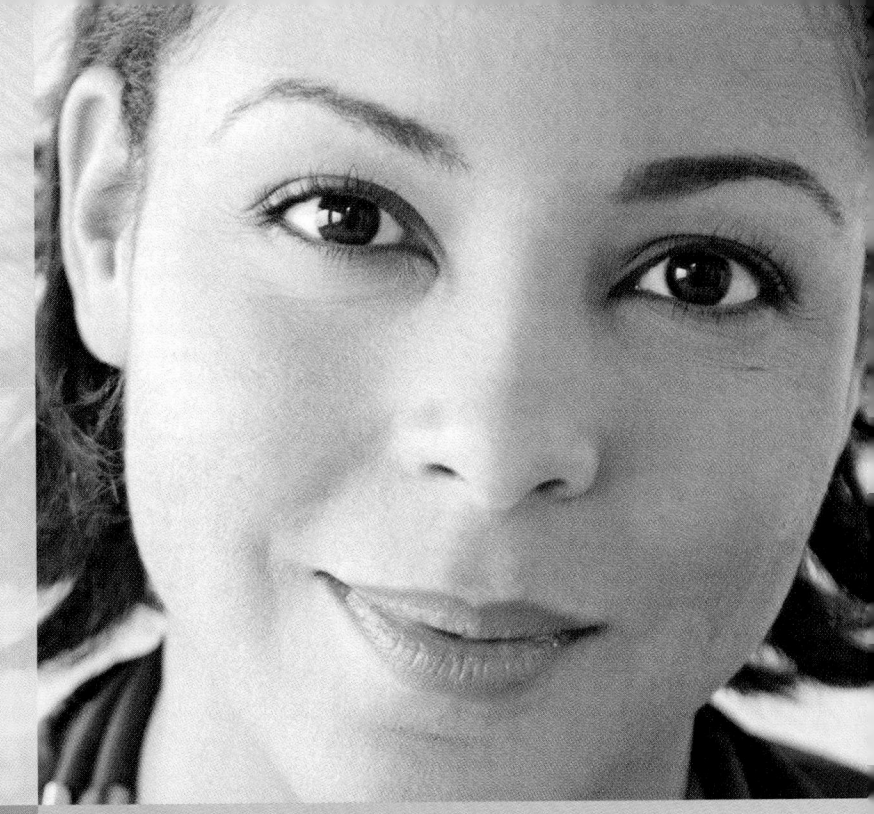

Unit One

Unit Two

Unit Three   Anatomy and Physiology

Unit Four

Unit Five

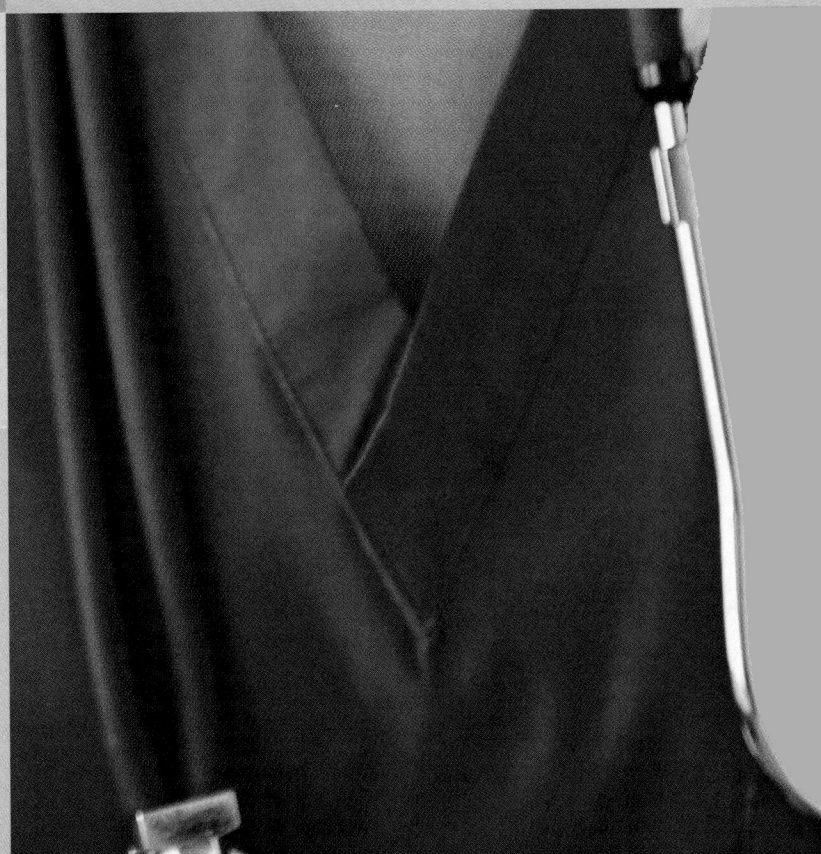

21

Body Structure and Function

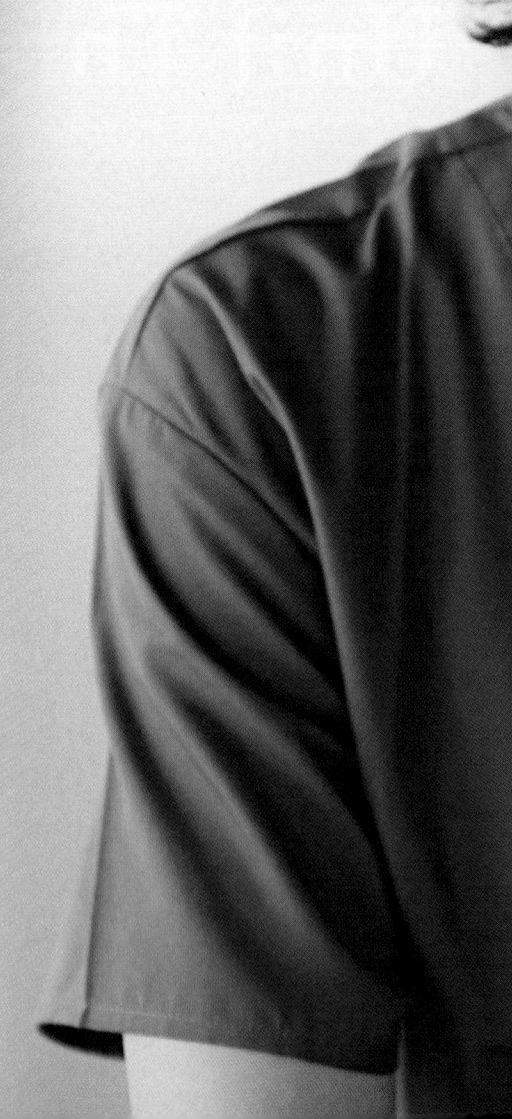

LEARNING OBJECTIVES

After completing this chapter, you should be able to:

- Define and spell the terms to learn for this chapter.

- List the organizational levels of the human body.

- Discuss the structural unit of the cell and briefly explain the function of each of its components.

- Discuss the various types of tissue in the human body.

- List the systems of the body and identify the organs located in each system.

- List and explain the major functions of the organ systems that comprise the human body.

- Explain the differences between passive and active transport.

- Discuss genetics, genetic engineering, genetic fingerprinting, and the role genetics plays in disease.

- Identify common genetic and congenital disorders.

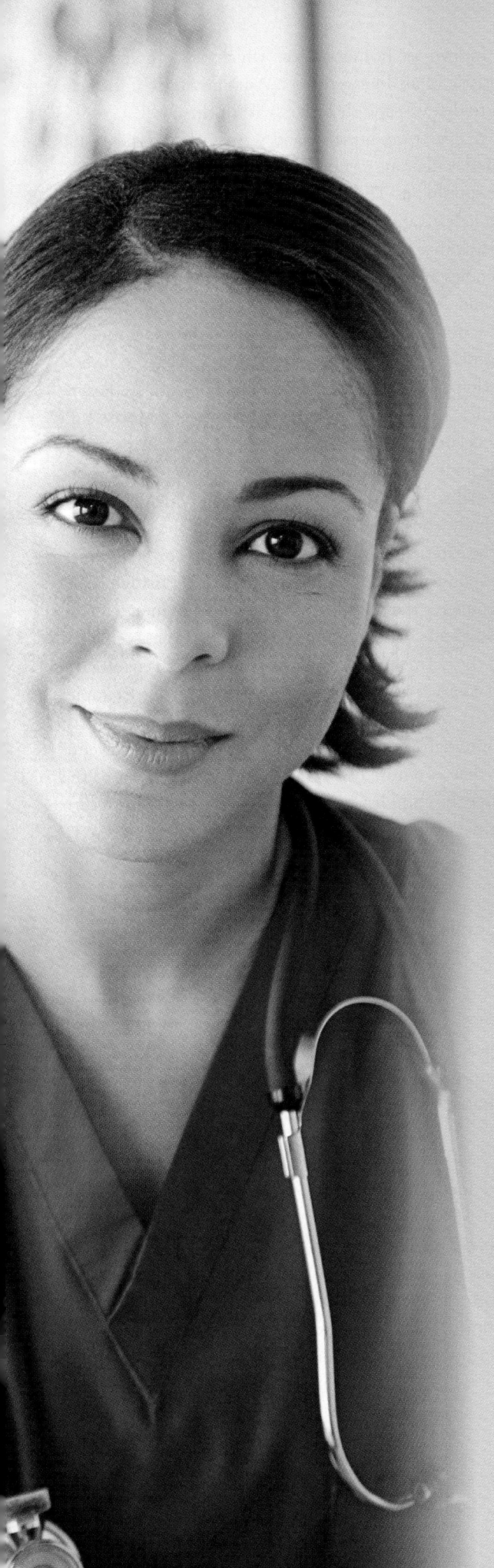

CHAPTER OUTLINE

CASE STUDY

Lucy Gutierrez is completing her medical assisting practicum and has the opportunity to shadow a medical assistant who works in a genetics clinic that is a part of Pearson General Hospital. This shadowing opportunity will last for 2 weeks. Lucy is very excited about this possibility because genetically acquired diseases have always intrigued her.

417

CERTIFICATION LINK

CMA (AAMA)
Anatomy and
physiology
  Structural Units

RMA
Anatomy and
physiology
  Body systems
  Disorders and
  diseases of
  the body

CMAS (AMT)
Medical assisting
foundation
  Anatomy and
  physiology

The human body is a complicated and intricate organism composed of millions and millions of cells. To understand the workings of the human body, it is important to understand its **anatomy** (the study of the structure of an organism) as well as its **physiology** (the study of the function of an organism). Various factors, including age, genetic predisposition, and environmental influences, can lead to the development of diseases and disorders within the body. The study of these diseases and disorders is termed **pathophysiology**.

The body is composed of increasing levels of organization, which are discussed later in this chapter. All these parts are intended to function in a normal unified state. By adjusting for constant changes in the environment, the body and its systems work together to maintain a constant balance.

This is known as **homeostasis**, which is a fundamental characteristic of all living things. A homeostatic imbalance can lead to diseases and disorders within the body.

Body temperature, nutrient and waste concentrations, and salinity and acidity are examples of mechanisms that our bodies use to sustain life. These properties each have chemical reactions that keep us alive as our bodies have built-in physiological mechanisms that maintain them at desirable levels.

Our bodies are equipped to respond to changes from both internal and external stimuli through two possible actions. The first action is negative feedback. When the body responds with **negative feedback** to external stimuli, it acts to reverse the direction of change, thus maintaining homeostasis. For instance, on a hot day your body temperature may rise and sweating occurs. The sweat formed by the body helps to decrease the body's temperature. The body's response to the hot day (external stimuli) was to produce sweat, which is used to cool the body, thus reversing the direction of the change created by the external stimuli. The other action our bodies may take in response to stimuli is positive feedback. **Positive feedback** encourages the stimuli to continue, or even accelerate, which also results in homeostasis. For instance, the accelerated release of the hormone oxytocin during childbirth enables the uterus to contract and the cervix to stretch. In this example, the body is responding to the stimulus of the childbirth process (internal stimuli). The body will increase the level of oxytocin that is released in order to enable the birth of the child. After the child has been delivered, the body will return to its normal state and maintain homeostasis.

The Human Body: Levels of Organization

The human body is organized in increasingly more complex levels of organization. The units of organization from simplest to most complex include atoms, molecules, organelles, cells, tissues, organs, organ systems, and the complete organism (Figure 21-1). The organ systems within the body are dependent on each other for maintaining a homeostatic balance.

ATOMS

Atoms are found at the most basic level of organization. An **atom** consists of at least one proton, which is a positively charged particle (+); at least one neutron, which is without an electrical charge; and at least one electron, which is a negatively (−) charged particle that revolves around the nucleus of the atom. Protons and neutrons constitute the majority of the atomic mass and reside within the nucleus. Protons, neutrons, and electrons form together to create elements. Table 21-1 lists elements found in the human body.

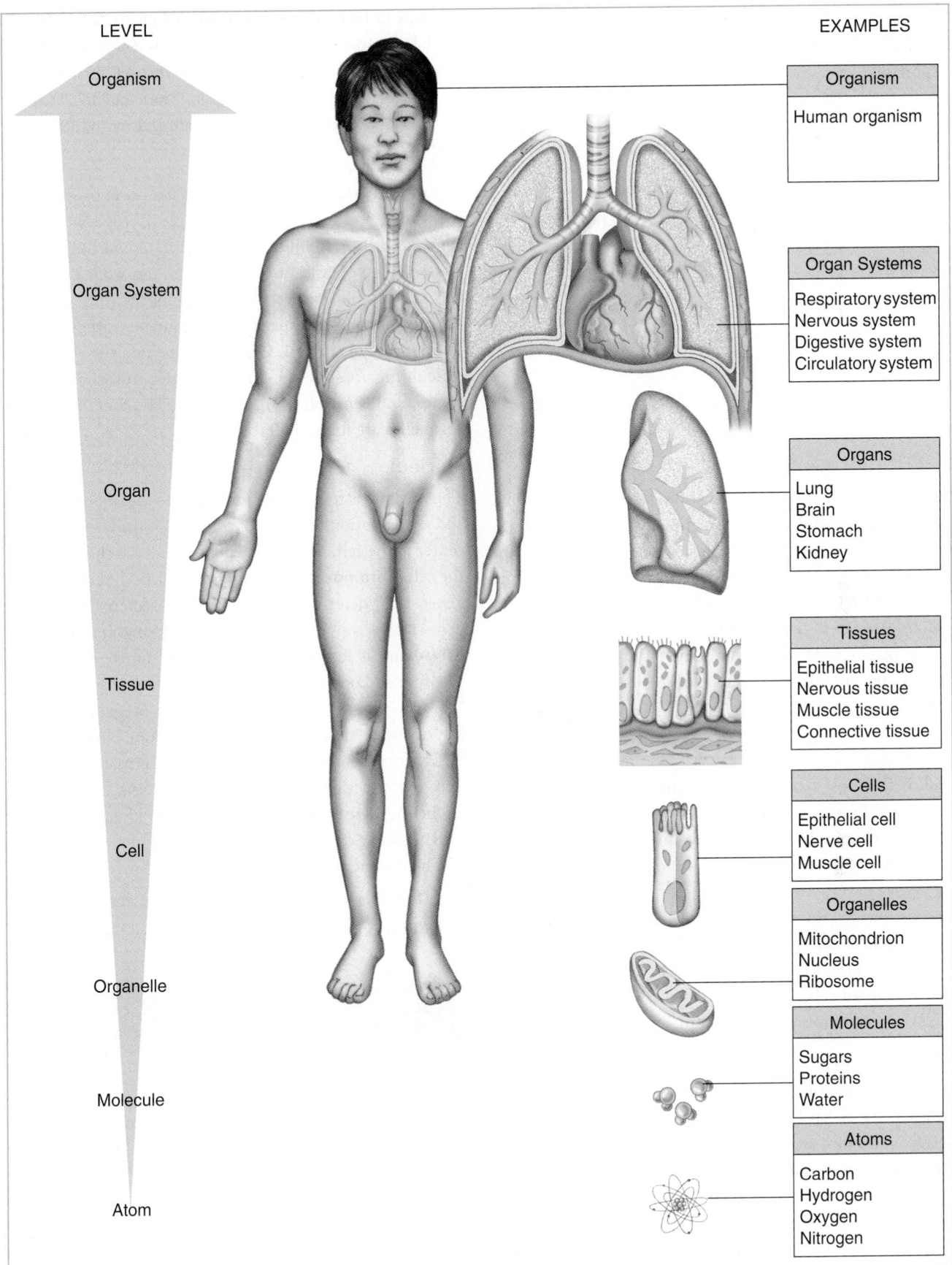

LEVEL

Organism

Organ System

Organ

Tissue

Cell

Organelle

Molecule

Atom

EXAMPLES

Organism
Human organism

Organ Systems
Respiratory system Nervous system Digestive system Circulatory system

Organs
Lung Brain Stomach Kidney

Tissues
Epithelial tissue Nervous tissue Muscle tissue Connective tissue

Cells
Epithelial cell Nerve cell Muscle cell

Organelles
Mitochondrion Nucleus Ribosome

Molecules
Sugars Proteins Water

Atoms
Carbon Hydrogen Oxygen Nitrogen

FIGURE 21-1 Organization of the human body.

TABLE 21-1 Elements Found in the Human Body

Symbol	Element	Symbol	Element
Al	Aluminum	Mn	Manganese
C	Carbon	Mg	Magnesium
Ca	Calcium	N	Nitrogen
Cl	Chlorine	O or O_2	Oxygen
Co	Cobalt	P	Phosphorus
Cu	Copper	K	Potassium
F	Fluorine	Na	Sodium
H	Hydrogen	S	Sulfur
I	Iodine	Zn	Zinc
Fe	Iron		

MOLECULES

A **molecule** is a chemical combination of two or more atoms that forms a specific chemical compound. In water molecules (H_2O), two hydrogen atoms and one oxygen atom are chemically joined together. A single drop of water is composed of millions of water molecules.

Molecules can move and thus can take the form of solids, liquids, or gases. Molecules are farthest apart in the form of gases and are closest together, moving slowly, in solid formation.

CELLS

A **cell** is the most basic unit of life and is often considered the building block of the human body. There are millions of different types of cells. Some are organisms unto themselves, whereas others function only as part of a larger organism. Our bodies have bone cells, nerve cells, fat cells, reproductive cells, skeletal muscle cells, blood cells, and smooth muscle cells, just to name a few (Figure 21-2). Though each cell has a unique function and feature, many features are recognized among all cells. Every cell has three common components: the cell membrane, cytoplasm, and the nucleus.

Cell Membrane

The outer covering of the cell is called the **cell membrane**. Cell membranes have the capability of allowing some substances to pass into and out of the cell while denying passage of other substances, making it selectively permeable. This selectivity allows cells to receive nutrition and dispose of waste just as the human being eats food and disposes of waste. The cell membrane also helps maintain the cell's shape.

The surface of some cells, as in the respiratory system, is covered with small hairlike projections called **cilia**. These cilia aid in increasing the overall surface area of a cell. Cilia work by propelling substances along a cell's surface which increases the cell's ability to absorb water and nutrients. Similar in structure to cilia are **flagella**. These tail-like structures enable a sperm cell to move through the reproductive tract.

Cytoplasm

Cytoplasm is a jellylike substance found between the cell membrane and the nuclear membrane. Cytoplasm is 80 percent water and generally clear in color, resembling the white of an egg, cytoplasm provides storage and work areas for the cell. **Organelles** are structures found within cytoplasm. Each organelle has a specific function and purpose to maintain vitality of the cell. Organelles include the endoplasmic reticulum, ribosomes, Golgi apparatus, mitochondria, lysosomes, and centrioles (Figure 21-3). The functions of these organelles are found in Table 21-2.

Nucleus

The **nucleus** is responsible for the cell's metabolism, growth, and reproduction. Because of this, it is considered the control center of the cell. Within the nucleus are the chromosomes of the cell. **Chromosomes** are microscopic bodies that carry the genes that determine hereditary characteristics. A single gene makes up each segment of **deoxyribonucleic acid (DNA)** and is located in a specific site on the chromosome. The human body contains 23 pairs of chromosomes.

DNA provides the cell's blueprint or genetic makeup. DNA is shaped in a double helix: two long chains of nucleic acid that twist around each other. DNA is mandatory for cellular reproduction. **Ribonucleic acid (RNA)** is a single chain of chemical bases. RNA takes the form of messenger RNA (mRNA) and transfer RNA (tRNA).

The nucleic functions include the following:

- Storage and organization of genes and chromosomes
- Transport of genetic productions

PROFESSIONALISM

THE LAW

Before beginning documentation of a procedure, be sure that you have the correct patient's chart. Documentation should always be done after the procedure has been completed, never before. This will ensure accurate charting and will allow you to describe the response of the patient to the procedure. The patient's chart is a legal document and can be requested in a court of law. Be sure all documentation is legible and accurate.

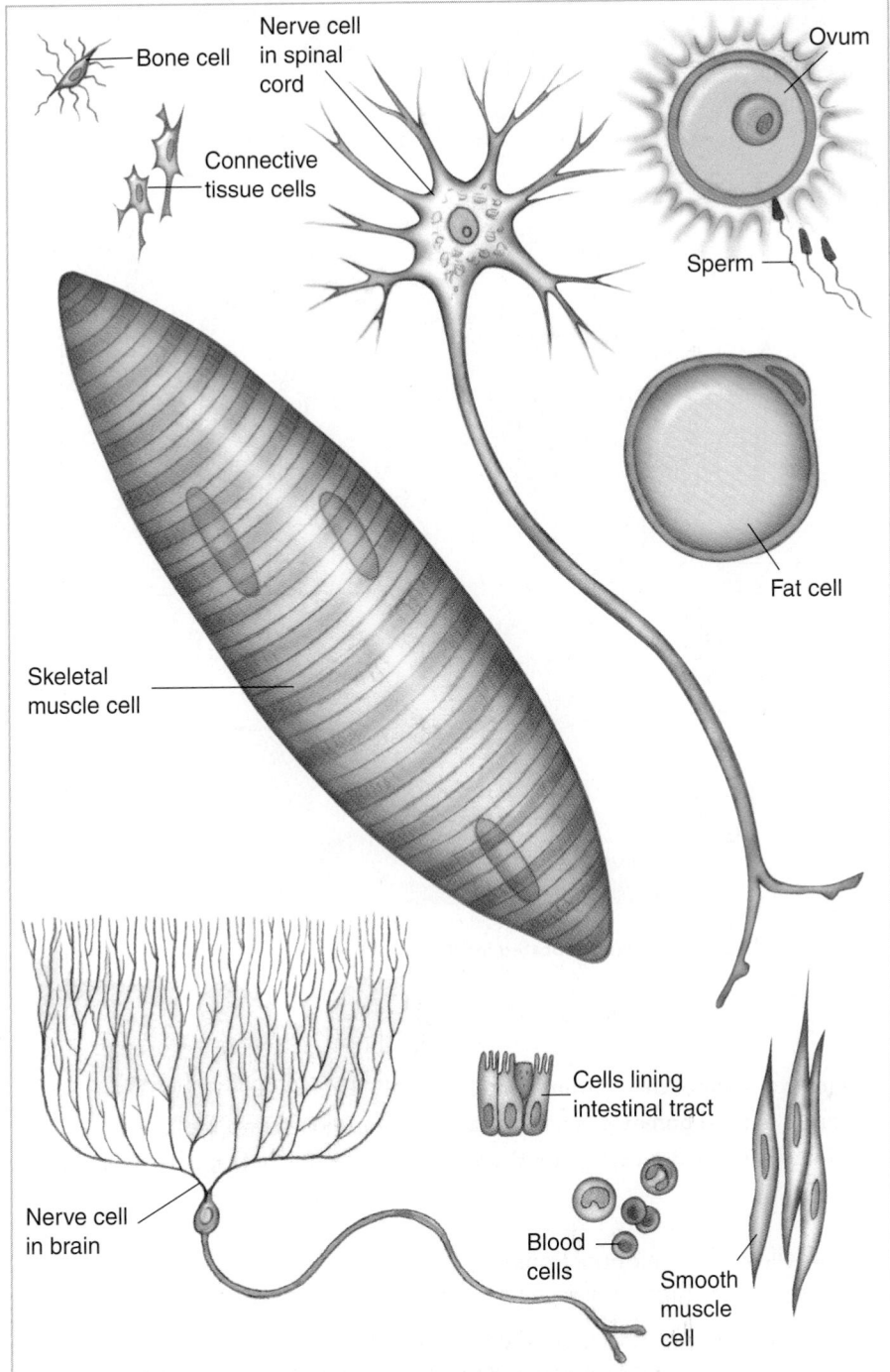

FIGURE 21-2 Cells are often described as the basic building blocks of the human body. There are millions of different cells.

- Production of messages through RNA (via mRNA and tRNA)
- Production of ribosomes
- Uncoiling of DNA to replicate key genes

Mitosis and Cell Division

A cell divides its chromosomes into two daughter cells via the processes of mitosis and cytokinesis. After cell division, each cell has 23 pairs of, or 46 chromosomes. During **mitosis** the nucleus of the cell divides. The stages of mitosis are prophase, prometaphase, metaphase, anaphase, and telophase (Figure 21-4). During **cytokinesis**, which follows mitosis, the cytoplasm divides into the two identical daughter cells. As cells tend to have a very short duration, mitosis and cytokinesis allow them to be renewed on a regular basis.

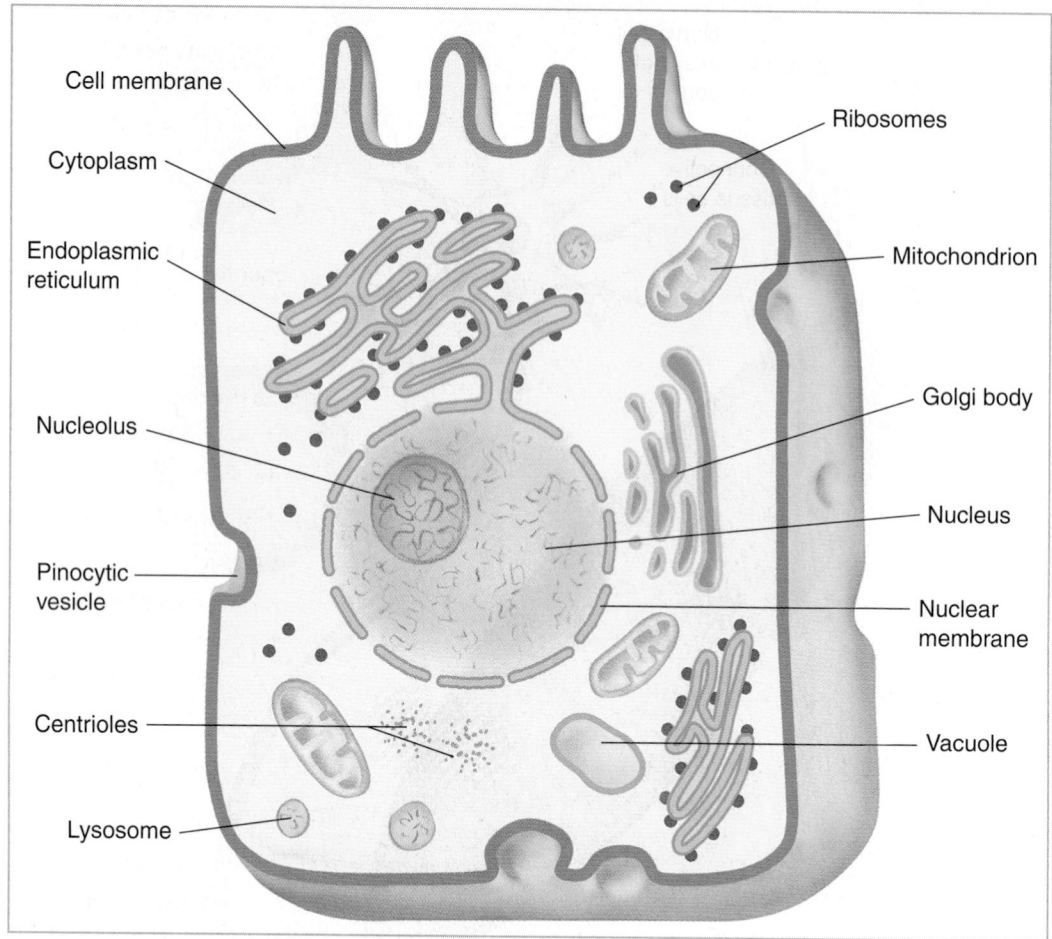

FIGURE 21-3   **Major parts of the cell and the structures located inside the cell.**

Meiosis

Meiosis is a process in which cells reduce their chromosomal number from 46 to 23 in order to form **gametes**, such as ova and sperm. When two gametes (one from each parent) are combined, a zygote is formed. The process of meiosis includes two complete phases:

- **Meiosis I**—Prophase I, Anaphase I, prometaphase I, Metaphase I, and Telophase I

TABLE 21-2 Cellular Organelles and Their Functions

Endoplasmic reticulum	A tubular network that is attached to the nuclear membrane. Rough endoplasmic reticulum has ribosomes embedded within; smooth endoplasmic reticulum does not.
Ribosomes	Location for the production of protein that is essential to the vitality of the cell.
Golgi apparatus	A saclike membranous structure that sorts, modifies, and transports various proteins throughout the cell.
Mitochondria	Considered the powerhouse of the cell, it is responsible for the production of adenosine triphosphate (ATP), a form of cellular energy.
Lysosomes	Sometimes considered the "stomach" of the cell, the lysosomes are the sites of digestion of proteins, lipids, and carbohydrates. Anything that is not digested by the lysosome is sent to the cellular membrane for removal from the cell.
Centrioles	These paired organelles are found lying at 90-degree angles near the nucleus. Centrioles are involved in cellular division.

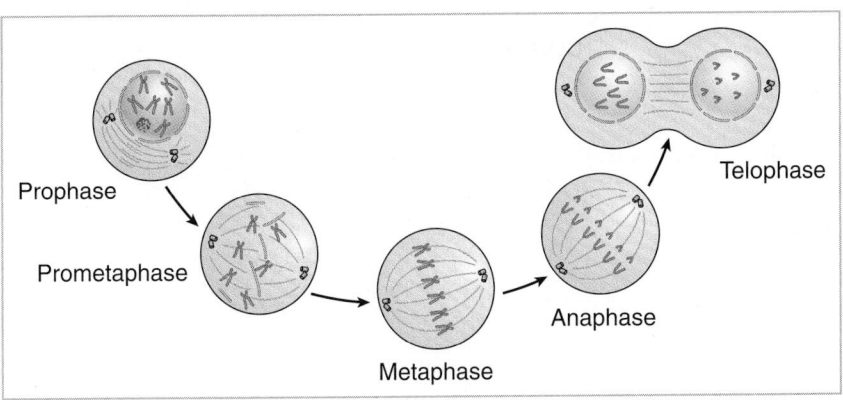

FIGURE 21-4 **Stages of mitosis.**

- Meiosis II—Prophase II, Anaphase II, Prometaphase II, Metaphase II and Telophase II

TISSUES

The next level of organization is the formation of tissues. **Tissues** result from the grouping of specialized cells that share the same function and purpose. The human body contains four types of tissue: epithelial, connective, muscle, and nerve (Figure 21-5).

Epithelial Tissue

Epithelial tissue is found on the outer layer of skin, covering the surface of organs, and lining the walls of body cavities. It also forms ducts, tubes, and parts of certain glands. Sheetlike in appearance, epithelial tissue is arranged in a flat formation, sometimes several layers thick. Functions of this tissue include absorption, secretion, excretion, and protection.

Connective Tissue

Of the four body tissues, connective tissue is most abundant. Connective tissue can be liquid or gel-like and fills spaces between cells. It has a vast assortment of functions, which include forming a support network for organs of the body, covering muscles, and connecting muscles to bones and bones to joints. In fact, bone is an extremely dense form of connective tissue.

Muscle Tissue

There are three unique types of muscle tissue in the human body:

- Voluntary or **striated** muscle tissue forms voluntary muscles such as skeletal muscle. They are striated, or striped, in appearance. Voluntary muscles are controlled by a person's will.

- Involuntary or smooth muscle tissues are controlled by the autonomic nervous system. A person's will does not control movement of involuntary muscles.

- Cardiac muscle tissue, which forms the heart muscles, is a specialized form of striated muscle and is under the control of the autonomic nervous system.

Nerve Tissue

Nerve tissue, composed of **neurons** (nerve cells), acts as the functional unit of the nervous system. Nerve tissue has two properties: excitability and conductivity. Nervous cells, and in turn nervous tissue, are active, which demonstrates the excitability property. Because nerve cells transmit impulses and coordinate activities in the body, nerve tissue is said to be conductive.

BODY ORGANS AND SYSTEMS

Just as a group of similarly functioning cells form tissue, similarly functioning tissues form **organs**. Together, organs that work together for a common purpose form body **systems**. All body systems work together to support and maintain homeostasis of the human body (Figure 21-6).

Chemistry

For cells to receive nourishment and eliminate wastes, materials must be transported both to and from the cell. This can be done via passive or active transport.

Passive transport does not require the cell to use energy; however, it does involve a number of processes, including diffusion, osmosis, and filtration. **Diffusion** involves moving dissolved particles from an area of greater concentration to an area of lesser concentration until they are evenly distributed. **Osmosis** is a form of diffusion whereby water is pulled through a semipermeable membrane, once again moving from areas of greater to lesser concentration. **Filtration** requires mechanical pressure to diffuse dissolved particles through membranes.

On the other hand, **active transport** requires cellular energy to carry materials from an area of lesser concentration to an area of greater concentration. The cellular energy used in active transport is adenosine triphosphate (ATP). Through active transport, cells are able to obtain what they need through tissue fluid. This can be done through two methods:

- **Phagocytosis**—In this method, the cell engulfs a solid particle, such as bacteria.

- **Pinocytosis**—In this method, the cell "drinks" the fluid required.

ELECTROLYTES

An **electrolyte** is a molecule that conducts electricity. When dissolved in water or other bodily fluids, electrolytes break down into ions that move to either a negative (cathode) or

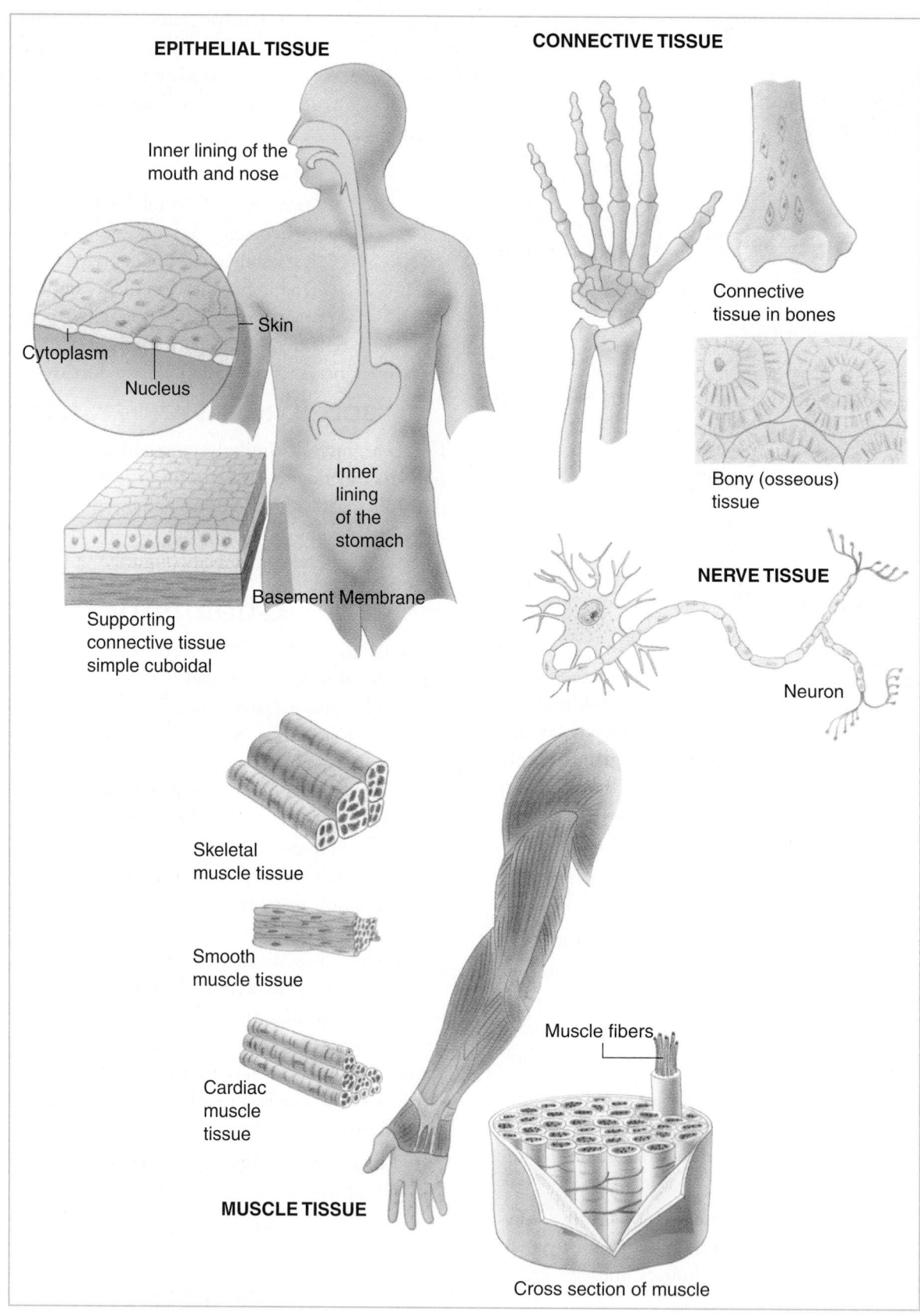

EPITHELIAL TISSUE

Inner lining of the mouth and nose

Cytoplasm

Nucleus

Skin

Inner lining of the stomach

Basement Membrane

Supporting connective tissue simple cuboidal

CONNECTIVE TISSUE

Connective tissue in bones

Bony (osseous) tissue

NERVE TISSUE

Neuron

Skeletal muscle tissue

Smooth muscle tissue

Cardiac muscle tissue

Muscle fibers

MUSCLE TISSUE

Cross section of muscle

FIGURE 21-5 Types of tissue in the human body.

Organ System		Major Functions
Integumentary system	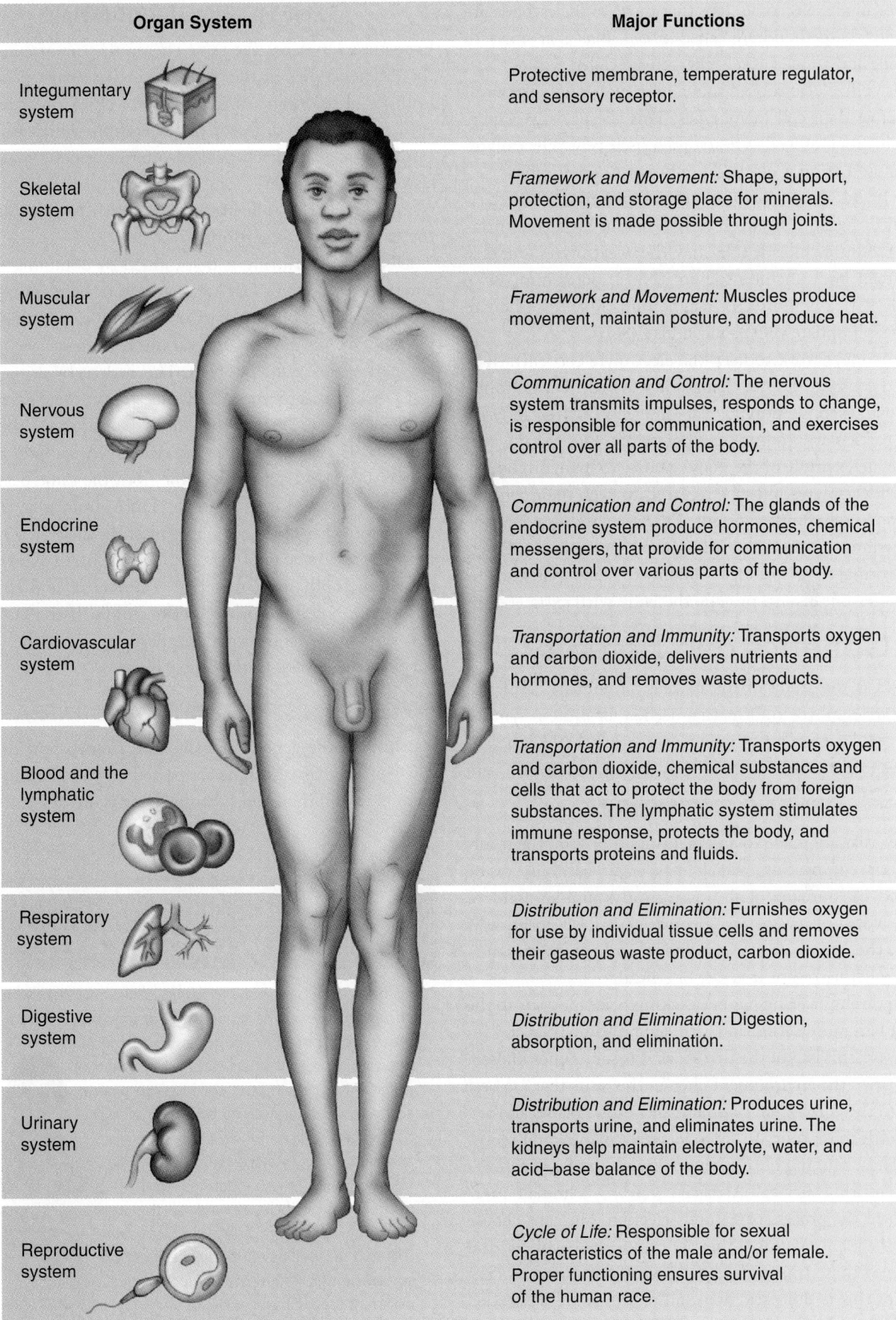	Protective membrane, temperature regulator, and sensory receptor.
Skeletal system		*Framework and Movement:* Shape, support, protection, and storage place for minerals. Movement is made possible through joints.
Muscular system		*Framework and Movement:* Muscles produce movement, maintain posture, and produce heat.
Nervous system		*Communication and Control:* The nervous system transmits impulses, responds to change, is responsible for communication, and exercises control over all parts of the body.
Endocrine system		*Communication and Control:* The glands of the endocrine system produce hormones, chemical messengers, that provide for communication and control over various parts of the body.
Cardiovascular system		*Transportation and Immunity:* Transports oxygen and carbon dioxide, delivers nutrients and hormones, and removes waste products.
Blood and the lymphatic system		*Transportation and Immunity:* Transports oxygen and carbon dioxide, chemical substances and cells that act to protect the body from foreign substances. The lymphatic system stimulates immune response, protects the body, and transports proteins and fluids.
Respiratory system		*Distribution and Elimination:* Furnishes oxygen for use by individual tissue cells and removes their gaseous waste product, carbon dioxide.
Digestive system		*Distribution and Elimination:* Digestion, absorption, and elimination.
Urinary system		*Distribution and Elimination:* Produces urine, transports urine, and eliminates urine. The kidneys help maintain electrolyte, water, and acid–base balance of the body.
Reproductive system		*Cycle of Life:* Responsible for sexual characteristics of the male and/or female. Proper functioning ensures survival of the human race.

FIGURE 21-6 Organ systems of the human body.

positive (anode) electrode. Ions that move to the cathode are positively charged and are called *cations*. Ions that move to the anode and are negatively charged are called *anions*.

Cells utilize electrolytes to maintain voltage or electrical force across their cell membranes. This is especially important in neurons, as well as heart and muscle cells. Electrolytes are also used to carry electrical impulses to other cells.

The body's fluids, including blood, plasma, and interstitial fluid (the fluid between cells), contain high concentrations of sodium chloride (NaCl). Other electrolytes found in the human body include sodium (Na^+), potassium (K^+), chloride (Cl), calcium (Ca), magnesium (Mg), bicarbonate (HCO_3), phosphate (PO_4), and sulfate (SO_4).

The kidneys work to keep the electrolyte concentrations in blood constant despite changes in the body. For example, when you exercise heavily, you lose electrolytes in your sweat, particularly sodium and potassium. Once again, this provides an example of the body's ability to maintain homeostasis. Electrolytes must be replaced to keep their concentrations in body fluids constant. Therefore, sodium chloride or potassium chloride is added to many sports drinks. Sugar and flavorings are also added, not only to make sports drinks taste better but also to provide the body with extra energy.

Genetics and Heredity

Genetics is the study of the makeup of animals or plants. DNA carries all the information needed for protein synthesis and replication of cells. In living organisms, DNA is organized in chromosomes and located in the nucleus of each cell.

GENETIC ENGINEERING

Changes that are made to an organism's DNA are the result of genetic engineering, which may occur naturally or be achieved by humans. This increasingly popular field of science is still relatively new. Because genetic engineering is so new, the effects are not yet known and controversy surrounds whether or not it is safe or ethical.

Genetic engineering has been taking place for years in the form of natural selection and artificial breeding. Natural selection, or "survival of the fittest" as it is sometimes known, occurs when the environment chooses the traits that are best suited to the current environment and allows plants and animals with those traits to reproductively mature and reproduce. This changing of the genes within a species is nature's way of ensuring survival. Artificial breeding is human intervention in the process of natural selection. Humans choose traits for a plant or animal that they think are beneficial and then breed those traits into the organism's offspring. An example of this is domestic dogs, all of which are descended from the wolf family through artificial breeding.

GENETIC FINGERPRINTING

Everyone's DNA has the same chemical structure; however, the difference lies in the order of the base pairs. There are millions of base pairs in each person's DNA, meaning that each person has a different sequence from which he or she can be identified. Each person's unique genetic makeup is also known as genetic, or DNA, fingerprinting. Identical twins provide the only instance in which two people carry the same genetic fingerprint.

DNA fingerprinting is determined by obtaining a small amount of a person's DNA, usually from hair, sexual fluid, blood, or saliva, but any part of a human can be used. This piece of DNA is put through various tests to extract and isolate part of the strand of DNA. This is done by using chemicals, such as enzymes, and electricity to separate the different parts of DNA. The sample analysis shows the DNA patterns. If two patterns from two DNA samples match, they are very likely to have come from the same person. In the case of proving parentage, DNA from the child is matched to that of the people requesting the test. The tests show the relationship of the people to the particular child by matching both the maternal (mother's) and paternal (father's) DNA fingerprints to the child's. If the DNA fingerprint shows significant similarities, then the people participating in the test are the parents.

GENETICS, HEREDITY, AND DISEASE

Heredity is the genetic transmission from parent to child. The genes for certain traits are passed down in families from parents to children, and hereditary traits are determined by specific genes.

PROFESSIONALISM
THE WORKPLACE

Perhaps the best way to build skills and review for a certification exam is to select a practicum or externship that is very broad in scope, such as a family practice, internal medicine, or pediatric office. After passing the certification exam, some medical assistants prefer to work in a specialty office. Once a medical assistant works in a specialty office, unused skills may become antiquated. A periodic review of the anatomy and physiology chapters in this text, as well as continuing education opportunities, can help a medical assistant stay current and versatile.

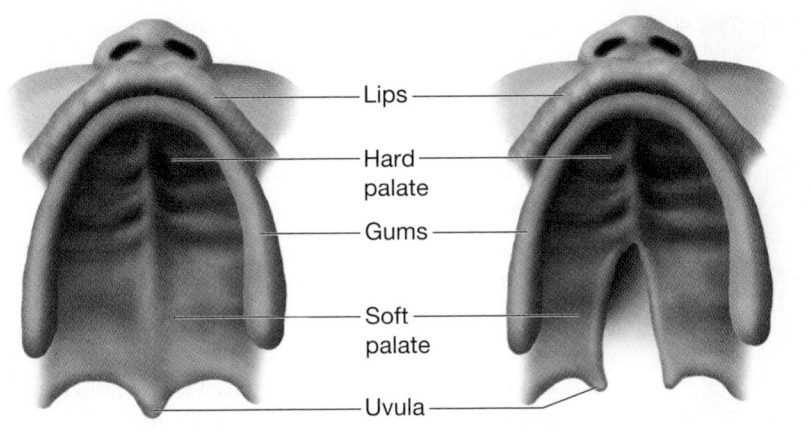
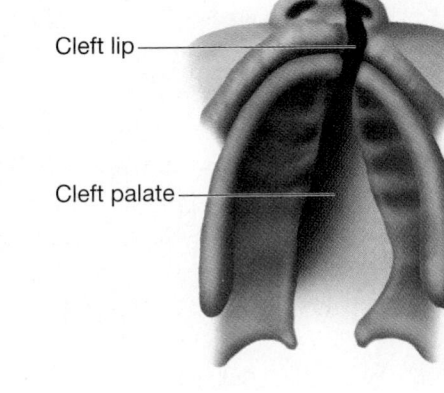

| Normal palate in infant | Partial cleft palate | Complete cleft palate and cleft lip |

FIGURE 21-7 **Cleft palate.**

Individuals carry two genes for each trait: one from the mother's egg and one from the father's sperm. When an individual reproduces, the two genes split up (segregate) and end up in separate gametes.

GENETIC DISORDERS

Genetic disorders are considered medical conditions and are caused by mutations in a single gene or a set of genes. Mutations are changes in the DNA sequence of a gene. Genetic mutations can occur at any point during life. It is important to differentiate that it is not a gene or genes that cause the illness but rather a mutation that causes the normal genes to operate improperly. A genetic disorder that is present at birth is frequently referred to as a **congenital disorder**. It may also be called a *birth defect*. The following are some of the more common congenital disorders:

- Albinism is a congenital, but nonpathological disorder. A recessive gene mutation causes hereditary lack of pigment in the skin, hair, and eyes. The patient may complain of photophobia and is prone to sunburn because protective melanin is not present.

- Attention-deficit/hyperactivity disorder (ADHD) is a disease that can affect both children and adults. It is characterized by the person having difficulty organizing and completing a task. The cause may be due to genetic factors, and it is ten times more prevalent in boys than in girls. No cure is known, but treatment often includes medications or counseling. Abstinence from certain foods or food additives may be recommended if these are determined to be part of the cause of hyperactivity. Symptoms of ADHD may subside or even disappear with time.

- Cleft palate (Figure 21-7) is a congenital defect in the roof of the mouth that occurs when the palatine bones

of the skull do not close properly. The cleft causes a passageway between the mouth and nasal cavities. It may also be associated with a cleft upper lip, and it affects females more often than males. Initially, the infant has special needs for feeding. Surgical repairs are usually performed within the first year of life and are generally successful in repairing the defect.

- Color deficiency is a disorder that was previously called color blindness. It often entails difficulty in distinguishing between reds and greens. It is an inherited, sex-linked disorder, usually passed from mother to son. In total color deficiency, the person is unable to perceive any color at all due to a defect in or absence of cones in the retina.

- Cystic fibrosis (CF) is a chronic and progressive disease usually diagnosed in childhood that causes mucus to become thick, dry, and sticky. The mucus builds up and clogs passages in many of the body's organs, primarily the lungs and the pancreas. In the lungs, the mucus can lead to serious breathing problems and lung disease. In the pancreas, the mucus can lead to malnutrition and problems with growth and development. People with CF have an average life expectancy of about 32 years, although new treatments offer hope for longer and healthier lives.

- Down syndrome (trisomy 21) is a disorder caused by the person having an extra chromosome, usually number 21 (hence, the name). A few of the major features seen include marked sloping of the forehead, a short broad hand with a single palmer crease (known as a simian crease), and a flat nose. A mother who gives birth after the age of 40 has a higher risk of delivering an infant with Down syndrome. Amniocentesis is generally used as a tool for diagnosing this disorder. See Figure 21-8 for a photo of someone with this anomaly.

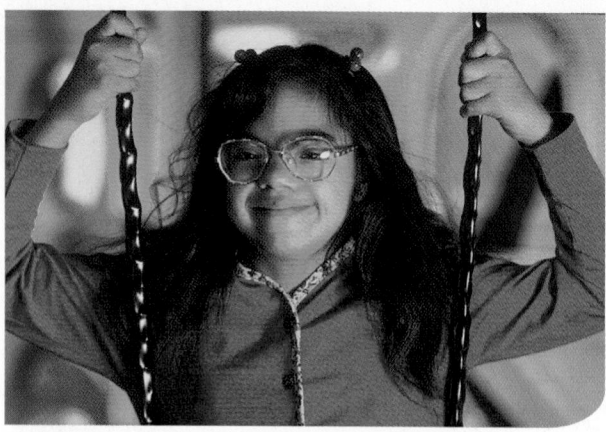

FIGURE 21-8 Girl with Down syndrome. © Beebe/Custom Medical Stock Photo.

- Fragile X syndrome, also known as Martin-Bell syndrome, Marker X syndrome, and FRAXA syndrome, is the most common form of inherited mental retardation. Individuals with this condition have developmental delays, variable levels of mental retardation, and behavioral and emotional difficulties. They may also have characteristic physical traits. Generally, males are affected with moderate mental retardation and females with mild mental retardation. Fragile X is caused by a mutation in the FMR-1 gene, located on the X chromosome. The role of this gene is unclear, but it is probably important in early development.

- Hemochromatosis is an inherited disorder of excessive body accumulation of iron. It is common among the Caucasian population, affecting approximately 1 in 400 individuals of European ancestry. Hemochromatosis patients are believed to absorb excessive amounts of iron from the diet. Since the human body has limited ways of eliminating the absorbed iron, the iron accumulates over time in the liver, bone marrow, pancreas, skin, and testicles. This accumulation of iron in these organs causes them to function poorly. Patients with early hemochromatosis have no symptoms and are unaware of their condition. The disease may be discovered when elevated iron blood levels are noted as a result of routine blood testing. In males, symptoms may not appear until 40 to 50 years of age. Iron deposits in the skin cause darkening of the skin. Because females lose iron through menstrual blood loss, they develop organ damage from iron accumulation 15 to 20 years later than men on average.

- Hemophilia is a hereditary, sex-linked disorder in which the blood coagulation time is greatly increased. It is due to a recessive gene mutation in the X chromosome. Females carry the recessive gene and transmit the disorder to their male offspring.

- Klinefelter's syndrome is a congenital endocrine disorder. Primary testicular failure occurs that usually is not evident until puberty. The testes are small and firm, and gynecomastia may be present. Boys with this disorder will have abnormally long legs. This disorder also can lead to subnormal intelligence.

- Muscular dystrophy is a genetic disease characterized by a gradual atrophy and weakening of the muscle. It is more frequent in males. The most common type is Duchenne muscular dystrophy, which accounts for

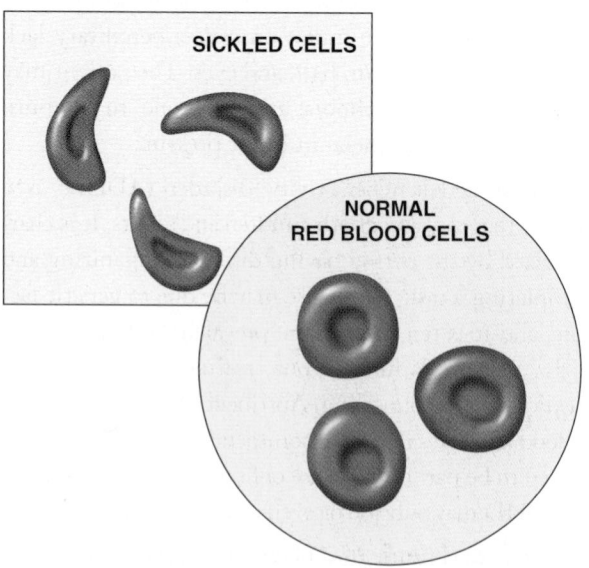

FIGURE 21-9 Sickled and normal red blood cells.

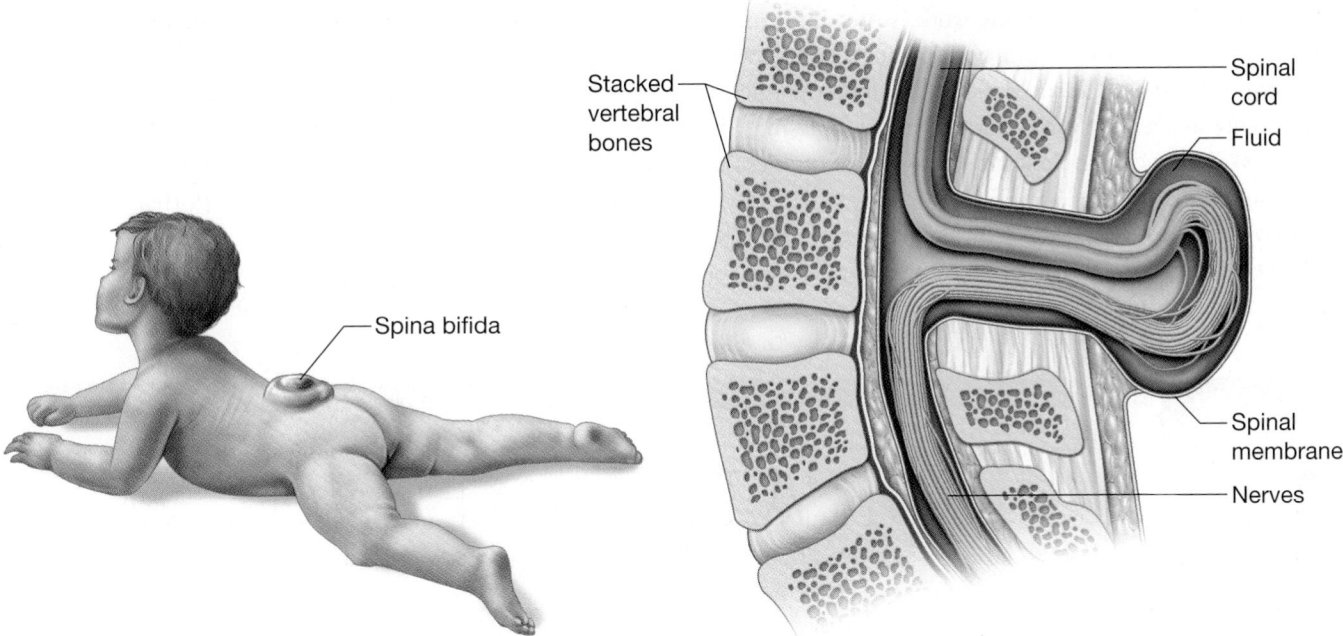

FIGURE 21-10 (A) An infant with spina bifida; (B) the spinal cord protrudes from the body.

50 percent of all cases. The onset is at an early age, and the patient is usually confined to a wheelchair by the age of 12. Death often occurs within 10 to 15 years of onset of symptoms. Unfortunately, there is no successful treatment, although physical therapy and exercise are recommended to prevent more atrophy of muscles.

- Phenylketonuria (PKU) is due to a recessive gene mutation. A defective enzyme causes the body to be unable to oxidize the amino acid phenylalanine into tyrosine. If the condition is not treated early, mental retardation occurs due to brain damage. Many states require testing at birth to detect PKU.

- Sickle cell anemia (Figure 21-9) is a hereditary, chronic form of anemia that is due to a recessive gene mutation. This disorder is discussed in Chapter 27.

- Spina bifida (Figure 21-10) is a congenital neural tube defect. The posterior vertebral arch has a developmental anomaly. In some cases, the spinal cord and its membranes may protrude. Most often the abnormality occurs in the lumbar region.

- Talipes (clubfoot) is a congenital deformity of the foot. Treatment may include casting of the foot or use of special orthopedic shoes to assist with walking.

- Tay-Sachs disease (TSD) is an inherited disorder that tends to affect people of central and northern European Jewish (Ashkenazi) or French-Canadian ancestry. The faulty gene targets the nervous system. Symptoms first appear in a previously healthy baby at around 6 months of age. Over a short period of time, the baby stops moving and smiling, becomes paralyzed, and eventually dies. Most children with TSD die before their fifth birthday. There is no cure.

- Turner syndrome is a congenital disorder caused by failure of the ovaries to respond to the stimulation of pituitary hormones. Intelligence may be impaired, amenorrhea may be present, and the patient is usually short in stature.

SUMMARY

In this chapter, you have learned of the organizational components of the body. As with most matter in the world, our bodies are made up of atoms that form molecules. These in turn form cells. A group of cells with similar functions forms tissues, and tissues with similar functions form organs. These organs then form systems that make up the human body. As each of these systems performs its function, the body can remain in homeostasis. Although disease processes may occur, the body is remarkable in its ability to fight off infections or, in some cases, as in cellular development, even to regenerate.

The systems of the body (as discussed in future chapters) are the integumentary, skeletal, muscular, nervous, circulatory, immune, respiratory, digestive, urinary, endocrine, and reproductive systems.

The cell, like a city, performs work, stores information, and uses molecules to perform work, thus creating waste that requires disposal. Parts of the cell include the nucleus, cell membrane, endoplasmic reticulum, cytoplasm, ribosomes, lysosomes, centrioles, mitochondria, ribosomes, and Golgi apparatus.

Body processes can be active or passive. Active transport uses energy, whereas passive transportation happens without energy consumption.

Genetics is a relatively new science with a lot of potential to help patients. Each person, unless a twin, has unique genetics. Understanding familial and inherited characteristics and disease risk can help the medical assistant to gather appropriate data from patients. Knowledge of congenital disorders can help predict the risk that a child may inherit one.

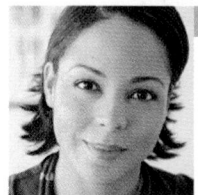 21 CHAPTER REVIEW

COMPETENCY REVIEW

1. Define and spell the terms to learn for this chapter.
2. List the organization of the body from atom to organism.
3. List five parts of the cell and their function.
4. What are the three types of muscle tissue?
5. What are the four functions of epithelial tissue?
6. What are the two properties of nerve tissue?
7. Which part of the cell is known as the control center and why?
8. Select five genetic disorders and describe their pathology.

PREPARING FOR THE CERTIFICATION EXAM

1. Which part of the cell allows for selective permeability?
   a. cytoplasm
   b. cell membrane
   c. vacuole
   d. Golgi body
   e. endoplasmic reticulum

2. Which of the following systems is responsible for elimination of waste products?
   a. reproductive
   b. respiratory
   c. cardiovascular
   d. musculoskeletal
   e. nervous

3. Talipes is also known as
   a. PKU
   b. anemia
   c. club foot
   d. Fragile X syndrome
   e. cleft palate

4. This organelle is considered the "power house" of the cell:
   a. Golgi apparatus
   b. nucleus
   c. lysosome
   d. mitochondria
   e. ribosome

5. This is the term for a positively charged particle:
   a. atom
   b. proton
   c. electron
   d. molecule
   e. neutron

6. Which cell structure is responsible for the production of ribosomes?
   a. nucleus
   b. cytoplasm
   c. endoplasmic reticulum
   d. Golgi bodies
   e. mitochondria

7. Which phase directly follows prophase during mitosis?
   a. prophase II
   b. cytokinesis
   c. anaphase
   d. metaphase
   e. telophase

8. Which genetic disorder is a hereditary, sex-linked disorder that affects blood coagulation?
   a. Klinefelter's syndrome
   b. muscular dystrophy
   c. hemochromatosis
   d. Fragile X
   e. hemophilia

9. The lung is considered a/an
   a. organ system
   b. organelle
   c. cell
   d. tissue
   e. organ

10. What is responsible for carrying electrical impulses to other cells?
    a. ions
    b. cations
    c. electrolytes
    d. anions
    e. plasma

CRITICAL THINKING

1. Lucy finds that many patients have a variety of genetically related diseases and disorders. She is particularly interested in the patient cases that deal with trisomy 21, as her younger cousin was born with it. What is the more common term for trisomy 21, and how is it generally diagnosed prior to birth?

2. If you were in Lucy's position, what would you like or dislike about having the opportunity to shadow and work in a genetic clinic of a hospital?

3. Lucy is learning that the genetic clinic at Pearson General Hospital has had an unusually high number of cases of children with Tay-Sachs disease (TSD) over the past 15 years. Which cultural groups are most often afflicted with TSD?

ON THE JOB

Kara is a medical assistant for an OB/GYN office. Kara is working with Dr. Miller, who is about to tell his patient Barbara Klemens that the results of her amniocentesis are not favorable. The test reveals a chromosomal anomaly that is present in patients with Down syndrome.

1. What is the alternate term for Down syndrome that is commonly used in the medical field? Why is it given this name?
2. What are some physical characteristics of Down syndrome?
3. Who has a higher risk of delivering an infant with Down syndrome?

INTERNET ACTIVITY

Use the Internet to find information pertaining to an amniocentesis procedure.

MEDMEDIA

Additional interactive resources and activities for this chapter can be found:

On your student DVD: View applicable procedure videos on the DVD-ROM found in the back of this book.

MyHealthProfessionsKit.com: Test your knowledge of this chapter with games and activities. MyHealthProfessionsKit also includes resources, helpful links, and a Spanish audio glossary.

Medical Assisting Interactive: Practice your procedures as a medical assistant in this simulated doctor's office. This can be accessed through MyHealthProfessionsKit.com.

22

The Integumentary System

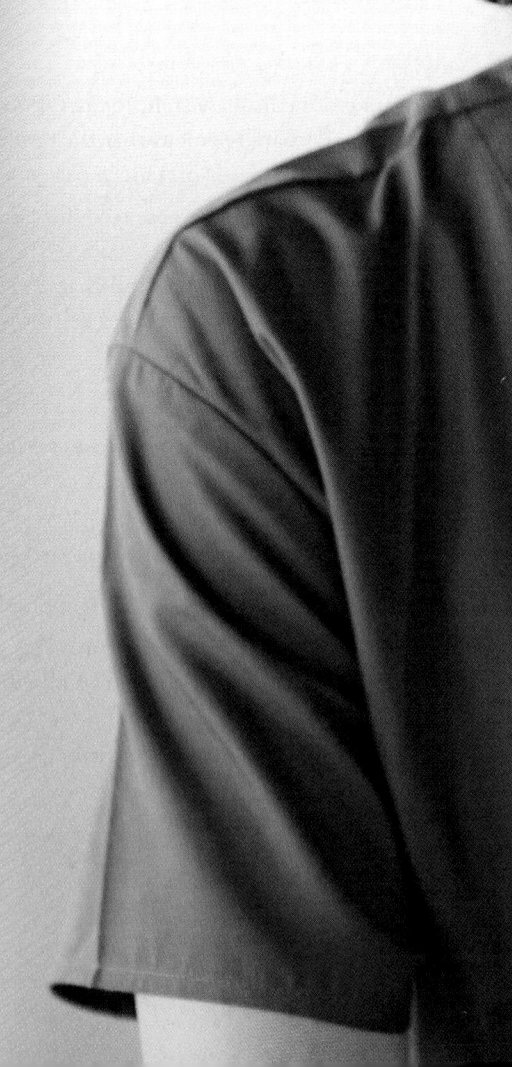

LEARNING OBJECTIVES

After completing this chapter, you should be able to:

- Define and spell the terms to learn for this chapter.

- List and describe the functions of the skin.

- Discuss the layers of the epidermis.

- Discuss the layers of the dermis.

- List and discuss the accessory structures of the skin.

- Differentiate between basal cell carcinoma, squamous cell carcinoma, and malignant melanoma.

- Explain skin differences of the child and the older adult.

- Identify and explain common disorders associated with the integumentary system.

- Identify and describe forms of skin care treatments that are used to help reverse the signs of aging.

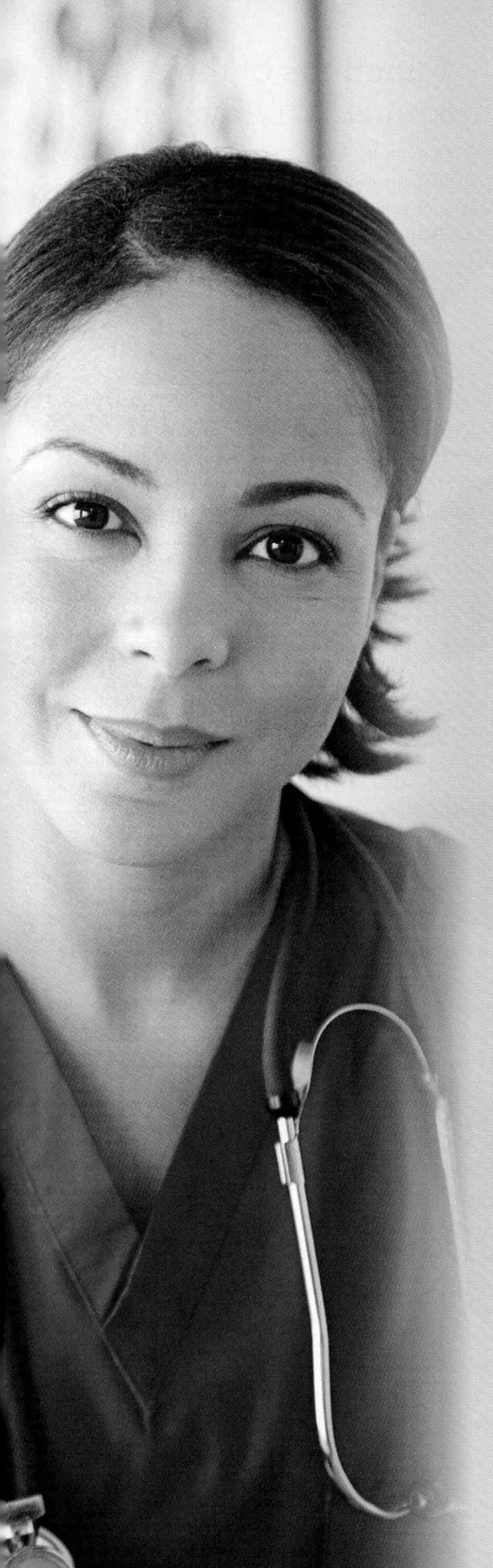

CHAPTER OUTLINE

CASE STUDY

Julie Yeung is a 29-year-old patient of Pearson Physicians Group. Julie, of Italian descent, and her husband Lou, of Chinese descent, have not been successful conceiving a child. She has recently been diagnosed with an ovarian disorder known as polycystic ovarian syndrome. Today, she is seeing Dr. Miller for increased dark-hair growth on her face and chin.

433

CERTIFICATION LINK

CMA (AAMA)	RMA	CMAS (AMT)
Anatomy and physiology	Anatomy and physiology	Medical assisting foundation
Systems (including structure, function, related conditions and diseases, and their relationships)	Body systems	Anatomy and physiology
	Disorders and diseases of the body	Medical terminology

Weighing more than 6 pounds and covering more than 3,000 square inches, the skin is the largest organ of the human body. Skin and its accessory structures comprise the integumentary system. Accessory structures of the integumentary system include hair, nails, sebaceous (oil) glands, and sudoriferous (sweat) glands.

Functions of the Integumentary System

The skin works in multiple ways to provide homeostasis for the body. The five main functions of the integumentary system include protection, regulation, sensation, absorption, and secretion. By providing these functions, the integumentary system, along with the other body systems, can maintain the internal conditions that are essential to the function of the body.

PROTECTION

Intact skin serves as a protective barrier to the internal structures and compartments of the body. The skin prevents harmful agents (such as bacteria, viruses, and pollution) from entering the body. Cuts and abrasions, which cause the skin not to be intact, allow harmful bacteria to enter the body. The skin guards the body against the sun's ultraviolet rays by producing a protective pigmentation called melanin. Vitamin D, which is essential to our body, is also produced by the skin.

REGULATION

The skin also regulates body temperature. When the body temperature rises and requires cooling, the blood vessels in the skin dilate. This allows more blood to be brought to the surface of the skin. The heat within the blood is then more easily released because it is closer to the surface. At the same time this is occurring, the body's sweat glands begin to secrete sweat to cool the body.

If the body needs to conserve heat, the blood vessels will constrict, allowing the heat-carrying blood to circulate to the muscles and vital organs. Both the constriction and the dilation of the blood vessels are due to a reflex reaction initiated by the nervous system. The regulation of body temperature is an example of how the integumentary system and nervous system work together to maintain homeostasis.

SENSORY RECEPTION

The skin contains millions of microscopic nerve endings that act as sensory receptors. Once again, the integumentary system and the nervous system work together for the function of sensation. Each nerve ending is specialized according to a type of sensory reaction. Sensory reactions include responses to pressure, traction, heat, cold, pain, and more. The nerve endings and their sensory receptors send information to the cerebral cortex of the brain. When the message reaches the brain, an appropriate response is triggered. For example, if the hand touches a hot plate, a message is sent to the brain signaling that the hand is on the hot plate. Next,

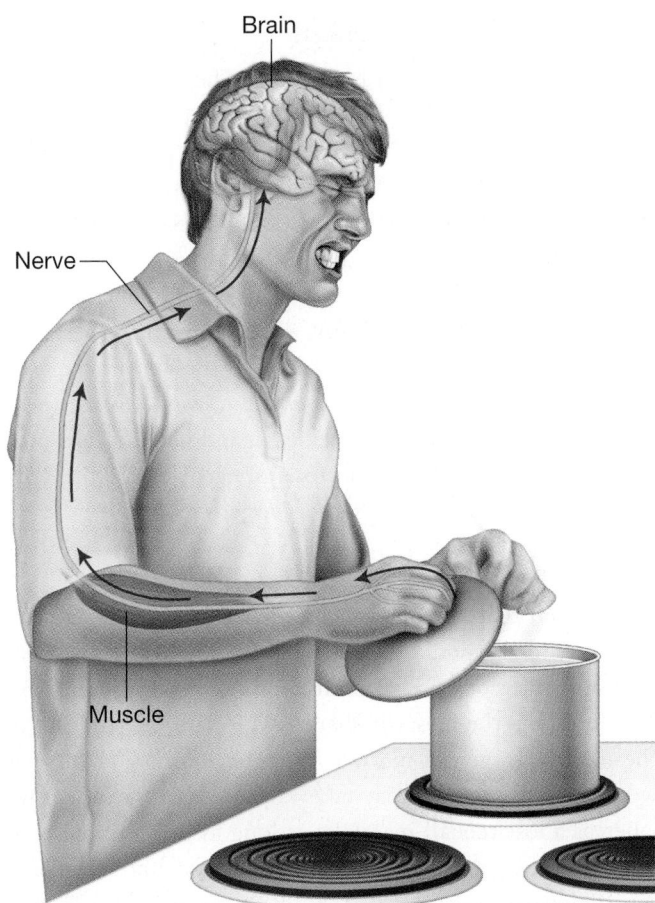

Brain

Nerve

Muscle

FIGURE 22-1 **The integumentary and nervous systems work together to recognize specific sensations, such as heat and pain.**

the brain sends back a response to remove the hand from the hot plate because the sensory reaction is hot and painful (Figure 22-1).

ABSORPTION

Based on new advances in medication, the skin also functions through absorption. Transdermal medication is administered through the use of a medicated patch. These patches are placed on various parts of the body, depending on the desired function of the medication. Common transdermal medications include those to prevent motion sickness, as well as hormonal therapy, including birth control patches. Another medication, nitroglycerin paste, is applied to the chest to regulate certain heart conditions.

Both the transdermal patch and medicated pastes have time-release properties that allow the medication to be absorbed through the skin and into the bloodstream.

SECRETION

The skin contains millions of sweat glands, which secrete perspiration or sweat, and sebaceous glands, which secrete oil for lubrication. Perspiration is composed mostly of water with small amounts of salt and other chemical compounds. If the secretions are allowed to accumulate, especially around body hair in the axillary region, bacteria will begin to grow, creating body odor. Sebaceous glands produce sebum, which acts to protect the body from dehydration and the possible absorption of harmful substances.

Structure of the Skin

The skin is composed of three layers: the epidermis, the dermis, and the subcutaneous layer (Figure 22-2).

THE EPIDERMIS

The **epidermis** is divided into four layers or strata: the stratum corneum, stratum lucidum, stratum granulosum, and stratum germinativum.

Stratum Corneum

The stratum corneum is the outermost layer of skin and consists of dead cells filled with the protein keratin. It forms a protective covering for the body, and the thickness of the layer depends on the part of the body. Because of the ongoing pressure on their surfaces, the soles of the feet and the palms of the hands have thicker layers than do the eyelids or forehead.

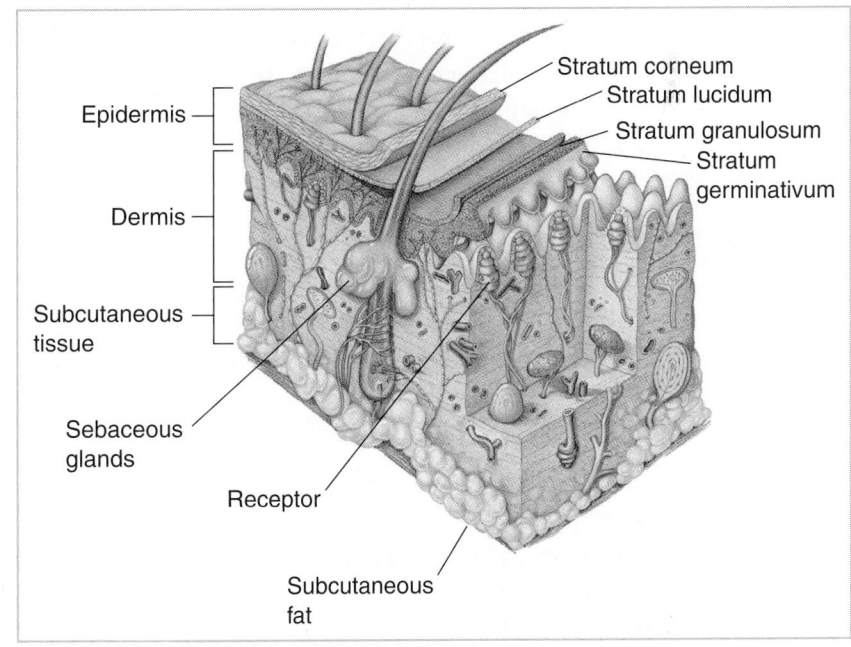

Epidermis

Dermis

Subcutaneous tissue

Sebaceous glands

Receptor

Subcutaneous fat

Stratum corneum
Stratum lucidum
Stratum granulosum
Stratum germinativum

FIGURE 22-2 **The integument: the epidermis, dermis, subcutaneous tissue, and its appendages.**

Stratum Lucidum

The stratum lucidum is a translucent layer lying directly beneath the stratum corneum. In thinner skin, it is often absent. Cells in this layer are either dead or dying.

Stratum Granulosum

The stratum granulosum consists of several layers of living cells that are becoming part of the stratum lucidum and stratum corneum. These cells are actively becoming keratinized or hardened, after they lose their nuclei.

Stratum Germinativum

The stratum germinativum contains several layers of living cells, still capable of mitosis, or cell division. This layer, occasionally referred to as the mucosum, is most responsible for the regeneration of the epidermis. If damage, such as a severe burn, occurs to this layer, the skin is unable to regenerate itself, and skin grafting must be done. This layer also contains the **melanocytes**, the cells that produce **melanin**, the pigment that gives the skin its color. The amount of melanin that is produced allows individuals to have varying shades of skin tones. The absence of melanin in the skin, hair, and eyes is an inherited disorder known as **albinism**.

THE DERMIS

The **dermis** is the middle layer of the skin and is often referred to as the "true skin." It is composed of connective tissue containing nerves and nerve endings, blood vessels, sebaceous and sweat glands, hair follicles, and lymph vessels. The dermis is further divided into two layers: the papillary layer and the reticular layer. The papillary layer is the upper layer and is made up of layers of papillae, which form the ridges that are fingerprints. The reticular layer is the lower layer and is made of white fibrous tissues that support blood vessels.

THE SUBCUTANEOUS LAYER

The subcutaneous layer of the skin is composed of subcutaneous tissue. This tissue helps support, nourish, insulate, and cushion the skin. Medical assistants must be familiar with the subcutaneous layer of the skin as many medications are administered via injection here. Medication administration is discussed in Chapter 54.

Accessory Structures of the Skin

The accessory structures of the skin include the hair, nails, sebaceous glands, and sweat glands.

HAIR

The visible portion of hair is the shaft. The root of the hair is embedded within the follicle. A loop of capillaries enclosed in connective tissue is the hair papilla. The papilla is found at the base of each hair follicle. The pilomotor muscle is attached to the side of each follicle. Contraction of the pilomotor muscle causes goose bumps, or the sensation of the hair standing on end. This is the result of both an emotional reaction and the skin's attempt at self-warming. With the exception of the palms of the hands and the soles of the feet, the entire body is covered by a very thin layer of hair.

Hairs that surround the eyes, ears, and nose act as a protective barrier by filtering out foreign particles and preventing their entrance into the sensory organs.

NAILS

Fingers and toenails are horny cell structures of the epidermis and are composed of hard keratin. The nail consists of the body, the root, and the **matrix**, or nail bed (Figure 22-3). The **lunula** is the crescent-shaped white area at the base of the nail. Average nail growth is about 1 mm (.04 in.) per week. A lost fingernail may take 3½ to 5½ months to regrow, whereas a lost toenail may take as long as 6 to 8 months to regrow. Nail growth is affected by disease and hormonal insufficiencies.

SEBACEOUS GLANDS

Located in the dermis, the **sebaceous glands**, or oil glands, secrete sebum. Sebum is made of fat and the debris of dead fat-producing cells. The function of sebum is to protect and waterproof hair and skin. The endocrine system regulates the amount of secretion of the sebaceous glands; however, amounts tend to vary with age, pregnancy, and puberty.

Sebaceous glands can usually be found in hair-covered areas where they are contained in hair follicles but can also be found in the hairless areas of the lips, eyelids, penis, labia minora, and nipples. At the hairless areas, sebum rises to the surface through ducts. The sebaceous glands of a fetus in utero secrete vernix caseosa, a "waxy" or "cheesy" white substance found coating the skin of the newborn baby.

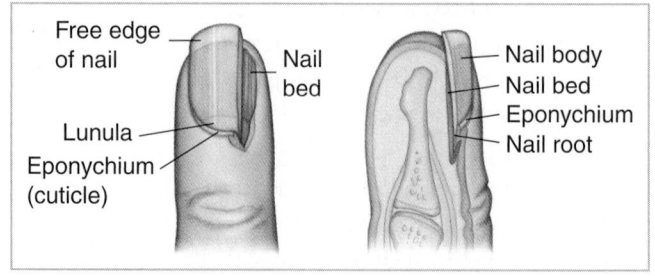

FIGURE 22-3 The fingernail, an appendage of the integument.

SUDORIFEROUS GLANDS

Predominant in the palms of the hands and the soles of the feet, **sudoriferous glands**, or **sweat glands**, occur in nearly all regions of the skin. Sweat glands are coiled, ball-shaped structures that are located in the dermis or subcutaneous layers. Sweat glands secrete perspiration, which helps to cool the body by evaporation. It is estimated that the body loses 0.5 L of fluid per day via sweat.

Common Disorders of the Integumentary System

Skin is vulnerable to many disorders because it is the most exposed of all the body systems. Skin disorders have multiple signs. Some common signs are illustrated in Figure 22-4.

SKIN CANCER

Accounting for the most common of all cancers, skin cancer affects more than one million people each year in the United States. These cancers occur when normal skin cells undergo a change during which they grow and multiply without normal controls.

As the cells multiply, they form a mass called a tumor. Tumors of the skin are often referred to as lesions. Malignant tumors encroach on neighboring tissues, especially lymph nodes, due to their uncontrolled growth. The three major types of skin cancers are these:

- Basal cell carcinoma
- Squamous cell carcinoma
- Malignant melanoma

The vast majority of skin cancers are either basal cell or squamous cell carcinomas. Although malignant, these are unlikely to spread, or metastasize, to other parts of the body. A small but significant number of skin cancers are malignant melanomas. Malignant melanoma is a highly aggressive cancer that tends to spread to other parts of the body. These cancers may be fatal if not treated early.

Like many cancers, skin cancers start as precancerous lesions that can develop into cancer due to skin changes. Health care professionals often refer to these changes as dysplasia. One example of this is a **dysplastic nevus**, or an abnormal mole. People with dysplastic nevi often have a lot of

them, perhaps one hundred or more. They are usually irregular in shape, with notched or fading borders. Dysplastic nevi may be either flat or raised, and the surface may be smooth or rough ("pebbly").

Basal Cell Carcinoma

Basal cell carcinoma, the most common form of skin cancer, is most often caused by overexposure to the sun. It may often appear as a change in the skin, such as a growth, irritation, or

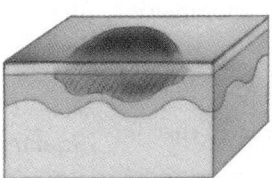

A macule is a discolored spot on the skin; freckle

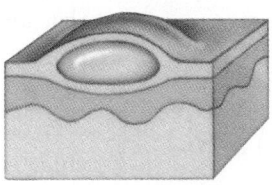

A wheal is a localized, evanescent elevation of the skin that is often accompanied by itching; urticaria

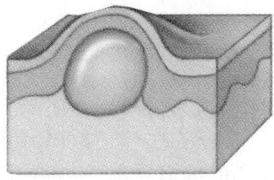

A papule is a solid, circumscribed, elevated area on the skin; pimple

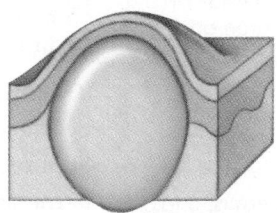

A nodule is a larger papule; acne vulgaris

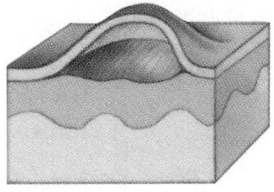

A vesicle is a small fluid filled sac; blister. A bulla is a large vesicle.

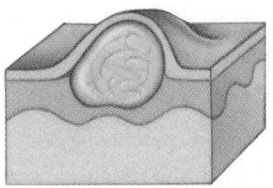

A pustule is a small, elevated, circumscribed lesion of the skin that is filled with pus; varicella (chickenpox)

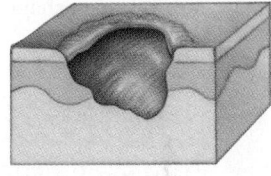

An erosion or ulcer is an eating or gnawing away of tissue; decubitus ulcer

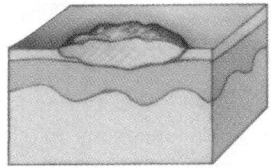

A crust is a dry, serous or seropurulent, brown, yellow, red, or green exudation that is seen in secondary lesions; eczema

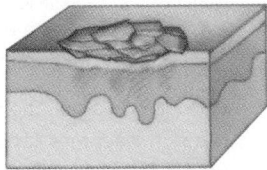

A scale is a thin, dry flake of cornified epithelial cells; psoriasis

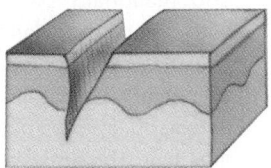

A fissure is a crack-like sore or slit that extends through the epidermis into the dermis; athlete's foot

FIGURE 22-4 Common skin signs are often evidence of an illness or disorder.

sore that does not heal or as a change in a wart or mole. Though the nose is the most common site, it also affects the head, neck, back, chest, or shoulders. Exposure to sunlight is the most common cause of this, and most, cancers.

Signs and Symptoms. Signs of basal cell carcinoma can vary and may include skin changes such as the following:

- Firm, pearly bump with visible and spiderlike tiny blood vessels (telangiectasias)
- Red, tender, flat spot that bleeds easily
- Small, fleshy bump with a smooth, pearly appearance, often with a depressed center
- Smooth, shiny bump that may look like a mole or cyst
- Scarlike patch of skin, especially on the face, that is firm to the touch
- Bump that itches, bleeds, crusts over, and then repeats the cycle and has not healed in 3 weeks
- Change in the size, shape, or color of a wart or mole

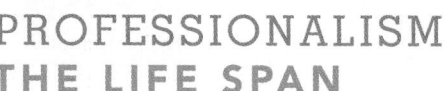

PROFESSIONALISM THE LIFE SPAN

The Child

- In children, skin conditions can be acute or chronic, local or systemic, and some can be congenital. Age-related skin conditions include milia (the white pimples occurring in newborns) and acne.
- Skin infections in children present as systemic infections with symptoms such as fever and malaise. Because the sebaceous glands do not produce sebum until the child is about 8 to 10 years old, a child's skin is drier and chaps more easily. For that reason, it is important to teach children good hygiene habits at an early age.

The Older Adult

- As a person ages, the papilla grow less dense, and the skin becomes looser. Less collagen and fewer elastic fibers are present in the upper dermis, and the skin loses its elastic tone, causing wrinkles to occur more easily. The occurrence of premalignant and malignant skin lesions may also increase with aging, especially on the nose, eyelids, and cheeks. Among skin cancers found in older adults, 80 percent are basal cell carcinomas.
- By age 50, approximately half of adults have some gray hair. The scalp hair continues to thin in men and women as aging progresses, and the hair becomes dry and brittle. The nails may flatten and become more discolored, dry, and brittle.

Treatment. Because skin cancer usually grows slowly, it often can be detected and successfully treated in its early stages of development. The most common treatment is surgery to destroy or remove the entire skin growth, including a margin of cancer-free tissue around the growth. A relatively newer treatment option is a type of surgery called Mohs micrographic surgery, originally known as chemosurgery. This microscopically controlled surgery to remove skin cancer is very effective, with cure rates higher than 90 percent. Overall treatment for skin cancer varies depending on the size and location of the cancer, as well as the age and overall health of the patient.

Squamous Cell Carcinoma

Squamous cell carcinoma is a malignant tumor that affects the middle layer of the skin. Changes to an existing wart, mole, or other skin lesion could indicate skin cancer. Another skin cancer indicator is the development of a new growth that ulcerates and does not heal well. Squamous cell carcinoma has a high cure rate if it is treated early, but neglect can allow the cancer to spread, causing great disability or even death. Along with exposure to sunlight, risk factors include genetic predisposition (skin cancers are more common in those who have light-colored skin, blue or green eyes, and blond or red hair), chemical pollution, and overexposure to X-rays or other forms of radiation. Exposure to arsenic, which may be present in some herbicides, presents another risk for development of skin cancers.

Signs and Symptoms. Similar to basal cell carcinoma, symptoms include any skin lesion, growth, or bump that is small, firm, reddened, nodular, coned, or flat in shape. Also, if the surface is scaly or crusted and the lesion or growth is located on the face, ears, neck, hands, or arms, it is likely to be a squamous cell carcinoma. Occasionally the growth may occur on the lip, mouth, tongue, or genitals.

Treatment. The treatment varies with the tumor's size, depth, location, and how much it has spread or metastasized. Surgical removal of the tumor, which may include removal of the skin around the tumor (wide excision), is often recommended. Microscopic shaving (Mohs micrographic surgery) may remove small tumors. Skin grafting may be needed if wide areas of skin are removed. The tumor may also be reduced in size by radiation treatments. Chemotherapy tends to be minimally effective; however, it can be used if surgery and radiation fail.

Malignant Melanoma

Originating in the melanocytes of the skin, **malignant melanoma** develops when melanocytes do not respond to the normal control mechanisms of cellular growth. They

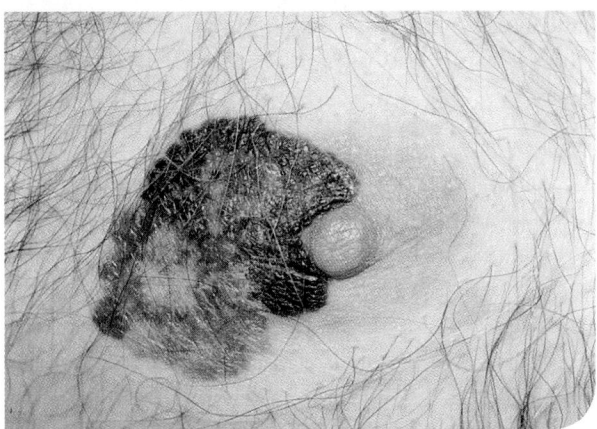

FIGURE 22-5 Melanoma.

may then invade nearby structures or spread to other organs in the body (metastasis), invading and compromising the function of that organ. The primary tumor begins in the skin, often from the melanocytes of a preexisting mole. Once it becomes invasive, it may progress beyond the site of origin to the regional lymph nodes or travel to other organ systems in the body and become systemic in nature (Figure 22-5).

Signs and Symptoms. Malignant melanomas are usually diagnosed by using the ABCDE rule (Table 22-1), which is an excellent way of identifying changes of significance in a mole. This includes checking the mole for the following: asymmetry, border irregularity, color variegation, diameter greater than 6 mm (0.24 in.), and elevation above surrounding tissue.

The Glasgow 7-point scale also identifies signs and symptoms of melanoma. The symptoms and signs (see the following) can occur anywhere on the skin, including the palms of the hands, soles of the feet, and the nail beds. In this scheme, change is emphasized along with size. Bleeding and sensory changes are relatively late symptoms:

- Change in size
- Change in shape
- Change in color
- Inflammation
- Crusting and bleeding
- Sensory change
- Diameter greater than 7 mm (0.28 in.)

Treatment. The key to successful treatment of melanoma is early diagnosis. Patients identified with localized, thin, small lesions nearly always survive. For those with advanced lesions, the outcome is poor in spite of progress in systemic therapy.

ACNE VULGARIS

Acne vulgaris (acne) is a common skin condition that occurs when oil and dead skin cells clog the skin's pores (Figure 22-6). It most often affects teens, with more than 85 percent of them developing at least a mild form of this condition. Whereas mild acne is merely annoying, severe acne can lead to emotional and physical scars. Most people outgrow acne by the time they are in their 40s and 50s.

Signs and Symptoms. The skin blemishes of acne vulgaris are often red and swollen. Severe acne can mean hundreds of pimples or sores that can cover the face, neck, chest, and back. With mild cases of acne, only whiteheads and blackheads may be present. At times, these may develop into an infection in the skin pore (pimple). Severe acne can produce hundreds of pimples that cover large areas of skin. Cystic lesions are pimples that are large and deep. These lesions are often painful and can leave scars on your skin.

TABLE 22-1 The ABCDEs of Melanoma Changes in a Mole

A—Asymmetry	The mole does not have two halves that match each other.
B—Border	The border is ragged, notched, or blurred together.
C—Color	Color is uneven; shades of black, brown, or tan are present; areas of white, red, or blue may be present.
D—Diameter	There may be a change in size, and the mole is typically greater than 6 mm in diameter.
E—Elevation	The mole sits above the surrounding tissue.

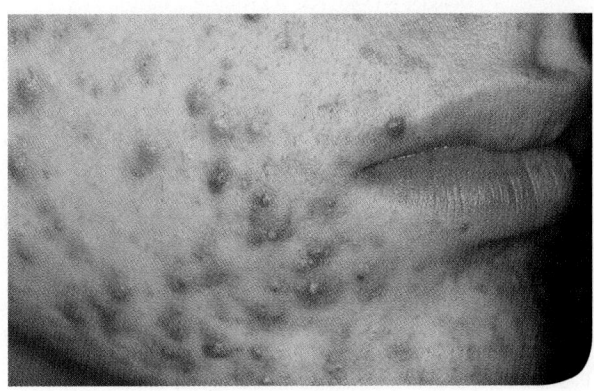

FIGURE 22-6 Acne vulgaris. *Courtesy of Jason L. Smith, MD.*

Treatment. The severity of acne will determine the most useful and beneficial treatment. Treatment could include lotions or gels applied to blemishes or sometimes entire areas of skin, such as the chest or back (topical medications) and oral antibiotics. Sometimes the health care provider will combine treatments to get the best results and to avoid the development of bacteria that are resistant to antibiotics.

ALOPECIA

Alopecia is baldness or loss of hair. The most common form is male-pattern baldness, also known as androgenic alopecia. Women may also experience alopecia. Alopecia areata is another type of hair loss, involving patches of baldness that may come and go. Alopecia areata affects about 1 in 100 people, mostly teenagers and young adults (Figure 22-7).

Signs and Symptoms. Alopecia areata causes patches of baldness that are about the size of a large coin. They usually appear on the scalp but can occur anywhere on the body, including the beard, eyebrows, and eyelashes. There are usually no other symptoms.

Male-pattern baldness is hereditary. It is called male-pattern baldness because it tends to follow a set pattern. The first stage is usually a receding hairline, followed by thinning of the hair on the crown and temples. When these two areas meet in the middle, a horseshoe shape of hair remains around the back and sides of the head. Eventually the person may be completely bald. Women's hair gradually thins with age, but women tend to lose hair only from the top of the head. This usually becomes more noticeable after menopause.

Treatment. Drugs are available to treat male- and female-pattern baldness, but they do not work for everyone and effects are not long lasting. Lotions are available that can be rubbed on the scalp, although these do not work for everyone; nor do they have long-lasting effects. Shampoos and formulas are available for improving circulation to the scalp, and some people try herbal treatments. Unfortunately, hair loss can lead to problems with confidence and self-esteem.

CELLULITIS

Cellulitis is an acute spreading bacterial infection below the surface of the skin. A cut, an abrasion, or ulceration may precede cellulitis, as it commonly appears at a break in the skin. It can also be due to local trauma, such as an animal bite. Very rarely is cellulitis caused by the **bacteremic** spread of infection (i.e., bacteria arriving from a distant source via the bloodstream). Risk factors for cellulitis include diabetes and impairment of the immune system. Cellulitis is not contagious because it is an infection of the skin's deeper layers: the dermis and subcutaneous tissue. The skin's top layer (the epidermis) provides a cover over the infection.

Signs and Symptoms. Cellulitis is characterized by **erythema** (redness), warmth, swelling, and pain. Fever, chills, and enlarged lymph nodes may also accompany this infection (Figure 22-8).

Treatment. Antibiotics, such as derivatives of penicillin, that are most effective against the staph germ are used to treat cellulitis. If other bacteria, as determined by culture tests, turn out to be the cause, or if patients are allergic to penicillin, other appropriate antibiotics are substituted.

CONTACT DERMATITIS

Contact dermatitis is an allergic reaction of the skin caused by irritating substances coming in contact with it. Causes of contact dermatitis often include exposure to poison ivy (Figure 22-9), poison oak, nickel (especially on jewelry or jean snaps), lotions, detergents, or other chemicals.

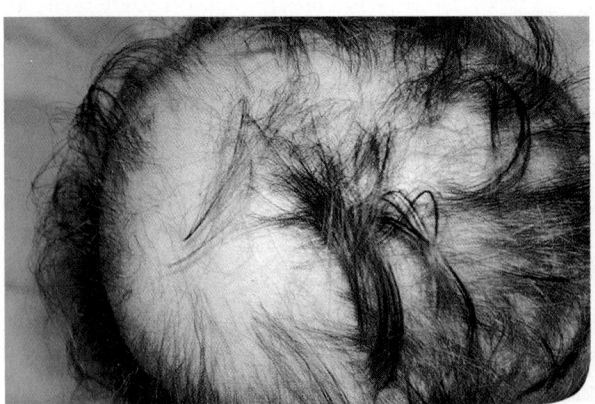

FIGURE 22-7 Alopecia. *Courtesy of Jason L. Smith, MD.*

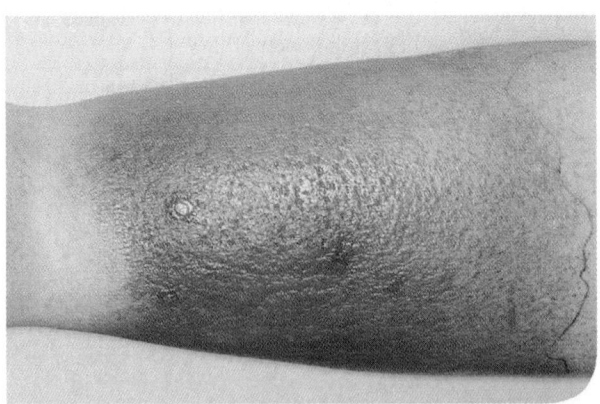

FIGURE 22-8 Cellulitis. *Courtesy of Jason L. Smith, MD.*

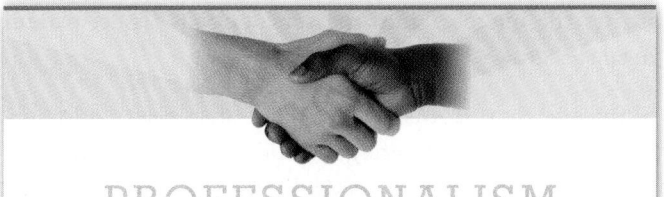
Signs and Symptoms.   With contact dermatitis, the obvious response is red, irritated skin, but **vesicles** (small blisters) and rash may also result. Oftentimes, itching and pain may be present. Serious allergic reactions may result in urticaria, or hives.

Treatment.   Most of these allergic reactions are treated with antihistamines (antiallergy medicines) and topical corticosteroid creams to reduce the inflammation. Widespread

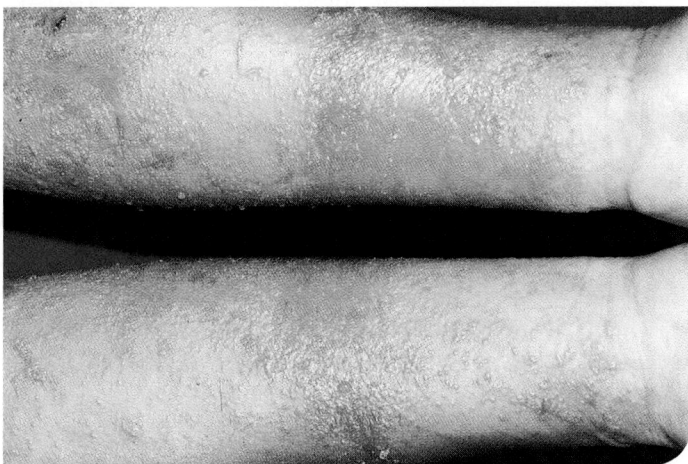

FIGURE 22-9   Contact dermatitis resulting from poison ivy. *Courtesy of Jason L. Smith, MD.*

or excessively uncomfortable reactions may also be treated with systemic corticosteroids (oral medications) that help to further decrease the inflammation caused by the allergic reaction.

CALLUSES AND CORNS

Calluses and corns are excessive growths of the stratum corneum layer of the epidermis. They often occur on the hands and feet. Both calluses and corns can be caused by physical bone deformities; however, they also can be caused by such other factors as ill-fitting shoes and unprotected hands during manual labor.

Signs and Symptoms.   A **callus** is an area of thickened skin that does not have an identifiable border. It may appear grayish-yellow, brown, or even red. It may cause no pain, or it may produce tenderness, throbbing, or burning. A **corn**, on the other hand, has a distinct border with various textures. Corns appear most often on the feet. Though corns may be hard or soft, they are generally painful.

Treatment.   Treatment becomes necessary when corns or calluses become burdensome or painful. Although patients with diabetes must be treated by a podiatrist to decrease the chance of infection and maximize wound healing, most patients can treat these conditions by themselves. Placing a bandage on the corn or callus to reduce friction is beneficial, as is applying lotions or creams to rough or hardened corns or calluses.

DECUBITUS ULCER

A **decubitus ulcer**, also called a pressure sore or bedsore, is an area of skin and tissue that breaks down. Such ulcers typically occur when constant pressure is maintained on a specific area of the skin, such as on the coccyx. The constant pressure on the area decreases the blood supply, causing death to the affected tissue. Patients who have been lying in bed for too long without being repositioned or patients who are in wheelchairs may be susceptible to these skin conditions. In addition to the coccyx, common locations for a decubitus ulcer include hips, heels, ankles, shoulders, back, and the back of the head.

Signs and Symptoms.   Signs and symptoms of decubitus ulcers vary with their stages. According to the National Pressure Ulcer Advisory Panel, the following are the four stages of decubitus ulcers:

- **Stage I**—A reddened area on the skin that does not blanch (turn white) when pressed. This is an early stage, and if the pressure is kept off of the area, healing may occur.

- Stage II—The skin has a blister or an open sore. The area around the site may be red and irritated.
- Stage III—The skin breakdown looks like a crater with damage to the tissue below the skin.
- Stage IV—The wound becomes so deep that damage occurs to the tissues beneath the initial ulcer, including damage to bone and muscle.

Treatment. Treatment of decubitus ulcers begin with relieving pressure. Special pillows, cushions, and sheepskin are frequently used to keep pressure off the area. Repositioning must be routine. Decubitus ulcers are typically debrided (i.e., cleaned of all toxins and then medicated and covered with special gauze dressings to help in healing). Protecting the wound from any further injury is essential in order to protect the patient from infections, systemic sepsis, and other serious complications.

ECZEMA

Eczema, or atopic dermatitis, is a chronic skin condition caused by an allergic-type reaction on the skin. Heredity tends to play a role as, typically, a family history of allergies and eczema is present. Eczema is most common in infants, and about half of the cases disappear by age three.

Signs and Symptoms. Eczema is characterized by scaling, itching, and rashes. Adults may also suffer from chronic episodes of eczema. The patient may also suffer from other allergic conditions.

Treatment. Treatment depends on the stage, or appearance, of the lesions that have formed on the skin. Lesions may be dry or scaly or have a "weeping" appearance. Weeping lesions are treated with mild soaps and dressings, whereas severe cases and dry scaly lesions may be treated with mild, anti-itch lotions or low-potency topical corticosteroids. Very severe cases may require treatment with systemic corticosteroids and topical immunomodulators (TIMs). Sometimes short periods of time in a tanning bed are useful to dry up lesions, but this treatment should always be under a physician's supervision.

FURUNCLES AND CARBUNCLES

A **furuncle,** or boil, is actually an abscess of a hair follicle and the adjacent subcutaneous tissues. A **carbuncle** is a collection of furuncles. The microbe involved in the disease process is usually *Staphylococcus aureus,* which lives harmlessly on the skin. When an opening in the integument invites the microbes into the subcutaneous tissue, painful furuncles grow.

Signs and Symptoms. Furuncles can appear red to purple in appearance and are generally painful. The area surrounding the furuncle tends to become tender to the touch. The center is generally white or yellow, and is filled with pus. Carbuncles can be anywhere from the size of a pea to the size of a golf ball and are similar in color to furuncles.

Treatment. The customary treatment for these disorders is incision and drainage followed by application of an antibiotic. Patients must be taught not to squeeze furuncles as that will cause the microbes to spread further. Hand washing is the best prevention.

FOLLICULITIS

An infection or inflammation of the hair follicles is known as **folliculitis.** Although folliculitis can occur anywhere body hair is present, it most often appears in areas that become irritated by shaving or the rubbing of clothes or where follicles and pores are blocked by oils and dirt. Common sites of folliculitis include the face, scalp, armpits, and legs (Figure 22-10).

Signs and Symptoms. General symptoms of folliculitis include a reddened rash; raised, red, often pus-filled lesions around hair follicles (pimples); pimples that eventually crust over and occur in areas of a high concentration of hair follicles, such as the face (especially in men's beards and moustaches), armpits, scalp, and groin; and itching at the site of the rash and pimples.

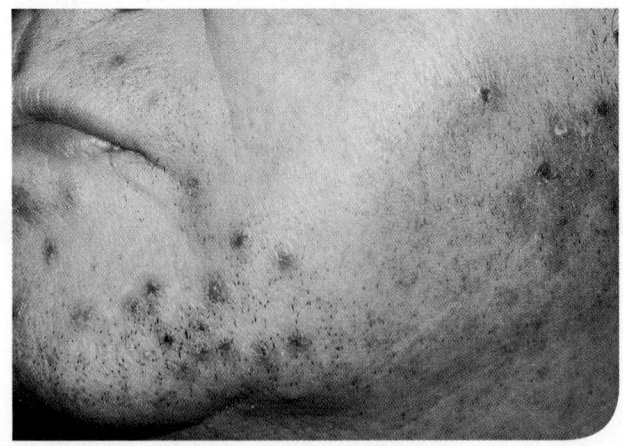

FIGURE 22-10 Folliculitis. *Courtesy of Jason L. Smith, MD.*

Treatment. Treating folliculitis generally involves taking steps to minimize damage to hair follicles by avoiding clothing that will rub against the skin, shaving with an electric razor as opposed to a blade razor, and keeping the skin clean using soap and water and skin cleansers. When folliculitis is present, treatment usually includes the application of antibiotic ointments.

HERPES SIMPLEX

Herpes simplex primarily affects the mouth or genital area. There are two strains of herpes simplex viruses:

- Herpes simplex virus type 1 (HSV-1) usually affects the face, including the lips and mouth. Acquired during childhood, it is the most common herpes simplex virus. HSV-1 is characterized by lesions inside the mouth or on the lips, including fever blisters. Antibodies are acquired by 90 percent of individuals by the time they reach adulthood (Figure 22-11).

- Herpes simplex virus type 2 (HSV-2) is sexually transmitted. Oral and genital lesions are common. Some people do not display any signs or symptoms. However, left untreated, the virus can also lead to complications such as meningoencephalitis (infection of the lining of the brain and the brain itself) or an infection of the eye. Cross-infection of type 1 and 2 viruses may occur from oral–genital contact.

The herpes virus can infect a fetus and cause congenital abnormalities. A newborn may acquire the virus if he or she is birthed vaginally. A newborn born vaginally to a mother with an active genital herpes infection is highly susceptible to the virus.

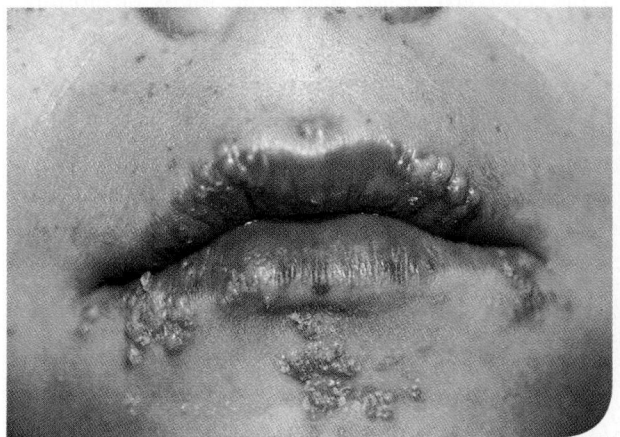

FIGURE 22-11 Blisters caused by HSV-1. *Courtesy of Jason L. Smith, MD.*

Signs and Symptoms. General signs and symptoms of herpes simplex include the following:

- Mouth sores
- A burning or tingling sensation followed by the development of genital lesions
- Blisters or ulcers on the mouth, lips, gums, or genitalia
- Fever blisters
- Fever—may be present especially during the first episode
- Lymph node enlargement in the neck or groin

Treatment. Mild cases of herpes simplex may not require any form of treatment. In prolonged cases, however, antiviral medications may be used. In situations of prolonged occurrence or frequent recurrence, individuals may become immunosuppressed.

HERPES ZOSTER

Herpes zoster, which is also known as shingles, is a viral infection that causes a painful rash. It is caused by the varicella zoster virus, which also causes chickenpox. Once a person has been infected with chickenpox, the virus lies dormant in the nerves. After the virus reactivates, it is diagnosed as shingles or herpes zoster.

Signs and Symptoms. Herpes zoster can be very painful. Often along with pain, a burning, tingling, and itchy feeling may be exhibited. A red rash with fluid-filled blisters begins to develop, and numbness or sensitivity in a certain part of the body may also occur. In serious conditions the skin can remain painful and sensitive to the touch; this is known as postherpetic neuralgia. Most of these symptoms occur on one side of the body, wrapping around from the back to the sternum, following the path of the nerve where the virus had been dormant. Headache, fever, and chills are also common symptoms.

Early treatment can help shorten a shingles infection and reduce the risk of complications.

Treatment. Oral antiviral medications are generally prescribed, preferably within 48 to 72 hours of the first sign of the rash. Corticosteroids are sometimes prescribed in order to reduce swelling and pain. If the pain is severe—particularly if the patient develops postherpetic neuralgia—the health care provider may prescribe oral analgesics or a skin patch that contains a pain-relieving medication.

HIRSUTISM

Hirsutism is a condition of thick abnormal hair growth that affects men and women, though women are more commonly affected by and diagnosed with the disorder. Often with this skin disorder, women have a pattern of hair growth that is typically found on males.

Signs and Symptoms. Women will develop thick and dark-hair growth. Common areas for the excessive hair growth include the face and chest. It is common for women of certain cultural descent, such as those from the Mediterranean region, to naturally have darker and more hair growth than lighter and fairer-skinned women. However, hirsutism is often linked to endocrine disorders, such as problems with the ovary or adrenal glands.

Treatment. Treatment consists of removing the unwanted hair through either shaving, plucking, waxing, or using depilatory creams. Electrolysis and laser hair removal are more permanent forms of hair removal; however, they are more costly. Physicians may also prescribe medications that block androgen hormones, helping to decrease the amount of hair growth. These medications may take 6 to 8 months to begin working.

IMPETIGO

Impetigo is a skin infection caused by bacteria. It is most common in children and is very contagious. Impetigo can originate in intact skin but also can be secondary to a preexisting skin condition or trauma.

Signs and Symptoms. Impetigo is characterized by round, crusted, oozing spots that grow larger day by day (Figure 22-12). It may affect the skin anywhere on the body but commonly occurs in the area around the nose and mouth. A honey-colored crust often develops from blisters that burst and ooze fluid.

Treatment. The treatment for impetigo varies depending on the severity. Mild cases of impetigo often resolve through the use of mild cleansing, removal of crust formations, and topical antibiotic ointment. More severe cases of impetigo may require the use of oral antibiotics.

KELOIDS

A **keloid** is often referred to as a hypertrophic scar. Keloids typically appear following a surgery or injury; however, they are also known to spontaneously appear after minor inflammation. Burns and piercings have also been known to produce keloids.

Signs and Symptoms. These unsightly skin blemishes can appear thickened and raised while being red or pink in color (Figure 22-13). Keloids also tend to be itchy and bothersome, as well as tender to the touch.

Treatment. Various treatments are available for keloids. Some of the most common include cortisone injections, surgery, and laser removal. Additional forms of treatment include cryosurgery, interferon injections, and application of silicone sheets.

PEDICULOSIS

Pediculosis is an infestation of lice in the form of eggs, larvae, or adults. Under suitable conditions of exposure, anyone may become louse infested as pediculosis is easily transmitted from person to person during direct contact. The various forms of pediculosis include *Pediculus humanus capitis* (head louse), *Pediculus humanus corporis* (body louse), and *Pthirus pubis* (pubic louse). Head lice are commonly found in school and instituitional settings. They are often transmitted with the sharing of hats, combs, or clothing. Body lice generally reside along the seams of clothing.

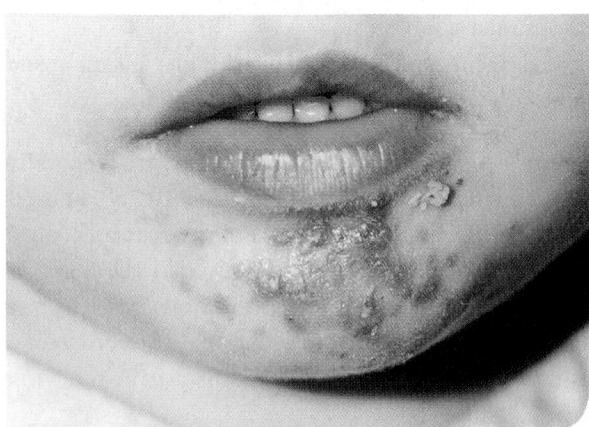

FIGURE 22-12 Impetigo. *Courtesy of Jason L. Smith, MD.*

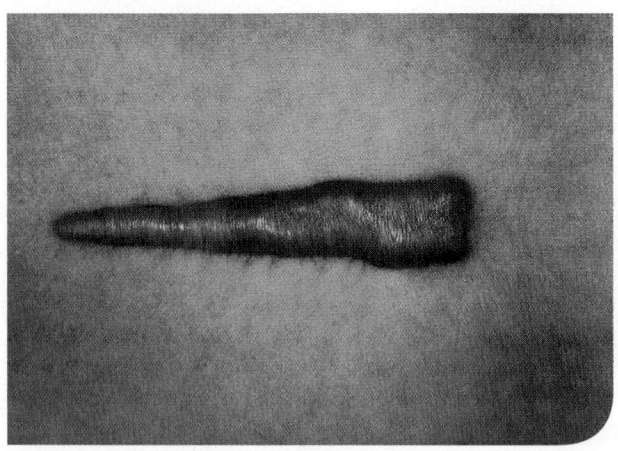

FIGURE 22-13 Keloid. *Courtesy of Jason L. Smith, MD.*

This form of lice is commonly found in places that are both crowded and unsanitary. Pubic lice, also known as crabs, are usually sexually transmitted.

Symptoms. The most common symptom among all forms of lice is itching. Head lice tend to cause itching around the back of the head or around the ears. Itching surrounding the genitals is an indicator of pubic lice. Body lice tend to travel to the body to feed on skin and then return to clothing.

Treatment. Two treatments are commonly used for pediculosis. Pyrethrins are found in medicated shampoos and cream rinses. This is preferred for the treatment of head lice. These products are available over the counter; therefore a prescription is not necessary.

Nit combs are available to help remove nits (lice eggs) from hair. Lindane-based shampoos provide another form of medicated treatments. Unlike pyrethrin-based shampoos, lindane-based shampoos require a prescription. To ensure that nits have not survived, retreatment after 7 to 10 days is recommended.

PSORIASIS

Psoriasis affects an estimated 7.5 million Americans. Though it can develop at any age, psoriasis develops most commonly between ages 30 and 50. This condition has genetic and autoimmune characteristics. Psoriasis is thought to be caused by a buildup of dead skin cells that, rather than shed off, pile and form scaly patches. Though it can be unsightly, psoriasis is not contagious.

Signs and Symptoms. Psoriasis is characterized by episodes of redness, itching, and thick dry scales on the skin. Its onset can be gradual or abrupt. Flare-ups have been attributed to infections, obesity, lack of sunlight as well as sunburn, stress, poor health, and cold climate. When the case is severe and widespread, large quantities of fluid can be lost, causing dehydration and severe secondary infections that can be serious.

Treatment. The extent and severity of psoriasis will determine the course of treatment. Treatment involves analgesics, sedation, intravenous fluids, retinoids, and antibiotics. Mild cases are treated at home with topical medications such as prescription or nonprescription dandruff shampoos, cortisone or other corticosteroids, and antifungal medications. Severe lesions may require hospitalization for proper treatment.

ROSACEA

Rosacea is a disorder primarily of the facial skin, often characterized by flare-ups and remissions. This condition affects an estimated fourteen million Americans—and most of them do not know they have it.

Signs and Symptoms. Symptoms of rosacea include redness on the cheeks, nose, chin, or forehead. Other symptoms include small visible blood vessels on the face, bumps on the face, and watery or irritated eyes. Over time, the redness becomes ruddier and more persistent.

Treatment. Therapies and medications are available to treat the symptoms associated with rosacea. Currently, a cure is not available for rosacea.

SCABIES

Scabies is a highly contagious disorder of the skin. It is caused by the human or scabies itch mite. Scabies is spread by personal contact, such as by shaking hands, sleeping together, or having close contact with infected articles such as clothing, bedding, or towels. Common among schoolchildren, roommates, and sexual partners, scabies is usually found where people are crowded together.

Signs and Symptoms.   As the female lays her eggs, a very small zigzag blister marks her trail. It is fairly difficult to see this; however, more obvious symptoms of scabies include intense itching and a red rash that occurs around the area. The sides of the fingers, backs of the hands, wrists, heels, elbows, armpits, inner thighs, and waistline are common locations for scabies (Figure 22-14).

Treatment.   Since Roman times, sulfur has been used as a scabicide. Sulfur is most often used in a lotion or cream with a 6 to 10 percent concentration. Corticosteriods and antihistamines are often used to relieve itching.

SEBORRHEIC DERMATITIS

Seborrheic dermatitis is an inflammatory condition of sebaceous or oil glands caused by an increase in sebum. This disorder is most common in infants and children and is frequently known as cradle cap.

Signs and Symptoms.   Some of the classic symptoms of seborrheic dermatitis include yellow or white scales that attach to the hair shaft, thick or patchy crusts on the scalp, itching or soreness, and dandruff.

Treatment.   This form of dermatitis is treated with low-strength creams. Although there is no prevention, shampooing the scalp daily with medicated shampoo can alleviate this problem.

TINEA

Tinea is any of several fungal infections of the skin. **Tinea corporis**, sometimes called ringworm, is not actually a worm but an integumentary disorder. Caused by a fungus, it can appear anywhere on the body. If the fungus is on the head, it is called **tinea capitis**. On the foot, it is known as **tinea pedis** or athlete's foot. When found in the genital area, it is referred to as **tinea cruris**, more commonly referred to as jock itch. Elsewhere on the body, the fungus is called tinea corporis (Figure 22-15).

Signs and Symptoms.   Tinea usually presents in the form of a ring, often with itchy, red, scaly patches.

Treatment.   Tinea is treated with antifungal creams or oral antifungal agents. Since the combining form for fungus is *myco,* that form frequently appears in the names of antifungal drugs.

URTICARIA

Urticaria, also known as hives, is a severe itching due to acute hypersensitivity to medications or environmental stimuli (Figure 22-16). The major concern related to urticaria is that

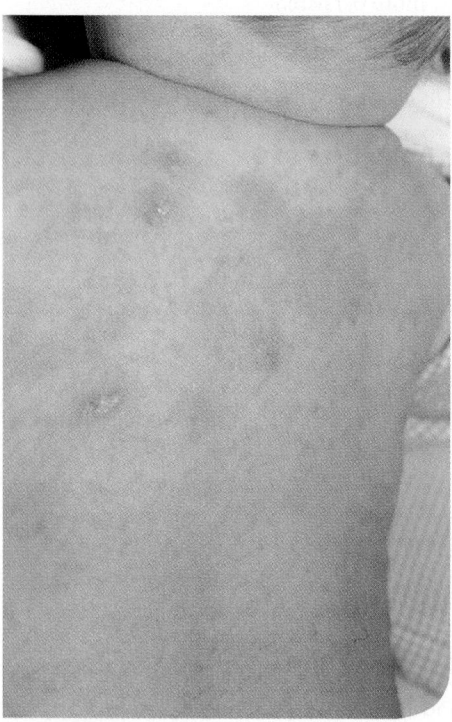

FIGURE 22-14   Scabies. *Courtesy of Jason L. Smith, MD.*

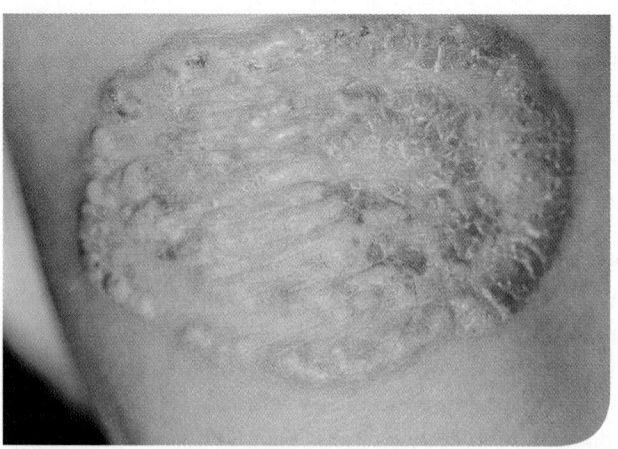

FIGURE 22-15   Tinea corporis. *Courtesy of Jason L. Smith, MD.*

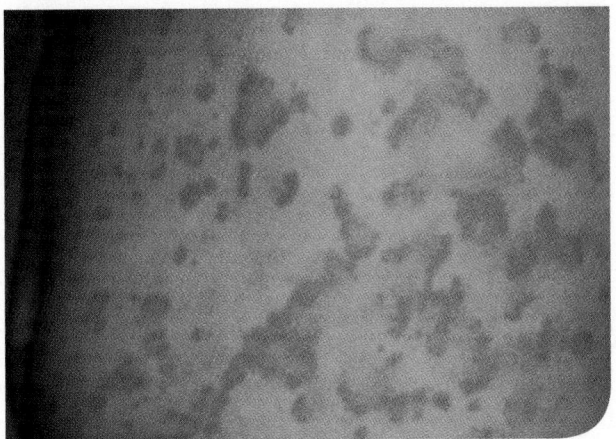

FIGURE 22-16 Urticaria (hives). *Courtesy of Jason L. Smith, MD.*

it can obstruct the pharyngeal airway. Because of the possibility of airway constriction, it is important to observe all patients after an injection or allergy tests.

Signs and Symptoms. Signs include localized areas of pink, itchy, swollen patches of skin. It is common for burning or stinging sensations also to be felt. Hives may vary in size from the diameter of a pencil eraser to the diameter of a cereal bowl. Many times, the hives may overlap, forming even larger areas of irritation and swelling.

Treatment. Treatment consists of removing the causitive allergens and treating with antihistamine and epinephrine.

VITILIGO

Vitiligo, also known as leukoderma, is a disorder that causes white patches and large areas of decreased pigmentation to form on the skin. These patches form due to the destruction of melanocytes, which are cells that produce melanin for pigmentation. This disease is often linked to immune system disorders, such as Addison's disease or pernicious anemia. Vitiligo also affects those with thyroid disorders.

Signs and Symptoms. Vitiligo is marked by the early or premature graying or whitening of body hair or by the depigmentation of skin or mucous membranes. When the skin is affected, it generally begins to appear on the neck, armpits, elbows, genitals, hands, or knees.

Treatment. The treatment of vitiligo is aimed at evening skin tone and color. This may be done by cosmetic, medical, or surgical means. Using sunscreen and avoiding tanning help make the depigmentation less noticeable. Makeup and self-tanning lotions may also be used to even out the skin tone. Medical treatments may include the use of topical corticosteroid therapy as well as a form of topical ultraviolet

therapy. Skin grafting as well as a form of tattooing called micropigmentation may also be successful.

WARTS

Warts, or verrucae, are a type of infection caused by viruses in the human papillomavirus (HPV) family. There are at least 60 types of HPV viruses. Warts can grow on all parts of the body, including the skin, the inside of the mouth, the genitals, and the rectal area. A common wart is the plantar wart, which is always located on the soles of the feet.

Signs and Symptoms. The appearance and texture of a wart will vary based on its location. Warts may appear grainy, fleshy, and varied in color from flesh toned to red, pink, or white. Warts may also appear as raised or flat skin lesions.

Treatment. Depending on the size, location, and type, various wart treatments are available. Over-the-counter medicines containing salicylic acid are available for purchase and treatment. A physician may perform cryotherapy, which freezes the wart; generally, liquid nitrogen is used in this procedure. Physicians may also prescribe various prescription medications. In severe cases, minor surgery may be an option.

Skin Care Treatments

Advancing medical technology and the desire to capture a youthful skin radiance and appearance have led to the surging popularity of medical skin care treatments. Many of the procedures that are discussed next are performed by trained and experienced professionals in a dermatologist's office or in a medical spa setting. Along with researching these procedures, patients should always use discretion when choosing a health care professional who specializes in this area of expertise.

BOTOX

Botox is a popular procedure that is indicated for reducing wrinkle lines. Most often, botox is used for frown lines, forehead lines, and wrinkles around the eyes, which are commonly referred to as crow's feet. A very small, diluted amount of the toxin *Clostridium botulinum* is injected into the wrinkle lines. This toxin will cause wrinkles to relax and soften, thereby diminishing their visibility. For maintenance reasons, this procedure is usually repeated every 4 to 6 months. Side effects of the treatment include headaches, bruising, and eyelid drooping, all of which are temporary.

CHEMICAL PEEL

A chemical peel is a type of chemical surgery that utilizes various acid concentrations to remove old and damaged layers of skin cells. A chemical peel can be performed at one of three levels.

- **Light chemical peel**—The purpose of this peel is to reduce the size of pores, make the skin appear softer, and produce more coloring in the skin. During a light chemical peel only the top layer of the skin is stripped. The procedure is complete in about an hour and leaves the skin mildly red, which disappears as time progresses.
- **Medium chemical peel**—The purpose of a medium chemical peel is to reduce wrinkles and result in much smoother skin than the light chemical peel can produce. The medium peel will result in the top layer and some underlying cells being stripped, causing collagen and elastin to be stimulated. Recovery from a medium chemical peel can last up to 10 days due to the peeling, swelling, and redness that occur after the treatment.
- **Deep chemical peel**—This is an aggressive treatment that can affect the layers of skin down to the dermal layer. The results are aimed at reducing all signs of aging with the exception of certain areas of the face. With this level of chemical peel, skin conditions such as pigmentation disorders and precancerous lesions can be removed. The healing process includes considerable pain, often felt up to 12 hours post surgery. Analgesic medications are required. It may take weeks for additional peeling, swelling, and redness to subside.

LASER RESURFACING

Laser resurfacing is one of the newer treatments available to reduce the signs of aging. Short, pulsated laser beams are used to vaporize damaged or troublesome areas of the skin. Full-face laser resurfacing takes approximately 1 to 2 hours, whereas a partial-face resurfacing lasts 30 to 45 minutes. The resurfacing results in the stimulation and production of new collagen and skin cells, which results in younger- and tighter-looking skin. Immediately following the procedure, antibiotic ointment and sterile dressings are applied to reduce the incidence of infection. The patient returns to the office 1 to 3 days after the procedure to have the sterile dressings removed. Analgesics are prescribed for pain relief. Complete healing following laser resurfacing takes approximately 10 to 21 days.

MICRODERMABRASION

During microdermabrasion, the top layer of dead skin cells is removed to provide the skin with a rejuvenated look. Tiny crystals are used to work with abrasion and suction devices to produce healthier-looking skin. This noninvasive and nonchemical approach is appealing to many patients who do not wish to pursue more aggressive skin-freshening treatments. Candidates for microdermabrasion include those who wish to erase signs of aging, including fine lines, wrinkles, and sun-damaged skin. As with other skin care treatments, it is important to find qualified professionals to perform these procedures.

DERMABRASION

Historically, dermabrasion preceded microdermabrasion. Though very similar in its action, dermabrasion is a much more forceful procedure than its counterparts. Because of newer technologies and techniques, dermabrasion is rarely used today.

SUMMARY

The skin provides many protective functions for the body, including preventing infection and preserving the internal environment. Skin also helps to promote optimum temperature levels. Disorders of the skin can be uncomfortable, but most can be treated without too much discomfort.

The integumentary system is comprised of the skin and accessory organs. The skin is the largest organ of the body and serves protective, regulatory, sensory reception, absorptive, and secretory functions for the body.

The protective function of the skin is supported by several layers: the epidermis (stratum corneum, stratum lucidum, stratum granulosum, stratum germinativum) and the dermis. Accessory organs that support the skin are the hair, nails, sebaceous glands, and udoriferous glands.

The large integumentary system is prone to disorders. Several types of skin cancer can develop: basal cell carcinoma, squamous cell carcinoma, and melanoma. Other disorders include acne vulgaris, alopecia, cellulitis, contact dermatitis, corns and callluses, decubitus ulcers, eczema, furuncles and carbuncles, folliculitis, herpes simplex and herpes zoster, impetigo, keloids, pediculosis, psoriasis, rosacea, scabies, seborrheic dermatitis, tinea, urticaria, vitiligo, and warts.

New techniques in skin care treatments help reverse the signs of aging, including wrinkles and sun damage. Some of the more common treatments include chemical peels, laser resurfacing, and microdermabrasion.

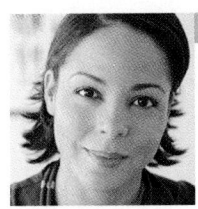 22 CHAPTER REVIEW

COMPETENCY REVIEW

1. Define and spell the terms to learn for this chapter.

2. What is the primary organ of the integumentary system?

3. Name the four accessory structures of the integumentary system.

4. Name the four functions of the skin.

5. Name the two layers of the skin.

6. What is the protein substance in the dead cells of the epidermis that serves as a protective mechanism?

7. Name the four layers of the epidermis.

8. What is the name of the cresecent-shaped area of the nail?

9. What is the name of the cell that gives color to the skin?

10. What are the ABCDEs of skin cancer?

PREPARING FOR THE CERTIFICATION EXAM

1. Which layer is the innermost layer of the skin?
   a. stratum corneum
   b. stratum granulosum
   c. stratum germinativum
   d. stratum lucidum
   e. lunula

2. Which of the following is a form of skin cancer?
   a. acne vulgaris
   b. psoriasis
   c. urticaria
   d. melanoma
   e. alopecia

3. If a patient has baldness, this is known as
   a. psoriasis
   b. vitiligo
   c. alopecia
   d. cellulitis
   e. seborrheic dermatitis

4. If a patient spends too much time in the same position in bed, she might develop
   a. eczema
   b. decubitus ulcer
   c. furuncle
   d. impetigo
   e. pediculosis

5. Herpes zoster is known to cause
   a. alopecia
   b. impetigo
   c. pediculosis
   d. psoriasis
   e. shingles

6. Which skin care treatment utilizes various concentrations of acid to remove layers of dead skin?
   a. microdermabrasion
   b. dermabrasion
   c. chemical peel
   d. laser resurfacing
   e. use of medicated lotions and ointments

7. Which of the following skin conditions is contagious?
   a. rosacea
   b. vitiligo
   c. scabies

   d. alopecia
   e. keloids

8. Excessive scarring is known as
   a. keloids
   b. furuncles
   c. rosacea
   d. tinea
   e. scabies

9. A fungal infection causes
   a. furuncles
   b. urticaria
   c. rosacea
   d. tinea
   e. pediculosis

10. Infestation with lice is known as
    a. tinea
    b. pediculosis
    c. furuncles
    d. psoriasis
    e. eczema

CRITICAL THINKING

1. Dr. Miller diagnoses Julie with hirsutism. What factors listed in the case study support his diagnosis?

2. After discussing treatment options, Julie has decided that she does not want to deal with shaving, waxing, or plucking on a daily basis, but she also doesn't want to undergo surgical treatment. What might be a viable treatment option for Julie that addresses her ideals?

INTERNET ACTIVITY

Several organizations have been established to help in the prevention and treatment of diseases affecting the integumentary system. Perform an Internet search to learn more about these organizations and what each provides to people afflicted with specific skin disorders.

Additional interactive resources and activities for this chapter can be found:

On your student DVD: View applicable procedure videos on the DVD-ROM found in the back of this book.

MyHealthProfessionsKit.com: Test your knowledge of the chapter with games and activities. MyHealthProfessionsKit also includes resources, helpful links, and a Spanish audio glossary.

Medical Assisting Interactive: Practice your procedures as a medical assistant in this simulated doctor's office. This can be accessed through MyHealthProfessionsKit.com.

23

The Skeletal System

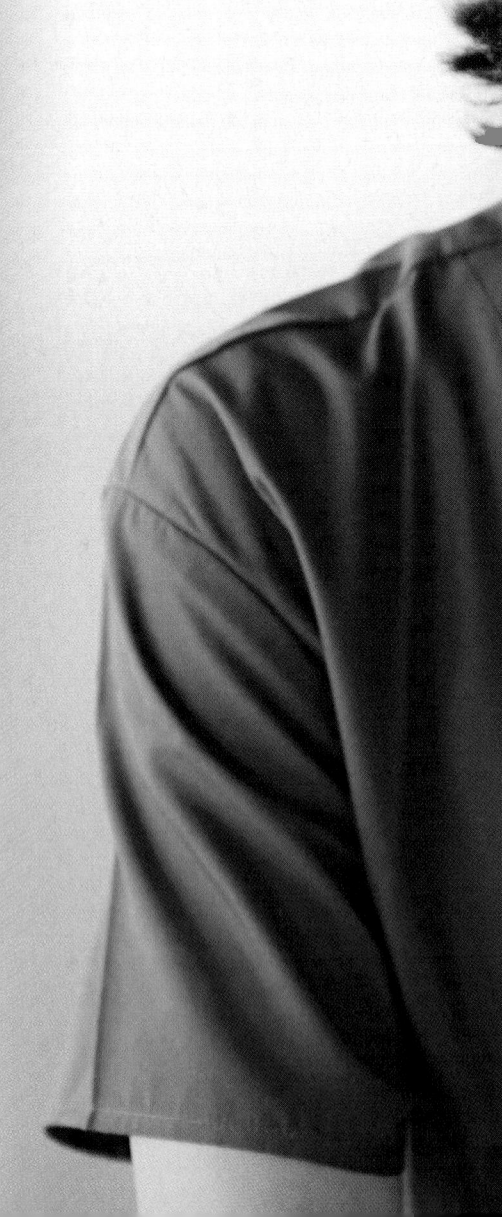

LEARNING OBJECTIVES

After completing this chapter, you should be able to:

- Define and spell the terms to learn for this chapter.

- List the various types of bones in the body.

- Identify specific bones for each bone classification

- Discuss the functions of the bones of the human skeleton.

- Explain various types of joints and body movements.

- Describe the axial skeleton.

- Describe the appendicular skeleton.

- List and explain common disorders of the skeletal system.

- Identify abnormal curvatures of the spine.

- Identify various types of fractures.

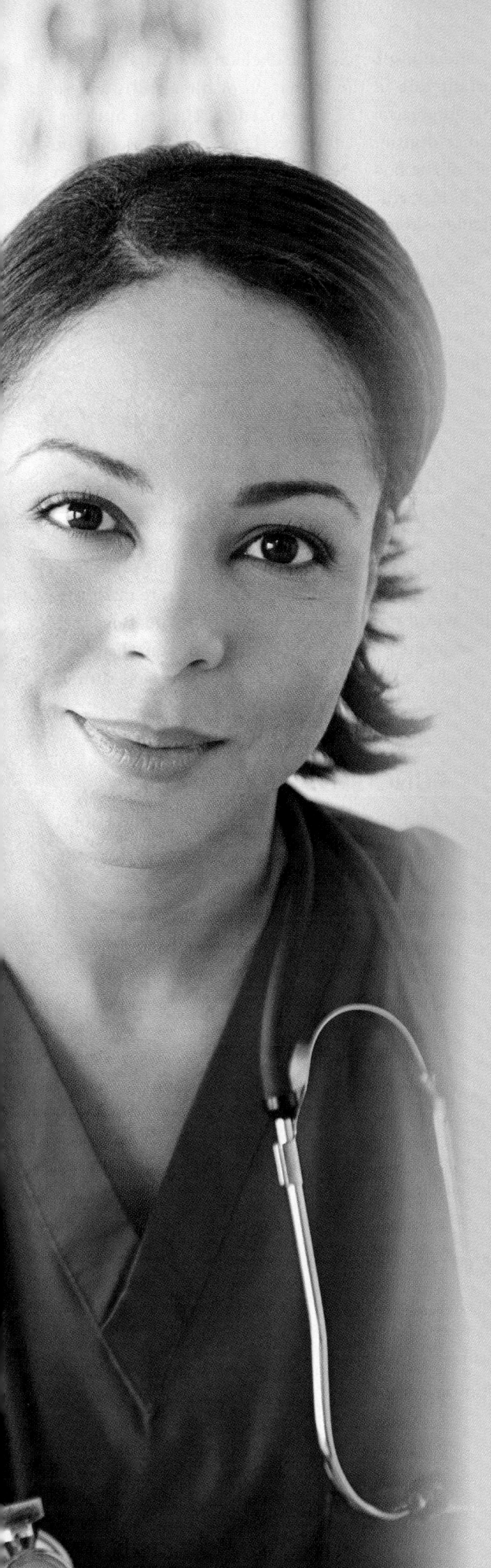

CHAPTER OUTLINE

CASE STUDY

Seventeen-year-old Charlie Baker was pitching during a high-school baseball game when he suddenly experienced a sharp pain in his right shoulder after striking out a player of the opposing team. Because of his intense pain, the coach had him taken to the emergency department at Pearson General Hospital. Charlie explained to the emergency department physician that the pain occurred immediately after he pitched the ball to the batter while trying to throw a fastball.

453

abduction	flexion
adduction	gout
amphiarthrotic joint	hallux valgus
appendicular skeleton	hammertoe
arthritis	inversion
articulation	kyphosis
atlas	lordosis
axial skeleton	medullary canal
axis	orthopedic physician
bursa	osteoarthritis
bursitis	osteomalacia
cancellous (spongy) bone	osteoporosis
chondrocytes	periosteum
circumduction	pronation
compact bone	protraction
diaphysis	reduction
diarthrotic joint	retraction
dislocation	rheumatoid arthritis
dorsiflexion	rickets
endosteum	rotation
epiphysis	scoliosis
etiology	supination
eversion	synarthrotic joint
extension	

CERTIFICATION LINK

CMA (AAMA)
Anatomy and physiology

   Systems (including structure, function, related conditions and diseases, and their relationships)

RMA
Anatomy and physiology

   Body systems
   Disorders and diseases of the body

CMAS (AMT)
Medical assisting foundation

   Anatomy and physiology
   Medical terminology

The skeletal system makes up the framework of the human body. It is responsible for providing shape and support, protecting internal organs, and serving as a storage place for mineral salts, calcium, and phosphorus. The skeletal system also plays an important role in the formation of blood cells and in providing an area for the attachment of skeletal muscles. Two distinct divisions comprise the skeletal system. The 206 bones of the body are divided into the **axial skeleton** (Figure 23-1), which is made of 80 bones, and the **appendicular skeleton**, which consists of the remaining 126 bones. The principal bones of the axial skeleton include the skull, vertebral system, and rib cage. The appendicular skeleton includes the shoulder and pelvic girdles, as well as the extremities. In addition, cartilage, tendons, and ligaments are also integral parts of the skeletal system.

Bones and Their Classification

It may be surprising to learn that bones are made of 50 percent water. The remaining 50 percent of bones are made of a rigid, calcified substance known as osseous tissue. Bones are classified according to shape. The six common shapes of bones are long, short, flat, irregular, sesamoid, and sutural (wormian) (Figure 23-2).

FUNCTIONS OF BONES

The bones of the human skeleton have six main functions:

- Providing shape, support, and the framework of the body

- Providing protection for the body's internal organs

- Serving as a storage place for mineral salts, calcium, and phosphorus

- Playing an important role in the formation of blood cells as hemopoiesis (formation of blood cells) takes place in the bone marrow

- Providing an area for the attachment of skeletal muscle

- Helping to make movement possible through articulation

STRUCTURE OF A LONG BONE

Long bones, such as the tibia, femur, humerus, and radius, have most of the features found in all bones (Figure 23-3). These features include the following:

- **Epiphysis**—the ends of a developing bone

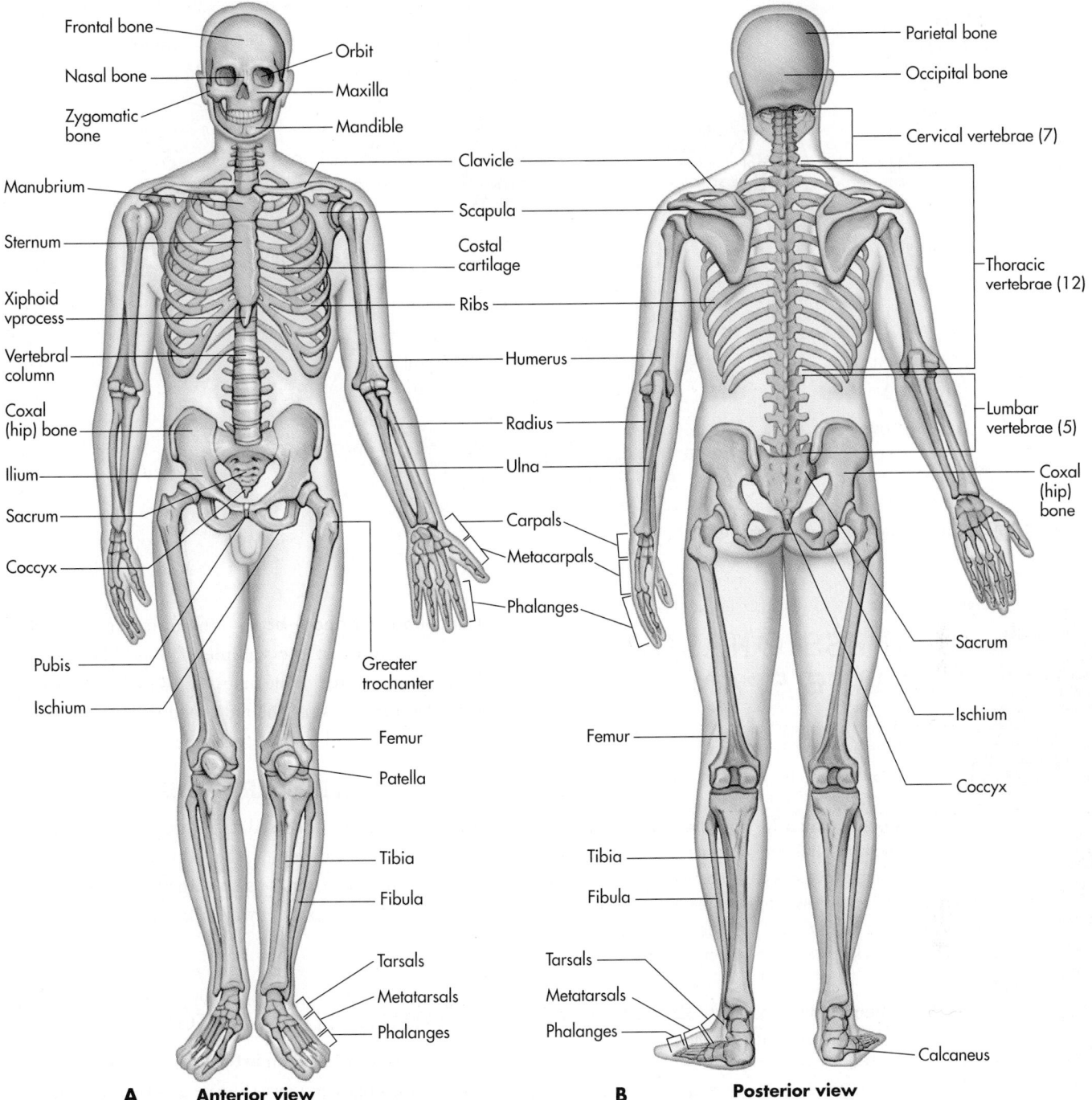

FIGURE 23-1 Anterior and posterior human skeleton.

- **Diaphysis**—the shaft of the long bone
- **Periosteum**—membrane that forms the covering of bones, except at their articular (of or relating to a joint) surfaces
- **Compact bone**—the dense, hard layer of bone tissue

- **Medullary canal**—the narrow space or cavity throughout the length of the diaphysis (The medullary canal contains yellow bone marrow, which is made of fat cells.)
- **Endosteum**—the tough, connective tissue membrane lining the medullary canal and containing the bone marrow

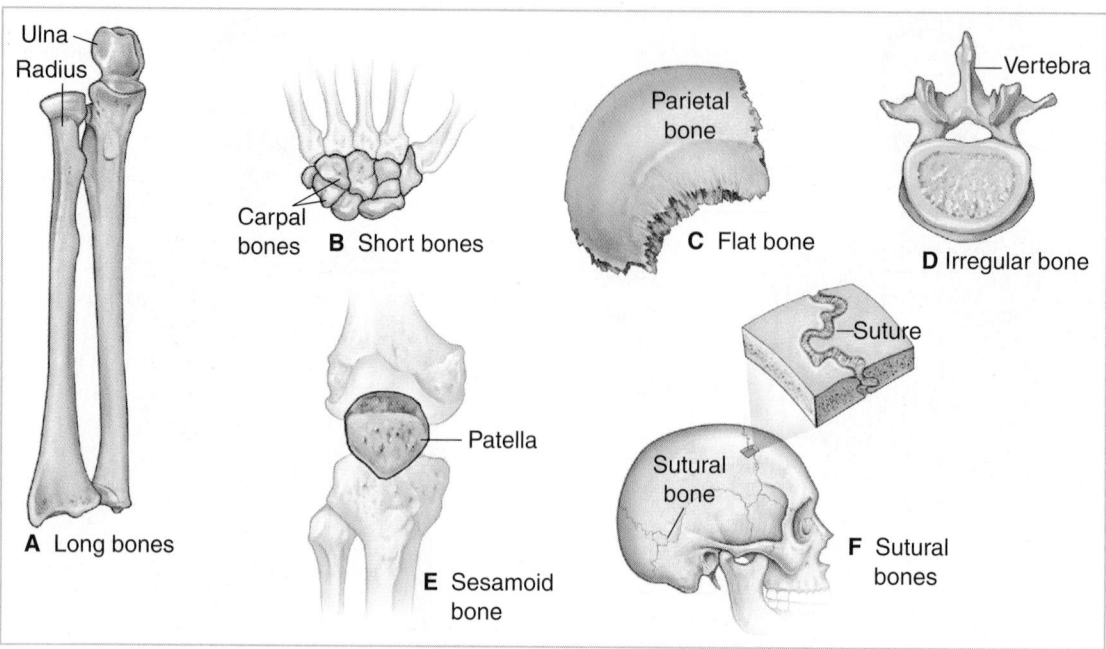

FIGURE 23-2 **Classification of bones by shape.**

- **Cancellous (spongy) bone**—the reticular tissue that makes up most of the volume of bone (The spongy bone contains red bone marrow. Red bone marrow manufactures most of the red blood cells found in the body and is found in the long bone.)

BONE MARKINGS

The markings of bones are used to indicate the position of different structural features of the bones. These features mark the attachment of tendons and ligaments to muscles, joining of bones, and passageways for blood vessels and nerves (Table 23-1).

Joints and Movement

A joint, which is also called an **articulation**, is located at the place where two bones connect (Figure 23-4). The positioning of the bones at the joint determines the type of move-

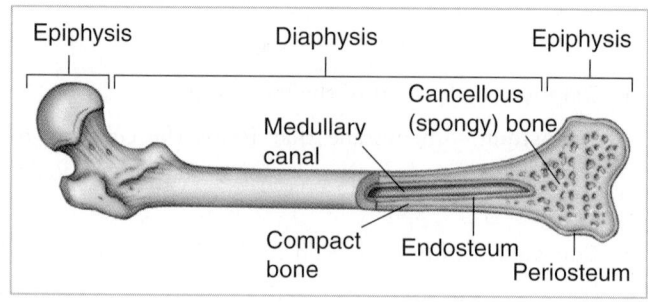

FIGURE 23-3 **The features found in a long bone.**

TABLE 23-1 Bone Markings

Crest	Narrow, usually prominent, ridge of bone
Epicondyle	Raised area on or above a condyle
Line	Narrow ridge of bone that is less prominent than a crest
Process	Bony projection
Spine	Sharp, slender, often pointed process
Trochanter	Very large, blunt, irregularly shaped process
Tubercle	Small rounded process
Tuberosity	Large rounded projection that may be roughened

ment that the joint performs. Because of this, joints are always classified according to the type of movement they provide. A joint that produces no movement is called a **synarthrotic joint**. Although the bones may actually touch, there is no joint cavity. An example of a synarthrosis is a cranial suture. An **amphiarthrotic joint** permits very slight movement. An example of this joint is the vertebrae. A **diarthrotic joint** allows for free movement in a variety of directions; examples of this type of joint are the elbow, wrist, hip, and knee.

The diarthrotic joint allows for several types of body movement. These movements, which can be seen in Figure 23-5, include the following:

- **Abduction**—the process of moving a body part *away from* the midline
- **Adduction**—the process of moving a body part *toward* the midline
- **Circumduction**—the process of moving a body part in a circular motion
- **Dorsiflexion**—the process of bending a body part backward
- **Eversion**—the process of turning outward
- **Extension**—the process of straightening a flexed limb or the spine
- **Flexion**—the process of bending (or curving) a flexed limb or the spine
- **Inversion**—the process of turning inward
- **Pronation**—the process of lying prone or face down; the process of turning the hand so that the palm points downward
- **Protraction**—the process of moving a body part forward
- **Retraction**—the process of moving a body part backward
- **Rotation**—the process of moving a body part around a central axis
- **Supination**—the process of lying supine or face upward; the process of turning the palm or foot upward

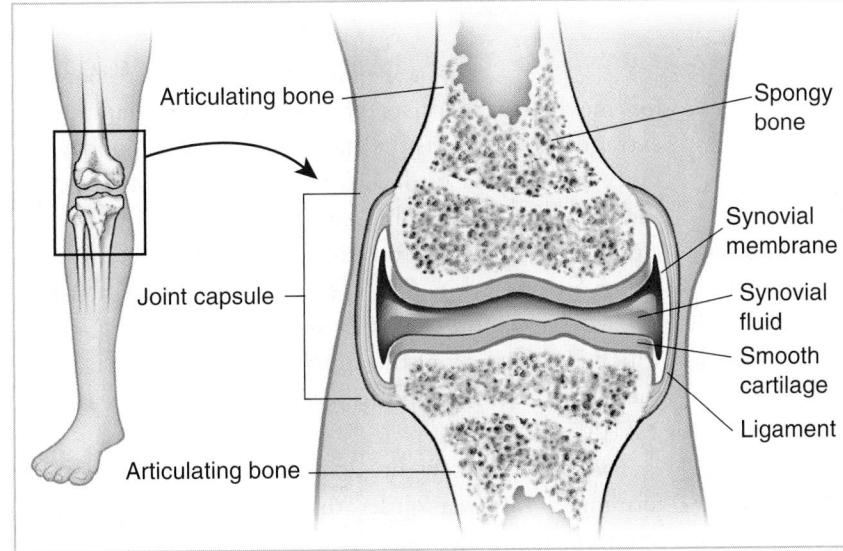

FIGURE 23-4 A typical joint.

Labels: Articulating bone, Joint capsule, Articulating bone, Spongy bone, Synovial membrane, Synovial fluid, Smooth cartilage, Ligament

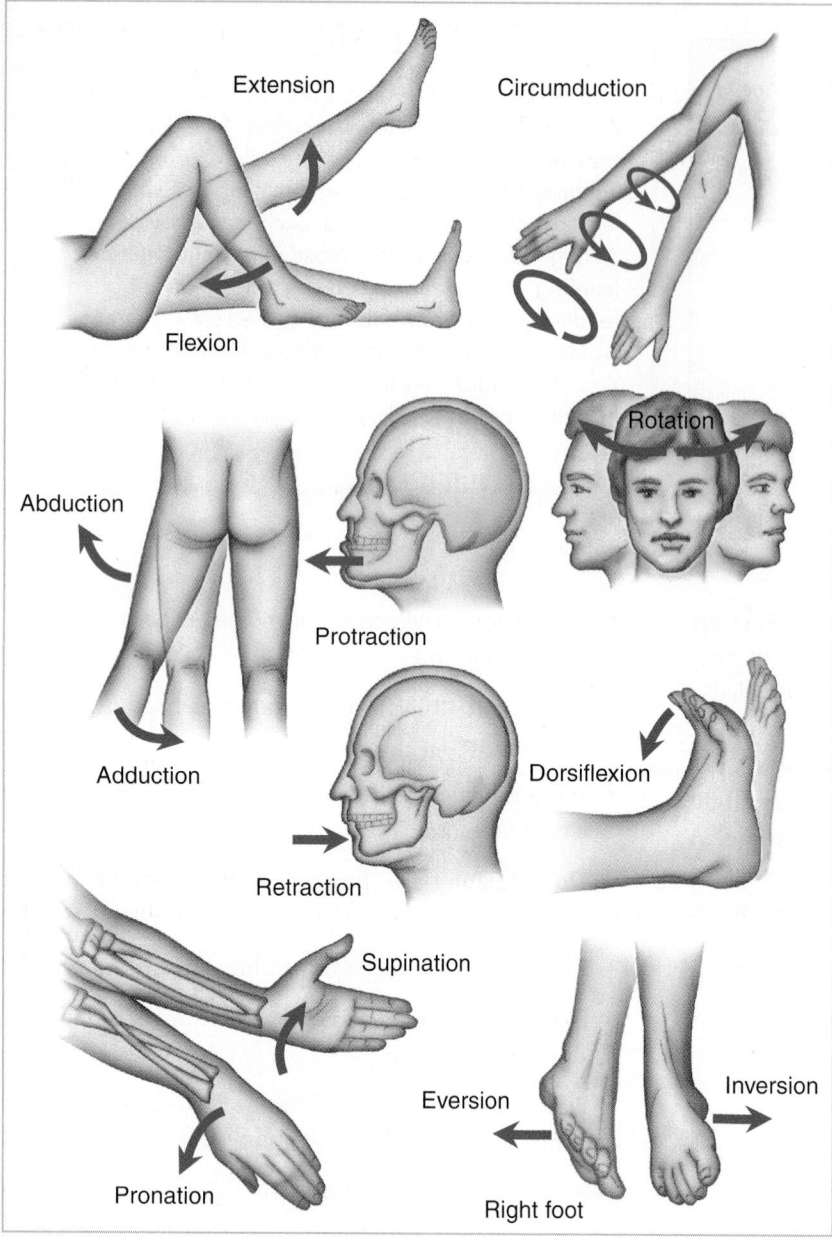

FIGURE 23-5 **Types of body movements.**

Labels within figure:
Extension
Circumduction
Flexion
Abduction
Rotation
Adduction
Protraction
Dorsiflexion
Retraction
Supination
Eversion
Inversion
Pronation
Right foot

The Axial Skeleton

The axial skeleton is the central portion of the skeleton (Figure 23-6). As mentioned, it consists of the skull, the sternum, the ribs, the vertebrae, the sacrum, and the coccyx. The head is composed of 22 bones; the skull has 8 bones, and the bones of the face total 14 (Figure 23-7).

The vertebral column, which houses the spinal cord, consists of a series of vertebrae that are connected in such a way as to form four spinal curves (Figure 23-8). These curves are referred to as cervical, thoracic, lumbar, and

sacral. The vertebrae are divided into five regions: the cervical, consisting of the first 7 vertebrae; the thoracic, the next 12 vertebrae; the 5 lumbar vertebrae; the sacral; and the coccyx, or tailbone. The first cervical vertebra is termed the **atlas** and attaches the spine to the occipital bone at the base of the skull. The **axis** is the second cervical vertebra and has a pivoting characteristic, allowing the head to turn from side to side.

The rib cage is also classified as part of the axial skeleton. This formation of ribs forms a protective cage that houses the heart, lungs, and other vital components of the human body. The rib cage consists of 12 pairs of ribs, which are divided into three categories; true ribs, false ribs, and floating ribs (Figure 23-9). There are 7 pairs of true ribs, which connect posteriorly to the spinal column and anteriorly to the sternum via small strips of cartilage. Three pairs of false ribs follow the true ribs by attaching to the spine in the back, but rather than attach to the sternum in the front, they are attached to the very last true ribs. Finally, the last two pairs of ribs are the floating ribs. These ribs are attached only to the spinal column, without any point of anterior articulation.

The Appendicular Skeleton

The appendicular skeleton, responsible for movement, consists of both the upper and lower extremities, as well as the clavicles and the scapula, which form the pectoral girdle. Upper extremity bones include the humerus, radius, ulna, carpals, metacarpals, and phalanges. The bones of the lower extremities include the femur, patella, tibia, fibula, tarsals, metatarsals, and phalanges (see Figure 23-10A and B). The pelvic girdle, which is also a part of the appendicular skeleton, includes the ileum, ischium, pubis, sacrum, and coccyx (Figure 23-10C).

The male pelvis (Figure 23-11A) is shaped like a funnel, forming a narrower outlet than the female's. It is both stronger and heavier than the female pelvis and therefore is

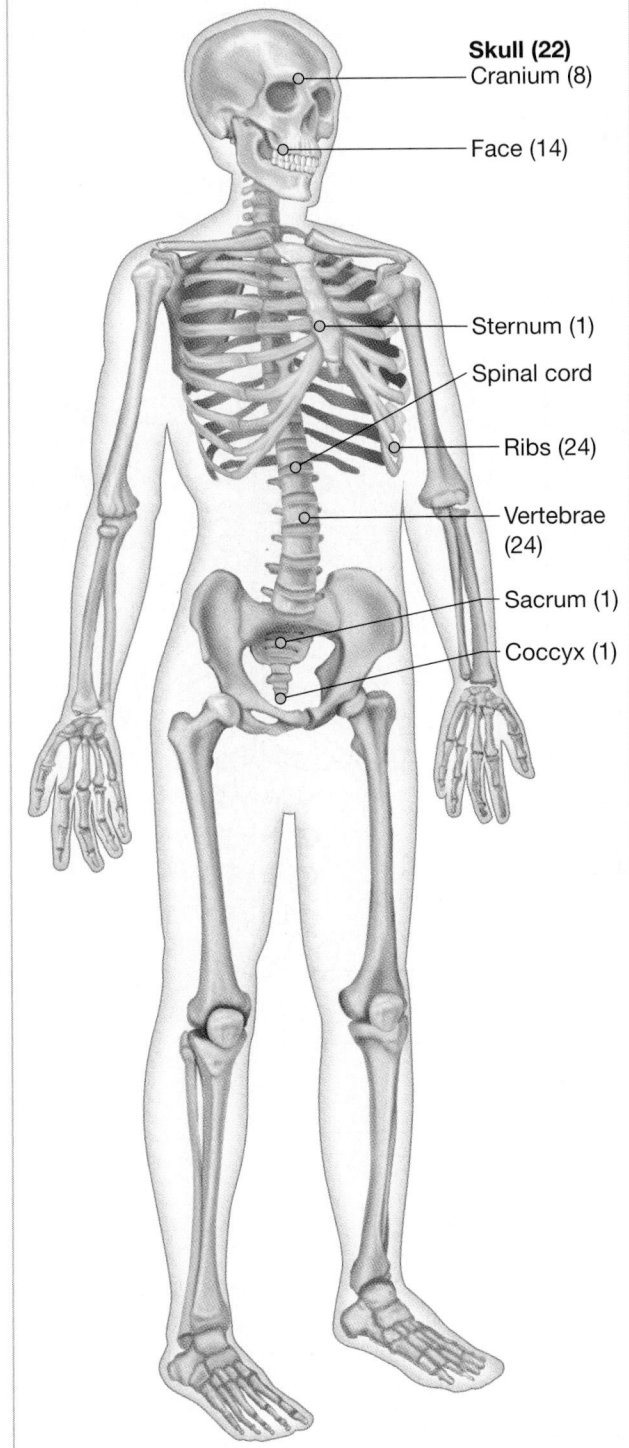

FIGURE 23-6 The axial skeleton.

Skull (22)
Cranium (8)

Face (14)

Sternum (1)

Spinal cord

Ribs (24)

Vertebrae (24)

Sacrum (1)

Coccyx (1)

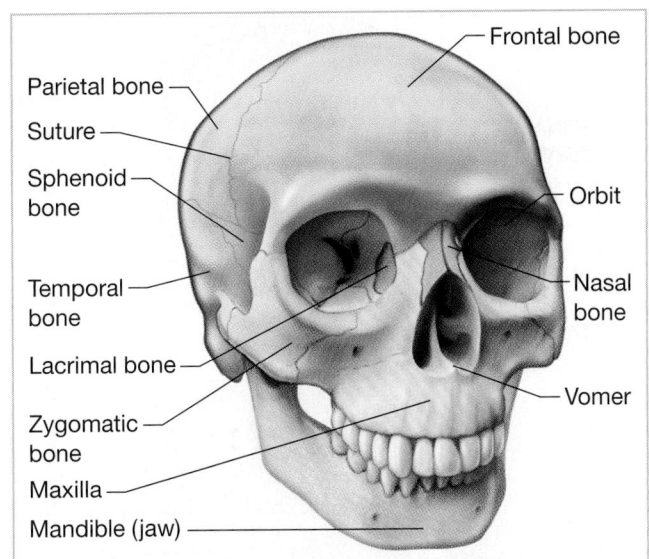

FIGURE 23-7 The cranial and facial bones.

Parietal bone

Suture

Sphenoid bone

Temporal bone

Lacrimal bone

Zygomatic bone

Maxilla

Mandible (jaw)

Frontal bone

Orbit

Nasal bone

Vomer

Common Disorders Associated with the Skeletal System

Many diseases and disorders are associated with the skeletal system. Many of these are discussed in the following pages. Table 23-2 lists additional disorders associated with the skeletal system.

ABNORMAL CURVATURE OF THE SPINE

Abnormal curvature of the spine, a portion of the axial skeleton, is often diagnosed as scoliosis, lordosis, or kyphosis (Figure 23-12).

Scoliosis

Scoliosis is an abnormal lateral curvature of the spine that is often diagnosed early in toddlers, children, and adolescents.

Signs and Symptoms. Many times, a scoliatic spine appears to have an S or C shape. Generally, a spine must have a curvature of at least 10 degrees, which is measurable on an X-ray. Those afflicted with scoliosis may often appear as if either their shoulders or legs are uneven.

Treatment. Orthopedic braces often are used to reduce the progression of the abnormal spinal curvature. In cases of severe curvature or a continual progression of the disease, surgical treatment may be required.

suited for lifting and running. The female pelvis (Figure 23-11B) is formed to be able to support pregnancy and childbirth. Often described as having a basin-like appearance, the female pelvis is much broader, rounder, and lighter than the male pelvis.

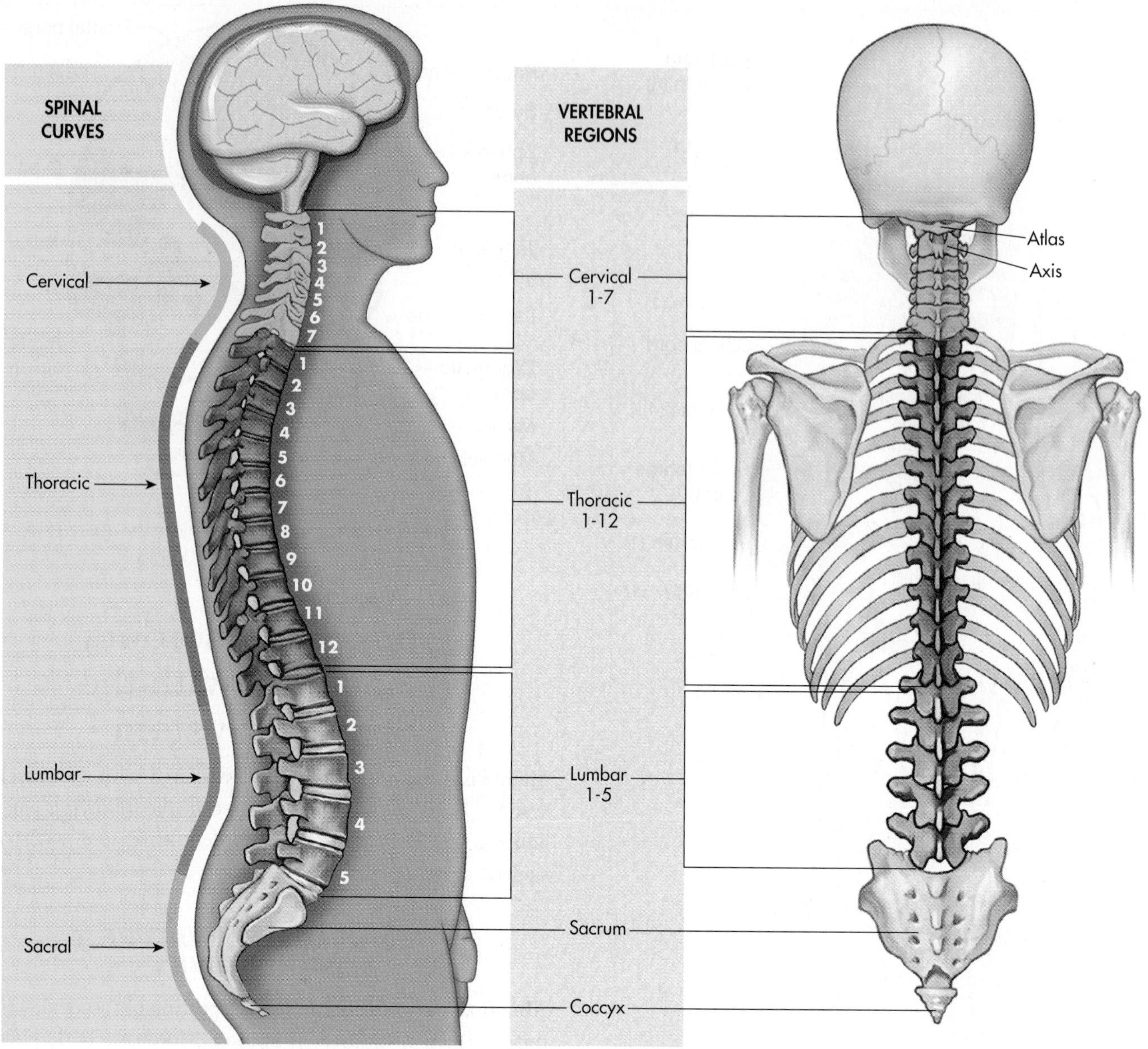

SPINAL CURVES
VERTEBRAL REGIONS
Cervical
Thoracic
Lumbar
Sacral
Cervical 1-7
Thoracic 1-12
Lumbar 1-5
Sacrum
Coccyx
Atlas
Axis
1
2
3
4
5
6
7
1
2
3
4
5
6
7
8
9
10
11
12
1
2
3
4
5

FIGURE 23-8 Vertebral regions showing the four spinal curves.

Lordosis

Lordosis is often called swayback. It is an exaggerated inward curvature of the lumbar spine.

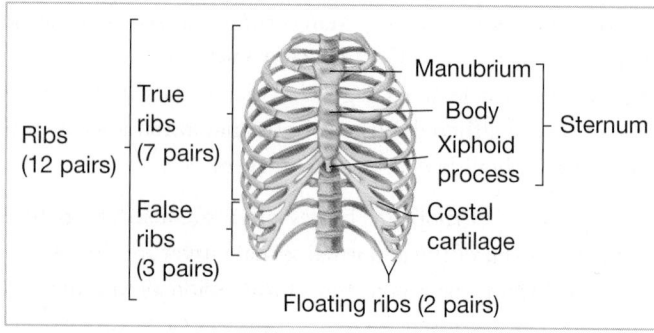

Ribs (12 pairs)
True ribs (7 pairs)
False ribs (3 pairs)
Manubrium
Body
Xiphoid process
Sternum
Costal cartilage
Floating ribs (2 pairs)

FIGURE 23-9 The rib cage.

Signs and Symptoms. When diagnosed in adults, lordosis is commonly found in men and women who are overweight, and pregnant women. When diagnosed in children, a prominently protruding abdomen and/or buttocks constitute the most common symptom.

Treatment. Treatment for lordosis will depend on the patient's overall health, age, and severity of the condition. The overall goal of treatment is to stop the curvature and prevent spinal deformity.

Kyphosis

Kyphosis is most often known as humpback and results from an exaggeration of the thoracic curvature. The normal thoracic curvature may become exaggerated due to a con-

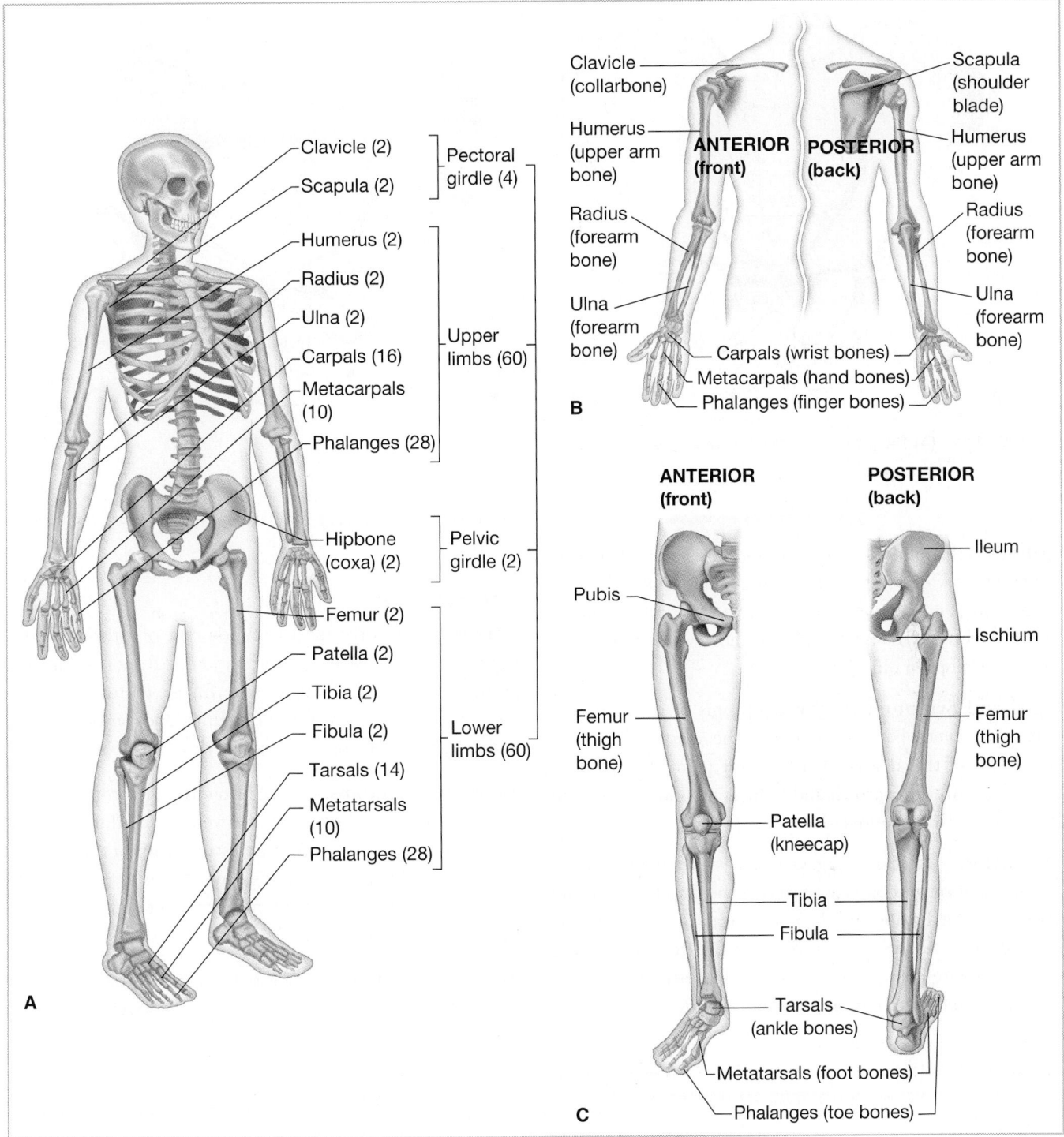

FIGURE 23-10 (A) The appendicular skeleton; (B) bones of the upper extremities; (C) bones of the lower extremities.

genital defect, disease process (such as tuberculosis, syphilis, or malignancy), compression fracture, faulty posture, osteoarthritis, rheumatoid arthritis, rickets, osteoporosis, or other condition.

Signs and Symptoms.   The most telling symptom of kyphosis is the rounded back appearance. In addition, symptoms may include fatigue, mild back pain, and either a tender or stiff feeling within the spine. In severe cases, shortness of breath may be apparent.

Treatment.   As with lordosis, the overall health and age of the patient will be taken into consideration when developing a treatment plan. In addition, the **etiology**, or the cause or source of the patient's disease or disorder, also will be considered.

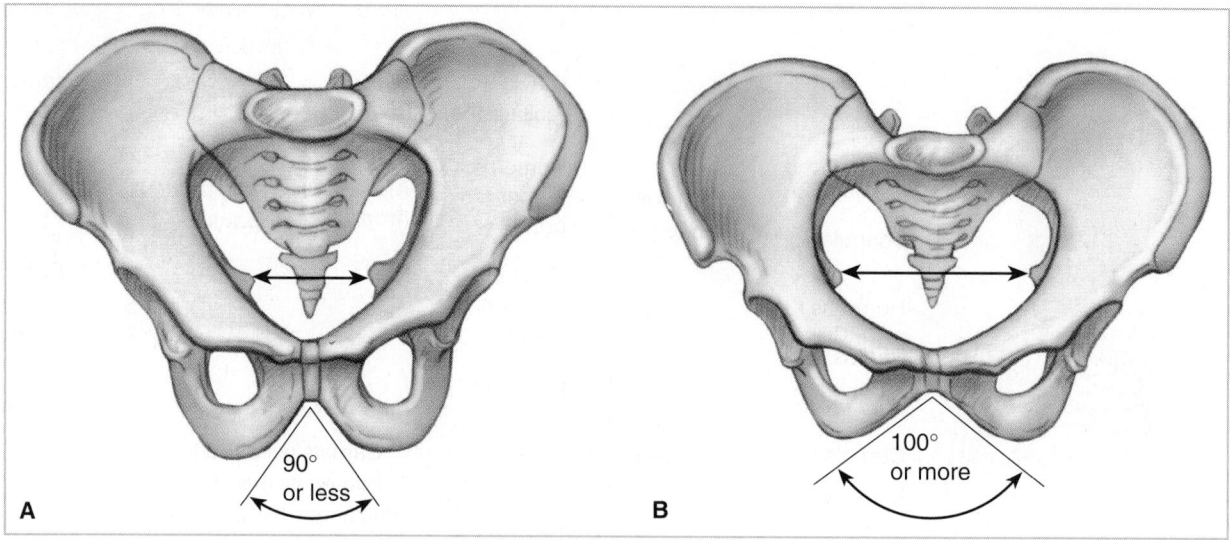

FIGURE 23-11 **(A) The male pelvis; (B) the female pelvis.**

ARTHRITIS

Arthritis is the inflammation of one or more joints. There are various causes of arthritis, including joint injury, autoimmune disorders, and normal to excessive wear and tear on the joints. Arthritis can occur at any age; however, it most commonly develops in older adults.

Signs and Symptoms. The symptoms of arthritis will vary with every patient; however, the classic signs and symptoms of this disease include joint pain and swelling, morning stiffness, warmth and redness around a joint, and decreased ability to move the joint.

Treatment. Treatment for arthritis is dependent on the age, occupation and other activities of the patient, cause and severity of the disease, and the joint affected. A modification to daily activities and low-impact aerobic exercise (such as swimming) are helpful in treatment. Medications to reduce joint pain and swelling, application of heat or cold, joint protection, and surgery may also be used in treating various levels of arthritis.

Osteoarthritis

Osteoarthritis is the most common type of arthritis resulting from years of wear and tear on joints. It most frequently occurs in the hips, knees, and finger joints of elderly patients. Obesity, a history of trauma, and various genetic and metabolic diseases increase the risk of osteoarthritis.

Signs and Symptoms. In addition to pain, symptoms associated with osteoarthritis include swelling and fluid accumulation around the joints. An interesting symptom that occurs with osteoarthritis is an aching pain that is associated with changes in the weather. Permanent joint deformity may occur in some cases (Figure 23-13).

Treatment. Treatment of osteoarthritis requires the use of nonsteroidal anti-inflammatory drugs (NSAIDs), steroid

TABLE 23-2 Additional Disorders of the Skeletal System

Disorder	Description
Epicondylitis	Commonly referred to as tennis elbow; characterized by elbow pain that is a result of repetitive grasping and rotating of the forearm
Osteomyelitis	Inflammation of the bone and bone marrow due to infection; can be difficult to treat
Paget's disease	A fairly common metabolic disease of the bone from unknown causes; usually attacks middle-aged and elderly people; characterized by bone destruction and deformity
Ruptured intervertebral disk	Herniation or outpouching of a disk between two vertebrae; also called a slipped or herniated disk
Spinal stenosis	Narrowing of the spinal canal causing pressure on the spinal cord and nerves

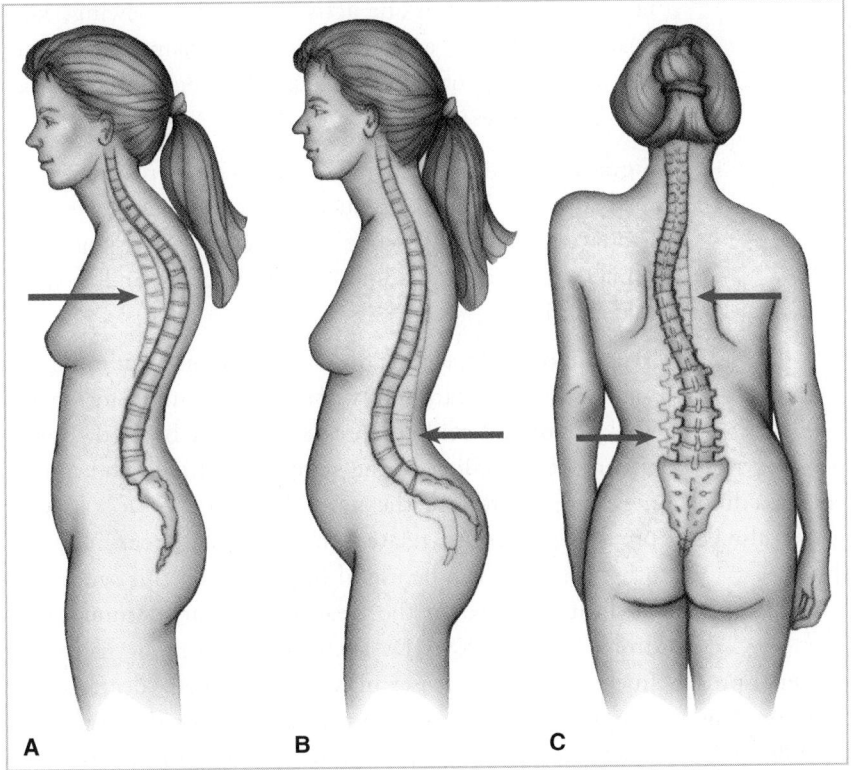

FIGURE 23-12 Abnormal curvatures of the spine: (A) kyphosis; (B) lordosis; (C) scoliosis.

Signs and Symptoms. Rheumatoid arthritis is marked by inflammation, joint swelling, and joint deformity (Figure 23-14). Morning joint stiffness is very common as joints have had limited movement during sleep. Fatigue and loss of appetite are also associated with this disease. In addition to the hands, other parts of the body can also be affected. The medical assistant must be aware of possible symptoms in order to obtain relevant information for the physician; this is accomplished by asking patients useful questions and correctly documenting their answers.

Treatment. There is no cure for rheumatoid arthritis. However, early detection, diagnosis, and treatment may deter pain and joint decay. In addition to rest, eating a balanced diet, and taking corticosteroids, disease-modifying antirheumatic drugs can be helpful in decreasing joint deformation. In severe cases, surgery may be required.

injections to the affected joint, and, in severe cases, joint replacement.

Rheumatoid Arthritis

Rheumatoid arthritis is an autoimmune disorder causing joints to become deformed due to inflammation. In addition to inflammation, increased growth of both cartilage and bone is associated with this autoimmune disorder.

BURSITIS

A **bursa** is a small sac of fluid that cushions and lubricates an area where joint-related tissues rub against one another. **Bursitis** is inflammation of the bursa.

Signs and Symptoms. The most common signs and symptoms of bursitis include joint pain, limited joint mobility, swelling, and tenderness surrounding the joint. Bursitis occurs most frequently in the elbow, knee, shoulder, and hip and is generally the result of overuse and trauma to joints.

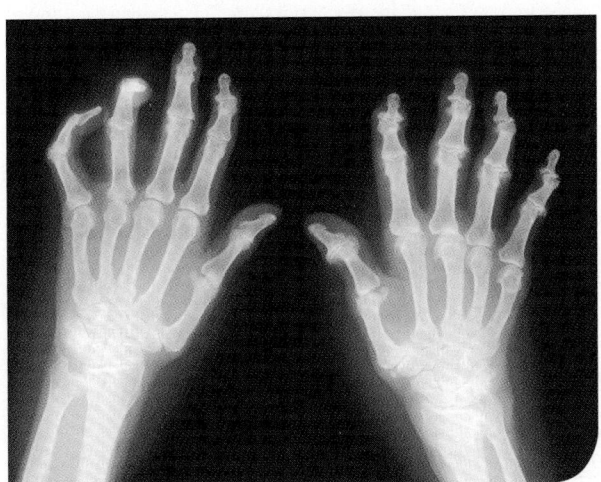

FIGURE 23-13 X-ray showing typical joint changes with osteoarthritis.

PROFESSIONALISM

THE LAW

When obtaining a medical history from a patient, it is important to check the patient's past medical history. Sometimes, the source of a current condition could be a result of a past disease or medications that the patient took many years previously. Although the final responsibility for diagnosis lies with the physician, the medical assistant can also ask questions that may trigger the patient to remember taking certain medications or experiencing diseases in the past. This information will help the physician to consider all possible diagnoses.

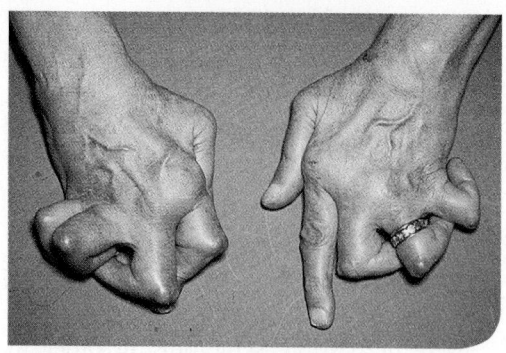

FIGURE 23-14 Typical hand deformities associated with rheumatoid arthritis.

racquetball or tennis, or activities such as sewing, keyboarding, driving, assembly-line work, painting, typing, writing, the use of hand tools or vibrating tools, or other similar activities.

Signs and Symptoms. When pressure is placed on the median nerve, pain is produced along with numbness and hand weakness. Certain conditions increase the risk of carpal tunnel syndrome, including obesity, diabetes, and rheumatoid arthritis.

Treatment. Treatment of bursitis usually involves rest, pain medication, steroid injections, aspiration of excess fluid from the bursa, and antibiotics. Physical therapy may also be utilized to increase and promote joint movement.

Treatment. Treatment for carpal tunnel syndrome can include the application of wrist splints at night for several weeks. Hot and cold compresses also may be used. Proper treatment can alleviate the symptoms of pain and numbness and can restore the normal use of the wrists. Also, proper ergonomics related to typing, keyboarding, and other activities can be useful in preventing this syndrome. Medications used in the treatment of carpal tunnel syndrome include NSAIDs such as ibuprofen or naproxen. Injections of corticosteroids can also help decrease the symptoms. If these measures do not provide significant relief, then a surgical procedure that decreases the pressure on the median nerve is about 85 percent effective in relieving carpal tunnel symptoms.

CARPAL TUNNEL SYNDROME

The carpal tunnel is a narrow passageway. The tunnel protects the median nerve to the hand and the nine tendons that bend the fingers (Figure 23-15). This disorder becomes present when pressure is placed on the median nerve. Repetitive movements might be caused by sports, such as

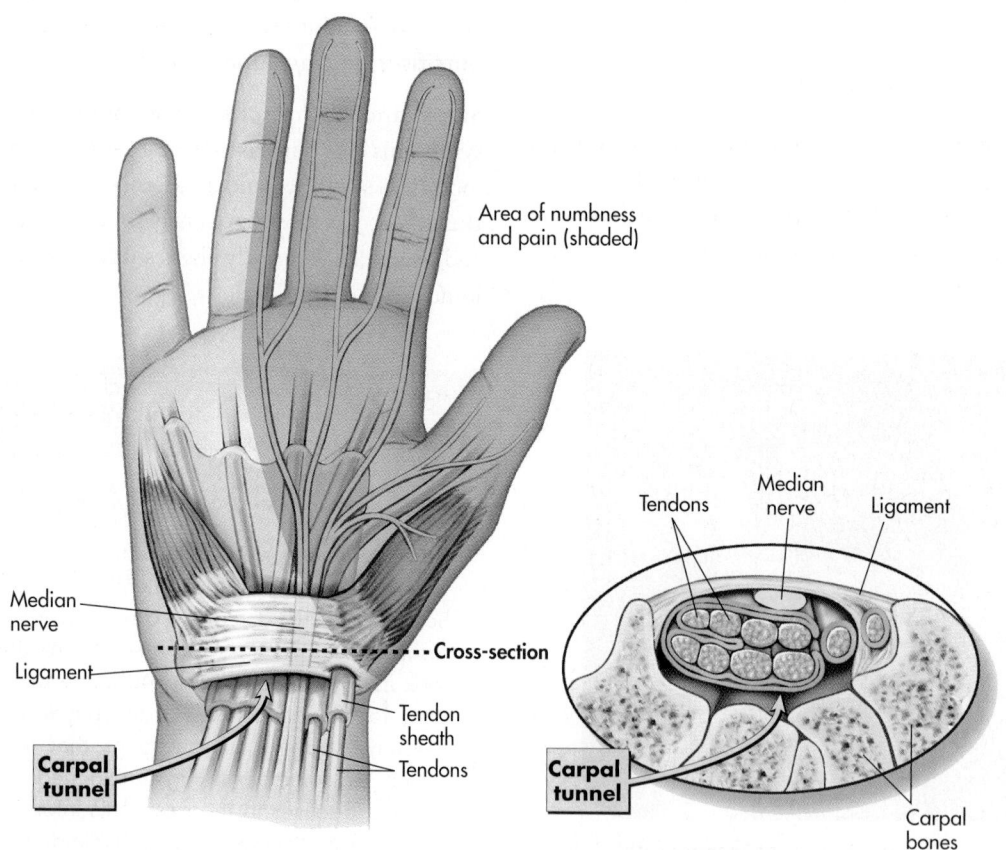

FIGURE 23-15 Cross-section of the wrist showing tendons and nerves involved in carpal tunnel syndrome.

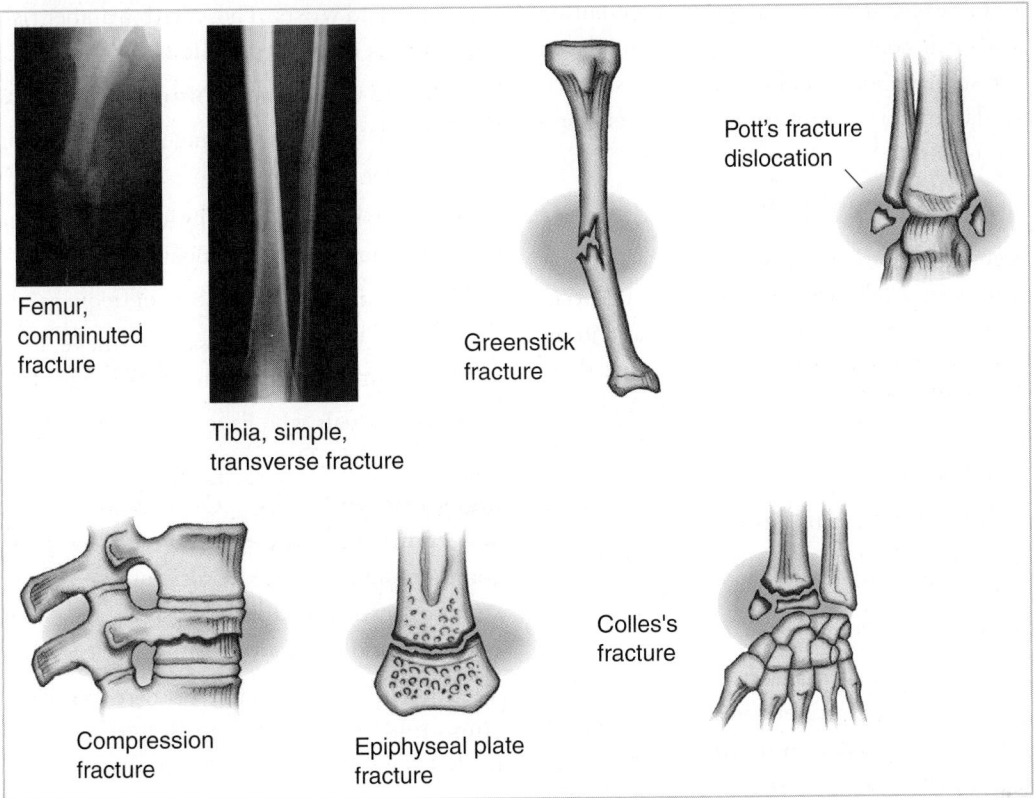

FIGURE 23-16 Various types of fractures.

FRACTURES

Fractures are bone cracks or breaks of various types. Fractures are classified based on their external appearance, the site of the fracture, and the nature of the crack or break in the bone.

Signs and Symptoms. The different types of fractures, some of which are illustrated in Figure 23-16, include the following:

- **Closed**—Also known as a simple fracture, this type of fracture does not involve a break in the skin. It is completely internal.

- **Open (compound)**—These are more dangerous fractures because of the projection of the fracture through the skin. Because the integrity of the skin and other tissues is damaged in this type of fracture, the risk of infection or hemorrhage is greater than with a closed fracture.

- **Comminuted**—In this type of fracture, part of the bone is shattered into a multitude of bony fragments.

- **Transverse**—These fractures break the shaft of the bone across its longitudinal access.

- **Greenstick**—This type of fracture usually occurs in young children, whose bones are still relatively soft.

Only one side of the shaft is broken; the other side is bent, similar to breaking a green plant stick.

- **Spiral**—Spiral fractures are spread along the length of a bone, and are produced by twisting stresses.

- **Colles's**—Colles's fracture is frequently the result of reaching forward to stop or cushion a fall. This fracture is exemplified by a break in the distal portion of the radius. Colles's fractures are most frequently seen in children and the elderly.

- **Pott's**—These fractures occur in the ankle and affect both bones of the lower leg (the tibia and fibula).

- **Compression**—Compression fractures occur in the vertebrae after severe stress, such as when someone falls and lands with a significant amount of force.

- **Epiphyseal**—These fractures are commonly seen in children in areas where the matrix (a special part of the bone near the growth plate) is undergoing calcification (a hardening process of the calcium in the bones) and the **chondrocytes** (cartilage-forming cells) are dying.

Treatment. Fractures are generally casted by a physician. An **orthopedic physician** is a physician who treats musculoskeletal conditions. The cast that is applied limits the movement of the bone affected, allowing proper healing to occur. At times, in severe fractures, surgical intervention must be performed. It is common that both pins and metal plating are used to stabilize joints and bones during surgery. Pain and anti-inflammatory medications are often prescribed for patient comfort.

DISLOCATIONS

A **dislocation** occurs when a bone slips out of the joint. A dislocation usually occurs following a blow, fall, or other trauma. Because two or more bones come together at a joint, if a sudden impact injures a joint the bones that meet there may become dislocated. Usually the joint capsule and ligaments tear when a dislocation occurs, and often the nerves are injured.

Signs and Symptoms.   Dislocated joints may be visibly out of place, discolored, misshapen, limited in movement, bruised or swollen, and intensely painful. It is generally very difficult to move the affected joint.

Treatment.   If a dislocation is suspected, patients generally should seek emergency department treatment, as many physician offices are not equipped to handle this injury. A procedure known as **reduction** is used to align and reposition the joint. Pain relievers and anti-inflammatory medications are often prescribed for patients. At times, general anesthesia is given for reduction procedures that are difficult and must be relocated in the operating room.

OSTEOPOROSIS

Osteoporosis is characterized by progressive loss of bone density and thinning of bone tissue. Osteoporosis affects more than twenty-five million Americans, mostly women ages 50 to 70 years old. Individuals with osteoporosis are subject to increased fracture potential, especially in the hips, vertebrae, and wrists. Those with a higher risk of developing osteoporosis include the following:

- Those with a family history of osteoporosis
- Those who do not engage in weight-bearing exercise as part of their lifestyle
- Caucasian women who have never been pregnant and experience early menopause
- Individuals with a history of frequent corticosteroid use
- Individuals who excessively smoke, drink alcohol, and consume diets high in salt, fat, and caffeine
- Individuals who have an insufficient intake of calcium or vitamin D

Signs and Symptoms.   Osteoporosis generally has gradual and sometimes hard-to-recognize symptoms. The most common signs of osteoporosis are decreased height and a stooped posture. Additional signs and symptoms include back pain and frequent fractures.

Treatment.   Treatment of osteoporosis includes calcium and vitamin D supplementation, medications to help preserve calcium, hormone replacement, and exercise.

GOUT

Gout, also referred to as gouty arthritis, is a disease caused by the formation and accumulation of urate crystals in the joints that result from high levels of uric acid, leading to inflammation. The most frequent joint affected is the great toe; however, fingers and hands can also be affected.

Signs and Symptoms.   A gouty joint is often very warm and very sore to the touch. After joints have been

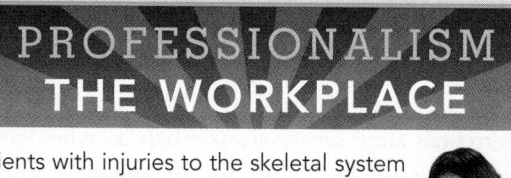

PROFESSIONALISM
THE WORKPLACE

Patients with injuries to the skeletal system may have trouble walking. It is important to have the wheelchairs and railings necessary to facilitate movement. The medical assistant may need to walk closely with the patient to ensure safety. If at all possible, place a patient who has trouble walking in an examination room near the reception area to reduce the amount of walking that is necessary.

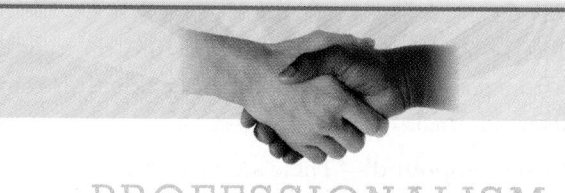

PROFESSIONALISM
CULTURAL CONSIDERATIONS

Although Caucasian women have a higher risk of osteoporosis, the disease also affects other races. It is important to teach all women, and men, the risk factors and preventive measures for osteoporosis. Any individual who is slender is at a greater risk for osteoporosis, but larger individuals may also be at risk. It is also important to double-check the patient's past medical history. For example, any individual who has taken steroids over a long period of time is at risk, and the physician should be alerted.

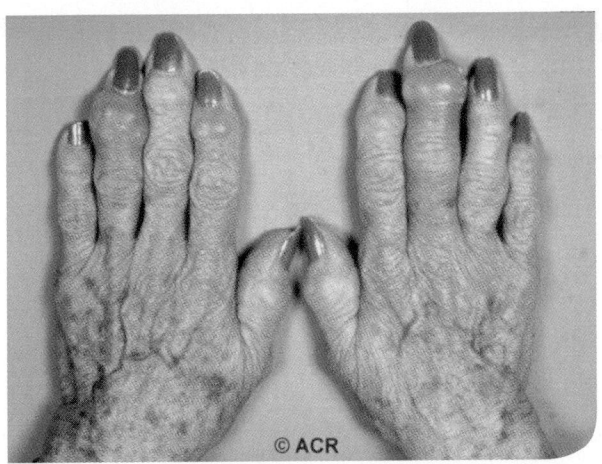

FIGURE 23-17 Gout of the finger joint. © 1972–2004 American College of Rheumatology Clinical Slide Collection. Used with permission.

persistently affected by gout, they may become disfigured (Figure 23-17).

Treatment. Medications are available to treat gout, and a diet rich in colorful fruits and vegetables such as kale, cabbage, leafy green vegetables, red peppers, strawberries, cherries, and blueberries helps to decrease the symptoms of gout. Dietary restrictions include the avoidance of caffeine, alcohol, liver, and other purine-rich foods are also advised.

HALLUX VALGUS

Hallux valgus, also called a bunion, is the enlargement of the inner portion of the metatarsophalangeal joint at the base of the big toe.

Signs and Symptoms. Reddened skin surrounds the inflamed joint of the big toe in hallux valgus. In addition, the joint may be filled with fluid and feel tender to the touch.

Treatment. Properly fitting shoes should be worn. Also, proper padding and cushioning of the joint should be considered. Foot surgery and pain medications may be required for severe cases. The patient may need to be fitted with special adaptive shoes made by a specialist in orthopedic shoes.

HAMMERTOE

Hammertoe is produced when the toe bends upward like a claw because of the abnormal flexion of the proximal interphalangeal joint.

Signs and Symptoms. Pain and visible joint deformation are classic symptoms of this skeletal disorder.

Treatment. Treatment for hammertoe consists of analgesics, splinting, and wearing specially designed footwear. In severe cases, surgical straightening of the toe may be required.

OSTEOMALACIA

Osteomalacia is the adult onset of rickets. As with rickets, deficiencies in calcium and vitamin D are causes for the disease. Additional causes for development of osteomalacia include cancer, liver disease, kidney failure, and side effects associated with antiseizure medications.

Signs and Symptoms. Symptoms of osteomalacia include bone pain, bowing legs, and frequent fractures.

Treatment. The treatment for osteomalacia is very similar to the treatment for rickets, including increasing vitamin and mineral intake and comfort measures to relieve symptoms.

RICKETS

Rickets is an early childhood disease caused by a deficiency in calcium, vitamin D, and phosphate. This disease results in bone deformities, especially bowed legs. Genetics may increase the risk of developing rickets.

Signs and Symptoms. Symptoms include pain and tenderness of the bones, an increased likelihood of bone breakage, impaired growth and decreased height, as well as muscle cramps.

Treatment. Treatment for rickets includes increasing vitamin and mineral intake as well as comfort measures, including rest and heat and ice applications, to relieve the symptoms.

SUMMARY

The skeletal system is divided into the axial skeleton and the appendages (arms and legs) that attach to it. Bones not only store essential minerals but also assist with joints and movement. Therefore, disorders of the skeletal system can seriously impair mobility and the ability to perform activities of daily living. Arthritis is a crippling degeneration of joints. Bursitis is an inflammation of the bursa that lubricates the joints. Carpal tunnel syndrome is caused by excessive repetitive use of the wrists. Fractures can occur from trauma or weakness in the bone. Dislocations occur when a bone slips out of the joint. Gout is caused by an accumulation of urate crystals. Hallux valgus, also known as a bunion, is an overgrowth of the great toe. Hammertoe occurs when the toe bends upward like a claw. Osteomalacia and rickets are caused when bone softens, sometimes from lack of vitamin D. Osteoporosis is damage to the bone caused when the bone becomes porous and weak.

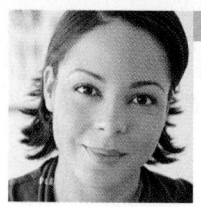

23 CHAPTER REVIEW

COMPETENCY REVIEW

1. Define and spell the terms to learn for this chapter.

2. Name the two main divisions of the skeletal system.

3. Name the six classifications of bone, and give an example of each.

4. Discuss the six main functions of the skeletal system.

5. Name the three classifications of joints.

6. Contrast the difference between the three abnormal curvatures of the spine.

7. Describe how the female pelvis differs from the male pelvis.

8. Draw pictures of the 13 types of body movements found in Figure 23-5.

9. Describe what kind of fracture could occur in a child that falls down the stairs, and explain your choices.

10. What is arthritis?

PREPARING FOR THE CERTIFICATION EXAM

1. Which of the following is also known as a bunion?
   a. hallux valgus
   b. hammertoe
   c. toe dislocation
   d. toe fracture
   e. bursitis

2. Which of the following is caused by a formation of urate crystals in the joints?
   a. gout
   b. scoliosis
   c. rickets
   d. lordosis
   e. osteoporosis

3. Which of the following is an abnormal lateral curvature of the spine?
   a. gout
   b. lordosis
   c. kyphosis
   d. scoliosis
   e. rickets

4. Which of the following is not part of the axial skeleton?
   a. ribs
   b. coccyx

   c. femur
   d. sternum
   e. vertebrae

5. Which of the following is the process of moving a body part around a central axis?
   a. flexion
   b. extension
   c. pronation
   d. rotation
   e. protraction

6. Which of the following is the process of bending the toes upward to relieve a cramp in the calf muscle?
   a. abduction
   b. adduction
   c. dorsiflexion
   d. extension
   e. circumduction

7. What type of fracture does twisting cause?
   a. comminuted
   b. spiral
   c. greenstick
   d. epiphyseal
   e. compound

8. Rickets is caused by a lack of which vitamin?
   a. A
   b. B
   c. C
   d. D
   e. E

9. Which of the following is an inflammation of the bone and bone marrow?
   a. osteoporosis
   b. osteoarthritis
   c. osteomalacia
   d. osteomyelitis
   e. epicondylitis

10. Which bone is on the side of the face?
   a. maxilla
   b. mandible
   c. lacrimal
   d. sphenoid
   e. zygomatic

CRITICAL THINKING

1. The emergency department physician suspects that Charlie may have dislocated his shoulder. What would be some additional signs and symptoms of a dislocation?

2. The physician informs Charlie he will have to have a reduction to his shoulder; however, it may be painful due to the severity of the injury. Charlie is very apprehensive about the procedure. What is an option that could be considered regarding the reduction?

3. Months after the successful reduction, Charlie developed bursitis in the same shoulder. What are some possible treatment methods for bursitis?

INTERNET ACTIVITY

Find the website of the National Osteoporosis Association. Determine what information the organization provides for patients and for health care providers. Utilize this information to learn how to teach a patient about osteoporosis.

MEDMEDIA

Additional interactive resources and activities for this chapter can be found:

On your student DVD: View applicable procedure videos on the DVD-ROM found in the back of this book.

MyHealthProfessionsKit.com: Test your knowledge of this chapter with games and activities. MyHealthProfessionsKit also includes resources, helpful links, and a Spanish audio glossary.

Medical Assisting Interactive: Practice your procedures as a medical assistant in this simulated doctor's office. This can be accessed through MyHealthProfessionsKit.com.

24

The Muscular System

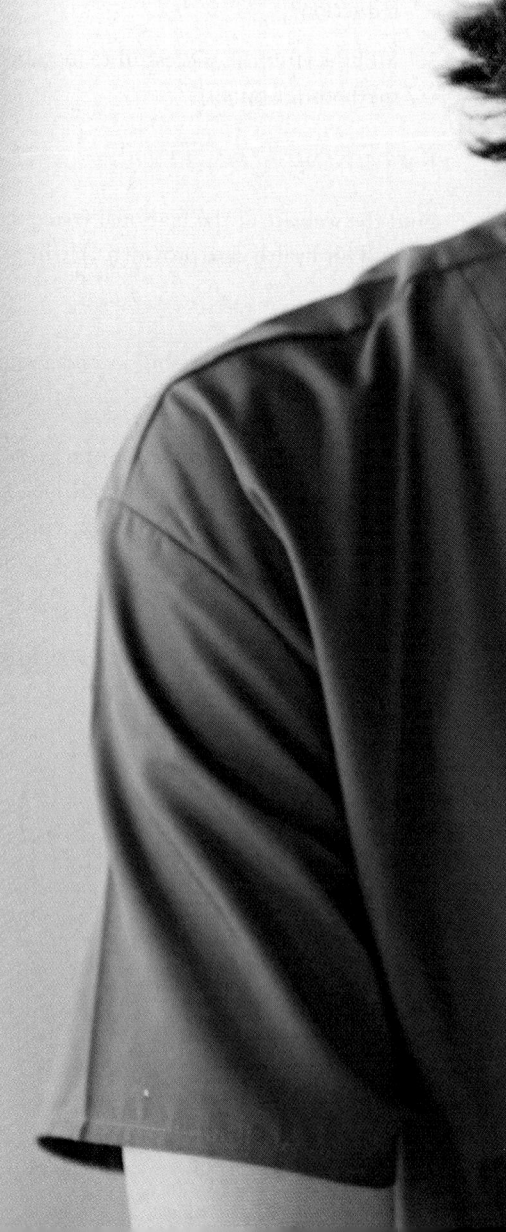

LEARNING OBJECTIVES

After completing this chapter, you should be able to:

- Define and spell the terms to learn for this chapter.

- Explain the functions of muscle.

- Identify and discuss types of muscle tissue.

- Describe the muscular system of the body.

- Discuss the energy requirements for muscles

- Explain the structure of skeletal muscles

- List and discuss the three types of skeletal muscle movements

- Identify the major skeletal muscle groups of the body.

- Identify and explain common disorders of the muscular system

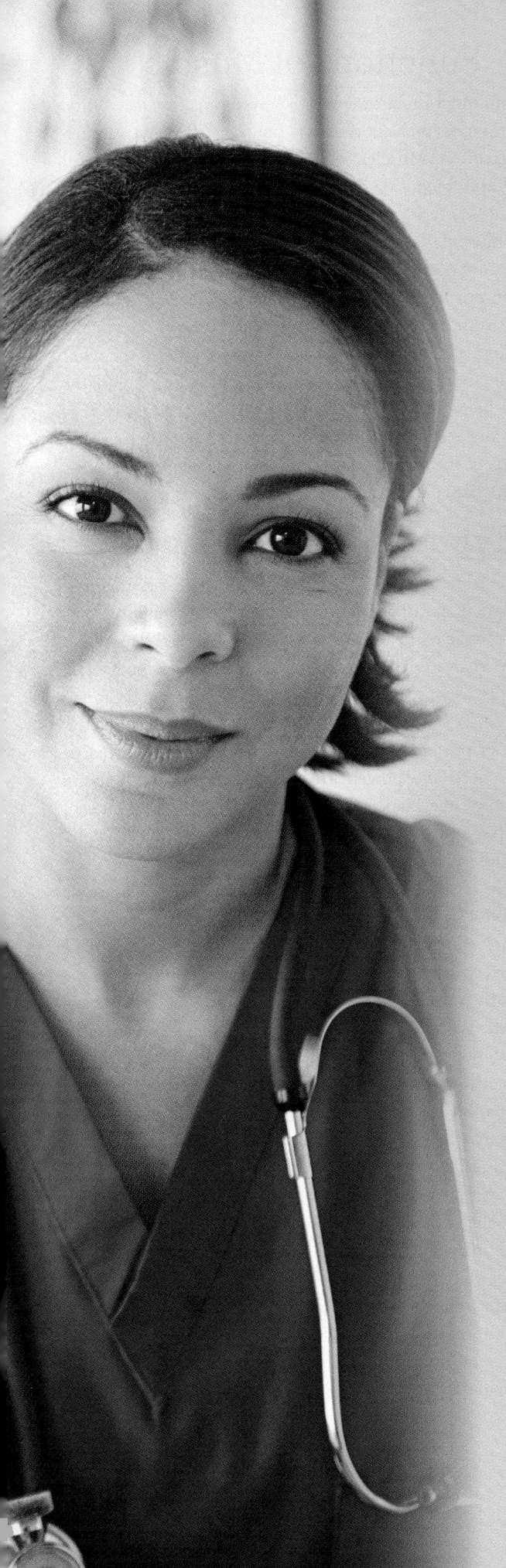

CHAPTER OUTLINE

CASE STUDY

On returning home from a camping trip, 12-year-old Felix Gutierrez noticed a small black bump near his left ankle. He showed his mother, Rosa, who immediately recognized that the black bump was in fact a tick. She immediately attempted to remove the tick but was not sure if she was completely successful.

471

The muscular system is composed of all the muscles within the body. In fact, muscles make up about 42 percent of a person's total body weight. Each muscle is made of specialized cells called muscle fibers. Muscle fibers are made of different lengths and shapes and vary in color from white to deep red. The muscle fibers are held together by connective tissue. The connective tissue is held together by a fibrous sheath called **fascia**. Each fiber within a muscle also has its own nervous system connection with a stored supply of energy in the form of glycogen. Muscle must be supplied with proper nutrition and oxygen to perform properly. The muscular system is well permeated by vessels from both the circulatory system and the lymphatic systems.

Functions of Muscle

The main function of the muscular system is contractibility. Nearly all movement in the body can be attributed to a muscle contraction. Muscles, where attached to bones, internal organs, and blood vessels, are responsible for movement (Figure 24-1).

The muscular system is also responsible for heat production, stability, and **tonicity**, which is the body's ability to maintain posture through a continual partial contraction of skeletal muscles. Muscles produce heat through the chemical changes involved in muscular activity. This is what helps the body maintain a normal temperature. Finally, muscles help the body to maintain stability, meaning that muscles are responsible for holding bones together so that the joints of the body remain stable. Our posture and stability often change as we age.

Types of Muscle Tissue

As discussed in Chapter 21, groups of cells that work together form tissue. Three different types of muscle cells work together to form muscle tissue. Each muscle cell is designed for specific functions that are needed by a certain area in the body. The three types of muscle tissues are skeletal, smooth, and cardiac (Figure 24-2). The various muscles of our bodies serve as the engines, or powerhouses, of the body and are constructed to provide speed and power. Muscles are composed of about 75 percent water, 20 percent protein, and about 5 percent carbohydrates, lipids, inorganic salts, and nonprotein nitrogenous compounds. The composition varies in the different muscles.

Muscle tissue has the ability to contract or to shorten, thus producing movement of internal and external body parts. Breathing, speaking, walking, talking, eating, and almost every other function require muscle tissue.

Smooth muscle, or involuntary muscle, is composed of elongated, spindle-shaped cells. The nucleus is centrally located. Smooth muscle cells contain no striations. Smooth muscle cells are located throughout the body and are commonly involved with involuntary motions, or contractions. Involuntary muscle contractions are movements that cannot be consciously controlled. Muscles made from these types of cells are also called visceral muscles because they are found in the body's organs, including those organs found in the respiratory tract, the urinary bladder, and the digestive system, as well as the walls of blood vessels.

Skeletal muscle, sometimes called voluntary or striated muscle, allows movement by being attached to bones in the body. Skeletal muscle controls voluntary movements, which are consciously controlled. Skeletal muscle is made up of

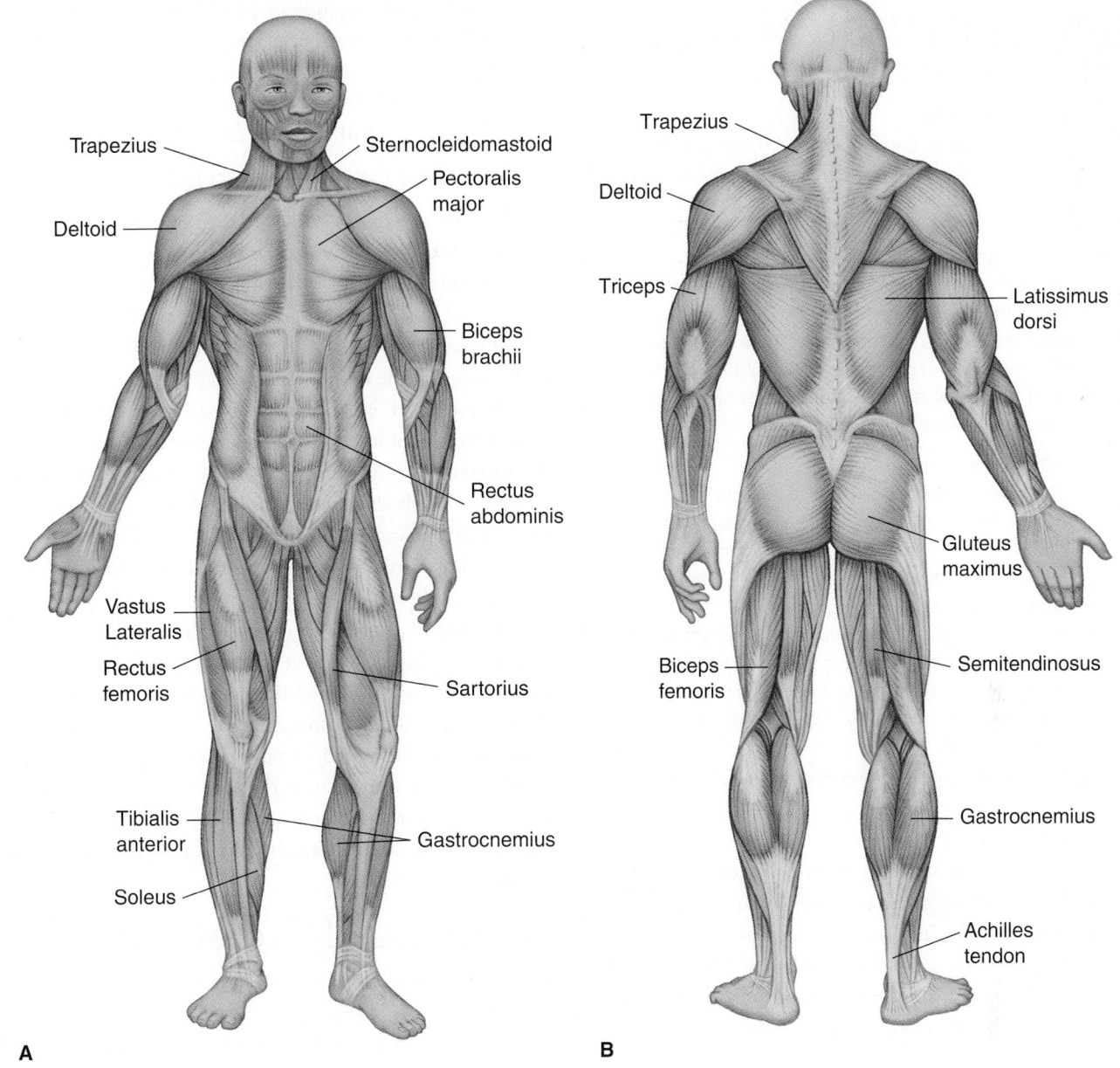

FIGURE 24-1 (A) Selected skeletal muscles (anterior view); (B) selected skeletal muscles and the Achilles tendon (posterior view).

cylindrical fibers. The nucleus tends to be toward the edge of each **striated** (striped in appearance) cell. Because all skeletal cells are striated, the skeletal muscle itself tends to have an overall striped look.

Cardiac muscle has a single central nucleus and is found in the heart. It is roughly quadrangular in shape. Cardiac muscle cells form a network of branching fibers. The cardiac muscle cells are cross striated and involuntary. Cardiac muscle tissues are supplied with nerve fibers that carry messages to and from the central nervous system (brain and spinal cord). Each involuntary contraction and relaxation of cardiac muscle results in a heartbeat. The average human heart beats 60 to 80 times a minute.

Energy Production for Muscle

Muscles use energy in the form of adenosine triphosphate (ATP), which is a type of chemical energy needed for sustained or repeated muscular contractions. ATP can be produced by either aerobic or anaerobic (without oxygen) means:

- Aerobic production of ATP—In the presence of oxygen, the body can utilize carbohydrates, fats, and proteins to make energy (ATP) that is utilized by the muscles. When the body uses ATP that is produced aerobically, more energy will be available to use. This is the type of energy required for endurance.

The Child

- From the time of fetal development and as a child continues to develop, the muscles and bones continue to grow. Although the movements of a newborn are uncoordinated and random, muscular development continues to proceed from head to toe and from the center of the body to the periphery. The head and neck muscles are the first muscles that can be controlled, so a baby will hold his or her head upright before he or she can sit up. Babies need freedom of movement to help develop those muscles in the proper order.

The Older Adult

- The changes related to mobility are the most obvious in the older adult. There can be measurable differences in muscle strength, endurance, range of motion, coordination, elasticity, and flexibility of connective tissue.
- The prevention of decreases in strength is fully dependent on regular exercise. Thus, exercise helps to strengthen muscles and keeps joints, tendons, and ligaments more flexible, allowing for a more active lifestyle.

- Anaerobic production of ATP—The body utilizes stored glucose, which is actually glycogen, to make ATP without oxygen. The glucose, which is the usable form of carbohydrate in the body, breaks down into ATP and lactic acid simultaneously. Generally, this form of energy production is useful for small bursts of energy, rather than endurance.

Because some patients—and physicians—are going to be unhappy in any medical practice, it is important to realize that, most of the time, individuals who complain about service are not attacking the person responding to their call but are instead venting their frustration because they do not understand something. As a professional, it is important for you to understand that listening and learning go hand in hand. If a patient is upset or concerned about his or her health, take the time to "listen" instead of getting angry, and try to focus on how you can best meet that patient's needs.

- Breaking down creatine phosphate is another method of acquiring muscular energy (ATP), which is also done without the use of oxygen. This is limited to skeletal muscles and, because it is anaerobic in nature, is used for small bursts of energy.

OXYGEN DEBT AND MUSCLE FATIGUE

The amount of oxygen "owed" to the body to recover is called **oxygen debt**. Oxygen debt may occur when the skeletal muscles are used for more than 1 or 2 minutes. This means that if your body is working hard it may not be able to absorb enough oxygen to cope with the level of activity. When oxygen is lacking, the body is unable to produce energy through aerobic means, thus the anaerobic method of creating energy is activated. Unfortunately, as mentioned, anaerobic energy production is only short term, not enough for endurance. Therefore, the body can only utilize this energy for about 60 seconds, depending on the individual, before severe fatigue sets in, making it very difficult to recover. To recover from oxygen debt, the body must increase respiration to allow more oxygen into the bloodstream to reach the muscles.

Muscle fatigue usually develops as a result of an accumulation of lactic acid. This accumulation of lactic acid decreases the muscle's ability to contract. This causes the muscle to become incredibly fatigued, and muscle cramps may occur. Muscle fatigue may also occur if the blood supply to a muscle is stopped or interrupted, or if a motor neuron loses its ability to release a neurotransmitter substance called acetylcholine into the muscle fibers.

Structure of Skeletal Muscles

As mentioned, skeletal muscle attaches to bone and is voluntarily controlled (Figure 24-3). More than 600 different skeletal muscles are responsible for the movement of the body through contractility, extensibility, and elasticity. Various sizes, shapes, and fiber arrangements create a variety of muscles that can each perform a specific function in the body.

Several coverings made up of connective tissue are associated with skeletal muscle. The fascia is the connective tissue covering each skeletal muscle and separating the muscles from one another. Muscles are surrounded by a thin fascia covering called the **epimysium** and are attached to bones by structures called tendons. The **aponeurosis** is a wide, thin, sheetlike tendon, made up of fibrous connective tissue, that typically attaches muscles to other muscles. The **perimysium**, also made up of connective tissue, is responsible for dividing a muscle into sections called **fascicles**. The **endomysium** is the covering of connective tissue that surrounds the individual muscle cell.

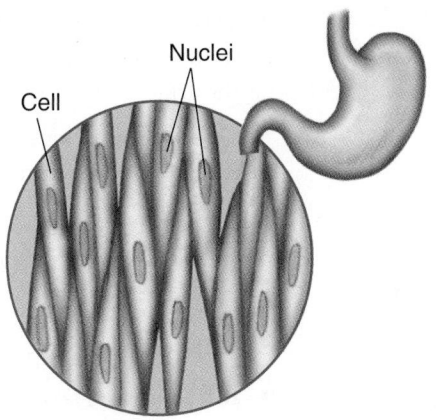

Cell

Nuclei

Smooth muscle tissue

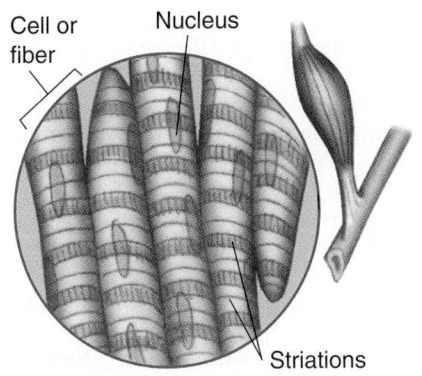

Cell or fiber

Nucleus

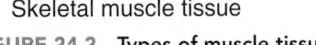

Striations

Skeletal muscle tissue

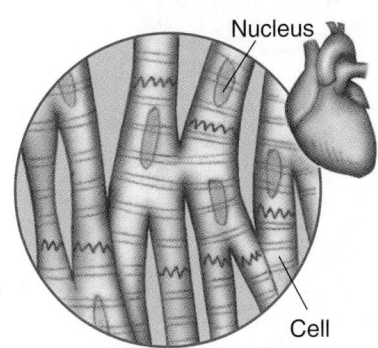

Nucleus

Cell

Cardiac muscle tissue

FIGURE 24-2 **Types of muscle tissue.**

ATTACHMENTS TO SKELETAL MUSCLES

Actions of skeletal muscles depend greatly on where the skeletal muscles are attached. The origin and the insertion are the points at which skeletal muscles attach to given structures. The **origin** is the attachment to the bone that is more fixed or still; the **insertion** is the attachment point on the bone that moves. For example, the biceps muscle has its origin at the shoulder, whereas its insertion point is in the forearm, close to the elbow. This insertion point near the elbow enables the forearm to flex during muscle contraction.

Muscles and nerves function together as a motor unit. For skeletal muscles to contract, it is necessary to have stimulation by impulses from motor nerves. Muscles perform in groups and are classified in the following categories:

- **Antagonist**—a muscle that counteracts, or opposes, the action of another muscle. For example, when the biceps contracts, the triceps relaxes; this is an antagonist pair.

- **Prime mover** or **agonist**—a muscle that is the primary actor in a given movement. This is the muscle that produces the movement in muscle contraction. When the knee extends, the prime mover is the quadriceps.

- **Synergist**—a muscle that acts with another muscle, most often a prime mover, to produce movement

Major Skeletal Muscles

When describing the major skeletal muscles, it is important to remember that these muscles are often identified according to their location, size, action, shape, or number of attachments to the muscle. They are usually listed in the following groups:

- Muscles of the head
- Muscles of the arm, wrist, hand, and fingers
- Respiratory muscles
- Abdominal muscles
- Muscles of the pectoral girdle
- Muscles of the leg, ankle, and foot.

MUSCLES OF THE HEAD

The muscles of the head include those that move the head, provide facial expressions, and move the jaw (see Figure 24-4). They include the following muscles:

- **Sternocleidomastoid**—pulls the head from side to side and to the chest

- **Splenius capitis**—rotates the head and allows it to bend to the side

The muscles that provide for facial expression include the following:

- **Frontalis**—raises the eyebrows
- **Orbicularis oris**—allows the lips to pucker
- **Orbicularis oculi**—allows the eyes to close
- **Zygomaticus**—pulls up the corners of the mouth
- **Platysma**—pulls down the corners of the mouth

The muscles of the jaw allow for chewing, or mastication. They include the following:

- **Masseter and temporalis**—close the jaw

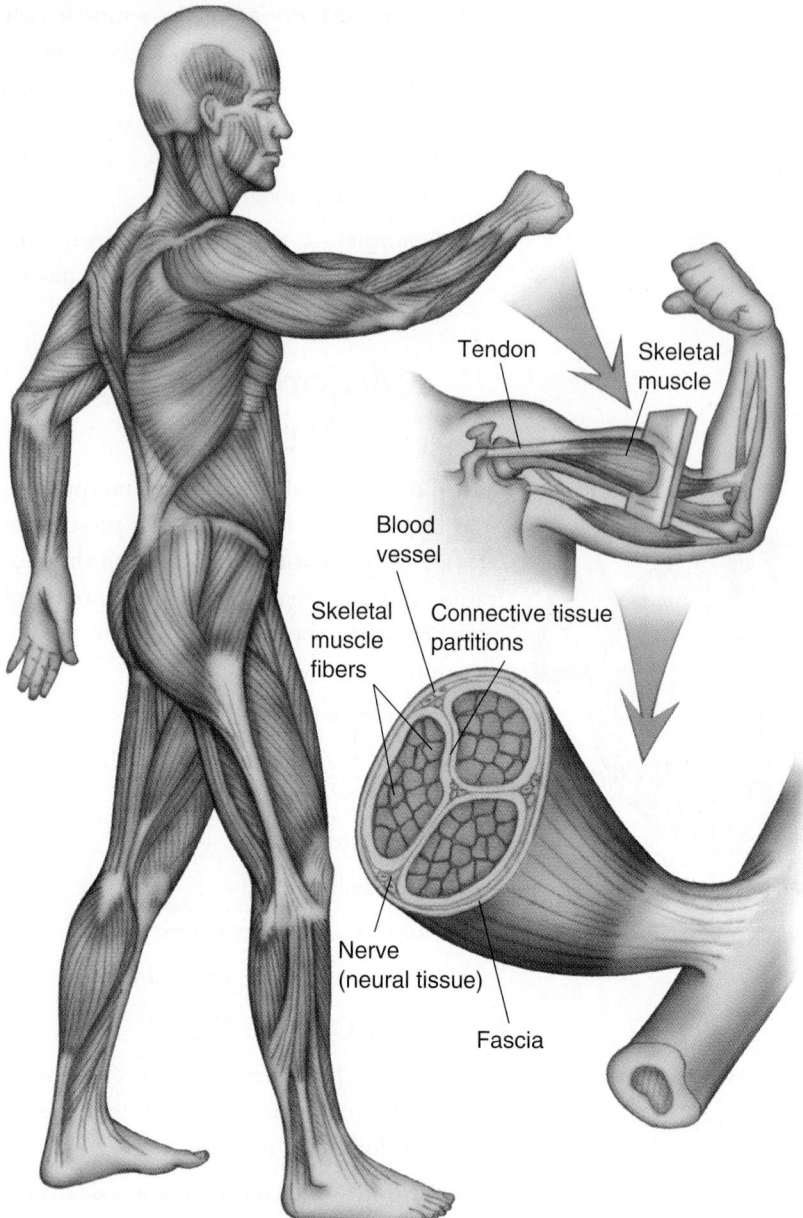

Tendon

Skeletal muscle

Blood vessel

Skeletal muscle fibers

Connective tissue partitions

Nerve (neural tissue)

Fascia

FIGURE 24-3 A skeletal muscle consists of a group of fibers held together by connective tissue. It is enclosed in a fibrous sheath (fascia).

- **Latissimus dorsi**—provides for extension, adduction, and inward rotation of the arm
- **Deltoid**—provides for abduction and extension of the arm at the shoulder
- **Serratus anterior**—also known as the "boxer's muscle," pulls the scapula forward
- **Subscapularis**—rotates the arm medially
- **Infraspinatus**—rotates the arm laterally
- **Biceps brachii**—flexes the arm at the elbow and rotates the hand laterally
- **Brachialis**—flexes the arm at the elbow
- **Brachioradialis**—flexes the forearm at the elbow
- **Triceps brachii**—extends the arm at the elbow
- **Supinator**—rotates the forearm laterally
- **Pronator teres**—rotates the forearm medially

Muscles that move the wrist, hand, and fingers include the following:

- **Flexor carpi radialis and flexor carpi ulnaris**—flex and abduct the wrist
- **Palmaris longus**—flexes the wrist
- **Flexor digitorum profundus**—flexes the distal joints of the fingers but not the thumb
- **Extensor carpi radialis longus and extensor carpi radialis brevis**—extend the wrist and abduct the hand
- **Extensor carpi ulnaris**—extends the wrist
- **Extensor digitorum**—extends the fingers but not the thumb

MUSCLES OF THE ARM, WRIST, HAND, AND FINGERS

Figures 24-5 and 24-6 illustrate many of the muscles of the arm, wrist, hand, and fingers.

Muscles that move the upper extremity include those in the arm and forearm:

- **Pectoralis major**—pulls the arm across the chest and also rotates and adducts the arms

RESPIRATORY MUSCLES

The muscles of respiration include the following:

- **Diaphragm**—separates the thoracic cavity from the abdominal cavity; its contraction causes the process of inspiration

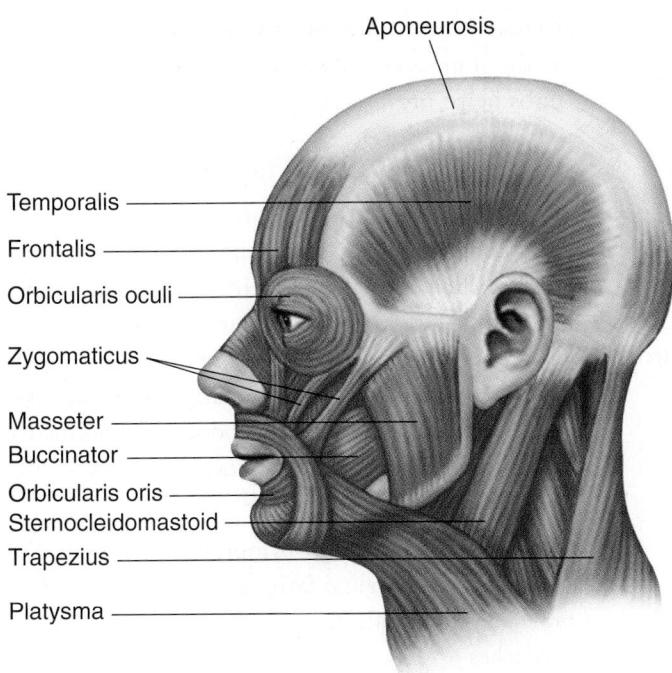

Aponeurosis

Temporalis

Frontalis

Orbicularis oculi

Zygomaticus

Masseter

Buccinator

Orbicularis oris

Sternocleidomastoid

Trapezius

Platysma

FIGURE 24-4 Muscles of the head, neck, and face.

- **External and internal intercostals**—contraction expands and lowers the ribs during breathing

ABDOMINAL MUSCLES

The muscles of the abdominal wall include the following (Figure 24-7):

- **External and internal obliques**—compress the abdominal wall

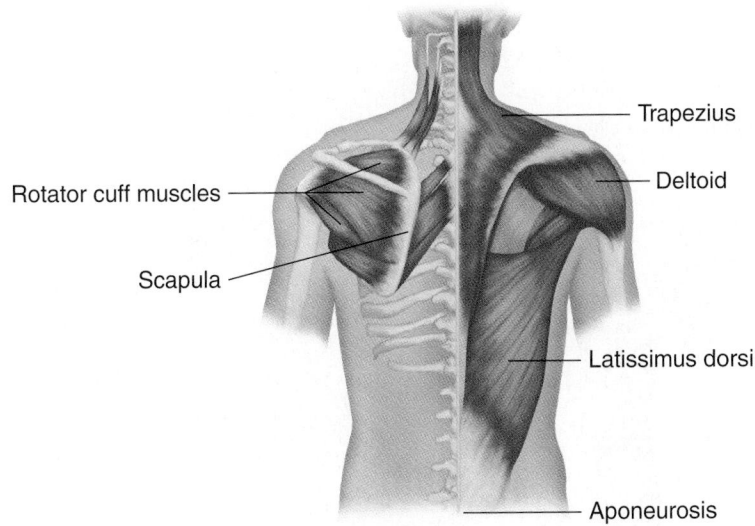

Rotator cuff muscles

Scapula

Trapezius

Deltoid

Latissimus dorsi

Aponeurosis

posterior

FIGURE 24-5 Muscles of the posterior torso that are responsible for arm movements.

- **Transversus abdominis**—also compresses the abdominal wall
- **Rectus abdominis**—flexes the vertebral column and compresses the abdominal wall

MUSCLES OF THE PECTORAL GIRDLE

The muscles that move the pectoral girdle, or shoulder, include the following:

- **Trapezius**—raises the arms and pulls the shoulders downward
- **Pectoralis minor**—pulls the scapula downward and raises the ribs

MUSCLES OF THE LEG, ANKLE, AND FOOT

The muscles that move the leg include the following (Figure 24-8):

- **Psoas major**—flexes the thigh
- **Iliacus**—also flexes the thigh
- **Gluteus maximus**—extends the thigh
- **Vastus lateralis**—extends the knee

The muscles that move the ankle and foot include the following:

- **Gastrocnemius**—flexes the foot and aids in pushing the body forward
- **Tibialis anterior**—causes dorsiflexion and inversion of the foot
  - **Peroneus**—everts the foot and helps bring about plantar flexion
  - **Flexor digitorum longus and extensor digitorum longus**—flexes and extends the toes, respectively, and assist in other movements of the feet

Common Disorders Associated with the Muscular System

Due to the sheer number of muscles, the diseases and disorders associated with the muscular system are quite numerous. Muscular disorders are characterized by abnormalities of muscle fibers. In addition, many neurological disorders, such as lesions of the central or peripheral nervous system and abnormalities of neuromuscular transmission, can also

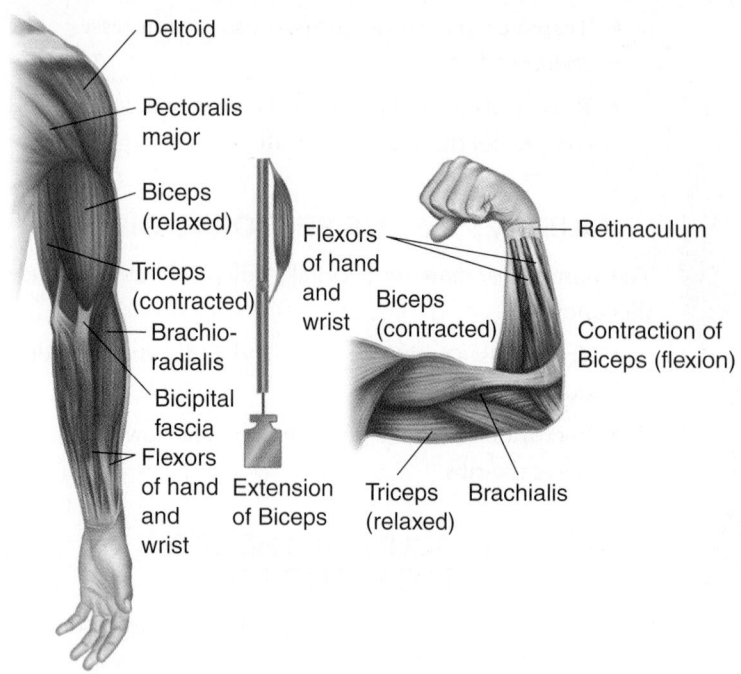

FIGURE 24-6 **Muscles of the arm and hand.**

Labels in figure: Deltoid; Pectoralis major; Biceps (relaxed); Triceps (contracted); Brachioradialis; Bicipital fascia; Flexors of hand and wrist; Flexors of hand and wrist; Biceps (contracted); Extension of Biceps; Triceps (relaxed); Brachialis; Retinaculum; Contraction of Biceps (flexion)

produce symptoms that are primarily muscular. Other systemic disorders, including those that are frequently seen in conditions of the cardiovascular, respiratory, and endocrine systems, frequently mimic muscular disorders but do not directly affect muscular function. These systemic disorders account for more than half of muscular complaints.

ATROPHY

Atrophy is the loss of muscle mass and strength that occurs with the disuse of muscles over a long period of time. Oftentimes, atrophy is caused by bed rest and immobility. Lipoatrophy (also known as lipodystrophy) is atrophy of fat tissue. It is common for lipoatrophy to occur at a site of insulin or corticosteroid injections.

Signs and Symptoms. The most common sign of atrophy is the apparent "wasting away" appearance of a muscle group. Frequently, patients will have extreme weakness and fatigue associated with atrophic muscle groups.

Treatment. If the atrophy is caused by a specific treatment (such as a cast or traction), performing isometric exercises of the immobilized muscle can decrease the level of atrophy due to immobilization. Isometric exercise uses active muscle contractions performed against stable re-

sistance (e.g., tightening the muscles of the thighs or the buttocks). Active exercise of uninjured limbs helps prevent atrophy.

FIBROMYALGIA

Fibromyalgia is a widespread musculoskeletal pain and fatigue disorder affecting an estimated three million individuals in the United States. Fibromyalgia occurs more often in women than men. There is no obvious known cause of fibromyalgia, but evidence points to a genetic predisposition that creates a neuromuscular or neuroendocrine abnormality that disturbs the usual sensory perception, especially to pain signals.

Signs and Symptoms. Symptoms include mild to severe muscle pain and fatigue, sleep disorders, irritable bowel syndrome, depression, and chronic headaches.

The American College of Rheumatology (ACR) has identified specific criteria for fibromyalgia. The ACR states that a patient must show pain at 11 of 18 trigger or tender points to be considered for a diagnosis of fibromyalgia (see Figure 24-9). The patient must also have a history of widespread pain lasting at least 3 months.

Treatment. Treatment is geared toward improving the quality of sleep and reducing pain. Sleep is important for many body functions, including tissue repair and antibody production, so the disruption of sleep will directly affect the quality of life in a patient with fibromyalgia. Frequently, the medications prescribed for

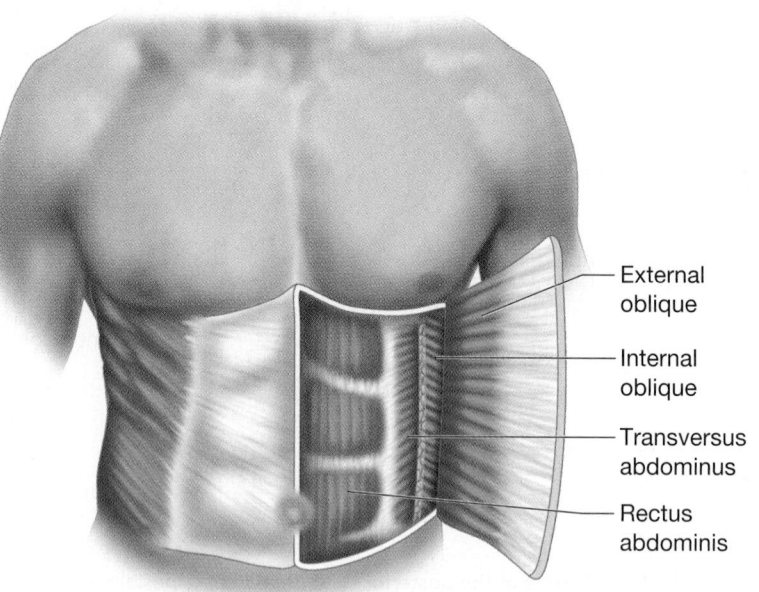

FIGURE 24-7 **Abdominal muscles.**

Labels in figure: External oblique; Internal oblique; Transversus abdominus; Rectus abdominis

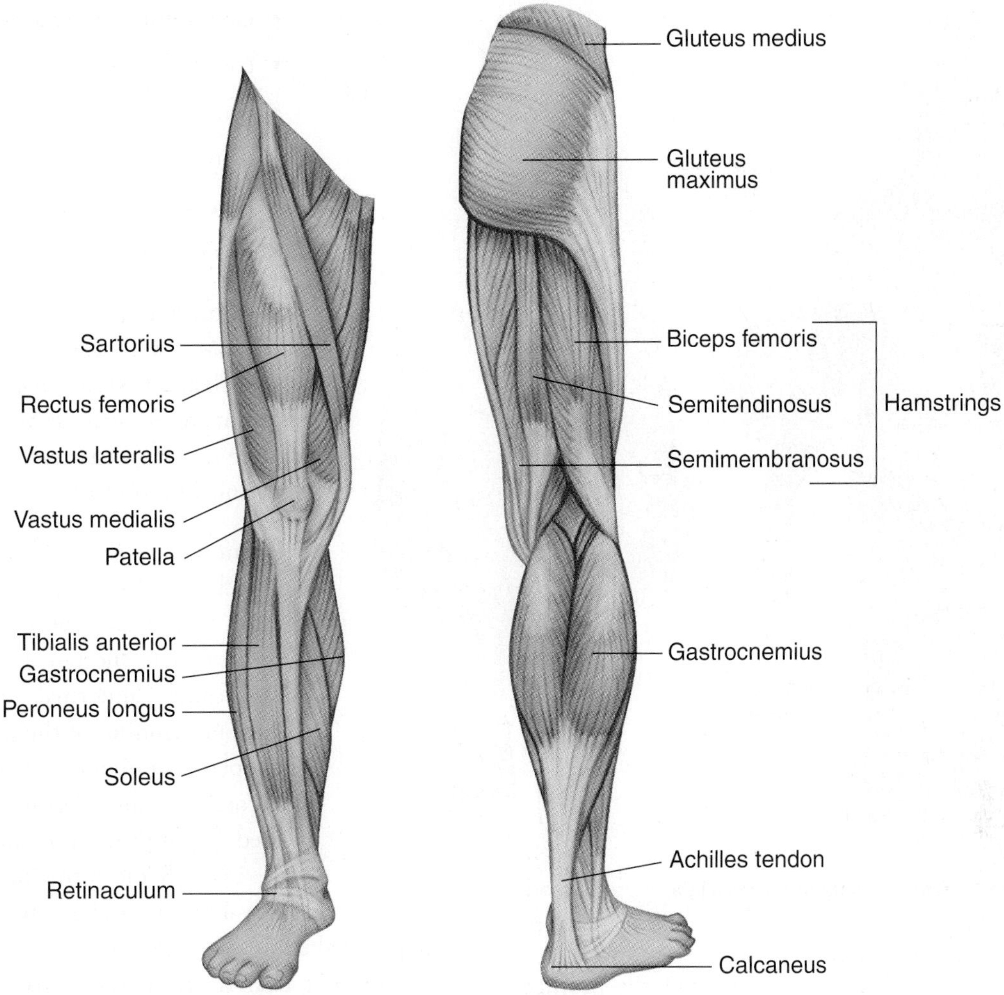
Sartorius
Rectus femoris
Vastus lateralis
Vastus medialis
Patella
Tibialis anterior
Gastrocnemius
Peroneus longus
Soleus
Retinaculum
Gluteus medius
Gluteus maximus
Biceps femoris
Semitendinosus
Semimembranosus
Hamstrings
Gastrocnemius
Achilles tendon
Calcaneus

FIGURE 24-8 **Muscles of the buttocks, leg, and foot.**

fibromyalgia include muscle relaxants, pain relievers, anti-inflammatory drugs, antidepressants, and antianxiety drugs. Other treatments frequently employed include chiropractic, acupuncture, acupressure, relaxation techniques, and massage.

GANGLION CYST

A **ganglion cyst** is a benign saclike swelling or cyst. Typically the cysts develop over a joint or tendon. Ganglion cysts occur more frequently in women than in men. There is no known cause for their development.

Signs and Symptoms. A ganglion cyst can be very painful. Typically these masses occur on the hands, feet, wrist, and ankles. Swelling may occur, although it is often erratic, developing and disappearing without cause.

Treatment. Anti-inflammatory drugs can be used to reduce swelling and pain. Often **aspiration** (removal by suction of fluid from within the cyst) is performed. This treatment is about 74 percent effective against recurrence of the cyst. If pain or decreased range of motion occurs, surgery may be performed. Even surgical removal of a ganglion cyst is not always 100 percent effective against recurrence.

LYME DISEASE

Lyme disease is caused by the *Borrelia burgdorferi* bacterium. It is carried by ticks, frequently found on deer and other wild animals. The bacterium is transmitted through the bite of an infected tick. Prevention of Lyme disease is the best medicine.

Signs and Symptoms. In addition to the telltale round bull's-eye rash, additional symptoms of Lyme disease include headache, fatigue, and fever. Prevention measures include wearing long sleeves and long pants while in heavily wooded

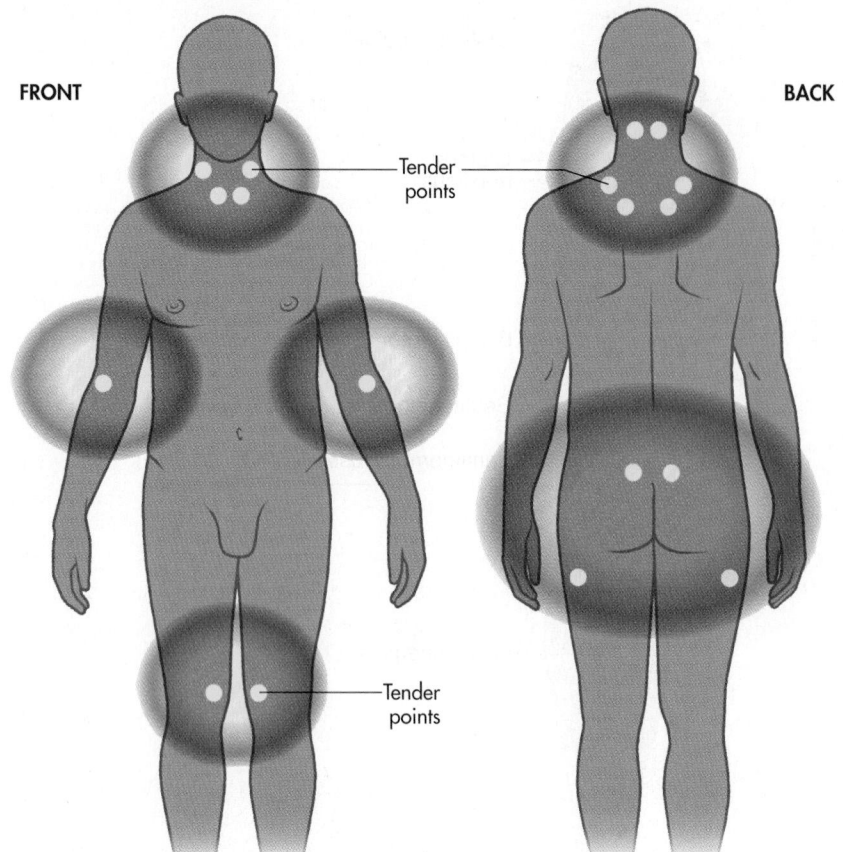

FRONT   Tender points   BACK

Tender points

FIGURE 24-9 The 18 tender points of fibromyalgia

areas, the proper use of insect repellent, and the prompt removal of any tick that may be lodged in the skin.

Treatment. If Lyme disease is detected early, full recovery is possible. This is accomplished by taking the prescribed round of antibiotic medications. Antibiotics often prescribed include erythromycin, penicillins, or doxycycline. If not detected early, Lyme disease can result in skin, joint, heart, and nervous system disorders.

MUSCULAR DYSTROPHY

Muscular dystrophy (MD) is one of a group of genetic diseases characterized by progressive weakness and degeneration of the skeletal or voluntary muscles that control movement. The muscles of the heart and some other involuntary muscles are also affected in some forms of MD, and a few forms involve other organs as well. The major forms of MD include the following:

- Duchenne MD
- Becker MD
- limb-girdle MD
- facioscapulohumeral MD
- congenital MD
- oculopharyngeal MD
- distal MD
- Emery-Dreifuss MD
- myotonic MD

Signs and Symptoms. Signs and symptoms of MD will vary based on the specific form. General signs and symptoms are apparent in all forms of MD. Some of these include muscle weakness, loss of coordination, and immobility.

Treatment. There is no specific treatment for any of the forms of MD. Physical therapy to prevent **contractures** (a condition in which shortened muscles around joints cause abnormal and sometimes painful positioning of the joints), **orthoses** (orthopedic appliances used for support), and corrective orthopedic surgery may be needed to improve the quality of life in some cases. Some forms of MD, including Emery-Dreifuss and myotonic, may necessitate a pacemaker due to the cardiac problems associated with them. The overall prognosis of MD depends on the type and progression of the disease.

MYASTHENIA GRAVIS

Myasthenia gravis (MG) is a chronic autoimmune neuromuscular disease characterized by varying degrees of weakness of the skeletal or voluntary muscles of the body. MG most commonly occurs in young adult women and older men but can occur at any age. Although MG may affect any voluntary muscle, certain muscles, including those that control eye movements, eyelids, chewing, swallowing, coughing, and facial expressions, are more often affected.

Signs and Symptoms. The primary symptom of MG is muscle weakness. The muscle weakness increases during periods of activity and improves after periods of rest. Weakness may also occur in the muscles that control breathing and arm and leg movements. The muscles involved in MG vary from one individual to the next.

Treatment. Though there is no cure for MG, people living with this disease are not only able to control it but also lead full and productive lives. Both corticosteroids and anti-cholinesterase (prevents destruction of the neurotransmitter acetylcholine) medications are often prescribed. Surgery, including removal of the thymus gland, may be required. Physicians will determine individualized treatment based on the patient's age, overall health, and general prognosis of the disease.

ROTATOR CUFF TEARS

The rotator cuff is the area that enables people to reach above their heads and lift with the arms. Rotator cuff tears are increasingly common in the muscles that form the shoulder and their tendons (supraspinatus, infraspinatus, teres minor, and subscapularis). Most rotator cuff tears occur due to many years of overuse of the muscles and tendons; however, one single traumatic injury can also cause a rotator cuff tear.

Signs and Symptoms. These tears can cause considerable pain and limit the function and range of motion of the patient. In addition, symptoms include atrophy of the shoulder muscle and a crackling sensation when moving the shoulder in certain positions.

Treatment. Treatment for a torn rotator cuff includes rest, narcotic and nonsteroidal anti-inflammatory drugs (NSAIDs), splinting, physical therapy, and performing range-of-motion exercises. More severe rotator cuff tears may require steroid injections and possibly surgery.

SHIN SPLINTS

Shin splints are caused by inflammation of the periosteum of the extensor muscles of the lower leg and surrounding tissues. The condition is usually caused by overuse or improper conditioning of the leg muscles. Shin splints commonly occur with running sports, military training, and high-impact dancing and in people with flat feet or rigid arches.

Signs and Symptoms. General symptoms of a shin splint include increased pain, tenderness, and possible swelling in the shin area.

Treatment. Shin splint treatment includes rest and applying ice or cold compresses to the shin area. Medication such as aspirin and NSAIDs may be used for pain management. Treatment also includes the use of proper footwear, which can prevent future episodes.

SPRAINS AND STRAINS

A **sprain**—a stretching or tearing—is an injury to a **ligament** (connective tissue that connects bones or connects cartilage to a joint), whereas a **strain** is an injury to either a muscle or a tendon. Depending on the severity of the injury, a strain may be a simple overstretching of the muscle or tendon, or it can result in a partial or complete tear.

Sprains

Sprains are very common injuries, especially among athletes. Often a sprain will occur after a ligament has been overstretched or torn, especially in ligaments of major joints such as elbows, knees, wrists, ankles, and feet. Ankle sprains are the most common injury in the United States.

Signs and Symptoms. Typically, the signs and symptoms associated with a sprain include pain, swelling, bruising, and loss of joint mobility and function. Depending on the severity of the sprain, these signs and symptoms will vary in intensity.

Treatment. Sprains are generally treated using the RICE method:

- **Rest**—If the injured joint is a weight-bearing joint, such as the ankle, it is important to utilize canes, crutches, or other walking devices.
- **Ice**—Ice the sprain with an ice pack or cold compress.
- **Compression**—Compression bandages should be worn around the sprain to encourage proper healing.
- **Elevation**—Elevate the affected sprain as soon as possible after an injury. It is most beneficial to have the strained muscle either above or at the same level as the heart.

Additional treatments may include range-of-motion exercises, physical therapy, and NSAIDs. Surgery, which is a rarity, may be performed when a sprain has been classified as chronic and other forms of treatment are not effective.

Strains

The twisting or pulling of a muscle often results in a strain. Prolonged, repetitive movements generally result in a chronic strain, whereas an acute strain may be caused by improperly lifting a heavy object. In addition, sports including soccer, football, hockey, tennis, gymnastics, and many others tend to place individuals at higher risk for muscle strains.

Signs and Symptoms. Common symptoms associated with a strain include pain, muscle weakness, muscle spasm, and loss of muscle function. Inflammation and cramping, accompanied by swelling, may also be associated with a strain.

Treatment. The treatment for a strain is very similar to that of a sprain. Rest, cold compressions, anti-inflammatory medication, and gentle stretching are often helpful. Heat application, as with a heating pad, is also beneficial. At times, a physician may recommend the application of a brace to limit mobility of the injured muscle.

TENDONITIS

A **tendon** is the band of connective tissue found at each end of a muscle that attaches the muscle to a bone. Excessive and repetitive movements are often associated with **tendonitis** (also spelled *tendinitis*), an inflammation of the tendon, which occurs when the tiny fibers of the tendon begin to tear. The following are the common areas associated with tendonitis:

- Elbow and wrist
- Biceps and shoulder
- Hip, leg, and knee
- Achilles tendon

Signs and Symptoms. Pain and stiffness commonly surround the affected area. Also, this condition has been known to cause a burning sensation that surrounds the joint and inflamed tendon. Generally, pain is worst during and immediately after activity, whereas the following day the tendon tends to become stiffer, though it still causes a significant amount of pain.

Treatment. With proper care, tendonitis should lessen over 3 weeks. However, healing of the area continues and does not peak until at least 6 weeks following the initial injury. The initial approach to treating tendonitis is to support and protect the tendons by bracing any areas of the tendon that are being pulled during use. It is important to loosen up the tendon, reduce the pain, and minimize any inflammation. Physical therapy, including exercises to increase range of motion, has proven to be a very beneficial treatment for tendonitis.

TETANUS

Tetanus is an often fatal infectious disease caused by the bacteria *Clostridium tetani,* which usually enters the body through a puncture, cut, or open wound. *Clostridium tetani*

PROFESSIONALISM THE WORKPLACE

It is important to know the main muscles in the body, but it is especially important to be familiar with those in which injections are frequently given. Children do not have well-developed arm or buttocks muscles, so their injections are usually given in the vastus lateralis. In adults, the deltoid muscle in the arm is used for small amounts of fluid. However, if the fluid is thick (viscous) or a large amount must be injected, the gluteus maximus in the buttocks may be preferred.

releases a toxin that affects the motor nerves (which stimulate the muscles).

Signs and Symptoms. Tetunus is characterized by profoundly painful muscle spasms, including locking that results in the mouth being unable to open (lockjaw). Difficulty swallowing due to neck stiffness is experienced, along with stiffness of the chest, abdominal, and back muscles. Fevers are also common with tetanus.

Treatment. Preventing tetanus is the best course of treatment. All children should be immunized against tetanus by receiving a full series of five diphtheria, pertussis, and tetanus (DPT, or Tdap) vaccinations, which generally are started at 2 months of age and are completed around 5 years of age. The tetanus and diphtheria (Td) vaccination is now recommended at 11 to 12 years of age if at least 5 years have elapsed since the last dose of a tetanus and diphtheria toxoid-containing vaccine. Follow-up booster vaccination is recommended every 10 years thereafter (i.e., 21 years old, 31 years old, etc.). In adult patients, it is recommended that the patient receive one dose of Tdap as a booster for tetanus, diphtheria, and pertussis during adulthood. It is recommended that the Tdap booster be given at least 2 years after a Td booster has been administered. Should an unvaccinated person contract tetanus, the likely course of treatment would include the administration of antitoxin, such as tetanus immune globulin, administration of antibiotics, and vaccination.

SUMMARY

The muscular system is composed of specialized cells called muscle fibers. These fibers, when brought together, form muscle, which makes up about 42 percent of a person's total body weight. The purpose of muscles is to create movement, maintain posture and stability, and aid in heat production. To achieve this, muscles must be supplied with proper nutrition and oxygen.

The three types of muscle are smooth, skeletal, and cardiac. Voluntary muscles, which are striated, move in coordination with decisions from the nervous system, either from the brain or spinal column. Involuntary muscles, which are smooth, are regulated by a complex endocrine system interacting with nerves and muscles. Cardiac tissue is both smooth and striated.

Thus, a person does not voluntarily control whether the heart contracts but can influence the rate of rhythm.

Muscles are named by their purpose, structure, or location. Antagonists counteract the action of another muscle. Prime movers (agonists) are the primary actor in a given movement. Synergists act with another muscle to produce movement.

Muscles receive a lot of wear and tear, and thus many disorders can develop. Among the disorders associated with the muscular system are atrophy, fibromyalgia, ganglion cysts, Lyme disease, muscular dystrophy, myasthenia gravis, rotator cuff tears, shin splints, sprains and strains, tendonitis, and tetanus.

24 CHAPTER REVIEW

COMPETENCY REVIEW

1. Define and spell the terms to learn for this chapter.

2. Name the three types of muscle tissue.

3. What are the two points of attachment for muscles?

4. What are the other names for skeletal muscle?

5. What are the three types of skeletal muscle units?

6. What are other names for smooth muscle?

7. Give examples of internal organs with smooth muscle.

8. What is the name and special property of heart muscle?

9. Why is the rotator cuff especially important to the patient's range of motion?

10. What are the four primary functions of muscle?

PREPARING FOR THE CERTIFICATION EXAM

1. Which of the following muscles is located in the arm?
   a. rectus abdominis
   b. gastrocnemius
   c. rectus femoris
   d. triceps
   e. pectoralis major

2. A muscle that is considered a prime mover, may also be termed a/an
   a. synergist
   b. primary muscle
   c. antagonist
   d. agonist
   e. synergist mover

3. Which muscle pulls the head from side to side and pulls the head to the chest?
   a. gastrocnemius
   b. biceps femoris
   c. gluteus maximus
   d. deltoid
   e. sternocleidomastoid

4. Which muscle(s) flexes the foot and aids in pushing the body forward?
   a. tibialis anerior
   b. gastrocnemius
   c. gluteus maximus
   d. extensor carpi ulnaris
   e. external obliques

5. Which of the following diseases is caused by *Borrelia burgdorferi*?
   a. fibromyalgia
   b. muscular dystrophy
   c. myasthenia gravis
   d. Lyme disease
   e. plantar fasciitis

6. Which of the following diseases has a preventative vaccine?
   a. muscular dystrophy
   b. ganglion cyst
   c. fibromyalgia
   d. tetanus
   e. myasthenia gravis

7. Which of the following is a genetic disorder?
   a. muscular dystrophy
   b. Lyme disease
   c. myasthenia gravis
   d. tetanus
   e. ganglion cyst

8. Which of the following separates the thoracic cavity from the abdominal cavity?
   a. peroneus
   b. trapezius
   c. supinator
   d. pronator teres
   e. diaphragm

9. Which of the following is in the pectoral girdle?
   a. gluteus maximus
   b. deltoid
   c. trapezius
   d. internal oblique
   e. frontalis

10. Which of the following is caused by twisting or pulling a muscle or tendon?
    a. sprain
    b. tendonitis
    c. strain
    d. myasthenia gravis
    e. cramping

CRITICAL THINKING

1. Should Rosa seek medical care for Felix? Explain why or why not.

2. What would be some signs and symptoms Rosa should be looking for if she is concerned that her son may have been bitten by a tick infected with the *Borrelia burgdorferi* bacterium?

3. What measures can be taken to prevent being bit by infected ticks?

INTERNET ACTIVITY

Do an Internet search to learn about resources for families who have members with muscular dystrophy.

MEDMEDIA

Additional interactive resources and activities for this chapter can be found:

On your student DVD: View applicable procedure videos on the DVD-ROM found in the back of this book.

MyHealthProfessionsKit.com: Test your knowledge of this chapter with games and activities. MyHealthProfessionsKit also includes resources, helpful links, and a Spanish audio glossary.

Medical Assisting Interactive: Practice your procedures as a medical assistant in this simulated doctor's office. This can be accessed through MyHealthProfessionsKit.com.

25

The Nervous System

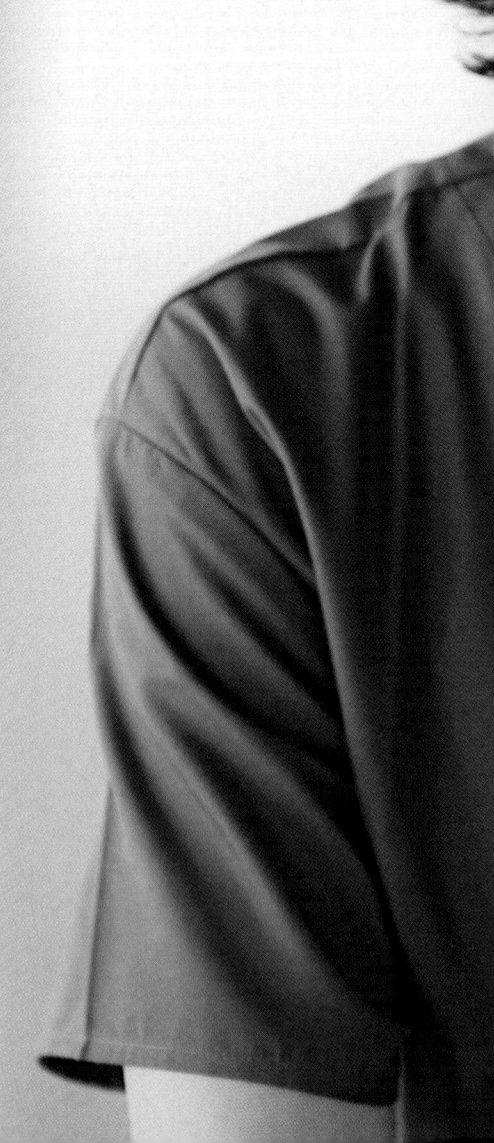

LEARNING OBJECTIVES

After completing this chapter, you should be able to:

- Define and spell the terms to learn in this chapter.

- List the functions of the nervous system.

- Identify and discuss the structures that make up the central nervous system.

- Explain how nerve impulses are transmitted.

- State the functions of the the peripheral nervous system, and the somatic nervous system and the autonomic nervous system, and distinguish the differences between each.

- Explain the delicate balance between the sympathetic and parasympathetic nervous system.

- Identify and explain common disorders associated with the nervous system.

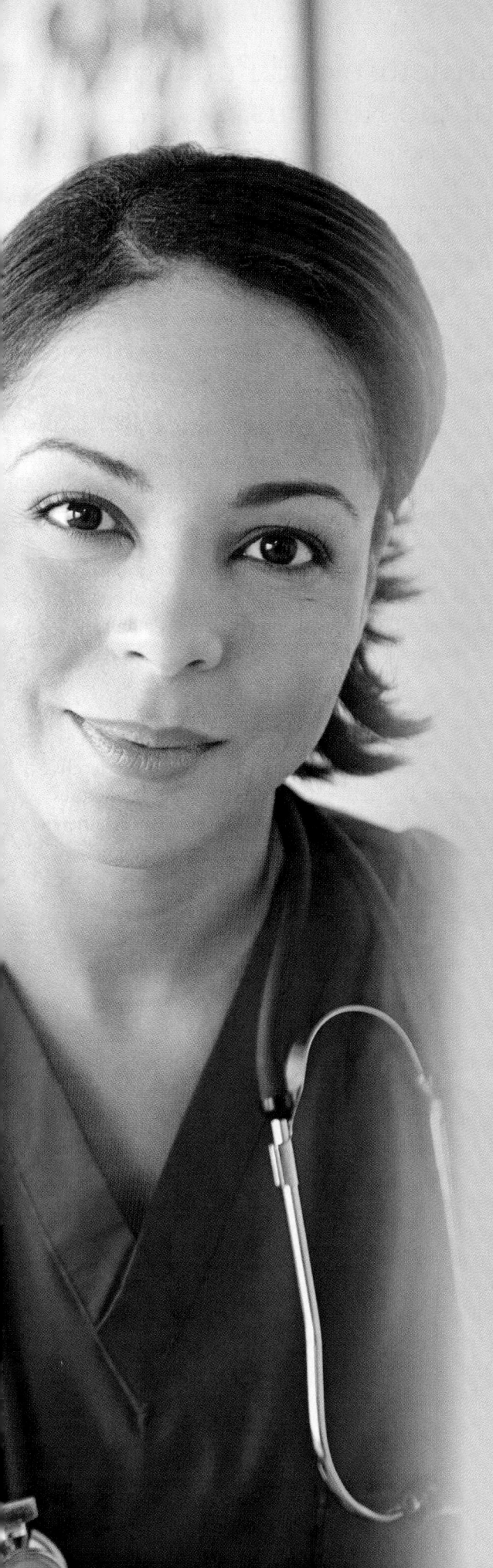

CHAPTER OUTLINE

CASE STUDY

Elena Bramatovich is 67 years old and has been a patient of Pearson Physicians Group for the past 7 years. According to her family, Elena's memory and cognitive functions have been decreasing over the past couple of years. Her daughter, Svetlana, has written a letter to Dr. Miller regarding more drastic changes in her mother's behavior. Svetlana informs Dr. Miller that she is concerned that her mother is developing dementia.

The nervous system is an essential and integral component of the human body. It acts to correlate both external and internal factors that affect our bodies (Figure 25-1). For this to occur, the nervous system must gather, store, and decipher both external and internal information. Through careful analysis of this information, the nervous system decides how to respond and react in an appropriate manner to satisfy certain needs. Of these needs, the most important is the need for survival. Various systems comprise the nervous system, and although most are interrelated some are able to function on their own.

Structure and Function of the Nervous System

The brain and spinal cord make up the **central nervous system (CNS)**. The **peripheral nervous system (PNS)** is made up of nerves that connect the CNS to the other parts of the body. Subsections of the peripheral nervous system include the somatic nervous system (SNS) and the autonomic nervous system (ANS). The ANS is further divided into the sympathetic and parasympathetic nervous systems. Each of these divisions of the nervous system is discussed in further detail later in this chapter. Figure 25-2 illustrates the components of the nervous system.

The nervous system transfers information via electrical impulses that travel along the length of the cells. The cell processes information from the sensory nerves and initiates an action within milliseconds.

The nervous system is responsible for three separate functions: (1) It detects and interprets sensory information. (2) It then takes that information and makes decisions about how it is being received. (3) Finally, it carries out a motor function based on the decisions made.

Neurons

Nervous system tissue is made up of specialized nerve cells called **neurons** as well as supporting tissue structures known as neuroglia. As the specialized units of the nervous systems, neurons are both structural and functional in nature. There are three types of neurons: motor neurons, sensory neurons, and interneurons. These cells enable the body to interact with its ever-changing internal and external environments.

MOTOR NEURONS

Motor neurons control most of the body's functions as they cause muscles to contract, glands to secrete, and organs to function properly. Motor neurons are considered **efferent nerves** because the impulse is transmitted from the neural cell body to stimulate the target muscle or organ. Motor neurons have processes known as the axon and dendrites that extend away from it in various directions. Neurons usually have several dendrites and only one axon. The axon is covered with a fatty insulating substance called the myelin sheath. Axons may be several feet long and reach entirely from the cell body to the area that is to be activated. Dendrites resemble tree branches and are unsheathed (Figure 25-3).

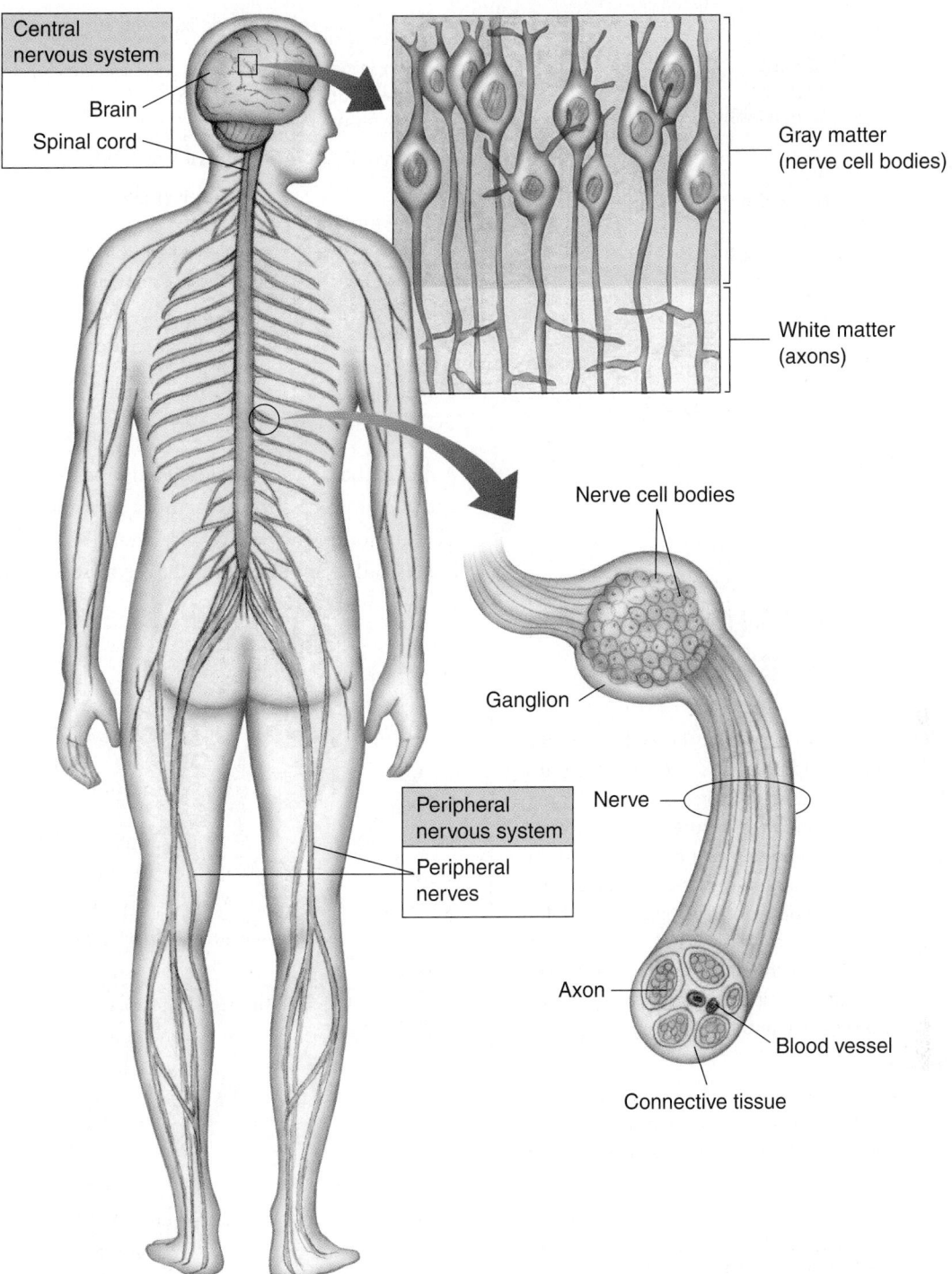

FIGURE 25-1 The nervous system.

SENSORY NEURONS

Sensory neurons transmit sensory information through a peripheral process. These specific neurons lack true dendrites, are sheathed, and more closely resemble axons. Attached to the sensory receptors, sensory neurons transmit impulses directly to the central nervous system. The CNS then activates motor neurons to respond to the sensory information.

Sensory neurons are also different from motor neurons because they are often referred to as **afferent nerves**, meaning they carry impulses from the sensory receptor to the CNS.

INTERNEURONS

Interneurons are often referred to as associative neurons because they are located entirely within the CNS. These cells

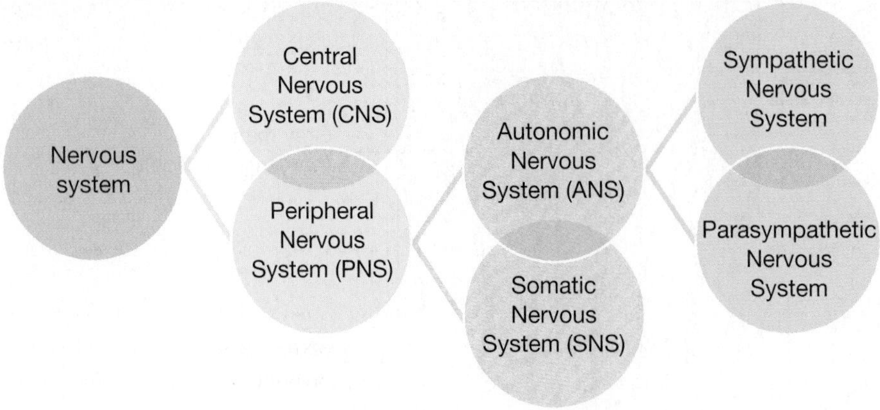

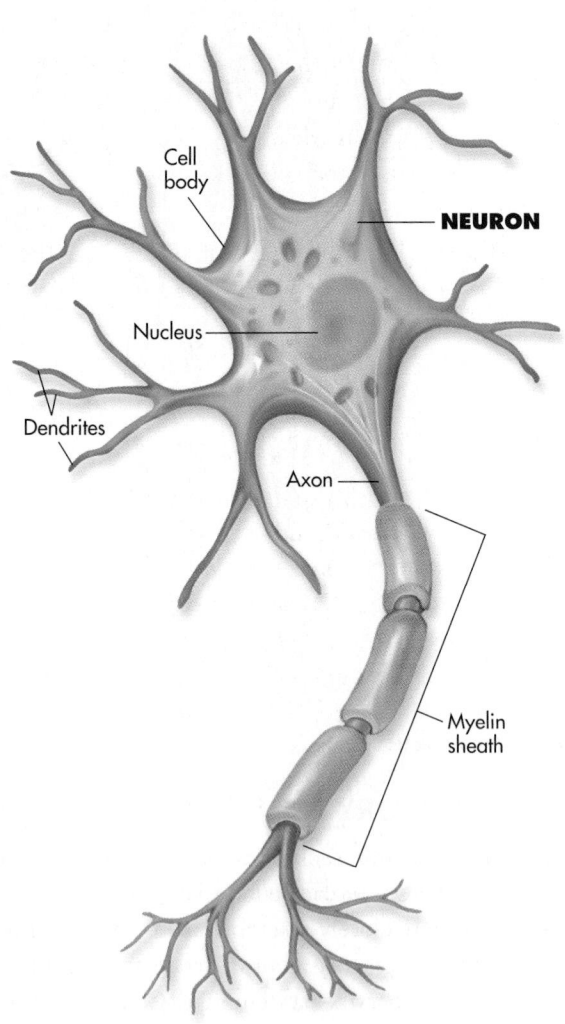

FIGURE 25-2 Components of the nervous system.

PROFESSIONALISM THE LIFE SPAN

The Child

- The development of the child's nervous system begins at about 6 weeks. By the time the child is born, the baby's brain waves can be measured. As the child grows, regular neurological testing can provide the physician with important information that indicates various neurological disorders. Testing of the child's nervous system includes testing the newborn's reflexes, as well as testing the child as he or she grows. This includes testing of mental status, motor functions and balance, and the sensory system.

The Older Adult

- In individuals who do not have neurological disease, intellectual performance tends to be maintained until at least age 80. However, tasks may take longer to perform because of some slowing in central processing. Verbal skills are well maintained until age 70, after which some healthy elderly persons gradually develop a reduction in vocabulary, a tendency to make semantic errors, and abnormal pronunciation. Other age-related changes are subtle but can be detected as difficulty learning, especially languages, and forgetfulness in noncritical areas. However, this mild forgetfulness is unlike dementia in that it does not impair recall of important memories or affect function.
- With normal aging, the number of nerve cells in the brain decreases. From age 20 or 30 to age 90, brain weight declines by about 10 percent, and the area of the cerebral ventricles (cavities) relative to the entire brain may increase three to four times.

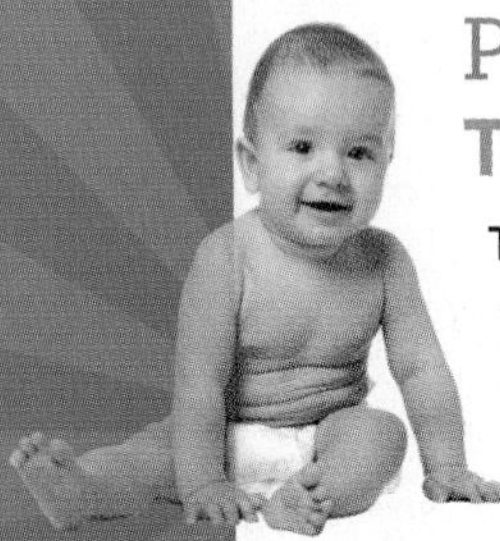

work as a liaison between sensory and motor neurons by mediating their impulses.

Nerve Fibers, Nerves, and Tracts

It is necessary to have an understanding of the correlation between nerve fibers, nerves, and their tracts because these components are all necessary in conducting an impulse.

NERVE FIBERS

A nerve fiber is a single elongated process, usually an axon or peripheral process from a sensory neuruon. The nerve fibers that are found in the PNS are wrapped in protective membranes called **sheaths**. Sheaths are formed by accessory cells

FIGURE 25-3 Motor neuron showing the axon, dendrite, and myelin sheath.

and are classified as either myelinated or unmyelinated. Myelin is a thick fatty substance, and myelinated sheaths have both an inner sheath of myelin and an outer sheath, or **neurilemma**, composed of Schwann cells. (Schwann cells are needed for the process of regenerating a damaged nerve fiber.) Unmyelinated sheaths are wrapped only in the neurilemma and lack myelin. On the other hand, nerve fibers of the CNS do not contain Schwann cells, and thus damage to the CNS is permanent, whereas damage to a peripheral nerve can be reversed.

NERVES

A nerve is a bundled unit of nerve fibers found outside the CNS. As noted, nerves are often described as being afferent (conducting impulses to the CNS) or efferent (conducting impulses to muscles, organs, and glands). Some nerves possess the fibers of both afferent and efferent nerves. These special nerves are called mixed nerves.

TRACTS

A group of nerve fibers within the CNS is often referred to as a **tract**. All nerve fibers that are housed within the nerve tract must have the same origin, function, and termination. This means that all the nerve cells within the tract have the same starting and ending points and work toward the same purpose. The spinal cord contains sensory tracts that are afferent, which ascend to the brain, and efferent tracts that descend from the brain. The largest nerve tract is the **corpus callosum**, which joins the right and left hemispheres of the brain.

Nerve Impulses and Synapses

A nerve impulse begins with stimulation, and stimulation of a nerve occurs at the receptor. Sensory receptors vary in complexity from the simple, such as sensing pain, to the very complex, such as the receptors that are found in the retina of the eye and collect the input necessary for sight. All sensory receptors are specialized to respond to certain stimulations, such as heat, cold, light, pressure, and pain. When the receptor is stimulated, it reacts by initiating a chemical change or impulse. The transmission of an impulse by a nerve fiber is based on the "all or none" principle, meaning that either there is a response or there is not. The receptor must receive sufficient stimulation to send the impulse, or else the impulse is not transmitted to the brain. Each receptor has its own threshold at which it will react to a stimulus, and each will only respond when its threshold is reached. The impulse is then transmitted via a synapse, which is a knob-shaped branch ending. The process is similar to a

domino effect; the end of the knob-shaped axon releases specialized cells known as neurotransmitters (nerve system chemicals); these transmitters travel across the synapse to the dendrites of the next nerve. This process repeats itself until it reaches its final destination, such as a motor plate that is attached to a muscle that will initiate a movement.

Central Nervous System

The CNS is solely comprised of the brain and spinal cord. This portion of the nervous system receives impulses from the entire body, requiring it to process information and respond with appropriate actions. These resulting actions or activities may be conscious or unconscious, depending on the sensory stimuli.

Both the brain and the spinal cord are divided into gray matter and white matter. The gray matter consists of unsheathed cell bodies and true dendrites, whereas the white matter consists of the myelinated nerve fibers. In the spinal cord, the arrangement of the gray and white matter in cross-section is H-shaped, with the gray matter forming the core of the spinal cord, surrounded by the white matter. In the brain, the reverse arrangement is true. The white matter forms the core of the brain with the gray matter surrounding the cortex (surface layer).

BRAIN

The brain is considered to be the largest mass of nervous tissue in the body. It is estimated that the male brain weighs just over a half pound, and the female brain weighs just slightly less. The brain is encompassed by three membranes, which are also known as **meninges**. These include the pia mater, the arachnoid, and the dura mater. In addition, the brain is divided into the cerebrum, the diencephalon, and the brainstem. The brainstem consists of the midbrain and the hindbrain. The hindbrain is further divided into the cerebellum, the pons, the medulla oblongata, and the reticular formation (Figure 25-4).

Cerebrum

The cerebrum is the largest portion of the mature brain. It governs all sensory and motor activity, including sensory perception, emotions, consciousness, memory, and voluntary movements; these are considered higher brain functions. The cerebrum is divided in half, forming two mirror-like images called cerebral hemispheres. As mentioned, the corpus callosum connects these two halves of the brain. The surface of the cerebrum is marked by numerous ridges or convolutions, called gyri, that are separated by grooves. This surface is known as the cerebral cortex. A deep groove in the brain is called a **fissure**, and a shallow groove is referred to as

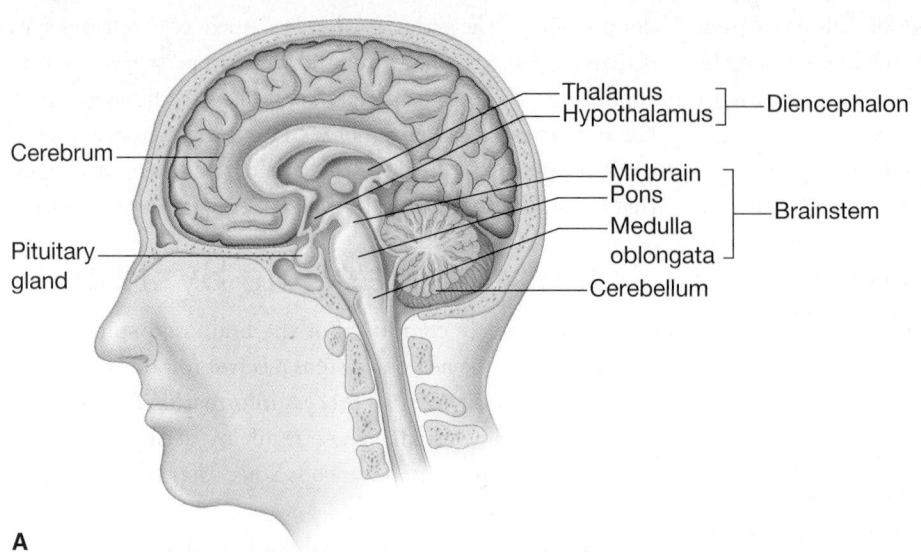

A

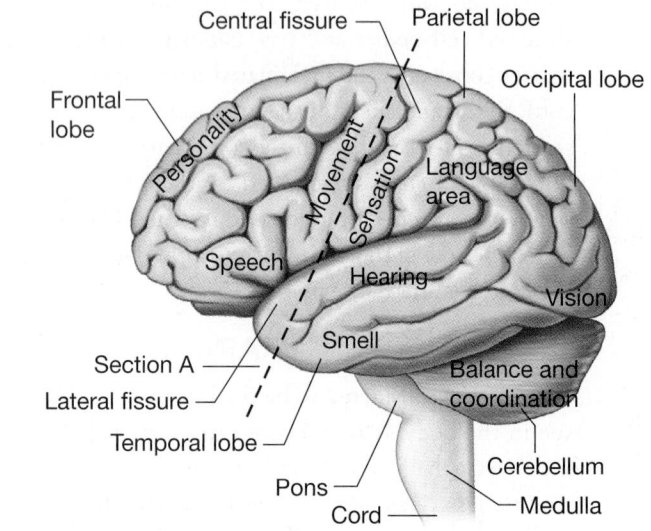

B

FIGURE 25-4 **(A) Sagittal section of the brain; (B) lateral view of the brain.**

Cerebral Cortex. The cerebral cortex houses 75 percent of all the neurons of the entire nervous system. Similar to the cerebrum, the cortex is also composed of gray matter as well as the white matter that lies directly below it. Responsible for interpreting sensory information and initiating body movements, the cerebral cortex also acts to store memories and create emotions.

Diencephalon

Literally translated, *diencephalon* means "second portion of the brain." Both the thalamus and hypothalamus make up the diencephalon. The thalamus is two large masses of gray cell bodies that are connected by a third mass. This portion of the brain serves as a relay center for all sensory impulses, with the exception of smell.

As its name implies, the hypothalamus lies beneath the thalamus and primarily regulates autonomic nervous activity associated with behavior and emotional expression. The hypothalamus also is responsible for a variety of metabolic functions that occur throughout the body as it produces neurosecretions for the control of water balance, sugar and fat metabolism, and regulation of body temperature.

a **sulcus.** A longitudinal fissure separates the right and left hemispheres of the cerebrum, and a transverse fissure separates the cerebrum from the cerebellum.

Lobes of the Cerebrum. Scientists have divided the cerebral cortex (see next section) into lobes as a means of identifying certain locations in the brain. The lobes have been named to correspond to the overlying bones of the skull and include the frontal, parietal, temporal, and occipital lobes. Following is a list of the lobes of the brain and their specific functions:

- **Frontal lobe**—deals with reasoning, emotions, problem solving, planning, and parts of speech and movement.
- **Parietal lobe**—perceives stimuli related to touch, pain, temperature, and pressure.
- **Temporal lobe**—perceives and recognizes auditory stimuli (hearing) and memory.
- **Occipital lobe**—primarily is concerned with the aspects of vision.

Brainstem

Structurally resembling a stem, as its name would suggest, the brainstem contains the midbrain, the pons, and the medulla oblongata. Together these structures relay important information to the cerebrum, including visual, auditory, and other sensory data.

Midbrain. The midbrain is located just below the cerebrum and above the pons. It is associated with visual reflexes and tracking visual movements of the eyes. The two lower segments are associated with the sense of hearing.

Pons. The pons is a broad band of white matter anterior to the cerebellum and between the midbrain and medulla oblongata. The pons contains fiber tracts that link the cerebellum and medulla to higher cortical areas. It plays a vital role in voluntary and involuntary motor control.

Medulla Oblongata. This highly important area of the brain connects the pons, as well as the rest of the brain, to the spinal cord. Here, nerve centers vital to the body's survival exert control over the circulation of blood by regulating both the heartbeat and arterial blood pressure. Different areas of the medulla oblongata are also responsible for involuntary bodily functions, including breathing, swallowing, coughing, sneezing, and vomiting.

Cerebellum

The cerebellum, which is located in the back of the skull below the cerebrum and behind the pons and medulla oblongata, is the second largest portion of the brain. The surface of the cerebellum has a large cortex of gray cell bodies with nerve fibers and white matter on its interior. The cerebellum plays an important part in the coordination of voluntary and involuntary patterns of movement and adjusts muscles to automatically maintain posture.

SPINAL CORD

Measuring approximately 43 to 45 centimeters (17 to 18 inches) long in adults, the spinal cord extends from the base of the medulla oblongata to the junction between the first (L1) and second (L2) lumbar vertebrae. The function of the spinal cord is to conduct sensory impulses from the rest of the body to the brain and to send motor impulses from the brain to the rest of the body; this occurs in the white matter. The spinal cord also serves as a reflex center for nerve impulses that do not need to pass through the brain.

CEREBROSPINAL FLUID

Although it is colorless in appearance, **cerebrospinal fluid (CSF)** is often considered to be the "blood" of the nervous system. Produced by the choroid plexus, which is located in the ventricles (cavities) of the brain, the CSF moves from the ventricles into the connecting canal, and then through the spinal canal and the subarachnoid space that surround the brain. CSF has several functions, including serving as a cushion to protect the brain and spinal cord, which float in the fluid, and nourishing the brain and spinal cord with oxygen and glucose. It also contains several neurotransmitters, including monoamines, acetylcholine, and neuropeptides.

Peripheral Nervous System

The PNS, which is further divided into the somatic nervous system and the autonomic nervous system, is one of the two major divisions of the nervous system. The nerves in the PNS connect the CNS to sensory organs (such as the

eye and ear), other organs of the body, muscles, blood vessels, and glands.

SOMATIC NERVOUS SYSTEM

The **somatic nervous system (SNS)** is made up of 12 pairs of cranial nerves that are arranged symmetrically (12 to each side of the brain) and named for the function or area in which they serve. The 12 pairs of cranial nerves and their functions are listed in Table 25-1. Figure 25-5 shows the relationship of the 12 cranial nerves to specific regions of the brain. The SNS also contains 31 pairs of spinal nerves that are connected to the spinal cord and named for the region of the vertebral column where they exist: 8 pairs of cervical spinal nerves, 12 pairs of thoracic spinal nerves, 5 pairs of lumbar spinal nerves, 5 pairs of sacral spinal nerves, and 1 pair of coccygeal spinal nerves (Figure 25-6).

AUTONOMIC NERVOUS SYSTEM

The **autonomic nervous system (ANS)** is responsible for controlling involuntary bodily functions such as sweating, secretion of glands, arterial blood pressure, smooth muscle tissue, and the heart. It is within the ANS where the final division of the nervous system is found. Here, the ANS divides into the sympathetic and parasympathetic nervous systems. These two systems counteract each other's activity to keep the body in a state of homeostasis.

Sympathetic Division

Branches from the 12 thoracic and first 3 lumbar spinal nerves form the first part of the sympathetic division of the ANS. The cell bodies of these nerve fibers are located in the gray matter of the spinal cord. Just outside the spinal cord, axons of these nerve cells leave the spinal nerves and enter almost immediately into masses of nerve cell bodies, which are called sympathetic ganglia.

TABLE 25-1 Cranial Nerves and Functions

Nerve/Number	Function
Olfactory (I)	Provides sense of smell
Optic (II)	Provides vision
Oculomotor (III)	Conducts motor impulses to four of the six external muscles of the eye and to the muscle that raises the eyelid
Trochlear (IV)	Conducts motor impulses to control the superior oblique muscle of the eyeball
Trigeminal (V)	Provides sensory input from the face, nose, mouth, forehead, and top of the head; motor fibers to the muscles of the jaw (chewing)
Abducens (VI)	Conducts motor impulses to the lateral rectus muscle of the eyeball
Facial (VII)	Controls the muscles of the face and scalp; the lacrimal glands of the eye and the submandibular and sublingual salivary glands; input from the tongue for the sense of taste
Vestibulocochlear (Acoustic) (VII)	Provides input for hearing and equilibrium
Glossopharyngeal (IX)	Provides general sense of taste; regulates swallowing; controls secretion of saliva
Vagus (X)	Controls muscles of the pharynx, larynx, thoracic, and abdominal organs; swallowing, voice production, slowing of heartbeat, acceleration of peristalsis
Accessory (XI)	Controls the trapezius and sternocleidomastoid muscles, permitting movement of the head and shoulders
Hypoglossal (XII)	Controls the tongue; tongue movements

Spinal nerves that synapse with the sympathetic ganglia tend to produce widespread innervation when activated. This occurrence is thought to prepare the body for fight or flight. During fight or flight, a person experiences increased alertness in conjunction with an increase in metabolic rate and other bodily functions. At this point, the SNS stimulates the adrenal gland to release epinephrine (adrenaline), the hormone that causes the familiar adrenaline rush.

Parasympathetic Division

Long fibers that branch from cranial nerves III, VII, IX, and X in conjunction with the long fibers of sacral nerves II, II, and IV form the first stage of the parasympathetic division. Cranial nerve fibers extend via the vagus nerve to ganglia serving the thoracic, abdominal, and pelvic viscera (internal organs). The fibers of the sacral spinal nerves form the pelvic nerve, which branches to synapse with small ganglia near or within the organs to be innervated. The cell bodies of these ganglia serve the lower colon as well as the rectum, bladder, and reproductive organs.

The parasympathetic division works to conserve energy and innervate the digestive system, earning it the nickname "Rest and Digest." Here, rather than the adrenaline rush that is felt with the SNS, a decrease in metabolism and bodily functions occurs.

Common Disorders Associated with the Nervous System

Like its endocrine counterpart, the nervous system initiates and regulates body functions and ensures its owner of an awareness of his or her surrounding environment. Nervous system disorders encompass a wide range of complexity and include simple ailments such as headaches and more complex conditions such as Alzheimer's disease.

PROFESSIONALISM
THE WORKPLACE

It is the responsibility of the medical assistant to be courteous, professional, and understanding while providing the neurological patient with care. Each office should have a routine for determining what type of care and treatment is necessary for patients afflicted with neurological disorders. Knowing prior to the patient coming into the office what these tasks are and what is expected is paramount to the medical assistant's role.

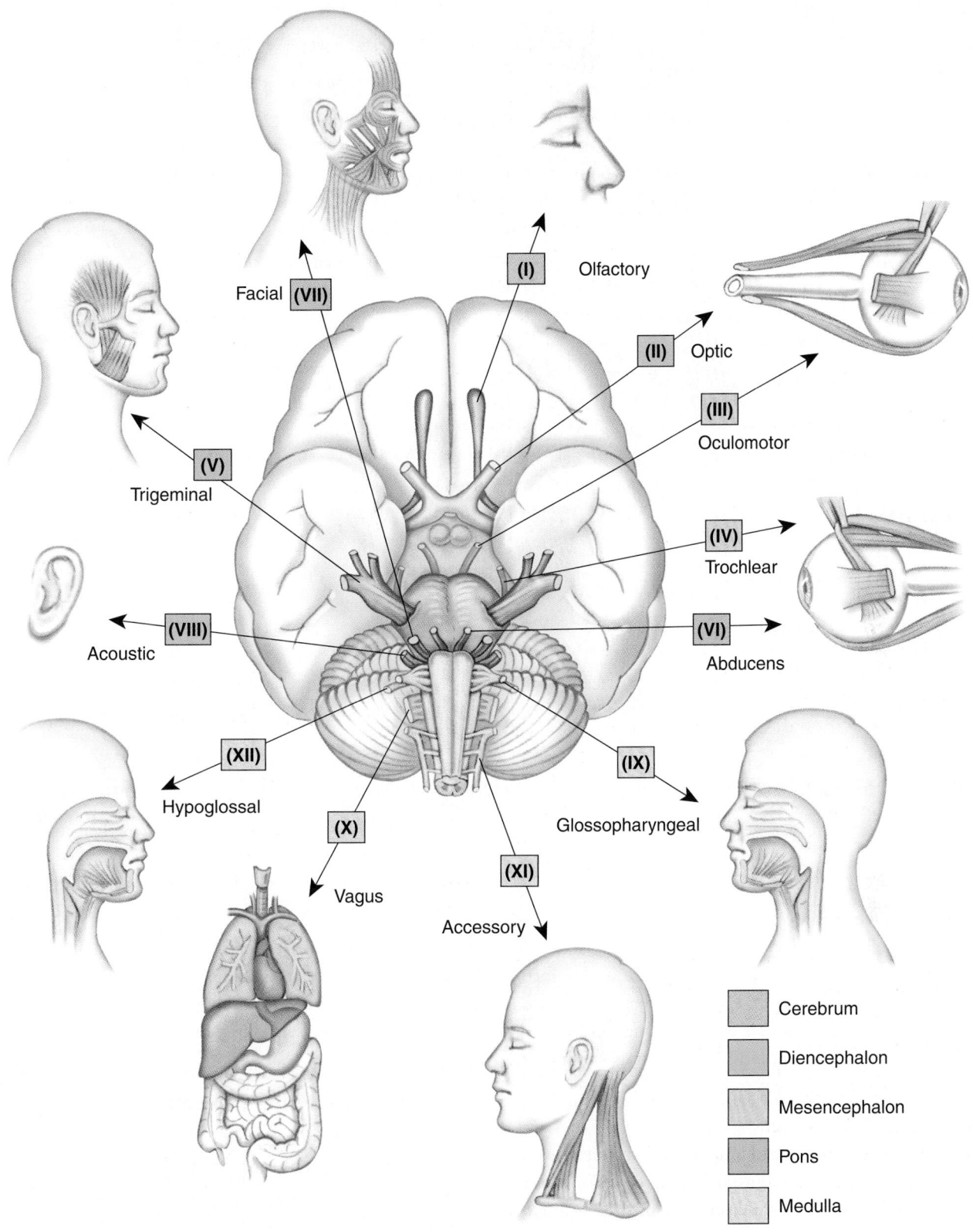

FIGURE 25-5   The relationship of the 12 cranial nerves to specific regions of the brain.

Facial (VII)

Olfactory (I)

Optic (II)

Oculomotor (III)

Trigeminal (V)

Trochlear (IV)

Acoustic (VIII)

Abducens (VI)

Hypoglossal (XII)

Glossopharyngeal (IX)

Vagus (X)

Accessory (XI)

Cerebrum

Diencephalon

Mesencephalon

Pons

Medulla

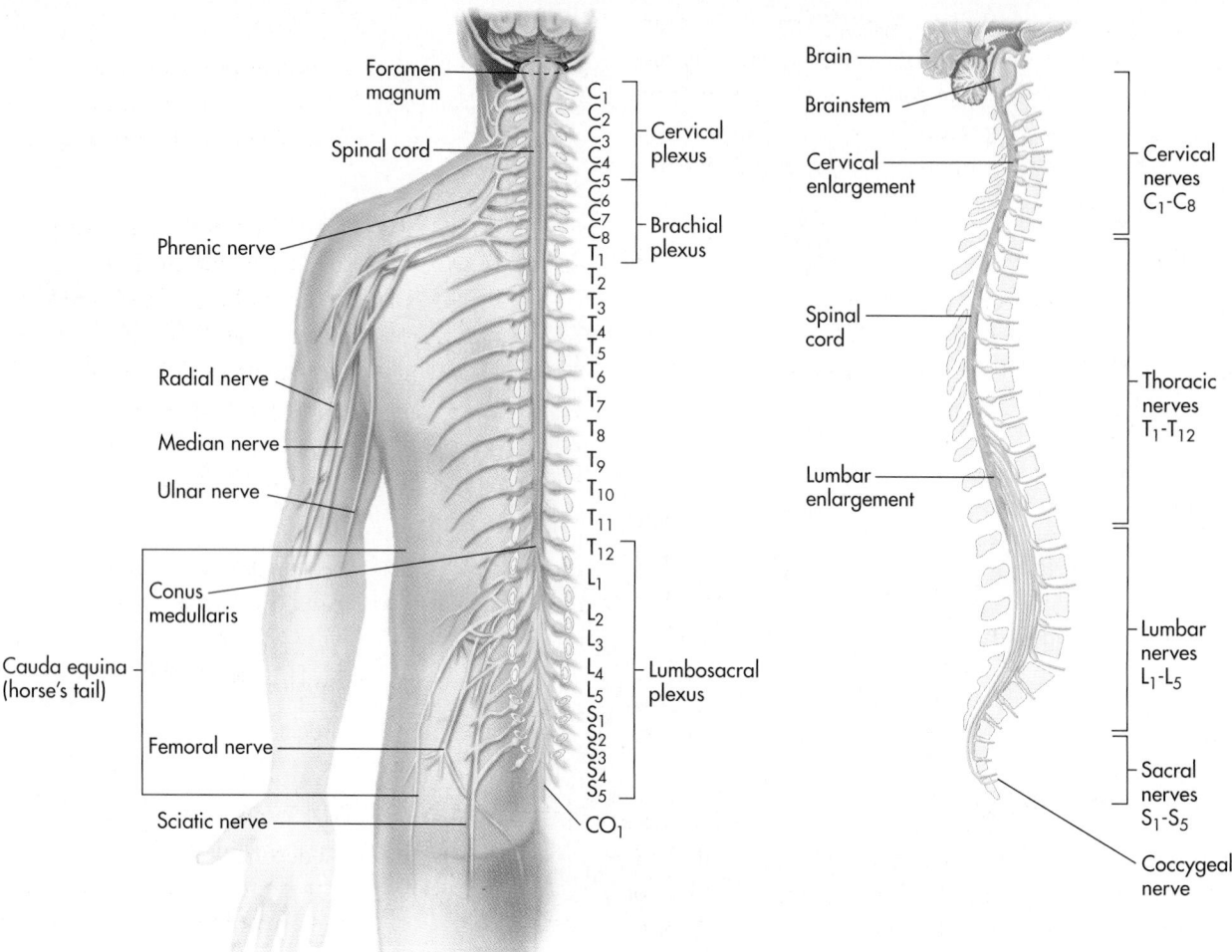

FIGURE 25-6 The 31 pairs of spinal nerves.

ALZHEIMER'S DISEASE

Alzheimer's disease is a progressively, degenerative disease that attacks the brain and its cognitive function. More than four million people are affected by this disease, and unfortunately there is no known cure. Family history often plays a role in the development of this disease, along with activity and age. The onset is generally in the later stages of life; the ages between 65 and 70 seem to be when Alzheimer's most frequently develops.

Signs and Symptoms. Mild forgetfulness of recent events commonly marks the first signs and symptoms. During its progression the ability to think and rationalize begins to diminish, thought processes are interrupted, speech may become difficult to understand, and reading and writing skills also begin to dissipate. Behavioral patterns may also change during the later stages. Patients may become agitated, depressed, and even aggressive or violent. The nervous

system will continue to deteriorate, rendering patients unable to speak, eat, or care for themselves.

Treatment. During the early stages of Alzheimer's disease, medications are available to slow its progression. Medication must continue throughout the patient's remaining life so as not to reverse progression.

AMYOTROPHIC LATERAL SCLEROSIS

Amyotrophic lateral sclerosis (ALS) has an unknown etiology. The disease acts by breaking down the nerves in the nervous system that are responsible for movement. This disease is also known as motor neuron disease and as Lou Gehrig's disease.

Signs and Symptoms. The motor neurons are greatly affected in ALS. As the motor neurons die (cause is unknown), individuals begin to lose control of voluntary muscle movement, including that of the arms, legs, and trunk. Involuntary muscle movement, such as that associated with the contraction of the heart and the smooth muscle of the internal organs, is not generally affected. Various forms of ALS may be associated with a loss of intellectual function (dementia) or sensory symptoms.

Treatment

There is no known cure for ALS. The only treatment available is to utilize medications that are able to lessen the symptoms associated with the disease and improve or maintain the quality of life.

BELL'S PALSY

Bell's palsy is weakness or paralysis of the muscles that control expression on one side of the face. It affects the appearance of the face but is not generally considered a serious condition. Bell's palsy is caused by damage to a facial nerve, one of which runs beneath each ear to the muscles on the same side of the face. Also known as facial palsy, it is named after Dr. Charles Bell of Edinburgh, Scotland, who first documented the disorder in 1882.

Signs and Symptoms.   Often, Bell's palsy is characterized by unilateral paralysis of the face that causes more problems with self-image than anything else. Facial drooping and lack of facial expression on the afflicted side are common symptoms.

Treatment

Doctors may prescribe corticosteroids within the first few days of onset. This is done to help ensure a good recovery. Most often, Bell's palsy will resolve on its own within either weeks or months of onset.

DISK DISORDERS

Disk disorders occur when the intervertebral disks between each of the spinal vertebrae deteriorate, creating pain and shortening of stature.

Signs and Symptoms.   Pain can often be very severe with disk disorders and is often located around or near the location of the problematic disk. This may include neck, back, and leg pain. Leg weakness and other muscle weakness may occur. Incontinence is also associated with disk disorders.

Treatment.   Treatment usually includes bed rest, application of heat or cold, and prescriptions of muscle relaxers along with analgesics. In some cases, surgery may also be recommended. Physical therapy can be prescribed for a ruptured or slipped disk. Massage therapy, acupuncture, and biofeedback are other therapies used for disk orders.

ENCEPHALITIS

Encephalitis is inflammation of the brain often caused by a viral infection. Infants and the elderly comprise the majority of the 1,500 cases per year of encephalitis that occur in the United States.

Signs and Symptoms.   Many signs and symptoms are associated with encephalitis, including headache, sudden fever, vomiting, sensitivity to light, stiff neck and back, confusion, drowsiness, clumsiness, and irritability. Emergency care is required should a patient exhibit any of the following: loss of consciousness, poor responsiveness, seizures, muscle weakness, or impaired judgment. These symptoms may indicate that the disease has made a life-threatening turn.

Treatment.   Those who suffer from encephalitis generally are hospitalized. Their treatments may include antibiotics, antiviral medications, anticonvulsants, steroids to decrease inflammation, and sedatives to control irritability and agitation.

EPILEPSY AND SEIZURES

Epilepsy is a disorder associated with misfiring or interference of electrical impulses within the brain. The cause of epilepsy is often unknown. However, it is often the result of another condition, such as head injury, stroke, brain infection, or brain tumor. A disorder known as a **seizure** can be associated with epilepsy. Seizures occur when abnormal and often intense bursts of electrical activity are produced within the brain. Seizure disorders affect about 0.5 percent of the population.

Signs and Symptoms.   Seizures temporarily interfere with muscle control, movement, speech, vision, or awareness. Having seizures is often terrifying if they are severe. Some individuals only have one seizure in a lifetime, whereas others may have repeated episodes.

Treatment.   Medication often is used to reduce the occurrence and the severity of seizures in patients. In almost all cases, medication must be taken for life. In very severe cases of epilepsy, surgery may be required.

HEADACHES

Headaches may possibly be the most common reason for visiting a doctor in the United States. They account for more than ten million visits to the physician each year. Researchers are not exactly sure why headaches occur or which people are more susceptible. Likewise, doctors cannot always tell what kind of headache an individual has and therefore what kind of medicine would be best. In 1988, the International Headache Society (IHS) developed the criteria most often used to differentiate the various types of headaches from one another. They are based on clinical features of the headache, including the number of attacks per month, length of time per attack, pain characteristics, and accompanying symptoms. The types of headaches include migraine, tension, cluster, and post-traumatic.

Migraine Headaches

Migraine headaches tend to be more common among women. It is thought that female hormones cause this higher frequency.

Signs and Symptoms. The pain associated with migraine headaches is usually very intense. It is typical for patients to complain of pain on one side of the head, with a focal point behind the eye. In addition to pain, additional symptoms include sensitivity to light and noise, and possibly nausea and vomiting.

Treatment. Patients will generally opt for over-the-counter medications such as acetaminophen, ibuprofen, and naproxen sodium. When these analgesics fail to help, physicians may prescribe prescription medications to relieve the symptoms and prevent the occurrence of future headaches.

Tension Headaches

A tension headache may also be referred to as a muscle contraction headache, stress headache, ordinary headache, psychomyogenic headache, and idiopathic headache. Tension headaches may be episodic or chronic in nature.

Signs and Symptoms. Common symptoms associated with tension headaches include a pressing or squeezing pain on both sides of the head, neck, or even facial areas. Generally, these pressure headaches are not throbbing in nature. Patients may also experience sensitivity to light and sound.

Treatment. As with all headaches, treatment for tension headaches includes both prescription and nonprescription analgesics. In addition, treatment is aimed at reducing stress. This may include such activities as biofeedback, yoga, and meditation. Finally, medications including antidepressants and antianxiety medications may also be prescribed.

Cluster Headaches

Cluster headaches, unlike migraines, are more common in men than women. Those who drink excessively and smoke are at the highest risk of developing these headaches.

Signs and Symptoms. Cluster headaches are defined by a penetrating, intense burst of pain that is commonly felt behind the eyes or temples. These headaches commonly afflict sufferers during the seasons of spring and autumn. Attacks can last from 45 minutes to 2 hours and tend to occur at night.

Treatment. In addition to the conventional analgesics that are used, those suffering from cluster headaches have found relief through use of oxygen masks that provide 100 percent pure oxygen, as well as prescription medications indicated for migraine headaches. In severe cases, as well as for those who cannot tolerate the side effects of medication, surgical treatment may be an option.

Post-Traumatic Headaches

Post-traumatic headaches often occur after a head or neck injury has healed. Unfortunately, as many as half of all those who suffer a head or neck injury will experience post-traumatic headaches.

Signs and Symptoms. Symptoms of a post-traumatic headache are very similar to those of migraine and tension headaches. Generally these symptoms will develop 24 to 48 hours after the initial injury; however, they also can develop later.

Treatment. Analgesics are often used for post-traumatic headaches. The focus of treatment is generally based on preventing the occurrence of these headaches. This is often accomplished by using anti-inflammatory medications as well as muscle relaxants and antidepressants.

HUNTINGTON'S CHOREA

Huntington's chorea is a hereditary degenerative disorder of the cerebral and basal ganglia. This disease is also referred to as Huntington's disease (HD).

Signs and Symptoms. Generally the onset of this disease begins during the mid to late thirties, although it may also develop in juveniles. Initial symptoms of the disease include changes in physical and emotional patterns. Involuntary movement, rigidity, problems with balance and coordination, difficulty swallowing, and slurred speech are also common symptoms.

Treatment. Analgesics and benzodiazepines are used to regulate pain, spasms, and seizures. There is, at present time, no cure for the disorder, and most patients die within 15 years of being diagnosed.

HYDROCEPHALUS

Commonly occurring in infants, this disorder is characterized by an excessive amount of CSF that collects within the ventricles of the brain. This causes the brain to compress against the skull. Without proper treatment, this can result in brain damage.

Signs and Symptoms. The most common symptom associated with hydrocephalus is an enlarged head. Additional symptoms include large scalp veins, irritability, and vomiting.

Treatment. A shunt that is surgically inserted into a ventricle is the only treatment available. This shunt creates an exit through which excessive CSF can drain off the brain.

MENINGITIS

Meningitis is an infection of the meninges that surround and protect the brain and spinal cord. Similar to encephalitis, meningitis may be caused by a virus or bacteria. If untreated, bacterial meningitis has a high death rate, killing 70 to 100 percent of all patients.

Signs and Symptoms. The general characteristics of meningitis include neck stiffness, headache, vomiting, high fever, and chills.

Treatment. Immediate medical treatment is necessary as this disease is often fatal. Generally, treatment will include antibiotics, anti-inflammatory medications to reduce brain swelling, general analgesics, and anticonvulsants. To prevent the spread of this disease, isolation may be required.

MULTIPLE SCLEROSIS

Multiple sclerosis (MS) is a chronic, potentially debilitating disease that affects the brain and spinal cord, and there is no known cure. MS is an autoimmune disease, in which the body actually attacks itself. In MS, the body directs the antibodies and white cells to attack the myelin sheath surrounding the nerves in the brain and spinal cord. This causes inflammation and injury to the sheath and the nerves, and scarring may result later. Because of these effects, the transmission of nerve impulses is impeded, resulting in difficulty with movement, vision, or sensation.

Signs and Symptoms. Symptoms may include double vision, dizziness, paralysis, loss of balance, and problems with speech and vision. In addition, symptoms may also include pins-and-needles sensations, bladder incontinence, numbness, and either muscle stiffness or uncontrollable tremors. Figure 25-7 lists the multisystem effects of multiple sclerosis.

Treatment. Treatment of MS depends on the type and severity of the disease. Often drug therapy is utilized to minimize the effects of the symptoms and improve the overall quality of life.

NEURALGIA

Neuralgia is a term used for general nerve pain.

Signs and Symptoms. The pain associated with neuralgia is usually brief but may be severe. It often feels as if it is shooting along the course of the affected nerve. The causes of neuralgia are varied; however, chemical irritation, trauma (including surgery), inflammation, and infections may all lead to neuralgia.

Treatment. Treatment varies depending on the cause, location, and severity of the pain and other factors. Rest, stretching, and heat are used to aid in the patient's relief. Mild over-the-counter analgesics such as aspirin, acetaminophen, or ibuprofen may be helpful for mild pain. Other treatments may include the use of narcotic painkillers, nerve blocks, and anesthetic agents that are administered via local injection, or surgical procedures to decrease sensitivity of the nerve.

PARKINSON'S DISEASE

Parkinson's disease is a progressive disorder, with no known cure, caused by degeneration of the nerve cells in the parts of the brain that control movement. Because of the degeneration, there is a shortage of the neurotransmitter dopamine, causing the movement impairments that characterize the disease.

Signs and Symptoms. Parkinson's typically presents as a tremor of a limb, especially when the body is at rest. The tremor usually begins on one side, is localized to one limb, and is usually seen in the hand. Other common symptoms include slow movement (bradykinesia) or an inability to

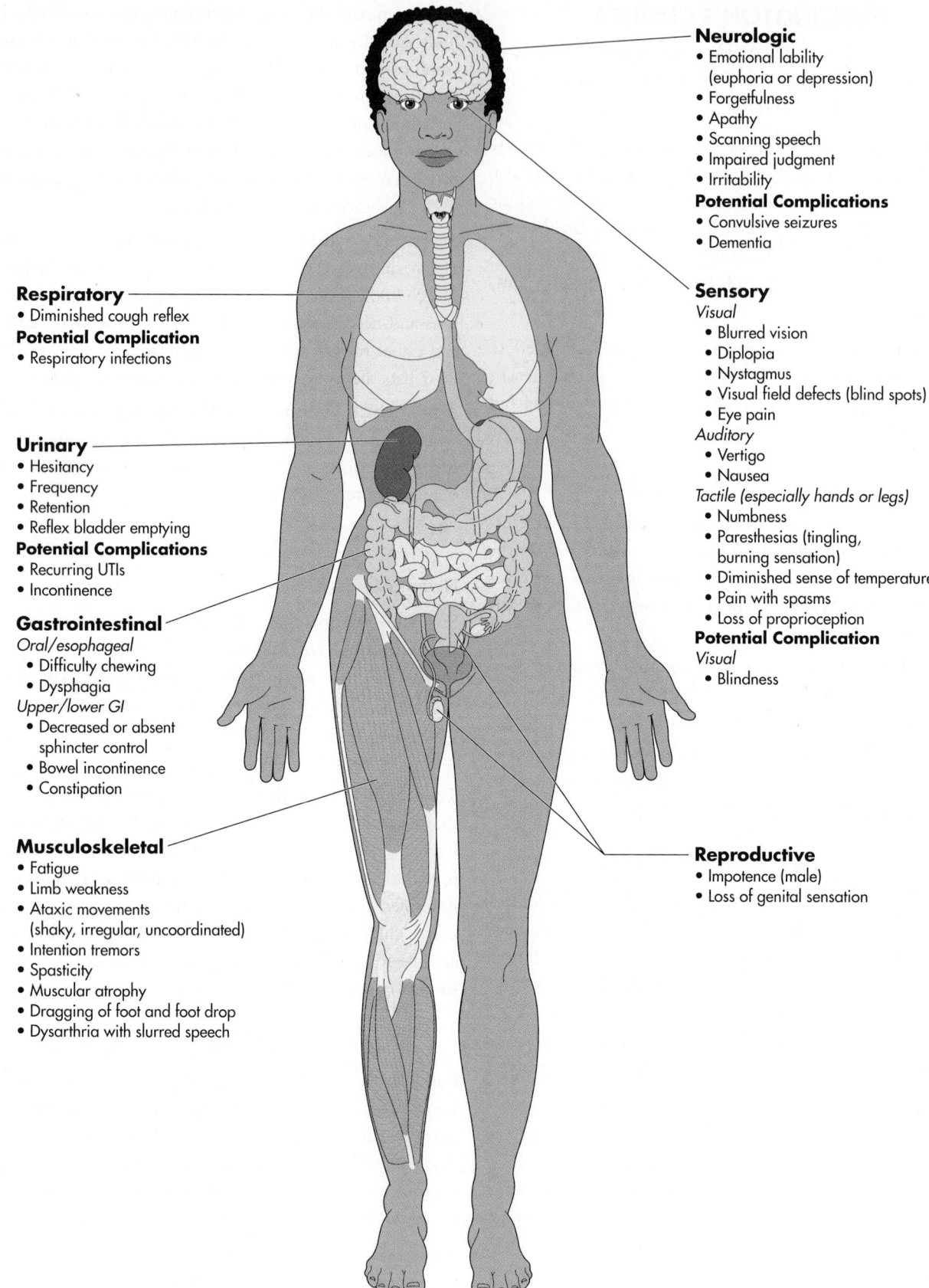

Neurologic
- Emotional lability
  (euphoria or depression)
- Forgetfulness
- Apathy
- Scanning speech
- Impaired judgment
- Irritability

Potential Complications
- Convulsive seizures
- Dementia

Sensory
Visual
- Blurred vision
- Diplopia
- Nystagmus
- Visual field defects (blind spots)
- Eye pain

Auditory
- Vertigo
- Nausea

Tactile (especially hands or legs)
- Numbness
- Paresthesias (tingling,
  burning sensation)
- Diminished sense of temperature
- Pain with spasms
- Loss of proprioception

Potential Complication
Visual
- Blindness

Respiratory
- Diminished cough reflex

Potential Complication
- Respiratory infections

Urinary
- Hesitancy
- Frequency
- Retention
- Reflex bladder emptying

Potential Complications
- Recurring UTIs
- Incontinence

Gastrointestinal
Oral/esophageal
- Difficulty chewing
- Dysphagia

Upper/lower GI
- Decreased or absent
  sphincter control
- Bowel incontinence
- Constipation

Musculoskeletal
- Fatigue
- Limb weakness
- Ataxic movements
  (shaky, irregular, uncoordinated)
- Intention tremors
- Spasticity
- Muscular atrophy
- Dragging of foot and foot drop
- Dysarthria with slurred speech

Reproductive
- Impotence (male)
- Loss of genital sensation

FIGURE 25-7 Multisystem effects of multiple sclerosis.

move (akinesia), rigid limbs, a shuffling gait, and a stooped posture. Other frequent signs of Parkinson's include reduced facial expression (the "mask"), and a soft voice. The disease may also cause depression, personality change, dementia, sleep disturbances, speech impairment, and sexual difficulties. Parkinson's tends to worsen over time.

Treatment. Levodopa is a medication that is commonly used to treat the symptoms of Parkinson's as there is not a known cure for the disease. Eventually, levodopa must be discontinued due to the side effects caused after regularly increasing the dosage amount. Few patients are eligible for surgical intervention that can help to minimize the effects of involuntary motions caused by this disease.

SCIATICA

Sciatica refers to a pain that runs along the sciatic nerve. It is often caused by inflammation due to a pinched root of the sciatic nerve. Sciatica usually occurs on one side of the body.

Signs and Symptoms. The most common symptom associated with sciatica is a sharp pain that runs from the lower back and down the back of the thigh. Pain may be worse during periods of activity, as well as at night. Many patients complain of increased pain when the weather changes.

Treatment. Patients generally are advised to rest and restrict activities that cause pain and discomfort. Analgesics and cold or heat therapy may be beneficial. Gentle stretching exercises as prescribed by a physician are also helpful in increasing tolerable movements. In extreme cases, surgical intervention may be necessary. Surgery is most common in instances when sciatica is caused by pressure that is placed on the sciatic nerve from a slipped disk.

SPINA BIFIDA

Spina bifida is the most frequently occurring, permanently disabling, and devastating of all birth defects. It affects approximately 1 out of every 1,000 newborns in the United States. More children have spina bifida than have muscular dystrophy, MS, and cystic fibrosis combined. It results from the failure of the spine to close properly during the first

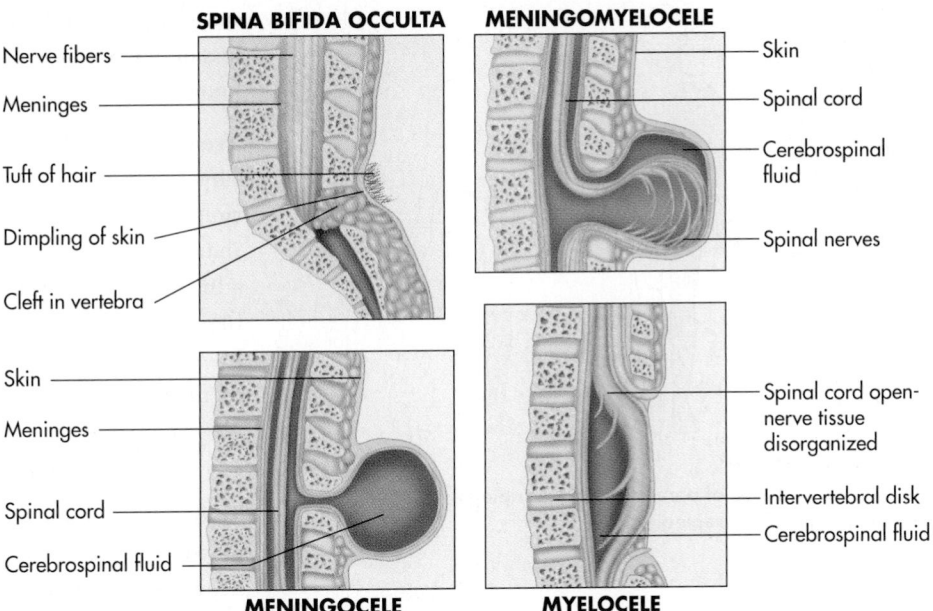

FIGURE 25-8 The various forms of spina bidida.

month of pregnancy. The various forms of spina bifida include spina bifida occulta, meningomyelocele, meningocele, and myelomeningocele.

Signs and Symptoms. Signs and symptoms will vary based on the form of spina bifida that is present. Spina bifida occulta causes malformation of one or two vertebrae, and the affected spinal area is covered by skin and not visible. Symptoms are rare with this form of the disorder. Closed neural tube defects are varied, as in some individuals no symptoms are present whereas others experience paralysis causing urine and bowel dysfunction. A meningocele is characterized by the meninges protruding from the spinal opening. Symptoms may or may not be present, and those present are similar to closed neural tube defects. Myelocele is the most severe form of spina bifida as the entire spinal cord is exposed through an opening. Paralysis may be partial or complete below the area of the myelocele (Figure 25-8).

Treatment. As with many other nervous system disorders, spina bifida does not have a cure. Any and all nerve damage that occurs as a result of spina bifida is permanent. Though some children may need surgical intervention as they grow and develop, children with milder forms of spina bifida may not require any treatment at all. Recent treatments have involved doctors performing surgery on the fetus in utero. However, in those cases, complications can be great for both the mother and fetus.

SPINAL CORD INJURIES

Damage, lesions, or a break in the spinal cord can result in paralysis of the body. It is most common for the paralysis to

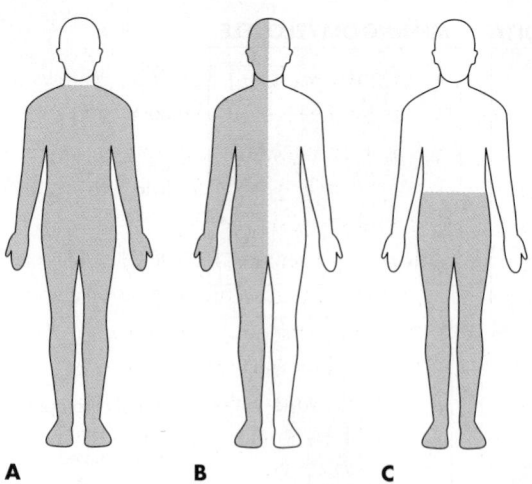

FIGURE 25-9   Types of paralysis: (A) quadriplegia; (B) hemiplegia; (C) paraplegia.

affect the injured area of the spinal cord and everything below that point. **Quadriplegia** refers to paralysis from approximately the shoulders down. **Paraplegia** refers to paralysis from approximately the waist down. **Hemiplegia** occurs when paralysis affects one side of the body (Figure 25-9).

Signs and Symptoms.   Complete lack of movement from the point of injury and below is the most common symptom of paralysis. Complications associated with paralysis include pressure sores (decubitus), blood clots (thrombosis), muscle atrophy, and pneumonia.

Treatment.   Treatment is aimed at reducing complications associated with paralysis by effective and careful care of the patient. Physical therapy may also be helpful, especially in patients who are hemiplegic due to complications associated with a stroke.

STROKE

A **stroke**, known in medicine as a cerebrovascular accident (CVA), is the third leading cause of death in the United States. Death occurs to brain tissue when the blood supply to a part of the brain is decreased, either by a clot or by hemorrhage. Brain cells can die when their oxygen supply is interrupted for more than a few minutes, so speed in diagnosis and treatment is extremely important.

Signs and Symptoms.   The following symptoms are often sudden and require emergency intervention: numbness or weakness on one side of the body, confusion or trouble speaking, vision disturbances in one or both eyes, dizziness, loss of balance or coordination, and severe headache with no known cause.

Treatment.   As stated, emergency intervention is vital. Physicians will attempt to stabilize the patient's condition by either dissolving blood clots or stopping hemorrhage. Surgery may be necessary, and physicians will administer medications to control the swelling of the brain and control blood pressure. Medications and treatments are given after the incident to reduce the chance of recurrence.

TRANSIENT ISCHEMIC ATTACK

Transient ischemic attacks (TIAs) are frequently precursors of strokes. In fact, these "ministrokes" can last anywhere from a few seconds to hours.

Signs and Symptoms.   Temporary sudden weakness, numbness, and change of consciousness are common signs. Signs and symptoms will depend on the portion of the brain affected.

Treatment.   Patients must seek medical attention during a TIA. Anticoagulants and aspirin therapy often may be used to reduce the risk of blood clot formation. The following may help in reducing the risk of future TIAs: cease smoking, stop overeating, decrease alcohol consumption, lower blood pressure, and control diabetes.

TRAUMA

Trauma to the nervous system can be devastating. Epidural and subdural hematomas can develop when the head receives a blow. Subdural hematomas can cause pressure in the brain that must be relieved with shunting. Trauma can also cause **concussion**—an injury caused by sharp jarring or a blow to the head that may result in a loss of consciousness—or the more serious **contusion,** which is a bruising of the brain. Skull fractures are known as depressions and can cause brain injury.

Signs and Symptoms.   Signs and symptoms related to trauma will vary depending on the injury that causes the trauma. Common symptoms associated with neurological trauma include loss of consciousness, headache, confusion, dizziness, blurred vision, and ringing in the ears. Behavioral, mood, and sleep pattern changes may also be indicative of neurological trauma to the brain.

Treatment.   Treatment depends on the type of trauma. Rehabilitation exercises are usually needed. Medications to suppress seizures, such as benzodiazepines and barbiturates, are frequently prescribed following brain trauma.

SUMMARY

The nervous system is a very complex communication system that affects all functions in the body. The structure and function of the nervous system provide for an efficient system of stimulus recognition and motor reaction for the entire body. The brain and the CNS collect, interpret, and coordinate all sensory input and responses performed by the PNS. Nerves do not form a continuous chain but instead fire across synapses through the work of neurotransmitters. The lack of neurotransmitters at the synapse can cause serious disorders, such as depression. The destruction of the myelin sheath that coats the spinal cord is detrimental to the functioning of the entire system. An intricate fight-or-flight system prepares the body for neurological decisions. However, reaction to chronic stress can fatigue the nervous system.

Because the system is so complex, a disorder can be devastating. Disorders of the nervous system include Alzheimer's disease, amyotrophic lateral sclerosis, Bell's palsy, disk disorders, encephalitis, epilepsy, and seizure disorders, headaches, Huntington's chorea, hydrocephalus, meningitis, multiple sclerosis, neuralgia, Parkinson's disease, sciatica, spina bifida, spinal cord injuries, stroke, TIAs, and trauma. Neurological disorders must be recognized and reported to appropriate professionals in a very timely manner to prevent long-lasting disability.

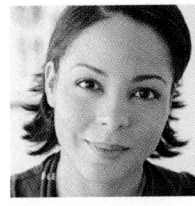

25 CHAPTER REVIEW

COMPETENCY REVIEW

1. Define and spell the terms to learn for this chapter.

2. What are the two divisions of the nervous system?

3. What are the functions of the nervous system?

4. What is the myelin sheath?

5. What is a neuron?

6. What are the parts of the central nervous system?

7. What are the functions of the hypothalamus?

8. What are the functions of the medulla oblongata?

9. What are three functions of the spinal cord?

10. What are the symptoms of a transient ischemic attack?

PREPARING FOR THE CERTIFICATION EXAM

1. The eighth cranial nerve (acoustic) is responsible for:
   a. sense of taste
   b. sense of smell
   c. sense of hearing and equilibrium
   d. sensation in the face and head
   e. sense of sight

2. Olfactory senses are those of
   a. taste
   b. sight
   c. smell
   d. touch
   e. hearing and equilibrium

3. A myelocele is a form of
   a. spina bifida
   b. Down syndrome
   c. meningitis
   d. epilepsy
   e. CVA

4. Which of the following is a hereditary degenerative disorder?
   a. TIA
   b. CVA
   c. Huntington's chorea
   d. spina bifida
   e. spinal cord injuries

5. Which word means half the body is paralyzed?
   a. quadriplegia
   b. hemiparesis
   c. paraplegia
   d. hemiplegia
   e. paraparesis

6. Bradykinesia, akinesia, and shuffling gait are symptoms of:
   a. Alzheimer's disease
   b. Huntington's chorea
   c. Bell's palsy
   d. spina bifida
   e. Parkinson's disease

7. If the spine does not close properly in fetal development, the infant will have
   a. sciatica
   b. spina bifida
   c. Huntington's chorea

   d. Bell's palsy
   e. multiple sclerosis

8. Which of the following is an example of the work of the parasympathetic nervous system?
   a. heart rate increases
   b. intestinal mobility decreases
   c. pupils constrict
   d. bladder sphincter closes
   e. bronchial muscle relaxes

9. Which of the following is an example of the work of the sympathetic nervous system?
   a. heart rate decreases
   b. intestinal digestion increases
   c. bladder sphincter relaxes
   d. heart force increases
   e. pupils constrict

10. Which disease causes the loss of memory?
   a. Bell's palsy
   b. Huntington's chorea
   c. Parkinson's disease
   d. Alzheimer's disease
   e. spina bifida

CRITICAL THINKING

1. After examining Elena, Dr. Miller diagnoses her with Alzheimer's disease in its early stages. Svetlana asks the physician how her mother can be treated. What might Dr. Miller say to Svetlana?

2. Svetlana asks Dr. Miller for information related to Alzheimer's disease. Dr. Miller decides to send Mary Ellen, an RMA, into the room to review a patient education brochure that discusses the progression of the disease. What information should this brochure include?

3. Alzheimer's disease affects memory, reasoning, and problem-solving skills. Which lobe(s) of the brain pertain to these aspects of cognitive functioning?

INTERNET ACTIVITY

Do an Internet search to learn about Alzheimer's support groups.

MEDMEDIA

Additional interactive resources and activities for this chapter can be found:

On your student DVD: View applicable procedure videos on the DVD-ROM found in the back of this book.

MyHealthProfessionsKit.com: Test your knowledge of this chapter with games and activities. MyHealthProfessionsKit also includes resources, helpful links, and a Spanish audio glossary.

Medical Assisting Interactive: Practice your procedures as a medical assistant in this simulated doctor's office. This can be accessed through MyHealthProfessionsKit.com.

26

The Special Senses

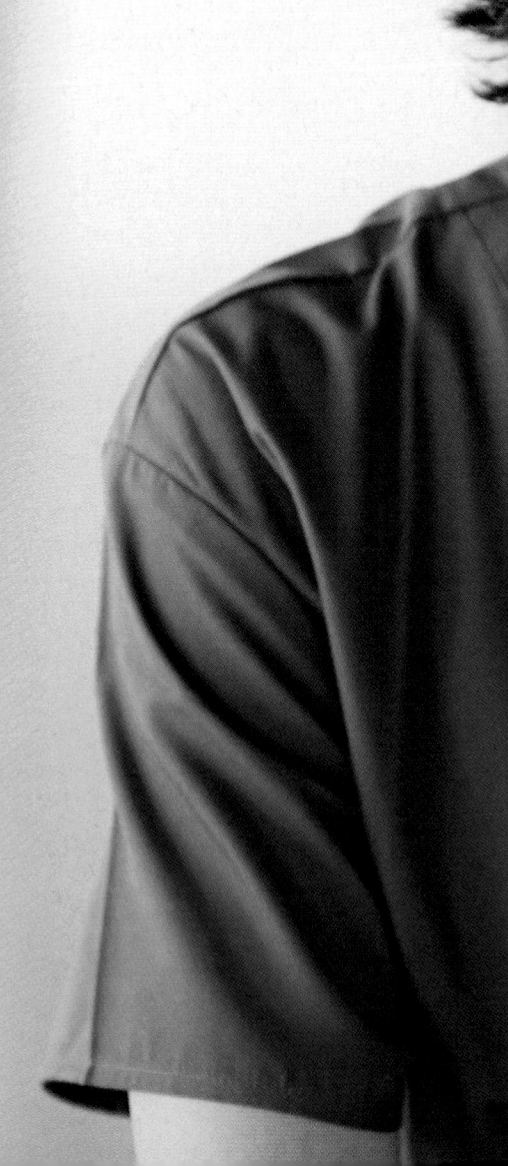

LEARNING OBJECTIVES

After completing this chapter, you should be able to:

- Define and spell the terms to learn for this chapter.

- Describe the anatomy of the eye, and briefly explain the function of each structure.

- Discuss common disorders associated with the eye.

- Describe the anatomy of the ear, and briefly explain the function of each structure.

- Explain common disorders associated with the ear.

- Describe the anatomy of the nose, and explain how the sense of smell occurs.

- Identify the anatomical structures that make up the special senses.

- Discuss the sense of taste, and briefly explain the function of taste buds.

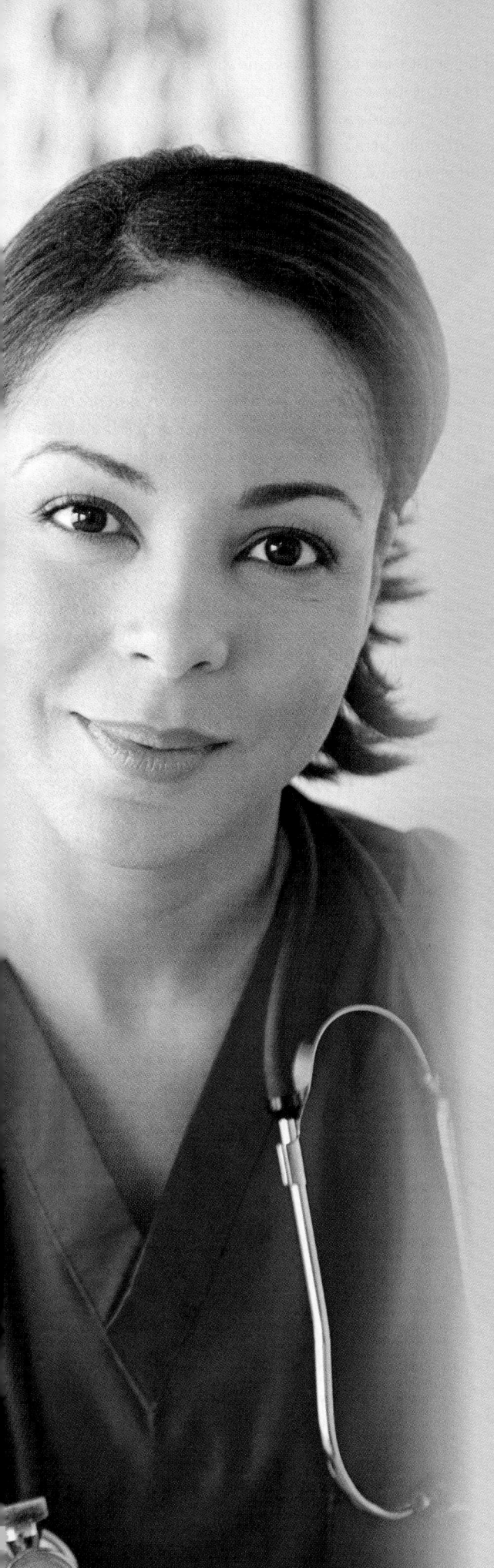

CHAPTER OUTLINE

CASE STUDY

Carmine DiStefano is visiting Dr. Salpega today with his 1½-year-old son, Lucas. Lucas has been very restless and has not been sleeping very well during the past few nights. During the day, he hardly eats and is constantly tugging on his left ear. Mr. DiStefano is concerned because his 5-year-old daughter, Sophia, struggles with chronic otitis media and has recently had tubes placed in her ears. He is certain that Lucas has an ear infection.

507

The senses are structures and organs that make it possible for us to see, hear, smell, taste, and feel. This chapter presents the five special senses, with particular attention to the organs of seeing and hearing and the disorders that may affect them.

The Eye and the Sense of Vision

The eye is a spherical, fluid-filled organ composed of specialized structures that work together to facilitate vision. Light rays pass through the cornea, pupil, lens, and vitreous humor to the retina, where they stimulate sensory receptors. Nerves in the eye control the amount of light entering the eye through the pupil, the focusing of the light by the lens on the retina, and the transmission of the resulting images to the brain.

ANATOMY OF THE EYE

The eye is made up of the eyeball and its internal structures, which perform the complex process of translating light into images, and external structures that support and protect the eyeballs.

THE STRUCTURES OF THE EYEBALL

The eyeball is housed in a cavity in the skull called an **orbit**. The eyeball itself can be divided into two cavities: a front, or anterior, cavity filled with a watery fluid called the **aqueous humor** and a posterior, or back, section located behind the lens and filled with a very thick fluid in the **vitreous chamber**, called the **vitreous humor** (Figure 26-1).

The surface of the eyeball is made up of three distinct layers. The outer layer is comprised of the **sclera**, or "white" part of the eye, and the **cornea**, which is frequently referred to as the "window" of the eye because it allows the light to enter.

The middle layer is composed of the following structures:

- **Choroid**—lines the sclera and absorbs extra light entering the eye

- **Ciliary body**—responsible for holding and moving the lens; secretes aqueous humor, which provides nutrients to the cornea, lens, and other tissues

- **Iris**—contains the pigment, or eye color, and has a "hole" in the center called the **pupil**, which controls the amount of light entering the eye

The innermost layer of the eye is the **retina**. Photosensitive cells in the retina called **rods** and **cones** translate light rays into nerve impulses that are transmitted to the brain.

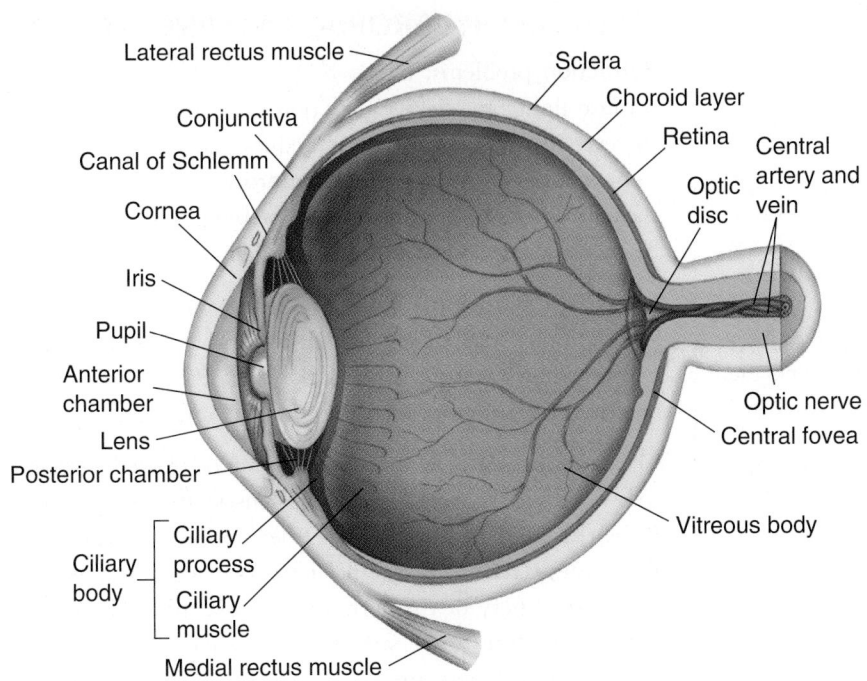

FIGURE 26-1   The eyeball and its anatomical structures.

incoming information from the eye to the brain. Inflammation at the optic nerve, known as **papilledema**, is usually caused by a tumor that increases pressure in the eye.

The **lens**, a colorless structure behind the iris, sharpens the focus of light rays onto the retina. A reflexive process called **accommodation** adjusts the eye's optical powers to maintain a clear image at various distances.

The External Structures of the Eye

Other important structures of the eye serve the primary functions of protection and support: the eyelids, conjunctiva, lacrimal apparatus, and extrinsic eye muscles.

The eyelids, or **palpebrae**, close over the eyeballs, protecting them from intense light, foreign matter, and impacts. They also keep the eyes moist by preventing tears from evaporating. Light enters through the **palpebral fissure**, the opening between the eyelids. Eyelashes in the margins (edges) of the eyelids further protect the eye from foreign matter. The superior and inferior palpebrae meet at the **canthus** at each corner of the eye.

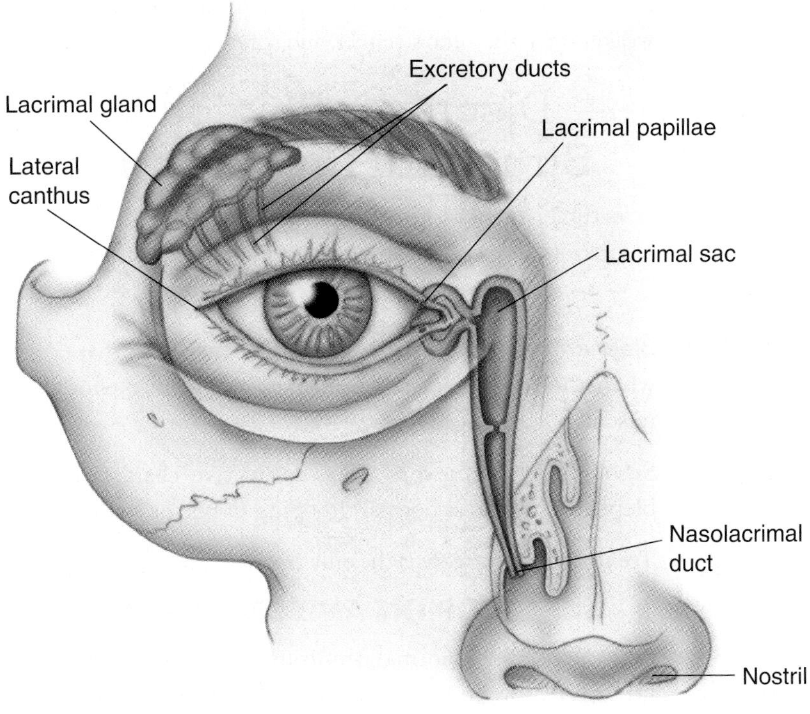

The **conjunctiva** is a mucous membrane that lines the underside of the eyelids and the anterior part of the eyeball. It serves a protective function.

Tears are a fluid the body produces to cleanse the eyes and keep them moist. Tears are produced, stored, and removed by the structures that make up the **lacrimal apparatus**. Above the outer corner of each eye is the **lacrimal gland**, which secretes tears through ducts on the surface of the conjunctiva of the upper lid. At the inner corner of each eye are two ducts, the **lacrimal canaliculi**, which collect and drain the tears into the **lacrimal sac**. The lacrimal sac empties into the **nasolacrimal duct**, which empties into the nasal cavity (Figure 26-2).

Six short extrinsic eye muscles connect the eyeball to the orbital cavity. These muscles provide the eyeball with support and rotary movement. Four of these muscles, the rectus muscles, are straight, and two are oblique, or slanted.

Rods react to dim light and are used in night vision; cones are sensitive to bright light and are used to see color. The **fovea centralis retinae** contains only cones and is located in the middle of the **macula lutea**, a yellow spot on the back of the eye. The **optic nerve** enters at the **optic disk** and carries

FIGURE 26-2   The lacrimal apparatus.

Common Refractive Disorders

The most common disorders of the eye are refractive errors, which are characterized by the inability of the eye to focus correctly. They are caused by factors such as aging and changes in the shape of the eyeball and various eye muscles.

ASTIGMATISM

Astigmatism is a condition caused by irregularities in the curvature of the cornea and lens that cause light to focus not on the retina but to spread out over an area.

Signs and Symptoms. Astigmatism is characterized by blurry near or distant vision. It may be accompanied by squinting and headaches.

Treatment. Treatment generally consists of corrective lenses or surgery to reshape the cornea.

MYOPIA, HYPEROPIA, AND PRESBYOPIA

Refraction problems, the inability to focus correctly, occur because light rays change direction when they pass through the eye. In **myopia**, or nearsightedness, the lens focuses the light in front of the retina. In **hyperopia**, or farsightedness, the lens focuses behind the retina. **Presbyopia** is characterized by the loss of elasticity in the lens, usually as a result of aging.

Signs and Symptoms. In myopia, objects that are farther away appear fuzzy or blurred. In hyperopia, distant objects are seen more clearly than closer objects. Presbyopia is characterized by difficulty focusing on close objects.

Treatment. Most refractive errors can be treated with corrective lenses (glasses or contact lenses) to help properly focus the light on the retina. Other options include radial keratotomy (RK) (surgical incisions are made from the pupil to the periphery of the cornea in a radial pattern) and the Lasik procedure (laser surgery that reshapes and corrects imperfections in the cornea).

STRABISMUS

Another common refractive disorder is **strabismus**, also called crossed eyes or wall eyes. In this condition, the eyes do not focus on the same image, as one eye turns in, out, up, or down. It is caused by weakness in the external eye.

Signs and Symptoms. Patients with strabismus may experience poor depth perception and double vision.

Treatment. Treatment for strabismus includes eyeglasses, eye exercises, wearing a patch over the stronger eye to force the weaker eye to become stronger, and surgery to realign the eyes.

Disorders Related to Structural Irregularities

Structural irregularities, defects, or underlying disorders cause blepharoptosis, ectropion, entropion, and exophthalmos.

BLEPHAROPTOSIS

Blepharoptosis is a usually congenital condition that occurs when the muscles of the eyelid are not strong enough to raise it.

Signs and Symptoms. The distinctive characteristic of blepharoptosis is abnormal drooping of one or both eyelids.

Treatment. Surgery is the only treatment for blepharoptosis.

ECTROPION AND ENTROPION

Ectropion is an abnormal condition in which the lower eyelid everts, or turns outward. In **entropion**, the eyelid inverts, or folds inward.

Signs and Symptoms. Both conditions are very uncomfortable, and the patient may exhibit redness of the eyes, tearing, sensitivity to light, and decreased vision.

Treatment. Both ectoprion and entroprion can be treated with surgery.

EXOPHTHALMOS

Exophthalmos is usually caused by hyperthyroidism or Graves' disease. Unilateral exophthalmos may also be caused by an orbital tumor.

Signs and Symptoms. The most distinctive characteristic of exophthalmos is the outward bulging of one or both eyeballs.

Treatment. The goal of treatment is to address the underlying hyperthyroidism with surgical ablation and radiation. Eyedrops may be used to keep the eyes well lubricated.

Infectious Eye Disorders

Infection and inflammation cause a number of common and often contagious eye disorders, such as blepharitis, conjunctivitis, and hordeolums.

BLEPHARITIS

Blepharitis is an inflammation of the eyelids.

Signs and Symptoms. Symptoms include redness, itching, and swelling of the eyelids.

Treatment. Blepharitis is treated with warm compresses and ophthalmic antibiotic therapy.

CONJUNCTIVITIS

Conjunctivitis is one of the most common and treatable eye infections, affecting both children and adults. Commonly known as pink eye, this highly contagious condition is an inflammation of the conjunctiva, the tissue lining the inside of the eyelid. Causes include a virus, bacteria, sexually transmitted infections (STIs), allergens, and irritants such as chlorine, dirt, or smoke.

Signs and Symptoms. Early recognition of symptoms is extremely important. The most common symptoms include redness in the sclera, increased tear production, a thick yellow discharge that crusts over the eyelashes, itchy eyes, burning eyes, blurred vision, and greater sensitivity to light.

Treatment. Early treatment of conjunctivitis is equally important. Topical or oral antibiotics, or eyedrops containing antihistamines or nonsteroidal anti-inflammatory agents, may be administered. The cure rate is almost always 100 percent.

HORDEOLUMS

Also known as sties, **hordeolums** are very common and frequently contagious. They are often caused by bacteria, generally *Staphylococcus,* and may accompany blocked or infected eyelid glands or inflamed eyelids. Contaminated fingers that touch the eye area may also cause the infection. Painful hordeolums can also occur under the eyelids.

Signs and Symptoms. Early symptoms include redness and tenderness, followed by itching, swelling, and discomfort in the upper or lower eyelid. The sty or hordeolum develops as a pus-filled swelling at the base of an eyelash.

Treatment. Hordeolums often resolve on their own. A warm, wet compress applied to the area may help relieve the pain. Antibiotics may be taken orally or applied topically to accelerate healing.

Age-Related Eye Disorders

As we age, the muscles and other structures in the eye weaken and vision declines. Eye disorders commonly seen in older adults are cataracts, retinal detachment, and macular degeneration, which is one of the leading causes of blindness in this population.

CATARACTS

A **cataract** is a clouding or opacity of the lens that prevents light from entering. Although the cause is unclear, there may be a correlation between the formation of cataracts and smoking, diabetes, and excessive exposure to sunlight.

Over time, and without proper treatment, images begin to look fuzzy. Night vision suffers. The patient may also experience double vision or problems with bright lights. The cataract may cloud the lens severely enough to block vision completely.

For early or immature cataracts, eyeglasses, magnifying lenses, and stronger lighting may be sufficient. If this is not successful, surgery is the recommended treatment. Cataract removal is a very common surgery; it is also extremely safe and effective, with a cure rate of 90 percent.

RETINAL DISORDERS

Among the disorders that affect the retina, two of the most severe are retinal detachment and macular degeneration. These disorders are fairly rare and primarily age-related.

Retinal Detachment

Retinal detachment occurs when a retina has separated from the underlying choroid layer. When such a separation occurs, vision is damaged. However, if the detachment is detected early, it can be repaired and the vision saved. If the retina has already detached, vision can frequently be restored by surgery and laser therapy.

Signs and Symptoms. Symptoms of retinal detachment include an increase in floaters (particles that float slowly within the viewer's eyes), or flashes of light in the field of vision. The individual may feel as if a curtain has obscured part of the vision.

Treatment. Anyone experiencing the symptoms of retinal detachment should seek professional help as soon as possible. Treatment for small holes or tears is usually laser surgery or cryotherapy (application of intense cold to induce a scar); for retinal detachment, surgery requiring a hospital stay is generally recommended.

MACULAR DEGERNATION

Macular degeneration is the deterioration of the macula, which is the central portion of the retina. It is an incurable disease that affects more than ten million Americans and is one of the leading cause of blindness among people over the age of 55.

Signs and Symptoms. The two types of macular degeneration are dry and wet. The dry (atrophic) type affects 85–90 percent of cases. In the dry type, small yellow deposits called drusen form under the macula, causing it to thin and dry out and leading to a loss of central vision. This form of macular degeneration has a slower progression than does the wet type but sometimes turns into the wet type.

Symptoms of dry macular degeneration include a decline in central vision, increasing haziness of overall vision, and a need for brighter illumination for reading and close work. Symptoms of wet macular degeneration include visual distortions and a blurry spot in the central vision.

In wet macular degeneration, abnormal new blood vessels grow under the retina and the macula. They may then bleed and leak fluid, which causes the macula to bulge or lift up, impairing or destroying the central vision. Vision loss may be rapid and severe.

Treatment. There is no known treatment or cure for dry macular degeneration. If performed early, laser surgery may halt the progression of wet macular degeneration, thus preventing a total loss of vision. Although this outcome cannot be guaranteed, laser surgery is currently the best treatment.

NYCTALOPIA

Nyctalopia is the inability to see well in a faint light. This condition occurs in patients with retinitis pigmentosa and choroidoretinitis, or it may be due to a vitamin A deficiency. It can also be provoked by smoking tobacco. Hypoxia (deficiency of oxygen reaching the tissues) associated with being above sea level in an aircraft may also decrease night vision.

Other Eye Disorders

Problems with the eyes and with vision may be caused by factors other than those already described. These include amblyopia, glaucoma, corneal abrasions, and nystagmus.

AMBLYOPIA

Amblyopia, or lazy eye, is a disorder seen in children that occurs when the muscles are weaker in one eye than in the other.

Signs and Symptoms. Many people with mild amblyopia are unaware of the condition. Children are often diagnosed only when their eyes are examined at the doctor's office. People with more severe amblyopia may suffer from various vision-related disorders, such as poor depth perception.

Treatment. The primary treatment for amblyopia is a patch worn over the stronger eye to strengthen the muscles of the weaker eye. Early diagnosis and treatment are essential.

CORNEAL ABRASION

A **corneal abrasion** is a lesion or abrasion on the cornea that can result from injury, infection, or both.

Signs and Symptoms. A corneal abrasion can be very painful. The patient will be very sensitive to light and will have difficulty opening the affected eye.

Treatment. The usual treatment consists of mild analgesics and resting the eyes. If the abrasion becomes infected, antibiotic eyedrops or ointments are given, and the use of an eye patch is recommended.

DIPLOPIA

Diplopia is double vision. Frequently it follows trauma to the eye or head. It can also be caused be a disease of the lens, retina, cranial nerve, cerebellum, cerebrum, or meninges.

GLAUCOMA

Glaucoma affects people of all ages and all races. It is characterized by increased pressure in the eye brought on by an excessive amount of aqueous humor. Left untreated, the pressure can lead to damage of the optic nerve and eventually blindness.

There are two basic types of glaucoma. In open-angle (acute) glaucoma, pressure builds up very slowly, causing a slow drainage of aqueous humor from the anterior segment of the eye. In closed-angle (chronic) glaucoma, which is considered more serious, the space between the iris and the cornea narrows, causing a greater degree of pressure to build. Approximately 80,000 people are totally blind as a result of glaucoma, another 250,000 are blind in one eye, and over 1.2 million people have some degree of visual loss.

Signs and Symptoms. Glaucoma has no symptoms, so it must be diagnosed by pressure testing in a doctor's office.

Treatment. Glaucoma is treated with medications, such as eyedrops to lower intraocular pressure, as well as with laser and conventional surgery.

NYSTAGMUS (NYSTAXIS)

Nystagmus (nystaxis) is characterized by involuntary, repetitive, rhythmic eye movements. It may be inherited or acquired and usually results in some loss of vision.

Signs and Symptoms. Uncontrolled eye movements may be lateral, horizontal, or even circular.

Treatment. Treatment must address the underlying cause, which might be a tumor, a lesion, alcohol abuse, or retinal maldevelopment.

RETINOPATHY

Patients with diabetes are prone to **diabetic retinopathy** which is a disease of the retina. Nerve damage can result from **hypertensive retinopathy** caused by hypertension, and can lead to permanent blindness.

PHOTOPHOBIA

Photophobia, or sensitivity to light, is a side effect of many medications. Sometimes it is caused by measles, rubella, meningitis, or inflammation of the eyes.

The Ear and the Sense of Hearing

The ear is the organ responsible for hearing and equilibrium, or balance. Specialized anatomical structures in the ear are sensitive to sound vibrations, gravity, and head movements. The eighth cranial nerve connects these structures to the brain.

ANATOMY OF THE EAR

The ear can be divided into three sections: the external, middle, and inner ears (Figure 26-3). Each section plays a distinct role in the hearing process.

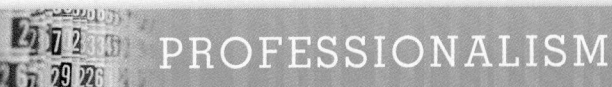

The External Ear

The external ear is the visible portion of the ear. It consists of the following structures:

- Pinna, or auricle—funnels sound waves through the auditory canal to the tympanic membrame
- Auditory canal, or auditory meatus—S-shaped, about 2.5 cm long; secretes **cerumen**, or earwax
- **Tympanic membrane**, or eardrum—separates the external ear from the middle ear
- The **fundus**—the floor of the tympanic cavity

The Middle Ear

The middle ear is a tiny cavity in the temporal bone of the skull. It contains three small bones, or **ossicles**, whose

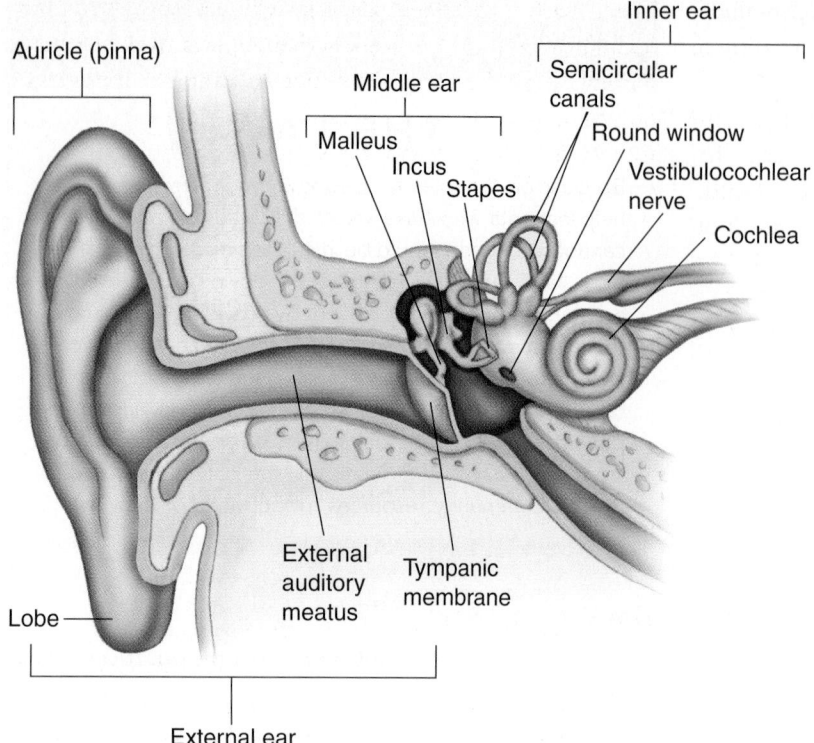

FIGURE 26-3 **The ear and its anatomical structures.**

names describe their shapes: the **malleus** (hammer), **incus** (anvil), and **stapes** (stirrup). The function of the middle ear is to transmit sound vibrations, equalize the air pressure on both sides of the tympanic membrane, and protect the ear from potentially damaging loud noise. Sound vibrations are transmitted by the ossicles from the tympanic membrane to the oval window and into the inner ear.

The Inner Ear

The inner ear is a maze of canals within a bony labyrinth in the temporal bone. The **cochlea**, **vestibule**, and three **semicircular canals** make up the **labyrinth**. The bony and membranous labyrinths are separated by a fluid called perilymph. Tiny hair cells in the inner ear function as receptors for hearing and balance.

The cochlea is a bony spiral structure that resembles a snail's shell (Figure 26-4). Three tubelike channels run the entire length of the spiral; between the upper and lower channels is the cochlear duct.

The vestibule is the fundus of the internal auditory meatus. The vestibular nerve is a main division of the acoustic or eighth cranial nerve. The organ of Corti, located in the cochlear duct, contains nerve endings that

transmit sound vibrations received from the stapes to the auditory region of the brain via the eighth cranial nerve,

The **Eustachian tube**, or auditory tube, extends 3 to 4 cm from the middle ear to the nasopharynx. If blocked, the patient may get an infection in the middle ear.

Hearing Loss

Audiology is the study of hearing disorders. The following are the two most common types of **hearing loss**:

- **Conductive**—temporary condition in which sound is not conducted efficiently through the auditory canal to the eardrum and the ossicles in the middle ear. Conductive hearing loss can be medically or surgically corrected.

- **Sensorineural**—permanent hearing loss caused by damage to the cochlea or to nerve pathways from the inner ear to the brain. Sensorineural hearing loss cannot be medically or surgically corrected.

Many of the following disorders either involve or result in hearing loss. See "Professionalism: Cultural Considerations" for a brief discussion of sensitivity toward patients with hearing difficulties.

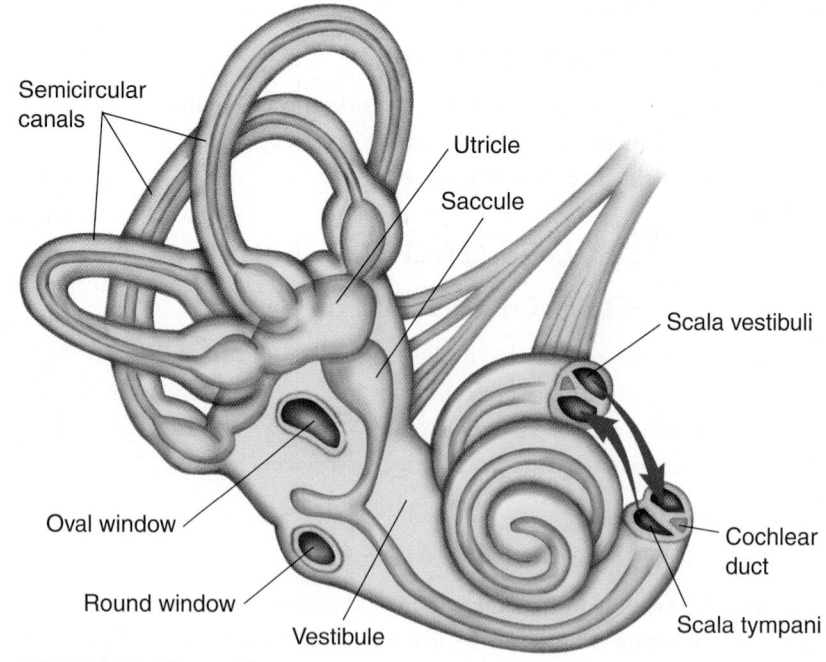

FIGURE 26-4 **The cochlea.**

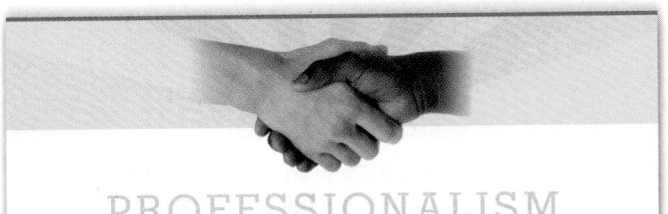
Common Disorders Associated with the Outer Ear

Two disorders of the outer ear involve cerumen, or earwax, and injury to the tympanic membrane.

IMPACTED CERUMEN

Cerumen or earwax is a complex mixture of lipids produced by the sebaceous glands of the auditory canal to lubricate the ear. **Impacted cerumen** is earwax that has hardened to the point that it obstructs the auditory canal. It generally affects older adults.

Signs and Symptoms. The patient with impacted cerumen may complain of blocked or muffled hearing, a plugged feeling in the ear, and even pain.

Treatment. Treatment includes softening the wax and removing it by flushing the ear with an ear syringe. Left untreated, impacted cerumen can lead to hearing loss or tinnitus.

RUPTURED TYMPANIC MEMBRANE

The tympanic membrane is vulnerable to injury, such as rupture or tearing, from objects entering the ear or from unequal air pressure on both sides of the membrane.

Signs and Symptoms. A sharp, sudden pain in the affected ear may be followed by drainage of fluid, tinnitus, and hearing loss.

Treatment. Treatment usually includes antibiotic medications to prevent infection and analgesics to reduce pain. Patients should be instructed not to clean their ears with objects such as swabs but instead to flush the ears with earwax softeners or room-temperature saline solution. Cold solutions should never be introduced into the ear.

Common Disorders Associated with the Middle Ear

Many disorders that affect hearing are inflammatory and often occur in the middle and inner ears. The most common inflammatory disorder affecting the middle ear is otitis media.

OTITIS MEDIA

Otitis is an inflammation of any part of the ear. Otitis externa (swimmer's ear) is an inflammation of the outer ear, whereas **otitis media** is an inflammation of the middle ear. It can be caused by viral or bacterial infections, often secondary to sore throats and colds. It occurs in children more frequently than in adults. Any swelling in the tissues that surround the Eustachian tube can close it, decreasing the ability of the ear to drain. Naturally occurring fluids that cannot drain from the ear become a source of infection. The Eustachian tube in children is also straighter than that in adults, so if a child drinks from a bottle while lying down, the fluid is more likely to flow backward up the tube and into the middle ear.

Signs and Symptoms. Children with otitis media may tug at the affected ear, be unusually irritable or fussy, have a fever and fluid drainage from the ear, and have difficulty sleeping. Fluid drainage and exhibiting a loss of balance are more serious symptoms.

Treatment. The main goal of treatment is to eliminate the cause of infection before more serious complications set in. Oral antibiotics help to kill bacteria and boost the immune system, and decongestants such as pseudoephedrine help reduce swelling in the Eustachian tubes. A pain reliever may also be prescribed. If the condition is more acute and there is thick effusion and poor Eustachian tube function, tubal **insufflation** (introduction of gas, vapor, or powder into a cavity) every 1 to 2 days may be in order. Recurrent ear infections may be treated with myringotomy to remove unwanted fluids and insertion of a drainage tube through the eardrum.

OTOSCLEROSIS

Otosclerosis is a frequently hereditary condition in which the tissue surrounding the stapes grows abnormally around it.

This overgrowth of tissue prevents the stapes from transmitting sound vibrations to the inner ear.

Signs and Symptoms. The overgrowth causes gradual hearing loss in one or both ears. Some people may also experience tinnitus and dizziness.

Treatment. Mild cases of otosclerosis may be treated with a hearing aid. In more severe cases surgery may be recommended.

Common Disorders Associated with the Inner Ear

The inner ear plays a large role in maintaining the body's equilibrium and balance. Many of the disorders specific to the inner ear are characterized by severe dizziness (vertigo), tinnitus, and loss of balance.

TINNITUS

Tinnitus is a symptom associated with many forms of hearing loss. It can also be a symptom of other health problems. At least 12 million Americans are estimated to have tinnitus, in some cases so severely that they have trouble hearing, working, or even sleeping. Tinnitus may be caused by hearing loss, loud noise, certain medications, and other health problems such as allergies and tumors.

Signs and Symptoms. The main symptom of tinnitus is ringing or roaring in one or both ears.

Treatment. There is no cure for tinnitus, but many patients have found relief with hearing aids, maskers (small electronic devices worn like a hearing aid to help mask the tinnitus), and medications such as antiarrhythmics and antidepressants.

MÉNIÈRE'S DISEASE

Ménière's disease is named after the French physician who first described the syndrome in 1861. It is believed that changes in fluid volume in the labyrinth of the inner ear cause the symptoms of Ménière's disease. Other possible causes include bacterial or viral infections, environmental factors, and noise pollution.

Signs and Symptoms. Symptoms include vertigo, tinnitus, headache, nausea, vomiting, and diarrhea, as well as hearing loss and the feeling of pressure or pain in the affected ear. Symptoms often occur suddenly, without warning, and they may occur daily or infrequently. Hearing returns after an attack but usually worsens over time.

Treatment. Although there is no known cure for Ménière's disease, symptoms can be controlled by reducing

fluid retention with a low-salt diet and by avoiding caffeine and alcohol. Diuretic drugs may be administered. Other medications, such as those that control allergies and improve blood circulation in the inner ear, may be beneficial. Eliminating tobacco use and reducing stress levels may also reduce the severity of symptoms.

PRESBYCUSIS

Presbycusis is a type of hearing loss involving the gradual deterioration of the sensory receptors in the cochlea. It is seen most frequently in older adults—approximately 25 percent are affected by the time they reach the age of 60 to 70—and affects more men than women. Factors that lead to presbycusis include prolonged exposure to loud noises, infection, injury, and side effects caused by certain medications.

Signs and Symptoms. Presbycusis generally occurs in both ears, causing problems with hearing both the normal and high-pitched tones of conversation.

Treatment. Treatment is generally a hearing aid.

The Senses of Taste and Smell

The nose is the primary organ for the sense of smell. Olfactory cells high in the roof of the nasal cavity respond to changes in volatile chemical concentrations. Once a smell receptor is activated, it sends the information to the brain via the olfactory nerves (Figure 26-5). See Chapter 29 for more information about the nose.

The sense of taste and the sense of smell function together to create a combined effect that is interpreted by the brain.

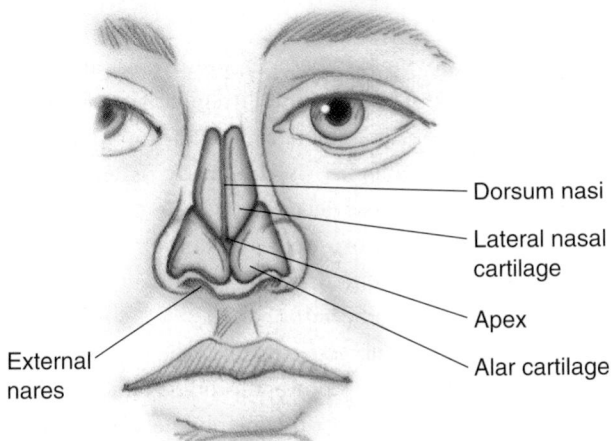

FIGURE 26-5 Nasal cartilage and external structures.

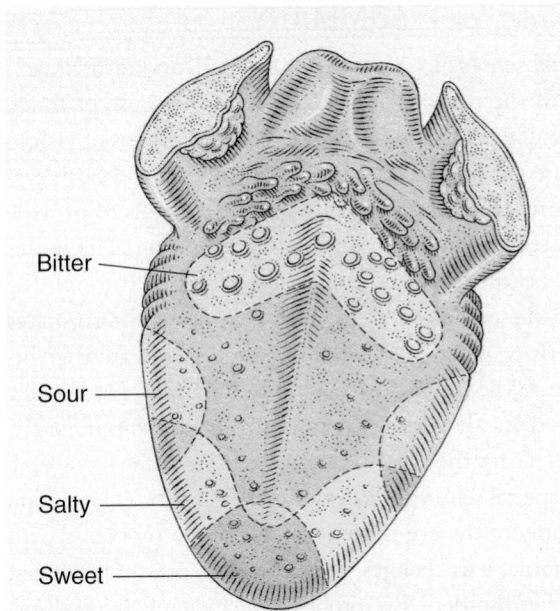

FIGURE 26-6 Tongue and taste buds.

When you smell something, some of the tiny molecules given off by that object move from the nose down into the mouth region and stimulate the taste buds. In actuality, part of what we refer to as smell is really taste.

Taste buds are microscopic bumps on the tongue (Figure 26-6), the roof of the mouth, and the walls of the throat. The cells in each taste bud serve as taste receptors. The four types of taste cells are sweet, located on the tip of the tongue; sour, on the sides of the tongue; salty, on the tip and sides of the tongue; and bitter, at the back of the tongue.

The Sense of Touch

Touch is our oldest, most primitive sense. It is the first sense we experience in the womb and the last one we lose before death. Unlike the other four senses (sight, hearing, smell, and taste), the sense of touch is found over the entire body. It originates in the dermis, the deepest layer of the skin. Nerve endings in the dermis, called receptors, transmit information to the spinal cord, which in turn sends messages to the brain, where the feeling is registered (Figure 26-7). See Chapter 22 for more information about the sense of touch.

The more nerve endings there are in a given area of the body, the more sensitive it is. The sides of the tongue, for example, have numerous nerve

endings; hence the pain that results from accidentally biting down on the tongue. However, the tongue is not as good at sensing hot or cold, which explains why it is so easy to burn the mouth when eating or drinking something especially hot.

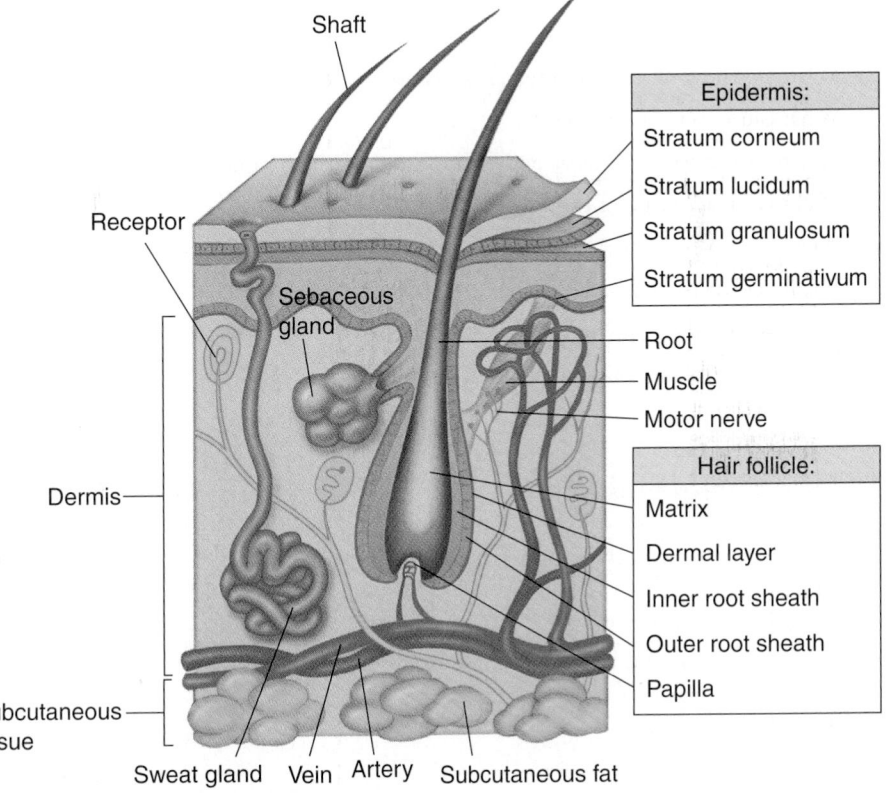

FIGURE 26-7 Layers of the skin, showing receptors.

SUMMARY

The special senses of vision, hearing, smell, and taste are extensions of the nervous system, whereas the sense of touch functions all over the body. The eyes are the organs of vision, the ears are the organs of hearing and balance, and both systems require the collaboration of specialized cells to provide appropriate input to the brain for interpretation. The senses of vision, hearing, taste, and smell are activated through the brain and the nervous system. The sense of touch originates in the dermis, where nerve endings process and transfer information to the spinal cord and on to the brain. During the aging process, all these systems can decline significantly, greatly affecting the activities and quality of life.

These special senses are also prone to disorders. The position and anatomy of the eye make it vulnerable to problems with fluids, trauma, lens changes, retinal disease, pressure changes, and vascular disorders. Eye problems include refraction disorders (astigmatism, myopia, hyperopia, presbyopia, and strabismus; disorders related to structural irregularities of the eye (blepharoptosis, ectroprion, entroprion, and exophthalmos); infectious eye disorders (blepharitis, conjunctivitis, and hordeolums); age-related eye disorders (cataracts, retinal detachment, macular degeneration, and nyctalopia); and others (amblyopia, corneal abrasion, diplopia, glaucoma, nystagmus [nystaxis], retinopathy, and photophobia).

Because infection and objects can enter the ear, the ear is also vulnerable to disorders. Common problems include impacted cerumen, ruptured tympanic membrane, otitis media, otosclerosis, tinnitus, Ménière's disease, and presbycusis.

The tongue is the sensory organ for the sense of taste. Different parts of the tongue sense different tastes (sweet, sour, salty, bitter). The skin is the primary organ for the sense of touch. The nose is the primary organ for the olfactory sense (smell).

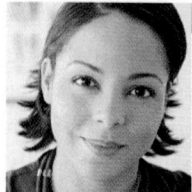

26 CHAPTER REVIEW

COMPETENCY REVIEW

1. Define and spell the terms to learn for this chapter.
2. What are the symptoms of Ménière's disease?
3. What causes refractive errors?
4. Where are sweet, sour, salty, and bitter tasted on the tongue?
5. What is the function of the aqueous humor?
6. What are the functions of the ear?
7. What are the three ossicles of the ear?
8. What structures make up the bony labyrinth?
9. What is the role of rods and cones in vision?
10. How should patients clean their ears?

PREPARING FOR THE CERTIFICATION EXAM

1. What is the name of the substance that fills the posterior cavity of the eyeball?
   a. vitreous humor
   b. nasolacrimal fluid
   c. aqueous humor
   d. lacrimal gland
   e. lacrimal fluid

2. The structure of the eye in which the rods and cones determine color perception is called the
   a. pupil
   b. aqueous humor
   c. retina
   d. ciliary body
   e. choroids

3. Which of the following is the term for farsightedness, in which the patient cannot focus well on objects close at hand?
   a. hyperopia
   b. astigmatism

c. presbyopia

d. myopia

e. glaucoma

4. A condition of the eye in which the lens clouds over and prevents light from entering is

a. glaucoma

b. cataracts

c. retinal detachment

d. astigmatism

e. corneal ulcers

5. A highly contagious condition of the eye also known as a sty is

a. corneal abrasion

b. astigmatism

c. hordeolum

d. conjunctivitis

e. macular degeneration

6. The apparatus that comprises all the structures that produce, store, and remove the tears that cleanse and lubricate the eye is called the

a. retina

b. sclera

c. lacrima

d. conjunctiva

e. iris

7. The ear bone that is shaped like a stirrup is called the

a. malleus

b. stapes

c. incus

d. hammer

e. anvil

8. Which of the following is an ear disorder?

a. blepharitis

b. glaucoma

c. Ménière's disease

d. strabismus

e. macular degeneration

9. Which of the following is a condition in which the eyeballs bulge outward?

a. entropion

b. ectropion

c. exophthalmos

d. eczema

e. nystagmus

10. Which taste cell is located on the back of the tongue?

a. bitter

b. sour

c. sweet

d. salty

e. bittersweet

CRITICAL THINKING

1. When Dr. Salpega sees Lucas, he asks his father if Lucas has had any cough or cold symptoms lately and if Lucas still uses a bottle. Why would Dr. Salpega be interested in the answers to these questions?

2. Dr. Salpega diagnoses Lucas with acute otitis media. Through some diagnostic assessment, the doctor determines that Lucas has some mild hearing loss. Mr. DiStefano is very concerned about this. He wonders if the hearing loss will be permanent. How will Dr. Salpega likely respond?

3. What is the likely course of treatment for Lucas? Would he likely want Lucas to follow up? Explain why or why not.

INTERNET ACTIVITY

Do an Internet search on Lasik surgery to learn more about the procedure.

MEDMEDIA

Additional interactive resources and activities for this chapter can be found:

On your student DVD: View applicable procedure videos on the DVD-ROM found in the back of this book.

MyHealthProfessionsKit.com: Test your knowledge of the chapter with games and activities. MyHealthProfessionsKit also includes resources, helpful links, and a Spanish audio glossary.

Medical Assisting Interactive: Practice your procedures as a medical assistant in this simulated doctor's office. This can be accessed through MyHealthProfessionsKit.com.

27

The Circulatory System

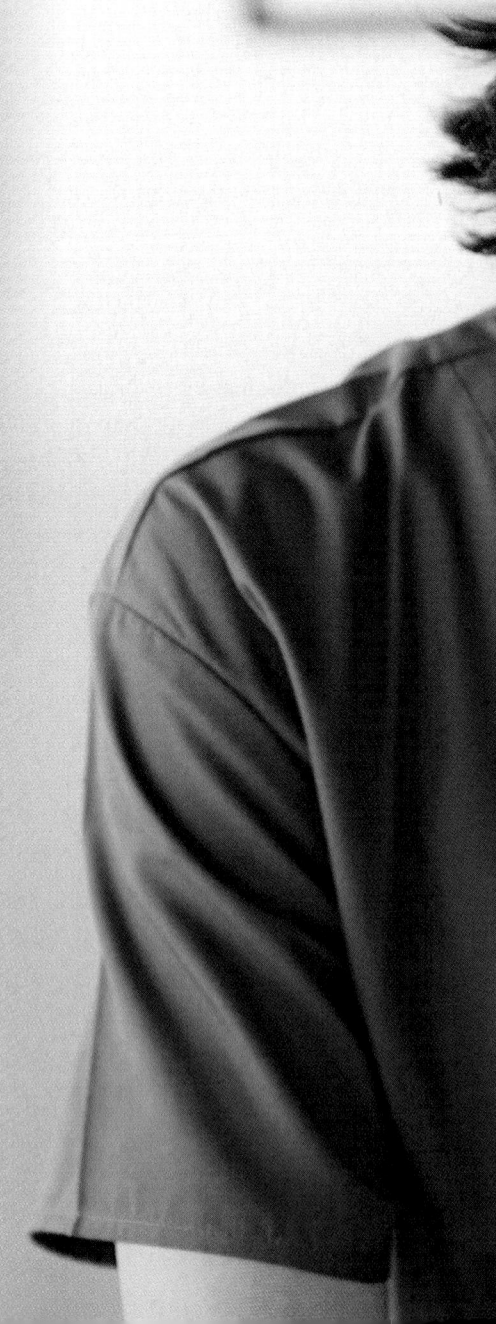

LEARNING OBJECTIVES

After completing this chapter, you should be able to:

- Define and spell the terms to learn for this chapter.

- Identify the organs that make up the circulatory system.

- Identify the structures that make up the heart and briefly explain the function of each.

- Explain the conduction system of the heart.

- Explain the functions of the arteries, veins, and capillaries.

- List and describe the components of blood.

- Discuss the importance of blood typing and cite which blood types are compatible.

- State the difference between Rh-positive blood and Rh-negative blood.

- Identify the organs of the lymphatic system, their location in the body, and the function of each.

- Describe lymph and explain how it is circulated throughout the body.

- Discuss common disorders associated with the circulatory system.

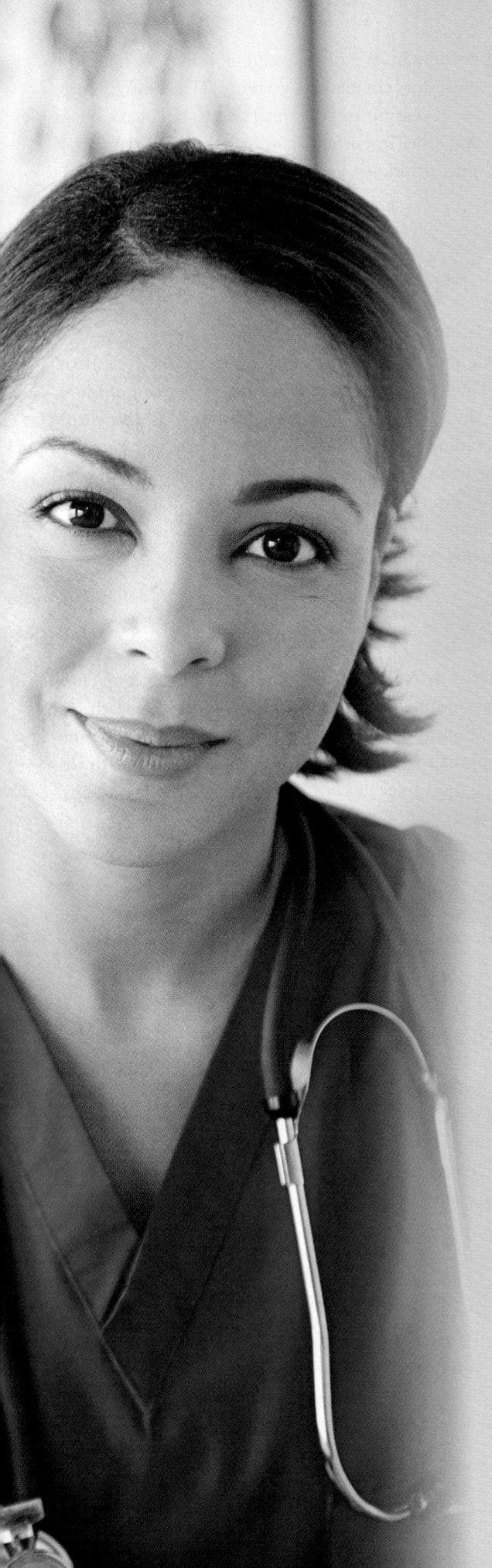

CHAPTER OUTLINE

CASE STUDY

Jamal Washington has made an appointment to see Dr. Miller at Pearson Physicians Group. He was reluctant to make the appointment and only made it because his wife, Tania, urged him. Now he does not want to go to the doctor. Jamal has been complaining of intense headaches and has had frequent episodes of epistaxis.

TERMS TO LEARN

agglutination

anemia

aneurysm

angioplasty

aorta

arrhythmia

arteriosclerosis

atherosclerosis

atria

atrioventricular (AV) node

auscultation

bicuspid valve

blood pressure

bradycardia

bruit

buffers

bundle of His

cardiac arrest

cardiac tamponade

cardiogenic shock

cardiomegaly

cardiomyopathy

carditis

carotid artery

cerebrovascular accident
(CVA)

congestive heart failure

coronary arteries

coronary heart disease

cor pulmonale

cyanosis

diastole

diastolic blood pressure

dyspnea

endocardium

erythrocytes

fibrillation

flutter

heart

heart murmur

hemoglobin

hemophilia

hemostasis

hypertension (HTN)

hypotension

hypoxia

infarction

inferior vena cava

ischemia

leukemia

leukocytes

lymph

mitral valve

myocardial infarction (MI)

myocardium

occlusion

pericardium

petechiae

plasma

platelets

prehypertension

pulmonary artery

pulmonary vein

pulse pressure

Purkinje fibers

RhoGAM

septum

sinoatrial (SA) node

sphygmomanometer

systole

systolic blood pressure

superior vena cava

tachycardia

thoracentesis

thrombophlebitis

tricuspid valve

venipuncture

ventricles

CERTIFICATION LINK

CMA (AAMA)
Anatomy and
physiology

Systems (including
structure, function,
related conditions
and diseases, and
their relationships)

RMA
Anatomy and
physiology

Body systems
Disorders and
diseases of
the body

CMAS (AMT)
Medical assisting
foundation

Anatomy and
physiology
Medical
terminology

The human organism could not live without the powerful circulatory system. The heart pump, never ceasing to beat until death, circulates blood and other important materials through a system of arteries, veins, arterioles, and capillaries.

Overview of the Circulatory System

The circulatory system consists of the heart, the blood vessels, the blood, and the structures that make up the lymphatic system. The heart is responsible for the movement of blood through the cardiovascular system throughout the entire body, providing oxygen and removing waste. The lymphatic system, which is a subsystem of the circulatory system, acts as the body's transportation system. The lymphatic system is also responsible for defending the body against disease-causing agents, called pathogens.

The Heart

The **heart** is a four-chambered muscular pump lying just left of the midline of the chest (mediastinum), beneath the sternum (Figure 27-1). It is about the size of a fist and weighs approximately 9 ounces. It is cone shaped, with the apex at the most inferior point, and consists of three linings, or layers (Figure 27-2):

- **pericardium**—the outer lining

- **myocardium**—the middle layer, or heart muscle

- **endocardium**—the innermost lining

Most of the heart is cardiac muscle, whose contractions are controlled by the autonomic nervous system.

The left and right sides of the heart are separated by a wall called the **septum**. The right side moves blood from the body to the lungs, and the left side pumps the blood back to the body (Figure 27-3). Four chambers make up the heart. The two upper chambers, the **atria** (singular is *atrium*), are receiving chambers. The **ventricles**, the two lower two chambers, pump blood out of the heart.

BLOOD FLOW THROUGH THE HEART

The blood enters the heart through two large veins. The **superior vena cava** brings blood from the head and upper chest to the heart. The **inferior vena cava** brings blood from below the heart to the atrium.

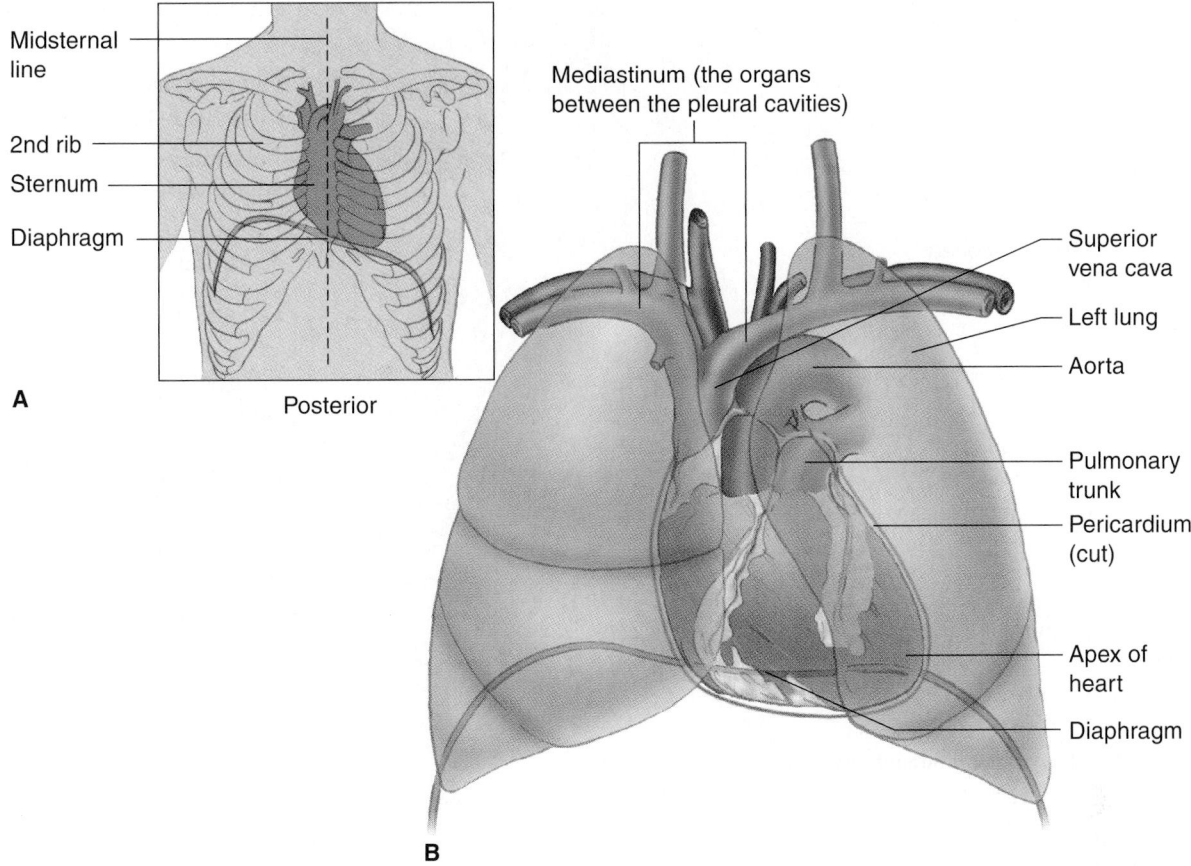

Midsternal line

2nd rib

Sternum

Diaphragm

A

Posterior

Mediastinum (the organs between the pleural cavities)

Superior vena cava

Left lung

Aorta

Pulmonary trunk

Pericardium (cut)

Apex of heart

Diaphragm

B

FIGURE 27-1 Location of the heart in the chest cavity.

The right atrium is the first chamber that blood flows into as it enters the heart. It is the smallest chamber with the thinnest wall, and it receives all the blood from the body via the two cardiac veins: the superior vena cava and the inferior vena cava. The valve (or entryway) from the right atrium to the right ventricle is the **tricuspid valve**.

After going through the tricuspid valve, the blood enters the right ventricle. This chamber is more muscular than the right atrium. Blood leaves the right ventricle through the pulmonary valve to go to the lungs, via the **pulmonary artery**, where carbon dioxide in the blood is exchanged for oxygen.

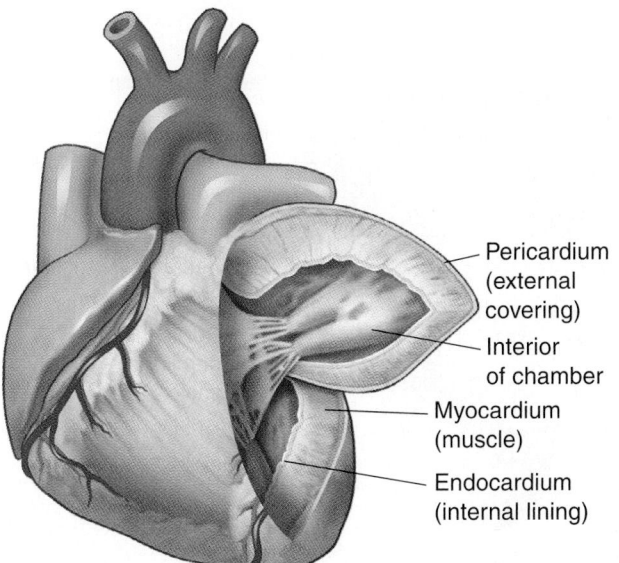

Pericardium (external covering)

Interior of chamber

Myocardium (muscle)

Endocardium (internal lining)

FIGURE 27-2 Linings of the heart.

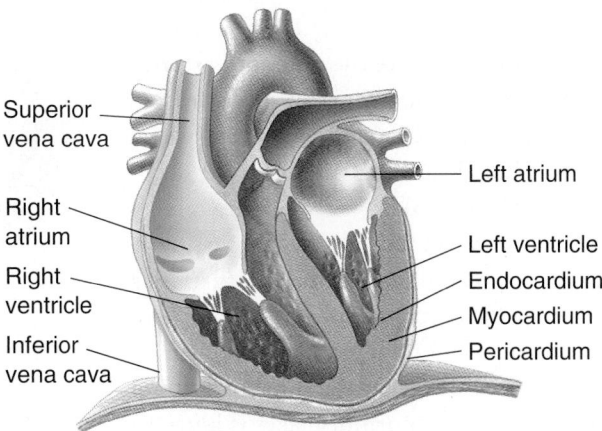

Superior vena cava

Right atrium

Right ventricle

Inferior vena cava

Left atrium

Left ventricle

Endocardium

Myocardium

Pericardium

FIGURE 27-3 The heart: interior view of the heart chambers.

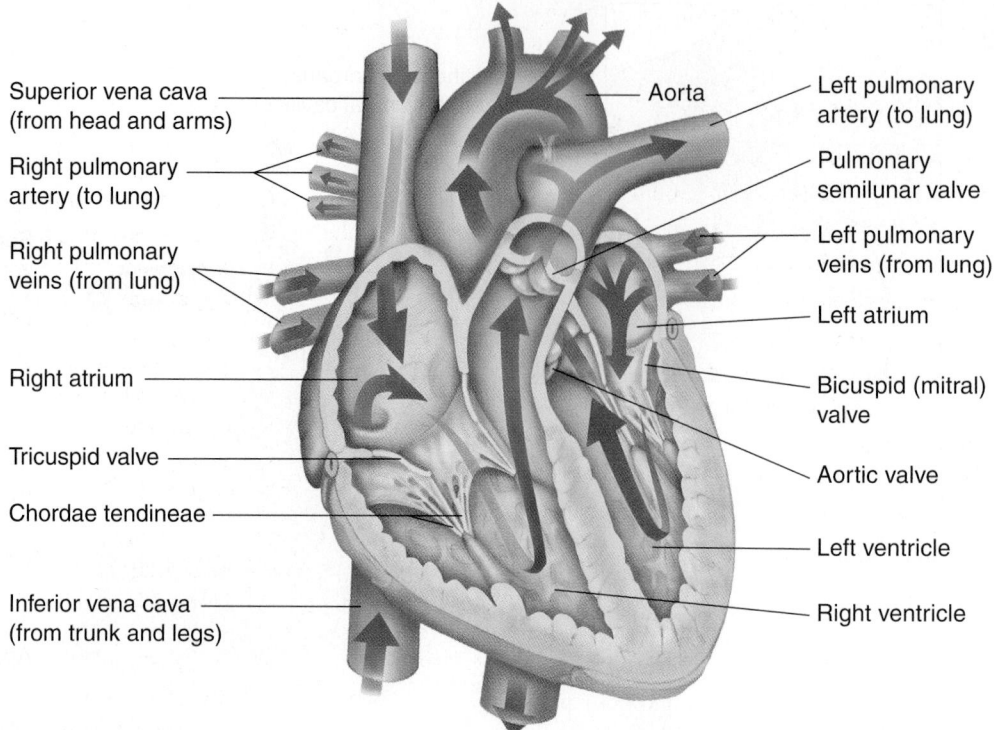

FIGURE 27-4 The flow of blood through the heart.

Labels (clockwise from top left):
- Superior vena cava (from head and arms)
- Right pulmonary artery (to lung)
- Right pulmonary veins (from lung)
- Right atrium
- Tricuspid valve
- Chordae tendineae
- Inferior vena cava (from trunk and legs)
- Aorta
- Left pulmonary artery (to lung)
- Pulmonary semilunar valve
- Left pulmonary veins (from lung)
- Left atrium
- Bicuspid (mitral) valve
- Aortic valve
- Left ventricle
- Right ventricle

On its return from the lungs, the oxygenated blood enters the left atrium via the **pulmonary vein**. This atrium is more heavily muscled than the right atrium. The blood leaves the left atrium through the **bicuspid valve (mitral valve)**.

The blood's final stop within the heart is the left ventricle, the powerhouse chamber. The highly muscular walls of this chamber pump blood out from the heart to the farthest reaches of the body. When the blood leaves the left ventricle through the aortic valve, it enters the **aorta**, the largest artery in the body, and begins its journey to the different regions of the body. The first arteries that the blood enters are the **coronary arteries**, a crown of arteries that supplies the heart with freshly oxygenated blood. Figure 27-4 shows the flow of blood through the heart.

As the blood makes its way through the chambers, the valves function as gateways, never allowing the blood to flow backward (Figure 27-5). A damaged or diseased valve can allow blood to escape and flow backward through the valve in a condition known as a **heart murmur**. The sound that this murmur makes is known as a **bruit**.

PHYSIOLOGY OF THE HEART

The heart is a strong muscle, pumping blood out from the left ventricle to the entire body with very little obvious effort. The mechanical, or pumping, action of the heart occurs with the contraction of the cardiac muscle. The opening of the valves allows the chambers to pump out the blood and receive the next flow of blood between contractions. When

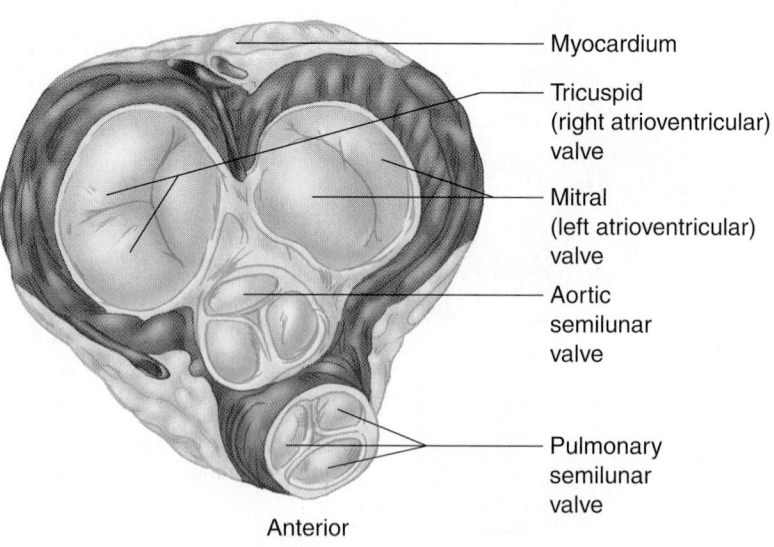

Labels:
- Myocardium
- Tricuspid (right atrioventricular) valve
- Mitral (left atrioventricular) valve
- Aortic semilunar valve
- Pulmonary semilunar valve
- Anterior

FIGURE 27-5 The valves of the heart.

the chamber is full, the valves close, impeding backflow of blood into the previous chamber.

VASCULAR SYSTEM OF THE HEART

The dense muscularity of the heart requires its own vascular system. The coronary arteries, illustrated in Figure 27-6, supply blood to the heart. The blood is drained into the coronary sinus by the coronary veins and then back into the right atrium for oxygenation. **Occlusion** (blockage) of these vessels deprives the heart muscle of oxygen, causing chest pain. Over a long period of time the lack of oxygen to the heart leads to heart muscle damage or death. Lack of blood flow to the heart is known as **ischemia**, but death of heart muscle is known as an **infarction**. When the occlusion leads to the heart stopping, it is known a **cardiac arrest**. The lack of oxygen to the tissues caused by ischemia and infarction is known as **hypoxia**.

CONDUCTION SYSTEM OF THE HEART

Cardiac muscle has the property of automaticity. This means that the heart's rate and rhythm are determined by way of the autonomic nervous system. Three areas of specialized neuromuscular tissue initiate the heartbeat. They are the sinoatrial node, the atrioventricular node, and the atrioventricular bundle, also known as the bundle of His. Figure 27-7 shows the conduction system of the heart.

The **sinoatrial (SA) node**, the pacemaker of the heart, is located in the upper wall of the right atrium. The SA node is responsible for initiating the heartbeat. It discharges the

electrical impulses to the right and left atria, causing the atria to contract. In a healthy adult at rest, heart rates initiated by the SA node are normally 60 to 80 beats per minute.

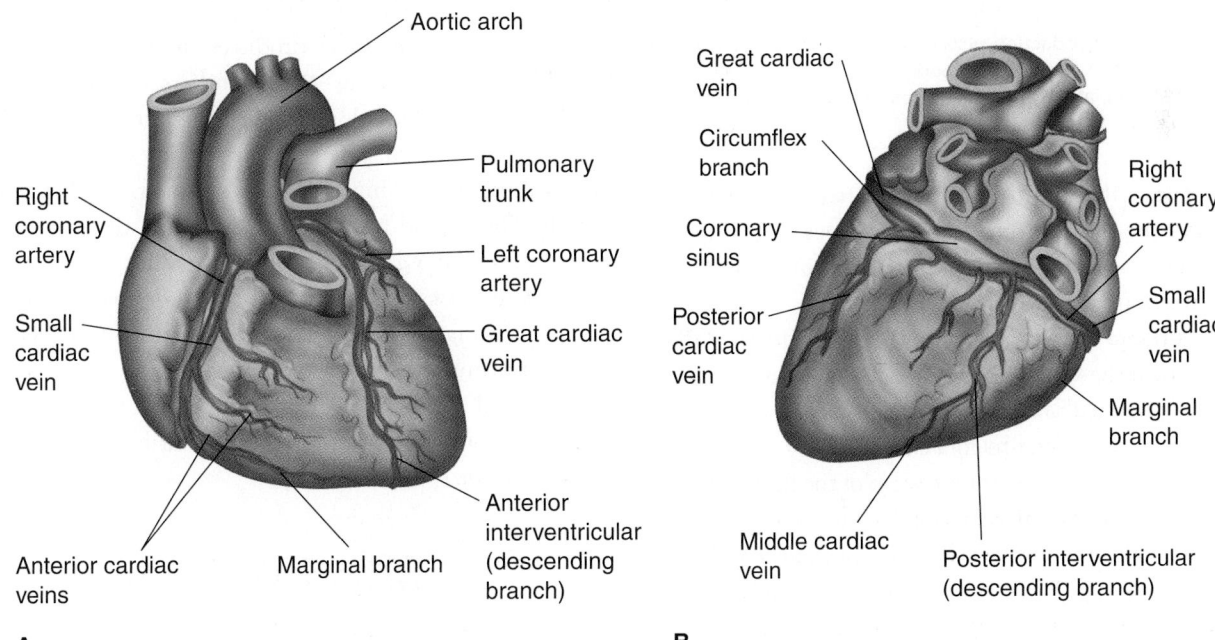

FIGURE 27-6 Coronary circulation: (A) coronary vessels portraying the complexity and extent of the coronary circulation; (B) coronary vessels that supply the anterior surface of the heart.

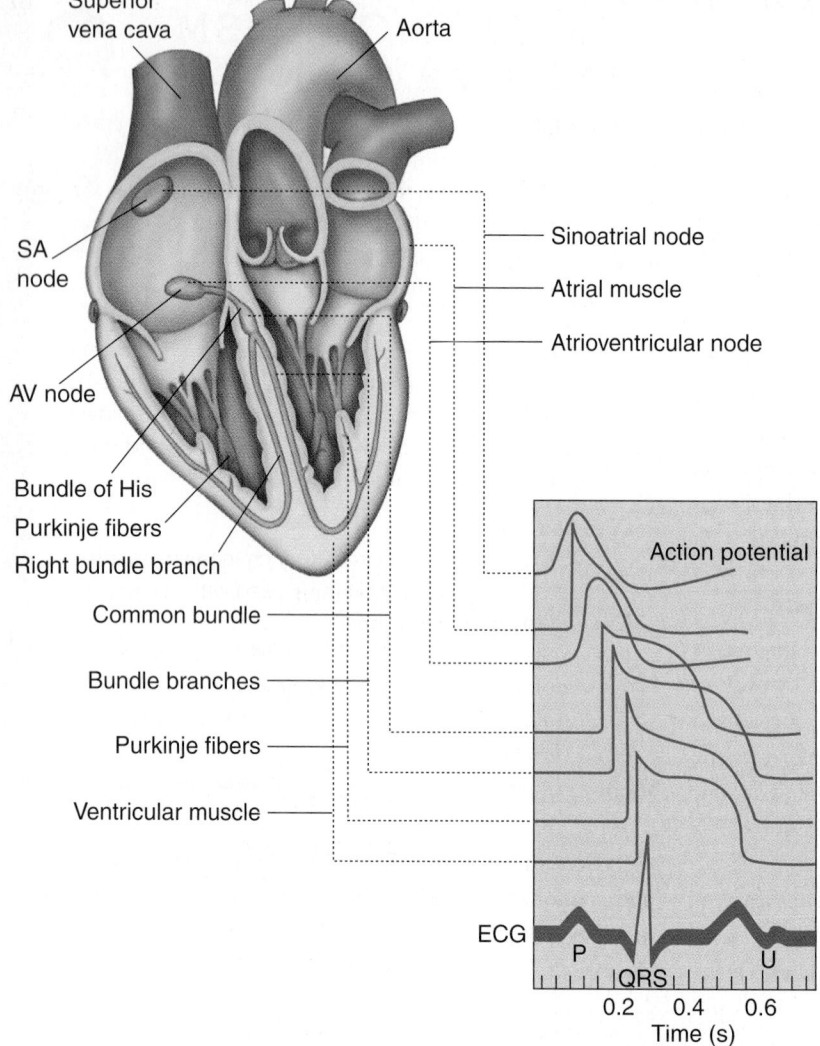

Superior vena cava

Aorta

SA node

AV node

Bundle of His

Purkinje fibers

Right bundle branch

Common bundle

Bundle branches

Purkinje fibers

Ventricular muscle

Sinoatrial node

Atrial muscle

Atrioventricular node

Action potential

ECG

P

QRS

U

0.2   0.4   0.6

Time (s)

FIGURE 27-7   The conduction system of the heart. Action potentials for the SA and AV nodes, other parts of the conduction system, and the atrial and ventricular muscles are shown, along with the correlation to recorded electrical activity (ECG).

When the electrical system has problems, **fibrillation**, or quivering, can occur. Automated external defibrillation equipment can be used to stop the shaking and restore normal sinus rhythm. If the heart trembles, it is known as **flutter**.

THE CARDIAC CYCLE

The cardiac cycle consists of all the events that occur during one complete heartbeat. On average, the heart beats about 70 times per minute, although adult heart rates can vary from 60 to 110 beats per minute. Exercise, smoking, or excitement can temporarily elevate heart rates.

The cardiac cycle has three phases:

Phase 1, atrial **systole**—the atria are contracted and ventricles are relaxed.

Phase 2, ventricular systole—both ventricles are contracted and the atria are relaxed.

Phase 3, atrial and ventricular **diastole**—longest phase; both atria and ventricles are relaxed, and pressure in the heart chambers is low. Blood returning to the heart from the superior and inferior venae cavae and the pulmonary veins fills the right and left atria and flows passively into the ventricles.

Heart Sounds

A heartbeat produces the familiar "lub-dup" sounds as the chambers contract and the valves close. The first heart sound, "lub," is heard when the ventricles contract and the AV valves close. This sound lasts longer and has a lower pitch. The second heart sound, "dup," is the sound of the ventricles relaxing and the semilunar valves closing.

In some cases, the valves may become ineffective, causing a clicking or swishing sound after the "lub." This is a heart murmur, and these "leaky" valves do not close completely and allow blood to pass back into the atria or into the ventricles. Listening for the flow of blood is known as **auscultation**.

The **atrioventricular (AV) node**, located under the endocardium of the right atrium, is a gatekeeper. It is responsible for transmitting impulses from the SA node to the inferior portions of the heart.

The **Purkinje fibers** are specialized conductive fibers located within the walls of the ventricles. They are responsible for relaying cardiac impulses to the cells of the ventricles, prompting the ventricles to contract.

The final part of the electrical system of the heart is the AV bundle, or the **bundle of His**. The AV bundle extends from the AV node into the intraventricular septum (the wall separating the right and left ventricles), where it sends a branch into each ventricle (the right and left bundle branches). The Purkinje system includes the bundle of His and the peripheral fibers. These fibers end in the ventricular muscles where they cause the strong ventricular muscle contractions.

Blood Vessels

Blood vessels—arteries, arterioles, veins, venules, and capillaries—form a closed pathway that carries blood from the heart to all the cells of the body and back to the heart again.

THE ARTERIES

The vessels that carry the blood away from the heart are the arteries (Figure 27-8). Arteries are elastic tubes that expand with pressure (during the contraction of the heart) and then relax between beats. Because of this expansion and recoil, arteries are an easy place to palpate the pulse for purposes of recording the heart rate. Some of the most common sites for palpating an artery to obtain an accurate pulse rate include the following (Figure 27-9):

- **Radial artery**—in the lateral wrist, just proximal to the thumb
- **Brachial artery**—in the antecubital space of the elbow; also between the biceps and triceps muscles in pediatric and thinner adult patients
- **Carotid artery**—in the lateral neck; most commonly used site to check for a pulse
- **Temporal artery**—in the temple area
- **Femoral artery**—in the groin

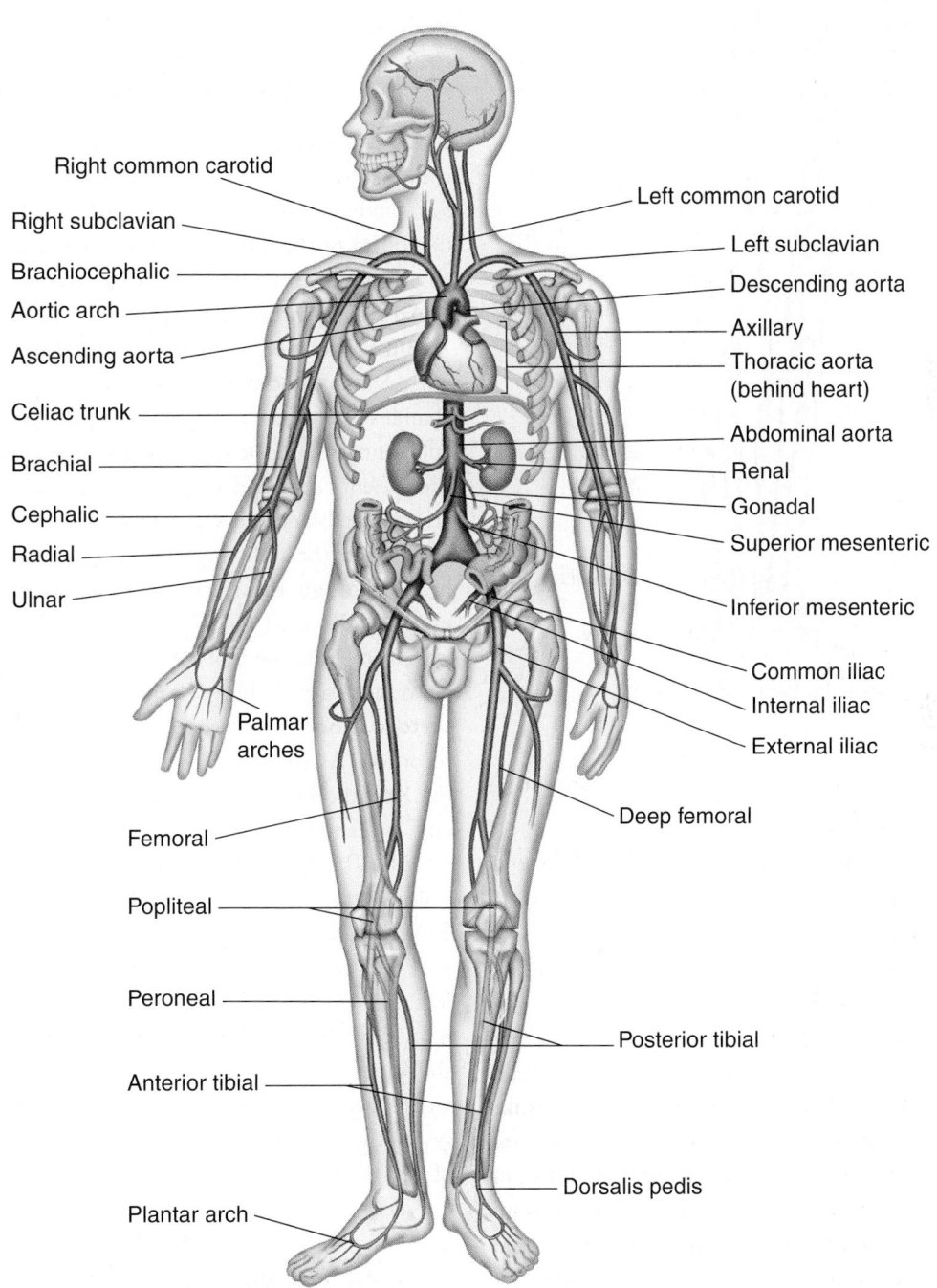

FIGURE 27-8 An overview of the arterial system.

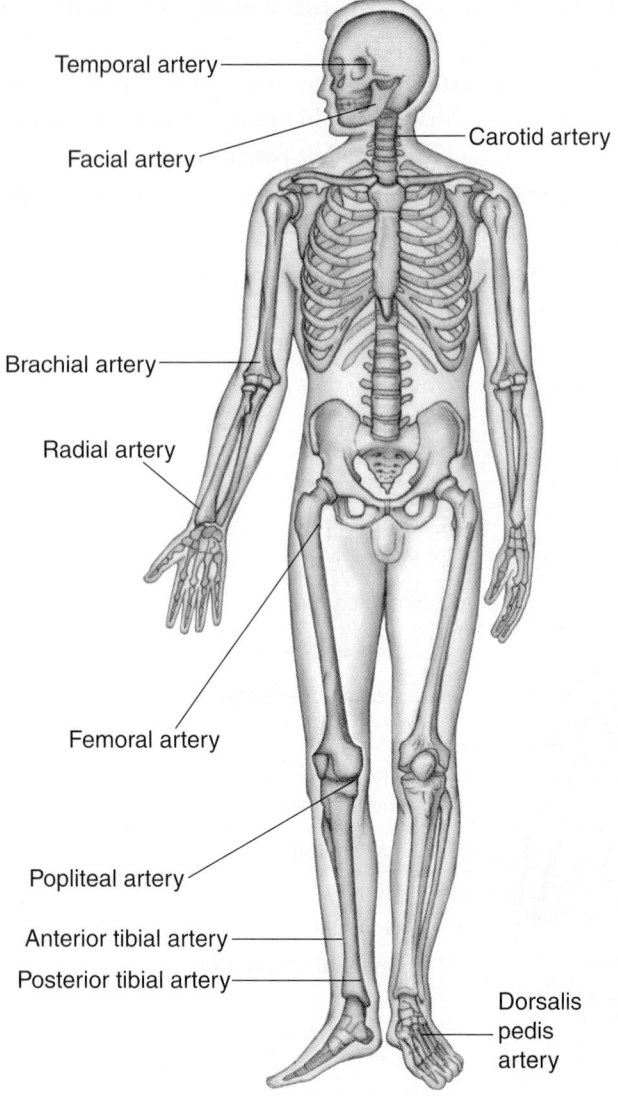

Temporal artery

Facial artery

Carotid artery

Brachial artery

Radial artery

Femoral artery

Popliteal artery

Anterior tibial artery

Posterior tibial artery

Dorsalis pedis artery

FIGURE 27-9 The primary pulse points of the body.

- **Popliteal artery**—behind the knee on the posteromedial (inside rear) aspect
- **Dorsalis pedis artery**—on the upper surface of the foot
- **Anterior tibial artery**—in the ankle medial (inside) the Achilles tendon.

VEINS

Veins are thin-walled vessels that transport blood from peripheral tissues to the heart (Figure 27-10). Veins contain valves that prevent blood from flowing backward. Like arteries, veins have elastic walls, but the pressure in the veins is significantly lower than in the arteries. **Venipuncture**, or phlebotomy, is the process of removing blood from the veins for examination. It is easier to draw blood and administer intravenous (IV) medications through veins because they are under less pressure and are more superficial than arteries.

CAPILLARIES

Capillaries are microscopic blood vessels located in the tissues (Figure 27-11). Oxygenated blood travels through arterioles (small arteries) to capillaries and on to the tissue cells, where oxygen and nutrients are deposited and waste material is picked up. The capillaries transport carbon dioxide and waste material in the blood to the venules (small veins) and on to the veins returning to the heart. The single-celled walls of capillaries facilitate this exchange of gases and nutrients. Small breaks in the capillaries can lead to **petechiae**, or tiny broken blood vessels on the surface of the skin, especially in the presence of clotting disorders.

Blood Pressure

Blood pressure is defined as the force exerted by the blood on the walls of the arteries. This pressure is determined by the force and amount of blood pumped as well as by the size and flexibility of the arteries. A person's blood pressure continually changes depending on activity, temperature, diet, emotional state, posture, physical condition, and medication use.

Blood pressure is usually measured in the brachial artery with a **sphygmomanometer**, an instrument that records changes in terms of millimeters of mercury. A blood pressure cuff connected to the sphygmomanometer is wrapped around the patient's arm, and a stethoscope is placed over the brachial artery. The blood pressure cuff is inflated until it diminishes circulation through the artery and, thus, no sounds can be heard through the stethoscope. The cuff pressure is then gradually lowered. *Korotkoff sounds* are the sounds heard during the measurement of blood pressure, and up to five phases or sounds may be heard. The first phase heard is when the **systolic blood pressure**—the left ventricle contracting—is recorded. As the pressure in the cuff is lowered still more, the Korotkoff sounds change in tone and volume. When the cuff pressure no longer constricts the brachial artery, no sound is heard. The cuff pressure at which the Korotkoff sounds disappear is the **diastolic blood pressure**, when the left ventricle relaxes.

The average resting blood pressure for a young adult is below 120/80 mmHg (millimeters of mercury). The higher number is the systolic blood pressure, and the lower number is the diastolic blood pressure. The recorded measurement is written with the systolic number on top and the diastolic number on the bottom. For example, a blood pressure measurement of 120/80 mmHg is expressed verbally as "120 over 80."

PULSE PRESSURE

The **pulse pressure** is the difference between the systolic and diastolic blood pressures. Normal pulse pressure is 30 to

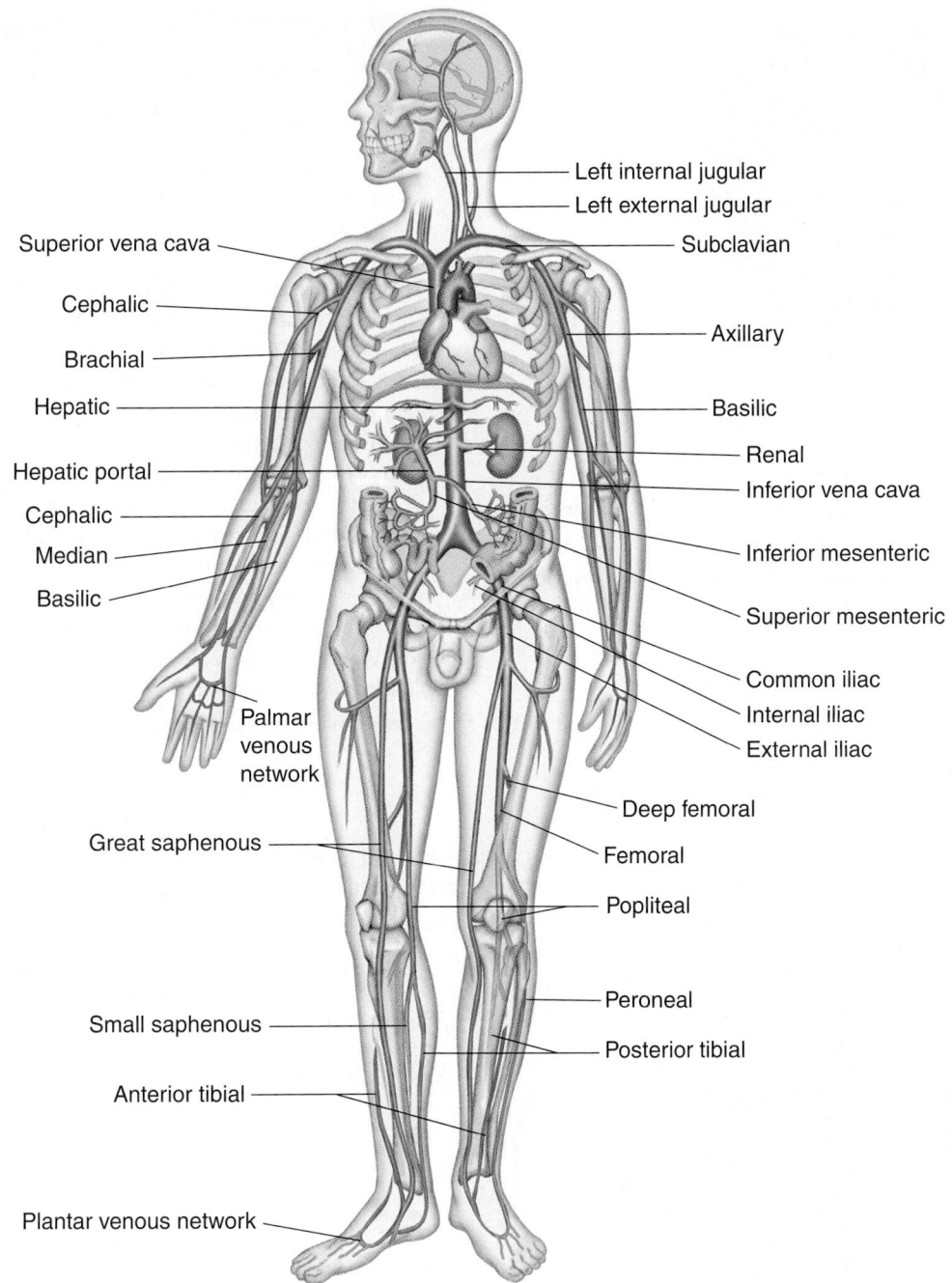

Left internal jugular
Left external jugular
Subclavian
Superior vena cava
Cephalic
Brachial
Hepatic
Axillary
Basilic
Hepatic portal
Renal
Cephalic
Inferior vena cava
Median
Inferior mesenteric
Basilic
Superior mesenteric
Common iliac
Internal iliac
External iliac
Palmar venous network
Deep femoral
Great saphenous
Femoral
Popliteal
Peroneal
Small saphenous
Posterior tibial
Anterior tibial
Plantar venous network

FIGURE 27-10 **An overview of the veins in venous circulation.**

50 points. The pulse pressure is an indication of the tone of the arterial walls. It can be helpful when assessing a patient's risk profile for heart disease.

Pulmonary and Systemic Circulation

The circulatory system can be divided into the pulmonary system and the systemic system (Figure 27-12). Pulmonary circulation is the route the blood takes from the heart to the lungs via the pulmonary artery and back to the heart via the pulmonary vein. The function of pulmonary circulation is to reoxygenate the blood going to the heart while carrying the waste product carbon dioxide to the lungs to be exhaled. The blood that returns to the left side of the heart from the lungs is oxygen rich and is moved to the cells needing oxygen by the systemic circulation.

Systemic circulation is the route the blood takes around the body: It leaves the heart through the aorta; travels through the body in arteries, capillaries, and veins; and

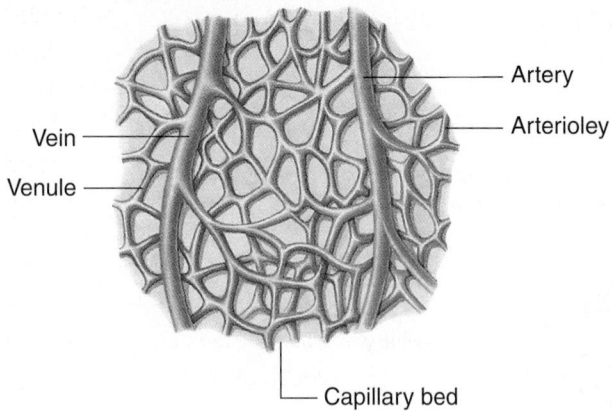

FIGURE 27-11 **The capillaries.**

returns to the heart through the vena cava. Two large veins comprise the vena cava. The superior vena cava brings blood to the heart from the head. The inferior vena cava carries blood to the heart from the lower areas of the body. The function of systemic circulation is to deliver oxygen and other nutrients to body cells and to carry carbon dioxide and waste products away from the cells for elimination from the body.

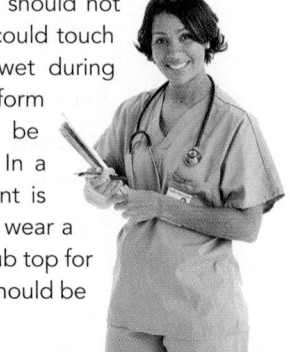
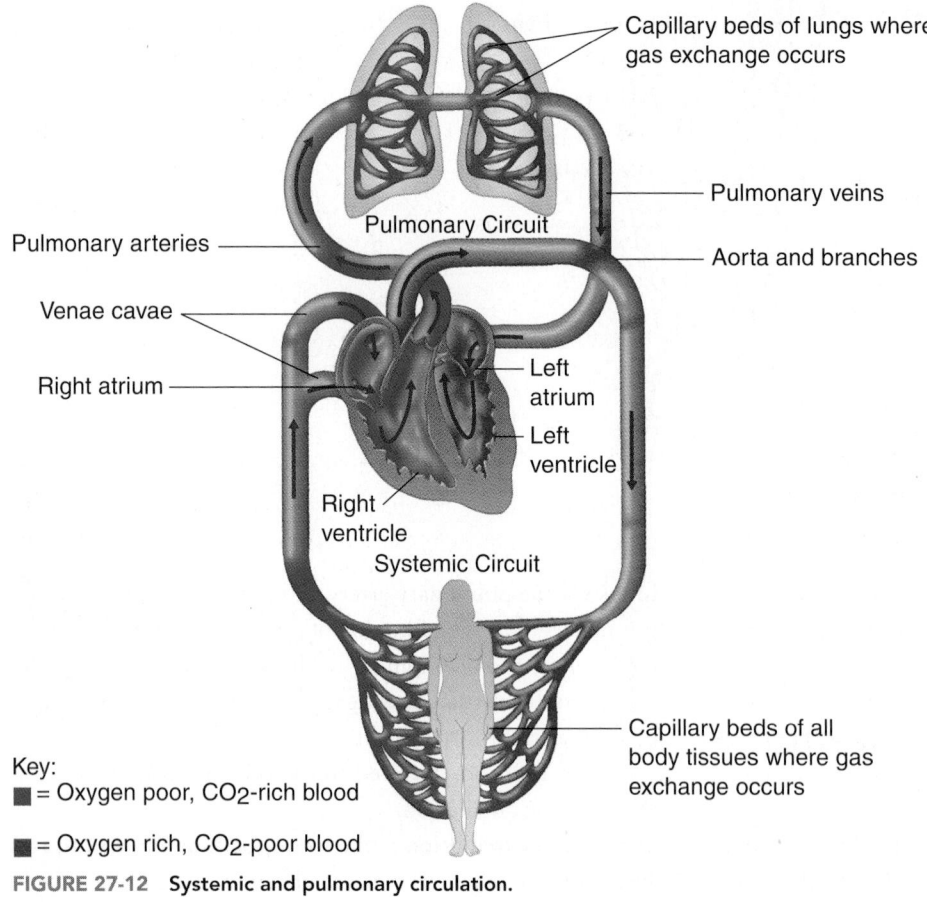

Key:
■ = Oxygen poor, CO₂-rich blood

■ = Oxygen rich, CO₂-poor blood

FIGURE 27-12 **Systemic and pulmonary circulation.**

Blood

Blood is a type of connective tissue composed of cells and plasma. The following are the three types of blood cells:

- erythrocytes, or red blood cells
- leukocytes, or white blood cells
- thrombocytes, or platelets

The fluid part of the blood is **plasma**. A person's blood volume may vary depending on his or her size, amount of adipose tissue, and degree of hydration. The average adult has approximately 5 liters of blood. In adults, the formation of blood cells (hematopoiesis) takes place primarily in the bone marrow.

COMPOSITION OF BLOOD

When a fresh blood sample is spun in a centrifuge tube, the blood separates

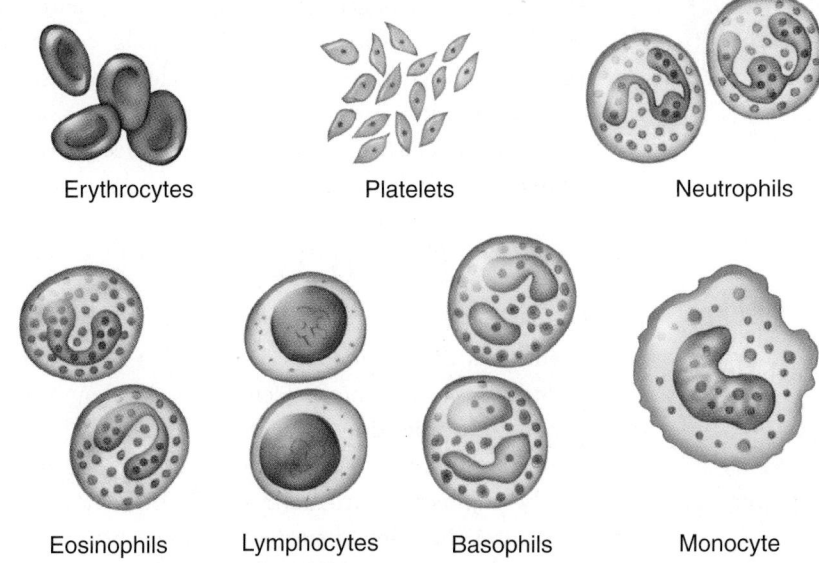

Erythrocytes   Platelets   Neutrophils

Eosinophils   Lymphocytes   Basophils   Monocyte

FIGURE 27-13 The formed elements of blood: erythrocytes, leukocytes (neutrophils, eosinophils, basophils, lymphocytes, and monocytes), and thrombocytes (platelets).

into three layers. The lower layer is composed of red blood cells, the middle *buffy coat* layer contains white blood cells and platelets, and the top layer is plasma. The *hematocrit* is the percentage of blood volume made up of red blood cells. Figure 27-13 shows the formed elements of blood: erythrocytes, leukocytes (neutrophils, eosinophils, basophils, lymphocytes, and monocytes), and thrombocytes (platelets). This is further discussed in Chapter 47.

Red Blood Cells

Red blood cells (RBCs), or **erythrocytes**, are produced in the red bone marrow. They are biconcave cells that are small enough to pass through capillary walls. Mature red blood cells do not contain nuclei but do contain **hemoglobin**, a red, iron-containing pigment. The function of hemoglobin is to carry oxygen from the lungs to cells throughout the body.

An RBC count refers to the number of red blood cells in 1 cubic mm of blood. This count is normally between 4 million and 6.5 million. A low RBC count indicates a decreased ability of the RBCs to carry oxygen, a condition referred to as anemia.

White Blood Cells

White blood cells (WBCs), or **leukocytes**, differ from RBCs in that they are usually larger, have a nucleus, lack hemoglobin, and are translucent unless stained. They are also not as numerous as RBCs; there are normally only 5,000 to 11,000 per cubic mm of blood. WBCs fight infection and in this function are important contributors to homeostasis.

The five types of leukocytes are divided into two categories. *Granulocytes* have granules in their cytoplasm, are visible after staining, and include neutrophils, eosinophils, and basophils. Monocytes and lymphocytes are *agranulocytes,* which do not contain granules.

A differential WBC count measures the number of each of the five types of leukocytes. An increase or decrease in percentages may be indicative of infection or disease.

Blood Platelets

Platelets, or thrombocytes, are cells that are fragments of larger cells formed in the red bone marrow. They are smaller than erythrocytes. Thrombocytes control the loss of blood by congregating to form a clot (coagulation) at the point of injury. A normal platelet count is 130,000 to 360,000 per cubic mm of blood.

Blood Plasma

Plasma is the liquid portion of the blood, consisting of 91 percent water. The other 9 percent is a mixture of proteins, nutrients, gases, electrolytes, fats, hormones, enzymes, and waste products. Plasma constitutes about 55 percent of the total volume of whole blood. Albumin, the most abundant protein found in plasma, helps maintain the fluid volume in the blood, thereby controlling blood pressure. Other major proteins are fibrinogen (which plays a role in clot formation), globulin, and prothrombin.

FUNCTIONS OF BLOOD

Blood has three major functions: transportation, regulation, and defense.

Transportation

Blood moves from the heart to all the tissues, where gas and nutrient exchange takes place across thin capillary walls. The blood transports oxygen from the lungs and nutrients from the digestive tract and delivers these to the tissues. Various organs and tissues also secrete hormones into the blood, which transports them to other organs and tissues, where they serve as signals that influence cellular metabolism. The blood also picks up waste materials from the cells that is later excreted by the kidneys.

Regulation

Blood helps to regulate body temperature by picking up heat, mostly from active muscles, and then distributing it

PROFESSIONALISM

THE LAW

When providing care and treatment to a patient with a disorder of the circulatory system, it is important for the medical assistant to be mindful of the patient's privacy. Patient privacy is a serious issue and, as such, the government has enacted HIPAA regulations that provide for patient rights and protection. In the office, when you are talking to a patient either directly or on the telephone, you must ensure that other patients cannot hear your conversation. Charts should always be turned so that no one walking by can see any patient's personal information. Never leave schedules or charts where nonemployees might be able to see them.

throughout the body. If the blood is too warm, the heat dissipates from dilated blood vessels in the skin, and the skin becomes flushed as heat is released. The salts and plasma proteins in blood act to keep the liquid content of blood high. In this way, the blood plays a key role in maintaining the body's water–salt balance. The blood contains **buffers**, which are mechanisms within the blood that balance the pH level, thus preventing blood from becoming too acidic or too alkaline.

Defense

Leukocytes defend the body against invasion by pathogens such as bacteria and viruses. This is accomplished in several ways:

- Neutrophils and monocytes engulf and destroy pathogens (*phagocytosis*).

- Lymphocytes secrete antibodies into the blood. Antibodies incapacitate the pathogens, making them vulnerable to destruction.

- When an injury occurs, platelets form a clot, thus preventing blood loss. **Hemostasis** is the term for this stoppage of bleeding. When a blood vessel breaks, the smooth muscle at the site of the break causes the vessel wall to contract, which in turn causes the blood vessel to spasm. The spasm reduces the amount of blood lost through the break. Platelets then begin to attach themselves to the broken area and to each other to form a "plug" that eventually stops the bleeding. After a period of time, a blood clot forms and replaces the platelet plug. During this process, *coagulation,* the plasma protein fibrinogen is converted to fibrin. Fibrin

sticks to the damaged area of the vessel, eventually creating a meshwork that entraps blood cells and platelets. The end result is the blood clot, which stops the bleeding until the vessel has time to repair itself. Without this clotting capacity we could bleed to death from even a tiny cut.

Blood Types

Blood type is determined by the presence or absence of certain antigens and antibodies (Figure 27-14). Whether these protein molecules are present or not is genetically determined. **Agglutination**, or clumping, occurs when an antigen on the surface of RBCs binds to antibodies in the plasma. The presence of anti-A and anti-B antibodies in the plasma requires that blood be typed and cross-matched for transfusions. If a patient is given the wrong blood type, the new blood may clump with the patient's blood, causing occlusion and shock. For this reason, blood banks carefully type and match blood before it is given to the patient.

Blood typing is performed by adding antiserum to drops of blood and observing for agglutination. If the blood clumps for anti-A serum, it is either an A or AB blood type. If the blood clumps for anti-B serum, the blood is either A or AB blood type. If the blood clumps with both drops, the type is AB. If the blood does not clump with either drop, the type is O.

The ABO blood group system identifies four blood types (Table 27-1):

- **Type A**—Type A antigen on the surface of the red blood cells and anti-B antibody in the plasma

- **Type B**—antigen B and anti-A antibody

- **Type AB**—both antigens A and B and neither anti-A nor anti-B antibody (People with type AB blood are universal recipients because the majority of them can receive all ABO blood types.)

- **Type O**—no A or B antigens but both anti-A and anti-B antibody (People with type O blood are universal donors because their blood can be administered to most people regardless of the recipient's blood type.)

THE Rh FACTOR

The Rh factor is based on an antigen first discovered on RBCs of the Rhesus monkey (hence the name *Rh*). Someone who is Rh-positive has RBCs that contain the Rh antigen. A person who is Rh-negative does not have the Rh antigen. If someone who is Rh-negative is given Rh-positive blood, the Rh-negative blood will form antibodies on exposure to

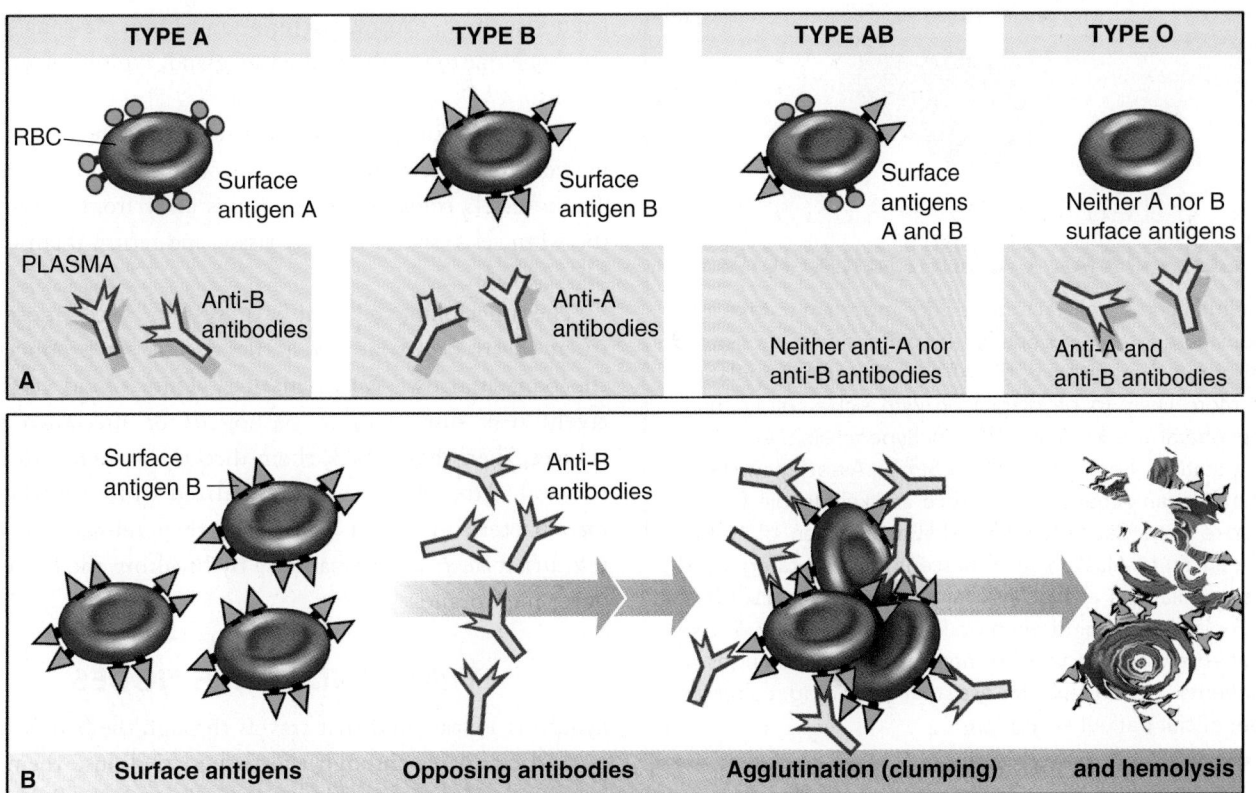

FIGURE 27-14 Blood typing and cross-reactions: The blood type depends on the presence of surface antigens (agglutinogens) on RBC surfaces. (A) The plasma antibodies (agglutinins) that will react with foreign surface antigens; (B) in a cross-reaction, antibodies that encounter their target antigens lead to agglutination and hemolysis of the affected RBCs.

TABLE 27-1 Blood Group Identification by Antigen and Antibody and Routine ABO Blood Typing

Blood Group Identification		
Blood Group	Antigen	Antibody
A	A	anti-B
B	B	anti-A
AB	A and B	neither
O	neither anti-A nor anti-B	anti-A, B

A

Routine ABO Blood Typing					
Reaction of Cells Tested with Group		Red Cell ABO	Reaction of Serum Tested Against Group		Reverse ABO
Anti-A	Anti-B		A1 Cells	B Cells	
O	O	O	+	+	O
+	O	A	O	+	A
O	+	B	+	O	B
+	+	AB	O	O	AB

B

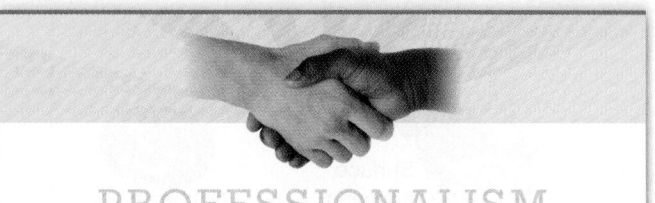
the Rh antigens. If the Rh-negative person is given Rh-positive blood on a second occasion, the antibodies will bind to the donor cells and agglutination will occur, precipitating a transfusion reaction.

The Rh factor plays an important role during pregnancy, so it is vital that a woman know her Rh type. If an Rh-negative female conceives a child with an Rh-positive male, there is a 50–50 chance that the fetus will be Rh-positive. When the blood of an Rh-positive fetus mixes with the mother's Rh-negative blood, the mother will develop antibodies against the fetus's RBCs. Because of the length of time it takes for the mother's body to generate these antibodies, the first Rh-positive fetus generally does not suffer any effect. However, if a second Rh-positive fetus is conceived, the fetus's blood will be attacked by the antibodies almost immediately. This can lead to a serious condition, erythroblastosis fetalis, in which the baby is born severely anemic. The condition can be prevented by giving the drug **RhoGAM** to the Rh-negative mother to inhibit the production of antibodies against the Rh antigen.

The Lymphatic System

The lymphatic system is a subsystem of both the circulatory system and the immune system. Its primary responsibility is to defend the body from foreign invasion by disease-causing agents such as viruses, bacteria, and fungi. It consists of the bone marrow, spleen, thymus gland, lymph nodes, and tonsils.

The lymphatic system, illustrated in Figure 27-15, is a network of vessels that assists in circulating body fluids. These vessels transport excess fluids away from interstitial (between cells) spaces in body tissue and return them to the bloodstream.

The function of the lymphatic system is seen most easily at the microscopic level. Blood cells are produced in the bone marrow. When mature, white blood cells actively seek out possible pathogens or unknown substances, then they attack them directly or facilitate their removal. After the T cells (specialized white blood cells) trap bacteria or other pathogen, they release a deadly toxin that destroys the bacteria by breaking the bacteria's outer membrane.

LYMPH AND LYMPH NODES

Lymph is a clear fluid that travels through the body's arteries and circulates through the tissues to cleanse them and keep them firm. It then drains away through the lymphatic system. Lymph nodes are the filters along the lymphatic system. Their job is to filter out and trap bacteria, viruses, cancer cells, destroyed microorganisms, and other unwanted substances, as well as to make sure they are safely eliminated from the body (Figure 27-16).

When lymph enters the lymphatic vessels, which contain valves that prevent lymph's backflow, it is pushed through the vessels by the skeletal muscles. If a leakage occurs in a lymphatic vessel, the surrounding tissue will swell and eventually result in the condition *edema*.

THYMUS AND SPLEEN

The thymus, which lies just above the heart, and the spleen, are located in the upper left portion of the abdominal cavity. The thymus, also an endocrine gland, carries out many of the same functions as the lymph nodes and is also responsible for the production of lymphocytes and the hormone thymosin, which stimulates the development of mature lymphocytes.

The spleen also plays an important part in the immune system and helps the body fight infection. Like lymph nodes, the spleen contains antibody-producing lymphocytes. These antibodies weaken or kill bacteria, viruses, and other organisms that cause infection. Also, if the blood passing through the spleen carries damaged cells, white blood cells in the spleen (macrophages) destroy and clear them from the bloodstream.

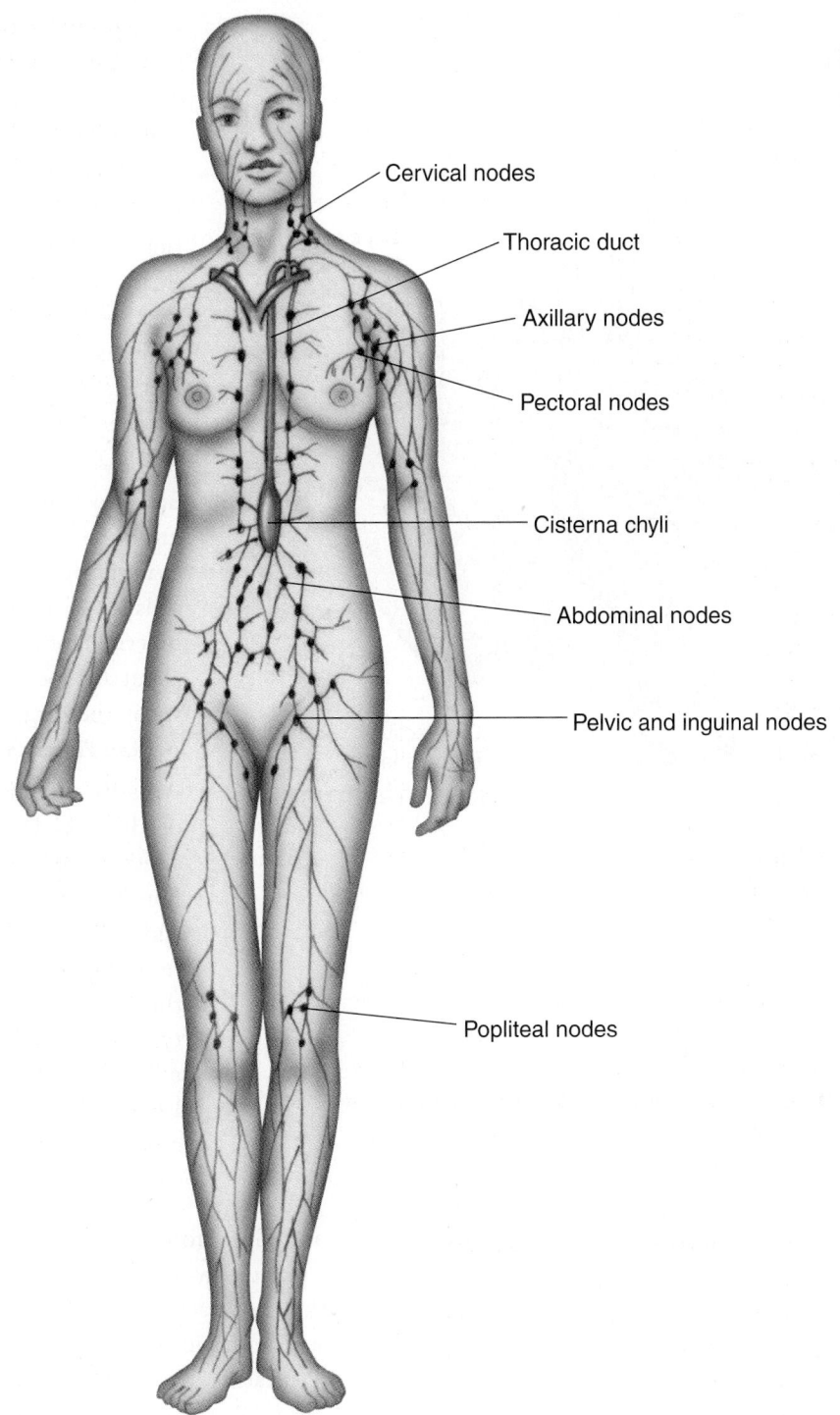

FIGURE 27-15 The lymphatic system.

Common Disorders Associated with the Circulatory System

Disorders of the circulatory system are very common in the United States. Many are the result of a combination of lifestyle factors (lack of exercise, stress, obesity) and genetics.

ANEMIA

Anemia is a condition characterized by abnormally low numbers of healthy RBCs circulating in the body—more specifically, low amounts of hemoglobin or abnormal hemoglobin in the RBCs. Often considered the most common dysfunction of RBCs, anemia affects about 3.5 million Americans.

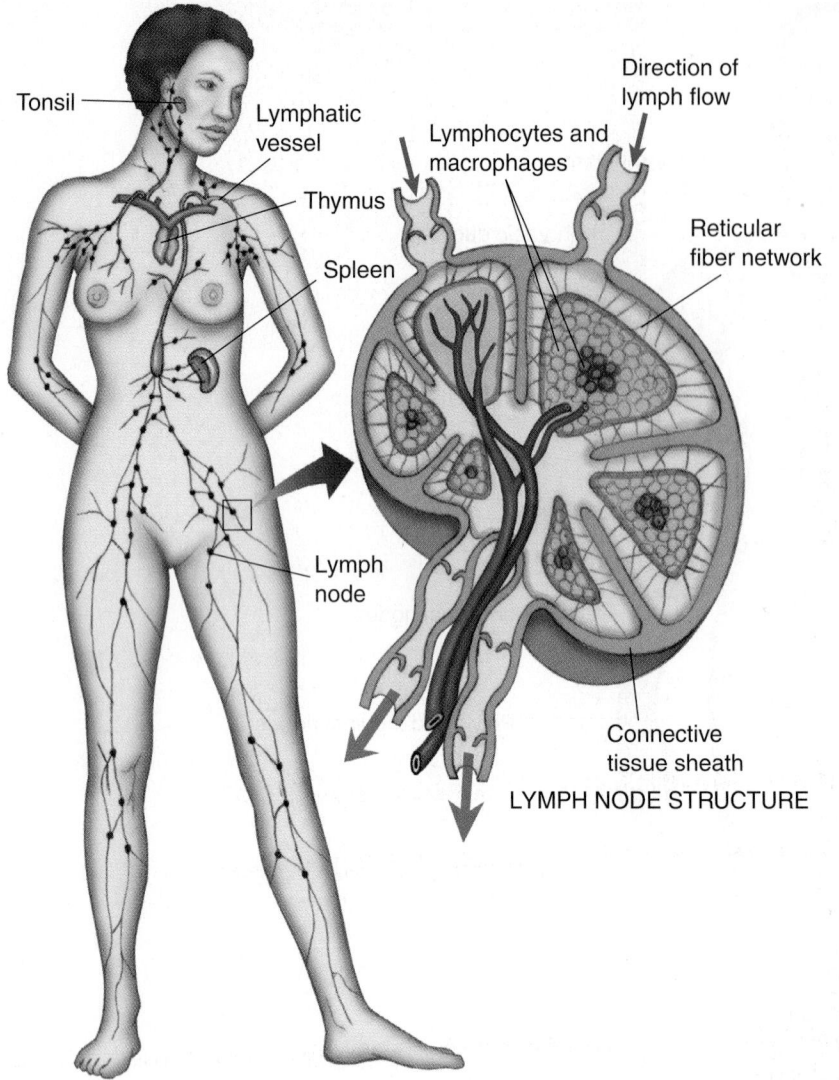

Tonsil

Lymphatic
vessel

Thymus

Spleen

Lymph
node

Direction of
lymph flow

Lymphocytes and
macrophages

Reticular
fiber network

Connective
tissue sheath

LYMPH NODE STRUCTURE

FIGURE 27-16 **The tonsils, lymph nodes, thymus, spleen, and lymphatic vessels with an expanded view of a lymph node.**

The three general causes of anemia are (1) decreased production of healthy red cells by the bone marrow, (2) increased erythrocyte destruction (hemolysis), and (3) blood loss from heavy menstrual periods or internal bleeding. Vitamin and mineral deficiencies in the diet can also slow the production of hemoglobin.

There are several types of anemia. Some may be inherited, whereas others are brought on by poor nutrition or toxins.

- **Iron-deficiency anemia**—The body needs iron for hemoglobin production. Low hemoglobin results in pale RBCs with a reduced capacity to transport oxygen. In general, most people need just 1 mg of iron daily. Menstruating or pregnant women may require iron supplements.

- **Vitamin-deficiency anemia**—Vitamin B_{12} is also essential for normal hemoglobin production. However,

some people have difficulty absorbing B_{12}. The result is a vitamin B_{12} deficiency, a condition known as *pernicious anemia*.

- **Hemolytic anemia**—This type of anemia is caused by the premature destruction of RBCs by antibodies produced by the immune system. This condition is sometimes associated with disorders such as lupus or lymphoma. Toxic materials such as lead, copper, and benzene can also lead to the destruction of RBCs.

- **Sickle cell anemia**—This anemia, also known as hemoglobin S disease, is characterized by sickle-shaped red blood cells. It is a serious, life-threatening, inherited form of anemia that occurs in about 0.6 percent of the population, with the highest incidence among African Americans.

- **Aplastic anemia**—This is one of the deadliest and rarest forms of anemia, affecting only 1 to 6 people per million. It is usually found in adolescents and young adults. The condition results from an unexplained failure of the bone marrow to produce certain types of blood cells. Instead, the bone marrow is replaced with fat cells. Injury to the bone marrow, or chemicals such as benzene and certain pesticides, can cause this type of anemia.

Signs and Symptoms. Common symptoms of anemia include fatigue, weakness, fainting, breathlessness, heart palpitations and tachycardia (see "Arrhythmia"), dizziness, headache, ringing in the ears, difficulty sleeping, and trouble concentrating. Sickle-cell anemia is characterized by pain in the joints and bones. Infections and heart failure may also occur. Symptoms of aplastic anemia can include bleeding in the mucous membranes, infections with high fevers, pallor, and dyspnea.

Treatment. The treatment for anemia depends on the type and cause. In some cases, injections of vitamin B_{12} may be necessary. Elimination of specific medications that suppress the body's immune system may be needed. Blood transfusions, analgesics, and antibiotics may also be required.

ANEURYSM

An **aneurysm** is an abnormal widening or ballooning of a portion of an artery, related to weakness in the vessel wall. Common locations for aneurysms include the aorta (aortic aneurysm), brain (cerebral aneurysm), leg (popliteal artery aneurysm), and intestine (mesenteric artery aneurysm).

Aneurysms can be congenital or acquired. The cause is unknown; however, defects in the artery wall may be a factor. High blood pressure and atherosclerotic disease may also contribute to the formation of certain types of aneurysms.

Signs and Symptoms. The symptoms of an aneurysm will vary, depending on its location. An aneurysm near the body's surface may be distinguished by a swelling, throbbing mass. Unfortunately, aneurysms within the body or brain often have no symptoms and frequently go undetected until it is too late.

Treatment. Surgical intervention may be required to repair the vessel and prevent rupturing. Some people may also be candidates for stent (a tube) placement within the affected vessel.

ARRHYTHMIA

An **arrhythmia** is an irregular heartbeat caused by a disturbance of the normal electrical activity of the heart. There are two types of arrhythmias:

- **Tachycardia** is an abnormally fast heartbeat of more than 100 beats per minute. The rhythm may be regular or irregular, but if it is too fast it may not allow the ventricles of the heart to fill properly, depriving the brain and body of oxygen. Extremely rapid tachycardia can be fatal if not treated immediately.

- **Bradycardia** is an abnormally slow heart rate, less than 60 beats per minute, which may be regular or irregular.

Figure 27-17 shows examples of normal heart rhythm and two examples of arrhythmias: sinus bradycardia and ventricular tachycardia.

Arrhythmias can be life threatening, especially when they significantly impact the pumping function of the heart. If the oxygen supply to the brain and major organs is interrupted for more than a few minutes, death can occur. Most arrhythmias are caused by heart diseases, including coronary artery disease (CAD), heart valve disease, heart failure, and infections such as endocarditis.

Signs and Symptoms. Both tachycardias and bradycardias produce similar symptoms, including dizziness, palpitations, shortness of breath, fatigue, weakness, angina, and fainting.

Treatment. Arrhythmias are usually treated with medications. Many patients can tolerate arrhythmias for years; however, the heart functions much better with a strong, metered rhythm.

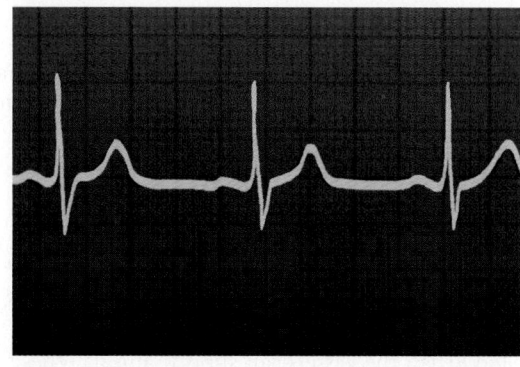

A

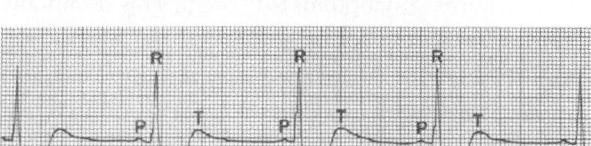

B

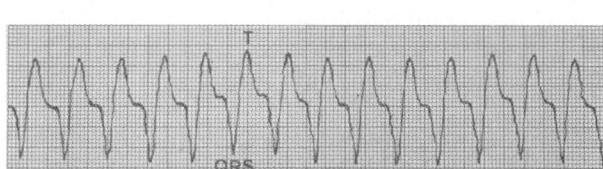

C

FIGURE 27-17 Examples of heart rhythms: (A) normal; (B) sinus bradycardia; (C) ventricular tachycardia.

ARTERIOSCLEROSIS

Often referred to as hardening of the arteries, **arteriosclerosis** is the thickening and loss of elasticity of the arteries. Over a period of many years, the artery walls develop areas that are hard and brittle because of calcium deposits. Arteries of the brain, kidneys, and upper and lower extremities may be affected. Causative factors include hypertension, diabetes mellitus, smoking, and obesity.

Signs and Symptoms. As this disease occurs within the body where it cannot be seen, it is not always recognized early or easily. However, a series of signs and symptoms should alert the individual and his or her physician: high blood pressure, recurrent kidney infections, and impaired circulation, particularly to the fingers and toes, due to peripheral vascular disease.

Treatment. Treatment consists of relieving symptoms and causes. Although there are several drugs for arteriosclerosis on the market, addressing the causative factors is crucial.

ATHEROSCLEROSIS

Atherosclerosis, or the narrowing and hardening of the vessel lumen of the arteries, results from a buildup of fatty material and plaque within the vessel (Figure 27-18). It is the leading cause of CAD. As the coronary arteries become more constricted, the flow of blood within the arteries may slow or even stop. The arteries can narrow to the point of total blockage. Plaque that breaks loose forms an embolus that can move and occlude a narrow vessel, causing death to the area supplied by that vessel.

Signs and Symptoms. The heart may not always be impacted by small blockages. When the heart needs more oxygen-rich blood than the vessels can supply, angina (chest pain) or other warning symptoms may occur. This commonly occurs during exercise or other activity. If the blockage is large, angina can occur with little or no activity. With unstable angina, the flow of blood to the heart is so limited as to restrict daily activities because of the risk of chest pain.

Treatment. Typically, angina decreases with rest and oxygen, but unrelieved angina is a common symptom of impending myocardial infarction.

CARDIAC TAMPONADE

Cardiac tamponade, or cardiac compression, is congestion of the heart muscle and restriction of heart movement caused by blood or fluid trapped in the pericardial sac.

Signs and Symptoms. Shortness of breath and the feeling of impending doom are common symptoms of cardiac tamponade.

Treatment. Treatment includes diuretic medications and possibly **thoracentesis** (or thoracocentesis) to draw fluid out of the chest.

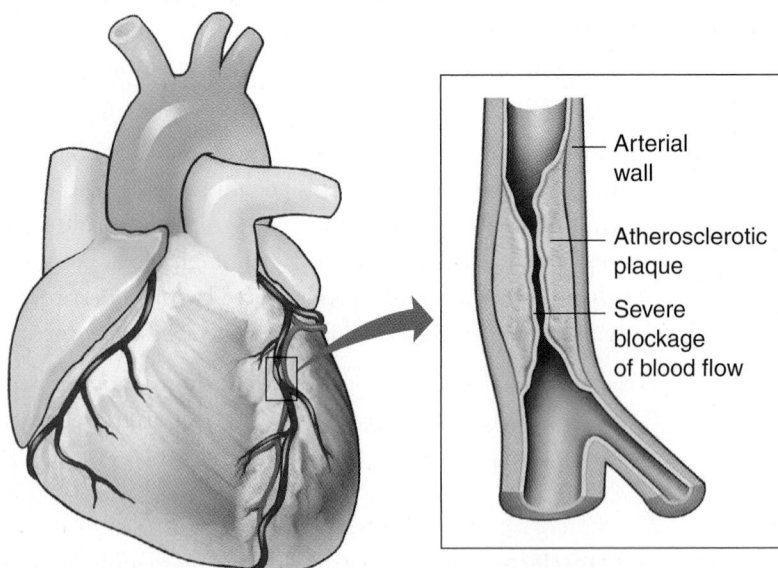

FIGURE 27-18 An atherosclerotic artery.

- Arterial wall
- Atherosclerotic plaque
- Severe blockage of blood flow

CARDIOGENIC SHOCK

Cardiogenic shock is a collapse of the cardiovascular system. It is characterized by vasodilation and fluid shifting away from the heart. Shock leads to inefficient cardiac function.

Signs and Symptoms. Symptoms of shock include restlessness, flushing, disorientation, and inability to adapt to temperature changes.

Treatment. Treatment includes placing the patient supine, with legs elevated, and keeping the patient warm but not overheated. Homeostasis should be reestablished and vital signs checked frequently. Cardiopulmonary resuscitation may be needed.

CARDIOMYOPATHY

Cardiomyopathy is a disease of the myocardium, or heart muscle, resulting in ventricular dysfunction. It is thought to be genetic and idiopathic (of undetermined cause).

Signs and Symptoms. The heart will enlarge, and the condition will be visible on chest X-rays and electrocardiograms (ECGs).

Treatment. Treatment consists of controlling the congestive heart failure (see "Congestive Heart Failure") that usually causes cardiomyopathy. Anticoagulant (anticlotting) medications are frequently prescribed, as well as medications that reduce blood pressure (antihypertensives).

CARDITIS (ENDOCARDITIS, MYOCARDITIS, PERICARDITIS)

Carditis is an inflammation of the heart. It is more accurately referred to as endocarditis, myocarditis, or pericarditis, depending on the layer of the heart that is affected.

Endocarditis

Endocarditis is an inflammation of the lining of the heart, including the heart valves. It is most commonly caused by a bacterial infection and frequently affects patients with existing abnormal conditions of the heart valves.

Signs and Symptoms. Persons who suffer from this life-threatening condition may experience weakness, fever, diaphoresis (excessive sweating), **dyspnea** (difficulty breathing), and the formation of embolisms that lodge in other organs.

Treatment. Treatment generally consists of antibiotics given intravenously followed by oral antibiotics over a 6-week period.

Myocarditis

Myocarditis is inflammation of the muscular layer of the heart. Myocarditis is a relatively uncommon and very serious condition that, left untreated, can lead to death. The most common cause of myocarditis is a viral infection; however, exposure to bacteria and certain drugs, chemicals, and allergens may also lead to its development.

Signs and Symptoms.   Symptoms generally include palpitations or chest pains that closely resemble a heart attack, fever, dyspnea, general fatigue and malaise, fainting, and decreased urine output.

Treatment.   The best treatment for myocarditis is reduction of the inflammation with anti-inflammatory medications, bed rest, and a low-sodium diet.

Pericarditis

Pericarditis is inflammation of the pericardium—the membrane that surrounds the heart. It is most commonly seen as a complication of a viral or bacterial infection.

Signs and Symptoms.   Symptoms of this deadly condition frequently include sharp, stabbing chest pain, fatigue, fever, and dyspnea, especially while lying down.

Treatment.   Treatment often includes analgesics, diuretics to help reduce the amount of fluid around the heart, and antibiotics to decrease the inflammation. Chronic cases may require pericardiocentesis to remove fluid around the heart.

CEREBROVASCULAR ACCIDENT

A **cerebrovascular accident (CVA)**, or stroke, occurs when the blood supply to part of the brain is suddenly interrupted by an occlusion of a blood vessel (ischemia or embolism) or a ruptured blood vessel (hemorrhage) in the brain. Brain cells die when they no longer receive oxygen and nutrients from the blood.

Signs and Symptoms.   The symptoms of a CVA generally occur suddenly: numbness or weakness on one side of the body, confusion or trouble speaking, vision problems, severe dizziness, loss of balance or coordination, or severe headache.

Treatment.   Therapies to prevent a first or recurrent CVA are based on managing underlying risk factors, such as hypertension, atrial fibrillation, and diabetes. Permanent neurological damage may be avoided with prompt treatment of the underlying cause. Post-CVA rehabilitation helps individuals overcome speech and mobility disabilities. Drug therapy includes the administration of antithrombotics and thrombolytics.

CONGESTIVE HEART FAILURE

Congestive heart failure (CHF), or heart failure, is a condition in which the heart is unable to pump sufficient blood to the body's other organs. This can result from several other conditions, including coronary artery disease, past heart attack, hypertension, heart valve disease due to past rheumatic fever or other causes, primary diseases of the heart muscle itself, heart defects present at birth, and any infection of the heart valves or heart muscle, such as endocarditis or myocarditis.

Signs and Symptoms.   As the "failing" heart functions less efficiently than it should, exertion causes shortness of breath and fatigue. As blood flow out of the heart slows, blood returning to the heart through the veins backs up, causing congestion in the tissues. Often swelling, or edema, results, usually in the legs and ankles, but sometimes in other parts of the body as well. Fluid may collect in the lungs and interfere with breathing, causing shortness of breath that becomes more pronounced when the person is lying down. Heart failure also affects the kidneys' ability to dispose of sodium and water. The retained water increases the edema.

Treatment.   A treatment program for CHF usually consists of rest, proper diet, modified daily activities, and medications such as angiotensin-converting enzyme (ACE) inhibitors, beta blockers, digitalis, diuretics, and vasodilators. When the specific cause of CHF is discovered, it should be treated or, if possible, corrected. For example, some cases can be treated by addressing high blood pressure. If an abnormal heart valve is the cause, the valve can be surgically replaced.

COR PULMONALE

Cor pulmonale, also known as right-sided heart disease, causes the right ventricle to enlarge. It is a result of primary lung disease.

Signs and Symptoms.   **Cardiomegaly**, or enlarged heart is a sign of col pulmonale. This can be seen with echocardiography.

Treatment.   Treatment seeks to relieve the pulmonary problems that precipitate the disease. Medications that improve pulmonary function are usually prescribed.

PROFESSIONALISM

Patients with heart disease seek to understand their illness. Although chest pain provides a great opportunity to teach the patient life changes (stop smoking, get exercise, lose weight, eat a low-fat/low-salt diet, etc.), the medical assistant should be careful to explain the disease process in terms that the patient can understand. For example, using the terms *chest pain* for *angina* or *blood thinner* for *anticoagulant* might be more helpful than using the more formal medical terms.

CORONARY ARTERY DISEASE

Coronary artery disease (CAD), also known as coronary heart disease (CHD), is the narrowing of the coronary arteries that supply blood to the heart. Left untreated, this progressive disease raises the risk of myocardial infarction, or heart attack, and possibly sudden death.

CAD is the most common form of heart disease as well as the leading cause of death in the United States. According to the American Heart Association, at least two people per minute—men and women—suffer from a CAD-related event, and one person dies every minute. Middle-aged men have about a 50 percent risk of a cardiac event, and women have a 32 percent risk. After menopause, the risk increases for women to the same level as men.

CAD affects people of all races. Lifestyle factors, including obesity, unhealthy diet choices, lack of exercise, and stress, are possible causes; genetic factors may play a role as well. High levels of lipoproteins or LDL cholesterol are associated with a higher risk of CAD. Risk can be lowered by maintaining a total cholesterol level below 200 mg/dL and an HDL cholesterol (good cholesterol) level above 35 mg/dL. Daily aerobic exercise, increasing dietary intake of vegetables and grain products, weight loss, and smoking cessation are all steps people can take to reach healthier cholesterol levels.

Signs and Symptoms. Shortness of breath and edema (swelling) in the ankles can be signs of CAD.

Treatment. Diuretic medications are used to decongest the body of extra fluid and relieve stress on the heart.

HEART ATTACK (MYOCARDIAL INFARCTION)

A heart attack or **myocardial infarction (MI)** occurs when the blood supply to a part of the myocardium is severely reduced or stopped (Figure 27-19). Atherosclerosis is usually

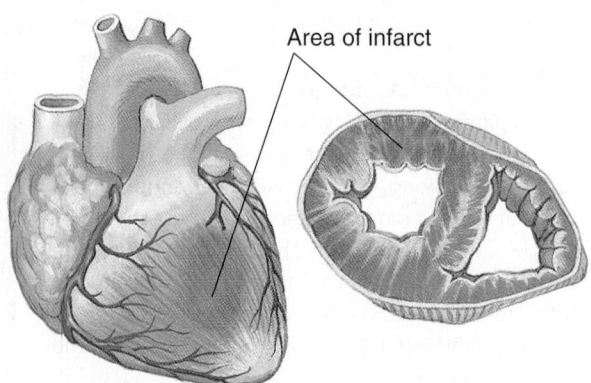

FIGURE 27-19 **Cross-section of myocardial infarction.**

the cause. In a coronary thrombosis or coronary occlusion, the accumulated plaque tears loose or ruptures and triggers a blood clot that blocks the artery. If the blood supply is cut off, the muscle tissues fed by that artery suffer irreversible damage and die. Depending on the extent of the damage, disability or death can result.

Signs and Symptoms. The most common symptom of an MI is chest pain. Angina pectoris is often described as a crushing or squeezing pain, with a feeling of fullness, heaviness, or aching in the center of the chest that may radiate down the left arm or into the neck or back. Men experience chest pain as a symptom of an MI more frequently than do women. However, women do experience the other symptoms— shortness of breath; diaphoresis; pain or discomfort in the arms, back, or jaw; dizziness or fainting; nausea; and a sense of impending doom. If any of these symptoms are present for more than 2 minutes, emergency treatment must be started immediately. Waiting to treat the symptoms increases the chances of serious disability or death. **Cyanosis**, or blue skin, is a sign that oxygenated blood is not being perfused (forced through) by the heart.

Treatment. Treatment for an MI, when administered quickly, can benefit most patients. Cardiopulmonary resuscitation (CPR) and defibrillation within the first few minutes increase the survival rate. Thrombolytics (clot busters) can stop some heart attacks in progress. **Angioplasty**, which is surgical vessel repair, is frequently performed to reopen blocked coronary arteries, and stents are used to hold the arteries open. If more conservative measures fail or if the heart attack is too severe, a coronary artery bypass graft (CABG), a form of open heart surgery, will be attempted to bypass the blocked artery using a vein from the leg or arm.

The key to heart attack survival is immediate intervention. Patients must be educated on the necessity of seeking medical assistance immediately when they have any symptoms of a heart attack. Delay because "It's just indigestion" only decreases the patient's chance of survival.

HEMOPHILIA

Hemophilia is a hereditary deficiency of clotting factors that affects male children more frequently than females.

Signs and Symptoms. Hemophilia predisposes the patient to hemorrhaging (bleeding heavily) when cut or injured. Hemophiliacs also tend to bruise easily.

Treatment. The only treatment for hemophilia is transfusion of healthy blood-clotting factors from another donor.

HYPERTENSION

Hypertension (HTN) (high blood pressure) is blood pressure that is higher than 140/90 mmHg. Systolic pressure of greater than 120 is considered borderline hypertension. By diagnosing the patient with borderline hypertension or prehypertension (see "Prehypertension"), treatment can be initiated earlier. If the blood vessels become rigid and constricted, the pressure within the vessels increases. When this force stays high for a period of time, the diagnosis of hypertension is made.

Sometimes hypertension is caused by congestion in the peripheral arteries. Peripheral artery disease occurs when the arteries that move blood away from the heart become diseased. These arteries can narrow, causing arteriostenosis. They can also become hardened and filled with fatty plaque and give rise to atherosclerosis. When blood does not flow easily through the blood vessels, blood pressure rises.

Signs and Symptoms. Because HTN has few, if any, symptoms, it is called the "silent killer." Symptoms that are present may include intense headaches, fatigue, and changes in vision. In severe cases of hypertension, nosebleeds (epistaxis) and possibly blood in the urine may also be symptomatic. If left untreated, hypertension can lead to serious conditions such as kidney failure, stroke, heart attack, peripheral artery disease, and eye damage.

Treatment. HTN can be controlled in a variety of ways, including antihypertensive and diuretic medications, dietary changes, and exercise.

HYPOTENSION

Hypotension, or low blood pressure, is an abnormal condition in which a person's blood pressure is much lower than usual, generally below 90/60 mmHg. If blood pressure drops significantly, blood flow to the heart, brain, and other vital organs is inadequate.

Low blood pressure can also be a sign of a well-conditioned heart in those who get regular aerobic exercise, such as running. In these individuals, the myocardium is able to produce strong contractions to easily pump the blood through the body.

Causes of hypotension include dehydration, heart failure, heart attack, changes in the heart's rhythm (arrhythmias), syncope (fainting), anaphylaxis, and drug overdose. Another common cause is orthostatic hypotension, which results from a sudden change in body position, usually from lying down to an upright position.

Signs and Symptoms. A sudden, significant drop in blood pressure is a warning that the body is not receiving enough oxygen and is in danger of shutting down. Normal body functions such as breathing, movement, and brain function can be im-paired, and permanent damage can occur. Blood pressure may drop to life-threatening levels due to loss of blood, shock, severe infection, or low body temperature caused by exposure to cold.

Treatment. Emergency treatment for hypotension raises blood pressure to a more normal level. This may include the use of vasoconstrictors to help raise blood pressure, and increasing the amount of fluid and sodium intake. If the patient suffers from orthostatic hypotension, slowly changing body positioning is often beneficial.

LEUKEMIA

Leukemia is a malignant cancer of the bone marrow and blood and, like all cancers, involves the uncontrolled growth of abnormal cells, in this case WBCs. Leukemia can be acute or chronic. Acute leukemias progress rapidly and cause a marked increase of cells that do not develop normally and never become functional. These cells crowd out the healthy blood cells, increasing the risk of anemia and infection. Patients with acute leukemia also lack platelets that help blood to clot, so they may bleed extensively. Chronic leukemias worsen gradually because the abnormal cells accumulate over time and affect other body tissues.

Leukemia is classified by the type of leukocyte affected. When it strikes lymphoid cells (cells containing lymphocytes), it is called lymphocytic leukemia. Myeloid or myelogenous leukemia strikes myeloid (bone marrow) cells.

Signs and Symptoms. The symptoms of the disease are broad. They include excessive bruising, fatigue, weakness, dyspnea, bleeding of the mucous membranes, bone and joint pain, abdominal pain, weight loss, abdominal bleeding, and enlargement of the lymph nodes, spleen, and/or liver. Anemia and frequent infections are common.

Treatment. The three major approaches to treating leukemia depend on the severity and phase of the disease: chemotherapy to kill leukemia cells using strong anticancer drugs, radiation therapy to kill cancer cells by exposure to high-energy radiation, and bone marrow transplantation.

PREHYPERTENSION

A newer classification of hypertension is **prehypertension**. This diagnosis is applied to individuals who are over 18 years old with blood pressure that ranges from 120/80 to 139/89 mmHg. According to a study by the Joint National Committee of the National Institutes of Health National Heart, Lung, and Blood Institute (NHLBI), adults at the upper end of the prehypertension blood pressure range are twice as likely to progress to hypertension as those with lower blood pressure.

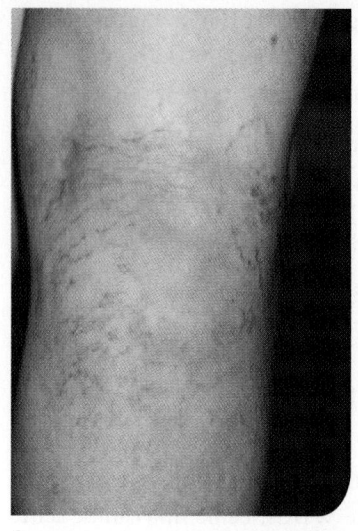

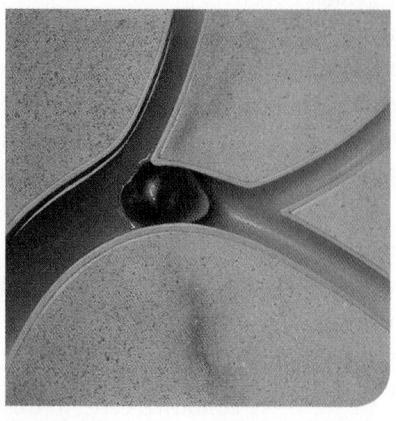

A   B

FIGURE 27-20 A-B Example of thrombophlebitis: (A) superficial thrombophlebitis of the leg; (B) cross-section of vein where thrombophlebitis is present.

Signs and Symptoms. Blood pressure ranging from 120/80 to 139/89 is a symptom of prehypertension.

Treatment. The committee report recommends lifestyle changes such as reducing dietary fat and sodium, increasing exercise, and limiting alcohol consumption.

THROMBOPHLEBITIS

Thrombo means "clot"; *phlebitis* is the inflammation of a vein. **Thrombophlebitis** occurs when a blood clot causes inflammation in one or more veins, typically in the lower extremities (Figure 27-20). On rare occasions, thrombophlebitis can also affect veins in the upper extremities. The affected vein may be near the surface of the skin (superficial thrombophlebitis) or deep within a muscle (deep venous thrombosis). A clot in a deep vein increases the risk of serious health problems, such as a pulmonary embolism (a dislodged clot that moves through the blood vessels and travels to the lungs where it blocks a smaller artery).

Thrombophlebitis is often caused by prolonged inactivity, such as a long journey in an airplane or automobile; by trauma; or by lengthy bed rest following surgery. Such inactivity decreases blood flow through the veins and may cause a clot to form. Other causes include paralysis and the use of oral contraceptives or hormone replacement therapy. A history of varicose veins or an inherited tendency for blood clots can also place someone at higher risk for thrombophlebitis.

Signs and Symptoms. The most common signs and symptoms of thrombophlebitis are redness, swelling, warmth, tenderness, and a dull ache or pain in the affected area. When a superficial vein is affected, a red, hard, tender cord may also be present just under the surface of the skin. If a deep vein is affected, the leg may become swollen, tender, and painful, particularly when the person stands or walks.

Treatment. For thrombophlebitis in a superficial vein, the physician generally recommends self-care steps such as applying heat to the painful area, elevating the affected limb, and using nonsteroidal anti-inflammatory drugs, such as aspirin. The condition usually subsides within a week or two. In more severe cases, as in deep venous thrombosis, an injection of a blood-thinning (anticoagulant) medication often prevents the clot from growing. Additional treatments may include the application of support stockings to constrict the superficial veins and increase blood flow in the deep veins, and varicose vein ligation or stripping, in which the doctor surgically removes the varicose veins that cause pain or recurrent thrombophlebitis. In the most severe cases, a thrombectomy or bypass surgery may be required to remove an acute clot blocking a pelvic or abdominal vein.

TRANSFUSION INCOMPATIBILITY REACTION

If blood of the wrong type is administered to a patient, a severe transfusion reaction can occur. The two blood types will create an antigen-versus-antibody reaction (as seen in Figure 27-14), and severe agglutination can occur.

Signs and Symptoms. Symptoms of transfusion incompatability arise rapidly with collapse of the circulatory system. Symptoms of shock, such as confusion, restlessness, and shortness of breath, are dramatic.

Treatment. If an incompatibility reaction occurs, immediately stop the flow of the donor blood and instead infuse normal saline intravenously. Administer antihistamines by physician order and monitor vital signs frequently. If the reaction is more aggressive, administration of epinephrine may be needed. Two people should always double-check the compatibility of the donor blood with the patient's blood type.

VALVULAR HEART DISEASE

Mitral stenosis, or valvular heart disease, is caused by insufficient closing of the valve. This leads to prolapse, or a protruding backward. The heartbeat is not as efficient in pumping, as some blood regurgitates upward into the atria, and the patient cannot exert him- or herself as easily.

Signs and Symptoms. This disease can produce a heart murmur that is audible with a stethoscope.

Treatment. Treatment includes medication to strengthen heart function.

VARICOSE VEINS

Varicose veins are gnarled, enlarged veins. The varicosity usually involves the superficial veins in the legs. It may be caused by prolonged periods of standing, pregnancy, or aging.

Varicose veins develop when the valves in the veins malfunction. As one gets older, the veins tend to lose elasticity and stretch. Blood pools in the veins, which become engorged with deoxygenated blood.

Signs and Symptoms. These visible, bulging veins are often linked with symptoms such as tired, heavy, or aching limbs. In severe cases, varicose veins can rupture or form open sores (varicose ulcers) on the skin.

Treatment. Treatment for varicose veins falls into two categories: relief of the symptoms and removal of the affected veins (ligation). Symptom relief includes such measures as moderate exercise, avoiding long periods of standing, elevating the legs, and wearing support stockings, which compress the veins and hold them in place. Cosmetic treatments may decrease the size and visibility of the affected veins.

For more a summary and additional information on disorders of the cardiovascular system, see Table 27-2.

TABLE 27-2 Disorders of the Cardiovascular System

Disorder	Description
Anemia	A reduction in the number of circulating red blood cells per cubic millimeter of blood. It is not a disease but a symptom of disease.
Aneurysm	An abnormal dilation of a blood vessel, usually an artery, due to a congenital weakness or defect in the wall of the vessel.
Angina pectoris	Condition in which there is severe pain with a sensation of constriction around the heart. It is caused by a deficiency of oxygen to the heart muscle.
Angioma	Tumor, usually benign, consisting of blood vessels.
Angiospasm	Spasm or contraction of blood vessels.
Aortic aneurysm	Localized, abnormal dilation of the aorta, causing pressure on the trachea, esophagus, veins, or nerves. This is due to a weakness in the wall of the blood vessels.
Aortic insufficiency	A failure of the aortic valve to close completely, which results in leaking and inefficient heart action.
Aortic stenosis	Condition caused by narrowing of the aorta.
Arrhythmia	An irregularity in the heartbeat.
Arterial embolism	Blood clot moving within an artery. This can occur as a result of arteriosclerosis.
Arteriosclerosis	Thickening, hardening, and loss of elasticity of the walls of arteries.
Atherosclerosis	The most common form of arteriosclerosis. It is caused by the formation of yellowish plaques of cholesterol building up on the inner walls of the arteries.
Bradycardia	An abnormally slow heart rate (under 60 beats per minute).
Cardiac tamponade	Congestion of the heart muscle and restriction of heart movement caused by blood or fluid being trapped in the pericardium.
Cardiogenic shock	Shock caused by the collapse of the cardiovascular system, characterized by fluid shifting and vasodilation.
Cardiomyopathy	A disease of the myocardium, or heart muscle, and resulting ventricular dysfunction.
Cerebrovascular accident	Also called stroke, a lack of blood flow to blood vessels in the head.
Congenital heart disease	Heart defects that are present at birth, such as patent ductus arteriosus, in which the opening between the pulmonary artery and the aorta fails to close at birth. This condition requires surgery.
Congestive heart failure	Pathological condition of the heart in which outflow of blood from the left side of the heart is reduced. This results in weakness, breathlessness, and edema.
Cor pulmonale	Also known as right-sided heart disease. Causes the right ventricle to enlarge. It is a result of primary lung disease.

(continued)

TABLE 27-2 (*continued*)

Disorder	Description
Coronary artery disease	A narrowing of the coronary arteries that is sufficient enough to prevent adequate blood supply to the myocardium.
Coronary thrombosis	Blood clot in a coronary vessel of the heart causing the vessel to close completely or partially.
Embolus	A blood clot that moves from one area to another and obstructs a blood vessel.
Endocarditis	Inflammation of the membrane lining the heart. May be due to microorganisms or to an abnormal immunological response.
Fibrillation	Abnormal quivering or contractions of heart fibers. When this occurs within the fibers of the ventricle, arrest and death can occur. Emergency equipment to defibrillate, or convert the heart to a normal beat, will be necessary.
Hemophilia	A hereditary disease of deficient clotting.
Hypertensive heart disease	Heart disease as a result of persistently high blood pressure that damages the blood vessels and ultimately the heart.
Hypotension	A decrease in blood pressure. This can occur in shock, infection, anemia, cancer, or as death approaches.
Infarct	Area of tissue within an organ or part that undergoes necrosis (death) following the cessation of the blood supply.
Ischemia	A localized and temporary deficiency of blood supply due to an obstruction to the circulation.
Mitral stenosis	Narrowing of the opening (orifice) of the mitral valve, which causes an obstruction in the flow of blood from the atrium to the ventricle on the left side of the heart.
Mitral valve prolapse (MVP)	Common and serious condition in which the cusp of the mitral valve drops back (prolapses) into the left atrium during systole.
Murmur	A soft blowing or rasping sound heard on auscultation of the heart.
Myocardial infarction	Condition caused by the partial or complete occlusion or closing of one or more of the coronary arteries. Symptoms include a squeezing pain or heavy pressure in the middle of the chest. A delay in treatment could result in death. This is also referred to as MI or heart attack.
Myocarditis	An inflammation of the myocardial lining of the heart resulting in an extremely weak and rapid beat and an irregular pulse.
Patent ductus arteriosus	Congenital presence of a connection between the pulmonary artery and the aorta that remains after birth. This condition is normal in the fetus.
Pericarditis	Inflammatory process or disease of the pericardium.
Phlebitis	Inflammation of a vein.
Reynaud's phenomenon	Intermittent attacks of pallor or cyanosis of the fingers and toes associated with cold or emotional distress. Numbness, pain, and burning may also occur during the attacks. It may be caused by decreased circulation due to smoking.
Rheumatic heart disease	Valvular heart disease as a result of having had rheumatic fever.
Tetralogy of Fallot	Combination of four symptoms (tetralogy), resulting in pulmonary stenosis, a septal defect, abnormal blood supply to the aorta, and hypertrophy of the right ventricle. A congenital defect that is present at birth and needs immediate surgery to correct.
Thrombophlebitis	Inflammation and clotting of blood within a vein.
Thrombus	A blood clot.
Valvular heart disease	Mitral stenosis, or valvular heart disease that causes insufficient closure of the valves, leading to prolapse.
Varicose veins	Swollen and distended veins, usually in the legs, resulting from pressure, such as occurs during a pregnancy.

SUMMARY

The circulatory system is made up of structures that circulate blood, oxygen, nutrients, and other substances throughout the body. These structures include the heart and the blood vessels. The heart is a pump that moves oxygen- and nutrient-rich blood to the body and carries waste and carbon dioxide back to the lungs for excretion from the body. Arteries carry blood away from the heart to the body; the exchange of oxygen and nutrients for carbon dioxide and waste takes place in the capillaries; then the veins carry the blood back to the heart and lungs.

Blood pressure keeps the heart functionally pumping blood to all the organs and cells. Blood is connective tissue that circulates through the body. Blood cells include red blood cells (erythrocytes), white blood cells (leukocytes), and clotting cells (platelets). The four blood types are A, B, AB, and O. The lymphatic system acts as a defense system for the body. Being an intricate system, many problems and diseases may arise in the circulatory system. Disease can occur in the heart, the blood vessels, or the blood cells.

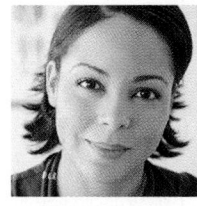

27 CHAPTER REVIEW

COMPETENCY REVIEW

1. Define and spell the terms to learn for this chapter.

2. Name the components of the circulatory system.

3. Name the three layers of the heart.

4. Name the upper chambers of the heart.

5. Name the lower chambers of the heart.

6. What role do the arteries play in circulation?

7. What role do the veins play in circulation?

8. Name the heart's pacemaker.

9. Describe how blood pressure is recorded in the patient's chart.

10. Define pulse pressure.

PREPARING FOR THE CERTIFICATION EXAM

1. Which of the following is a valve?
   a. tricuspid
   b. vena cava
   c. sinoatrial node
   d. pacemaker
   e. intraventricular septum

2. Blood enters the left atrium of the heart through the
   a. pulmonary artery
   b. superior and inferior venae cavae
   c. pulmonary veins

d.   descending aorta

e.   coronary artery

3.   What are the upper chambers of the heart called?

   a.   superior and inferior venae cavae
   b.   right and left pulmonary arteries
   c.   right and left pulmonary veins
   d.   right and left ventricles
   e.   right and left atria

4.   The muscular layer of the heart is called the

   a.   pericardium
   b.   myocardium
   c.   apex
   d.   endocardium
   e.   mediastinum

5.   Valvular heart disease is also known as

   a.   cor pulmonale
   b.   mitral stenosis
   c.   varicose veins
   d.   cardiac tamponade
   e.   anemia

6.   Which of the following is a blood pressure within normal limits?

   a.   90/60
   b.   120/40
   c.   110/80
   d.   130/105
   e.   160/90

7.   Tachycardia means

   a.   abnormally fast heartbeat
   b.   abnormally slow heartbeat
   c.   abnormally high blood pressure
   d.   abnormally low blood pressure
   e.   normal cardiac function

8.   The artery in the neck where the pulse is taken is the

   a.   radial artery
   b.   temporal artery
   c.   carotid artery
   d.   facial artery
   e.   femoral artery

9.   What is the term for a right-sided heart disease?

   a.   anemia
   b.   embolus
   c.   coronary artery disease
   d.   cor pulmonale
   e.   phlebitis

10.   What is the term for a clot that travels in blood vessels?

   a.   platelets
   b.   hemophilia
   c.   thrombus
   d.   phlebitis
   e.   embolus

CRITICAL THINKING

1.   David, a CMA (AAMA) obtains Jamal's vital signs after he has escorted him to the examination room. David notes Jamal's vital signs as follows: Wt: 235 lbs, T: 97.6°F, P: 94 bpm, rapid and bounding, BP: 148/92. What can you ascertain from these findings?

2.   Jamal is an African American. How does this impact his health status relating to circulatory system disorders?

3.   What might Dr. Miller suggest to help Jamal take control of his blood pressure?

INTERNET ACTIVITY

Access one of the many "healthy heart" websites and see what type of education they provide for their readers. What are some good features of the sites you access?

MEDMEDIA

Additional interactive resources and activities for this chapter can be found:

On your student DVD: View applicable procedure videos on the DVD-ROM found in the back of this book.

MyHealthProfessionsKit.com: Test your knowledge of this chapter with games and activities. MyHealthProfessionsKit also includes resources, helpful links, and a Spanish audio glossary.

Medical Assisting Interactive: Practice your procedures as a medical assistant in this simulated doctor's office. This can be accessed through MyHealthProfessionsKit.com.

28

The Immune System

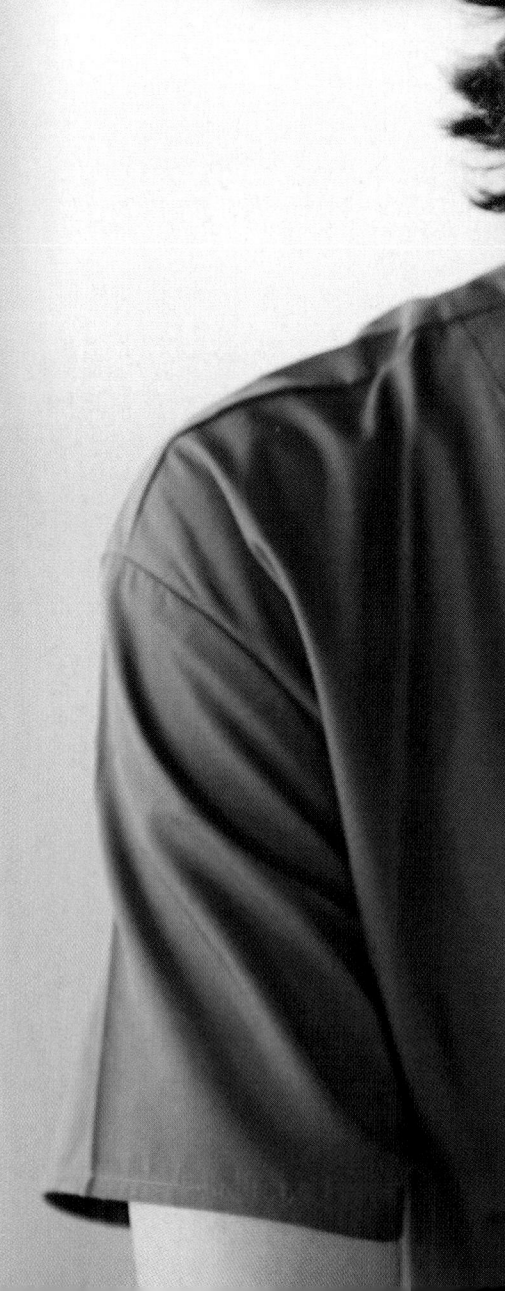

LEARNING OBJECTIVES

After completing this chapter, you should be able to:

- Define and spell the terms to learn for this chapter.
- Identify and discuss the anatomy of the immune system.
- Discuss the functions of the immune system.
- Explain the immune system and its response.
- List and briefly discuss disorders of the immune system.

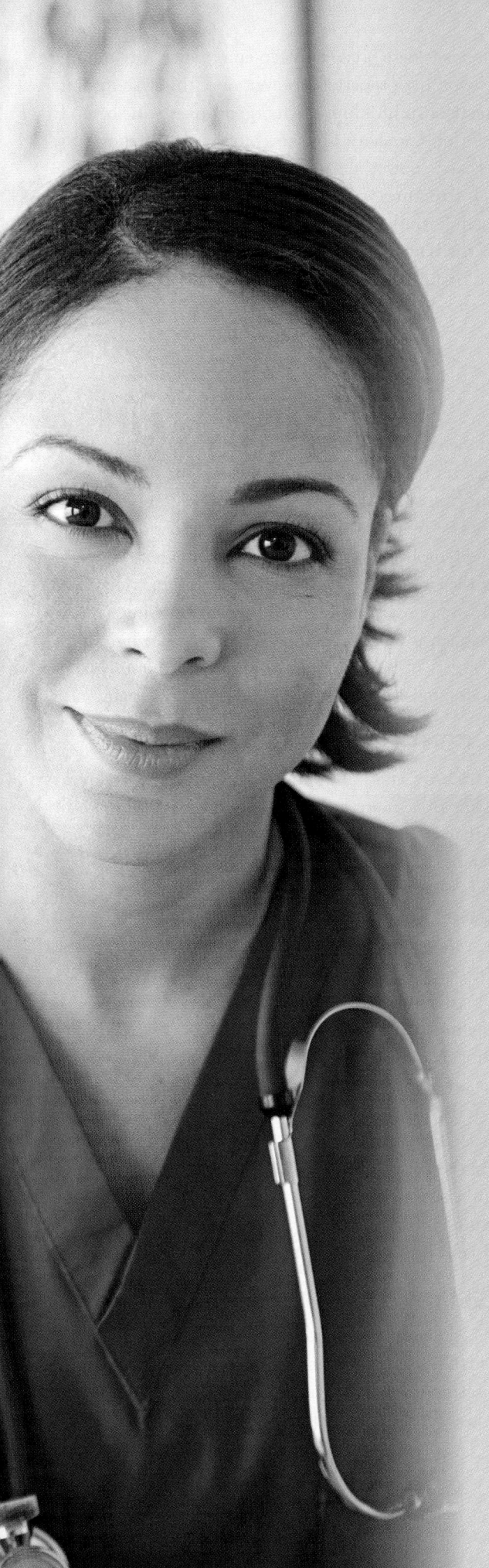

CHAPTER OUTLINE

CASE STUDY

Rosa Gutierrez, age 49, is being seen today by Dr. Bahjat. She has been suffering from what appears to be a multitude of individual problems including low blood pressure, cold and flulike symptoms, extreme fatigue, and what she describes as "hot and cold flashes." Following a thorough physical exam, which includes a complete blood cell count and an evaluation of her entire treatment history, Rosa is diagnosed with chronic fatigue syndrome. As part of her care, Dr. Bahjat has informed her that she must take an active role in her treatment. This includes getting plenty of rest and being monitored for any additional viral infections.

CERTIFICATION LINK

CMA (AAMA)	RMA	CMAS (AMT)
Anatomy and physiology	Anatomy and physiology	Medical assisting foundation
Systems (including structure, function, related conditions and diseases, and their relationships)	Body systems Disorders and diseases of the body	Anatomy and physiology

Inside the body is an amazing protection mechanism called the immune system. The **immune system** consists of tissues, organs, and physiological processes that identify abnormal cells, foreign substances, and foreign tissues, such as transplants, and defend against substances that might be harmful to the body. Those substances may be bacteria, microbes, viruses, toxins, or parasites.

To understand the power of the immune system, all one has to do is look at what happens after death. When a person dies, the immune system shuts down. In a matter of hours, the body is invaded by all sorts of bacteria, microbes, and par-

asites. None of these organisms can enter when the immune system is working properly; however, once this system shuts down, the door to invading microorganisms is wide open. It takes them only a short time to completely dismantle the body and carry it away, until all that is left is a skeleton.

Several structures are central to the immune system. These include the central lymphoid tissue, which is comprised of the bone marrow and thymus, and the peripheral lymphoid tissue, consisting of the lymph nodes, spleen, and mucosa-associated lymphoid tissue.

Anatomy of the Immune System

The immune system operates throughout the body. However, at certain sites the cells of the immune system are organized into specific structures, classified as central lymphoid tissue and peripheral lymphoid tissue. All these structures are also part of the lymphatic system (Figure 28-1), which is a subsystem of the circulatory system. The primary function of the lymphatic system is to defend the body against invasion by pathogens such as viruses, bacteria, and fungi. The lymphatic system consists of the bone marrow, spleen, thymus gland, lymph nodes, tonsils, appendix, and a few other organs.

CENTRAL LYMPHOID TISSUE

The bone marrow and the thymus comprise the central lymphoid tissue. Bone marrow contains stem cells that create all the cells that make up the tissues and structures of the immune system. It is also where red blood cells, white blood cells, and platelets are produced. In a process called hematopoiesis, these cells become either mature cells of the immune system or precursors of cells that will mature in a part of the body other than the bone marrow. The bone marrow also produces B cells and natural killer cells.

The **thymus gland** is located posterior to the sternum, in the anterior mediastinum. It enlarges during childhood but shrinks again after maturity, continuing to function throughout life. It is divided into two distinct compartments, an outer cortex and an internal medulla. Immature lymphoid cells enter the cortex, reproduce and mature, then move to the medulla where they reenter the circulation. The thymus manufactures infection-fighting T cells and helps distinguish normal T cells from those that attack the body's own tissues.

PERIPHERAL LYMPHATIC SYSTEM

The peripheral lymphatic system consists of the lymph nodes, spleen, and other lymphoid tissue (see Figure 27-16 in Chapter 27). Lymphatic capillaries, lymphatic vessels, and lymphatic ducts are also part of the peripheral lymphatic system.

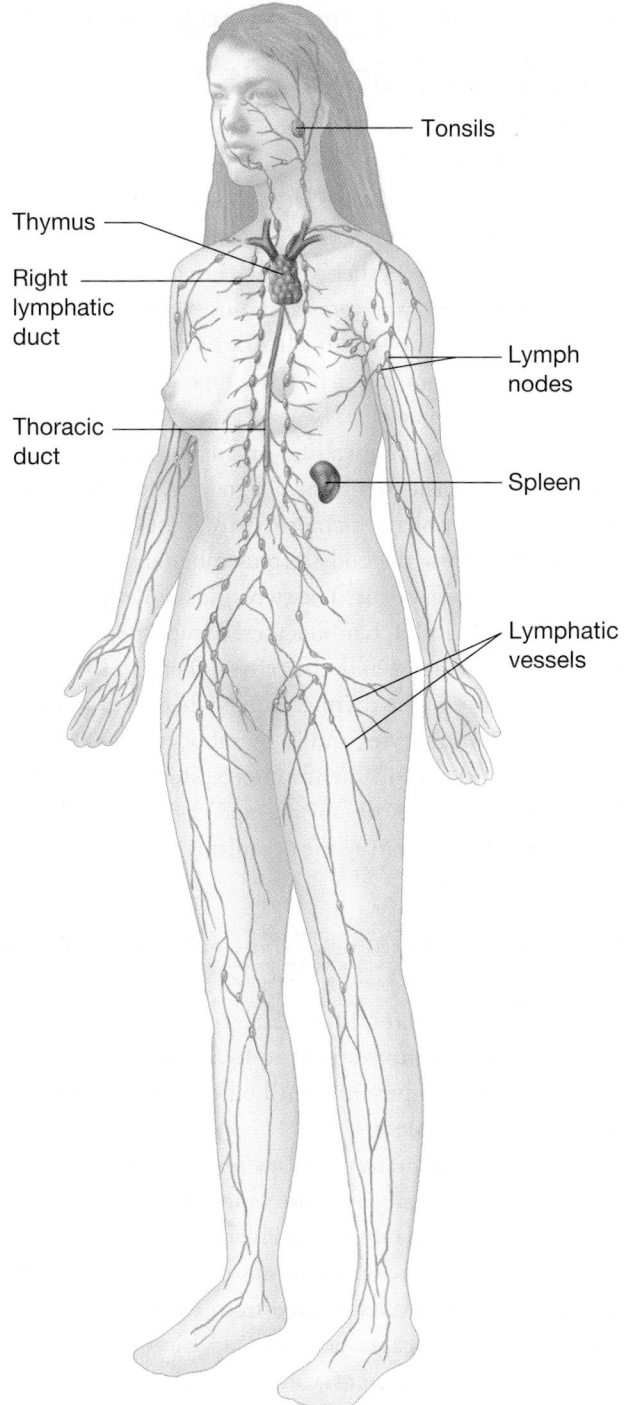

FIGURE 28-1 **Components of the lymphatic system.**

Labels on figure:
- Tonsils
- Thymus
- Right lymphatic duct
- Thoracic duct
- Lymph nodes
- Spleen
- Lymphatic vessels

cytes. The **germinal centers** are the primary locations where B lymphocytes reproduce quite prolifically.

B lymphocytes are the cells responsible for production of circulating **antibodies** which are specialized proteins that lock onto specific antigens. Each unique type of B cell produces only one type of antibody. When an **antigen** (a foreign substance that invades the body) enters the body, these B lymphocytes rapidly undergo mitosis and divide, thereby producing large quantities of a specific antibody to seek out and help destroy the antigen by enveloping the antigen and eating the enemy antigen. The rest of the cortex contains **T lymphocytes**, which are cells that circulate through the lymph nodes, bloodstream, and lymphatic ducts to seek out any infection. The **medulla** of the lymph node is primarily made up of macrophages attached to reticular fibers.

Lymph Nodes

Lymph nodes are many different sizes and shapes, but most are bean shaped and about 1 inch long. Covered with a thick fibrous capsule, each node is subdivided into different compartments by inward-pointing **trabeculae**. As with many organs, the lymph node has two basic parts, the **cortex** and the medulla. The cortex is populated mainly with lympho-

Spleen

Located in the upper left quadrant of the abdomen, the spleen receives blood from an artery that branches off the aorta. After passing through an intricate meshwork of tiny blood vessels in the spleen, the blood continues to the liver. These blood vessels are surrounded by nests of B lymphocytes, mainly of the memory type. As the blood slowly

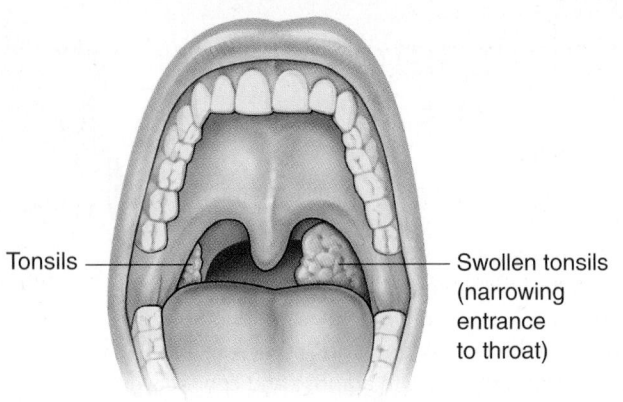

Tonsils

Swollen tonsils (narrowing entrance to throat)

FIGURE 28-2   Tonsils—normal and enlarged.

moves through the spleen, it is monitored by T cells for any non-self invaders. If a suspicious cell or molecule is detected, it is presented to the B cells for a match to an appropriate memory B cell. Once a matching B cell is activated, it divides rapidly and begins producing antibodies specific to the invading antigen.

The spleen's blood vessels are also lined with macrophages. In a disease such as mononucleosis, the macrophages in the spleen become overactive and trap a higher number of white blood cells. In the process, the spleen becomes swollen and may even rupture.

Tonsils

The **tonsils** are located in the depressions of the mucous membranes of the throat and pharynx (Figure 28-2). There are three sets: the palatine, the pharyngeal (**adenoids**), and the lingual. The function of the tonsils is to filter bacteria and aid in the formation of white blood cells.

PROFESSIONALISM
THE WORKPLACE

As a medical assistant, you work under the license of the physician. You and the physician are both team members, but you are still subordinate to physicians and their levels of education. Always address physicians by their title and name (e.g., "Dr. Morales"). Even if the physician has invited you to call him or her by a first name, never do so in front of a patient. This can undermine the doctor–patient relationship. Physicians refer to each other as "Dr. So-and-So" when talking to their patients, and the staff should take their cue from the physician. They have earned the right to be called "Dr.," and the medical assistant should honor that right.

The Immune System and the Body's Defenses

As previously noted, the immune system is the body's defense against infectious organisms and other pathogenic invaders. Through a series of steps called the **immune response**, the cells, tissues, and organs comprising the immune system work together to attack organisms and substances that invade body systems and cause disease.

Leukocytes, or white blood cells (WBCs), seek out and destroy harmful organisms. The two types of WBCs are phagocytes and lymphocytes.

Phagocytes attack the invading organism. A number of different cells are considered to be phagocytes, but the most common are **neutrophils**, which primarily fight off bacteria.

Lymphocytes allow the body to remember and recognize previous invading organisms. The two kinds of lymphocytes are B lymphocytes and T lymphocytes. Lymphocytes originate in the bone marrow and either stay there and mature into B cells or move to the thymus gland, where they mature into T cells. B lymphocytes and T lymphocytes have separate responsibilities within the immune system. B lymphocytes seek out invading organisms and send defenses to attach to them; T cells destroy the organisms that the B lymphocytes have identified.

HOW IMMUNITY WORKS: ANTIGENS VERSUS ANTIBODIES

When an antigen is detected, several types of cells work together to recognize and respond to it. These cells trigger the B lymphocytes to produce antibodies. This process is known as *humoral immunity*.

The terms *antibody* and *immunoglobulin* (glycoproteins that function as antibodies) are often used interchangeably. They are found in blood, tissue fluids, and many secretions. Structurally they are globulins, which means they are synthesized and secreted by plasma cells derived from the B cells of the immune system. B cells are activated on binding to their specific antigen and differentiating into plasma cells. In some cases, the interaction of the B cell with a T cell is also necessary.

Once antibodies have been produced, they remain in the body. If the same antigen is presented to the immune system again, the antibodies are already there to neutralize it. That is why if a person becomes ill with a specific disease, such as chickenpox, that person typically will not get sick from it again. It is also the reason immunizations, or vaccinations, are given to protect against specific diseases. A vaccine contains fragments of a disease organism or small amounts of a weakened disease organism. It stimulates the immune system to develop antibodies that can subsequently recognize and attack the same organism if the body is exposed to it. Although an immunization may not always completely prevent the disease, it will significantly reduce its severity. More information on immunizations is covered in Chapter 34.

Although antibodies can recognize an antigen and lock onto it, they are not capable of destroying it alone. That is the job of the T cells. T cells are part of the system that destroys antigens that have been tagged by antibodies or cells that have been infected or somehow changed. T cells also assist other cells, such as phagocytes. Antibodies can also neutralize toxins produced by different organisms. Finally, antibodies can activate a group of proteins called **complement** that are also part of the immune system. Complement assists in destroying bacteria, viruses, or infected cells.

Immunosuppressants are medications that suppress the immune system. These are usually given after an organ transplant to prevent rejection of the organ. However, these medications render the patient very vulnerable to illness because the natural immune process is impeded. Extreme stress can also suppress the immune system.

All these specialized cells and parts of the immune system protect the body against disease. This protection is called *immunity*. The three types of immunity are innate, active, and passive.

Innate Immunity

Everyone is born with innate, or natural, immunity. This immunity renders many of the viruses and bacteria that affect other species incapable of harming human beings. For example, the viruses that cause leukemia in cats or distemper in dogs do not affect humans. The reverse is also true. For example, the HIV/AIDS virus is not capable of infecting cats or dogs.

Innate immunity is provided in part by the external barriers of the body, including the skin and mucous membranes that line the nose, throat, and gastrointestinal tract, all of which constitute the body's first line of defense. If this outer defensive wall is broken, such as by a cut in the skin, special immune cells on the skin attack any invading microorganisms.

Active Immunity

The introduction of immunity by infection or with a vaccine is called **active immunity**. Active immunity is permanent, meaning that the individual has lifelong protection against the disease. **Acquired active immunity** occurs when the person is exposed to a live pathogen, develops the disease, and becomes immune as a result of the primary immune response. **Artificially acquired active immunity** is induced by a **vaccine**, a substance that contains the antigen and

stimulates a primary response against the antigen without causing symptoms of the disease.

Passive Immunity

Passive immunity is "borrowed" from another source and lasts for only a short time. For example, antibodies in breast milk provide an infant with temporary immunity to diseases to which the mother has been exposed. This immunity helps protect the infant against infection during the early years of childhood. **Natural immunity** is an inherited immunity to certain diseases. For example, certain people are naturally immune to the plague.

It is important to remember that everyone's immune system is different. Some people rarely get infections, whereas others seem to be sick all the time. As people mature, they are exposed to a wider variety of germs and develop immunity against them. That is why adults and teens tend to get fewer colds than children do; their bodies have learned to recognize and immediately attack many of the viruses that cause colds.

Common Disorders Associated with the Immune System

Immune system disorders occur when the immune response is inappropriate, excessive, or absent. A lack of one or more components of the immune system can result in a number of immunodeficiency disorders. Disorders may be inherited, acquired through infection or other illness, or produced as an inadvertent side effect of certain drug treatments (Table 28-1).

ALLERGIES

An **allergy** is a hypersensitivity to a normally harmless substance. An *allergen* is any substance capable of causing an allergic reaction. Most allergic reactions are a result of an immune system that responds to a "false alarm." When a harmless substance such as dust, mold, or pollen is encountered by a person who is allergic to that substance, the immune system may react dramatically by producing antibodies that "attack" the allergen. **Anaphylaxis** is an extreme, often life-threatening, response to an antigen. It is sometimes seen in a physician office after a vaccine or medication is introduced into the patient. For this reason, it is prudent to observe patients for 15 to 30 minutes after injections.

Signs and Symptoms. Symptoms of an allergic reaction may include wheezing, itching, runny nose, watery or itchy eyes, headache, nausea, and other reactions. During anaphylaxis, swelling on the neck can cause breathing to be

TABLE 28-1 Disorders of the Lymphatic System

Disorder	Description
Acquired immune deficiency syndrome (AIDS)	A disease that involves a defect in the cell-mediated immunity system. A syndrome of opportunistic infections occurs in the final stages of infection with the human immunodeficiency virus (HIV). This virus attacks T4 lymphocytes and destroys them, which reduces the person's ability to fight infection.
AIDS-related complex (ARC)	A complex of symptoms that appears in the early stages of AIDS. This is a positive test for the virus but only mild symptoms of weight loss, fatigue, skin rash, and anorexia.
Elephantiasis	Inflammation, obstruction, and destruction of the lymph vessels, which results in enlarged tissues due to edema.
Epstein-Barr virus	Virus believed to be the cause of infectious mononucleosis.
Hodgkin's disease	Lymphatic system disease that can result in solid tumors in any lymphoid tissue.
Lymphadenitis	Inflammation of the lymph glands. Referred to as swollen glands.
Lymphangioma	A benign mass of lymphatic vessels.
Lymphoma	Malignant tumor of the lymph nodes and tissue.
Lymphosarcoma	Malignant disease of the lymphatic tissue.
Mononucleosis	Acute infectious disease with a large number of atypical lymphocytes. Caused by the Epstein-Barr virus. There may be abnormal liver function and spleen enlargement.
Multiple sclerosis	Autoimmune disorder of the central nervous system in which the myelin sheath of nerves is attacked.
Non-Hodgkin's lymphoma	Malignant, solid tumors of lymphoid tissue.
Peritonsillar abscess	Infection of the tissues between the tonsils and the pharynx. Also called quinsy sore throat.
Sarcoidosis	Inflammatory disease of the lymph system in which lesions may appear in the liver, skin, lungs, lymph nodes, spleen, eyes, and small bones of the hands and feet.
Splenomegaly	Enlargement of the spleen.
Systemic lupus erythematosus (SLE)	A chronic autoimmune disorder of connective tissue that causes injury to the skin, joints, kidneys, mucous membranes, and nervous system.
Thymoma	Malignant tumor of the thymus gland.

impeded, and that can lead to hypoxia and death. Therefore, it is vital to react quickly to any complaint of swelling on the throat.

Treatment. Allergies are rarely cured, but many medications, supplements, and other treatment options are available to help relieve symptoms. The best strategy for a person with an allergy is to avoid the offending allergen. If that is not possible, treatment may include the use of antihistamines or decongestants to help combat allergy symptoms. Reactions to certain airborne allergens may be treated by the use of air filters and dehumidifiers. Alternative treatments include acupressure and chiropractic treatments. In severe cases, optimal treatment may be identified only through specific allergy testing and desensitization. If anaphylaxis occurs, it is important for the physician to immediately order medications (such as epinephrine) that will stop the process. Of great concern is swelling in the neck during anaphylaxis because it can cause breathing to stop. See Chapter 37 for more information on allergies.

CANCER

Cancer is actually a group of many related diseases that all have to do with cells. Cancer cells do not appear or act as normal cells; rather, they grow and spread very rapidly. Normal body cells grow and, through mitosis, divide and know when to stop growing. Over time, they also die. Unlike normal cells, cancer cells continue to grow and divide erratically and do not die. Cancer cells are also not well differentiated, so they do not work on behalf of the body. Instead, they make use of the body's resources at the expense of healthy cells.

Cancer cells usually clump together to form tumors. A growing tumor can destroy the normal cells around it and damage the body's healthy tissues. Sometimes cancer cells break away from the original tumor and travel to other areas of the body, where they keep growing and form new tumors. This process is called **metastasis**.

Cancer and the Immune System

When the immune system is operating at its peak, it recognizes, attacks, and destroys the cancerous cells before potentially deadly growth and multiplication can occur. However, if those cells are not destroyed immediately by the immune system, the new cancer cells avoid the usual controls on growth and multiplication in normal cells. The growth begins when **oncogenes**, the genes controlling cell growth and multiplication, are transformed by cancer-causing agents, called carcinogens, into cancer-producing cells. These abnormal cancer cells divide more rapidly than the normal surrounding cells. The fast multiplication results in invasion and destruction of normal body cells.

Cancerous cells act as uncontrollable parasites, consuming needed nutrients while contributing nothing except malnutrition. If they are not killed and removed, these cancerous cells can metastasize from their original site via the bloodstream and lymphatic system to other parts of the body and are potentially fatal if they cause vital organs to fail.

The immune response is critical to eliminating or controlling cancer. A healthy immune response recognizes cancerous cells and responds quickly to kill them. A suppressed or impaired immune response fails to respond in a timely manner when overwhelmed by a massive number of corrupted cancer cells that have multiplied rapidly and undetected. An impaired immune response exposes the body to the development and spread of, too-often, deadly cancer cells in the body.

Whereas the causes of cancer are relatively unknown, certain risk factors may predispose a person to cancer. These include the presence of a suppressed immune system; exposure to radiation, tobacco, toxins, or environmental stressors; and some viruses.

Signs and Symptoms. Cancer signs and symptoms depend on the site of the tumor and include, but are not limited to, tissues that change color and shape (melanoma), lumps that form (breast cancer, uterine cancer, prostate cancer), shortness of breath (lung cancer), hoarse speech (throat cancer), and depressed organ function (thyroid).

Treatment. Cancer may be treated with surgery, chemotherapy, radiation, or a combination of all three. The choice of treatment generally depends on the type of cancer and the stage (i.e., the extent to which the cancer has spread within the body) of the tumor. For thyroid cancer, for example, radiation and surgery are the preferred treatment. For blood cancers, chemotherapy might be best. If the cancer is in the later stages, more drastic treatment (such as chemotherapy) might be necessary. Surgery is the oldest form of cancer treatment.

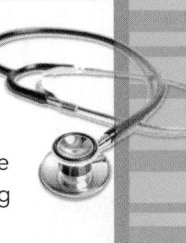
Three out of every five people with cancer may require surgery to remove it. During surgery some healthy cells or tissue may also be removed to make sure that all the cancer is removed.

In **chemotherapy**, anticancer drugs are used to treat the cancerous growth or tumor. These medicines are sometimes taken in pill form but more often are given intravenously. Chemotherapy usually is given over a number of weeks or months. Often, a port-a-cath, a permanent intravenous (IV) catheter, is placed under the skin into one of the larger blood vessels of the upper chest. This method allows the administration of several courses of chemotherapy and other medicines through the catheter without the need to insert a new IV needle each time. The catheter remains under the skin until the cancer treatment is completed.

Radiation therapy uses high-energy waves, such as X-rays, to damage and destroy cancer cells. This form of treatment causes tumors to shrink and, in some cases, disappear completely. Radiation therapy is one of the most common treatments for cancer.

The most modern form of cancer therapy involves creating mutated defense cells that are "programmed" to specifically target cancer cells. This empowers the body's own immune system to target only cancer cells, rather than also destroying healthy cells. This process is known as immunotherapy.

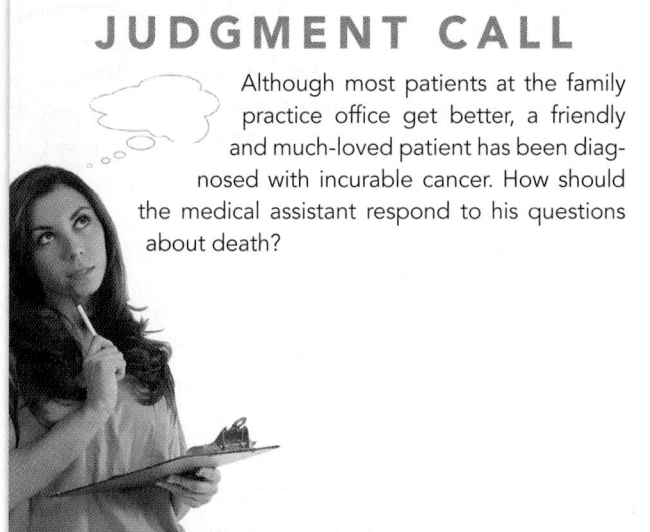
CHRONIC FATIGUE SYNDROME

Although there is no single known cause of **chronic fatigue syndrome (CFS)**, some authorities believe it is a condition shared by many different underlying diseases rather than a separate disorder. Others believe it is caused by a defect of the immune system. Hormonal deficits, low blood pressure, and viral infections have also been studied as possible causes or contributors. There is some correlation between chronic single and multiple viral infections, but CFS has also been identified in the absence of any apparent viral infection. Food allergies, candidiasis, intestinal parasites, and exposure to toxic chemicals are all commonly associated with this disorder.

Signs and Symptoms. Signs and symptoms include depression, sleep disorders, and lack of energy.

Treatment. Any treatment regimen for CFS generally begins with a thorough evaluation of the patient's prior treatment history. Both the quality and quantity of sleep are important factors. Educating the patient with emphasis on

becoming an active participant in the treatment regimen is extremely important in the treatment of CFS.

INFECTIOUS MONONUCLEOSIS

Infectious mononucleosis is a viral infection caused by the Epstein-Barr virus (EBV), which is part of the herpes family of viruses. It is characterized by an increase of white blood cells that are mononuclear (i.e., they contain only a single nucleus); hence the common slang term for the disease, *mono*. Because it often develops in young adults between the ages of 15 and 24 and is frequently spread through saliva, mono is also commonly referred to as the *kissing disease*. The illness is less severe in young children. The incubation period for mono is generally between 4 and 8 weeks.

Signs and Symptoms. Symptoms of mono include fever, fatigue, sore throat, and swollen lymph glands.

Treatment. There is usually no treatment for this disorder other than getting plenty of rest, gargling with saltwater or using throat lozenges to soothe a sore throat, and taking antipyritic and analgesic medications to reduce fever and relieve sore throat and headache. If neglected, mono can lead to liver inflammation, or hepatitis, as well as enlargement of the spleen. Recovery from mono generally takes several weeks. However, for some individuals, it may be several months before they regain their normal energy levels.

LYMPHEDEMA

Lymphedema is a condition that results from a damaged or dysfunctional lymphatic system (Figure 28-3). There are two different types of lymphedema. The first, primary lymphedema, can be hereditary and has several stages. Secondary lymphedema is generally caused by an obstruction of or damage to the lymph system that interrupts the normal lymphatic flow.

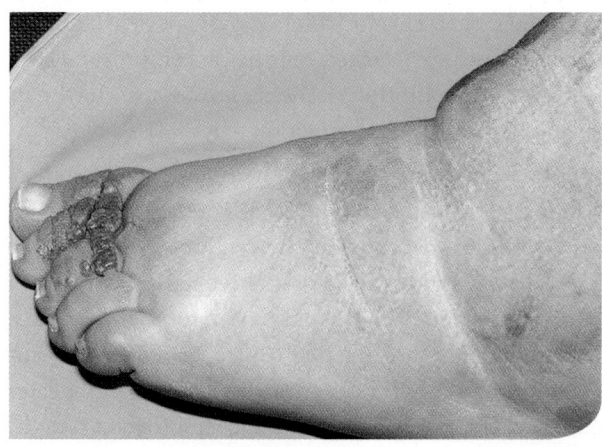

FIGURE 28-3 Chronic lymphedema.

A developmental disorder of the lymphatics, in utero infection or injury, and difficulties during delivery are among the likely causes of congenital primary lymphedema. The causes of secondary lymphedema are multiple. Infections from insect bites, serious wounds, or burns can damage or destroy lymphatics, as can any type of serious injury. Radiation for cancer treatments is also a cause. Outside the tropics the leading cause of secondary lymphedema is the removal of lymph nodes for cancer biopsies. Through improved techniques for small-needle biopsies, advances in diagnostic radiology, and site-specific node biopsies, there has been a marked decrease in secondary lymphedema.

Signs and Symptoms.   Swelling at the lymph nodes is the primary sign.

Treatment.   The preferred treatments for lymphedema are complete decongestive therapy (CDT) and manual decongestive therapy (MDT). CDT is used primarily in the treatment of lymphedema. CDT is a combination of MDT, bandaging exercises, and skin care, and it also may involve breathing exercises, compressive garments, and a dietary regimen. For lymphedema caused by irradiation or surgery for cancer, CDT can relieve edema, fibrosis, and the accompanying pain and discomfort. Other treatments include the use of compression pumps, surgery, and newer approaches such as lasers, liposuction, and even acupuncture.

RHEUMATOID ARTHRITIS

Rheumatoid arthritis (RA) is a chronic autoimmune disease. One of the ways in which the immune system works is by producing antibodies that destroy invading organisms such as viruses and bacteria. Sometimes, the immune system produces antibodies that stick to the body's own cells. These antibodies, called *autoantibodies,* cause an inflammatory reaction that results in damage to the body's own cells. This creates **autoimmune diseases**, in which the body attacks itself. RA is one of these diseases.

RA causes a great deal of suffering, reduced quality of life, major financial burden, and loss of income due to functional impairment and the prospect of becoming an invalid. Out of every 100 persons, 1 suffers from chronic RA. Individuals with a family history of RA are four times more likely to develop the disease than others.

RA occurs when the body's immune defenses attack tissue in the joints, leading to pain and degeneration of the articular cartilage. The disease and its treatment also increase mortality, and patients often have a shorter life expectancy than their healthy peers.

Signs and Symptoms.   Symptoms include pain and stiffness in the joints.

Treatment.   The treatment of RA is based on medication regimens and educating the patient on how to facilitate daily activities. Drugs are used to treat and reduce the symptoms and to help the patient to function at a more productive level. However, since drugs are only effective symptomatically they do not actually treat or cure the disease. That being said, treating the symptoms is only part of the regimen for the RA patient. Maintenance of joint function is equally important.

SYSTEMIC LUPUS ERYTHEMATOSUS

Systemic lupus erythematosus (SLE) is another autoimmune disorder. Patients suffering from SLE produce abnormal antibodies in their blood that target tissues within their own body rather than foreign infectious agents. SLE is called a systemic disorder because its effects may appear in many parts of the body—that is, it is systemwide. *Lupus* refers to a type of skin rash, and *erythematosus* means "red."

Women constitute 90 percent of patients with SLE, and they are generally diagnosed before menopause. There is a genetic component as well, as the risk of developing SLE rises if a close family member has it.

Signs and Symptoms.   SLE can produce many different symptoms and imitate many other diseases. Many patients with SLE have pain and swelling in the joints. They may also suffer from general fatigue, fever, chills, and headache.

Round (discoid) lesions that are raised and scaly affect about 20 percent of patients with SLE. This condition is known as discoid lupus erythematosus. If left untreated, these lesions expand and can cause severe scarring.

A condition that may be present with lupus is vasculitis, or inflamed blood vessels, characterized by red marks in any area of the body. Sometimes deep red lumps appear, especially on the leg, where they may develop into ulcers. In some people, the tips of the fingers and toes may develop reddish-purple lesions.

Treatment.   Unfortunately, there is no cure for most autoimmune diseases, and SLE is no exception. Treatment is usually aimed at reducing the immune response by using drugs such as steroids. SLE is a chronic, lifelong condition with periods of remission and relapse. The course for a given individual is difficult to predict, but with immediate treatment, most patients can expect to have a normal life span.

SUMMARY

The immune system is the body's defense against infectious organisms and other pathogenic invaders. The organs that function together in the immune system are the bone marrow, spleen, thymus gland, lymph nodes, tonsils, appendix, and a few others. There are three types of immunity: innate, active, and passive. When the immune system is functioning properly, it attacks antigens by forming antibodies. Immune system disorders occur when the immune response is inappropriate, excessive, or absent.

Disorders may be inherited, acquired through infection or other illness, or produced as an inadvertent side effect of certain drug treatments. An allergy is an overreaction of the immune system to an allergen. Many cancers appear to have a genetic component, but cancer production is usually a combination of predisposing genetic makeup and environmental carcinogenic factors that trigger the inappropriate immune response. Treatment for cancer includes surgery, radiation, chemotherapy, and measures that boost the correct immune response.

Viral infections can cause infectious mononucleosis. Chronic fatigue syndrome has many possible causes. A dysfunctional immune system may lead to lymphedema. When the immune system inappropriately attacks joints, rheumatoid arthritis results. Systemic lupus erythematosus is an autoimmune disease that causes systemic problems.

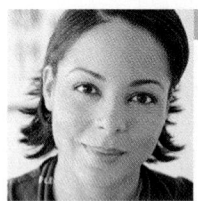

28 CHAPTER REVIEW

COMPETENCY REVIEW

1. Define and spell the terms to learn for this chapter.
2. What is the function of leukocytes?
3. What is the most common type of leukocyte?
4. What is the main function of the immune system?
5. Name the three accessory organs of the lymphatic system.
6. What is the difference between innate immunity and active immunity?
7. Explain what causes allergies.
8. List four causes of cancer.
9. List four treatments for cancer.
10. List five symptoms of systemic lupus erythematosus.

PREPARING FOR THE CERTIFICATION EXAM

1. What structures are foreign substances that invade the body?
   a. neutrophils
   b. lymphocytes
   c. phagocytes
   d. antigens
   e. antibodies

2. An autoimmune disorder in which the myelin sheath of nerves is attacked is
   a. sarcoidosis
   b. thymoma
   c. elephantiasis
   d. multiple sclerosis
   e. mononucleosis

3. Immunity conferred to a breast-feeding infant by his mother is
   a. innate immunity
   b. active immunity
   c. passive immunity
   d. vaccination immunity
   e. immunosuppression

4. An autoimmune viral disease that is believed to be the cause of infectious mononucleosis is
   a. allergies
   b. Epstein-Barr virus
   c. Hodgkin's disease
   d. acquired immune deficiency syndrome
   e. elephantiasis

5. Which immune system organ is found in the pharynx?
   a. thymus
   b. bone marrow
   c. spleen
   d. tonsils
   e. liver

6. Which of the following is the usual treatment for systemic lupus erythematosus?
   a. chemotherapy
   b. radiation
   c. surgery
   d. steroidal medications
   e. diet and exercise changes

7. If the medical assistant works for Dr. Charles Cole, who goes by the name "Chuck," how should the medical assistant address him in front of patients?
   a. Dr. Cole
   b. Doc
   c. Charles
   d. Chuck
   e. Cole

8. All of the following are believed to be risk factors for cancer in predisposed patients EXCEPT
   a. immunosuppression
   b. tobacco
   c. radiation
   d. bacteria
   e. viruses

9. All of the following are malignant tumors EXCEPT
   a. hematoma
   b. thymoma
   c. lymphoma
   d. lymphosarcoma
   e. adenocarcinoma

10. Which disorder affects the joints, has familial risk factors, and affects 1 in 100 people?
   a. lymphedema
   b. mononucleosis
   c. chronic fatigue syndrome
   d. rheumatoid arthritis
   e. allergies

CRITICAL THINKING

1. Why was it important to note that Rosa was having many cold and flulike symptoms?

2. Why did the physician order a complete blood cell count?

3. Why did the physician tell Rosa to get plenty of rest and decide to monitor her for any other viral infections?

INTERNET ACTIVITY

Do an Internet search for chronic fatigue syndrome services in your hometown. What resources are available in your area?

MEDMEDIA

Additional interactive resources and activities for this chapter can be found:

On your student DVD: View applicable procedure videos on the DVD-ROM found in the back of this book.

MyHealthProfessionsKit.com: Test your knowledge of this chapter with games and activities. MyHealthProfessionsKit also includes resources, helpful links, and a Spanish audio glossary.

Medical Assisting Interactive: Practice your procedures as a medical assistant in this simulated doctor's office. This can be accessed through MyHealthProfessionsKit.com.

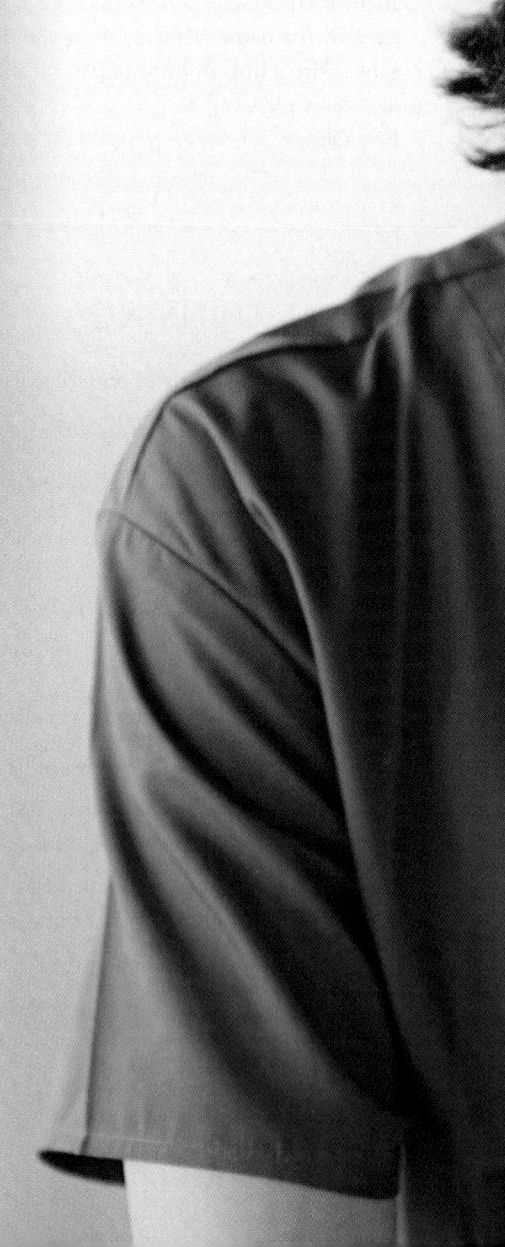

29

The Respiratory System

LEARNING OBJECTIVES

After completing this chapter, you should be able to:

- Define and spell the terms to learn for this chapter.

- Explain the purpose and function of the respiratory system.

- List and explain the structures and functions of the organs of the respiratory system.

- Explain the different respiratory volumes and capacities.

- Identify and discuss common disorders associated with the respiratory system.

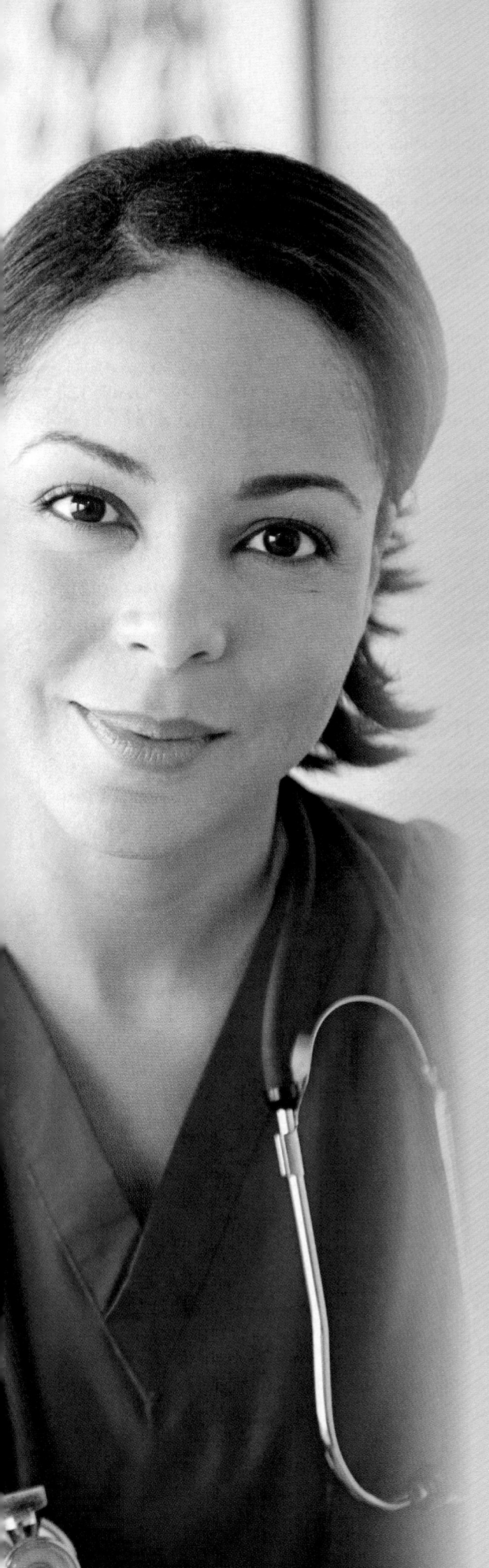

CHAPTER OUTLINE

CASE STUDY

Collin McConnley is a 57-year-old businessman who travels 80 percent of his work week. It is a hot summer day, and he has an appointment with Dr. Miller because he believes that he has the flu. His symptoms include severe headache, blood-stained mucus, high fever with cold sweats, and diarrhea.

alveoli	larynx
apnea	Legionnaires' disease
arterial blood gases (ABGs)	lung cancer
asphyxia	lungs
asthma	nares
bronchi	orthopnea
bronchitis	pertussis (whooping cough)
bronchodilators	pharynx
carbon dioxide (CO_2)	pleura
chronic obstructive pulmonary disease (COPD)	pleurisy
cilia	pneumonia
common cold	pneumothorax
cyanosis	pulmonary edema
diaphragm	pulmonary embolism (PE)
dyspnea	septum
emphysema	severe acute respiratory syndrome (SARS)
epiglottis	sinuses
expiration	sinusitis
hay fever	tonsils
hemoptysis	trachea
hila	tuberculosis (TB)
influenza	visceral pleura
inspiration	

CERTIFICATION LINK

CMA (AAMA)
Anatomy and physiology

   Systems (including structure, function, related conditions and diseases, and their relationships)

RMA
Anatomy and physiology

   Body systems
   Disorders and diseases of the body

CMAS (AMT)
Medical assisting foundation

   Anatomy and physiology
   Medical terminology

The primary function of the respiratory system is to supply oxygen to the blood, which delivers it to all parts of the body. It does this through breathing. When we breathe, we inhale oxygen and exhale carbon dioxide. This exchange of gases is the respiratory system's means of getting oxygen to—and carrying carbon dioxide, a waste product, away from—the cells of the body.

Overview of the Respiratory System

Respiration is achieved through the mouth, nose, trachea, lungs, and diaphragm. Oxygen enters the respiratory system through the mouth and the nose. The oxygen then passes through the larynx (where speech sounds are produced) and the trachea, which is a tube that enters the chest cavity. In the chest cavity, the trachea splits into two smaller tubes, the bronchi. Each bronchus then divides again, forming the bronchial tubes. The bronchial tubes lead directly into the lungs, where they divide into many smaller tubes called bronchioles that connect to tiny sacs, the alveoli. The **alveoli** perform the gas exchange between oxygen and carbon dioxide for the lungs. The inhaled oxygen passes into the alveoli and then diffuses through the capillaries into the arterial blood. Meanwhile, the waste-rich blood from the veins releases carbon dioxide into the alveoli. The diaphragm helps pump air into, and carbon dioxide out of, the lungs. On exhalation, the carbon dioxide follows the same path out of the lungs by which oxygen flowed into the lungs.

Organs of the Respiratory System

The organs of the respiratory system extend from the nose to the lungs The system is divided into the upper and lower respiratory tracts (Figure 29-1). The upper respiratory tract consists of the nose, paranasal sinuses, and pharynx (or throat). The lower respiratory tract includes the larynx (or voicebox); the trachea (which splits into two main branches called bronchi); tiny branches of the bronchi called bronchioles; and the lungs, a pair of saclike, spongy organs. The nose, pharynx, larynx, trachea, bronchi, and bronchioles move air to and from the lungs. The lungs interact with the circulatory system to deliver oxygen and remove carbon dioxide. The sinuses drain into the nose.

NOSE

The nose is the organ of smell and also part of the apparatus of respiration and voice (Figure 29-2). It also performs several other functions:

- Serving as a passageway for air
- Warming and moistening inhaled air
- Trapping dust, pollen, and other foreign matter with hairlike projections (**cilia**)
- Assisting in the making of sounds for speaking and singing

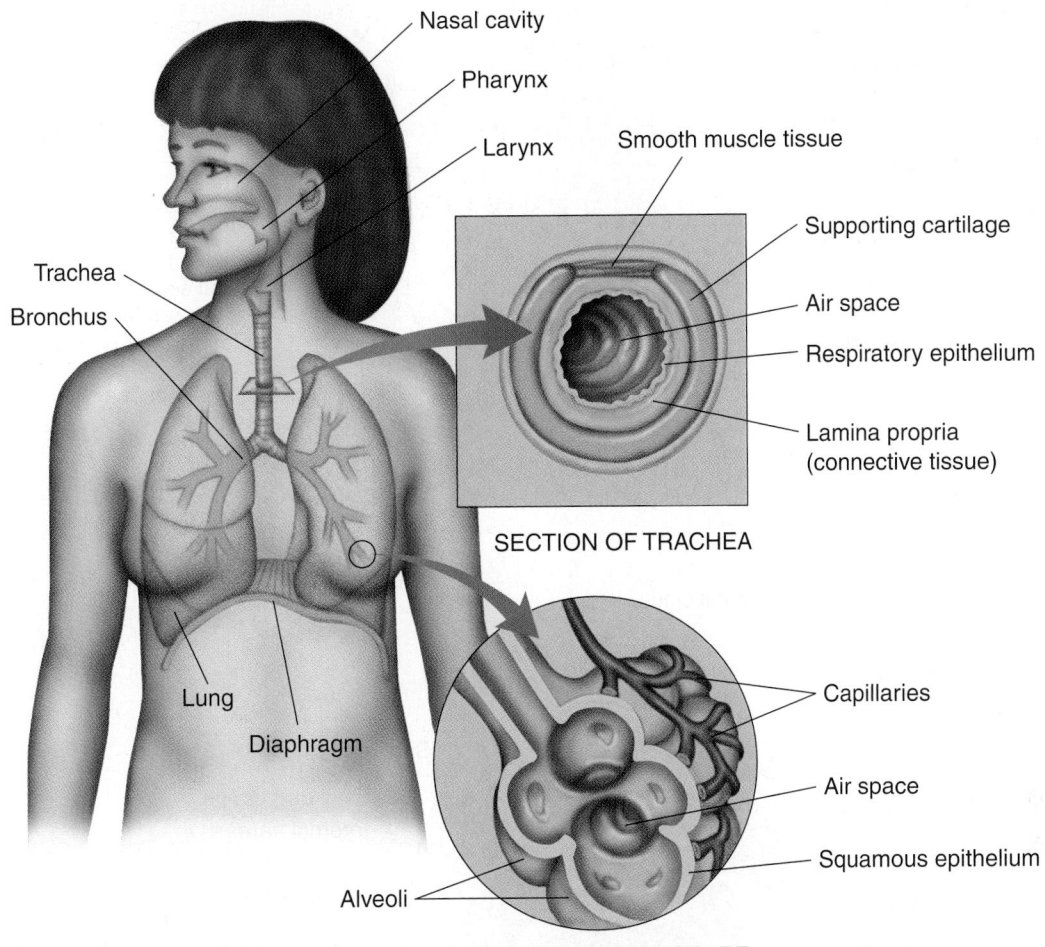

FIGURE 29-1 **The respiratory system: nasal cavity, pharynx, larynx, trachea, bronchi, and lungs with expanded views of the trachea and alveolar structure.**

Anatomically, the nose is divided into external and internal portions. The external portion, the visible projection to which the term *nose* is popularly applied, is made up of bone and cartilage and is lined with mucous membrane. The external entrances are the nostrils, or **nares**.

The internal portion of the nose consists of two principal cavities, or nasal fossae, separated by the **septum**, a cartilaginous wall also lined with mucous membrane. Each side of the nose is divided into three air passageways—conchae (inferior, middle, and superior) or turbinates—that connect to the Eustachian tube (to the ear), the paranasal sinuses (also known as "the sinuses"), and the nasolacrimal ducts. The conchae form a "maze" in which air moves around, which allows for warming of the air and removal of foreign particles by the mucus secreted by the mucous membranes (mucosae). The nasal mucosae produce about one quart of mucus per day, which moistens the air moving through the nose and traps pollen, dust, and other foreign matter traveling through the nose. The nose is separated from the mouth by the palatine bones of the skull.

The nasolacrimal ducts drain fluid from the eyes into the nose, which explains why your nose runs when you cry. The nose also drains the four pairs of paranasal **sinuses** (cavities)—the maxillary sinuses over the medial portion on the cheekbones; the frontal sinuses over the eyebrows; the ethmoidal sinuses in the area between and behind the eyes; and the sphenoidal sinuses behind the ethmoidal sinuses. The sinuses decrease the weight of the skull by creating air pockets, aid in phonation, and provide protection and insulation.

PHARYNX

The **pharynx** is a musculomembranous tube approximately 5 inches long that stretches from the base of the skull to the cervical spine and connects to the trachea and esophagus. The major functions of the pharynx include serving as a passageway for air and food and assisting in the production and sound of speech.

The pharynx consists of three parts: the nasopharynx, which connects with the nose; the oropharynx, which connects with the back of the mouth; and the laryngopharynx,

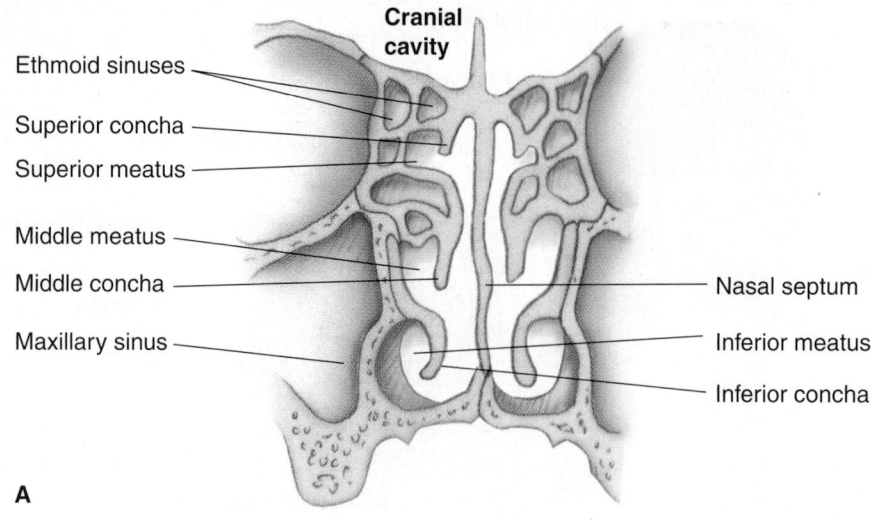

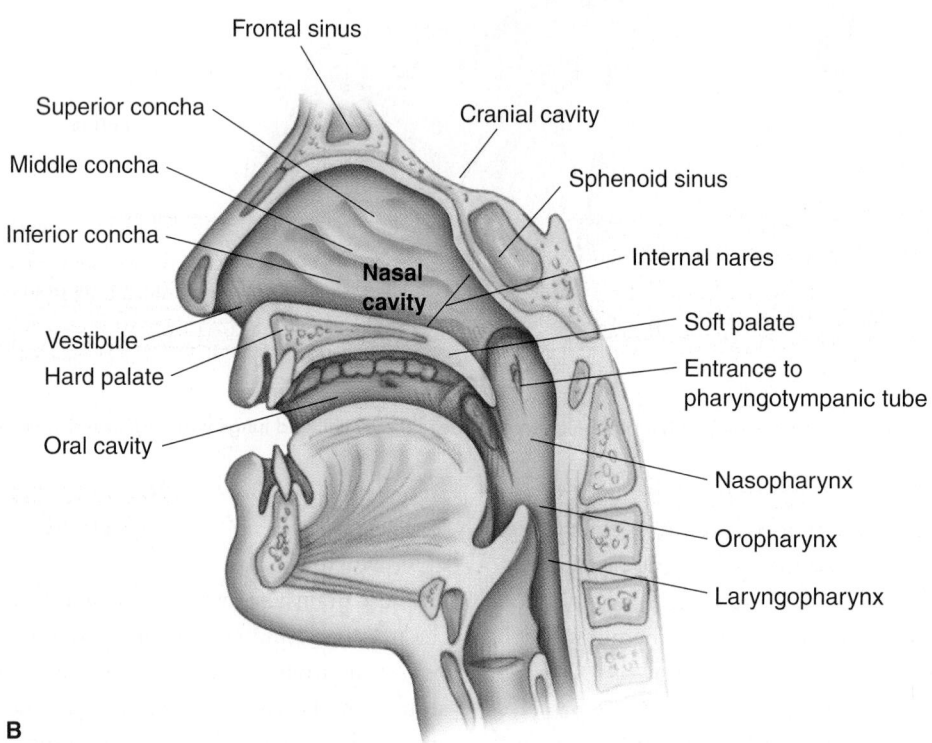

FIGURE 29-2 The nasal cavity and pharynx: (A) meatuses and positions of the entrance to the ethmoid and maxillary sinuses; (B) sagittal section of the nasal cavity and pharynx.

behind the larynx, where the pharynx is located. Three pairs of **tonsils** reside in the pharynx:

- **Pharyngeal tonsils (adenoids)**—located behind the nose and often blamed for snoring, especially in children
- **Palatine tonsils**—often referred to as "the tonsils," located on either side of the throat on the anterior portion of the oropharynx
- **Lingual tonsils**—located at the base of the tongue

The tonsils are part of the immune system and help in infection control.

LARYNX

The **larynx** is also known as the voicebox (Figure 29-3). It is a muscular, cartilaginous structure lined with mucous membrane and connected to the inferior (lower) end of the pharynx. The larynx has several cartilaginous structures, three of which help protect it from trauma:

- The thyroid cartilage, or Adam's apple, is the largest of the cartilage structures.
- The epiglottic cartilage, or epiglottis, covers the trachea (windpipe) during swallowing so that food is directed

down the esophagus to the stomach rather than down the trachea and into the lungs.

- The C-shaped cricoid cartilage, the lowest cartilage in the larynx, wraps around it to protect it from pressure. The "opening" in the "C" allows for large boluses of food to be swallowed down the esophagus.

The interior of the larynx contains the false and true vocal folds and the entrance of the glottis, the opening between the true vocal folds through which air passes. The larynx functions in the production of vocal sounds. When the vocal cords are long and relaxed, low sounds are produced. Short, tense vocal cords produce higher-pitched notes. The nose, mouth, pharynx, and bony sinuses impact other aspects of sound production.

TRACHEA

The **trachea** or windpipe, is a cartilaginous tube about 1 inch wide and 4.5 inches long that extends between the larynx and the main bronchi (Figure 29-3). As with the larynx, C-shaped rings of cartilage protect its structure and shape. The interior of the trachea is lined with mucous membrane and cilia that trap foreign matter. The most important function of the trachea is to serve as an open passageway through which air reaches the lungs. The **epiglottis** is a flap of tissue that covers the trachea when swallowing occurs to prevent food from entering the trachea.

BRONCHI

The **bronchi** are the two main branches of the trachea that extend into the lungs (Figure 29-3). These structures are the passageway for air between the trachea and the lungs. The right bronchus is the longer, larger branch moving down the right side of the heart. The left bronchus is shorter and more vertical, as it makes room for the heart in the chest cavity. After entering the lungs at the hilum, the bronchi subdivide into the bronchial tree, which continues to branch into smaller and smaller branches, or bronchioles.

LUNGS

Eventually, the bronchioles terminate at the alveoli in the lungs, the small air sacs that support a network of capillaries that perform oxygen and carbon dioxide transfer (Figure 29-4). In healthy individuals, the alveoli resemble small balloons that inflate and deflate as air moves in and out. The average adult's lungs contain about 600 million of these spongy, air-filled sacs.

The **lungs** are large, conical, lobed, spongy organs in the chest (see Figure 29-3). At birth the lungs are pinkish in color, but as adulthood approaches they turn a dark, slate-gray. The lungs are porous and spongy in texture and highly elastic. The

right lung is made up of three lobes: the upper, middle, and lower lobes. The right lung has three lobes, but the left lung only has two—an upper and a lower lobe—because the heart takes up that chest space. Each lung is between 10 and 12 inches in length. The two lungs are separated by the mediastinum, a space that contains the heart, trachea, esophagus, and blood vessels. The bases of the lungs are called **hila**.

The **pleura**, made up of thin sheets of epithelium sometimes referred to as pleural membranes, covers the outer surface of the lungs and the inside of the thoracic cavity. The pleural space separates two layers of the pleura: the parietal pleura and the **visceral pleura**. The pleura produces surfactant,

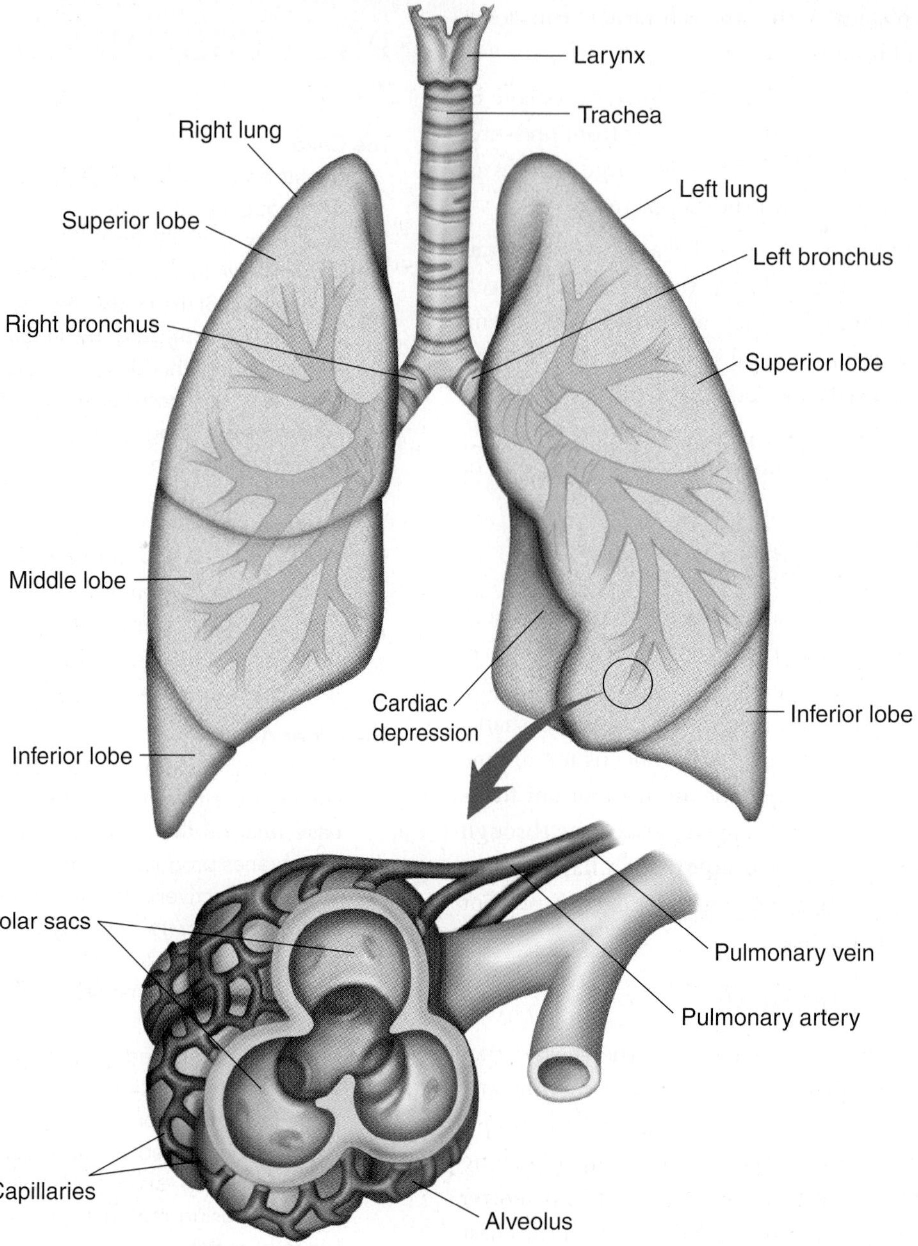

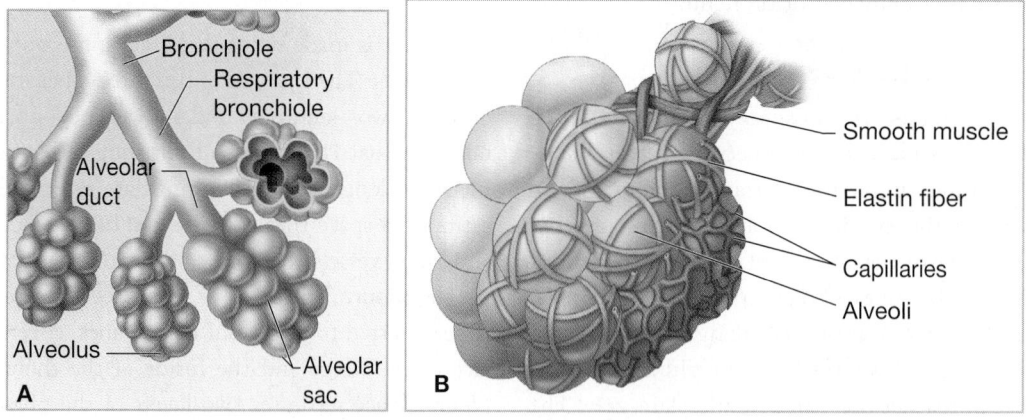

FIGURE 29-3 The larynx, trachea, bronchi, and lungs with an expanded view showing the structures of an alveolus and the pulmonary blood vessels.

FIGURE 29-4 (A) Alveolar sac; (B) alveoli with capillaries.

a lubricating fluid that helps the lungs glide smoothly in the chest cavity during inhalation and exhalation.

The lungs are made up of three dozen distinct types of cells. Some of these cells scavenge foreign matter. Others have cilia that sweep the mucous membranes lining the smallest air passages. Some cells act on blood pressure control, whereas others spot infectious invaders. The most important function of the lungs is to bring air into contact with the blood in order to facilitate the exchange of gases in the alveoli.

Mechanism of Breathing

Ventilation is the term for the movement of air to and from the alveoli. The two processes of ventilation are inhalation and exhalation, which are brought about by the nervous system and the respiratory muscles. The respiratory centers are located in the brainstem, specifically in the medulla oblongata and the pons. The respiratory muscles are the diaphragm and the internal and external intercostal muscles.

The **diaphragm** is the dome-shaped muscle below the lungs that separates the thoracic cavity from the abdominal cavity. The intercostal muscles are located between the ribs. The external intercostal muscles pull the ribs upward and outward, and the internal intercostal muscles pull the ribs downward and inward. Ventilation is the result of changes in pressure within the alveoli and bronchial tree brought about by the respiratory muscles.

Difficulty breathing is known as **dyspnea**. The absence of breathing for more than 19 seconds is termed **apnea**. If a patient has trouble breathing unless a certain position is maintained (such as with head elevated), it is termed **orthopnea**.

INHALATION

Inhalation, or **inspiration**, involves a precise sequence of events. The nervous system sends an impulse to the diaphragm and external intercostal muscles. The diaphragm contracts and flattens, which increases the top-to-bottom length of the thorax. This contraction elevates the ribs and increases the size of the thorax from the front to the back and from side to side. The increase in the size of the chest cavity reduces pressure within it, and what follows is an active process through which air moves into the lungs.

EXHALATION

Quiet *exhalation,* or **expiration**, is ordinarily a passive process. During expiration the diaphragm relaxes and the thorax returns to its resting size and shape. The elastic recoil of lung tissues aids in quiet expiration. Forceful expiration involves the internal intercostals and abdominal muscles. The reduction in the size of the thoracic cavity builds pressure and causes air to leave the lungs. Figure 29-5 illustrates the mechanism of breathing.

Respiratory Volumes and Capacities

During the act of breathing, different volumes of air move in and out at different capacities, which can be calculated by adding together specific respiratory volumes. We can assess lung flexibility and capacity by doing respiratory function testing. These tests are also used for baseline measurement to determine over time the effects of certain occupations such as coal mining or cleaning asbestos from walls. For example, when measuring lung volume, the following volumes would be used:

- Tidal volume (V_T) = volume of air entering or leaving the lungs during a single breath. Although the individual being tested may have more air in the lungs (residual volume), the actual amount moving in and out (like a tidal wave) is called the tidal volume.

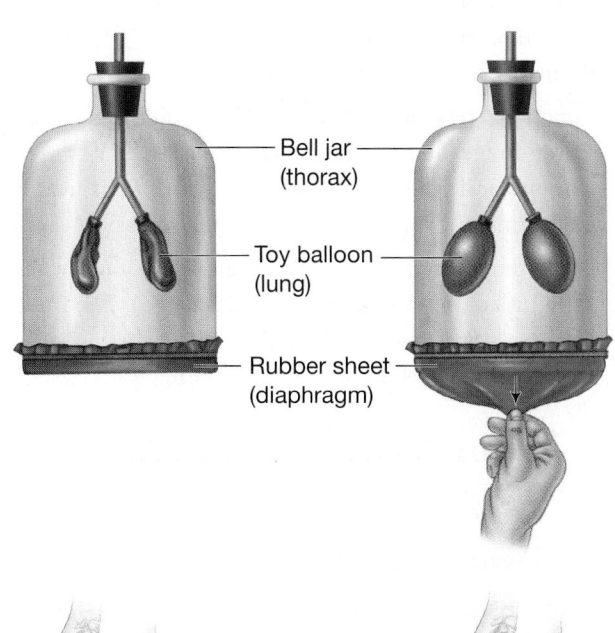

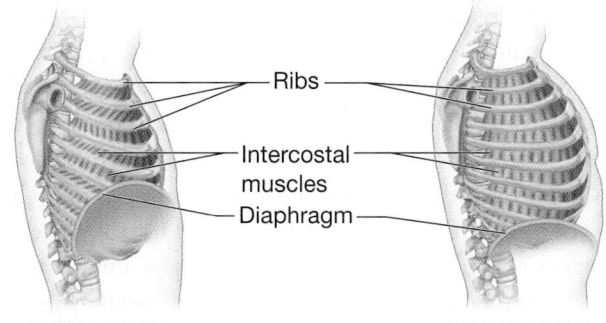

EXPIRATION   **INSPIRATION**

FIGURE 29-5 **Mechanism of breathing.**

- Inspiratory reserve volume (IRV), or complemental air = volume of air that can be inspired over and above the resting tidal volume. If the individual being tested forces the lungs to suck in more air than usual, this measurement is not valid.

- Expiratory reserve volume (ERV), or supplemental air = volume of air that can be expired after a normal expiration. The individual being tested is asked to blow out as completely as possible after normal expiration.

- Residual volume (RV) = volume of air remaining in the lungs after a maximal expiration, which can be estimated as 25 percent of the vital capacity. This is what is left in the lungs after the individual being tested has truly forced out as much air as possible.

When measuring lung capacities, the following measurements would be used:

- Inspiratory capacity (IC) = maximum volume that can be inspired after a normal expiration = VT + IRV. The medical assistant should say, "Breathe out. . . . Now breathe in as much as you can."

- Vital capacity (VC) = maximum volume that can be expired after a maximal inspiration = VT + IRV + ERV. The medical assistant should say, "Breathe in deeply. . . . Now breathe out deeply."

- Functional residual capacity (FRC) = volume of air left in the lungs after a normal expiration = ERV + RV. The medical assistant should say, "After you breathe out normally, breathe out again as much air as you can."

- Total lung capacity (TLC) = volume of the lungs when fully inflated = VC + RV (or 1.25 × VC). The medical assistant computes this figure using the measurements gained with the preceding commands.

Common Disorders Associated with the Respiratory System

Pulmonary diseases have a wide range of presentation, from life threatening to mildly irritating. Many are present in childhood, whereas others develop during the aging process. Any lack of oxygen, known as hypoxia, can be serious. It can lead to **asphyxia** or suffocation. **Arterial blood gases (ABGs)** are drawn by drawing blood out of the arteries. Unlike venipuncture, arterial blood draws are usually done by physicians. If ordered, they must be processed immediately to truly ascertain the level of oxygen and carbon dioxide (CO_2) in the blood because these gases evaporate quickly.

Carbon dioxide is a compound of carbon and oxygen, given off in the process of metabolism in the cells, and expired from the body through the lungs.

ASTHMA

Asthma is a chronic inflammatory disease of the bronchi. It is typically caused when allergens or other irritating substances cause swelling in the lining of the trachea and bronchial tubes, aggravating sensitive tissues. The tissues create mucus in an attempt to trap the offending intruder, which can cause coughing or a sense of struggling to breathe, which, in turn, causes more swelling and more mucus production. A vicious cycle results.

Asthma is related to the same process that causes allergic reactions, so the two disorders are usually related. Asthma can begin during childhood, but adult-onset asthma is also common.

Signs and Symptoms. Difficult respirations, or dyspnea, and cough are classic signs of asthma.

Treatment. Bronchodilators, which open the bronchial passages, are the treatment of choice for asthma. Most individuals with asthma carry an inhaler of a beta-2 medication, either albuterol or pirbuterol. This type of medication is a rescue medicine used during an asthma episode.

Long-term, preventive medications include long-acting beta-2 medications such as salmeterol (Serevent); eicosanoid lipid mediators such as leukotrienes (Singulair); and inhaled corticosteroids such as Flovent, Intal, and beclomethasone. These medications do not stop an already occurring asthma episode but are taken every day to keep medication levels in the tissues at an effective level for preventing asthma attacks. In response to a severe asthma attack, a course of

PROFESSIONALISM

THE LAW

Many children may require a second supply of their asthma medication to be kept at school for administration by the school nurse. Be aware of the medication requirements of the local school district. Most do not allow students to self-administer or carry any prescription or over-the-counter medications on school grounds. Be ready to write a special note for the physician to sign, giving the school nurse an explanation of the physician's orders so that medications may be given appropriately at school.

treatment with steroids such as prednisone may be prescribed to help reduce the inflammation, speed healing, and reduce complications.

CHRONIC OBSTRUCTIVE PULMONARY DISEASE

Chronic obstructive pulmonary disease (COPD) consists primarily of two related diseases: chronic bronchitis and emphysema. Both diseases are characterized by chronic obstruction of the flow of air through the airways and out of the lungs, and the obstruction is generally permanent and progressive over time. Air pollution and certain occupational pollutants, such as cadmium and silica, may increase the risk of COPD, but smoking is responsible for 90 percent of cases in the United States. Although not all cigarette smokers develop COPD, it is estimated that 15 percent do, and smokers with COPD have higher death rates than nonsmokers with COPD. Smokers also suffer more frequent respiratory symptoms, such as coughing and shortness of breath, and more deterioration in lung function than nonsmokers.

A medical history that includes many of the symptoms of COPD and a physical examination that detects signs of COPD are usually the basis for diagnosis. Tests used to make or confirm the diagnosis include chest X-ray, computed tomography (CT or CAT scan) of the chest, pulmonary function tests, and the measurement of oxygen and carbon dioxide levels in the blood.

Signs and Symptoms.   Signs include moderate to severe dyspnea, air hunger, pursed lips, and the use of accessory muscles in order to breathe.

Treatment.   The goals of COPD treatment are to prevent further deterioration in lung function, alleviate symptoms, and improve the patient's performance of daily activities and quality of life. Treatment strategies include smoking cessation, medications to dilate airways (bronchodilators) and decrease airway inflammation, vaccination against influenza and pneumonia, regular oxygen supplementation, and pulmonary rehabilitation.

Bronchitis

Bronchitis is a respiratory disease in which the mucous membrane in the bronchial passages becomes inflamed. As the irritated membrane swells and grows thicker, it narrows or shuts off the tiny airways in the lungs. The disease occurs in two forms: acute (lasting less than 6 weeks) and chronic (recurring frequently for more than 2 years). In asthmatic bronchitis the lining of the bronchial tubes is also inflamed.

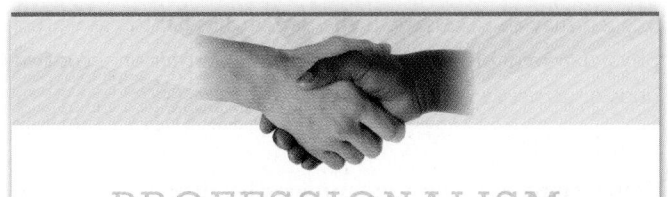

Acute bronchitis is generally caused by lung infections, usually viral but occasionally bacterial in origin. Chronic bronchitis may be caused by repeated attacks of acute bronchitis, which irritate and weaken the bronchial airways over time, and by industrial pollution. Coal miners, grain handlers, metal molders, and others who are continually exposed to dust develop chronic bronchitis at higher-than-normal rates. However, the chief cause is heavy, long-term smoking, which irritates the bronchial tubes and causes them to produce excess mucus. The symptoms of chronic bronchitis are also worsened by air pollution.

Signs and Symptoms.   Symptoms of acute bronchitis include a hacking cough; yellow, white, or green phlegm, usually appearing 24 to 48 hours after the cough begins; fever and chills; soreness and tightness in the chest; pain below the breastbone during deep breathing; and shortness of breath. Chronic bronchitis is characterized by a persistent cough that produces yellow, white, or green phlegm (for at least 3 months of the year and for more than two consecutive years) and sometimes wheezing and breathlessness.

Treatment.   Conventional treatment for acute bronchitis may consist of simple measures such as getting plenty of rest, drinking lots of fluids, avoiding smoke and fumes, and possible use of an inhaled bronchodilator and/or cough syrup. In severe cases of chronic bronchitis, inhaled or oral steroids to reduce inflammation of the airways or supplemental oxygen may be necessary. If the patient has COPD as well, a physician may prescribe oxygen therapy, either on a continuous or as-needed basis.

Emphysema

Emphysema is a long-term, progressive disease of the lung in which the tissues that support the physical shape and function of the lung are destroyed. It is considered an obstructive lung disease because, with the destruction of lung tissue around the bronchioles, these tiny airways are unable to hold their shape properly on exhalation.

Tobacco smoking is by far the most common cause of emphysema—but also the most preventable. Other risk factors include a deficiency of the enzyme alpha$_1$-antitrypsin, air pollution, airway reactivity, heredity, gender (male), and age.

Signs and Symptoms. Shortness of breath is the most common symptom of emphysema. Coughing, sometimes caused by the production of mucus, and wheezing may also be symptoms. Tolerance for exercise may also decrease over time.

Emphysema usually develops slowly. Acute episodes of shortness of breath may not occur. Slow deterioration is the rule, and it may go unnoticed.

Treatment. Treatment for emphysema can take many forms. Smoking cessation is a treatment that most doctors require of patients as it may halt the progression of the disease and improves lung function to some extent. Bronchodilating medications, which cause the air passages to open more fully and allow better air exchange, are usually the first medications prescribed. Steroids and antibiotics may also be prescribed. If the patient experiences shortness of breath, oxygen therapy may be given. In very severe cases, surgery to remove a lung may be required.

PROFESSIONALISM
THE WORKPLACE

Any facility in which a medical assistant works should orient the assistant to where vital supplies such as oxygen and the crash cart are kept. It is a good idea for the working team to rehearse what to do when a patient needs oxygen, so all members are prepared in the event of an emergency.

COMMON COLD

A **common cold** is a viral infection of the upper respiratory tract. Although more than 200 viruses can cause a common cold, the rhinovirus is the most common culprit. Many cold viruses are highly contagious. The common cold can be spread by droplets. These droplets can be transmitted through sneezing and coughing, hand-to-hand contact with someone who has a cold, or the use of shared objects, such as utensils, towels, toys, or telephones.

Signs and Symptoms. Because any one of over 200 viruses can cause a common cold, symptoms can vary greatly. Signs and symptoms usually appear 1 to 3 days after exposure to a cold virus. They may include a runny or stuffy nose, itchy or sore throat, cough, congestion, slight body aches, mild headache, sneezing, watery eyes, low-grade fever of less than 102°F, and mild fatigue. Nasal discharge may become thicker and turn yellow or green as the cold runs its course. What makes a cold different from other viral infections is that it is generally not accompanied by a high fever. Significant fatigue is also unlikely.

Treatment. There is no cure for the common cold. Antibiotics are useless against cold viruses, and over-the-counter cold preparations do not cure a common cold or shorten its duration. However, over-the-counter medications can relieve some symptoms. For fever, sore throat, and headache, mild pain relievers may be helpful. For runny nose and nasal congestion, antihistamines or decongestants may be useful. Because so many different viruses can cause a common cold, no effective vaccine has been developed. However, some measures can help to slow the spread of cold viruses: washing the hands; scrubbing countertops clean, especially when someone in the household has a cold; sneezing and coughing into tissues and discarding them immediately; and not sharing drinking glasses or other utensils with family members who may be sick.

HAY FEVER

Hay fever, or seasonal allergic rhinitis or pollinosis, is a seasonal allergy in which the mucous membranes of the nose and eyes become inflamed. About 26 million Americans experience hay fever symptoms each year. When plants are actively pollinating, vulnerable people breathe in the pollen and have an allergic reaction to it.

Signs and Symptoms. Some of the symptoms of hay fever are repeated and prolonged sneezing; a stuffy and watery nose; redness, swelling, and itching of the eyes; itching of the nose, throat, mouth, and ears; and other ear problems.

Patients may have difficulty breathing at night. Coughing in response to postnasal dripping of clear mucus is sometimes a symptom. Loss of smell is common, and sometimes the sense of taste is impaired. In severe cases nosebleeds occur.

Treatment. Hay fever is best controlled by avoiding the substance that causes the reaction, usually by removing pollen from the air with air conditioners and filters. Certain medications counteract the histamine released during the reaction. In more severe cases, corticosteroids may be taken.

INFLUENZA

Influenza, commonly called the flu, is an illness caused by viruses that infect the respiratory tract. Compared with most viral respiratory infections, such as the common cold, influenza is often a more severe illness. Influenza viruses continually change over time, usually by mutation, and they evade the immune system, rendering the host susceptible to influenza virus infection throughout life.

Signs and Symptoms. Typical symptoms of influenza include fever (usually 100°F to 103°F in adults, often higher in children); respiratory symptoms such as cough, sore throat, and runny or stuffy nose; headache; muscle aches; and extreme fatigue. Although nausea, vomiting, and diarrhea can sometimes accompany influenza, especially in children, gastrointestinal symptoms are rarely prominent. The term *stomach flu* is a misnomer sometimes used to describe gastrointestinal illnesses caused by other microorganisms.

Treatment. Antiviral medications can shorten the course of influenza, but only if taken early in the disease process. Most people affected by the flu recover completely in 1 to 2 weeks, but some people develop serious and potentially life-threatening medical complications such as pneumonia. The best defense against influenza is an annual influenza vaccination. Because there are many strains of influenza, the three most lethal strains found in Asia during the spring season are used to prepare the annual vaccinations given in the United States during the fall. The patient who receives an influenza vaccination may succumb to other strains, but the immune system will be more efficient from having developed a defense against the strains in the vaccination. Health care workers, the elderly, those who are immunosuppressed, and children have the highest risk of contracting this sometimes fatal disease and should be vaccinated on an annual basis.

LEGIONNAIRES' DISEASE

Legionnaires' disease is a type of pneumonia or lung infection that causes 2 percent of pneumonia cases requiring hospital treatment. The disease came to be known as Legionnaires' disease, or legionellosis, in 1976 after numerous attendees at an American Legion convention became ill in a Philadelphia hotel. The microbe causing the illness was isolated, identified, and named. More than 40 different strains of the *Legionella* bacteria have since been identified. Outbreaks of the disease tend to occur in healthy people staying in hotels or other buildings in which the cooling systems or showers have been contaminated by *Legionella* microbes. About three-quarters of all cases in the United States occur as isolated instances in which the source of the microbe is unclear, rather than as epidemics. Legionnaires' disease usually affects middle-aged or elderly people and more commonly affects smokers or people with other respiratory problems. The mortality rate in previously healthy people is about 10 percent.

Signs and Symptoms. The symptoms of the disease generally start 2 to 10 days after a person has been infected. They include high fever with sweating, severe headache, shortness of breath, a worsening cough with thick, greenish mucus that can be bloodstained, and muscle aches and pains. In severe cases, other body systems may be affected, leading to diarrhea, vomiting, mental confusion, and kidney and liver damage. But the most serious effects are on the lungs. After recovery, many people experience fatigue, lack of energy, difficulty concentrating, joint pain, and muscle weakness. These symptoms may last for several months up to 2 years.

Treatment. Treatment normally consists of administration of antibiotics. In severe cases, if the patient experiences difficulty breathing, intensive care with ventilation may be necessary.

LUNG CANCER

Lung cancer affects the lung tissue. It is the leading cause of cancer deaths in both women and men in the United States and throughout the world. Smoking is the most significant factor in the development of lung cancer. About 85 percent of lung cancers occur in smokers or former smokers. The risk of developing lung cancer is related to the number of cigarettes smoked, the age at which a person started smoking, and how long a person has smoked (or smoked before quitting). Another cause of lung cancer is secondhand smoke. The presence of other lung diseases, as well as asbestos exposure and air pollution from motor vehicles and factories, may increase the risk for lung cancer.

Signs and Symptoms. Shortness of breath is a key indicator, as a cancerous tumor grows in the chest.

Treatment. The most widely used therapies for lung cancer are surgery, chemotherapy, and radiation therapy.

PERTUSSIS

Even though there is an effective vaccination against **pertussis (whooping cough)**, some people choose not to vaccinate their children against it. If they decide against vaccination, their child may not be able to enter public schools. Since most children have been immunized, pertussis used to be very rare. Recently more cases of pertussis are arising in unvaccinated adults and children.

Signs and Symptoms. Persistent and severe coughing is the cardinal sign of whooping cough.

Treatment. Patients are usually hospitalized, medicated, and carefully monitored.

PLEURISY

Pleurisy, or pleuritis, is an inflammation of the membrane that surrounds and protects the lungs (the pleura). A variety of conditions can give rise to pleurisy, including infections, such as pneumonia, tuberculosis, and other bacterial or viral respiratory infections; immune disorders, including systemic lupus erythematosus (SLE), rheumatoid arthritis (RA), and sarcoidosis; and other diseases, including pancreatitis, liver cirrhosis, and heart or kidney failure. Pleurisy may also result from an injury. In people who are otherwise healthy, respiratory infections or pneumonia are the main causes of pleurisy.

Signs and Symptoms. The chief symptom of pleurisy is sudden, intense chest pain, usually over the area of inflammation. Although the pain may be constant, it is usually most severe when the lungs move during breathing, coughing, sneezing, or even talking. In some cases the pain may be referred—that is, felt in other areas, such as the neck, shoulder, or abdomen. Another indication of pleurisy is that holding one's breath or exerting pressure against the chest relieves the pain.

Pleurisy is also characterized by certain respiratory symptoms. A rapid, shallow breathing pattern may be the patient's response to the pain. If severe breathing difficulties persist, the patient's complexion, lips, or nail beds may turn bluish in appearance. This is called **cyanosis** and occurs as a result of a lack of oxygen in the tissues.

Treatment. The pain of pleurisy is usually treated with analgesic and anti-inflammatory drugs, such as acetaminophen. Relief may also be obtained by lying on the painful side. Sometimes a painful cough can be controlled with codeine-based cough syrups. However, as the pain eases, the patient should try to breathe deeply and clear any congestion by coughing; otherwise pneumonia may occur.

PNEUMONIA

Pneumonia is an inflammation of the lung or lungs, caused by bacteria, viruses, fungi, or chemical irritants. *Streptococcus pneumoniae* (pneumococcus) is the most common bacterial cause of pneumonia in the United States. Pneumonia often occurs following influenza in the debilitated (those who are weakened by age or disease) and the elderly.

Signs and Symptoms. Symptoms include a productive cough with greenish mucus or puslike sputum, fever, chills, fatigue, chest pain, and muscle aches. Diagnostic indicators include chest auscultation with a stethoscope, sputum cultures, and chest X-rays.

Treatment. Pneumonia is treated with fluids, rest, antibiotics, and nonprescription drugs for pain relief. Oxygen therapy and respiratory treatments can be administered to thin out and remove secretions as necessary.

PNEUMOTHORAX

A **pneumothorax** occurs when air enters the chest outside the lungs. It occurs most frequently when the lung has been punctured from trauma.

Signs and Symptoms. Air hunger, extreme dyspnea, cyanosis, restlessness.

Treatment. Treatment must be quick to prevent compression of the heart and lungs. Normally surgery is required. Before surgery, a temporary flap is made to allow air to exit but not reenter.

PULMONARY EDEMA

Pulmonary edema is a condition in which fluid accumulates in the lungs. It can be a chronic condition, or it can develop suddenly and quickly become life threatening. Most cases of pulmonary edema are caused by failure of the heart's main chamber, the left ventricle, to pump adequately. It also can be brought on by an acute heart attack, severe ischemia, volume overload of the left ventricle, and mitral stenosis. Non-heart-related pulmonary edema is caused by lung problems such as pneumonia, an excess of intravenous fluids, some types of kidney disease, severe burns, liver disease, nutritional problems, and Hodgkin's disease.

Signs and Symptoms. Early symptoms of pulmonary edema include shortness of breath on exertion, sudden respiratory distress after sleep, difficulty breathing (except when sitting upright), and coughing. In severe cases, the symptoms may worsen: labored and rapid breathing; frothy, bloody sputum containing pus; a fast pulse and possibly serious disturbances in the heart's rhythm; cold, clammy, cyanotic skin; and a drop in blood pressure resulting in a thready pulse.

Treatment. Pulmonary edema requires immediate emergency treatment. Treatment includes placing the patient in a sitting position and, in some cases, administering oxygen, assisted or mechanical ventilation, and drug therapy. The goal of treatment is to reduce the amount of fluid in the lungs, improve gas exchange and heart function, and, where possible, correct the underlying disease.

PULMONARY EMBOLISM

A **pulmonary embolism (PE)** is a blood clot in the lung. The clot usually comes from smaller vessels in the leg, pelvis, arm, or heart and travels through smaller and smaller vessels of the lung until it becomes wedged in a vessel that is so narrow it cannot pass through it. The wedged clot prevents blood flow to that section of the lung. Deprived of oxygen, that portion of the lung suffers an infarct (necrosis of the tissue), referred to as a pulmonary (or lung) infarct.

The risk of clot formation is higher when a person is immobilized because of illness, injury, or prolonged sitting, such as on an airplane or a long car trip, which allows the blood to pool in the legs. Other factors that contribute to the risk are recent surgery, trauma or injury (especially to the legs), obesity, heart disease, burns, and a previous history of blood clots in the legs.

Signs and Symptoms. Specific symptoms may indicate that a PE has occurred: chest pain that is sharp and stabbing, has a sudden onset, and is worse when taking a deep breath; shortness of breath; anxiety or apprehension; dry cough; sweating; and passing out.

Treatment. For the critically ill patient who has severe shortness of breath, low blood pressure, and low oxygen concentrations, treatment may be much more aggressive and often includes medications to elevate the blood pressure and raise blood oxygen levels. Thrombolytics, which are clot-buster medications, may be used to help dissolve the emboli, and medications used to raise the blood pressure are often administered. In less severe cases, oxygen therapy and blood-thinning medications are generally sufficient.

SEVERE ACUTE RESPIRATORY SYNDROME

Severe acute respiratory syndrome (SARS) is a recently identified respiratory illness that first infected people in parts of Asia, North America, and Europe in early 2003. SARS is caused by a previously unknown strain of coronavirus, a family of viruses that often cause mild to moderate upper respiratory illness, including the common cold. This new virus is known as SARS-CoV. It is possible that outbreaks of SARS are seasonal, appearing during winter months. Experts believe SARS may have first developed in animals, as the virus has been found in civets, a catlike wild animal that is eaten as a delicacy in China.

The World Health Organization (WHO) reported that 8,096 people became ill with SARS during the first outbreak, 774 of whom died. In 2004, China reported 5 confirmed and 4 possible cases of SARS on April 30. By May 18 of the same year, WHO reported that the outbreak had been contained.

Like most respiratory illnesses, SARS is spread mainly through contact with infected saliva or droplets from coughing. SARS cannot be contracted from brief, casual exposure to an infected person, such as passing that person on the street. Close proximity—less than 3 feet—or contact is probably necessary to become infected. Close contact includes living with, caring for, or having direct contact with saliva or respiratory droplets from an infected person.

Signs and Symptoms. Cough and difficulty breathing are key signs of SARS.

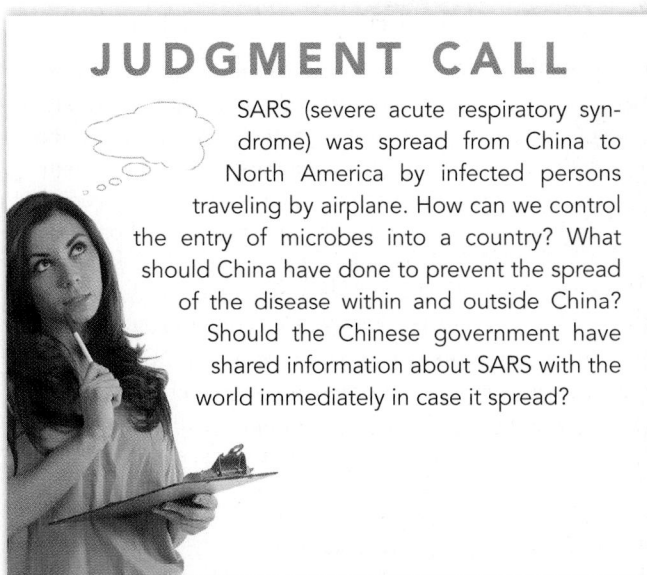

JUDGMENT CALL

SARS (severe acute respiratory syndrome) was spread from China to North America by infected persons traveling by airplane. How can we control the entry of microbes into a country? What should China have done to prevent the spread of the disease within and outside China? Should the Chinese government have shared information about SARS with the world immediately in case it spread?

Treatment. Treatment of SARS usually consists of antibiotics, antiviral medications, and the use of corticosteroids.

SINUSITIS

Sinusitis is an infection or inflammation of the mucous membranes that line the inside of the nose and sinuses. Sinuses are hollow spaces, or cavities, located around the eyes, cheeks, and nose. When a mucous membrane becomes inflamed, it swells, blocking the drainage of fluid from the sinuses into the nose and throat and causing pressure and pain in the sinuses. Sinuses that do not drain properly are more vulnerable to bacterial and fungal growth.

Sinuses can become blocked during a viral infection such as a cold, and sinus inflammation and infection can develop as a result. One key distinction between a cold and sinusitis is that cold symptoms begin to improve within 5 to 7 days. Sinusitis symptoms last longer and worsen after 7 days. There are two types of sinusitis: acute (sudden) and chronic (long term). A person with chronic sinusitis is never completely symptom free.

Signs and Symptoms. Pain and pressure in the face and a stuffy or runny nose are the main symptoms of sinusitis. There may also be a yellow or greenish discharge from the nose. Leaning forward or moving the head often increases facial pain and pressure. The location of pain and tenderness may depend on which sinus is affected. Pain over the cheeks and upper teeth is often caused by maxillary sinus inflammation. Pain in the forehead, above the eyebrows, may be caused by frontal sinus inflammation. Pain behind the eyes, on top of the head, or in both temples may be caused by sphenoid sinus inflammation. Ethmoid sinus inflammation may cause pain around or behind the eyes.

Treatment. Sinusitis is generally treated with medications and home treatment measures, such as applying moist heat to the face. The goals of treatment are to improve mucus drainage, reduce swelling in the sinuses, relieve pain and pressure, clear up any infection, prevent the formation of scar tissue, and avoid permanent damage to the tissues lining the nose and sinuses. Medications are particularly effective against sinusitis caused by a bacterial infection. Length of treatment with medications ranges from 3 days to several weeks or longer. The medications most commonly used are a combination of antibiotics, decongestants, analgesics, corticosteroids, and mucolytics.

TUBERCULOSIS

Tuberculosis (TB) is a contagious disease caused by the bacillus *Mycobacterium tuberculosis.* The bacteria are spread when droplets infected with the bacteria are inhaled from an infected person into a susceptible host. The bacteria may leave an infected person through coughing, spitting, sneezing, or laughing. TB bacteria is most commonly found in the lungs, where they produce granulomas (granular tumors), but they can be found elsewhere in the body. Individuals who are immunosuppressed, such as the homeless, those with AIDS, infants, the elderly, and individuals on chemotherapy, have the highest risk of developing TB.

Signs and Symptoms. Symptoms of tuberculosis include coughing, **hemoptysis** (coughing up blood), white or gray frothy sputum, and night sweats. Other symptoms can include fatigue, chills, weakness, and anorexia.

Diagnosis is made by chest X-ray and sputum culture. The Purified Protein Derivative (PPD) skin test, also known as the Tuberculin Sensitivity Test, is done to check if an individual has ever been exposed to the bacteria and if it is lying dormant; however, this test does not indicate whether the person has an active case of TB.

Treatment. Treatment of this disease is long term, as it usually takes 9 to 12 months to eradicate the bacteria. The first period requires that the patient take respiratory precautions to prevent the spread of the bacteria. Antibiotics—usually rifampin, isoniazid, and ethambutol HCl—are used to begin eradication of the bacteria. After the patient shows negative sputum cultures, he or she must continue antibiotic treatment for another 6 to 9 months to prevent multidrug-resistant TB, which is more difficult to treat.

PROFESSIONALISM

Teamwork is one of the most important aspects of working in the medical field. Always remember that no matter how different the personalities of staff members are, each member's purpose is to help the patients. Never verbalize frustrations with team members in front of patients. Always treat team members even better than you want to be treated. Always remember that not everybody gets along with everybody else, but personal differences must be set aside at work. Learn your own strengths and the strengths of your teammates so that work can be fairly divided, but also so that each team member can take on responsibilities at which they excel. This helps the team to be more successful. If everyone is working for the benefit of the team, then the whole team will succeed.

SUMMARY

The respiratory system consists of a system of tubes lined with mucous membranes and cilia, which serve a protective function. Through the lungs, the cellular waste product (carbon dioxide) is expelled and oxygen (the fuel for the cells) is drawn in. Respiratory volumes and capacity can affect the system's ability to function effectively. Multiple disease processes can result from infection and inflammation within the system. Among the often debilitating diseases of the respiratory system are asthma, chronic obstructive pulmonary disease, shay fever, pleurisy, and lung cancer. Microbes cause the common cold, influenza, Legionnaires' disease, pertussis, pneumonia, some sinusitis, severe acute respiratory syndrome, and tuberculosis. Pulmonary edema, pneumothorax, and emboli can also cause the system to malfunction.

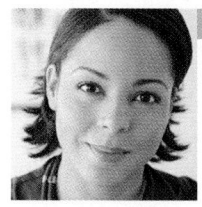

29 CHAPTER REVIEW

COMPETENCY REVIEW

1. Define and spell the terms to learn for this chapter.

2. List the organs of the respiratory system.

3. What is the primary function of the respiratory system?

4. Which two gases are exchanged in the lungs?

5. What are the five functions of the nose?

6. What are the functions of the pharynx?

7. What is the function of the epiglottis?

8. Describe the bronchi. What are the differences between the left and right bronchi?

9. What are the alveoli?

10. What does tidal volume represent?

PREPARING FOR THE CERTIFICATION EXAM

1. What organ is shared by both the respiratory and digestive systems and connects the nose, mouth, and voicebox?
   a. pharynx
   b. nares
   c. trachea
   d. bronchi
   e. epiglottis

2. Which of the following breaths per minute would be considered normal for a newborn?
   a. 5
   b. 10
   c. 20
   d. 40
   e. 100

3. Which organ has the specific function of preventing aspiration of food into the lungs?
   a. bronchial tube
   b. trachea
   c. alveolus
   d. pharynx
   e. epiglottis

4. The function of the larynx is primarily to
   a. aid in swallowing
   b. aid in speaking
   c. prevent swallowing
   d. prevent aspiration
   e. aid in aspiration

5. A chronic inflammatory disease caused by allergens or other irritating substances is:
   a. asthma
   b. pneumonia
   c. cystic fibrosis
   d. Legionnaires' disease
   e. tuberculosis

6. The volume of air entering or leaving the lungs during a single breath is called
   a. tidal volume
   b. inspiratory reserve volume
   c. expiratory reserve volume
   d. residual volume
   e. vital capacity

7. High fever is a symptom of
   a. sinusitis
   b. lung cancer
   c. common cold

d. influenza
e. pulmonary edema

8. A PPD test is done to detect which of the following?
   a. cystic fibrosis
   b. tuberculosis
   c. lung cancer
   d. asthma
   e. emphysema

9. Which of the following is the measurement of the volume of air left in the lungs after a normal expiration?
   a. inspiratory capacity
   b. vital capacity
   c. functional residual capacity
   d. total lung capacity
   e. tidal volume

10. An attack of hay fever is triggered by
    a. touching the infected person
    b. breathing in an allergen
    c. breathing in infected droplets
    d. a casual handshake
    e. smoking

CRITICAL THINKING

1. Mr. McConnley has some flulike symptoms. What other respiratory disorders do these symptoms mimic?

2. Dr. Miller asks Mr. McConnley if he has recently stayed at a hotel with an air conditioning system. Why would he be asking this question?

3. Mr. McConnley states that he returned 4 days ago from a convention in Florida where he both lodged and attended conference meetings at the same hotel. Does this support Dr. Miller's suspicions? Why or why not?

INTERNET ACTIVITY

Do an Internet search for COPD services in your hometown and see what resources are available in your area.

MEDMEDIA

Additional interactive resources and activities for this chapter can be found:

On your student DVD: View applicable procedure videos on the DVD-ROM found in the back of this book.

MyHealthProfessionsKit.com: Test your knowledge of this chapter with games and activities. MyHealthProfessionsKit also includes resources, helpful links, and a Spanish audio glossary.

Medical Assisting Interactive: Practice your procedures as a medical assistant in this simulated doctor's office. This can be accessed through MyHealthProfessionsKit.com.

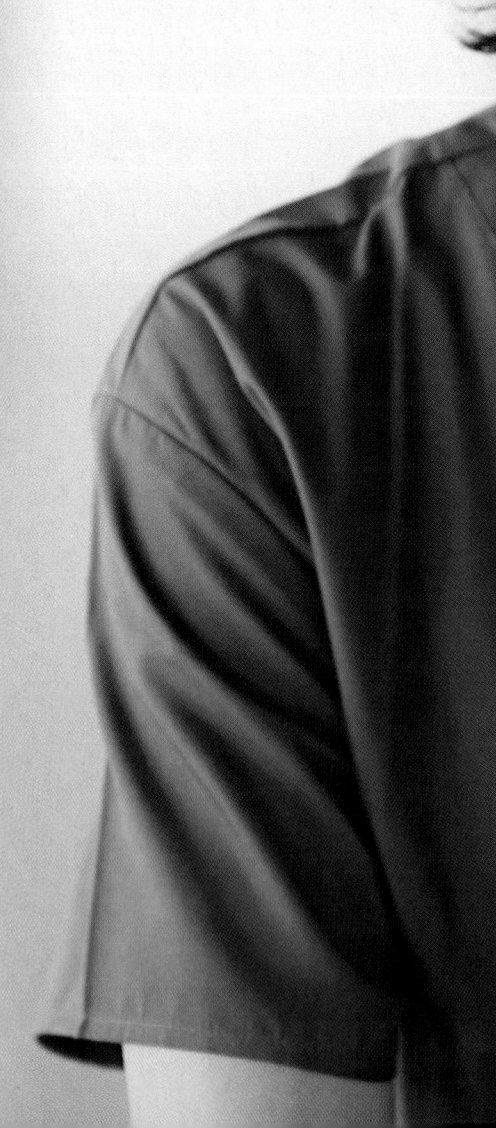

30

The Digestive System

LEARNING OBJECTIVES

After completing this chapter, you should be able to:

- Define and spell the terms to learn for this chapter.

- Describe the purpose and function of the digestive system.

- Identify the primary organs of the digestive system and briefly explain the function of each.

- Describe the three main portions of a tooth.

- Identify the accessory organs of the digestive system and briefly explain the function of each.

- Briefly explain common disorders associated with the digestive system.

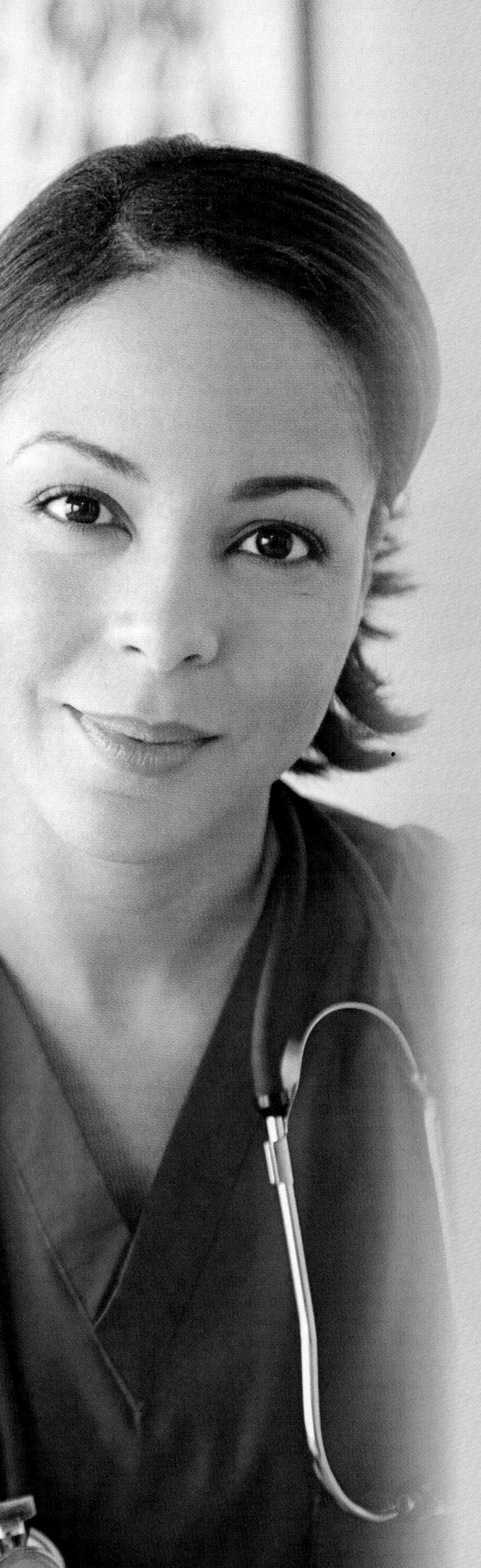

CHAPTER OUTLINE

CASE STUDY

Susan Schultz, CMA (AAMA), is working as a clinical medical assistant today with Dr. Penningworth. The doctor's next patient is a new patient, Marshall Raines. Susan immediately notices a yellowish tint to his eyeballs, and because he is wearing shorts she can see that his legs are slightly swollen and very bruised. She also notices a faint odor of alcohol. When Susan asks Marshall what has brought him to the office, he informs her that he has recently succumbed to alcohol after being sober for 3 months. Also, for the past few days he "hasn't been feeling right."

579

TERMS TO LEARN

appendicitis
appendix
bile
cecum
cementum
cholelithiasis
chyme
cirrhosis
colitis
colon
colorectal cancer
constipation
Crohn's disease
dentin
diarrhea
diverticulitis
diverticulosis
enamel
esophagus
gallbladder
gastroesophageal reflux disease (GERD)

gingivae
hemorrhoid
hernia
hiatal hernia
inguinal hernia
irritable bowel syndrome (IBS)
large intestine
liver
mastication
oral cancer
pancreas
pancreatic cancer
peptic ulcer disease (PUD)
peristalsis
pharynx
pyloric stenosis
rectum
salivary glands
small intestine
stomach
stomach ulcer

CERTIFICATION LINK

CMA (AAMA)
Anatomy and physiology

> Systems (including structure, function, related conditions and diseases, and their relationships)

RMA
Anatomy and physiology

> Body systems
> Disorders and diseases of the body

CMAS (AMT)
Medical assisting foundation

> Anatomy and physiology
> Medical terminology

The digestive system consists of organs that are responsible for getting food into and out of the body and for making use of it. These organs include the salivary glands, mouth, esophagus, stomach, small intestine, liver, gallbladder, pancreas, colon, rectum, and anus. The main part of the digestive system is the digestive or gastrointestinal tract, which is also known as the alimentary canal. This tract is essentially a long, continuous tube (some 30 feet long in adults) that starts at the mouth, where

food and drink enter the body, and ends at the anus, where waste products leave the body. The three main functions of the digestive system are digestion, absorption, and elimination. Each of the various organs commonly associated with digestion is described in this chapter, and the organs of digestion are shown in Figure 30-1.

Organs of the Digestive System

The digestive system is a series of hollow organs joined in a long, twisting tube from the mouth to the anus. Inside this tube is the mucosal lining (mucosa). In the mouth, stomach, and small intestine, the mucosa contains tiny glands that produce juices to help digest food.

MOUTH

The mouth is a cavity formed by the palate, the lips and cheeks, and the tongue (Figure 30-2). The cheeks form the lateral walls and are continuous with the lips. The hard and soft palates form a roof for the oral cavity, and the tongue is connected to the floor of the mouth by the lingual frenulum. The vestibule is the space between the cheeks and the teeth. The combining form for mouth, as mentioned in Chapter 4, is stom/o.

The oral cavity (the mouth) contains the teeth and the salivary glands. The **gingivae**, or gums, hold the teeth in place. Three pairs of salivary glands secrete saliva into the oral cavity: the parotid, sublingual, and submandibular glands.

The tongue is made of skeletal muscle and is covered with mucous membrane. It can be divided into the rear portion (the root), the central body, and the pointed tip. Papillae (elevations) and taste buds are located on the surface of the tongue. There are four types of taste buds: sweet, salt, sour, and bitter.

The posterior margin of the soft palate supports the muscular pharyngeal arches, which function in swallowing and phonation, and the uvula, which is the tissue dangling from the center of the pharyngeal arches. The line formed by the pharyngeal arches and the uvula separates the oral cavity from the pharynx.

Digestion begins in the mouth with the process of **mastication** (chewing) and the secretion of saliva, which moistens the food and begins its chemical breakdown. The combination of the chewing action and the saliva helps to form the food into a bolus (ball) for swallowing.

TEETH

Humans have two sets of teeth: 20 deciduous teeth (the baby teeth) and 32 permanent teeth (Figure 30-3). The deciduous teeth are smaller than the permanent teeth but generally resemble the permanent teeth, though on a much smaller scale. The set of deciduous teeth include 8 incisors, 4 canines

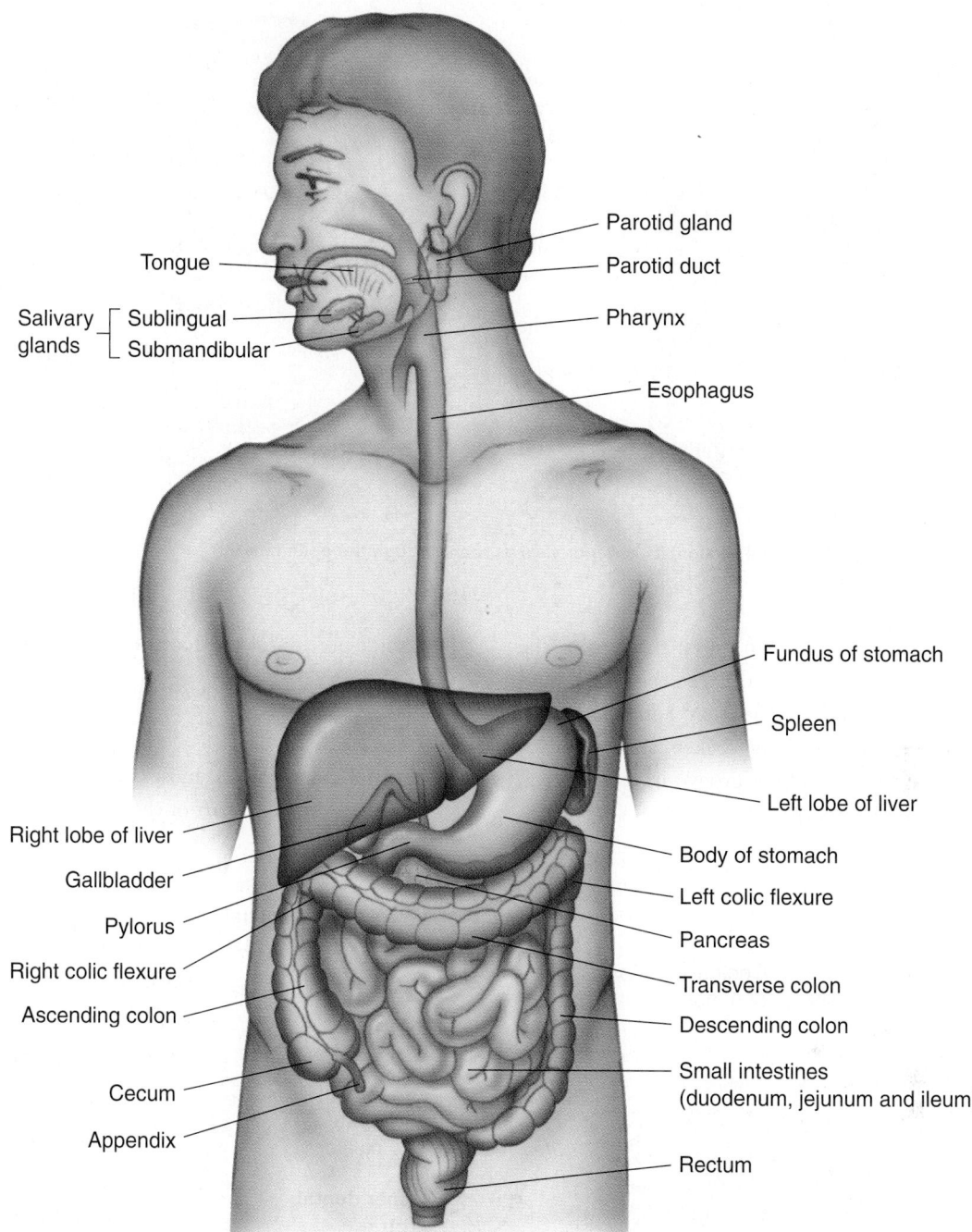

FIGURE 30-1 The digestive system.

(cuspids), and 8 molars. The permanent teeth include 8 incisors, 4 canines, 8 premolars, and 12 molars, which can be differentiated as follows:

- The incisors are the four front teeth of the dental arch. They have a sharp, cutting edge, used for biting into food. The upper incisors are larger and stronger than the lower ones.

- The canine teeth, or cuspids, have roots that reach deep into the bones of the jaw. The upper canines are also

known as the *eye teeth* and are larger than the lower canines. The lower canines are often called the *stomach teeth.*

- The premolar teeth are behind the canine teeth. Also known as *bicuspid teeth,* they are smaller and shorter than the canines. There are four premolars in each arch.

- The molar teeth are the largest teeth in the permanent set and are adapted to grinding and pounding food. An adult has 12 molars, 6 in each arch, posterior to the premolars.

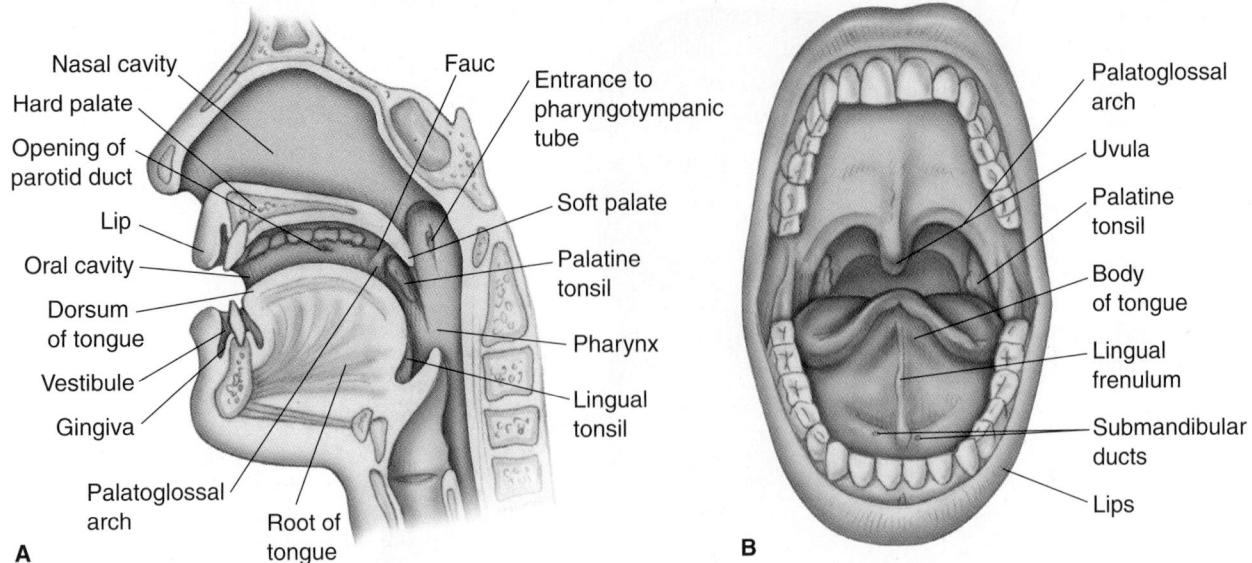

FIGURE 30-2 The oral cavity: (A) sagittal section; (B) anterior view as seen through the open mouth.

Each tooth consists of three main parts: the crown (the part above the gum); the root (embedded in the gums); and the neck, the portion between the root and the crown (Figure 30-4). The root sits in a bony socket called the alveolus. The gingival sulcus, a shallow groove in the gingiva, surrounds the neck of each tooth.

The solid portion of the tooth consists of the following:

- **Dentin**—calcified, largely mineral tissue that forms the bulk of the tooth

- **Enamel**—hardest and most compact part of the tooth; covers the exposed part of the crown

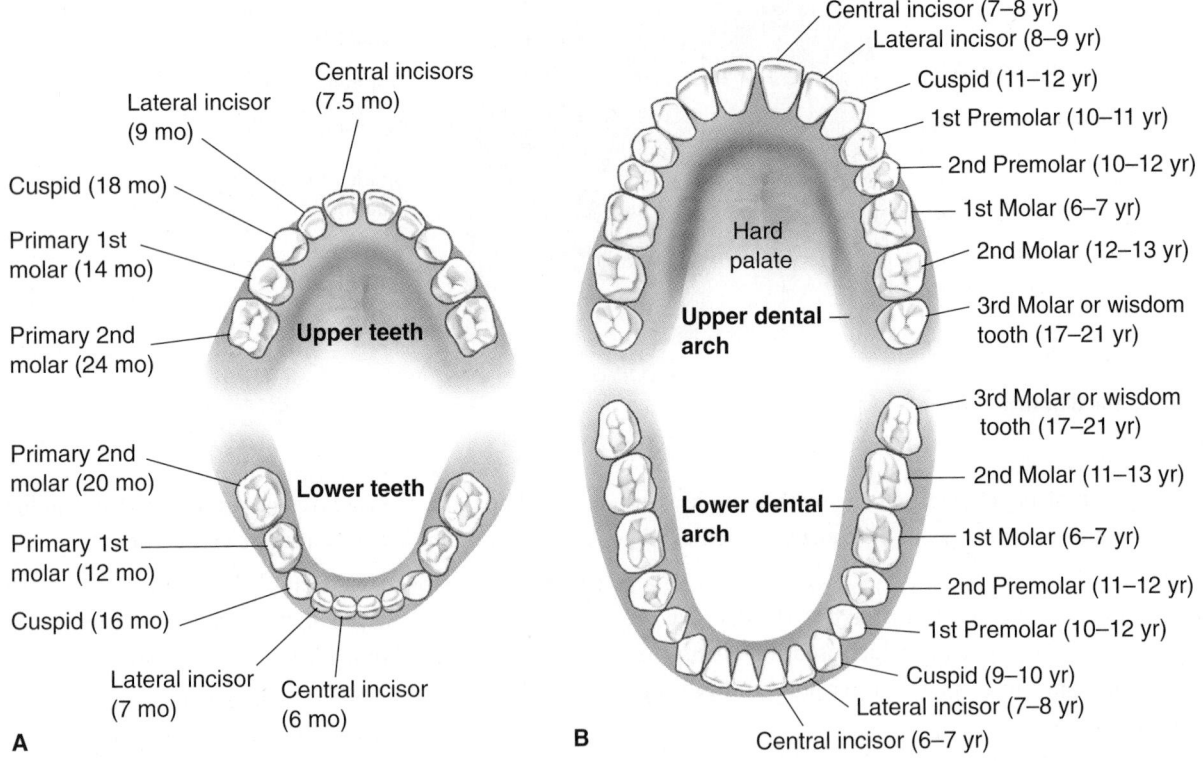

FIGURE 30-3 Deciduous and permanent teeth: (A) deciduous teeth, with the age at eruption given in months; (B) permanent teeth, with the age at eruption given in years.

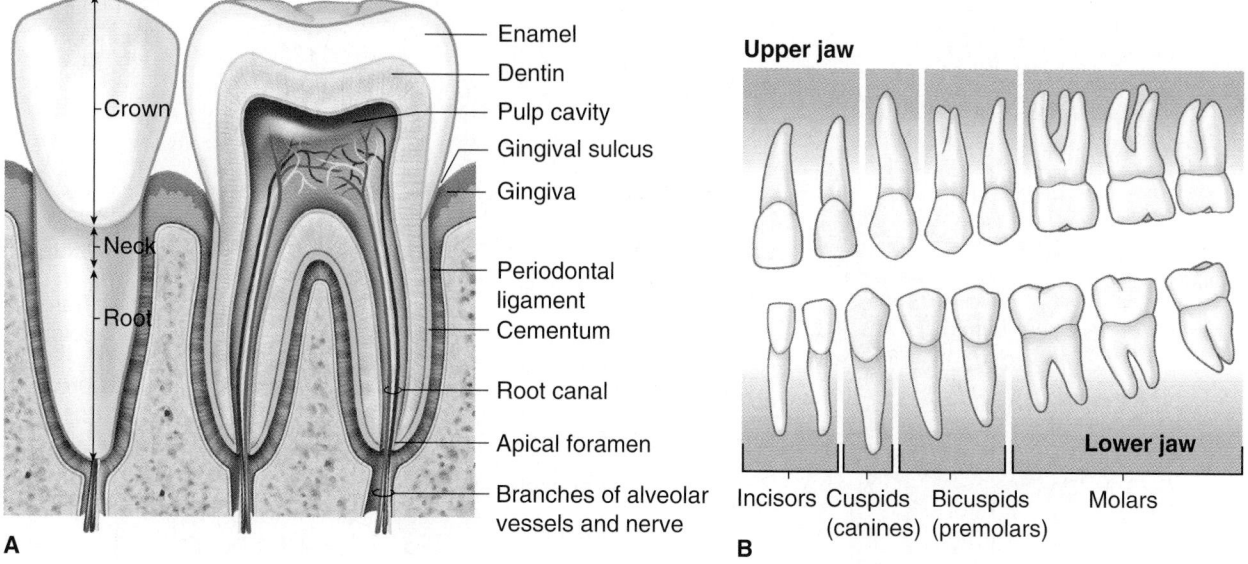

FIGURE 30-4 Teeth: (A) a diagrammatic section through a typical adult tooth; (B) the adult teeth.

Labels for image A: Enamel, Dentin, Pulp cavity, Gingival sulcus, Gingiva, Periodontal ligament, Cementum, Root canal, Apical foramen, Branches of alveolar vessels and nerve; Crown, Neck, Root.

Labels for image B: Upper jaw, Lower jaw, Incisors, Cuspids (canines), Bicuspids (premolars), Molars.

- **Cementum**—thin layer of bone that covers the dentin of the root, providing protection and anchoring the periodontal ligament

The teeth are bound to the bony sockets in the maxillary bone and mandible by fibers of the periodontal ligament. Teeth erupt through the gums when they are sufficiently calcified to tolerate the stress they will be subjected to later. Deciduous teeth erupt from the gums from the age of about 7 months to about $2\frac{1}{2}$ years of age. The permanent teeth erupt at about the following ages:

First molars	6th to 7th years
Two central incisors	7th to 8th years
Two lateral incisors	8th to 9th years
First premolars	10th to 11th years
Second premolars	10th to 12th years
Canines	11th to 12th years
Second molars	12th to 13th years
Third molars	17th to 21st years

PHARYNX

The **pharynx** lies posterior to the mouth and is the beginning of the tube that leads to the stomach. It is a passageway for both air and food and therefore belongs to both the respiratory and the digestive systems. Both the larynx and the esophagus begin in the pharynx. Once food is swallowed, it passes through the pharynx into the esophagus reflexively. Muscular contractions move the bolus of food into the esophagus while closing the larynx to prevent food from entering the trachea.

ESOPHAGUS

The **esophagus** is a collapsible tube about 10 inches long that starts at the pharynx and ends at the stomach. Food and liquids are carried down the esophagus by the muscular contractions of **peristalsis**. These involuntary wavelike contractions move the bolus of food through the entire digestive system.

STOMACH

The **stomach** is a large, muscular, saclike organ in which the early stages of the digestive process take place (Figure 30-5). The stomach can hold 1 to 1.5 liters of food and fluid. It secretes hydrochloric acid and gastric juices that convert food into **chyme**, a semiliquid, that is then passed into the small intestine for further digestion. The cardiac sphincter at the superior end and the pyloric sphincter at the inferior end close to facilitate passage into and out of the stomach.

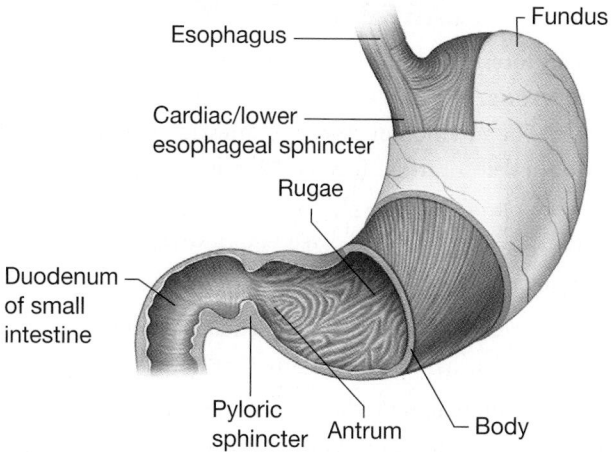

Labels: Esophagus, Fundus, Cardiac/lower esophageal sphincter, Rugae, Duodenum of small intestine, Pyloric sphincter, Antrum, Body.

FIGURE 30-5 Stomach.

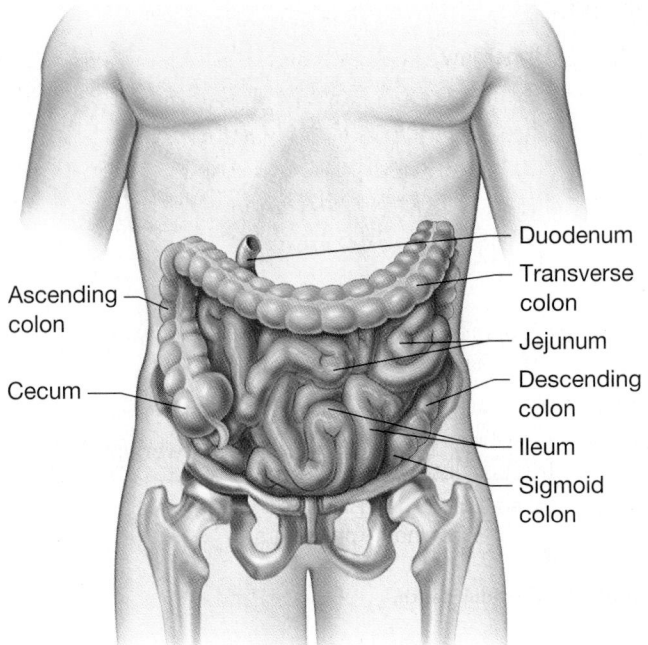

FIGURE 30-6 Small intestine.

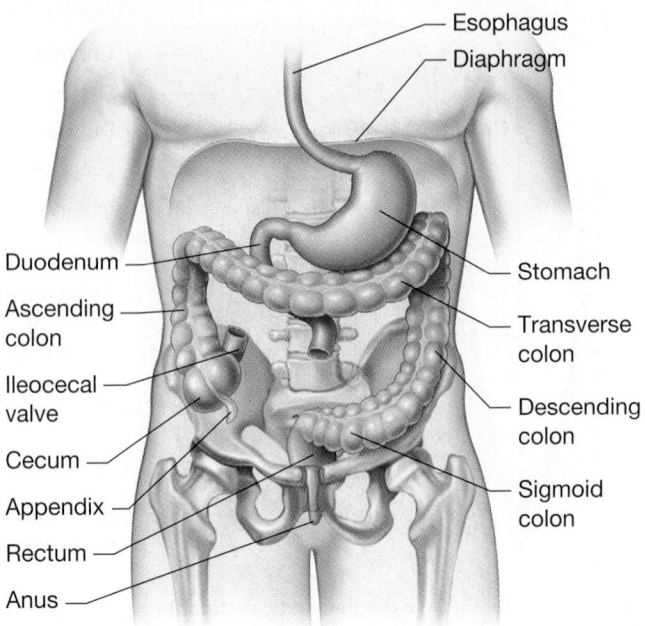

FIGURE 30-7 Large intestine (colon).

SMALL INTESTINE

The **small intestine** is 21 feet long and about 1 inch in diameter (Figure 30-6). The opening of the small intestine, the pyloric sphincter, is at the base of the stomach. The first 12 inches of the small intestine comprise the duodenum, the next 8 feet of the small intestine comprise the jejunum, and the last 12 feet comprise the ileum.

Chyme moves into the small intestine from the stomach through the pylorus. There it mixes with bile from the liver and gallbladder and with pancreatic juice from the pancreas. Nutrients are absorbed into tiny capillaries and lymph vessels in the walls of the small intestine and then transmitted to body cells via the circulatory system. Absorption of nutrients takes place in the small intestines.

LARGE INTESTINE

The small intestine terminates at the ileocecal orifice of the **large intestine**, which is about 5 feet long and 2.5 inches in diameter. The function of the large intestine is to complete digestion and absorption. It can be divided into several parts (Figure 30-7):

- The **cecum** is a small pouch about 3 inches long that forms the beginning of the large intestine.
- The **appendix** is a small appendage attached to the cecum that has no known function in humans.
- The **colon** makes up the bulk of the large intestine and is divided into the ascending colon (on the right side of the abdomen), the transverse colon (moves across the

body transversely from right to left), the descending colon (on the left side of the abdomen), and the sigmoid colon, which leads to the rectum.

- The waste products of digestion are eliminated from the body via the **rectum** and the anus.

ACCESSORY ORGANS

The accessory organs that are important in the role of digestion are the salivary glands, the gallbladder, the liver, and the pancreas (see Figure 30-8). They are not part of the digestive tract but perform functions closely related to it.

Salivary Glands

The **salivary glands** are located in and near the mouth and produce saliva in response to the sight, smell, taste, or mental image of food. There are three pairs of salivary glands. The parotid glands are located on either side of the face, just below the ear. The submandibular glands are located in the floor of the mouth. The sublingual glands are located below the tongue. All these glands secrete saliva through openings into the mouth. Saliva contains amylase, an enzyme that helps to break down carbohydrates.

Liver

The **liver** is located in the upper right quadrant of the abdomen. It is the largest glandular organ and weighs about 3.5 pounds. The liver plays an essential role in the metabolism of carbohydrates, fats, and proteins. In carbohydrate metabolism, it changes glucose to glycogen and stores that glycogen for future use by the body's cells. To metabolize fat,

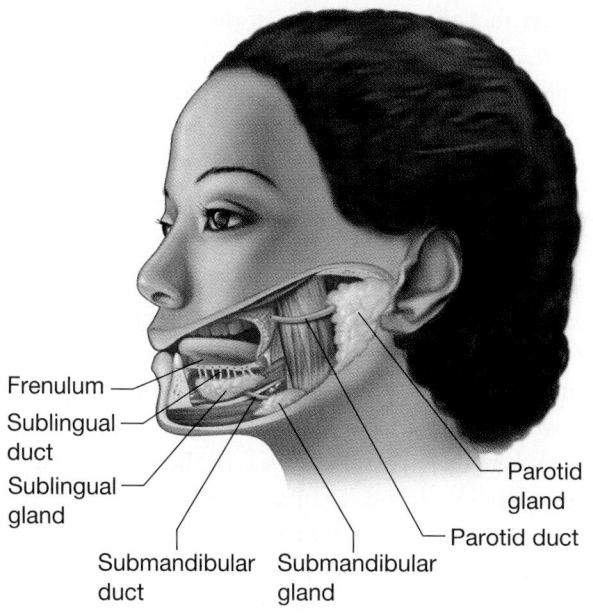

Frenulum
Sublingual duct
Sublingual gland
Submandibular duct
Submandibular gland
Parotid gland
Parotid duct

A

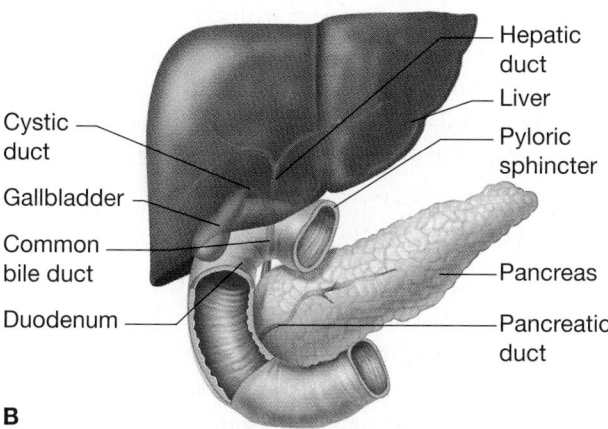

Cystic duct
Gallbladder
Common bile duct
Duodenum
Hepatic duct
Liver
Pyloric sphincter
Pancreas
Pancreatic duct

B

FIGURE 30-8 (A) Salivary glands; (B) gallbladder, liver, and pancreas.

the liver produces bile, which emulsifies fats before releasing the products into the bloodstream. In protein metabolism, the liver stores the components of proteins so the body can break down or build up proteins as required.

The liver produces four substances important for body functioning:

- **Bile**—digestive juice that emulsifies fats
- **Fibrinogen and prothrombin**—essential for blood clotting
- **Heparin**—prevents the clotting of blood
- **Blood proteins**—albumin, gamma globulin

The liver also stores iron and vitamins B_{12}, A, D, E, and K. It produces body heat and detoxifies the body from substances such as drugs and alcohol.

Gallbladder

The **gallbladder** is a membranous sac in which bile is stored and concentrated. Any bile stored in the gallbladder is six to ten times more concentrated than bile that comes from the liver. Because of this high concentration of bile, gallstones can form (**cholelithiasis**) and the gallbladder can become inflamed.

Pancreas

The **pancreas** is an elongated gland, 6 to 9 inches in length, that is situated behind the stomach and secretes pancreatic juice into the small intestine. It contains cells that produce digestive enzymes and other cells that secrete the hormones insulin and glucagon, which lower and raise glucose levels in the blood.

Common Disorders Associated with the Digestive System

Digestive disorders range from the occasional upset stomach, heartburn, and nausea to the more serious and life-threatening colorectal cancer. These disorders involve the gastrointestinal tract as well as the liver, gallbladder, and pancreas. Most digestive disorders and diseases are complex, with subtle symptoms and often unknown causes (see Table 30-1). Some may be genetic or develop from multiple factors such as stress, fatigue, diet, smoking, and alcohol abuse. A thorough medical history and physical examination are crucial for accurate diagnoses. More extensive diagnostic evaluations may be necessary, including laboratory tests, endoscopic procedures, and imaging techniques.

APPENDICITIS

The appendix is a small, tubelike structure attached to the colon (at the cecum), in the lower right portion of the abdomen. It has no known function, and removal appears to cause no change in digestive function. **Appendicitis** is an inflammation of the appendix. Blockage of the inside of the appendix, or lumen, leads to increased pressure, impaired blood flow, and inflammation. Anyone can get appendicitis, but it occurs most often between the ages of 10 and 30.

Signs and Symptoms. Acute pain at the McBirney point on the abdomen is the key symptom. This pain will not be relieved by over-the-counter pain relievers, rest, or change of position.

Treatment. Appendicitis is the most common acute surgical emergency of the abdomen. Because there is no effective medical therapy, appendicitis is considered a medical

The Child

- A child's digestive system continues to develop throughout the first year of life. Many environmental factors can stress a child's digestive system. Aside from the dietary factors, children are exposed to heavy metals, pollutants, solvents, and carcinogens found in food, water, air, medicine, and plastics that can injure the digestive system.
- Digestive disorders affecting infants and children range from simple problems that most children experience from time to time, such as vomiting or diarrhea, to more serious (and possibly life threatening) birth defects, such as tracheoesophageal fistula or illnesses such as appendicitis.
- Digestive and liver disorders can have significant effects on the health of a child. A healthy digestive system processes the foods and liquids that we eat, replenishing vitamins, minerals, proteins, carbohydrates, and fats that are vital for the body to function properly. Occasional vomiting or diarrhea may lead to dehydration; however, long-term problems with the digestive system or liver can deplete these important nutrients, causing malnutrition that affects a child's physical and mental growth and development.

The Older Adult

- The digestive system becomes less motile with aging as muscle contractions become weaker. Glandular secretions decrease, causing a drier mouth and a lower volume of gastric juices. Nutrient absorption decreases due to the atrophy of the mucosal lining. Because of age and continued use, the gums recede and the tooth surfaces wear down. A loss of taste may occur, and food preferences may change.
- Gastric motor activity slows, causing delayed gastric emptying and a decrease in hunger contractions. Although there are no significant changes in the small intestine, the muscle layer and the blood flow through the large intestine begin to decline. Constipation can be a frequent problem, especially because of a decrease in dietary and fluid intake.

emergency. When treated promptly, most patients recover without difficulty. If treatment is delayed, however, the appendix can burst, causing infection and even death.

The appendix is almost always removed, even if it is found to be normal. With complete removal, any later episodes of pain cannot be attributed to appendicitis. If the diagnosis is uncertain, or if the doctor suspects a nonsurgical or treatable cause, the patient may be watched and sometimes treated with antibiotics. If the cause of the pain is infectious, intravenous antibiotics and intravenous fluids are used to resolve symptoms.

CIRRHOSIS

Cirrhosis is a potentially life-threatening condition that occurs when scarring damages the liver. This scarring (also called *fibrosis*) replaces healthy tissue and prevents the liver from functioning normally. Cirrhosis usually develops after years of liver inflammation.

Cirrhosis has many possible causes. In the United States, the major causes of cirrhosis are many years of excessive alcohol consumption and certain forms of viral hepatitis (mainly hepatitis B or C). Other causes include excessive amounts of fat stored in the liver, as well as inflammation and blockage of the ducts that transport bile out of the liver. The latter condition may be related to a problem with the immune system. Another type of cirrhosis, autoimmune hepatitis, results when the immune system attacks the liver. Sometimes cirrhosis can be caused by an inherited disease, such as cystic fibrosis. A condition called cryptogenic cirrhosis has no obvious cause.

Signs and Symptoms. In many cases, symptoms develop only after the disease has progressed. They include fluid buildup in the legs (edema) and abdomen (ascites), fatigue, yellowing of the skin (jaundice), itching, nosebleeds, redness of the palms, bleeding from enlarged veins in the digestive tract, easy bruising, weight loss and muscle loss, abdominal pain, frequent infections, and confusion.

Treatment. The patient with cirrhosis must avoid substances that can further damage the liver, especially alcohol and nonsteroidal anti-inflammatory drugs. Treatment may also include dietary changes and using medications and surgery to prevent and treat complications. A liver transplant may be considered when liver damage is severe.

COLITIS

Colitis is an inflammation of the large intestine. Many different disease processes may cause colitis, including acute and chronic infections, primary inflammatory disorders (ulcerative colitis, Crohn's colitis, lymphocytic and collagenous colitis), impaired blood flow (ischemic colitis), and history of radiation exposure to the large bowel.

Signs and Symptoms. Symptoms can include abdominal pain, diarrhea, dehydration, abdominal bloating, increased intestinal gas, and bloody stools. The disorder may be identified by flexible sigmoidoscopy or colonoscopy. In both

TABLE 30-1 Disorders and Pathology of the Digestive System

Disorder/Pathology	Description
Anorexia	Loss of appetite that can accompany other conditions such as a gastrointestinal (GI) upset
Ascites	Collection or accumulation of fluid in the peritoneal cavity
Bulimia	Eating disorder that is characterized by recurrent binge eating followed by purging of the food with laxatives and vomiting
Cholecystitis	Inflammation of the gallbladder
Cholelithiasis	Formation or presence of stones or calculi in the gallbladder or common bile duct
Cirrhosis	Chronic disease of the liver
Cleft lip	Congenital condition in which the upper lip fails to come together; often seen along with cleft palate; corrected with surgery
Cleft palate	Congenital condition in which the roof of the mouth has a split or fissure; corrected with surgery
Constipation	Difficult or infrequent defecation
Crohn's disease	Form of chronic inflammatory bowel disease affecting the ileum or colon; also called regional ileitis
Diarrhea	Passing of frequent, watery bowel movements; usually accompanies gastrointestinal (GI) disorders
Diverticulitis	Inflammation of a diverticulum or sac in the intestinal tract, especially in the colon
Dyspepsia	Indigestion
Emesis	Vomiting, usually with some force
Enteritis	Inflammation of only the small intestine
Esophageal stricture	Narrowing of the esophagus that makes the flow of foods and fluids difficult
Fissure	Cracklike split in the rectum or anal canal or roof of mouth
Fistula	Abnormal tubelike passage from one body cavity to another, or between an organ and the exterior of the body
Gastritis	Inflammation of the stomach, which can result in pain, tenderness, nausea, and vomiting
Gastroenteritis	Inflammation of the stomach and small intestine
Halitosis	Bad or offensive breath, which is often a sign of disease
Hepatitis	Inflammation of the liver
Ileitis	Inflammation of the ileum of the small intestine
Inflammatory bowel syndrome	Ulceration, of unknown origin, of the mucous membranes of the colon; also known as ulcerative colitis
Inguinal hernia	Hernia or outpouching of intestines into the inguinal region of the body; may require surgical correction
Intussusception	Result of the intestine slipping or telescoping into another section of intestine just below it; more common in children
Irritable bowel syndrome	Disturbance, from unknown causes, in the functions of the intestine; symptoms generally include abdominal discomfort and an alteration in bowel activity
Malabsorption syndrome	Inadequate absorption of nutrients from the intestinal tract; may be caused by a variety of diseases and disorders, such as infections and pancreatic deficiency
Peptic ulcer	Ulcer occurring in the lower portion of the esophagus, stomach, or duodenum thought to be caused by the acid of gastric juices; some now successfully treated with antibiotics
Pilonidal cyst	Cyst in the sacrococcygeal region due to tissue being trapped below the skin

(continued)

TABLE 30-1 (continued)

Disorder/Pathology	Description
Polyphagia	Eating excessively
Polyps	Small tumors that contain a pedicle or footlike attachment in the mucous membranes of the large intestine (colon)
Reflux esophagitis	Acid from the stomach backing up into the esophagus, causing inflammation and pain
Regurgitation	Return of fluids and solids from the stomach into the mouth; similar to emesis but without the force
Ulcerative colitis	Ulceration, of unknown source, of the mucous membranes of the colon; also known as inflammatory bowel disease
Volvulus	Condition in which the bowel twists on itself and causes an obstruction; painful and requires immediate surgery

tests, a flexible tube is inserted into the rectum and used to evaluate specific areas of the colon. Biopsies taken during these tests may show changes related to inflammation. Other studies, such as barium enema, abdominal CT scan, abdominal MRI, and abdominal X-ray may be used to identify colitis.

Treatment. Treatment of colitis is directed at the underlying cause—infection, inflammation, lack of blood flow, or another cause.

COLORECTAL CANCER

Colon cancer is cancer of the large intestine (colon), the lower part of the digestive system. Rectal cancer is cancer of the rectum, which is the last 8 to 10 inches of the colon. To-gether, they are often referred to as **colorectal cancer**, the second-leading cause of cancer-related deaths in the United States after lung cancer.

Most cases of colon cancer begin as adenomatous polyps, which are small, noncancerous (benign) clumps of cells. Over time some of these polyps become cancerous.

Signs and Symptoms. Because the polyps are small and produce few, if any, symptoms, regular screening tests are important to help prevent progression to end-stage cancer. If signs and symptoms of cancer do appear, they may include a change in bowel habits, bloody stools, persistent cramping, gas, or abdominal pain. Screening tests and a few simple changes in diet and lifestyle can dramatically reduce a person's overall risk of developing colon cancer.

Treatment. The three primary treatment options are surgery, chemotherapy, and radiation; the physician's choice depends largely on the stage of the cancer. Surgery is the main treatment for colorectal cancer. How much of the colon is removed and whether other therapies, such as radiation or chemotherapy, are an option is determined by the extent to which the cancer has penetrated into the wall of the bowel and whether it has spread to the lymph nodes or other parts of the body. If part of the colon is removed, sometimes the colon is brought to the surface so stool comes out of a stoma (colostomy) instead of the rectum.

PROFESSIONALISM

Ensuring that patients and their families understand instructions and explanations can present difficulties. Never address any patient with nicknames such as "Sweetie" or "Honey." Many individuals consider these terms derisive and unprofessional. Instead, address all adults as Mr. or Ms. or Mrs. unless otherwise instructed. If you are working in an office where English is the primary language and your first language is not English, or if you have a heavy regional accent not native to your office, practice speaking very clearly so that those who have hearing difficulties can still understand your instructions. Supplement verbal instructions with clearly written instructions to help increase understanding. Be sure all explanations are not in medical terminology, but do not oversimplify so that the patients feel "talked down to."

CONSTIPATION

Constipation is the term for difficult defecation. Constipation is said to be present if a person has two or fewer bowel movements a week or has two or more of the following problems at least 25 percent of the time: straining, a feeling of not completely emptying the bowels, and hard or pelletlike stools. Lack of dietary fiber and dehydration are common causes of constipation. Other causes include irritable bowel syndrome, travel or other changes in one's daily routine, lack of exercise, immobility caused by illness or aging, medication use, overuse of laxatives, and pregnancy.

Signs and Symptoms.   Constipation may be accompanied by cramping and rectal pain caused by straining to pass hard, dry stools. Bloating and nausea may be present. Bleeding hemorrhoids or a slight tearing of the anus (anal fissure) as the stool is pushed through may leave small amounts of bright red blood on the stool or on the toilet tissue. This should clear up when the constipation is controlled.

Treatment.   Constipation can usually be treated effectively at home, through exercise, good nutritional habits, and scheduling a certain time each day for bowel movements. Laxatives may also be used.

CROHN'S DISEASE

Crohn's disease is a chronic inflammatory disease of the intestines. It can affect the digestive system anywhere from the mouth to the anus but primarily causes ulcerations or breaks in the lining of the small and large intestines. Crohn's disease is closely related to ulcerative colitis, a chronic inflammatory condition that involves only the colon. Together, the two diseases are frequently referred to as inflammatory bowel disease (IBD). They affect 0.5 million to 2 million people in the United States. Crohn's disease may have a genetic component, as it tends to be more common in relatives of patients with Crohn's disease or ulcerative colitis.

Crohn's disease is not contagious, and the exact cause is unknown. Some scientists suspect that certain bacteria, such as strains of mycobacterium, may be the cause. Although diet may affect the symptoms, it is unlikely that diet is responsible for the disease.

Signs and Symptoms.   Common symptoms of Crohn's disease are abdominal pain, diarrhea, and weight loss. Less common symptoms are poor appetite, fever, night sweats, rectal pain, and rectal bleeding. Patients with Crohn's disease typically experience periods of relapse (worsening of inflammation) followed by periods of remission (reduced inflammation) lasting months to years.

Treatment.   There is no cure for Crohn's disease. The goals of treatment are to induce remission, maintain remission, minimize side effects of treatment, and improve quality of life. Patients with mild or no symptoms or whose disease is in remission (symptoms are absent) may not need treatment. Treatment of both Crohn's disease and ulcerative colitis with medications is similar, though not always identical. These medications may include anti-inflammatory agents such as

5-ASA compounds, corticosteroids, antibiotics, and immunomodulators. Severe Crohn's disease may lead to a colostomy, temporarily or permanently.

DIARRHEA

Diarrhea is an increase in the frequency of bowel movements or a greater looseness in stool formation. Although changes in frequency or in stool formation can vary independently of each other, they usually occur in conjunction with each other.

Diarrhea can be acute or chronic. Acute diarrhea lasts from a few days up to a week. Chronic diarrhea can be defined in several ways but almost always lasts more than 3 weeks. It is important to distinguish between acute and chronic diarrhea because they usually have different causes, require different diagnostic tests, and require different treatment.

Infection—viral, bacterial, or parasitic—is the most common cause of acute diarrhea. Another important cause of acute diarrhea is the side effect of medications. Food containing infectious microbes can lead to the colon not functioning properly and not retaining fluid, thus causing the loose stools of diarrhea.

Signs and Symptoms.   Increase in frequency of stool from the patient's normal amount is one symptom. Runny stool is another symptom.

Treatment.   Diarrhea is usually treated with absorbents and antimotility medications. Absorbents are compounds that absorb water. Taken orally, they bind with water in the small intestine and colon and make the stools less watery. They also may bind toxic chemicals produced by bacteria that cause the small intestine to secrete fluid; however, the importance of toxin binding in reducing diarrhea is unclear. Antimotility medications relax the muscles of the small intestine or the colon, slowing the flow of intestinal contents. A slower flow provides more time for water to be absorbed from the intestine and colon, thereby reducing the water content of stool. Cramps caused by spasm of the intestinal muscles also are relieved by muscular relaxation.

DIVERTICULITIS

Diverticulitis is an inflammation or infection of a diverticulum, a small pouch or sac in the wall of the colon (Figure 30-9). The exact cause of diverticulitis is not known, but the inflammation generally begins when stool lodges in a diverticulum. Infection can lead to complications such as swelling or rupture.

Signs and Symptoms.   Symptoms include pain, fever, chills, cramping, bloating, constipation, and diarrhea.

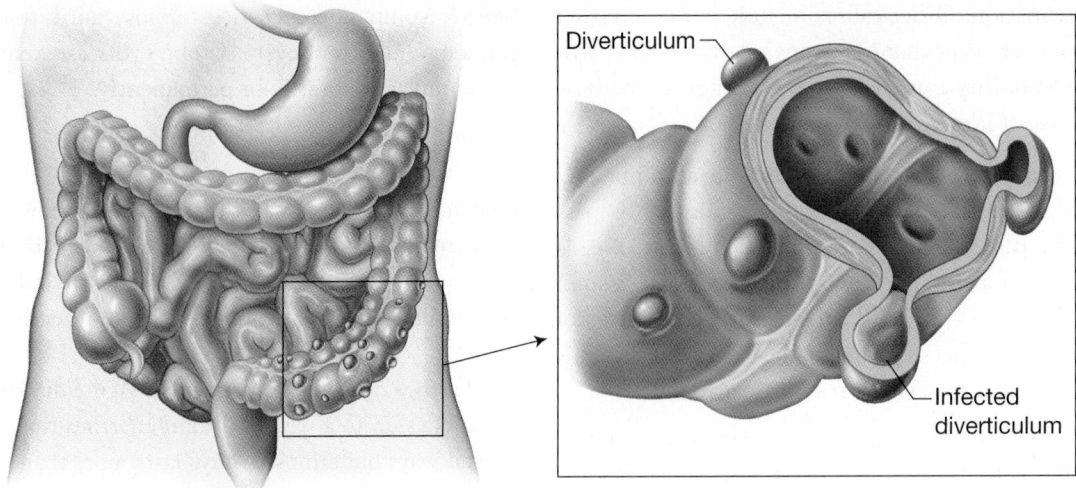

FIGURE 30-9 Colon with diverticulosis. An inflamed or infected diverticulum is called diverticulitis.

Treatment. Treatment depends on the severity of the condition and ranges from a liquid diet and oral antibiotics to hospitalization and surgery.

DIVERTICULOSIS

Diverticulosis is characterized by the presence of diverticula, or small outpouchings, from the colon (see Figure 30-9). It can occur anywhere in the colon but typically appears in the sigmoid colon, the S-shaped segment of the colon in the left lower part of the abdomen. The incidence of diverticulosis increases with age as the walls of the colon weaken and diverticula form more easily. By age 80, most people have diverticulosis. Another key factor in the formation of diverticula is elevated pressure within the colon brought on when a person is constipated and has to push down to expel hard, dry stool.

Signs and Symptoms. Most patients with diverticulosis have few or no symptoms; mild symptoms include abdominal cramping and bloating. However, this condition sets the stage for inflammation and infection of the diverticula (diverticulitis).

Treatment. Eating a high-fiber diet is the best way to avoid developing diverticulosis. Fiber keeps the bowels moving, helps maintain normal pressure within the colon, and slows or stops the formation of diverticula. Treatments include relaxing the colon with IV therapy and a soft diet. Surgery to remove the diverticula is sometimes needed.

GASTROESOPHAGEAL REFLUX DISEASE

Gastroesophageal reflux disease (GERD) occurs when the muscle at the superior portion of the stomach (the cardiac sphincter) does not close tightly, or relaxes inappropriately, allowing for gastric fluids and stomach contents to back up into the esophagus and the throat. If not treated, the patient with GERD may develop reflux esophagitis, a potentially serious inflammation of the esophagus caused by the acidic fluids from the stomach. GERD may also lead to Barrett's esophagitis, a precancerous condition that must be treated. Other possible results of long-term, untreated GERD are perforation of the esophagus, esophageal cancer, esophageal stricture (abnormal narrowing of the esophagus), and esophageal ulcers.

Signs and Symptoms. Symptoms include heartburn, sore throat, a hoarse voice, a bad taste in the mouth, belching, and regurgitation of food. Some patients are symptom free.

Treatment. Treatment of GERD relies on medications that block the production of hydrochloric acid (the chief

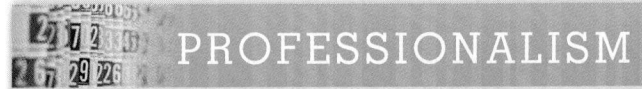

PROFESSIONALISM

THE LAW

Some digestive disorders, such as stomach ulcers, IBS, and GERD, may be associated with a person's lifestyle. As a member of the health care profession, your role is to provide care and assist with the treatment of your patients, and it is never acceptable, nor appropriate, to judge or make reference to how a person chooses to live his or her life. However, when required, you are expected to provide patients with information and education regarding how they can best manage their conditions and, at the same time, live a long and productive life.

digestive acid) and protect the mucosa of the esophagus. Patients may incorporate simple measures such as not lying down until at least 3 hours after eating, losing weight, sleeping on a bed that has the head raised 6 inches, and sleeping on the left side. If medications and basic treatments do not work, fundoplication, a surgical procedure that tightens the cardiac sphincter and its surrounding tissues, can be performed. Strictures are treated with dilation, or expansion, of the narrowed area.

HEMORRHOIDS

A **hemorrhoid** is a dilated, or enlarged, vein in the walls of the anus and sometimes the rectum, usually caused by untreated constipation but occasionally associated with chronic diarrhea.

Signs and Symptoms. The major symptom is bleeding after defecation. If untreated, hemorrhoids can worsen and protrude from the anus. Fissures may develop and cause intense discomfort.

Treatment. Treatment involves changing the diet to prevent constipation and avoid further irritation, using topical medication and sometimes surgery or sclerotherapy (injection of a solution such as saline to shrink the hemorrhoid). In their worst stage, external hemorrhoids must be returned to the anal cavity manually.

HERNIA

A **hernia** is the abnormal protrusion of an organ or part of an organ through the wall of the body cavity that contains it. The most common types of abdominal hernias are hiatal hernias and inguinal hernias.

Hiatal Hernia

Hiatal hernia is a condition in which the upper portion of the stomach protrudes into the chest cavity through an opening in the diaphragm called the esophageal hiatus (Figure 30-10). This opening is normally large enough to accommodate the esophagus alone. With weakening and enlargement, however, the opening (or herniation) can allow the passage or even entrapment of the upper stomach above the diaphragm. Hiatal hernia is a common condition.

Suspected causes or contributing factors of hiatal hernia include obesity, poor seated posture (such as slouching), frequent coughing, straining with constipation, frequent bending over or heavy lifting, heredity, smoking, and congenital defects.

Signs and Symptoms. Symptoms include chest pain or pressure, heartburn, difficulty swallowing, coughing, belching, and hiccups. Hiatal hernia also causes discomfort when it is associated with gastroesophageal reflux disease. GERD is characterized by the backing up of stomach acids and digestive enzymes into the esophagus through a weakened sphincter that normally acts as a one-way valve between the esophagus and stomach. Hiatal hernia is thought to contribute to the weakening of this sphincter muscle.

Treatment. Remaining in an upright position or sleeping in an upright chair might ease the reflux. Some medications help with the reflux and with healing the esophagus. Weight loss can reduce pressure on the stomach. Ultimately the only cure is surgery.

Inguinal Hernia

An **inguinal hernia** occurs when tissue or part of the intestine pushes through a weak spot in the abdominal wall in

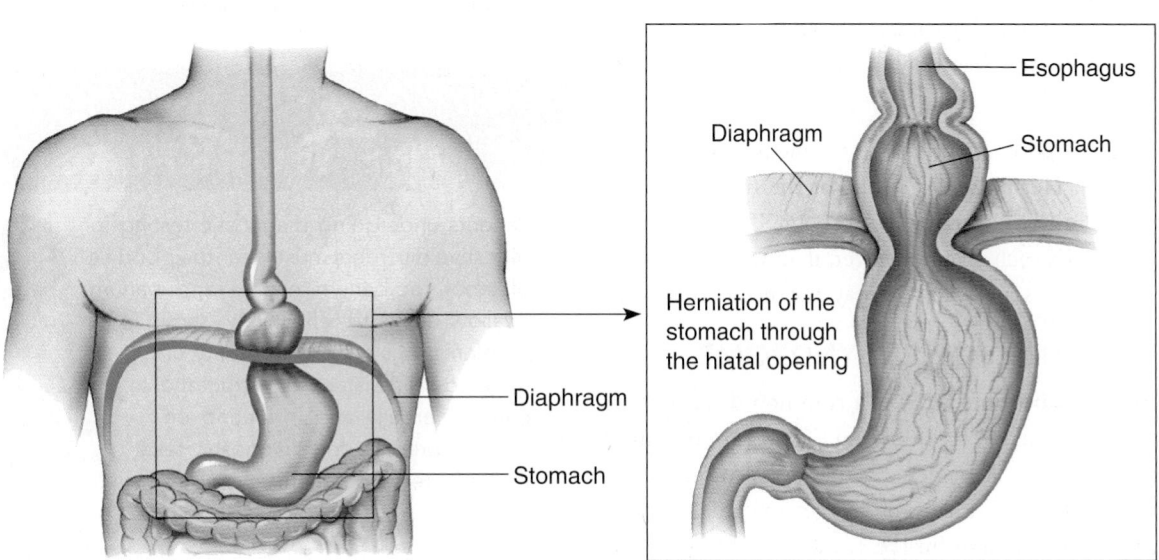

FIGURE 30-10 Hiatal hernia.

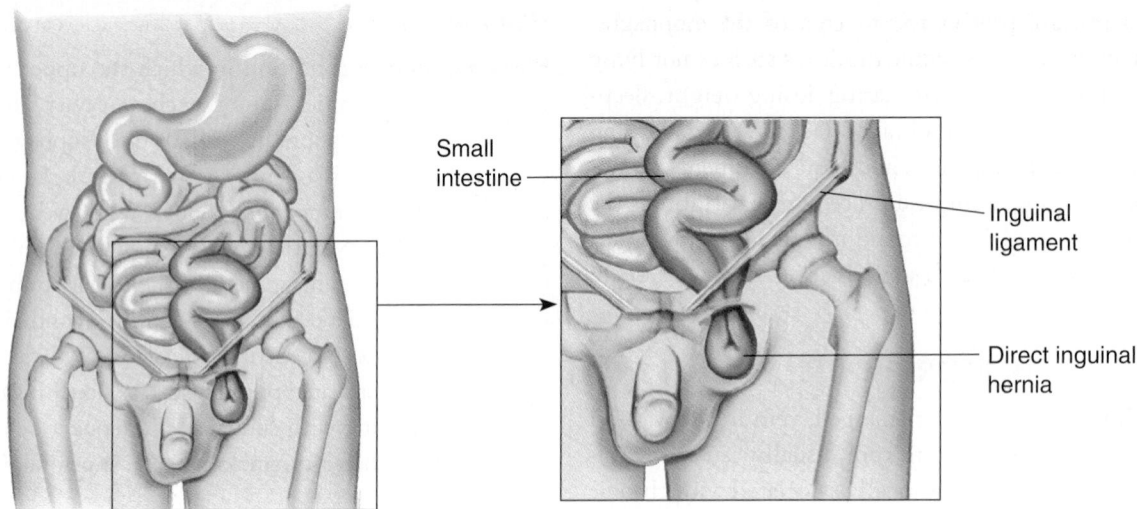

FIGURE 30-11 Inguinal hernia.

the groin area, causing a bulge in the groin or scrotum (Figure 30-11). The bulge may appear gradually over a period of several weeks or months, or it may form suddenly after the patient has been lifting heavy weights, coughing, bending, straining, or even laughing. Many hernias flatten when the patient lies down.

Signs and Symptoms. Many hernias do not cause any pain. If pain and discomfort are present, they are usually worse when the person bends or lifts an object. Nausea and vomiting may also be present if part of the intestine bulges outside the abdomen and becomes trapped (incarcerated) in the hernia.

Other symptoms of a hernia include heaviness, swelling, and a tugging or burning sensation in the area of the hernia, scrotum, or inner thigh. Males may have a swollen scrotum, and females may have a bulge in the large fold of skin (labia) surrounding the vagina. Discomfort and aching are relieved only when the person lies down, especially as the hernia grows larger.

Treatment. Surgery is the only treatment and cure for inguinal hernia. Hernia repair is one of the most common surgeries done in the United States. About 750,000 people have hernia repairs each year. However, if an inguinal hernia does not cause any symptoms, it may not need treatment.

IRRITABLE BOWEL SYNDROME

Irritable bowel syndrome (IBS) is a common disorder that interferes with normal colon function. The cause or causes remain unclear. IBS is considered a functional disorder because it is thought to result from changes in colon activity. Stress is an important factor in IBS because of the close nervous system connections between the brain and the intestines.

Just as healthy people under stress can feel nauseated or have an upset stomach, people with IBS react the same way, but to a greater degree. Finally, IBS symptoms sometimes intensify during menstruation, which suggests that female reproductive hormones are another trigger.

Signs and Symptoms. IBS is characterized by abdominal pain and cramps, changes in bowel movements (diarrhea, constipation, or both), gassiness, bloating, and nausea. Other symptoms, which vary from person to person, include an uncontrollable urge to defecate (urgency), passage of a sticky fluid (mucus) during bowel movements, and the feeling after finishing a bowel movement that the bowels are still not completely empty. The symptoms of IBS tend to rise and fall in intensity rather than worsen over time.

Treatment. There is no cure for IBS, and much about the condition remains poorly understood. However, dietary

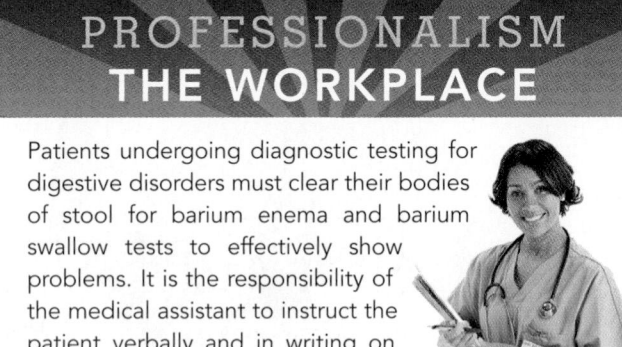

PROFESSIONALISM THE WORKPLACE

Patients undergoing diagnostic testing for digestive disorders must clear their bodies of stool for barium enema and barium swallow tests to effectively show problems. It is the responsibility of the medical assistant to instruct the patient verbally and in writing on how to prepare for diagnostic tests that require preparation.

changes, drugs, and psychological treatment are often sufficient to eliminate or substantially reduce symptoms.

ORAL CANCER

Almost all cases of **oral cancer** start in the flat squamous
cells that line the mouth. Squamous cell carcinoma can start
on the lips, the inside of the lips and cheeks (buccal mucosa),
the gums, the front two-thirds of the tongue, the tissue under the tongue, the tissue behind the wisdom teeth, and the
bony roof of the mouth (hard palate).

Oral cancer has no single cause, but several factors appear
to increase the risk of developing it:

- Aging, particularly after 50
- Gender—more men develop oral cancer
- Smoking, particularly if combined with heavy alcohol
  consumption
- Using chewing tobacco or snuff, or chewing betel nut
- Heavy alcohol consumption, particularly if combined
  with smoking
- Excessive sun exposure to the lips
- Certain medical problems in the oral tissues

Signs and Symptoms.   The signs and symptoms of oral
cancer can be seen and felt quite early. Pain is very rare in the
early stages, but any sore, irritation, or swelling in the
mouth or lump on the neck that lasts longer than 2 weeks
should be checked by a doctor or dentist. Velvety red or
white patches in the mouth may also indicate a precancerous
condition. Other symptoms are sores or wartlike patches on
the lip; a persistent sore throat; sores under dentures; a lump
in the lip, tongue, or neck; and trouble chewing, swallowing, or speaking.

Treatment.   Treatment of oral cancer depends on the
extent of the condition. Surgery to remove part or all of
the tumor and some surrounding tissue may be required.
Radiation and chemotherapy, which interfere with the
cancer cells' ability to grow and spread, are other treatment
options.

PANCREATIC CANCER

The most common type of **pancreatic cancer** develops in
the exocrine glands and is called adenocarcinoma of the
pancreas. The endocrine glands of the pancreas can give rise
to a completely different type of cancer, a very rare form
called pancreatic neuroendocrine carcinoma, or islet cell
tumor. In 2004, approximately 31,800 people in the
United States were diagnosed with pancreatic cancer; of
these, approximately 31,200 people died. These numbers

reflect the challenge in treating pancreatic cancer and the
relative lack of curative options.

Signs and Symptoms.   The symptoms of pancreatic cancer are generally vague and can easily be attributed to other
less serious and more common conditions. Because of the
lack of specific symptoms, a large number of people are not
diagnosed until the disease is in an advanced stage. The
main symptoms are pain in the abdomen, the back, or both;
weight loss, often associated with loss of appetite; bloating;
diarrhea or fatty bowel movements that float in water; and
jaundice or yellowing of the skin.

Treatment.   Complete surgical removal of the cancer is
the only known cure for pancreatic cancer. Unfortunately,
only 15 to 20 percent of pancreatic cancers can be surgically
removed at the time of diagnosis. Depending on how
advanced the cancer is, chemotherapy and radiation therapy
may be included in the treatment.

PEPTIC ULCER DISEASE

Peptic ulcer disease (PUD) is characterized by a disruption
in the lining of the esophagus, stomach, or duodenum
(Figure 30-12). PUD appears most frequently in the duodenum (the upper part of the small intestine). Ulcers in the
stomach are also common. The stomach produces acid that
breaks food down during the digestive process. The stomach
and upper part of the small intestine (duodenum) are protected from the acid by a lining of sticky fluid (mucus).
Damage to the lining exposes the sensitive tissue underneath to acid, and further irritation may cause a **stomach
ulcer** to form. Bacteria may also cause stomach ulcers.

An imbalance between acid and pepsin (an enzyme) secretion
and the defenses of the mucosal lining results in inflammation,
which may be caused or aggravated by aspirin or nonsteroidal
anti-inflammatory drugs (NSAIDs) such as ibuprofen. Infection
with the bacterium *Helicobacter pylori* can cause erosion of the
stomach mucosa, further aggravating the condition.

Ulcers can be prevented by avoiding alcohol and tobacco
and limiting the use of NSAIDs and aspirin. Spicy foods do
not cause ulcers but can aggravate the condition.

Signs and Symptoms.   The most common symptoms of
PUD are abdominal pain, nausea, vomiting, and weight
loss. Esophageal ulcers often cause heartburn and chest pain.
Other symptoms include tarry black or maroon stools (indicating old blood), fresh blood in the stools (which is normally bright red in appearance), and a burning or gnawing
pain in the stomach or the back.

Stomach or gastric ulcers are more common in people
over the age of 50. Mild symptoms may be mistaken for

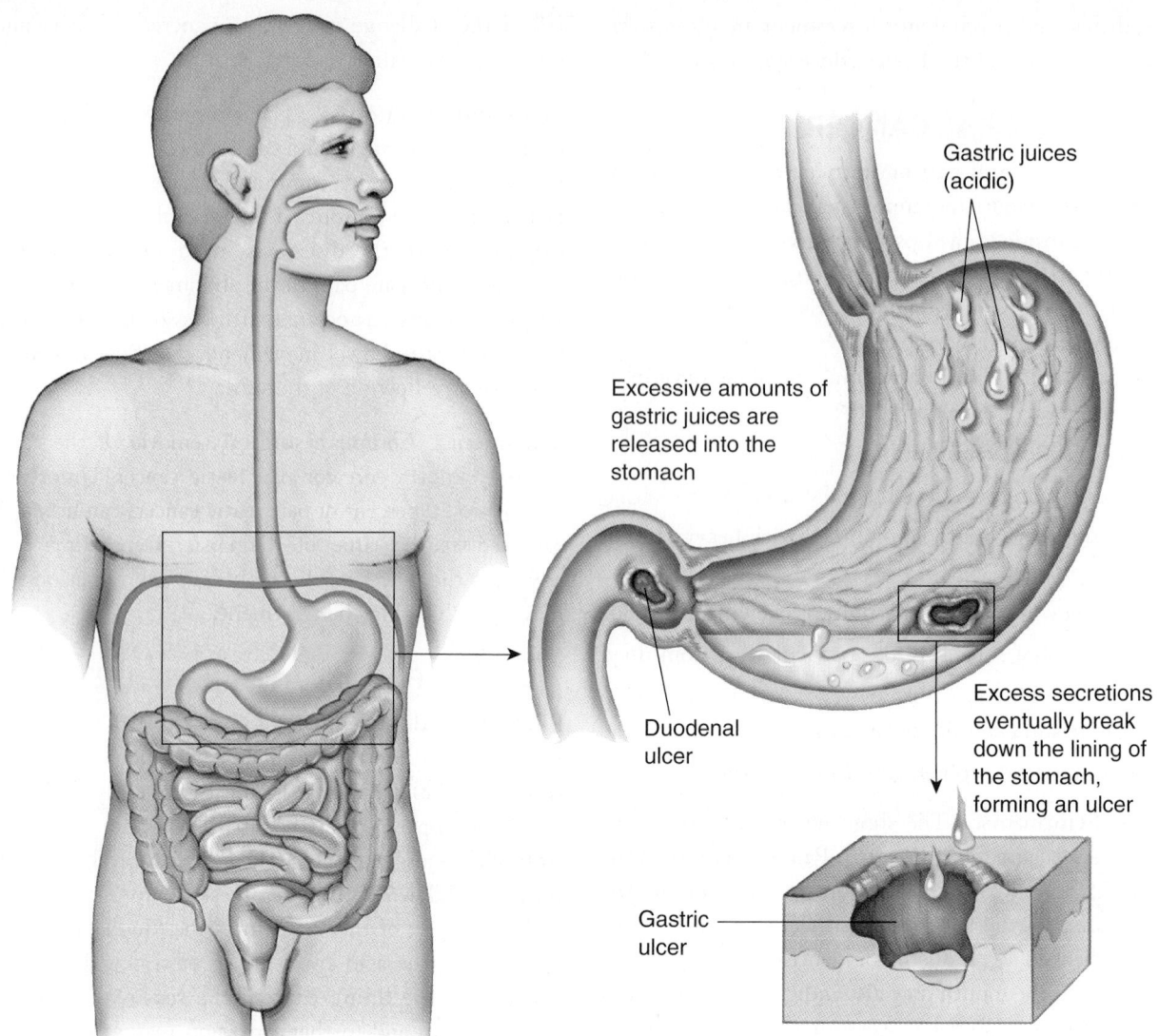

Gastric juices
(acidic)

Excessive amounts of
gastric juices are
released into the
stomach

Duodenal
ulcer

Excess secretions
eventually break
down the lining of
the stomach,
forming an ulcer

Gastric
ulcer

FIGURE 30-12   Peptic ulcer disease (PUD).

indigestion or heartburn. Symptoms include any or all of the following:

- Pain or a burning sensation (similar to indigestion) in the upper abdomen and sometimes the lower chest. The pain from a duodenal ulcer can be worse when the stomach is empty and is relieved by eating, but then recurs a few hours afterward
- Pain that is made worse by eating
- Difficulty swallowing or regurgitation (bringing up swallowed food into the mouth)
- Bloating, retching, and feeling ill, particularly after eating
- Vomiting and nausea
- Loss of appetite and weight loss

Severe ulcers may have the tendency to bleed and be very painful. Bleeding may indicate a serious problem; the ulcer

may have burrowed through the stomach or duodenal wall, or it may be blocking the path of food trying to leave the stomach. Sometimes the stomach acid or the ulcer itself breaks a blood vessel in the lining of the stomach or duodenum.

Treatment.   Treatment of PUD depends on the cause. Any medications that may cause or aggravate the condition must be changed. Tobacco and alcohol should be avoided because they delay healing. Medications are prescribed to protect the stomach by decreasing or stopping the secretion of stomach acids. If long-term treatment with aspirin or another NSAID is the cause of the stomach ulcer, ulcer-healing drugs and additional drugs to protect the lining of the stomach and duodenum are recommended. Antibiotics may be given to treat *H. pyloric* infections. Occasionally surgery may be required if the ulcer does not respond to medication. Surgical options include the following:

- **Vagotomy**—cutting the vagus nerve that links the stomach to the brain, reducing acid production

- **Antrectomy**—removing the lower part of the stomach that produces the hormone that controls the production of digestive juices
- **Pyloroplasty**—enlarging the opening into the duodenum and small intestine to allow the contents of the stomach to move more freely

PYLORIC STENOSIS

The pylorus is the connection between the stomach and the first part of the small intestine (duodenum). In **pyloric stenosis**, a baby's pylorus gradually swells and thickens, interfering with the flow of food into the intestine. This disorder can occur anytime between birth and 5 months of age but most commonly develops about 3 weeks after birth.

Signs and Symptoms.   Vomiting all or most of feedings repeatedly is the main symptom of pyloric stenosis. The vomiting usually starts gradually and worsens over time. As the pylorus constricts, the vomiting becomes more frequent and more forceful. The baby loses weight, develops symptoms of dehydration, is sleepier than normal, and is very fussy when awake.

Treatment.   Pyloric stenosis is always treated with surgery (pyloromyotomy). After surgery, the disorder usually does not develop again.

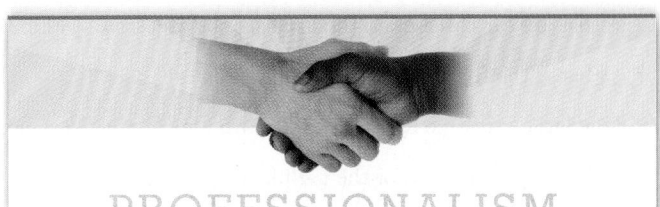

PROFESSIONALISM
CULTURAL CONSIDERATIONS

Culture seems to play a major role in how people eat and view disorders of the digestive system. Hindus, for example, believe in fasting and in eating a specific way. Americans may believe such a lifestyle could lead to digestive problems, whereas Hindus believe their dietary practices are part of what makes them one with God. Other cultures, such as those in the Far East, believe that alternative medicine therapies, such as acupuncture, homeopathy, meditation, and biofeedback, are frequently more useful than Western medicine in treating disorders of the digestive system. Whereas there may appear to be many cultural stereotypes regarding specific diseases of the digestive system, it is important for all members of the health care team to always respect a person's beliefs and focus on supporting and treating the patient. When asking questions or assisting in a treatment, make sure that the questions are not disrespectful and that your care is directed at the "total" patient, not just the disease.

SUMMARY

The digestive system consists of a single tube starting at the mouth and ending at the rectum. Its three main functions are digestion, absorption, and elimination. The primary organs of the digestive system are the mouth, pharynx, esophagus, stomach, small intestine, large intestine, and rectum. The accessory organs of digestion are the salivary glands, pancreas, liver, and gallbladder. Disorders of the digestive system involve the organs of the gastrointestinal tract and the accessory organs. Among the diseases of the gastrointestinal system are appendicitis, cirrhosis, colitis, colorectal cancer, constipation, Crohn's disease, diarrhea, diverticulitis, diverticulosis, gastroesophageal reflux disease, hemorrhoids, hernias, irritable bowel syndrome, oral cancer, pancreatic cancer, peptic ulcer disease, and pyloric stenosiss.

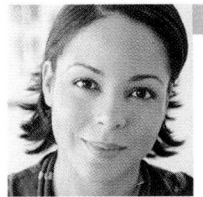

30 CHAPTER REVIEW

COMPETENCY REVIEW

1. Define and spell the terms to learn for this chapter.

2. Name the primary organs associated with digestion.

3. What are the four accessory organs of digestion?

4. What are the three main functions of the digestive system?

5. What is the first portion of the intestine called?

6. The large intestine can be divided into four distinct sections. Name them.

7. What is the function of the gallbladder?

8. What saclike organ converts food into a semiliquid form called chyme?

9. With how many deciduous teeth is a person born?

10. What essential role does the liver play?

PREPARING FOR THE CERTIFICATION EXAM

1. Which of the following is found on the right side of the abdomen?
   a. ascending colon
   b. descending colon
   c. pancreas
   d. stomach
   e. cardiac sphincter

2. The muscle at the most inferior portion of the stomach is the
   a. pyloric sphincter
   b. esophageal sphincter
   c. cardiac sphincter
   d. gallbladder
   e. fundus

3. Which vitamin is NOT stored by the liver?
   a. A
   b. K
   c. C
   d. D
   e. E

4. Which of the following is part of the large intestine?
   a. jejunum
   b. ileum
   c. duodenum
   d. pancreas
   e. sigmoid

5. What is the function of the liver?
   a. production of bile
   b. storage of bile
   c. production of pepsin
   d. production of insulin
   e. storage of insulin

6. By what age do most children have all their deciduous teeth?
   a. 6 months
   b. 1 year
   c. 2 years
   d. 3 years
   e. 10 years

7. Which of the following is a disease of the mouth?
   a. pancreatitis
   b. cirrhosis
   c. cholecystitis
   d. colitis
   e. stomatitis

8. A chronic disease of the liver is
   a. pancreatitis
   b. cirrhosis
   c. cholecystitis
   d. colitis
   e. stomatitis

9. The abbreviation GERD stands for is
   a. generalized enteritis recurrent disease
   b. gastrointestinal reflux disease
   c. gastrointestinal recurrent disease
   d. gastroesophageal reflux disease
   e. gastroesophageal recurrent disease

10. Which of the following is an adenocarcinoma?
    a. cirrhosis
    b. diverticulosis
    c. pancreatic cancer
    d. oral cancer
    e. GERD

CRITICAL THINKING

1. Dr. Penningworth speaks with Marshall and then excuses himself from the examination room. Meanwhile, Dr. Penningworth tests Susan's knowledge and asks her if she has any idea what might be afflicting Marshall. Based on what is known, what might be Susan's response?

2. Dr. Penningworth asks Marshall how long he has struggled with his addiction to alcohol. Marshall informs him that he has had a drinking problem since he was 18, for more than 28 years. Does this strengthen or weaken your suggestion regarding Susan's response to Dr. Penningworth in the preceding question?

3. Assuming the preceding questions have been answered correctly, which quadrant of Marshall's abdomen would be affected?

INTERNET ACTIVITY

Do an Internet search on peptic ulcer disease.

MEDMEDIA

Additional interactive resources and activities for this chapter can be found:

On your student DVD: View applicable procedure videos on the DVD-ROM found in the back of this book.

MyHealthProfessionsKit.com: Test your knowledge of this chapter with games and activities. MyHealthProfessionsKit also includes resources, helpful links, and a Spanish audio glossary.

Medical Assisting Interactive: Practice your procedures as a medical assistant in this simulated doctor's office. This can be accessed through MyHealthProfessionsKit.com.

31

The Urinary System

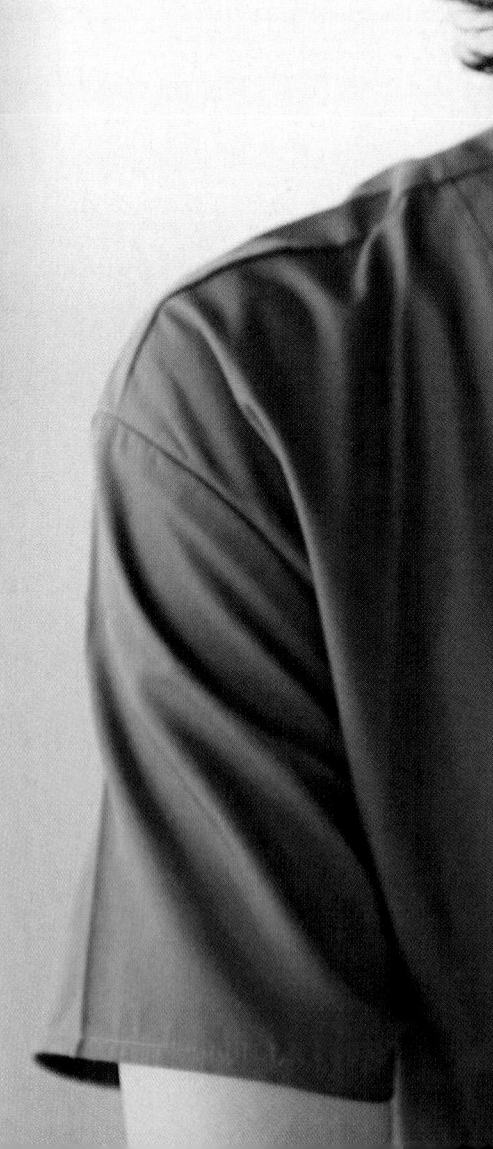

LEARNING OBJECTIVES

After completing this chapter, you should be able to:

- Define and spell the terms to learn for this chapter.

- Describe the purpose and function of the urinary system.

- Identify the structure and function of the individual organs of the urinary system.

- List and discuss the three processes involved in the formation of urine.

- Explain the normal constituents of urine.

- List and briefly explain common disorders associated with the urinary system.

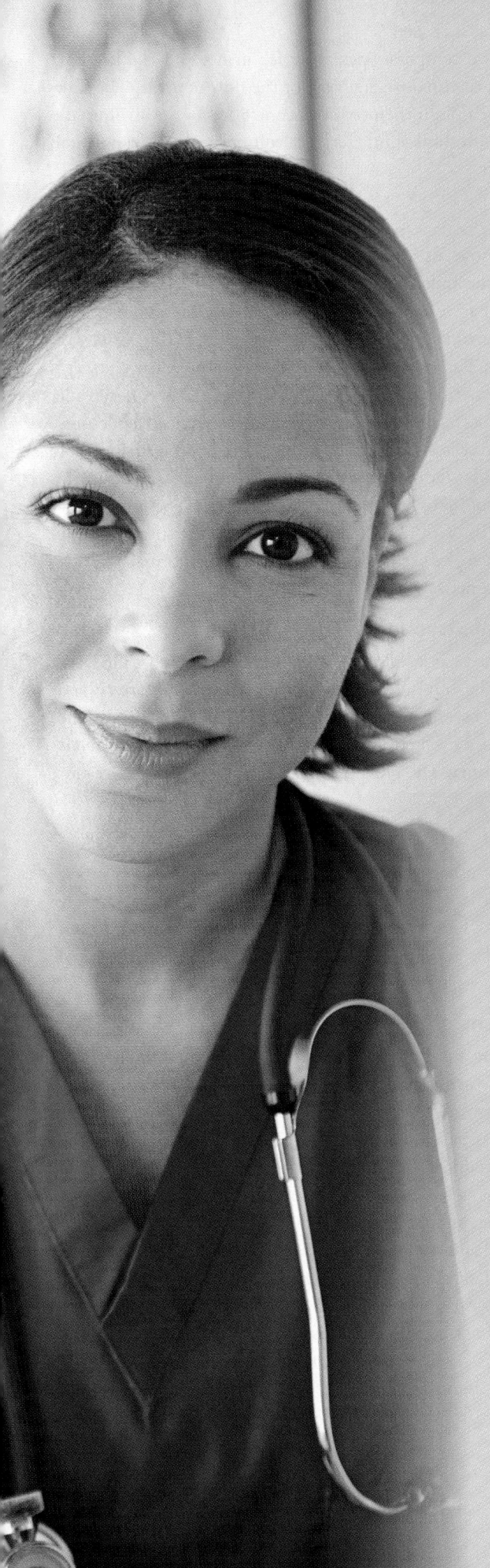

CHAPTER OUTLINE

CASE STUDY

Martin Wilkinson was seen at the emergency room of Pearson General Hospital. He had complaints of severe right-side flank pain. He did not have a previous history of kidney problems and had no pelvic pain or difficulty urinating. He presented to the ED with the following symptoms: sweating, nausea, and complaints of extreme pain. Mr. Wilkinson is diagnosed with a kidney stone (renal calculus) in the right renal ureter.

599

CERTIFICATION LINK

CMA (AAMA)	RMA	CMAS (AMT)
Anatomy and physiology	Anatomy and physiology	Medical assisting foundation

Systems (including structure, function, related conditions and diseases, and their relationships)	Body systems
	  Disorders and diseases of the body
		Anatomy and physiology
		  Medical terminology

The urinary system, also called the genitourinary system, consists of organs that produce and excrete urine from the body (Figure 31-1). Urine is a transparent yellow fluid containing unwanted wastes, mostly excess water, salts, and nitrogen compounds. The primary organs of the system are the kidneys, which continuously filter substances from the blood and produce urine. Urine flows from the kidneys through two long, thin tubes, the ureters. With the aid of gravity and wavelike contractions, the ureters transport the urine to the bladder, a muscular vessel. The normal adult bladder can store up to about 0.5 liter (1 pint) of urine, which it excretes through the tubelike urethra.

Organs of the Urinary System

The kidneys are the primary organs of the urinary system. The other components are the ureters, which transport urine from the kidneys to the urinary bladder; the urinary bladder, which is a temporary reservoir for urine; and the urethra, which is the final passageway for the flow of urine. The flow of urine through the urethra is controlled by an involuntary internal urethral sphincter and voluntary external urethral sphincter.

KIDNEYS

The **kidneys** are a pair of bean-shaped organs located at the back of the abdominal cavity, between the 12th thoracic and 3rd lumbar vertebrae (Figure 31-2). They lie on either side of the spinal column in the flank area, against the muscles of the back. Three capsules surround each kidney: the true capsule, the perirenal fat, and the renal fascia. The true capsule is a smooth, fibrous connective membrane that loosely adheres to the surface of the kidney. Surrounding that is the perirenal fat (adipose capsule), which embeds the kidney in fatty tissue, providing a layer of protection. The renal fascia is a sheath of fibrous tissue that anchors the kidney to the surrounding structures and ensures that the normal position is maintained.

External Structure of the Kidney

The concave border of each kidney has a notch called the **hilum**. The hilum is the entrance for the renal artery and vein, nerves, and the lymphatic vessels. The hilum is also the opening for the ureter, which connects with the **renal pelvis** in the kidney. The renal pelvis is a saclike collecting area for urine.

Internal Structure of the Kidney

Two distinct parts of the kidney are visible on a cross-section: the **cortex** (outer layer) and the **medulla** (middle portion). The arteries, veins, convoluted tubules, and glomerular capsules are found in the cortex, and the renal pyramids are found in the medulla.

Nephrons

Nephrons are the functional units of the kidney. There are about one million nephrons (Figure 31-3), and they are visible only by microscopic examination. Each nephron contains a renal corpuscle and a tubule. The nephron removes the waste products of metabolism from the blood plasma. Nephrons help the body to maintain fluid balance by regulating the amount of fluid and electrolytes reabsorbed into the blood and the amount excreted. Approximately 1,000 to 1,200 mL of blood pass through each kidney per minute, or about 1.5 million mL each day.

The renal corpuscle consists of the glomerulus and the Bowman's capsule. As blood flows into the glomerulus, the nephron removes materials to be discarded. A tubule extending from the Bowman's capsule consists of a proximal

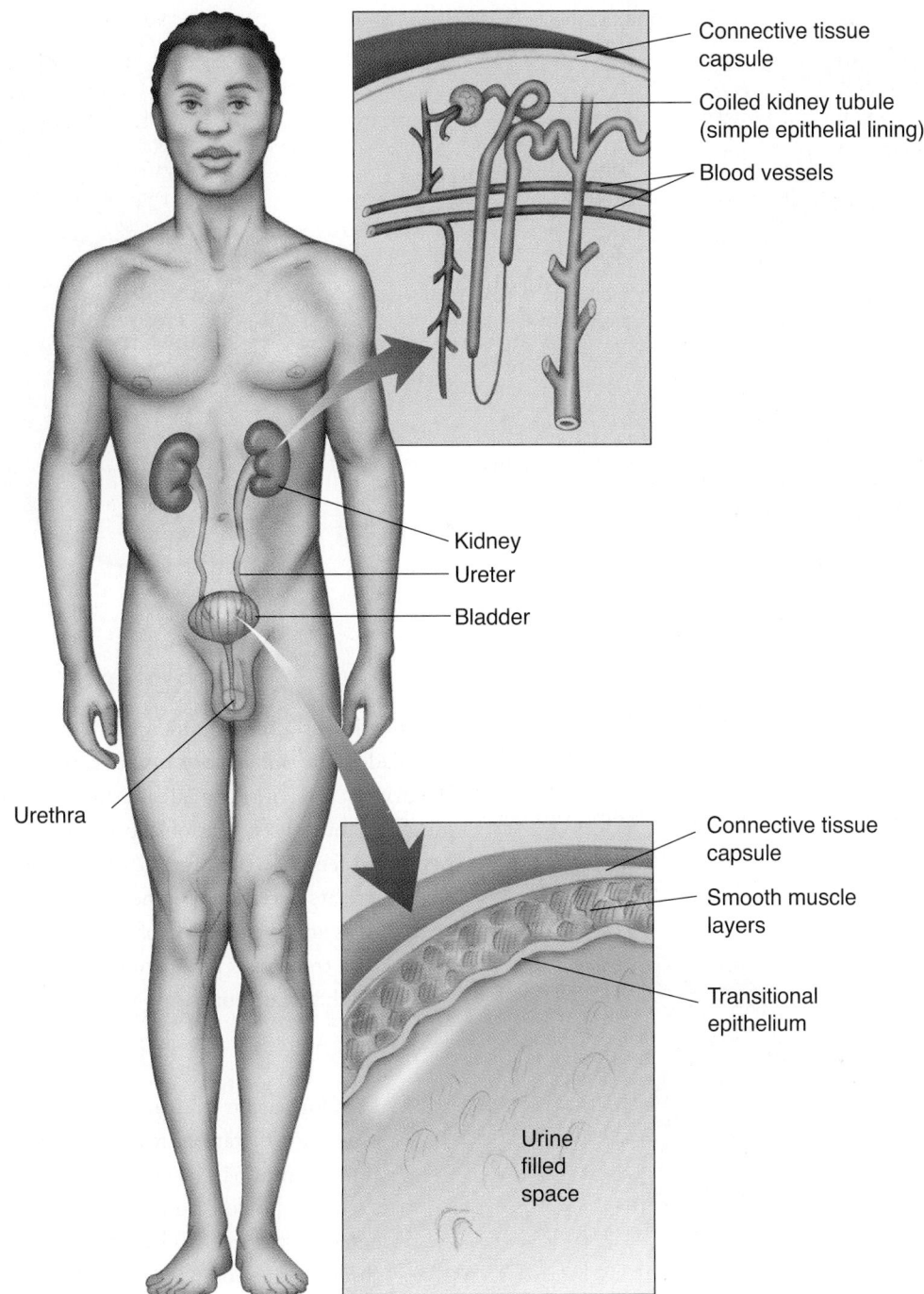

FIGURE 31-1 The urinary system: kidneys, ureters, bladder, and urethra with expanded view of a nephron and the urine-filled space within a bladder.

convoluted portion, the loop of Henle, and a distal convoluted portion, which opens into a collecting tubule. In these tubes, some materials are reabsorbed and others are discarded—depending on the body's need at that time.

URETERS

The **ureters** are two muscular tubes that carry the newly formed urine from each kidney down to the bladder. Each

ureter is 28 to 34 cm long, with a diameter of 1 mm to 1 cm. The ureter wall has three layers: an inner coat of mucous membrane, a middle coat of smooth muscle, and an outer layer of fibrous tissue.

URINARY BLADDER

The **urinary bladder** is a muscular sac in the pelvic cavity that serves as a reservoir for urine. The wall of the bladder is

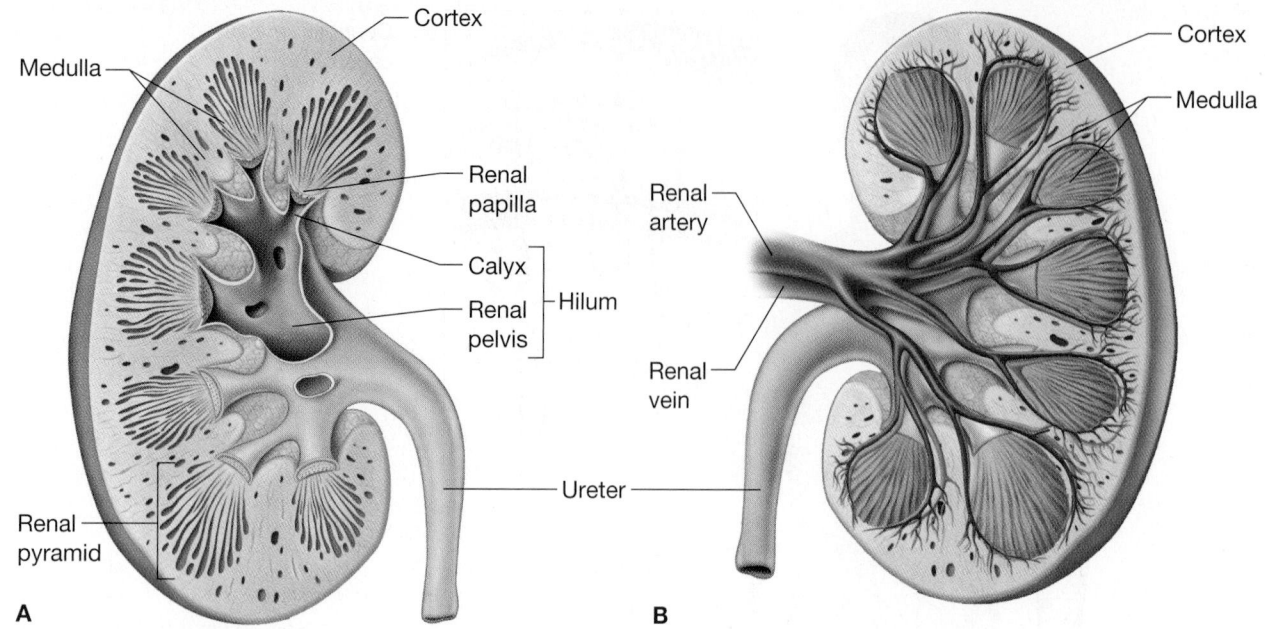

FIGURE 31-2 (A) Sectioned kidney; (B) renal artery and vein.

made up of four layers: an inner layer of epithelium, a muscular coat of smooth muscle, an outer layer of longitudinal muscle, and a fibrous layer. When the bladder is empty, it feels firm because the walls are thick. As the bladder becomes fuller, it stretches and the walls become thinner. The capacity of the bladder is 500 mL of urine.

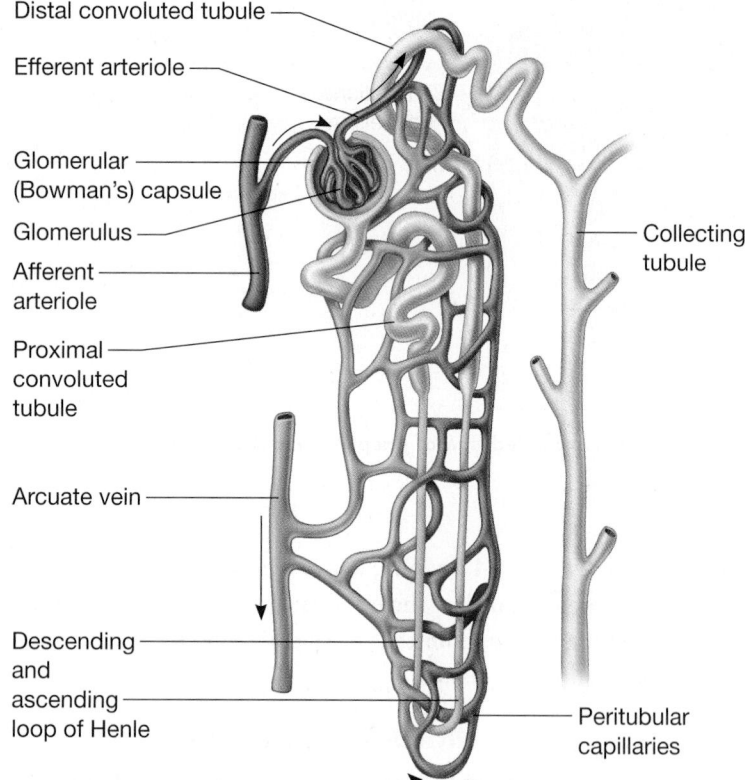

FIGURE 31-3 The structure of a nephron.

URETHRA

The **urethra** is a musculomembranous tube extending from the bladder to the **urinary meatus**, the external opening of the urinary system. The male urethra is approximately 20 cm long and has three sections: prostatic, membranous, and penile. In females, the urethra is approximately 3 cm long, and its external opening is situated between the clitoris and the opening of the vagina. In males, the urethra transports both urine and semen. In females, the urethra transports only urine.

Urine

The formation of urine can be divided into three processes: filtration, reabsorption, and tubular secretion (Figure 31-4). During filtration, or glomerular excretion, blood pressure forces all the small molecules in the blood into the lumen of the nephron through the pores in the walls of both the glomerular capillaries and the Bowman's capsule. As the filtrate passes through the tubules of the nephron, water and many dissolved materials are reabsorbed by the blood. In fact, up to 99 percent of the water is reabsorbed. In addition, the tubules also remove substances from the blood. This process—tubular secretion—supplements the initial glomerular filtration. Water and some selected substances are reabsorbed from the filtrate by the capillaries surrounding the nephrons. Other substances, such as hydrogen ions and uric acid, are transported into the filtrate, now known as urine.

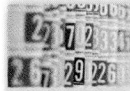

PROFESSIONALISM

THE LAW

Patient privacy is always of utmost concern in any part of the medical field. Never leave a telephone message stating the results of any test, or even stating the type of test a patient had. All messages should simply request that the patient call you back during office hours. Never leave any more information, even on a cell phone. By following this procedure, you will avoid violating HIPAA regulations.

PROFESSIONALISM THE LIFE SPAN

The Child

- At about the 10th week of gestation, the kidneys begin forming urine. By the 3rd months of gestation, the fetus actually begins to secrete small quantities of urine. Quantities continue to increase during the rest of fetal development. However, a newborn's kidneys cannot concentrate urine. Because of this, newborns and even older infants are more prone to fluid volume excess or dehydration. Extreme changes in temperature and fluid intake must be avoided until childrens' kidneys are better able to adjust for fluid needs. Because of the lack of fat pads in the flank, the kidneys of small children are more susceptible to trauma.
- Small children, especially those wearing diapers, are susceptible to urinary tract infections. It is especially important that the diaper area be cleaned regularly and appropriately to prevent urinary tract infections.

The Older Adult

- As people age, the kidneys begin to lose mass as the blood vessels degenerate. The kidneys lose their ability to filter as well, and their ability to conserve water and sodium declines. This means that dehydration can happen more quickly. In addition, the tubules' ability to balance both body pH and electrolytes decreases. As a result, acid–base imbalances are more likely. There is also a loss of muscle tone in the ureters, bladder, and urethra. Bladder capacity is reduced by as much as 50 percent, causing more frequent trips to the bathroom. In some adults, urge incontinence (the inability to voluntarily retain urine) is a big concern.

Urine consists of 95 percent water and 5 percent solid substances. The average adult feels a need to **void**, or urinate, when the bladder contains 300 to 350 mL of urine. The medical term for urination is **micturition**. Typically, 1,000 to 1,500 mL of urine is voided daily, depending on fluid intake. Normal urine is clear (not cloudy), straw colored, and has a mildly aromatic odor, with a specific gravity of 1.003 to 1.030 and a slightly acidic pH of about 6. Specific gravity measures the kidney's ability to concentrate or dilute urine in relation to plasma. Because urine is a solution of minerals, salts, and compounds dissolved in water, the specific gravity is greater than 1.000. The more concentrated

the urine, the higher the specific gravity. An adult's kidneys have a remarkable ability to concentrate or dilute urine. In infants, the range for specific gravity is narrower because immature kidneys cannot concentrate urine as effectively as mature kidneys.

Common Disorders Associated with the Urinary System

Compromised kidneys, and even healthy kidneys, can suffer from a variety of conditions that can affect an individual's lifestyle and activities of daily living (Table 31-1).

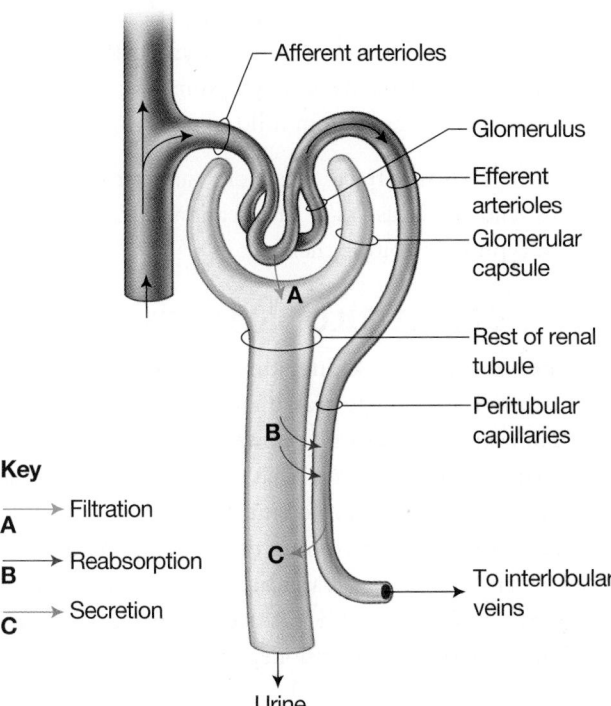

Key

→ **A** Filtration

→ **B** Reabsorption

→ **C** Secretion

FIGURE 31-4 Schematic view of the three stages of urine production: (A) filtration; (B) reabsorption; (C) secretion.

TABLE 31-1 Disorders of the Urinary System

Disorder	Description
Anuria	No urine formed by the kidneys and a complete lack of urine excretion
Bladder neck obstruction	Blockage of the bladder outlet
Dysuria	Painful or difficult urination
Enuresis	Involuntary discharge of urine after the age by which bladder control should have been established; usually occurs by age 5 years; called bed-wetting at night
Glomerulonephritis	Inflammation of the kidney (primarily of the glomerulus); glomerular membrane is inflamed, becomes more permeable, resulting in protein (proteinuria) and blood (hematuria) in the urine
Hematuria	A condition of blood in the urine; usually a symptom of a disease process
Hypospadias	A congenital opening of the male urethra on the underside of the penis
Interstitial cystitis	Disease of an unknown cause in which there is inflammation and irritation of the bladder; most commonly seen in middle-aged women
Nocturia	Excessive urination during the night; may or may not be abnormal
Pyelitis	Inflammation of the renal pelvis
Pyelonephritis	Inflammation of the renal pelvis and the kidney; one of the most common types of kidney disease; may be the result of a lower urinary tract infection that moves up to the kidney via the ureters; large quantities of white blood cells and bacteria may be present in the urine; hematuria may also be present; can result from an untreated or persistent case of cystitis
Pyuria	Presence of pus in the urine
Renal colic	Pain caused by a kidney stone; can be excruciating pain and generally requires medical treatment

CYSTITIS

Cystitis is an inflammation of the bladder, usually secondary to ascending urinary tract infections. Cystitis occurs when bacteria infect the lower urinary tract, causing irritation and inflammation. Most cases of cystitis are caused by *Escherichia coli* (*E. coli*), a bacterium found in the lower gastrointestinal tract.

Urinary tract infections are a common condition that can affect anyone, but particularly sexually active women between the ages of 20 and 50. Women are more frequently affected, in large part because of the anatomy of the perineum, the short length of the urethra, and improper personal hygiene. Sexual activity can introduce bacteria into the urethra. Bacteria in the bladder are often removed through urination, but occasionally they reproduce more quickly than they are washed away, causing an infection. In men, cystitis is usually secondary to another infection, such as epididymitis, prostatitis, gonorrhea, syphilis, or kidney stones.

Interstitial cystitis (IC) is a painful inflammation of the bladder wall. Ninety percent of the 450,000 people who suffer from this condition are women. The cause is unknown.

Signs and Symptoms. The most common symptoms of cystitis are urgency (the need to void immediately) and frequency (the need to void often). Another common symptom is painful urination. Occasionally, the patient may suffer from chills and fever. In chronic cystitis, **dysuria** (burning or painful urination) may be the only symptom. The symptoms of interstitial cystitis range from mild to severe.

Treatment. Urinary tract infections are treated with antibiotics and antispasmodic medications. IC does not respond to typical antibiotic therapy.

GLOMERULONEPHRITIS

Glomerulonephritis is a kidney disease that hampers the kidneys' ability to remove waste and excess fluids. Also called glomerular disease, glomerulonephritis is an inflammation of the kidneys that primarily affects the glomeruli. It can be acute, referring to a sudden attack of inflammation, or chronic, coming on gradually. Glomerular disease can be part of a systemic disease, such as lupus or diabetes, or it can be a disease by itself (primary glomerulonephritis). Glomerulonephritis can lead to kidney failure.

There are many causes of glomerulonephritis, including infections, autoimmune diseases, inflammation of the blood vessels (vasculitis), and conditions that scar the glomeruli. Chronic glomerulonephritis sometimes develops after a bout of acute glomerulonephritis. Infrequently, chronic glomerulonephritis runs in families. In many cases, the specific cause is unknown.

Signs and Symptoms. Specific signs and symptoms of glomerulonephritis vary, depending on the cause and whether the patient has the acute or chronic form. The first indication that something is wrong may be the appearance of symptoms or the results of a routine urinalysis. Signs and symptoms include urine, dark amber in appearance, the color of cola or iced tea. This occurs due to the presence of red blood cells (hematuria); foam in the toilet water from protein in the urine (proteinuria); high blood pressure (hypertension); fluid retention (edema) with swelling evident in the face, hands, feet, and abdomen; fatigue from anemia or kidney failure; and less frequent urination than usual.

Treatment. Some cases of acute glomerulonephritis, especially those that follow a *Streptococcus* infection, often improve on their own and require no specific treatment. In other cases treatment may include the use of diuretics, angiotensin-converting enzyme (ACE) inhibitors, calcium channel blockers, and beta blockers.

INCONTINENCE

More common in women who have had children, **incontinence** is the involuntary and unpredictable flow of urine.

Signs and Symptoms. There are several types of incontinence:

- *Stress incontinence,* the most common form, occurs when sneezing, laughing, or other causes of intra-abdominal pressure cause the involuntary release of urine.

- With *urge incontinence,* the bladder contracts without warning, and leakage occurs if the patient is not able to respond to that need to void immediately.

- *Overflow incontinence* occurs when a blockage prohibits normal emptying. The bladder simply overflows.

- Incontinence while sleeping is known as **enuresis**. Although enuresis is common in small children, by the age of 8 years the pituitary gland should be secreting antidiuretic hormone to stop bed-wetting at night (see Chapter 32).

Treatment. Incontinence is diagnosed by a urologist, and treatment may include medications, surgery, and pelvic floor exercises. Enuresis usually responds well to behavioral modification training, but antidiuretic hormone and medications to control the bladder can also be effective.

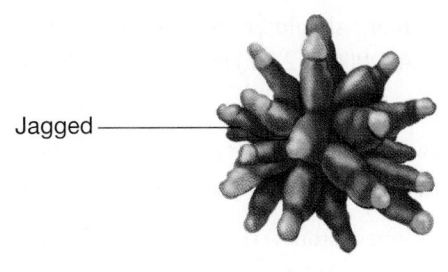

Jagged

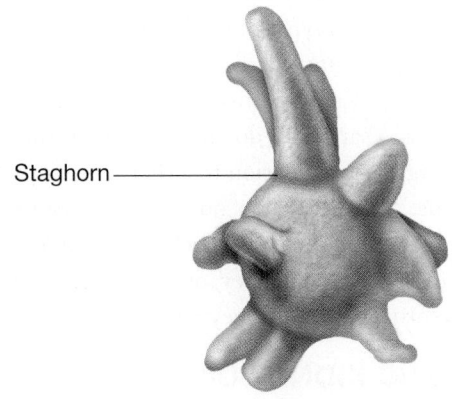

Staghorn

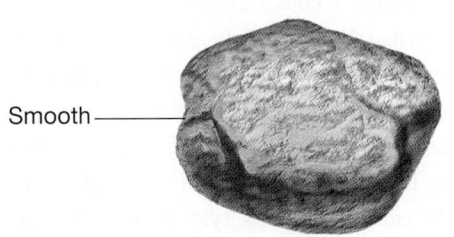

Smooth

FIGURE 31-5 Types of kidney stones found in an adult.

KIDNEY STONES

Kidney stones, or **renal calculi**, are caused by deposits of mineral salts in the kidney (Figure 31-5). The stones are usually benign while still in the kidney, but when they pass into the ureter, they slow or block urine flow. Because the stones have a rough surface, they irritate and scratch the ureters, causing bleeding. The bleeding and decreased urine flow irritate the kidney, causing pain (often very intense) and spasms.

Kidney stones afflict about 10 percent of the people in the United States, and men are more often afflicted than women. Those with a familial history of calculi are more likely to be afflicted. Urinary tract infections, kidney disorders, and metabolic disorders such as hyperparathyroidism are linked to kidney stones.

Most kidney stones are made of calcium oxalate. Excess calcium is absorbed from food and excreted into the urine, where it combines with oxalates to create the stones. Individuals who are prone to this type of stone are advised to control their intake of foods containing calcium and oxalate. Foods high in oxalate include beets, chocolate, tea, coffee, cola, nuts, rhubarb, strawberries, wheat bran, and spinach. To prevent stone formation, fluid intake should be sufficient to produce at least 2 quarts or at least 1,800 to 2,000 mL of urine each day.

Signs and Symptoms. A person suffering from a kidney stone usually presents with flank pain along with possible nausea and vomiting. On urinalysis, hematuria is usually present.

Treatment. Many kidney stones pass out of the body without physician intervention. Stones that cause lasting symptoms or other complications may require treatment, including **lithotripsy**. The two types of lithotripsy are extracorporeal shock wave lithotripsy and percutaneous ultrasonic lithotripsy. Both procedures involve passing shock waves through the body that break down the stone. Other procedures require surgical intervention to either retrieve or disintegrate the stone. Stones that do not pass may cause infection or, if they completely block the ureter, hydronephrosis (swelling of the kidney due to backup of urine), which can eventually cause kidney damage.

POLYCYSTIC KIDNEY DISEASE

Polycystic kidney disease (PKD) is a disorder in which clusters of cysts develop primarily within the kidneys. Cysts are noncancerous (benign) round sacs filled with a waterlike fluid. The disease is not limited to the kidneys, although they are usually the most severely affected organs. Cysts may develop in the liver, pancreas, membranes that surround the brain and central nervous system, ovaries, and seminal vesicles.

PKD affects more than 12 million people worldwide. The disease varies greatly in its severity, and some complications are preventable. Developing high blood pressure is the greatest risk for people with PKD, but regular checkups can help reduce damage to the kidneys. Kidney failure is also common with PKD.

Signs and Symptoms. Signs and symptoms of polycystic kidney disease include high blood pressure, back or side pain related to enlarged kidneys, abdominal pain, an increase in the size of the abdomen, blood in the urine, kidney stones, kidney failure, kidney infections, and headache.

Treatment. Treating polycystic kidney disease involves dealing with and treating the signs, symptoms, and complications of high blood pressure, pain, bladder and kidney infections, blood in the urine, and kidney failure.

PYELONEPHRITIS

Pyelonephritis is an infection of the kidney and renal pelvis. It may have a sudden onset or be a chronic condition. Bacteria entering the kidneys from the bladder, usually *E. coli,* cause pyelonephritis. This may result from the same mechanisms seen in cystitis. Pyelonephritis may be caused by an indwelling urinary catheter, cystoscopy (visualization of the urinary bladder and urethra with a special telescopic instrument), prostate enlargement, and kidney stones.

Signs and Symptoms. Symptoms of pyelonephritis include back, side, and groin pain; urgency and frequency; pain and burning during urination; fever; nausea and vomiting; and blood and pus in the urine.

Treatment. Antibiotics are used to treat pyelonephritis. If it is left untreated, scarring may result that could cause permanent kidney damage.

RENAL FAILURE

When the kidney ceases to function properly, the condition is called renal failure. Renal failure may be acute or chronic.

Acute Renal Failure

Acute renal failure occurs when something causes a change in the filtering function of the kidneys, impairing the kidneys' ability to maintain normal body function. A blockage, toxins, or a sudden loss of blood flow to the kidneys can cause acute renal failure. People who have other kidney diseases are at greater risk for the condition.

Signs and Symptoms. Acute kidney failure has no immediate signs, but, over time, urine output is decreased, resulting in increased fluid buildup in the tissues. Common symptoms include irregular heart rate, **ascites** (fluid in the abdomen), and swelling in the extremities.

Treatment. The treatment of choice for acute renal failure is dialysis. The patient will depend on the dialysis machine

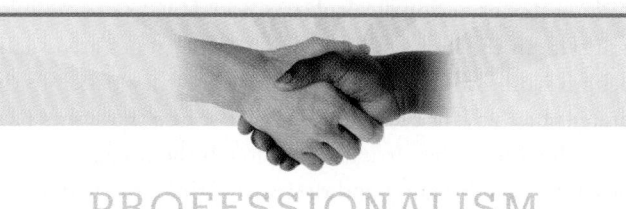

PROFESSIONALISM
CULTURAL CONSIDERATIONS

Be very alert to the modesty requirements of different cultures when discussing urinary tract issues. It may be advisable, and even required in some medical offices, to have a female medical assistant present during examinations of female patients. Female medical assistants should provide the patient education for female patients, and male medical assistants should attend to male patients. Some cultures will not discuss the urinary tract at all, and others may require extensive education and sensitivity to deal with these issues. Be cognizant of patients' body language to help identify issues with which they are uncomfortable.

regained, **dialysis** may be necessary (Figure 31-6). Dialysis uses a filter other than the kidneys to remove toxins and maintain water balance. The two types of dialysis are hemodialysis and peritoneal dialysis.

In hemodialysis, a machine cleans the blood outside of the body. A specialized catheter (a shunt) is inserted into the patient's arm or leg. The shunt is accessed with special tubing that carries the blood to the dialysis machine, where it is

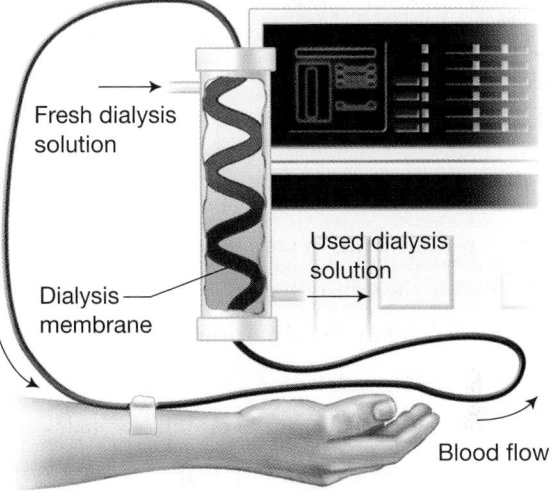

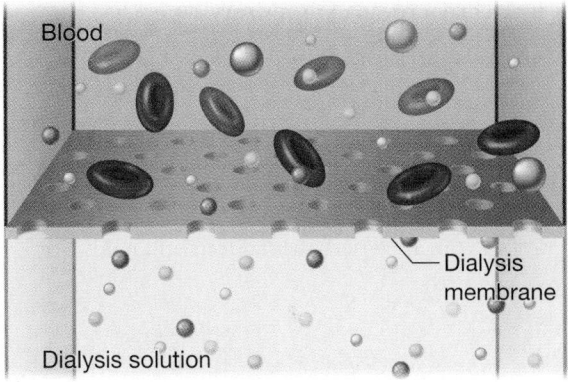

FIGURE 31-6 Dialysis machine showing diffusion of concentrations, which are the same, between the patient's blood and the dialysis solution.

until the kidneys function again. However, if the kidneys do not function on their own again, chronic renal failure is the diagnosis, and three-times-per-week dialysis is required until a kidney transplant is possible or the patient dies.

Chronic Renal Failure

In **chronic renal failure**, there is a gradual and progressive loss of kidney function. Renal failure may be mild or severe and typically takes a period of years to progress. Diabetes and hypertension are the two most common causes of chronic renal failure in the United States. About 2 out of every 1,000 people in the United States have the disorder.

Signs and Symptoms.   Symptoms may be mild or nonexistent until at least 10 percent of kidney function is lost. In chronic renal failure, oliguria (scanty urination) leads to anuria (no urination) and the kidneys cease productive functioning.

Treatment.   The goal of treatment for chronic renal failure is to identify and treat the reversible causes if the kidney fails. Then treatment focuses on preventing fluid volume excesses while the kidneys have a chance to heal and resume their normal function. If normal function cannot be

filtered and cleaned, and then returns the blood to the body. Patients receiving hemodialysis must go to a special center three times a week for 2 to 3 hours at a time.

Peritoneal dialysis is done through the tissues of the abdomen, where a dialysis fluid is instilled in the stomach, left for a period of time while abdominal membranes filter toxins, and then removed. These patients can be dialyzed at home or in any environment.

Some patients may receive a kidney transplant, in which a donor kidney is inserted into the patient's body and the blood vessels and ureters are attached to the patient's already existing structures. Kidney transplant recipients must take antirejection drugs for the rest of their lives in order to live with the transplanted kidney. Kidney transplants are the second most common transplant procedure in the United States.

SUMMARY

The urinary tract can present many challenges for both the patient and the medical assistant. One of the most common reasons patients come into the medical office is to seek help for a urinary tract infection. The urethra's position near the rectum, trauma, and poor hygiene contribute to the frequency of infections. The function of the urinary system, or excretory system, is to extract certain wastes from the bloodstream and transport those wastes as urine outside the body via the kidneys, bladder, ureters, and urethra. Urine is formed by filtration, reabsorption, and tubular secretion. Common disorders of the urinary system include cystitis, glomerulonephritis, kidney stones, and pyelonephritis. Incontinence can also pose a problem, both medically and socially. Polycystic kidney disease can severely impair kidney function. Renal failure is the result of acute or chronic kidney problems and is treated with dialysis.

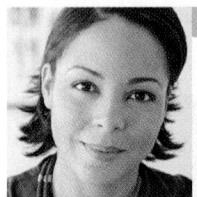

31 CHAPTER REVIEW

COMPETENCY REVIEW

1. Define and spell the terms to learn for this chapter.
2. List the organs of the urinary system.
3. What are the vital functions of the urinary system?
4. Where are the kidneys located?
5. In what portion of the kidney is the medulla located?
6. What is the vital function of the nephrons?
7. What are the three processes of urine formation?
8. What is the major organ of the urinary system?
9. How is renal failure treated?
10. How much urine is formed daily?

PREPARING FOR THE CERTIFICATION EXAM

1. The part of the urinary tract that collects and holds urine for expulsion is the
   a. ureter
   b. bladder
   c. urethra
   d. jejunum
   e. renal pelvis

2. The condition in which an individual experiences an involuntary and unpredictable flow of urine while sleeping is
   a. constipation
   b. enuresis
   c. dysuria
   d. nocturia
   e. anuria

3. A urinary disease characterized by clusters of noncancerous round sacs of waterlike fluid is
    a. pyelonephritis
    b. glomerulonephritis
    c. polycystic kidney disease
    d. cystitis
    e. renal calculus

4. Pain caused by a kidney stone is known as
    a. cystitis
    b. enuresis
    c. incontinence
    d. renal colic
    e. nocturia

5. The anatomical structure of the urinary system that is responsible for carrying urine from the bladder to outside the pelvis is
    a. nephron
    b. ureter
    c. collecting tubule
    d. urethra
    e. renal pelvis

6. An abnormal condition of stones in the bladder is known as
    a. cholelithiasis
    b. cystitis
    c. colitis
    d. cystolithiasis
    e. polycystic disease

7. Which organ is 28 to 34 cm long?
    a. kidney
    b. bladder
    c. urethra
    d. ureter
    e. nephron

8. The usual pH of urine is
    a. 4
    b. 5
    c. 6
    d. 7
    e. 8

9. The normal capacity of a bladder is
    a. 100 mL
    b. 250 mL
    c. 500 mL
    d. 1,000 mL
    e. 1.5 L

10. Which of the following is NOT controlled by the kidneys?
    a. blood sodium
    b. blood pressure
    c. blood clotting
    d. blood potassium
    e. blood chloride

CRITICAL THINKING

1. Mr. Wilkinson had a urinalysis performed that showed a substantial amount of blood in his urine. Why is hematuria common with kidney stones?

2. Due to the size and number of kidney stones present, Mr. Wilkinson was unable to pass the kidney stones. Explain an alternate treatment available for Mr. Wilkinson.

3. When Mr. Wilkinson was discharged from the hospital he was given a list of dietary limitations. What might this list have included?

INTERNET ACTIVITY

Use the Internet to learn about types of incontinence and their treatment.

MEDMEDIA

Additional interactive resources and activities for this chapter can be found:

On your student DVD: View applicable procedure videos on the DVD-ROM found in the back of this book.

MyHealthProfessionsKit.com: Test your knowledge of this chapter with games and activities. MyHealthProfessionsKit also includes resources, helpful links, and a Spanish audio glossary.

Medical Assisting Interactive: Practice your procedures as a medical assistant in this simulated doctor's office. This can be accessed through MyHealthProfessionsKit.com.

32

The Endocrine System

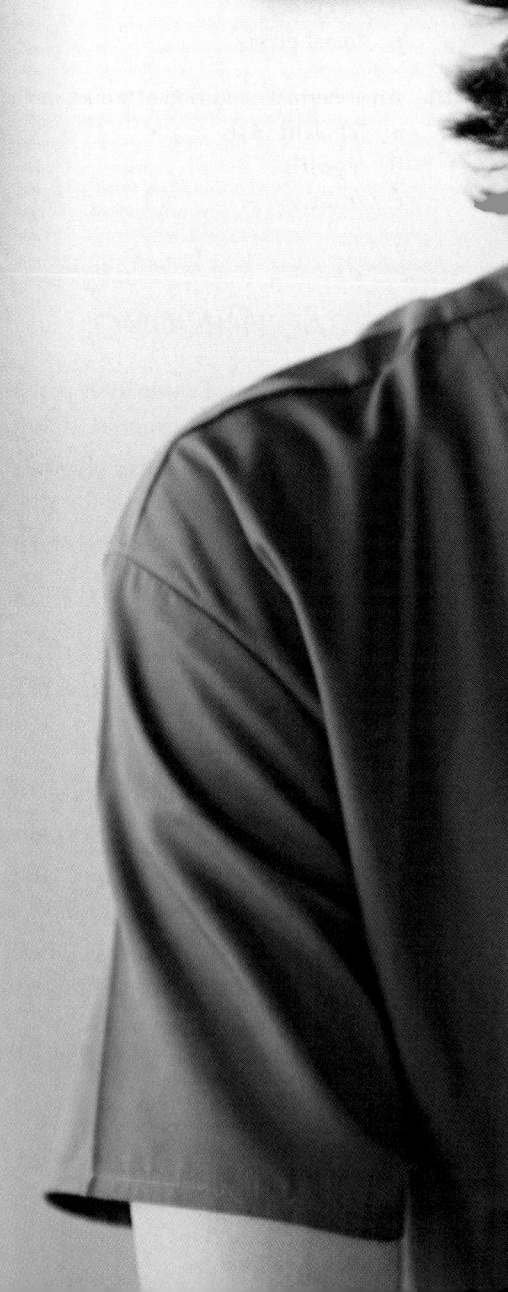

LEARNING OBJECTIVES

After completing this chapter, you should be able to:

- Define and spell the terms to learn for this chapter.

- Describe the primary glands of the endocrine system.

- Explain the vital function of the endocrine system.

- State the structure and primary functions of the endocrine glands.

- Identify and state the functions of the various hormones secreted by the endocrine glands.

- Identify and explain common disorders associated with the endocrine system.

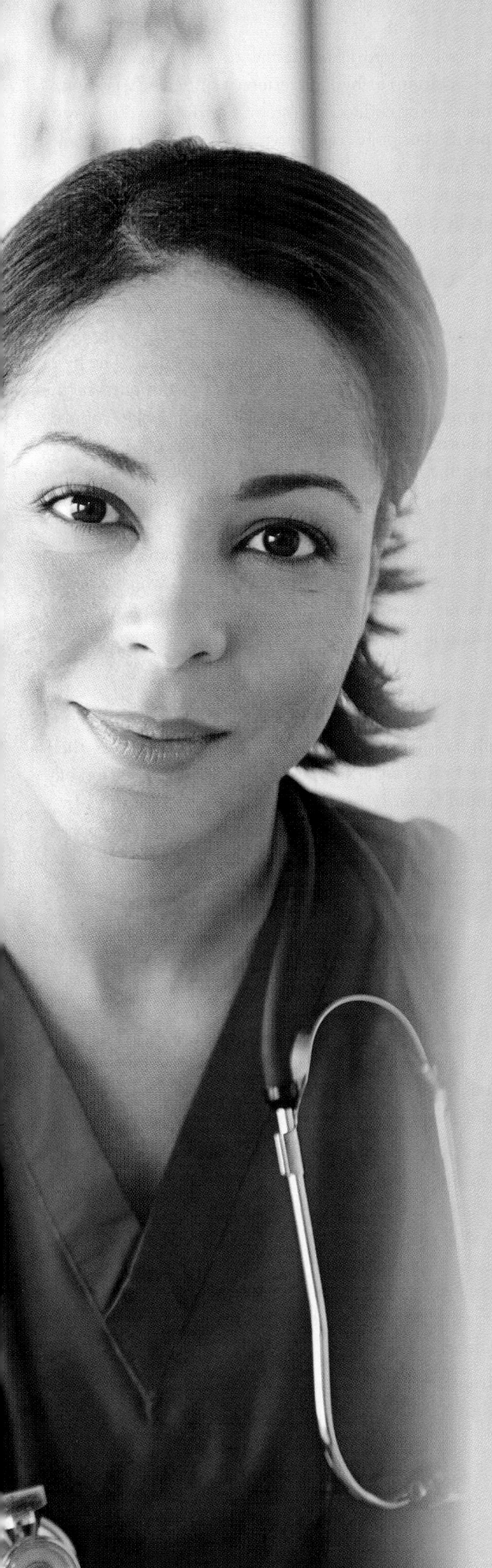

CHAPTER OUTLINE

CASE STUDY

Rosa Gutierrez was just seen by Dr. Bahjat. Her laboratory tests have come back, and she has been diagnosed with type 2 diabetes. She is a Mexican immigrant who has lived in the United States for the past 32 years. She is very worried about how the disease will affect her life.

TERMS TO LEARN

acromegaly

Addison's disease

adrenal glands

cardiomegaly

Cushing's disease

diabetes mellitus

dwarfism

exophthalmos

gestational diabetes

gigantism

goiter

Graves' disease

Hashimoto's thyroiditis

hyperthyroidism

hypothyroidism

insulin-dependent diabetes mellitus (IDDM)

islets of Langerhans

lipolysis

myxedema

non–insulin-dependent diabetes mellitus (NIDDM)

parathyroid glands

pineal gland

pituitary gland

thymus gland

thyroid gland

CERTIFICATION LINK

CMA (AAMA)
Anatomy and physiology

  Systems (including structure, function, related conditions and diseases, and their relationships)

RMA
Anatomy and physiology

  Body systems

  Disorders and diseases of the body

CMAS (AMT)
Medical assisting foundation

  Anatomy and physiology

  Medical terminology

T he endocrine system is made up of glands, which are organized clusters of cells that secrete hormones. Endocrine glands secrete hormones that circulate within the body. Exocrine glands (e.g., salivary glands), secrete hormones to an epithelial surface, but those hormones do not circulate into the bloodstream. The primary glands of the endocrine system include the pituitary, pineal, thyroid, parathyroid, pancreas, adrenals, ovaries in the female and testes in the male, and thymus. Figure 32-1 illustrates the primary glands of the endocrine system.

Function of the Endocrine System

The vital function of this system is the production and regulation of hormones. Hormones are chemical transmitters that regulate different body functions: growth, development, mood, tissue function, metabolism, and sexual function in both males and females.

Many disorders are associated with the hypersecretion (excessive secretion) or hyposecretion (insufficient secretion) of hormones of the endocrine system. Controlling the secretion of specific hormones can help treat many hormonal conditions or disorders.

The nervous system works closely with the endocrine system in the maintenance of homeostasis. For example, the hypothalamus, which is located in the lower central part of the brain, is the link between the endocrine and nervous systems. The nerve cells in the hypothalamus control the pituitary gland by producing chemicals that either suppress or stimulate hormone secretions from the pituitary. The hypothalamus synthesizes and secretes releasing hormones, such as thyrotropin-releasing hormone (TRH) and gonadotropin-releasing hormone (GTRH), and releasing factors, such as corticotropin-releasing factor (CRF), growth hormone-releasing factor (GHRF), prolactin-releasing factor (PRF), and melanocyte-stimulating hormone-releasing factor (MRF). The secretion of the hormones norepinephrine and epinephrine is also controlled by the hypothalamus, which exerts direct nervous control over the anterior pituitary and the adrenal medulla.

Pituitary Gland

The **pituitary gland** (see Figure 32-2) is located near the base of the brain in the sella turcica, a small depression of the sphenoid bone. It is attached to the hypothalamus by the infundibulum stalk and consists of an anterior lobe and a posterior lobe. The pituitary is called the "master gland" because it regulates all of the other endocrine glands.

ANTERIOR LOBE

The adenohypophysis or anterior lobe (Figure 32-3) secretes several hormones that are essential for the growth and development of bones, muscles, organs, sex glands, the thyroid gland, and the adrenal cortex. The hormones produced in the anterior lobe include the following:

- **Growth hormone (GH) (also called somatotrophic hormone)**—essential for the growth and development of bones, muscles, and other organs. GH enhances protein synthesis, decreases glucose use, and promotes the destruction of fats (**lipolysis**). Hyposecretion of this hormone results in dwarfism; conversely, hypersecretion leads to gigantism during early life and acromegaly in adults.

- **Adrenocorticotropic hormone (ACTH)**—essential for the growth and development of the middle and inner

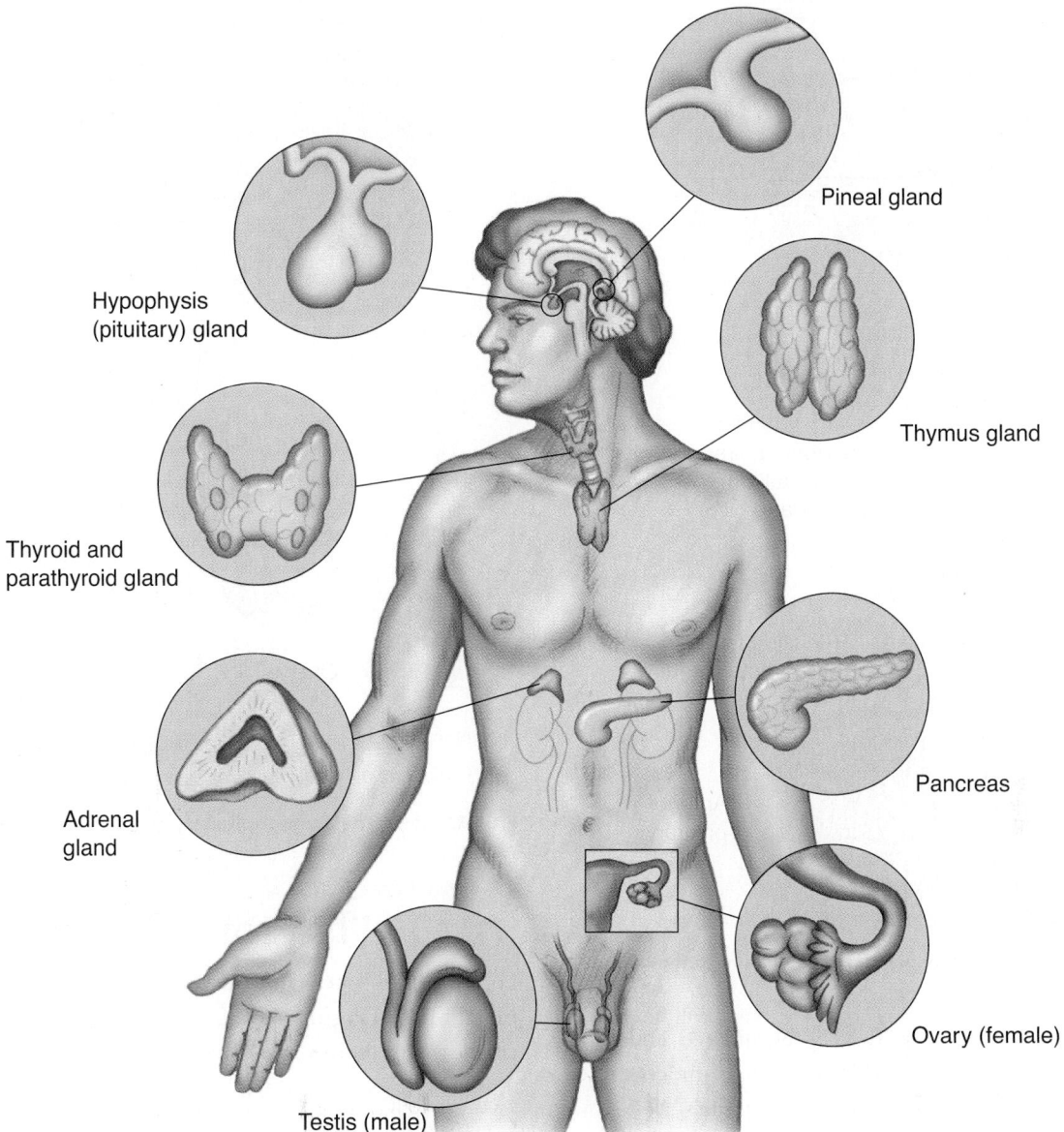

FIGURE 32-1 The primary glands of the endocrine system.

parts of the adrenal cortex. The glucocorticoids cortisol and corticosteroid are secreted by the adrenal cortex.

- **Thyroid-stimulating hormone (TSH)**—controls the growth and development of the thyroid gland. It also stimulates the production of thyroxine and triiodothyronine, influencing the body's metabolic processes and metabolism.

- **Follicle-stimulating hormone (FSH)**—gonadotropic hormone that stimulates the growth of ovarian follicles in females and the production of sperm in males.

- **Luteinizing hormone (LH)**—gonadotropic hormone that plays an essential role in the maturation process of the ovarian follicles and in stimulating the development of the corpus luteum (progesterone-secreting

endocrine tissue) in the female. In the male, LH is responsible for the production of testosterone.

- **Prolactin (PRL) (also known as lactogenic hormone)**—gonadotropic hormone that stimulates the mammary glands to produce milk after childbirth.

- **Melanocyte-stimulating hormone (MSH)**—controls skin pigmentation. The deposit of melanin helps protect skin after exposure to sunlight.

POSTERIOR LOBE

The posterior lobe of the pituitary gland, also known as the neurohypophysis, secretes two hormones:

- **Antidiuretic hormone (ADH)**—also known as vasopressin, it stimulates the reabsorption of water by the

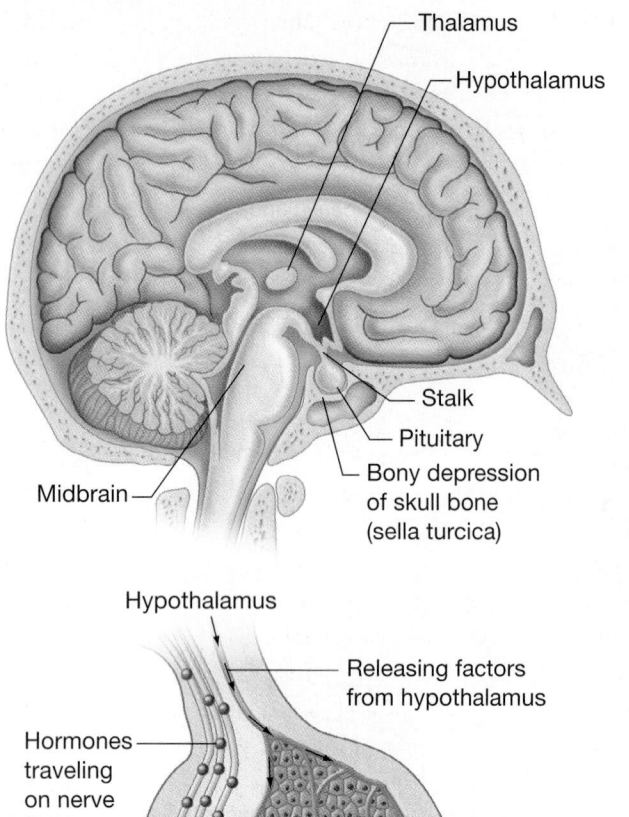

FIGURE 32-2   The pituitary gland and its relation to the brain.

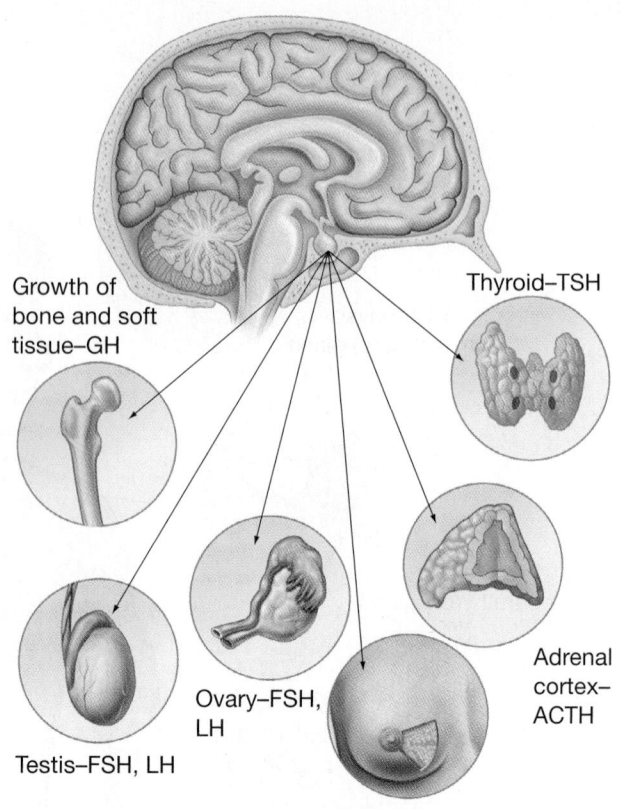

FIGURE 32-3   The anterior pituitary gland and its target organs.

kidneys, so that less fluid is eliminated and blood pressure is elevated. If this hormone is undersecreted, the condition known as diabetes insipidus results.

- **Oxytocin**—stimulates the uterus to contract during labor and childbirth and the mammary glands to release milk after delivery.

Pineal Gland

The **pineal gland** is located at the posterior end of the corpus callosum in the brain. It secretes melatonin and serotonin. Melatonin is released at night and helps with sleep and the release of gonadotropin. Serotonin is a neurotransmitter, vasoconstrictor, and smooth muscle stimulant. Depression is commonly associated with disorders related to the hormone serotonin.

Thyroid Gland

Located in the neck, the **thyroid gland** is responsible for metabolism (Figure 32-4). It is located anterior to the trachea, just below the thyroid cartilage. The thyroid is

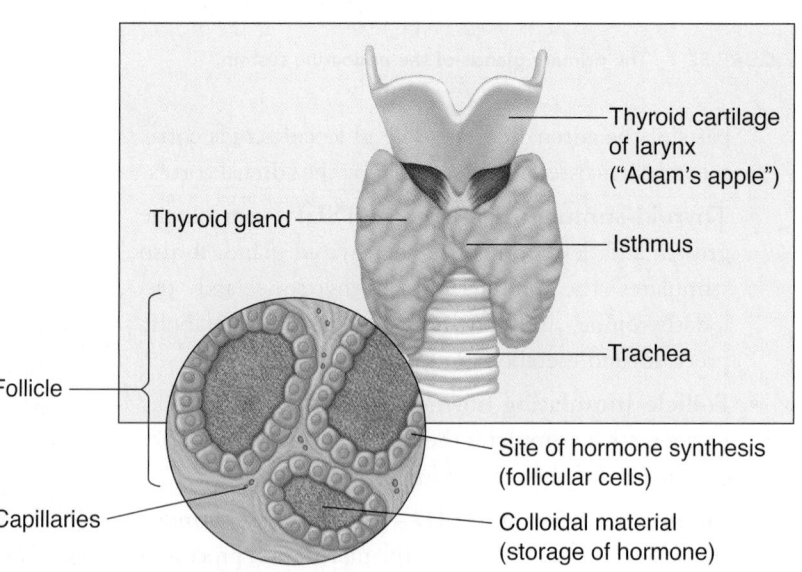

FIGURE 32-4   The thyroid gland.

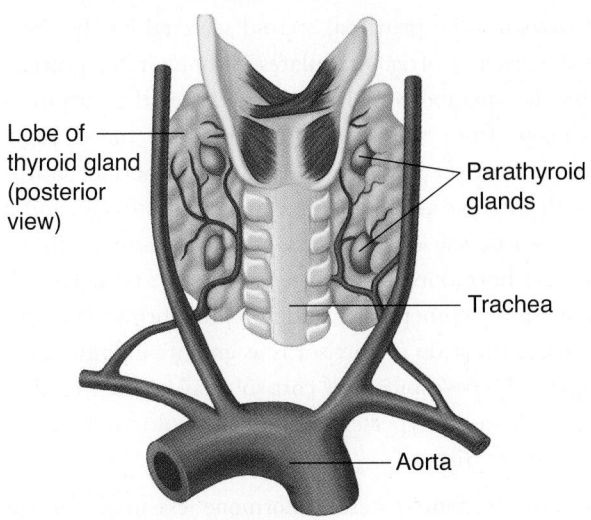

FIGURE 32-5   Parathyroid glands.

approximately 5 cm long and 3 cm wide and weighs about 30 grams. The thyroid gland is responsible for secreting three hormones:

- **Thyroxine (T_4)**—essential for the maintenance and regulation of the basal metabolic rate (BMR). Thyroxine influences growth and development, both physical and mental, as well as the metabolism of fats, proteins, carbohydrates, water, vitamins, and minerals. In thyroid dysfunction, it can be replaced with medications. Disorders resulting from hyposecretion of thyroxine include cretinism, myxedema, and Hashimoto's disease.

- **Tri-iodothyronine (T_3)**—influences the BMR.

- **Calcitonin**—influences bone and calcium metabolism. During infancy, a deficiency of calcitonin may result in cretinism, with arrested physical and mental development. Myxedema and Hashimoto's disease also result from hyposecretion of calcitonin and its companion hormones, T_3 and T_4.

Hypersecretion of T_3 and T_4 results in hyperthyroidism (thyrotoxicosis). Other disorders resulting from hypersecretion of T_3 and T_4 are Graves' disease, exophthalmic goiter, and toxic goiter.

Parathyroid Glands

The four **parathyroid glands** are located around the dorsal and lower aspects of the thyroid gland (Figure 32-5). Each parathyroid gland is about 6 mm in diameter and weighs about 0.033 gram. The parathyroids secrete parathyroid hormone (PTH, or parathormone). PTH is responsible for the maintenance of normal serum calcium levels and the metabolism of phosphorus. Hyposecretion of PTH may result in hypoparathyroidism, causing tetany (twitching of muscles or nerves). Hypersecretion of PTH may result in hyperparathyroidism, which may lead to osteoporosis, kidney stones, and hypercalcemia.

Pancreas

The **islets of Langerhans** are small clusters of cells within the pancreas (Figure 32-6). Three types of cells make up the islets of Langerhans: alpha, beta, and delta cells.

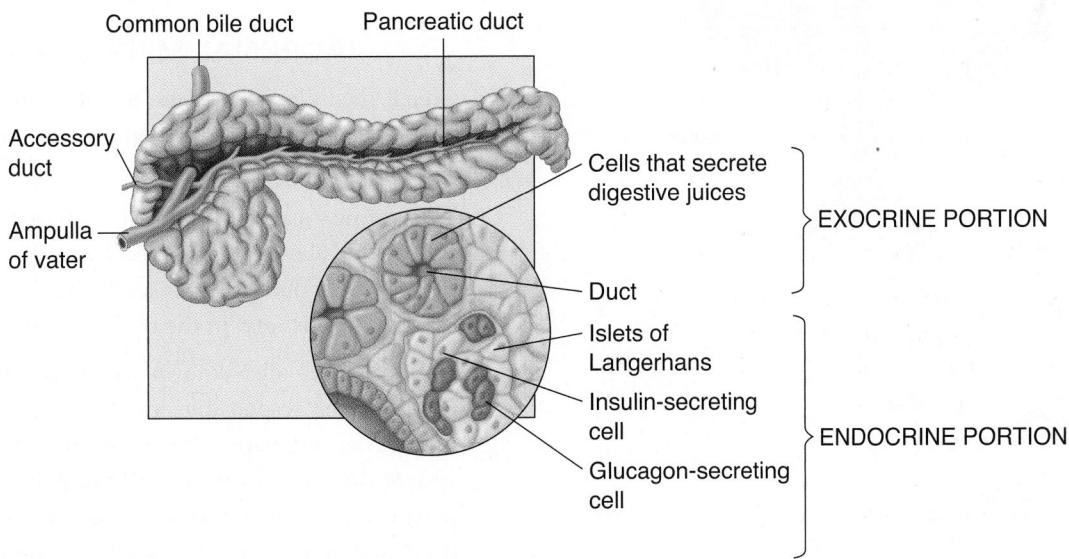

FIGURE 32-6   The pancreas, an endocrine and exocrine gland.

The *alpha cells* secrete the hormone glucagon, which helps break down glycogen into glucose, which causes an increase in blood sugar. The *beta cells* secrete the hormone insulin, which has an adverse reaction and lowers blood sugar. Normal fasting blood sugar is 70 to 110 mg/dL. A synthetic insulin can be injected subcutaneously in individuals who do not produce enough insulin. These patients are considered insulin-dependent diabetics and require insulin to help control their blood sugar levels. (Diabetes, and its different forms, are discussed later in this chapter.) The *delta cells* secrete somatostatin, which suppresses the release of glucagon and insulin.

Adrenal Glands

The **adrenal glands** are located on top of each kidney (Figure 32-7). Each triangular gland consists of an outer portion (cortex) and an inner portion (medulla).

ADRENAL CORTEX

The adrenal cortex secretes groups of hormones called glucocorticoids (cortisol and corticosterone), mineralocorticoids (aldosterone), and androgens. These hormones are essential to life:

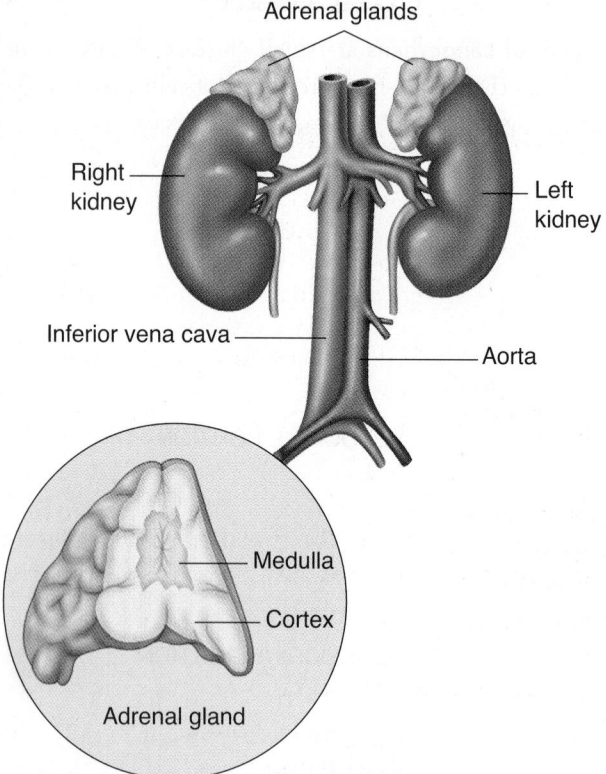

FIGURE 32-7 **The adrenal glands.**

- **Cortisol**—the principal steroid secreted by the adrenal cortex. Cortisol regulates carbohydrate, protein, and fat metabolism. It also stimulates the output of glucose from the liver, increasing the blood sugar level. Cortisol also promotes the transport of amino acids into extracellular tissue for energy storage, and it influences the effectiveness of catecholamines (function as hormones or neurotransmitters or both) such as dopamine, epinephrine, and norepinephrine. The final critical function of cortisol is as an anti-inflammatory agent. Hyposecretion of cortisol may result in Addison's disease. Hypersecretion of cortisol may result in Cushing's disease.

- **Corticosterone**—steroid hormone essential for the normal use of carbohydrates, the absorption of glucose, and gluconeogenesis (formation of glucose by the liver from substances other than carbohydrates).

- **Aldosterone**—the principal mineralocorticoid secreted by the adrenal cortex. Aldosterone is essential in regulating electrolyte and water balance by promoting sodium and chloride retention and potassium excretion. A reduced plasma volume may result from hyposecretion of aldosterone. Hypersecretion may result in primary aldosteronism (a condition characterized by loss of body potassium, muscular weakness, and elevated blood pressure).

- **Androgens**—Androgens are hormones that promote the development of male characteristics. The two main androgens are testosterone and androsterone. These hormones play an essential role in the development of secondary sex characteristics.

ADRENAL MEDULLA

The adrenal medulla synthesizes, secretes, and stores catecholamines. The primary catecholamines are dopamine, epinephrine, and norepinephrine:

- **Dopamine**—causes vasoconstriction, so that the blood pressure is elevated. As a result, cardiac output and urine production are increased. Synthetic dopamine can be administered in the treatment of shock.

- **Epinephrine**—also known as adrenaline, this catecholamine is responsible for the fight-or-flight syndrome, as regulated by the sympathetic nervous system. In times of stress or threat, epinephrine causes peripheral vasoconstriction, dilation of the pupils, decreased salivation, decreased gastrointestinal (GI) motility, and increased heart rate. It also elevates the

Female Secondary Sex Characteristics
- Sexual desire
- Body hair growth
- Breast development
- Feminine body features

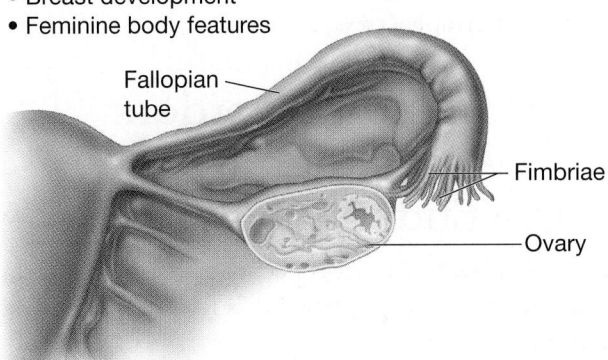

Fallopian tube

Fimbriae

Ovary

FIGURE 32-8 Structure and functions of the ovary.

blood pressure and dilates the bronchial tubes. Epinephrine can be synthetically produced and administered in emergency situations, such as cardiac arrest or allergic reaction.

- **Norepinephrine**—also acts on the sympathetic nervous system by causing vasoconstriction, elevating systolic and diastolic blood pressure, and increasing the heart rate and cardiac output, while also increasing glycogenolysis (the breakdown of glycogen).

Ovaries

The ovaries produce estrogens and progesterone (Figure 32-8). Estrogen is the female sex hormone secreted by the Graafian follicles of the ovaries. Progesterone is secreted by the corpus luteum and is a steroid hormone. These hormones promote the growth, development, and maintenance of secondary female sex organs and characteristics. Other functions of these hormones are preparation of the uterus for pregnancy and promotion of mammary gland development. They also play a vital role in a woman's emotional well-being and sexual drive.

Testes

The testes are located in the male scrotum and produce the male hormone testosterone, which is essential for the normal growth and development of the male accessory sex organ (Figure 32-9). Testosterone is necessary for the act of copulation.

Placenta

In addition to acting as an endocrine gland, the placenta is the spongy structure that joins mother and fetus and provides

the blood supply between the two. Present only during pregnancy, the placenta produces chorionic gonadotropin hormone, estrogen, and progesterone.

Gastrointestinal Mucosa

The mucosa of the pyloric area of the stomach secretes the hormone gastrin. Gastrin stimulates gastric acid secretion in the stomach, gallbladder, pancreas, and small intestine.

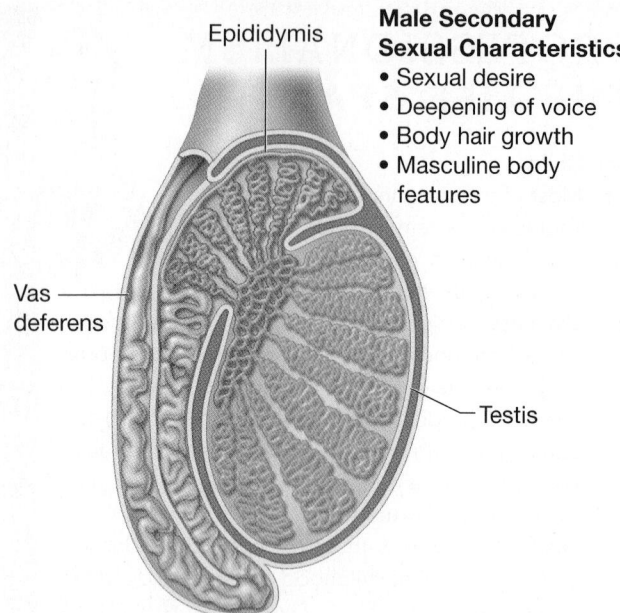

Epididymis

Male Secondary Sexual Characteristics
• Sexual desire
• Deepening of voice
• Body hair growth
• Masculine body features

Vas deferens

Testis

FIGURE 32-9 Structure and functions of the male testes.

Secretin is secreted by the mucosa of the duodenum and jejunum. Secretin stimulates pancreatic juice, bile, and intestinal secretions. Pancreozymin-cholecystokinin, which stimulates the pancreas, is also secreted by the duodenal mucosa, as is enterogastrone, a hormone that regulates gastric secretions.

Thymus Gland

The **thymus gland** is composed of lymphoid tissue and is located in the mediastinal cavity, in front of and above the heart (Figure 32-10). The thymus is part of the lymphatic system but also functions as an endocrine gland by releasing thymosin and thymopoietin. Thymosin promotes the maturation of T lymphocytes. Thymopoietin influences the production of lymphocyte precursors and aids in their process of becoming T lymphocytes.

Common Disorders Associated with the Endocrine System

A variety of diseases affect the endocrine system (Table 32-1). Most are treated medically; however, a few surgical options are appropriate.

ACROMEGALY

Acromegaly is a hormonal disorder that results from the overproduction of GH by the pituitary gland. It most commonly affects middle-aged adults. The most serious health consequences of acromegaly are diabetes mellitus, hypertension, increased risk of cardiovascular disease, and premature death. It also can be caused by a pituitary tumor.

Signs and Symptoms. Acromegaly is commonly characterized by the abnormal growth of the hands and feet. Swelling of the soft tissues of the hands and feet is often an early feature, as patients notice a change in ring or shoe size. Gradually, bony changes alter the facial features: The brow and lower jaw protrude, the nasal bone

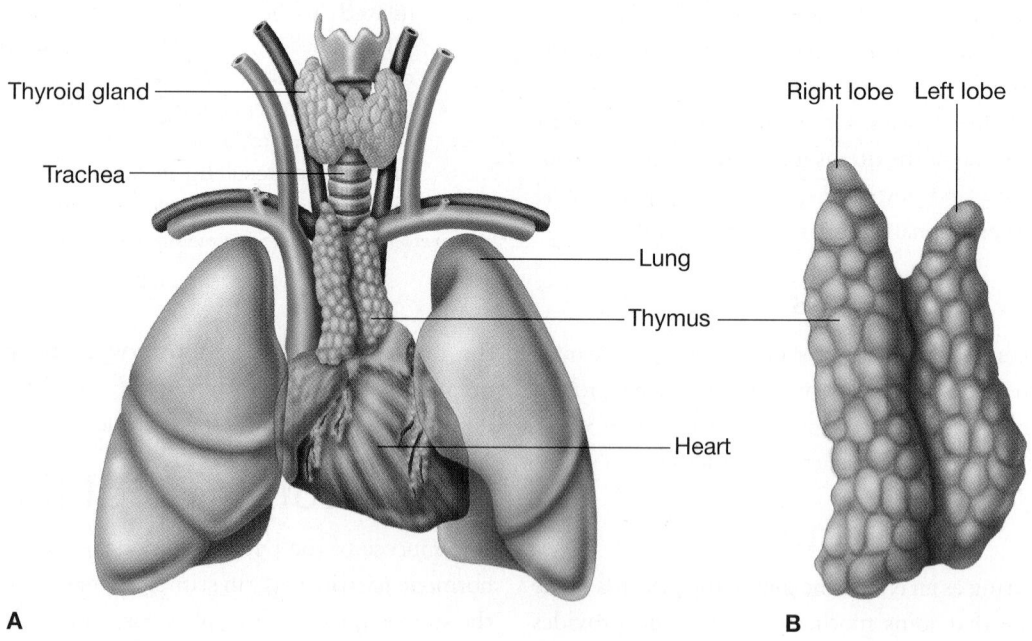

Thyroid gland

Trachea

Lung

Thymus

Heart

A

Right lobe   Left lobe

B

FIGURE 32-10 The thymus gland: (A) appearance and position; (B) with anatomical structures.

TABLE 32-1 Disorders of the Endocrine System

Disorder	Description
Acidosis	Excessive acidity of bodily fluids due to the accumulation of acids, as in diabetic acidosis
Acromegaly	Chronic disease of middle-aged persons that results in an elongation and enlargement of the bones of the head and extremities; mood changes possible
Addison's disease	Disease resulting from a deficiency in adrenocortical hormones; increased pigmentation of the skin, generalized weakness, and weight loss possible
Adenoma	A neoplasm or tumor of a gland
Cretinism	Congenital condition due to a deficiency in the secretion of thyroid hormones; may result in arrested physical and mental development
Cushing's syndrome	Set of symptoms that result from hypersecretion of the adrenal cortex; may result from a tumor of the adrenal glands; may present symptoms of weakness, edema, excess hair growth, skin discoloration, and osteoporosis
Diabetes insipidus (DI)	Disorder caused by the inadequate secretion of antidiuretic hormone (ADH) by the posterior lobe of the pituitary gland; polyuria and polydipsia are symptoms
Diabetes mellitus (DM)	Chronic disorder of carbohydrate metabolism; results in hyperglycemia and glycosuria; type 1 diabetes mellitus (IDDM): involves insulin dependency, requires daily injections of insulin; type 2 (NIDDM): may not be insulin dependent
Diabetic retinopathy	Secondary complication of diabetes mellitus (DM); affects the blood vessels of the retina, resulting in visual changes and even blindness
Dwarfism	Condition of being abnormally small; may be the result of a hereditary condition or an endocrine dysfunction
Gigantism	Excessive development of long bones of the body due to overproduction of the growth hormone by the pituitary gland
Goiter	Enlargement of the thyroid gland
Graves' disease	Disease that results from an overactivity of the thyroid gland; can result in a crisis situation; also called hyperthyroidism
Hashimoto's disease	A chronic form of thyroiditis
Hirsutism	Condition of having an excessive amount of hair on the body; term that describes females who have the adult male pattern of hair growth; can result from hormonal imbalance
Hypercalcemia	Condition of having an excessive amount of calcium in the blood
Hyperglycemia	Having an excessive amount of glucose (sugar) in the blood
Hyperkalemia	Condition of having an excessive amount of potassium in the blood
Hyperthyroidism	Condition that results from overactivity of the thyroid gland; also called Graves' disease
Hypoglycemia	Condition of low amount of glucose (sugar) in the blood
Hypothyroidism	Result of a deficiency in secretion of hormones by the thyroid gland; results in a lowered basal metabolism rate (BMR) with obesity, dry skin, slow pulse, low blood pressure, sluggishness, and goiter; treated with synthetic thyroid hormone
Ketoacidosis	Acidosis due to an excess of ketone bodies (waste products); can result in death for the diabetic patient if not reversed
Myasthenia gravis	Condition characterized by great muscular weakness and progressive fatigue; may be difficulty in chewing and swallowing and drooping eyelids; if thymoma is causing the problem: can be treated with removal of the thymus gland
Myxedema	Condition resulting from hypofunction of the thyroid gland; possible symptoms: anemia, slow speech, enlarged tongue and facial features, edematous skin, drowsiness, and mental apathy
Thyrotoxicosis	Condition that results from overproduction of hormones by the thyroid gland; symptoms: rapid heart action, tremors, enlarged thyroid gland, exophthalmos, and weight loss
von Rechlinghausen's disease	Excessive production of parathyroid hormone; results in degeneration of the bones

enlarges, and spacing between the teeth increases. The overgrowth of bone and cartilage often leads to arthritis. Thickened tissue may trap nerves and cause carpal tunnel syndrome, with its characteristic numbness and weakness of the hands. Other symptoms include thick, coarse, oily skin; skin tags; enlarged lips, nose, and tongue; a deeper voice that results from enlarged sinuses and vocal cords; snoring due to upper airway obstruction; excessive sweating and skin odor; fatigue and weakness; headaches; impaired vision; abnormal menstrual cycle and, sometimes, breast discharge in women; and impotence in men. Body organs, such as the liver, spleen, kidneys, and heart, may also enlarge.

Treatment. The goals of treatment for acromegaly are to reduce GH production to normal levels, to relieve the pressure exerted by the growing pituitary tumor on the surrounding brain areas, to maintain normal pituitary function, and to reverse or alleviate symptoms. Current treatment options include surgical removal of the tumor, drug therapy, and radiation therapy of the pituitary.

ADDISON'S DISEASE

In **Addison's disease**, the cortex of the adrenal gland is damaged, decreasing the production of adrenocortical hormones. It is an autoimmune disease, in which the body attacks itself. It may also be caused by infection of the adrenal glands, cancer, or hemorrhage into the glands. Addison's disease is rare, occurring in 1 in 100,000 Americans. It can occur at any age, including infancy, and is equally prevalent in men and women.

Signs and Symptoms. Signs and symptoms of Addison's disease include weight loss, anorexia, weakness and lethargy, increased pigmentation of the skin and mucous membranes, hypoglycemia, joint and muscle aches, persistent fever, nausea, vomiting, diarrhea, and abdominal discomfort. Most symptoms occur over several months; occasionally, however, they may appear quite suddenly. Addison's disease is diagnosed by blood and urine tests that measure corticosteroid hormone levels. With Addison's disease, the level of corticosteroids is very low.

Treatment. Replacement of adrenocortical hormones and supplemental sodium comprise the usual course of treatment for Addison's disease. The patient and family are taught the importance of lifelong treatment and intramuscular hydrocortisone injections. The patient must always carry medical identification.

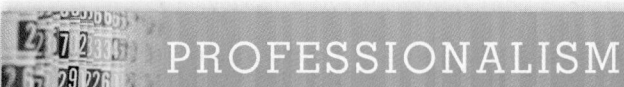
CUSHING'S DISEASE

Cushing's disease is a rare disorder that develops when there is a hypersecretion of cortisol. (Figure 32-11). ACTH releases cortisol as a result of stimulation of the pituitary. Cushing's disease is usually a side effect of the pharmacological use of steroids in the management of inflammatory illnesses. Glucocorticoid excess that results from tumors of the pituitary or adrenal glands, or from excess levels of ACTH, is very rare.

Signs and Symptoms. Symptoms of Cushing's disease include muscular weakness, thinning of the skin, easy bruising, rounding of facial features ("moon faces"), weight gain, and fatigue. Results of the disease include diabetes, high blood pressure, depression, and osteoporosis. Cushing's disease can cause death if it is not treated.

Treatment. Treatment for Cushing's disease include surgery and radiation. If caused by overuse of steroids, the patient should wean himself or herself from the steroids by taking them with increasingly less frequency. Adenomas, or tumors, may need to be removed.

DIABETES MELLITUS

In **diabetes mellitus** the body is unable to produce enough insulin to properly control blood sugar levels. Insulin is a hormone that converts sugar and starches into the energy the body needs.

Diabetes, especially adult-onset diabetes, is a silent disease that may not be detected until it is in an advanced stage. According to the American Diabetes Association, approximately 13 million people have been diagnosed with diabetes, but an estimated 5.9 million are undiagnosed.

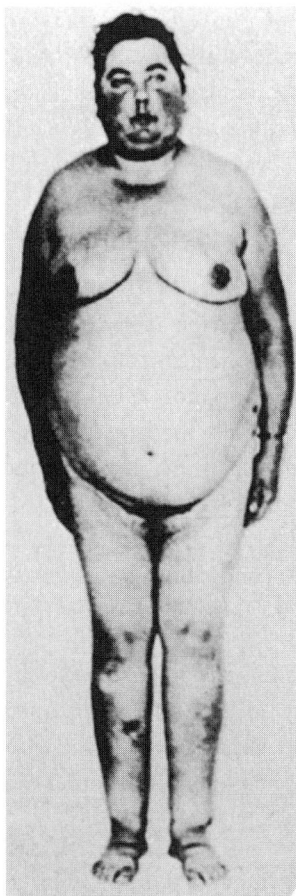
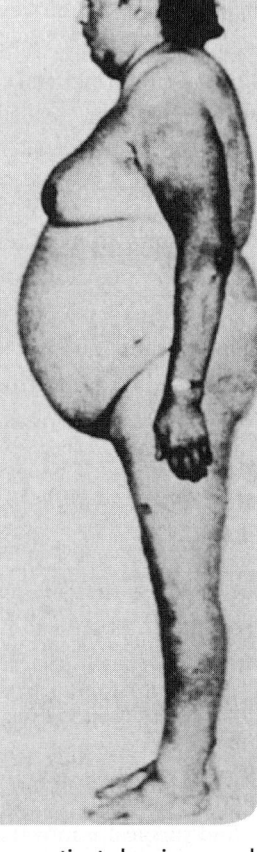

FIGURE 32-11 Cushing's syndrome patient showing round, red face; stocky neck; and marked obesity of the trunk with protruding abdomen. Note bruises on trunk and legs and also stretch marks. Note fat pads above the collarbone and on the back of the neck, which produce the "buffalo hump."

Gestational diabetes is pregnancy related. Typically, this type of diabetes disappears after the pregnancy is completed, but occasionally it precipitates ongoing type 2 diabetes.

Signs and Symptoms. Classic symptoms of diabetes are polyuria (frequent urination), polydipsia (excessive thirst), and polyphagia (excessive hunger). Other symptoms include weakness, weight loss, lethargy, anorexia, irritability, dry skin, recurrent infections, abdominal cramps, and vaginal yeast infections in women.

Treatment. Type 1 diabetes can usually only be treated by a pancreatic transplant. However, recent studies with stem cell research have led to promising hope that stem cells can be used to replace the defective pancreas.

Type 2 diabetes is treated with diet, exercise, and oral hypoglycemic medications to help control blood sugar levels. Unfortunately, with uncontrolled diabetes, as time progresses with the disease, many Type 2 diabetics must also administer insulin injections in addition to oral medications. Type 2 diabetes may be preventable with modest lifestyle changes, including healthy diet choices, exercise, and weight management.

During pregnancy the patient with gestational diabetes may have to monitor her diet and blood sugar and may need to give herself daily insulin injections.

There are three types of diabetes. Juvenile diabetes is also known as type 1 diabetes or **insulin-dependent diabetes mellitus (IDDM)**. It is typically diagnosed in children who cannot produce sufficient quantities, if any, of insulin. These children are typically dependent on insulin injections for the duration of their lives.

Type 2 diabetes is also known as **non–insulin-dependent diabetes mellitus (NIDDM)** or adult-onset diabetes. Type 2 diabetes is the most common form of the disease and is typically diagnosed later in life. It results from insulin resistance combined with a relative insulin deficiency. There is a very strong correlation between obesity and type 2 diabetes. People who are overweight may make sufficient insulin for their ideal body weight but cannot make enough to compensate for extra weight.

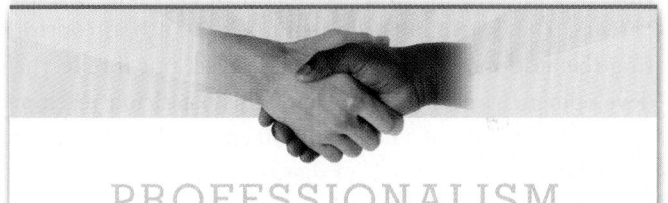

PROFESSIONALISM
CULTURAL CONSIDERATIONS

Many cultures are at much higher risk for developing type 2 diabetes. Take for instance, the Native American Pima tribe in Arizona. The Pimas are 19 times more likely to develop type 2 diabetes. Latino and African Americans are also more likely than the Caucasian population to develop the disease. Because food is a major part of any given ethnic group or culture, it can be helpful to have a dietician who is familiar with the cultural environment of the patient consult with the patient regarding modification of the diet to fit the practices of the family. Education and reinforcement are necessary in these situations.

DWARFISM

Dwarfism refers to a group of conditions characterized by shorter-than-normal skeletal growth in the arms and legs or the trunk. More than 300 conditions can cause abnormal skeletal growth and dwarfism.

Achondroplasia is the most common type of short-limb dwarfism, occurring in 1 in 25,000 children, with males and females at equal risk. This type of abnormal skeletal growth (skeletal dysplasia) is usually diagnosed at birth. Most children born with the disorder have average-size parents. The development of motor skills, such as controlling the head movements, may be delayed, but intellectual development is normal. Men with this condition reach an average full height of 51 inches (130 cm), and women reach 49 inches (125 cm). People of short stature lead normal, fulfilled lives, achieving high levels of education and career and personal ambitions.

Signs and Symptoms. The physical characteristics of achondroplasia are a trunk of normal length; disproportionately short arms and legs; bowed legs; reduced joint mobility in the elbow, although loose ligaments make other joints seem overly flexible or double jointed; shortened hands and feet; a large head; a flat midface; crowded teeth (because of a small upper jaw); a prominent forehead; and a flattened bridge of the nose.

Treatment. There is no cure for achondroplasia. In addition to social and family support, treatment focuses on the prevention, management, and treatment of medical complications.

Surgery may be performed to relieve pressure on the nervous system, generally at the base of the skull and lower back, or to open obstructed airways by removing the adenoids. Dental and orthodontic work may be necessary to correct malocclusion (abnormality in the way the teeth meet) and preserve dental health.

GIGANTISM

Gigantism results from excessive secretion of GH during childhood, before the closure of the bone growth plates.

The cause of excess GH secretion is most often a pituitary gland tumor. Gigantism may also be caused by an underlying medical condition such as multiple endocrine neoplasia. Pituitary tumors are rarely ever malignant (cancerous). If excessive secretion of GH occurs after normal bone growth has stopped, the condition is known as acromegaly.

Signs and Symptoms. Gigantism is characterized by overgrowth of the long bones and very tall stature, accompanied by growth in the muscles and organs. Children with gigantism are extremely large for their age. The disorder can also delay puberty.

Treatment. Treatments for gigantism include radiation therapy and surgical removal of the tumor.

HYPERTHYROIDISM

Hyperthyroidism is characterized by elevated thyroid hormone levels. **Graves' disease** is the most common form of hyperthyroidism; it is an autoimmune disorder; antibodies produced by the immune system stimulate the thyroid to produce too much thyroxine. Other forms of hyperthyroidism may be caused by thyroiditis (inflammation of the thyroid gland) or benign or malignant tumors.

Signs and Symptoms. The symptoms of hyperthyroidism include nervousness, restlessness, heart palpitations, tremors, sweating, increased activity in the intestinal tract, menstrual changes, weight loss, and changes in the fingernails and hair. The heart may be enlarged. A condition known as **exophthalmos** is another possible symptom, in which the eyeballs protrude beyond their normal protective orbit when the tissues behind them swell (Figure 32-12). Hyperthyroidism can lead to a rapid heart rate, atrial fibrillation, and congestive heart failure. Other complications include osteoporosis (weak, brittle bones), sensitivity to light, and blurring and double vision.

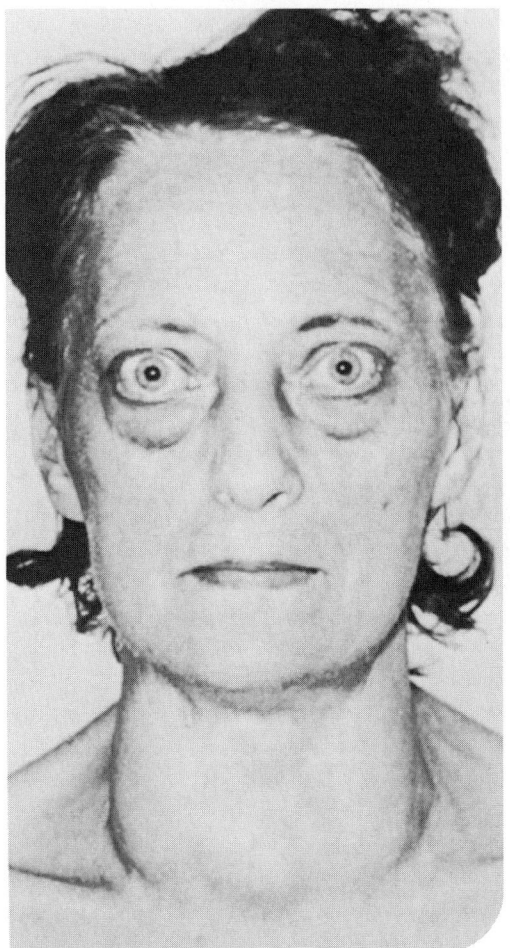

FIGURE 32-12 A patient with exophthalmos.

also associated with a higher risk of heart disease because of the high levels of low-density lipoproteins (LDL, the "bad" cholesterol) that can develop. **Cardiomegaly** (enlarged heart) can also occur.

Treatment.   Hyperthyroidism is treated with antithyroid medications, radioactive iodine to destroy the thyroid, or surgery (thyroidectomy). If the thyroid is removed or destroyed, lifelong thyroid replacement therapy must be initiated.

HYPOTHYROIDISM

In **hypothyroidism**, the thyroid produces inadequate amounts of the thyroid hormones. Because hypothyroidism develops slowly, only about half of the seven million cases in the United States are diagnosed early. Figure 32-13 shows a child born with hypothyroidism.

Untreated hypothyroidism can lead to other conditions because the constant stimulation to release more thyroid hormones can cause the thyroid gland to enlarge, a condition called a **goiter** (see Figure 32-14). The most common cause of a goiter is **Hashimoto's thyroiditis**, an autoimmune inflammation of the thyroid. Untreated hypothyroidism is

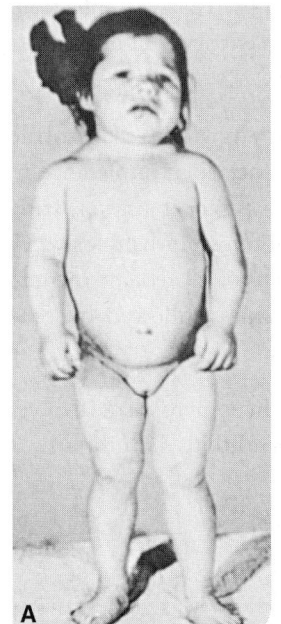 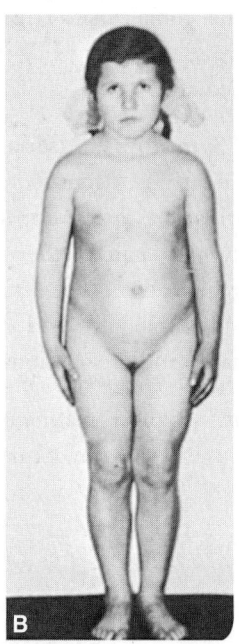

FIGURE 32-13 (A) A 6-year old child with congenital hypothyroidism, cretinism, exhibiting marked mental and physical retardation; (B) the same patient after 3 years of thyroxine therapy, which resulted in a spurt of growth and regression of pathological manifestations. Mental retardation is delayed.

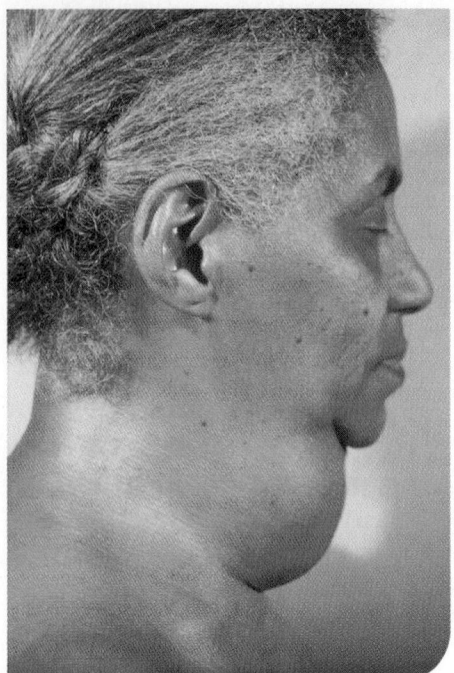

FIGURE 32-14 A goiter.

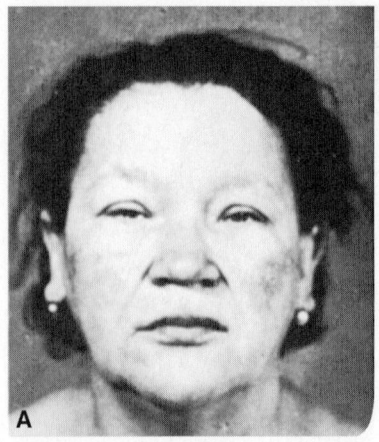

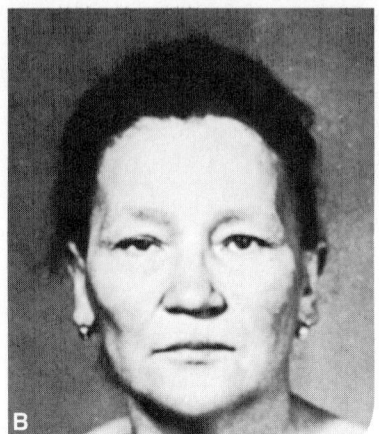

FIGURE 32-15 (A) A 62-year-old patient with myxedema exhibiting marked edema of the face and a somnolent look. The hair is stiff and without luster; (B) the same patient after 3 months of treatment with thyroxine.

Other complications of hypothyroidism are depression, decreased sexual desire, and slowed mental functioning. **Myxedema** is a rare, life-threatening condition that results from long-term, untreated hypothyroidism (see Figure 32-15). A myxedema coma can be triggered by sedatives, infection, or other stress, and emergency treatment should be administered immediately.

Signs and Symptoms. Initial symptoms tend to be subtle and include fatigue, decreased concentration, intolerance to cold, constipation, loss of appetite, muscle cramping, stiffness, and weight gain. Other symptoms are hair loss, dry skin, and nail changes. The symptoms of myxedema include intense cold intolerance and drowsiness followed by profound lethargy and unconsciousness.

Treatment. Typical treatment for hypothyroidism involves the daily use of levothyroxine (Synthroid, Levothroid), a synthetic thyroid hormone. This oral hormone reduces symptoms, particularly fatigue, weight loss, and increased LDL. This medication must be taken on a routine basis. It should be monitored regularly with blood work and the dosage should be adjusted as necessary. Thyroid supplementation is a lifelong therapy.

SUMMARY

The endocrine system releases hormones that keep the body in proper balance, or homeostasis. Working closely with the nervous system, these hormones regulate growth, development, mood, tissue function, metabolism, and sexual function. The organs of the endocrine system include the pituitary gland, pineal gland, thymus gland, thyroid and parathyroid glands, adrenal glands, pancreas, ovaries, and testes. The anterior lobe of the pituitary gland secretes growth hormone, follicle-stimulating hormone, adrenocorticotropin, thyroid-stimulating hormone, luteinizing hormone, prolactin, and melanocyte-stimulating hormone. The posterior lobe secretes antidiuretic hormone and oxytocin. Melatonin is released by the pineal gland. Thyroxine, tri-iodothyronine, and calcitonin are secreted in the thyroid glands. The parathyroid glands produce parathormone. Insulin and glucagon are secreted by the pancreas. The adrenal cortex secretes cortisol, corticosterone, aldosterone, and androgens. The adrenal medulla secretes dopamine, epinephrine, and norepinephrine. The ovaries secrete estrogens and progesterone. The testes secrete testosterone. The placenta controls pregnancy hormones: chorionic gonadotropin hormone, estrogen, and progesterone. Secretin is secreted by the gastrointestinal mucosa, and the thymus gland releases thymosin and thymopoietin. Common disorders of the endocrine system include acromegaly, Addison's disease, Cushing's disease, diabetes mellitus, dwarfism, gigantism, hyperthyroidism, and hypothyroidism.

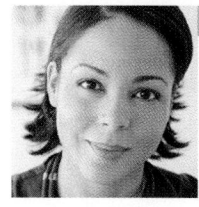

32 CHAPTER REVIEW

COMPETENCY REVIEW

1. Define and spell the terms to learn for this chapter.

2. What is the vital function of the endocrine system?

3. Why is the pituitary gland known as the master gland of the body?

4. What hormones are secreted by the thyroid gland?

5. What is the function of insulin?

6. What are the four functions of cortisol?

7. Name three functions of the hormone epinephrine.

8. Name the catecholamines synthesized, secreted, and stored by the adrenal medulla.

9. What hormones do the ovaries secrete?

10. Name two hormones secreted by the thymus.

PREPARING FOR THE CERTIFICATION EXAM

1. Which of the following organs/structures is/are NOT found in the endocrine system?
   a. pineal
   b. ovaries
   c. thymus
   d. testes
   e. liver

2. Cushing's disease is a result of the dysfunction of what structure?
   a. pituitary
   b. thymus
   c. ovary
   d. thyroid
   e. adrenal gland

3. The endocrine gland that is responsible for calcitonin secretion is the
   a. parathyroid
   b. pancreas
   c. ovary
   d. thyroid
   e. adrenal cortex

4. The result of hypersecretion of thyroid hormones is
   a. diabetes insipidus
   b. diabetes mellitus
   c. tetany
   d. exophthalmos
   e. Addison's disease

5. A disease caused by the hypofunction of the thyroid gland is
   a. myasthenia gravis
   b. myxedema
   c. Graves' disease
   d. Cushing's disease
   e. Addison's disease

6. Which of the following is NOT one of the cardinal signs of diabetes mellitus?
   a. polyphagia
   b. polyuria
   c. polypharmacy
   d. hyperglycemia
   e. polydipsia

7. The most common cause of a goiter is
   a. neck tumor
   b. Graves' disease
   c. Hashimoto's disease
   d. Cushing's disease
   e. Addison's disease

8. An excessive amount of hair on the body because of a hormone imbalance is known as
   a. Hashimoto's disease
   b. hirsutism
   c. myxedema
   d. von Rechinghausen's disease
   e. myasthenia gravis

9. Testosterone affects all of the following EXCEPT
   a. sexual desire
   b. body hair growth
   c. deepening of voice
   d. masculine body features
   e. gastric secretions

10. Undersecretion of growth hormone (GH) results in
    a. exophthalmos
    b. dwarfism
    c. Simmonds' disease
    d. Cushing's syndrome
    e. gigantism

CRITICAL THINKING

1. One of the laboratory tests that was performed was an FBS (fasting blood sugar) ordered by Dr. Bahjat. Give an example of what Rosa's FBS level may have been that would have helped Dr. Bahjat arrive at the diagnosis of type 2 diabetes.

2. List some signs and symptoms that Rosa may have had, which would have indicated to Dr. Bahjat that she should be tested for type 2 diabetes mellitus.

3. How does Rosa's ethnicity play a role in her diagnosis? What should be considered regarding patient education?

INTERNET ACTIVITY

Do an Internet search to learn about support groups for individuals with diabetes. What kind of support is available for people with this disorder?

MEDMEDIA

Additional interactive resources and activities for this chapter can be found:

On your student DVD: View applicable procedure videos on the DVD-ROM found in the back of this book.

MyHealthProfessionsKit.com: Test your knowledge of the chapter with games and activities. MyHealthProfessionsKit also includes resources, helpful links, and a Spanish audio glossary.

Medical Assisting Interactive: Practice your procedures as a medical assistant in this simulated doctor's office. This can be accessed through MyHealthProfessionsKit.com.

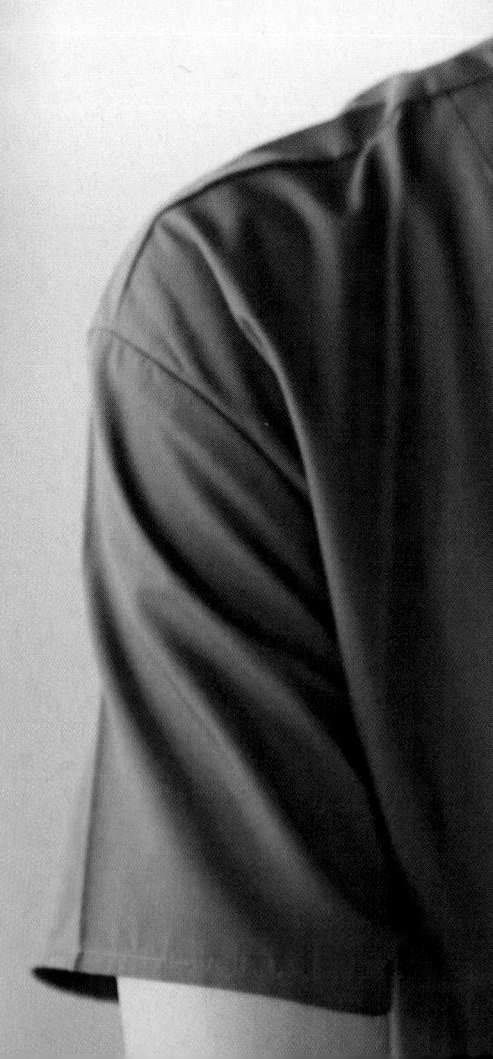

33

The Reproductive System

LEARNING OBJECTIVES

After completing this chapter, you should be able to:

- Define and spell the terms to learn for this chapter.

- Identify the structures of the female reproductive system and briefly explain the function of each.

- Explain the menstrual cycle.

- Explain the purpose and function of the male reproductive system.

- Identify the male external organs of reproduction and explain the function of each.

- Identify and state the function of the testes, epididymis, ductus deferens, seminal vesicles, prostate gland, bulbourethral glands, and the urethra.

- List common disorders associated with the female and male reproductive systems.

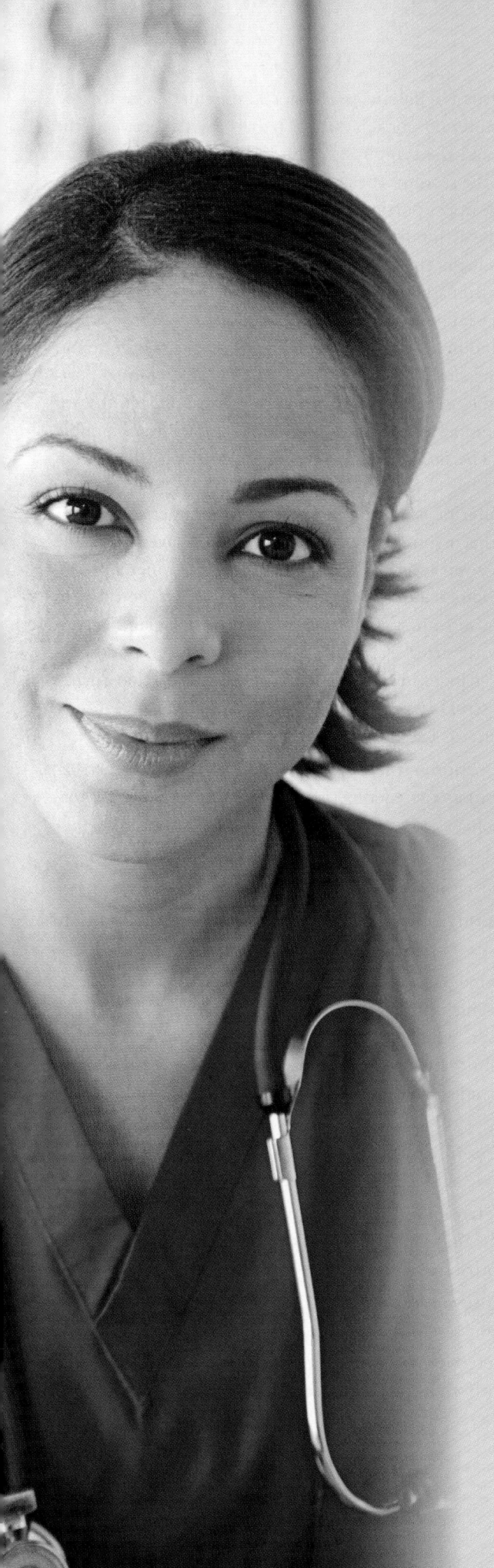

CHAPTER OUTLINE

CASE STUDY

Nabiel Hamsi is a 21-year-old male being seen by Dr. Bahjat. He is being seen in the office today because of a swollen left testicle. Nabiel noticed the swelling a week ago but is now unable to bear the pain. Dr. Bahjat diagnoses Nabiel with epididymitis. During the examination, Dr. Bahjat asks Nabiel if he is sexually active. Nabiel answers, "No, I am waiting until I am married."

The Female Reproductive System

The female reproductive system consists of the ovaries, which are the primary sex organs, and the accessory sex organs, which include the fallopian (uterine) tubes, the uterus, the vagina, the vulva, and the breasts (Figure 33-1). The vital function of the female reproductive system is to perpetuate the species through sexual (germ cell) reproduction.

UTERUS

The **uterus** is a hollow, pear-shaped, muscular organ located in the anterior portion of the pelvic cavity, between the sacrum and the symphysis pubis, above the bladder and in front of the rectum. It can be divided into three identifiable areas: the upper portion, called the body; the central portion, called the isthmus; and the neck, or cervix (Figure 33-2). The fundus is the bulging surface of the uterine body that extends from the internal os (mouth) of the cervix upward above the fallopian tube. A number of ligaments support the uterus and hold it in place: two broad ligaments, two round ligaments, and two uterosacral ligaments. The normal position of the uterus is tilted, with the cervix pointing toward the sacrum and the fundus pointing toward the suprapubic region. The normal uterus is about 8 cm long and 2.5 cm thick.

The uterine wall has three layers: the perimetrium (outer layer), the myometrium (muscular middle layer), and the endometrium (mucous membrane lining the inner surface). The endometrium is composed of columnar epithelium (columns of lining tissue) and connective tissue and is supplied with arterial blood. The endometrium undergoes marked changes in response to hormonal stimulation during the menstrual cycle.

The uterus has three primary functions:

- It performs the cyclic discharge of blood (menstruation) as the endometrium is shed in response to hormonal changes.

- It provides nourishment and protection to the fetus during pregnancy.

- During labor, the myometrium contracts rhythmically to expel the fetus from the uterus.

In some circumstances, the uterus may become displaced. This is often a result of weakness in the supporting ligaments, which may be the result of trauma, a disease process in the uterus, or multiple pregnancies. The following are some of the more common abnormal positions of the uterus:

- **Anteflexion**—the bending forward of the uterus at its body and neck

- **Retroflexion**—the bending backward of the uterus at any angle with the cervix unchanged from its normal position

- **Anteversion**—the turning of the fundus toward the pubis, with the cervix tilted up toward the sacrum

- **Retroversion**—the turning backward of the uterus, with the cervix pointing forward toward the symphysis pubis.

funnel-shaped opening (the ostium) at the infundibulum (end of the tube). Each ostium is surrounded by fimbriae, fingerlike processes that help propel the ovum toward the tube after it is discharged from the ovary.

OVARIES

The two **ovaries**, located on either side of the uterus, are almond-shaped organs attached to the uterus by the ovarian ligaments (Figure 33-3). They lie close to the fimbriae of the fallopian tubes. The anterior border of each ovary is connected to the posterior layer of the broad ligament by the mesovarium. On the sides, they are attached by the suspensory ligaments. Each ovary is about 4 cm long, 2 cm wide, and 1.5 cm thick.

The ovary has two distinct microscopic divisions: the cortex (the outer layer) and the medulla (inner layer). The cortex contains small secretory sacs called follicles, which hold the ova in different stages of development: primary, growing, and Graafian (mature). The ovarian medulla contains connective tissue, nerves, blood and lymphatic vessels, and some smooth muscles at the hilus.

The ovaries have two functions:

- To produce ova (plural of *ovum*)
- To produce hormones

The activity of the ovaries is controlled by the anterior lobe of the pituitary, which produces the gonadotropic hormones follicle-stimulating hormone (FSH) and luteinizing hormone (LH). FSH is instrumental in the development of the follicle nurturing the ovum. LH stimulates the development of the corpus luteum, a small mass of cells that develops after the release of the ovum. Each month, a Graafian follicle ruptures on the ovarian cortex, and an ovum is released into the pelvic cavity and into one of the fallopian tubes. This process is known as **ovulation**. In the average woman more than 400 ova may be produced during the reproductive years.

The hormones estrogen and progesterone are also produced by the ovaries. These two hormones play key roles in the reproductive system. Estrogen is the female sex hormone secreted by the follicles. Progesterone is a steroid hormone secreted by the corpus luteum. These hormones also prepare the uterus for pregnancy, promote development of the mammary glands, and play a major role in a woman's

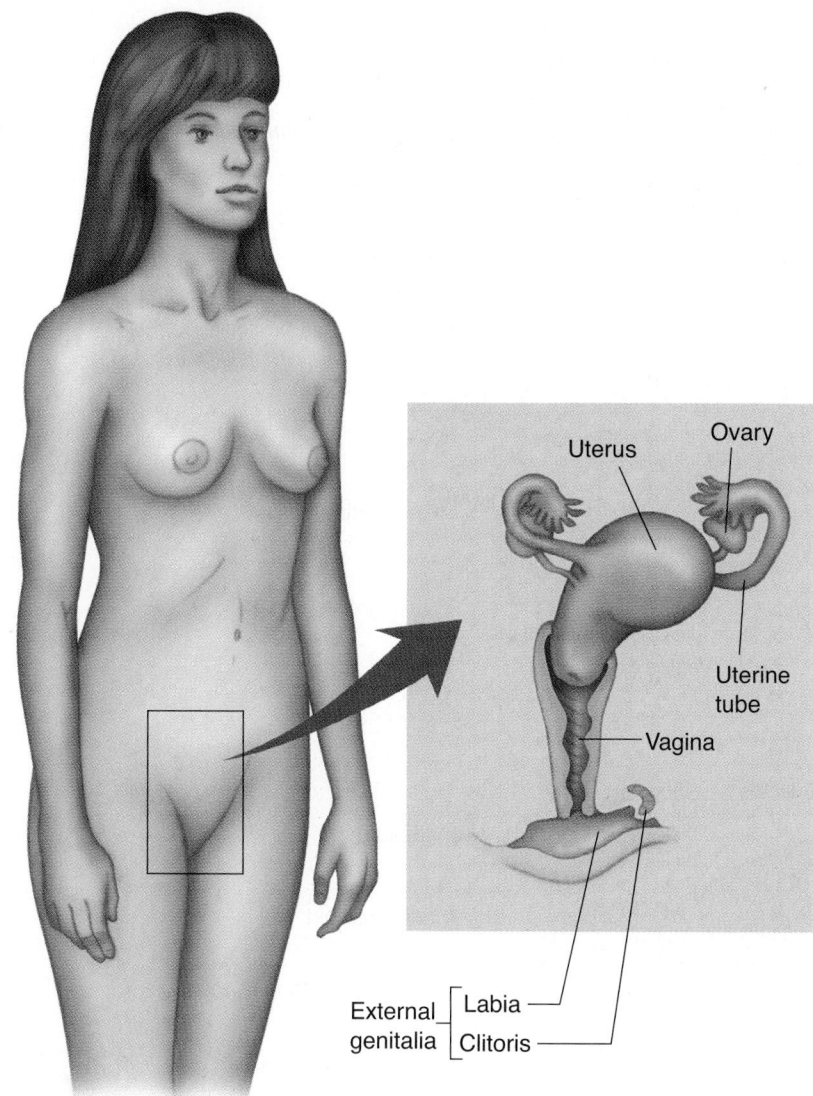

FIGURE 33-1 The female reproductive system.

FALLOPIAN TUBES

The **fallopian tubes**, also referred to as the uterine tubes or the oviducts, extend laterally from each side of the uterus closest to the ovary. Their function is to serve as ducts to move the **ovum** (egg or reproductive cell) from the ovary to the uterus and to move **spermatozoa (sperm)**, the male reproductive cell, from the uterus toward the ovary. Each tube is about 11.5 cm long and 6 mm wide and is composed of three layers. The serous layer is outermost and made of connective tissue. The middle layer is muscular and made of circular and longitudinal smooth muscle. The mucosa is innermost and consists of simple columnar epithelium.

The isthmus is the constricted portion of the tube nearest the uterus. The tube continues laterally from the isthmus to the ampulla, where it widens until it forms a

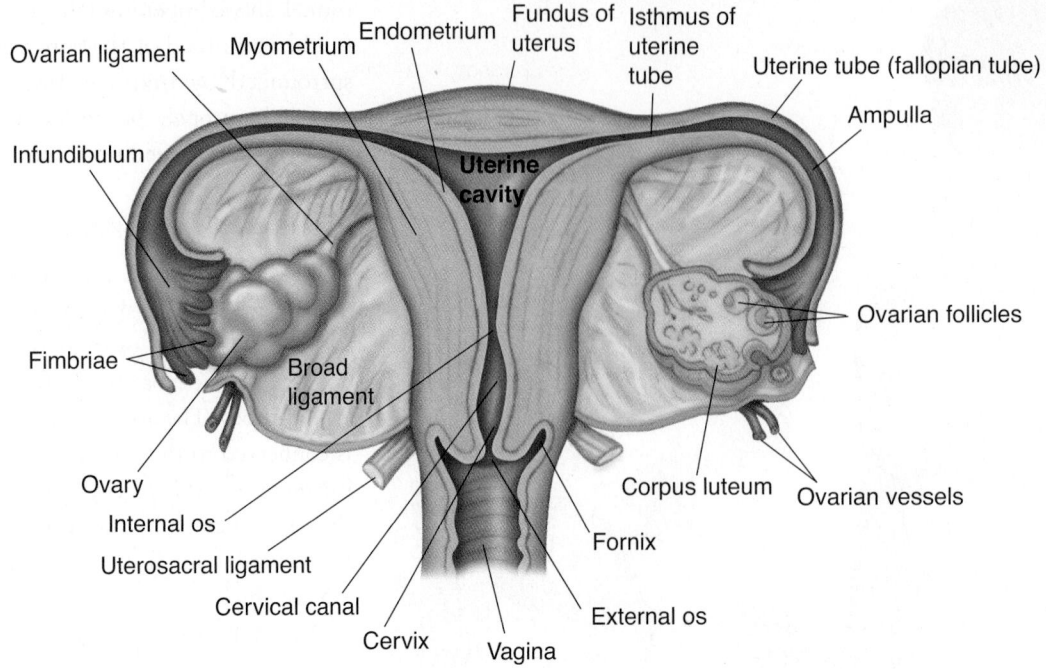

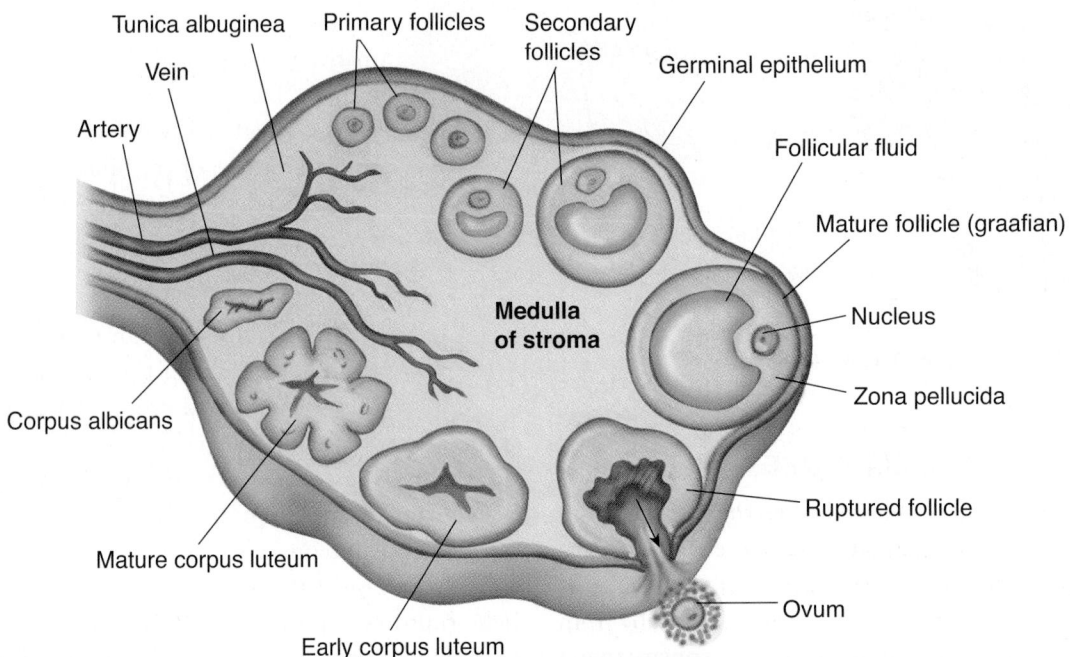

FIGURE 33-2 The uterus, ovaries, and associated structures, with expanded view of a mammalian ovary showing stages of Graafian follicle and ovum development.

emotional well-being and sexual drive. Both hormones are responsible for promoting growth, development, and maintenance of the female secondary sex characteristics and organs.

Secondary sex characteristics are physical features that are not specific to the function of reproduction but differentiate men from women. Secondary sex characteristics in women include enlarged breasts, less facial hair, functional mammary glands, and smoother skin texture. Primary sex characteristics are organs that are specific to reproduction and are present at birth. At puberty, secondary sex characteristics become visible.

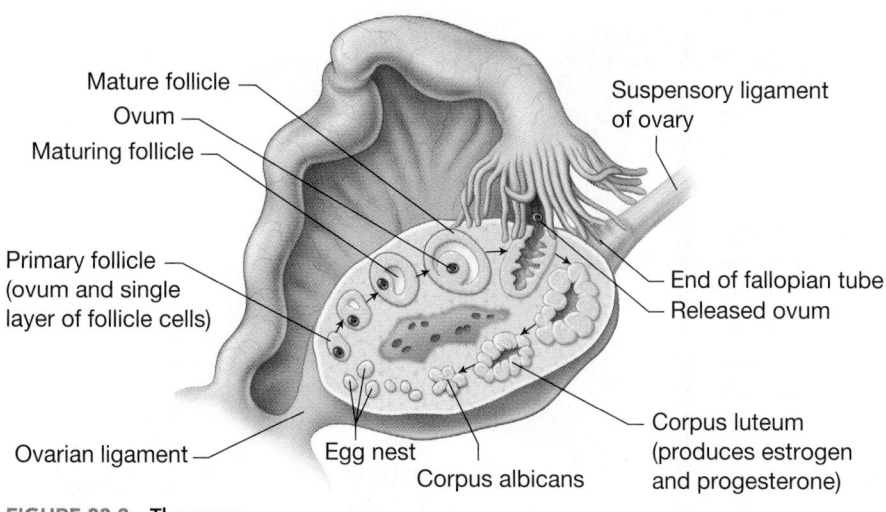

Mature follicle
Ovum
Maturing follicle
Primary follicle
(ovum and single
layer of follicle cells)
Ovarian ligament
Egg nest
Corpus albicans
Suspensory ligament
of ovary
End of fallopian tube
Released ovum
Corpus luteum
(produces estrogen
and progesterone)

FIGURE 33-3 The ovary.

VAGINA

The **vagina** is a musculomembranous tube extending from the vestibule to the uterus. It is typically 10 to 15 cm in length and is situated between the bladder and the rectum. It is lined by mucous membrane and squamous epithelium. The hymen, a fold of membrane, partially covers the external opening of the vagina.

The vagina has three basic functions:

- It is the organ of female copulation.
- It is the passageway for discharge of menstruation.
- It is the passageway for the birth of the fetus.

VULVA

The **vulva** is made up of the five organs that comprise the external female genitalia:

- **Mons pubis**—the pad of fatty, triangular-shaped fatty tissue that is covered with hair after puberty. It is the rounded area over the symphysis pubis.
- **Labia majora**—the two liplike folds of adipose tissue on either side of the vaginal opening.
- **Labia minora**—the two thin folds of skin within the labia majora enclosing the vestibule.
- **Vestibule**—the cleft between the labia minora. There are four structures in the vestibule: the urethra (the external opening of the urinary system), the vagina, and the two excretory ducts of the Bartholin's glands.
- **Clitoris**—the small organ of sensitive erectile tissue that is analogous to the penis of the male.

Between the vulva and the anus is the **perineum**, an external region that is composed of muscle covered with skin. Sometimes during labor, this area is incised by the physician in an **episiotomy**, a procedure that is performed to prevent tearing of the perineum during delivery.

BREAST

The breasts, or mammary glands, are compound alveolar structures consisting of 12 to 15 glandular tissue lobes separated by septa of connecting tissue (Figure 33-4). The areola is the dark, pigmented circular area of skin found on each breast, and the nipple is the elevated area in the center of the areola. During pregnancy, the areola often becomes darker in color. The areola is supplied with a row of small sebaceous glands that secrete an oil that keeps it resilient. During lactation, milk flows from the lobes of the mammary glands through lactiferous ducts in the areola to the suckling infant. Prolactin, a hormone produced by the anterior lobe of the pituitary, stimulates the mammary glands to produce milk after childbirth. The other hormones that play a role in milk production are insulin and glucocorticoids.

The Menstrual Cycle

The onset of the menstrual cycle, **menarche**, occurs at the age of puberty. Cessation of the menstrual cycle is menopause. Typically, the menstrual cycle lasts about 28 days, with a repetitive series of changes to the uterine tissue, breasts, and vagina. There are four phases in the menstrual cycle:

- Menstruation phase—characterized by the discharge of bloody fluid from the uterus as the endometrium is shed. This phase averages 4 to 5 days. The first day of the blood discharge is considered the first day of the cycle.
- Proliferation phase (also called the postmenstrual phase)—characterized by the thickening and vascularization of the endometrium and the maturing of the ovarian follicle. This phase begins on about the fifth day of the cycle and lasts until the eruption of the Graafian follicle, about day 14.
- Luteal or secretory phase (also called the ovulatory stage)—characterized by the continued thickening of the endometrium, and by the appearance of coiled arteries in the tissue. The endometrium becomes edematous (swollen and fluid filled). During this phase, the body is preparing for a possible pregnancy by preparing

The Child

- Every child develops according to his or her own biological clock. Puberty is triggered when the pituitary gland signals the body to release hormones. Hormones in turn stimulate the growth and development of the reproductive organs. Estrogen and testosterone spur the development of the child's secondary sex characteristics, such as breast development in girls and the growth of facial hair in boys. Fluctuating levels of hormones may also bring on adolescent mood swings.

The Older Adult

- The most dramatic age-related changes in the reproductive system occur with women at menopause, when their estrogen production ceases and they lose their capacity to reproduce. Menopause, in which the cycle of ovulation ceases, generally occurs between the ages of 45 and 52 years.
- Lower estrogen levels also cause atrophic changes in the uterus and vagina. The uterine lining thins and elasticity decreases. Common symptoms include hot flashes, palpitations, irritability, headaches, depression, fatigue, weight gain, insomnia, night sweats, forgetfulness, and inability to concentrate. The vaginal walls become thinner and less elastic, and lubrication decreases.
- In the years following menopause, the circulating follicle-stimulating hormone (FSH) and luteinizing hormone (LH) are greatly increased. Over subsequent years, FSH and LH levels fall slowly before leveling off about 30 years after menopause. These hormonal changes cause a relaxation of ligaments and a loss of muscular tone that alter the contour of the breast. At this time, women also face an increased risk for osteoporosis, heart attack, stroke, and possibly Alzheimer's disease.
- In men, the decline in reproductive ability is more gradual. The testes secrete testosterone and produce spermatozoa. With aging, the rate of sperm production slows, although there are few changes in sperm number so fertility is not affected. However, there may be an increase in chromosomal abnormalities. By the age of 85 there is a 35 percent decrease in the level of testosterone and a reduction in the size of the testes. The amount of fluid ejaculated remains the same. Declining levels of testosterone may be partly responsible for losses in muscle strength.

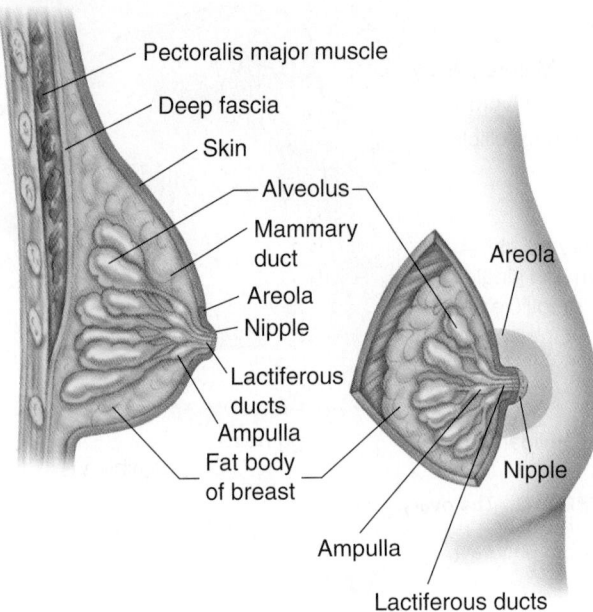

FIGURE 33-4 **The breast.**

the endometrium to support the early developmental phase of an embryo. The corpus luteum in the ovary is developing and secreting progesterone at this time. The progesterone level is at its highest during this phase, and the estrogen level begins to decrease.

- During the premenstrual phase, the coiled arteries become constricted, the endometrium begins to shrink and the corpus luteum decreases in functional activity. This phase lasts about 2 days and ends with the onset of menstruation.

The Male Reproductive System

The male reproductive system consists of the testes; various ducts; the urethra; accessory glands, which include the bulbourethral, prostate, and seminal vesicles; and the supporting structures and accessory sex organs, the scrotum and the penis (Figures 33-5 and 33-6). The vital function of the male reproductive system is to provide the sperm cells necessary to fertilize the ovum and perpetuate the species.

EXTERNAL ORGANS

In the male, the scrotum and the penis are the external organs of reproduction. The **scrotum** is a pouchlike structure behind the penis. It is suspended from the perineal region and is divided into two sacs by a septum. Each sac contains one of the two testes along with the epididymis, a connecting tube. The tissues of the scrotum have fibers of smooth muscle that

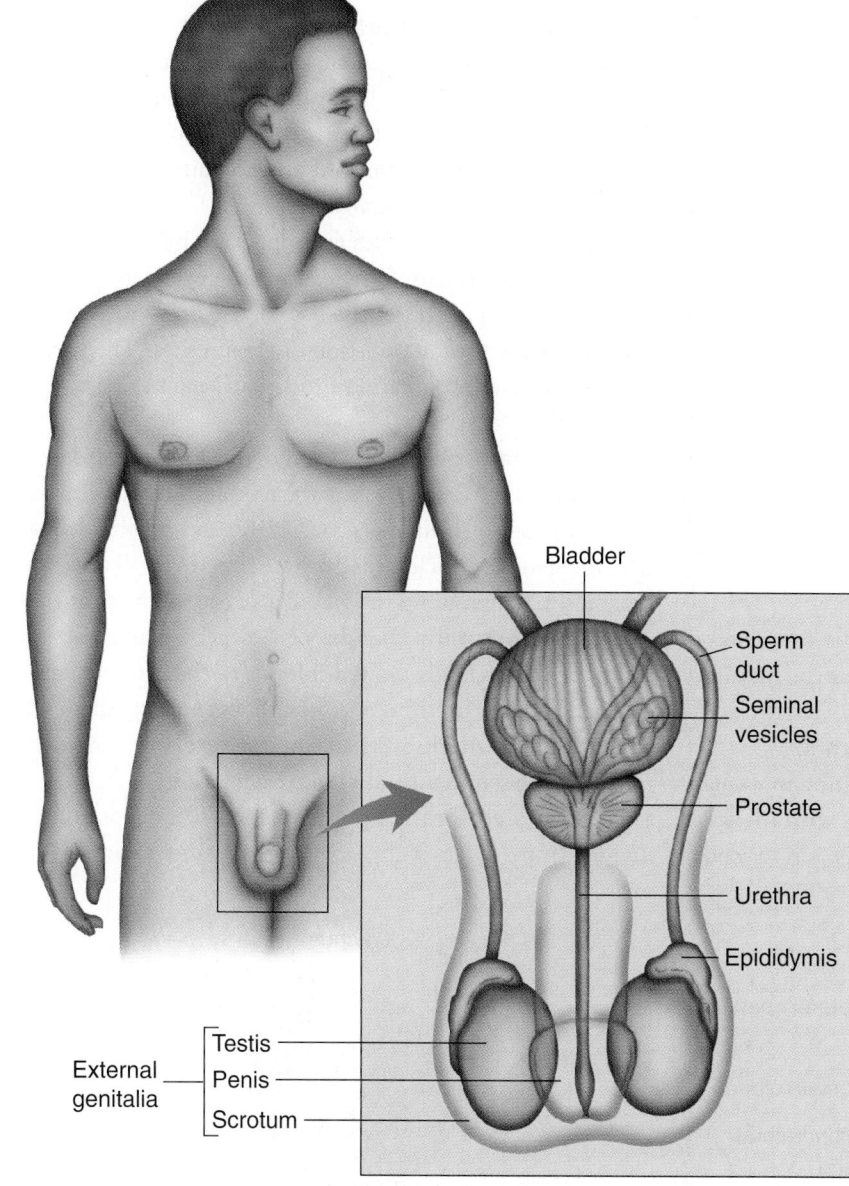

urethral orifice. The penis is covered with a loose fold of skin called the foreskin or prepuce. The foreskin contains glands that secrete a lubricating fluid called smegma. During a procedure called **circumcision**, the foreskin is removed. This is often performed for medical, cultural, or religious reasons.

The erectile state in the penis occurs when sexual stimulation causes large quantities of blood from dilated arteries supplying the penis to fill the cavernous spaces in the erectile tissue. When the arteries constrict, the pressure on the veins in the area is reduced, allowing more blood to leave the penis than can enter it, and the penis returns to its normal size. The functions of the penis are to serve as the male organ for intercourse or copulation, and as the site of the orifice through which urine and semen are eliminated from the body.

INTERNAL ORGANS

The internal organs of the male reproductive system are the testes, the epididymis, the ductus deferens (vas deferens), the seminal vesicles, the prostate gland, the bulbourethral glands, and the urethra. The two oval-shaped organs in the scrotum are called the **testes**. Each testis is about 4 cm long and 2.5 cm wide. Fibrous tissues divide the interior of each into about 250 wedge-shaped lobes. The seminiferous tubules are coiled within each lobe and are the site of the development of the spermatozoa (Figure 33-7). Other cells within the testes produce the male sex hormone testosterone. Testosterone is responsible for the development of the normal secondary sex characteristics during puberty. Male secondary sex characteristics include chest and abdominal hair, more facial hair, vocal timbre, fat deposits around the abdomen, and coarse skin texture. Testosterone also plays a vital role in the erection process and thus is necessary for the reproductive act. The network of seminiferous tubules in the testes connects with the efferent ductus, which leaves the testes and opens into the epididymis.

The epididymis is a coiled tube lying on the posterior aspect of the testes. Although each epididymis is between 13 and 20 feet in length, it is coiled into a space less than 5 cm

FIGURE 33-5 The male reproductive system: sperm duct, seminal vesicles, prostate, urethra, epididymis, and external genitalia.

contract in the absence of sufficient heat, giving the scrotum a wrinkled appearance. This contractile action brings the testes closer to the perineum, helping them to absorb sufficient body heat to maintain the viability of the sperm.

The **penis** is composed of erectile tissue covered with skin. The size and shape of the penis vary; the average erect penis is about 15 to 20 cm in length. Three longitudinal columns of erectile tissue in the penis are capable of significant enlargement when engorged with blood, such as during sexual stimulation. Two of these columns constitute the corpora cavernosa penis. The third column, the corpus spongiosum, extends at its distal end into the glans penis, the cone-shaped head at the end of the penis and the site of the

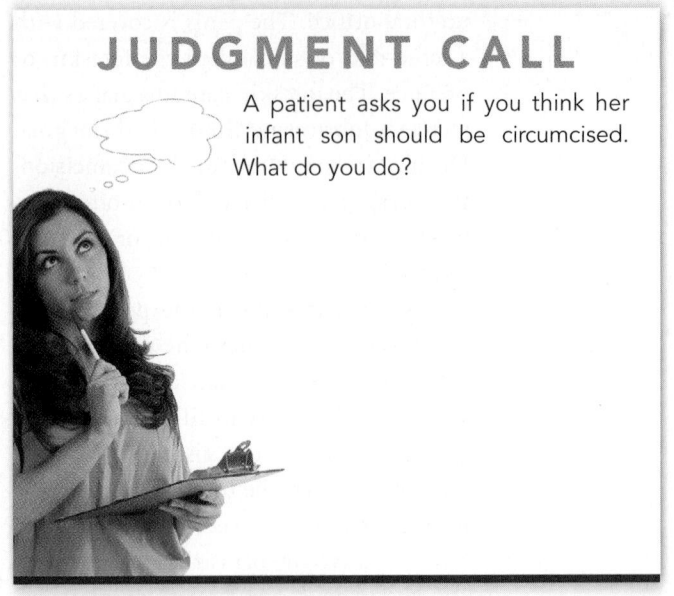
from a point adjacent to the testes and enters the abdomen at the inguinal canal. A duct from the seminal vesicle joins the ductus deferens at the inguinal canal. Between the testes and the internal inguinal ring (part of the abdomen), the ductus deferens is contained within a structure known as the spermatic cord. The spermatic cord also contains arteries, veins, lymphatic vessels, and nerves.

The two seminal vesicles are connected by a narrow duct to the ductus deferens, which forms the ejaculatory duct, a short tube that penetrates the base of the prostate gland and opens into the prostate portion of the urethra. The seminal vesicles produce an alkaline fluid that becomes part of the seminal fluid or semen.

The **prostate gland** lies behind the urinary bladder. It wraps around the first 2.5 cm of the urethra. About 4 cm wide, it is composed of glandular, connective, and muscular tissue. Like the seminal vesicles, the prostate secretes an alkaline fluid that aids in maintaining the viability of the spermatozoa.

The **bulbourethral glands**, or Cowper's glands, are two small, pea-size glands located inferior to the prostate and on either side of the urethra. A 2.5-cm duct connects them with the wall of the urethra, where they secrete a mucous secretion into the seminal fluid before ejaculation.

The male **urethra** is approximately 20 cm long and is divided into three sections: prostatic, membranous, and

in length that ends at the ductus deferens. The function of the epididymis is to serve as the storage site for the maturation of sperm and as the first part of the duct system through which the sperm pass as they travel to the urethra.

The ductus deferens (vas deferens) is a slim, muscular tube about 45 cm in length that is continuous with the epididymis. It is the excretory duct of the testes and extends

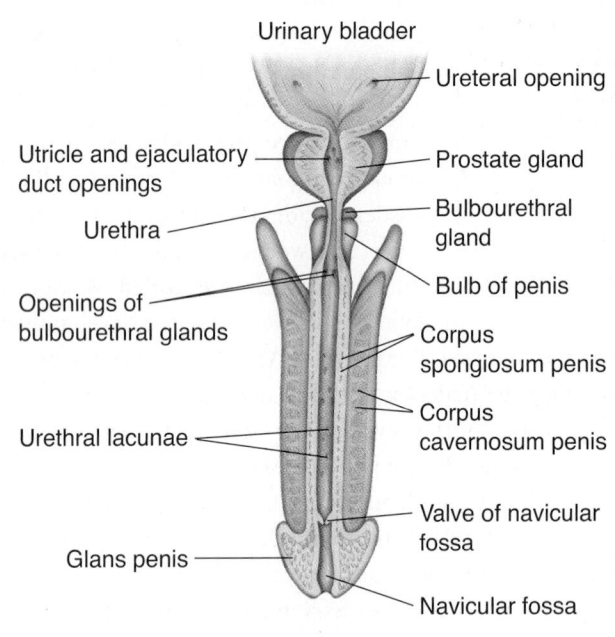

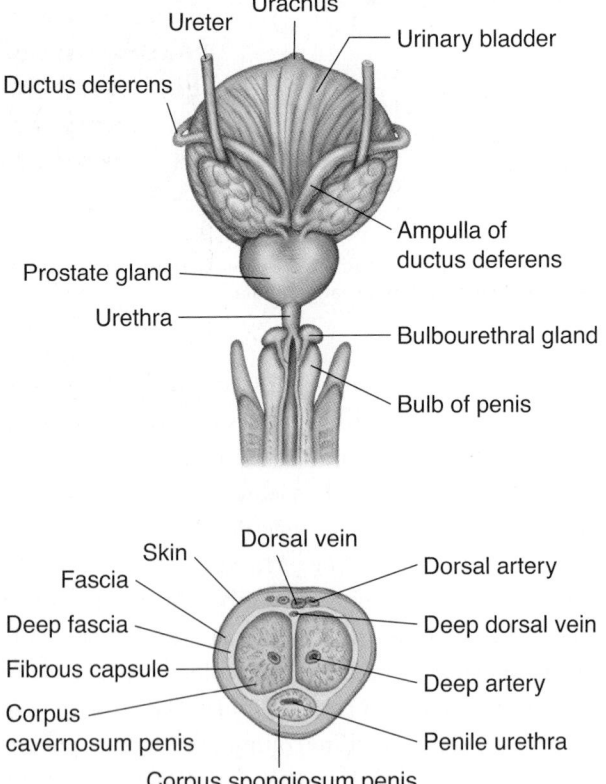

FIGURE 33-6 The structures of the bladder, prostate gland, and penis.

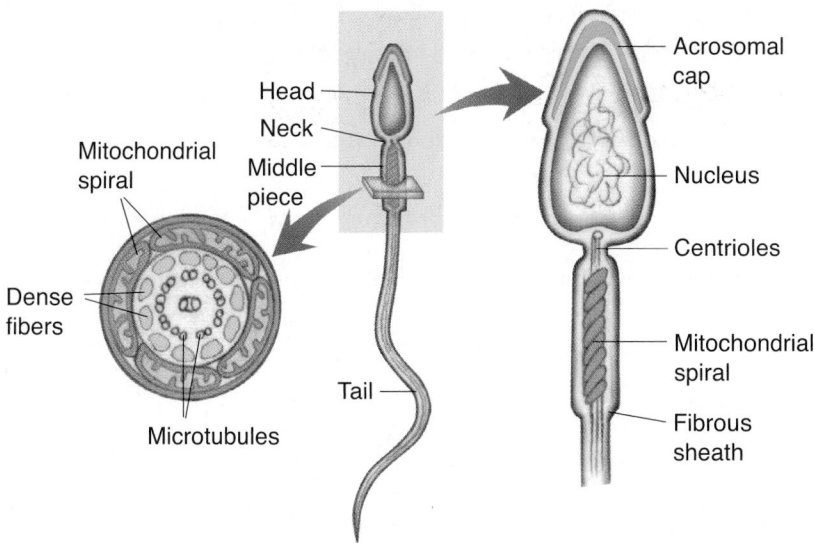

FIGURE 33-7 The basic structure of a spermatozoan (sperm).

penile. The urethra extends from the bladder to the urethral orifice at the end of the penis. The functions of the urethra in the male are the expulsion of urine and semen from the body.

Common Disorders Associated with the Female Reproductive System

Disorders that may affect the proper functioning of the female reproductive system cover a wide range, including abnormal hormone secretion, breast diseases, sexually transmitted infections (STIs), cancer, inflammations, infections, and other disorders. Many of these disorders frequently affect fertility and the mechanics of reproduction. Table 33-1 lists common disorders and pathology of the female reproductive system.

BREAST CANCER

Breast cancer is cancer arising in breast tissue (Figure 33-8). Although it affects women primarily, about 1 percent of breast cancers occur in men. It is the most common type of cancer in women and the second leading cause of death by cancer in women, second only to lung cancer.

About 80 percent of breast cancers develop in the tiny ducts that run from the lobules of the mammary glands and end in the nipple. Cancer may also develop in the lobules. Another type of breast cancer is inflammatory breast cancer. The most serious cancers are metastatic cancers, which spread from their origin into other tissues. Breast cancer metastasizes most commonly into the lymph nodes under the arm or above the collarbone on the same side as the

cancer. Other common sites of breast cancer metastasis are the brain, the bones, and the liver.

Family history is an important risk factor for breast cancer, particularly if the affected relative developed breast cancer at a young age or is a close relative such as a mother, sister, daughter, or aunt. Hormonal influences also play a role in the development of breast cancer. Women who begin menstruating at an early age or experience a late menopause have a higher risk of developing breast cancer. Conversely, having one's first menstrual period at a later age or having an early menopause often has a protective effect.

Signs and Symptoms. Breast cancer in the early stages has no symptoms and is not painful. Most breast cancer is discovered before symptoms occur, usually when an abnormality is detected on a mammogram or a breast lump is felt. A lump under the arm or above the collarbone that does not go away may indicate the presence of breast cancer.

Other possible symptoms are breast discharge, nipple inversion, and changes in the skin overlying the breasts. Of note is the fact that most breast lumps are not cancerous; however, all breast lumps should be evaluated by a physician. Breast discharge is a common problem and rarely a symptom of cancer. Like breast lumps, though, all breast discharge should be evaluated, particularly if it is from only one breast or is bloody. Nipple inversion is a common variation of normal nipples, but if it is a new development the physician should be informed. Any changes in the skin of the breast such as redness, changes in texture, and puckering also should be evaluated.

Treatment. Patient preference plays a major role in decisions regarding treatment for breast cancer. Several factors are considered: the type of breast cancer, the hormone receptor status of the tumor, the stage of the tumor, the size of the breast, and the woman's general health, age, and menstrual status (pre- or postmenopausal).

Surgery is the standard and often the best form of therapy for breast cancer. When choosing the type of surgery, a number of factors are taken into consideration, including the type, size, and location of the tumor as well as the woman's overall health and personal wishes. Surgery that saves the breast, such as lumpectomy, is often possible. More radical treatment includes simple mastectomy, modified radical mastectomy, and, in the most severe cases, radical mastectomy, which is complete removal of the breast.

TABLE 33-1 Disorders of the Female Reproductive System

Disorder	Description
Abruptio placenta	An emergency condition in which the placenta tears away from the uterine wall after the 20th week of pregnancy; requires immediate delivery of the baby
Amenorrhea	An absence of menstruation, which can be the result of many factors, including pregnancy, menopause, and dieting
Breech presentation	Position of the fetus within the uterus in which the buttocks or feet are presented first for delivery rather than the head
Carcinoma in situ	Malignant tumor that has not extended beyond the original site
Cervical cancer	A malignant growth in the cervix of the uterus; especially difficult to treat; causes 5 percent of cancer deaths in women; Pap test for possible early detection
Cervical polyp	Fibrous or mucous tumor or growth found in the cervix of the uterus; removed surgically if they may become malignant
Cervicitis	Inflammation of the cervix of the uterus
Choriocarcinoma	A rare type of cancer of the uterus that may occur following a normal pregnancy or abortion
Condyloma	A wartlike growth on the external genitalia
Cystocele	Hernia or outpouching of the bladder that protrudes into the vagina; may cause urinary frequency and urgency
Dysmenorrhea	Painful cramping associated with menstruation
Eclampsia	Convulsive seizures and coma occurring between the 20th week of pregnancy and the first week postpartum
Ectopic pregnancy	A fetus that is abnormally implanted outside the uterine cavity; known as a tubal pregnancy if implanted in a fallopian tube; requires immediate surgery
Endometrial cancer	Cancer of the endometrial lining of the uterus
Fibroid tumor	Benign tumor or growth that contains fiberlike tissue; uterine fibroid tumors are the most common tumors in women
Mastitis	Inflammation of the breast; common during lactation but can occur at any age
Menorrhagia	Excessive menstrual bleeding (total number of days, amount of blood, or both)
Ovarian carcinoma	Cancer of the ovary
Ovarian cyst	Sac filled with fluid or semisolid material that develops within the ovary
Pelvic inflammatory disease (PID)	Any inflammation of the female reproductive organs, generally bacterial in nature
Placenta previa	Condition in which the placenta is attached to the lower portion of the uterus, blocking the birth canal
Preeclampsia	Toxemia of pregnancy that if untreated can result in true eclampsia; symptoms include hypertension, headaches, albumin in the urine, and edema
Premature birth	Delivery in which the infant (neonate) is born before the 37th week of gestation (pregnancy)
Premenstrual syndrome (PMS)	Symptoms that develop just prior to the onset of a menstrual period and can include irritability, headache, tender breasts, and anxiety
Prolapsed uterus	A fallen uterus that can cause the cervix to protrude through the vaginal opening; generally caused by weakened muscles from vaginal delivery or as a result of pelvic tumors pressing down
Rh factor	A condition that can develop in a baby when the mother's blood type is Rh negative and the father's is Rh positive; baby's red blood cells can be destroyed as a result of this condition; treatment is early diagnosis and blood transfusion (See Chapter 27 for more about the Rh factor.)
Salpingitis	Inflammation of the fallopian tube or tubes
Spontaneous abortion	Loss of a fetus without any artificial aid; also called miscarriage
Stillbirth	Birth in which the fetus dies before or at the time of delivery
Toxic shock syndrome	Rare and sometimes fatal *Staphylococcus* infection that generally occurs in menstruating women
Vaginitis	Inflammation of the vagina, generally caused by a microorganism

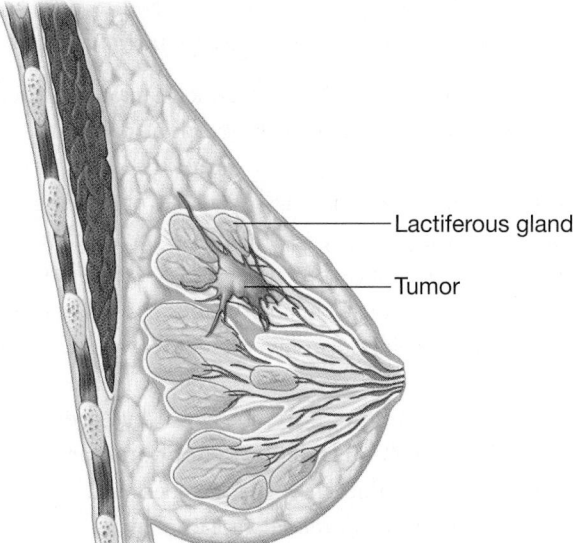

FIGURE 33-8 Breast cancer. Tumor is growing within a milk gland.

Radiation therapy is used to kill any tumor cells left after surgery. Chemotherapy may also be used to kill the cancer cells or stop them from growing. Hormonal therapy is another option.

CERVICAL CANCER

Cervical cancer is the rapid, uncontrolled growth of severely abnormal cells on the cervix. There are two main types: squamous cell (epidermoid) cervical cancer and adenocarcinoma cervical cancer. If detected at an early stage, cervical cancer is highly curable. Regular Pap test screening is the single most important tool for preventing cervical cancer because it can detect abnormal cervical cell changes when treatment is most effective: before they become cancerous.

Several factors may contribute to the development of cervical cancer: smoking or a history of smoking; an impaired immune system, such as from having human immunodeficiency virus (HIV) or human papillomavirus (HPV); and taking birth control pills for more than 5 years.

Signs and Symptoms. Abnormal changes in cervical cells rarely cause symptoms, so regular Pap test screening is critical. As these cell changes progress to cervical cancer, symptoms may develop, such as abnormal vaginal bleeding, a significant unexplained change in the menstrual cycle, pain during sexual intercourse, and abnormal vaginal discharge containing mucus that may be tinged with blood. Once cervical cancer has progressed, symptoms may include anemia caused by abnormal vaginal bleeding; ongoing pelvic, leg, or back pain; urinary problems because of a blocked kidney or ureter; an abnormal opening (fistula) developing between the vagina and the bladder or rectum, leading to leakage of urine or fecal content into the vagina; and weight loss.

Treatment. Cervical cancer detected in its early stages can be cured with treatment and close follow-up. Treatment may include surgery to remove the cancer, radiation therapy to treat other organs affected by the cancer, or chemotherapy to treat cancer that has spread or metastasized. The treatment plan may consist of a single therapy or a combination of any of these. Both the choice of treatment and the long-term outcome depend on the type and stage of cancer. The woman's age, overall health, quality of life, and desire to have children are usually taken into consideration.

CERVICITIS

Cervicitis is inflammation of the cervix. Most cases are caused by STIs such as gonorrhea and chlamydia.

Signs and Symptoms. There are generally no signs and symptoms, and the patient may first learn she has the condition as a result of a Pap test or a biopsy for another condition. If symptoms are present, they may include grayish or yellow vaginal discharge, possibly with an odor; frequent, painful urination; pain during intercourse; and vaginal bleeding after intercourse, between menstrual periods, or after menopause.

Treatment. Successful treatment of cervicitis involves addressing the cause of the inflammation. In most cases, antibiotics are used to clear an underlying bacterial infection. If the cause is viral, such as genital herpes, an antiviral medication is given. However, antiviral medication does not cure herpes, which is a chronic condition. The person's sexual partner may also be treated to prevent reinfection.

DYSMENORRHEA

More than half of all girls and women suffer from some form of **dysmenorrhea**, or painful abdominal cramps during menstruation.

Signs and Symptoms. Dysmenorrhea is generally characterized by a dull or throbbing pain usually centered in the lower abdomen and radiating toward the lower back or thighs. Menstruating women of any age can experience cramps, and whereas the pain may be only mild for some women, for others the discomfort may be severe enough to significantly interfere with everyday activities. Cramps usually last for 2 or 3 days at the beginning of each menstrual period. Some women may also experience nausea and vomiting, diarrhea, irritability, sweating, or dizziness. For many women, painful periods disappear after they have their first child, probably because the opening of the uterus has been stretched or because the uterine blood supply and muscle activity improve.

Treatment. Dysmenorrhea is controlled by treating the underlying disorder. Nonsteroidal anti-inflammatory drugs (NSAIDs) such as aspirin and ibuprofen, are used to help with pain. For more severe pain, prescription-strength ibuprofen (Motrin) may be given. These drugs are usually begun at the first sign of the period and taken for a day or two. There are many different types of NSAIDs, and a woman may need to experiment to find the one that works best for her.

Recent studies suggest that a drug patch containing glyceryl trinitrate may also ease pain. Other possible treatments include simply changing the position of the body; altering dietary intake of fibers, fats, calcium, and carbohydrates; and using visualization and guided imagery to help relieve the cramps. Aromatherapy and massage are helpful for some women. Others find that imagining a white light hovering over the painful area can actually lessen the pain briefly. Acupuncture and Chinese herbs are other popular alternative treatments for cramps.

ENDOMETRIOSIS

Endometriosis occurs when endometrial tissue is found outside the uterus, usually in the pelvis or abdominal cavity. This tissue reacts to changing levels of estrogen, thickening, breaking down, and bleeding each month, but is not sloughed off with the tissues inside the uterus. It also forms scars and adhesions. Typically, this is what causes daily or monthly cyclic pain.

Although the cause of endometriosis is unknown, one theory suggests that delayed childbearing increases the risk. Another theory is that during menstruation, some of the endometrial tissue backs up through the fallopian tubes into the abdomen. Endometriosis may also have a genetic component.

Signs and Symptoms. Symptoms of endometriosis include blood in the urine, difficulty urinating, dyspareunia (painful intercourse), heavy menstrual bleeding, irregular periods, nausea and vomiting, pelvic pain after intercourse

or exercise, and dysmenorrhea. Symptoms tend to decrease after menopause, when the involved tissues shrink.

Treatment. Early diagnosis and treatment may limit cell growth and help prevent adhesions. Pregnancy, oral contraceptives, and other hormones appear to delay the onset of endometriosis. Treatment with medication focuses on treating the discomfort. Surgery is generally reserved for women with severe endometriosis. The goal of conservative surgery is to remove or destroy all endometrial tissue outside the uterus, remove adhesions, and restore the pelvic anatomy. More extensive surgery is performed on women with severe symptoms of the disease and no desire to bear children. Typically, a **hysterectomy** (removal of the uterus) and **salpingo-oophorectomy** (removal of ovaries and fallopian tubes) are performed. After the ovaries are removed, hormonal replacement is lifelong.

FIBROCYSTIC BREAST DISEASE

Fibrocystic breast disease involves common, benign changes in the tissues of the breast (Figure 33-9). Because the condition is so common in normal breasts, it is considered a normal variant. It is also referred to as mammary dysplasia, benign breast disease, and diffuse cystic mastopathy. The cause is not completely understood, but the changes appear to be associated with ovarian hormones because the condition usually subsides with menopause and may vary in consistency during the menstrual cycle.

Fibrocystic breast disease is estimated to affect more than 60 percent of all women. It is common in women ages 30 to 50 but rare in postmenopausal women. Risk factors may include family history and diet.

Signs and Symptoms. Symptoms of fibrocystic breast disease may range from mild to severe and frequently include a

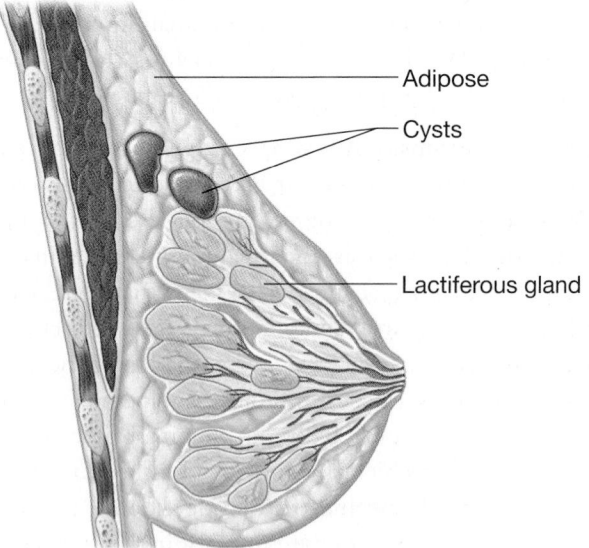

FIGURE 33-9 Fibrocystic breast disease.

dense, irregular, "cobblestone" consistency in the breast tissue; persistent or intermittent breast discomfort; and a feeling of fullness in the breasts. Premenstrual tenderness and swelling and nipple sensations, such as itching, may also be present.

Treatment.   Treatment of this disorder often involves self-care, eliminating caffeine from the diet, performing a monthly breast self-exam, and wearing a well-fitted bra that provides good breast support. Oral contraceptives, which often decrease the symptoms, may also be prescribed.

OVARIAN CANCER

Ovarian cancer begins in the cells of one or both ovaries. It can be classified into three main types, depending on where the cancer starts:

- Epithelial cell cancer—starts in the outer covering of the ovary and is the most common type of ovarian cancer.
- Germ cell tumor—starts in the egg cells within the ovary and generally occur in younger women, even in children.
- Stromal tumor—starts in the cells that form the structural framework of the ovary.

Signs and Symptoms.   Ovarian cancer can develop over a long time without causing any signs or symptoms. When symptoms do appear, they are often vague and easily mistaken for more common illnesses. By the time it is diagnosed, the cancer is usually at an advanced stage.

Early-stage symptoms frequently include mild abdominal discomfort or pain, abdominal swelling, changes in bowel habits, feeling full after a light meal, indigestion, gas, an upset stomach, a feeling that the bowel has not completely emptied, nausea and vomiting, chronic fatigue, pain in the lower back or leg, abnormal menstrual or vaginal bleeding, more frequent urination, and pain during intercourse. Symptoms of advanced ovarian cancer often include a buildup of fluid in the abdomen, shortness of breath, dry persistent cough, nausea and vomiting, abdominal tumors, and weight loss.

Treatment.   Treatment is based on the type, grade, and stage of the cancer and may include surgery to remove the tumor and some surrounding tissue, radiation therapy, and chemotherapy. Complementary therapies, such as meditation and supportive therapies, are also encouraged. Alternative therapies, such as traditional Chinese medicines or special diets, are sometimes used; however, their effectiveness has not been definitively proven.

OVARIAN CYSTS

Ovarian cysts are sacs filled with fluid or a semisolid material that develop on or within the ovary. Ovarian cysts are not disease related and typically disappear on their own. In

PROFESSIONALISM THE WORKPLACE

Patients in a gynecologist's office include both pregnant women and women with fertility problems. If a woman has recently lost a baby or had trouble getting pregnant, she may not want to see pictures of the physician holding newborns, surrounded by happy new mothers. Ensure that the office examination rooms are decorated separately for pregnant women and for those who would prefer not to see photos of babies.

the days preceding ovulation, a follicle grows in the cortex of the ovary. At the time of expected ovulation, however, the follicle fails to rupture and release an egg. Instead of being reabsorbed, the fluid within the follicle forms a cyst. Most of these cysts are harmless and cause no symptoms. Functional cysts are relatively common and usually disappear within 60 days without treatment. They occur most often during the childbearing years but may occur at any time. Functional ovarian cysts are different from other disease conditions involving ovarian cysts, specifically benign cysts of different types that require treatment; true ovarian tumors, including ovarian cancer; and hormonal conditions such as polycystic ovary disease in which the ovary is filled with numerous small cysts.

Signs and Symptoms.   Ovarian cysts are often asymptomatic. If symptoms are present, they generally include constant, dull pelvic pain; pelvic pain during movement, with intercourse, or shortly after the beginning or end of a menstrual period; and abdominal bloating or distention.

Treatment.   Functional ovarian cysts generally disappear within 60 days without treatment. Oral contraceptive pills may be prescribed to help establish normal cycles and impede the development of functional ovarian cysts. Ovarian cysts that are not functional may require surgical removal by laparoscopy or exploratory laparotomy. Cysts larger than 6 cm or persisting for longer than 6 weeks may require surgical removal. If other disorders, such as polycystic ovary disease, are causing the cysts, other medical options may merit exploration.

PELVIC INFLAMMATORY DISEASE

The most common and serious complication of STIs among women is **pelvic inflammatory disease (PID)**, an infection of the upper genital area. It is caused by disease-carrying organisms that migrate upward from the urethra and cervix. Among the many different organisms that can cause PID, the bacteria responsible for gonorrhea and chlamydia are the most common. PID can affect the uterus, ovaries, and fallopian tubes. Untreated, PID can cause scarring, which can lead to infertility, tubal pregnancy, chronic pelvic pain, and other serious complications.

Signs and Symptoms. The major symptoms of PID are lower abdominal pain and abnormal vaginal discharge. Other possible symptoms are fever, pain in the right upper quadrant, painful intercourse, and irregular menstrual bleeding. PID may be very painful or may have few if any symptoms, in spite of the serious damage it can do to the reproductive organs.

Treatment. Treatment for PID begins with treating the underlying infection. If the pelvic organs are too scarred for pregnancy to result, surgery to remove the scarred tissue and connect the opened tubes to the uterus may be necessary.

PREMENSTRUAL SYNDROME

It is estimated that 85 percent of women who menstruate are affected by **premenstrual syndrome (PMS)**, or premenstrual dysphoric disorder. However, only 5 to 10 percent of menstruating women are severely impaired by PMS. It is unknown why some women are affected and others are not. Although no specific cause has been determined, it is believed that PMS is associated with the amount of hormones produced (Figure 33-10).

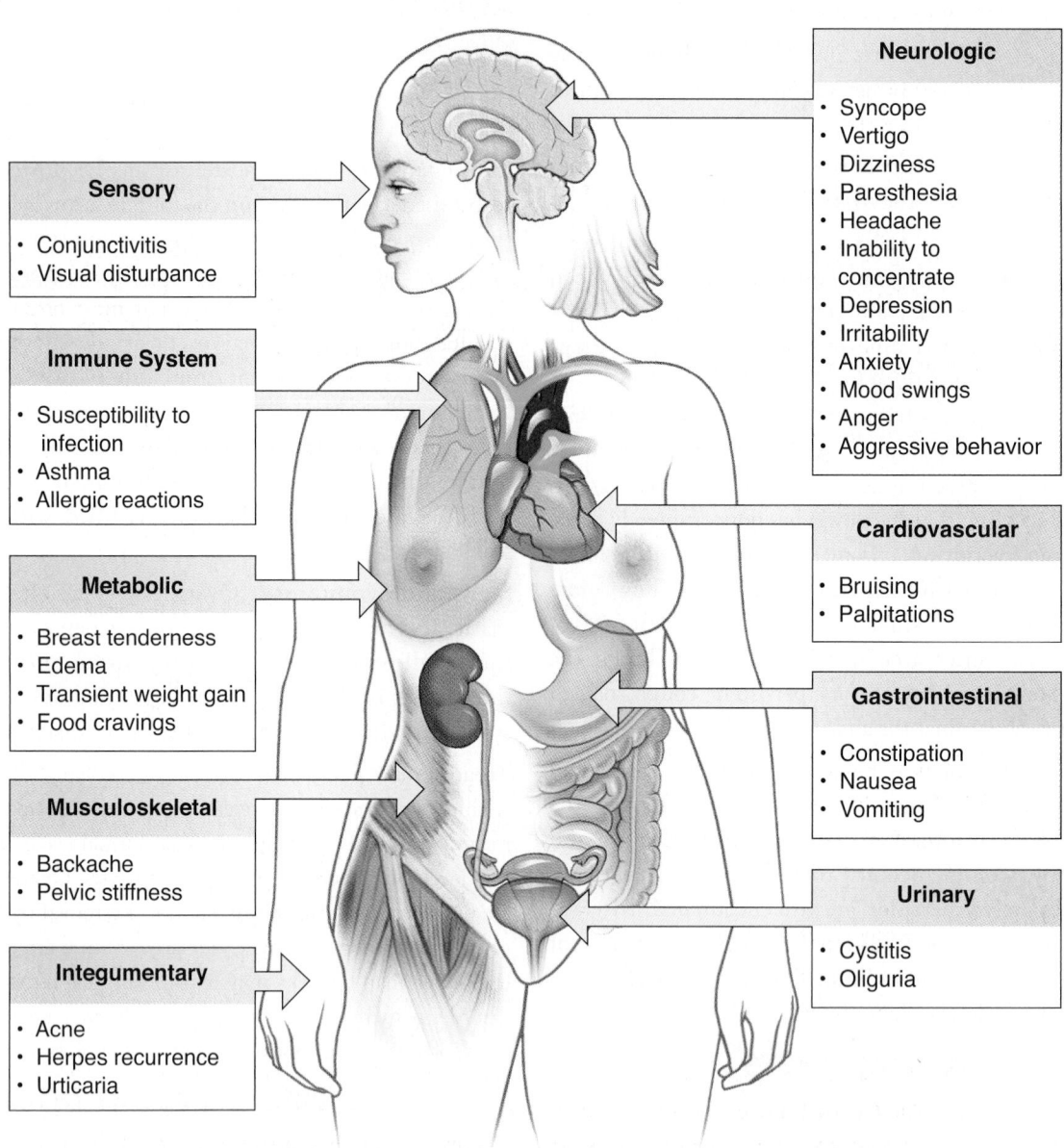

FIGURE 33-10 Multisystem effects of premenstrual syndrome.

Signs and Symptoms. Symptoms of PMS include constipation, diarrhea, nausea, anorexia, appetite cravings, headache, backache, muscular aches, edema, insomnia, clumsiness, malaise, irritability, indecisiveness, mental confusion, and depression.

Treatment. The severity of PMS symptoms may be alleviated by a healthy diet high in vegetables and fruits; low in starches, sugars, sodium, fat, caffeine, and alcohol; and sufficient in vitamins and minerals, especially B vitamins, calcium, and magnesium. Regular aerobic exercise, relaxation therapy, and stress management techniques also may be of benefit. Certain herbal products, such as chasteberry and black cohosh, have been helpful to some women. Medications that may help decrease and control the symptoms of PMS also are available.

SEXUALLY TRANSMITTED INFECTIONS

Sexually transmitted infection (STI) is the term for more than 20 different infections that are transmitted via the exchange of semen, blood, and other body fluids or by direct contact with the affected body areas of people with STIs. STIs are also called venereal diseases. Some of the most common and potentially serious STIs in the United States are chlamydia, HPV, genital herpes, gonorrhea, syphilis, and HIV infection.

The Centers for Disease Control and Prevention (CDC) has reported that 85 percent of the most prevalent infectious diseases in the United States are sexually transmitted. The rate of occurrence for STIs in the United States is 50 to 100 times higher than that of any other industrialized nation. One in four sexually active Americans will be affected by an STI at some point in their lives.

STIs can have very painful long-term consequences in addition to causing immediate health problems. They can cause birth defects, blindness, bone deformities, brain damage, cancer, heart disease, infertility and other reproductive abnormalities, mental retardation, and death.

Signs and Symptoms. The incubation period varies among different STIs. In some STIs, symptoms appear fairly soon after sexual contact, often in less than 48 hours. In others the incubation period is longer, so that the patient may not realize the early symptoms are those of an STI.

The symptoms of STIs vary somewhat according to the disease agent, the sex of the patient, and the body systems affected. Some are easy to identify, whereas others may go unnoticed for some time or may be confused with other diseases. Syphilis in particular can be confused with disorders ranging from infectious mononucleosis to allergic reactions to prescription medications.

Symptoms of STIs that affect the genitals and reproductive organs include bleeding not associated with menstruation, abnormal vaginal discharge, vaginal burning, itching, and pelvic pain during sexual intercourse. Male symptoms include discharge from the penis and swelling of the lymph nodes near the groin area. Both males and females may experience pain or burning during urination and may also develop skin rashes, sores, bumps, or blisters near the mouth or genitals. Systemic symptoms (affecting the body as a whole) include fever, chills, and other flulike symptoms, skin rashes over large parts of the body, arthritislike pains or aching in the joints, and throat swelling and redness lasting 3 weeks or longer.

Treatment. Some of the pain and symptoms of STIs can be alleviated through self-care. Others require medical attention, such as the administration of antibiotics, which are used to treat gonorrhea, chlamydia, syphilis, and other STIs caused by bacteria.

The risk of contracting an STI can be reduced or eliminated by adopting certain personal behaviors. Abstaining from sexual relations or maintaining a mutually monogamous relationship with a partner are legitimate options. Avoiding sexual contact with people who are known to be infected with an STI, whose health status is unknown, who abuse drugs, or who are involved in prostitution are also considered ways of reducing or eliminating altogether the risk of infection with an STI. See Table 33-2 for more information about STIs.

UTERINE CANCER

Uterine cancer (endometrial cancer or adenocarcinoma) generally develops in the glandular tissue of the endometrium. If the cancer is detected and treated early, treatment is usually very successful. There is no one single cause of uterine cancer; however, some factors appear to increase the risk of developing it: age, particularly in women over 50; obesity; childlessness; menopause that begins later than average; prolonged use of medications with the hormone estrogen; and use of the drug tamoxifen.

Signs and Symptoms. Many of the signs and symptoms of uterine cancer may be associated with other disorders of the female reproductive system. These include bleeding between menstrual periods, heavy bleeding or spotting during periods or after menopause, bleeding after intercourse, and a foul discharge. Other symptoms are a watery yellow discharge; cramping pain; pressure in the abdomen, pelvis, back, or legs; and discomfort over the pubic area.

Treatment. Treatment of uterine cancer depends on the type, grade, and stage of the cancer. Treatments may include surgery, radiation therapy, chemotherapy, or a combination of them.

TABLE 33-2 Sexually Transmitted Infections

Disease	Description
Acquired immune deficiency syndrome (AIDS)	The final stage of infection from the human immunodeficiency virus (HIV); no cure at present
Candidiasis	A yeastlike infection of the skin and mucous membranes that can result in white plaque on the tongue and vagina
Chancroid	Highly infectious nonsyphilitic ulcer
Chlamydia infection	Genital infection in males and females caused by the bacterium *Chlamydia trachomatis*; can lead to pelvic inflammatory disease (PID) in females and eventual infertility
Genital herpes	Painful vesicles on the skin and mucosa that erupt periodically and can be transmitted through the placenta or at birth
Genital warts	Growths and elevations on the genitalia of both males and females that can lead to cancer of the cervix in females; currently no cure
Gonorrhea	Sexually transmitted inflammation of the mucous membranes of either sex; can be passed on to an infant during the birth process
Hepatitis	Infectious, inflammatory disease of the liver; hepatitis B and C spread by contact with blood and bodily fluids of an infected person
Syphilis	Infectious, chronic venereal disease that can involve any organ; may exist for years without symptoms
Trichomoniasis	Genitourinary infection caused by a parasite that is usually asymptomatic (without symptoms) in both males and females; can produce itching and/or burning and a foul-smelling discharge and result in vaginitis in women

UTERINE FIBROIDS

Uterine fibroids are benign growths or tumors made up of muscle cells and other tissues that grow within the wall of the uterus (Figure 33-11). Fibroids can grow as a single growth or as a cluster of tumors. They can be the size of an apple seed or larger than a grapefruit. They are common in women of childbearing age, and African-American women are the most susceptible of all racial groups. African-American women also tend to get fibroids at an earlier age. There also appears to be a higher risk for fibroids among women who are overweight or obese. Women who have given birth appear to be at a lower risk. Although the cause of fibroids is unknown, they may result due to a combination of hormones, genetics, and environmental factors. Fibroids usually, but not always, shrink or disappear after menopause.

Signs and Symptoms. Symptoms of uterine fibroids include heavy bleeding or painful periods, bleeding between periods, feeling of fullness in the pelvic area, frequent urination, pain during sex, lower back pain, and reproductive problems, including infertility and early onset of labor.

Treatment. Patients with mild symptoms may only require over-the-counter medications for relief of pain and inflammation. Those who require more relief may require gonadotropin-releasing hormone agonists (GnRHa), which decrease the size of the fibroids. Side effects can include hot flashes, depression, insomnia, decreased libido, and joint pain. Antihormonal agents may stop or slow the growth of fibroids. These drugs only offer temporary relief from symptoms, which return as soon the therapy is discontinued.

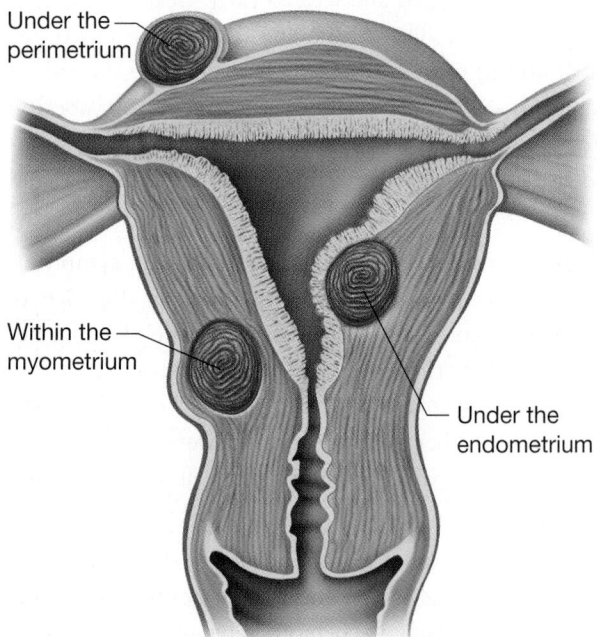

Under the perimetrium

Within the myometrium

Under the endometrium

FIGURE 33-11 Types of uterine fibroid tumors.

Two types of surgery are used to treat fibroids. A **myomectomy** removes the fibroids without taking any healthy tissue of the uterus, either by laparotomy or as an open surgery. A hysterectomy removes the entire uterus.

VAGINITIS

Vaginitis is an inflammation of the vagina that can result in discharge, itching, or pain. The most common cause is a change in the normal balance of vaginal bacteria or an infection. Reduced estrogen levels after menopause are another contributing factor. The most common types of vaginitis are bacterial vaginitis, yeast infections, trichomoniasis, and atrophic vaginitis.

Signs and Symptoms. The signs and symptoms of vaginitis include any change in color, odor, or amount of discharge from the vagina, vaginal itching or irritation, pain during intercourse, painful urination, and light vaginal bleeding.

Treatment. Treatment depends on the type of vaginitis. For bacterial vaginitis, vaginal gels or creams may be prescribed. Yeast infections are usually treated with antifungal creams or suppositories. Trichomoniasis is frequently treated with metronidazole (Flagyl); atrophic vaginitis results from decreased levels of estrogen after menopause and is treated with estrogen.

Common Disorders Associated with the Male Reproductive System

The male reproductive system is essential to reproduction and is also related to the urinary system. Many disorders affect both systems. Conditions range from inflammatory disorders, such as epididymitis, to infectious diseases, such as those classified as STIs, to life-threatening conditions such as prostate and testicular cancer. See Table 33-3 for more information about disorders of the male reproductive system.

BENIGN PROSTATIC HYPERPLASIA

Benign prostatic hyperplasia (BPH), or benign prostatic hypertrophy, is an enlargement of the prostate gland that may occur in men 50 years of age and older (Figure 33-12). By age 60, four out of five men have an enlarged prostate. As the prostate enlarges, it compresses the urethra, restricting the normal flow of urine. The restriction generally causes a number of symptoms collectively known as prostatism.

Prostatism is any condition of the prostate gland that interferes with the flow of urine from the bladder.

Signs and Symptoms. Symptoms usually include a weak or difficult-to-start urine stream; a feeling that the bladder is not empty; a need to urinate often, especially at night; a feeling of urgency (sudden need to urinate); abdominal straining; interruption of the stream; acute urinary retention; and recurrent urinary infections.

Treatment. Treatment for BPH includes drug therapy, nonsurgical procedures, and surgery. Medications work either by reducing the size of the prostate or by relaxing the smooth muscle of the prostate and the bladder neck to improve urine flow and reduce bladder outlet obstruction.

EPIDIDYMITIS

Epididymitis is an inflammation or infection of the epididymis, the long coiled tube attached to the upper part of each testicle, where mature sperm are stored before ejaculation. It is the most common cause of pain in the scrotum. The most severe pain and swelling are usually associated with the acute form. If symptoms last for more than 6 weeks after treatment begins, the condition is considered chronic.

Epididymitis can occur anytime after the onset of puberty but is most common between the ages of 18 and 40. Risk factors include infection of the bladder, kidney, prostate, or urinary tract; other recent illness; a narrowing of the urethra; and use of a urethral catheter.

Although epididymitis can be caused by the same organisms that cause some STIs or as a result of prostate surgery, it is generally caused by pus-generating bacteria associated with infections in other parts of the body. It can also be caused by injury or infection of the scrotum or by irritation from urine that has accumulated in the vas deferens.

TABLE 33-3 Disorders of the Male Reproductive System

Disorder	Description
Anorchism	A congenital absence of one or both testes
Aspermia	The lack of, or failure to eject, sperm
Azoospermia	Absence of sperm in the semen
Balanitis	Inflammation of the skin covering the glans penis
Benign prostatic hyperplasia (benign prostatic hypertrophy)	Enlargement of the prostate gland, commonly seen in males over age 50
Carcinoma of the testes	Cancer of one or both testes
Cryptorchidism	Failure of the testes to descend into the scrotal sac before birth (generally descend permanently before age 1 year); may result in sterility; orchidopexy (surgical procedure) may bring the testes down into the scrotum and secure them permanently
Epididymitis	Inflammation of the epididymis that causes pain and swelling in the inguinal area
Epispadias	Congenital opening of the male urethra on the dorsal surface of the penis
Hydrocele	Accumulation of fluid within the testes
Hypospadias	Congenital opening of the male urethra on the underside of the penis
Impotence	Inability to copulate due to inability to maintain an erection or to achieve orgasm
Phimosis	Narrowing of the foreskin over the glans penis that results in difficulty with hygiene; can lead to infection or difficulty with urination; treated with circumcision (surgical removal of foreskin)
Prostate cancer	A slow-growing cancer that affects a large number of males after age 50; PSA (prostate-specific antigen) test used for early detection
Prostatitis	An inflamed condition of the prostate gland that may be the result of infection
Varicocele	Enlargement of the veins of the spermatic cord that commonly occurs on the left side of adolescent males; seldom needs treatment

Signs and Symptoms.   Epididymitis is characterized by sudden redness and swelling of the scrotum. The affected testicle is hard and sore, and the other testicle may feel tender. Chills, fever, and acute **urethritis** (inflammation of the urethra) usually accompany those symptoms. Enlarged lymph nodes in the groin may cause scrotal pain that inten-sifies throughout the day, sometimes to the point that walking becomes impossible.

Treatment.   This disorder, which can affect both testicles, causes sterility. It is because of this concern that antibiotic therapy must be initiated as soon as symptoms appear. To prevent reinfection, medication must be taken exactly as prescribed, even if symptoms disappear or the patient begins to feel better. If approved by a family physician or urologist, over-the-counter anti-inflammatories can be used for pain relief. Bed rest is also recommended until symptoms subside, and patients are advised to wear an athletic supporter upon resuming normal activities. To alleviate more severe pain, a local anesthetic such as lidocaine (Xylocaine) may be injected directly into the spermatic cord.

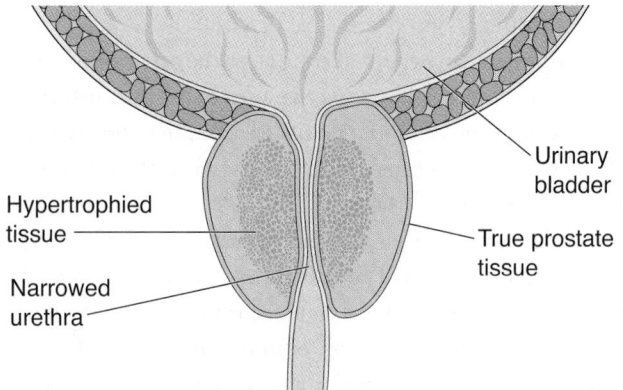

FIGURE 33-12   Benign prostatic hyperplasia.

Hypertrophied tissue

Narrowed urethra

Urinary bladder

True prostate tissue

ERECTILE DYSFUNCTION

Erectile dysfunction (ED) is the inability to achieve or maintain an erection sufficient for sexual intercourse. It occurs when not enough blood is supplied to the penis, when the smooth muscle in the penis fails to relax, or when the penis does not retain the blood that flows into it. According to studies at the National Institutes of Health, 5 percent of men have some degree of erectile dysfunction at age 40, and by age 65 and older that figure rises to 15 to 25 percent. But erectile dysfunction is not an inevitable part of aging. About 80 percent of erectile dysfunction has a physical cause that can be addressed.

Risk factors for ED include hypertension, hyperlipidemia, endocrine disorders, low testosterone, thyroid disease, diabetes, coronary artery disease, peripheral vascular disease, anemia, smoking, alcohol abuse, and certain medications, surgical procedures, neurological conditions, and psychiatric illnesses.

ED can affect relationships, and men should discuss the issue with their partners as well as their physicians. A medical evaluation is usually done to explore any underlying causative factors. Patients may be uncomfortable talking about ED, as they may feel that a loss of erection affects how they are perceived as men. Care must be taken by the medical assistant to ensure confidentiality and reassure the patient that medical treatments are available.

Signs and Symptoms. The penis may achieve, but not maintain, an erection.

Treatment. Treatment options are medication therapy, medication changes, the vacuum constriction device, urethral and penile injection therapies, and surgery, including penile prostheses.

HYDROCELE

A **hydrocele** is a painless buildup of watery fluid around one or both testicles that causes swelling in the scrotum or groin area. Although it may be unsightly and uncomfortable, this swelling is not painful and generally not dangerous. A hydrocele can be congenital (present at birth) or acquired (develops after birth). A congenital hydrocele develops when, after the normal process of testicle migration, the space around the testicles does not close or the closure is delayed. Fluid from the abdominal cavity fills this space, creating the hydrocele.

Signs and Symptoms. The main symptom of a hydrocele is a swollen scrotum or groin area. The scrotum may have a bluish tinge. The swelling is painless, may be soft or firm, and cannot be reduced by changing its position or gently pushing it up. The swelling may change size, starting out small in the morning and gradually increasing in size throughout the day, and the skin on the scrotum may appear to be translucent. Any pain accompanying the swelling may indicate the presence of an inguinal hernia, injury to the testicles, or some other problem.

Treatment. For a congenital hydrocele that does not grow in size or gets smaller, aggressive treatment is not recommended, as it generally will disappear by age 1 or 2. However, surgery generally is necessary if the hydrocele varies in size, does not go away by the age of 1 or 2, comes and goes, or feels firm.

PROSTATE CANCER

Prostate cancer is a malignant tumor that grows in the prostate gland. It is the most common cancer among American men and the second leading cause of death as a result of cancer in men, exceeded only by lung cancer. By age 50, one in four American men have some cancerous cells in the prostate gland. By age 80, the ratio increases to one in two. The average age of diagnosis is 70. However, only 1 in 32 men with this diagnosis actually dies from prostate cancer.

Some risk factors associated with prostate cancer are advanced age, a diet high in animal fats, being of African or Northern European origin, a family history of cancer, and a history of vasectomy, smoking, or cadmium exposure.

Signs and Symptoms. Prostate cancer can grow slowly for many years, but it occasionally grows quickly and spreads (metastasizes) to other parts of the body. Symptoms may or may not be present. When they are, the most common include dull pain in the lower pelvic area; general pain in the lower back, hips, and upper thighs; blood in the urine or semen; dribbling when urinating; erectile dysfunction; frequent urination, especially at night; painful urination or ejaculation; smaller stream of urine or urgent need to urinate; and loss of appetite and weight. If the cancer has spread to other parts of the body, there may be persistent bone pain, occasional nerve loss, or loss of bladder function.

Treatment. Depending on the type and stage of the prostate cancer, treatment options include any one or a combination of the following: chemotherapy, cryosurgery to freeze cancer cells, external radiation to the prostate and pelvis, hormone therapy, radioactive implants in the prostate, surgery to remove part or all of the prostate and the surrounding tissue, surgical removal of the testes to block testosterone production, and watchful waiting and monitoring. Hormones and chemotherapy are used for advanced cancer. The focus of hormone therapy is to reduce the body's production of testosterone, which should slow the growth of the cancer.

SUMMARY

The reproductive system functions both for reproduction and for maintaining the secondary sex characteristics of both males and females. The organs of the female reproductive system are the uterus, fallopian tubes, ovaries, vagina, vulva, and breasts. The female body prepares for reproduction with an approximate 28-day menstrual cycle. The organs of the male reproductive system include the penis, testes, scrotum, epididymis, ductus deferens, prostate gland, bulbourethral glands, urethra, and seminal vesicles. The male reproductive system produces sperm on a regular basis and does not depend on a reproductive cycle. Many diseases can develop in the reproductive organs.

Common female reproductive disorders include cancers of the breast, cervix, ovaries, and uterus, as well as cervicitis, dysmenorrhea, endometriosis, fibrocystic breast disease, ovarian cysts, pelvic inflammatory disease, premenstrual syndrome, STIs, uterine fibroids, and vaginitis. Complications of pregnancy include abruptio placenta, breech presentation, eclampsia, ectopic/tubal pregnancy, placenta previa, preeclampsia, premature birth, spontaneous abortion, and stillbirth.

Common disorders of the male reproductive system include anorchism, aspermia, azoospermia, balanitis, benign prostatic hyperplasia (benign prostatic hypertrophy), carcinoma of the testes, cryptorchidism, epididymitis, epispadias, hydrocele, hypospadias, impotence, phimosis, prostate cancer, prostatitis, and varicocele.

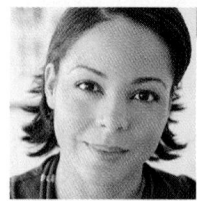

33 CHAPTER REVIEW

COMPETENCY REVIEW

1. Define and spell the terms to learn for this chapter.

2. What is another term for fallopian tubes?

3. What are the three identifiable areas of the uterus?

4. What are the two functions of the ovaries?

5. What are the three functions of the vagina?

6. What are the two principal hormones in the female reproductive system?

7. What is the most vital function of the male reproductive system?

8. What are the two functions of the penis?

9. What are the two functions of the male urethra?

10. What is the function of the seminal vesicles?

PREPARING FOR THE CERTIFICATION EXAM

1. The triangular-shaped pad of fatty tissue that is rounded over the symphysis pubis is known as
   a. clitoris
   b. mons pubis
   c. labia minora
   d. labia majora
   e. perineum

2. Which of the following is NOT a sexually transmitted infection?
   a. syphilis
   b. endometriosis
   c. trichomoniasis
   d. candidiasis
   e. genital warts

3. The female reproductive system does NOT include the
   a. breasts
   b. urethra
   c. follicles
   d. corpus luteum
   e. fundus

4. The lower portion of the uterus is called the
   a. fundus
   b. corpus
   c. ovum
   d. cervix
   e. vulva

5. All of the following are pregnancy complications EXCEPT
   a. placenta abruptio
   b. dysmenorrhea
   c. eclampsia
   d. pre-eclampsia
   e. placenta previa

6. All of the following are symptoms of premenstrual syndrome EXCEPT
   a. diarrhea
   b. backache
   c. mood swings
   d. depression
   e. herpes recurrence

7. Which of the following terms means failure of the testes to descend into the scrotal sac before birth?
   a. epispadias
   b. hypospadias
   c. cryptorchidism
   d. circumcision
   e. anorchism

8. The sterilization of the male reproductive system is done with surgery to what organ?
   a. ductus deferens
   b. prostate
   c. penis
   d. scrotum
   e. urethra

9. The ovaries produce
   a. progesterone
   b. growth hormone
   c. testosterone
   d. oxytocin
   e. prolactin

10. The hormone that stimulates the uterus to contract is
   a. progesterone
   b. estrogen
   c. testosterone
   d. oxytocin
   e. prolactin

CRITICAL THINKING

1. Why would Dr. Bahjat ask Nabiel if he is sexually active?

2. Dr. Bahjat next asks Nabiel if he has had any recent injuries. Nabiel informs him that he was injured in the groin during a soccer game a couple of weeks ago. Could this injury be related to Nabiel's diagnosis?

3. Because Nabiel has been in pain for almost 2 weeks, would his condition be considered acute or chronic epididymitis?

INTERNET ACTIVITY

Do an Internet search of the National Breast Cancer Foundation and other breast cancer awareness organizations. Research the following regarding breast cancer: cancer myths, early detection, and up-and-coming research.

MEDMEDIA

Additional interactive resources and activities for this chapter can be found:

On your student DVD: View applicable procedure videos on the DVD-ROM found in the back of this book.

MyHealthProfessionsKit.com: Test your knowledge of the chapter with games and activities. MyHealthProfessionsKit also includes resources, helpful links, and a Spanish audio glossary.

Medical Assisting Interactive: Practice your procedures as a medical assistant in this simulated doctor's office. This can be accessed through MyHealthProfessionsKit.com.

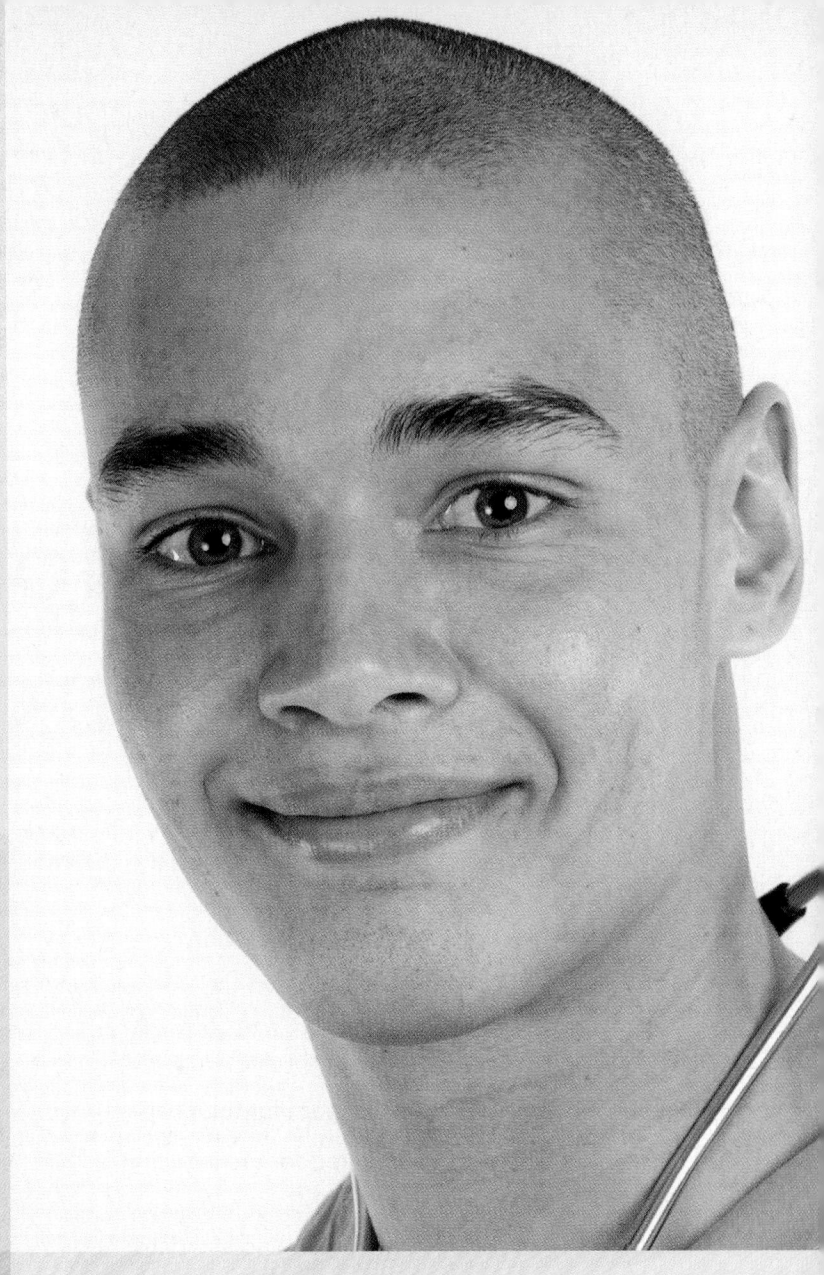

Unit One

Unit Two

Unit Three

Unit Four

Clinical Medical Assisting

Unit Five

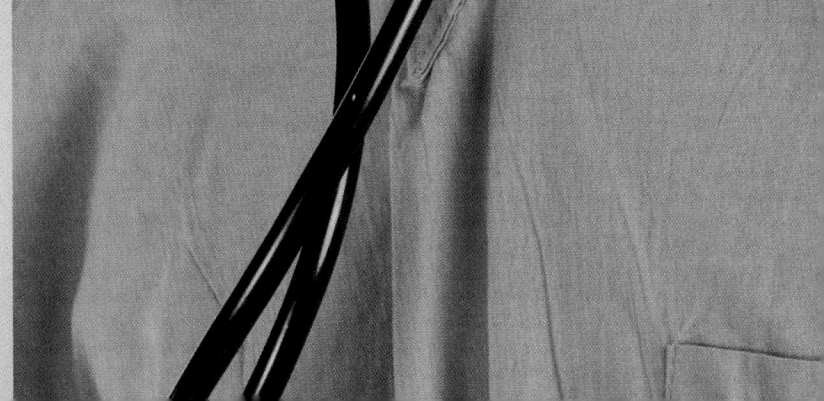

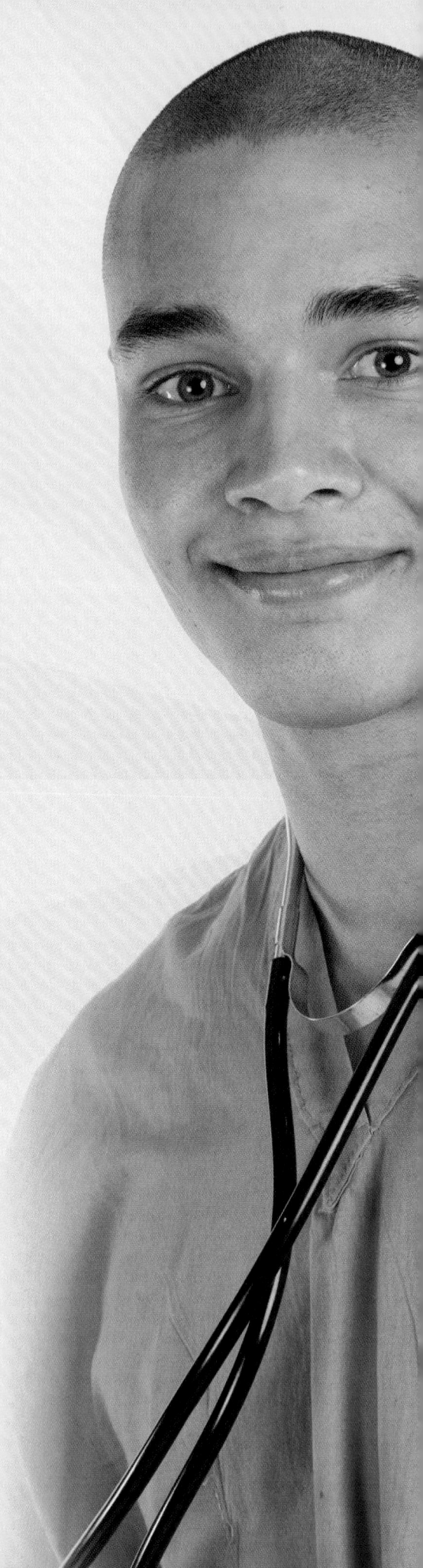

34

Infection Control

LEARNING OBJECTIVES

After completing this chapter, you should be able to:

- Define and spell the terms to learn for this chapter.

- Describe the conditions required for the infection process to occur.

- Perform the steps to follow concerning standard precautions.

- Define medical asepsis.

- Perform the correct procedure for hand washing.

- Define surgical asepsis.

- Explain the difference between sanitization, disinfection, and sterilization.

- Discuss the modes of transmission for the different types of hepatitis.

- Describe the means of transmission for HIV.

- Explain the term MRSA and the repercussions in health care today.

- Define bioterrorism and list two examples of possible biological agents.

CHAPTER OUTLINE

CASE STUDY

Dr. McWalters asks David, RMA, to perform venipuncture on the 34-year-old female in examination room 4. The physician explains that the patient needs to have routine blood work performed, including a liver function test (LFT), to evaluate the progression of hepatitis B, which the patient was diagnosed with over 2 years ago.

Pathogens, which are disease-producing organisms, are everywhere. Healthy individuals have some measure of resistance to pathogens. Patients already suffering from a disease are more susceptible to new infections. Therefore, controlling pathogens is especially important in the medical office setting. The medical assistant must be aware of how easily pathogens can be spread from one person to another or from an inanimate object to a person.

History of Asepsis

Methods for controlling the spread of infection were used before early humans understood the infection process. About five hundred years ago, certain microorganisms (bacteria, viruses, protozoa, and fungi) were suspected to be the cause of some diseases and were termed germs. But it was not until about a hundred years ago that Semmelweiss, Lister, and Pasteur contributed solid research to our understanding of germ theory. Their contributions to the medical field are discussed in Chapter 2.

Today, we have a better understanding of disease-causing germs with the aid of high-powered microscopes and more specific laboratory procedures. Sophisticated equipment is used to disinfect and sterilize equipment and materials. However, sterilization (to render an object free of all microorganisms) is meaningless if good aseptic technique is not practiced. **Asepsis** is the state of being free from germs, infection, and any form of microbial life. With the advent of communicable diseases such as hepatitis, acquired immunodeficiency syndrome (AIDS), and tuberculosis (TB), the need to adhere to aseptic technique has become critical.

Microorganisms

Microorganisms are small, living substances that can only be seen with the aid of a microscope. Microorganisms that are normally found on the skin and in the urinary, gastrointestinal, and respiratory tracts are known as **normal flora**. They do not cause disease as long as they are not transferred to another part of the body.

The sizes of microorganisms (also called microbes) can be expressed in micrometers. A micrometer is one-millionth of a meter or one-thousandth of a millimeter. (Refer to Figure 34-1 for an illustration of pathogens.) The study of each type of microorganism represents a separate scientific field:

- **Bacteriology**—the study of bacteria
- **Mycology**—the study of fungi
- **Protozoology**—the study of protozoa
- **Virology**—the study of viruses

HOW MICROORGANISMS GROW

Microorganisms exist everywhere in nature. They have several growth requirements: food, moisture, darkness, and a suitable temperature. In addition, some bacteria are **aerobic** (require oxygen to live), and some are **anaerobic** (do not require oxygen to live). Refer to Table 34-1 for the conditions that are necessary for the growth of bacteria.

Some microorganisms, such as certain types of fungi and bacteria, are necessary for normal body functions. For example, normal types of flora within the digestive system break down food and convert unused food into waste products. In some cases these will invade areas of the body where they do not belong and, thus, they become pathogens. For example, *Escherichia coli,* a normal bacteria within the colon, aids in food digestion. When *E. coli* moves into the

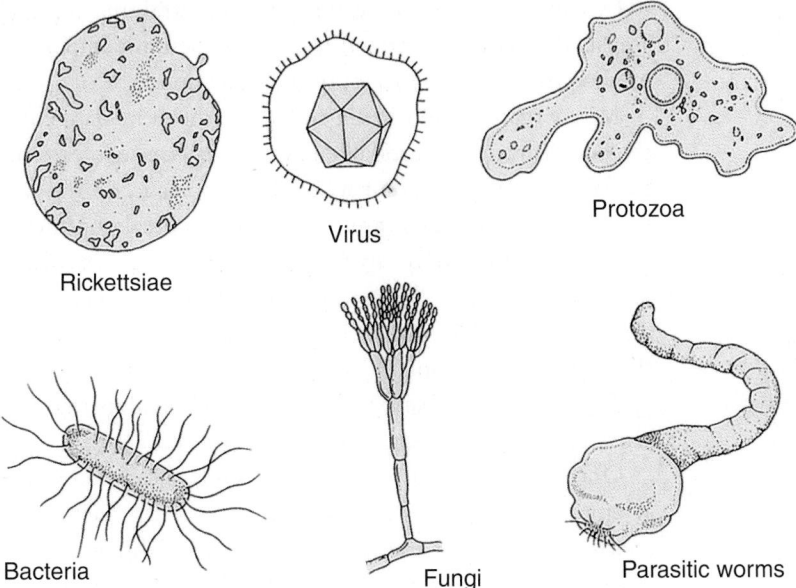

Rickettsiae

Virus

Protozoa

Bacteria

Fungi

Parasitic worms

FIGURE 34-1 **Examples of pathogens.**

bladder or bloodstream, through such poor habits as improper (or lack of) hand hygiene, it can cause urinary tract and blood infections. Those microorganisms that are capable of producing disease (pathogens) grow best at a body temperature of 98.6°F/37°C, destroy and use human tissue as food, and excrete waste toxins that are absorbed by and poison the body.

TRANSMISSION OF INFECTION

Scientists have determined that microorganisms are capable of multiplying very rapidly. If not controlled, germs may spread infection and diseases rapidly from one person to another.

The principles of asepsis are applied in the hospital setting to prevent the spread of **nosocomial infections**. These are infections acquired while in a medical facility. The pathogens were not in the body at the time the patient came into the facility but were introduced into the body due to poor aseptic technique in the facility. Regardless of the medical setting, a dedicated emphasis on halting the spread of infection must take place.

The presence of a pathogenic organism, or microorganism, is not enough to cause an infection to occur. Several factors must be in place for infection to occur. These are referred to as the chain of infection:

1. The pathogen present in the **reservoir host** is the beginning of the chain of infection. This host not only is infected with the pathogen but also is the source of transfer of that pathogen. The host (unknowingly) provides nourishment and sustenance for the microorganism, allowing it to grow.

2. For the pathogen to spread there must be a **portal of exit** from the reservoir host. The means of exit include the respiratory, gastrointestinal, urinary, and reproductive tracts of the body. An open wound is also an excellent portal of exit.

3. Next, there must be a means of transmission for the pathogen from one person to another. This may be through direct contact, either with the infected person or with the discharge or **excreta** (waste products) of the infected person. The transmission can also occur by indirect contact, such as air droplets from a cough or sneeze, or even by touching a contaminated object. Other methods of indirect contact are through contaminated food or insects.

4. A **portal of entry** into a new host is required. This is the means by which the pathogens enter the body. These portals include, for example, the respiratory,

TABLE 34-1 Conditions Required for Bacterial Growth

Condition	Explanation
Moisture	Bacteria grow best in moist areas: skin, mucous membranes, wet dressings, wounds, dirty instruments.
Temperature	Bacteria thrive at body temperature (98.6°F). Low temperatures (32°F and below) retard, but do not kill, bacterial growth. A temperature of 107°F and higher will kill most bacteria.
Oxygen	Aerobic bacteria require an oxygen supply to live. Anaerobic bacteria can survive without oxygen.
Light	Darkness favors the growth of most bacteria. Some bacteria will die if exposed to direct sunlight or light.

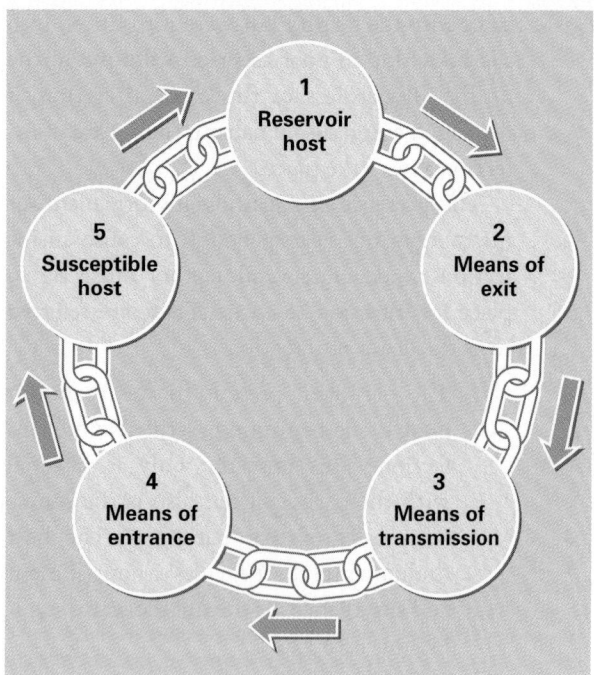

FIGURE 34-2 The chain of infection.

or by using standard precautions. In fact, attaining medical asepsis through proper hand hygiene is the most important method for decreasing the spread of infections.

Microorganisms normally found on the skin may enter the body through a portal of entry and may cause infections. Portals of entry may occur when the skin is cut, as in a surgical incision; when an injury causes a skin break; or during any invasive procedure, such as the insertion of a needle in venipuncture. The stages of the infection process are described in Table 34-2. These stages include invasion by the pathogen, multiplication (reproduction) of the pathogens, an incubation period, a prodromal period, an acute period, and finally, the recovery period.

Once the infection process has begun, it can be broken at any point, thus preventing the spread of the bacteria to another person. For example, effective hand hygiene after coughing may prevent the spread of microorganisms to another person or to an inanimate object that might become a means of transmission.

The Infection Control System

The body has several natural defense mechanisms to prevent the spread of infection. These include the following:

- Dietary intake of sufficient nutrients to promote health
- Age of the person—the young and aged are more susceptible to diseases due to immaturity of the immune system in the young and decrease in effectiveness of the immune system in the aged
- Adequate amount of rest

Mechanisms that promote the spread of infection include the following:

- Presence of other disease processes in the body—diseases such as diabetes and pneumonia may weaken the system.

urinary, and reproductive tracts, skin and mucous membranes, or blood.

5. A **susceptible host** must be available and capable of being infected by the pathogen. For a host to be susceptible, it must be unable to fight off the infection. Some situations that lead to susceptibility include poor health, poor hygiene, or poor nutrition. Stress may also be a factor.

When another reservoir host is found, the chain begins again. Figure 34-2 illustrates the chain of infection.

Fortunately, if the chain is broken, infection does not occur. For instance, the chain may be broken at the reservoir by using medical asepsis, good employee hygiene practices,

TABLE 34-2 Stages of the Infection Process

Stage	Description
Invasion	Pathogen enters the body through the portal of entry: respiratory, digestive, reproductive, urinary tracts, and skin.
Multiplication	Reproduction of pathogens.
Incubation period	May vary from several days to months or years during which time the disease is developing but no symptoms appear.
Prodromal period	First mild signs and symptoms appear; a highly contagious period.
Acute period	Signs and symptoms are evident and most severe.
Recovery period	Signs and symptoms begin to subside.

- Genetic inheritance of a disease, such as cystic fibrosis, may leave the body in a more susceptible state.

The spread of infection can be prevented in two ways: by preventing the spread of the causative microorganism and by destroying the microorganism itself.

PREVENTION

The human body has several natural barriers to infection. These include the skin, mucous membranes, the gastrointestinal tract, and the lymphatic and blood systems. The largest natural barrier to infection is the intact skin. The acid pH of the skin inhibits bacterial action. Mucous membranes lining the body's orifices and its respiratory, digestive, reproductive, and urinary tracts also assist in repelling microorganisms. The gastrointestinal tract, containing hydrochloric acid (HCl), causes a **bactericidal** action that destroys disease-producing bacteria.

The Lymphatic System and the Blood

The lymphatic system and the blood produce antibodies that protect the body from disease. The composition of the lymph varies in different parts of the body. Leukocytes (white blood cells) actively fight pathogenic microorganisms with the process of **phagocytosis**. The process of phagocytosis is shown in Figure 34-3. During the process of inflammation, phagocytes engulf, digest, and destroy pathogens. Lymphocytes produce antibodies during the antigen–antibody reaction.

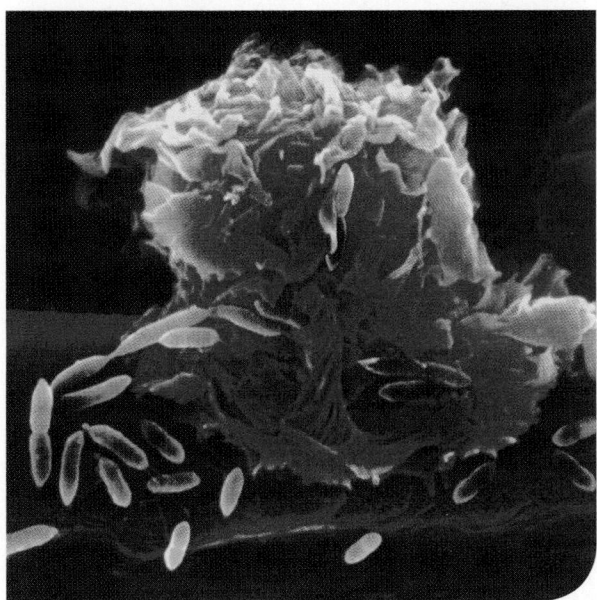

FIGURE 34-3 This illustration shows the process of phagocytosis: a phagocyte engulfing bacteria or other foreign material.

Antigen–Antibody Reaction

Lymphocytes produce antibodies during the antigen–antibody reaction. **Antibodies**—protein substances produced by lymphocytes in the spleen, lymph nodes and tissue, and the bone marrow—react in response to antigens (foreign substances). Antibodies have the ability to neutralize antigens or make them more susceptible to phagocytosis. The antigen–antibody reaction then occurs in response to an invasion of antigens.

Immunity

The body has a natural protective mechanism called immunity. **Immunity**, a resistance to disease, is said to have occurred when enough antibodies have been produced to provide protection for weeks, months, or years.

Immunity can be either genetic or acquired. Genetic immunity does not involve antibodies. Species immunity is passed on genetically and protects humans from certain animal diseases such as chicken cholera. It also protects animals from certain human diseases such as measles and influenza. Acquired immunity, on the other hand, does involve the development of antibodies. This type of immunity may be acquired through active or passive means. The two types of active immunity are natural (person is born with this immunity) and artificial (from an immunization or having had the disease, such as with measles). Active immunity provides long-term immunity because the body produces its own antibodies. Passive immunity develops when antibodies are artificially introduced into the body and provides only temporary immunity.

Active and passive immunity can be produced by both natural and acquired methods. Natural active immunity develops as a result of having recovered from a disease, such as measles, or being exposed to disease and becoming a carrier, such as in TB.

Artificial active immunity is the result of receiving vaccinations with inactivated (dead) or attenuated (weakened) organisms. Examples of inactivated vaccines include the influenza, whooping cough, typhoid, and polio (Salk) vaccines. Examples of attenuated vaccines are measles, polio (Sabin), smallpox, German measles (rubella), and mumps. Natural passive immunity is produced when a mother's antibodies cross the placental barrier and protect the fetus in the womb. Mothers also pass natural passive immunity to their children through breastfeeding. Artificial passive immunity is produced by injecting a commercially prepared product to produce antibodies; gamma globulin, used to prevent viral hepatitis, is an example. The various types of acquired immunity are described in Table 34-3.

TABLE 34-3 Acquired Immunity

Type of Immunity	Description
Active acquired natural	Acquired by having the disease, which results in production of antibodies and "memory cells" that respond when the antigen reappears again
Active acquired artificial	Acquired by administration of a vaccine that stimulates production of antibodies and "memory cells" to prevent that disease from occurring
Passive acquired natural	Acquired from someone else's antibodies, such as from the mother to the fetus through the placenta or through breast milk
Passive acquired artificial	Temporary protection acquired from gamma globulin (examples: tetanus immune globulin, rabies antiserum)

The Inflammatory Process

The body may react to the invasion of a foreign substance, such as bacteria or a virus, with an acute inflammatory process. This process results in the dilation of blood vessels due to an increased blood flow, production of watery fluids and materials (exudates), and invasion of monocytes and neutrophils into the injured tissues to produce phagocytosis. This action of phagocytosis is necessary for repair of tissues. The signs and symptoms of the inflammatory process may be local or systemic.

The four cardinal signs of inflammation are redness, heat, swelling, and pain. These signs are localized at the site of injury and may also be accompanied by hardening or stiffness at the site. Systemic symptoms may vary according to the part of the body that is affected. See Table 34-4 for a description of the inflammatory process.

Universal Precautions

Over time guidelines have been developed by several government agencies to protect patients and health care workers from exposure to pathogens. In 1970 the Centers for Disease Control and Prevention (CDC) published a manual of isolation techniques for hospitals. This was updated in 1975. In

1985 universal precautions were developed to help prevent the transmission of hepatitis B, human immunodeficiency virus (HIV), and other diseases resulting from bloodborne pathogens. In 1996 the CDC developed and published new guidelines for isolation precautions in hospitals, and these were called standard precautions. Standard precautions combine the major features of universal precautions and body substance isolation precautions into one set of recommendations. In 1985, and again in 1988, guidelines for hand hygiene and antisepsis were published by the Association for Professionals in Infection Control and Epidemiology (APIC). These were similar to the CDC guidelines. In 1996 the Healthcare Infection Control Practices Advisory Committee (HICPAC) recommended that antimicrobial soap or waterless **antiseptic** agents be used for hand hygiene when leaving rooms of patients infected with multidrug-resistant organisms (MDROs).

Universal precautions is a method used in infection control that treats all human blood and body fluids as if infected with high-risk diseases such as HIV or hepatitis B. Bloodborne pathogens such as *Staphylococcus* (staph), *Streptococcus* (strep), and malaria can also cause disease. Other potentially infectious materials (OPIM) that may also carry microorganisms include all body fluids and secretions except sweat. The

PROFESSIONALISM THE LIFE SPAN

Infants, especially those under 3 months of age, and the elderly are more prone to infection. Infants' immune systems are underdeveloped, and the immune systems in the elderly are slowing down. In addition, the elderly often do not eat nutritionally sound meals and this further weakens their resistance.

TABLE 34-4 Acute Inflammatory Process

Cardinal Sign	The Body's Response
Redness	Leukocytosis
Heat	Fever
Swelling/edema	Increased pulse rate
Pain	Increased respiration rate
Stiffness	—

Occupational Safety and Health Administration (OSHA) developed bloodborne pathogen standards that require the following:

- All employees must follow universal precautions to impede contact with infectious material.
- If body fluids cannot be differentiated, all are to be considered contagious.
- All blood and infectious material must be handled with precautions such as gloves, mask, gowns, and work place controls to limit exposure.

STANDARD PRECAUTIONS

OSHA allows hospitals to use alternatives to universal precautions such as body substance isolation (BSI) and standard precautions (all body fluids are infectious), if all other provisions of the standards are followed completely.

The CDC recommends using standard precautions when caring for all patients, whatever their diagnosis. The guidelines for standard precautions apply to all blood, body fluid secretions, and excretions except sweat, whether blood is visible or not. These guidelines include hand washing and use of **personal protective equipment (PPE)** such as gloves, gowns, and masks whenever touching or exposed to patients' body fluids.

Hand sanitizing is one of the best means of reducing the spread of microorganisms in a health care facility and at home. Hand hygiene recommendations include not wearing artificial fingernails or extenders when having direct contact with high-risk patients such as those in intensive care or operating rooms. Natural fingernails should be kept short: less than one-quarter inch long.

In 2007 the CDC issued several new elements of standard precautions. These guidelines involve three areas of practice:

1. Respiratory hygiene/cough etiquette—Respiratory hygiene/cough etiquette is aimed at patients, family members, friends, and any other persons entering a health care facility with signs of illness, cough, congestion, or rhinorrhea (runny nose). The guidelines suggest that signs be posted reminding people to cover their mouth or nose when coughing, to dispose of tissues appropriately, to perform hand hygiene after contact with respiratory secretions, to use a mask when appropriate, and whenever possible to provide at least 3 feet of space between persons with respiratory infections.

2. Safe injection practices—Safe injection practices include the use of aseptic technique and the use of single-use items (needles, syringes, and whenever possible single-dose vials for parenteral medication). No

multidose vials should be kept in the immediate treatment area.

3. Do not use bags or botilees of intravenous (IV) solutions among several patients.

4. Use masks for insertion of catheters or injection of material into spinal or epidural spaces during lumbar puncture procedures.

Standard precautions equipment and examples of situations in which they must be used are found in Box 34-1.

TRANSMISSION-BASED PRECAUTIONS

The second tier of CDC guidelines focuses on infected patients or those suspected of being infected. These guidelines require transmission–based precautions. Transmission-based precautions are used in addition to standard precautions to further interrupt the spread of pathogens in hospitals. Transmission-based precautions fall into three categories: airborne precautions, droplet precautions, and contact precautions.

- Airborne precautions are designed to reduce the transmission of certain diseases, such as TB, measles, or chicken pox. In addition to practicing standard precautions, use airborne precautions for patients who are known to be infected with microorganisms that are transmitted via airborne droplet nuclei (smaller than 5 microns), that can remain suspended in the air, and that can be widely dispersed throughout a room by air currents. Airborne precautions often involve patient isolation in a private room if hospitalized and require use of mask and gown by all health care personnel who come in contact with the patient. By using these precautions the risk of transmitting diseases such as TB and chicken pox is reduced. Hand washing and gloves are required as well. The transport of the patient should be as limited as possible, with the patient wearing a mask during transport. All reusable patient care equipment should be cleaned and disinfected before use on another patient. Disposable items should be used if available.

- Droplet precautions are used for patients suspected of being infected with organisms spread by droplets during sneezing, coughing, and talking. Some examples are diseases such as *Haemophilus influenzae* type b, meningitis, pneumonia, pertussis, and *streptococcal* pneumonia. A mask should be worn if the caregiver is within 3 feet of an infected patient. Gown and gloves are worn if there is a chance of coming into contact with blood or body fluids of suspected patents. Transport of the patient should be limited. All reusable equipment should be cleaned and disinfected.

Box 34-1 Summary of Standard PRECAUTIONS

1. Wear gloves when there is any potential for exposure to blood or body fluids, secretions, excretions, or contaminated items. This includes performing routine clinical work, touching mucous membranes and the nonintact skin of patients, and handling tissue and clinical specimens. (See Figure 34-4)
2. Wear gloves when drawing blood, including finger-stick and heel-stick on infants, and during preparation of blood smears.
3. Wear protective barrier equipment (e.g., face mask, eye shield, or goggles) when there is any risk of splashing, splattering, or aerosolization (becoming airborne in small particles) of potentially infectious body fluids.
4. Change gloves after each patient. Perform hand sanitation before putting on gloves and after removing them.
5. Change gloves if they become contaminated with blood or other body fluids, and discard them in a biohazards collection container.
6. Wash hands and other skin surfaces immediately or as soon as possible if they become contaminated with potentially infectious blood or body fluids.
7. Care for linens and equipment that are contaminated with blood, blood products, body fluids, excretions, and secretions in a manner that avoids contact with your skin and mucous membranes or cross-contamination to another person.
8. Wear a mask if the patient has an airborne disease. A special mask is recommended if a patient has an active case of TB.
9. Use care with needles, scalpels, and other sharp instruments to avoid unintentional injury.
10. Dispose of needles and other sharp items in a rigid, puncture-proof sharps container.
11. Do not recap or handle used needles.
12. Store reusable sharp instruments and needles in a puncture-proof container.
13. Avoid the direct mouth-to-mouth resuscitation technique in all but life-threatening situations. Use a mechanical device or mask barrier instead.
14. Use a solution of household bleach (1:10 dilution) to disinfect environmental surfaces and reusable equipment.
15. Use hazardous waste containers for contaminated materials.

STANDARD PRECAUTIONS
For all patient care

PROCEDURE	🚰	🧤	👤	😷	👓
Talking to patient					
Adjusting IV fluid rate or non-invasive equipment					
Examining patient *without* touching blood, body fluids, mucous membranes	X				
Examining patient *including* contact with blood, body fluids, mucous membranes	X	X			
Drawing blood	X	X			
Inserting venous access	X	X			
Suctioning	X	X			
Inserting body or face catheters	X	X			
Handling soiled waste, linen, other materials	X	X			
Intubation	X	X	X	X	X
Inserting arterial access	X	X	X	X	X
Endoscopy	X	X	X	X	X
Operative and other procedures which produce extensive splattering of blood or body fluids	X	X	X	X	X

FIGURE 34-4 Standard precautions.

Note: Adapted from *Guidelines for Isolation Precaution in Hospitals*, developed by the Centers for Disease Control and Prevention and the Hospital Infection Control Practices Advisory Committee, January 2002.

- Contact precautions are used when infections are difficult to treat and the likelihood of microorganism transmission among patients and health care providers is high. Conditions such as intestinal infections, hepatitis, open wounds, respiratory infections, herpes, scabies, and pediculosis are all treated using contact precautions. These precautions include isolating patients and wearing gowns and gloves. If there is a chance of coming in contact with body fluids, mask and eyewear should be worn. Health care providers should be aware that some diseases are transmitted by several routes, and all precautions should be taken.

Some patients may be latex sensitive. Before touching a patient while wearing latex gloves, ask the patient if he or she has a history of latex sensitivity. High-risk patients, such as those with congenital defects and indwelling catheters, must always be assessed for latex sensitivity. Patients with allergies to bananas, chestnuts, kiwi, and avocados may have cross sensitivity to latex. It is prudent to ask about those allergies as well. Symptoms to latex sensitivity include contact dermatitis, swelling, itching, and rhinitis and may include anaphylaxis in some cases. Latex-free gloves, syringes, IV tubing, and solution bags should be available to meet the needs of the patients and the health care providers.

Implementing OSHA Guidelines

The CDC precautions are enforced by OSHA. As previously mentioned, OSHA directives are aimed at minimizing exposure of health care workers to the hepatitis B virus (HBV) and HIV. The OSHA guidelines apply to facilities in which the employees could be "reasonably anticipated" to come into contact with potentially infectious materials. An exposure control program must be implemented in each facility and must include the following:

- **Exposure determination**—job classifications and probability of exposure
- **Method of compliance**—documentation of safety measures that would decrease the risk of exposure
- **Postexposure evaluation**—specification of procedures in the event of exposure

For protection of employees, engineering controls are the responsibility of the employer. These would include items such as availability of gloves (sterile and nonsterile of various sizes), safety needles, disposable cannula, sharps containers, sinks and running water, and biohazard containers. Work practice controls are the responsibility of the employee. See Procedure 34-1 and Figures 34-5A–D about proper disposal of infectious waste.

PHYSICAL AND CHEMICAL BARRIERS

Effective physical and chemical barriers are used to maintain infection control. The development of a nosocomial infection, or health care–associated infection (HAI), is prevented when careful medical and **surgical asepsis** (sterile equipment and procedures) are maintained. Surgical asepsis refers to the destruction of organisms before they enter the body.

Medical Asepsis

Medical asepsis refers to the destruction of organisms after they leave the body. Techniques such as hand hygiene, using disposable equipment, and wearing gloves can help reduce the transfer of pathogens. Aseptic techniques are the fundamental means of providing a safe environment in medical facilities.

Ordinary hygiene habits of everyday life are a form of medical asepsis. These include hand washing when handling food, or after using the bathroom, and covering one's mouth during a cough or sneeze. One of the most effective means of reducing pathogen transmission is through hand hygiene. This is considered the first step of infection control since the hands are a primary means of transferring infection from the host to the receiver. To keep the skin free of harmful organisms, frequent hand hygiene is necessary—either with soap, friction, and warm running water or with alcohol-based hand sanitizers. Jewelry should be removed prior to performing hand hygiene or applying gloves. Artificial nails, chipped fingernail polish, or polish left on more than 4 days may impede infection control practices.

Situations involving medical asepsis include but are not limited to taking oral, aural, and rectal temperatures; obtaining throat or vaginal cultures or smears; obtaining urine, stool, or sputum specimens; administering medications; and cleaning treatment rooms.

Aseptic techniques that can cause a break in the chain of infection include the following:

- Washing hands before and after any contact with patients or equipment
- Handling all specimens and materials as though they contain pathogens
- Using gloves for protection when handling contaminated articles or materials, such as specimens
- Not wearing jewelry that can attract and harbor bacteria
- Using disposable equipment whenever possible (Dispose of all equipment properly after use.)
- Cleaning all nondisposable equipment as soon as possible after patient use, using an approved disinfectant

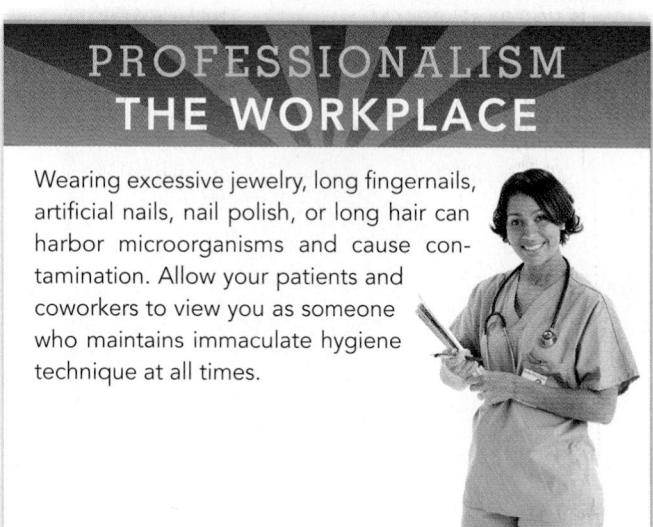

PROFESSIONALISM
THE WORKPLACE

Wearing excessive jewelry, long fingernails, artificial nails, nail polish, or long hair can harbor microorganisms and cause contamination. Allow your patients and coworkers to view you as someone who maintains immaculate hygiene technique at all times.

DISPOSAL OF INFECTIOUS WASTES AND SUBSTANCES

Objective: Student will perform the procedure without errors.

EQUIPMENT AND SUPPLIES

infectious waste container with lid marked appropriately with universal biohazard symbol and label; red disposable plastic liners

METHOD

1. Check to ensure that the infectious waste container is lined with a red disposal plastic bag (Figure 34-5A).
2. Discard any infectious waste into the infectious waste container.
3. Make sure that all liquid waste is already contained in a closable device before putting it into the infectious waste container.
4. Do not put contaminated glass into the infectious container. Instead, all glass should be placed into a puncture-proof or very highly puncture-resistant container for disposal; small glass items can be deposited into a sharps container for disposal.

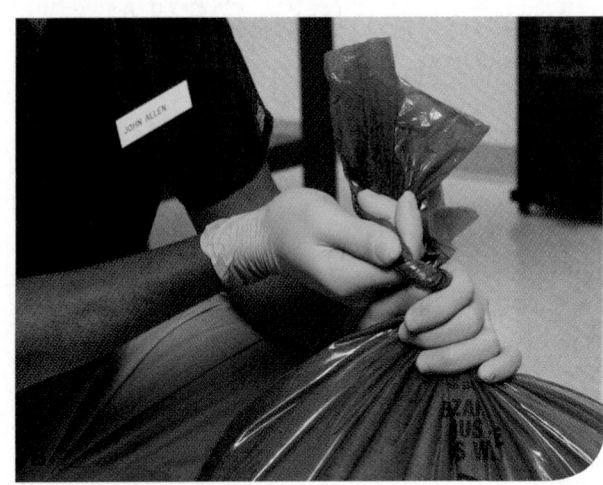

5. When the infectious waste container becomes full, close the red trash bag, either by tying with a securing knot, twist-tying, or otherwise securing it (Figures 34-5B, C).

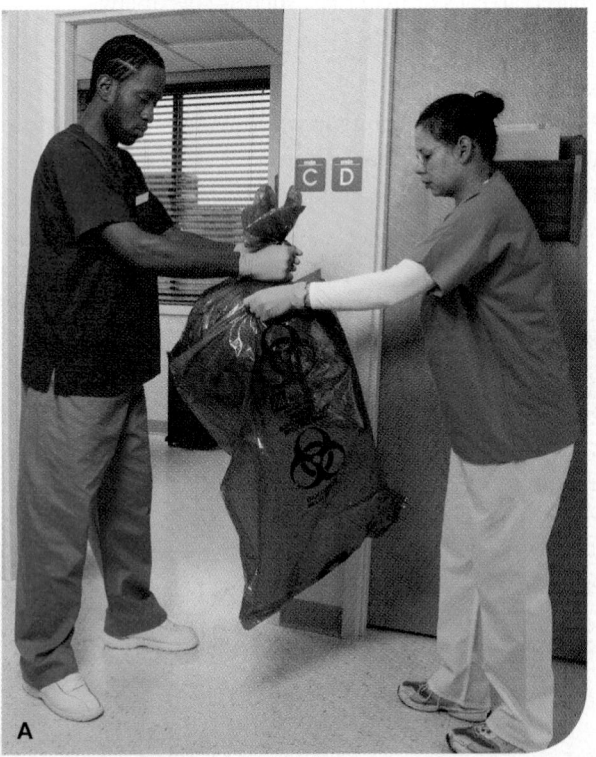

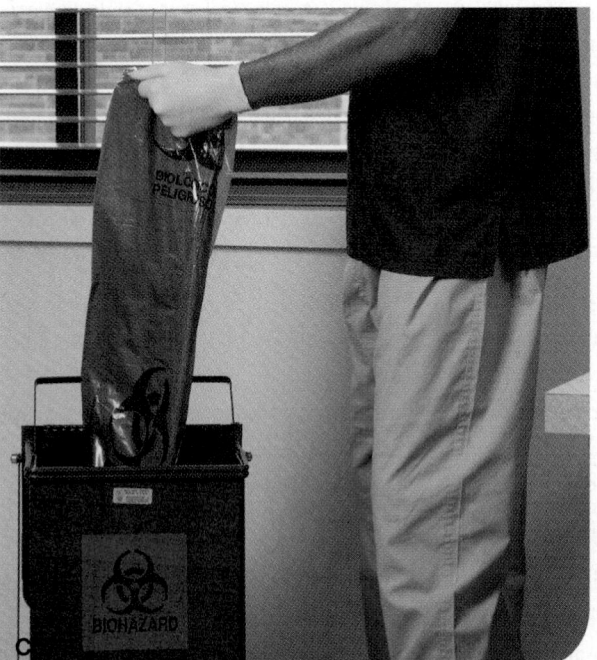

FIGURE 34-5   (A) Place the hazardous waste bag into another bag held open, outside the examining room or the patient's room; (B) close the hazardous waste bag securely; (C) place a new hazardous waste bag in the container after the full one is removed.

6. Make sure that the contents of the red bag are completely contained inside the closed bag.

7. Make sure the red bag is not overstuffed so that it cannot be closed, ruptured when handled or lifted, opened, or leak.

8. Do not mix noninfectious trash in the same large bin, container, or dumpster with infectious waste or trash.

9. Make sure that no sharps are put into the infectious bag without being contained in a separate designated sharps container.

10. Make sure no glass of any kind is placed into the infectious bag.

11. Closed red bags should be transported from the point of waste generation to a dirty utility room or area and stored in a designated holding area that cannot be accessed by other than authorized staff until they are transported away from the facility. Never store trash in hallways, entrances, corridors, or other areas accessible to and used by the public (Figure 34-5D).

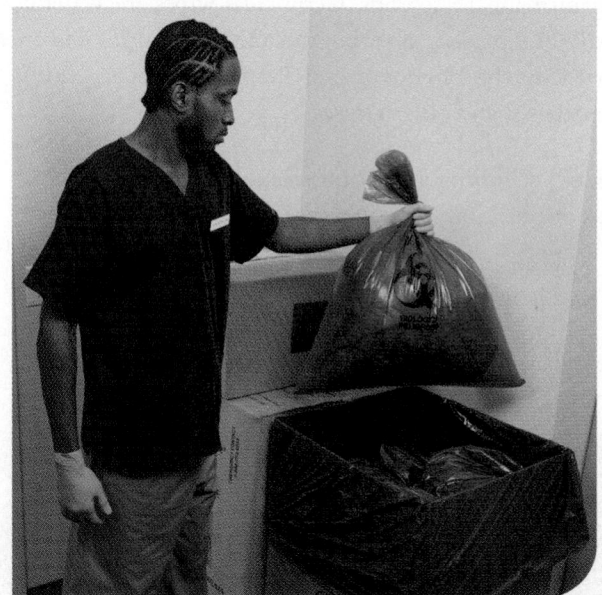

FIGURE 34-5 (D) Place properly secured red biohazard waste bag in the specified area for disposal.

- Using only clean or sterile supplies for each patient

- Using a protective covering over clothes if there is any danger of contaminated materials or supplies coming into contact with it

- Discarding items that fall on the floor if they cannot be cleaned (Any item dropped on the floor must be resterilized or redisinfected prior to use. All floors are considered contaminated. If in doubt, throw it out!)

- Placing all wet or damp dressings and bandages in a waterproof bag to protect the persons handling the waste removal

Medical asepsis also relates to other aspects of the facility, not just to the equipment and instruments. Having proper ventilation in all areas of the medical office will also assist in decreasing the transfer of microorganisms. All examination rooms should be cleaned with an approved disinfectant after each patient contact. Checking and emptying trash cans, replacing sharps containers in a timely manner, and observing for any insect infestation are also means of maintaining medical asepsis.

Some medical offices have one seating area for well patients and another for sick patients. For example, a patient who is returning for a follow-up visit is seated in one area, while a patient with symptoms of the flu is seated in another area. This helps to decrease the chance of cross-contamination.

Hand Hygiene. Frequent and diligent hand hygiene provides the first defense against the spread of disease and should be done often. Refer to Procedure 34-2 and Figures 34-6A–D for a demonstration of proper hand washing procedure and technique.

Alcohol-Based Hand Rubs. The CDC has presented some new guidelines concerning the use of alcohol-based (waterless) hand rubs. These rubs have the advantage of not requiring rinsing, and many contain emollients that prevent drying of the skin. A disadvantage, however, is that they may be more expensive than hand soaps and may cause stinging if there is an abrasion on the skin.

The guidelines suggest that the alcohol-based hand rubs can be used at the times usually required for hand washing. However, the hands should be washed with soap and water every third time hand hygiene is performed or if they are visibly soiled with dirt or body fluids, before eating, and after using the restroom. Manufacturers' instructions regarding the use of alcohol-based hand rubs should be followed exactly.

As with regular hand washing, jewelry should be removed prior to using the hand rubs. Approximately 2 to 3 mL of the gel should be placed in the palm of the hand and thoroughly spread over the surface of both hands up to one-half inch above the wrist (Figure 34-7). Continue to rub the hands together until dry, approximately 15 to 30 seconds.

Waterless hand sanitizers kill 99.9 percent of common microorganisms in 15 seconds. Germicidal wipes are available that kill 99.9 percent of pathogenic microorganisms and are approved by the Environmental Protection Agency (EPA) for hepatitis B and other viruses.

Protective Clothing and Equipment. Protective clothing, such as gowns, gloves, and masks, are worn for two reasons:

1. To protect the patient from any microorganisms that might be present on the health care worker's street clothing

2. To protect the health care worker from carrying microorganisms away from the patient

In addition, protective devices, such as gloves and masks, assist in protecting the health care worker from contamination with **bloodborne pathogens**, which are microorganisms capable of causing disease in blood. Nonsterile gloving technique is used for procedures such as drawing blood, specimen collection, infant handling, and when in contact with a patient who is in isolation. Wearing each piece of PPE will not be needed for every procedure. PPE should be chosen in consideration of the possibility of contamination.

procedure 34-2

PERFORMING HAND WASHING
Objective: Perform hand washing procedure without error.

EQUIPMENT AND SUPPLIES
soap in liquid soap dispenser; nail cleaner (brush or orange cuticle stick); warm running water; paper towels; waste container

METHOD
1. Remove any jewelry (includes rings with the exception of a wedding band). Artificial nails must be removed to maintain infection control practices.
2. Stand at the sink without allowing clothing to touch the sink. Turn the water on with the foot or knee pedal or faucet (Figures 34-6A, B). Adjust the running water to a moderately warm temperature.

3. Wet hands under running water and place liquid soap (1 teaspoon, or about the size of a nickel) into the palm of hand. Work soap into a lather by moving it over the palms, sides, and backs—the entire surface—of both hands for 15 to 30 seconds. Use a circular motion and friction. Interlace the fingers and move soapy water between them (Figure 34-6C).
4. Keep the hands pointed down with hands and forearms below elbow level during the entire hand washing procedure.
5. Use nail cleaner to clean under fingernails at the start of each day and if hands are heavily soiled.

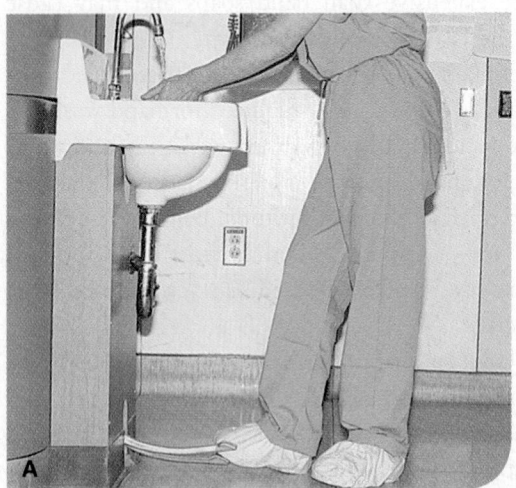
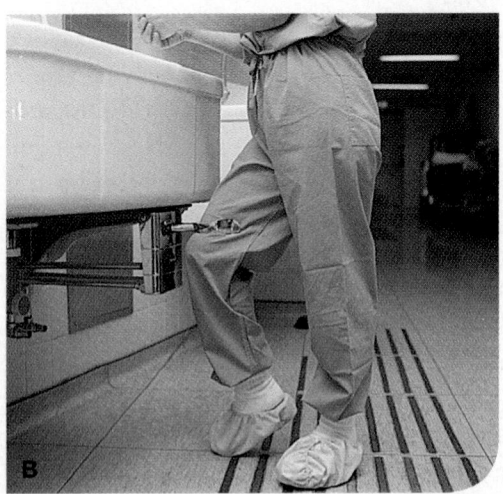

FIGURE 34-6 (A) To perform hand hygiene, use foot pedal to turn on water whenever possible; (B) using a knee pedal to turn on water.

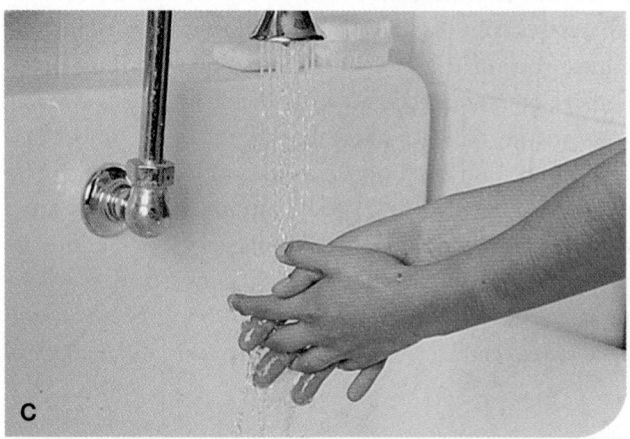

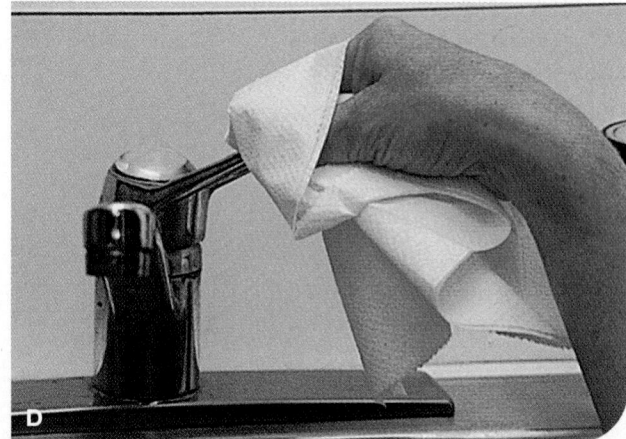

FIGURE 34-6 (C) Keep fingers pointed downward during hand washing to prevent contaminating the arms; (D) if foot or knee pedal is not available, turn off water using a paper towel.

6. Rinse hands under running water with fingers pointed down, using care not to touch the sink or faucets.
7. If hands are heavily soiled, reapply soap and wash them again.
8. Rinse hands under running water.

9. Dry hands thoroughly with a paper towel. Discard the paper towel.
10. Use a dry paper towel to turn the faucet off if the foot or knee pedal is not available (Figure 34-6D).

When wearing a mask, it should fit snugly over the nose, mouth, and chin.

If wearing more than one piece of PPE, maintain medical asepsis when removing it. Untie the gown and remove the gloves. After removing the gloves, then remove the gown, and lastly, remove the mask. Wash your hands after completion of any procedure, including removal of PPE.

The proper step-by-step technique for applying and removing gloves is explained in Procedure 34-3, and performing transmission-based precautions is explained in Procedure 34-4.

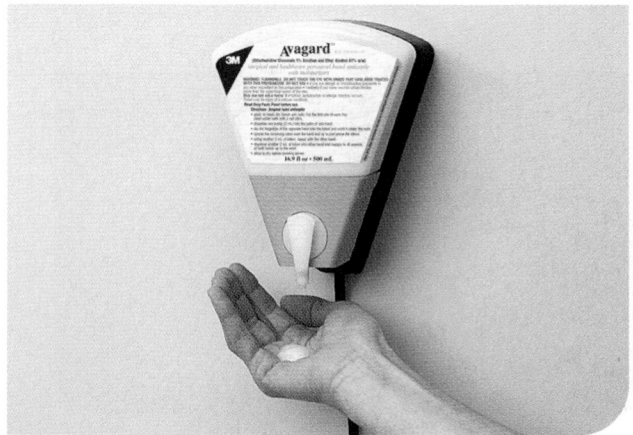

FIGURE 34-7 Dispense 2 mL of hand scrub into palm of hand.

In Figure 34-10 the medical assistant is wearing a mask and other PPE to prevent exposure to body fluids or the patient's coughing.

Surgical Asepsis

Surgical asepsis refers to the techniques practiced to maintain a sterile environment. It involves the destruction of organisms before they enter the body. Three important methods are used to reach sterility (the absence of microorganisms). These methods for preventing the spread of disease in the medical facility are sanitization, disinfection, and sterilization. Sanitization inhibits or inactivates pathogens by scrubbing and washing items. Disinfection destroys most or all pathogens on inanimate objects with the use of chemicals such as iodine, chlorine, alcohol, and phenol. Sterilization is the destruction of all living organisms and spores with the use of pressurized steam, extreme temperatures, or radiation.

Sanitization. **Sanitization** is a cleaning process that inhibits or inactivates pathogens by means of careful scrubbing of equipment and instruments using a brush and detergent with a neutral pH, such as a soapless soap, and then rinsing in hot water and air drying. Although sanitization cleans items, microorganisms and bacteria are not destroyed. This process can be used for supplies and equipment that do not come into direct contact with the patient or that touch only the skin surface. If a contaminated material cannot be sanitized immediately, then it should be soaked in detergent and water according to the manufacturer's instructions.

Another means of sanitizing equipment is with the use of ultrasound. In this case the instruments and equipment are placed into a bath tank in which sound waves vibrate to break up the contamination. The articles are then rinsed thoroughly. Always follow the instructions of the facility procedure manual regarding the proper procedure for sanitizing instruments. See Procedure 34-5 for one method of sanitizing instruments.

Disinfection. **Disinfection** involves a soaking and wiping process. Disinfection destroys or inhibits the activity of disease-causing organisms. Disinfecting agents include chemical germicides, flowing steam, and boiling water. Chemical germicides are used to disinfect heat-perishable objects in the medical office, including some rubber and plastic items, and to clean floors and office furniture. Two common disinfectants are benzalkonium chloride (Zephiran Chloride) and chlorophenol. Disinfectants can eliminate many organisms but are not effective against spores (the dormant stage of some bacteria), spore-forming bacteria, and some viruses. Some disinfectants, however, although effective

procedure
34-3

APPLYING AND REMOVING NONSTERILE GLOVES

Objective: Apply nonsterile gloves and remove them appropriately to prevent the spread of pathogens.

EQUIPMENT AND SUPPLIES

gloves; biohazard waste container

METHOD

1. Perform hand hygiene (see Procedure 34-2).
2. Choose the appropriate size gloves for your hands (Figure 34-8A). Hold a glove at the wrist opening and insert fingers, pulling the glove up to wrist.
3. Apply the second glove in the same manner, checking for holes and other flaws (Figure 34-8B). If any flaws are found, discard the gloves and obtain new gloves.
4. To remove gloves, grasp the glove covering your non-dominant hand at the palm and pull it away (Figure 34-8C).

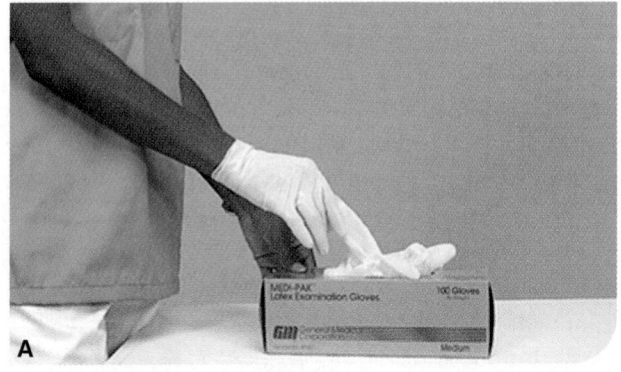

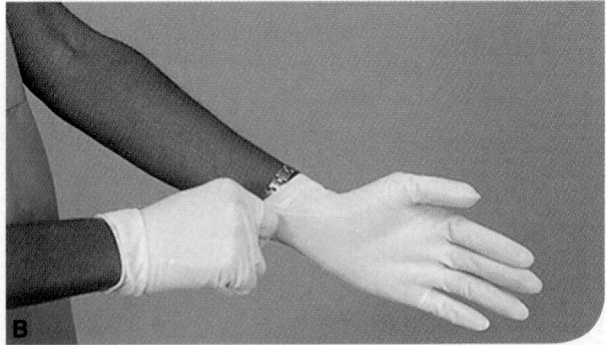

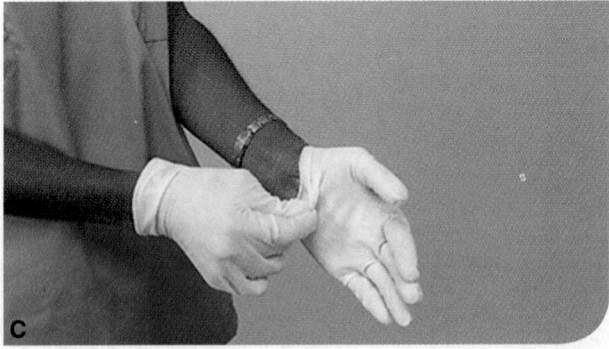

FIGURE 34-8 (A) Use a clean pair of gloves for each patient contact; (B) grasp glove just below the cuff; (C) pull glove over hand while turning glove inside out.

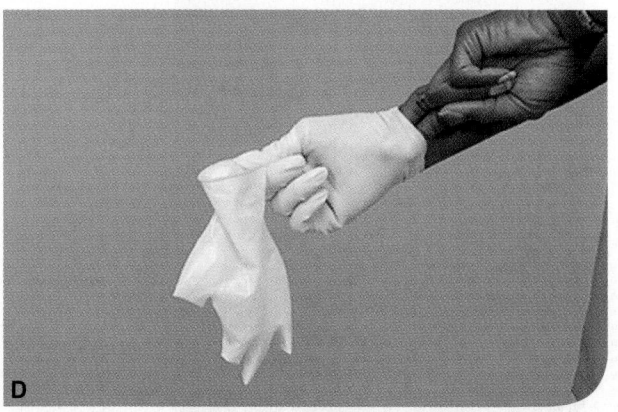

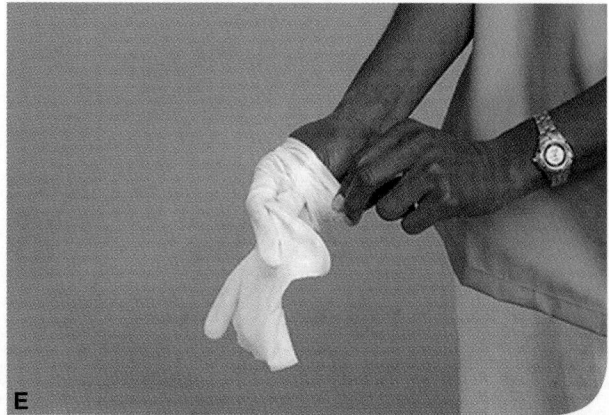

FIGURE 34-8 (D) Place the ungloved index and middle fingers inside the cuff of the glove, turning the cuff downward; (E) pull down the cuff and turn the glove inside out as you remove your hand.

5. Pull the glove off and hold it in the palm of the gloved dominant hand (Figure 34-8D).
6. While holding the soiled glove in your gloved hand, slide the index finger of the ungloved hand below the cuff of the remaining glove and peel it down, inverting it over

the first glove (Figure 34-8E). Both gloves will be in a ball and inside out.
7. Dispose of the gloves in a biohazard container.
8. Perform hand hygiene.

procedure
34-4

PERFORMING TRANSMISSION-BASED PRECAUTION: ISOLATION TECHNIQUES

Objective: Provide barrier protection for caregivers to prevent the spread of infectious diseases.

EQUIPMENT AND SUPPLIES

disposable gowns, masks, caps, nonsterile gloves, sterile gloves; sink and running water; paper towels

METHOD

1. Review orders and agency protocols regarding isolation procedures.

Note: Office-based health care personnel may not use transmission-based precautions often, but they should be familiar with the necessary PPE and how to put them on appropriately. Figure 34-9A shows examples of four types of personal protective equipment.

2. Assemble the necessary equipment that is appropriate for the type of protection required.
3. Remove lab coat and jewelry.

4. Perform hand hygiene (see Procedure 34-2).
5. Apply the appropriate disposable apparel.
6. Apply the cap to cover hair and ears completely.
7. Apply the gown over outergarments as follows: Hold the gown in front of the body and place arms through the sleeves. Pull the sleeves on, covering the wrists. Tie the gown securely at the neck and waist.
8. Apply the mask by placing the top of mask over the bridge of the nose and pinching the metal strip to secure a snug fit on the nose, tying it if needed. Apply protective eyewear.
9. Apply nonsterile gloves and pull up over the cuffs of the gown to cover the wrists completely.
10. Perform patient tasks as needed, then exit the isolation area.

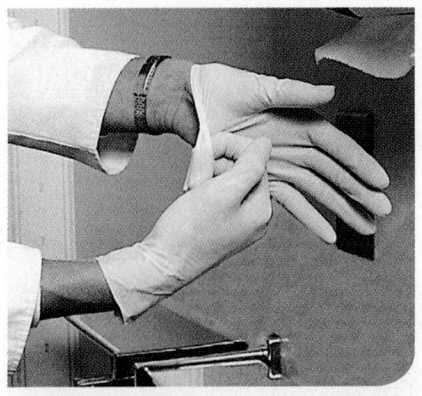
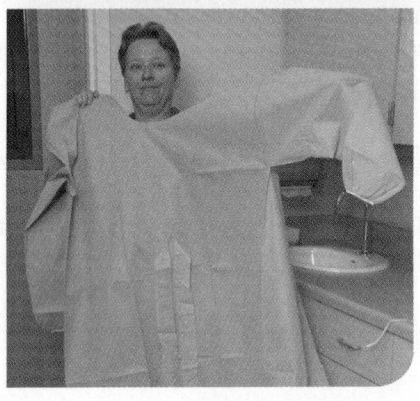
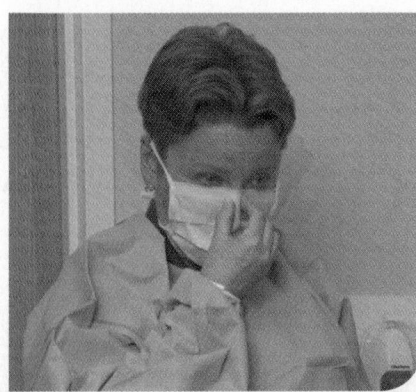
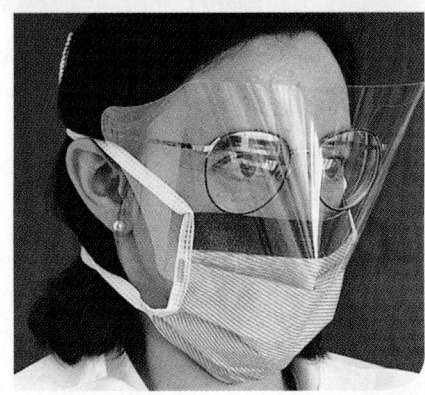

A

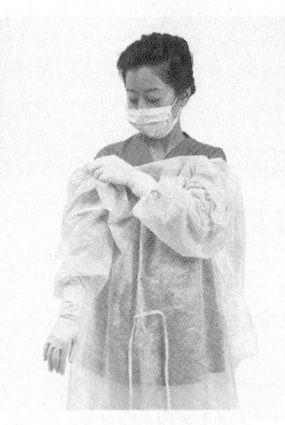

B

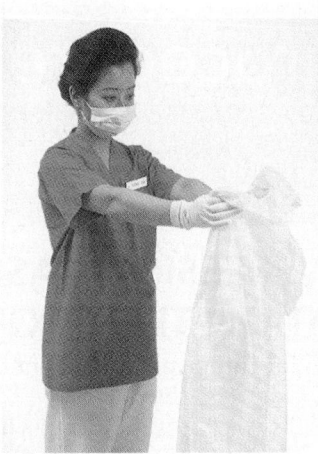

C

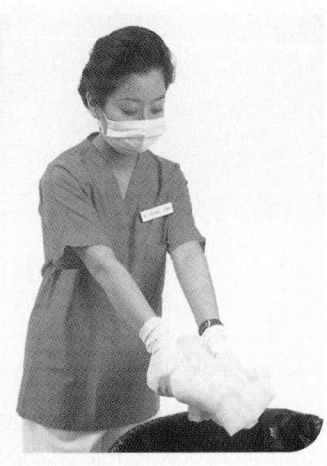

D

FIGURE 34-9 (A) Examples of personal protective equipment: gloves, mask, face shield, and glasses; (B) to remove the gown, pull from the shoulders, then down over the arms; (C) after pulling the gown off, hold it away from the body and roll it inside out; (D) roll the gown inside out and discard.

11. Remove barrier protections in the following order:
    - Untie waist of the gown.
    - Remove gloves (see Procedure 34-3).
    - Wash hands (see Procedure 34-2).
    - Untie the neck of the gown. Remove the gown by pulling it down from the shoulders. Turn the gown inside out and remove arms from the sleeves (Figure 34-9B). The inside of the gown is not contaminated.

    - Holding the gown away from the body with contaminated area on the inside, fold and place it in a biohazard container (Figures 34-9C and D).
12. Remove protective eyewear.
13. Remove mask and discard.
14. Perform hand hygiene.

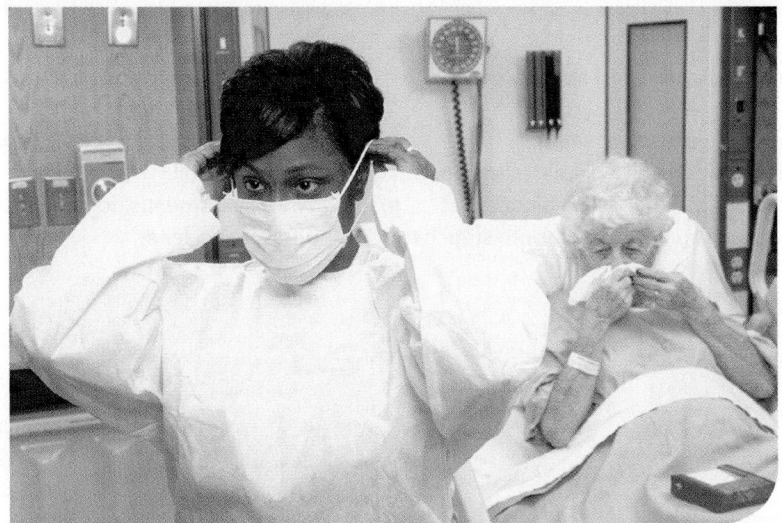

FIGURE 34-10 The mask covers both the mouth and nose to prevent exposure to body fluids and blood or to the patient's excessive coughing.

on objects, may be too strong to use on patients (e.g., formaldehyde). Antiseptics such as alcohol and povidine–iodine are used when preparing a patient's skin for surgical procedures or injections because they prevent the growth of some microorganisms.

Contaminated instruments and equipment are completely immersed in a germicidal solution according to the manufacturer's instructions for a period of 1 to 10 hours. They are then rinsed in water. (Instruments are rinsed in distilled water to prevent rust and corrosion.) Instruments must be dried after disinfection and rinsing. Objects that come into contact with mucous membranes, such as vaginal speculums, laryngoscopes, or thermometers, should be disinfected (or even sterilized, if possible). Instruments that cannot be soaked, such as scopes, computers, and electrical instruments, should be wiped thoroughly with a germicidal solution. Germicidal solutions must be changed frequently according to the manufacturer's instructions. The chemical disinfection process is referred to as a "cold" process since no heat is used or generated. Chemical

procedure
34-5

SANITIZING INSTRUMENTS

Objective: Learn to clean and sanitize instruments with no visible contamination remaining.

EQUIPMENT AND SUPPLIES

disposable gloves; rubber (utility) gloves; plastic brush; towel; sink; running water; container to hold all the instruments; low-sudsing (low-pH) detergent or germicidal agent

Note: Instruments should be rinsed under warm running water immediately after surgery to remove gross blood, body fluids, and tissue. If it is not possible to clean them immediately, instruments should be submerged in water containing a low-pH detergent.

METHOD

1. Apply both disposable and rubber gloves.
2. Place a low-sudsing (low-pH) detergent or germicidal agent in a large container with water. Rinse all instruments (Figure 34-11A).
3. Rinse instruments in clear water in either a sink or other container. Delicate and sharp instruments should be separated from general instruments.
4. Scrub each instrument individually with a brush and detergent under running water. Open instruments to

thoroughly scrub all serrated edges and hinge areas (Figure 34-11B).

5. Rinse instruments thoroughly under hot water.
6. If instruments cannot be cleaned immediately after use, then soak them in a solution of water and a blood solvent. When ready to wash instruments begin with step 1.

7. After thoroughly rinsing cleaned instruments, roll them in a towel to dry them.
8. Check the condition of all instruments for defects or remaining soil.
9. Wrap instrument(s) for sterilization or place them in an ultrasonic cleaner.

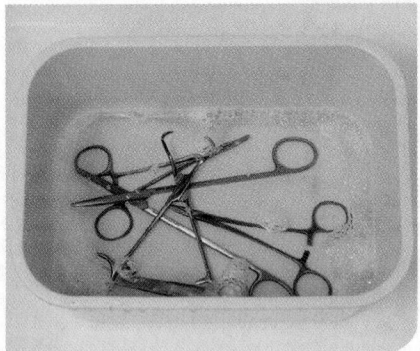

A

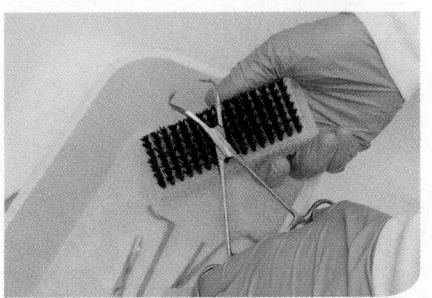

B

FIGURE 34-11   (A) Dirty instruments are placed in a basin immediately after use; (B) scrub instruments individually and check for defects.

disinfectants used for soaking and wiping include soap, alcohol, phenol, acid, alkalines (such as bleach), and formaldehyde (Table 34-5).

Ultraviolet rays are a means of disinfection used in operating rooms. Equipment that cannot be soaked is placed under ultraviolet lamps for a specified period of time. This kills microorganisms.

Although not effective for viruses (such as hepatitis) or for destroying spores, boiling water can be used as a means of disinfection. Moist heat of up to 212°F will kill most pathogens. However, sterilization cannot occur at this temperature. Stainless steel, glassware, and instruments can be boiled without damage. The articles are submerged in a container filled with cold water. (Distilled water should be used

TABLE 34-5 Disinfection Methods

Method	Description and Use
Alcohol (70% isopropyl)	Used for skin surfaces, equipment such as stethoscopes and thermometers, and table surfaces Causes damage to rubber products, lenses, and plastic Flammable
Chlorine (sodium hypochlorite or bleach)	Use in dilution of 1:10 (1 part bleach to 10 parts water) Used to eliminate a broad spectrum of microorganisms Has a corrosive effect on instruments, rubber, and plastic products Can cause skin irritation Inexpensive
Formaldehyde	Used to disinfect and sterilize Dangerous product that is regulated by OSHA—must have clearly marked labels
Hydrogen peroxide	Effective disinfectant for use only on nonhuman surfaces and products May damage rubber, plastics, and metals
Glutaraldehyde	Effective against viruses, bacteria, fungi, and some spores Regulated by OSHA—must have clearly marked labels and be used only in well-ventilated area Must wear gloves and masks when using

when boiling instruments or stainless steel to prevent sediment or deposits from forming.) The water must completely cover the articles to be disinfected. The water is then brought to the boiling point and continues to boil for 20 to 30 minutes for disinfection. When the boiling time has elapsed, the disinfected materials are allowed to cool. To maintain disinfection, they must be touched only with sterile forceps.

Sterilization. **Sterilization** kills all microorganisms, both pathogenic and nonpathogenic. The use of heat (steam or dry), chemicals, high-velocity electron bombardment, or ultraviolet-light radiation are used for this process. Heat sterilization (produced by an autoclave under steam pressure) can kill spores, bacteria, and other microorganisms. Dry heat is used for sterilizing dense ointments, such as petroleum jelly.

All supplies—including dressings, needles, and instruments that come into contact with internal body tissue or an open wound—must be sterile. Once a sterile article is touched by hands or another unsterile object, it is considered contaminated. Sterile gloves must be used when touching sterilized items. The procedure for applying gloves (whether sterile or nonsterile) is sometimes referred to as donning.

Autoclave. The methods used for sterilization include the autoclave (steam and pressure) and chemical (cold) sterilization. The autoclave process is an effective means of sterilization in the medical office. Types of autoclaving include steam under pressure, dry heat (320°F for 1 hour), dry gas, or radiation.

Autoclaving destroys organisms by the condensation of steam on each of the items, causing them to explode, not by the heat produced. This method of sterilization requires 15 pounds of pressure per square inch (PSI) and a temperature of 250°F to 270°F, depending on the manufacturer's recommendations. Heat is actually transferred to the items by way of the steam condensation. Steam sterilization of surgical packs is not effective if air pockets are present within them. Distilled water must be used in the steam autoclave.

The autoclave consists of an outer chamber (jacket) that creates a buildup of steam that is forced into an inner chamber. Items that are to be sterilized are placed inside the inner chamber. (Figure 34-12 is an example of an autoclave.)

Depending on the model, an autoclave may have three gauges (some have only one): (1) a jacket pressure gauge to indicate pressure in the outer chamber, (2) a chamber pressure gauge to indicate the steam pressure in the inner chamber, and (3) a temperature gauge to indicate the temperature in the inner chamber in which items are placed.

A pump within the autoclave will first remove air from the chamber. The pressure level and temperature levels within the

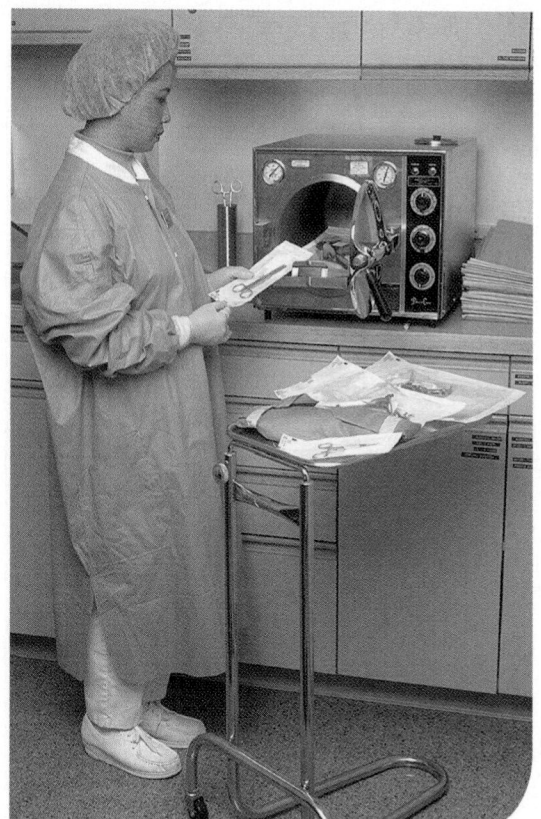

FIGURE 34-12 An autoclave.

autoclave chamber can be built up only after the air is removed. Therefore, the gauges indicating pressure and temperature must be monitored by the medical assistant. Table 34-6 describes autoclave sterilization time requirements. Always read and follow the manufacturer's instructions for use and maintenance prior to using any piece of electrical equipment.

The autoclave should be thoroughly cleaned (sanitized) and free of any materials or lint before using. If detergent or other cleaner is used for cleaning, the autoclave should be completely rinsed before placing objects into it. The air exhaust valve must be cleaned and free of lint after each use.

The wrappings in which the instruments and materials are sterilized must be **permeable** (allowing steam to pass through) and strong enough to hold together during the steam process. Wrapping materials include heavy paper, muslin, plastic, and stainless steel containers. The wrapping generally consists of two layers of permeable materials. All items must be completely covered with the wrapping material and fastened with autoclave tape, which looks similar to masking tape. Autoclave indicator tape is used to fasten the autoclave package securely. The lines on the tape change color during the autoclaving process and indicate that exposure to the high temperature has occurred, but that is not necessarily an indication that the proper time and temperature for sterilization have been reached (Figure 34-13).

TABLE 34-6 Sterilization Time Requirements

Time	Article
15 minutes	Glassware Metal instruments—open tray or individual wrapping with hinges open Syringes (unassembled) Needles
20 minutes	Instruments—partial metal in double-thickness wrapper or covered tray Rubber products: gloves, tubing, catheters wrapped or unwrapped Solutions in a flask (50–100 mL)
30 minutes	Dressings—small packs in paper or muslin Solutions in a flask (500–1,000 mL) Syringes—unassembled, individually wrapped in gauze Syringes—unassembled, individually wrapped in glass tubes Needles—individually packaged in paper or glass tubes Sutures—wrapped in paper or muslin Instrument and treatment trays—wrapped in paper or muslin Gauze—loosely packed
60 minutes	Petroleum jelly—in dry heat

Sterilization pouches or bags are often used to hold individual instruments. Careful inspection must be made to make sure the bag has not ruptured or been punctured during the autoclave process. Small, lightweight instruments are suitable for pouches. The pouches have sterilization indicators both inside and outside the bag.

Each package should be labeled with the date of sterilization, the items within the packet, and the initials of the individual who prepared the pack. Instruments with hinges should be in the open position, the tubing should be free of any kinks, and syringes should be unassembled before wrapping. (Refer to Procedure 34-6 and Figure 34-14A–D for how to wrap and label instruments for the autoclave.)

Instruments that will be used immediately can be placed in perforated trays and autoclaved unwrapped. The lid for the tray is placed next to the open tray of instruments. The lid is immediately placed over the instruments after sterilization. A towel is usually placed under the instruments to absorb moisture during autoclaving.

Items should be wrapped in individual packs that can be handled by their outer wrapping for storage and use without contaminating the inner items. When the autoclaved package is opened, the contents must be removed without contaminating them.

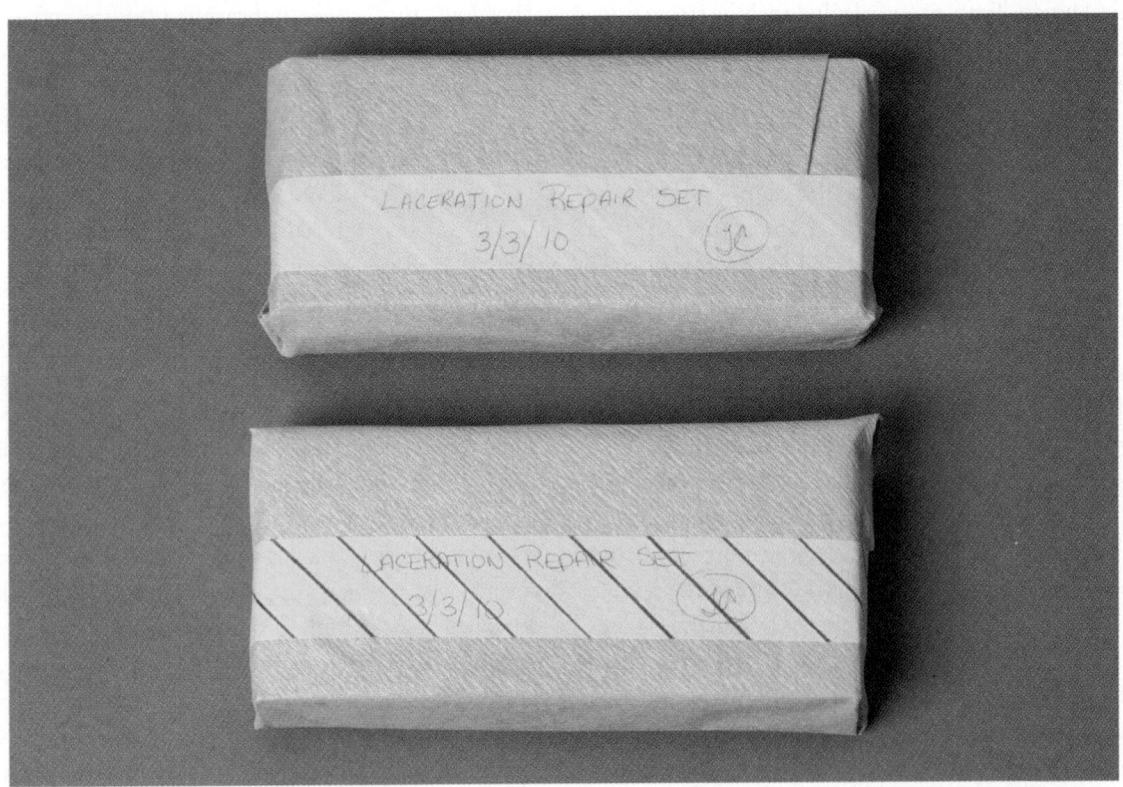

FIGURE 34-13 **(A) Autoclave tape before sterilization; (B) autoclave tape after sterilization.**

WRAPPING AND LABELING INSTRUMENTS FOR AUTOCLAVING

Objective: Wrap and label instruments properly.

EQUIPMENT AND SUPPLIES

wrapping material; instrument(s) for autoclaving; sterilization indicator strips; autoclave tape; indelible pen; label

METHOD

1. Wash your hands.
2. Place a square of wrapping material on the table so that it appears as a "diamond" shape when you look at it. Be sure the wrapping material is large enough to cover the entire article being wrapped.
3. Place the item in the center of the wrapping material. If hinged items are included, be sure the instrument is in the open position. If sharp instruments are being autoclaved, place the tip in a piece of gauze to prevent puncture through the material.
4. Place the indicator strip in the center of the packet.
5. Fold the bottom point of the wrapping material up and over the instruments. Fold a small portion of the point back over so that it can be used to pick up the paper when it is unwrapped (Figure 34-14A).
6. Fold the right side of the wrapping paper over until it covers the instrument(s). Fold a small portion of the point back over as in the previous step.
7. Fold the left side of the wrapping paper over until it covers the instrument(s). Fold a small portion of the point back over as in the previous step (Figure 34-14B).
8. Now fold up the bottom of the package. Continue folding until you have reached the top point (Figure 34-14C).
9. Be sure the pack is folded snugly.
10. Secure the package with a piece of autoclave tape (Figure 34-14D).
11. Label the package with the name of the item(s) inside, your initials, and the date.
12. If bags are used for the autoclaving procedure, place the item and an indicator strip inside the bag. (If the item has a sharp point, wrap the point in a piece of gauze.)
13. Seal the bag. Label the bag with the name of the item(s) inside, your initials, and the date.

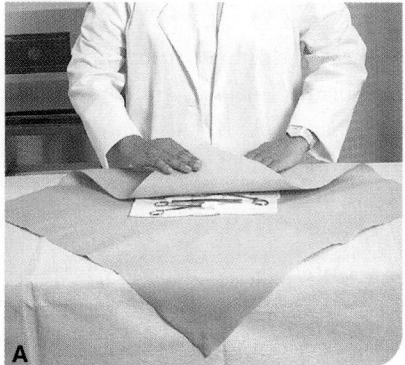

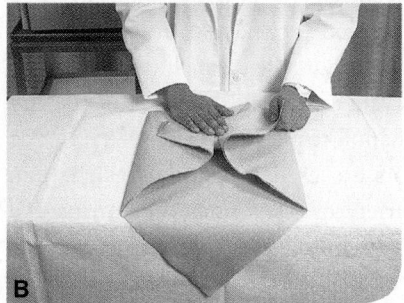

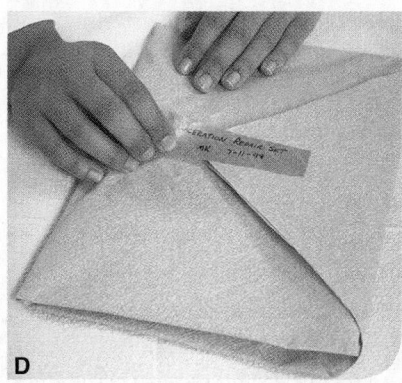

FIGURE 34-14 (A) Place item in center of wrapping material with the hinges open, and fold the bottom up over instrument; (B) fold the right side of the paper until it covers the item and make a small flap; next, proceed in the same way with the left side; (C) fold up the bottom of the package; (D) use a piece of autoclave tape to secure the package.

Containers and jars of supplies should be placed on their sides for full sterilization to occur. Solutions should be autoclaved separately since they may boil over during autoclaving. The lids of plastic containers and bags will become sealed during sterilization.

The autoclave chamber must not be overloaded or the steam will not be able to penetrate the wrapping and sterilize the instruments and materials. Items should be placed on their edges to permit the proper penetration with moisture and heat.

The time or pressure required for autoclaving, according to the manufacturer's recommendations, must never be shortened. If proper timing and pressure are not observed when autoclaving, the items will not be sterilized.

At intervals, an independent company should check the operation of the autoclave. Your medical office can continue to autoclave items as usual, but one item is chosen to be sent to an outside lab where it is checked for sterility. These checks are necessary to determine that the autoclave is working properly. For example, if the steam levels or temperatures being used are inadequate, autoclaved items might not be completely sterilized.

After the autoclave process is complete, the drying process takes place. This process is almost as important as achieving the correct temperature and pressure during autoclaving. Wetness on items ("wet packs") can cause a break in sterility since moisture will allow bacteria to grow and be transmitted into the inside of the package. Wet packs can be avoided by allowing for a drying period at the end of autoclaving. To do this, open the door of the autoclave $\frac{3}{4}$ inch (but no more) just before the drying cycle on the autoclave. Run the dry cycle according to the manufacturer's directions.

Sterilization indicators are used to signify sterilization. Indicators come in a variety of types, including strips and tape. The strip is placed inside the wrapper or in the chamber. The color changes or dots that appear on an indicator denote that the inner contents have been exposed to the conditions for sterility: correct temperature, correct time, and exposure to moisture. Figure 34-15 displays examples of sterility check strips.

Autoclaved packages are stored according to the date and type of item(s) visible. The oldest dated packs are placed in front of the stack so that they can be used first. Instruments are considered sterile for 21 to 30 days (21 days in plastic bags, 30 days in muslin), with a shelf life of approximately 1 month. Shelf life is dependent on the type of wrapper used. The individual manufacturer's guidelines should be followed concerning when to resanitize and resterilize the item. Autoclaved items cannot be reautoclaved in the same packages without washing, rinsing, drying, and rewrapping

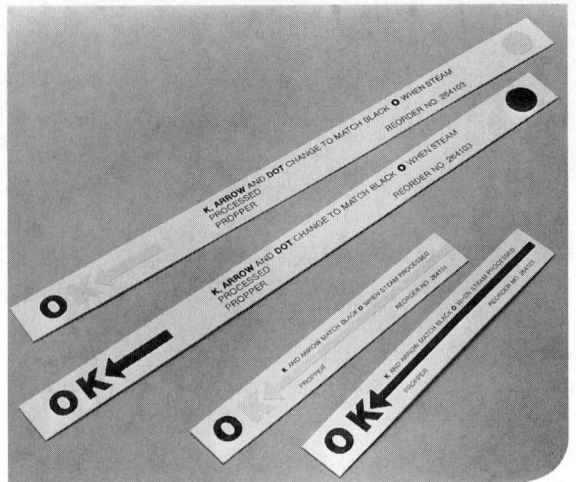

FIGURE 34-15   **Sterility check strips.**

each item. See Procedure 34-7 for the steps when using an office-size autoclave and Procedure 34-8 for chemically sterilizing instruments.

Hepatitis

Several diseases require special attention during a discussion of infection control. They are hepatitis, HIV, AIDS, and methicillin-resistant *Staphylococcus aureus* (MRSA) because these diseases affect several million people each year. Each is discussed in the following sections.

Hepatitis is a viral disease of the liver resulting in inflammation and infection. Forms of hepatitis include A, B, C, D, E, and G. Of these, hepatitis A, B, and C are considered the major forms of hepatitis in the United States.

HEPATITIS A VIRUS

Hepatitis A virus (HAV), or acute infective hepatitis, is transmitted by the fecal–oral route and sexual contact. Fecal contamination of food or the water supply is the most common source of infection. This occurs when food or water become contaminated with the fecal waste products of animals or humans. Poor hand hygiene and sanitation are the main causes of contamination. The **incubation** period, or period of time between exposure to a pathogen and the appearance of the first symptoms, is from 14 to 50 days with a very slow onset of symptoms. Symptoms include fever, loss of appetite, jaundice, nausea, vomiting, malaise, dark urine, and whitish stools. There is no chronic long-term infection, and once an individual has had HAV it cannot be contracted again. Vaccination is available that prevents infection by HAV. It is recommended for individuals 12 months of age and older. Short-term protection is possible with immunoglobulins that may be given within 2 weeks of coming in contact with HAV.

STERILIZING INSTRUMENTS IN AN AUTOCLAVE

Objective: Sterilize instruments in an autoclave to prevent the spread of pathogens.

EQUIPMENT AND SUPPLIES

autoclave; instruments sanitized and wrapped for autoclaving; distilled water; autoclave directions

METHOD

1. Check the level of water in the autoclave reservoir. Add distilled water as needed to the fill line (Figure 34-16A).
2. Load the autoclave. Trays and packs should be loaded on their sides. Containers should be loaded on their sides with lids off or ajar. Mixed loads are loaded with hard objects on bottom racks and softer items on top racks. Keep large packs 2 to 4 inches apart and smaller packets 1 to 2 inches apart.
3. Read the manufacturer's instructions and follow them exactly. Most autoclaves follow similar protocols.
   a. Turn the control knob to FILL and observe carefully with the door open until the water reaches the chamber fill line.
   b. Turn the knob to autoclave position (Fig 34-16B). This shuts off the water.
   c. Close and lock the door.
   d. When pressure reaches 15 to 17 pounds per square inch and the temperature reaches 250°F to 270°F, set the timer for the required time. Typical timing is 30 minutes for wrapped trays and packages and 15 minutes for unwrapped items. Always check the manufacturer's suggested times and facility protocol.
4. When timing is complete turn the control knob to VENT.
5. When the pressure reaches zero, open the chamber door about 1 inch and allow items in the autoclave to dry completely before removing them (about 30 to 45 minutes).
6. Turn the autoclave knob to OFF.
7. Remove the wrapped items and check the autoclave tape on the outside for color change. Store in a dry closed cabinet for use. Unwrapped items must be removed using sterile transfer forceps and must be placed on a sterile field or in a sterile storage area (Fig 34-16C).
8. Record date, time, and types of items autoclaved in log and initial.

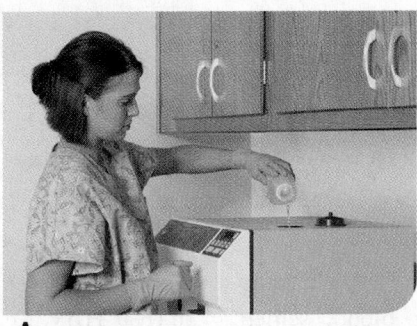

A

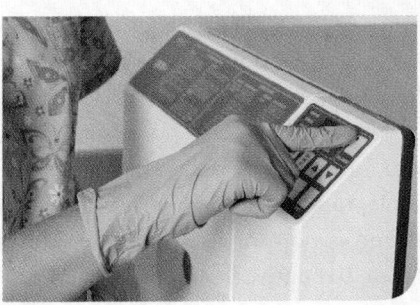

B

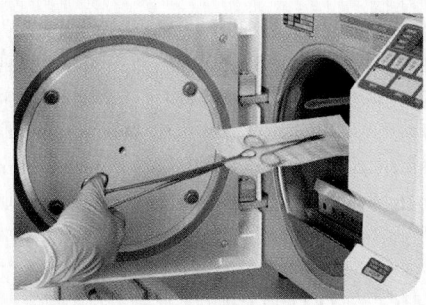

C

FIGURE 34-16 **(A) Check the level of water in the autoclave, and add water as needed; (B) properly set the autoclave according to the manufacturer's instructions; (C) remove instruments to a clean container using the sterile transfer forceps.**

procedure
34-8

CHEMICALLY STERILIZING INSTRUMENTS

Objective: Chemically sterilize heat-sensitive instruments to prevent the spread of pathogens.

EQUIPMENT AND SUPPLIES

chemical disinfectant; goggles, disposable gloves, utility (rubber) gloves; sink; glass or stainless steel container with cover; sterile towels; sterile transfer forceps; sterile basin; sanitized articles

Note: Before anything can be chemically sterilized, it must be sanitized properly as described in Procedure 34-5. Always read and follow the manufacturer's directions on the original container of the chemical agent.

METHOD

1. Sanitize instruments appropriately.
2. Select the type of chemical needed for the instruments to be sterilized.
3. Read the directions on the original germicidal agent label. If opening the germicide for the first time, write the date on the container and follow directions to prepare the chemical agent. See Figure 34-17 for an example of a cold chemical sterilizer.
4. Place the chemical agent in an appropriate container that is large enough to submerge the instrument completely.
5. Cover tightly and record the time, date, and your initials.
6. Do not open the container during the sterilization process.
7. When sterilization timing is complete, remove the instrument from the container using sterile gloves or transfer

forceps, and rinse thoroughly with sterile water over a sterile basin. Hold the instruments over the basin for a few moments to drain excess sterile water.
8. Dry the instruments thoroughly with a sterile towel and place on a sterile field for use.
9. Change the chemical agent every 7 to 14 days, or as recommended by the manufacturer.
10. Remove gloves and perform hand hygiene.

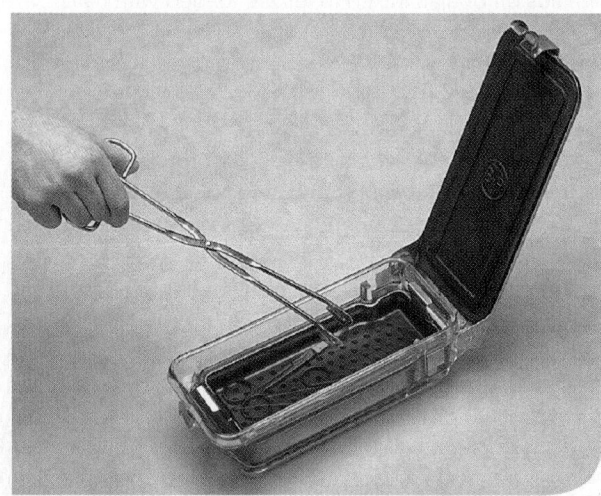

FIGURE 34-17 Cold chemical sterilization.

HEPATITIS B VIRUS

Hepatitis B (serum hepatitis), also called HBV, is transmitted through body fluids, including blood, semen, saliva, and breast milk contaminated with the virus. This potentially fatal disease can be passed from one drug user to another when sharing a contaminated needle. HBV can also be transmitted during sexual intercourse. The efficacy of latex condoms is unknown. Infection with HVB increases the risk of contracting HIV and HAV. The incubation period for this liver infection is 60 to 90 days with a rapid onset of symptoms. About 30 percent of individuals have no signs or symptoms. HBV symptoms include symptoms similar to HAV. HBV can cause a lifelong infection, scarring of the liver, liver cancer, or liver failure and death.

Treatment for all forms of hepatitis is a high-protein diet and rest for several weeks. Several drugs are presently in use to treat HBV. Relapse is a possibility.

Hepatitis B vaccine has been available since 1982. Routine vaccines are recommended for ages birth to 18 years. Vaccination is recommended for high-risk groups, such as health care workers and public safety workers, persons with multiple sexual partners, IV drug users, and persons in a household with others who are infected with HBV. Two types of vaccines are available for HBV: Recombivax HB and Energix-B. HBV vaccine is administered in three doses; the second dose is given 1 month after the first, and the third dose is given 5 months later.

Any personnel with a high risk of contact with blood and body fluids should be encouraged to receive the vaccination against hepatitis B. However, it is not required. If the employee decides not to receive the vaccination, a disclaimer must be signed and placed in the employee file. The disclaimer allows for the possibility that the employee might decide at a later date to receive the vaccine.

Some individuals should not receive the vaccine. Those who are sensitive to yeast or any of the other components found in the vaccine should not receive it. If a woman is pregnant, or plans to attempt to become pregnant within the next 6 months, she should not receive the vaccine. Others, such as breast-feeding mothers or people with heart diseases, should also be cautious about receiving the vaccine. Occasionally side effects occur and usually include swelling, pain or redness at the injection site, and flulike symptoms.

HEPATITIS C VIRUS

Hepatitis C, previously referred to as non-A and non-B hepatitis, is the most common form of new hepatitis cases every year. HCV is spread when the blood from an infected person enters a noninfected individual. Commonly HCV is spread through sharing needles, exposure to infected sharps on the job, or being passed from an infected mother to the baby at birth. The symptoms and treatment are similar to those of hepatitis B. A patient may be a carrier of hepatitis C and not be aware of it. The CDC reports that chronic infection occurs in 75 to 85 percent of infected individuals. Treatments are available, yet liver damage, liver failure, and cancer can occur. There is no vaccine for HCV. Treatment with interferon and ribavirin are presently the treatments of choice. As with other forms of hepatitis, drinking alcohol may make the disease worse.

HEPATITIS D VIRUS

Hepatitis D, also called delta hepatitis, is one of the most recently identified forms of hepatitis. The symptoms of hepatitis D can be more severe than those of other forms of hepatitis. Hepatitis D is spread through the use of IV drugs and intimate contact. This form of hepatitis is rapidly on the rise as it is being identified in an increasing number of HIV and AIDS cases.

HEPATITIS E AND G VIRUSES

Hepatitis E is the result of exposure to food contaminated with human feces. It is a major infectious disease in developing countries due to poor sanitary conditions. This form of hepatitis is uncommon in the United States. Recently hepatitis G has been isolated as a bloodborne infection transmitted via needlesticks or contaminated blood.

HIV and AIDS

HIV is the virus that causes AIDS. AIDS was first identified in the United States in 1981. From 1981 through 2006 it is thought that more than 1 million people are living with HIV in the United States and that 24 to 27 percent of those are unaware of their HIV status. In the United States between 500,000 and 600,000 people have died after developing AIDS. At the present time, AIDS is considered the second leading cause of death in the United States in men between the ages of 25 and 44 and the fifth leading killer of women in that age bracket. In 2006 African Americans made up half the diagnosed cases of HIV/AIDS. It is estimated that more than 47 million people worldwide have been infected with HIV since the start of the epidemic. The CDC reports that between the mid and late 1990s treatment advances slowed the progression of HIV to AIDS and led to a decrease in the number of deaths from AIDS. It has recently been noted that resistance to HIV drugs has increased and that a new strain of HIV may have developed.

AIDS is the severe form of a range of illnesses linked to HIV. The CDC defines AIDS as an HIV infection and a CD4 (cluster of differentiation) + T lymphocyte count of fewer than 200 cells per microliter of blood, or a CD4+ percentage under 14. This virus causes the immune system—the body's shield against infection—to break down. Eventually the HIV virus invades the body's T cells, which fight disease. When the T cells are invaded, they render the macrophages useless for fighting off pathogenic invasions.

The various means by which the AIDS virus can enter the body are as follow:

- Vaginal, anal, or oral intercourse with a person who has the virus
- Sharing needles or syringes with a person who has the virus
- Receiving transfusions of blood or blood products donated by someone who has the virus
- Receiving organ transplants from a donor who has the virus
- Contaminating open wounds or sores with blood, semen, or vaginal secretions infected with the virus
- Receiving artificial insemination with the sperm of a man who has the virus
- Being born to a mother who is infected with the virus
- Being an infant who is breast-fed by a woman who is infected with the virus

HIV cannot survive on inanimate objects. The virus can, however, survive well in body fluids such as blood, semen, and vaginal secretions. The virus can stay in cells for months, even years. During this time the cells will replicate (reproduce) themselves. The body's defensive T cells eventually are destroyed by the new viral cells.

Some HIV victims will develop AIDS-related complex (ARC), the symptomatic stage of infection before the onset of AIDS. The clinical signs of ARC include loss of appetite, weight loss, diarrhea, skin rash, fatigue, night sweats, swollen lymph glands, poor resistance to infection, the presence of HIV antibodies, and a decreased CD4+ count.

Not all HIV patients develop AIDS or any other HIV-related condition. It may take 8 to 10 years for symptoms of HIV infection to develop and 12 years or more for symptoms of AIDS to develop. Initial infection with HIV sometimes causes mononucleosis-type symptoms with fever, sore throat, swollen glands, and muscle aches. After antibodies develop, the person will test positive for HIV, and another period with no symptoms may occur. This incubation period can last several years. Even without observable symptoms, the immune system becomes increasingly damaged during this time. A person with HIV may experience a long period of swelling of the lymph glands in the throat, armpits, and groin. This condition is called persistent generalized lymphadenopathy and may last a number of years. When HIV has seriously damaged the immune system, other symptoms may occur. These symptoms can include a white coating of the mouth and throat (thrush), similar infections of the skin and mucous membranes of the anus and genital area, and severe viral infections such as herpes. The final stage of an HIV infection (AIDS) includes a variety of viral, fungal, bacterial, and parasitic infections; nervous disorders; and cancers.

When these infections are present in the healthy body, they can be overcome by the immune system. However, in the AIDS patient, the immune system is no longer effective and, hence, the infections become life threatening. The immune system can be suppressed for many reasons, including stress, poor nutrition, or an infection such as HIV. During this time, the patient is more susceptible to infections. These are known as **opportunistic infections**. This means the infection, having the advantage of the suppressed immune system, has had the opportunity to make the patient sick. Opportunistic diseases for AIDS patients include the following:

- *Pneumocystis carinii* pneumonia (PCP)
- Kaposi's sarcoma, a type of skin cancer
- Toxoplasmosis, an infestation of parasites that infect the brain and central nervous system

TB is seen with increasing frequency among persons infected with HIV. HIV infection is one of the most high-risk factors known for the progression of TB from infection to disease. However, of the diseases associated with HIV infection, TB is one of the few that is transmissible, treatable, and preventable.

AIDS is diagnosed based on several factors: functioning ability of the immune system determined by tests such as T-cell counts; the presence of one or more opportunistic infections; and the presence of HIV antibodies. The United States Food and Drug Administration (FDA) has approved a point-of-care HIV test that provides results in 5 minutes. The HIV or AIDS antibody test—the enzyme-linked immunosorbent assay (ELISA)—is also used as a screening test. With a point-of-care test or a positive ELISA, a patient is said to be HIV positive or HIV antibody positive. The Western blot test is used to confirm the results of any test. Once a positive Western blot test is determined, the patient is referred for postexposure prophylaxis (PEP).

HIV does not survive well outside the human body, and it is not transmitted through air, food, water, pets, or bugs. HIV is destroyed by a 1:10 household bleach solution or an application of heat treatment at 132°F (56°C) for 10 minutes. Standard precautions, which include the use of aseptic technique, proper hand hygiene, gloving, and careful handling of needles and syringes to avoid puncture wounds, can protect health care workers from contracting the virus.

People at the highest risk for HIV infection include men and women who engage in unprotected sex, IV drug users who share needles, sexual partners of those who engage in high-risk activity, infants born to HIV-positive mothers, and people who received blood transfusions or clotting factors between 1977 and 1985 (prior to current screening processes for blood).

The following are the symptoms of AIDS:

- CD4 + T lymphocyte count of fewer than 200 cells per microliter of blood, or a CD4+ percentage under 14
- Unexplained weight loss of 10 to 15 pounds in less than 2 months that is not associated with diet or exercise
- Long-lasting occurrences of diarrhea
- Unexplained fever, chills, and drenching night sweats for more than 2 weeks
- Unexplained extreme fatigue
- Swelling or hardening of lymph glands located in the throat, groin, or armpit
- Periods of continued deep, dry coughing that are not due to other illnesses or smoking

- Increased shortness of breath

- Appearance of discolored or purplish growths on the skin or inside the mouth

- Unexplained bleeding from growths on the skin, mucous membranes, or from any opening on the body

- Severe numbness or pain in the hands and feet, loss of motor control and reflex, paralysis, or loss of muscular strength

- Altered state of consciousness, personality change, or mental deterioration

There is currently no cure for AIDS. However, several treatment regimens are used that can help delay the progression of the disease and improve the quality of life for those living with the symptoms. These include the main form of treatment, antiviral therapy, which suppresses the replication of the HIV virus in individuals. Supportive measures to improve the quality of life for the AIDS patient include delivery of home meals, nutritional supplements, and hospice care.

When patients come in for HIV or AIDS testing, they should receive counseling from the physician before and after the test. The counseling should include information on methods for safer sex. The medical assistant may be asked to provide information to a caregiver regarding caring for an AIDS patient. Such recommendations are presented in Box 34-2.

Multidrug-Resistant Organisms

Multidrug-resistant organisms (MDROs) are bacteria and other microorganisms that have developed resistance to antimicrobial drugs. Some examples include **methicillin-resistant Staphylococcus aureus (MRSA)**, **vancomycin-resistant Staphylococcus aureus (VRSA)**, **vancomycin-resistant Enterococci (VRE)**, multidrug-resistant tuberculosis (MDR TB), extended-spectrum beta-lactamases (ESBLs) that are resistant to cephalosporins and monobactam, and penicillin-resistant *Streptococcus pneumonia* (PRSP). Among those listed, the most common MDROs detected in nonhospital settings are MRSA and VRE.

MRSA and VRE are often found in patients in long-term care facilities. PRSP infections are most common in outpatient facilities such as clinics, child care facilities, and physicians' offices. Several factors increase the risk of acquiring these organisms: severe illness, previous treatment with antimicrobial medications, underlying health considerations, invasive procedures such as dialysis and catheterization, and advanced age.

The health care costs associated with MDROs is staggering. Increased length of hospital stays, increased cost of treatments, and death are associated with these organisms.

METHICILLIN-RESISTANT STAPHYLOCOCCUS AUREUS

MRSA is another name for methicillin-resistant *S. aureus,* an organism that is highly resistant to antibiotics. There are two forms of MRSA: hospital-associated MRSA and community-based MRSA. The first, as the name implies, occurs mostly in health care facilities to individuals with weakened immune systems. This organism is one of the most common agents responsible for nosocomial infections.

S. aureus is a gram-positive coccid (round shaped) found in grapelike clusters. It is normally found on the skin and may be found in the nasal passages. *S. aureus* is the causative agent in boils, acne, some forms of septicemia, and pneumonia. Infection may occur from cuts, sores, and through catheters or breathing tubes. Symptoms of *Staphylococcus* (staph) infection include pus formation, fever, swelling, and tenderness around the area of infection. Individuals with weakened immune systems are more susceptible to this type of infection. Serious staph infections may lead to endocarditis (inflammation of the lining of the heart), cellulitis (inflammation of subcutaneous and connective tissue), pneumonia, and toxic shock syndrome.

According to the CDC, in 2005 just under a million people developed MRSA and approximately 18,650 people died during their hospital stay from conditions related to a MRSA infection. About 85 percent of all MRSA infections are related to health care, and 14 percent of all MRSA infections occur in persons not associated with health care exposure.

PROFESSIONALISM

THE LAW

The medical assistant has the grave responsibility of maintaining aseptic technique. Every break in aseptic technique must be reported and corrected immediately. Even when one cannot see a needle puncture in a glove, the wearer of the glove may know there has been a puncture, resulting in a break in the barrier to infection. The medical assistant must readily admit if a barrier has been broken so that corrective action can be taken.

The identity of an employee or patient who is HIV positive or has AIDS or hepatitis is confidential and must be kept confidential.

Box 34-2 Caring for Someone with AIDS

To protect themselves from infection, caregivers should be reminded to do the following:

- Handle all needles with care. Never recap needles or remove needles from syringes. Dispose of all needles in puncture-proof containers out of the reach of children.
- Wear gloves when in contact with blood, blood-tinged body fluids, urine, feces, or vomit.
- Perform hand hygiene after removing gloves.
- Cover with a bandage any cut, open sore, or breaks on exposed skin of either the patient or the caregiver.
- Flush down the toilet all liquid waste containing blood. using care to avoid splashing during pouring. Nonflushable items such as paper towels, sanitary pads and tampons, wound dressings, or items soiled with blood, semen, or vaginal fluid should be enclosed in a plastic bag and tightly sealed. Check with your local health department or physician to determine trash disposal regulations for your area.
- Use a disinfection solution of 1 part bleach to 10 parts water to disinfect such items as floors, showers, tubs, and sinks. Discard the solution in the toilet after using.

To protect the person with AIDS from infection:

- If the caregiver has a cold or flu, and no one else is available to care for the AIDS patient, a surgical-type mask should be worn.
- Hands should be washed before touching the AIDS patient.

- Anyone with boils, fever blisters (herpes simplex), or shingles (herpes zoster) should avoid close contact with the patient.
- Gloves should be worn if the caregiver has a rash or sores on the hands.
- Persons living with or caring for an AIDS patient should have received all the recommended childhood immunizations and booster shots, including the hepatitis vaccine.
- The AIDS patient should not be in the same room with a person who has, or is recovering from, chicken pox.

The caregiver should also do the following:

- Call the local AIDS service organization for support.
- Seek the help of clergy, counselors, and other health care professionals to help cope with feelings of frustration and stress.
- Be comfortable touching the person with AIDS.
- Encourage the patient to become involved in his or her own care and assist the patient in being active as long as possible.
- Freely discuss the disease with the patient.

For more information on HIV or AIDS, write to the CDC National AIDS Clearinghouse, P.O. Box 6003, Rockville, MD 20849-6003; CDC Control and Prevention, 1600 Clifton Road, N.E., Atlanta, GA 30333; or call 1-800-CDC-INFO (1-800-232-4636).

The American Academy of Orthopedic Surgeons (AAOS) reports that in 2005 in the United States about 370,000 hospital admissions were due to MRSA. The number of deaths (18,650) surpassed the number of deaths from Hurricane Katrina and AIDS combined and is higher than deaths related to polio at the peak of the polio epidemic. The AAOS states that reimbursement for treating nonsurgical hospital-acquired infections is being eliminated based on the concept that proper infection control guidelines can reduce these infections. Also, it has been reported that legislative elimination of payment for treating hospital-acquired surgical site infections has been proposed.

MRSA has evolved as a result of decades of antibiotic treatments that saved millions of lives. The "superbugs" that were feared are here. MRSA is unpredictable as far as resistance to antibiotics and epidemiology patterns. Serious MRSA infections are treated with two or more antibiotics—namely, vancomycin, rifampin, and others—given intravenously. The AAOS also reports that data suggest that *S. aureus* that is resistant to vancomycin and rifampin may cause even greater problems.

As many as 11 to 40 percent of the world population is estimated to be **colonized** or carry the bacteria in the nose, throat, armpit, and groin. Most of these individuals do not develop an infection unless there is injury to the skin or elsewhere. Diagnosis of *S. aureus* is established by culture from the infected individual. A sensitivity test determines which antibiotics are most effective in killing the organism. If the organism grows in the presence of methicillin, it is classified as MRSA. The physician then prescribes the medication that most readily kills the microorganism.

Community-based MRSA (CA-MRSA) occurs in healthy individuals, not recently hospitalized, who share personal items or equipment such as towels or razors. This form of the microorganism is often found in schools, military facilities, or day care centers. The AAOS reports that community-based MRSA is genetically distinct from hospital-associated MRSA (HA-MRSA) and clinically different as well.

The best way to avoid MRSA infection is to use good hygiene practices, including hand washing and wearing gloves and other PPE when treating a patient with MRSA. Using an antiseptic cream and covering any skin breaks with adhesive bandages also will help prevent MRSA. When MRSA infections occur EPA-registered disinfectants should be used to clean surfaces that have come in contact with infected areas.

VRSA is a type of *S. aureus* organism that is resistant to the antibiotic vancomycin. The CDC reports that as of September 2006 six VRSA infections had been reported in the United States.

VANCOMYCIN-RESISTANT ENTEROCOCCI (VRE)

Enterococci are bacteria normally present in human intestines, the female genital tract, and the environment. Individuals more at risk are those who are immune compromised, have recently had abdominal or chest surgery, have indwelling medical devices, or have been treated with vancomycin long term. According to the CDC, during 2006–2007 1 in 8 infections in hospitals were caused by *Enterococci,* and 30 percent of those were VRE. Some individuals are colonized with VRE but have no symptoms. VRE infections are treated with antibiotics other than vancomycin.

VRE is spread by direct contact, usually by caregivers who have not practiced hand hygiene appropriately. It can be spread by touching contaminated inanimate objects. To prevent VRE at home or work, wash after each use of the bathroom and before preparing food. Wash or use alcohol-based hand rubs after contact with persons with VRE. As always, use gloves when in contact with any body fluids such as stool or infected wounds. If you have or carry VRE, make the caregiver aware of the condition.

MULTIDRUG-RESISTANT TUBERCULOSIS

TB is caused by an airborne microorganism (*Mycobacterium tuberculosis*) that usually affects the lungs. The germ particles can remain in the air for hours after coughing, sneezing, and talking. It may also affect other organs such as the brain, kidneys, or spine. Multidrug-resistant tuberculosis (MDR TB) is an organism that is resistant to at least two of the major medications used to treat TB—isoniazid and rifampin—as well as at least one of the injectable second-line drugs: kanamycin, amikacin, or capreomycin. Another multiresistant form, extensively drug-resistant TB (XDR TB) is resistant to both the first and second line of drugs. Thus the patient is left with few treatment options. The XDR TB form is of special concern to HIV persons with a weakened immune system. All individuals infected with HIV should be tested for TB.

Drug-resistant forms are believed to occur because TB patients fail to complete the whole course of treatment or the administered drugs are of poor quality. There is a vaccine for TB, bacillus (or bacille) Calmette-Guérin (BCG), which is used in some countries (not in the United States) but has limited effectiveness. After exposure to TB, a TB skin test should be performed.

Bioterrorism

Bioterrorism is defined as the deliberate release of bacteria, viruses, other agents that can cause illness and death in humans, animals, or plants. Biological agents can be spread through air, water, or food. Some biological agents are difficult to detect; thus, if a terrorist spread the agent, its effects may not be felt for several hours or days. Biological terrorism agents are classified by the CDC into categories A, B, and C, with A being the agents of highest risk. The Category A agents or toxins are easily spread, cause the highest death rates, may cause public disruption, and require public health preparedness:

- Anthrax
- Botulism
- Plague
- Smallpox
- Tularemia
- Viral hemorrhagic fevers

Since September 11, 2001, the awareness of other possible terrorist attacks has been on the minds of all Americans. The term *agents of mass destruction* is all too familiar as well. The CDC Special Pathogens Branch and the CDC National Center for Preparedness, Detection, and Control of Infectious Diseases (NCPDCID) monitor outbreaks of the category illnesses. Their goals include developing rapid diagnostic tests, gathering information, and offering assistance in control and prevention during outbreaks. Each of the Category A agents is briefly discussed in the following paragraphs. For further information, see the CDC website.

ANTHRAX

Anthrax is a disease caused by the spore-forming organism *Bacillus anthracis.* This acute infectious disease can be passed from animal to human by contact with animal hair or waste. This disease can attack the lungs, skin, and gastrointestinal tract, causing symptoms from respiratory distress to coma. In 2001 anthrax was spread in the United States through the U.S. Postal Service system, causing 22 cases of anthrax infection. The first symptoms of anthrax contracted through inhalation are the same as for the flu. Respiratory anthrax is the most severe, with half the cases ending in death. Penicillin, tetracycline, and erythromycin are antibiotics of choice for treatment.

Contaminated materials should be incinerated. The CDC and other government agencies are developing plans for anthrax attack with training and education programs for health care providers, public service personnel, and media. A vaccine to prevent anthrax has been developed but is not yet available for the general public.

BOTULISM

Botulism is a paralytic condition caused by the neurotoxin produced by the spore-forming bacteria *Clostridium botulinum.* The three types of botulism are food-borne botulism, wound botulism, and infant botulism. Food-borne botulism is caused by eating foods containing the toxin. Improperly prepared canned foods are often a source. Wound botulism is caused by a wound infected with *C. botulinum.* Infant botulism is caused by consumption of spores that grow and release toxins. All forms may be fatal and should be considered a medical emergency.

Botulinum toxin is one of the most poisonous substances known. One gram of toxin evenly dispersed and inhaled would kill more than a million people. It is the first biological toxin to be licensed in the United States for treatment of disease. It is used to treat conditions such as eyelid spasms, dystonia (abnormal, repetitive muscle movements), and strabismus (squinting). A weakened form of the botulinum toxin (Botox) is widely used to reduce facial wrinkles.

The CDC reports that cases of botulism are rare in the United States. Most of these cases are infant botulism. The signs and symptoms of food-borne illness appear as early as 6 hours and as long as 10 days after eating contaminated food. Double vision, slurred speech, difficulty breathing, and paralysis due to the toxin occur unless treated. Recovery may take weeks and necessitate use of a ventilator. Food-borne and wound types may respond to horse antitoxin if given early enough. Human antitoxin is available from the state of California Public Health Department for treatment of infant botulism.

PLAGUE

Plague, an infectious disease that affects humans and animals, has several forms. All forms of the plague are caused by the bacteria *Yersinia pestis,* which are found in rodents and their fleas in the United States and many other areas of the world. A person may develop one form or may develop a combination of pneumonic plague, which affects the lungs; bubonic plague, which affects the lymph glands and causes swelling; and septicemic plague, which occurs when the organism enters the bloodstream. Symptoms include fever, chills, and pneumonia, and if

not treated, death can occur in a matter of a few days. Wearing a mask and early treatment with antibiotics such as gentamycin or tetracycline within 24 hours are suggested.

SMALLPOX

Smallpox is caused by the *Variola* virus. It causes an acute, contagious disease that can be quickly spread from person to person. Signs and symptoms of smallpox include fever, macules, papules, vesicles, pustules, and crusts.

Smallpox outbreaks have been occurring for thousands of years according to historians. The CDC reported that the last case of smallpox in the United States occurred in 1949, and the last case in the world was in Somalia in 1977. Until 1972, smallpox vaccinations were recommended for the general public. Eventually it seemed that smallpox had been eradicated, as no new cases have been reported. Recently there has been the possibility of heightened danger of the use of the *Variola major* virus as a bioterrorism weapon.

According to the CDC, as of 2004 the United States has enough vaccine stockpiles to inoculate every citizen in the event of a smallpox emergency. Vaccinations are available and have been given to military personnel and to medical personnel who might come into contact with the virus.

TULAREMIA

Tularemia is a serious illness caused by the bacterium *Francisella tularensis.* This organism is found in rabbits and rodents. The symptoms of tularemia include fever, chills, headache, cough, weakness, and diarrhea.

Tularemia is spread by the bite of a tick or flea infected with the organism; by contact with an infected animal carcass, food, or water contaminated with *F. tularensis;* or by inhaling the organism. It is not spread from person to person and can be treated with antibiotics. To protect against tularemia, practice good personal hygiene and hand washing, and use insect repellent containing N,N-diethyl-meta-toluamide (DEET).

VIRAL HEMORRHAGIC FEVERS

Viral hemorrhagic fevers are a group of illnesses caused by several different groups of viruses. These viruses have a number of similar features, such as the following:

- They are RNA viruses.
- They must live in either an animal or insect host (ticks, mosquitoes, certain types of rats, mice).
- They are usually restricted to areas where the hosts live.
- Humans can transmit viruses to one another but are not natural hosts.
- There are no vaccines or cures for the most part, with a few exceptions.

Some examples of VHFs are Ebola-hemorrhagic fever and Lassa fever. The signs and symptoms vary but include fever, fatigue, and loss of muscle strength; bleeding under the skin and from the mouth, eyes, and ears; delirium; and coma.

Death is possible. Precautions include controlling rodent populations, proper cleaning of rodent nests and droppings, good personal hygiene, isolation of affected people, and use of PPE.

SUMMARY

Good aseptic technique is everybody's business. The medical assistant is often the first line of defense against the spread of infection in the medical office. A thorough understanding of universal and standard precautions and isolation techniques is important to maintain a safe patient environment. The meticulous attention given to sterilization of all reusable materials and equipment is often the full responsibility of the medical assistant and is a serious responsibility. All who handle waste products must be trained in safety measures such as standard precautions. When practicing an aseptic technique, one should learn the correct method and then never deviate from it. Health care professionals need to have a basic understanding of the major diseases threatening our world today. Illnesses such as hepatitis, HIV/AIDS, and MRSA have major impacts on health care today. The awareness of biological agents of bioterrorism gives the health care provider a broader understanding of global health care struggles.

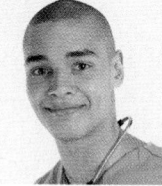

34 CHAPTER REVIEW

COMPETENCY REVIEW

1. Define and spell the terms to learn for this chapter.
2. How does the age of the person affect susceptibility to infections?
3. List three natural barriers to infection.
4. List the four cardinal signs of infection.
5. List three examples of body fluids included in standard precautions.
6. A sterilized package has reached its expiration date. What should you do?
7. What solution of household bleach has been found to be effective in destroying HIV?
8. What test would be ordered after the ELISA test shows a patient is HIV positive?
9. List three examples of PPE.
10. Define *multidrug-resistant organism (MDRO)* and give on example.

PREPARING FOR THE CERTIFICATION EXAM

1. The term asepsis means
   a. contaminated
   b. needs oxygen
   c. free of pathogens
   d. soap
   e. needs sanitizing
2. Most sterilization indicators operate on what principle?
   a. Color change will revert back when an item is contaminated.
   b. Original color reappears after 6 weeks.
   c. Color change indicates the package has been properly sealed.
   d. Color change indicates sterilization is complete.
   e. Color change occurs at the beginning of the process.
3. An organism that is infected with a pathogen and is a source of the infection to others is
   a. a reservoir host
   b. a carrier
   c. an anaerobe

d. not an infectious risk to others

e. an inanimate object

4. Which of the following procedures are covered by standard precautions?
   a. Change gloves between patients.
   b. Dispose of needles in sharps container.
   c. Wash environmental surfaces with soapy water.
   d. Never recap needles.
   e. Perform hand hygiene every third time you change gloves.

5. Bacteria require which of the following to grow?
   a. disinfectants
   b. cool temperature
   c. light
   d. no nutrition
   e. moisture

6. MRSA is a/an
   a. disinfectant
   b. type of microorganism
   c. oxygen source
   d. physician's credential
   e. drug

7. How long is it necessary to wash hands prior to assisting a new patient?
   a. 1 minute
   b. 6 minutes

c. 2 to 3 minutes

d. 45 minutes

e. 15 seconds

8. Which of the following is an opportunistic infection associated with AIDS?
   a. cold
   b. measles
   c. antibody
   d. *Pneumocystis carinii*
   e. hives

9. Which of the following is listed as a possible bioterrorism agent on the CDC Class A list?
   a. smallpox virus
   b. *Streptococcus*
   c. *Staphylococcus aureus*
   d. hepatitis virus
   e. mumps virus

10. HIV is spread mainly by
    a. sharing needles
    b. sexual intercourse
    c. tears
    d. sitting on toilet seats
    e. Both A and B

CRITICAL THINKING

1. What type of PPE would David need to wear when performing venipuncture on this patient?

2. Why would the physician include a liver function test as part of the patient's routine blood work?

3. Which particular groups of individuals are encouraged to receive the vaccination to guard against HBV?

ON THE JOB

Emma Brown, 70 years old, is caring for her 78-year-old husband, George Brown. Mr. Brown, a diabetic, has been hospitalized with a recurring infection that may lead to amputation of his right leg. Mr. Brown's physical condition may not be able to withstand another massive leg infection. He has been placed on antibiotics, and his leg is now healing. Mrs. Brown will require instructions on irrigating the leg wound and changing her husband's dressing. When the leg wound was cultured, *E. coli* was present. Mrs. Brown mentioned to the medical assistant that she is concerned about her own health since she has a colostomy.

1. What patient education is required for Mrs. Brown regarding the procedure to be used in caring for her husband?

2. Is it possible that the *E. coli* was transmitted from Ms. Brown's colostomy site to her husband's leg wound? Explain.

INTERNET ACTIVITY

Research Kaposi's sarcoma on the Internet.

MEDMEDIA

Additional interactive resources and activities for this chapter can be found:

On your student DVD: View applicable procedure videos on the DVD-ROM found in the back of this book.

MyHealthProfessionsKit.com: Test your knowledge of this chapter with games and activities. MyHealthProfessionsKit also includes resources, helpful links, and a Spanish audio glossary.

Medical Assisting Interactive: Practice your procedures as a medical assistant in this simulated doctor's office. This can be accessed through MyHealthProfessionsKit.com.

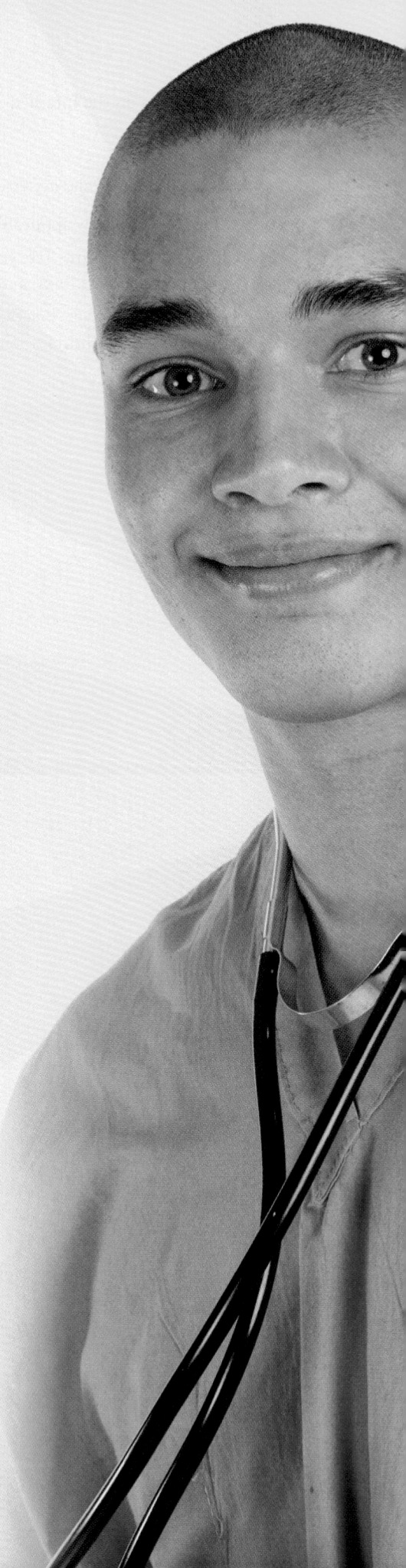

35

Vital Signs

LEARNING OBJECTIVES

After completing this chapter, the student will be able to:

- Define and spell the terms to learn for this chapter.

- List and describe the components of a medical history.

- Convert weight in pounds to kilograms (and vice versa).

- Convert height from inches to centimeters (and vice versa).

- Convert temperature readings from degrees Fahrenheit (F) to degrees Centigrade (C) (and vice versa).

- State the normal values of temperature, pulse, respiratory rates, and blood pressure.

- List ten conditions that cause the body temperature to increase or decrease.

- State three situations in which measuring an oral, rectal, and axillary temperature should be avoided.

- List and describe the nine pulse sites.

- Describe the respiratory rate range for the various age groups.

- Discuss the five phases of the Korotkoff sounds.

- Explain the four physiological factors that affect blood pressure.

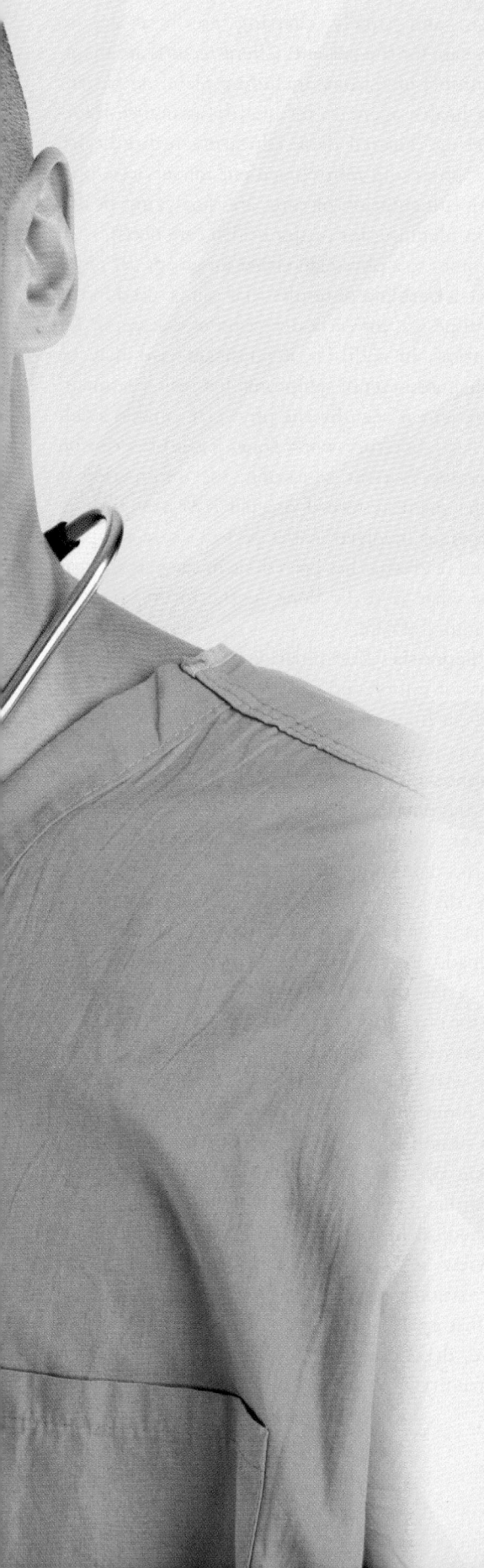

CHAPTER OUTLINE

CASE STUDY

Elanya Jordan, age 13, is seeing Dr. Salpega for persistent headaches. David, RMA, obtains her vital signs, which are T: 98.6°F, P: 88 bpm, R: 20 rpm, BP: 110/74. Elanya is 5 feet, 1 inch tall and weighs 104 pounds. Her mother, Mary Ellen, states that she has lost 6 pounds during the past 3 weeks, as she has lost her appetite since the headaches began.

TERMS TO LEARN

acute pain	intermittent pulse
afebrile	intractable pain
anthropometry	Korotkoff sounds
apical	manometer
apnea	medical diagnosis
arrhythmia	metabolism
asymptomatic	orthostatic hypotension
basal metabolism	palpatory method
baseline	phantom pain
bounding pulse	prognosis
bradycardia	pulse deficit
bradypnea	pulse pressure
chronic pain	pyrexia
clinical diagnosis	radiating pain
cyanosis	referred pain
diagnosis	respiratory cycle
diastolic blood pressure	rhythm
differential diagnosis	sphygmomanometer
dysrhythmia	subjective symptom
eupnea	syncope
febrile	systolic blood pressure
frenulum linguae	tachycardia
hyperpyrexia	tachypnea
hypertension (HTN)	thready pulse
hyperthermia	tympanic membrane thermometer
hyperventilation	
hypotension	vital signs
hypothermia	volume
hypoventilation	

CERTIFICATION LINK

CMA (AAMA)
Patient preparation and assisting the physician

CMAS (AMT)
Vital signs and measurements

RMA
Vital signs and mensurations

Various members of the health care team record information and submit test results that become a permanent part of the medical history. Confidentiality of patient information must be safeguarded at all levels. Accuracy in testing, clear documentation, and timely charting are necessary to ensure quality care for the patient. Client records are maintained for a number of reasons, including planning patient care, auditing health agencies for quality assurance information, gathering research data, educating future health care providers, obtaining reimbursement for services, providing legal documentation of care, and analyzing health care to assist in planning for future health care needs.

A patient comes to a physician either for an annual physical to establish a **baseline** of results that can be used in the event of later illnesses, for early detection of disease, or for disease prevention. In addition, a physician visit may be scheduled to diagnose a set of symptoms and seek treatment. Each time a patient is seen by the physician, makes a call to the office, has laboratory work done, has a prescription ordered, or receives patient education, the information is recorded in the medical record or chart. At any time, a health care provider involved in the patient's care can pick up the chart and read what has been done in the past to treat the patient or what is to be done in the future, thereby ensuring continuity of care.

Although **diagnosis** (determination of the cause and nature of a disease or injury) and treatment of the problem are the main goals, a final or **medical diagnosis** is arrived at after all examinations, tests, and procedures are complete. A **clinical diagnosis** or working diagnosis is a preliminary presumptive diagnosis made by the physician based on the health history and physical examination. A **differential diagnosis** is the determination of which one of multiple possibilities is the cause of a problem. Once the medical diagnosis is made (and sometimes this is not possible), the **prognosis** is made. Prognosis is the prediction of the course of the condition and the recovery rate. During the course of the condition, the physician will monitor the patient's progress and adjust treatment as needed.

Interaction with the patient begins with making the appointment. From this point on the medical assistant has the chance to establish a positive, empathetic relationship with the patient by acting in a professional, warm manner. Before a patient has a physical examination or is seen by the physician, a medical history must be obtained. The initial patient interview is conducted by the medical assistant, and the information gathered becomes part of the permanent medical history. Health history forms vary from brief to comprehensive, depending on the physician specialty and choice of the facility.

Patient care depends on effective communication. The patient's medical history is a formal, enduring legal document that makes available information that is necessary to provide quality health care.

After initial data have been gathered, the patient's vital signs, height, and weight are assessed. Then the physician examines the patient and records the information obtained. In this chapter the components of taking a medical history and interviewing patients, as well as rules for charting, measuring vital signs, and recording height and weight, are discussed. Chapter 36 includes a more detailed discussion of assisting with physical examinations, along with more detail about types of medical records.

Interviewing the Patient

A patient's medical history provides information about current and past illnesses and treatments that the physician utilizes to provide care. Figure 35-1 is an example of a health history form. Information gathered during the initial interview forms the basis of this vital document.

PRIVACY

The patient is entitled to privacy during the interviewing process. The federal government's Health Insurance Portability and Accountability Act (HIPAA) mandates that facilities make every effort to preserve confidentiality of patient information. The Patient's Bill of Rights reminds health care workers that patients have the right to respectful, considerate care. The interview should be done in an area that ensures privacy and freedom from interruption. Patients may feel more comfortable sharing details about their health and private life if they have a sense of confidentiality and privacy.

EFFECTIVE COMMUNICATION

The goal of the patient interview is to obtain information about the patient's condition while establishing rapport and

Pearson Physicians Group
123 Michigan Avenue
Parker Heights, IL 30310
(312)-123-1234

Patient Health History

Name: _____   Date: _____
SSN: _____   Birth date: _____

What is the reason for your visit today? (Please describe problem in detail including history of present illness):
_____
_____

Medical History: Please check all that apply to you:

❑ Arthritis	❑ Epilepsy/seizures	❑ Kidney disease	❑ Psychiatric disease
❑ Cancer	❑ Heart problems	❑ Liver disease	❑ Stroke
❑ Depression	❑ Heart surgery	❑ Measles	❑ Thyroid
❑ Diabetes	❑ High blood pressure	❑ Mumps,	❑ Hepatitis
❑ AIDS	❑ Chicken pox	❑ Rheumantic fever	❑ HIV positive
❑ Anemia bleeding disorder	❑ Gall bladder disease	❑ Scarlet fever	❑ Other
❑ Tuberculosis	❑ Typhoid fever		

Please list any medications you are taking with done and frequency:

Drug	Dose/Frequency
_____	_____
_____	_____
_____	_____
_____	_____

Please list any allergies that you have: _____
_____

Please list past surgeries with approximate date: _____
_____

Please describe any serious injuries you have had: _____
_____

FIGURE 35-1   Patient health history form.

Patient Health History

Please check any problems or conditions, that you are experiencing or have experienced.

General Health
❑ Good general health
❑ Recent weight change
❑ Loss of appetite
❑ Fatigue
❑ Fever/chills

Allergy
❑ Drug allergies
❑ Food allergies
❑ Hay fever
❑ Other:

Ears, Nose, Mouth, Throat
❑ Difficulty swallowing
❑ Earaches
❑ Loss of hearing/deafness
❑ Loss of smell
❑ Loss of taste
❑ Painful chewing
❑ Ringing in ears
❑ Sinus infection
❑ Sores in mouth
❑ Other:

Skin
❑ Rash or itching
❑ Sun sensitivity
❑ Hair loss
❑ Color changes
❑ Other:

Genitourinary
❑ Blood in urine
❑ Female: irregular periods
❑ Female: #pregnancies
   #miscarriages
❑ Female: vaginal discharge
❑ Kidney stones
❑ Male: prostate disease
❑ Male: testicle pain
❑ Painful or burning urination
❑ Sexual difficulty
❑ Sexually transmitted disease
❑ Urgency with urination
❑ Urine retention/incontinence
❑ Other:

Gastrointestinal
❑ Blood in stools
❑ Increasing constipation
❑ Nausea
❑ Painful bowel movements
❑ Persistent diarrhea
❑ Stomach or abdominal pain
❑ Ulcer
❑ Vomiting
❑ Other:

Heart and Lungs
❑ Pain in chest
❑ High blood pressure
❑ High cholesterol
❑ Irregular heart beat
❑ Other:

Muscle/Joints/Bones
❑ Back pain
❑ Difficulty walking
❑ Joint pain
❑ Joint stiffness or swelling
❑ Muscle pain or tenderness
❑ Neck pain

Psychiatric
❑ Depression
❑ Anxiety
❑ Eating disorder
❑ Other:

Eyes
❑ Blind spots
❑ Blurred vision
❑ Double vision
❑ Loss of vision
❑ Glaucoma
❑ Injury
❑ pain
❑ Other:

Neurofogical
❑ Balance problems
❑ Black outs/loss of
   consciousness
❑ Difficulty speaking
❑ Difficulty walking
❑ Facial drooping
❑ Headaches
❑ Injury to the brain or spine
❑ Light-headed or dizziness
❑ Memory loss
❑ Mental confusion
❑ Migraines
❑ Mini stroke
❑ Neuropathy
❑ Numbness or tingling
❑ Paralysis
❑ Stroke
❑ Tremors
❑ Weakness
❑ Other:

Pulmonary
❑ Asthma
❑ Blood in cough
❑ Cancer
❑ Chronic or frequent cough
❑ Emphysema
❑ Pneumonia
❑ Shortness of breath
❑ Other:

Social History:
Do you drink alcohol? ❑ Yes ❑ No   If yes, how much/week? _____

Do you smoke? ❑ Yes ❑ No   If yes, how many cigarettes/day? _____

Do you consume caffeine? ❑ Yes ❑ No   If yes, how many cups/week? _____

Do you use recreational drugs? ❑ Yes ❑ No   If yes, what type and frequence? _____

Are you on a special diet? ❑ Yes ❑ No   If yes, please describe? _____

Family History: Do you know of any blood relative who has or had:
❑ Asthma
❑ Aneurysm
❑ Brain Tumor
❑ Cancer, Type:
❑ Diabetes
❑ Epilepsy/Seizures

❑ Headaches
❑ Heart Problems
❑ High blood pressure
❑ Kidney disease
❑ Lung Disease
❑ Migraine

❑ Multiple Sclerosis
❑ Psychiatric Disease
❑ Stroke
❑ Thyroid

FIGURE 35-1 (Continued)

a positive relationship. Review Chapter 5 regarding communication techniques, styles, barriers, and questioning skills before continuing with this chapter.

Follow these steps in interviewing a patient:

- Review the patient's chart before meeting the patient and plan the interview.
- Greet the patient by name (Mrs. Jones) and give your name.
- Maintain a professional demeanor.
- Ask permission to interview the patient to help him or her feel more in control.
- Use icebreaker comments to help put the patient at ease (e.g., about the weather, sports, etc.).
- Provide privacy during the interview.
- Be aware of verbal and nonverbal cues.
- Avoid making judgmental responses.
- Avoid providing medical assurances.
- Treat sensitive topics with respect, keeping in mind cultural and personal biases.
- Summarize important points.
- Document the interview according to facility policy.

Correct Documentation

A patient's chart is a vital document and an integral part of their health care. Chapter 13 presented different methods for documentation. Regardless of the method used, the following guidelines must be followed when recording information in a patient's medical record. Refer to Box 35-1 for the six C's of charting and a summary of charting guidelines.

- Record the date and time of every entry (although the time may not be required in the medical office, it is in hospital and ambulatory care settings).
- Write legibly.

- Use permanent dark ink.
- Use medical terminology and accepted abbreviations.
- Use correct spelling.
- Sign every entry.
- Accurately document information (stick to facts, not opinions).
- Document the proper sequence in which events occurred.
- Document appropriate information concerning health and care given.
- Be concise.
- Correct errors only by drawing a single line through the incorrect entry and initialing it. Then record the corrected entry.

Measuring Weight and Height

Weight and height are two important measurements, even though they are not considered vital signs in the true sense of the term. Weight and height are anthropometric measurements since they relate to **anthropometry**, the science of size, proportion, weight, and height.

Weight and height can provide indications of a person's general health. Infants who fail to gain weight or fail to thrive need close supervision of weight gains and losses. The diagnosis of hormonal imbalances in children resulting in abnormal growth patterns can be picked up through routine comparisons of the child's height and weight against national growth charts. See Chapter 40 for measuring height, weight, chest, and head circumference in infants and small children.

Diabetic patients, pregnant women, cardiac patients, patients with fluid retention, and patients suffering from eating disorders such as bulimia and obesity also need to be monitored frequently for weight gain and loss.

Box 35-1 The Six C's of CHARTING

To better recall the guidelines for charting, remember the six C's:

1. *Client's* own words must be used exactly and in quotes.
2. *Clarity* must be achieved when recording information, using proper spelling and medical terminology and abbreviations.
3. *Completeness* is essential for all information recorded in the medical record.
4. *Conciseness* of the entry saves writing and reading time and chart space.
5. *Chronological* order of information is imperative.
6. *Confidentiality* of patient information is mandatory in every aspect of patient care.

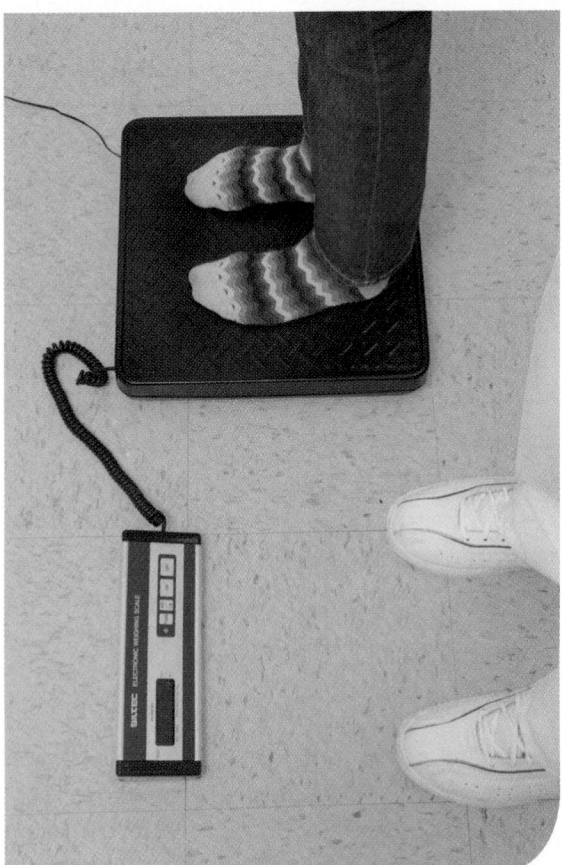

FIGURE 35-2 Upright scale.

WEIGHT

Patients prefer privacy when having their body measurements taken. They can remain fully clothed for this procedure. Indicate on the medical record if measurements were taken with clothes on or off. Patients are weighed and measured with shoes off. A paper towel is placed on the scale to protect the patient's feet.

Scales may be calibrated in either kilograms (metric weight) or pounds (Figure 35-2). In some cases, a scale will have a ruled panel that can be flipped up to reveal both pounds and kilograms. However, the medical assistant must know how to do conversions from pounds into kilograms and vice versa. Table 35-1 contains conversion charts to be used when converting a weight from kilograms to pounds or from pounds to kilograms. Patients who cannot stand may be weighed on a chair or bed scale (Figure 35-3). Procedure 35-1 lists the steps for obtaining the weight and height of a patient.

HEIGHT

The patient's height is measured without shoes with the heel, buttocks, and back of head touching the measuring stick or bar. The L-shaped arm is raised and lowered until it rests on the top of the head, not on the top of the hair. The

TABLE 35-1 Conversion Chart for Pounds and Kilograms

TO CONVERT KILOGRAMS TO POUNDS (kg to lbs)

1 kilogram (kg) = 2.2 pounds (lbs)

Multiply the number of kilograms by 2.2 lbs. *Example:* If a patient weighs 64 kilograms, multiply 64 by 2.2.

64 × 2.2 = 140.8 or 141 pounds

TO CONVERT POUNDS TO KILOGRAMS (lbs to kg)

1 pound = 0.45 kilograms

Multiply the number of pounds by 0.45. *Example:* If a patient weighs 130 pounds, multiply 130 by 0.45.

130 × 0.45 = 58.5 or 59 kilograms

---

height is then taken and may be recorded in inches and feet or centimeters. To convert inches and feet to centimeters, multiply by 2.5. To convert centimeters to inches, divide by 2.5. Older patients and women should be measured yearly to observe for signs of osteoporosis.

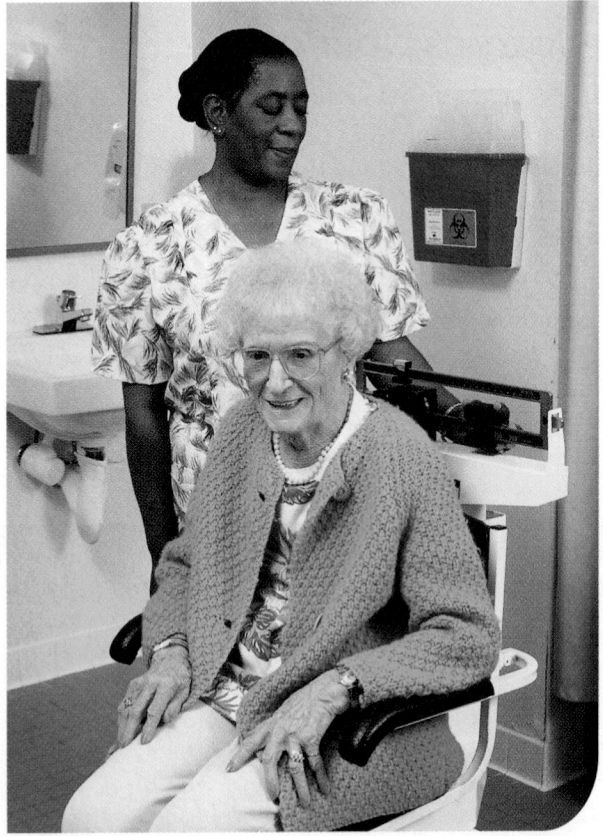

FIGURE 35-3 Patients unable to stand are often weighed while seated in a chair.

procedure
35-1

MEASURING ADULT WEIGHT AND HEIGHT
Objective: Obtain height and weight measurements and perform math conversions.

EQUIPMENT AND SUPPLIES
balance scale with bar to measure height; paper towel; pen; patient record

METHOD
1. Perform hand hygiene.
2. Identify the patient.
3. Explain the procedure to the patient.
4. For patients who wish to remove shoes, place a paper towel on the scale. Heavy objects such as keys should be removed, and female patients should set aside their purses.
5. Set all the weights to zero. Balance the scale by adjusting the small knob at one end until the balance bar pointer floats in the center of the frame. (A coin can be used to make this adjustment.)
6. Assist the patient onto the scale.
7. Ask the patient to stand still.
8. First move the large weight into the groove closest to the weight you estimate for the patient. If the balance bar pointer touches the bottom of the bar, then move the large weight back one notch. Move the small weight by tapping it gently until it reaches a point in which the pointer floats in the center of the frame.
9. Leave the weights in place.

CONTINUE WITH HEIGHT
10. Ask the patient to place his or her back to the scale, stand erect, and look straight ahead.
11. Raise the height bar in a collapsed position making sure the tip is over the patient's head.
12. Open the bar into the horizontal position and bring it down gently to touch the top of the patient's head. Leave this setting in place (Figure 35-4).
13. Assist the patient in stepping off the scale.
14. Read the weight scale by adding the number at the large weight to the number behind the small weight to the nearest $\frac{1}{4}$ pound. For example, 150 pounds at the large weight and $23\frac{1}{2}$ pounds at the small weight totals $173\frac{1}{4}$ pounds.
15. Record this measurement on the patient's record.
16. Read the height as marked behind the movable level of the ruled bar. Record this measurement to the nearest

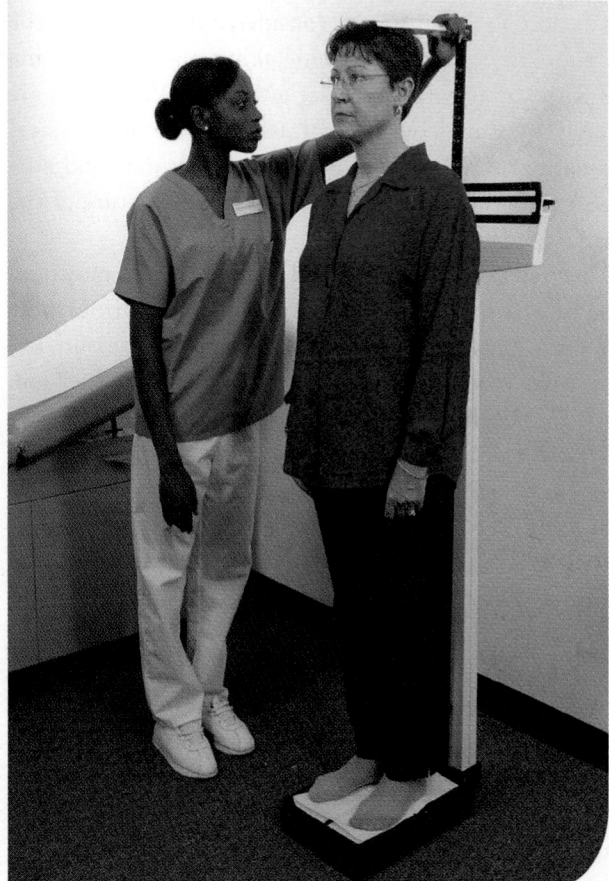

FIGURE 35-4 The height bar attached to the scale is used for measuring adult and child height.

$\frac{1}{4}$ inch on the patient's record. (Chart height in feet and inches. Convert inches to feet by dividing by 12.)
17. Return the weights to zero and the height bar to the normal position.
18. Discard paper towel.
19. Perform hand hygiene.

CHARTING EXAMPLE
2/14/XX 8 A.M. wt. $140\frac{1}{4}$ lbs with shoes; ht. 5'7" = 67 inches · · ·
· M. King, CMA (AAMA)

Vital Signs

A healthy human body regulates itself. **Vital signs** are indicators of the body's ability to maintain homeostasis. Temperature (T), pulse (P), respiration (R), and blood pressure (BP) measurements are considered vital signs because they measure some of the body's vital functions and provide necessary information about the patient's physical well-being. These measurements demonstrate the healthy functioning of the body. Vital signs must be calculated with utmost accuracy. Pain is considered by many to be the fifth vital sign, with assessment taking place at the same time as the other vital signs are evaluated. Vital signs are routinely measured by medical assistants before physical examinations. Care must be taken to be accurate and efficient so the reading or results reflect a true picture of the patient's condition.

When temperature, pulse, and respirations are measured at the same time, it is referred to as *TPR*. During some office visits, only one of the vital signs may be measured—for example, blood pressure in a patient with hypertension. Factors influencing readings and procedures with step-by-step instructions for accurately and efficiently measuring vital signs are thoroughly presented.

All health care professionals are required to use standard precautions to maintain infection control while measuring vital signs. The details of standard precautions are not repeated for each procedure in this text. The medical assistant is expected to know and continually apply the techniques recommended by the Centers for Disease Control and Prevention (CDC), as discussed in Chapter 34.

Along with the physiology behind body temperature, pulse rate, respirations, blood pressure, and measurement of weight and height, this chapter presents the normal or average readings for all vital signs at varying ages. Different methods and types of equipment for measuring temperature, pulse rate, respirations, and blood pressure are addressed, along with guidelines and ways for choosing the best methods and equipment.

Temperature

An understanding of the way the body maintains a balance between the amount of heat produced and the amount of heat lost is important for the medical assistant. Other factors that inform and assist the medical assistant to measure temperature accurately include knowledge of normal readings, factors that influence readings, how to select and use the proper thermometer, and how to clean and care for equipment.

PHYSIOLOGY OF BODY TEMPERATURE

Body temperature is regulated through balancing the amount of heat produced in the body with the amount of heat lost from the body. **Metabolism** is the sum of all biochemical and physiological processes that take place in the body. These processes produce heat and are needed to grow and maintain life. The hypothalamus, a portion of the brain that controls autonomic nervous system functions, is able to adjust the body temperature as the need for more or less heat production occurs during the day. For example, when a jogger is running on a hot day, the body's cooling mechanism reacts to this by creating perspiration, which evaporates and removes some of the excess heat the jogger experiences. Heat is also lost from the body through radiation, the transfer of heat from one object to another; by convection, the dispersion of heat by air currents; and by conduction, transfer of heat from a hotter molecule or body to a cooler molecule or substance (e.g., a patient with high fever is placed in cool water).

TEMPERATURE: NORMAL VALUES AND TERMS

The average body temperature of a healthy person is 98.6°F (37°C), and may vary by 1°F (0.6°C) either up or down during the day. There is normally only a 1°F to 2°F variance throughout the day. Although a slight variance in body temperature (diurnal rhythm) is not a cause for alarm, it is important to remember that greater variations from normal body temperature are often the first sign of illness or disease. Body temperature is lowest on rising in the morning and rises in late afternoon. Table 35-2 describes some causes of variations in body temperature.

Always be alert for all causes of changes in body temperature. For example, an infant's elevated temperature during an examination may be due to the infant's crying and not due to an illness. Always ask whether the patient has taken aspirin or Tylenol, both of which lower the temperature. Older adults who normally have body temperatures below normal may be ill even when their temperature is within a normal range for adults.

FAHRENHEIT AND CELSIUS CONVERSIONS

The Fahrenheit (F) scale of temperature measurement is widely used throughout the United States. However, some physicians use the Celsius (or centigrade) (C) scale. Figure 35-5 shows examples of Fahrenheit and Celsius in nonmercury thermometers. To convert degrees Fahrenheit to Celsius, subtract 32 and then multiply by 5/9. To convert

TABLE 35-2 Factors Affecting Body Temperature

Cause	Description
Time of day	Body temperature is lower in the morning on waking, when metabolism is still slow. The lowest body temperature is between 2:00 A.M. and 6:00 A.M. The highest body temperature usually occurs in the evening between 5:00 P.M. and 8:00 P.M. Daily variation in oral temperature can range from 97.6°F to 99.6°F (36.4°C to 37.3°C).
Age	Infants and children normally have a higher body temperature than adults due to immature heat regulation. Children often spike a fever late in the day. Older adults usually have lower-than-normal body temperature.
Gender	Women may experience a slight increase in body temperature at the time of ovulation.
Physical exercise	Body temperature will rise with exercise due to increased muscle contraction.
Emotions	Emotions such as crying and anger can cause an increase in body temperature.
Pregnancy	An increase in metabolism during pregnancy may cause the body temperature to rise.
Environmental changes	Hot weather can cause serious consequences in older adults whose bodies are unable to regulate body temperature due to a decreased metabolism. Exposure to cold may lower body temperature.
Infection	An elevated temperature may be one of the first signs of an infection. A fever is the body's way of fighting or killing off infectious organisms.
Drugs	Drugs may increase muscular activity or metabolism, which in turn increases temperature. Antipyretic (fever-reducing) drugs such as aspirin lower the above-normal temperature.
Food	The process of eating may also raise the body temperature. Fasting decreases metabolism, which will lower body temperature.

degrees Celsius to Fahrenheit, multiply by 9/5, and then add 32. See Figure 35-6 for a Fahrenheit/Celsius conversion chart and Table 35-3 for temperature scale conversion formulas and examples.

Fever

Fever or **pyrexia** is a body temperature above 100.4°F (38°C), at which point the body is producing greater heat than it is losing and is **febrile**. Absence of a fever is **afebrile**. When the body temperature exceeds 105.8°F (41°C), a serious condition known as **hyperpyrexia** or **hyperthermia**

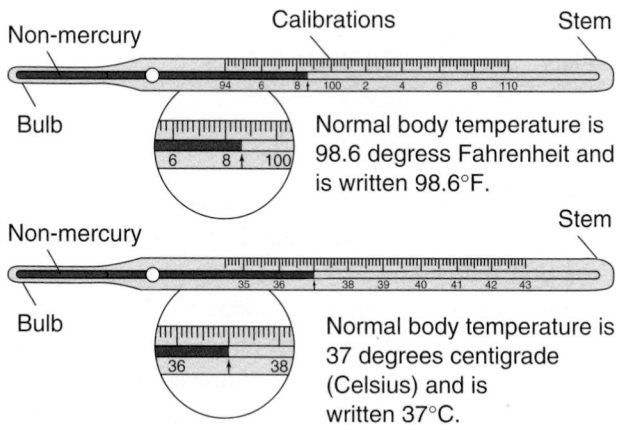

FIGURE 35-5 Fahrenheit and centigrade thermometers.

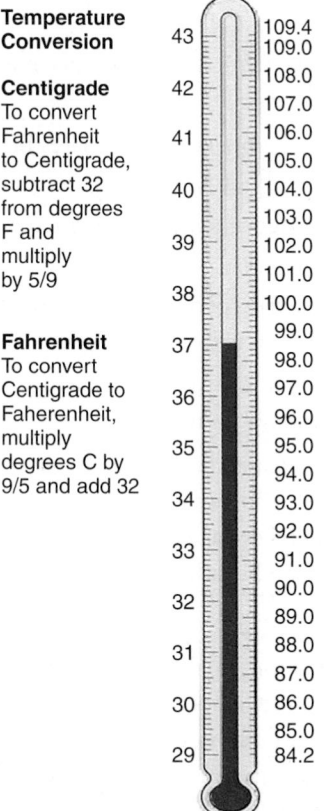

FIGURE 35-6 Fahrenheit/centigrade conversion.

Table 35-3 Temperature Conversions

- To convert Celsius to Fahrenheit:
  Fahrenheit degrees = (Celsius degrees × 9/5) + 32
- To convert Fahrenheit to Celsius:
  Celsius degrees + (Fahrenheit degrees − 32) × 5/9
Examples of Celsius and Fahrenheit readings in degrees:

Celsius (C)	Fahrenheit (F)
35.0	95.0
35.5	95.9
36.0	96.8
36.5	97.7
37.0	98.6 (normal oral)
37.5	99.5
38.0	100.4
38.5	101.3
39.0	102.2
39.5	103.1
40.0	104.0
40.5	104.9
41.0	105.8

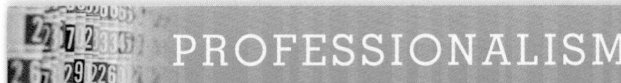

PROFESSIONALISM

THE LAW

The medical assistant has an ethical responsibility to use careful, proper technique when performing procedures to measure vital signs since an incorrect reading could lead to misdiagnosis and result in serious consequences for the patient. Proper technique, to name just a few specifics, includes allowing enough time for the temperature to register, using a watch with a second hand when taking pulse and respiration, and never guessing the time when measuring pulse and respirations. Incorrect documentation of vital signs can lead to serious complications for the patient and legal consequences for the physician and the medical assistant.

develops. Temperatures at this level may result in seizures in infants and small children. Body temperature above 109.4°F (43°C) is usually fatal. It can be a result of hyperthermia. There are four common types of fevers:

- **Intermittent fever**—body temperature alternates between fever and normal or subnormal
- **Remittent fever**—wide range of temperature fluctuations over a 24-hour period
- **Relapsing fever**—short febrile periods of a few days with a few days of normal temperature readings
- **Constant fever**—body temperature fluctuating a small amount but always above normal

Clinical signs of fever include increased heart rate, increased respiratory rate, shivering, chills, and sweating. Hyperthermia symptoms include cessation of sweating, loss of coordination, drowsiness, convulsions, and death.

Hypothermia

The reverse of a fever is a subnormal temperature or **hypothermia**. This occurs when the temperature falls below 97°F (36°C). At this point, the body is losing more heat than it is producing. This occurs in cases of exposure and near-drowning in cold water. In general, a temperature below 93.2°F (34°C) is fatal. Clinical signs of hypothermia

are decreased pulse and respirations; pale, waxy, cool skin; lack of muscle coordination; and drowsiness progressing to coma and death.

SITES FOR MEASURING BODY TEMPERATURE

Body temperature can be measured in a variety of ways, including oral (mouth), aural (ear) or tympanic membrane, axillary (under the arm), rectal (rectum), and temporal artery (forehead). Oral and rectal temperatures measure the body's core temperature, whereas tympanic membrane, axillary, and temporal artery are more variable but are acceptable for tracking significant changes.

Normal Values

The normal temperature based on statistical averages for each of the sites where temperature can be measured is:

Oral	98.6°F (37°C)
Rectal	99.6°F (37.6°C)
Axillary	97.6°F (36.4°C)
Ear (aural)	98.6°F (37°C)
Temporal artery	98.6°F (37°C)

As these figures indicate, the temperature obtained through the rectal method registers 1°F (or 0.6°C) higher than the oral temperature. Axillary temperatures register 1°F (0.6°C) lower than oral temperatures. The medical assistant must document where the temperature was measured—for example, rectally by the abbreviation "R," axillary by the abbreviation "AX," or temporal artery by the abbreviation "TA."

Oral

The oral method of temperature measurement is commonly used. Some facilities do not require the designation "O" when documenting this measurement, and others do require it. There is a potential for error with this method, however, because the patient may not form a tight closure over the thermometer. This allows air to enter the mouth and give a false temperature reading. The thermometer is inserted under the tongue on either side of the **frenulum linguae**, the longitudinal fold of mucous membrane. For an accurate measurement, the patient must be advised not to talk during the procedure. Oral temperature should only be measured if 15 minutes have passed since the patient has taken fluids or smoked.

Aural (Eardrum)/Tympanic Membrane

One of the newer technologies for accurate temperature measurement involves the aural site. This method uses the tympanic membrane area at the end of the external auditory canal for an instantaneous temperature measurement. The tympanic membrane thermometer provides a closed cavity within the easily accessible ear. The aural method is considered to be an accurate means of temperature measurement. Tympanic membrane thermometers are able to detect heat waves in the ear canal and calculate body temperature from the data. This method also poses fewer problems with standard precautions.

Axillary

The axillary (under the arm) method has proven to be the least accurate of the temperature measurement sites. It is the recommended site for small children unable to understand how to hold an oral thermometer in their mouth if a tympanic membrane thermometer is not available. The axillary site is recommended for patients who have had oral surgery, any situation in which the patient may bite the oral thermometer, and mouth-breathing patients. The axillary temperature reading is affected by perspiration. The underarm area should be dry for an accurate reading.

Rectal

The rectal method is considered more reliable than the oral method. The mucous membrane lining of the rectum does not come into contact with air, which could interfere with accuracy, as do the oral and axillary routes. The rectal route is advised for unconscious patients, infants, small children, and mouth-breathing patients. The rectal method should be avoided when there is a danger of rectal wall perforation.

Temporal Artery

Temporal artery measurement is a new noninvasive procedure involving a device that measures the temperature over the temporal artery. The temporal artery is located close to the skin surface on the forehead and temple area. When the temporal artery probe/scanner is passed over the surface of the forehead toward the temple it can read the peak arterial temperature value, which is then recorded as the body temperature. It is fast and fairly accurate. A number of commercial devices are available to measure the temporal artery temperature.

Use the guidelines given in Table 35-4 to determine which method to use when measuring a patient's body temperature.

TABLE 35-4 Selecting a Method for Measuring Body Temperature

Method	Advisable	Inadvisable
Oral	Most adults and children who are able to follow instructions	Patients who have had oral surgery, mouth sores, dyspnea; uncooperative patients; patients on oxygen; infants and small children; patient's with facial paralysis or nasal obstruction
Rectal	Infants and small children; patients who have had oral surgery; mouth-breathing patients; unconscious patients	Active children; fragile newborns
Axillary	Small children	Patients who cannot form an airtight seal around the thermometer
Tympanic (aural)	Small children	Patient with in-the-ear hearing aids or ear infections
Temporal artery	Infants and small children; patients who have had oral surgery; mouth-breathing patients; unconscious patients	Active children; fragile newborns

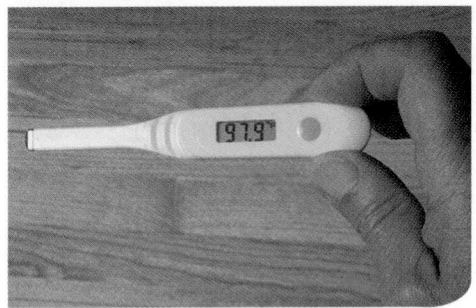

FIGURE 35-7 Digital electronic thermometer.

TYPES OF THERMOMETERS

Several types of thermometers are available for measuring body temperature: non-mercury glass, electronic, tympanic membrane, temporal artery, and chemical disposable thermometers. Figure 35-7 is an example of an electronic digital thermometer.

Mercury thermometers are no longer widely used in the health care environment due to the potential danger of mercury and the frequency of breakage. Mercury is toxic and can be harmful to humans and animals. In 2002 the American Hospital Association (AHA) agreed to eliminate mercury from the health care environment. Many hospitals have either replaced mercury containing devices or labeled them for proper handling. Some cities have banned the sale of mercury thermometers and some areas have thermometer exchange programs, in which an individual brings in a mercury thermometer and is given a non-mercury one in exchange. This book uses non-mercury thermometers in its discussion of assessing body temperatures.

Non-Mercury Thermometers

Though electronic thermometers are most widely used, non-mercury thermometers may still be utilized in some office settings. Non-mercury thermometers are available in two shapes to measure temperature using the oral, rectal, and axillary methods. Mercury has been replaced by safer chemicals, and glass has been replaced by plastic in many cases.

The oral thermometer has a long, slender tip that fits easily under the tongue. A thermometer with a stubby or pear-shaped tip is available that can be used for taking oral, axillary, and rectal temperatures. Some thermometers may have a blue dot that indicates the thermometer is for oral use or a red dot that indicates for rectal use.

The shaft or stem of the thermometer is calibrated in tenths (0.2, 0.4, 0.6, and so on) of degrees, with each short line representing two-tenths (0.2) of a degree. A whole degree is marked with a long line. The even-numbered degrees are printed on the thermometer. The average normal body

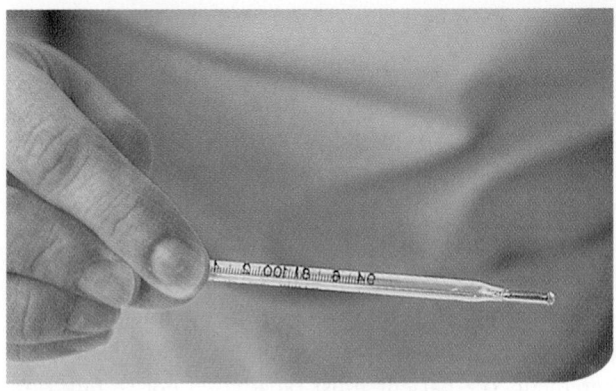

FIGURE 35-8 Non-mercury clinical thermometer.

temperature (98.6°F or 36°C) is indicated by an arrow on the thermometer.

When reading the thermometer, it should be held between the thumb and index finger, at eye level, by the stem end (Figure 35-8). While looking at the edge of the thermometer, keep the lines at the top of the edge and the numbers at the bottom. The stem is then gently rotated until the silver column can be seen in the middle of the lines and numbers. The point where the silver line stops is read for the body temperature at each 0.2 of a degree. When the silver line appears between two markings, the temperature is read at the next higher 0.2 of a degree.

The temperature reading is then recorded. The temperature must be carefully charted with absolute accuracy. Always record tenths of degrees of temperature in even numbers when using a non-mercury thermometer.

Thermometer Sheaths. Plastic disposable slip-on sheaths are available to use with both oral and rectal non-mercury thermometers (Figure 35-9). The sheath comes in a small

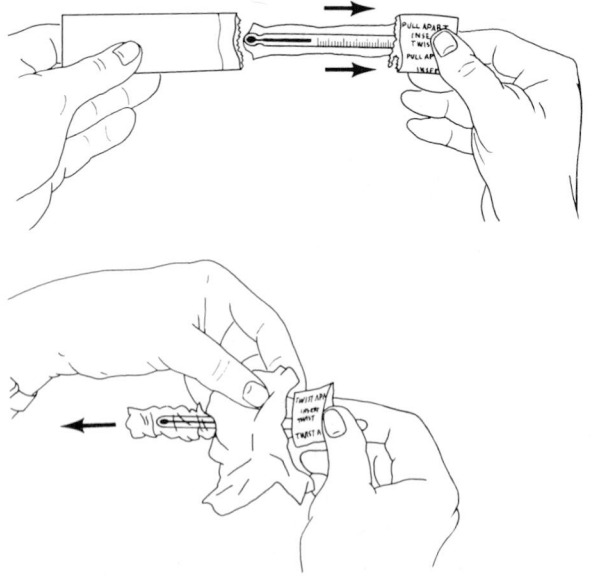

FIGURE 35-9 Thermometer sheath.

Date	TPR	Initials
9/9/09	100⁶ Ⓡ - 72 - 20	BF

FIGURE 35-10 Charting temperature.

paper envelope and slips over the tip of the thermometer. The sheath provides a sanitary protective covering and is discarded after use. When using a rectal thermometer, a lubricant is always used over the sheath for ease of insertion into the rectum. The sheath is removed from the thermometer by pulling on the tear tab, which inverts the plastic and thus protects the medical assistant's hands from coming into contact with contamination. Remove and properly dispose of the sheath in a hazardous waste container. After the temperature is read, clean and disinfect the thermometer.

A rectal thermometer has a small, round bulb that is inserted gently into the rectum. This thermometer may be marked "For Rectal Use" on its stem and have a red dot to indicate that the rectal route should be used. It is not safe to use an oral thermometer to take a rectal temperature because the long slender tip may injure tender rectal mucous membranes or may break off in the rectum. Figure 35-10 provides an example of how to chart temperature readings.

Cleaning and Storing Non-Mercury Thermometers. The non-mercury thermometer must be cleaned and soaked in a disinfectant after each use. The thermometer is then stored in a proper container.

Electronic or Digital Thermometers

The electronic thermometer is considered accurate, easy to read, sanitary, and fast, and it requires no cleaning or disinfection. Electronic thermometers are battery operated with

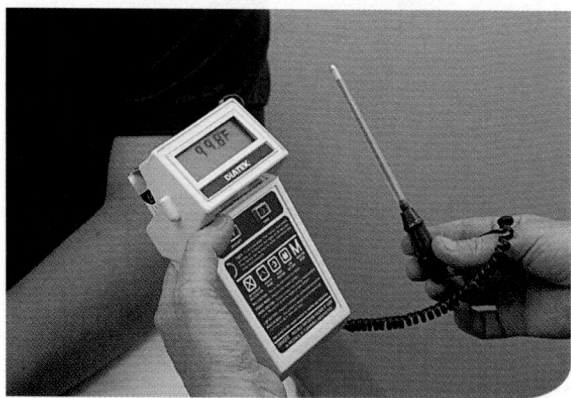

FIGURE 35-11 Electronic thermometers have a large window, making them easy to read.

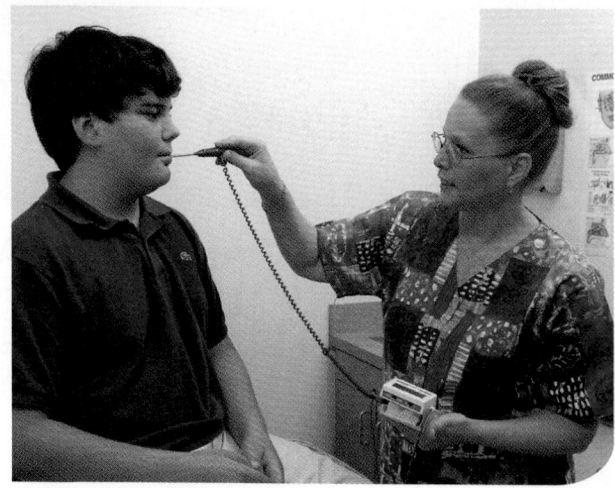

FIGURE 35-12 The disposable cover or sheath provides sanitary protection for the patient.

digital windows for easy viewing and reading (Figure 35-11). This type of thermometer plugs into a base receptacle and has an electronic metal probe containing a heat sensor that can accurately register body temperature within a few seconds.

The metal probe is color coded: blue for oral, and red for rectal. The probe is attached to the battery unit by a flexible cord. A nonflexible plastic disposable cover fits over the probe to provide each patient with a sanitary thermometer (Figure 35-12). This plastic-covered probe is inserted under the patient's tongue or rectally like a non-mercury thermometer. The medical assistant will hold the thermometer in place since the reading is performed quickly. The unit will emit a signal when the temperature has registered. The plastic probe shield is then popped into a biohazard waste container and the probe is replaced into the battery-powered storage unit. Procedure 35-2 provides the steps for measuring an oral temperature with a electronic or digital thermometer.

The electronic thermometer can be used for oral, rectal, and axillary body temperature readings. The blue oral probe is generally used for taking oral and axillary temperatures. Rectal temperatures, taken using the red probe, require lubrication on the tip of the probe. The electronic method of obtaining a rectal temperature is the most widely used form. The rectal probe is inserted $\frac{1}{2}$ inch into the adult rectum and $\frac{1}{4}$ inch into a child's rectum. The probe may have to be angled slightly to ensure contact with the rectal mucosa.

These units are time saving but expensive. They are used in medical offices, hospitals, and clinics, but rarely by patients in their homes due to cost. The battery-operated unit must be readjusted at intervals to maintain accuracy.

MEASURING ORAL TEMPERATURE USING AN ELECTRONIC OR DIGITAL THERMOMETER

Objective: Accurately perform all steps of the procedure and provide an accurate temperature reading.

EQUIPMENT AND SUPPLIES

electronic or digital thermometer (rechargeable); probe cover; waste container; pen; patient's chart

METHOD

1. Perform hand hygiene.
2. Assemble equipment.
3. Identify the patient and explain the procedure.
4. Remove the thermometer unit from the base and attach the probe (blue for oral).
5. Remove the thermometer probe from the holder.
6. Insert the thermometer probe into the disposable tip box to secure the tip (Figure 35-13A).
7. Insert into the patient's mouth on either side of the frenulum linguae and instruct the patient to close mouth.
8. When temperature signal is seen or heard, remove the thermometer from the patient's mouth and read the result in the LED window.
9. Dispose of the thermometer tip in a waste container. (Figure 35-13B)

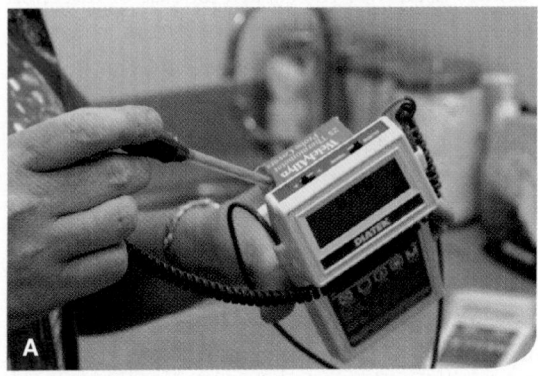

10. Return the thermometer probe to the storage place (Figure 35-13C).
11. Replace the unit on the rechargeable base.
12. Perform hand hygiene.
13. Document the results.

CHARTING EXAMPLE

07/25/XX 4 P.M. T 99.6R · · · · · · · · · · · · · · · · E. Leonard, RMA

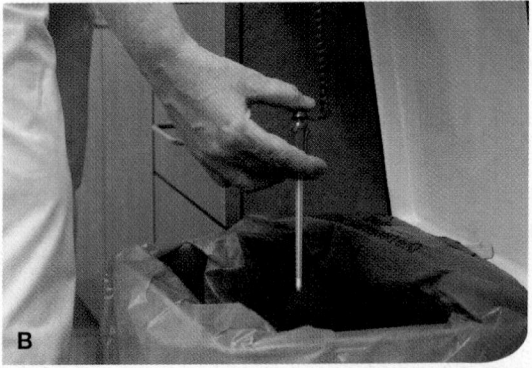

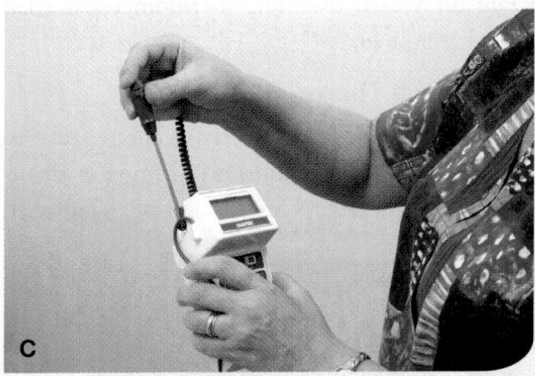

FIGURE 35-13 (A) Insert the thermometer probe into the disposable tip box to secure a tip; (B) after measuring temperature, press to eject the probe cover; (C) replace the probe in the holder.

The unit should always be returned to the charging stand after each use to maintain the battery. Procedure 35-3 provides the steps for measuring a rectal temperature with a digital or electronic thermometer.

Axillary Temperature

The axillary area under the arm is easily accessible and offers no possibility of rectal perforation or broken oral thermometers. It is used in assessing body temperature in newborns,

procedure
35-3

MEASURING RECTAL TEMPERATURE USING AN ELECTRONIC THERMOMETER

Objective: Accurately perform all steps of the procedure and provide an accurate temperature reading.

EQUIPMENT AND SUPPLIES

electronic thermometer; red (rectal) probe; disposable thermometer sheath; disposable gloves; patient's record; paper and pen/pencil; tissue; watch with second hand; water-soluble lubricant; biohazard waste container

METHOD

1. Perform hand hygiene.
2. Apply gloves.
3. Identify the patient.
4. Explain the procedure. If the patient is a child, explain the procedure to both the parent and child.
5. Instruct the patient to remove appropriate clothing so that the rectal area can be accessed. Provide privacy for the patient.
6. Assist the patient onto the examining table and cover with a sheet or drape.
7. Instruct the patient to lie on the left side with top leg bent (Sim's position).
8. Remove the electronic thermometer from the base and place a cover on the probe.
9. Place a small amount of lubricant on a tissue. Dip the probe in the lubricant.
10. With one hand raise the upper buttock to expose the anus or anal opening.
11. If unable to see the anal opening, ask the patient to bear down slightly. This will expose the opening.
12. With the other hand, gently insert the lubricated thermometer $1\frac{1}{2}$ inches into the anal canal (Figure 35-14). Do not force the thermometer into the anal canal. Rotating the thermometer may make insertion easier.
13. Hold the thermometer in place until the result is signaled.

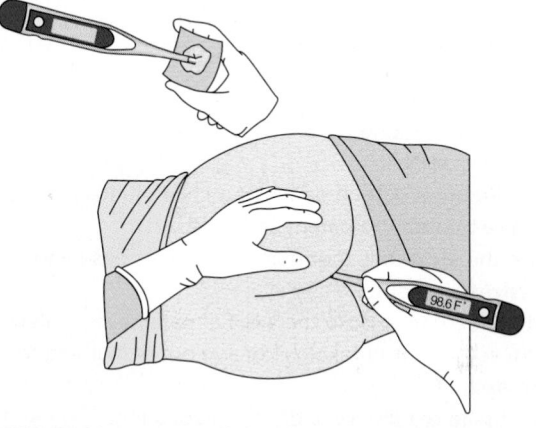

FIGURE 35-14 **Insert the probe cover approximately $1\frac{1}{2}$ inches into the anus.**

14. Withdraw the thermometer.
15. Dispose of the probe cover in a biohazard waste container.
16. Wipe the anus from front to back to remove any excess lubricant.
17. Assist the patient from the examination table. Instruct the patient to dress, and assist the patient if necessary.
18. Remove gloves and place in a biohazard waste container.
19. Perform hand hygiene.
20. Record the temperature in the patient's record using (R) to indicate a rectal reading.

CHARTING EXAMPLE

2/14/XX 4:00 P.M. Temp. 99.6°R · · · · · · · M. King, CMA (AAMA)

---

infants, children, and adults with jaw impairments or surgery and those who are irrational. The process for measuring axillary temperature is given in Procedure 35-4.

Tympanic Membrane Thermometers

The tympanic membrane thermometer is used for an aural temperature. The **tympanic membrane thermometer** or aural thermometer is so named because it is able to detect heat waves within the ear canal and near the eardrum. The thermometer calculates the body temperature from the energy generated by these heat waves. Figure 35-16 shows an example of a tympanic membrane thermometer, and Procedure 35-5 lists the steps required to obtain a temperature reading using such a thermometer. It is important to note that the ear canal

MEASURING AXILLARY TEMPERATURE

Objective: Accurately perform all steps of the procedure and provide an accurate temperature reading.

EQUIPMENT AND SUPPLIES

electronic thermometer and probe; paper and pen/pencil; patient's record; tissue; watch with second hand; biohazard waste container

METHOD

1. Perform hand hygiene.
2. Identify the patient.
3. Explain the procedure. If patient is a child then explain procedure to both the parent and child.
4. Remove the electronic thermometer from its base and place cover on probe.
5. Ask the patient to expose the axilla. If patient is an infant or child, ask parent to take child's arm out of clothing to expose axilla.
6. Using a tissue pat the axilla dry of perspiration.
7. Place the probe with cover into the axillary space (Figure 35-15A).
8. Ask the patient to remain still and hold the arm tightly next to the body while the temperature registers.
9. When the thermometer beeps, remove thermometer and discard the probe in a waste container (Figure 35-15B).
10. The medical assistant can take pulse and respirations while the patient is holding the thermometer under the axilla.
11. Return the thermometer to the storage base.
12. Record the temperature in patient's record.
13. Perform hand hygiene.

CHARTING EXAMPLE

2/14/XX 4:00 P.M. Temp. 97.0° AX · · · · · M. King, CMA (AAMA)

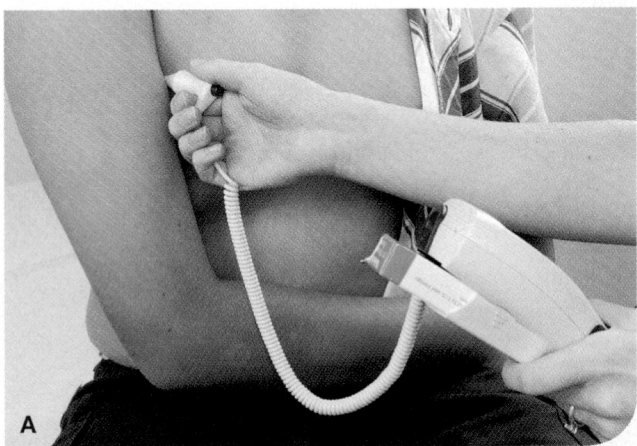
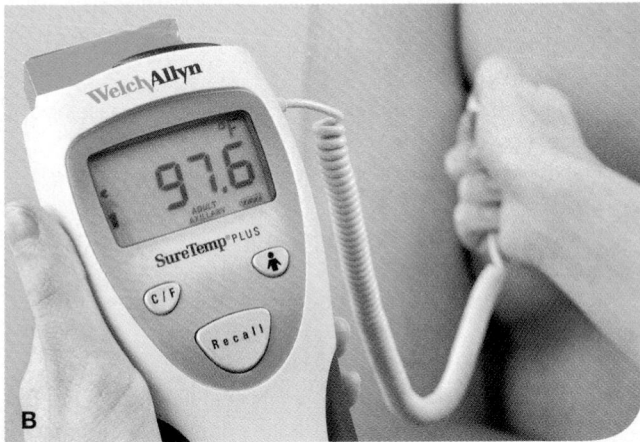

FIGURE 35-15 (A) With the thermometer in the axilla, the arm should be down and the forearm should be crossed on the chest; (B) axillary temperatures are generally 1°F below the average body temperature.

---

should be straightened when using a tympanic membrane thermometer. This is done by pulling the outer ear upward and out for adult patients or pulling the outer ear downward and back for young children.

Disposable Thermometers

There are several types of disposable thermometers. A chemical disposable thermometer uses liquid dots or heat-sensitive bars or patches applied to the forehead. They change color to indicate body temperature. Some are single use and others may be reused several times. Procedure 35-6 lists the steps to measure body temperature using a heat-sensitive wearable thermometer. Figure 35-18 shows an example of a disposable thermometer with chemical dots. The reading is taken by noting the highest reading among the dots that have changed color. Figure 35-19 shows

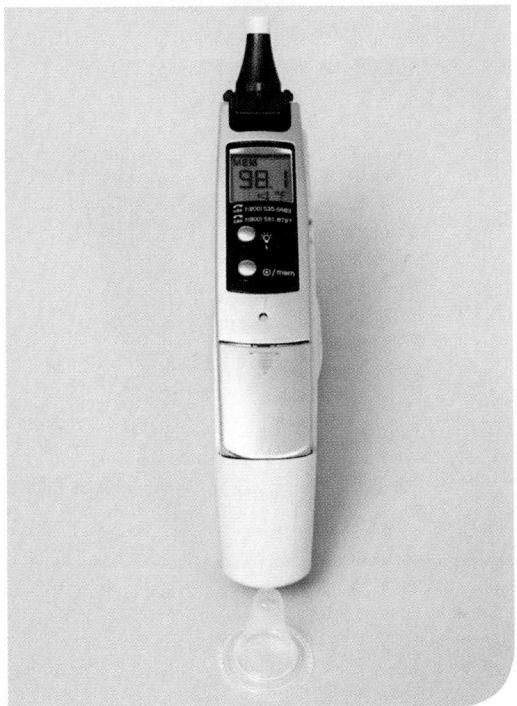

FIGURE 35-16 An infrared tympanic membrane thermometer used to measure the tympanic membrane temperature.

temperature-sensitive tape being used to measure temperature. It is held in place for about 15 seconds and is read by the color change on the strip. Both of these methods are excellent when dealing with small children or large numbers of patients who need to be evaluated.

Temporal Artery Thermometers

A temporal artery (TA) thermometer is a scanner that when stroked gently across the forehead measures the heat emitted through the skin from the temporal artery below. The instrument actually takes a large number of readings per second and selects the most accurate. These devices are being used in facilities to replace the tympanic membrane thermometer, which tends to be inaccurate if positioning in the ear canal is inconsistent. TA thermometers are available commercially for home use.

Arterial temperature is close to rectal temperature, about one degree higher than oral temperature, and two degrees higher than axillary temperature. TA readings are not affected by factors such as smoking, drinking, or coughing that may interfere with oral measurement.

When measuring TA temperature assess the side of the head that is exposed, not the side covered by hair or resting on a

procedure 35-5

MEASURING TEMPERATURE USING AN AURAL (TYMPANIC MEMBRANE) THERMOMETER

Objective: Accurately perform all steps of the procedure and provide an accurate temperature reading.

EQUIPMENT AND SUPPLIES

tympanic membrane thermometer; disposable protective probe cover; paper and pen/pencil; patient record; biohazard waste container

METHOD

1. Perform hand hygiene.
2. Identify the patient.

Note: To avoid error, call the patient by name and check against the name on the patient's record.

3. Explain the procedure to patient.
4. Remove the thermometer from its base. The display will read "Ready."
5. Attach a disposable probe cover to the earpiece.

6. With one hand, gently pull upward on the patient's outer ear if an adult or pull back and downward if an infant or child (Figure 35-17A).
7. Gently insert the plastic-covered tip of the probe into the ear canal (Figure 35-17B).
8. Press the scan button, which activates the thermometer.
9. Observe the temperature reading in the display window.
10. Gently withdraw the thermometer.
11. Eject the used probe cover into a biohazard waste container by pressing the eject button.
12. Record the temperature using the designation indicating a tympanic membrane temperature (T).
13. Return the tympanic membrane thermometer to its base.

CHARTING EXAMPLE

10/23/XX 4:00 P.M. Temp. 99.2°F(T) · · · · M. King, CMA (AAMA)

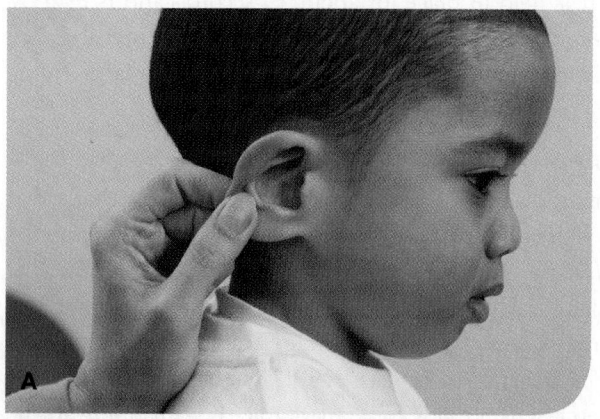
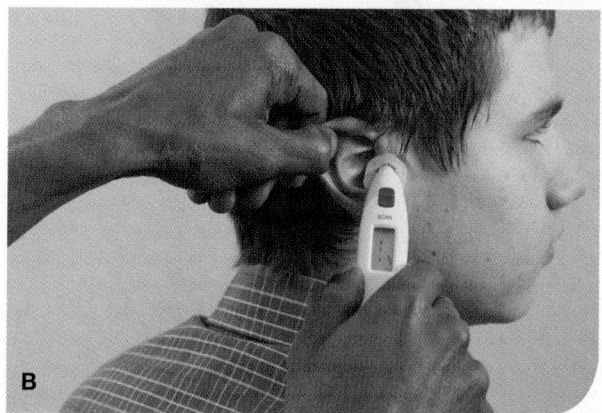

FIGURE 35-17 (A) Pull the pinna back and down for a child under age 3; (B) place probe in client's ear and advance into ear canal to make a firm seal.

procedure

35-6

MEASURING TEMPERATURE USING A HEAT-SENSITIVE WEARABLE THERMOMETER

Objective: Accurately perform all steps of the procedure and provide an accurate temperature reading.

EQUIPMENT AND SUPPLIES

wearable heat-sensitive thermometer (chemical strip, liquid crystal); paper and pen/pencil; patient's record; tissue; watch with second hand; biohazard waste container

METHOD

1. Perform hand hygiene.
2. Assemble the equipment.
3. Identify the patient.
4. Explain the procedure.
5. Dry the patient's forehead.
6. Place the thermometer strip on the forehead.
7. Read the correct temperature by reading color changes. See Figure 35-18 and Figure 35-19 for examples of heat-sensitive thermometers.

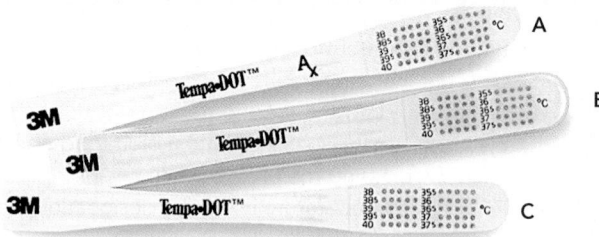
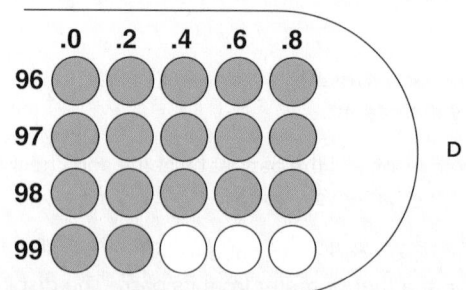

FIGURE 35-18 Disposable thermometers with chemical dots. (A) Axillary (marked with "AX"); (B) Rectal (with plastic cover); (C) Oral; (D) enlargement showing a reading of 99.2°F. *Courtesy of 3M Medical Division—3M Health Care.*

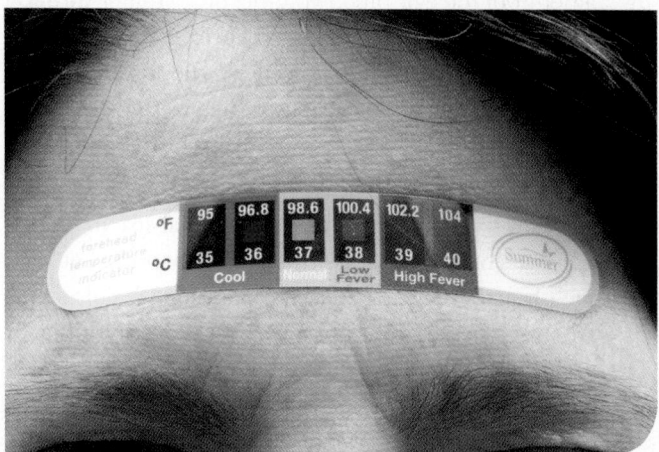

FIGURE 35-19 Temperature-sensitive skin tape.

8. Record the temperature.
9. Discard strip.
10. Perform hand hygiene.

CHARTING EXAMPLE
07/11/XX 9:08 A.M. 99.0°F (chemstrip). ·······L Kenney, RMA

pillow. The latter may cause a higher reading because heat is not allowed to dissipate. Slide the thermometer in a fairly straight line across the forehead midway between the eyebrows and the upper hairline. At this point the TA is less than two millimeters below the surface of the skin. Do not slide it down the side of the face. The TA thermometer is quick, accurate, noninvasive and easy to use. Procedure 35-7 lists the steps to measure body temperature using a TA thermometer.

procedure 35-7

MEASURING TEMPERATURE USING A TEMPORAL ARTERY THERMOMETER

Objective: Accurately measure body temperature using a temporal thermometer.

EQUIPMENT AND SUPPLIES
paper and pen/pencil; patient's record; temporal artery thermometer

METHOD
1. Perform hand hygiene.
2. Assemble the equipment.
3. Identify the patient.
4. Explain the procedure.
5. Brush aside the patient's hair.
6. Place the probe flush on the center of the forehead and depress the red button. See Figure 35-20 for placement of the probe at the start and at the conclusion of the procedure.
7. Keep the button depressed and slowly slide the probe on the midline across the forehead to the hairline.
8. Lift the probe from the forehead and touch it on the neck just behind the earlobe.
9. Release the button and read the temperature.
10. Record the results in the patient's record.
11. Perform hand hygiene.

CHARTING EXAMPLE
12/18/XX 10 A.M. T 100°F (TA) ······ L. Cohen, CMA (AAMA)

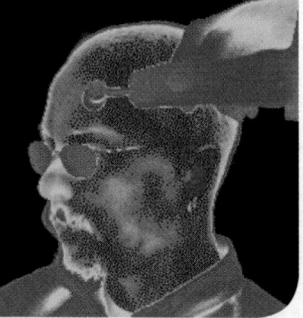 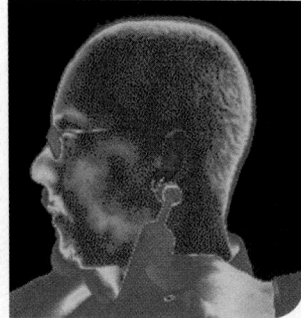

FIGURE 35-20 Positioning the temporal artery thermometer to start on the left; position at the conclusion of the procedure on the right. *Copyright © Exergen Corporation. All rights reserved.*

Pulse

Pulse rate is a measurement of the number of times the heart beats per minute (bpm). It is the wave of blood created each time the left ventricle of the heart contracts. Between contractions the heart rests. Each pulse beat represents one cardiac cycle or one heartbeat. In a healthy person the heart normally beats around 70 times per minute. An increased oxygen requirement will cause an increase in heart rate and result in a faster pulse rate. For instance, a jogger starts out at a slow pace; as the pace increases, muscles will need more oxygen to produce energy, thus the heart rate (pulse) will increase as will the rate of breathing (respiratory rate). A pulse rate above 100 bpm is **tachycardia**; a rate below 60 bpm is referred to as **bradycardia**.

FACTORS INFLUENCING PULSE RATE

The pulse rate is influenced by numerous factors, including exercise, age, gender, size, physical conditions, disease states, medications, and feelings such as depression, fear, anxiety, and anger. Table 35-5 describes factors that influence pulse rate, and Table 35-6 lists average pulse rates for different age groups.

CHARACTERISTICS OF PULSE RATE

Four characteristics must be noted and recorded when observing pulse rate: rate, volume, rhythm, and compliance of the arterial wall:

1. Rate describes the number of pulse beats per minute.
2. **Volume**, or force, refers to the strength of the pulse. This is noted as a full or **bounding pulse**, indicating an increase in blood volume; a strong or normal amount of force or blood volume; or a weak or **thready pulse**, indicating a barely perceptible force or blood volume. Volume is influenced by the forcefulness of the heartbeat, the condition of the arterial walls, and dehydration. A variance in intensity of the pulse may indicate heart disease.
3. **Rhythm** refers to the regularity, or equal spacing, of all the beats of the pulse. Normally, the intervals between each heartbeat are of the same duration. A pulse with an irregular rhythm is known as a **dysrhythmia** or **arrhythmia**. The irregular rhythm may be random irregular beats or a predictable pattern of irregular beats. It is not considered abnormal if the heart occasionally skips a beat. This is referred to as an **intermittent pulse**. Exercise or drinking a caffeine-rich beverage may cause this to occur. When arrhythmia occurs on a consistent basis, it may indicate heart disease and should be brought to the attention of the physician. If an irregular pulse is detected, the apical pulse should be assessed. In addition, the physician may want to order an electrocardiogram (ECG) to further assess the arrhythmia.
4. Compliance of the arteries refers to their ability to expand and relax. The condition of the arterial wall should be felt as elastic and soft. With age, arteries lose their elasticity and greater force is required to pump the blood into the arteries. A pulse taken in a blood vessel that feels hard and ropelike is considered abnormal and may indicate heart disease such as arteriosclerosis.

TABLE 35-5 Factors That Influence Pulse Rate

Exercise	Activity increases body's requirements. Rate may increase 20–30 bpm.
Age	As age increases, pulse rate decreases. Infants and children have a faster pulse rate than adults.
Gender	Female pulse rate is about 10 bpm higher than a male of the same age.
Size	Pulse rate is proportionate to the size of the body. Heat loss is greater in a small body, resulting in the heart pumping faster to compensate. Larger males will have slower pulse rates than smaller males. During sleep and rest, the pulse rate may drop to 50–60 bpm.
Physical condition	Athletes and people in good physical condition have lower pulse rates. The lower rate is due to a more efficient circulatory system. Pulse rate of 60 or below can be normal for athletes.
Disease conditions	Pulse rate is increased in thyroid disease, fever, and shock due to increased metabolism.
Medications	Many medications can either raise or lower the pulse rate. Medications such as digoxin are given to regulate the heartbeat. Caffeine and nicotine can increase the heart rate in certain people. Drugs used recreationally, such as cocaine and methamphetamine, increase the pulse rate.
Depression	May lower the pulse rate.
Fear, anxiety, anger	May raise the pulse rate.

TABLE 35-6 Average Pulse Rates by Age

Less than 1 year	120–160 bpm
2–6 years	80–120 bpm
6–10 years	80–100 bpm
11–16 years	70–90 bpm
Adult	60–80 bpm
Older adult	50–65 bpm

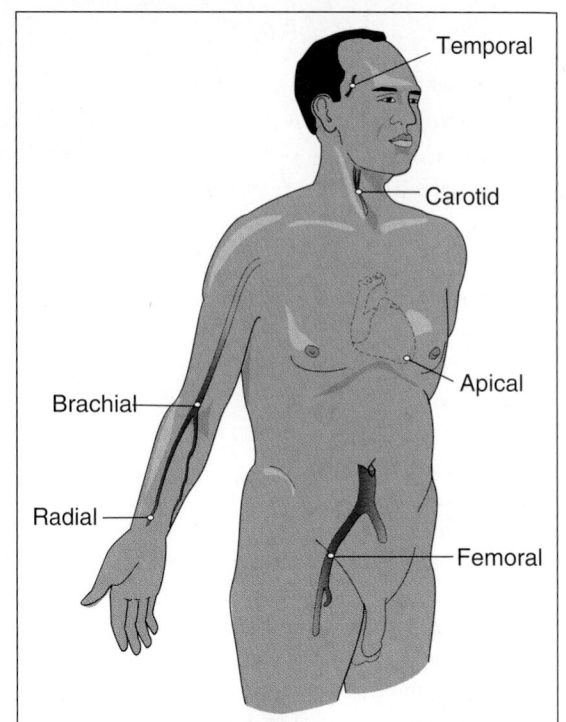

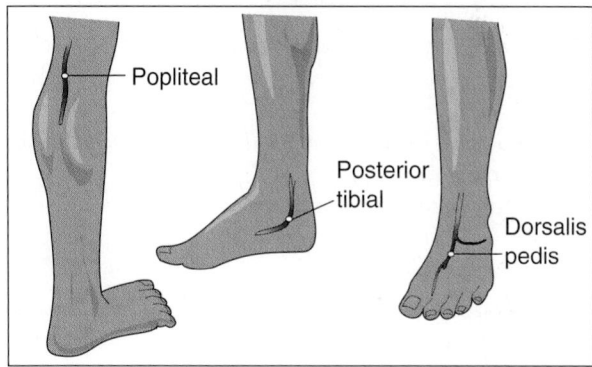

FIGURE 35-21 **Nine pulse sites on the human body.**

PULSE SITES

There are nine areas in the body where the pulse can be measured easily. These pulse sites are at the radial, brachial, carotid, temporal, femoral, popliteal, posterior tibial, dorsalis pedis, and apical arteries (Figure 35-21). Table 35-7 describes the nine common pulse sites.

Procedure 35-8 provides the steps for accurately measuring a radial pulse. Figures 35-23A–G illustrate the location of pulse sites on an actual patient.

APICAL HEART RATE

The **apical** heart rate is counted at the apex of the heart. It can only be heard with a stethoscope placed over the apex. This is considered to be a very accurate heart rate. The apical rate is taken in infants and young children. The physician may also request an apical rate be taken when a patient is on heart medications.

An apical–radial pulse rate may be taken to determine if there is a difference between the pulse rates taken at the two sites. An apical–radial pulse must be taken for a full minute.

TABLE 35-7 Location of Common Pulse Sites

Site	Location
Radial	Thumb side of wrist about 1 inch below base of thumb (most frequently used site)
Brachial	Inner (antecubital fossa/space) aspect of the elbow (pulse heard when taking BP)
Carotid	At side of neck between larynx and sternocleidomastoid muscle (pulse used in CPR; pressing both carotids at the same time can cause a reflex drop in BP and pulse)
Temporal	At side of head just above the ear
Femoral	In groin where femoral artery passes to leg
Popliteal	Behind the knee; pulse located deeply behind the knee and felt when knee is slightly bent
Posterior tibial	On medial surface of ankle near ankle bone
Dorsalis pedis	On top of foot slightly lateral to midline; helps assess adequate circulation to foot
Apical	At apex of heart left of sternum 4th or 5th intercostal space below the nipple

procedure
35-8

MEASURING RADIAL PULSE

Objective: Accurately perform all steps of the procedure and provide an accurate radial pulse reading.

EQUIPMENT AND SUPPLIES

paper and pen/pencil; patient's record; watch with second hand

METHOD

1. Perform hand hygiene.
2. Identify the patient.
3. Explain the procedure.
4. Ask the patient about any recent physical activity or smoking.
5. Ask the patient to sit down and place the arm in a comfortable, supported position. The hand should be at chest level with the palm down.
6. Place fingertips on the radial artery on the thumb side of the wrist (Figure 35-22).
7. Check the quality of the pulse.
8. Start counting pulse beats when second hand on watch is at 3, 6, 9, or 12.
9. Count the pulse for 1 full minute. The number will always be an even number.
10. Immediately write the pulse beats per minute on a piece of paper.
11. Perform hand hygiene.

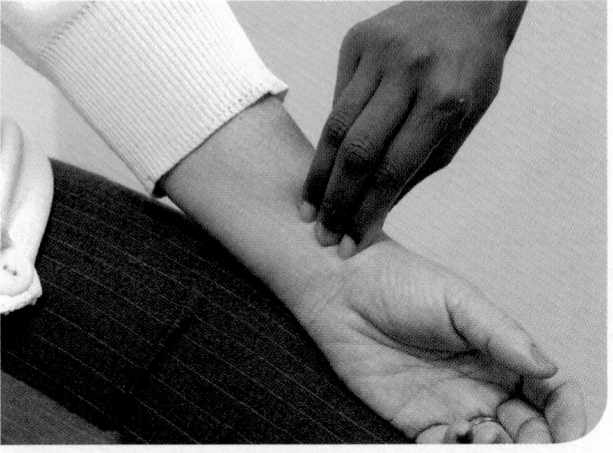

FIGURE 35-22   **Measuring a patient's radial pulse.**

12. Record the pulse beats per minute in patient's record, describing any abnormalities in pulse rate.

CHARTING EXAMPLE

2/14/XX 4:00 P.M. Pulse 72 (R) Regular and strong · · · · · · · · · ·
· M. King, CMA (AAMA)

Normally the pulse rates should be the same. The radial pulse is never greater than the apical pulse. The difference between the two readings is called the **pulse deficit**. Refer to Procedure 35-9 for taking an apical–radial pulse. This measurement requires two people: one to take the radial pulse and one to take the apical pulse. When only one person is doing the procedure, the apical pulse rate is taken first, then the radial pulse rate. When taking an apical–radial pulse, have only one person responsible for using the watch. This person will raise one finger or nod the head when counting begins and lower the finger or nod again when a minute has passed. Coordination of timing is good when using this method.

Respiration

Respiration, or the act of breathing, is the exchange of oxygen and carbon dioxide (CO_2) between the atmosphere and the body's cells. It consists of one expiration or exhalation

and one inspiration or inhalation. This is called the **respiratory cycle**. Respiratory rates indicate how well oxygen is provided to the tissues of the body.

PHYSIOLOGY OF RESPIRATION

During the process of inspiration, oxygen, which is necessary for body cells and life, is taken into the lungs. The diaphragm moves downward, intercostal muscles move outward, and the lungs expand in order to take oxygen into the lungs. During expiration, air containing carbon dioxide is expelled from the lungs as a waste product. The diaphragm moves upward, and the lungs deflate.

The respiratory process is both external and internal. The external respiratory process is an exchange of oxygen and carbon dioxide between the alveoli (the minute air sacs of the lungs) and the blood. The internal respiratory process takes place when blood in the capillaries comes into contact with

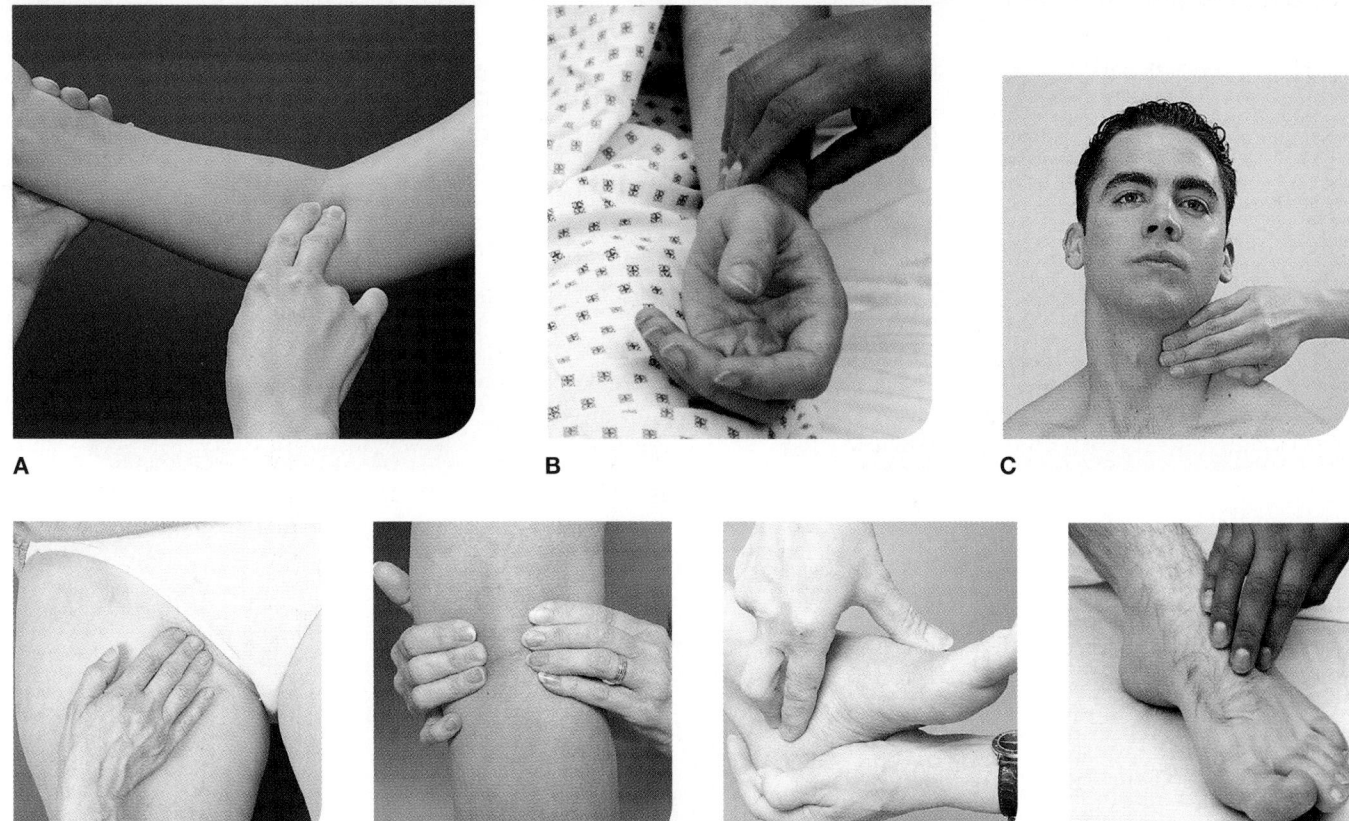

FIGURE 35-23 (A) Brachial pulse; (B) Radial pulse; (C) Carotid pulse; (D) Femoral pulse; (E) Popliteal pulse; (F) Posterior tibial pulse; (G) Dorsalis pedis pulse.

procedure 35-9

MEASURING APICAL–RADIAL PULSE (TWO PERSONS)

Objective: Accurately perform all steps of the procedure and provide an accurate apical–radial pulse reading.

EQUIPMENT AND SUPPLIES

stethoscope; alcohol wipe/cotton balls with 70 percent isopropyl alcohol; paper and pen/pencil; patient's record; watch with second hand

METHOD

1. Perform hand hygiene.
2. Prepare the stethoscope using alcohol wipe or cotton balls with alcohol on earpieces and diaphragm of scope.
3. Identify the patient.
4. Explain the procedure. If the patient is a child, explain the procedure to both the parent and child.
5. Uncover the left side of the patient's chest. Provide privacy with a drape, if necessary.

6. The first person places the earpieces of stethoscope in his or her ears, with opening in tips forward.
7. Locate the apex of patient's heart by palpating to the left fifth intercostal space (between fifth and sixth ribs) at the midclavicular line. This is found just below the nipple (Figure 35-24A).
8. Warm the chest piece by holding it in the palm of the hand before placing onto patient's chest.
9. The second person locates the radial pulse in the thumb side of wrist, 1 inch below base of thumb (Figure 35-24B).
10. The first person places the chest piece of the stethoscope at the apex of the heart. When the heartbeat is heard, a nod is made to the second person and counting

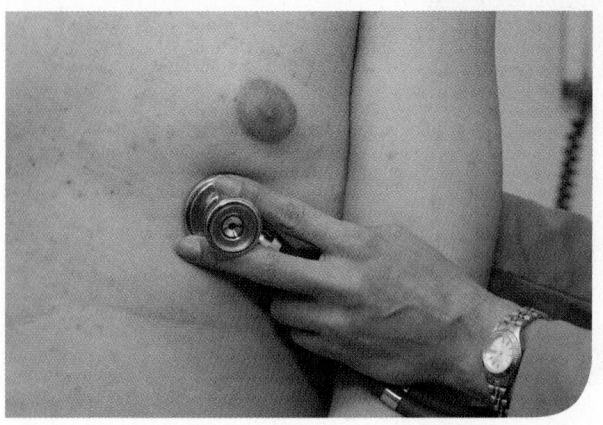

A

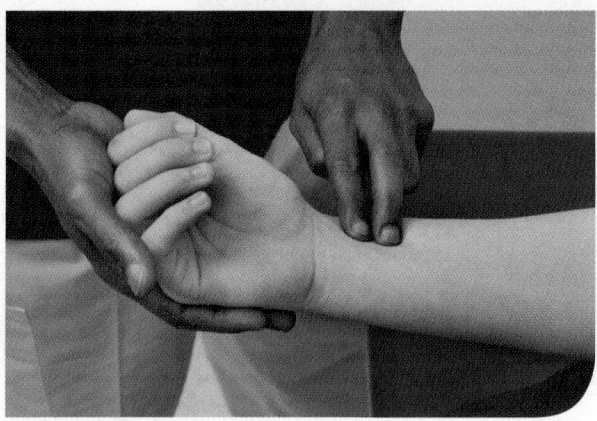

B

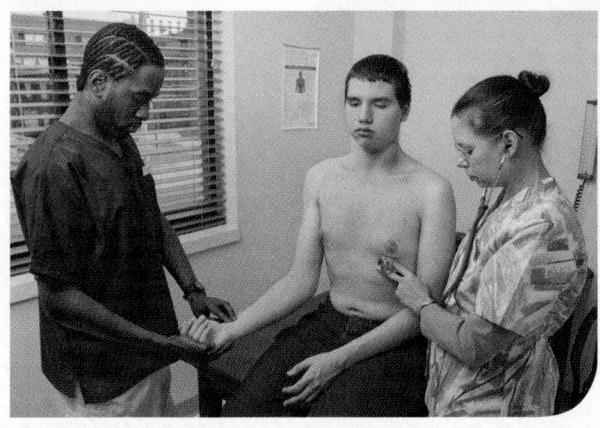

C

FIGURE 35-24 (A) The first medical assistant locates the apical pulse; (B) The second medical assistant locates the radial pulse site; (C) The counting begins when the heartbeat is heard.

begins. Ideally, the count should begin when the second hand is at 3, 6, 9, or 12 (Figure 35-24C).

11. Count for 1 full minute.

Note: Both systole and diastole (or lub/dub) count as one beat.

12. Remove the stethoscope and earpieces.
13. Record the rate and quality of heartbeats. Include both apical and radial rates using the designation "AP." Calculate the pulse deficit by subtracting the radial pulse rate from the apical pulse rate.

Note: A pulse deficit may indicate that the heart contractions are not strong enough to produce a palpable radial pulse.

14. Assist the patient with replacement of clothing, if necessary. Assist the patient from the examining table.
15. Wipe the earpieces and chest piece of the stethoscope with alcohol wipes or cotton balls and alcohol.
16. Perform hand hygiene.

CHARTING EXAMPLE
2/14/XX 4:00 P.M. 82/78 AP Pulse deficit 4. Quality of beat strong.
.... M. King, CMA (AAMA)

the alveoli, where it picks up oxygen and carries it to cells throughout the body. Carbon dioxide is thrown off as a waste product and then carried back to the lungs, where it is exhaled. The process then begins all over again with inhalation.

The medulla oblongata located in the base of the brain contains the respiratory, cardiac, and vasomotor centers.

When the medulla oblongata receives a message indicating there is a buildup of carbon dioxide, this message is translated by the brain into a need for increased respiration to occur. Breathing is actually controlled by the involuntary nervous system. However, breathing is also under some control of the voluntary nervous system.

Respirations are counted by watching, listening, or feeling the movement of inspiration and expiration on the patient's back, stomach, or chest. A stethoscope also may be used to assist with counting respirations.

CHARACTERISTICS OF RESPIRATION

When counting a patient's respiration rate, watch or feel the rise and fall of the chest. Each rise and fall constitutes one respiration. Do not take respiration measurements immediately after the patient has experienced exertion, such as climbing stairs, unless so ordered. Because patients have some control over their respiration, it is advisable to take a respiratory count without the patient's awareness. It is recommended that respirations be counted while appearing to count the pulse. This will result in a more accurate indication of the true respiratory rate.

The pulse and respiratory rate are usually taken at the same time. However, it is never permissible to take the respiratory rate and multiply it by four to estimate a pulse rate. Likewise the respiratory rate cannot be determined by dividing the pulse rate by four. When counting respirations several characteristics should be noted: rate, rhythm, depth, and quality or characteristics of breathing. Procedure 35-10 describes how to measure the patient's respirations.

Respiratory Rate

Rate refers to the number of respirations per minute and can be described as normal, rapid, or slow. The adult normal

procedure 35-10

MEASURING RESPIRATIONS

Objective: Accurately perform all steps of the procedure and provide an accurate respiration measurement.

EQUIPMENT AND SUPPLIES
watch with sweep second hand

METHOD
1. Perform hand hygiene.
2. Identify the patient.
3. Assist the patient into a comfortable position.
4. Place your hand on the patient's wrist in position to take the pulse, or place your hand on the patient's chest (Figure 35-25).
5. Count each breathing cycle by observing and/or feeling the rise and fall of the chest or upper abdomen.
6. Count for 1 full minute using a watch with a sweep second hand. If the rate is atypical or unusual in any way, take it for another minute.
7. Record the respiratory rate in the patient's record, noting the date, time, any abnormality in rate, rhythm, and depth, and your signature.

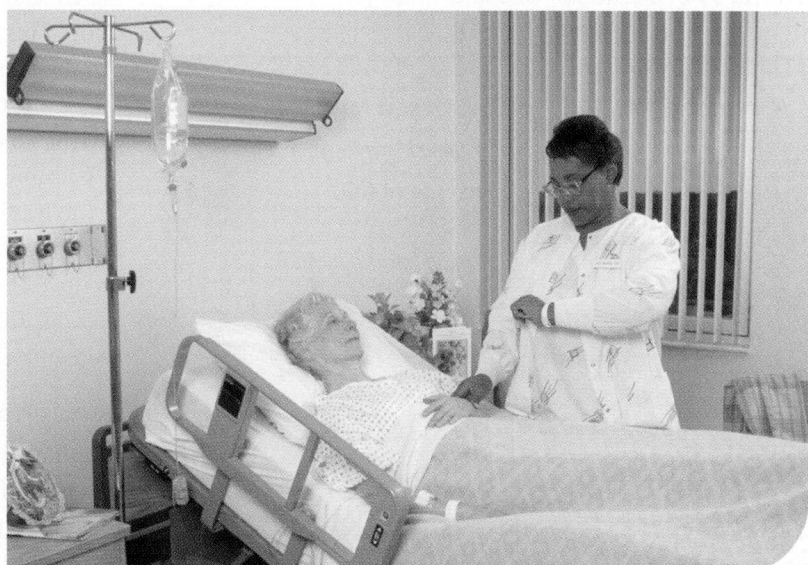

FIGURE 35-25 Place a hand on the chest when respirations are difficult to count. Patient must be unaware you are counting respirations.

CHARTING EXAMPLE
2/14/XX 4:00 P.M. Resp. 20 and regular · · · M. King, CMA (AAMA)

TABLE 35-8 Respiratory Rate Ranges of Various Age Groups

Newborn	30–50
1 year old	20–40
2–10 years old	20–30
11–18 years old	18–24
Adult	14–20

range of respirations is 14 to 20 cycles per minute. A respiratory rate of below 12 (**bradypnea**) or above 40 (**tachypnea**) in an adult should be considered a serious symptom. Rapid respirations are usually shallow in depth. **Apnea** means the absence of breathing for longer than 19 seconds, and **eupnea** means normal breathing.

Children, with an average of 30 to 50 cycles per minute, have a much more rapid rate of breathing than adults. Table 35-8 lists respiratory rates for various age groups. The respiratory rate is usually one-quarter of the pulse rate. Many factors affect the respiratory rate. Some of these include an elevated temperature, age, pain, and medical conditions such as asthma. An elevated temperature in both adults and children can result in an elevated respiratory rate. Extreme

TABLE 35-9 Situations Causing Changes in Respiratory Rate

Increased Rate	Decreased Rate
Allergic reactions	Certain drugs (e.g., morphine)
Certain drugs (e.g., epinephrine)	Decrease of CO_2 in blood
Disease (e.g., asthma, heart disease)	Disease (stroke, coma)
Exercise	
Excitement/anger	
Fever	
Hemorrhage	
High altitudes	
Nervousness	
Obstruction of air passage	
Pain	
Shock	

pain may also cause respirations to increase. The respiratory rate is also affected by both emotional and physical conditions. Table 35-9 lists situations that may cause an alteration in the respiratory rate.

Rhythm

Rhythm is the breathing pattern that occurs at either regular or equal spacing of breaths. In regular rhythm, inspirations and expirations should be the same in rate and depth. In an irregular breathing pattern, the amount of air inhaled and exhaled, and the rate of respirations per minute, will vary.

If the breathing rhythm appears irregular after 1 minute of observation, then respirations should be observed for several more minutes for comparison purposes. Patients with emphysema, an abnormal pulmonary condition, may experience no difficulty with inhalation but may struggle to fully exhale. Asthma may also cause an irregularity in breathing rhythm.

Depth

The depth of respiration refers to the volume of air inhaled and exhaled. It is described as either shallow or deep. Shallow respirations with a rapid rate occur in some disease conditions such as high fever, shock, and severe pain. **Hyperventilation** refers to deep rapid respirations, and **hypoventilation** refers to shallow respirations.

When a patient is unable to take in enough oxygen during inhalation, the skin and nail beds may appear bluish in color. This is called **cyanosis** and is due to the increase of carbon dioxide (CO_2) in the blood. In this situation, both the depth of respiration and cyanosis must be noted in the patient's record.

Chronic obstructive pulmonary disease (COPD) is one of the leading causes of disability and affects approximately 17 million Americans. Cigarette smoking, air pollution, and occupational exposure to dust and fumes are some of the leading causes of this disease. COPD results from chronic bronchitis, asthma, emphysema, or heart disease.

Respiratory Quality

Respiratory quality or character refers to breathing patterns that differ from normal effortless breathing. Labored breathing refers to respirations that require greater effort from the patient.

Breath Sounds

Normal respirations have no noticeable sound. Breath sounds occur in some disease conditions. Terms for describing breath sounds include the following:

Stridor—a shrill, harsh sound, heard more clearly during inspiration. This sound may be heard in children with croup and patients with laryngeal obstruction.

Stertorous sounds—noisy breathing sounds such as those heard in snoring.

Crackles or rales—crackling sounds resembling crushing tissue paper, caused by fluid accumulation in the airways and heard with some types of pneumonia.

Rhonchi (gurgles)—rattling, whistling sounds made in the throat; may be heard in a patient with a tracheostomy who requires suctioning of mucus.

Wheezes—high-pitched, whistling sounds made when airways become obstructed or severely narrowed, as in asthma or COPD.

Cheyne-Stokes breathing—irregular breathing that may be slow and shallow at first, then becomes faster and deeper, and may stop for a few seconds and begin the pattern again. This type of breathing may be seen in certain patients with cerebral, cardiac, or pulmonary diseases.

Bubbling breathing sounds—like gurgling sounds, as if air is passing through moist secretions in the respiratory tract.

PROFESSIONALISM THE LIFE SPAN

As a medical assistant you will be assessing vital signs on patients at either end of the age spectrum. The following are a few considerations to keep in mind when dealing with infants:

- If an infant is crying, all vital signs will be increased. Try to calm the infant with a pacifier.
- Always take the apical pulse in infants before taking the temperature. It is important to have an apical pulse baseline.
- In assessing the respiratory rate, try to calm the infant. Place your hand on the abdomen to feel inhalation and exhalation.
- To obtain BP readings, use a pediatric stethoscope with a small diaphragm; use the palpatory method if you cannot hear with the stethoscope.
- To obtain the temperature reading, use the axilla while holding the arm across the chest. If no ear infection is present, use the tympanic thermometer, remembering to pull the ear down and back to straighten the ear canal.

Blood Pressure

The measurement of blood pressure (BP) is an important vital sign to aid in diagnosis and treatment, and therefore it is taken routinely. Many medical conditions can be indicated by either a rise or fall in blood pressure. The condition of high blood pressure known as **hypertension (HTN)** is often **asymptomatic** (without any symptoms). An abnormal blood pressure reading can be the first indication of this condition. It is also known as essential HTN, whereas secondary HTN is due to an underlying cause such as renal disease, pregnancy, or an endocrine disorder. Symptoms of HTN are headache, blurred vision, chest pain, or no symptoms at all, which is why it is known as the silent killer. **Hypotension** is low blood pressure and may be due to emotional shock, trauma, and central nervous system disorders. Symptoms of hypotension are dizziness and **syncope** (fainting).

PHYSIOLOGY OF BLOOD PRESSURE

Blood pressure is actually caused by the action of the blood moving against the walls of the arteries. Blood is pushed out of the heart and into the aorta and pulmonary arteries as the ventricles contract. This, in turn, exerts continuous pressure on the walls of the arteries. Refer to Figure 35-26 to review the blood flow of the heart.

BLOOD PRESSURE READINGS

Blood pressure levels are taken at two different points called *readings.* The two blood pressure readings are **systolic blood pressure**, or the highest pressure that occurs as the left ventricle of the heart is contracting, and **diastolic blood pressure**, which is the lowest pressure level that occurs when the heart is relaxed (the ventricle is at rest). The pulse beat is felt at the systolic pressure level and is absent at the diastolic pressure level.

Blood pressure is read in millimeters (mm) of mercury (Hg). The abbreviations *mm* and *Hg* are not necessary when recording the blood pressure readings. The actual blood pressure is recorded using just the systolic or highest pressure reading, over the diastolic or lowest reading. For example, 120/80 would be considered a normal blood pressure reading for an adult.

Generally, a range of normal is used for blood pressure readings since slight variations can occur among normal healthy adults. A deviation, either a rise or fall, from the patient's baseline measurement of 20 to 30 mmHg can be significant for that patient.

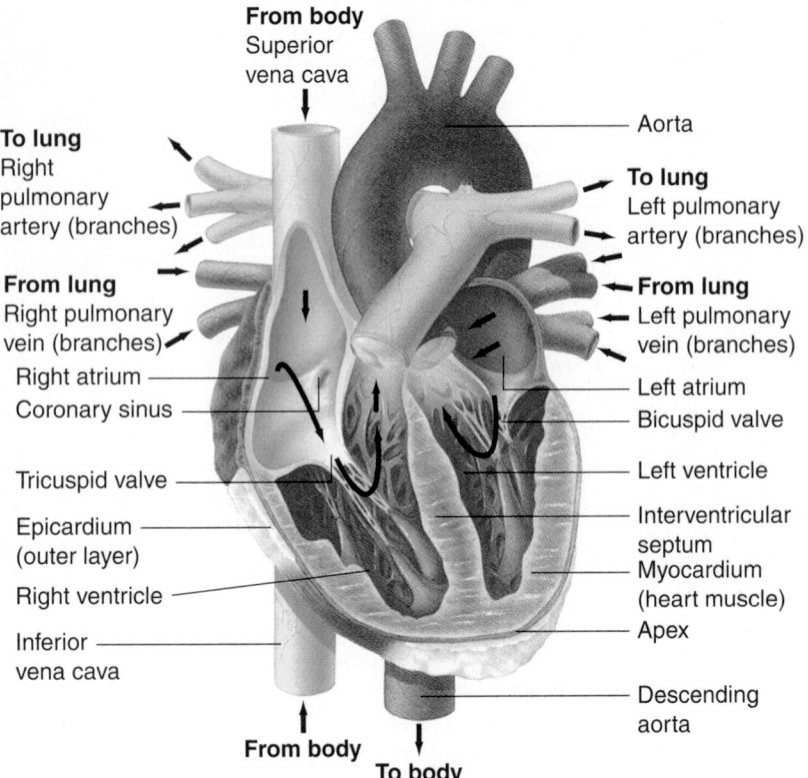

FIGURE 35-26 Circulation of blood through the heart.

Labels on figure:

From body
Superior vena cava

To lung
Right pulmonary artery (branches)

From lung
Right pulmonary vein (branches)

Right atrium

Coronary sinus

Tricuspid valve

Epicardium (outer layer)

Right ventricle

Inferior vena cava

From body

Aorta

To lung
Left pulmonary artery (branches)

From lung
Left pulmonary vein (branches)

Left atrium

Bicuspid valve

Left ventricle

Interventricular septum

Myocardium (heart muscle)

Apex

Descending aorta

To body

Pulse pressure is the difference between the systolic and diastolic readings. This is found by subtracting the diastolic reading from the systolic reading. A pulse pressure that is greater than 50 mmHg or less than 30 mmHg is considered to be abnormal. For instance, if the blood pressure is 130/82, the pulse pressure would be 48, which is still within the range considered normal. Extremes of pulse pressure can result in stroke or shock.

PROFESSIONALISM
THE WORKPLACE

Each medical assistant must have his or her own stethoscope to prevent the spread of infection among coworkers. A watch with a second hand is essential also.

Blood pressure readings should routinely be started at age 5 as part of the school physical or earlier if medically necessary. Patients should have a complete physical to see why their blood pressure is elevated. Patients with a sustained high blood pressure measurement may require further diagnostic evaluation for the presence of other disease conditions, as well as medication to lower the blood pressure. Controlling blood pressure can lower the incidence of stroke and heart attack.

If a patient's blood pressure deviates from the normal range, he or she should be tested again. Many patients experience "white coat syndrome." They are so apprehensive about visiting the physician and having blood pressure taken that the results are extremely elevated. Often these same individuals, when tested at home, are within the normal range. Being empathetic and sensitive to their problems may help you obtain a better reading. Ideally, blood pressure is taken while the patient is sitting with both feet flat on the floor because crossed knees may result in elevated readings. If the patient's condition warrants, blood pressure may be measured with the patient lying down but should be charted as such.

KOROTKOFF SOUNDS

Korotkoff sounds are the sounds actually heard as the arterial wall distends during the compression of the blood pressure cuff. The sounds were first classified into five different phases by Russian neurologist Nicolai Korotkoff.

When the blood pressure cuff is first inflated, no sound can be heard because the brachial artery is compressed. As air is slowly removed from the cuff during deflation, the Korotkoff sounds become audible. The deflation of air should be at the rate of 2 to 3 mmHg per heartbeat. The medical assistant should practice taking blood pressure readings slowly in order to be able to identify each phase. The systolic pressure is the first distinct clear tapping sound that is heard, and the diastolic pressure is the pressure at which the last sound is heard. Some facilities and physicians measure the diastolic pressure at the fourth Korotkoff phase where the sound changes from a clear tapping or thumping sound to a more muffled softer sound. When the fourth sound is used as the diastolic pressure, three readings are often made: systolic, first diastolic (fourth Korotkoff sound),

TABLE 35-10 Five Phases of Korotkoff Sounds

Phase I	This is the first faint sound heard as the cuff is deflated. Record this reading as the systolic pressure reading. The cuff must be inflated to a level high enough to hear this first sound during relaxation.
Phase II	The second phase occurs as the cuff continues to be deflated and blood flows through the artery. This sound has a swishing quality. The cuff has to be slowly deflated in order to hear this soft sound. An auscultatory gap is said to have occurred if there is a total loss of sound at this stage that reoccurs later. An auscultatory gap can occur in certain cases of heart disease and hypertension. An auscultatory gap should be reported to the physician.
Phase III	During this phase the sound will become less muffled and develop a crisp tapping sound as the blood flow moves easily through the artery. If the BP cuff was not inflated enough to hear the Phase I sound, then the Phase III sound may be heard and incorrectly stated as the systolic reading.
Phase IV	The sound will now begin to fade and become muffled. The American Heart Association, which believes Phase IV is the best indicator of the diastolic pressure, recommends the reading at this phase be recorded as the diastolic pressure for a child.
Phase V	Sound will disappear at this phase. Some physicians want both phase IV and phase V recorded for the diastolic pressure reading (e.g., 120/78/74 rather than 120/74).

and second diastolic (last sound). Korotkoff sounds are described in Table 35-10.

NEW GUIDELINES FOR BLOOD PRESSURE

In 2003 new guidelines for blood pressure were established in the Seventh Report of the Joint National Committee on the Prevention, Detection, Evaluation and Treatment of High Blood Pressure (JCN 7) published by the National Institutes of Health, U.S. Department of Health and Human Services. The normal blood pressure range for an adult should be 119/79 or below. Refer to Table 35-11 for the complete list of new values recommended by the JCN 7.

Average normal blood pressure readings are listed in Table 35-12. Although an average blood pressure is listed for a newborn, blood pressure readings are not generally taken on infants. Monitors are used on the very young.

FACTORS AFFECTING BLOOD PRESSURE

Physiological factors affecting blood pressure include volume or amount of blood in the arteries, peripheral resistance of the vessels, condition of the heart muscle, and elasticity of vessels. These four factors are discussed in Table 35-13.

Many other factors may affect blood pressure. Two of these are gender and age. Women generally have a lower blood pressure than men. Blood pressure is lowest at birth and tends to increase as people age. The time of day can also cause blood pressure variations. For example, blood pressure is usually at its lowest point early in the morning just before awakening. Activities such as standing, sitting, or lying down can affect blood pressure. When blood pressure is measured while the patient is in an erect position, it is referred to as an orthostatic blood pressure reading. **Orthostatic hypotension** refers to the lowered blood pressure that occurs when

TABLE 35-11 Blood Pressure Guidelines

New Classification (2003)		Previous Classification
140/90 or above	Hypertension	High blood pressure > 140/90
120/80 to 139/89	Prehypertension	Borderline 130–139/85–89
119/79 or below	Normal	Normal 129/84 or below
		Optimal 120/80 or below

TABLE 35-12 Average Normal Blood Pressure Readings

Newborn	75/55
6–9 years of age	90/55
10–15 years of age	100/65
16 years to adulthood	118/76
Adult	120/80

a patient moves from a lying down to an erect position. Sudden movement or a sudden change in position with a resulting fall in blood pressure is referred to as postural hypotension.

The pressure reading in the right arm is usually 3 to 4 mmHg higher than in the left arm. Numerous situations that cause changes in blood pressure readings are listed in Table 35-14. Terms relating to abnormal blood pressure readings are described in Table 35-15.

TABLE 35-13 Physiological Factors Affecting Blood Pressure

Volume of blood	Increase of blood volume increases the BP. Decrease of blood volume decreases BP. *Example:* Hemorrhage causes volume and BP to drop.
Peripheral resistance	Relates to the size of the lumen (the cavity or space) within blood vessels and amount of blood flowing through it. *Example:* The smaller the diameter of the lumen, the greater the resistance to blood flow. Fatty cholesterol deposits result in high BP due to narrowing of the lumen.
Condition of heart muscle	Strength of heart muscle affects volume of blood flow. The pumping action of the heart and how efficiently it does the job affect the BP. *Example:* A weak heart muscle can cause an increase or decrease in BP.
Elasticity of vessels	The ability of blood vessels to expand and contract decreases with age. *Example:* Nonelastic blood vessels, as in arteriosclerosis, cause an elevated BP.

TABLE 35-14 Causes of Blood Pressure Variations

Elevated/Increased BP	Lowered/Decreased BP
Anger	Anemia
Certain drug therapies, nicotine, caffeine	Approaching death
Endocrine disorders (hyperthyroidism)	Cancer
Exercise	Certain drug therapies (antihypertensives, narcotics, analgesics, diuretics)
Fear, excitement	Decreased arterial blood volume (hemorrhage)
Heart and liver disease	Decreased arterial BP
Increased arterial BP	Dehydration
Late pregnancy	Massive heart attack
Lying down position with legs elevated	Middle pregnancy
Obesity	Pain
Renal disease	Shock
Rigidity of blood vessels	Starvation
Smoking	Sudden postural changes
Stress, anxiety	Thyroid and adrenal disorders
Taking pressure at the right arm	Time of day (during sleep and early morning)
Vasoconstriction or narrowing of peripheral blood vessels	Weak heart

TABLE 35-15 Terms Related to Abnormal Blood Pressure Readings

Benign	Slow-onset elevated blood pressure without symptoms.
Essential	Primary hypertension of unknown cause. It may be genetically determined.
Hypertension	A condition in which the patient's blood pressure is consistently above the norm for his or her age group. Also called high blood pressure. Below 120/80 is the baseline.
Hypotension	Condition of abnormally low blood pressure that may be caused by shock, hemorrhage, and central nervous system (CNS) disorders.
Malignant	Rapidly developing elevated blood pressure that may become fatal if not treated immediately.
Orthostatic	A temporary fall in blood pressure that occurs when a patient moves rapidly from a lying to a standing position. Dizziness and blurred vision can also be present.
Postural	A temporary fall in blood pressure from standing motionless for extended periods of time.
Renal	Elevated blood pressure as a result of kidney disease.
Secondary	Elevated blood pressure associated with other conditions such as renal disease, pregnancy, arteriosclerosis, and obesity.

Blood pressure is a routinely taken vital sign. It is especially important when the following characteristics or conditions are present:

1. Patient is on antihypertensive drugs.

2. Patient has a history of heart disease, kidney disease, stroke, or hypertension.

3. Patient (including children) is receiving a complete physical examination.

4. Patient is pregnant.

5. Patient is receiving preoperative or postoperative care.

6. Patient is bleeding or in shock.

7. Patient has symptoms of a neurological disorder.

8. Patient is experiencing allergic reactions

As with all vital signs, blood pressure readings should be interpreted in relation to the patient's baseline measurement. This means that a blood pressure reading taken previously when the patient was not ill is used as that patient's "normal" measurement. All subsequent readings are then compared to that patient's "normal" baseline reading.

EQUIPMENT FOR MEASURING BLOOD PRESSURE

Two pieces of equipment are necessary for measuring blood pressure: a sphygmomanometer and a stethoscope. The **sphygmomanometer** is the instrument used for measuring the pressure the blood exerts against the walls of the artery (Figure 35-27). The stethoscope is a diagnostic instrument that amplifies sound. It is used to detect sounds produced by blood pressure as well as the heart and other internal organs such as the stomach.

Sphygmomanometers

The components of a sphygmomanometer are manometer, inflatable rubber bladder, cuff, and bulb. The **manometer** is a scale that registers the actual pressure reading. The core of the blood pressure cuff is the rubber bladder, which, when inflated, distends to temporarily constrict blood circulation

MERCURY SPHYGMOMANOMETER

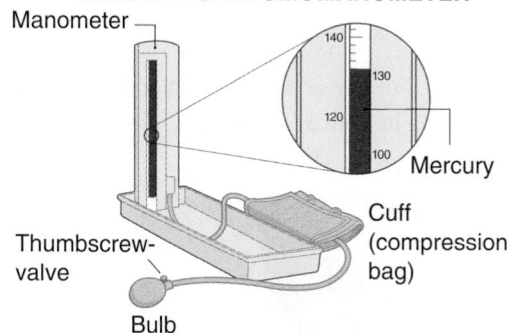

ANEROID SPHYGMOMANOMETER

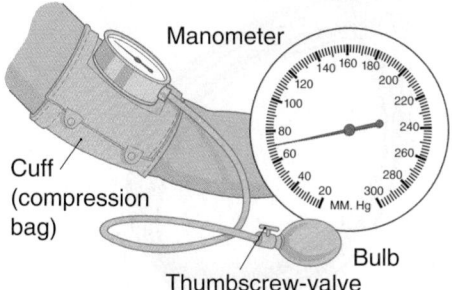

FIGURE 35-27 Sphygmomanometers are used to measure blood pressure and may be either mercury or aneroid.

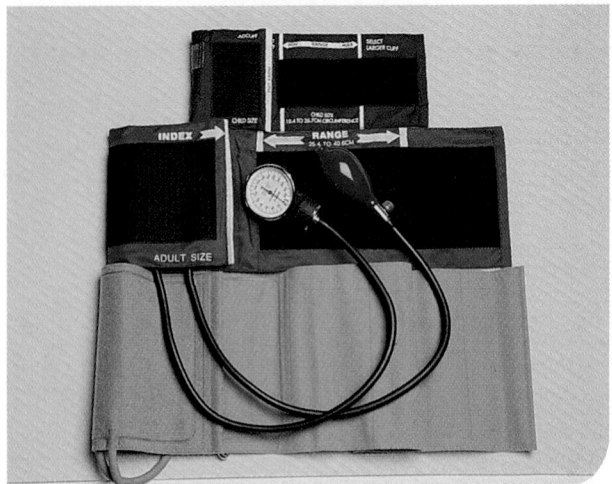

FIGURE 35-28 Three standard sizes of cuffs: a small size for a child or frail adult; a normal adult size; and a large size for measuring blood pressure on the leg (thigh) or on the arm of an obese adult.

in the arm. A soft material cuff covers the bladder and is placed next to the skin of the patient. The pressure bulb has a thumbscrew attached to a control valve that allows for inflation and deflation of the cuff.

The size of the blood pressure cuff is important. Three sizes are available: a small cuff for a child or a frail or small-limbed adult; a normal adult size; and a large size for measuring blood pressure on the leg (thigh) or on the arm of an obese adult (Figure 35-28). Blood pressure cuffs are not generally used on infants. When using a leg cuff, the popliteal artery is palpated for a pulse.

The three types of sphygmomanometers are mercury, aneroid, and electronic. The electronic version provides a digital readout on a lighted display, is easy to use, and does not require a stethoscope. Discussions of the mercury and aneroid sphygmomanometers follow with illustrations of portable and wall-mounted versions of each type (Figure 35-29A and Figure 35-29B).

Mercury Sphygmomanometer. The mercury sphygmomanometer is not as widely used as the aneroid version. Mercury is a toxic substance, and these sphygmomanometers are being replaced for safety reasons. However, mercury instruments may be found on the walls in many physicians' offices. They contain a column of mercury that rises as the pressure bulb is pressed and the rubber bladder inflated. A calibrated scale runs down both sides of the mercury column. The reading is taken at eye level at the top of the mercury line next to a calibrated scale. This type of instrument must be placed vertically on the wall or on a flat, level surface so that the mercury will rise in a vertical position. Periodic recalibration is necessary to maintain accuracy.

Aneroid Sphygmomanometer. The aneroid sphygmomanometer has a round dial that contains a scale calibrated in millimeters (mm) and a needle to register the reading. The needle must be at zero before starting the procedure. The aneroid sphygmomanometer should be recalibrated for accuracy every year by using a mercury manometer as the model. This instrument is easily portable. Some facilities and many individuals use electronic blood pressure devices. The home units are relatively inexpensive and easy to use.

Stethoscope

The stethoscope is used to detect sounds produced by blood pressure. This instrument consists of a chest piece contain-

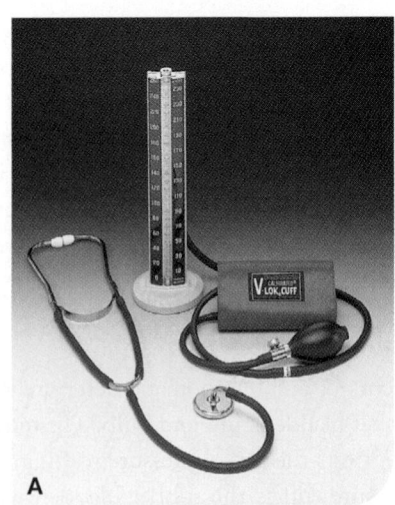
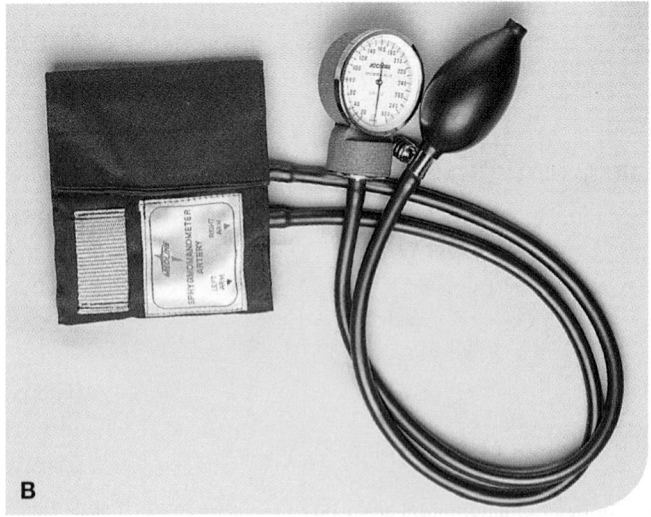

FIGURE 35-29 (A) Portable mercury sphygmomanometer; (B) Portable aneroid sphygmomanometer.

TABLE 35-16 Components of the Stethoscope

Chest piece	Portion of the instrument that is placed over the site where the sound is to be heard. May consist of a diaphragm or a bell or both.
Diaphragm	A disclike sound sensor that picks up both low- and high-pitched sound frequencies. More useful for high sounds such as bowel and lung sounds.
Bell	A hollow, curved bell or cup-shaped sound sensor that may have one, two, or three "heads" that are useful in picking up sounds of the cardiovascular system.
Flexible tubing	Rubber or plastic tubing to carry the sound from the patient to the binaurals. The usual length of tubing is 12 to 14 inches. Some people prefer using longer tubing up to 22 inches. However, some of the sound clarity is lost as the tubing becomes longer.
Binaurals	Rigid, small metal tubes that connect the tubing to the earpieces.
Spring mechanism	Flexible external metal spring that holds the binaural steady so that the earpiece will remain in the ear.
Earpieces	Molded plastic tips that attach to the end of the binaurals and are placed in the medical assistant's ears.

ing a diaphragm and/or bell, flexible tubing, binaurals, a spring mechanism, and earpieces. The American Heart Association recommends the use of the bell of the stethoscope for greater accuracy. The key components of the stethoscope are described in Table 35-16 and shown in Figure 35-30A and 35-30B. Stethoscopes are also used to measure apical pulse and listen to chest sounds.

MEASURING BLOOD PRESSURE

After greeting the patient, attempt to relax him or her by explaining in a calm, quiet manner what the procedure will entail and that the procedure is not painful. Most patients have had BP measured previously. Ask the patient if he or she knows what the previous reading was or if there is have a history of hypertension. This will guide you when you have to inflate the cuff (30 mmHg over systolic pressure). If this is this first time taking a reading on a new patient, you should take a BP reading on each arm. After inflating the cuff to the level recommended by your physi-

cian (180 mmHg in some offices) and the pulse beat is audible, deflate the cuff and begin inflating again 20 to 30 mmHg higher than previously. Do not comment on the BP reading to the patient unless the physician has instructed you to do so. Remember that it is the physician's duty to explain the results. Procedure 35-11 lists the steps to correctly measure a systolic and diastolic blood pressure.

Estimated Systolic Pressure

The **palpatory method** of feeling the radial pulse while the blood pressure cuff is deflating can be used to determine systolic pressure. This method cannot be used to determine the diastolic pressure or to hear the Korotkoff sounds. However, it is useful when a student is learning to take blood pressure readings. The level of inflation necessary to hear the first sound in phase I can be determined by using the palpatory method, which is explained in Procedure 35-12.

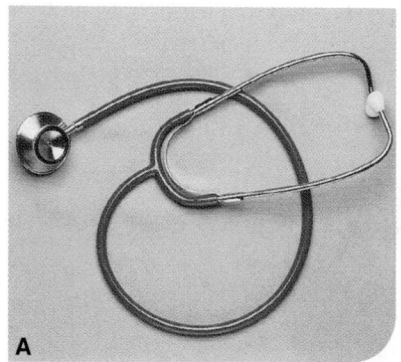

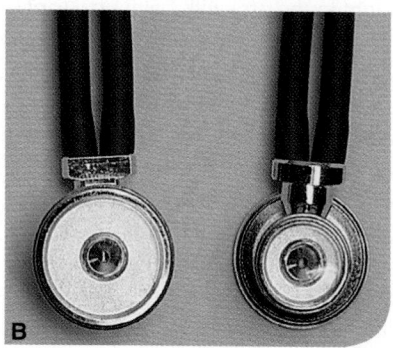

FIGURE 35-30 (A) Stethoscope with both a bell and a flat disc amplifier; (B) Close-up of a flat disc amplifier on the left and a bell amplifier on the right.

MEASURING BLOOD PRESSURE

Objective: Obtain an accurate systolic and diastolic reading.

EQUIPMENT AND SUPPLIES

sphygmomanometer; stethoscope; 70 percent isopropyl alcohol; alcohol sponges or cotton balls; paper and pen/pencil; patient's record

METHOD

1. Perform hand hygiene.
2. Assemble the equipment. Thoroughly cleanse the earpieces, bell, and diaphragm pieces of the stethoscope. Use an alcohol sponge or cotton ball with 70 percent isopropyl alcohol. Allow the alcohol to dry.
3. Identify the patient verbally and explain the procedure.
4. Assist the patient into a comfortable position. BP may be taken with the patient in a sitting or lying position. The patient's arm should be at heart level. If the patient's arm is below heart level the BP reading will be higher than normal; if the arm is higher than heart level, the BP will be lower than normal. Patients should be reminded not to cross their legs or talk during the procedure.

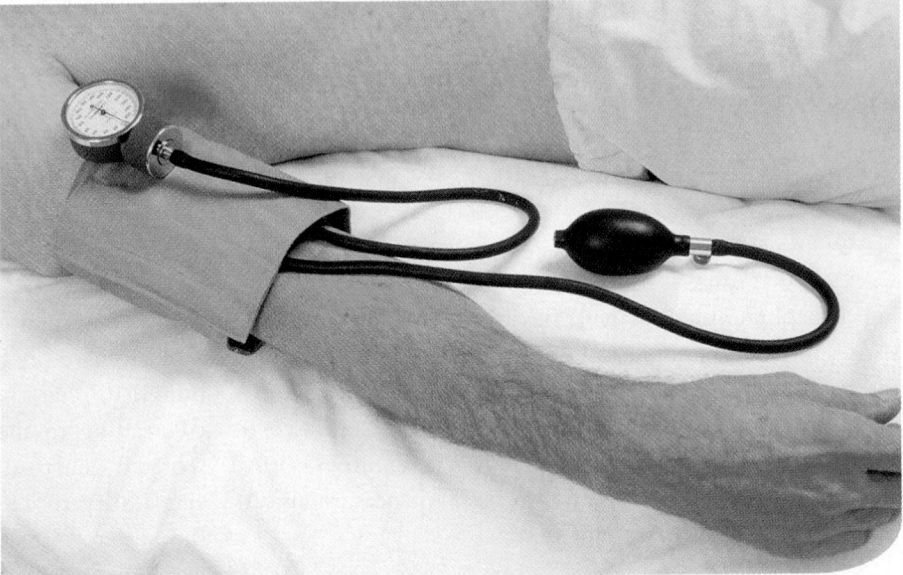

5. Place the sphygmomanometer on a solid surface with the gauge within 3 feet for easy viewing.
6. Uncover the patient's arm by asking the patient to roll back his or her sleeve 5 inches above the elbow. If the sleeve becomes constricting when rolled back, ask the patient to slip the arm out of the sleeve. Never take a BP reading through clothing.
7. Have the patient straighten the arm with palm up. Apply the proper-size cuff of the sphygmomanometer over the brachial artery 1 to 2 inches above the antecubital space (bend in the elbow). Many cuffs are marked with arrows or circles to be placed over the artery. Hold the edge of the cuff in place as you wrap the remainder of the cuff tightly around the arm. If the cuff has a Velcro closure, press it into place at the end of the cuff (Figure 35-31A).
8. Palpate with your fingertips to locate the brachial artery in the antecubital space (Figure 35-31B).
9. Pump air into the cuff quickly and evenly until the level of mercury is 20 to 30 mmHg above the point at which the radial pulse is no longer palpable. Note the level and rapidly deflate and wait 60 seconds. The manometer should be at eye level for a more accurate reading.
10. Place the earpieces in your ears and the diaphragm (or bell) of the stethoscope over the area where you feel the brachial artery pulsing. Hold the diaphragm in place with one hand on the chest piece without placing your thumb over the diaphragm (Figure 35-31C). The stethoscope tubing should hang freely and not touch any object or the patient during the reading.
11. Close the thumbscrew on the hand bulb by turning clockwise with your dominant hand. Close the thumbscrew just enough so that no air can leak out. Do not close so tightly that you will have difficulty reopening it with one hand.
12. Slowly turn the thumbscrew counterclockwise with your dominant hand. Allow the pressure reading to fall only 2 to 3 mmHg at a time.

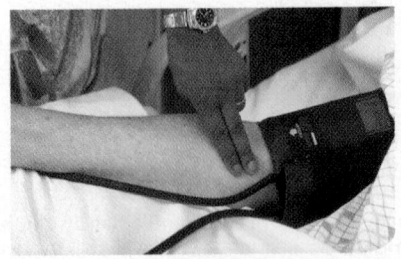

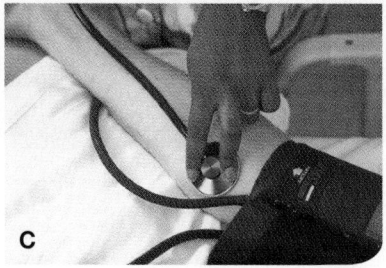

C

13. Listen for the point at which the first clear sound is heard (phase I of the Korotkoff sounds). Note where this occurred on the manometer. This is the systolic pressure.

14. Slowly continue to allow the cuff to deflate. The sounds will change from loud to murmur and then fade away (phases I, II, III, and IV of the Korotkoff sounds). Read the mercury column (or spring gauge scale) at the point where the sound is no longer heard. This is the diastolic pressure (phase V of the Korotkoff sounds).

15. Many physicians will want both phase IV and phase V reported for the diastolic reading (Figure 35-31D).

16. Quickly open the thumbscrew all the way to release the air and deflate the cuff completely.

17. If you are unsure about the BP reading, wait at least a minute or two before taking a second reading. Never take more than two readings in one arm since blood stasis may have occurred, resulting in an inaccurate reading.

18. Immediately write the BP as a fraction on paper. You may inform the patient of the reading if this is the policy in your office.

19. Remove the cuff.

20. Clean the earpieces of the stethoscope with an alcohol sponge.

21. Perform hand hygiene.

22. Chart the results, including the date, time, BP reading, and your name.

CHARTING EXAMPLE

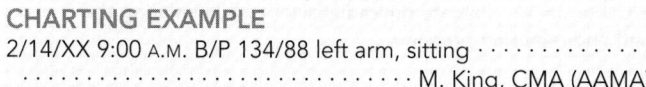

2/14/XX 9:00 A.M. B/P 134/88 left arm, sitting · · · · · · · · · · · · ·
· M. King, CMA (AAMA)

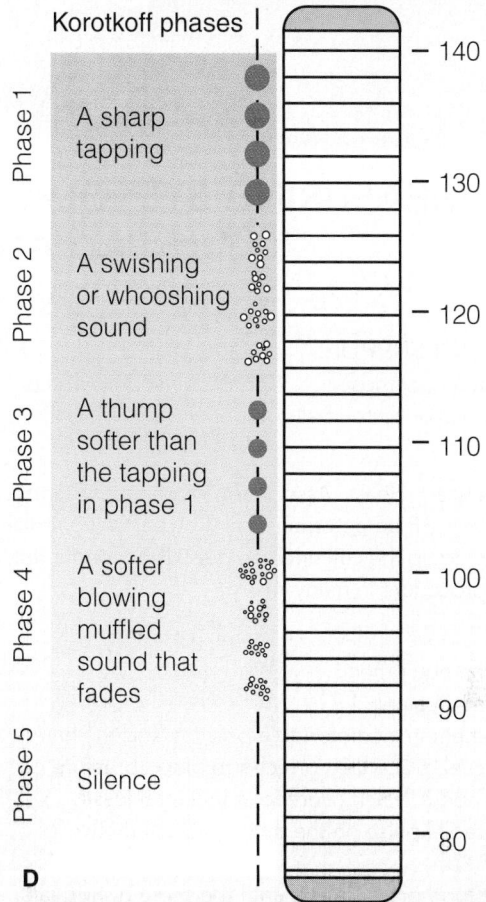

Korotkoff phases

Phase 1 — A sharp tapping — 140, 130

Phase 2 — A swishing or whooshing sound — 120

Phase 3 — A thump softer than the tapping in phase 1 — 110

Phase 4 — A softer blowing muffled sound that fades — 100, 90

Phase 5 — Silence — 80

D

FIGURE 35-31 **(A) Wrap a blood pressure cuff snugly around the upper arm; (B) Palpate the brachial artery on the medial antecubital fossa; (C) Place a stethoscope on the medial antecubital fossa; (D) Korotkoff sounds can be differentiated into five phases. In the illustration the blood pressure is 138/90 or 138/102/90.**

Causes of Error in Blood Pressure Measurements

Accuracy is very important in the evaluation of blood pressure. Many conclusions about a patient's health are made based on a BP assessment. Being in a hurry and failing to allow sufficient time to elapse before retaking a reading are common errors. Table 35-17 describes causes of errors in taking BP readings. BP measurement is not used solely to determine if hypertension exists. Abnormal BP measurements are found with other conditions, including kidney disease and stress.

Pain

Pain is often considered the fifth vital sign. Many patients will not mention pain unless they are specifically asked about it. Pain is a universal symptom we all have experienced. It is extremely subjective and personal, and it can overpower and

procedure

35-12

MEASURING SYSTOLIC BLOOD PRESSURE USING THE PALPATORY METHOD

Objective: Obtain an accurate systolic reading.

EQUIPMENT AND SUPPLIES

sphygmomanometer; stethoscope; 70 percent isopropyl alcohol; alcohol sponges or cotton balls; paper and pen/pencil; patient's record

Note: The American Heart Association recommends that approximate systolic BP be determined first by palpating radial pulse, then pumping up the cuff until the pulse is no longer felt. This is standard procedure in many cases.

METHOD

1. Assemble the equipment.
2. Perform hand hygiene.
3. With the patient in a comfortable position and the hand is at heart level, place the correct-size blood pressure cuff on the arm about 1 inch over the antecubital fossa.
4. Locate the radial pulse on the thumb side of the wrist (Figure 35-32).
5. Inflate the blood pressure cuff until the pulse disappears, being sure to note the reading on the manometer; continue to inflate about 30 mmHg above the point at which the radial artery pulse disappeared.
6. Slowly deflate the cuff 2 to 3 mmHg per second while keeping the fingers on the pulse. The point at which the pulse is felt is the systolic blood pressure.
7. Remove the cuff and perform hand hygiene.
8. Record the systolic pressure as "palpated systolic pressure."

CHARTING EXAMPLE

07/24/XX 7:00 P.M. Palpated systolic pressure 170 mmHg. · · · ·
· H. Martinez, CMA (AAMA)

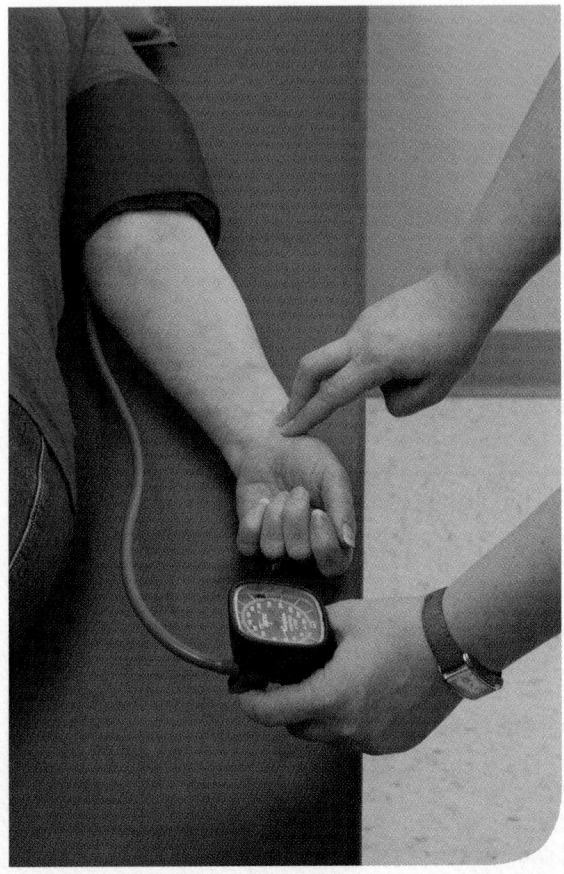

FIGURE 35-32 Palpate the radial artery while inflating the cuff and releasing pressure.

change one's life. No two individuals experience pain in the same way. If the patient says he or she is in pain, the caregiver must accept his or her word because pain is a **subjective symptom**. When documenting a patient's description of pain, the caregiver must use the patient's own words. For example, if the patient complains of a "sharp, knifelike stabbing pain in the belly," that is how it should be written in the chart. Common words to describe pain are listed in Table 35-18.

Pain is difficult to describe. It is important for medical personnel to have a vocabulary of terms and to observe for nonverbal signs when discussing pain with a patient. Signs such as grimacing or moaning or grasping a particular body part are forms of nonverbal communication. Use of a numerical pain measurement scale, with 1 being no pain and 10 being extreme pain, can be useful. For children and non–English-speaking patients, scales with happy and sad faces are avail-

TABLE 35-17 Causes of Error in Blood Pressure Readings

Equipment	Cuff is improper size. The cuff bladder should be 20 percent wider than the diameter of the extremity where the cuff is placed. Large cuffs for obese arms and small cuffs for children should be available in all offices. Air leaks around the valve may cause mercury to drop suddenly. Air leaks in the cuff bladder delay the inflation rate and could give a false high reading. Air leaks may also occur along the tubing if it is old or worn. Mercury column is not calibrated to the zero point. Velcro may be worn and does not hold.
Procedure	Patient's arm is not uncovered. Medical assistant is too far away from manometer to accurately read gauge. Cuff is improperly applied (too loose or too small). Cuff is not centered over the brachial artery, 1 to 2 inches above bend in the elbow. End of the cuff is not secured tightly Part of stethoscope tubing or chest piece touches the blood pressure cuff while taking the pressure reading. Failure to locate brachial pulse before placing stethoscope in position. The rubber bladder in the cuff was not deflated completely before beginning the procedure. Valve on bulb is not completely closed before beginning to pump air into cuff. Cuff was not inflated to a level 20 to 30 mmHg above the palpated or previously measured systolic pressure or 200 mmHg. Deflation occurs too rapidly to accurately determine the sounds. The arm used for the reading is not at the same level as the heart. The arm was held above the level of the heart. Failed to wait 1 to 2 minutes before taking second reading. Failed to notice the auscultatory gap.
Patient	Patient is nervous or anxious, resulting in a false high reading. Patient's arm is too large for accurate reading with available equipment.

able. See Figures 35-33A and 35-33B for examples of pain scales. The goal of assessing pain is to find a treatment or means to relieve the discomfort. Assessment of pain is also important after treatment plans have been initiated.

JOINT COMMISSION PAIN STANDARDS

In 2000 and 2001 the Joint Commission on Accreditation of Healthcare Organizations (JCAHO; now known simply as the Joint Commission) recommended standards for managing pain for all health care facilities. These include the following:

- Recognize that patients have the right to appropriate pain assessment and management.

TABLE 35-18 Common Words Used to Describe Pain

• Stabbing	• Intractable
• Sharp	• Unbearable
• Cutting	• Colicky
• Tearing	• Excruciating
• Burning, Stinging	• Radiating
• Dull	• Penetrating
• Intermittent	• Aching
• Continuous	• Nagging, gnawing
• Throbbing	• Fleeting

- Pain levels should be assessed and recorded regularly.
- Facilities will have policies in place so patients can be treated with opioids to relieve pain and with patients being involved in their own pain management.
- Facilities should monitor the effectiveness of pain management.
- Data for pain management must be collected and monitored.
- Patients and families must be informed about pain management, and arrangements for pain control must be made when patients are discharged.

Many states have passed laws requiring that pain be assessed as the fifth vital sign. All patients are entitled to treatment according to their needs.

TYPES OF PAIN

Pain may be acute or chronic. **Acute pain** is expected pain associated with trauma or surgery that lasts through the recovery of that condition. **Chronic pain** is long-term pain

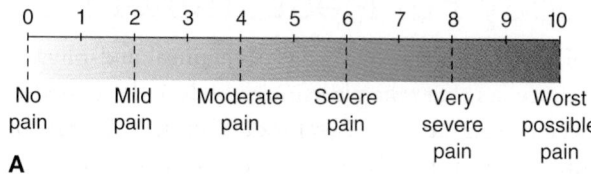

FIGURE 35-33 **(A) Numerical pain level chart with word modifiers.**

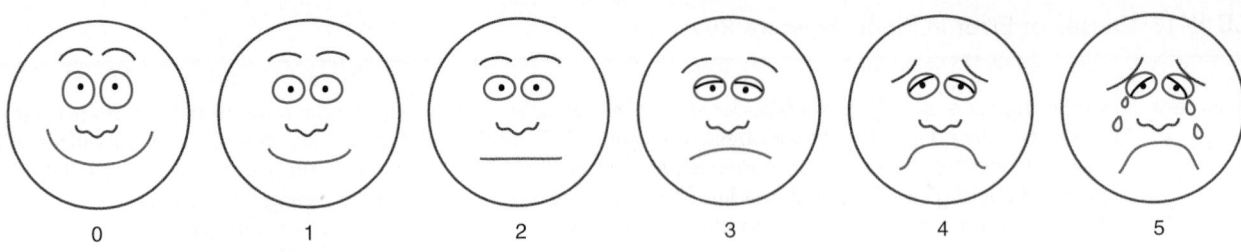

1. Explain to the child that each face is for a person who feels happy because he or she has no pain (hurt, or whatever word the child uses) or feels sad because he or she has some or a lot of pain.

2. Point to the appropriate face and state,"This face..." :
   0—"is very happy because he (or she) doesn't hurt at all."
   1—"hurts just a little bit."
   2—"hurts a little more."
   3—"hurts even more."
   4—"hurts a whole lot."
   5—"hurts as much as you can imagine, although you don't have to be crying to feel this bad."

3. Ask the child to choose the face that best describes how he or she feels. Be specific about which pain (e.g., "shot" or incision) and what time (e.g., Now? Earlier before lunch?)

B

FIGURE 35-33   (B) The Wong/Baker FACES Rating Scale.
Source: From Hockenberry MJ, Wilson D, Winkelstein ML: Wong's Essentials of Pediatric Nursing, ed. 7 St. Louis, 2005 p. 1259. Used with permission. Copyright, Mosby.

that persists for 6 months and interferes with functions of life. Pain can be categorized by where it seems to be coming from—for example, from deep in the organs or from the surface of the body. Pain is also described by where it is felt in the body. **Radiating pain** spreads out from an area. For instance, pain from a heart attack is felt in the chest and down the right arm. **Referred pain** is pain that is felt at a site away from the injured or diseased body part. An example of this is gallbladder pain, which may be felt in the right shoulder. **Intractable pain** is overwhelming, difficult to relieve, and all consuming like the pain associated with end-stage cancer. **Phantom pain** is a sensation felt in a missing body part after it has been removed. Other terms, such as *dull, achy, throbbing, cramping,* or *stabbing* may be used by patients to describe their pain.

Pain threshold is the amount of pain stimulation required for an individual to feel pain. It is generally fairly consistent from person to person, but it can change with other circumstances. For example, a sprained ankle hurts, but if the patient is emotionally upset and depressed it may be more bothersome than normal. Pain tolerance is the amount and duration of pain a person can experience before requiring intervention and relief. This also varies with the individual and cultural and psychological circumstances.

Body Fat Measurement

Metabolism is the sum of all the biochemical and physiological processes that take place in the body and are needed to grow and maintain life. **Basal metabolism** is the rate of metabolism when the body is awake and at rest. The amount of calories one takes in should equal the number of calories of energy expended; otherwise, a weight gain will result. The ideal weight is the weight at which the individual maintains optimal heath. The ideal weight values vary with age, sex, body build, and standardized charts. Many methods are avaialble for measuring the percentage of body fat. Some are expensive and time consuming—for example, underwater weighing or X-ray absorptiometry methods. Two easier and more practical methods are the skin-fold test and the calculation of body mass index (BMI) method.

SKIN-FOLD FAT MEASUREMENT

The skin-fold measurement of body fat involves using special skin calipers to measure the thickness of fat folds in three areas: triceps, suprailiac, and subscapular areas. See Procedure 35-13 for the steps on using calipers to measure skin-fold fat. After the designated area is measured, a reading from the instrument is taken. After the reading is complete, calculations are made and the results are recorded. For example, an acceptable result in the triceps area for a woman would be 12 to 25 percent body fat or 9 to 17 mm.

BODY MASS INDEX

Body mass (BMI) index is calculated using the following:

- Patient's height in meters (1 m = 3.3 ft or 39.6 in.)
- Patient's weight in kilograms (1 kg = 2.2 lbs)
- The following formula: BMI = weight in kilograms/ height in meters squared

A BMI of 19 to 22 is most desirable. A reading over 30 is considered obese. See Procedure 35-14 for instructions on calculating the body mass index.

DETERMINING THE FAT-FOLD MEASUREMENT IN AN ADULT

Objective: Accurately determine and record body fat measurement.

EQUIPMENT AND SUPPLIES

fat-fold body calipers; patient's record; pen and paper

METHOD

1. Gather equipment and supplies.
2. Perform hand hygiene.
3. Read caliper directions.
4. Identify the patient and explain the procedure.
5. Grasp the triceps in the upper arm with the thumb and index finger (Figure 35-34). Do not pinch too hard.
6. Place the calipers over the fold and measure.
7. Record the measurement.
8. Grasp the subscapular region beneath the shoulder blade and obtain the caliper reading and record.
9. At the suprailiac area (located posterior and immediately superior to the fanning of the hip bone), obtain a caliper reading and record it.
10. Determine the total percentage of body fat, using a table provided by the manufacturer of the calipers.
11. Perform hand hygiene.
12. Document the result in the patient's record.

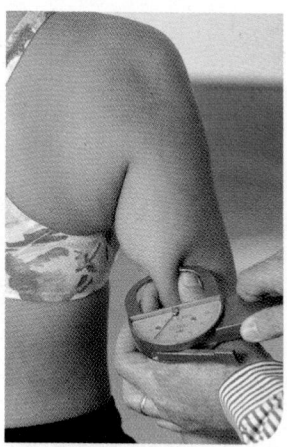

FIGURE 35-34 Calipers are used to measure body fat on the triceps of a patient.

CHARTING EXAMPLE

7/24/XX 2:00 P.M. Triceps 9 mm; scapula 12 mm; abdomen 40 mm. Results are within acceptable ranges (7 to 15 percent).
· D. Martinez, RMA

CALCULATING ADULT BODY MASS INDEX

Objective: Accurately calculate adult body mass index following the steps in the procedure.

EQUIPMENT AND SUPPLIES

patient's record; paper and pen; scale for height and weight; BMI formula or nomogram or chart for BMI

METHOD

1. Perform hand hygiene.
2. If the recent height and weight measurements are not available, follow the steps in Procedure 35-1 for measuring adult height and weight.
3. Insert the patient's height and weight into the formula, using pounds and inches or kilograms and meters according to facility policy.
4. Formula for pounds and inches:
   BMI = Weight in pounds ÷ (Height in inches × Height in inches) × 703
5. Example: Wt. 175 lbs; Ht 64 inches
   175 ÷ (64 × 64) = 0.0427 × 703 = 30.0 BMI
   A BMI between 19 and 25 is considered a healthy weight; 25–30 is considered overweight; over 30 is considered obese. See Figure 35-35 for a Body Mass Index Table.
6. Record results in the patients' record.

CHARTING EXAMPLE

07/24/XX Ht. 64 inches; Wt. 175 lb; BMI 30.0 · · · · · · · · · · · · ·
· N. McPhillips, CMA (AAMA)

Body Mass Index Table

Height (inches)	Normal						Overweight					Obese										Extreme Obesity														
BMI	19	20	21	22	23	24	25	26	27	28	29	30	31	32	33	34	35	36	37	38	39	40	41	42	43	44	45	46	47	48	49	50	51	52	53	54
												Body Weight (pounds)																								
58	91	96	100	105	110	115	119	124	129	134	138	143	148	153	158	162	167	172	177	181	186	191	196	201	205	210	215	220	224	229	234	239	244	248	253	258
59	94	99	104	109	114	119	124	128	133	138	143	148	153	158	163	168	173	178	183	188	193	198	203	208	212	217	222	227	232	237	242	247	252	257	262	267
60	97	102	107	112	118	123	128	133	138	143	148	153	158	163	168	174	179	184	189	194	199	204	209	215	220	225	230	235	240	245	250	255	261	266	271	276
61	100	106	111	116	122	127	132	137	143	148	153	158	164	169	174	180	185	190	195	201	206	211	217	222	227	232	238	243	248	254	259	264	269	275	280	285
62	104	109	115	120	126	131	136	142	147	153	158	164	169	175	180	186	191	196	202	207	213	218	224	229	235	240	246	251	256	262	267	273	278	284	289	295
63	107	113	118	124	130	135	141	146	152	158	163	169	175	180	186	191	197	203	208	214	220	225	231	237	242	248	254	259	265	270	278	282	287	293	299	304
64	110	116	122	128	134	140	145	151	157	163	169	174	180	186	192	197	204	209	215	221	227	232	238	244	250	256	262	267	273	279	285	291	296	302	308	314
65	114	120	126	132	138	144	150	156	162	168	174	180	186	192	198	204	210	216	222	228	234	240	246	252	258	264	270	276	282	288	294	300	306	312	318	324
66	118	124	130	136	142	148	155	161	167	173	179	186	192	198	204	210	216	223	229	235	241	247	253	260	266	272	278	284	291	297	303	309	315	322	328	334
67	121	127	134	140	146	153	159	166	172	178	185	191	198	204	211	217	223	230	236	242	249	255	261	268	274	280	287	293	299	306	312	319	325	331	338	344
68	125	131	138	144	151	158	164	171	177	184	190	197	203	210	216	223	230	236	243	249	256	262	269	276	282	289	295	302	308	315	322	328	335	341	348	354
69	128	135	142	149	155	162	169	176	182	189	196	203	209	216	222	229	236	243	250	257	263	270	277	284	291	297	304	311	318	324	331	338	345	351	358	365
70	132	139	146	153	160	167	174	181	188	195	202	209	216	222	229	236	243	250	257	264	271	278	285	292	299	306	313	320	327	334	341	348	355	362	369	376
71	136	143	150	157	165	172	179	186	193	200	208	215	222	229	236	243	250	257	265	272	279	286	293	301	308	315	322	329	338	343	351	358	365	372	379	386
72	140	147	154	162	169	177	184	191	199	206	213	221	228	235	242	250	258	265	272	279	287	294	302	309	316	324	331	338	346	353	361	368	375	383	390	397
73	144	151	159	166	174	182	189	197	204	212	219	227	235	242	250	257	265	272	280	288	295	302	310	318	325	333	340	348	355	363	371	378	386	393	401	408
74	148	155	163	171	179	186	194	202	210	218	225	233	241	249	256	264	272	280	287	295	303	311	319	326	334	342	350	358	365	373	381	389	396	404	412	420
75	152	160	168	176	184	192	200	208	216	224	232	240	248	256	264	272	279	287	295	303	311	319	327	335	343	351	359	367	375	383	391	399	407	415	423	431
76	156	164	172	180	189	197	205	213	221	230	238	246	254	263	271	279	287	295	304	312	320	328	336	344	353	361	369	377	385	394	402	410	418	426	435	443

FIGURE 35-35 Body Mass Index Table. *Adapted from Clinical Guidelines on the Identification, Evaluation, and Treatment of Overweight and Obesity in Adults: The Evidence Report, 1998, National Institutes of Health, National Heart, Lung, and Blood Institute.*

SUMMARY

Patient interviewing and correct documentation in a medical history or record are of vital importance to the health of the patient and the quality of health care provided by the physician. Privacy, empathy, and confidentiality are important goals to keep in mind when interviewing and assisting patients.

Vital signs are an important objective indication of the patient's overall physical condition. One vital sign measurement taken alone does not necessarily provide a complete picture. The medical assistant must be able to skillfully take all vital measurements and be able to assess what she or he is observing, such as the rate, rhythm, and depth of respirations. Other factors such as age, gender, nervousness, and physical condition of the patient may affect vital sign read-

ings. Measurements such as height and weight are an important part of patient examination. At times additional assessments of BMI or skin-fold fat percentage may be requested. Assessing pain, the fifth vital sign, helps provide additional information to aid in the delivery of health care.

The accuracy of obtaining and recording vital sign measurements is critical for the ultimate diagnosis and treatment of the patient. Communication skills, although important in all aspects of medical assisting work, are essential when obtaining vital measurements. A positive and sincere approach in interacting with the patient may be enough to put the patient at ease and may result in obtaining more valid vital sign measurements.

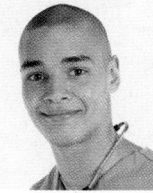

35 CHAPTER REVIEW

COMPETENCY REVIEW

1. Define and spell the terms to learn for this chapter.

2. Name five factors that affect body temperature.

3. Name four types of fever.

4. What is hypothermia?

5. What is the desirable range for blood pressure in an adult?

6. List the six C's of charting.

PREPARING FOR THE CERTIFICATION EXAM

1. An abnormally slow pulse rate is
   a. extrasystole
   b. tachycardia
   c. thready pulse
   d. pulse volume
   e. bradycardia

2. Systolic pressure of 140 or above is referred to as
   a. bradycardia
   b. tachycardia
   c. hypertension
   d. hypotension
   e. pulse pressure

3. Normal pulse rate for an adult is
   a. 40–60
   b. 60–90
   c. 80–100
   d. 90–100
   e. More than 100

4. The normal rate of respiration per minute for adults is
   a. 6–10
   b. 10–13
   c. 14–20
   d. 18–22
   e. 22–28

5. Which of the following would NOT be included in the vital signs?
   a. weight
   b. respiration
   c. pulse
   d. temperature
   e. blood pressure

6. Which of the Korotkoff sounds represents the systolic pressure?
   a. absence of sound
   b. the muffled sound
   c. the first distinct sound
   d. the change of sound
   e. the light tapping sound

7. The term used to describe difficult or labored breathing is
   a. apnea
   b. eupnea
   c. orthopnea
   d. tachypnea
   e. dyspnea

8. The normal rectal temperature reading, which is higher than the normal oral or axillary temperature, is
   a. 97.6°F
   b. 99.6°F
   c. 30.0°C
   d. 35.0°C
   e. 36.8°C

9. If pulse is taken at the wrist the artery used is the
   a. temporal artery
   b. carotid artery
   c. popliteal artery
   d. femoral artery
   e. radial artery

10. An increase in one's pulse rate may be caused by
    a. fever
    b. poisons
    c. mental depression
    d. rest
    e. chronic disease

CRITICAL THINKING

1. Elanya's vital signs are almost normal based on her age; however, one vital sign is out of range. Identify the vital sign that is out of range and indicate what it should be, based on Elanya's age.

2. The physician would like to prescribe Elanya a medication for her headaches. The medication dosage is based on body weight in kilograms. What is Elanya's body weight in kilograms?

3. Would the pain that Elanya is experiencing due to her headaches be considered acute or chronic? Explain your answer.

ON THE JOB

Lakisha Smith is working in an OB/GYN clinic affiliated with a major teaching hospital. Her general responsibilities include registering patients, handling phone calls when the receptionist is on a break, escorting patients into the examination room, taking vital signs, running selected laboratory tests, setting up the clinic examination rooms for gynecological examinations, and providing patient education.

The following is the morning's schedule of patients and visitors:

9:00 Adele Bishop	New mother checkup
9:15 Amy Campbell	First OB visit
9:30	
9:45 Maria Lopez	OB patient in last month of pregnancy
10:00 Meg Rivers	Regular OB checkup
10:15 Vanessa Brown	New gynecology patient w/ovarian cyst
10:30	
10:45 Tiffany Baker	Regular OB checkup
11:00 Vern Simmons	Pelvic inflammatory disease

11:15 Latonya Pike   1st visit after miscarriage

11:30 Emma Thompson   Yearly checkup, gynecology patient

12:00 Lunch break

During the morning, the following occurs:

When Maria Lopez arrives, she tells Lakisha that she has been bleeding since the weekend.

A pharmaceutical representative comes in at 10:00 A.M. and asks to see the doctor.

Supplies are delivered that must be signed for.

Dr. Williams is called away to perform a delivery at 11:00 A.M.

Vital signs including TPR, BP, and weight are taken for all OB patients.

Urinalysis is performed by another medical assistant assigned to the clinic laboratory.

What are your responses to the following?

1. How should Lakisha handle the pharmaceutical representative?
2. Should Maria Lopez's bleeding be considered an emergency? If so, what is Lakisha's responsibility?
3. What is the correct procedure for signing for and checking in medical supplies?
4. Since Dr. Williams was called away for a delivery, how should the patients be rescheduled? What about the patients who are already in the waiting room?

INTERNET ACTIVITY

Go to the American Heart Association website and look for dietary guidelines for hypertension.

MEDMEDIA

Additional interactive resources and activities for this chapter can be found:

On your student DVD: View applicable procedure videos on the DVD-ROM found in the back of this book.

MyHealthProfessionsKit.com: Test your knowledge of the chapter with games and activities. MyHealthProfessionsKit also includes resources, helpful links, and a Spanish audio glossary.

Medical Assisting Interactive: Practice your procedures as a medical assistant in this simulated doctor's office. This can be accessed through MyHealthProfessionsKit.com.

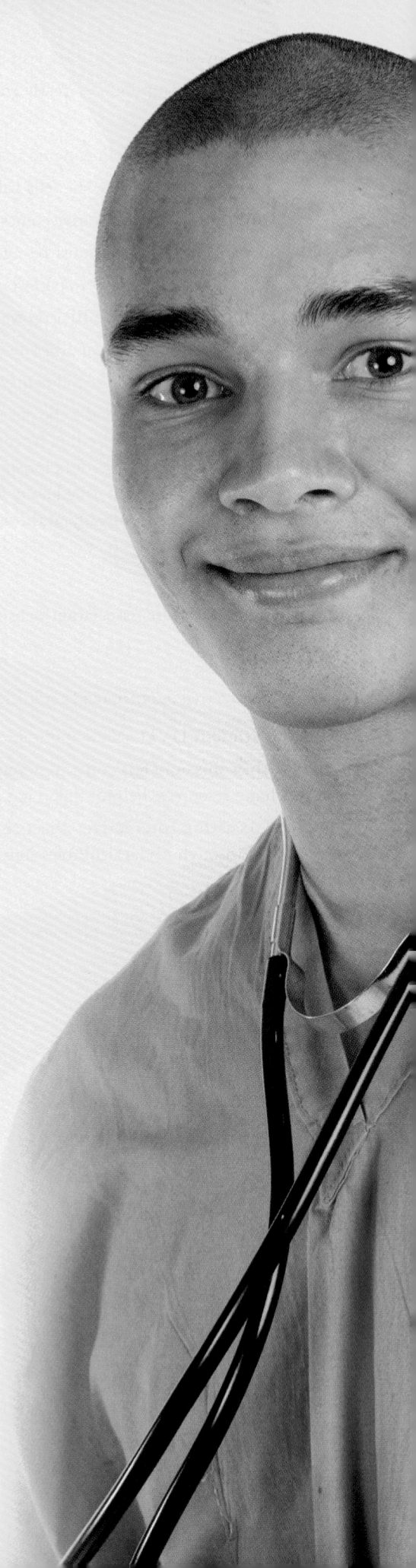

36

Assisting with Physical Examinations

LEARNING OBJECTIVES

After completing this chapter, you should be able to:

- Define and spell the terms to learn for this chapter.

- Recognize six pieces of equipment commonly used during a physical examination.

- Describe the six examination methods used by physicians.

- Discuss the steps to take in preparing a patient for a physical examination.

- Explain concepts of properly draping patients.

- List and describe nine patient examination positions that are used during a physical examination.

- List laboratory and diagnostic tests that may be ordered as part of a complete physical examination.

- Explain the sequence of a routine physical examination.

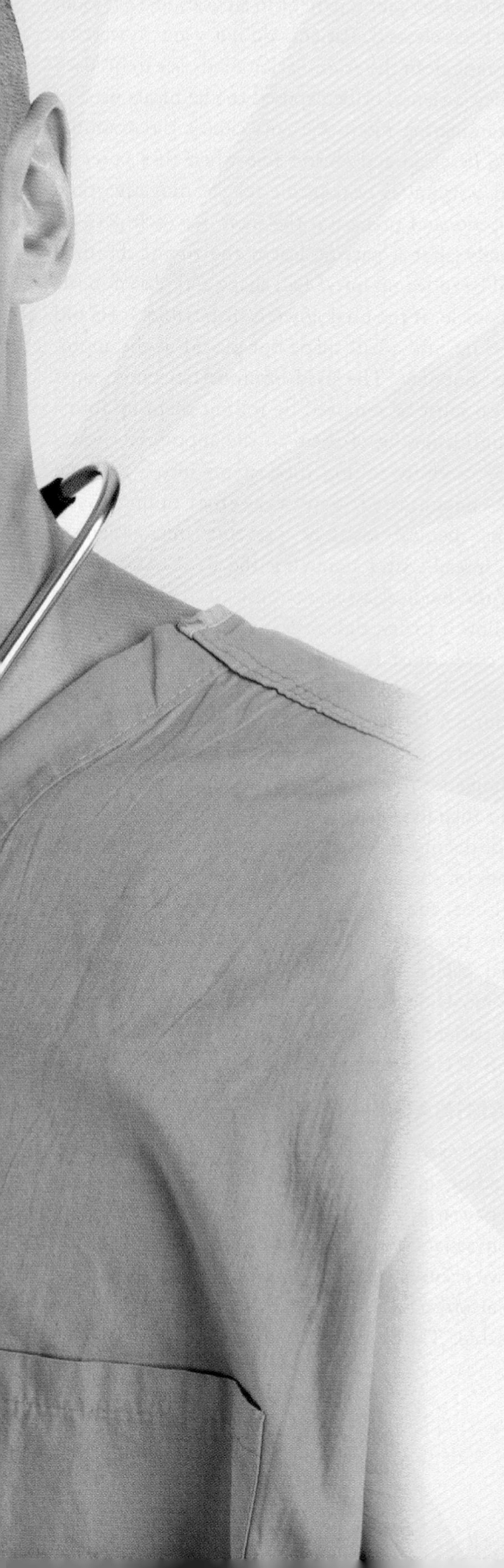

CHAPTER OUTLINE

CASE STUDY

Molly McConnley has arrived at Pearson Physicians Group for her appointment with Dr. Miller. Susan, CMA (AAMA), escorts Molly to the examination room and asks what brings her to the medical office today. Molly responds by saying, "I am here for my annual physical and Pap smear."

TERMS TO LEARN

amplify

auscultation

bimanual

chief complaint (CC)

goniometer

inspection

laryngeal mirror

manipulation

mensuration

objective symptom

ophthalmoscope

otoscope

palpation

patella

percussion

present illness (PI)

reflex hammer

review of systems (ROS)

speculum

subjective symptom

tongue depressor

tuning fork

turgor

vaginal speculum

CERTIFICATION LINK

CMA (AAMA)
Patient history interview

Patient preparation and assisting the physician

RMA
Vital signs and mensurations

Physical examinations

CMAS (AMT)
Basic health history interview

Vital signs and measurements

Examination preparation

One of the key responsibilities of the medical assistant is assisting the physician with a patient's physical exam. The medical assistant's role in the patient physical exam includes interviewing the patient, documenting patient information, preparing the exam room prior to the patient visit, positioning and draping the patient, assisting the physician during the examination, cleaning the room after the visit, and instrument care. Other duties include maintaining supplies, ensuring the safety of patient and coworkers through adherence to infection control standards, observing confidentiality and patient privacy, and performing these functions in a professional, competent, empathetic manner. Chapter 35 presented information regarding patient interviewing, an overall discussion of the main components of a medical history, and guidelines for charting. This chapter expands that information and the process of patient physical examination.

Preparing the Examination Room

Preparing for the next patient begins immediately after the previous patient leaves the examining room. A medical assistant should never take a patient to an examination room that has not been cleaned. Patients do not want to watch a medical assistant clean the examination room, see items used on or by other patients, or be exposed to chemicals used to clean the examination room. Patients expect the examination room to be clean and clutter free when they enter it. The medical assistant is responsible for cleaning the room between patients and preparing the room for each patient.

Immediately after a patient leaves the room, the used gown should be rolled up into a ball shape and placed in the laundry receptacle. If the used gown is disposable, it should also be rolled up into a ball shape but placed in the appropriate waste container. The used examination table paper and drape also must be removed by rolling them up into a ball shape and disposing of them in the appropriate waste container. By carefully rolling these items into a ball and keeping the contaminated items away from uniforms and clothing, the medical assistant prevents microorganism from being spread. After removing the used examination table paper, the medical assistant must clean the examination table, allow it to dry, and cover it with clean, new paper. The pillow cover must be disposed of following universal precautions and replaced with a new one. Disposable equipment used during the examination must be discarded in the appropriate containers. Reusable equipment must be taken (following universal precautions) to the appropriate area for cleaning and disinfection. All surfaces in the examination room must be disinfected with an appropriate cleaner to prepare the room for the next patient. All biohazard containers should be closed, and, if full, the bag should be sealed and removed from the room to the appropriate holding area per Occupational Safety and Health Administration (OSHA) regulations. No evidence of any other patient should remain when a new patient is taken into an examination room. See Procedure 36-1: Cleaning the Examination Room.

EXAMINATION ROOM FEATURES

The number of examination rooms available to a physician varies, depending on the medical office. If a physician has his or her own practice, there may be two to four examination rooms. A physician who belongs to a group practice may have only two examination rooms designated to him or her. Each medical office may have different types and sizes of rooms available. The standard examination room is most often used and is furnished with an examination table (with stirrups in a practice performing pelvic exams), a pillow, a footstool, a supply cupboard, a trash can, hazardous waste and sharps containers, a rolling stool, and a chair. Sometimes, a writing surface and a sink are also present. For specialist physicians, special chairs or other diagnostic equipment specific to the practice may also be present. Physicians in specialized practices such as ophthalmology will require specialized furniture and equipment. All instruments and equipment needed for the examination should be ready for the physician. This equipment should not be left within reach of the patient. If an examination light is present, the medical assistant is responsible for positioning the light so that it provides correct illumination for the physician, but not so that it could fall on the patient or cause a burn. Gooseneck lamps are especially prone to tipping over, so caution should be exercised.

The size of the examination room varies from medical office to medical office. Renting office space can be very expensive for a medical office, so rooms are often designed to be just big enough for the patient, the physician, the medical assistant, and the equipment. The examination room, however, should be spacious enough that the patient, the physician, and the medical assistant do not feel confined.

EXAMINATION ROOM SAFETY

Examination rooms must follow the standards required by the Americans with Disabilities Act (ADA). These standards address the width of doorways and hallways; placement of

PROFESSIONALISM
THE LIFE SPAN

Care and consideration should be used when dealing with all patients; however, children, adolescents, and older adults may need additional assistance.

The Child
Children require a little extra time and understanding. Explain in very simple, age-appropriate terms exactly what you want them to do, and plan to talk to the child during any special procedures.

The Adolescent
Adolescents may also require a little extra time. It is important for the medical assistant to take the time to ask adolescents questions and to get them involved with their medical care. Never use "baby talk" with adolescents because it offends them.

The Older Adult
Older adults tend to accept examinations as "necessary." Be sure to carefully explain the examination, in terms they understand so that they are comfortable with what is expected. If older adults need help disrobing, be sure to protect their privacy while assisting them, and be very respectful of their need for modesty. Be sure there is a safe step when they need to climb up on the examination table. Providing a supporting hand will help to stabilize the patient when getting up and down from the table.

procedure 36-1

CLEANING THE EXAMINATION ROOM
Objective: Clean an examination room to instructor specifications.

EQUIPMENT AND SUPPLIES
disinfectant; paper towels; disposable gloves; examination table; pillow; disposable gown

METHOD
1. Perform hand hygiene.
2. Apply a clean pair of disposable gloves.
3. Roll the soiled disposable gown into a ball shape and dispose of it in the appropriate waste container.
4. Roll the soiled examination table paper into a ball shape and dispose of it in the appropriate waste container.
5. Remove the soiled pillow cover and dispose of it in the appropriate waste container.

6. Remove any other soiled items or equipment from the examination room.
7. Clean the examination table and cabinet surfaces with disinfectant and paper towels (Figure 36-1).
8. Dispose of the soiled paper towels in the appropriate waste container.
9. Remove the soiled gloves and dispose of them in the appropriate waste container.
10. Perform hand hygiene.
11. Put clean paper on the examination table.
12. Put a new pillow covering over the pillow.
13. Make sure the examination room is clean and clutter and odor free.

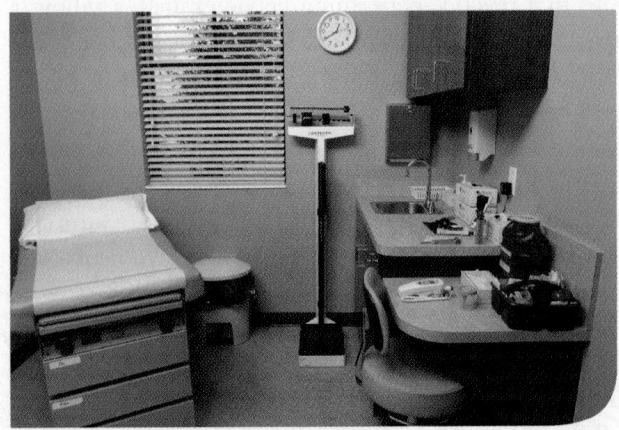

FIGURE 36-1 Examination room.

door handles, grab bars, and handrails; spatial accommodations for patients in wheelchairs; floor surfaces; and much more. For further information about the ADA Standards for Accessible Design, visit the ADA website.

If a medical assistant witnesses any unsafe situation, he or she should take care of the situation immediately. Examples of unsafe situations include clutter in the hallway or examination room, a spill on the floor, and an extension cord lying in the middle of a dirty utility room. A patient or staff member of the medical office could trip or slip on any of these items and be injured. All furniture in the examination room should be checked routinely. Any item such as a broken drawer, a sharp edge on the countertop, or a broken hinge on a door should be reported immediately. If it cannot be repaired immediately, the medical assistant must document the situation in the maintenance log book.

Most examination rooms have electrical cords running from an outlet to a piece of medical equipment. Cables also can be running to a computer or medical devices. It is important for the medical assistant to make sure all electrical cords and cables are secured to the floor or wall. Unsecured electrical cords or cables are unsafe for patients and medical office staff.

Medical assistants should ensure their own safety by using proper body mechanics when moving or assisting patients. Proper body mechanics should be used in all aspects of patient care, including front office work.

PATIENT COMFORT

Patients often change into thin, disposable gowns while waiting for the physician, so the medical assistant must make sure the room is warm enough for the patient. Most medical offices keep the thermostat around 71°F to 73°F. If the thermostat is set on the reading established by the physician or office manager and the patient is still cold, the medical assistant can give the patient a sheet, a disposable sheet, or a blanket to help keep warm. A patient may already be uncomfortable being in a thin, disposable gown, and he or she can become anxious and agitated if also feeling cold. This does not lead to a pleasant experience for the patient and is poor customer service.

When the patient enters the examination room, it should smell both fresh and clean. A well-ventilated examination room can help decrease offensive odors. Offensive odors can come from sweat, urine, feces, vomit, blood, and infectious wounds. If an offensive odor is sensed in the examination room after the patient leaves, the medical assistant must find the item causing the offensive odor and properly dispose of it. If a chair smells from sweat, it must be removed from the examination room and replaced with a new chair until the soiled chair is clean and ready to be used again. Items soaked in urine, feces, blood, or infectious waste must be double bagged and taken to the dirty utility room to be stored. When the medical assistant eliminates the sources of offensive odors, he or she can then concentrate on removing any offensive odor that may linger in the air. This can be accomplished by disinfecting all surfaces and using a room deodorizer and air freshener.

PATIENT PRIVACY

Patients expect privacy, especially when in the examination room. If a patient must wear a gown during the examination, the medical assistant must make sure one is available and must explain to the patient whether it should open to the front or back. The medical assistant also should tell the patient where his or her clothes can be kept during the examination. Properly draping patients to protect their sense of modesty is vitally important to their sense of well-being during an examination. (Draping techniques are discussed fully later in this chapter.) Professional etiquette demands that the medical assistant and other office personnel always knock and wait for a response before entering a patient room. This prevents surprising a patient and ensures patient comfort at all times. Be sure to keep the doors of examination rooms closed to provide for patient privacy and respect while patients are waiting.

If a patient is in the middle of getting dressed and the medical assistant knocks and walks into the examination room without permission, the patient may become very upset or embarrassed; again, this is poor customer service.

Patient History

Before the physician can adequately assess the patient's condition, a past medical history is obtained from the patient. This history assists the physician in assessing the patient's general health status and helps determine a diagnosis of the patient's present problem or condition. See Figure 35-1 in Chapter 35 for an example of a Patient Health History form. Although each office or facility has preferences regarding the specific format of the health history form, the following information is standard:

- **Intake or registration form**—demographic information, name, address, sex, age, DOB, education, occupation, Social Security number, insurance information, racial or ethnic background, marital status, number of children, and nearest relative (Figure 36-2); HIPAA form; and any financial agreements the facility requires for payment.
- **Medical history**—chief complaint, present illness, past medical history, family history (FH), social history (SH) or personal history (PH), review of systems or systems assessment, result of a general physical examination.
- **Test results**—requested by the physician and performed in the office or elsewhere (blood, urine, X-rays, scans, etc.).
- **Records from other physicians or facilities**—received with the patient's written permission.
- **Diagnosis and detailed treatment plan**—determined by the physician.
- **Operative reports**—on all procedures and surgeries, including treatment and follow-up care information.
- **Informed consent forms**—signed by the patient and indicating understanding of and granting permission for specific treatments, including possible outcomes.
- **Hospital discharge summary**—if the patient was hospitalized, includes pertinent information about the hospital stay, including reason for admission, procedures, treatments, medications, care plans, and outcomes.
- **Correspondence**—written information stamped with the date received in office.

Many medical offices give new patients the history form to complete upon arrival for the first visit with the physician. If the patient is expected to complete a history form,

PATIENT REGISTRATION FORM
(Please Print)

Date: ________

Patient's Name: ______________________ DOB: ____ ____ ____
First Middle Last Month Day Year

Address: ______________________ Phone: ____ ____-____
Street City State Zip (Area code)

Patient's SS#: ____-____-____ Driver's License #: ________ Occupation: ________

Method of payment (circle): cash check credit card insurance co-payment

Primary Insurance Co.: ______________ Policy/Group #: ________

Medicare #: ______________ Medicaid #: ______________

Person Responsible For Payment: ______________________ ________
First Middle Last Relationship

Address: ______________________ Phone: ____ ____-____
Street City State Zip (Area code)

Employer Name: ______________________ Dept: ________
First Middle Last

Address: ______________________ Phone: ____ ____-____
Street City State Zip (Area code)

Spouse or Nearest Relative: ______________________ ________
First Middle Last Relationship

Address: ______________________ Phone: ____ ____-____
Street City State Zip (Area code)

How were you referred to this office? ______________________

____

Statement of Financial Responsibility: I, ______________________
do hereby agree to pay all medical charges incurred by the above listed patient. I further understand that these charges are my responsibility, regardless of insurance coverage.

Responsible Person's Signature: ______________________

FIGURE 36-2 Patient registration form.

then the medical assistant is responsible for making sure that the patient understands the terminology and how to answer the questions.

Some medical offices send the health history form to the patient's residence with a request that the form be completed and submitted when the patient comes for the first visit. This allows patients the opportunity to check their own records for important dates and the names and dosages of medications they are taking. When the form is sent to the patient ahead of time, many offices request patients come to the office a half hour before the actual examination by the physician. This permits the medical assistant to verify that the form is complete, to get information required for billing and insurance, and to help patients who require assistance completing the form.

Some physicians prefer to take all the components of the medical history directly from the patient. On some medical history forms, specific questions are geared to the physician's specialty. A cardiologist, for example, may require a more extensive history relating to the cardiovascular system. Whether the patient completes the form at home or in the office, it is important to mark any sections the patient is not supposed to fill in. Particular care should be taken to assist patients who may be embarrassed that they are unable to complete the form themselves due to frailty, disability, or illiteracy. The medical assistant must stress the importance of filling out the form completely.

The patient history should include the following six areas:

1. Chief complaint
2. Present illness
3. Past medical history
4. Family medical history
5. Social history or personal history
6. Assessment of body systems (review of systems) performed by the physician in the office

CHIEF COMPLAINT

The **chief complaint (CC)** is also referred to as the presenting problem. The chief complaint is the reason for the office visit. It usually consists of one or two signs or symptoms. Symptoms are either subjective or objective. A **subjective symptom** is felt by the patient but not apparent to an observer, such as vertigo or pain, and cannot be measured. An **objective symptom** is felt by the patient and is apparent to observers, such as a rash or fever, and can be measured. The chief complaint is usually stated in the patient's own words, such as "I'm having trouble sleeping" or "I'm out of breath after climbing only two or three stairs."

It is important to ask the following questions to obtain more complete information:

- *What?* What is the patient experiencing? What makes it worse or relieves it?
- *When?* When did it start (onset)? How long does it last (duration)?
- *Where?* Where is the symptom located? How intense is it?

Because only the physician is able to diagnose the patient's problems, the medical assistant does not use diagnostic terms when recording the chief complaint. The patient's own words are used to describe the problem.

- *Correct documentation:* 10/23/XX Pt. c/o "dying of thirst all the time" and unusual weight loss during past month.
- *Incorrect documentation:* 10/23/XX Pt. experiencing excessive thirst and unusual weight loss indicative of diabetes.

See Procedure 36-2: Documenting a Chief Complaint During a Patient Interview.

PRESENT ILLNESS

The **present illness (PI)** provides a more complete, expansive description of the chief complaint. The PI component of the health history must contain a detailed description of the symptom(s), including the onset, duration, and intensity of each. Each symptom should be documented as to its relationship to the chief complaint. For example, a patient who came to the office with a chief complaint of "dull aching pain in left side of belly" may add that it happens every time she eats popcorn or nuts and has occurred monthly for the past 6 months. This information amplifies the CC. See Procedure 36-3: Interviewing a New Patient to Obtain Medical History Information and Preparing for a Physical Examination.

PAST MEDICAL HISTORY

This part of the medical history includes all diseases and medical problems the patient has experienced in the past. Past illnesses or injuries can affect present health. Dates of major illnesses, hospitalizations, surgeries, and current medications are noted whenever possible. Patients often forget to tell the physician how much aspirin or other over-the-counter (OTC) drugs they take. Remind patients that aspirin is considered a drug even though it may be purchased OTC. Aspirin can duplicate other medication the physician may prescribe or can interfere with the treatment of conditions such as gastric ulcers. Today, herbal supplements are used by many, and patients should be queried about what vitamins and supplements they are taking.

DOCUMENTING A CHIEF COMPLAINT DURING A PATIENT INTERVIEW

Objective: Accurately document the chief complaint using correct charting format and abbreviations while interviewing a patient.

EQUIPMENT AND SUPPLIES

problem list or progress notes form; black or blue pen

Note: Instructor may provide a variety of patient scenarios for students to role-play for this procedure.

METHOD

1. Gather supplies, including the medical record with problem list or progress notes form.
2. Review briefly the patient's medical history form before greeting the patient.
3. Greet and identify the patient, and escort the patient into examination room.
4. Ask open-ended questions to gather information about why the patient is being seen today. Maintain eye contact and actively listen to patient responses.
5. Gather information about the PI by asking questions: e.g., What makes the problem better or worse? When did it start? Where does it hurt? Ask the patient to rate pain on a scale of 0 to 10.
6. Document the CC and the PI correctly on the correct form in the patient's own words where necessary.
7. Thank the patient and explain that the physician will enter shortly to examine him or her.
8. Make sure the patient is comfortable before leaving the room.

CHARTING EXAMPLE

03/03/XX 11 A.M. CC: Pt c/o N&V × 3 days. "Pounding headache not relieved by Tylenol. Unable to eat or drink." PI: Pt states N&V started after eating fried clams at home. T 101 × 2 days. "Has pain all over belly." T 99.8°F (O), P 84, R 20, BP 110/68 (L) Sitting. · A. Martinez, CMA (AAMA)

INTERVIEWING A NEW PATIENT TO OBTAIN MEDICAL HISTORY INFORMATION AND PREPARING FOR A PHYSICAL EXAMINATION

Objective: Obtain pertinent patient information for a medical history that will assist the physician in establishing cause and treatment of the present illness (PI). Include CC, past history, social or personal history, and family history.

Note: This may be performed on a fellow student.

EQUIPMENT AND SUPPLIES

medical history form; clipboard; pen (black and red); scale; equipment for vital signs; urine container; gown; drape

METHOD

1. Identify the patient, greet the patient warmly, and identify yourself.
2. Explain what you are going to do and what you want the patient to do and why.
3. Provide a private area to conduct the interview.
4. Ask the patient to fill in the patient demographics and data portions of the form. Be sure to speak in a clear voice and use terminology the patient can understand.

Be ready to assist if the patient seems unable to complete the form.

5. Review the portion of the form completed by the patient, and ask for any additional necessary information.
6. Ask why the patient has come to the physician's office that day (the CC).
7. Record the CC in the patient's own words, as appropriate.
8. Ask the patient other open-ended questions to gather more information about the CC to record under PI. Use observation skills during the interview.
9. Gather other information on the patient's PH and SH or PH, and document in the patient's record.
10. Ask the patient about allergies. Record in red ink as required by office policy (usually on the first page of the medical history). If the patient states they do not have any allergies, record NKA (no known allergies) according to the office policy, which may be in red letters.

11. Note any other observations or information you feel are relevant (such as illness at home or loss of a loved one).
12. Record all information using correct charting guidelines.
13. Correct any errors by drawing one line through the error, and date and initial each one. Record the correct information.
14. Ask the patient to provide a urine specimen if required, or ask the patient to empty the bladder.
15. Explain what clothes you wish the patient to remove, where you want the opening of the exam gown to be, and where you want the patient to sit and wait.
16. Explain what procedures will follow ("The physician will be in shortly," etc.).
17. Place the patient history in the designated place for the physician to obtain.

Interactions between herbal supplements and medications are possible. A complete past medical history will include information about the following items:

- Childhood diseases
- Major illnesses
- Injuries
- Hospitalization
- Surgeries
- Allergies
- Immunizations
- Current and past medications (prescription and OTC)
- Last examination

FAMILY MEDICAL HISTORY

The family history is a record of the health problems of the patient's blood relatives. Blood relatives include the patient's mother, father, sisters, brothers, grandparents, aunts, and uncles related by birth. Information on blood relatives should include their current health, major health problems, and cause of death, as well as the age at which the individual died. Family medical histories focus on diseases that may be inherited, such as diabetes mellitus (DM), seizures, heart disease, hypertension or elevated blood pressure, and some types of cancer.

SOCIAL HISTORY OR PERSONAL HISTORY

Social or personal histories include lifestyle patterns that could affect the health status of the patient—for example smoking,

drinking, and using recreational drugs. The patient's occupation, marital status, and sexual preferences are also noted, along with the patient's diet choices, frequency of exercise, sleep habits, and other health habits. Information about the patient's previous occupation(s) (if the patient has had several occupations) and lifelong hobbies, or interests, often provide helpful information. Box 36-1 provides a list of questions that are included on the patient history form or might be asked to gain a good personal history from a patient.

Equipment and Supplies Used for Physical Examinations

The physician's hands are the primary tool used for the physical exam, but special instruments are also used to help with the exam and diagnosis. These include the ophthalmoscope, otoscope, reflex hammer, pinwheel, stethoscope, sphygmomanometer, tuning fork, laryngeal mirror, and tape measure. Supplies are generally considered disposable items that are replaced as they are used in the exam room. Refer to Figure 36-3 for examples of equipment and supplies necessary for a health examination.

EQUIPMENT

The following is a description of the equipment usually found in an examining room:

- **Ophthalmoscope**—The **ophthalmoscope** is used to examine the interior of the eye, especially the retina. Light is focused through a magnifying lens

1. What was the last grade you attended in school?
2. What is your occupation?
3. How long have you done that type of work?
4. Have you been exposed to any toxic or harmful substances such as dust, chemicals, cleaning fluids/fumes, smoke, radiation, pesticides, or paint at work? At home?
5. What do you usually eat for breakfast?
6. Have you gained or lost 10 or more pounds during the past year? Is there a reason?
7. Do you follow a low-fat diet? low-salt?
8. What do you do for exercise? how often?
9. How much alcohol do you drink a day? a month? What is your preferred drink?
10. Do you smoke cigarettes? If yes, how many packs a day? Filtered?
11. Do you smoke a pipe or cigars or chew tobacco? If yes, how much?
12. How many cups of coffee do you drink a day? tea? soft drinks with caffeine?
13. Have you ever used heroin, cocaine, or LSD? OTC drugs? laxatives? How often?
14. Do you have unusual stress at home or work?
15. What are your hobbies?

onto the inner surfaces of the eye to check for abnormalities. Position the patient in a sitting position and looking straight ahead during this examination. Chapter 39 of this text covers eye and ear examinations in detail.

- Otoscope—The **otoscope** is used to examine the ears. The light is focused through the disposable **speculum** to examine the outer ear, then the tympanic membrane (eardrum). A speculum is any instrument used to view a body cavity. The long, pointed speculum on the otoscope can be replaced with a short, wide disposable speculum for visualization of the lining of the nose and other internal structures of the nose.

- Reflex hammer and pinwheel—The **reflex hammer** is sometimes called a percussion hammer. It has a hard rubber, triangular head used for testing reflexes. This instrument is commonly used to check the patellar reflex of the knee and may also be used to check the reflex of the Achilles tendon (in the ankle) or the elbows. The pinwheel has sharp points and is used for testing sensory perception.

- Stethoscope—The stethoscope is used to **amplify** (make louder) sounds in the body, such as the heart, lungs, and abdomen. It is made of two earpieces connected by rubber tubing to a chest piece with a bell and/or diaphragm to amplify sound. Stethoscopes are discussed in more detail in Chapter 35.

- Sphygmomanometer—This is a blood pressure measuring device that may be portable or attached to the wall. Refer to Chapter 35 for further discussion of sphygmomanometers.

- Tuning fork—The **tuning fork** is a metal instrument that has two prongs extending from the handle that are designed to vibrate at a specific frequency. Tuning forks come in different sizes, and each size produces a different pitch level. The tuning fork makes a humming sound that can be heard and felt when struck. The patient's ability to hear the sound is a test of his or her hearing.

- Laryngeal mirror—The **laryngeal mirror** is a small mirror attached to a long handle that is used to visualize the larynx. Warming the laryngeal mirror can help prevent fogging. Warming can be done by using warmers, by running warm water over the mirror, or by briefly holding the mirror close to the exam light.

- Tape measure—A tape measure is used to measure a body part, such as the chest or head in an infant, or a lesion, and must be bendable and plastic. It should also indicate inches and centimeters.

SUPPLIES

Supplies are the disposable items used for patient examination and treatment. Supplies include examination table paper, drapes and various dressings and bandages, tongue depressors, disposable gloves (both sterile and nonsterile), syringes and needles, and alcohol pads, to name a few. A **tongue depressor** is a thin, flat, disposable wooden blade used to press down the tongue to observe the mouth and throat.

Supplies		Purpose
Flashlight or penlight	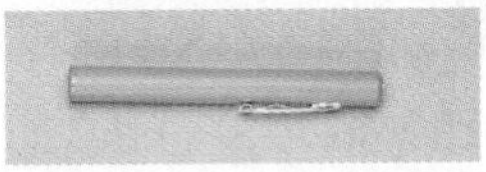	To assist viewing of the pharynx and cervix or to determine the reactions of the pupils of the eye
Laryngeal or dental mirror	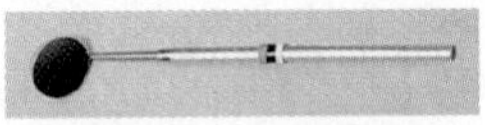	To observe the pharynx and oral cavity
Nasal speculum	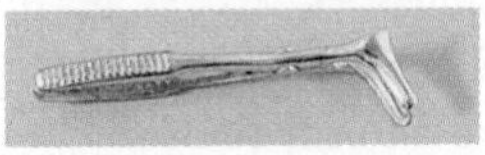	To permit visualization of the lower and middle turbinates; usually, a penlight is used for illumination
Ophthalmoscope	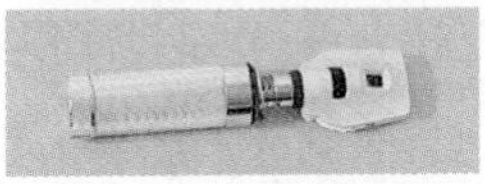	A lighted instrument to visualize the interior of the eye
Otoscope	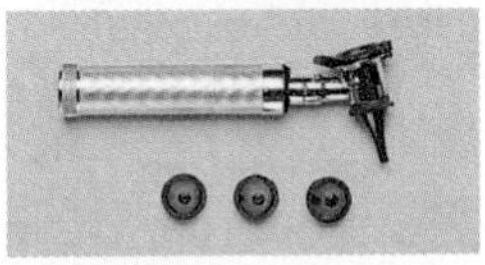	A lighted instrument to visualize the eardrum and external auditory canal (a nasal speculum may be attached to the otoscope to inspect the nasal cavities)
Percussion (reflex) hammer	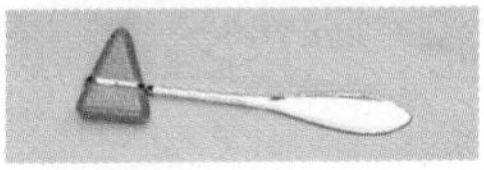	An instrument with a rubber head to test reflexes
Tuning fork	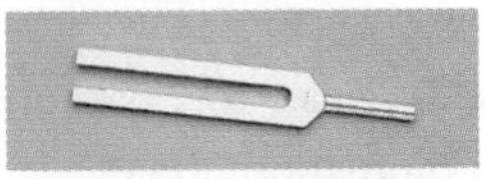	A two-pronged metal instrument used to test hearing acuity and vibratory sense
Vaginal speculum	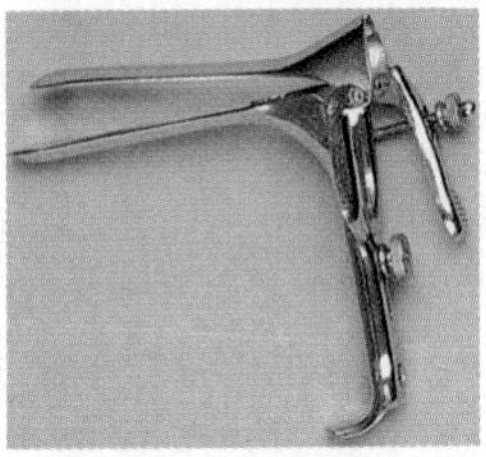	To assess the cervix and the vagina
Cotton applicators	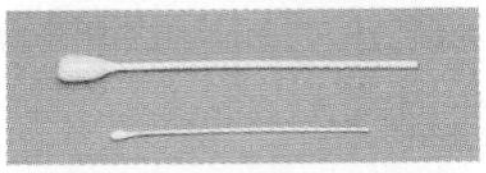	To obtain specimens
Disposable pads	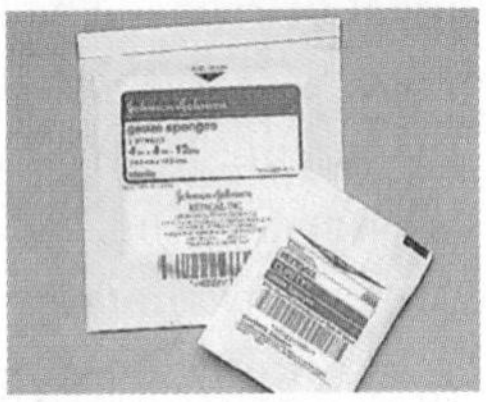	To absorb liquid
Gloves	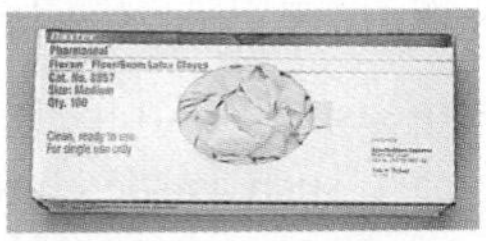	To protect the nurse
Lubricant	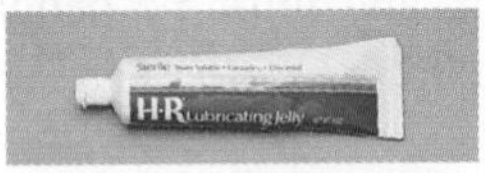	To ease insertion of instruments (e.g., vaginal speculum)
Tongue blades (depressors)	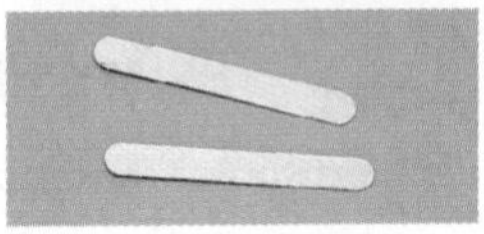	To depress the tongue during assessment of the mouth and pharynx

FIGURE 36-3 Equipment and supplies used for a health examination.

Ordering supplies and stocking the exam rooms are important to patient care and maintaining work flow. Delaying a procedure while you run for something that should have been there can put the patient at risk, delay schedules, and be annoying to all. An overall supply list is good office policy. Once an item is down to half a box or bottle, a new one should be placed in the exam room as a backup. An inventory system should contain the following information:

- List of supplies used in your facility
- Each supplier's name, addresses, telephone number, and contact person
- Amount of each supply used monthly
- How often to reorder

Refer to Table 36-1 for descriptions of additional supplies and equipment commonly present in exam rooms.

Examination Methods Used by the Physician

The hands of the physician are used during the various methods of examination. Some of these methods require pieces of equipment to be used as well. The six commonly

TABLE 36-1 Typical Examining Room Equipment and Supplies

Equipment/Supply	Use
Alcohol wipes	Disinfect and cleanse skin before injections and phlebotomy.
Balance scale	Take patient's weight and height.
Bandages (small)	Applied after taking blood sample and some injections.
Batteries and light bulbs	Extra batteries and light bulbs are required for lighted equipment.
Betadine (or other topical antiseptic)	Used to disinfect skin before minor surgery.
Biohazard waste container	Closed rigid container with biohazardous labeling and appropriate red waste bags.
Cotton balls (sterile and nonsterile)	Used to apply antiseptic or to clean the skin.
Cotton-tipped swabs (sterile and nonsterile)	Used to clean recessed areas, to apply medications and lubricant, and to obtain specimens from the throat and other orifices.
Drapes	Disposable paper or cloth sheet used to cover patient during examination.
Emesis basin	Kidney-shaped receptacle for body drainage, such as sputum, and for used instruments.
Fixative spray	Used to preserve slides.
Gauze dressings (4 × 4 or 3 × 4)	Applied to dress small wounds.
Gloves (nonsterile disposable)	Worn by all staff to protect against microorganisms and bloodborne pathogens.
Gloves (sterile disposable)	Worn when performing minor surgery and handling sterile materials.
Gooseneck lamp	Movable light used to focus on a body area for increased visibility.
Hydrogen peroxide (H_2O_2)	Used to clean open wounds.
Irrigation syringe	Used to wash cerumen (earwax) out of ear canal or to irrigate wounds.
Lubricant	Water-soluble gel applied to physician's glove, speculum, or rectal thermometer to reduce friction during insertion. Prevents damage to delicate mucous membranes.
Soap dispenser	Used to dispense germicidal soap for hand washing between each patient.
Sphygmomanometer	Machine used to measure blood pressure.
Tape	Used to secure dressings.
Tape measure	Measure lesions, head circumference, body measurements.
Thermometers of various types	Measure temperature.
Tissues	Wipe body secretions.
Tongue depressor	Wooden blade used to hold down patient's tongue while examining mouth and throat.
Vaginal speculum	Instrument used to expand vaginal opening to view cervix.

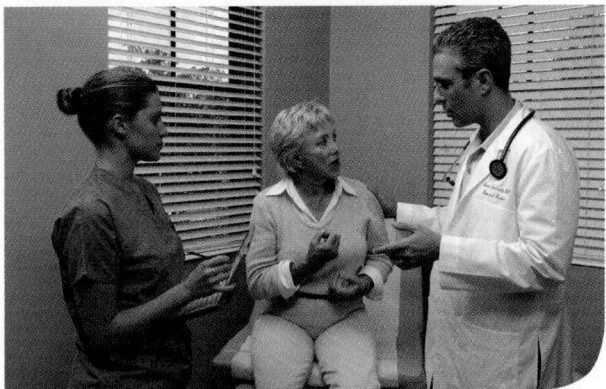

FIGURE 36-4 Inspection is one method of examination used in a health exam.

used methods of physical examination are inspection, palpation, percussion, auscultation, mensuration, and manipulation. As the physician enters the room, these methods of examination begin with inspection. As the physician is greeting the patient, he or she is evaluating speech, social response, and general behavior. Once the review of systems begins, many of the following examination methods are employed—some at the same time. All contribute salient information about the patient's general overall health.

INSPECTION

A physician performs **inspection** by visually examining the exterior surface of the body. At the same time the general state of health, overall demeanor, grooming, and social interactions are observed. Some interior portions of the body, including the throat, eyes, ears, vaginal wall, cervix, and rectum may be inspected using special instruments. Notes are made of any unusual color, size, shape, position, or symmetry of the areas being inspected (Figure 36-4).

PALPATION

Palpation is the process of using the hands to feel the skin and accessible underlying organs and other tissues. Other areas examined by palpation include the axilla (armpits), neck, and chest. Palpation is used to determine any unusual tenderness, size, shape, and texture. Oftentimes, abnormalities and masses in the abdomen can be discovered through palpation. Refer to Figures 36-5A and B for examples of light palpation using one hand and **bimanual**, or two-handed, deep palpation.

PERCUSSION

Percussion is the process of using the fingertips to tap the body lightly but sharply to gain information about the

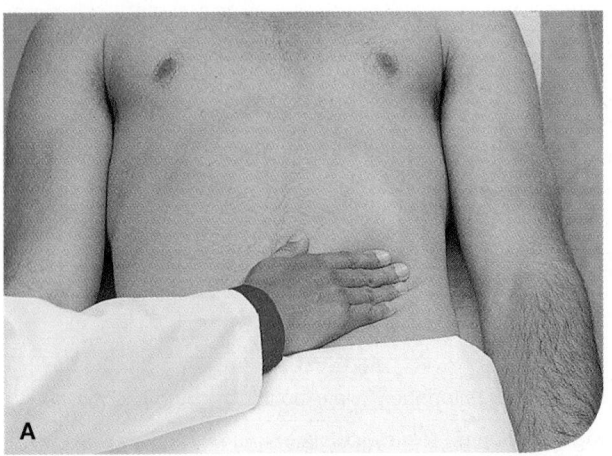

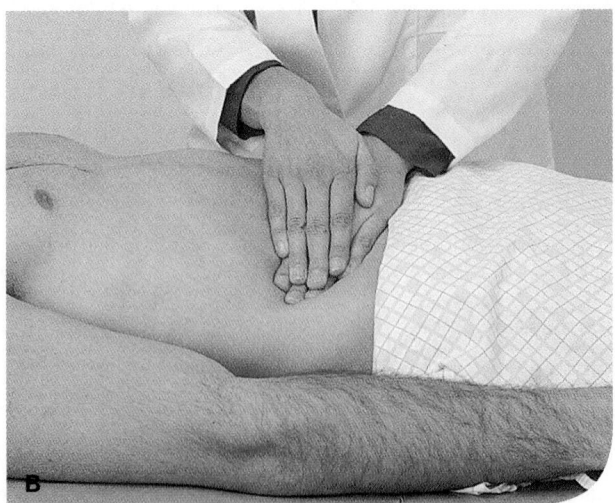

FIGURE 36-5 (A) An example of light palpation of the abdomen; (B) The physician uses two hands for deep bimanual palpation.

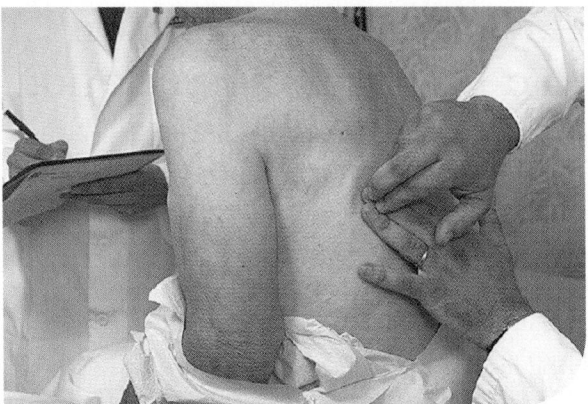

FIGURE 36-6 The physician uses percussion—tapping—to detect sound or vibration.

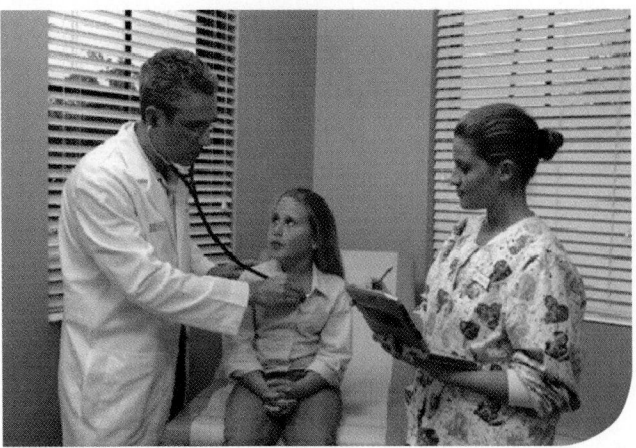

FIGURE 36-8 The physician uses auscultation to listen to a patient's heart.

position and size of the underlying body parts, To do this, two fingers of one hand are placed on the patient's skin and then struck with the index and middle finger of the other hand. The physician uses his or her fingers to percuss the chest wall and abdomen by gentle thumping or tapping, which produces a standard sound or vibrations. An alteration of this sound or vibration aids in determining the presence of fluid or pus in a cavity. Figure 36-6 illustrates percussion on a patient's back.

The physician uses the reflex hammer to test the reflexes of the body. As part of the neurological test, the physician gently taps the reflex hammer once against the tendon reflex at the bottom of the **patella** (kneecap) (Figure 36-7).

AUSCULTATION

Auscultation is the process of listening to sounds that are found within the body. Sounds made by the heart, lungs, stomach, and bowel are assessed for strength, presence or absence, and rhythm. These sounds must be differentiated

from normal body sounds by the physician. These sounds can be heard by using the auscultation method of examination (Figure 36-8). A stethoscope is usually used to amplify body sounds; however, auscultation can also be performed by placing the ear directly over the body surface.

MENSURATION

Mensuration is the use of special tools to measure the body or specific parts. These special tools include a scale, tape measure, and calipers. To determine a patient's weight, a scale is used. A tape measure is used to determine, for example, a patient's height; an infant's head and chest circumference; the diameter or length of a limb; or the length and width of a wound. A **goniometer** is used to measure the range of motion of a joint (Figure 36-9). Calipers are used to determine the amount of body fat.

MANIPULATION

Manipulation is the process of passively assessing the range of motion of a joint. While a physician is performing this examination method, he or she may palpate the joint for abnormalities and warmth. Neurologists and orthopedists may use this method to evaluate patients who want to return to work after injuries or illness or for insurance company records.

Adult Examination

Patient visits to physician offices are scheduled for a variety of reasons, including illness, emergency, and routine checkups. Typically a physical examination is done as part of each visit. The length, extent, and type of exam are determined

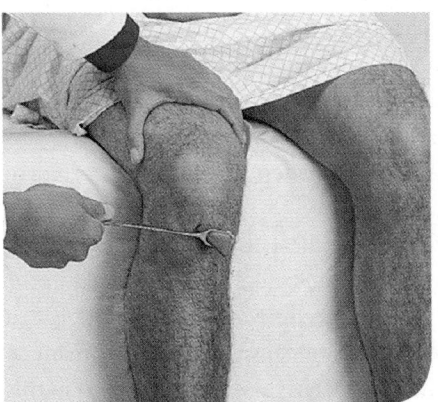

FIGURE 36-7 Testing the patellar reflex with a percussion hammer.

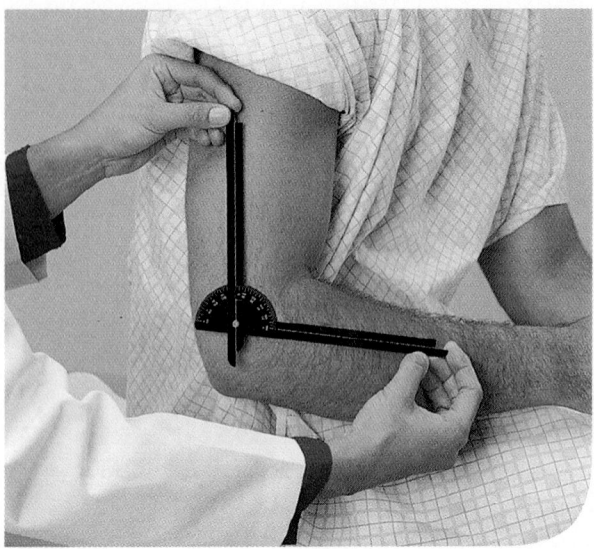

FIGURE 36-9 Mensuration—a physician uses a goniometer to measure range of motion in a joint.

by the reason for the visit and the specialty of the physician. The purpose of the physical examination is to assess as much of the body as possible during the visit to help diagnose new diseases and to measure the effectiveness of the current plan of care of previously diagnosed issues. The physical examination may also include laboratory and diagnostic tests, such as blood work and X-rays.

Oftentimes, patients will have a routine physical examination with no PI or CC. This is a time when it is especially important for the physician to have up-to-date medical records to compare the current physical examination with previous ones. The physician will be looking for weight changes, blood pressure variances, or other conditions requiring more frequent evaluations by the health care provider.

Other patients will be seen by the physician to diagnose a problem. The physician will analyze the information gained during the physical examination and combine it with the past medical history, laboratory findings, and other medical information to determine a diagnosis. Only the physician may actually diagnose a condition. The medical assistant's role in this process is to assist the physician in obtaining correct, current data.

Sometimes the symptoms a patient demonstrates can be indicative of more than one diagnosis. At this time, the physician will have to make a differential diagnosis. The physician will then begin to rule out (R/O) diagnoses in an attempt to determine the most correct one. It is important to remember that when coding for insurance purposes, the R/O diagnosis may not be used. The actual diagnosis must be used.

Assisting the Physician with a Physical Examination

The physician, not the medical assistant, will actually perform the physical examination, but the medical assistant will help the physician in the following ways:

1. Position and drape the patient for examination. If the patient is elderly or has a disability, then help the patient to maintain the correct position.

2. Hand instruments, equipment, and other medical supplies to the physician.

3. Document and label specimens.

4. Offer reassurance to the patient.

5. Act as a witness to the behavior of the physician and the patient.

6. Carry out treatment plans, such as providing patient education, applying dressings, and administering medications.

7. Schedule diagnostic tests as ordered by the physician.

Table 36-2 lists the methods and equipment used to examine the areas or parts of the body during a complete physical examination.

PATIENT PREPARATION

Patient preparation consists of obtaining the patient's medical history, acquiring the CC, measuring vital signs including height and weight, and assisting the patient to prepare for the visit with the physician. For specific information in obtaining vital signs, see Chapter 35. All vital signs should be entered on the chart prior to the time the physician sees the patient. As medical offices vary in their use of charting methods, it is important to know and understand the type of charting method being used. Refer to Chapters 13 and 14 to review various styles of medical charting.

The patient's level of anxiety should be assessed. If the patient seems extremely nervous or ill at ease, then the medical assistant must attempt to allow the patient to express these feelings. Unusual nervousness should be reported to the physician.

It is important for the medical assistant to prepare the patient for any task or procedure before it is performed in the medical office. Each task or procedure must be communicated to the patient in a warm, caring, simple, and direct manner. Patients are usually more cooperative when approached in this manner. Elderly, frail, and young patients should not be left unattended. If the medical assistant is unable to remain in the

TABLE 36-2 Body Part, Method of Examination, and Equipment Used during the General Physical Examination

Area	Body Part	Method/Equipment
Head	Skull, hair, scalp	Inspection and palpation
Ears	Ear canals, eardrum	Inspection with otoscope and tuning fork
Eyes	Visual acuity	Vision chart, Snellen eye chart Inspection with ophthalmoscope
Nose	Nasal passages	Inspection with otoscope and nasal speculum
Mouth and throat (pharynx)	Mucous membranes, lips, gums, teeth, tongue, pharynx	Inspection with laryngeal mirror, flashlight, tongue blade Palpation and inspection
Neck	Thyroid gland, trachea, and cervical lymph nodes; carotid artery	Palpation, auscultation, and inspection
Back and spine	Muscles, spinal cord	Inspection, palpation, and percussion
Chest and lungs	Heart, lungs	Stethoscope Inspection, percussion, palpation, and auscultation
Breasts	Breast tissue, nipples	Palpation
Heart	Heart sounds, apical pulse	Auscultation with stethoscope
Abdomen	Bowel sounds Symmetry Presence of air masses, enlargement Uterus	Auscultation Inspection Percussion, palpation Palpation Stethoscope
Inguinal area	Inguinal nodes hernia	Palpation
Genitalia	*Female:* cervix and vagina *Male:* penis, scrotum, prostate gland	Inspection using vaginal speculum Palpation
Rectal	Anus Rectum	Inspection Inspection using proctoscope
Legs	Circulation Pulse sites	Inspection Palpation
Musculoskeletal system	Muscle strength Gait abnormalities	Inspection Palpation
Neurological examination	Reflexes	Percussion hammer, pinwheel

room, a family member should be asked to sit with the patient until the doctor begins the examination.

Depending on the gender of the physician and the patient, a medical assistant may be requested during certain examinations. For example, if a male physician must perform a gynecological examination, he would request a female medical assistant to be in the examination room to serve as a witness. This method protects both the physician and patient from accusations of unethical behavior.

Patients should be asked to empty their bladder prior to undressing, and instructions for obtaining a urine sample should be given when required. (Obtaining urine specimens is fully discussed in Chapter 46 of this text.) Be sure that patients know how to find their way back to the appropriate exam room from the restroom. All specimen collection containers should be appropriately labeled before giving them to patients.

The medical assistant should provide a patient gown and drape for all examinations. Depending on the type of exam, all clothing, including underwear, should be removed, and the patient should wear the patient gown. It is especially important to be sure that the patient knows whether to leave the gown open at the front or the back. For problem-specific exams, only part of the clothing (such as all clothing above the waist) may need to be removed. In this case, patient gowns and drapes should still be provided. Depending on patient needs, the medical assistant may need to assist the patient with disrobing

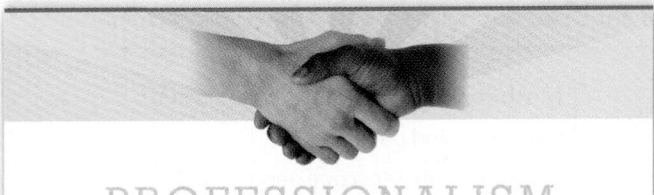

or climbing onto the examination table. Be especially cautious when assisting patients onto a step stool or other step to access the table because this is a time when falls may happen.

Draping the Patient

Drapes are sheets used to protect patient privacy and keep the patient warm. When used properly, they cover all but the part of the patient being examined. Typically, drapes are smaller than bed sheets, although they are often made of the same material or may be disposable. Protecting a patient's modesty as much as possible is important to ensure patient comfort and compliance with uncomfortable positions and examinations. However, the drape must not obstruct the visibility of the physician or interfere with the examination.

During sterile procedures, sterile drapes may be used to protect the surgical area from contamination and to provide a sterile surface for instruments, suture materials, and dressings. They also function to protect the patient from blood or drainage during the procedure. Sterile drapes will be placed around a surgical site in such a manner as to expose only the site of the incision using sterile surgical technique.

Positioning the Patient

The medical assistant will help the physician with the physical examination by positioning the patient. Nine standard positions are used for a variety of medical and surgical examinations and procedures. They are supine (or horizontal recumbent), dorsal recumbent, lithotomy, Fowler's, semi-Fowler's, prone, Sims', knee–chest, and Trendelenburg. Complete familiarity with each position is necessary. As a medical assistant you must give patients clear directions on how to assume each position while gently guiding them and protecting their safety. If a patient must turn from back to stomach or vice versa, the medical assistant should always stand alongside the examination table and have the patient turn toward him or her to prevent the patient from falling off the examination table. Each position will be considered in the following paragraphs. Procedures 36-4 through 36-11 list the steps for assisting a patient into the first seven positions. The final three—sitting, Trendelenburg and proctological—are variations of some of the others.

Supine Position. In the supine position, also known as the horizontal recumbent position, the patient lies flat on his or her back with hands at the sides. Be sure that the patient's feet are supported by extending the table. This position is used to examine anything on the anterior or ventral surface of the body (head, chest, stomach) and for certain types of X-rays. The patient should be draped from the chest, down over the feet. The medical assistant will expose any areas necessary during the examination as indicated by the physician. This position may not be comfortable for patients who are short of breath or who have lower back problems. Placing a pillow under the head and under the knees may be more comfortable for them. See Procedure 36-4: Positioning the Patient in the Supine Position.

Dorsal Recumbent Position. In this position the patient is lying flat on the back with knees bent and feet flat on the table This position relieves strain on the lower back and relaxes abdominal muscles. The dorsal recumbent position is used to inspect the head, neck, chest, and vaginal, rectal, or perineal areas. This position can be used for digital exams of the vagina and rectum. To drape the patient, place the drape at the patient's neck or underarms and cover the body down to the feet. Patients with leg problems may find this uncomfortable. Patients with severe arthritis may find this position more tolerable than the lithotomy position. See Procedure 36-5: Positioning the Patient in the Dorsal Recumbent Position.

Lithotomy Position. The lithotomy position is similar to the dorsal recumbent position, except the patient's feet are placed in stirrups attached to the side of the table. The stirrups must be locked in place. The patient may need assistance placing her feet in the stirrup. After the feet are in place in the stirrups, the patient is instructed to slide down until the buttocks are positioned at the edge of the table. The patient is draped from under the arms to the ankles. This position is used for vaginal examinations requiring the use of a **vaginal speculum** (an instrument used to hold open the walls of the vagina) and for obtaining Pap smears.

POSITIONING THE PATIENT IN THE SUPINE POSITION

Objective: Safely assist the patient into supine position for examination of the anterior surface of the body.

EQUIPMENT AND SUPPLIES
examination table; gown; drape

METHOD
1. Perform hand hygiene.
2. Provide a gown and assist the patient if necessary.
3. Assist the patient onto the table. If a separate step stool is used, stabilize it with your feet as the patient steps up to prevent the stool from sliding.
4. Ask the patient to lie back on the table while pulling out the foot extension. Support the patient's back.
5. Place a pillow under the patient's head.
6. Cover the patient with a drape from the chest to ankles (Figure 36-10).
7. After the examination, assist the patient to a sitting position. Allow the patient to remain seated to prevent dizziness.
8. Push the foot extension into place while supporting the patient's feet.

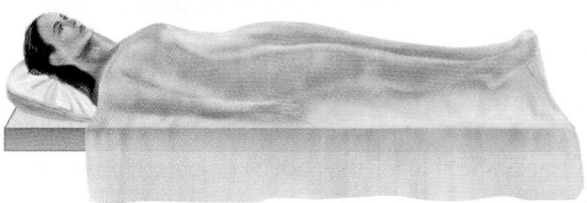

FIGURE 36-10   **The supine or horizontal dorsal recumbent position.**

9. When the patient is stable and the examination is complete, assist the patient to a standing position and hold the patient's arm while he or she steps down. Stabilize the step stool with your feet again. Give further instructions as needed.
10. Clean the examination room for the next patient following the steps in Procedure 36-1.
11. Perform hand hygiene.

POSITIONING THE PATIENT IN THE DORSAL RECUMBENT POSITION

Objective: Safely assist the patient into the dorsal recumbent position for examination of the anterior surface of the body, catheterization, or pelvic examination.

EQUIPMENT AND SUPPLIES
examination table; gown; drape

METHOD
1. Perform hand hygiene.
2. Have the patient disrobe and don a gown as appropriate for the examination. Assist the patient as needed.
3. Assist the patient to sit on the end of the table, stabilizing the step stool as needed.
4. Assist the patient to lie back, as you support the back while pulling out the foot extension.

5. Ask the patient to bend the knees and place the feet flat on the table (Figure 36-11). Push in the foot extension.
6. Cover the patient with a drape with the point of the drape between the patient's legs.
7. Place the pillow under the head if needed.
8. Place the light source and a rolling stool in place for the examiner.
9. After the procedure is complete, assist the patient to a sitting position using the foot extension to support the patient's feet.

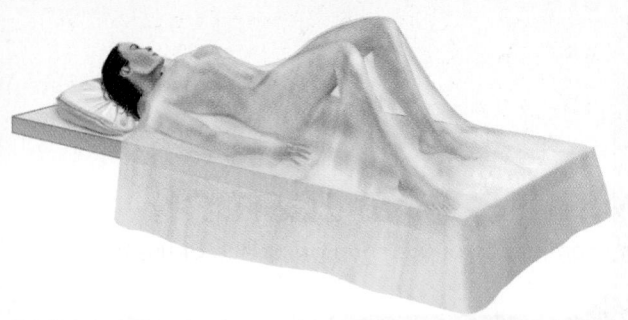

10. Ask the patient to remain seated a few moments to prevent dizziness.
11. Assist the patient off the table, stabilizing the step stool as needed.
12. Give other instructions as necessary.
13. Clean the examination room for the next patient following the steps in Procedure 36-1.
14. Perform hand hygiene.

FIGURE 36-11 **Dorsal recumbent position.**

It is uncomfortable for the patient to maintain this position for any length of time, therefore the patient's feet should not be placed in stirrups until the physician is in the room and ready to begin the vaginal examination. Patients with severe arthritis or those who are severely obese or at the end of pregnancy may find this position impossible. The dorsal recumbent position may be used instead with physician permission. See Procedure 36-6: Positioning the Patient in the Lithotomy Position.

Fowler's Position. In this position the patient sits on the examination table with the head of the table raised to a 90-degree angle. If the patient is able, he or she may be seated on the edge of the table with feet over the edge in an upright position. This position is useful for examinations of the head, neck, and upper body. Patients who have difficulty breathing in the supine position may find this position more comfortable. The drape should be placed over the patient's lap covering the legs. Procedure 36-7: Positioning the Patient in the Fowler's Position.

Semi-Fowler's Position. The semi-Fowler's position is similar to the Fowler's position, but the head of the table is at a 45-degree angle instead of 90. This position is used for postsurgical exams, patients with breathing difficulties or lower back injuries, or those suffering from general malaise. The drape should be placed over the patient's lap and covering the legs.

procedure 36-6

POSITIONING THE PATIENT IN THE LITHOTOMY POSITION

Objective: Safely assist the patient into and out of the lithotomy position for a pelvic examination or catheterization.

EQUIPMENT AND SUPPLIES
examination table with stirrups; gown; drape

METHOD
1. Perform hand hygiene.
2. Ask the patient to disrobe and don a gown, providing assistance as needed.
3. Assist the patient to sit on the end of the table.
4. Cover the patient's legs with a drape.
5. Ask the patient to lie back on the table while you support the feet and pull out the foot extension.
6. Position the stirrups level with the height of the table, about 1 foot from the side of the table, and lock them in place.
7. Ask the patient to slide down on the table until the buttocks are on the edge of the table end.
8. Assist the patient to bend the knees and place the feet in the stirrups. Position a drape for privacy with a point between the legs (Figure 36-12).
9. Position the light source and a rolling stool for the examiner.
10. Place a pillow under the patient's head as needed.
11. When the examination is complete, pull out the foot extension and help the patient remove the feet from the stirrups and place them on the foot extension.
12. Ask the patient to slide up on the table, assisting as necessary. Keep the drape in place to ensure privacy.

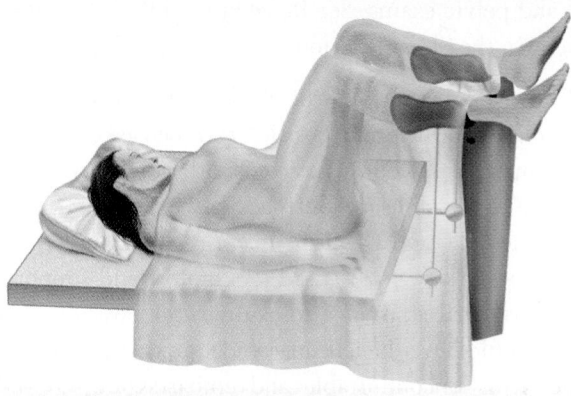

FIGURE 36-12   Lithotomy position.

13. Assist the patient to a sitting position and push in the foot extension. Allow time to prevent dizziness.
14. Assist the patient from the table, stabilizing the step stool if necessary, and provide further instruction for home care.
15. Clean the examination room for the next patient following the steps in Procedure 36-1.
16. Perform hand hygiene.

procedure
36-7

POSITIONING THE PATIENT IN THE FOWLER'S POSITION

Objective: Safely assist the patient into the Fowler's position for examination of the upper body and the head.

EQUIPMENT AND SUPPLIES
examination table; gown; drape

METHOD
1. Perform hand hygiene.
2. Provide a gown and assist the patient to don it as necessary.
3. Assist the patient up the step to sit on the end of the table. Stabilize the step stool as needed.
4. Cover the legs with a drape.
5. Assist the patient to slide back and lean on the raised end of the table.
6. Pull out the foot extension while supporting the patient's feet.
7. Raise the head of the table to a 90-degree angle for Fowler's position (Figure 36-13) and to a 45-degree angle for Semi-Fowler's position (Figure 36-14).
8. Place a pillow under the patient's knees to relieve strain on the lower back. Adjust the drape as needed.
9. When the examination is complete, push in the foot extension. Ask the patient to remain seated at the end of the table to prevent dizziness.
10. Inform patient before lowering the table. Ask the patient to lean forward while you support the patient's back and lower the table.
11. Assist the patient off the table, stabilizing the step stool as needed. Give further instructions as needed.
12. Clean the examination room for the next patient, following the steps in Procedure 36-1.
13. Perform hand hygiene.

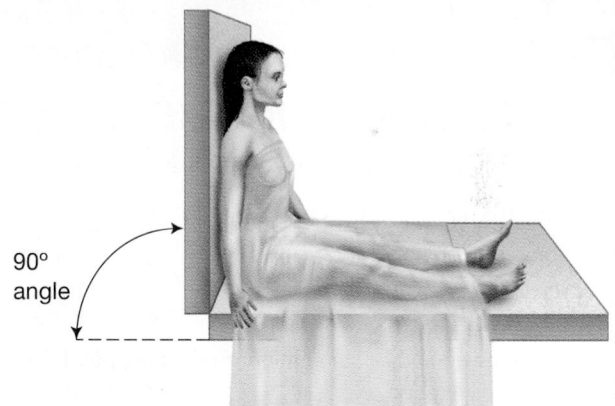

90°
angle

FIGURE 36-13   Fowler's position.

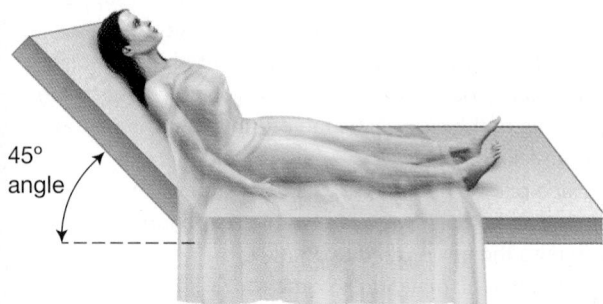

45°
angle

FIGURE 36-14   Semi-Fowler's position.

Prone Position. The prone position requires the patient to lie face down, flat on the stomach or the ventral surface of the body, with the head turned to the side and arms either alongside the body or crossed under the head. It is the opposite of the supine position. The drape should cover the patient from upper back to over the feet. This position is used for back exams and certain types of surgery. The prone position is unsuitable for patients with breathing problems, women in late-term pregnancies, or the elderly. In these cases the Sims' position may be more appropriate. See Procedure 36-8: Positioning the Patient in the Prone Position.

Sims' Position. The Sims' or lateral recumbent position requires the patient to be placed on the left side with the right leg sharply bent upward and the left leg slightly bent. The patient's weight is mainly on the chest area. The right arm is flexed next to the head for support. The patient is draped from under the arm to below the knees on an angle. This allows the physician to raise a small section of the drape while keeping the rest of the patient covered. This position is used for rectal exams, rectal temperatures, enemas, and perineal and pelvic exams. See Procedure 36-9: Positioning the Patient in the Sims' Position.

Knee–Chest Position. In the knee–chest position, the patient is placed in the prone position and then asked to pull the knees up to a kneeling position with thighs at a 90-degree angle to the table and buttocks in the air. The head is turned to one side, and the arms may be placed under the head or on either side of the head for comfort and support. Most patients need assistance to assume this position correctly and should never be left unattended in this position at any time. It is uncomfortable and embarrassing, so the patient should not be made to assume the knee–chest position until necessary during the examination. This position is used for proctologic exams, sigmoidoscopy procedures, and rectal and vaginal exams. The drape should be placed from the upper back at an angle covering the anal area. A fenestrated drape (a drape with a precut opening in the appropriate area) may be used.

procedure 36-8

POSITIONING THE PATIENT IN THE PRONE POSITION

Objective: Safely assist patient into the prone position for examination of the posterior of the body.

EQUIPMENT AND SUPPLIES
examination table; gown; drape

METHOD
1. Perform hand hygiene.
2. Provide a gown and ask the patient to disrobe, providing assistance as needed.
3. Assist the patient onto the end of the table, bracing the step stool as needed. Cover the patient's legs with a drape.
4. Ask the patient to lie back on the table while supporting the back and pulling out the foot extension.
5. Ask the patient to turn toward you onto his or her side, then onto the abdomen. Position yourself close to the middle of the side of the table to prevent the patient from falling.
6. Place pillows under the patient's head and feet as needed for comfort. Cover with a drape from the shoulders to the ankles (Figure 36-15).
7. When the examination is complete, ask the patient to turn toward you and help the patient to a sitting position.

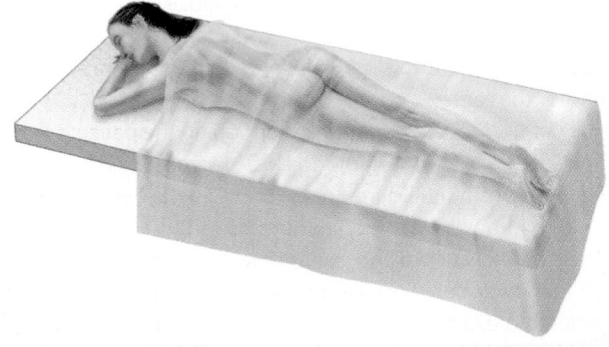

FIGURE 36-15 Prone position.

8. Have the patient stay seated a few moments to prevent dizziness from occurring.
9. Assist the patient from the table, stabilizing the step stool if needed, and provide further instructions.
10. Clean the examination room for the next patient following the steps in Procedure 36-1.
11. Perform hand hygiene.

procedure 36-9

POSITIONING THE PATIENT IN THE SIMS' POSITION

Objective: Safely assist the patient into the Sims' position for rectal exams, rectal temperatures, enemas, and perineal and pelvic exams.

EQUIPMENT AND SUPPLIES
examination table; gown; drape

METHOD
1. Perform hand hygiene.
2. Ask the patient to disrobe, provide a gown, and assist the patient to don the gown as needed.
3. Ask the patient to sit on the end of the table, stabilizing the step stool as needed.
4. Place the drape over the lap and legs.
5. Assist the patient to lie back, supporting the patient's back while extending the foot of the table.
6. Ask the patient to turn toward you onto his or her left side, placing the body weight on the chest with the left knee flexed slightly.
7. Ask the patient to flex the right knee to a 90-degree angle. Bend the patient's right arm at the elbow with the hand toward the head. Adjust the drape to cover the patient from the shoulders to the ankles (Figure 36-16).
8. When the examination or procedure is complete, ask the patient to turn toward you and onto his or her back.

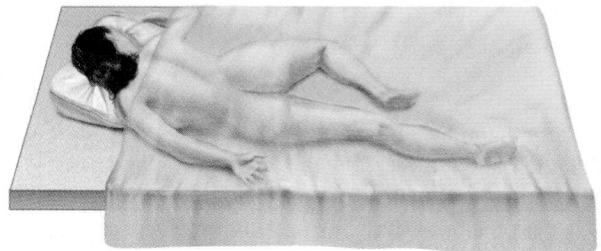

FIGURE 36-16 Sims' position.

Assist the patient to a sitting position. Ask the patient to remain seated at the end of the table a few moments to prevent dizziness.

9. Assist the patient from the table, stabilizing the step stool as needed, and provide further instruction as needed.
10. Clean the examination room for the next patient following the steps in Procedure 36-1.
11. Perform hand hygiene.

Many physicians have proctologic tables available for this type of exam. This specialized examination table can be elevated in the middle, which places the patient so he or she is bent at the hips with head and feet lowered. It is much easier on the patient than the knee–chest position. See Procedure 36-10: Positioning Patient in the Knee–Chest Position.

Trendelenburg Position. This position is not normally used in a physician's office except in cases of shock or low blood pressure. For this position the patient is placed in the supine position, the end of the table is raised to about a 30-degree angle. This position is also used for abdominal surgeries. The patient is draped from underarms to below the knees (Figure 36-17).

Proctologic Position. The proctologic (jack-knife) position is used for proctologic examinations with a sigmoido-

scope. It is similar to the knee–chest position but with a greater bend at the hips. Patients will lie face down with

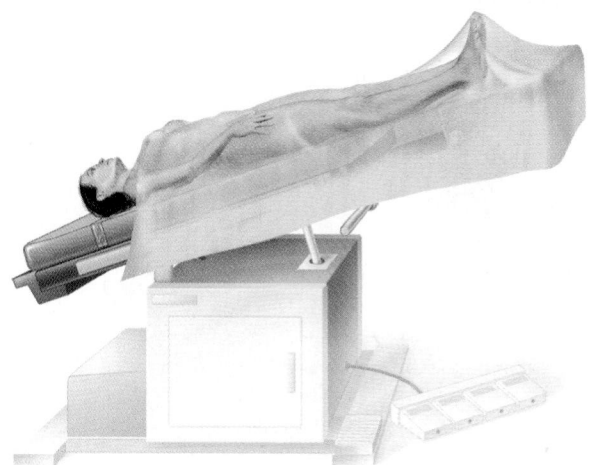

FIGURE 36-17 Trendelenburg position.

POSITIONING THE PATIENT IN THE KNEE–CHEST POSITION

Objective: Safely assist the patient into the knee–chest position for examination of the rectum, sigmoid colon, or vagina.

EQUIPMENT AND SUPPLIES

examination table; gown; drape

METHOD

1. Perform hand hygiene.
2. Ask the patient to disrobe, provide a gown, and assist the patient to don the gown as needed.
3. Ask the patient to sit on the end of the table, stabilizing step stool as needed.
4. Cover the legs with a drape.
5. Ask the patient to lie back while supporting the back and pulling out the foot extension.
6. Ask the patient to turn toward you onto the abdomen, providing assistance as needed. Position yourself in the center of the side of the table to prevent the patient from falling. Adjust the drape.
7. Assist the patient onto the knees, with hips bent and keeping the chest on the table. Buttocks will be raised in the air, arms bent, head turned to the side, and hands next to the head. The patient may rest his or her weight on the elbows if it is more comfortable (Figure 36-18).
8. Adjust the drape so the point of the drape is between the patient's legs.

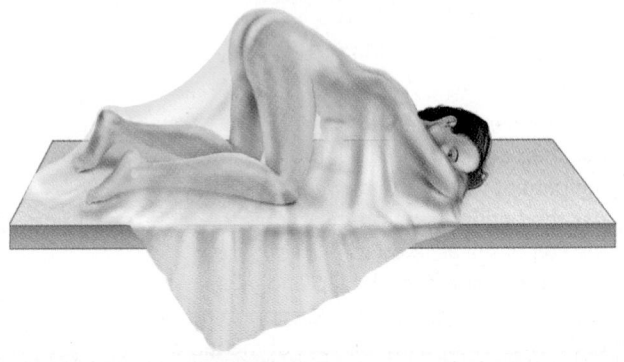

FIGURE 36-18   Knee–chest position.

9. When the examination is complete help the patient to lie flat on the abdomen. When the patient is ready, ask him or her to turn toward you and lie on the back. Help the patient to sit up and remain seated a few moments to prevent dizziness.
10. Assist the patient from the table, stabilizing the step stool as needed. Provide further instructions as needed.
11. Clean the examination table for the next patient, following the steps in Procedure 36-1.
12. Perform hand hygiene.

---

hips at the hinge of the table. A special examination table may then be tipped downward (Figure 36-19).

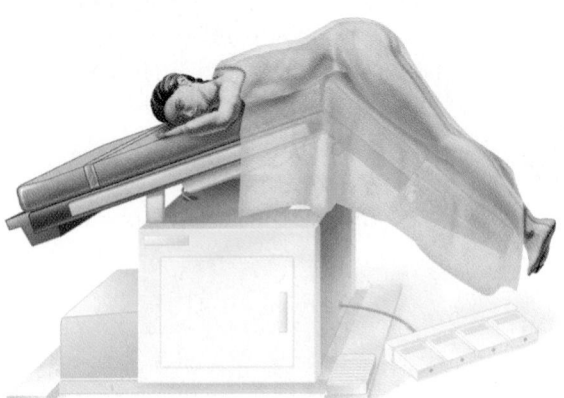

FIGURE 36-19   Proctologic (jack-knife) position.

Sitting Position.   This position is used to examine the head and chest (anterior and posterior). The patient sits upright with legs over the side of the examination table (Figure 36-20).

Patient Communication

Always explain to the patient why he or she is being placed in a specific position and the purpose of the drapes. Be sure that the patient is never left in an uncomfortable position any longer than is necessary, and assist the patient when a position change is required. Some of the positions can be very embarrassing to a patient. A medical assistant must be professional at all times to prevent the patient from being uncomfortable and self-conscious. A patient will be less embarrassed if the medical assistant explains why he or she must be in that particular position; therefore, it is essential

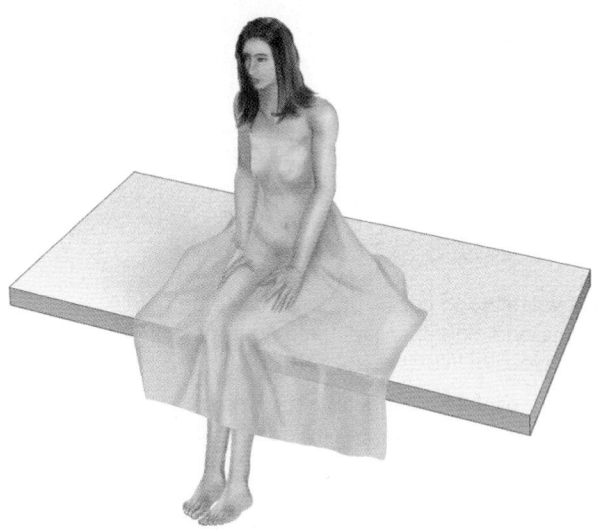

FIGURE 36-20 Sitting position.

for a medical assistant to understand the reason for placement in any position.

Physicians expect the medical assistant to have the patient in the correct position for a procedure. If the physician has to correct the medical assistant in front of the patient, the patient may think the medical assistant is incompetent. In turn this can cause the patient to lose trust and faith in the medical assistant and possibly cause the patient to become more apprehensive than he or she is already.

The medical assistant must always explain to the patient the events that will occur during the physical examination. This allows the patient time to prepare as well as to ask any questions. The medical assistant must also be truthful when preparing a patient for a physical examination. If a certain part of the physical examination is going to make the patient uncomfortable, the medical assistant must be honest and explain this to the patient so the patient can be prepared and more willing to cooperate. For example, if a female patient is having a Pap smear, the medical assistant must explain to the patient that when the physician inserts the vaginal speculum into the vagina she might feel some pressure in that area. How do you think the patient would feel if the medical assistant never told her that this might happen? The patient could feel angry and upset. The patient may not trust the medical assistant anymore because the medical assistant did not tell her what could be happening to her and her body. This is just one example of how a patient could be made uncomfortable when the medical assistant is not communicating effectively with the patient.

Some positions are also uncomfortable to patients because of health reasons. If a patient has low back pain, he or she may not be able to sit for a long time. If a patient with COPD is in the supine position and having difficulties breathing, the medical assistant should immediately help the patient to a semi-Fowler's position so he or she can breathe better. When a medical assistant is aware of the patient's medical history, he or she can make the patient more comfortable.

LABORATORY AND DIAGNOSTIC TESTS

Laboratory and other diagnostic tests may be ordered as an adjunct to the physician's exam. Some of these tests, such as a urinalysis or electrocardiogram, may be conducted in the office on the day of the examination, and others, such as X-rays, may be scheduled by appointment with a separate laboratory or diagnostic facility. Table 36-3 gives examples of tests that might be ordered as part of a complete examination.

Sequence of Examination Procedures

Individual physicians will instruct their medical assistant regarding the specific order of the physical examination. Typically, they will discuss the past medical history, CC, and the history of the PI first, and then do a **review of systems (ROS)**, or a head-to-toe exam; however, this will vary among physicians. The following is a common sequence for an examination:

skin→hair→nails→head→neck→eyes→ears→nose→mouth throat→arms→heart→chest→lungs→breasts→abdomen genitalia→rectum→legs→feet→neurological system

The ROS sheet will be documented by the physician as this portion of the exam is completed. During the examination the physician will wear the appropriate personal protective equipment (PPE). See Procedure 36-11: Assisting with a Complete Physical Examination.

A word about medical terminology and abbreviations is appropriate before considering individual sections of the ROS. Every medical assistant must have excellent medical terminology skills and be thoroughly familiar with correct usage and spelling of abbreviations. The proper usage, pronunciation, and spelling of medical terms are critical to your functioning professionally as a medical assistant. If you encounter words you are unsure of, look them up when time permits. Never guess at the meaning. When you are unsure of an abbreviation used in a physician's order, ask or look it up. Although many terms and abbreviations are fairly generic and widely used, others pertain to specific specialties and may be unfamiliar.

TABLE 36-3 Laboratory and Diagnostic Tests

Tests	Description
Blood chemistry profile	Package (or panel) of chemistry tests that provides overview of patient's body chemistries; less expensive than performing individual tests.
SMA-12 (or Chem 12)	Panel of 12 chemistry tests
SMAC (or Chem 20)	Panel of 20 tests
Complete blood count (CBC) including a differential count	Includes red blood cell (RBC) count, white blood cell (WBC) count, hemoglobin (Hg), hematocrit (Hct), RBC indices, platelets, and differential; the differential count indicates abnormalities of RBCs, platelets, and types of WBCs
Electrocardiogram (ECG)	Record of electrical activity of the heart; useful in diagnosis of heart muscle damage causing disruption of electrical activity of the heart and abnormal cardiac rhythm
Pulmonary function	Breathing equipment used to determine respiratory function and measure lung volume and gas exchange
Sedimentation rate (Sed rate, ESR)	Measures the rate at which erythrocytes (RBCs) settle out of blood in 1 hour; inflammatory conditions cause faster settling since they are heavier and the sed rate will be higher than normal
Visual acuity	Sharpness of vision
Vital signs	Measurements of signs of life, which include temperature, pulse, respirations, and blood pressure
Weight and height	Anthropometric measurements of the human body
X-rays	Radiology studies of body parts (e.g., chest and spine)

procedure 36-11

ASSISTING WITH A COMPLETE PHYSICAL EXAMINATION

Objective: Assist with a physical examination by preparing the necessary equipment, while observing proper sequencing and ensuring patient safety with limited direction.

EQUIPMENT AND SUPPLIES

alcohol swabs; drape; emesis basin; examination table with clean sheet; disposable gloves; laryngeal mirror; lubricant; nasal speculum; ophthalmoscope; otoscope; pillow (with clean cover); reflex hammer; scale with height rod; Snellen chart (vision); sphygmomanometer; stethoscope; tape measure; thermometer; tissues; tongue depressors; tuning fork; urine specimen container

Note: Equipment and supplies will vary, depending on the type and purpose of the examination and personal preferences of the physician.

METHOD

1. Perform hand hygiene.
2. Assemble all equipment in the examining room.
3. Identify the patient and explain the procedure. Patients should always be accompanied into the examining room.
4. For comfort and efficiency during the examination, the patient should have an empty bladder. If a urine sample is needed for testing, at this time provide the patient with a urine specimen container and instructions. Otherwise, simply offer the patient the opportunity to use the bathroom now.
5. Take vital signs and measurements (temperature, pulse, respirations, blood pressure, height, and weight). Document these data in the patient's record or on a complaint slip immediately.
6. Provide the patient with a gown and drape and give instructions on disrobing. Have the patient wear the gown with the opening in front if this is appropriate.

Ask the patient to sit on the side of the examination table, then leave the room to allow the patient to disrobe in privacy.

7. Return to the room, and place a drape sheet over the patient's legs.

Note: The physician may prefer to examine the female breasts and axilla when the patient is in a reclining position.

8. Tell the physician that the patient is ready. A female medical assistant should remain in the room if the patient is a female and the physician is a male or if the physician needs assistance.

9. Assist the physician as needed. The patient may require assistance during position changes.

10. Use gloves when handling used equipment that may contain biohazardous materials, such as the laryngeal mirror. The mirror and other contaminated equipment are placed in the emesis basin until they can be carried to the decontamination area. (In Figure 36-21 a physician is using an otoscope to examine a patient's ear.)

11. As the physician progresses from one section of the body to the next during the ROS, reposition the drape to expose only the portion of the patient's body being examined. Label all specimen slides as soon as possible. Use gloves when handling specimens.

12. When the examination is complete, assist the patient to sit up slowly.

Note: Some patients experience dizziness if they sit up suddenly. When removing legs from stirrups, take both legs down together to prevent strain on hips and back.

13. Assist the patient off the examination table if necessary.

14. Ask the patient if he or she requires help dressing. If no help is needed, allow the patient to dress in privacy.

15. Instruct the patient where to go after dressing.

16. After the patient has left the examination room, place all disposable materials in the appropriate sharps and waste containers. (Ideally, and to prevent injury to the patient, sharps should be disposed of one by one as they are used.) Remove soiled linens and place them in the laundry container. Reusable equipment is removed to a decontamination area to be cleaned and disinfected or sterilized.

17. Resupply the examination room.

18. Clean the examination table and replace the soiled linens and gowns.

19. Complete any documentation on the patient's record or the complaint slip. In some offices and hospitals, charting may be done electronically in the examination room or at the patient's bedside (Figure 36-22).

CHARTING EXAMPLE

2/14/XX 3:00 P.M. CPX by Dr. Williams. Pt. referred to clinic lab for CBC, UA, and mammogram. Pt. to return in 1 week to discuss results. Appointment made for 2/21/XX. · M. King, CMA (AAMA)

Note: The physician will document his or her findings from the CPX on the patient record.

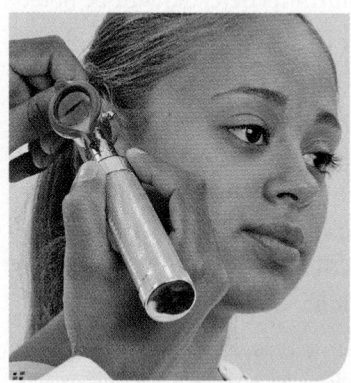

FIGURE 36-21 **Inspecting a patient's ear during a physical examination.**

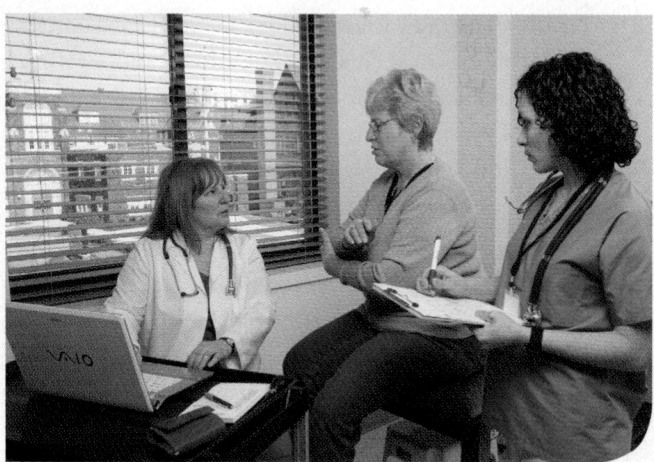

FIGURE 36-22 **Portable bedside computing aids in patient charting.**

REVIEW OF SYSTEMS

- **Skin**—The physician will inspect and palpate the skin, taking special note of the condition of the skin. This is an important aspect of the physical examination because it can indicate the patient's nutritional status and level of hydration. The color, temperature, texture, and turgor of the skin are assessed. **Turgor** refers to the resistance of the skin when grasped between fingers. Turgor is decreased in dehydration and increased in edema.

- **Hair**—The color, texture, distribution, quantity, and growth pattern of the hair are assessed. Certain diseases such as hyperthyroidism can cause alopecia (hair loss). Excessive facial hair in a female (hirsutism) may indicate hormonal imbalance.

- **Nails**—Color, texture, symmetry, shape, and size are assessed for possible circulation problem, fungus, or infections. Brittle, grooved, or lined nails may indicate local or systemic conditions.

- **Head**—The shape, size, and symmetry of the head are assessed. The scalp is also assessed for parasites (nits and lice), lesions, flakes, and irritations. The face of a patient reveals much about his or her state of health and stress level. Bruises or other signs of trauma may be indications of abuse. Specific questions by the physician during an examination may shed light on potential abuse problems.

- **Neck**—The neck is assessed for range of motion, texture, color, lumps, masses, pulsations, and swelling. The physician will also assess the carotid pulse, lymph nodes, thyroid gland, and trachea. Asking a patient to swallow while palpating the thyroid gland helps detect lumps or enlargement of the thyroid gland (goiter).

- **Eyes**—Prior to the physician seeing the patient, the medical assistant will test the patient's distance vision by using a Snellen chart, near vision using a Jaeger reading card, and color vision using the Ishihara test book. The physician will examine visual fields, pupils' reaction to light, and the internal and external structures of the eye. The internal examination is accomplished with an ophthalmoscope. The color of the sclera or white of the eye is evaluated for signs of jaundice. Eye movements are noted as well.

- **Ears**—The physician will examine the internal and external ear for color, size, shape, and position. The physician will use tuning forks and whispering to assess the patient's hearing. The ear canals are examined with an otoscope for signs of foreign bodies or excess cerumen or earwax.

- **Nose**—The internal and external nose will be examined for color and symmetry. The physician will also assess the patient's sense of smell. If drainage is observed, the physician will note the amount, color, and consistency. Red swollen mucosa with yellow to greenish discharge indicates infection.

- **Mouth**—The physician will assess the lips and inside the mouth for symmetry, moisture, color, and lesions. The tongue texture, color, size, shape, symmetry, movement, and position will be assessed. The number of teeth as well as the color and condition will be noted. Adequate oral hygiene is important to a patient's overall health. Patients should be reminded to schedule regular dental care and cleaning. Gums should be pink and healthy and not prone to bleeding.

- **Throat**—When the physician asks the patient to say "Ah," this gives the physician an opportunity to assess the uvula, tonsils, and throat for color, size, shape, symmetry, and movement, using the tongue depressor. The physician will also check the patient's gag reflex.

- **Arms**—The joints and pulses of the arms as well as the strength and range of motion will be assessed by the physician.

- **Heart**—Using a stethoscope the physician will auscultate the sounds of the heart, noting the rate, rhythm, pitch, and quality. The physician will then place the stethoscope over various areas of the patient's heart and listen. Any murmurs detected will be noted.

- **Chest**—The chest wall will be assessed for symmetry during inspiration and expiration. It will also be assessed for pain, tenderness, lesions, lumps, and temperature. Postural abnormalities such as scoliosis, or curvature of the spine, may be noted as well.

- **Lungs**—Using a stethoscope the physician will auscultate the patient's breath sounds, noting rate, rhythm, pitch, depth, and location.

- **Breasts**—The physician will assess the breasts of both males and females. The breasts will be assessed for size, shape, symmetry, and texture. Any discharge, lumps, masses, pain, or tenderness will be noted.

- **Abdomen**—The abdomen is assessed for symmetry, texture, temperature, and movement. Using a stethoscope the physician will auscultate the patient's bowel sounds for frequency, pitch, gurgling, and clicking sounds. The abdomen is visually divided into four quadrants: right and left upper quadrants and right and left lower quadrants. Next, the organs in each quadrant are percussed and palpated for signs of masses, position of organs, and muscle tone.

- **Genitalia**—The physician will assess the internal and external genitalia of a female patient. For the male patient the physician will assess the external genitalia and perform a testicular examination. These examinations will be discussed more fully in Chapter 38.
- **Rectum**—To assess the rectum for lesions or masses, the physician will perform a digital rectal examination. Most physicians require anyone over 40 years of age to have a digital rectal exam for early detection of colorectal cancer. A stool sample may be gathered for occult or hidden blood at the same time.

- **Legs and feet**—The joints and pulses of the legs and feet as well as the strength and range of motion will be assessed by the physician. Other postural problems may be noted.
- **Neurological system**—The physician will examine each reflex for the appropriate response. The physician will also observe the patient's gait, facial expressions, sensation response, speech, and movement.

Table 36-4 presents a synopsis of the ROS. Table 36-5 presents a typical sequence of procedures to be performed

TABLE 36-4 Review of Systems (ROS)

Head	Headaches, sinus pain, masses, alopecia (unusual hair loss), dizziness, injury, or trauma
Eyes	Visual acuity, blurred vision, burning, halo effect, tearing, photophobia (sensitivity to light), discharge, redness, jaundice (yellowing of skin and sclera), known eye diseases, date of last eye exam, prescription glasses, contact lenses
Ears	Tinnitus or ringing in the ears, dizziness, hearing loss, discharge, ear infections, exposure to loud noise on a regular basis
Nose	Allergies, obstruction, sense of smell, pain, discharge
Mouth	Dental work, dentures, gums, sense of taste, teeth, salivation (producing saliva), dryness of mouth, tongue, leukoplakia (white patches, possibly cancerous), gingivitis
Throat	Hoarseness, laryngitis (loss of voice), redness, speech defect, masses, pain
Neck	Tenderness, pain, swelling, difficulty swallowing, enlarged nodes
Respiratory	Dyspnea (labored breathing), cough, asthma, wheezing, allergies, hemoptysis (coughing up blood), chest pain, night sweats, orthopnea (difficulty breathing while lying down), shortness of breath (SOB)
Cardiovascular (CV)	Chest pain, hypertension, peripheral edema, cyanosis, fainting, dizziness, heart murmurs, palpitations, arrhythmias
Gastrointestinal (GI)	Nausea, vomiting, anorexia (loss of appetite), bulimia (eating disorder—binge eating followed by purging), indigestion, diarrhea, constipation, hemorrhoids, presence of blood in stool, number of bowel movements daily, hematemesis (vomiting blood)
Genitourinary (GU)	History of urinary tract infection, frequency, hesitation, oliguria (reduced urine), hematuria (blood in urine), dysuria (difficult or painful urination), renal colic (kidney pain), stones, discharge, nocturia (urination during the night)
Female reproductive	Menstrual history, obstetric history, leukorrhea (white discharge), itching, pain, discharge, date of last Pap smear, breast self-exam history, sexual habits, menopause symptoms, last mammogram (breast exam)
Male reproductive	Prostate problems, testicular self-exam, discharge, sexual habits, frequency of urination, decreased stream, nocturia, impotence
Endocrine	Growth and development, goiter, excessive thirst, intolerance to temperature change, hormone therapy, diabetes symptoms, irregular menses, symptoms of thyroid disorders
Skin	Rash, urticaria (hives), texture, moles, infection, redness, jaundice, cyanosis, allergies, dry/oily, acne
Musculoskeletal (MS)	Joint pain, swelling, weakness, stiffness, numbness, muscle pain, fractures, discoloration, edema
Neurologic	Fainting, loss of consciousness, headaches, tremor, nervousness, paralysis, pain, memory loss
Psychiatric	Mental health history, emotional stability, depression, stress
General	Weight gain or loss, sleep habits, fatigue, eating habits, smoking, work environment

TABLE 36-5 Sequence of Physical Examination Procedures

1. Registration	Receptionist/medical assistant
2. History	Receptionist/medical assistant
3. Urine specimen	Medical assistant or laboratory technician
4. Blood specimen	Medical assistant or laboratory technician
5. Vital signs	Medical assistant
6. Weight and height	Medical assistant
7. Visual acuity	Medical assistant
8. Electrocardiogram	Medical assistant
9. X-ray	X-ray technician (provided X-ray room is available; otherwise X-ray is completed before the patient's visit)
10. Preparation of the patient	Medical assistant

and the person responsible for completing the procedure. Guildelines 36-1 lists important guidelines for charting. It is important to remember the steps associated with accurately documenting information in the patient medical record. Information pertaining to correct documentation can be found in Chapters 13 and 14.

PROFESSIONALISM THE WORKPLACE

Be sure to practice driving to your externship or new position location several times prior to the start of your externship. It is especially important to do this during high traffic times and at the time of day you are scheduled to begin work. This will help you to plan your commute time appropriately. Have two or three alternate routes planned for traffic emergencies. Having a good map with the routes highlighted can be very helpful at this time.

GUIDELINES 36-1

CHARTING

1. Double-check to make sure that you have the correct patient chart.
2. Use dark ink, preferably black, and write legibly. Printing is preferred if one's handwriting is difficult to read.
3. The patient's name should appear on each page of the record. Many offices will have a device that stamps the patient's name and identification number onto paper.
4. Every entry must be dated and initialed by the person writing in the record. The full name of the person initialing the document should either be in the medical record or on file in the physician's office.
5. Entries should be brief but complete.
6. Use only accepted medical abbreviations known by the general staff, and correctly spell all medical terms. See Appendix IV for a list of commonly used medical abbreviations.
7. Never erase, use a liquid eraser, or in any way remove information from a medical record. The accepted method of correcting medical records is described fully in Chapter 13.
8. Document all telephone calls relating to the patient in the medical record as well as other correspondence.
9. Document any action(s) taken as a result of telephone conversations.
10. Document all missed appointments.
11. Document any incidences of noncompliance.
12. Document every circumstance of patient education.
13. Do not record personal opinion, speculations, or judgments.

SUMMARY

The atmosphere provided by the medical assistant, whose responsibilities include preparation of the exam room and the medical record, creates a patient's first impression of a physician's office. The ability to anticipate the physician's needs during the exam is acquired with experience. Patient safety and comfort during the exam are a priority because they allow the physician to efficiently complete the examination while obtaining the most accurate data. The medical assistant's role before, during, and after the examination is to ensure that the medical record, the patient, and the equipment are completely prepared and ready for the exam. Accuracy and thoroughness are imperative to providing quality medical care.

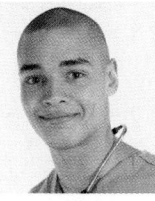

36 CHAPTER REVIEW

COMPETENCY REVIEW

1. Define and spell the terms to learn for this chapter.

2. Prepare an exam room for a physical examination.

3. Identify instruments and equipment used by the physician when completing a physical examination.

4. Prepare a patient for a physical exam.

5. Demonstrate knowledge of positions used for physical examinations.

6. List the six methods used in physical examinations.

PREPARING FOR THE CERTIFICATION EXAM

1. The position used for a patient in shock is
   a. lithotomy
   b. Fowler's
   c. supine
   d. Sims'
   e. Trendelenburg

2. To examine a patient vaginally the patient is usually placed in the
   a. lithotomy position
   b. Fowler position
   c. supine position
   d. anatomic position
   e. prone position

3. Listening to sounds produced through an instrument or with your ear is
   a. inspection
   b. auscultation
   c. percussion
   d. palpation
   e. examination

4. A general medical history is obtained preferably
   a. at the beginning of the first office visit
   b. whenever the need arises
   c. before admission to a hospital
   d. at the reception desk
   e. at a convenient time

5. Face down on an examination table with legs out straight is the
   a. supine position
   b. knee–chest position
   c. Sims' position
   d. dorsal recumbent position
   e. prone position

6. Listening to sounds when the body is struck in a definite manner is called
   a. auscultation
   b. percussion
   c. palpation
   d. mensuration
   e. manipulation

7. Distinguishing between two similar diseases by comparing their symptoms is called
   a. physical diagnosis
   b. laboratory diagnosis
   c. clinical diagnosis
   d. differential diagnosis
   e. radiologic diagnosis

8. The process of measuring is called
   a. inspection
   b. palpation
   c. palpitation
   d. mensuration
   e. manipulation

9. A patient with COPD struggling to breath in the sitting position should be changed to which position?
   a. lithotomy
   b. dorsal recumbent
   c. semi-Fowler's
   d. knee–chest
   e. prone

10. The instrument used to examine the eyes during a physical examination is the
    a. otoscope
    b. stethoscope
    c. proctoscope
    d. ophthalmoscope
    e. cystoscope

CRITICAL THINKING

1. How should Susan record Molly's chief complaint?

2. Susan obtains Molly's vital signs which are T: 98.8°F, P: 82 bpm, BP: 130/88. Pearson Physicans Group utilizes the SOAP method of charting. Which part of the SOAP note would be appropriate to include Molly's vital signs?

3. What should Susan instruct Molly to do prior to being seen by the physician?

ON THE JOB

Elizabeth Smith, CMA, just started working for Dr. Williams today. The first task he gave Elizabeth was to make sure each exam room had the correct supplies. After she completed that task, Dr. Williams had her prepare the examining room for his next patient.

1. What supplies should an examining room typically contain?
2. What is the function of the supplies in a typical examining room?
3. How should Elizabeth prepare the examining room for Dr. Williams's next patient?

INTERNET ACTIVITY

Perform an Internet search for examples of the various types of electronic medical record systems available for a medical office.

Additional interactive resources and activities for this chapter can be found:

On your student DVD: View applicable procedure videos on the DVD-ROM found in the back of this book.

MyHealthProfessionsKit.com: Test your knowledge of the chapter with games and activities. MyHealthProfessionsKit also includes resources, helpful links, and a Spanish audio glossary.

Medical Assisting Interactive: Practice your procedures as a medical assistant in this simulated doctor's office. This can be accessed through MyHealthProfessionsKit.com.

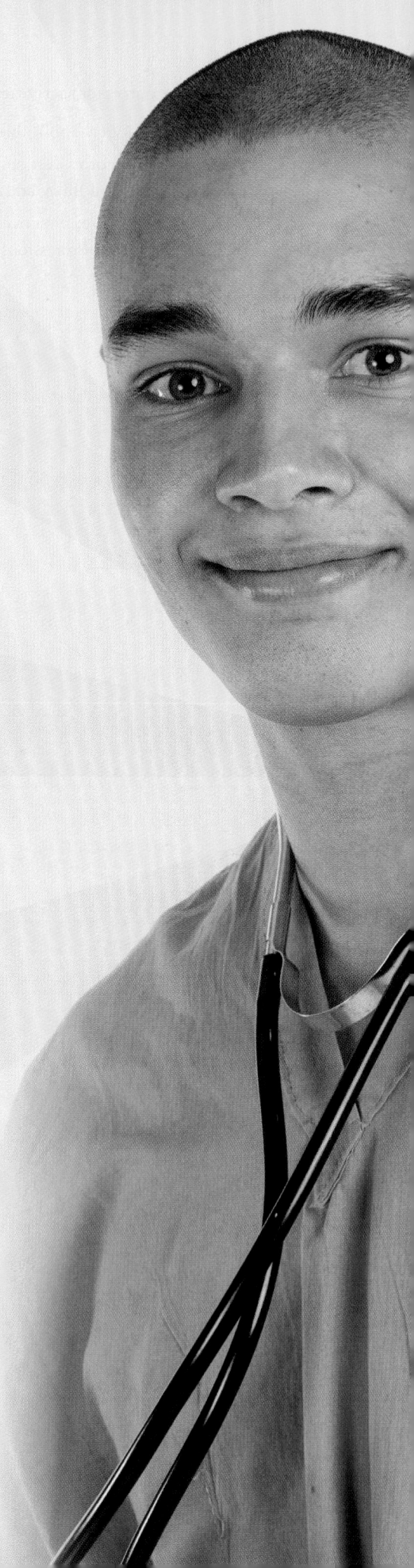

37

Assisting with Medical Specialties

LEARNING OBJECTIVES

After completing this chapter, you should be able to:

- Define and spell the terms to learn for this chapter.

- Prepare patients for examinations and diagnostic procedures.

- Assist the physician with examinations and treatments.

- Perform selected diagnostic tests.

- Instruct patients with special procedures.

- Document special procedures accurately.

CHAPTER OUTLINE

CASE STUDY

Benito Salvatore, a 65-year-old business executive, is scheduled to have a sigmoidoscopy with Dr. Bahjat. When David, RMA, escorts him to the procedure room, Benito confides that he is extremely nervous and is concerned he did not prepare well enough for the sigmoidoscopy.

allergen

anaphylactic shock

angina

arthritis

atherosclerosis

benign

colic

desensitizing injections

diaphoresis

embolus

eosinophil

histamine

hypersensitivity

ischemia

kyphosis

lordosis

malignant

myocardial infarction (MI)

neurology

nonsteroidal anti-inflammatory drugs (NSAIDs)

occult

oncology

orthopedics

polydipsia

polyuria

proctologist

Queckenstedt's sign

Romberg test

scoliosis

thrombus

venom

wheal

CERTIFICATION LINK

CMAS
Vital signs and measurements
Examination preparation

RMA
Vital signs and mensurations
Physical examinations

CMA (AAMA)
Patient preparation and assisting the physician

Special examinations and procedures related to specific body systems are commonly performed in the medical office. The most commonly performed examinations include pediatric, prenatal, gynecologic, cardiovascular, proctoscopic, and sigmoidoscopic. Discussion of some of these examinations and a review of procedures and tests related to specific body systems, are presented in this chapter. For additional information related to diseases and disorders associated with each body system, refer to Unit Three: Anatomy and Physiology.

The Role of the Medical Assistant

The role of the medical assistant is to assist the physician during special examinations and procedures and to instruct the patient before, during, and after many of these procedures. Though some of the procedures discussed throughout this chapter are performed in the hospital setting, the medical assistant, as one of the prime educators of the patient, must know and understand a vast amount of medical information regarding these procedures.

Working as a medical assistant will bring you into contact with a variety of conditions and diseases. Whether the conditions are acute (rapid onset) or chronic (long lasting or recurring) patients will exhibit a wide range of reactions, such as fear, anger, and frustration. They deserve your empathy and support.

Allergy

An allergy is an abnormal response or **hypersensitivity** to a substance (**allergen**), such as a medication or pollen that does not normally cause a reaction in most people. Allergens enter the body through inhalation, injection, swallowing, or contact with the skin. Any substance in the environment, such as pollen, certain foods, insect **venom** (poison), and animal dander or saliva, can cause an allergy in sensitive persons. Allergic reactions may be localized, such as a mosquito bite, or systemic, such as asthma or anaphylactic shock, both of which can be life threatening. An antigen is a substance, usually protein in nature, which induces the production of antibodies. An antibody is a protein substance produced in the body in response to a foreign invading substance (antigen). In a normal immune reaction, the foreign substance (antigen) and the specific antibody unite and are excreted from the body. The allergic interaction of an antigen and antibody causes the release of **histamine**, which is the substance that produces signs and symptoms of allergies. The symptoms of allergies consist of a local or systemic inflammatory reaction, which is characterized by redness, edema, and heat. Respiratory symptoms include wheezing, sneezing, coughing, and nasal congestion.

Allergic conditions include eczema, allergic rhinitis, hay fever, bronchial asthma, urticaria (hives), and food allergies. (See Table 37-1 for information on common allergies.) An increase in the blood eosinophil level may occur with allergies. An **eosinophil** is a granular white cell that captures invading microorganisms and antibody–anitgen reactions through phagocytosis (engulfing or eating).

The treatment for allergies consists of medications, such as the antihistamine diphenhydramine (Benadryl), allergy testing, and desensitization. **Desensitizing injections** involve administering minute amounts of the allergen into the patient's system over an extended period of time and are used to build and develop a tolerance for the allergen in the patient. Desensitization is necessary if the allergic reactions

TABLE 37-1 Common Types of Allergies

Allergy	Description
Allergic rhinitis	Inflammation of the nasal mucosa that results in nasal congestion, rhinorrhea (runny nose), sneezing, and itching of the nose. Seasonal allergic rhinitis, such as hay fever, occurs only during certain seasons of the year. Children suffering from this type of allergy may rub their nose in an upward movement, called the "allergic salute."
Asthma	Condition seen most frequently in childhood in which wheezing, coughing, and dyspnea are the major symptoms. Asthmatic attacks may be caused by allergens inhaled from air, food, or drugs. The patient's airway is affected by constriction of the bronchial passages. Treatment is medication and control of the causative factors.
Contact dermatitis	Inflammation and irritation of the skin due to contact with an irritating substance, such as soap, perfume, cosmetics, plastics, dyes, and plants, such as poison ivy. Treatment consists of topical and systemic medications and removal of the causative item.
Eczema	Superficial dermatitis accompanied by papules, vesicles, and crusting. The condition can be acute or chronic.
Urticaria	Skin eruption of pale reddish wheals with severe itching. It is usually associated with a food allergy, stress, or drug reactions. Also called hives.

significantly interfere with the patient's lifestyle or are life threatening. Figure 37-1 shows a young patient receiving an allergy injection.

ANAPHYLACTIC SHOCK

In some persons, a life-threatening allergic reaction called **anaphylactic shock** can occur. Insect stings (e.g., bees and wasps) and allergies to drugs (e.g., penicillin) or foods (e.g., peanuts or shellfish) can cause severe reactions. The symptoms include acute respiratory distress, edema, hypotension, rash, tachycardia, pale cool skin, convulsions, and cyanosis. This condition can result in circulatory and respiratory changes. It requires emergency treatment consisting of medication, such as epinephrine to relax smooth muscles in the airways, and in some cases requires endotracheal intubation and mechanical ventilation. (The terms adrenaline and epinephrine are used interchangeably.) If no treatment is received, unconsciousness and death may result in a short period of time.

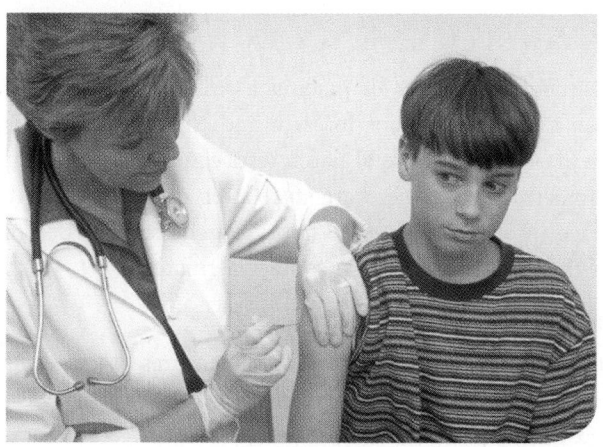

FIGURE 37-1 An allergy shot is used to desensitize an allergen.

Anaphylaxis is an emergency situation that requires medical intervention. Patients with hypersensitivity to insect venom or foods, such as peanuts, must carry an anaphylactic shock kit containing a self-injecting dose of epinephrine. The kit should be carried by the patient at all times. Should anaphylaxis occur, either the patient can self-administer or a witness may perform the intervention. Thus, patient and family education on the use of epinephrine for anaphylaxis is extremely important. All allergy patients should be instructed to read labels of foods, herbal products, and over-the-counter medications carefully. You should remind those with severe food allergies to check with their server or host about food ingredients that could be harmful if not fatal to them.

ALLERGY TESTING

Testing is ordered by the physician to determine a patient's sensitivities to allergens. The methods used include scratch or skin testing, intradermal tests, patch tests, and the radioallergosorbent test (RAST).

Scratch Test

The scratch method of allergy testing is usually performed on the patient's back or arm. The skin is divided into small squares, which are approximately 1 inch apart, and labeled with a ballpoint pen to indicate which allergen is being used. A drop of allergen is placed on the skin at the appropriately labeled site, then the skin is scratched with a needle or lancet. A new needle or lancet is used for each allergen tested. Many scratch tests using different allergens can be performed at the same time. See Procedure 37-1 for the steps to perform a scratch test. If a **wheal** forms within 15 minutes after placing an allergen on the skin, an allergy is indicated

PERFORMING A SCRATCH TEST

Objective: Determine specific substances that cause an allergic reaction in the patient.

EQUIPMENT AND SUPPLIES

allergen extracts; control solution; cotton balls; alcohol; disposable sterile needles or lancets; timer; tape; ruler; cold pack or ice bag; patient's record; disposable gloves; biohazard waste containers, including sharps container

METHOD

1. Perform hand hygiene.
2. Identify the patient, introduce self, and explain the procedure.
3. Assist the patient onto the examination table if necessary.
4. Apply gloves and swab the test site (either upper arm or back) with alcohol and allow it to air dry.
5. Label the skin surface with adhesive tape in rows about $1\frac{1}{2}$ to 2 inches apart.
6. Place a drop of allergen above or below the correct label. Be consistent.
7. Using a separate sterile lancet or needle for each extract, make a small scratch (no more than $\frac{1}{8}$ inch deep) on the skin below each drop.
8. Set the timer for the specified reaction time. Time is usually 10 to 30 minutes.
9. After the specified time period elapses, clean each site with alcohol and a cotton ball, taking care not to remove labels.
10. Examine and measure each site and record the results in the patient's record. Figure 37-2 shows examples of wheals resulting from allergy testing.
11. Have the physician check each site.

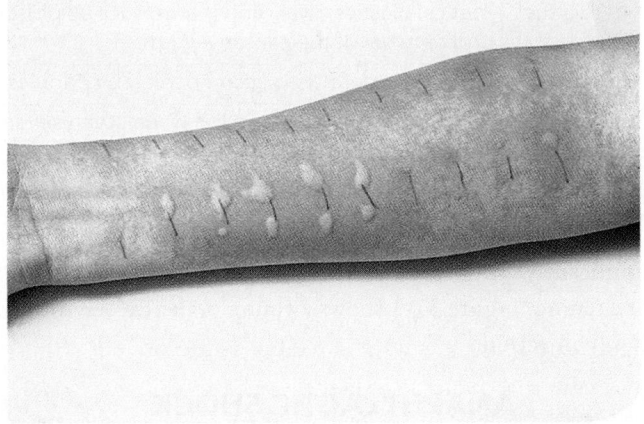

FIGURE 37-2 The patient's forearm shows a number of wheals formed after injection with an antigen. The size of the wheal corresponds to the degree of allergy to the specific antigen injected.

12. Apply cold packs or ice bag to relieve itching if necessary.
13. Dispose of used material properly.
14. Assist the patient off the examination table, and allow time and privacy for the patient to dress, offering aid as needed.
15. Clean the examination room. Record any further data in the patient's record.
16. Perform hand hygiene.

CHARTING EXAMPLE

03/13/XX 9:05 A.M. Scratch test performed. No positive reactions. Checked by Dr. Rosen · · · · · M. Dennehey, CMA (AAMA)

(Figure 37-3). A wheal is a small, round raised area that may be accompanied by itching. The patient should be advised to remain in the physician's office for at least 30 minutes after the testing has been completed in the event there is a delayed allergic reaction to the testing.

Intradermal Test

Intradermal allergy testing is performed by injecting 0.01 to 0.02 mL of an allergen extract into the anterior surface of the forearm. Several tests (10 to 18) can be performed on each arm. A red wheal is a positive sign. An intradermal test is considered more accurate than a scratch test. See Chapter 54 for a more detailed description of intradermal injections.

Patch Test

The patch test consists of placing a small amount of the allergen onto the anterior forearm and then covering this with a plastic wrap. Several patch tests can be performed at the same time, and these are read after the patches have remained in place for 24 to 48 hours. Patch tests are used to detect the causative agents in contact dermatitis.

Radioallergosorbent Test

The radioallergosorbent test (RAST) measures blood levels of antibodies to particular antigens. A venipuncture is performed on the patient, and the sample is sent to a laboratory where it is exposed to a variety of suspected allergens

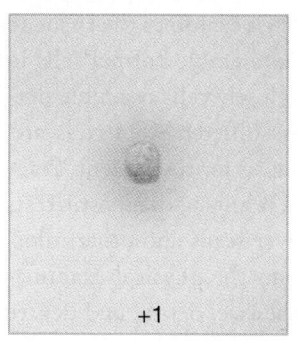
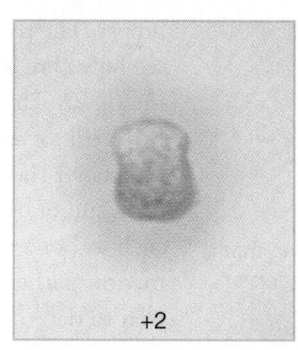
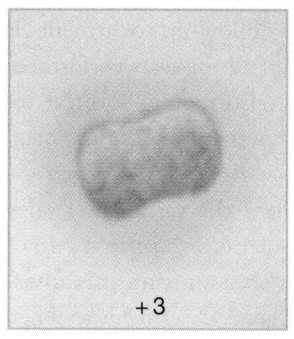
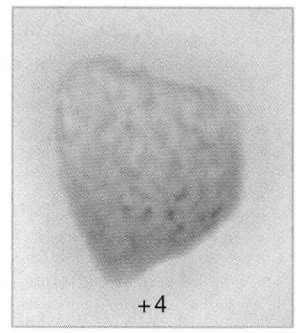

+1

+2

+3

+4

FIGURE 37-3 Wheals are formed in reaction to a scratch testing of allergens.

and the levels of antibodies are measured. This test is expensive but more sensitive and useful for patients who have dermatological problems or cannot stop taking allergy medication safely in order to have one of the other tests performed.

Dermatology

The skin and its accessory structures—sweat glands, oil glands, nails, and hair—are known as the integumentary system. The sense organs, which respond to changes in temperature, pain, touch, and pressure, are located in this system. The skin consists of the epidermis (thin outer membrane), the dermis (middle, fibrous layer), and subcutaneous (innermost layer containing fatty tissue) layers. Medical conditions related to this system occur in all three layers. Refer to Chapter 22 for additional information.

COMMON SKIN DISORDERS

Most skin conditions and diseases are diagnosed, in part, by observing the lesion. Skin lesions can occur whenever the normal surface of the skin is invaded or changed. A skin lesion is not always a sign of disease, as is seen with a noncancerous nodule. There is generally some discoloration or change from the normal coloration.

Some of the more common skin lesions are illustrated in Figure 37-4. These terms should be used when charting information related to any skin lesions.

Bacteria, viruses, and parasites can all invade the skin if its protective barrier is broken. Inflammatory skin disorders result in swelling, redness, and often itching over the affected site. These conditions include cellulitis, decubitus ulcers, psoriasis, acne vulgaris, and scleroderma:

- Cellulitis or erysipelas is an inflammation of the cellular or connective tissue caused by either *Staphylococcus* or *Streptococcus* infection of a cut or lesion. Treatment consists of antibiotics and application of warm compresses.

- Decubitus ulcers, or bedsores, are open sores caused by pressure over bony prominences on the body due to a lack of blood flow. These can appear in bedridden patients who lie in one position too long. Treatment consists of relieving the pressure through frequent turning and exercise of the patient, thorough cleansing of the wound, and topical antibiotics. Deep ulcers may require surgical debridement (removal of dead tissue).

- Psoriasis is a chronic inflammatory condition consisting of discrete red or pink lesions covered with silver scaling. Psoriasis is not contagious and is thought to be an autoimmune disease. Treatment consists of topical ointments and, in some severe cases, ultraviolet light therapy.

- Acne vulgaris is an inflammatory disease of the sebaceous glands and hair follicles that results in papules and pustules. Treatment consists of thorough cleansing and systemic and topical antibiotics.

- Scleroderma is a chronic, progressive autoimmune disease that affects the blood vessels and connective tissue of the skin and other organs. Integumentary symptoms include hardening of the skin, pallor, edema, and fixating of skin to subcutaneous tissues. There is no known cause and no cure.

DERMATOLOGICAL NEOPLASMS

Neoplasms or tumors can be either **benign** (noncancerous) or **malignant** (cancerous). Neoplasms are biopsied by surgically removing a small amount of tissue for testing. Benign growths may grow in size but are usually encapsulated. Malignant growths are invasive and tend to take over surrounding tissues. Invasion of area tissue takes place when malignant cells break through the basement membrane, separating epithelial cells from the connective tissue below. Cancer cells then may invade blood and lymphatic tissue and spread to other areas of the body. See

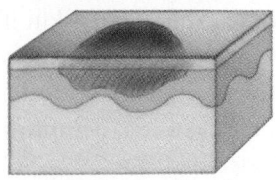

A macule is a discolored spot on the skin; freckle.

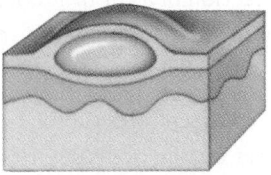

A wheal is a localized, evanescent elevation of the skin that is often accompanied by itching; urticaria.

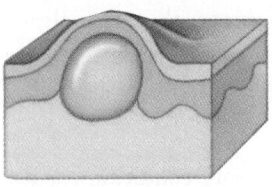

A papule is a solid, circumscribed, elevated area on the skin; pimple.

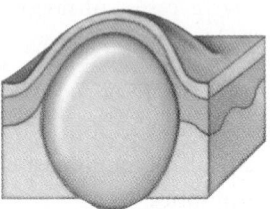

A nodule is a larger papule; acne vulgaris.

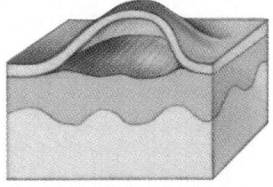

A vesicle is a small fluid filled sac; blister. A bulla is a large vesicle.

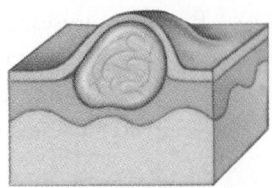

A pustule is a small, elevated, circumscribed lesion of the skin that is filled with pus; varicella (chickenpox).

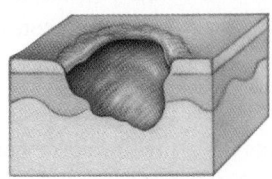

An erosion or ulcer is an eating or gnawing away of tissue; decubitus ulcer.

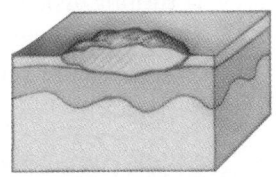

A crust is a dry, serous or seropurulent, brown, yellow, red, or green exudation that is seen in secondary lesions; eczema.

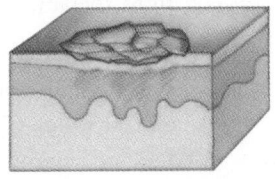

A scale is a thin, dry flake of cornified epithelial cells.

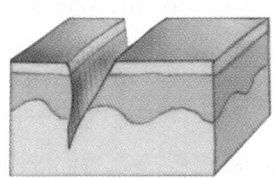

A fissure is a crack-like sore or slit that extends through the epidermis into the dermis; athlete's foot.

FIGURE 37-4 Skin lesions are objective signs of an illness or disorder. They can be seen, measured, and felt.

Table 37-2 for a list of different types of neoplasms and corresponding descriptions.

To determine a course of treatment, a physician must grade and stage the malignancy. Grading is done by a pathologist, who examines the tissue removed during biopsy. The pathologist examines the tissue to see how closely cells resemble normal cells in the tissue. The less closely cells resemble normal cells or the less differentiated cells are, the poorer the prognosis for the patient. Staging a tumor uses the results of diagnostic tests such as bone and liver scans and other information gathered from the physical examination to determine the size, depth, and degree of spread of the initial tumor. Treatment of a malignant tumor is usually surgical removal of the tumor, and follow-up treatment is based on the results of all the tests performed. Benign tumors may also require surgical removal if they impair normal functioning of an organ.

When patients hear the term *tumor* they immediately think of cancer. Since a tumor can be either benign or malignant, it is advisable not to use the general term *tumor* when talking to a patient. **Oncology** is the branch of medicine dealing with malignant neoplasms or tumors. Cancer therapy, consisting of some combination of chemotherapy (toxic drugs), radiation, cryotherapy, and radiotherapy, is used in the treatment of cancer.

Diagnostic Procedures

A variety of diagnostic tests and procedures are used when treating disorders of the integumentary system. These are described in Table 37-3. These procedures are performed by the physician with the assistance of the medical assistant. The physician may order a wound culture to determine the causative agent and best antibiotic to treat an infected wound. Procedure 37-2 provides the steps necessary to obtain a culture of a wound.

Cardiovascular System

Cardiology is the study of the cardiovascular or circulatory system. This system includes the heart and blood vessels. For a review of anatomy and physiology of the cardiovascular system, see Chapter 27. Cardiovascular disease is the most frequent cause of death and illness in the United States, regardless of gender. Working as a medical assistant in any specialty, you will care for patients with heart disease. It is important that you recognize the

TABLE 37-2 Dermatological Neoplasms

Benign (Noncancerous) Neoplasms	Description
Dermatofibroma	Fibrous tumor of the skin. It is painless, round, firm, red, and generally found on extremities.
Hemangioma	Benign tumor of dilated vessels.
Keloid	Formation of a scar after an injury or surgery that results in a raised, thickened, red area.
Keratosis	Overgrowth or thickening of cells in the epithelium located in the epidermis of the skin.
Leukoplakia	Change in the mucous membrane that results in thick, white patches on the mucous membrane of the tongue and cheek. It is considered precancerous and is associated with smoking.
Lipoma	Fatty tumor that generally does not metastasize (spread).
Nevus	Pigmented (colored) congenital skin blemish that is usually benign but may become cancerous. Also called a birthmark or mole.
Malignant (Cancerous) Neoplasms	**Description**
Basal cell carcinoma	Epithelial tumor of the basal cell layer of the epidermis. A frequent type of skin cancer that rarely metastasizes.
Karposi's sarcoma	Form of skin cancer frequently seen in acquired immune deficiency syndrome (AIDS) patients. It consists of brownish-purple papules that spread from the skin.
Malignant melanoma	Dangerous form of skin cancer caused by an overgrowth of melanin in the skin. It may metastasize.
Squamous cell carcinoma	Epidermal cancer that may go into deeper tissue but does not generally metastasize.

TABLE 37-3 Procedures and Diagnostic Tests Related to the Integumentary System

Procedure/Test	Description
Adipectomy	Surgical removal of fat.
Biopsy	Removal of a piece of tissue by syringe and needle, knife, punch, or brush to examine under a microscope as an aid to diagnosis.
Cauterization	Destruction of tissue with a caustic chemical, electrical current, freezing, or hot iron.
Chemobrasion	Abrasion of skin using chemicals; also called chemical peel.
Cryosurgery	Use of extreme cold to freeze and destroy tissue.
Curettage	Removal of superficial skin lesions with a curette or scraper.
Debridement	Removal of foreign material or dead tissue from a wound.
Dermabrasion	Abrasion or rubbing, using wire brushes or sandpaper.
Dermatoplasty	Transplantation of skin or skin grafting. May be used to treat large birthmarks (hemangiomas) and burns.
Electrocautery	Destruction of tissue with an electric current.
Exfoliative cytology	Scraping cells from tissue and then examining them under a microscope.
Frozen section	Taking a thin piece of tissue from a frozen specimen for rapid examination under a microscope. Often performed during a surgical procedure to detect cancer.
Fungal scrapings (FS)	Scrapings taken with a curette from lesions, placed on a growth medium and examined under the microscope to identify fungal growth.
Incision and drainage (I&D)	Making an incision to create an opening for the drainage of material, such as pus.
Laser therapy	Removal of skin lesions and birthmarks using a laser that emits intense heat and power at close range. The laser converts frequencies of light into one small beam.

(continued)

TABLE 37-3 *(continued)*

Procedure/Test	Description
Lipectomy	Surgical removal of fat.
Marsupialization	Creation of a pouch to promote drainage by surgically opening a closed area, such as a cyst.
Needle biopsy	Use of a sterile needle to remove tissue for examination under a microscope.
Plication	Taking tucks surgically in a structure to shorten it.
Rhytidectomy	Surgical removal of excess skin to eliminate wrinkles. Commonly referred to as a facelift.
Skin grafts	Transfer of skin from a normal area to cover another site. Used to treat burn victims and after some surgical procedures.
Sweat test	Test performed on sweat to see the level of chloride. There is an increase in skin chloride in some diseases, such as cystic fibrosis.
Tzanck test	Microscopic examination of a small piece of tissue that has been surgically scraped from a pustule. The specimen is placed on a slide and stained; then the type of viral infection can be identified.

procedure
37-2

TAKING A WOUND CULTURE

Objective: Obtain a sample from a wound by using a swab technique without error.

EQUIPMENT AND SUPPLIES

gloves; culture tube with sterile swab and transport media; tape for dressing; sterile water for cleansing wound; sterile 4 × 4 gauze dressing; hazardous waste container; bag for soiled dressing; prepared label for culture tube or pen for labeling tube

METHOD

1. Perform hand hygiene.
2. Assemble equipment.
3. Identify the patient and explain procedure.
4. Apply gloves.
5. Remove the dressing, noting amount and type of exudate, and place in bag.
6. Observe the wound for redness, crusting, swelling, and odor.
7. Using a sterile swab, place it in the wound and rotate swab back and forth. Place the swab in the sterile culture tube (Figure 37-5). Crush the ampoule of preservative that is in the culture tube and seal the tube. Label the culture tube with patient's name, identification number, source of specimen and date.
8. Remove gloves, perform hand hygiene, and apply sterile gloves.
9. Clean the wound using sterile water and 4 × 4 gauze squares.
10. Apply sterile dressing over the wound.
11. Instruct patient in wound care.

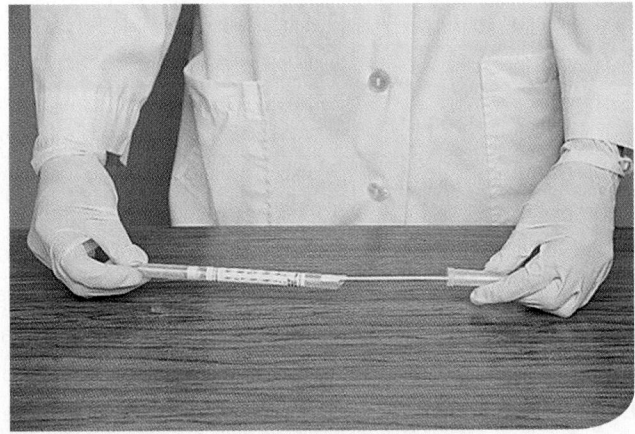

FIGURE 37-5 After obtaining the wound culture, push the tip of the swab into the liquid culture medium.

12. Remove gloves and dispose of them properly in hazardous waste container.
13. Chart the procedure.

CHARTING EXAMPLE

2/14/XX 3:30 P.M. Small amount of exudate obtained from open wound on L. ankle using sterile swab. Tube labeled and sent to lab. Wound cleaned and dressed. Erythema surrounding wound site. No odor noted. Home care instructions given. · · · · · · · · · · ·
· M. King, RMA

signs and symptoms of heart disease. You also must be able to explain and perform diagnostic procedures and tests associated with the circulatory system. Chapter 49 discusses performing routine tests such as ECG and Holter monitoring.

The symptoms of cardiovascular disease and disorders are varied due to the wide range of precipitating causes, such as poor circulation, defective heart valves, conduction defect, and blood clots in the heart layers or blood vessels. The most common symptoms of cardiovascular disorders are:

- Chest pain (crushing type of pain)

- Cyanosis—bluish skin color due to lack of oxygen in the tissues

- **Diaphoresis**—excessive sweating

- Dyspnea—difficulty breathing

- Edema

- Irregular heartbeat

Procedures and diagnostic tests related to the cardiovascular system are listed in Table 37-4.

TABLE 37-4 Procedures and Diagnostic Tests Related to the Cardiovascular System

Procedure/Test	Description
Aneurysmectomy	Surgical removal of an aneurysm, which is an abnormal dilation of a blood vessel.
Angiography	X-rays taken after the injection of opaque material into a blood vessel. They can be performed on the aorta as an aortic angiogram, on the heart as an angiocardiogram, and on the brain as a cerebral angiogram.
Angioplasty	Surgical procedure of altering the structure of a vessel by dilating the vessel using a balloon inside the vessel.
Arterial blood gases	Measurement of the amount of oxygen, carbon dioxide, and nitrogen in the blood, and a pH reading of the blood. Blood gases are measured in emergency situations and provide valuable evaluation of cardiac failure, hemorrhage, and kidney failure.
Artery graft	A piece of blood vessel that is transplanted from a part of the body to the aorta to repair a defect.
Artificial pacemaker	Electrical device that substitutes for the natural pacemaker of the heart. It controls the beating of the heart by a series of rhythmic electrical impulses. An external pacemaker has the electrodes on the outside of the body. An internal pacemaker has the electrodes surgically implanted within the chest wall.
Cardiac catheterization	Passage of thin tube (catheter) through an arm vein and the blood vessels leading into the heart. It is done to detect abnormalities, to collect cardiac blood samples, and to determine the pressure within the cardiac area.
Cardiac enzymes	Complex proteins capable of inducing chemical changes within the body. Cardiac enzymes are obtained by blood sample to determine the amount of heart disease or damage.
Cardiac magnetic resonance imaging (MRI)	Noninvasive procedure in which images of the heart and blood vessels are captured for examination to determine effects.
Cardiolysis	Surgical procedure to separate adhesions that involves a resection of the ribs and sternum over the pericardium.
Cardiorrhaphy	Surgical suturing of the heart.
Cardioversion	Converting a cardiac arrhythmia (irregular heart rhythm) to a normal sinus rhythm using a cardioverter to give countershocks to the heart.
Commissurotomy	Surgical incision to change the size of an opening. For example, in mitral valve commissurotomy, a stenosis or narrowing is corrected by cutting away at the adhesions around the mitral opening.
Coronary artery bypass surgery	Open heart surgery in which a shunt is created to permit blood to travel around the constriction in the coronary vessel(s).
Doppler ultrasonography	Measurement of sound waves as they bounce off tissues and organs to produce an image. Can assist in determining heart and blood vessel damage; also called an echocardiogram.
Electrocardiogram (ECG)	Record of the electrical activity of the heart. Useful in the diagnosis of abnormal cardiac rhythm and heart muscle (myocardium) damage. This procedure is explained fully in Chapter 49.

(continued)

TABLE 37-4 *(continued)*

Procedure/Test	Description
Electrolytes	Measurement of blood sodium (Na), potassium (K), and chloride (Cl).
Embolectomy	Surgical removal of an embolus or blood clot from a vessel.
Heart transplantation	Replacement of a diseased or malfunctioning heart with a donor's heart.
Holter monitor	Portable ECG monitor worn by the patient for a period of a few hours to a few days to assess the heart and pulse activity as the person goes through the activities of daily living. Used to assess a patient who experiences chest pain and unusual heart activity during exercise and normal activities when a cardiogram is inconclusive.
Lipoproteins	Measurement of blood to determine serum cholesterol and triglyceride levels.
Open heart surgery	Surgery that involves the heart, coronary arteries, or the heart valves. The heart is actually entered by the surgeon.
Percutaneous balloon valvuloplasty	Insertion through the skin of a balloon catheter across a narrowed or stenotic heart valve. When the balloon is inflated, the narrowing or constriction is decreased.
Percutaneous transluminal coronary angioplasty (PCTA)	Method for treating localized coronary artery narrowing. A balloon catheter is inserted through the skin into the coronary artery and inflated to dilate the narrow blood vessel.
Phleborrhaphy	Suturing of a vein.
Prothrombin time	Measurement of the time it takes for a sample of blood to coagulate.
Stress testing (treadmill test)	Method for evaluating cardiovascular fitness. The patient is placed on a treadmill or bicycle and then subjected to steadily increasing levels of work. An ECG and oxygen levels are taken while the patient exercises. The test is stopped if abnormalities occur on the ECG.
Valve replacement	Surgical procedure to excise a diseased heart valve and replace with an artificial valve.
Venography	X-ray of the veins in which the venous flow is traced. Also called phlebography.

CORONARY ARTERY DISEASE

Coronary artery disease (CAD) usually results from **atherosclerosis** (buildup of fatty material and plaque in the arteries), particularly the coronary arteries. See Figure 37-6 for an illustration of a heart showing an enlargement of an artery with arterial plaque. As the coronary arteries narrow, the blood flow to the heart muscle is lessened and **angina** (suffocating chest pain) may occur. If enough of the heart muscle is denied oxygen-rich blood supply, a **myocardial infarction (MI)** or heart attack may occur. Classic symptoms are pain in the left arm and jaw, sweating, and a crushing or squeezing sensation. In females, the symptoms vary widely and often go undetected because it has been commonly believed that CAD is a man's disease. One in ten American women ages 45 to 64 has some sort of heart disease, and the number affected increases over 65 years of age to one in four.

CONGESTIVE HEART FAILURE

Congestive heart failure (CHF) may result from **ischemia** (reduced blood supply) to the heart muscle. Symptoms of

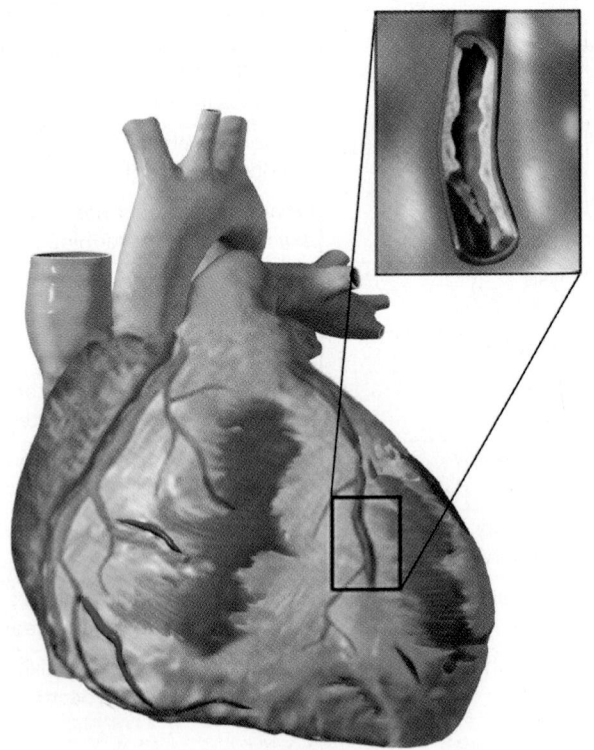

FIGURE 37-6 **Coronary artery disease due to atherosclerosis.**

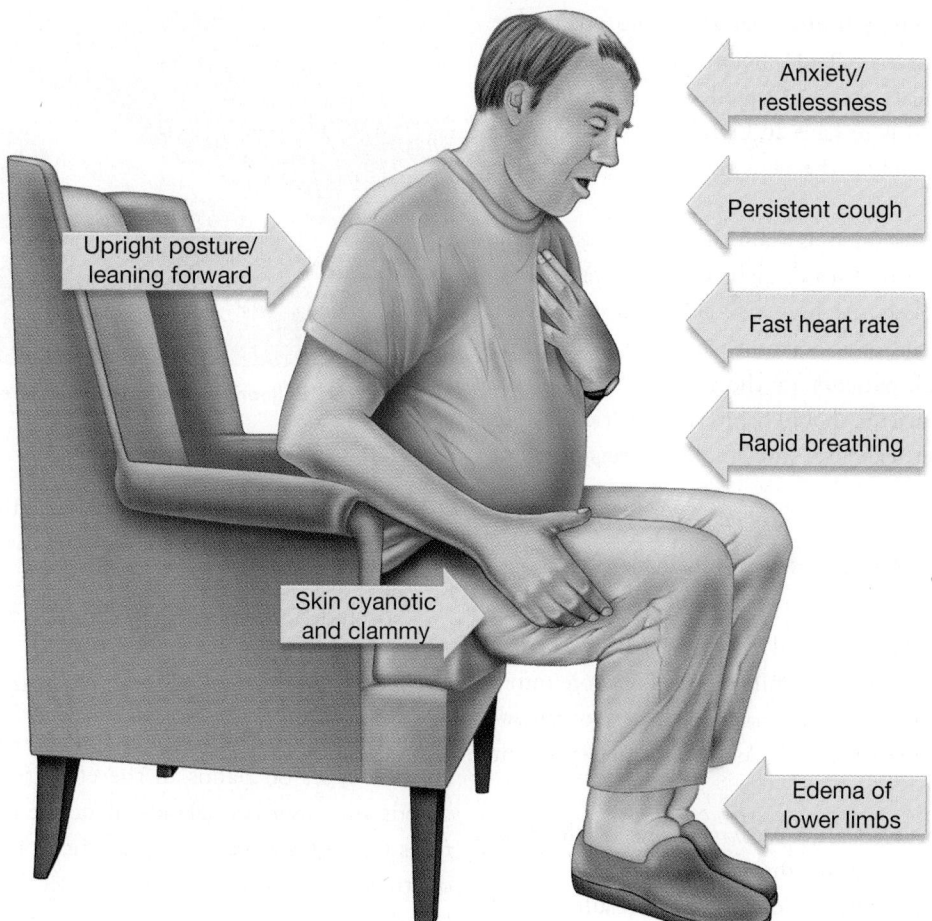

Anxiety/ restlessness

Upright posture/ leaning forward

Persistent cough

Fast heart rate

Rapid breathing

Skin cyanotic and clammy

Edema of lower limbs

FIGURE 37-7 Examples of symptoms of congestive heart failure.

CHF are shortness of breath and swollen feet and ankles (Figure 37-7). Figure 37-8 shows grading of peripheral edema. Excess fluid in soft tissues may occur in a patient with CHF. These symptoms occur because the heart muscle becomes weakened and is less able to pump blood to the rest of the body. The American Heart Association reports that every 29 seconds someone in the United States has a CHF-related event, and every minute someone dies from this event.

1+	2+	3+	4+
2 mm	4 mm	6 mm	8 mm

FIGURE 37-8 Peripheral edema may occur in patients with congestive heart failure. Swollen fluid-filled soft tissue in legs and feet can be demonstrated by pressing on the area. It is also known as pitting edema.

RISK FACTORS

Understanding the risk factors associated with heart disease will help you to educate your patients. Patients with multiple risk factors are not only at risk for heart attack but also for cerebrovascular accident (CVA) or stroke due to blood clots traveling to the brain. Evidence indicates that cardiac changes that were once associated with aging can be modified by changes in lifestyle and personal habits. Reducing fat intake, monitoring sodium intake, exercising regularly, refraining from smoking, moderating alcohol intake, and managing stress help to promote good cardiovascular health. Physicians monitor blood pressure and blood lipid levels of patients as part of annual physical examinations.

The National Cholesterol Education Program recommends more intensive treatment, such as drug therapy for individuals at a moderately high to high risk of having a heart attack. Research indicates that the more you lower low-density lipids (LDL or "bad" cholesterol), the less likely you are to have a heart attack. Overall, for very high-risk patients the new goal is to have an LDL below 100 mg/dL. In moderate-risk patients, the new goal is an LDL under 130 mg/dL.

Very high risk is defined as those who have just had a heart attack; have heart disease, diabetes, or hypertension; and are regular smokers. At high risk are those with heart disease, metabolic syndrome, and other multiple risk factors. Moderately high-risk patients are those with multiple risk factors. All at-risk patients should begin therapeutic lifestyle changes (low-fat diet, exercise, stop smoking), regardless of LDL level.

TREATMENT OF HEART DISEASE

Treatment of heart disease is varied because of the wide number of conditions associated with the cardiovascular system. Three treatments are examined here. For more information regarding heart disease and treatments, organizations such as the American Heart Association are excellent resources.

- *Hypertension* or *high blood pressure* is one of the first symptoms a patient may exhibit. Blood vessels become more rigid and constricted and, as a result, blood pushes on the vessel with more force. Treatment for hypertension includes making life changes to reduce risk factors such as obesity, smoking, and lack of exercise. A variety of medications are available to reduce blood pressure, including diuretics, which help eliminate excess fluid from the body. The cholesterol-lowering medications known as statins may be prescribed. Blood pressure should be monitored regularly.

- *Dysrhythmia* is an abnormality of the rhythm or rate of the heartbeat. Dysrhythmia is caused by a disturbance of the electrical system in the heart. Tachycardia is a rapid heartbeat over 100 beats per minute, and bradycardia is a slow heart rate under 60 beats per minute. A pacemaker to override the heart's rhythm and provide electrical impulses to regulate rhythm may be necessary. Pacemakers can either be attached externally or implanted internally.

- *Coronary artery blockage* occurs when plaque and fatty deposits occlude or block one or more of the coronary arteries (arteries that supply the heart muscle with oxygenated blood). Various methods are used to open the coronary vessels, including clot-breaking drugs, such as tissue-plasminogen activator (tPA), and bal-

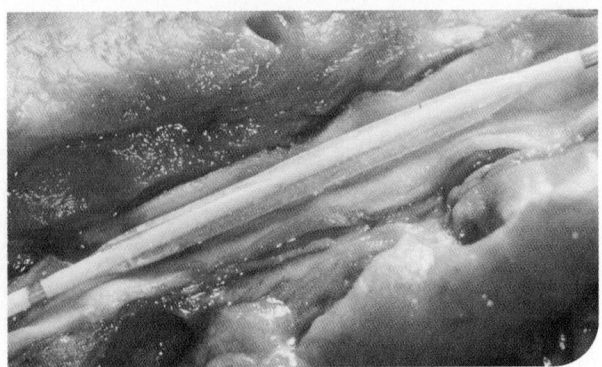

FIGURE 37-9 Balloon angioplasty is used to open coronary vessels.

loon angioplasty (Figure 37-9). If these efforts fail, coronary artery bypass surgery using a graft of the patient's vein or an artificial vein to bypass the occluded area of the heart muscle may be necessary.

Endocrinology

Endocrinology is the study of the endocrine system. There are two types of glands in the endocrine system: exocrine glands and endocrine glands. Exocrine glands release secretions through a duct or another organ. Endocrine glands are ductless, produce hormones, and secrete directly into the blood stream. The endocrine system includes the following organs: two adrenal glands, two ovaries in the female, two sets of parathyroid glands, the pancreas (islets of Langerhans), two testes in the male, the pituitary gland, the thymus gland, and the thyroid gland.

HORMONES

Hormones are chemical messengers produced by the endocrine glands and transported to target tissue by the blood stream. Hormones transfer information and instructions from one set of cells to another. They regulate growth, sexual development, mood, and metabolism and help maintain homeostasis. Each hormone targets specific cells in the body. For example, thyroxine produced by the thyroid gland targets all the cells in the body and regulates the basic metabolic rate of each cell and thus the body as a whole.

Hormones are regulated by the nervous system, endocrine control, and a feedback system. The under- or overproduction of even a small amount of a hormone can have drastic consequences for the patient. For instance, the underproduction of growth hormone from the pituitary gland in a child can result in dwarfism. In this condition, the body has normal proportions but attains a height of only 3 to 4 feet.

Overproduction of growth hormone can result in gigantism, and the person may grow to a height of 8 feet.

TREATMENTS USING HORMONES

Many conditions are treated with hormones. For example, diabetes mellitus is treated with insulin, which is now produced synthetically. Steroids, a type of hormone naturally produced in the body, can be used as anti-inflammatory agents to fight disease. Infertility may be treated with estrogens.

DIABETES MELLITUS

One of the most common hormonal imbalances the medical assistant will encounter is diabetes mellitus (DM). Approximately 17 million Americans have been diagnosed with DM, and nearly 200,000 die each year from the disease. DM is characterized by hyperglycemia (too much sugar in the blood) and results in a lack of insulin or resistance to the effects of insulin by cells. Without insulin to assist the transportation of glucose into the cells, a patient will experience adverse symptoms, including elevated blood glucose level, excessive thirst (**polydipsia**), excessive urination (**polyuria**), rapid weight loss, fatigue, itching, skin infections, and vision problems. If untreated, life-threatening conditions such as stroke, cardiovascular disease, loss of limbs due to infection and amputation, blindness due to retinal damage, kidney damage, and diabetic coma can result.

Types of Diabetes Mellitus

Type 1 DM, or insulin-dependent diabetes mellitus (IDDM), is characterized by the destruction of the beta cells of the islets of Langerhans in the pancreas and a complete lack of insulin. Type 1 DM has a rapid onset, is believed to be an autoimmune condition triggered by a virus, and occurs most often in children. Scientists believe there may be a genetic predisposition for this type of DM. Type 1 DM is treated by administration of insulin by injection. Blood glucose levels must be monitored carefully, sometimes as many as eight to ten times a day, to calculate the amount of insulin needed to maintain normal glucose levels.

In type 2 DM, or noninsulin-dependent diabetes mellitus (NDDM), the insulin that is produced by the islets of Langerhans in the pancreas has little or no effect on cells because of a deficiency of insulin receptors on cell membranes. The majority of diabetes cases fall into this category. Type 2 DM has a slow onset, and risk factors include obesity and family history of diabetes. Control of type 2 DM may not

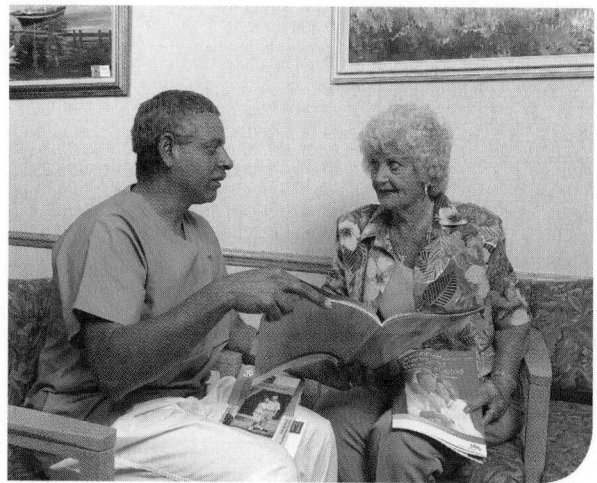

FIGURE 37-10 Using educational materials, a medical assistant discusses lifestyle changes with a diabetic patient.

require insulin injection but may be controlled with medications that enable the insulin to react with cell receptors. Careful food management and moderate exercise are also important for controlling type 2 DM. The American Diabetes Association notes that type 2 DM has increased by 33 percent in the past 10 years, and investigators relate the increase to the rapidly increasing rate of obesity. The National Institute of Health's diabetes mellitus statistics in 2007 estimate that 57 million adults over the age of twenty have impaired fasting glucose; 7.8 percent of the population of the United States has diabetes.

The medical assistant will be taking an active part in educating the patient on diabetes management, performing glucose monitoring, and helping the patient understand and comply with the treatment plan the physician has established (Figure 37-10). The newly diagnosed diabetic patient will have to make life changes to regulate his or her blood sugar to avoid the long-term complications of this devastating disease.

Table 37-5 lists procedures and diagnostic tests related to the endocrine system.

Gastrointestinal System

The gastrointestinal (GI) or digestive system includes the mouth, esophagus, stomach, small and large intestines, and accessory organs (liver, gallbladder, and pancreas). This system stores and digests food, eliminates waste, and utilizes nutrients. Table 37-6 lists procedures and diagnostic tests related to the digestive system.

The digestive system involves many organs, and similar symptoms may be present in a number of disorders and conditions. A patient who sees a gastroenterologist is usually

TABLE 37-5 Procedures and Diagnostic Tests Related to the Endocrine System

Procedure/Test	Description
17-hydroxycorticosteroids (17-OHCS)	Test performed on urine to identify adrenocorticosteroid hormones. It is used to determine adrenal cortical function.
17-ketosteroids (17-KS)	Test performed on urine to determine the amount of 17-KS present. 17-KS is the end product of androgens and is secreted from the adrenal glands and testes. It is used in diagnosing adrenal tumors.
2-hour postprandial glucose tolerance test	Blood test to assist in evaluating glucose metabolism. The patient fasts overnight and then eats a high-carbohydrate meal in the morning. A blood sample is then taken 2 hours after the meal.
Basal metabolic rate	Somewhat outdated test to measure the energy used when the body is in a state of rest.
Blood serum test	Blood test to measure the level of such substances as calcium, electrolytes, testosterone, insulin, and glucose. Used to assist in determining the function of various endocrine glands.
Fasting blood sugar	Blood test to measure the amount of glucose circulating throughout the body after fasting for 12 hours.
Glucose tolerance test (GTT)	Test to determine the blood sugar level. A measured dose of glucose is given to the patient either orally or intravenously. Blood samples are then drawn at certain intervals to determine the ability of the patient to utilize glucose. Used for diabetic patients to determine their insulin response to glucose.
Parathyroidectomy	Excision of one or more of the parathyroid glands. This is performed to halt the progress of hyperparathyroidism.
Protein bound iodine test (PBI)	Blood test to measure the concentration of thyroxine (T4) circulating in the bloodstream. The iodine becomes bound to the protein in the blood and can be measured.
Radioactive iodine uptake test (RAIU)	Test in which radioactive iodine is taken orally or intravenously and the amount of iodine eventually taken into the thyroid gland (uptake) is measured to assist in determining thyroid function.
Radioimmune assay test (RIA)	Test used to measure the levels of hormones in the plasma of the blood.
Serum glucose test	Blood test performed to assist in determining insulin levels and useful for adjusting medication dosage.
Thymectomy	Surgical removal of the thymus gland.
Thyroid echogram	Ultrasound examination of the thyroid that can assist in distinguishing a thyroid nodule from a cyst.
Thyroidectomy	Surgical removal of the thyroid gland. The patient is then placed on replacement hormone (thyroid) therapy.
Thyroid function tests	Blood tests used to measure the levels of T3, T4, and TSH in the bloodstream to assist in determining thyroid function.
Thyroparathyroidectomy	Surgical removal (excision) of the thyroid gland and parathyroid glands.
Thyroid scan	Test in which a radioactive element is administered that localizes in the thyroid gland. The gland can then be visualized with a scanning device to detect pathology such as tumors.
Total calcium	Blood test to measure the total amount of calcium to assist in detecting parathyroid and bone disorders.

referred by the primary care physician (PCP). Proctology is a subspecialty of gastroenterology. A **proctologist** treats disorders of the rectum and anus only.

Many of the examinations associated with the digestive system may be uncomfortable and embarrassing for the patient, such as a digital rectal examination or colonoscopy. The medical assistant must be prepared to provide reassurance to the patient before, during, and after procedures. Patients have the right to privacy, and every effort must be made to drape the patient to prevent him or her from being

JUDGMENT CALL

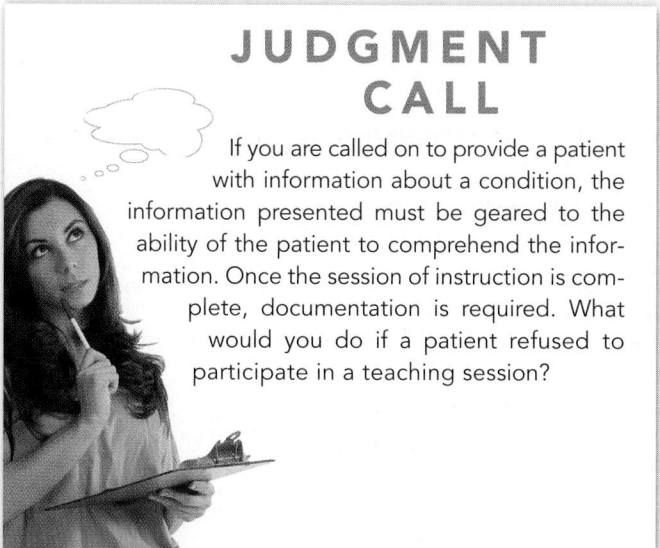

If you are called on to provide a patient with information about a condition, the information presented must be geared to the ability of the patient to comprehend the information. Once the session of instruction is complete, documentation is required. What would you do if a patient refused to participate in a teaching session?

unnecessarily exposed and further embarrassed. When gathering information from patients, listen carefully to their replies. If pain is involved, ask the patient to show you where the pain is located. Pain may be referred (appear somewhere else) and not over the involved organ. For example, gallbladder pain may be in the upper right back, not the abdomen (Figure 37-11).

Symptoms such as **colic** (acute abdominal pain) may be present in a number of conditions. Indigestion is a symptom of gastroesophageal reflux disease (GERD) and also may be present in some patients who are having a heart attack. Many of the procedures associated with the gastrointestinal system involve endoscopy (looking into an opening of the body with a lighted instrument); therefore, proper patient preparation is important to obtain valid results.

TABLE 37-6 Procedures and Diagnostic Tests Related to the Digestive System

Procedure/Test	Description
Abdominal ultrasonography	Ultrasound equipment produces sound waves used to create an image of the abdominal organs.
Air-contrast barium enema	Using both barium and air to visualize the colon on X-ray.
Anastomosis	Creating a passageway or opening between two organs or vessels.
Appendectomy	Surgical removal of the appendix.
Barium enema (lower GI)	Radiographic examination of the small intestine, large intestine, or colon, in which an enema containing barium is administered to the patient while X-ray pictures are taken.
Barium swallow (upper GI)	Barium mixture swallowed while X-ray pictures are taken of the esophagus, stomach, and duodenum. It is used to visualize the upper GI tract. Also called esophogram.
Colectomy	Surgical removal of the entire colon.
Cholecystectomy	Surgical excision of the gallbladder. Removal of the gallbladder through the laparoscope is a newer procedure with fewer complications than the more invasive abdominal surgery. The laparoscope requires a small incision into the abdominal cavity.
Cholecystogram	Dye given orally to the patient is absorbed and enters the gallbladder, and then an X-ray is taken.
Choledocholithotomy	Removal of a gallstone through an incision into the bile duct.
Choledocholithotripsy	Crushing of a gallstone in the common bile duct. Commonly called lithotripsy.
Colonoscopy	Flexible fiberscope passed through the anus, rectum, and colon is used to examine the upper portion of the colon. Polyps and small growths can be removed during the procedure.
Colostomy	Surgical creation of an opening of some portion of the colon through the abdominal wall to the outside surface.
Diverticulectomy	Surgical removal of a diverticulum.
Endoscopic retrograde cholangiopancreatography (ERCP)	Using an endoscope to X-ray the bile and pancreatic ducts.
Esophagoscopy	The esophagus is visualized by passing an instrument down the esophagus. A tissue sample for biopsy may be taken.

(continued)

TABLE 37-6 (*continued*)

Procedure/Test	Description
Esophagram	As barium is swallowed, the solution is observed traveling from the mouth into the stomach. Also called a barium swallow.
Esophagogastrostomy	Surgical creation of an opening between the esophagus and stomach.
Esophagostomy	Surgical creation of an opening into the esophagus.
Exploratory laparotomy	Abdominal operation for the purpose of examining the abdominal organs and tissues for signs of disease or other abnormalities.
Fistulectomy	Excision of a fistula.
Gastrectomy	Surgical removal of part or all of the stomach.
Gastrointestinal endoscopy	A flexible instrument or scope is passed either through the mouth or anus to facilitate visualization of the GI tract.
Gastric lavage	A sample of gastric contents is obtained by insertion of an orogastric tube through the mouth to the stomach.
Glossectomy	Complete or partial removal of the tongue.
Hemorrhoidectomy	Surgical excision of hemorrhoids from the anorectal area.
Hepatic lobotomy	Surgical excision of a lobe of the liver.
Ileostomy	Surgical creation of a passageway through the abdominal wall into the ileum. The fecal matter (stool) drains into a bag worn on the abdomen.
Intravenous cholangiogram	A dye administered to the patient allows for visualization of the bile vessels.
Intravenous cholecystography	A dye administered intravenously to the patient allows for visualization of the gallbladder.
Jejunostomy	Surgical creation of a permanent opening into the jejunum.
Lithotripsy	Crushing of a stone located within the gallbladder.
Liver biopsy	Excision of a small piece of liver tissue for microscopic examination. This is generally used to determine if cancer is present.
Liver scan	A radioactive substance is administered intravenously to the patient. This substance enters liver cells, and the organ can then be visualized to detect tumors, abscesses, and other hepatomegaly.
Occult blood	Test performed on feces to determine the presence of invisible amounts of blood. Positive results may indicate gastrointestinal bleeding.
Ova and parasites	Test performed on stool to identify ova and parasites. A positive result indicates protozoa infestation.
Proctoplasty	Plastic surgery of the anus and rectum.
Splenectomy	Surgical removal of the spleen.
Stool culture	Test performed on stool to identify the presence of organisms.
Ultrasonography, gallbladder	Test to visualize the gallbladder by using high-frequency sound waves. Used to detect gallbladder inflammation, biliary obstructions, or gallstones.
Ultrasonography, liver	Test to visualize the liver by using high-frequency sound waves. Used to detect hepatic tumors, cysts, abscesses, and cirrhosis.
Upper gastrointestinal fiberscopy	Direct visualization of the gastric mucosa via a flexible fiberscope. Used to detect gastric neoplasm.
Vagotomy	Surgical resection of the vagus nerve in an attempt to decrease the amount of acid secretion into the stomach. Used as a treatment for ulcer patients.

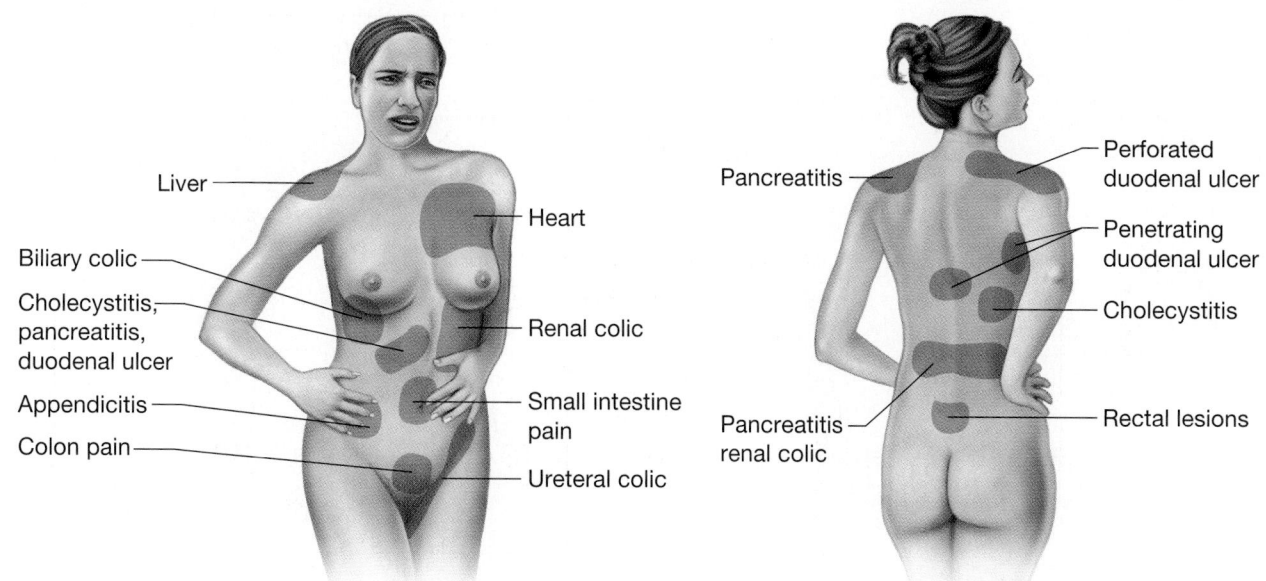

Liver

Heart

Biliary colic

Cholecystitis, pancreatitis, duodenal ulcer

Renal colic

Appendicitis

Small intestine pain

Colon pain

Ureteral colic

Pancreatitis

Perforated duodenal ulcer

Penetrating duodenal ulcer

Cholecystitis

Pancreatitis renal colic

Rectal lesions

FIGURE 37-11   Examples of sites of referred abdominal pain.

COMMON DISORDERS OF THE DIGESTIVE SYSTEM

One of the most commonly encountered GI disorders is GERD. Approximately one-third of Americans suffer from this common disorder. GERD is also known as acid reflux or acid indigestion and is caused by stomach acid flowing back up into the esophagus. Normally the sphincter muscle at the juncture of the stomach and esophagus prevents the reflux of acid. If this sphincter muscle is weak, acid reflux may occur. In some patients, the presence of hiatal hernia, eating spicy or greasy foods, or drinking alcohol may cause a local irritation. A hiatal hernia occurs when the upper portion of the stomach protrudes into the chest through the esophageal opening or hiatus of the diaphragm (Figure 37-12A). GERD symptoms include heartburn, burping, and a sour taste in the back of the throat. Persistent acid reflux increases the risk of esophageal cancer. To diagnose GERD, an upper GI series and barium swallow and gastroscopy are usually ordered. Treatment of GERD includes making some lifestyle changes, such as eating small meals six times a day, eating at least 2 to 3 hours before bedtime, modifying diet to avoid problem foods, losing weight, and moderating amounts of coffee and alcohol. If those measures fail, then a medication that reduces acid secretions can be ordered or purchased over the counter. Repeated use of antacids is not recommended because they can disrupt body chemistry and cause the stomach to increase acid secretions.

Another common GI disorder is diverticular disease. Diverticula are outpouching or small sacs found mainly in the lower part of the colon or large intestine and occasionally in other parts of the digestive tract. A diverticulum is a bulging of the inner lining of the intestinal wall through the muscular layers of intestines (Figure 37-12B). Chronic constipation and a diet low in fiber are thought to be causative factors. Diverticulosis, the presence of diverticula, is found in about half of those over 60 years of age in the United States. Many individuals with diverticula are asymptomatic. Diverticulitis is an inflammation of one or more diverticula, causing severe pain, muscle spasm, nausea, and fever. The patient may complain of cramping and tenderness on the left side of the abdomen, small round hard stools, and gas. Untreated diverticulitis may cause narrowing of the intestine; intestinal obstruction and peritonitis; or inflammation of the lining of the abdominal cavity if the diverticula burst.

Diagnosis of diverticular disease depends on patient history, X-ray of the lower GI tract, barium enema, and sigmoidoscopy or colonoscopy. Diverticular disease requires no treatment except to encourage the patient to avoid constipation and to increase dietary fiber intake. Diverticulitis requires treatment with antibiotics and possibly antispasmodic medication to relieve abdominal pain. In the case of intestinal blockage, hospitalization and intravenous fluids are necessary. A colectomy, surgical removal of all or part of the colon, may be necessary and possibly a colostomy, creation of an opening of the colon through the abdominal wall to allow for passage of stools. Dietary restriction of foods containing seeds, nuts, and corn is recommended by some physicians, whereas others say it is not necessary to avoid these foods because research has not shown them to be directly linked to diverticular disease.

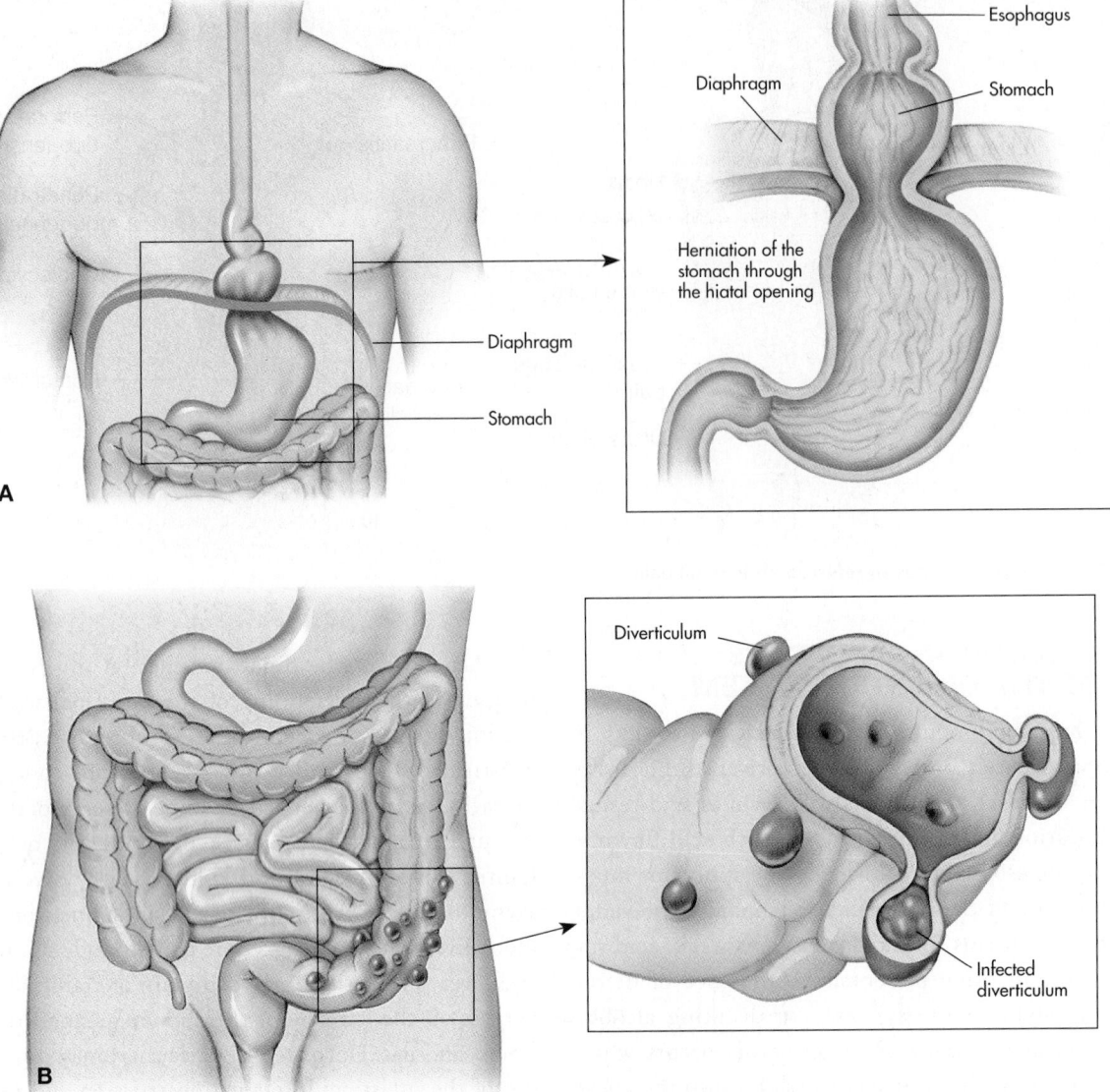

FIGURE 37-12   (A) Hiatal hernia; (B) Colon with diverticulosis. An infected diverticulum is called diverticulitis.

SIGMOIDOSCOPY

The sigmoidoscopy, also called a proctoscopic or proctosigmoidoscopic examination, is an examination of the interior of the sigmoid colon for diagnostic purposes. This is a useful procedure to assist in the detection of cancer of the colon, polyps, ulcerations, and other disorders of the lower intestinal tract.

The sigmoidoscope, a flexible, metal or plastic instrument with a light source and magnification lens, is used for the sigmoidoscopy. The flexible sigmoidoscope, more widely used by physicians, allows the physician to see farther into the colon and view the mucous membranes of the intestines. It is more comfortable for the patients as well. For this procedure the patient may be placed in the Sims' position or on a proctoscopic examination table (Figure 37-13).

Preparation for this examination is important. Patients should be told to empty their bowel and bladder before coming

in for the procedure. The physician will usually have the patient take a commercially prepared enema 2 hours before the examination. Patients should be advised to drink plenty of clear liquids and eat sparingly the day before the examination. Some physicians will ask the patient to refrain from eating raw fruits and vegetables, grains, and dairy products a few days prior to the examination so the colon will be easier to visualize. It is critical that every attempt be made to ensure the patient follows the instructions for the preparation because an improperly prepared bowel may result in having to reschedule the procedure.

This procedure can be uncomfortable for patients. It is made easier for patients if they are instructed to concentrate on breathing deeply through the mouth while trying to relax the abdominal muscles. Even though the procedure lasts only a few minutes, the patient will need encouragement throughout the procedure. It is helpful to inform patients

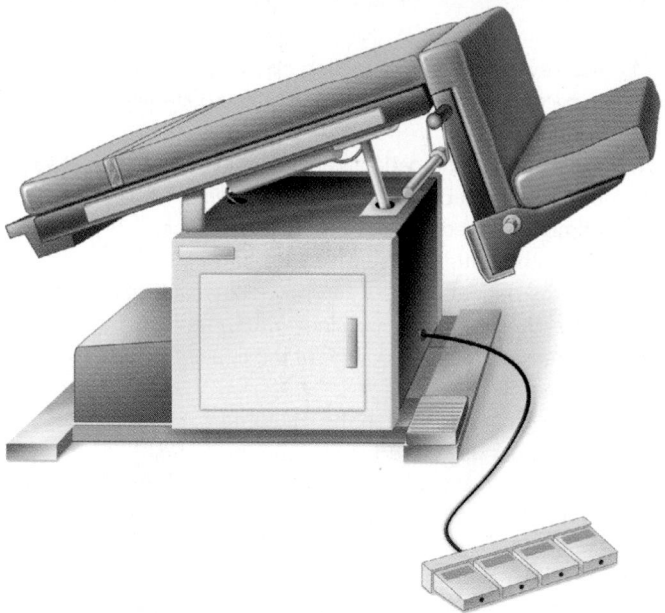

FIGURE 37-13 **Proctoscopic examination table.**

after the procedure that they might experience flatulence (gas) as a result of the air introduced during the procedure.

The physician may take several biopsy samples during the procedure, requiring that specimen containers be part of every sigmoidoscopy setup. The patient should sign a consent form for both the procedure and any biopsy of materials. Procedure 37-3 provides the steps for assisting with a sigmoidoscopic examination.

procedure
37-3

ASSISTING WITH A SIGMOIDOSCOPY

Objective: Assist the physician during the sigmoidoscopic examination by positioning the patient, handling all equipment and biopsy material, and providing support for the patient throughout the procedure without error.

EQUIPMENT AND SUPPLIES

sigmoidoscope with obturator; flexible or inflexible (metal or plastic); anoscope; rectal speculum; insufflator; suction equipment; sterile specimen container with preservative; sterile biopsy forceps; cotton applicators (long); lubricating jelly; basin of warm water; patient drape; gloves; patient gown; small towel or examination table pad; tissue; biohazard waste container

METHOD

1. Perform hand hygiene.
2. Prepare the equipment and supplies. Check all lights and light bulbs in equipment. Prepare a basin of warm water to receive used instruments. Test the suction equipment. Place the obturator within the sigmoidoscope. See Figure 37-14 for a flexible sigmoidoscope with parts labeled.
3. Identify the patient and explain the procedure. Verify that the patient has followed the enema and diet instructions. Check to make sure the consent form has been signed.
4. Ask the patient to undress, put on a patient gown, and empty the bladder.

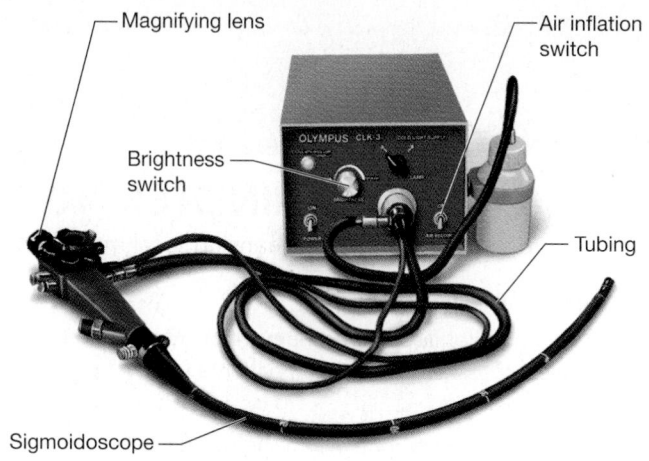

FIGURE 37-14 **The parts of a flexible sigmoidoscope.**

5. Assist the patient into the Sims', lateral, or knee–chest position or onto the proctology table.
6. Drape the patient and place a towel or disposable examination pad under the perineal area.
7. Apply gloves.
8. Place lubricant on the physician's gloved fingers for a digital examination.
9. Place metal scope in a basin of warm water to warm it before insertion into patient.
10. Lubricate the tip of the scope.
11. Attach the inflation bulb (for air inflation during the procedure) and attach the light source. Turn the scope on just before the physician is ready to use it.
12. Remind the patient to take deep breaths and relax the abdominal muscles. Observe the patient for any undue reactions.
13. Assist the physician by handing instruments and equipment such as suction and cotton-tipped applicators, as they are needed. Place used equipment, including suction tubing, into the basin of water.

14. Assist with biopsy by holding open specimen containers to receive specimen, while maintaining sterility of the container.
15. Clean around the patient's anal opening with tissue. Discard the tissue in a biohazard waste container.
16. Remove gloves and perform hand hygiene.
17. Assist the patient to slowly sit up.
18. Ask the patient to dress and provide assistance as needed.
19. Label the specimen container with the patient's name, address, date, time, source of the specimen, and ID number.
20. Apply gloves and clean the equipment, sterilize the equipment as needed, and clean the room.
21. Remove gloves and document the procedure. The physician will document the results of the procedure.

CHARTING EXAMPLE
2/14/XX 9:00 A.M. Assisted patient with sigmoidoscopic examination. Biopsy sent to lab. No dizziness or discomfort noted after procedure. · · · · · · · · · · · · · · · · · M. King, CMA (AAMA)

COLONOSCOPY

Colonoscopy procedures are performed in an office or hospital outpatient area because an IV sedative is administered prior to the procedure. Colonoscopy allows the physician to examine more of the large intestine than the sigmoidoscopy. The American Cancer Society recommends all individuals over the age of 50 have a colonoscopy to screen for cancer.

Sometimes the patient will not have complied with preparation instructions, and the physician may order an enema in the office in order to complete the examination. Procedure 37-4 lists the steps for administering a disposable

procedure
37-4

ADMINISTERING A DISPOSABLE ENEMA

Objective: To assist in cleansing fecal material from bowel in preparation for a diagnostic examination.

EQUIPMENT AND SUPPLIES
examination table; disposable enema; lubricant; Mayo tray; towel; gloves; tissues; drape; pen; patient's record

METHOD
1. Assemble equipment. Warm the disposable enema container prior to using to avoid causing abdominal cramping.
2. Identify the patient and explain the procedure.
3. Perform hand hygiene.
4. Instruct the patient to disrobe from the waist down. Assist the patient onto the examination table as needed.

5. Ask the patient to assume the Sims' position (left side with right knee at 90-degree angle). Drape for comfort and privacy.
6. Apply gloves.
7. Remove the tip from the enema container. Apply a small amount of lubricant (Figure 37-15).
8. Separate the buttocks to expose the anus and gently insert the lubricated tip about 2 inches into the anus, with tip pointing toward patient's navel (Figure 37-16).
9. Instruct the patient to take deep breaths while you slowly empty the contents of the container.

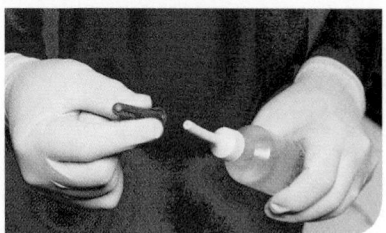

FIGURE 37-15 Remove the cap from the enema container, and lubricate the tip.

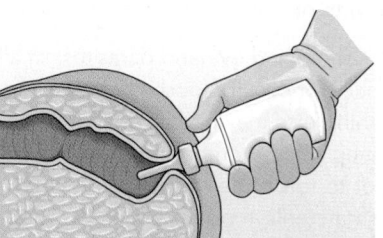

FIGURE 37-16 Insert the tip of the enema container into the rectum about 2 inches, and expel all the fluid.

10. Ask the patient to retain the liquid as a long as possible to ensure good results: 5 to 10 minutes should help the enema to work.
11. After withdrawing the tip, gently wipe the anal area with tissue to remove excess lubricant.
12. Provide a bedpan or direct the patient to the rest room, instructing the patient not to flush the toilet until you have checked the results.
13. Review instructions with the patient as necessary for the next test procedure.

14. Clean the room; discard disposable enema equipment in appropriate waste containers.
15. Remove gloves and perform hand hygiene.
16. Document the patient's record.

CHARTING EXAMPLE
03/21/XX 2:15 P.M. Pt. to have sigmoidoscopy. Bowel preparation at home not entirely successful. Administered disposable cleansing enema per Dr. Chang. Enema returned small amount of dark brown, hard stool. Pt. complained of stomach cramps but tolerated procedure.· · · · · · · · · · · R. Negri, CMA (AAMA)

enema to a patient. These steps will help you provide clearer instructions to your patients and ensure better compliance.

COLLECTING A STOOL SPECIMEN

Stool specimens (feces) may be collected to detect bacteria, viruses, parasites, and occult blood. The first three topics are discussed in Chapter 45. **Occult** or hidden blood in feces may be an indication of bleeding in the GI tract. Instructing

patients to collect a fecal specimen either at home or in the office is difficult and embarrassing for the patient. Bleeding may be intermittent; therefore, fecal specimens should be obtained on three separate days. Patients who have daily bowel movements should not find this a problem. Those who have bowel movements less regularly may take more than three days to collect specimens. Procedure 37-5 provides the steps for instructing patients how to collect stool specimens.

procedure

INSTRUCTING THE PATIENT IN COLLECTING A STOOL SPECIMEN

Objective: To instruct patients how to obtain an adequate stool specimen for laboratory testing.

Note: Check the physician's orders for the type of test to be performed prior to collecting the specimen.

EQUIPMENT AND SUPPLIES
sterile specimen container with lid (for culture or ova and parasite testing); three occult blood slides with envelope and applicator sticks (for testing for occult blood); lab request form; pen; patient's record; label; printed instructions; tongue depressor; biohazard transport bag; note pad; bedpan or or other container for the collection of stool.

METHOD
1. Assemble needed items next to the patient.
2. Label the specimen container or the occult blood slides and fill in the laboratory request form.
3. Identify the patient and explain the physician orders. Give the patient a copy of the printed instructions and review them together.

4. Instruct the patient how to obtain a small amount of stool.

Note: 3–4 tablespoons for culture and ova and parasites; small amount on the applicator stick for occult blood. For the culture and ova and parasites, nothing else may be placed in the container (no toilet paper, tissues, urine, or menses), and to maintain sterility patients are not to touch the inside of the cup or cover. The patient may use a sterile tongue depressor to obtain larger samples of stool from the bedpan, commode, or specipan (Figure 37-17). Patient compliance is difficult, and it is up to you to put the patient at ease as much as possible.

5. Instruct the patient to write the date and time of the specimen, place it in a biohazard transport bag, and bring it as soon as possible with the laboratory request form to the laboratory or office. Storage and time of delivery directions depend on the test performed and are specified in the testing facility manual. For example, specimens for culture and ova and parasites must be brought to the laboratory immediately. Sometimes specimens are refrigerated if it is not possible to drop them off within two hours. This depends on the test ordered. It is not necessary to refrigerate occult blood slides. See

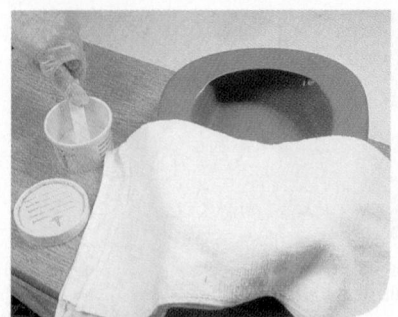

FIGURE 37-17 Equipment for collecting a stool specimen.

Procedure 37-6 for further instructions on testing for occult blood.
6. Have the patient or family member repeat instructions to you to verify comprehension.
7. Document that instructions were given to the patient.

CHARTING EXAMPLE
03/21/XX 9 A.M. Verbal & printed instructions given to pt. for collection of stool specimen for lab testing. Pt. repeated instructions · M. Blardo, CMA (AAMA)

TESTING FOR OCCULT BLOOD

Patients must be instructed to follow guidelines for preparation listed by manufacturer of testing kits. Guidelines should be observed two days prior to collecting specimens and continued until all three samples have been obtained. The following are the guidelines:

- Drink plenty of fluids.
- Do not collect samples during menses.
- Avoid red meats, liver, and processed meats.

- Avoid turnips, broccoli, cauliflower, and melons.
- Avoid aspirin, iron supplements, and large doses of vitamin C for 7 days before collecting specimens (unless otherwise instructed by physician).
- Eat a high-fiber diet. Store slides at room temperature away from sun and heat.

Procedure 37-6 provides the steps for testing feces for occult blood.

procedure 37-6

TESTING FOR OCCULT BLOOD
Objective: To test feces for occult blood.

EQUIPMENT AND SUPPLIES
3 occult blood slides; applicators; envelope; timer; patient's record; pen; gloves; color developer

Note: Many test kits are available on the market. Each one has its own set of directions, color developer, slides, and control monitors. The test kit directions should be followed exactly.

METHOD
1. Perform hand hygiene.
2. Apply gloves. Place a paper towel on the area to hold the slides.
3. Check the name and date on the occult blood slides.

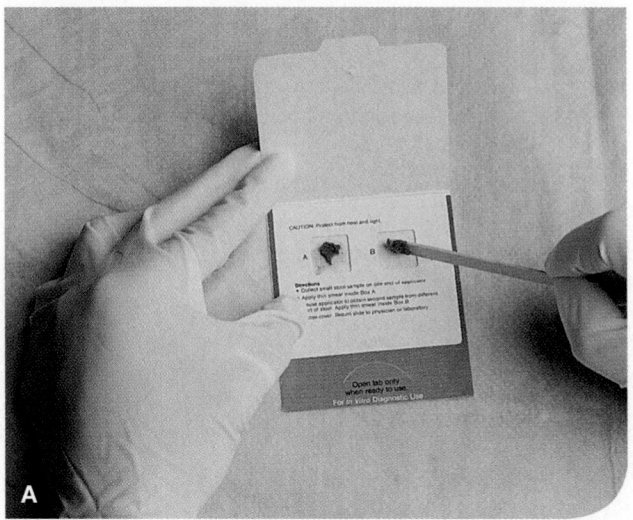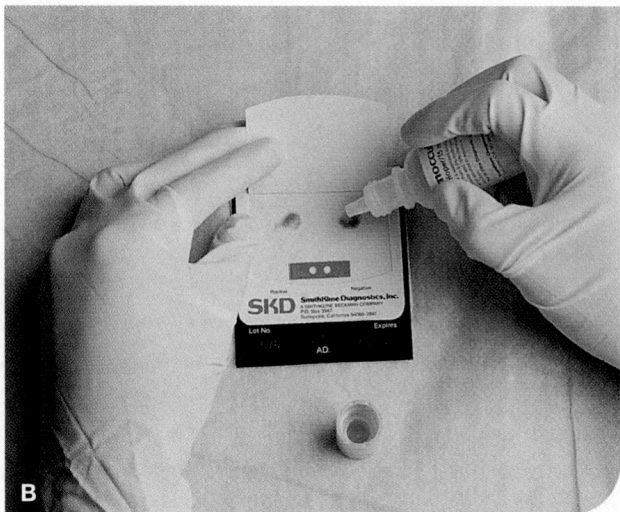

FIGURE 37-18 (A) Supplies needed for testing stool for occult blood; (B) Open the back flap of the slide and apply 2 drops of color developing fluid over each smear.

4. Check the expiration date on the color developer. See Figure 37-18A for the supplies needed for occult blood testing.
5. Open the window flap on the back of slide and apply 2 drops of the developer to Box A and Box B (Figure 37-18B).
6. Interpret the results in 30 to 60 seconds or according to the manufacturer's directions. A positive result will have blue color around the edge of the specimen; a negative result will have no color change visible. Any amount of blue color is positive.
7. Perform a test on positive and negative controls as required by the manufacturer for quality control purposes.
8. Test the remaining slides in the same manner.
9. Dispose of all materials in a biohazard waste container. Clean the work area.
10. Remove gloves.
11. Perform hand hygiene.
12. Document the results in the patient's record.

CHARTING EXAMPLE

03/21/XX 10:30 A.M. 3 occult blood rec'd. All tested neg. for occult blood. Dr. Chang notified of results. Pt. notified per Dr. Chang · B. Negri, CMA (AAMA)

Lymphatic System

The lymphatic system, which consists of lymph glands, ducts, nodes, tonsils, thymus gland, and spleen, is the basis of the body's defense or immune system. This system protects the body against the invasion of foreign microorganisms. It works in conjunction with the circulatory system to purify the blood and drain fluids throughout the body.

Immunity is the body's ability to defend itself against pathogenic organisms and toxic substances. Immunity is either natural or acquired. Natural immunity is nonspecific and does not require exposure to pathogenic microorganisms. An example of natural immunity is when macrophages (special cells) roam through the body ingesting bacteria and other foreign substances. Acquired immunity develops following exposure to a specific pathogenic microorganism. Immunizations are a type of acquired immunity where a weakened form of the pathogen is given to the patient and specific antibodies to that particular pathogen develop. For example, a child is given the polio vaccine to develop antibodies to the polio virus. The child is then immunized from getting polio.

In some diseases, such as acquired immune deficiency syndrome (AIDS), part of the body's immune system has been destroyed; therefore, the natural ability to fight off infection is lost. AIDS is discussed more fully in Chapter 28. Table 37-7 lists procedures and diagnostic tests related to the lymphatic system.

Musculoskeletal System

The prevention of or treatment for conditions of the musculoskeletal system (bones and muscles) is called **orthopedics**, and physicians who diagnose and treat conditions related to the musculoskeletal system are orthopedists. Figure 37-19 illustrates examples of three types of abnormal spinal

TABLE 37-7 Procedures and Diagnostic Tests Related to the Lymphatic System

Procedure/Test	Description
Bone marrow aspiration	Removing a sample of bone marrow by syringe for microscopic examination. Useful for diagnosing diseases such as leukemia. For example, a proliferation (massive increase of white blood cells) could confirm the diagnosis of leukemia.
CT scan (CAT)	Use of computerized tomography to diagnose disorders of the lymphoid organs.
Enzyme-linked immunosorbent assay (ELISA)	Blood test for an antibody to the AIDS virus. A positive test means that the person has been exposed to the virus. If a reading is determined to be a false-positive, then the Western blot test would be used to verify the results.
Lymphadenectomy	Excision of a lymph node. This is usually done to test for a malignancy.
Lymphangiogram	X-ray taken through the lymph vessels after the injection of dye into the foot. The lymph flow through the chest is traced.
Splenopexy	Artificial fixation of a movable spleen.
Tonsillectomy	Surgical removal of the tonsils. Usually adenoids are removed at the same time; if so, the procedure is known as T&A.
Western blot	Test used as a backup for the ELISA blood test to detect the presence of the antibody to HIV (AIDS virus) in the blood.

curvatures. **Scoliosis** is an abnormal C-shaped or S-shaped lateral curvature of the spine. A scoliosis check is routinely done for elementary schoolchildren by school nurses. **Kyphosis** is an abnormal curvature of the thoracic vertebrae, and **lordosis** is excessive forward curvature of the lumbar vertebrae.

Osteopaths treat the body by realigning the skeletal system to promote healing. They also use conventional medical methods. Rheumatologists see patients with joint inflammations and treat patients with autoimmune disorders, such as rheumatoid arthritis and lupus. Chiropractors use manual

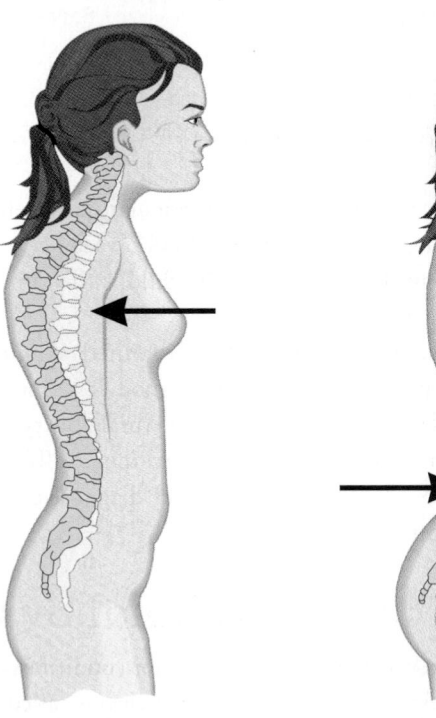
Excessive kyphosis
(slouch)

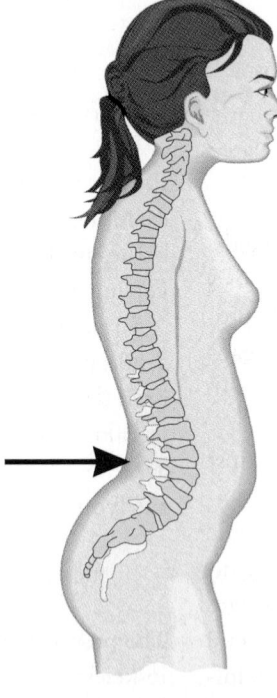
Excessive lordosis
(swayback)

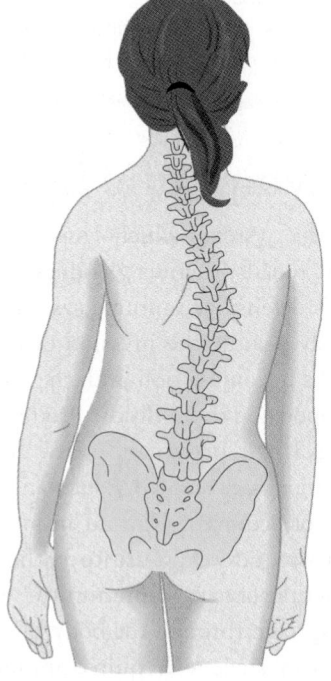
Scoliosis

FIGURE 37-19 Abnormal spinal curvatures.

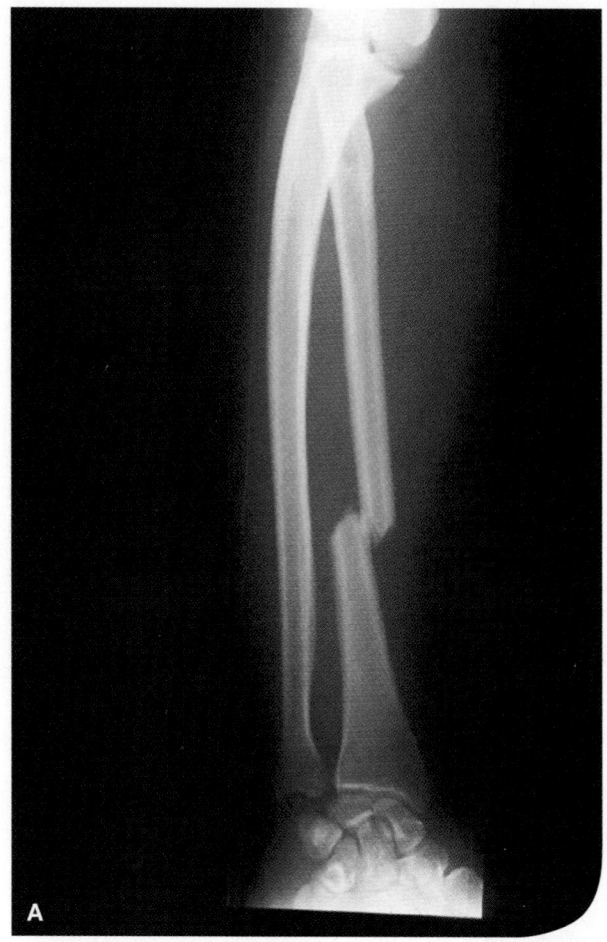

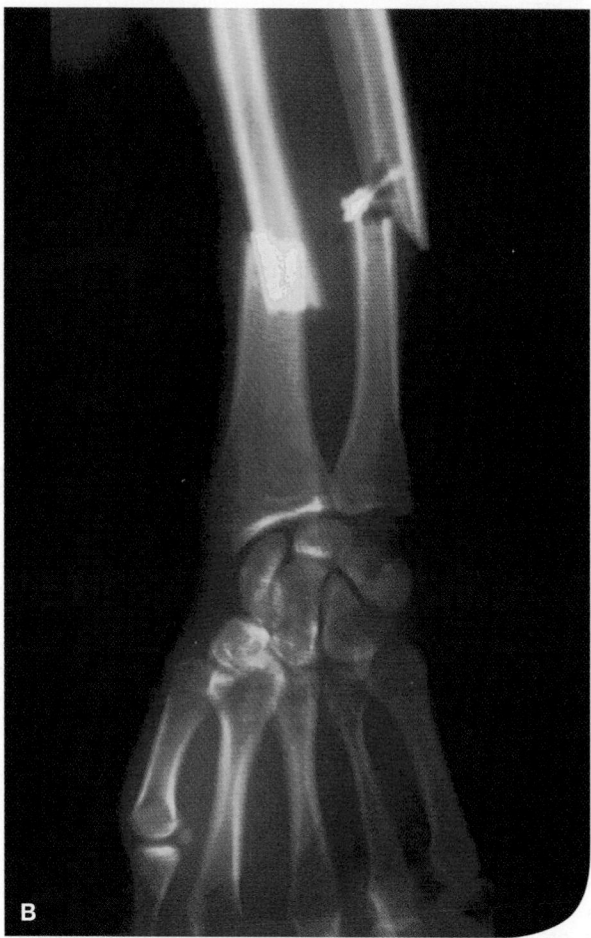

FIGURE 37-20 (A) An X-ray of a complete fracture of the radius; (B) An enhanced color X-ray of forearm fractures.

adjustment of the spine to promote healing and maintain homeostasis.

A medical assistant's training is comprehensive enough to permit employment in any of the specialties mentioned. Radiology and diagnostic imaging are usually needed to evaluate musculoskeletal conditions (Figures 37-20A and 37-20B). Many orthopedists, chiropractors, and osteopaths have X-ray equipment in or associated with their offices. Radiology is discussed in Chapter 48. In some states, medical assistants are not permitted to take X-rays; it is therefore important for you to be familiar with state regulations.

MUSCULOSKELETAL SYSTEM AND THE MEDICAL ASSISTANT

There are 206 bones and over 600 muscles in the body. Muscles account for approximately 50 percent of body weight. In addition to bones and muscles, the musculoskeletal system includes all the connective tissue, such as tendons, ligaments, and cartilage, which is necessary for proper functioning of this complex system. The functions of the musculoskeletal system are to provide movement, protect internal organs,

produce blood cells of all types, and store minerals. See Chapters 23 and 24 for a review of the skeletal and muscular systems. In your career as a medical assistant, regardless of which specialty you work in, you will encounter patients with musculoskeletal conditions.

The symptoms a patient may present related to this system are numerous and vary widely. Many of the symptoms patients experience have a great bearing on their quality of life. For example, the young woman suffering from rheumatoid arthritis may be so disabled and in so much pain she cannot work or care for herself. Consider the elderly patient who falls and fractures a hip, requiring a total hip replacement (THR), or the young child who suffers from muscle weakness and lack of motor control due to muscular dystrophy.

Your role includes listening carefully to the patient's description of the problem: When did it start? What was done to alleviate the problem? What are his or her concerns at present? Note carefully the exact location of pain, and ask the patient to quantify it on a scale of 1 to 10. Offer to assist the patient to the examining room and provide a wheelchair, if necessary. Once in the examining room, make any accommodations necessary to ensure that the patient is comfortable, such as providing a blanket for warmth or an extra pillow to support the injured part. When evaluating muscle strength, recall that it should be equal on both sides of the body. For instance, if you ask a patient to squeeze your hands, the amount of pressure the patient exerts with each hand should be equal. Observe the patient's gait and the range of motion of the affected area. All are important clues the physician needs to help make an accurate diagnosis.

Therapeutic modalities, such as application of heat and cold, are covered in Chapter 51. Table 37-8 lists procedures and diagnostic tests related to the musculoskeletal system.

ARTHRITIS

Arthritis means "inflammation of the joint." More than a hundred types of arthritis affect more than 40 million Americans. Chances are great that you will encounter patients with this painful and sometimes crippling disorder.

Osteoarthritis, also known as degenerative joint disease (DJD), is a natural consequence of aging. The articular cartilage in weight-bearing joints, such as the knee, hip, and ankle, wears away and the surface becomes rough. The result is a painful, stiff joint. Obesity, trauma, and genetic predisposition increase the risk of osteoarthritis. Treatment involves reducing pain with medication such as **nonsteroidal anti-inflammatory drugs (NSAIDs)** (e.g., ibuprofen) and maintaining normal motion.

Nervous System

The study of the nervous system is **neurology**. A neurologist specializes in treating and diagnosing conditions of the nervous system. A neurosurgeon performs surgical procedures on the nervous system that are are necessitated by disease or trauma. A psychiatrist treats mental and neurological conditions that affect behavior.

Patients with nervous system conditions exhibit many different types of symptoms. A neurological examination focuses on the state of consciousness of the patient reflex response, motor response, speech patterns, and patterns of behavior. If, as a medical assistant, you notice inappropriate responses or changes in grooming habits, the physician should be made aware of your observations. Your role in the neurological examination is to provide support and encouragement to patients and assist in positioning them as needed and to have all the necessary equipment set up for the physician, including the following:

- Otoscope
- Ophthalmoscope
- Percussion hammer
- Penlight
- Tuning fork

TABLE 37-8 Procedures and Diagnostic Tests Related to the Musculoskeletal System

Procedure/Test	Description
Aldolase	Blood serum test to measure ALD enzyme present in skeletal and heart muscle to diagnose Duchenne muscular dystrophy before symptoms appear.
Antinuclear antibody (ANA)	Antibodies present in a variety of immunologic diseases such as rheumatoid arthritis and systemic lupus.
Amputation	Partial or complete removal of a limb for a variety of reasons, including tumors, gangrene, intractable pain, crushing injury, or uncontrollable infection.
Anterior cruciate ligament (ACL) reconstruction	Replacing a torn ACL with a graft by means of arthroscopy.
Arthrocentesis	Removal of synovial fluid with a needle from a joint space, such as in the knee, for examination.
Arthrodesis	Surgical reconstruction of a joint.
Arthrography	Visualization of a joint by a radiographic study after injection of a contrast medium.
Arthroplasty	Surgical reconstruction of a joint.
Arthroscopic surgery	Use of an arthroscope, a lighted instrument with camera/video capabilities, to facilitate performing surgery on a joint.
Arthrotomy	Surgically cutting into a joint.
Bone graft	Piece of bone taken from the patient that is (a) used to take the place of a removed bone or a bony defect at another site or (b) wedged between bones for fusion of a joint.
Bone scan	Use of scanning equipment to visualize bones. It is especially useful in observing progress of treatment for osteomyelitis and cancer metastases to the bone.
Bunionectomy	Removal of the bursa at the joint of the great toe.

Calcium	Blood serum test to determine levels of calcium. Calcium is essential for muscular contraction, nerve transmission, and blood clotting.
Carpal tunnel release	Surgical cutting of the ligament in the wrist to relieve nerve pressure caused by the repetitive motion (e.g., typing) that results in carpal tunnel syndrome.
Computerized axial tomography	Computer-assisted X-ray used to detect tumors and fractures. Also referred to as CT scan.
Creatine phosphatase (CPK)	Blood serum test to measure the CPK level that is increased in necrosis or atrophy of skeletal muscle, traumatic muscle injury, strenuous exercise, progressive muscular dystrophy, and after heart attack.
C-reactive protein (CRP)	Positive result may indicate rheumatoid arthritis, acute inflammatory change, or widespread metastasis.
Electromyography (EMG)	Study and record of the strength of muscle contractions as a result of electrical stimulation. Used in the diagnosis of muscle disorders and to distinguish nerve disorders from muscle disorders.
Fasciectomy	Surgical removal of the fascia (fibrous membrane) covering and supporting muscles.
Goniometry	Measurement of joint movements and angles via a goniometer.
Lactic dehydrogenase (LDH)	Blood serum test to measure the level of the enzyme LDH. It is increased in muscular dystrophy, after damage to skeletal muscles, after pulmonary embolism, and during skeletal muscle malignancy.
Laminectomy	Removal of the vertebral posterior arch to correct severe back problems caused by compression of the lamina.
Magnetic resonance imaging (MRI)	Medical imaging that uses radio-frequency radiation as its source of energy. It does not require the injection of contrast medium or exposure to ionizing radiation. The technique is useful for visualizing large blood vessels, the heart, brain, and soft tissues.
Meniscectomy	Removal of all or part of a torn meniscus (knee cartilage).
Muscle biopsy	Removal of muscle tissue for pathological examination.
Myelography	Study of the spinal column after injecting opaque contrast material.
Phosphorous (P) blood test	Testing of the phosphorous level of the blood; level may be increased in osteoporosis and during fracture healing.
Photon absorptiometry	Measurement of bone density using an instrument for the purpose of detecting osteoporosis.
Reduction	Correcting a fracture by realigning the bone fragment. A closed reduction of the fracture is the manipulation of the bone into alignment and the application of a cast or splint to immobilize the part during healing process. Open reduction is the surgical incision at the site of the fracture to perform the bone realignment. This is necessary when there are bone fragments to be removed.
Serum glutamic oxaloacetic transaminase (SGOT)	Blood serum test to measure the level of the enzyme SGOT. It is increased in skeletal muscle damage and muscular dystrophy. This test is also called aspartate aminotransferase (AST).
Serum glutamic pyruvic transaminase (SGPT)	Blood serum test to measure the level of the enzyme SGPT. It is increased in skeletal muscle damage. This test is also called alanine aminotransferase (ALT).
Serum rheumatoid factor (RF)	An immunoglobulin present in the serum of 50 to 95 percent of adults with rheumatoid arthritis.
Spinal fusion	Surgical immobilization of adjacent vertebrae. This may be done for several reasons, including correction of a herniated disk.
Thermograph	Process of recording heat patterns of the body's surface. Used to investigate the pathophysiology of rheumatoid arthritis.
Total hip replacement (THR)	Surgical replacement of a hip by implanting a prosthetic or artificial joint.
Uric acid blood test	Measurement of uric acid in the blood; level is increased in gout, arthritis, multiple myeloma, and rheumatism.

- Cotton ball
- Pin
- Tongue depressor
- Small vials containing hot and cold liquid, vials with different scents, and vials with different-tasting liquids, per the physician's order

Many types of tests and procedures may be ordered as follow-ups to the initial examination. Table 37-9 discusses procedures and diagnostic tests related to the nervous system.

Assisting with a neurological examination entails handing equipment to the physician and monitoring patients for unusual patterns of behavior or speech. The procedures to

TABLE 37-9 Procedures and Diagnostic Tests Related to the Nervous System

Procedure/Test	Description
Babinski's sign	Reflex test developed by John Babinski, a French neurologist, to determine lesions and abnormalities in the nervous system. The Babinski reflex is present or positive when the great toe extends instead of flexes when the lateral sole of the foot is stroked.
Brain scan	Injection of radioactive isotopes into the circulation to determine the function and abnormality of the brain.
Carotid endarterectomy	Surgical procedure for removing an obstruction within the carotid artery. It was developed to prevent strokes but is found useful only in severe stenosis with a transient ischemic attack (TIA).
Cerebral angiogram	X-ray of the blood vessels of the brain after the injection of radioopaque dye.
Cerebrospinal fluid shunts	Surgical creation of an artificial opening to allow for the passage of fluid. Used in the treatment of hydrocephalus.
Cordectomy	Removal of part of the spinal cord.
Craniotomy	Surgical incision into the brain through the cranium.
Cryosurgery	Use of extreme cold to produce areas of destruction in the brain. Used to control bleeding and treat brain tumors.
Echoencephalogram	Recording of the ultrasonic echoes of the brain. Useful in determining abnormal patterns of shifting in the brain.
Electromyogram	Written recording of the contraction of muscles as a result of receiving electrical stimulation.
Laminectomy	Removal of a posterior vertebral arch.
Lumbar puncture	Puncture with a needle into the lumbar area (usually the fourth intervertebral space) to withdraw fluid for examination and for the injection of anesthesia.
Nerve block	Method of regional anesthetic to stop the passage of sensory stimulation along a nerve path.
Pneumoencephalography	X-ray examination of the brain following withdrawal of cerebrospinal fluid and injection of air or gas via spinal puncture.
Positron emission tomography (PET)	Use of positive radionucleotides to reconstruct brain sections. Measurement can be taken of oxygen and glucose uptake, cerebral blood flow, and blood volume.
Romberg's sign	Test developed to establish neurological function in which patients are asked to close their eyes and place their feet together. This test for body balance is positive if the patient sways when the eyes are closed.
Spinal puncture	Puncture with a needle into the spinal cavity to withdraw spinal fluid for microscopic analysis.
Sympathectomy	Excision of a portion of the sympathetic nervous system. Could include nerve or ganglion.
Transcutaneous electrical nerve stimulation (TENS)	Application of a mild electrical stimulation to skin electrodes placed over a painful area, causing interference with the transmission of painful stimuli. Can be used in pain management to interfere with the normal pain mechanism.
Trephination	Process of cutting out a piece of bone in the skull to gain entry into the brain to relieve pressure.
Vagotomy	Surgical incision into the vagus nerve. Medication can be administered into the nerve to prevent its function.

perform evaluation of patient's pupils and assisting with neurological examination follow.

The pupils of the eyes often display signs relevant to the functioning of the brain and nervous system. This straightforward noninvasive procedure is simple and quick. Procedure 37-7 lists the steps for evaluating patients' pupils. The pupils are checked for the following:

- Equal size
- Equal dilation in both eyes in darkness or dim light
- Rapid constriction to light in both eyes
- Equal reaction to light
- Accommodation to objects near or far

ASSISTING THE PHYSICIAN WITH A NEUROLOGICAL EXAMINATION

In evaluating neurologic disorders the physician uses all methods of examination previously described. Vision and hearing tests may be required and are discussed later in this textbook. Procedure 37-8 provides steps for assisting with a neurological examination.

CEREBROVASCULAR DISEASE

Cerebrovascular disease is any disease affecting the blood vessels of the brain. Because the brain requires about 20 percent of the body's blood supply, any decrease in blood and oxygen supply has major consequences and causes brain dysfunction. There are many causes of cerebrovascular disease: atherosclerosis, arteriosclerosis, hemorrhage, and **thrombus** (blood clot). Stroke or CVA is any situation that causes an interruption of the blood supply to the brain and is the third-leading cause of death in the United States. Risk factors for stroke are similar to those for coronary artery disease—namely hypertension, obesity, high cholesterol, smoking, diabetes, family history,

procedure 37-7

PERFORMING A PUPIL CHECK ON A PATIENT

Objective: To correctly check patients' pupils for size, dilation, constriction, accommodation, and equal reaction to light.

EQUIPMENT AND SUPPLIES
penlight; patient's record; pen

METHOD
1. Identify patient and introduce yourself.
2. Observe the patient for responsiveness to your introduction.
3. Explain the procedure. (It may help to partially darken the room.)
4. Ask the patient to look straight ahead.
5. Using a penlight or flashlight, approach from the side and shine light on one pupil at a time. Observe for constriction of the pupil. Figure 37-21 shows variations in pupil diameters in millimeters.
6. Shine the light on the pupil again and observe the other pupil for constriction.

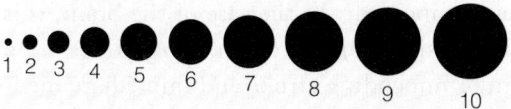

FIGURE 37-21 When testing a patient's pupils, move the light toward the patient's eye from the side position. This figure shows the variations in pupil sizes in millimeters.

7. Hold open the eyes and observe the pupils for size. They should be equal in size.
8. Hold an object, penlight, or pen about 10 cm (4 in.) from the bridge of the patient's nose. Ask the patient to look at the top of the object and then at an object on the wall across the room. Observe for pupil response. (Pupil should constrict when looking at close object and dilate when looking across the room).
9. Move the pen toward the patient's nose. Pupils should converge toward the patient's nose.
10. Observe the pupils for shape. They should be equal or similar in shape.
11. Explain to the patient what other tests will be performed.
12. Document the patient's record either using the abbreviation for Pupils Equal, Round, Reactive to Light and Accommodation (PERRLA) or with the details of whatever result was obtained.

CHARTING EXAMPLE
03/21/XX 11 A.M. T 99°; P 82; R 18; BP 168/80; HT 68"; WT 182 lb; F; PERRLA. · T. Blardo, RMA

procedure
37-8

ASSISTING WITH A NEUROLOGIC EXAMINATION

Objective: To assist the physician with a neurologic screening examination.

EQUIPMENT AND SUPPLIES

percussion hammer; safety pin; tongue depressor; Mayo tray; penlight; cotton ball; tuning fork; neurological wheel; ophthalmoscope; otoscope; hot and cold water; materials with different odors

METHOD

1. Perform hand hygiene.
2. Assemble equipment on the tray and cover the tray.
3. Identify patient and explain procedure.
4. Evaluate the patient's mental status while taking a medical history, paying attention to responses, memory, and coherence of thought, overall mood, and awareness.
5. If ordered, perform a visual acuity test.
6. Assist the patient onto the examination table and drape as needed for comfort.
7. The physician will test reflexes with percussion hammer.
8. Sensory abilities and skin sensations are tested using a safety pin, neurological wheel, and cotton ball and the patient's recognition of simple objects by touch (key, pen, coin).
9. The physician will check the cranial nerves by having the patient touch the finger to the nose, touch the heel to the shin, and move the heel down the opposite shin (Figure 37-22).
10. Assist the physician as needed during the remainder of the examination by handing equipment.

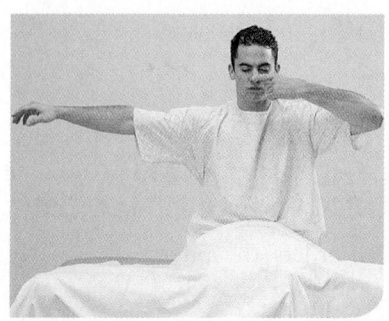

FIGURE 37-22 **Ask the patient to close the eyes, abduct and extend the arms at shoulder height, and touch the nose alternately with one index finger then the other several times in a row.**

11. Assist the patient off the table if the physician wants to evaluate gait or to have the patient perform the **Romberg test** successfully (patient closes eyes and stands with feet together without swaying).
12. Assist the patient off the table and instruct him or her to dress. Assist and provide privacy as needed.
13. Clean the examination room.
14. Perform hand hygiene.
15. Document the patient's record.

CHARTING EXAMPLE

03/21/XX 11 A.M. Assisted Dr. Young with neurologic screening. Scheduled pt. to see Dr. Black, neurologist on 04/04/XX at 11 A.M. · C. Negri, CMA (AAMA)

PROFESSIONALISM
THE WORKPLACE

Every health care facility depends on cooperation among employees. If a colleague is extra busy and you have a few minutes, offer to help clean up an examination room, escort a patient to the appointment desk, or set up for an upcoming examination. Use initiative and show dedication to your field of work.

sedentary lifestyle. Regardless of the cause, thrombus, **embolus** (thrombus that has moved from its place of origin), or hemorrhage, the resulting condition is referred to as a stroke. When blood is decreased to an area of the brain (ischemia) and is temporary, it is referred to as a transient ischemic attack (TIA). A prolonged decrease of blood to an area results in death (necrosis) of the tissue in the vicinity of the incident. In the case of the brain, this often means irreversible damage or death. A TIA is often a warning sign of impending stroke and immediate medical evaluation and possible treatment are important. Since signs of a TIA are temporary, often lasting only a few seconds or minutes to several hours, patients and family members often dismiss them as inconsequential.

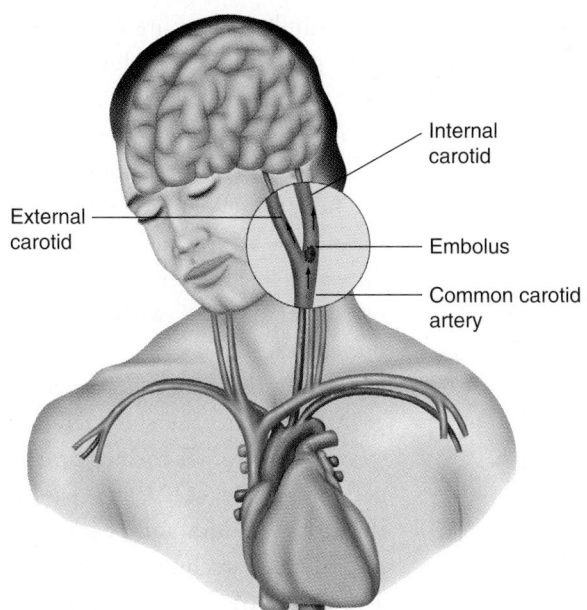

FIGURE 37-23 An embolus is a thrombus or blood clot that moves in the cardiovascular system.

Figure 37-23 depicts an embolus traveling through the carotid artery to the brain.

Recent research recommends that an individual seek medical assistance immediately if there is suspicion of a stroke. Some health care providers recommend these three simple tests:

- Ask the patient to smile

- Ask the patient to speak a simple sentence

- Ask the patient to raise both arms.

If the patient cannot perform any of these simple tasks, seek medical help immediately. Quick intervention with thrombolytic drugs and other medications may restore blood supply and prevent irreversible brain damage. Symptoms of a CVA include sudden severe headache, difficulty in speaking or loss of speech, confusion, one-sided numbness or paralysis, facial droop, memory loss, and blurred vision.

Many patients and family members are unaware that a stroke is in progress and delay seeking help. It is recommended that anyone who suspects they may be having a stroke seek help immediately at a facility prepared to administer clot-dissolving medications. According to the statistics from the American Stroke Association, 780,000 Americans will suffer a new or recurrent stroke. Someone will suffer a stroke every 40 seconds. The cost for stroke-related medical care and disability was about $65.5 billion in 2008.

Physical, occupational, and speech therapy for CVA patients also should begin as soon as conditions allow. It is possible for some patients (mainly those under age 50) to retrain the many extra neurons in the cerebral cortex that are not in use and recover some functions.

DEMENTIA

Dementia is a condition resulting in progressive loss of memory and intellectual ability. It can occur at any age and is not a normal result of aging. Approximately half of dementia patients suffer from Alzheimer's disease. No specific tests are available to obtain a definitive diagnosis. It is important to rule out possible underlying causes such as low thyroid function, alcohol abuse, depression, certain vitamin deficiencies, brain tumors, and drug interactions. If an underlying cause is found, treatment to correct the problem may be successful and progressive deterioration may cease. However, in most cases, dementia is irreversible. Dementia patients may require supervision to ensure their safety. Behavior problems make this devastating condition difficult for patients, family members, and health care providers. Dementia results ultimately in the need for 24-hour care and inevitably death for the patient.

ASSISTING WITH LUMBAR PUNCTURE

The physician may wish to examine spinal fluid for the presence of red cells, white cells, or pathogenic microorganisms. Examination of cerebrospinal fluid (CSF) is an important diagnostic tool to assist in determining conditions

PROFESSIONALISM
THE LIFE SPAN

Alzheimer's disease is a progressive, chronic mental disorder named for Alosi Alzheimer, a German neurologist. This disorder affects people between the ages of 40 and 80 and is characterized by deteriorating cognitive function (also referred to as dementia, sometimes rapid), progressive loss of memory, difficulty with word retrieval, gait problems, and apathy. It is important to keep an open mind when dealing with patients of all ages. Difficulty with word retrieval in an elderly patient does not automatically mean that the person has Alzheimer's disease. Conversely it is possible for relatively young patients to exhibit some Alzheimer's symptoms. It is important not to jump to conclusions based on a patient's age.

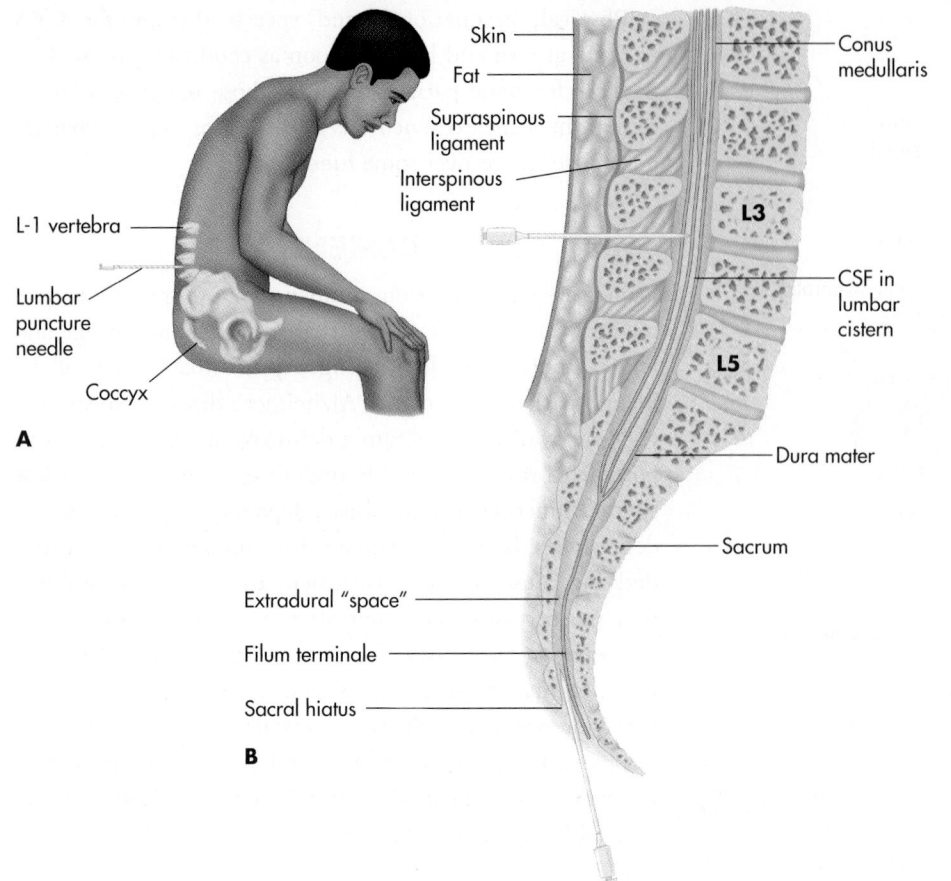

Skin

Fat

Supraspinous ligament

Interspinous ligament

L-1 vertebra

Lumbar puncture needle

Coccyx

A

Conus medullaris

L3

CSF in lumbar cistern

L5

Dura mater

Sacrum

Extradural "space"

Filum terminale

Sacral hiatus

B

FIGURE 37-24 Drawing shows the location of a lumbar puncture.

A lumbar puncture is an invasive procedure; therefore, extra care should be taken when handling the CSF tubes, and universal precautions should be carefully observed. All CSF tests should be treated as stat procedures. In some states only licensed personnel assist with lumbar punctures.

During this procedure a needle is inserted into the subarachnoid space of the spinal cord. A small-gauge needle (22) is passed through the dura and is inserted into the subarachnoid space at L 4–5 below the level of the spinal cord (Figure 37-24). When the stylet, or thin probe, is removed from the needle, CSF will escape and can be collected in tubes for microscopic examination. Patients are prone to headaches after this procedure due to leakage of fluid from the spinal spaces. Intracranial pressure may be evaluated by testing for the **Queckenstedt's sign**. This involves having the assistant press on the patient's jugular vein in the neck (right, left, or both) while the physician monitors the CSF pressure. The pressure should increase when the jugular vein is compressed. If there is no pressure increase, it signifies blockage of CSF flow. Headaches can be diminished if the patient is instructed to lie perfectly flat for several hours (6 to 12) after the procedure. This procedure is more commonly performed in a clinic setting than a medical office to allow the patient to remain flat for the prescribed time.

such as stroke, brain hemorrhage, meningitis, encephalitis, polio, and tumors of the brain and spinal cord. CSF normally is clear, colorless, and sterile, free of any microorganisms. Three tubes of CSF are sent to the laboratory for tests. They include a culture for the presence of microorganisms that are found in infectious diseases such as meningitis; cell count of red cells or white cells that would be present in cases of hemorrhage and infection, respectively; and chemical tests for glucose and protein that help to pinpoint the diagnosis.

SUMMARY

The topics presented in this chapter represent a variety of medical specialty areas. No physician's practice will include all of them. Since the profession of medical assisting is for the multiskilled individual, he or she is expected to have a general knowledge of medicine.

Much of the clinical role of the medical assistant involves assisting with procedures related to the body systems,

including digestive, musculoskeletal (orthopedics), respiratory, integumentary, endocrine, lymphatic, and cardiovascular. No matter what the task involves, the trademark of a good medical assistant should be careful attention to detail and respect for the rights of the patient.

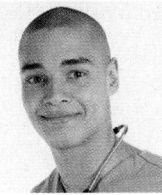

37 CHAPTER REVIEW

COMPETENCY REVIEW

1. Define and spell the terms to learn for this chapter.

2. Develop a teaching plan for a patient with diabetes mellitus.

3. List four types of allergy test used to determine a patient's sensitivities.

4. Describe at least four risk factors for developing coronary artery disease.

5. The physician tells you to schedule Mrs. Dunn for a sigmoidoscopy next week. What would you tell the patient to do to prepare for this procedure?

6. Why is it vital for the patient to follow the exact recommended preparations prior to a sigmoidoscopy?

7. What is CHF? Why does it occur?

8. Describe the signs and symptoms exhibited by a patient with CHF.

9. What instruments should you have ready prior to a neurological examination?

10. Define dementia. What symptoms might a patient with dementia exhibit?

PREPARING FOR THE CERTIFICATION EXAM

1. Which type of physical examination will reveal abnormalities of the nervous system?
   a. oncological
   b. urological
   c. neurological
   d. gynecological
   e. proctological

2. Diabetes mellitus type 2 (NIDDM) is the result of the impaired action of what hormone?
   a. thyroxine
   b. insulin
   c. adrenaline
   d. glucagon
   e. testosterone

3. To test a patient for allergies the physician would order
   a. fasting blood glucose
   b. lumbar puncture
   c. neurological evaluation
   d. RAST test
   e. colonoscopy

4. A fluid-filled lesion is called a
   a. wheal
   b. papule
   c. vesicle
   d. nodule
   e. macule

5. A life-threatening allergic reaction to bee stings or certain drugs or foods is
   a. prophylaxis
   b. diverticulitis
   c. antihistamine
   d. anaphylaxis
   e. GERD

6. One common symptom of coronary artery disease is
   a. dyspnea
   b. polydipsia
   c. dysphagia
   d. leucopenia
   e. digitalis

7. Some factors that lead to the development of heart disease are all of the following EXCEPT
   a. heredity
   b. obesity
   c. flatus
   d. smoking
   e. elevated cholesterol

8. Peripheral edema is seen in what condition?
   a. gastroenteritis
   b. allergic rhinitis
   c. pediculosis
   d. congestive heart failure (CHF)
   e. dermatitis

9. Diabetes mellitus type 2 may be controlled by the following:
   a. frequent ECGs
   b. diet and exercise
   c. removal of pancreas
   d. frequent weight and height evaluation
   e. taking antibiotics

10. Testing for occult blood is performed on what type of specimen?
   a. blood
   b. serum
   c. CSF
   d. vaginal secretions
   e. feces

CRITICAL THINKING

1. Dr. Bahjat wanted Mr. Salvatore to have a sigmoidoscopy to confirm his suspicion that Mr. Salvatore has diverticulitis. What symptoms are indicative of diverticulitis?

2. Mr. Salvatore expressed concern regarding his preparation for the procedure. What instructions should Mr. Salvatore have been given regarding proper preparation?

3. What can David do to help Mr. Salvatore's comfort level during the procedure?

ON THE JOB

Shelia Meyer, a medical assistant in Dr. Ryan's large cardiovascular practice, is taking the medical history of Edna Helm, an obese elderly woman with congestive heart disease. Edna states, "I'm always short of breath, and I perspire all the time. I guess I'm gaining weight, but the funny thing is that only my legs seem heavier. My heart is pounding when I lie down at night; it even seems to stop sometimes. I've even started to wear red nail polish to hide the funny blue color of my nails."

Edna gives you a copy of her medical history from an out-of-state physician. The medical history indicates that she has had the following conditions, tests, and procedures:

Conditions	Tests	Surgical Procedures
Positive Babinski sign	Holter monitor testing	Basal cell carcinoma removed in 1992
Allergic rhinitis	Radioimmunoassay test	Sebaceous cyst removed in 1982
Aortic insufficiency	Protein bound iodine test	Meniscectomy in 1978
Ascites	Glucose tolerance test	Rhytidectomy in 1970
Gastritis		
Osteoarthritis		

1. Using correct medical terms, chart Edna's presenting symptoms.
2. Define each of the procedures and conditions listed on her medical record.

INTERNET ACTIVITY

Radiologists are considered allied health professionals. Perform an Internet search and discover the types of facilities in which they are normally employed, their duties, educational requirements, employment opportunities, and licensure, certification, or registration requirements.

MEDMEDIA

Additional interactive resources and activities for this chapter can be found:

On your student DVD: View applicable procedure videos on the DVD-ROM found in the back of this book.

MyHealthProfessionsKit.com: Test your knowledge of this chapter with games and activities. MyHealthProfessionsKit also includes resources, helpful links, and a Spanish audio glossary.

Medical Assisting Interactive: Practice your procedures as a medical assistant in this simulated doctor's office. This can be accessed through MyHealthProfessionsKit.com.

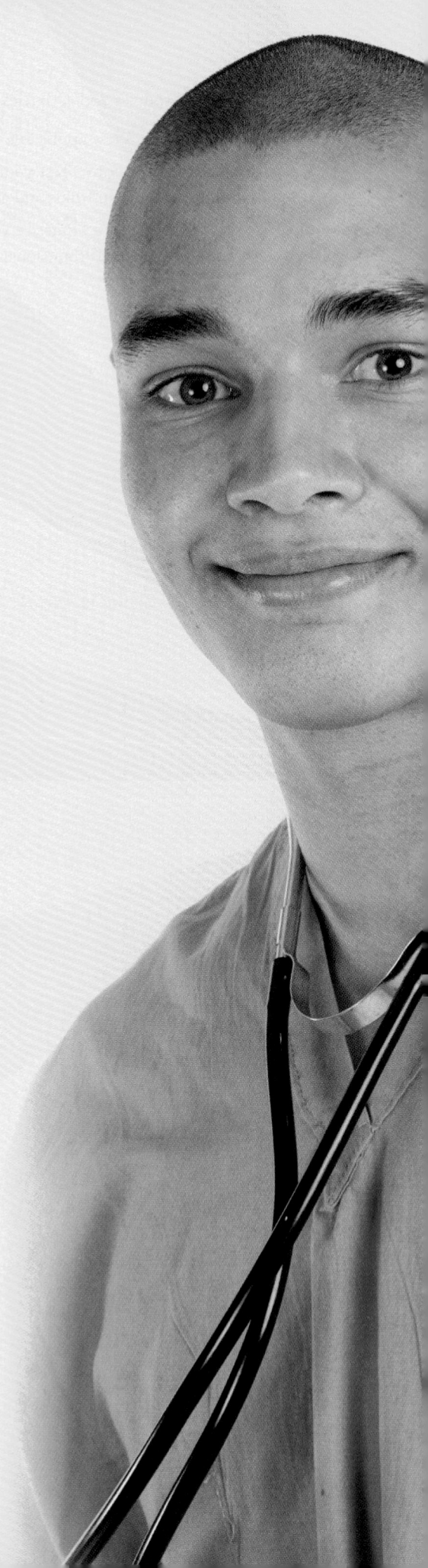

38

Assisting with Reproductive and Urinary Specialties

LEARNING OBJECTIVES

After reading this chapter, you should be able to:

- Define and spell the terms to learn for this chapter.

- Prepare patients for examinations and diagnostic procedures.

- Assist the physician with examination and treatments.

- Assist the physician in performing selected diagnostic tests.

- Instruct patients with special procedures.

- Document special procedures.

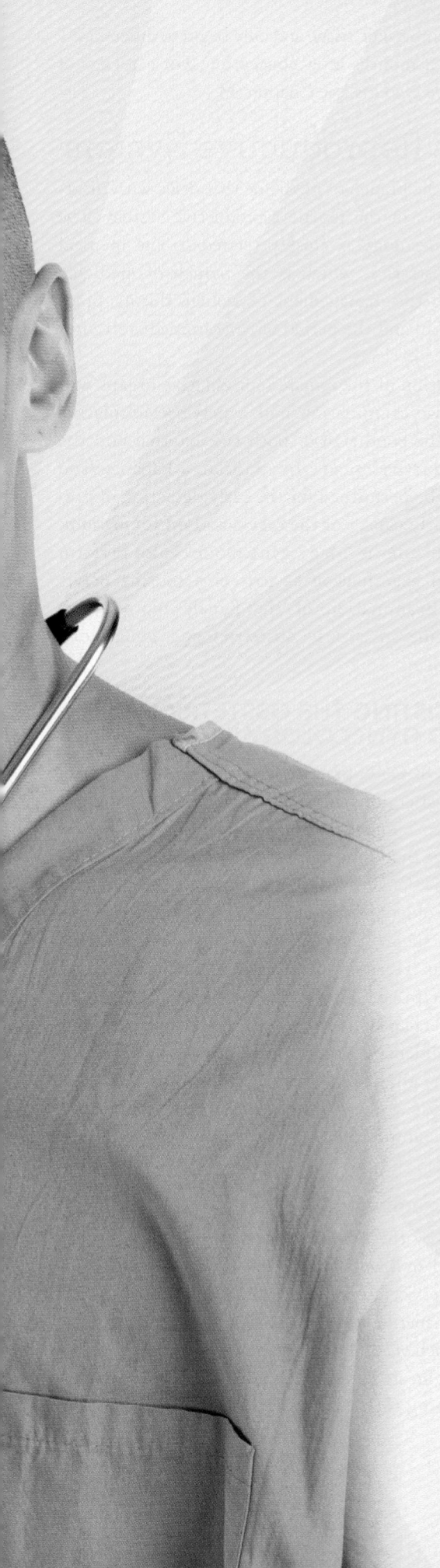

CHAPTER OUTLINE

CASE STUDY

Sonja Lufti is being seen by Dr. McWalters for her first prenatal visit. Sonja's last menstrual period was January 14, 2010. This is the third time that Sonja has been pregnant. She has one 5-year-old son and had a miscarriage at 14 weeks of pregnancy 2 years ago.

ssisting with special examinations related to the reproductive systems of both males and females is explored in this chapter. In addition, examinations related to the urinary systems of both males and females are covered. Sexually transmitted infections (STIs) and their affects on both sexes are discussed. Because of the nature of these situations, it is important to keep the privacy of the patient in mind.

Reproductive Systems

The main function of the male and female reproductive systems is to produce offspring to continue the human species. All of the male and female **gonads**, or sexual organs, develop from the same embryonic tissue and only begin to differentiate approximately 2 months after conception. For a review of the reproductive systems, see Chapter 33.

Female Reproductive System

Gynecology is the branch of medicine that deals with disorders and diseases of the female reproductive system. The practice of gynecology is closely related to the medical specialty of obstetrics, which is the branch of medicine concerned with the management of women during pregnancy, childbirth, and the period of time immediately after childbirth.

An examination of the female reproductive organs will include a breast examination and a pelvic examination to determine the condition of both the external and the internal reproductive organs. In addition, a Papanicolaou (Pap) test may be performed for the early detection of precancerous or early cancer of the cervix and **endometrium**, the lining of the uterus. Many gynecologists also perform a digital rectal examination as part of a routine pelvic examination. Examination of the female reproductive organs is routine in a busy obstetrics and gynecology (OB/GYN) office.

ASSISTING THE OBSTETRICS AND GYNECOLOGY PATIENT

Patients in an OB/GYN practice will cover a wide age span and present a variety of symptoms and conditions. Medical assistants may encounter the teenager having her first pelvic examination, the first-time mother, the mother of seven, the perimenopausal female, the middle-aged menopausal female, and the older postmenopausal female. Because all are in distinct life stages, their emotional and physical needs will be different. Hormones play a large part in the stages of development in the female and will have a bearing on the emotional status of your patients as well. One of your tasks is to help identify patients' problems and provide information to the physician. Using your listening skills and being empathetic will provide an environment in which the patient is comfortable enough to convey her feelings and discomforts.

The Breast Examination

It is estimated by the American Cancer Society (ACS) that over a lifetime 1 in 8 women will develop breast cancer. The American Cancer Society states that most physicians feel that early detection methods for breast cancer save many thousands of lives each year. Mammograms, clinical breast examinations (CBE), breast self-examinations (BSE), and magnetic resonance imaging (MRI) are tools for early detection. The

Gender—Females develop breast cancer 100 times more frequently than males, probably due to the effects of estrogen.

Aging—Risk increases with age: 1 in 8 women under age 45 develop invasive breast cancer, whereas 2 of 3 age 55 or older develop it.

Genetic factors—Between 5 and 10 percent of breast cancer cases are believed to be hereditary. BRCA1 and BRCA2 genes are the most common genes involved.

Family history—Risk is higher if a blood relative developed breast cancer. Occurrence in mother, sister, or daughter doubles a woman's risk.

Personal history of breast cancer—Women with cancer in one breast have a three- to fourfold increased risk of developing it in the same or other breast.

Race—White women are slightly more likely to develop breast cancer, but African-American women are more likely to die from it.

Abnormal breast biopsy results—Lesions with excessive growth in ducts or lobules of breast tissue increase the risk more than cysts and fibrosis.

Oral contraceptives—Studies suggest that using oral contraceptives may slightly increase the risk of breast cancer.

Postmenopausal hormone therapy (PHT)—Combined PHT (estrogen and progesterone) use does increase the risk of developing and dying from breast cancer. The risk levels return to those of the general population after cessation of PHT for 5 years. Estrogen alone does not increase the risk unless used for 10 years or more.

ACS suggests women in their twenties and thirties should have a CBE as part of a periodic regular health exam by a health professional every 3 years. At this time patients should be given information about the benefits of mammograms and BSE. Women at greater risk of developing breast cancer should have an MRI and mammogram every year. Yearly MRI screening is not recommended for women with a low risk of breast cancer. See Box 38-1 for a summary of risk factors for developing breast cancer.

A CBE by the physician precedes the pelvic examination. The patient lies in the supine position for this examination and is generally asked to place her hand behind her head on the side that is being examined first. This allows the physician to examine the lymph nodes under the axilla. The physician palpates the breast using his or her fingertips in a circular fashion around all the breast tissue to search for lumps, tenderness, or inflammation. In addition, any dimpling or puckering of the skin around the breast and nipple is noted. The nipples are checked for cracking, bleeding, or discharge.

BSE is encouraged for women starting in their twenties. Some women are comfortable performing a BSE, and others become stressed about performing it correctly. The overall goal should be for the patient to be familiar with her own breasts and to report any changes immediately to her physician.

The physician may advise the patient to perform BSE every month, usually 1 week after the menstrual period ends. Women who have reached menopause should examine their breasts on the same day each month. The medical assistant may have the responsibility of explaining the correct procedure for the BSE. If the woman notes any abnormality during self-examination, she should call her physician for an appointment and not wait for another month to see if the abnormality disappears. Procedure 38-1 illustrates the correct way of instructing a woman on how to perform self-examination of the breasts. Figure 38-2 illustrates a medical assistant using a prosthetic teaching model to instruct a patient on breast self-examination.

The American Cancer Society recommends the following:

- Women between the ages of 20 and 39 should have a breast examination performed by a physician every 3 years; a baseline mammogram should be done at the age of 35.

- Women over the age of 40 should have a yearly breast examination by a physician, and a mammogram every 1 to 2 years.

- Women over the age of 50 should have a yearly breast examination by a physician and a yearly mammogram.

The Pelvic Examination

The gynecologic or pelvic examination is included as part of a routine physical examination for the female. Although some family and internal physicians may perform these on their patients, other physicians prefer that the patient see a gynecologist for the examination. A pelvic examination alone may be conducted in order to diagnose a problem relating specifically to the female reproductive organ.

INSTRUCTING A PATIENT ON BREAST SELF-EXAMINATION

Objective: Instruct the patient how to do breast self-examination.

EQUIPMENT AND SUPPLIES

breast model (if available); pamphlets on breast self-examination

METHOD

1. Perform hand hygiene.
2. Assemble equipment.
3. Identify the patient and explain the necessity for performing the procedure correctly in three different positions each month. Use the breast model to explain the correct application of fingertips.
4. *In the shower* (Figure 38-1A):
   - Raise the right arm. Use the left hand to examine the right breast, then raise the left arm and use the right hand to examine the left breast.
   - Using flat fingertips, check breast tissue and underarm tissue, gently feeling for any lump or thickening. Touch every part of the breast when skin is wet; hands will move easily over the softened wet skin.
5. *Before a mirror* (Figure 38-1B):
   - Inspect the breasts for any irregularity in shape while arms are at the side of the body.
   - Look for swelling, dimpling, or puckering of the skin; lumps; or changes in the nipples, such as retracting. Gently squeeze both nipples and look for discharge.
   - Raise the arms overhead and look for size, shape, and contour changes in each breast.
   - With palms resting on hips, flex chest muscles to observe for any obvious differences in breasts.

Note: The left and right breasts on most females do not match exactly.

6. *Lying down* (Figure 38-1C):
   - To examine the right breast, place a pillow or folded towel behind the right shoulder and place the right hand behind the head. Examine the right breast with the left hand and the left breast with the right hand.
   - Using the hand with fingers flat, gently press the breast tissue using small circular motions starting at the outermost top of the breast in the 12:00 position and spiraling toward the nipple (Figure 38-1D). Cover all the breast tissue, feeling for lumps or any abnormal hanges in breast tissue. Gently squeeze the nipple of each breast between the thumb and index finger and note lumps or discharge.
   - Repeat the procedure for the left breast.
7. *With the arm resting on a firm surface* (Figure 38-1E):
   - Use the same circular motion to examine the underarm area. (This is breast tissue, too.) Repeat the procedure for both underarm areas.
8. Report any abnormalities to the physician. This self-examination is not a substitute for periodic examinations by a qualified physician.

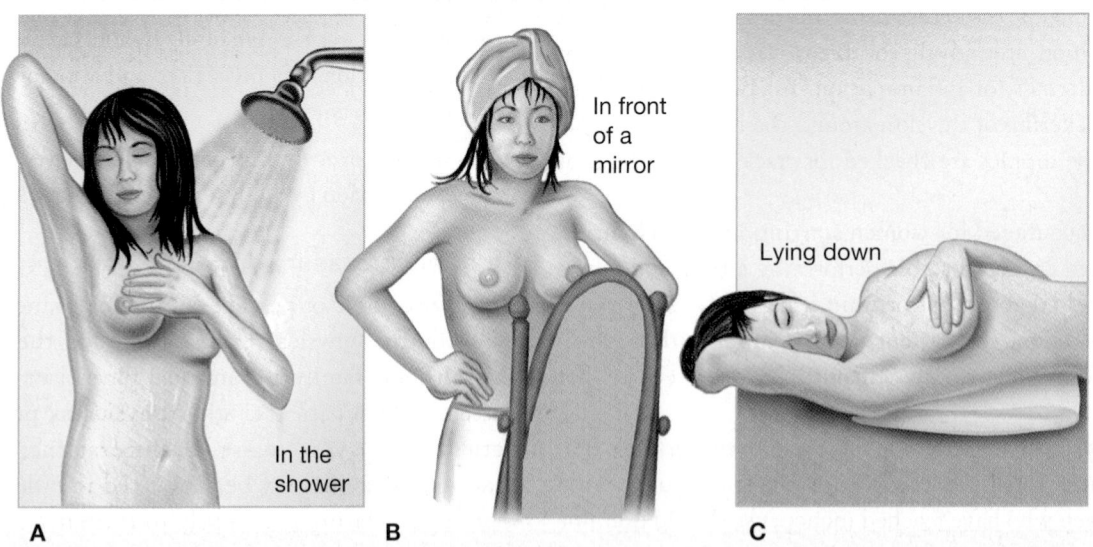

In front of a mirror

Lying down

In the shower

A   B   C

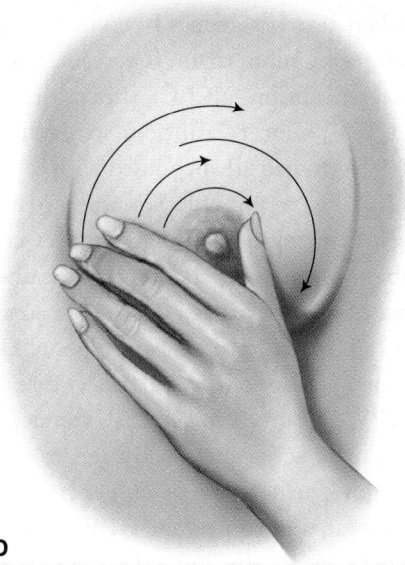

D

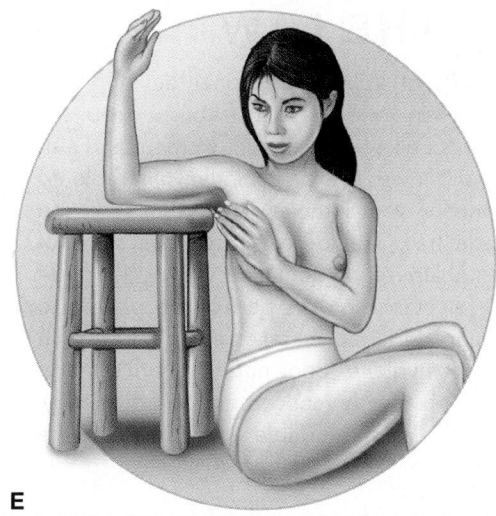

E

FIGURE 38-1   (A) In the shower; (B) In front of a mirror; (C) Lying down; (D) In concentric circles; (E) With arm raised.

CHARTING EXAMPLE

2/14/XX 2:00 P.M. Breast self-exam explained to patient using breast model. Pt demonstrated procedure satisfactorily. · · · · ·
· M. King, CMA (AAMA)

Prior to the patient scheduling a Pap test, the medical assistant should advise her of the following:

- Do not douche for 24 to 48 hours before the examination. Doing so may wash away cervical cells that should be obtained during a Pap smear.

- Avoid sexual intercourse for at least 48 hours before the examination.

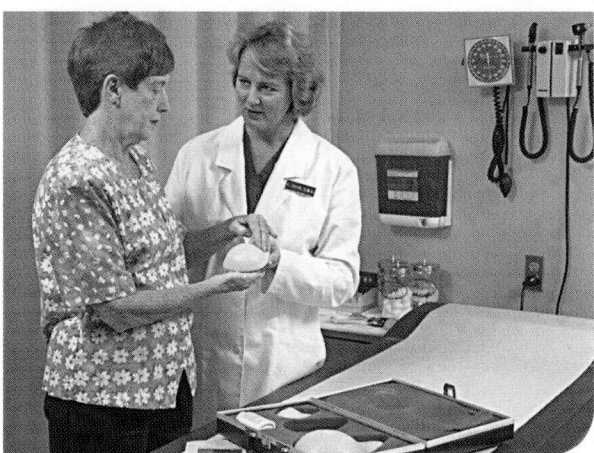

FIGURE 38-2   **A medical assistant using a breast model to instruct a patient on proper technique for performing self-examination of the breasts.**

- Do not schedule the Pap test for a time when you may be menstruating. It should be scheduled at least 5 days after the last day of menstruation.

The gynecologic examination begins with taking a thorough history from the patient. Questions about the menstrual cycle, past pregnancies, and discomfort during sexual intercourse are important in order to obtain a picture of the patient's overall health status. You should have knowledge of conditions and diseases affecting this system and a thorough understanding of the signs, symptoms, and treatments of STIs (see later in this chapter). Additional information related to the reproductive system can be found in Chapter 33. Bruises and other signs of physical abuse must be reported.

For legal reasons, a female medical assistant is usually present to assist with a gynecologic examination. Before beginning the pelvic examination, the physician will listen to the patient's heart and lungs. The pelvic examination begins with an examination of the **external genitalia** (external reproductive organs) for swelling, redness, or ulcerations. The vaginal speculum is inserted into the vagina to inspect the vagina and cervix for color, lacerations, nodules, or discharge. The size of the speculum selected will depend on the

THE LAW

An integral part of your professional development should include an awareness of abuse problems among patients of all ages. Children, women, and elderly women and men are particularly vulnerable to abuse. Vigilance in your interviewing and observation techniques will help you detect suspicious signs of abuse. Signs of abuse or domestic violence include bruising and reluctance on the part of the patient to explain the injury. Elder abuse takes many forms, such as neglect, poor hygiene, poor nutrition, bruises and sores, and being overly concerned about money. Establishing a secure comfortable environment in the office may help abused patients feel at ease to talk about their problems.

Many states mandate that suspicions of abuse be reported. How you go about reporting suspicions and to whom to report should be part of your office policy. Take the initiative and prepare a folder, including the names and numbers of state agencies, women's shelters, and domestic violence hotlines. If there is no clear-cut set of standards for you to follow, contact agencies in your state, such as the Department of Health, the Department of Aging, and the Department of Children and Family Services. All these agencies will have printed material and guidelines to help you understand what and how to report your suspicions. Any immediate concerns should be brought to the physician at once. Ignoring the situation helps no one.

examination. It is a cytological screening test named for a Greek physician, George Papanicolaou. Various experts agree that the Pap test has reduced cervical cancer rates in the United States by more than 70 percent. The National Cervical Cancer Coalition (NCCC), part of the Human Papillomavirus (HPV) Cancer Coalition, states that in the United States 10,000 women are diagnosed with cervical cancer each year and that 11 percent of U.S. women do not have Pap test screenings. In many developing countries cervical cancer is the number-one cause of cancer-related deaths in women.

Human papillomaviruses (HPVs) are actually a group of more than a hundred viruses. Four types of HPV are responsible for the majority of cervical cancer cases and for genital warts. HPV is spread by sexual contact. Women who become sexually active at an early age, as well as those who have multiple partners, are at higher risk of infection from HPV. The best way to prevent HPV infection is to refrain from sexual contact. In 2006 the United States Food and Drug Administration (FDA) approved the use of a new vaccine, Gardasil, to prevent infection from the four types of HPV. Gardasil vaccine is given in a series of three injections over a 6-month period. It is recommended that it be given before a female becomes sexually active. Because the vaccine is new, it is not known whether booster injections will be necessary. The National Cancer Institute (NCI) reports that about 30 percent of cervical cancers and 10 percent of genital warts will not be prevented by these vaccines. It is recommended that both vaccinated and unvaccinated women undergo cervical screenings.

PAP TEST PROCEDURE

The Pap test is a screening procedure that examines cells from the vaginal and cervical mucosa. A thin scraping of

sexual maturity and physical state of the patient. Vaginal specula may be either metal, requiring sanitization and sterilization after each use, or disposable and meant for one use only. Warming the speculum in warm water or keeping it warm in a drawer equipped with a heating pad will make the examination more comfortable for the patient. (Figure 38-3 illustrates the speculum and the manual pelvic examination for females.) The patient may need reassurance that the procedure is painless, especially if it is her first gynecologic examination.

Pap Test and Cervical Cancer. The Pap test is usually included as part of a pelvic

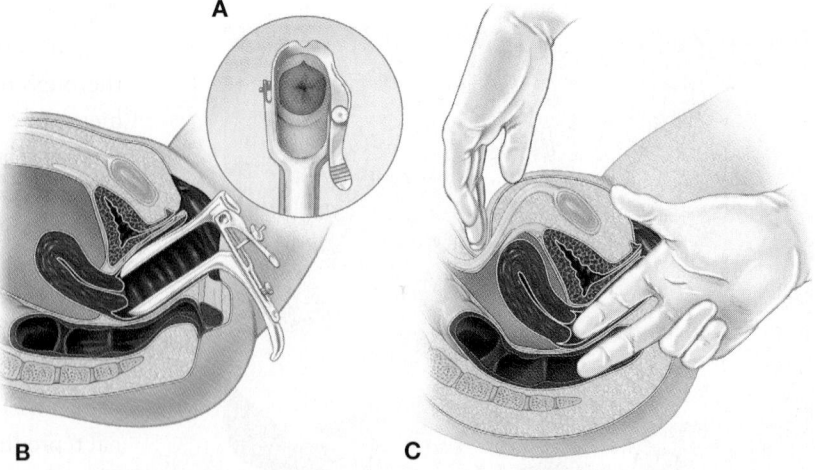

FIGURE 38-3 (A) and (B) Pelvic examination of female using a vaginal speculum; (C) a bimanual examination.

these exfoliated cells is taken from the cervix, vagina, and endocervical canal using a cervical spatula and cervical brush or broom. Presently, two methods of Pap specimen preparation are used. In the older "dry" method, separate slides are made by the physician; the medical assistant then labels the slides C, V, E, (cervix, vaginal, and endocervical canal), based on the source of the cells, and sprays them with a fixative to preserve the cells.

The newer more accurate liquid-based method requires the specimen to be collected in a similar fashion, but the plastic vaginal speculum and brush or broom that are used are swirled around several times in a liquid cytology medium in order to suspend and preserve the sample. With either method of collection, the properly labeled specimens are then sent to the laboratory for examination. A cytologist prepares, stains, examines, and evaluates the three slides for evidence of infection, **dysplasia** (abnormal cells), or cancerous cells. The laboratory requisition form has a specific field that requires the medical assistant to enter the first day of the patient's last menstrual period (LMP). The cytologist needs this information to make an accurate evaluation and to provide a maturation index (MI) if it is requested as part of the evaluation. An MI provides a hormonal evaluation of the patient that may assist in evaluating causes of infertility, menopausal or postmenopausal bleeding, or **amenorrhea** (absence of menstrual periods).

After collecting the specimens, a bimanual pelvic examination is performed. The physician inserts a gloved, lubricated finger into the vagina and palpates the lower abdomen. Between the physician's two hands, he or she can detect the size, shape, and position of the uterus and ovaries and also lumps or abnormalities.

A rectal examination usually follows. To perform a rectal examination the physician removes his or her gloves and dons a new pair. The medical assistant will lubricate one of the physician's gloved fingers, which is then inserted into the rectum to check for hemorrhoids, polyps, or other abnormalities.

Grading of Pap Specimens

Several methods of grading Pap specimens are used. One system provides a grading system for cervical changes, using cervical intraepithelial neoplasia (CIN) criteria of I, II, or III and the amount of dysplasia present. CIN I is mildly dysplastic, CIN II is moderate to moderately severe dysplasia, and CIN III indicates **carcinoma in situ** (cancer in that particular area that has not broken through the basement membrane).

The Pap smear is 95 percent accurate in detecting cervical carcinoma. The NCI and the ACS recommend that women who have become sexually active or are over the age of 18 have a Pap smear. Women who have had a total hysterectomy do not need cervical cancer screening unless they have a history of precancerous cells or cervical cancer. It is recommended that women with genital herpes or HPV have a Pap smear every 3 to 6 months.

A colposcope is used to identify abnormal tissue (Figure 38-4). Procedure 38-2 lists the steps for assisting with a pelvic examination and a Pap test.

PRENATAL CARE

Prenatal care includes care provided to pregnant women before delivery, including a series of visits and specific tests to promote the health of both mother and fetus. Postnatal or postpartum care covers the time from the delivery of the infant through the mother's 6-week postnatal follow-up appointment.

Many health practitioners recommend that anyone considering or wishing to become pregnant visit or call their health care provider to discuss the preconception health of the mother. Specific steps may be taken to help ensure the health of both mother and child. The U.S. Public Health Service recommends that women of childbearing age consume at least 400 micrograms of folic acid daily, either through food (especially green leafy vegetables) or supplements.

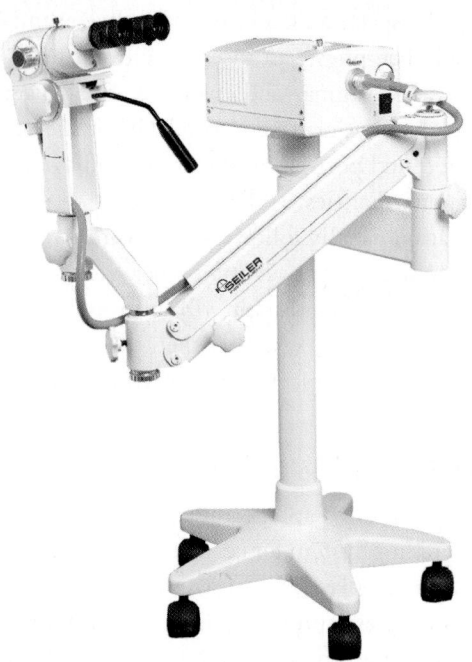

FIGURE 38-4 A colposcope.

Folic acid helps prevent neural tube defects, such as spina bifida. Folic acid should be taken 3 months prior to conception and for at least 3 months after conception.

Maintaining a healthy lifestyle prior to conception and during pregnancy can help reduce gestational problems. Health care providers recommend that expectant mothers refrain from smoking, drinking alcohol, and taking any medication. This includes both prescription and over-the-counter medications. Physicians may allow some medications to be taken during the pregnancy if failure to take the prescribed treatment would hinder the health of the mother.

A normal, full-term pregnancy lasts for 40 weeks. The pregnancy is divided into three trimesters, or stages of approximately 3 months each. The first trimester includes the period of time from implantation of the embryo in the uterus through the fourteenth week. This is a most critical stage of fetal life because most of the major organ systems develop during this period. It is also the period during

procedure
38-2

ASSISTING WITH A PELVIC EXAMINATION AND PAP TEST

Objective: Set up and assist with a gynecologic examination, including collection without error of dry or liquid-based prep method Pap smear.

EQUIPMENT AND SUPPLIES

vaginal speculum; water-soluble lubricant; cotton-tipped applicator; patient drape; Pap smear materials: Dry Prep—cervical spatula brush, glass slides, fixative spray or liquid slide holder, identification label; Liquid-Based Prep—plastic cervical spatula, broom or brush, cytology medium transport vial, identification label; laboratory request form; cleansing tissue; gloves; container for contaminated vaginal speculum; gooseneck lamp; biohazard waste container

METHOD

For dry prep collection:

1. Perform hand hygiene.
2. Assemble equipment.
3. Label the slides, and complete the laboratory form.
4. Identify the patient, and explain the procedure.
5. Direct the patient to the bathroom to empty her bladder.
6. Ask the patient to remove her clothing and put on the gown with the opening in front.
7. Drape the patient appropriately, and assist her into the supine position for breast and abdominal examination.

8. When the physician is ready to collect the Pap specimen, assist and instruct the patient to assume the dorsal lithotomy position with her buttocks at the edge of the table and her feet in the stirrups. Knees should be relaxed and rotated outward. Expose the genitalia by moving the drape away from this area while it still covers the legs.
9. Adjust the gooseneck lamp and place the physician's stool in the proper position at the end of examination table.
10. Assist the physician with the procedure (Figure 38-5):
    - Apply gloves.
    - Hand gloves and equipment to the physician as needed. Place lubricant onto the speculum as the physician holds it.
    - Hold the microscopic slides as the physician smears the slides. Mark the slides: C for cervical, V for vaginal, and E for endocervical.
    - Spray fixative from about 6 inches away from the slide.
    - Place the slide into a container with the appropriate label.

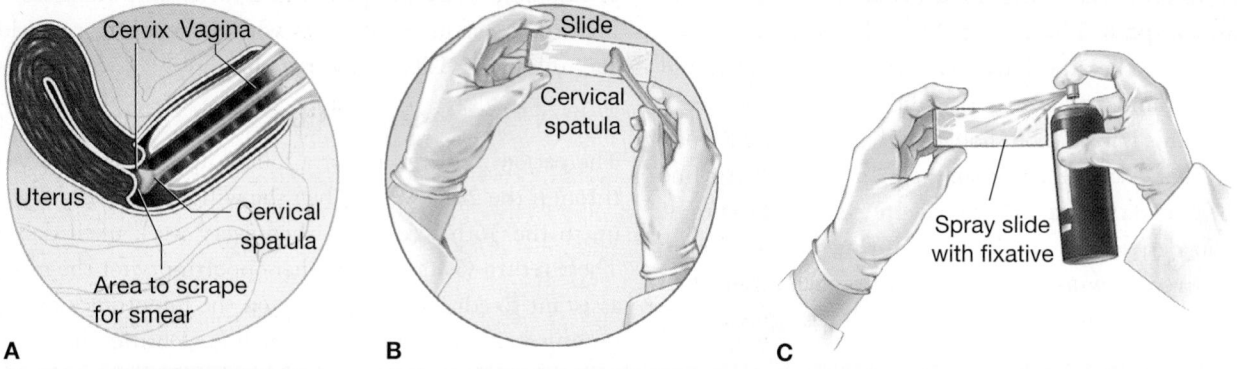

FIGURE 38-5 (A) Female reproductive organs showing the location for obtaining a scraping for a Pap smear; (B) making a Pap smear; (C) spray slide with fixative.

11. Hold the receptacle as the physician places the contaminated speculum into it. Set the container into the sink for later cleaning.
12. Apply lubricant to the physician's gloved fingers in preparation for the manual examination.
13. Properly dispose of gloves in a hazardous waste container and perform hand hygiene.
14. Assist the patient to sit up by (a) helping her move back on the table, (b) taking her feet out of the stirrups, and (c) helping her to a sitting position.
15. Sanitize and sterilize equipment as needed.
16. Perform hand hygiene.
17. Prepare the Pap specimen to be sent to the laboratory.

For liquid-based prep collection:
18. Proceed through steps 1–9 in previous page.
19. Open the vial of liquid transport medium and hold for the physician to place both the plastic spatula and either brush or broom containing the specimen in the vial.
20. Rinse the broom vigorously by pushing it to the bottom of the vial ten times.
21. Use the spatula to scrape cells from the brush and swirl both in the vial to mix before removing.
22. Label the vial and dispose of hazardous waste appropriately.
23. Proceed through steps 12 through 17 above.

Note: The physician will chart the procedure.

which the embryo is most vulnerable to substances that may cause birth defects, such as bacterial and viral infections, drugs, alcohol, and other chemical substances. After the eighth week, the embryo is referred to as a fetus. The second trimester begins at the end of the fourteenth week and continues to the end of the sixth month. During this period, refinement of all the organs takes place and fetal movement (**quickening**) may be felt. The third trimester is the period from the end of the sixth month to birth and is marked by an increase in the size and weight of the fetus. During this stage, the fetus usually assumes a head-down position and is said to have reached the age of **viability** (able to sustain life independently) at 7 months.

First Prenatal Visit

The first prenatal visit usually takes place after the patient has missed two menstrual periods. This visit requires more time than follow-up visits because a full history and prenatal assessment must be done. In addition, a complete physical examination, pelvic examination, including a Pap smear, and cultures (as needed) must be performed. Blood tests are ordered at this visit, and it is up to the medical assistant to reinforce the importance of the patient complying with the physician's orders. Blood tests include CBC, ABO/Rh, serology test for syphilis, and Rubella titer. Usually a complete urine analysis (UA) is ordered as well. These test results provide a baseline to compare with results obtained later in pregnancy.

The fundal height measurement is taken on the initial visit and is used as a guideline for all subsequent visits. It is the height from the top of the pubic symphysis to the **fundus** (top of the uterus) using a nonstretchable tape measure. Normally during pregnancy, the uterus enlarges and rises into the abdominal cavity, and the fundal height increases each month.

Prenatal History

Prenatal history includes recording the menstrual history including **menarche** (onset of menstruation), menstrual interval cycle, duration of menses, amount of flow, any menstrual cycle problems, and any types of contraception used currently or previously.

The past obstetrical history also is a component of the prenatal record. This includes **gravida** (total number of pregnancies), **para** (births after 20 weeks of gestation, regardless of whether the infant is born dead or alive), and **abortions** (number of fetuses that did not reach the age of viability). This information should be charted, using Roman numerals. For example, a woman pregnant for the first time would be gravida I, para 0. A woman pregnant at the current visit, who delivered a single child during her first pregnancy, delivered twins on her second pregnancy, and had one miscarriage would be charted as follows: gravida IV, para III, abs I.

After obtaining the patient's past history, it is important to gather information pertaining to her present pregnancy history. The patient is asked the following questions:

- Do you have any preexisting conditions? Heart disease, kidney disease, and diabetes are especially important.

- Do you have any symptoms, such as morning sickness, fatigue, headaches, vaginal bleeding, discharge, or breast changes?

- Are you taking any prescriptions, over-the-counter medications, vitamins, or herbal supplements?

- Do you drink, smoke, or use recreational drugs? If so, what and how much?

- Are you employed, a student, married, divorced, or single?

More often than not, the information most important to the patient during her first prenatal visit is the expected date of delivery. A gestation calculator may be used to predict the estimated date of delivery (EDD). Another method to calculate EDD is to use Naegele's rule, applying the following formula:

LMP (last menstrual period) + 7 days − 3 months + 1 year = EDD

Example: LMP was June 10, 2009

Add 7 days (= 17)

Subtract 3 months from June (= March)

Add 1 year (= 2010)

Thus, the EDD is March 17, 2010.

Prenatal Patient Education

The initial prenatal visit affords an opportunity to provide the patient with information about what to expect during each stage of pregnancy, nutritional guidelines, vitamin and mineral requirements, and substances to be avoided. Pamphlets and brochures should be available in the reception room and examining room. At this visit the physician will order blood tests and other diagnostic procedures, such as an ultrasound, to be completed at a later date. Reinforce the importance of prenatal visits when scheduling procedures and follow-up visits for the patients.

Follow-Up Prenatal Visits

The patient will return for a follow-up visit every 4 weeks through the 28th week. Then she will return every 2 weeks up to the 36th week, and then every week until delivery. These return visits offer another opportunity for the medical assistant to educate the patient on the importance of maintaining her follow-up visit schedule. During these visits, you can reinforce proper nutritional guidelines and answer any questions the patient may have.

The Medical Assistant's Role in Follow-up Prenatal Visits. On each subsequent visit you will do the following:

- Set up the examining room

- Obtain a urine specimen from the patient

- Weigh the patient

- Obtain patient's blood pressure

- Ask the patient to describe any problems

- Chart all information

- Assist the patient onto the examining table

- Drape the patient appropriately

The physician will review the findings, ask the patient to recline so the fundal height can be measured, check for signs of edema, use a fetoscope to listen to the fetal heart rate, and answer any questions the patient may have.

At 10 to 12 weeks the fetal heart tone (FHT) is audible with the use of a Doppler fetal pulse detector. The normal FHT is 120 to 160 beats per minute (Figure 38-6). If fetal

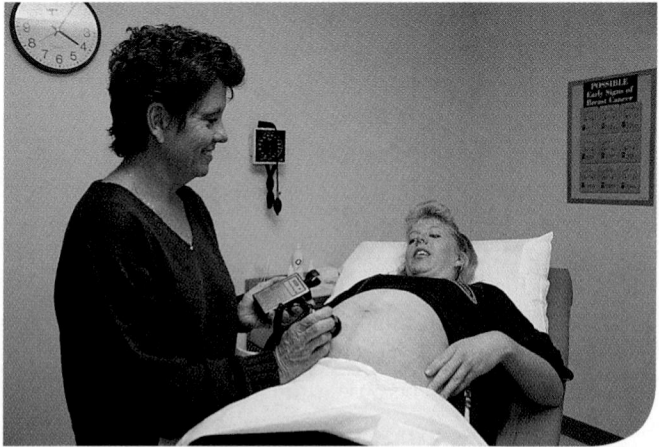

FIGURE 38-6 **Listening to the fetal heartbeat with a Doppler device.**

distress is indicated by extremely rapid or slow heart rate, fetal stress tests may be ordered to evaluate the condition of the fetus.

The physician will discuss delivery options with the patient. Closer to the date of delivery, the patient will attend classes on prepared childbirth, delivery, and breast-feeding. Classes are usually given at the facility chosen for delivery. Other procedures and diagnostic tests related to the female reproductive system are described in Table 38-1.

Screening Tests

Additional screening tests are performed during pregnancy to detect abnormalities and to be better prepared for a high-risk newborn. Some of these tests are offered to the mother, such as the following, and she may choose whether or not she wishes to have the test performed:

- Alpha-fetoprotein (AFP) test is a blood test taken between the 15th and 18th week of pregnancy to detect neural tube defects.

- Amniocentesis is performed between the 15th and 20th week of gestation. It involves using a fine nee-dle to take a sample of amniotic fluid from the sac

Table 38-1 Procedures and Diagnostic Tests Related to the Female Reproductive System

Procedure/Test	Description
Abortion	Termination of a pregnancy before the fetus reaches a viable point in development.
Amniocentesis	Puncturing the amniotic sac using a needle and syringe for the purpose of withdrawing amniotic fluid for testing. Can assist in determining fetal maturity, development, and genetic disorders.
Breast examination	Visual inspection and manual examination of the breasts for changes in contour, symmetry, dimpling of skin, retraction of the nipples, and the presence of lumps.
Cauterization	Destruction of tissue using an electric current, a caustic product, a hot iron, or freezing.
Cervical biopsy	Taking a sample of tissue from the cervix to test for the presence of cancer cells.
Cesarean section (C-section)	Surgical delivery of a baby through an incision into the abdominal and uterine walls.
Chorionic villus sampling (CVS)	Procedure that involves the insertion of a catheter into the cervix and into the outer portion of the membranes surrounding the fetus. A sample of the chorionic villi can be examined for chromosomal abnormalities and biochemical disorders. This procedure can be done 8 weeks into pregnancy.
Colposcopy	Visual examination of the cervix and vagina.
Conization	Surgical removal of a core of cervical tissue or a partial removal of the cervix.
Cryosurgery	Exposing tissue to extreme cold in order to destroy tissues. This procedure is used in treating malignant tumors, to control pain and bleeding.
Culdoscopy	Examination of the female pelvic cavity using an endoscope (or culdoscope).
Dilation and curettage (D&C)	Surgical procedure in which the opening of the cervix is dilated and the uterus is scraped or suctioned of its lining and tissue. A D&C is performed after spontaneous abortion and to stop excessive bleeding from other causes.

(continued)

TABLE 38-1 (continued)

Procedure/Test	Description
Doppler ultrasound	Using a Doppler instrument placed externally over the uterus to detect the presence of fibroid tumors and to outline the shape of the fetus.
Endometrial biopsy	Taking a sample of tissue from the lining of the uterus to test for abnormalities.
Episiotomy	Surgical incision of the perineum to facilitate the delivery process. Can prevent an irregular tearing of tissue during birth.
Estrogens	Urine or blood serum test to determine the level of estrone, estradiol, and estriol.
Fetal monitoring	Using electronic equipment placed on the mother's abdomen to monitor the fetus's heart and strength of uterine contractions during labor.
Human chorionic gonadotropin (HCG)	Urine or blood serum test to determine the presence of HCG. A positive result may indicate pregnancy.
Hymenectomy	Surgical removal of the hymen.
Hysterectomy	Surgical removal of the uterus.
Hysterosalpingography	Imaging with an X-ray after injecting radioopaque material into the uterus and oviducts.
Hysteroscopy	Inspection of the uterus using a special endoscopic instrument.
Intrauterine device (IUD)	Device inserted into the uterus by a physician for the purpose of contraception.
Kegel exercises	Exercises named after A. H. Kegel, an American gynecologist who developed them to strengthen female pelvic muscles. The exercises are useful in treating incontinence and as an aid in childbirth.
Laparoscopy	Examination of the peritoneal cavity with a laparoscope. The instrument is passed through a small incision made by the surgeon into the peritoneal cavity.
Laparotomy	Surgical incision through the abdominal wall to gain access into the abdominal cavity.
Mammography	X-ray imaging of the breast. This procedure is able to locate breast tumors before they grow to 1 cm. It is the most effective means of detecting early breast cancers.
Oophorectomy	Surgical removal of an ovary.
Panhysterectomy	Excision of the entire uterus, including the cervix.
Panhysterosalpingo-oophorectomy	Surgical removal of the entire uterus, cervix, ovaries, and fallopian tubes. Also called a total hysterectomy.
Pap (Papanicolaou) test	Test for the early detection of cancer of the cervix named after the developer of the test, George Papanicolaou. A scraping of cells is removed from the cervix for examination under the microscope.
Pelvic examination	Physical examination of the vagina and adjacent organs performed by a physician. A visual examination is performed using a speculum. A manual exam is performed by the doctor placing two gloved fingers of one hand in the vagina while the other hand presses gently on the abdomen.
Pelvimetry	Measurement of the pelvis to assist in determining if the birth canal will allow the passage of the fetus for a vaginal delivery.
Pelvic ultrasonography	Use of ultrasound waves to produce an image or photograph of an organ or the fetus.
Polypectomy	Surgical removal of a polyp.
Pregnancy test	Chemical test on urine that can determine pregnancy during the first weeks of pregnancy. This can be performed in the physician's office or with an at-home test. A blood serum test also can be performed at an outside laboratory.
Salpingo-oophorectomy	Surgical removal of the Fallopian tube and ovary.
Tubal ligation	Surgical tying off of the Fallopian tube to prevent conception from taking place. This results in the sterilization of the female.
Wet mount or wet prep	Examination of vaginal discharge for the presence of bacteria and yeast. A vaginal smear is placed on a microscope slide, wet with normal saline, and then viewed under a microscope by the physician.

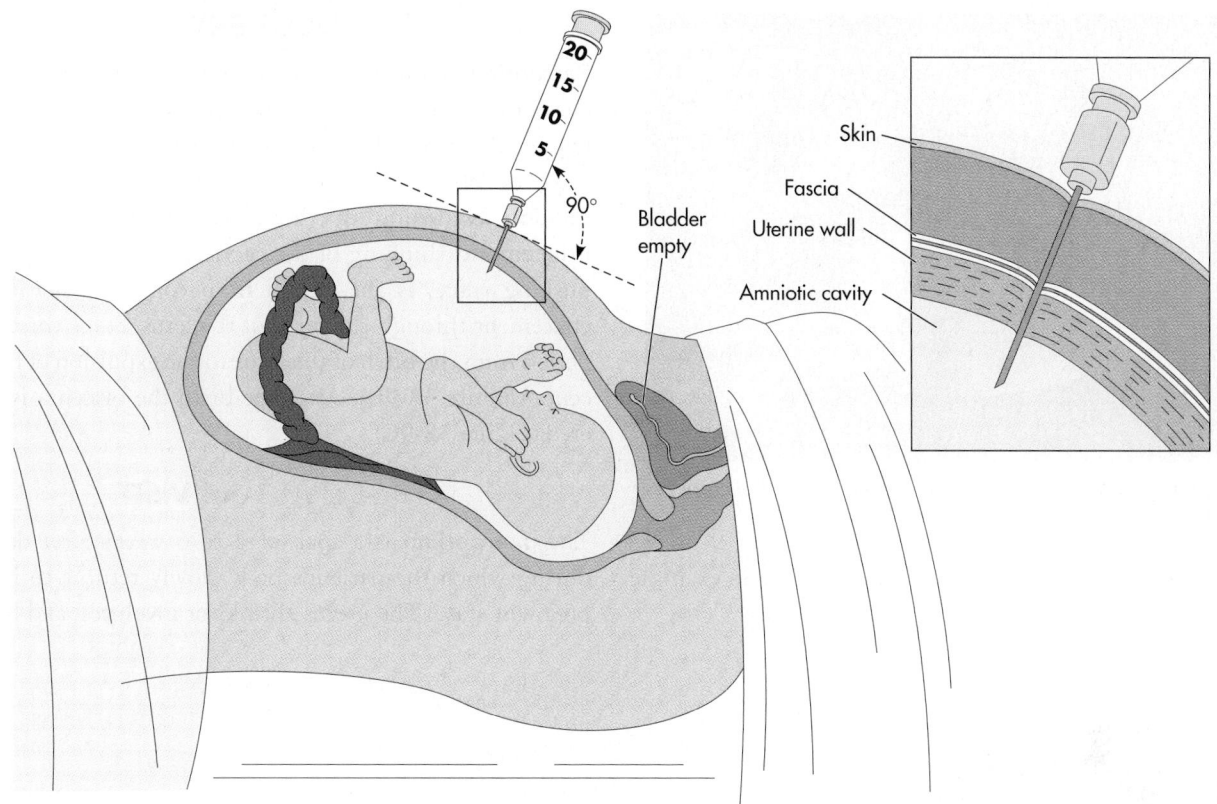

FIGURE 38-7 Amniocentesis. The patient is examined with ultrasound to determine the placental site and to locate the fluid. When the needle is in place within the amniotic cavity, amniotic fluid is withdrawn.

around the fetus (Figure 38-7). The fluid containing fetal cells will be cultured, grown in a laboratory, and screened to detect chromosomal defects such as Down syndrome. Amniocentesis is also used to assess fetal gender, maturity, and development. It is recommended that women over age 35 and women who have a family history of genetic defects have this test.

- **Chorionic villus sampling (CVS)** is a procedure in which a small sample of cells is taken from the placenta and examined for chromosomal abnormalities. It isperformed at 10 to 12 weeks of pregnancy. There is some risk to the fetus with this test.

- Genetic testing is recommended if there is a family history of certain diseases such as cystic fibrosis or hemophilia. However genetic disorders can occur in families with no history of genetic disorders.

- Glucose tolerance testing is performed to test for gestational diabetes. This blood test is performed between 24 and 28 weeks of pregnancy. After fasting, the patient is given a specific dose of glucose and blood is taken 1 hour later. An elevated test will

require an additional, more comprehensive 3-hour glucose tolerance test. Women who develop gestational diabetes are at higher risk of developing diabetes later in life.

A diet low in fat, moderate in carbohydrates, and high in fiber, and regular exercise are recommended. Insulin may be needed if diet and exercise are not sufficient to lower blood sugar.

- Group B *Streptococcus* is a common inhabitant of the urinary and reproductive tract and normally does not cause illness. A vaginal culture at 35 to 37 weeks is recommended. Between 1 and 2 percent of infants may be infected, and infection may be life threatening. A patient who tests positive will be treated with antibiotics during labor to prevent fetal infection.

- Nuchal translucency screening is a special ultrasound test of the fetus to screen for the risk of Down syndrome and other birth defects.

- Ultrasound is used to determine the age, growth rate, position of the fetus, and obvious birth defects. It is generally performed at 16 to 20 weeks and is generally painless. A vaginal ultrasound may be done to examine

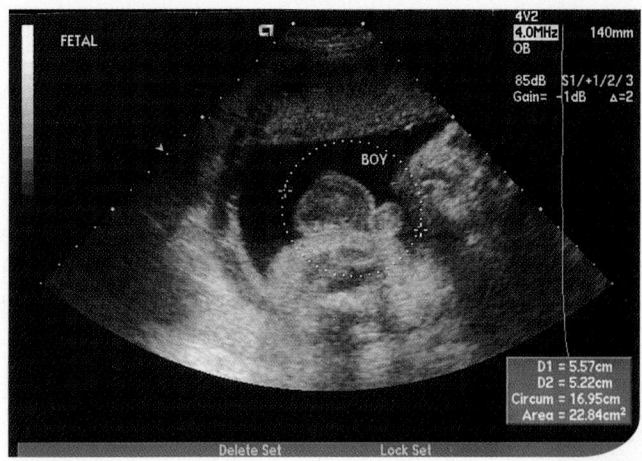

FIGURE 38-8 Ultrasonogram showing a male fetus. *Courtesy of Nancy West.*

the fetus more closely. See Figure 38-8 for an example of an ultrasonogram showing a male fetus.

DELIVERY

Parturition, or birth, occurs anytime from week 38 to 42 under normal circumstances. Labor involves three stages and is triggered by the release of the hormone **oxytocin**. The first stage of labor varies in length and ends with complete **dilation** (widening of the cervix) (Figure 38-9A) and **effacement** (thinning of the cervical walls). Stage two, the pushing stage, is the period from complete dilation and effacement through the birth of the fetus. Stage three is the period from the birth of the fetus to the expulsion of the placenta (Figure 38-9B). After the birth the placenta is delivered (Figure 38-9C).

POSTPARTUM VISIT

The **puerperium** is a span of 4 to 6 weeks after delivery, during which the patient's body slowly returns to its prepregnant state. The uterus shrinks or involutes, and healing

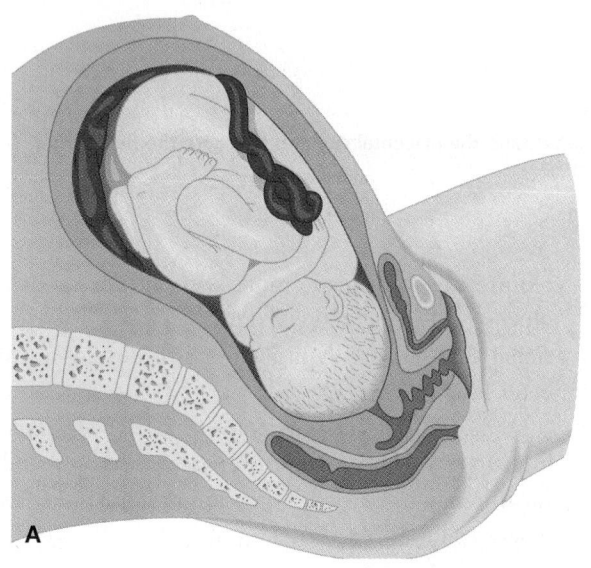

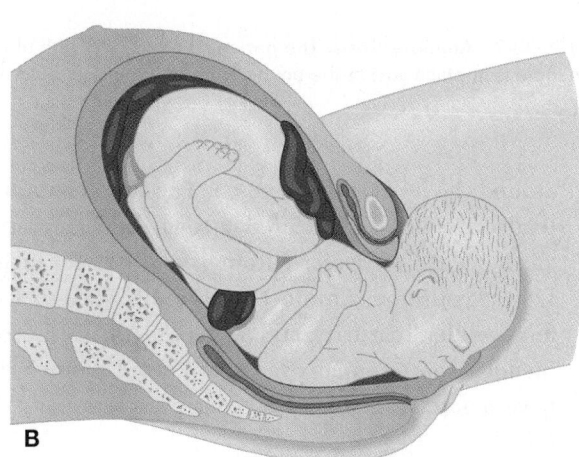

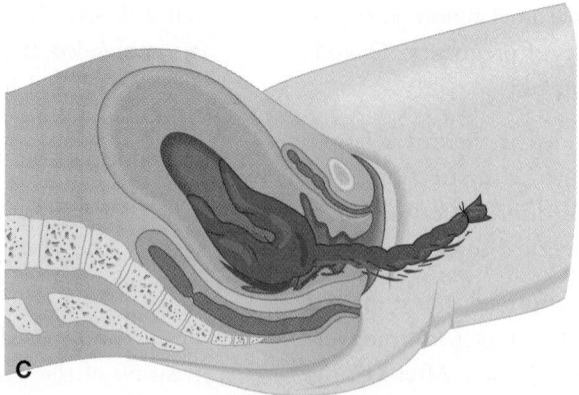

FIGURE 38-9 (A) Dilation stage: Uterine contractions cause dilation of the cervix; (B) Expulsion stage: Birth, or expulsion, of the baby; (C) Placental stage: Delivery of the placenta.

of the birth canal takes place. During this time, the patient experiences **lochia**, which is vaginal discharge from the uterus. This discharge consists of blood, tissue, mucus, and white blood cells. The color of lochia is an indication of healing in the uterus. Normally lochia is bright red until about the fourth day. The discharge then becomes brownish red by the tenth day; the discharge becomes yellow-white and disappears altogether after about 3 weeks. If at any time the discharge becomes bloody or foul smelling, the patient is instructed to call the physician because these may be symptoms of infection and bleeding. Menstruation should resume after about 8 weeks in the non-nursing mother and 6 months in the nursing mother.

During the puerperium, the patient should be encouraged to eat balanced meals, continue taking vitamins, and avoid fatigue and lifting heavy objects. A postpartum visit should be scheduled approximately 6 weeks after delivery. At this time, the overall health status of the patient is evaluated and information about contraceptive methods may be provided, if desired. This office visit includes measuring height, weight, and vital signs; performing pelvic and breast examinations and a rectal examination to detect hemorrhoids; and an anemia evaluation (hemoglobin and hematocrit).

COMPLICATIONS DURING PREGNANCY

Placenta previa is a complication in which the placenta develops in the lower portion of the uterus, blocking the opening in the cervix. During labor, the cervix is unable to dilate and efface completely. The result is oxygen deprivation for the fetus and maternal hemorrhage. Both can be life threatening, and an emergency Cesarean section (C-section) may be required. Ultrasound examination can detect the placental placement and a scheduled C-section may avoid an emergency situation. **Placenta abruptio** is a complication that occurs when the placenta tears away from the uterine wall, resulting in hemorrhage and fetal distress. Placenta abruptio occurs secondary to trauma, such as a fall, or because of vascular insufficiency resulting from hypertension or preeclampsia. This requires an emergency C-section.

Hypertension during pregnancy or gestational hypertension occurs in roughly 10 percent of pregnancies. If protein in the urine and edema occur as well, then preeclampsia exists. **Preeclampsia** develops in approximately 5 percent of pregnant women and usually occurs after the 20th week of pregnancy. Although the cause of preeclampsia is not definitively known, experts believe that blood vessel spasms in the placenta may elevate blood pressure. The blood flow to the placenta can be compromised, and if left untreated, the placenta can be damaged and the fetus will die. The high blood pressure can also affect the brain, kidneys, liver, and lungs. The symptoms of preeclampsia include agitation and confusion, changes in mental status, decreased urine output, headaches, nausea and vomiting, pain in the upper right quadrant, shortness of breath, sudden weight gain, swelling of the face or hands, and visual impairment. If seizures develop, then the condition is known as **eclampsia**.

There are no known ways to prevent preeclampsia. All pregnant women should have good prenatal care and should monitor their blood pressure closely.

CONTRACEPTION METHODS

Since the average woman in the United States is fertile for about half her life, it is fairly safe to assume that birth control will be discussed at some point in time. It is important for the medical assistant to have an understanding of the various methods of birth control and the effectiveness of each. The patient chooses the most suitable method, based on physical condition, cost, side effects, and effectiveness.

Contraceptive methods include barrier methods, hormonal methods, intrauterine devices (IUDs), natural family planning, and coitus interruptus or withdrawal of the penis during intercourse. A newer contraceptive method is the emergency contraception pill, commonly referred to as "the morning after" pill.

Barrier Methods

Barrier contraceptive methods include the use of male condoms, female condoms, diaphragms, shields, spermicides, sponges, and cervical caps. For extra protection all of these methods should be used with a spermicide.

- *Spermicides* substances that inactivate or kill sperm on contact. They are available in foam, gel, cream, tablet and suppository forms. They can be used alone (71 percent effectiveness rate) but are more effective when used with condoms or diaphragms or cervical caps.

- The *male condom* is worn over the penis during intercourse and prevents the sperm from entering the vagina. It is inexpensive, easy to use, and available without prescription. Condoms provide a measure of protection from sexually transmitted infections (STIs); however they are not foolproof. Condoms have an effectiveness rate of about 85 percent.

- The *female condom* is a polyurethane sheath that lines the vagina with an inner ring that fits over the cervix and an outer ring that permits entrance of the penis. The sheath is removed after ejaculation. It has an effectiveness rate of about 79 percent.

- The *cervical cap* is a small, reusable, flexible device that fits over the cervix and prevents the entry of sperm. It is obtained by prescription and requires a physician to determine the size needed. It is held in place by the cervix. It must be in place 30 minutes before intercourse and remain in place for 6 to 8 hours afterward. It has an effectiveness of about 71 percent.

- The *diaphragm* is a flexible dome of rubber that fits over the cervix and prevents the entry of sperm. An examination and physician's prescription are needed. It can be inserted 6 hours before intercourse and must be left in place 6 hours afterward. It is effective about 84 percent of the time when used correctly.

- The *shield* is a reusable one-size-fits-all, cup-shaped device that fits over the cervix and is held in place by suction and the vaginal wall. It must be left in place for a minimum of 8 hours after intercourse and is effective about 85 percent of the time when used correctly.

- The *contraceptive sponge* is a piece of polyurethane foam impregnated with spermicide that blocks the cervical opening. It can be inserted up to 24 hours before intercourse and must remain in place 6 hours afterward. The failure rate is high because of the tendency of the sponge to be displaced during intercourse.

Hormonal Methods

Hormonal methods of birth control are based on using hormones to change the levels of female hormones in the body to prevent ovulation or implantation of the fertilized ovum. They include birth control pills, hormone patches, the vaginal ring, hormonal implants, hormone injections, the minipill, and the morning-after pill and must be prescribed by a physician. These methods are easy to use and very effective:

- *Birth control pills* ("the pill"), the most widely used method, contain either a combination of estrogen and progestin or only small amounts of progestin. They are contraindicated—their use is not advised—in women who smoke, are over age 35, or have had a history of blood clots, high blood pressure, breast cancer, liver disease, or advanced diabetes. The pill has a 92 percent effectiveness rate. It does not protect against STIs. Side effects are similar to those for the patch.

- The *emergency or morning-after pill* consists of a series of pills containing estrogen and progestin that inhibit the possibility of implantation of a fetus and may be used in cases of rape and sexual abuse.

- *Implanon* is an implantable, matchstick-size contraceptive device that was approved in 2006 by the FDA. It may be left in place for up to 3 years or removed at any time. It is said to be 99 percent effective. Implants may stop menstruation, cause irregular bleeding, breast soreness and acne.

- *Injection* (Depo-Provera) is highly effective (97 percent). One injection is given every 3 months within the first 5 days of the menstrual cycle. Weight gain, irregular bleeding, and delayed return of menstrual cycle after stopping use are common side effects.

- The *progestin-only pill,* ("the minipill") is taken daily and is permissible for nursing mothers to take. Effectiveness is 92 percent, as are other hormonal methods; however, it may cause breakthrough bleeding.

- The *skin patch* is an adhesive square that slowly releases estrogen and progestin through the skin to the bloodstream. It is 98 percent effective. Side effects include headache, nausea, bloating, depression, and decreased sex drive.

- The *vaginal ring* is inserted into the vagina and impregnated with estrogen and progestin. It is used for the first 3 weeks of the menstrual cycle and removed for the 4th week for menstruation. It is 92 percent effective and has side effects similar to other hormonal methods.

Intrauterine Devices

An **intrauterine device (IUD)** is a small device with progestin that is placed in the uterus by the physician. IUDs are very effective, up to 99 percent. However, in some cases they may cause pain, bleeding, and infection. See Figure 38-10 for examples of IUDs.

Natural Family Planning

Natural family planning, also known as the rhythm method or most recently known as fertility awareness-

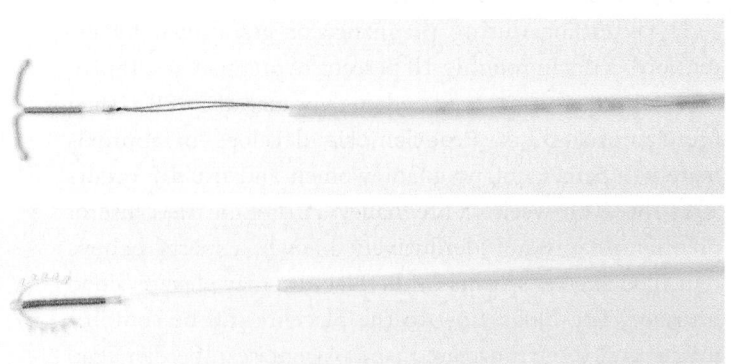

FIGURE 38-10 **Examples of intrauterine devices.**

based birth control, is based on avoiding intercourse around the time of ovulation. It relies on the woman having a relatively normal menstrual cycle and ovulating predictably. Other fertility awareness-based practices include measurement of basal body temperature, keeping an accurate menstruation calendar, and being aware of the viscosity of cervical mucus. The effectiveness of this method varies from 80 to 98 percent, depending on the thoroughness of diligence of the couple.

Coitus Interruptus

Coitus interruptus is the withdrawal of the male's penis before ejaculation in the vagina. It is unreliable because sperm may be released even before a male ejaculates.

Sterilization

Women are fertile for about 40 years of their adult lives, whereas healthy men are fertile throughout their adult lives. Since the 1960s sterilization has become more common as a permanent method of birth control. Several methods are available for women, including Essure coils and tubal ligation. (The sterilization method for a male requires vasectomy, which is discussed in the Male Reproductive System section of this chapter.)

- *Essure* is a permanent method of birth control in which tiny metal coils are placed in the fallopian tubes of a woman. Scar tissue forms in time over these coils and blocks the tubes, thus preventing sperm from reaching the ovum. It does not require surgical incision as does tubal ligation. This method is 99 percent effective. Side effects and risks are few. The coils are inserted by a physician.

- *Tubal ligation* is a permanent method of birth control effective 99 percent of the time. A small incision is made near the navel and a laparoscope is inserted. Instruments are inserted through the laparoscope to seal the tubes by cauterizing or closing them with clips or rings.

Male Reproductive System

The male reproductive system is a combination of the reproduction and urinary systems. The major male organs of reproduction are located outside the body in the scrotum and penis. The scrotum (scrotal sac) contains two testes and the seminal ducts. The penis contains the urethra, which carries both urine and sperm to the outside of the body. The internal organs of reproduction are the seminal vesicles, ejaculatory duct, and prostate gland. To review these systems, see Chapter 33.

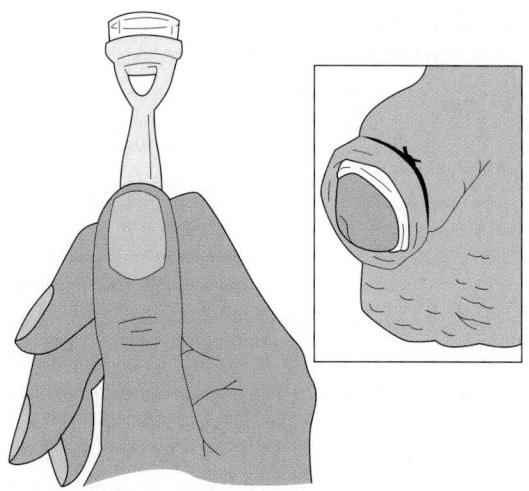

FIGURE 38-11 Circumcision using the Plastibell. The bell is fitted over the glans penis and a suture is tied around the bell's rim. The excess prepuce (foreskin) is cut away. The device is left in place for 3 to 4 days until healing occurs. It may be allowed to fall off or is removed after 8 days.

CIRCUMCISION

Circumcision is the removal of the foreskin of the penis. In the United States it was customary for most newborn male babies to have this procedure performed in the hospital shortly after birth. The American Academy of Family Physicians and the American Academy of Pediatrics do not recommend routine circumcision at this time. Studies about the benefits of circumcision are conflicting. It is believed to promote cleanliness and reduce the possibility of contracting genital warts and other infections. More recently, only about 50 percent of newborn males are having the procedure performed. See Figure 38-11 for an example of circumcision using the Plastibell device.

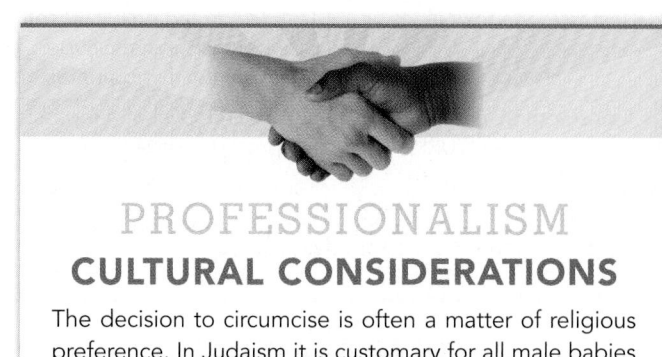

PROFESSIONALISM
CULTURAL CONSIDERATIONS

The decision to circumcise is often a matter of religious preference. In Judaism it is customary for all male babies to be circumcised when they are 8 days old. Regardless of your religious or personal beliefs associated with circumcision, you must never impose judgment or inject your opinion regarding a parent's right to have their child circumcised.

TABLE 38-2 Procedures and Diagnostic Tests Related to the Male Reproductive System

Procedure/Test	Description
Castration	Excision of the testicles in the male or the ovaries in the female.
Cauterization	Destruction of tissue with an electric current, caustic agent, hot iron, or freezing.
Circumcision	Surgical removal of the end of the prepuce (foreskin) of the penis. Generally performed on the newborn male at the request of the parents. The primary reason is ease of hygiene. Circumcision is also a ritual practiced in some religions.
Digital rectal examination	Manual examination for an enlarged prostate gland performed by palpating the prostate gland through the rectum wall.
Epididymectomy	Surgical excision of the epididymis.
Erickson sperm separation method	Process of separating the Y-chromosome sperm from the X-chromosome sperm. A sperm sample is taken and placed in a tube of albumin. Those sperm that survive are Y-chromosome sperm, which produce male infants. Females inseminated with these sperm have a 75 to 80 percent chance of producing a male child.
Fluorescent treponemal antibody absorption	Test performed on blood serum to determine the presence of *Treponema pallidum*, the microorganism that causes syphilis.
Orchidopexy	Surgical fixation to move undescended testes into the scrotum and attaching them to prevent retraction.
Orchiectomy	Surgical removal of the testes.
Paternity test	Test to determine whether a certain male could be the father of a specific child. The test can indicate only who is not the father. Types of tests that may be used are blood type, human leukocyte antigen (HLA), white blood cell, enzyme, protein, and genetic. The blood type of the child and the alleged father are analyzed for compatibility. For example, a parent with type O blood cannot be the parent of a child with type AB blood. HLA looks at the body's tissue compatibility system, and the white blood cell test looks at chemical markers (antigens) on the surface of the white blood cells. Enzyme and protein tests look at red blood cell enzymes. A new genetic test is being developed that uses molecular and protein biology to look at family-related genetic patterns.
Prostatectomy	Surgical removal of the prostate gland.
Prostate-specific antigen (PSA)	Blood test to screen for prostate cancer. Elevated blood levels of PSA are associated with prostate cancer.
Semen analysis	Procedure used when performing a fertility workup to determine if the male is able to produce sperm. Sperm is collected by the patient after he has abstained from sexual intercourse for a period of 3 to 5 days. Also used to determine if a vasectomy has been successful. After a period of 6 weeks, no further sperm should be present in a sample from the patient.
Sterilization	Process of rendering a male or female sterile, or unable to conceive children.
Testosterone toxicology	Test performed on blood serum to identify the level of testosterone. Increased level may indicate benign prostatic hyperplasia. Decreased level may indicate hypogonadism, testicular hypofunction, hypopituitarism, or orchidectomy.
Transurethral resection of the prostate (TURP)	Surgical removal of the prostate gland by inserting a device through the urethra and removing prostate tissue.
Vasectomy	Removal of a segment or all of the vas deferens to prevent sperm from leaving the male body.
Venereal disease research laboratory (VDRL)	Test performed on blood serum to determine the presence of *Treponema pallidum*. Used to detect syphilis.

TESTICULAR EXAMINATION

Procedures and diagnostic tests related to the male reproductive system are described in Table 38-2. Procedure 38-3 and Figure 38-12 provide an explanation of testicular self-examination for the male patient.

VASECTOMY

Vasectomy is a widely performed surgery to render the male sterile (Figure 38-13). It involves cutting the vas deferens and tying off the ends to prevent sperm from being transported out of the testes. This is a brief procedure

INSTRUCTING A MALE PATIENT HOW TO PERFORM A TESTICULAR SELF-EXAMINATION

Objective: Instruct a male patient how to correctly perform a testicular self-examination.

EQUIPMENT AND SUPPLIES

instruction sheet; testicular examination model or illustration

METHOD

1. Identify the patient and introduce yourself.
2. Explain to the patient that he should perform the examination in the shower or right after a warm shower, which causes the scrotal tissue to relax.
3. Using the testicular model or illustration, explain that he should place his middle and index fingers underneath the scrotum and thumb on top and use a gentle motion to roll the testes between the fingers.

   Indicate on the model or illustration the location of the epididymis, a soft tubular cord behind the testis, which stores and carries sperm. The patient should know what the epididymis feels like so he does not confuse it with a lump (Figure 38-12A–D).
4. The entire procedure should be repeated on the second testicle.
5. Encourage the patient to immediately report to his physician any lumps or thickening found during an examination. Early testicular cancer cases have a high cure rate.
6. Document the instruction in the patient's record.

CHARTING EXAMPLE

09/11/XX 3:30 P.M. Pt. given verbal and written instruction on testicular self-examination. Pt. verbalized understanding · · · · · · · · · · · · · · · ·
· J. Holloran, RMA

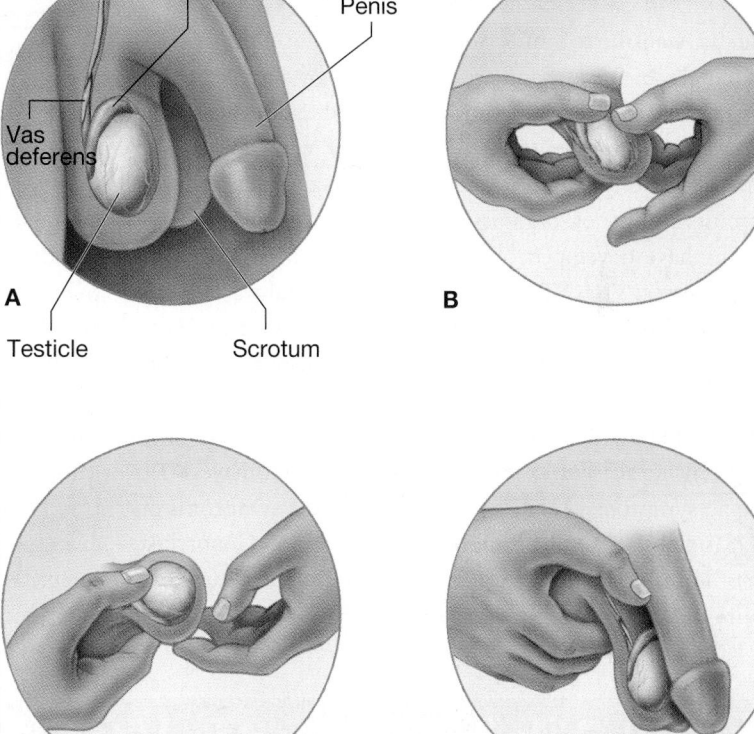

FIGURE 38-12 **Testicular self-examination: (A) male reproductive system; (B) begin by examining the testicles; (C) next examine the cord behind the testicles (epididymis); (D) continue by gently feeling the tube that runs from the epididymis (vas deferens).**

performed in the urologist's office with little or no discomfort associated with it. The patient can return home immediately after the procedure and resume work and regular activities the next day. After a vasectomy the man still achieves an orgasm and ejaculates minus the sperm.

Birth control methods should be used for 6 to 8 weeks afterward or until a postvasectomy sample confirms the absence of sperm. In some cases it is reversible, but vasectomy should be considered a permanent form of birth control.

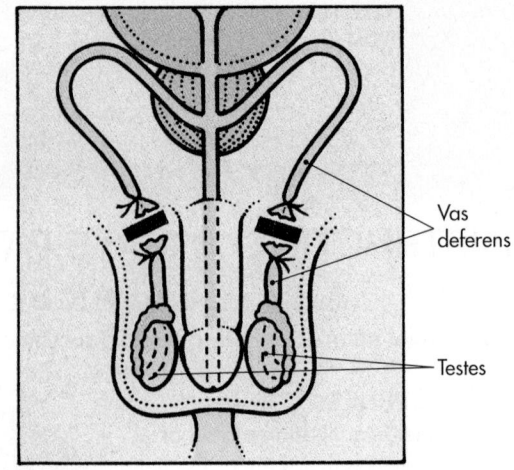

FIGURE 38-13 Illustration of a vasectomy.

Sexually Transmitted Infections

Sexually transmitted infections (STIs) can occur in males and females of any age and are transmitted by sexual contact from person to person or mother to child. STIs caused by bacteria are generally treated successfully with antibiotics such as penicillin and tetracycline. Recently, antibiotic-resistant strains of organisms that cause gonorrhea and syphilis have developed, making it more difficult to treat these diseases. Viral STIs, such as herpes, genital warts, hepatitis, and HIV, are incurable at this time. Some treatments that reduce the symptoms of these conditions do exist, however.

Individuals infected with an STI may not have any symptoms at all. For example, most people who have HIV have no symptoms. HIV may not produce the symptoms of AIDS until 10 years or more after infection. Gonorrhea symptoms do not appear in females until 2 months after exposure. Genital warts may not appear until 5 months after

exposure. Symptoms of the presence of STIs include sores, discharge, itching, and pain in both males and females. Women may develop pelvic inflammatory disease (PID), which causes abdominal pain, fever, malaise, and severe pain on manipulation of the cervix. In the male, additional symptoms, such as profuse discharge from the penis, swelling and pain in the testicles, and painful urination, may occur. Males frequently will seek help at this point because of the difficulty with urination. See Box 38-2 for information on infertility due to chlamydia infection and treatment of infertility with in vitro fertilization. Certain examinations and some laboratory procedures can identify infective organisms and symptoms. For many STIs, however, no diagnostic tests are completely accurate. Patients

Box 38-2 Infertility and In Vitro FERTILIZATION

In vitro fertilization (IVF) is one method of treating infertility in those who are unable or have a diminished capacity to conceive. There are many causes of infertility, and selecting the correct treatment depends on determining whether the cause is functional or a result of infection.

Repeated infections of sexually transmitted diseases, such as chlamydia, are often symptomless yet may cause scarring and occlusion (blockage) of the Fallopian tube. When this happens the ovum released during ovulation is unable to make its way to the uterus through the Fallopian tube. Normally conception occurs in the upper one-third of the Fallopian tube, and the zygote (fertilized ovum) then moves down the tube to implant into the uterus. If the Fallopian tube is blocked or scarred, conception and implantation cannot take place. Many women are unaware that they have ever had a chlamydia infec-

tion, and when they decide it is time to conceive, they find it is impossible.

IVF is fertilization outside the body, usually in a Petri dish in the laboratory. A woman who wishes to conceive may be given follicle-stimulating hormone (FSH) to stimulate the release of more than one ovum. The ova are then removed through laparoscopic surgery and put into the Petri dish. Sperm, from either the husband or a sperm donor, is added to the Petri dish. After fertilization and cleavage (cell division of the zygote) have taken place, the zygote is then placed in the woman's uterus. Since the birth of the "first test tube baby" in 1978, thousands of babies have been born through in vitro fertilization. It is not always successful, however, and it may be necessary to have this procedure repeated several times before being successful. Each attempt is very costly.

may have the disease but test negative until later in the cycle of the disease, as with HIV.

SEXUALLY TRANSMITTED INFECTIONS EDUCATION

Treating and preventing the spread of STIs begins with proper education, as well as identifying sexual partners who may have been exposed. The only foolproof means of preventing STIs is complete abstinence from sexual activity. Agreeing to a monogamous relationship goes a long way in reducing the chance of being infected. If individuals are going to be sexually active, there are strategies that will reduce the chance of exposure to STIs:

- Use a barrier device (condom) and spermicide during every act of sexual intercourse.

- Limit the number of sexual partners.

- Know your sexual partners well, as well as their history of sexual partners.

- Seek prompt treatment of any suspected STI.

- Complete all cycles of medication, and comply with follow-up testing.

- Cooperate in tracing sexual contacts.

Educating patients about STIs, their causes, symptoms, and treatments is very important. Often the medical assistant is the individual with whom the patient feels most comfortable discussing potentially embarrassing problems. You must feel comfortable yourself with the facts about STIs and be able to discuss these issues in an unemotional, nonjudgmental manner. Brochures and pamphlets should be readily available and easily accessed in your office. Patients may feel more comfortable picking up reading material they can review in the privacy of their own home rather than asking questions in the office.

REPORTING STIs

In your role as a medical assistant, you should understand the different types of STIs, recognize their symptoms, and comprehend your role in the legal ramifications of reporting patients with STIs to the proper state and national agencies. For example, in all fifty states, confirmed cases of HIV/AIDS are reportable conditions either by statute or administrative act. Other STIs, such as gonorrhea and syphilis, are reportable diseases in most states. Legally you need to be aware of your responsibility wherever you are employed. Confidentiality is extremely important when dealing with sensitive information such as testing positive for an STI. Many states require a post-treatment follow-up for certain diseases; therefore, your role in patient compliance is vital. Identifying partners of infected patients is one way to stop the spread of STIs and protect the health of unsuspecting persons. Office policy should spell out clearly your role in these sensitive matters.

TYPES OF SEXUALLY TRANSMITTED INFECTIONS

- **Bacterial vaginosis**—Bacterial vaginosis (BV) has no known cause and is the most common vaginal infection in women of childbearing age. Certain behaviors increase the risk of infection, such as multiple partners and douching. When BV occurs it is because the normal balance of "good" and "bad" bacteria has been disrupted. Symptoms include thin gray or white discharge with unpleasant fishy odor. Having BV increases susceptibility to other STIs. Treatment is important for pregnant women especially and includes metronidazole or clindamycin. In pregnant patients, BV may cause premature birth or low birth weight in their offspring.

- **Chlamydia Infection**—Chlamydia infection is caused by the bacterium *Chlamydia trachomatis*. It is the most frequently reported bacterial infection in the United States. The CDC reports that in 2006 more than a million cases were reported from fifty states. Underreporting is a problem because many individuals are asymptomatic. Chlamydia infection in males is characterized by urethritis and epididymitis, whereas in females there may be no initial symptoms. Because of the lack symptoms and delay in seeking treatment, chlamydia may lead to pelvic inflammatory disease (PID). Infected females have an increased risk of ectopic pregnancy and sterility. Infants born to infected mothers may develop conjunctivitis or pneumonia. Chlamydia infections can be successfully treated with azithromycin or doxycycline. The CDC recommends yearly testing for chlamydia for all sexually active women 25 years or younger, all pregnant women, and any older women who are at risk from having multiple partners.

- **Genital Herpes**—Painful lesions erupting within 2 weeks in the genital area is a primary symptom of genital herpes in both males and females. This disease is caused by herpes simplex viruses type 1 (HSV-1) and type 2 (HSV-2). HSV-1 herpes is associated with cold sore lesions, and HSV-2 causes most cases of genital herpes. HSV-1 infection of the genitals can be caused by oral genital contact with an individual with "cold sores." The CDC reports that about

45 million people in the United States have had genital herpes or 1 in 5 adolescents and adults. No cure is known for herpes at present. Antivirals may lessen the duration of symptoms. The lesions are usually self-limiting but reoccur during stressful situations. Recently new treatments have reduced the severity of the reoccurrences. Abstinence and careful use of condoms help to reduce chance of contracting genital herpes.

- **Genital Human Papillomavirus Infection**—Human papillomavirus (HPV) infection refers to a group of viruses that cause this common STI. Genital warts, or condylomas, are found in clusters on the external sexual organs of both males and females, internally in the female in the vagina and cervix, and in the anus and rectum of the male. Though the patient may not have visible signs of warts, HPV can be discovered in the female by a Pap test. It may take several months to several years after contact for the person to show signs of infection. Genital warts increase a female's risk of developing cervical cancer. There is no vaccine to prevent HPV-related diseases in men at this time.

- **Gonorrhea**—Gonorrhea is an STI caused by the organism *Neisseria gonorrhoeae,* a bacterium that grows well in warm, moist conditions. It can grow in the vagina, fallopian tubes, and uterus in the female and in the urethra, mouth, anus and eyes of both males and females. The rate of infection is high in the United States and is increasing after declining or remaining stable until 2006. It is estimated by the CDC that the rate of infection is about 120 infections per 100,000 people. It is estimated that only about half of the gonorrheal infections are reported to state departments of health.

In the male, gonorrhea is characterized by penile drainage, clear at first, becoming thick and milky, burning, itchy, and painful on urination. Females are often asymptomatic, and then they develop a yellowish-green discharge. Gonorrhea may possibly lead to PID. Other symptoms that may be experienced by both sexes include sore throat, swollen glands, anal discharge, and fever. Treatment includes large doses of penicillin or tetracycline with follow-up examinations because antibiotic-resistant strains of the organisms complicate treatment.

Untreated, gonorrhea can cause infertility in both males and females and can spread to the blood or joints. It is known to cause blindness, as well as joint or blood infection in an infant born to an infected mother.

Tests for gonorrhea can be diagnosed by smear and Gram stain. Many people who have gonorrhea also have chlamydia and must be treated for both. Condoms, abstinence, and long-term monogamous relationships reduce the chance of infection.

- **Human immunodeficiency virus**—Human immunodeficiency virus (HIV) causes acquired immunodeficiency syndrome or AIDS, the final stage of HIV infection. As mentioned it can take years to reach the AIDS stage. At this point the immune system—specifically the infection-fighting white blood cells known as T-cells or CD4 cells—is reduced, and opportunistic infections can ravage the body and cause death. Presently the CDC estimates that about 56,300 people were infected with HIV in 2006. About three-fourths of those cases were in males. The CDC reports further that about one million individuals are living with HIV/AIDS and one-fourth of them do not know they are infected.

Misconceptions are many about how HIV is or is not transmitted. It is a very delicate virus that does not survive outside the body. It is not spread by any type of casual contact or day-to-day activities such as shaking hands, kissing, or sitting on toilet seats. Nor is it transmitted by mosquitoes. HIV is spread by having oral, vaginal, or anal sex with someone infected with HIV; sharing needles or syringes with someone infected with HIV; and being exposed as a fetus or infant to HIV before or during birth or breast-feeding. It also can be spread through blood infected with the virus. All donated blood supplies since 1985 have been tested for HIV so there is little risk today from transfused blood supplies.

Preventing transmission depends on responsible sex, knowing your sexual partners, avoiding illegal drug use, using condoms with lubricant every time you have sex, getting tested, and having your partner (partners) tested. Many tests and testing places are available through local physicians, clinics, and state health departments.

- **Lymphogranuloma venereum (LGV)**—Lymphogranuloma venereum is an STI caused by three stains of the *Chlamydia trachomatis* bacterium. Although it is less common than other types of STIs, it is difficult to diagnose because the symptoms are similar to other conditions. LGV may cause papules on the genitals, swollen lymph glands, rectal ulcers, pain, bleeding, and discharge. It can be mistaken for ulcerative STIs such as syphilis and genital herpes. Untreated, LGV may cause lymphatic obstruction and elephantiasis (massive swelling of the scrotum).

Commercially available tests have limitations; therefore, diagnosis is mainly based on clinical findings. Treatment includes use of doxycycline, erythromycin, or azithromycin.

- **Pelvic inflammatory disease**—**Pelvic inflammatory disease (PID)** is the term used to describe inflammation of the vagina, cervix, uterus, and fallopian tubes. It may be caused by a number of STIs if they are left untreated. Untreated scar tissue may develop in the fallopian tubes, which then blocks the movement of the ovum in the tubes. If the tubes are completely blocked, sperm cannot reach the ovum to cause fertilization; if partially blocked, a fertilized ovum may begin to grow in the fallopian tube rather than in the uterus. This is known as an **ectopic pregnancy**. An ectopic pregnancy can rupture the fallopian tube, causing severe pain or even death.

PID is diagnosed by clinical symptoms and ultrasound of the abdomen. Because PID symptoms are similar to those of other abdominal conditions, such as appendicitis, diverticulitis, ectopic pregnancy, and ulcerative colitis, a thorough history and diagnostic tests are necessary. PID can result in blood clots, peritonitis and even death if untreated. Antibiotics can cure PID; however, treatment does not correct any damage already done to the reproductive organs. It is estimated by the CDC that more than a million women per year have an episode of PID. Prevention is the same as for other types of STIs.

- **Syphilis**—Syphilis is an STI caused by the bacterium *Treponema pallidum.* Its signs and symptoms are similar to other diseases, thus mimicking other conditions. About 36,000 cases of primary and secondary syphilis were reported in the United States in 2006, an almost 12 percent increase from the previous year. That same year, 64 percent of the cases reported were among men who had sex with men, according to U.S. health officials.

As with other STIs, syphilis is spread by direct person-to-person contact with a syphilitic **chancre**, or sore (Figure 38-14). Sores may occur on the genitals, anus, rectum, mouth, and lips. Syphilis also may be transmitted to a newborn by an infected mother, resulting in stillbirth or developmental delays or death after birth.

Signs and symptoms of syphilis may not appear for years in an infected person. A primary chancre occurs in about 3 weeks or up to 3 months after exposure. It may heal without treatment; however, the disease still progresses unless treated. Second-stage signs are skin rash on palms of hands and soles of feet and elsewhere on the body along with fever, swollen glands, weight loss, and fatigue. The signs and symptoms of the secondary stage may disappear without treatment also. The latent stages occur 10 to 20 years after the first two stages have disappeared, and an untreated person still has syphilis at that time. The disease will damage brain, heart, liver, and other internal organs, and it can cause paralysis, dementia, blindness, and death.

Syphilis is diagnosed by dark-field microscopic examination of chancre material or by blood tests for the presence of syphilis antibodies (RPR, VDRL). Treatment of syphilis is fairly simple. In the primary stage, a single large dose of penicillin may cure the patient. Additional penicillin doses may be necessary for those who have had syphilis longer than a year. Having syphilis puts an individual at greater risk of contracting HIV sexually. Responsible sexual behavior and proper hygiene after sexual contact lessens the chances of contracting syphilis. Some cases of penicillin-resistant syphilis have been reported.

- **Trichomoniasis**—Trichomoniasis is a protozoal infection caused by the organism *Trichomonas vaginalis,* resulting in an infection of the lower genitourinary tract. Trichomoniasis causes a white or yellow, foamy vaginal discharge with a foul odor in females. The male is usually asymptomatic, except for urethral itching. Diagnosis can be made by obtaining a sample of vaginal secretions and preparing a slide with normal saline. Microscopic examination will reveal the oval *Trichomonas* parasite with four hair-like flagella whipping across the field. Treatment for both males and females is a course of the antibiotic metronidazole or tinidazole taken orally.

Urinary System

The function of the urinary system is to filter and remove metabolic waste products from the blood, help maintain electrolyte and pH balance, excrete waste from the body in the form of urine, and help regulate red blood cell production and blood pressure. In your role as a medical assistant, it is important for you to comprehend the functions and

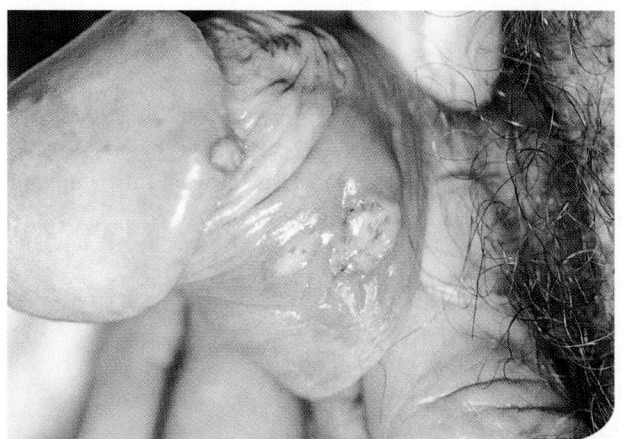

FIGURE 38-14 Syphilitic chancre. *Courtesy of Jason L. Smith, MD.*

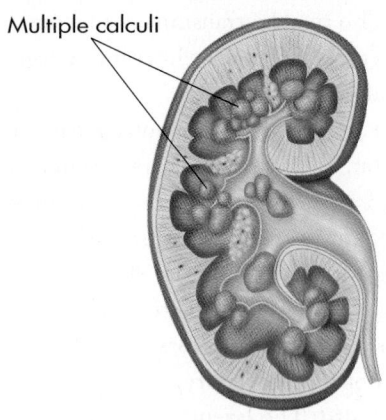

Multiple calculi

FIGURE 38-15 Multiple urinary calculi.

importance of the urinary system in the overall health of the patient. Symptoms of urinary tract disorders vary, as do the age-related problems of this intricate system. For example, increased urine production is seen in diabetes; frequency of urination is seen in urinary tract infection; severe pain is seen in episodes of kidney stone movement; swelling and weight gain are seen in congestive heart failure (CHF) and renal dysfunction; and decreased urinary output is seen in urinary obstructions. See Figure 38-15 for a drawing of renal calculi.

Most people urinate four to six times per day and excrete about 2,000 cc or 2 quarts of urine per day. The maximum volume of urine the bladder can hold declines with aging, leading to increased frequency of urination and, in some individuals, incontinence.

Urine specimens are an easily obtainable, noninvasive way to evaluate the homeostatic condition of the body and are among the most frequently ordered tests in the medical office. Collecting, processing, and testing urine specimens will be one of your duties. (This is further discussed in Chapter 46.) After the patient is greeted and escorted to the examining room, a urine sample may be requested. Give the patient an appropriately labeled container and clear directions on the type of sample required. Urine samples are potentially infectious, and gloves should be worn when handling patient samples. After the sample is obtained, it is tested or stored for later processing. Be sure to follow the processing guidelines to maintain the integrity of the specimen and ensure valid results.

The medical assistant must be sensitive to the abilities of the variety of patients, some with special needs. Offer assistance as needed and provide for patient privacy.

Procedures and diagnostic tests related to the urinary system are described in Table 38-3.

PROSTATE CONDITIONS

Benign prostatic hyperplasia (BPH) is an enlargement of the prostate gland that may occur after age fifty (Figure 38-16). As the prostate enlarges it presses on the urethra and causes restriction of the flow of urine. Restricted urinary flow can result in urinary retention, interruption of the urine stream, and difficulty starting to urinate. Medications are available that may relieve the symptoms in some men. Nonsurgical treatments may also be successful.

Prostate cancer is a slow-growing malignant tumor of the prostate gland affecting one in four men in the United States. Prostate cancer may spread to the adjacent urinary tract and male reproductive organs, as well as to the lymph nodes and bones. It is the second most common form of cancer in men. Because of its slow rate of growth, prostate cancer can be detected and treated in its early stages with regular medical examinations. The cause of prostate cancer is not known, but age, heredity, and a high-fat diet increase the risk of developing it. Symptoms include weak stream of urine, blood in the urine, erectile dysfunction, **nocturia** (frequency of urination at night), and pelvic pain. The protein-specific antigen (PSA) blood test and a digital rectal examination are used to screen for prostate cancer. The PSA test checks for a protein released by the prostate. If levels are elevated, then a biopsy of prostate tissue is done, usually in the office. If the results are positive for cancer cells, then a bone scan is done to detect possible spread of the disease. Treatments for prostate cancer vary from watching and waiting with regular checkups, to surgery, radiation, hormone therapy, and chemotherapy. PSA results of under 4 mg/dL are considered normal. The interpretation of these results and additional testing are required because a very high result may not mean prostate cancer, and very low results may not mean the individual is cancer free.

RENAL FAILURE

Renal failure (kidney failure) is the inability of the kidneys to adequately filter metabolic waste products from the blood. Many causes lead to the decline of renal function, and renal failure is classified as acute or chronic.

Acute Renal Failure

Acute renal failure has a rapid onset of a few days to a few weeks. It is caused by any condition that decreases blood supply to the kidney, obstructs the flow of urine anywhere in the urinary tract, or injures the kidney.

TABLE 38-3 Procedures and Diagnostic Tests Related to the Urinary System

Procedure/Test	Description
Blood urea nitrogen	A blood test to determine the amount of urea that is excreted by the kidneys. Abnormal results indicate urinary tract disease.
Catheterization	The insertion of a sterile tube through the urethra and into the urinary bladder for the purpose of withdrawing urine. This procedure is used to obtain a sterile urine specimen and also to relieve distension when the patient is unable to void on his or her own.
Clean catch specimen (CC)	To minimize contamination from the genitalia, urine sample is obtained after cleaning the urinary opening and catching or collecting a sample in midstream (halfway through the urination process).
Creatinine	A blood test to determine the amount of creatinine present. Abnormal results indicate kidney disease.
Creatinine clearance	A urine test to determine the glomerular filtration rate (GFR). Abnormal results indicate kidney disease.
Culture, urine	A urine test to determine the presence of microorganisms. Abnormal results indicate urinary tract infection.
Cystography	The process of instilling a contrast material or dye into the bladder by catheter to visualize the urinary bladder.
Cystoscopy	Visual examination of the urinary bladder using a cystoscope. The patient may receive general or local anesthesia for this procedure.
Dialysis	The artificial filtration of waste material from the blood. It is used when the kidneys fail to function.
Extracorporeal shockwave lithotripsy (ESWL)	Use of ultrasound waves to break up kidney stones. Process does not require invasive surgery.
Excretory urography	Injection of dye into the bloodstream followed by an X-ray, which traces the action of the kidney as it excretes the dye.
Hemodialysis	Use of an artificial kidney that filters a person's blood to remove waste products. Use of this technique in patients who have defective kidneys is lifesaving.
Intravenous pyelogram (IVP)	Injection of radioopaque dye into the bloodstream followed by an X-ray, which traces the action of the kidneys, ureters, and bladder as the dye is excreted.
Kidney, ureters, bladder (KUB)	A flat plate X-ray of the abdomen that indicates the size and position of the kidneys, ureters, and bladder.
Meatotomy	Surgical enlargement of the urinary opening.
Peritoneal dialysis	The removal of toxic waste substances from the body by placing warm, chemically balanced solutions into the peritoneal cavity. This is used in treating renal failure and in certain types of poisonings.
Renal biopsy	The removal of tissue from the kidney. Abnormal results may indicate kidney cancer, kidney transplant rejection, and glomerulonephritis.
Renal transplant	Surgical placement of a donor kidney.
Retrograde pyelogram	A diagnostic X-ray in which dye is inserted through the urethra to outline the bladder, ureters, and renal pelvis.
Sound	Metal rod curved at one end with a handle at the other end, used to treat stricture or an obstruction in the urethra. A physician will pass the sound up the urethra.
Urinalysis	A laboratory test that consists of the physical, chemical, and microscopic examination of urine.
Urography	The use of contrast medium to provide an X-ray of the urinary tract.
Ultrasonography, kidneys	The use of high-frequency sound waves to visualize the kidneys. The sound waves (echoes) are recorded on an oscilloscope and film. Abnormal results may indicate kidney tumors, cysts, abscesses, and kidney disease.

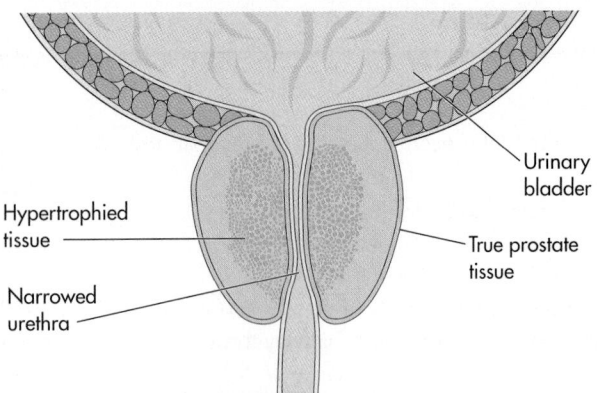

FIGURE 38-16 Benign prostatic hyperplasia.

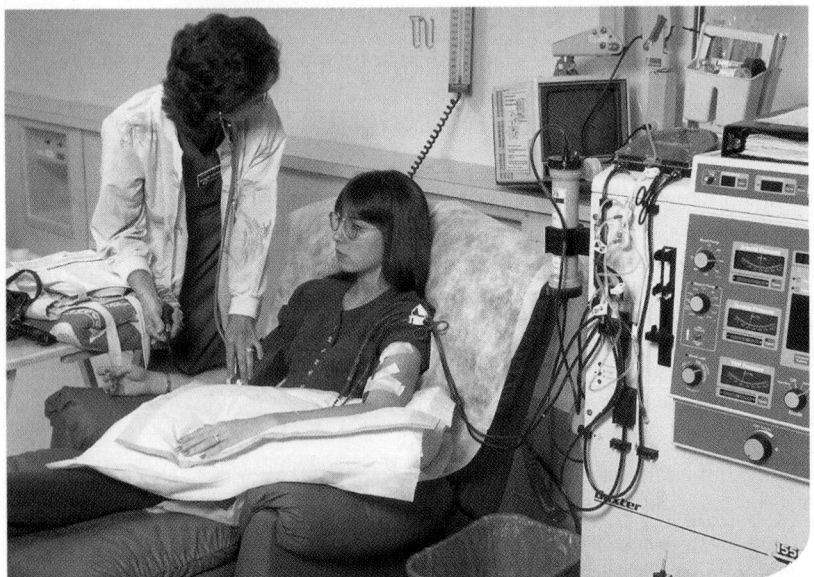

FIGURE 38-17 A patient undergoing hemodialysis.

The symptoms of renal failure vary with the cause and rate of onset and include fluid retention in the hands and feet, dark-colored urine, decrease in urinary output, fatigue due to increase in metabolic waste levels in the blood stream, nausea, and pruritis (itchiness). Diagnosis is made based on symptoms and blood tests, such as blood urea nitrogen, creatinine, electrolytes, and diagnostic tests such as CAT scan and ultrasound. Acute renal failure can affect people of any age; however, it is more common in older people. Dialysis and transplants have improved the survival rate greatly.

Chronic Renal Failure

Chronic renal failure is a slow progressive decline in renal function over a period of months to several years. Acute renal failure can become chronic if kidneys do not fully recover after treatment. Any condition that can cause acute renal failure can cause chronic renal failure. The most common causes of chronic renal failure are diabetes mellitus and hypertension. Other causes include kidney abnormalities, renal disease (e.g., glomerulonephritis), and autoimmune disorders (e.g., systemic lupus erythematosus).

The patient may experience mild symptoms including nocturia and elevated blood urea nitrogen. As the condition progresses, fatigue, lack of mental alertness, anemia, loss of appetite, and shortness of breath affect the patient's quality of life. Diagnosis is based on patient history,

Box 38-3 DIALYSIS

Dialysis is the process of removing waste products and excess fluids from the body. Hemodialysis is the use of an artificial kidney machine to perform the functions of the nephrons of the patient's kidneys. The patient's blood is passed through tiny tubules surrounded by fluid (dialysate), which has the same chemical composition as blood plasma. Waste products and excess fluids pass out of the patient's blood into the fluid of the machine. They are thus eliminated, and purified blood is returned to the patient. Hemodialysis must be repeated on average three times per week. To achieve this goal, easy access to the patient's bloodstream is necessary. This may be accomplished by a number of means such as creating an arteriovenous fistula or creating a synthetic graft between an artery and

vein. Either type of access requires a surgical procedure. Because of the tendency of the blood to clot, heparin is administered during hemodialysis.

Peritoneal dialysis involves the use of the peritoneum, the membrane that lines the abdomen and covers the abdominal organs, to function as a filter for dialysis (Figure 38-17). The peritoneum has a large surface and rich blood supply making filtration easier. Dialysate is put into the abdominal cavity through a catheter and left for a period of time (hours or overnight) to allow waste and excess fluids to be removed from the bloodstream, and then the filtrate is drained out and discarded. Several types of peritoneal dialysis are available; however, each requires varying amounts of time ranging from 10 to

(continued)

12 hours overnight, or every 3 to 4 hours four times a day. A catheter may be placed in the abdominal wall temporarily or permanently as needed. Choosing the type of dialysis depends on many factors such as age, physical condition, type of renal disorder, and lifestyle. Either type of dialysis restricts a patient's life in terms of loss of time, specialized diet, loss of mobility, and loss of independence. In children, renal disease may stunt their growth and cause feelings of isolation.

symptoms, and blood tests for levels of creatinine and blood urea nitrogen. Chronic renal failure is fatal if not treated. Survival for patients with end-stage renal disease is a few months.

Treatments of chronic renal failure include restriction of protein and calcium in the diet and administration of various medications to adjust blood pressure, regulate electrolyte balance, and counteract anemia. When these treatments are no longer effective, renal dialysis or transplants are the alternatives (Figure 38-17). Most patients with advanced renal failure die within 5 to 10 years, even with the benefits of improved dialysis. Box 38-3 discusses hemodialysis and peritoneal dialysis.

SUMMARY

The topics covered in this chapter include the male and female reproductive and urology specialties, methods of contraception, and STIs. These topics are presented to ensure that health care providers are up to date on information critical to the health of their patients. It is the responsibility of the health care provider to be nonjudgmental when discussing delicate issues with patients and to be certain that HIPAA regulations regarding privacy are carefully followed.

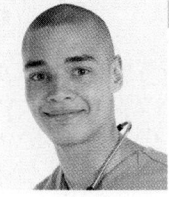

38 CHAPTER REVIEW

COMPETENCY REVIEW

1. Define and spell the terms to learn in this chapter.

2. Develop a brochure instructing female patients how to do a breast self-examination and male patients how to do a testicular self-examination.

3. List the equipment necessary for a Pap smear. What is the medical assistant's responsibility for assisting with this procedure?

PREPARING FOR THE CERTIFICATION EXAM

1. Health care workers who acquire HIV from occupational exposure are at greatest danger from
   a. unprotected personal care
   b. contaminated blood in an open wound
   c. accidental needlesticks
   d. using clean gloves with each patient
   e. not washing hands

2. The rule to calculate a woman's due date for delivery is
   a. rule of nine
   b. Clark's rule
   c. Snellen chart
   d. Naegele's rule
   e. West's nomogram

3. An exam tray that includes gloves, speculum, three glass slides, fixative, and sterile culture swabs with containers is ready for what type of examination?
   a. rectal
   b. pelvic
   c. gastroenterology
   d. neurological
   e. urological

4. The causative agent of syphilis is
   a. *Treponema pallidum*
   b. *Streptococcus pyogenes*
   c. *Staphylococcus aureus*
   d. *Trichomonas vaginalis*
   e. herpes simplex type 2

5. Which of the following tests is not required for prenatal testing?
   a. syphilis
   b. blood group, Rh type
   c. antibody for rubella
   d. glucose tolerance test
   e. alpha-fetoprotein test (AFP)

6. The STI that is caused by a protozoan is
   a. gonorrhea
   b. chlamydia
   c. candidiasis
   d. trichomoniasis
   e. genital warts

7. Barrier methods of contraception include all of the following EXCEPT
   a. morning-after pill
   b. contraceptive sponge
   c. condom
   d. cervical cap
   e. diaphragm

8. A condition that may cause urinary retention and weak stream of urine in men over age fifty is known as
   a. syphilis
   b. benign prostatic hyperplasia (BPH)
   c. renal calculi
   d. human papillomavirus
   e. gastroenteritis

9. Vasectomy involves the severing and tying off of the
   a. fallopian tubes
   b. scrotum
   c. urethra
   d. vas deferens
   e. epididymis

10. The term *parturition* refers to
    a. the duration of pregnancy
    b. stages of menstrual cycle
    c. birth
    d. discharge after delivery
    e. placenta

CRITICAL THINKING

1. Determine Sonja's EDD based on her LMP.

2. How would Sonja's past obstetrical history be recorded in the prenatal record?

3. What should Sonja expect to have completed during her first prenatal visit with Dr. McWalters?

ON THE JOB

A young male patient has an appointment but refuses to speak to you, the medical assistant, about his problem. He indicates that it is a "very personal matter." After asking some questions, you surmise that he has symptoms of an STI. What should you do? How should you respond to him?

INTERNET ACTIVITY

Look up online the newest statistics related to HIV/AIDS worldwide. Find the website in your state dealing with reportable STIs.

MEDMEDIA

Additional interactive resources and activities for this chapter can be found:

On your student DVD: View applicable procedure videos on the DVD-ROM found in the back of this book.

MyHealthProfessionsKit.com: Test your knowledge of this chapter with games and activities. MyHealthProfessionsKit also includes resources, helpful links, and a Spanish audio glossary.

Medical Assisting Interactive Practice your procedures as a medical assistant in this simulated doctor's office. This can be accessed through MyHealthProfessionsKit.com.

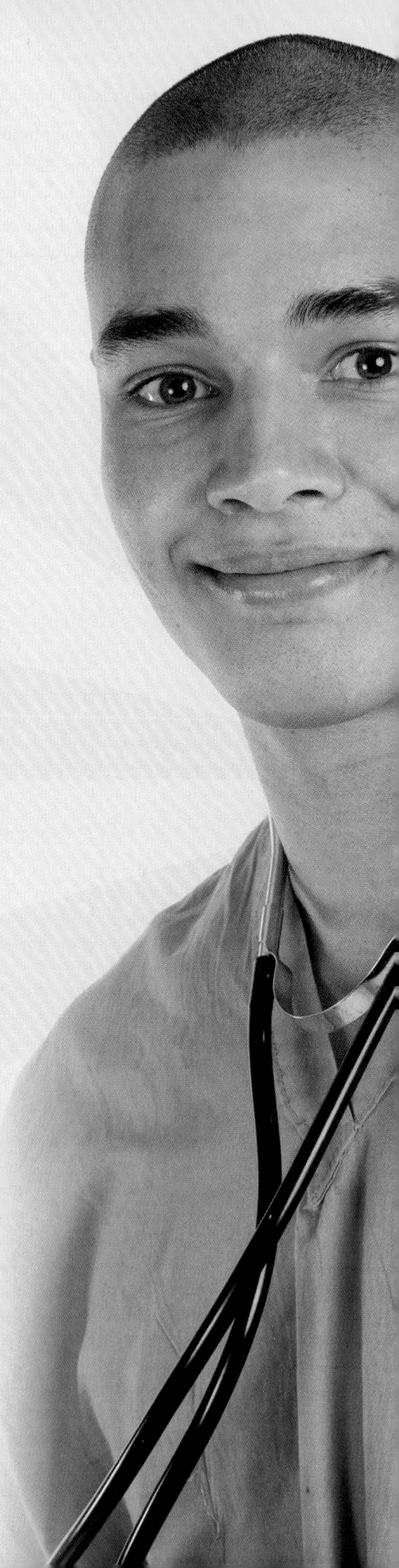

39

Assisting with Eye and Ear Care

LEARNING OBJECTIVES

After reading this chapter, you should be able to:

- Define the terms to learn in this chapter.

- Explain procedures to evaluate distance vision, near vision, color vision, and contrast sensitivity.

- Explain procedures to irrigate the eye and instill eye medications.

- Name three causes of blindness.

- Explain the procedure for assisting visually-impaired patients to prepare for physical examinations.

- List and explain five age-related changes in the eye.

- Name and explain two types of hearing impairment.

- Explain procedures to irrigate the ear and instill ear medications.

- Explain the procedure to evaluate hearing acuity using an audiometer.

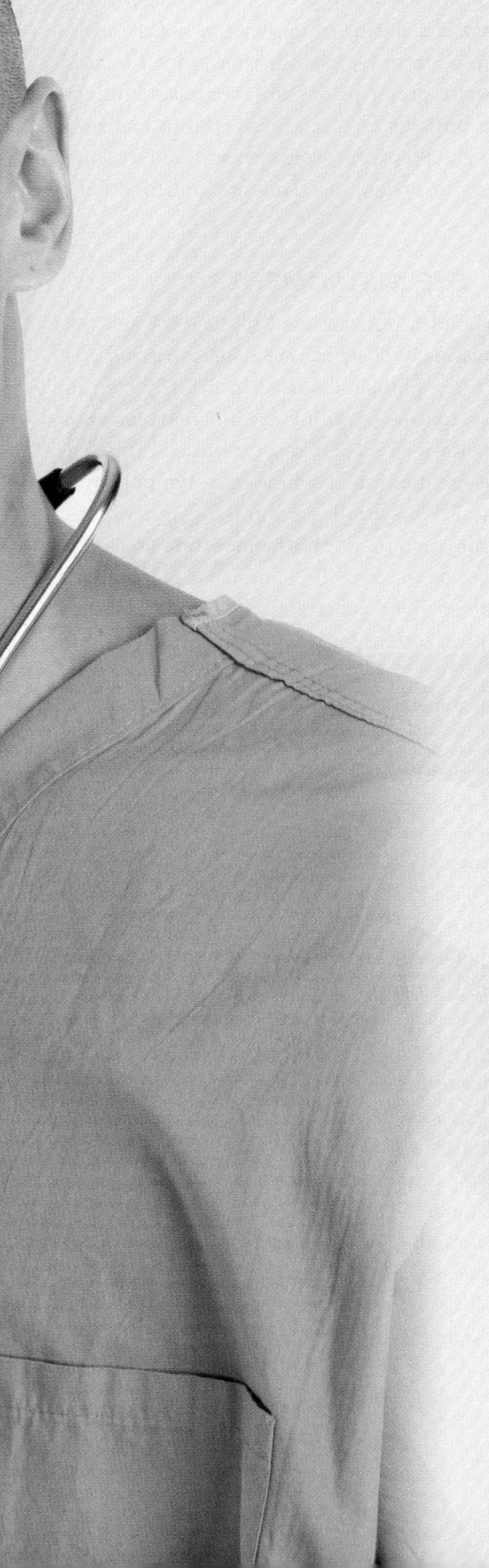

CHAPTER OUTLINE

CASE STUDY

Kyle Schultz is a nine-year-old boy whose parents are concerned that he is having trouble seeing the blackboard in school. Kyle is shy and will not ask the teacher to change his seat. Kyle's parents have both worn glasses since their teens. Samra is working with Dr. Miller. Dr. Miller asks Samra to perform a Snellen eye exam. The results are 20/80 OD and 20/60 OS. After Dr. Miller reviews the results, he orders a further eye exam that requires instillation of eyedrops in both eyes to dilate the pupils. Kyle does not want to have this procedure done.

829

Special examinations and procedures related to specific body systems are commonly performed in the medical office. In this chapter we consider examinations and procedures related to the eye and ear. The role of the medical assistant is to assist the physician during special examinations and procedures and to instruct the patient before, during, and after procedures. You will learn the procedures to perform visual and auditory **acuity** (sharpness) testing, to **instill** or put in eye and ear medications, and to **irrigate** or rinse both eyes and ears. Keep in mind that you are representing the physician and that you play an important role in setting a positive tone and atmosphere in the office. All patients should be treated with respect during all phases of the procedures.

The Study of the Eye

The eye is the organ of sight. The branch of medical science that deals with the structure, function, and diseases of the eye is **ophthalmology**. An **ophthalmologist** is a medical doctor who can perform eye examinations and eye surgery and prescribe medications, eyeglasses, and contact lenses. An **optometrist** is a doctor of optometry, not a medical doctor, who can perform eye examinations, prescribe medications and write prescriptions for eyeglasses and contact lenses. An **optician** is a technician who specializes in grinding lenses and preparing eyeglasses and contact lenses. (See Chapter 26 to review the structure and function of the eye.)

EYE INSTRUMENTS

A number of complex tests are used to diagnose and treat vision problems, many of which are done in the office of specialists, such as ophthalmologists. In primary care and pediatric offices, routine screening examinations for vision problems are performed as part of physical examinations. The **otoscope** is used to examine the **tympanum** or **myringa** (medical terms for the eardrum) for signs of infection and inflammation. The **ophthalmoscope** is used to view inner parts of the eye. The physician positions the ophthalmoscope so light penetrates the pupil of the patient's eye and then screens for retinal damage and vascular problems.

The care and maintenance of the otoscope and the ophthalmoscope is a routine task performed by the medical assistant. These instruments utilize batteries that must be recharged on a regular basis. The tiny bulbs used in both instruments must be replaced occasionally. Most physicians use disposable ear and nasal specula to examine the tympanic membrane and nose. A **speculum** (*specula,* pl.) is any instrument that holds open a body cavity to permit inspection. Monitoring supplies, including disposable specula, for the examining room is a routine task performed by the medical assistant.

Before every eye examination, the overall appearance of the eye is evaluated for symptoms such as redness, puslike discharge, and excessive tearing. In addition, the physician evaluates the status of the patient's pupils and ability to focus on objects at different distances. PERRLA is an acronym that stands for "Pupils Equal, Round, React to Light and Accommodation." Normally the pupils of the eyes are the same size and change or accommodate when a beam of light is focused on the eye and is then removed. Injuries to the brain may result in the patient having pupils of unequal size.

VISUAL ACUITY AND REFRACTIVE ERRORS

Normal **visual acuity**, or clarity of vision, is referred to as 20/20 vision, which means the eye should see an object 20 feet away clearly. Errors of refraction occur when the eyeball is either too long or too short, the lens loses its elasticity, or the lens or cornea has an irregular curvature. The **cornea** is the clear, transparent covering of the eye. Each of these refractive errors is discussed individually.

Myopia or nearsightedness means that the eye sees near objects well but distant objects appear blurry. This occurs either because the eyeball is too long or because the lens is too thick and the light rays do not reach the retina. The shape of the eyeball and lens are hereditary. The myopic eye requires a concave lens to correct vision. **Hyperopia** or farsightedness means that the eyes see distant objects well but near objects are blurry. In this case, the eyeball is too short or the lens too thin. The hyperopic eye requires a convex lens to correct the visual defect. **Presbyopia** is the term associated with farsightedness

that occurs with aging. The lens loses its elasticity and glasses are needed for reading. **Astigmatism** is a refractive disorder in which irregularities in the curvature of the cornea cause light to focus not on the retina but spread out over an area causing overall blurring of vision. Images may be clear in the center of the field and blurry at the outer edges of the visual field. Figure 39-1 shows how lenses correct visual problems.

Strabismus is an eye disorder caused by weakness in the external eye muscles resulting in the eyes looking in different directions. Normally the eyes focus on a subject in coordination; otherwise double vision occurs. Children with strabismus appear "cross-eyed" and may need to wear a patch over the "good" eye to strengthen the weaker eye. You may need to teach the patient basic eye exercises as part of the treatment plan. It is important that treatment begin at an early age to prevent permanent damage to the eye. If the patch and exercise plan are ineffective, surgery on the eye muscle may be necessary.

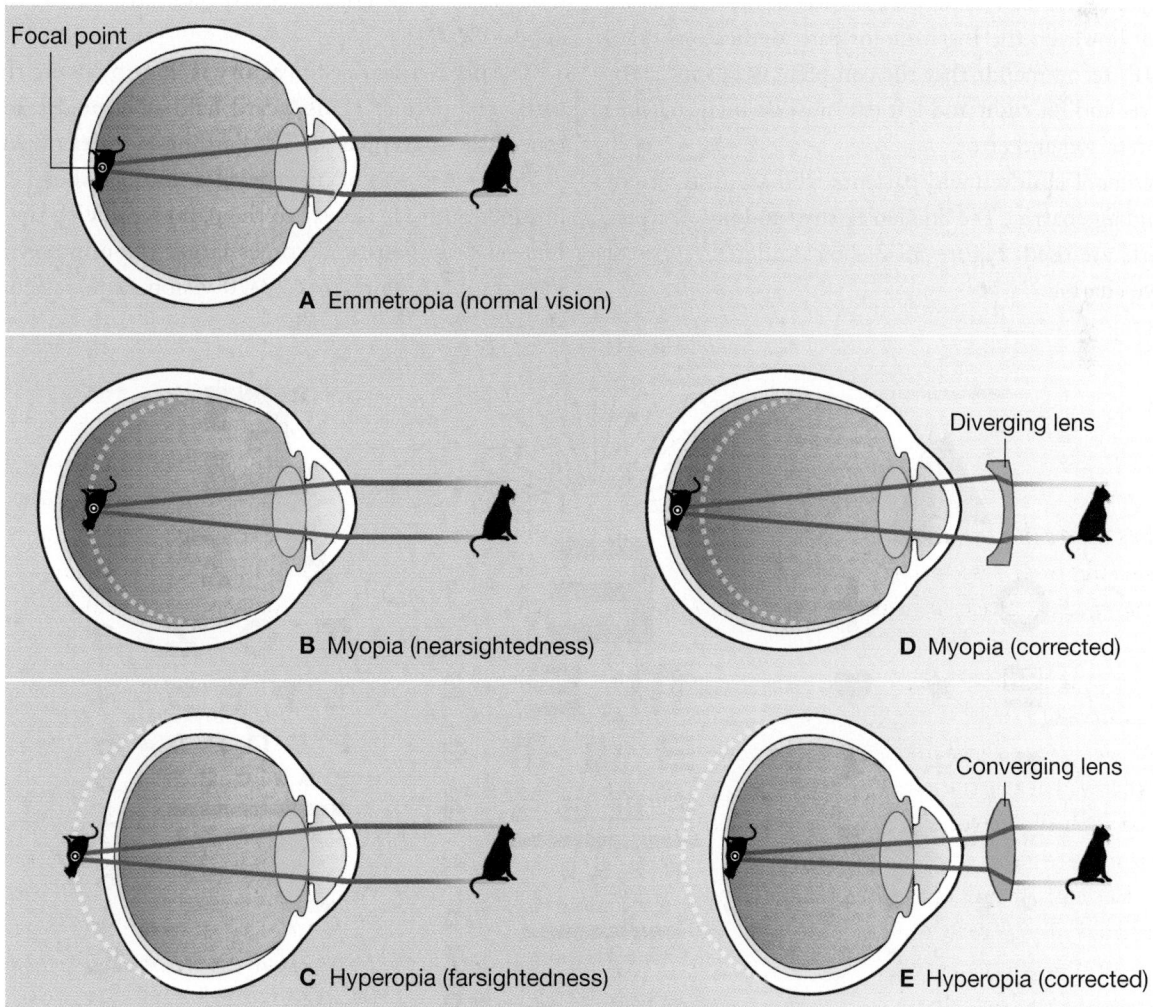

FIGURE 39-1 How lenses correct visual problems: (A) emmetropia; (B) myopia; (C) hyperopia.

Assessing Visual Acuity

As noted previously, visual acuity testing is frequently performed in a variety of medical settings. Performing these tests is usually the task of the medical assistant. Distance acuity testing, near vision acuity testing, and testing for color blindness will be discussed.

DISTANCE ACUITY

Distance acuity is measured using the **Snellen chart**. Snellen charts place the largest symbols on the top line, and each line after is of decreasing size. The person with normal vision would be able to read the top line at 200 feet. To the right of each line is a ratio indicating what a person with normal vision could read at decreasing distances of 100, 70, 50, 40, 30, and 20 feet. A result of 20/20 vision means that a person with normal distance acuity could read that line at a distance of 20 feet.

The abbreviation for the right eye is OD (oculus dexter), for the left eye it is OS (oculus sinister), and the abbreviation for both eyes is OU (oculus uterque). These abbreviations are often used; however, the Institute for Safe Medication Practices (ISMP) recommends that the complete words for right and left eye, and for right and left ear must be used to avoid misinterpretation and error.

For preschool children and patients who are illiterate or have a language barrier, the Snellen E, the Landolt C, or pictorial charts are used. Figure 39-2 shows different types of Snellen eye charts.

If you are unsure if the patient has the ability to recognize the Snellen eye chart letters, you should verify his or her ability by using a demonstration chart prior to testing. To do so, have the patient demonstrate by pointing his or her finger in the direction the E is pointing on the Snellen E Chart so you can determine whether or not the patient can follow your instructions. When dealing with young children, it may be helpful to make a game of it, showing them how to hold their hands to illustrate which direction the E is facing.

Procedure 39-1 presents the steps for performing a distance acuity test using the Snellen eye chart.

NEAR VISION ACUITY

Testing for near vision acuity should be done if the patient complains of difficulty reading or performing other close-range tasks. It is done to test for hyperopia or presbyopia. The lens of the eye loses its elasticity with age and cannot change from viewing distant objects to close work as readily as before. Close work appears blurry, and the individual tends to hold the book or newspaper farther away to make it appear clearer.

Testing for near vision acuity is done by using the Jaeger card. The patient reads a card held at normal reading distance (14 to 16 inches). The card has a series of paragraphs decreasing in size of print with a number above each. The number one (J1) is next to the paragraph with the smallest text, and as the text becomes larger the number increases. Paragraph J2 represents 20/20 vision. The patient's result

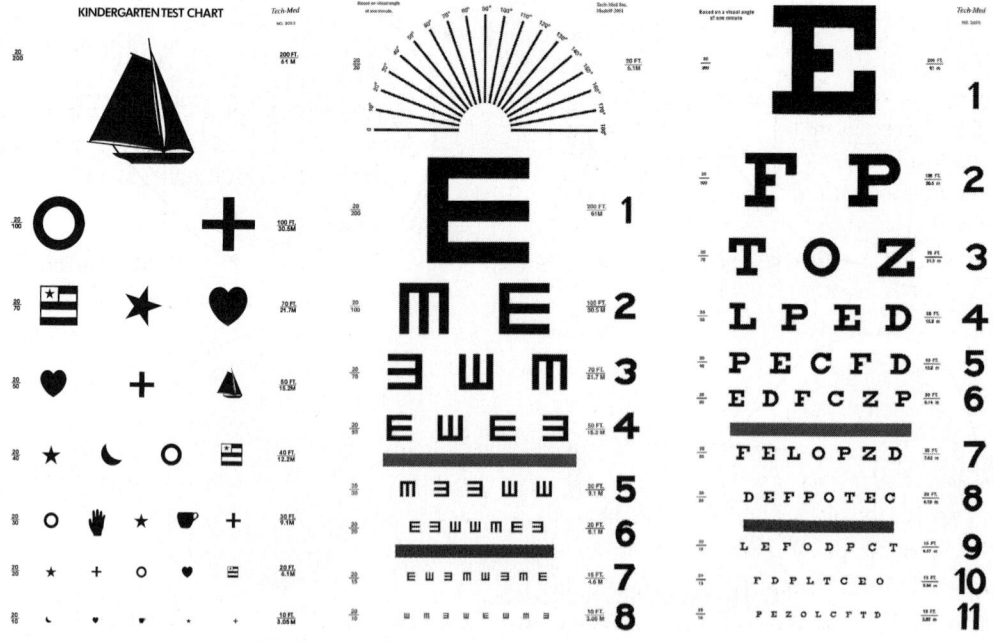

FIGURE 39-2 Different types of Snellen eye charts.

TESTING VISUAL ACUITY USING A SNELLEN EYE CHART

Objective: Screen a patient for distance acuity using a Snellen eye chart.

EQUIPMENT AND SUPPLIES

Snellen eye chart placed at a distance of 20 feet; eye shield or occluder; pointer; pen and paper; alcohol and gauze

METHOD

1. Assemble equipment.
2. Review physician's order.
3. Perform hand hygiene and identify the patient.
4. Explain the procedure.
5. Determine the patient's ability to recognize letters. If the patient is unable to read letters, use the necessary chart to accommodate the patient's abilities.
6. Place the patient 20 feet from the chart, either seated or standing, as long as the Snellen eye chart is at eye level (Figure 39-3).
7. Follow office policy regarding testing with or without corrective lenses.
8. Following office policies regarding which eye to test first, have the patient cover the other eye with a cup or occluder. The occluder should be held in such a way as not to interfere with the normal position of a patient's glasses.
9. Instruct the patient to keep both eyes open even though one eye is covered. Have patient read the lines with both eyes first at a distance of 20 feet.
10. Use pointer and point to letters or appropriate symbols in random order.
11. Starting with the 20/70 line ask the patient to identify each line and proceed down the chart to the last line the patient can read without error. Observe for signs of squinting or tilting the head, which indicate difficulty identifying letters.
12. Record the ratio numbers adjacent to the line the patient can read without error. If there is an error, note it (e.g., "Right

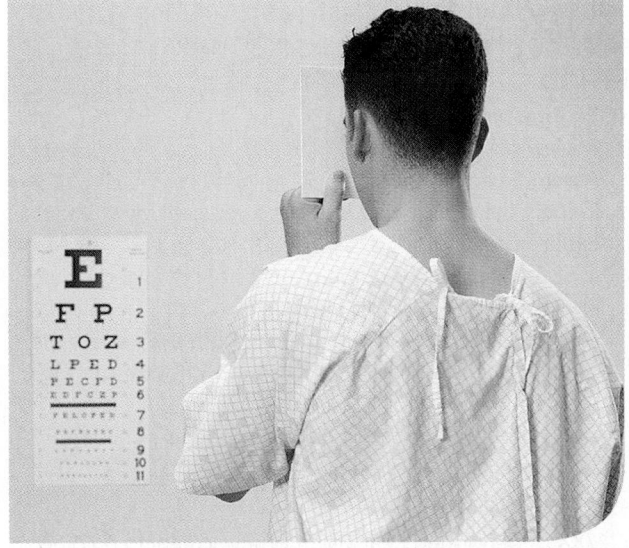

FIGURE 39-3 **Test of distance vision using the Snellen eye chart.**

eye 20/40—1"; or "Right eye 20/40—1 with correction," meaning glasses were worn during testing). ISMP recommends using words instead of abbreviations for eye designations to avoid misinterpretation. Follow office protocol regarding charting.
13. Repeat the procedure with the other eye and record the result, noting any unusual symptoms such as squinting or blinking excessively.
14. Clean the occluder with gauze and alcohol.
15. Remove gloves and perform hand hygiene.
16. Document the results accurately.

CHARTING EXAMPLE

2/14/XX 4:00 P.M. Snellen eye test. Rt eye 20/30. Lt eye 20/30. Both eyes 20/30. · · · · · · · · · · · · · · · · · M. King, CMA (AAMA)

---

is the number above the last paragraph he or she can read easily. This test should always be performed in a well-lit room. Office policies differ on whether or not to have patients wear corrective lenses during the test and whether to test each eye individually or both eyes together. As a medical assistant you will follow the policy in your facility.

Procedure 39-2 presents the steps to perform a near vision acuity test.

COLOR VISION IMPAIRMENT

Color vision impairment is the inability to distinctly differentiate colors of the spectrum. Defects in color vision

SCREENING FOR NEAR VISION ACUITY

Objective: Screen near vision acuity using the Jaeger system.

EQUIPMENT AND SUPPLIES

Jaeger near vision acuity chart; paper and pen

METHOD

1. Perform hand hygiene.
2. Review physician's order.
3. Assemble equipment.
4. Identify the patient and introduce yourself.
5. Explain procedure.
6. In a well-lit room, have the patient hold the Jaeger card at a distance of 14 to 16 inches.
7. Ask the patient to read aloud, with both eyes open, the smallest paragraph or line possible without error (Figure 39-4).
8. Document the results accurately, noting any unusual symptoms, such as squinting.

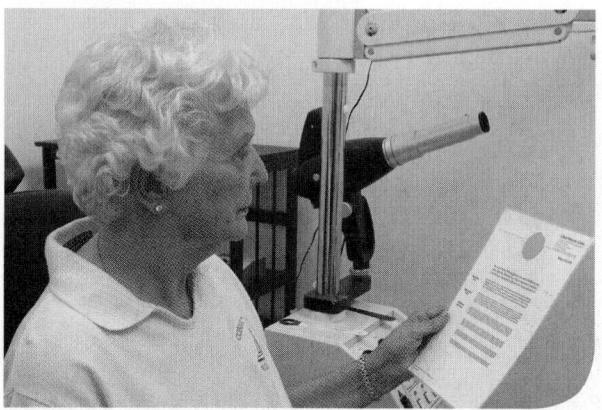

FIGURE 39-4 **A patient using a near vision acuity card.**

CHARTING EXAMPLE

09/11/XX pt performed near vision acuity screening reading without error—J2. · L. McKay, RMA

---

are either congenital (patient was born with the defect), inherited, or acquired through disease or injury. Congenital color blindness is more prevalent in males. It is important to test for color vision defects because changes in color vision may indicate diseases of the retina, optic nerve, or thyroid.

The ability to distinguish colors depends on the cones of the retina, which react to light and permit us to see shades of red, green, and blue. The inability to see any colors is rare and is most likely due to a defect or absence of the cones in the retina. The most common type of color vision defect, which is inherited, is the inability to distinguish red and green. Other types of color blindness prevent patients from distinguishing shades of various colors.

The **Ishihara test** is printed in either card or booklet form with a single color-dot illustration containing a number or curved lines and shapes. For instance, a person with normal color vision would be able to see the green number 27 on the red–orange background, as in Figure 39-5. The patient is shown 14 color plates or pages and must correctly identify 10 to be considered to have color vision within normal limits. The Ishihara booklet or cards should be stored out of direct light to prevent fading of the color plates. Procedure 39-3 presents the steps to perform a screening for color vision acuity using the Ishihara test.

CONTRAST SENSITIVITY

Contrast sensitivity measures the patient's ability to distinguish faint differences in shades of gray. Several new testing procedures and instruments are used to test for contrast sensitivity, such as the Vistech Consultant system and the Pelli-Robson chart. To perform a procedure for contrast sensitivity, adhere to the manufacturer's directions and observe the usual procedural steps for appropriate patient care, such as hand hygiene and correct documentation. It has been determined that contrast sensitivity is affected by most major eye conditions, such as macular degeneration, cataracts, glaucoma, and diabetic retinopathy.

SCREENING FOR COLOR VISION ACUITY

Objective: Screen a patient for color vision defects.

EQUIPMENT AND SUPPLIES

Ishihara screening book/cards; paper and pen

METHOD

1. Perform hand hygiene.
2. Review physician's order.
3. Assemble equipment.
4. Identify the patient and introduce yourself.
5. Explain the procedure.
6. Have the patient assume a comfortable position, and ask patient to keep both eyes open.
7. In a well-lit room, have the patient identify at a distance of 30 inches the number that is formed by the colored dots on each card or page within 3 seconds per page or card.
8. If the patient is unable to identify the numbers, have the patient trace the number with his or her finger.
9. Score each plate as it is read. (Figure 39-5 is an example of one color plate.) If the patient is able to identify the number, then record the number seen after the plate number (e.g., Plate 1:7). If the patient was unable to identify a number on a plate, record the plate number and mark an X next to it.
10. Note any unusual symptoms.
11. Document the results accurately.

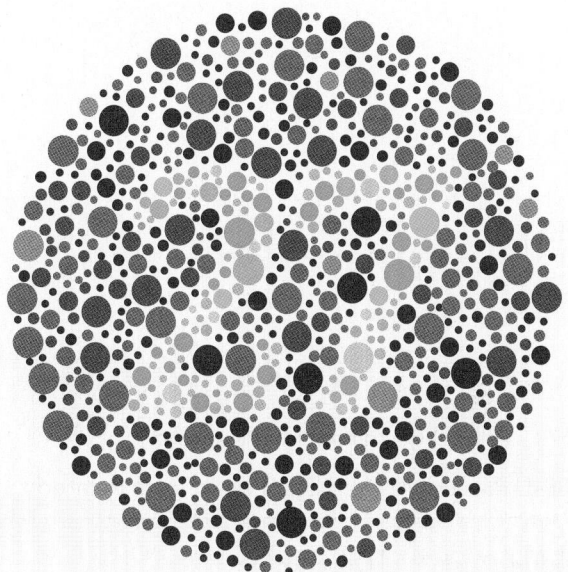

FIGURE 39-5 **One page of color vision chart.**

CHARTING EXAMPLE

2/14/XX 3:00 P.M. Ishihara eye chart normal. ··············
·································· M. King, CMA (AAMA)

Figure 39-6 shows a Pelli-Robson chart for testing contrast sensitivity. Figure 39-7 illustrates a patient being tested for glaucoma. Table 39-1 lists and explains tests and procedures related to the eye.

Irrigation of the Eye

Irrigation or lavage (rinsing) of the eye is necessary to remove foreign substances or chemicals. Eye irrigation requires the use of sterile technique and equipment. As with any procedure, the medical assistant must first explain the procedure to the patient and answer any questions. Never try to remove a foreign object from the eye using an applicator stick as this may cause corneal abrasions. Procedure 39-4 presents steps for irrigating the eye.

Instillation of Eye Medications

Instilling (putting in) eye medications may be one of your duties. Only ophthalmic or optic medications can be used in the eye, and they must be sterile. It is important that you reinforce the need for sterile medications with your patients. Encourage them to discard eye medications when the prescribed treatment time has been completed. In addition, instruct them that eye medications should never be shared with others or even used in the other eye if treatment is needed. The danger of contamination is great. Procedure 39-5 provides the steps for performing instillation of eye medication.

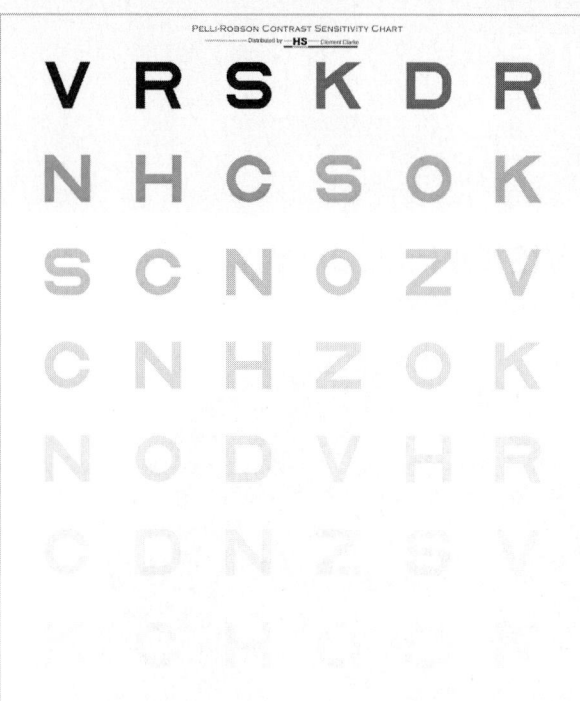

FIGURE 39-6　Pelli-Robson contrast sensitivity chart.

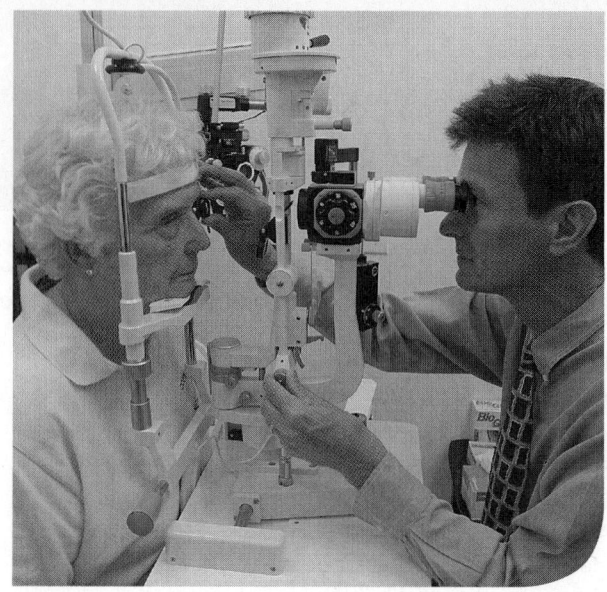

FIGURE 39-7　Patient having glaucoma test.

TABLE 39-1 Procedures and Diagnostic Tests Related to the Eye

Procedure/Test	Description
Corneal transplant	Surgical process of transferring the cornea from a donor to a patient.
Electroretinogram	Record of the electrical response of the retina to light stimulation.
Fluorescein angiography	Process of injecting fluorescein (a dye) followed by a series of photographs of the retina through dilated pupils. This test provides diagnostic information about the blood flow in the retina, detecting vascular changes in diabetic and hypertensive retinopathy, and identifies lesions in the macular area of the retina, determining if there is detachment of the retina.
Gonioscopy	Use of gonioscope to examine the anterior chamber of the eye to determine ocular motility and rotation.
Keratometry	Measurement of the cornea using a keratometer.
Keratoplasty	Surgical repair of the cornea (corneal transplant).
Laser surgery	Surgical procedure performed with a laser handpiece that transfers light into intense, small beams capable of destroying or fixing tissue in place.
Optomyometer	Instrument used to measure the strength of the muscles of the eye.
Phacoemulsification	Process of using ultrasonic vibrations to disintegrate a cataract. A needle is inserted through a small incision and the disintegrated cataract is aspirated. (The ophthalmic surgeon uses a small, self-sealing scleral-tunnel incision.)
Radial keratotomy	Surgical procedure that may be performed to correct nearsightedness (myopia). Delicate spokelike incisions are made in the cornea to flatten it, thereby shortening the eyeball so that light reaches the retina. Not all patients have their vision improved, and complications could lead to blindness.
Slit-lamp microscopy	Instrument used in ophthalmology for examining the posterior surface of the cornea.
Tonometry	Measurement of intraocular pressure (IOP) of the eye using a tonometer to check for glaucoma. An air puff tonometer records the cornea's resistance to pressure.
Visual acuity	Measurements of the sharpness of a patient's vision. Usually a Snellen eye chart is used, and the patient identifies letters from a distance of 20 feet.
Vitrectomy	Surgical procedure for replacing the contents of the vitreous chamber of the eye

IRRIGATION OF THE EYE

Objective: Cleanse or irrigate the eye.

EQUIPMENT AND SUPPLIES

nonsterile gloves; sterile basin; emesis basin; sterile solution; sterile irrigating syringe; sterile gauze; towel; tissues; pen and patient's chart

METHOD

1. Identify the patient and explain the procedure.
2. Review the physician's order.
3. Assemble the equipment: Check the label of the irrigating solution three times to ensure it is the correct solution and concentration ordered by the physician. Check the expiration date on the label to make sure the solution has not expired. The solution should be brought to room temperature by wrapping the bottle in a dry heating pad or standing the bottle in a warn water bath.
4. Perform hand hygiene and apply gloves.
5. Ask the patient which position he or she would prefer, sitting or lying down.
6. Place a towel over the patient's shoulder. If both eyes are to be irrigated, then two separate sets of equipment must be used to prevent cross-infection.
7. Open the irrigating solution and fill the syringe.
8. Ask the patient to tilt the head to the affected side if seated, and hold the basin.
9. Open the patient's eye using the index finger and thumb of the nondominant hand.
10. Hold a tissue on the patient's cheekbone below the lower lid and pull down and expose the conjunctiva.
11. Hold the syringe $\frac{1}{2}$ inch from the eye (Figure 39-8).
12. Gently irrigate from inner to outer canthus (corner of eye), aiming at the lower conjunctiva.

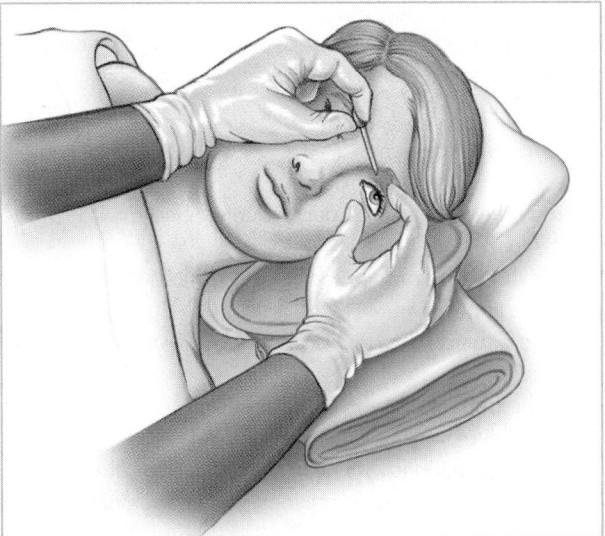

FIGURE 39-8 **Irrigation of the eye.**

13. Continue irrigating until the solution is used up.
14. Dry the area around the eye with sterile gauze.
15. Dispose of the equipment properly.
16. Perform hand hygiene.
17. Document information in the patient's chart in the appropriate manner.

CHARTING EXAMPLE

09/13/XX 10 A.M. Rt eye irrigated with 50 mL of 100°F normal saline. Eye sl. Red Pt. says "eye feels fine." · · · · · · · · · · · · · · · ·
· E. Zandri, CMA (AAMA)

Patient Safety Guidelines

Patients should be made aware of some general safety guidelines to protect their sight. Regular physical examinations on a yearly basis may discover conditions or diseases, such as diabetes or hypertension, that impact their vision. An eye examination every 1 to 2 years is important to monitor changing conditions in the patient's vision. Encourage patients to wear sunglasses to protect eyes from ultraviolet rays, which can damage the cornea. For minor eye problems, tell patients to avoid rubbing and apply cold compresses. Advise patients to wear protective eyewear when using tools or machinery that can cause flying objects. Make patients aware that when chemicals splash in the eye, they should flood the eye with water for 20 minutes and seek immediate medical attention. Remind patients of the importance of maintaining sterility of optic medications.

INSTILLING EYE MEDICATION

Objective: Instill eye medication following the physician's orders.

EQUIPMENT AND SUPPLIES
sterile medication; sterile eyedropper (if needed); tissues; sterile gauze squares; nonsterile gloves; drape or towel

METHOD
1. Perform hand hygiene.
2. Check the physician's orders.
3. Identify the patient, introduce yourself, and explain the procedure.
4. Check the name of the medication, expiration date, and concentration three times.
5. Ask the patient if he or she has any known allergies to the medication.
6. Give the patient a tissue to blot cheeks.
7. Put on gloves.
8. Position the patient with head tilted back and looking up.
9. Pull down the lower eyelid exposing the conjunctiva (Figure 39-9).
10. Place the dropper about $\frac{1}{2}$ inch above the eyeball with the dominant hand. Insert the proper amount of drops to the center of the conjunctiva, or if ointment is used apply as a thin strip from inner to outer canthus.
11. Do not touch the dropper or ointment tube to the eye.
12. Ask the patient to gently close the eye and rotate the eyeball.
13. Using sterile gauze, dry the excess medication from the inner canthus to the outer canthus.

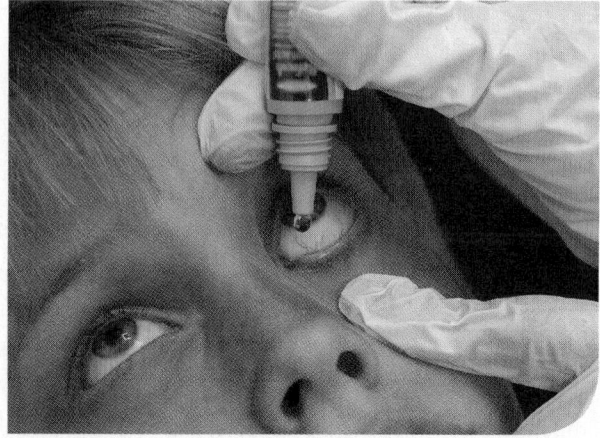

FIGURE 39-9   Instilling eye medication.

14. Explain to the patient that vision may be blurry.
15. Clean the area and dispose of unused medication.
16. Remove gloves and perform hand hygiene.
17. Document the procedure appropriately.

CHARTING EXAMPLE
09/12/XX 9:00 A.M. Instilled 2 gtt of 1 percent atropine sulfate to both eyes. Pt. complained of "stinging and blurry vision for a few minutes." · L. McKay, RMA

Changes in the Aging Eye

The eye ages just like the rest of the body. Because these changes may impair vision, care must be taken to instruct the elderly on safety issues. Their depth perception and difficulty seeing at night make them more vulnerable to falling. "Professionalism: The Life Span" lists some changes that occur in the structure and function of the eye with age.

Assisting the Visually-Impaired Patient

Blindness occurs due to accident, birth defect, injury, or disease. Some people are totally blind and have been that way since birth. Their frame of reference to the world depends on descriptions from others. Some individuals can sense light and dark but may not be able to discern anything else. Others have some vision but cannot read. To be declared legally blind, a person must only be able to see at 20 feet what a normal person would see at 200 feet. Those who have lost their sense of sight need special training and education. Blindness is a devastating impairment, both physically and psychologically.

The Study of the Ear

The study of hearing is known as **otology**. Physicians who specialize in the ear are otologists or **otorhinolaryngologists**, or ENT (ear, nose, and throat) doctors. Every physical examination includes an examination of the nose and throat as

inserted into the ear canal to examine the tympanic membrane. Figure 39-10 shows a physician performing an ear examination using an otoscope. A healthy eardrum should be pearly gray and concave. An infected eardrum appears reddened, swollen, and bulging. See Box 39-1 for an explanation of ear infections in children.

IRRIGATION OF THE EAR

Irrigation of the ear is necessary to remove impacted **cerumen** (earwax) or a foreign matter from the ear. Figure 39-11 shows irrigation of the ear. Patients may be apprehensive about the discomfort of the procedure, and it is your responsibility to put them at ease as much as possible. Procedure 39-6 outlines steps for irrigating the patient's ear.

INSTILLATION OF EAR MEDICATION

Instilling ear medication is also commonly performed by medical assistants. You may also be required to instruct a patient how to administer eardrops. You may use the same steps to instruct the patient that you would use performing instillation of medications in the office. Provide the patient with a printed list of instructions, and review the guidelines in the office. Ask the patient to demonstrate the steps prior to leaving the office to ensure that he or she

well as the ears. In patients, infections that affect the throat or nose may also affect the ear.

The ear is the organ of hearing and balance. Most parts of the ear are internal and are protected by the temporal bone of the skull. For a review of the structures and function of the ear, see Chapter 26.

INSTRUMENTS USED IN EAR EXAMINATIONS

The instruments used in the office for ear examinations are the otoscope, tuning fork, and audiometer. The otoscope is a lighted instrument with a small, disposable speculum that is

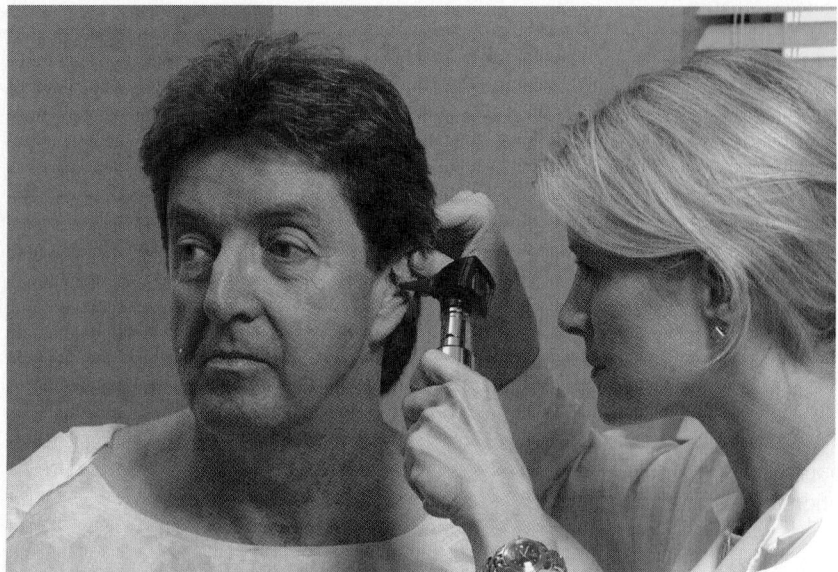

FIGURE 39-10 Examination of the ear using an otoscope.

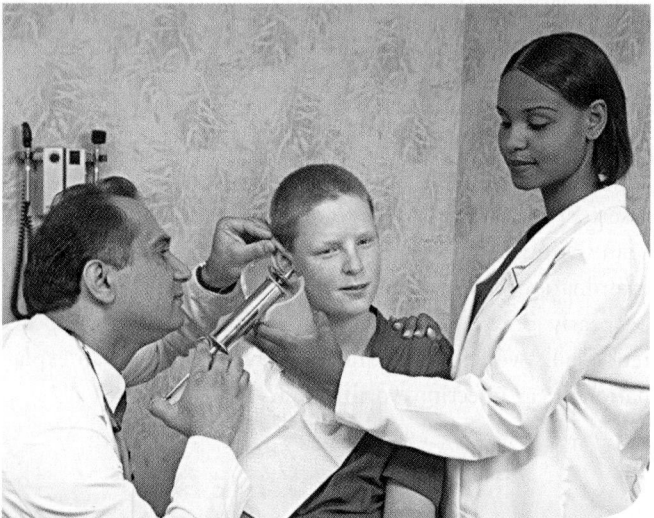

FIGURE 39-11 Ear irrigation.

understands the procedure. Procedure 39-7 provides the steps for performing instillation of eardrops.

Hearing Acuity

Hearing is essential in the process of learning to talk because speech is based on imitation of sounds and mimicking the way words are used to communicate. As with vision, there are many degrees of hearing loss. Various forms of hearing impairments fall into one of two main categories, sensorineural hearing loss and conduction hearing loss. **Sensorineural hearing loss**—nerve damage—is due to damage of the organ of Corti, or to the auditory nerve. The **organ of Corti**, located in the cochlea (part of the inner ear), contains hairlike fibers that convert the waves of sound that travel through the ear. The sound waves are then sent to the brain via the auditory nerve. When the sound waves reach the inner ear but are unable to be converted into electrical impulses that are sent to the brain, damage is present. Nerve deafness can be hereditary, or may be due to loud noises or viral infections. **Conduction hearing loss** is due to obstruction of sound waves; thus the sound waves never reach the organ of Corti. Foreign material or excess cerumen in the external ear canal, calcification of the bones in the middle ear, infection or fluid buildup in the middle ear, or a combination of these problems may cause conduction hearing loss.

A number of tests are used to evaluate **hearing acuity** (sharpness of hearing). The abbreviations AD (aurus dextra) for right ear, AS (aurus sinistra) for left ear, and AU (aurus

Box 39-1 Otitis Media in CHILDREN

Otitis media—middle ear infection or inflammation—is the most frequent ear problem in the pediatric patient, particularly those under 6 years of age. The several types of otitis media are acute, recurring, otitis media with effusion (fluid buildup in middle ear), and chronic otitis media.

Because of children's young age and their inability to explain how they feel, it is important to know the symptoms of earaches in children. In an upper respiratory infection, whether viral or bacterial, organisms may spread from the mucous membranes of the nose and throat through the Eustachian tube or auditory tube, which connects the nasopharynx and the middle ear. Allergies may also cause fluid buildup in the middle ear. When excess fluid or pus builds up in the middle ear, sound waves cannot be transmitted as easily and pressure on the tympanic membrane is

increased. The eardrum will become reddened and inflamed and bulging or convex. It may even rupture. In addition, ear pain can be intense. Signs that an infant or small child has an ear infection are pulling on ear, redness of external ear, drainage from ear, fever, crying, crankiness, and unsteadiness.

Treatment in the case of infection is usually antibiotics; if allergy related, an antihistamine will be prescribed. An analgesic to reduce fever and discomfort may also be necessary. Children who have frequent ear infections, regardless of the cause, run the risk of hearing impairment due to scarring of the eardrum. Scar tissue renders the tympanic membrane less flexible to incoming sound waves. In addition, chronic ear infections can lead to ossification of the tiny ear bones: The bones become fused together and cannot transmit sound waves effectively, leading to a form of conductive loss of hearing.

Surgical treatments for children with reoccurring ear infection are a myringotomy, or cutting of the eardrum to release pressure and insertion of a small plastic tube to permit drainage of the middle ear. After several months to a year, the tubes will fall out unassisted. When tubes are placed in the ear, it is important to restrict water from entering the ear canal. In such instances, earplugs should be used while shampooing and swimming.

procedure

39-6

IRRIGATION OF THE EAR

Objective: Irrigate ear following the physician's orders.

EQUIPMENT AND SUPPLIES

gloves; ear syringe; sterile basin; emesis basin; warm irrigation solution per physician's order; towels; cotton balls

METHOD

1. Check the physician's orders.
2. Perform hand hygiene.
3. Assemble the equipment.
4. Check the name, concentration, and expiration date of the irrigating solution three times.
5. Identify the patient, and explain the procedure.
6. Apply gloves.
7. Have the patient sit with the affected ear tilted slightly downward.
8. Place a towel over the patient's shoulder, and ask the patient to hold the emesis basin.
9. Clean the external ear with a moistened cotton ball.
10. Pour the warmed solution into a sterile basin and fill the syringe with 50 mL of solution.
11. For adults, pull the earlobe up and back to straighten the ear canal; for children under three years pull the earlobe down and back to straighten the ear canal.
12. Expel air from the syringe and insert the tip into the ear canal; aim the stream of flow toward the roof of the canal (Figure 39-12).
13. Repeat until the return from the ear is clear.
14. Remove the basin, dry the outer ear, and remove the towel.
15. Give the patient cotton balls to wipe any external drainage.

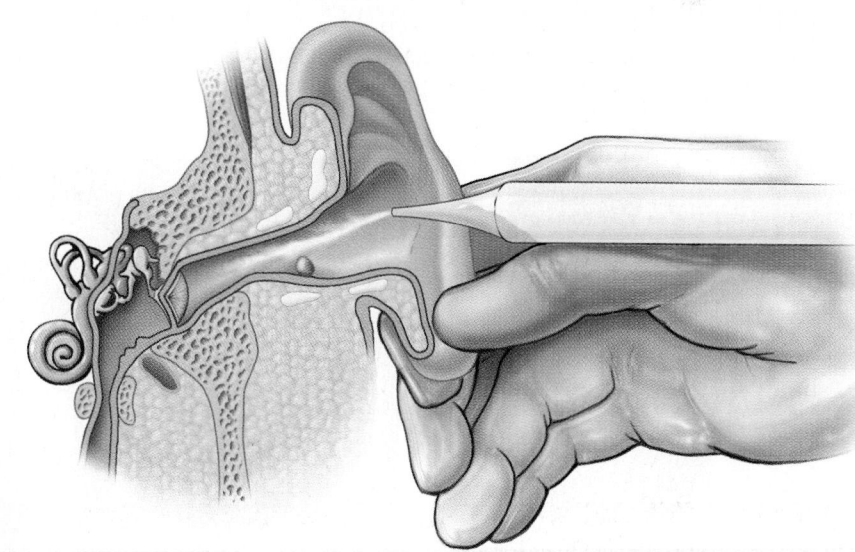

FIGURE 39-12 **Irrigating the ear to remove a foreign body.**

16. Instruct the patient about home care if needed. Ask the patient if he or she has any questions.
17. Dispose of any waste material properly.
18. Perform hand hygiene.
19. Document the procedure, noting the type of drainage and any patient symptoms such as pain or dizziness.

CHARTING EXAMPLE

2/14/XX 11:00 A.M. Ear irrigation to both ears. Cerumen plug removed from right ear. No pain or dizziness experienced. Patient remained lying on right side for 15 minutes.· M. King, CMA (AAMA)

INSTILLING EAR MEDICATION

Objective: Instill ear medication as ordered by physician.

EQUIPMENT AND SUPPLIES

otic drops in dropper bottle; cotton balls; disposable gloves

METHOD

1. Check physician's orders.
2. Perform hand hygiene.
3. Assemble the equipment.
4. Identify patient.
5. Check the medication label three times for the correct name, expiration date, and concentration.
6. If the medication is cold, warm it by rolling between the palms.
7. Have the patient tilt the head away from the affected ear or lie down with the affected ear facing up.
8. Pull the earlobe up and back for an adult (Figure 39-13), down and back for a child (Figure 39-14).
9. Place the dropper in the ear canal without touching the sides of the canal (Figure 39-15).
10. Instill the appropriate number of eardrops along the side of the canal.
11. Instruct the patient to remain in the same position for 3 to 5 minutes.
12. Give instructions for home care if needed. Ask the patient if he or she has any questions.
13. Dispose of the equipment and clean the area.
14. Perform hand hygiene.
15. Document the procedure appropriately.

CHARTING EXAMPLE

09/11/XX 7 P.M. 2 gtt Neosporin solution instilled in Rt ear. Pt verbally confirmed instruction for home instillation 2x days for 7 days. · C. Lynch, RMA

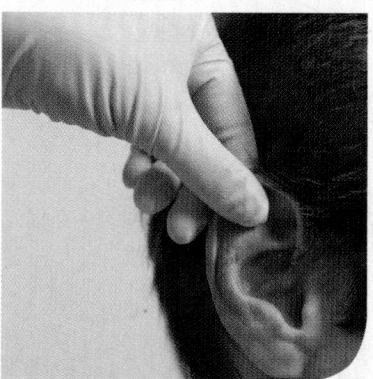

FIGURE 39-13 Straightening the ear canal of an adult by pulling the ear up and back.

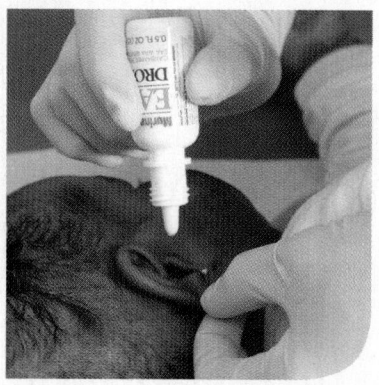

FIGURE 39-14 Straightening the ear canal of an infant by pulling the ear down and back.

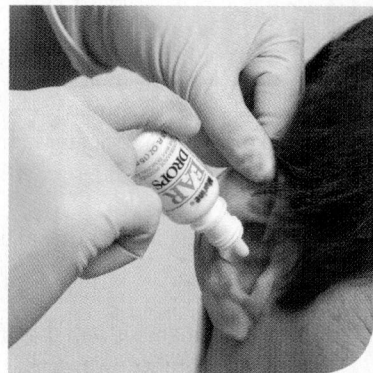

FIGURE 39-15 Instilling eardrops.

---

uterque) for both ears are used when charting results involving ears. However, it is recommended that whole words be used to designate each ear to avoid errors.

Hearing Assessment

A tuning fork is a metal, fork-shaped instrument that produces vibrations when struck. (Figure 39-16) The vibrating instrument is then held near the patient's ear or placed on various locations on the head to give a rough hearing assessment.

An **audiometer** (Figure 39-17) is an electronic instrument that measures more precisely the **frequencies** or the number of fluctuations per second of energy in the form of sound waves. The intensity of the sound, or **decibel** that patients hear is evaluated as well. When the patient indicates his or her ability to hear a sound, a recording is made. The **audiogram**, which is a record of patient responses, is then

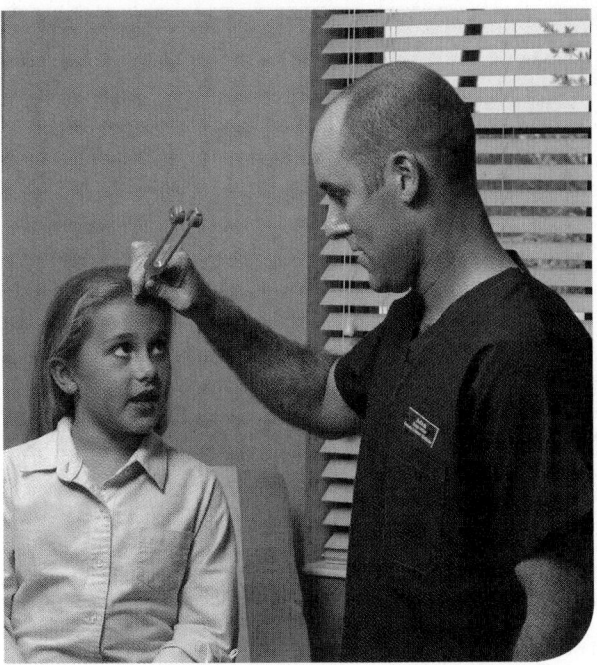

FIGURE 39-16 Testing hearing acuity using a tuning fork.

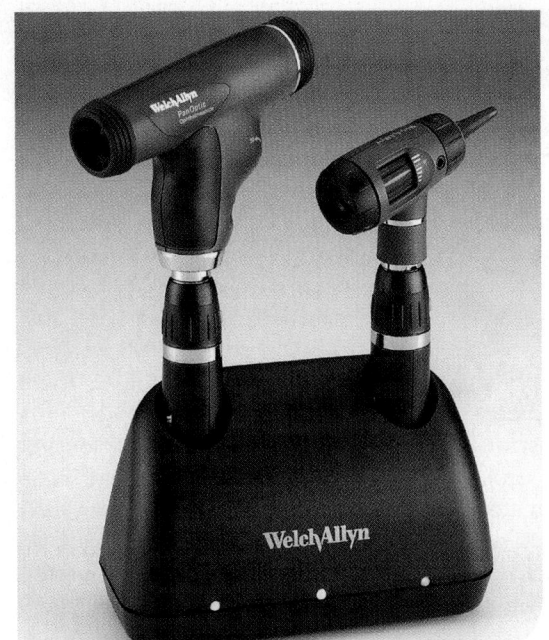

FIGURE 39-17 Audiometer.

used by the physician to evaluate the patient's hearing. A person with normal hearing should hear all frequencies up to 15 decibels under normal conditions. Prolonged exposure to loud noise over 85 decibels can cause temporary or permanent hearing loss. Figure 39-18 illustrates the decibel levels in various locations and associated with various conditions.

Many varieties of audiometers are in use today. Although most audiometers function in a similar way, it is important to follow the instructions provided by the manufacturer. Sales representatives often give in-service demonstrations to staff when an instrument is purchased. A procedure document should be drawn up based on the manufacturer's specifications for audiometer use and should be included in the office

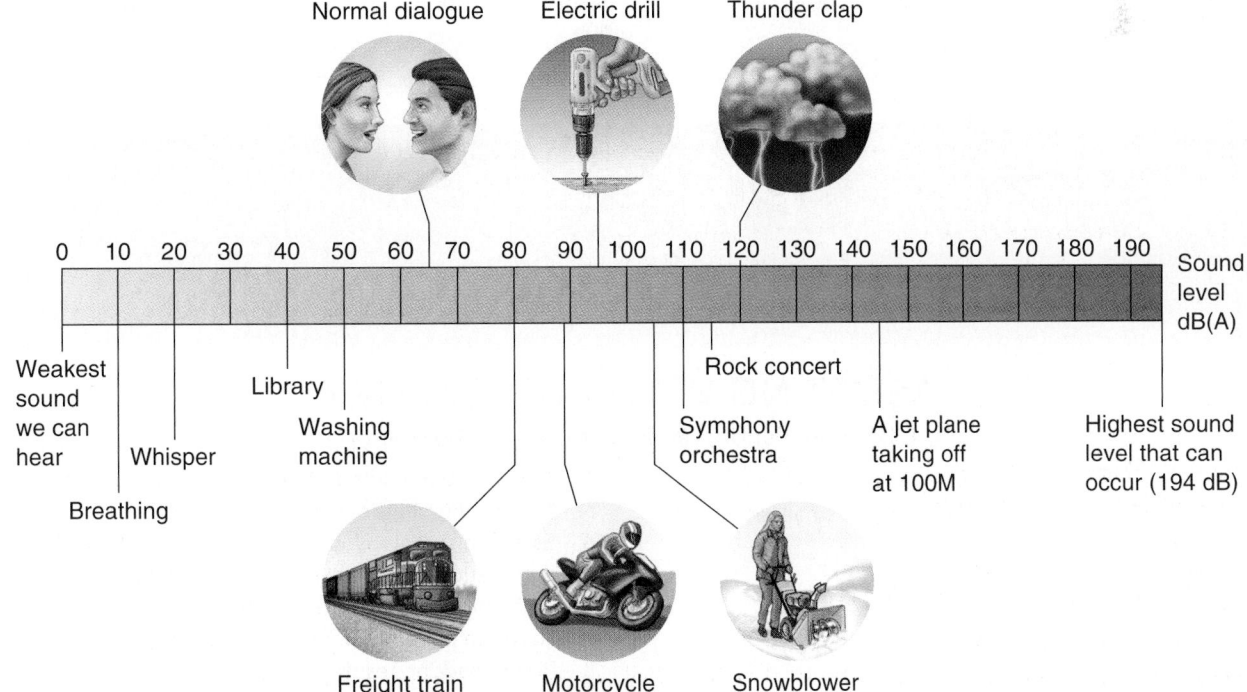

FIGURE 39-18 This illustration shows the decibel level in various locations and associated with different conditions.

Your occupation as a medical assistant often brings you into contact with other allied health professionals. To improve communication with other health care workers, it is important that you understand the duties and training of other members of the allied health team. Ophthalmic assistants work under the supervision of an ophthalmologist and work in offices or clinics. While some ophthalmologists hire medical assistants and train them on the job to perform the functions necessary in their office, others will only hire an ophthalmic assistant (OA). There are specific programs of training for the OA as there are for the medical assistant. The OA must have a high school diploma or equivalency and attend a clinical program approved by a review committee of ophthalmic medical personnel. An OA's duties include conducting acuity testing, tonometry, adjusting glasses, assisting during surgical procedures, and administering some eye medications. In addition, the OA may be trained in the use and care of more highly technical instruments. OA students who pass a national certification examination earn the title of certified ophthalmic assistant (COA). For information on this field, contact the Joint Commission on Allied Health Personnel in Ophthalmology, 2025 Woodlane Drive, St. Paul, MN 55125-2995, (800) 232-3937.

Another health professional you may encounter is the audiologist. An audiologist is an allied health professional who performs diagnostic hearing tests, assesses patient's hearing, fits hearing aids, teaches proper use of the hearing aid, and rehabilitates clients with hearing loss. To become an audiologist, one must graduate from an accredited, five-year master's degree program and pass a national certification examination. Audiologists work in hospitals, schools, and private offices. For further information on this profession contact the American Academy of Audiology.

policies and procedures manual. See Box 39-2 for information about dealing with other allied health professionals.

The medical assistant may be asked to perform an audiometer test and may do so if he or she has undergone the proper training. The physician will interpret the results and inform the patient of the outcome. You are not permitted to release results to a patient unless you have been specifically instructed to do so by the physician. Procedure 39-8 describes the steps for performing an audiometric test on a patient. Table 39-2 lists and explains some of the tests and procedures related to the ear.

ADDITIONAL DIAGNOSTIC TESTS

Tympanometry, a diagnostic test, is used to measure the ability of the myringa to move, thereby estimating the pressure in the middle ear. If the middle ear is filled with fluid, the tympanic membrane will be more rigid. A printout of the results is produced for the physician to evaluate.

procedure
39-8

ASSISTING WITH AUDIOMETRY
Objective: Perform audiometric test without error.

EQUIPMENT AND SUPPLIES
audiometer with headphones; quiet room or small, enclosed cubicle; patient's record; pen
METHOD
1. Check the physician's orders.
2. Perform hand hygiene.
3. Prepare the equipment.
4. Test the equipment and make sure the power is on.
5. Identify the patient, and explain the procedure.
6. Establish signal response that patient will give if no automatic button is available; nodding head or holding up a finger are acceptable signals (Figure 39-19).
7. Have the patient assume a comfortable position.
8. Place headphones over the patient's ears.

9. Begin with low frequency and watch the patient for indication that the sound is heard; push the button to record if the machine does not do it automatically.
10. Gradually increase the frequency until the test is completed in the first ear.
11. Proceed to the other ear and repeat the entire procedure.
12. Remove the headphones.
13. Clean the equipment following the manufacturer's instructions.
14. Perform hand hygiene.
15. Document the procedure appropriately.

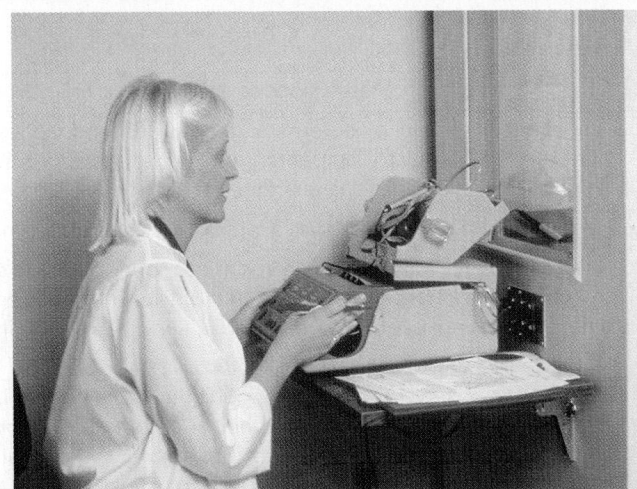
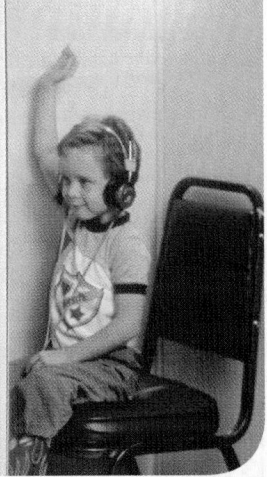

FIGURE 39-19 Performing a hearing test on a child.

CHARTING EXAMPLE

2/14/XX 9:00 A.M. Audiometry test administered in both ears. Results given to Dr. Williams. · · · · · · · M. King, CMA (AAMA)

The **electronystagmograph (ENG)** is a special examination that evaluates balance through measurement of the movement of the eyes. ENG is used to evaluate patients with vertigo (a false sense of spinning or motion that can cause dizziness) and other disorders that affect hearing and vision. Electrodes are placed above and below the eye to record electrical activity. By measuring electrical changes in the electrical field in the eye, an ENG can detect nystagmus (involuntary rapid eye movement) in response to stimuli.

There are several different types of ENG examinations. In the water caloric test, warm or cool water is placed into the ear canal so that it touches the tympanic membrane. Air can also be used in this procedure instead of water for patients who have a damaged eardrum. A normal response to the stimuli means no nystagmus. If nystagmus does occur on stimulation, a problem may exist within the ear, nerves associated with the ear, or certain parts of the brain.

Assisting the Hearing-Impaired Patient

It is important to provide for the comfort level of the hearing-impaired patient as much as possible in your office setting. Accommodations, such as having available telephones with hearing amplifiers, demonstrate that your care is patient centered. It is important not to lose patience with the patient who is having difficulty hearing your instructions. Remember to face the patient when speaking to him or her and to speak clearly without raising your voice.

Presbycusis is a decline in hearing acuity and a normal part of aging. Elderly patients may be reluctant to admit that they are having hearing problems, but the family will frequently volunteer the information. Signs like speaking louder, turning up the radio or television, and not hearing

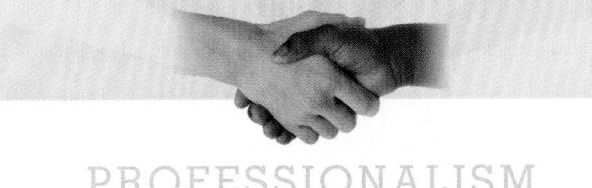

PROFESSIONALISM
CULTURAL CONSIDERATIONS

Though many hearing-impaired patients are able to read lips, some patients will bring along interpreters to assist with the appointment. When working with a patient via an interpreter, it is important to always direct your questions toward the patient. Consider learning a few common sign language signs, such as alphabetic letters and the sign for "Thank you."

TABLE 39-2 Procedures and Diagnostic Tests Related to the Ear

Procedure/Test	Description
Audiogram	Chart that shows the faintest sounds a patient can hear during audiometry testing.
Audiometric test	Test of hearing ability by determining the lowest and highest intensity and frequencies that a person can distinguish. The patient may sit in a soundproof booth and receive sounds through earphones as the technician changes the volume and tones.
Electrocochleography	Recording of the electrical activity produced when the cochlea is stimulated.
Electronystagmography	Recording of eye movement in response to specific stimuli, such as sound, water, or air. It is used to determine the presence and location of a lesion in the vestibule of the ear, to help diagnose unilateral hearing loss of unknown origin, and to help identify the cause of vertigo, tinnitus, and dizziness.
Falling test	Test used to observe balance and equilibrium. The patient is observed standing on one foot, then with one foot in front of the other, and then walking forward with eyes open. The same test is conducted with the patient's eyes closed. Swaying and falling with the eyes closed can indicate an ear and equilibrium malfunction.
Mastoid antrotomy	Surgical opening made in the cavity within the mastoid process to alleviate pressure from infection and allow for drainage.
Mastoid X-ray	X-ray taken of the mastoid bone to determine infection, which can be an extension of a middle ear infection.
Myringoplasty	Surgical reconstruction of the eardrum.
Myringotomy	Surgical puncture of the eardrum with removal of fluid and pus from the middle ear; it is used to eliminate a persistent ear infection and excessive pressure on the tympanic membrane. A tube is placed in the tympanic membrane to allow drainage of the middle ear cavity.
Otoplasty	Corrective surgery to change the size of the external ear or pinna. The surgery can either enlarge or decrease the size of the pinna.
Otoscopy	The use of a lighted instrument to examine the external auditory canal and the middle ear.
Rinne and Weber tuning fork tests	The physician holds a tuning fork, an instrument that produces a constant pitch when it is struck against or near the bones on the side of the head. These tests assess both nerve and bone conduction of sound, although in very different ways. *Rinne test:* The examiner places the base of the vibrating fork against the patient's mastoid bone and in front of the auditory meatus (air conduction). *Weber test:* The tuning fork is placed on the center of the forehead.
Stapedectomy	Removal of the stapes bone to treat otosclerosis (hardening of the bone). A prosthesis or artificial stapes is implanted.
Tympanometry	Measurement of the movement of the tympanic membrane that can indicate pressure in the middle ear.
Tympanoplasty	Another term for the surgical reconstruction of the eardrum. Also called myringoplasty.

what is said from another room are all indications that hearing loss has occurred. As a medical assistant, you must handle these situations with delicacy. Your responsibility is to act in the patient's best interest and speak to the physician about your concerns. Other signs of aging are narrowing of the ear canal, dryness of earwax, lessened flexibility of the eardrum, and sclerosis of the ear bones.

EAR SAFETY GUIDELINES

Remind patients never to put anything in the ear canal. Earwax is a protective substance produced by the body to prevent foreign objects and substances from getting to the eardrum. Attempting to remove earwax is a dangerous habit and could cause perforation of the tympanic membrane.

Patients must understand the connection between repetitive exposure to loud noise and deafness. Young people who listen to loud music on earphones or at concerts are particularly susceptible to this danger. Workers who must engage in duties that require them to be exposed to loud noise should wear protective ear gear.

Patients who are hearing impaired and cannot use devices such as hearing aids may need other strategies to help

Examination of the Nose and Throat

Examination of the nose and throat is part of a physical examination and is considered routine in most offices. The physician will use a nasal speculum to inspect the mucous lining of the nose for signs of irritation and infection. He or she will use a tongue depressor to examine the throat for signs of infection, enlarged tonsils, and abnormalities of the tongue or oral cavity. If signs of infection are present in the throat, a throat culture may be ordered to determine the infecting agent. An appropriate antibiotic will then be ordered for the patient. The most common cause of throat infection is the *Streptococcus* bacteria, group A. When untreated, this organism can cause secondary infections and possibly serious damage to the kidney, heart, and other organs. Signs and symptoms of nasal problems include nosebleeds or epistaxis, reduced sense of smell, congestion, and allergic rhinitis (inflammation of the lining of the nose). See Procedure 39-9 for steps to assist with instilling nasal medication.

increase their awareness of their surroundings at home. Devices such as doorbells that light up when rung, telephone amplifiers, and close-captioned television are accommodations that help the hearing impaired.

procedure

39-9

INSTILLING NASAL MEDICATIONS

Objective: Instill nasal medication as ordered by the physician.

EQUIPMENT AND SUPPLIES

physician's order; patient's record; nasal medication; sterile medicine dropper; tissues; gloves

METHOD

1. Check physician's orders
2. Perform hand hygiene.
3. Assemble the equipment. Apply gloves.
4. Identify the patient and explain the procedure.
5. Position the patient with head lower than the shoulders to instill medication into the ethmoid and sphenoid sinuses. To instill medication into the maxillary and frontal sinuses, have the patient assume the same back-lying

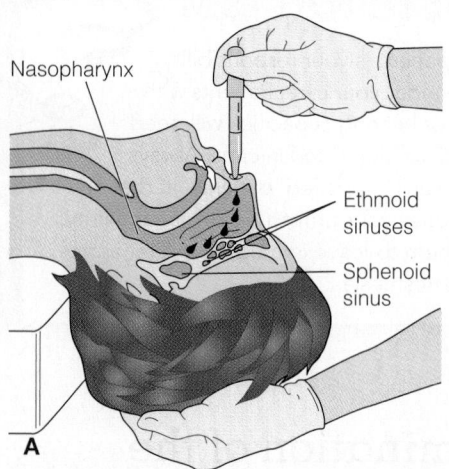

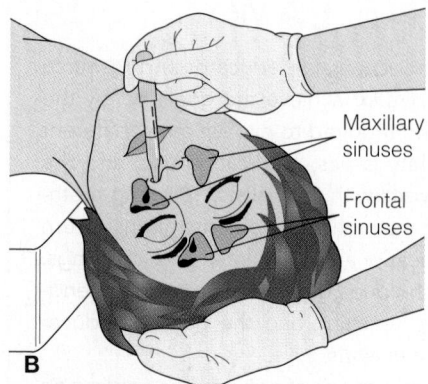

FIGURE 39-20 **(A) Instilling nosedrops into the ethmoid and sphenoid sinuses; (B) instilling nosedrops into the maxillary and frontal sinuses.**

position with the head turned toward the side to be treated (Figure 39-20A–B). Place patient in a supine position with a pillow under the neck to lower the head below the shoulders. Make the patient as comfortable as possible.

6. Check the medication three times for correct name, dosage, and expiration date. Draw the medication into a dropper and hold it over the center of the affected nostril, taking care not to touch the dropper to the inside of the nostril.

7. Administer the medication. Repeat in the other nostril if ordered.

8. Tell the patient to stay in that position for 5 minutes to prevent medication from running out of the nostril.

9. Provide tissues for the patient to wipe excess from the skin.

10. Discard the dropper in the biohazard waste container, recap the medication, and return it to the storage place.

11. Clean the area and remove gloves.

12. Provide home instruction if needed. Verify patient understanding.

13. Perform hand hygiene.

14. Document the procedure in patient's record.

CHARTING EXAMPLE

09/13/XX 9 A.M. Afrin nasal drops 3 gtt per nostril instilled per Dr. Schwartz. · N. Lynch, RMA

SUMMARY

In this chapter, we have considered signs and symptoms of disorders of the eye and ear. As a multiskilled health care professional, you will be expected to assist with or perform a number of technical functions while you aid the physician. The procedures in this chapter deal with irrigating the eye and ear and instilling medications in the eye and ear. You will be expected to be able to accomplish these independently and without error. In addition, you will be asked to assess both visual and hearing acuity using the procedures provided in this chapter. Dealing with special needs patients, such as children, the elderly, patients with dementia, or those who are illiterate, requires extra skills. Knowing the changes in vision and hearing that occur with age enables you to be more sensitive to these patients. Educating the patient to perform certain technical skills, such as administering eye and ear medications at home, is an important factor in his or her treatment. As a patient advocate, you can encourage eye and ear safety suggestions. At all times, it is your responsibility to provide the most respectful and empathetic care for the patient.

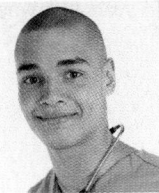

39 CHAPTER REVIEW

COMPETENCY REVIEW

1. Define and spell the terms to learn for this chapter.

2. Develop a teaching plan for a young child with strabismus.

3. What are several precautions the medical assistant should take in the office to assist the hearing-impaired elderly patient?

4. Explain how you would remove impacted cerumen from the ear canal of a 40-year-old male.

5. A patient has a visual acuity reading of 20/10 in the left eye. Using this information, answer the following questions:
   A. How far was the patient from the eye chart?
   B. At what distance would a person with normal acuity be able to read this line?

6. Mrs. Evans is 81 years old and has a contrast sensitivity test result below normal. List several conditions that could cause this abnormal result.

7. When measuring visual acuity, explain why you would not permit a patient to do the following:
   A. study the Snellen eye chart
   B. close his or her eye while testing using Snellen eye chart

8. A 2-year-old child must have a myringotomy and tympanoplasty performed because the child has had more than six bouts of otitis media within 1 year. Explain to the parents what these procedures entail.

PREPARING FOR THE CERTIFICATION EXAM

1. On the Snellen eye chart, the symbol on the top line can be read by people with normal vision at a distance of
   a. 100 feet
   b. 200 feet
   c. 150 feet
   d. 20 feet
   e. 50 feet

2. An illuminated instrument used to examine the ear is an
   a. ophthalmoscope
   b. anoscope
   c. otoscope
   d. cystoscope
   e. sigmoidoscope

3. To measure intraocular pressure the instrument used is the
   a. eye spud
   b. ophthalmoscope
   c. probe
   d. tonometer
   e. otoscope

4. Infection of the ear involving fluid buildup behind the ear drum is
   a. otitis externa
   b. otitis media
   c. pruritis
   d. ossicles
   e. rhinitis

5. Hearing loss associated with age is
   a. myopia
   b. myringa
   c. presbyopia
   d. presbycusis
   e. anacusis

6. Ear irrigations are performed
   a. daily
   b. to remove cerumen, foreign matter
   c. as part of every physical examination
   d. to relieve conjunctivitis
   e. to relieve retinitis

7. What chart is used to measure near vision acuity?
   a. Snellen
   b. Pelli-Robson
   c. Jaeger
   d. Ishihara
   e. nomogram

8. Impaired color vision
   a. is a factor of age
   b. is hereditary
   c. is more common in females
   d. is correctable with surgery
   e. is not important

9. To straighten the ear canal of a child under 3 years you would
   a. pull the earlobe down and back
   b. pull the ear lobe up and back
   c. leave the ear lobe untouched
   d. straighten the ear drum
   e. ask the parent to do it

10. The term used to describe someone who is nearsighted is
   a. emmetropic
   b. hyperopic
   c. myopic
   d. presbyopic
   e. astigmatic

CRITICAL THINKING

1. What do Kyle's results of the Snellen examination mean? What would you tell Kyle about his results?

2. What explanations would you use to convince Kyle to let you instill the eyedrops? What would you do if he still resisted?

3. What precautions should you use before using any eye medications, and why?

4. Dr. Sims gives Kyle's parents a prescription for eyeglasses. When they leave the room, he tells you that he is not going to wear them and look like a "geek" no matter what! How should you handle this?

5. Are you obligated to tell Kyle's parents and Dr. Sims about his feelings?

ON THE JOB

Agnes Jones, the medical assistant in a busy ENT office, is asked to transcribe the following ophthalmology report for the physician:

Reason for consultation—evaluation of progressive loss of vision in right eye.

History of present illness—Patient has noted a gradual deterioration of vision and increasing photophobia over the past year, particularly in the right eye. She states that it feels like there is a film over her right eye. She denies any change of vision in her left eye.

Results of physical examination—Visual acuity test showed no changes in this patient's long-standing hyperopia. The eye muscles function properly, and there is no evidence of conjunctivitis or nystagmus. The pupils react properly to light. Intraocular pressure is within normal limits (WNL). Ophthalmoscopy after application of mydriatic drops revealed presence of a large, opaque cataract forming in the right eye. There is no evidence of retinopathy, macular degeneration, or keratitis.

1. The results of the physical exam state that the patient's pupils react properly to light. What does this mean? How do pupils react in bright and dim light? Why is this important?
2. This patient wears corrective lenses for which condition?
   A. farsightedness
   B. nearsightedness
   C. abnormal curvature of the cornea
3. The patient history states that Ms. Jones does not have nystagmus or conjunctivitis. Explain these two conditions.

INTERNET ACTIVITY

LASIK surgery is a popular eye procedure. Research it on the Internet. If you were a candidate for this procedure, would you have it done? Why, or why not? How will the information you obtain help you in dealing with patients?

MEDMEDIA

Additional interactive resources and activities for this chapter can be found:

On your student DVD: View applicable procedure videos on the DVD-ROM found in the back of this book.

MyHealthProfessionsKit.com: Test your knowledge of this chapter with games and activities. MyHealthProfessionsKit also includes resources, helpful links, and a Spanish audio glossary.

Medical Assisting Interactive: Practice your procedures as a medical assistant in this simulated doctor's office. This can be accessed through MyHealthProfessionsKit.com.

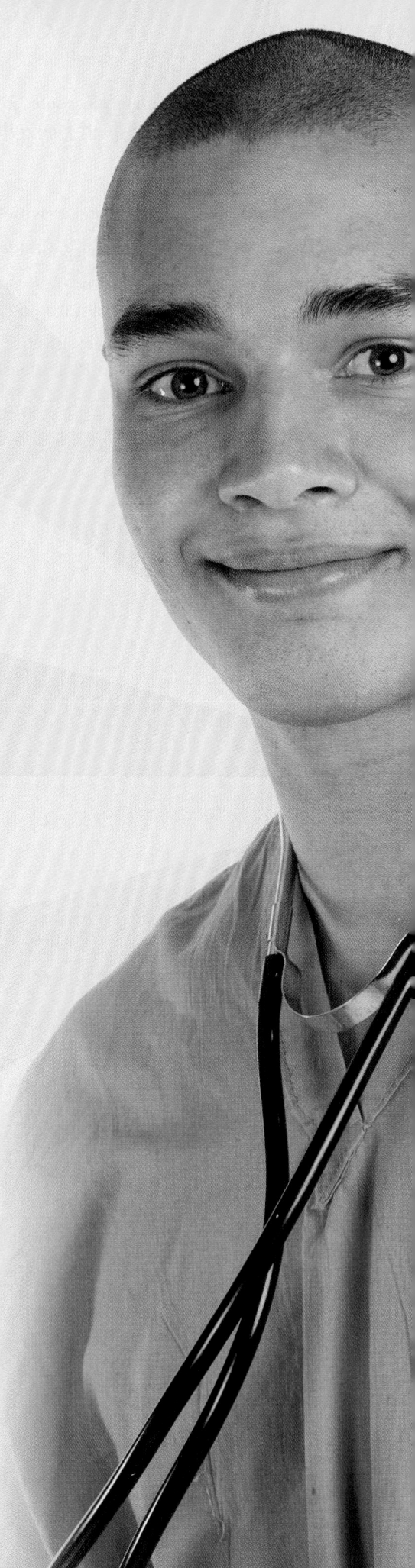

40

Assisting with Life Span Specialties: Pediatrics

LEARNING OBJECTIVES

After reading this chapter, you should be able to:

- Define and spell the terms to learn in the chapter.

- Identify and explain childhood growth and development patterns.

- Accurately measure a child's height, weight, and head and chest circumference.

- Calculate growth percentiles.

- Correctly apply a pediatric urine collection device.

- Describe some emotional and physical signs of adolescence.

- Distinguish among three types of eating disorders.

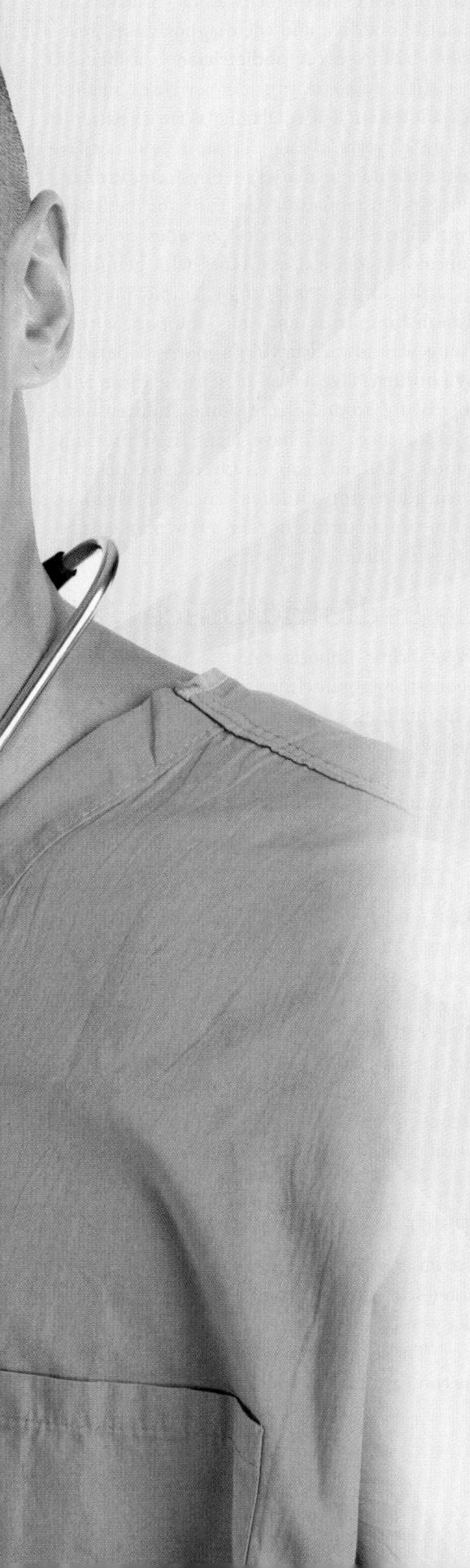

CHAPTER OUTLINE

CASE STUDY

Keyla Jefferson, age 18 months, is being seen by Dr. Penningworth for a well-child check. Dr. Penningworth is concerned about Keyla's size and developmental delays. He diagnoses her with failure to thrive.

adolescence

amenorrhea

anorexia nervosa

BRAT diet

bronchiolitis

bulimia nervosa

croup

excoriation

failure to thrive (FTT)

febrile seizures

genitalia

hydrocephalus

meatus

microencephaly

myringotomy

pediatrician

purging

respiratory syncytial virus (RSV)

rhinovirus

sleep apnea

stridor

sudden infant death syndrome (SIDS)

tonsillectomy

CERTIFICATION LINK

CMA (AAMA)
Communication
  Adapting communication according to an individual's needs
Patient preparation and assisting the physician
  Vital signs
  Examinations

RMA
General medical assisting knowledge
  Human relations
Clinical medical assisting
  Physical examinations
  Vital signs and mensurations

CMAS
Examination preparation

This chapter discusses assisting the pediatric population of patients. Pediatric office visits include well-child visits and sick-child visits. During well-child visits, medical assistants perform measurements such as height, weight, head and chest circumference, and vital signs, then record the information on growth charts. This chapter reviews childhood diseases and disorders, including such conditions as croup and upper respiratory infections, and their diagnoses and treatments. Inherited disorders such as cystic fibrosis and thalassemia, or conditions such as autism and sudden infant death syndrome (SIDS), also are included. Since injuries are the number-one cause of death in children, safety issues in the office and at home are discussed with an emphasis on educating caregivers. Physical and mental changes associated with puberty and dealing with eating disorders also are discussed.

Assisting in Pediatrics

Pediatrics is the branch of medicine dealing with the care and development of children and the diagnosis and treatment of childhood illnesses. A **pediatrician** is a medical doctor who specializes in the treatment of newborns, infants, children, and adolescents. Pediatricians treat patients from birth to age 20 years. At age 20 most pediatricians recommend patients find a primary care physician. Primary care physicians and osteopaths also care for pediatric patients. Subspecialties of pediatrics includes pediatric surgery and oncology. Medical assistants who genuinely like working with children may enjoy employment in pediatrics. Establishing trust and good rapport with a child goes a long way toward having a more cooperative patient. Many children have a way of sensing those who are comfortable being around them. Some children have had negative experiences and have fears from previous medical encounters. You may gain children's confidence if you smile when addressing children, speak to them at their level and in simple terms, or take a few moments to interact or play with them.

The Pediatric Office

Several factors of prime importance in a pediatric office include telephone triage guidelines, safety of infants and children, and maintaining a healthy environment for these young patients. Filling out the vast numbers of forms encountered in pediatrics (school physical, sports, and health insurance forms) correctly and in a timely fashion is also salient.

TELEPHONE TRIAGE

Telephone triage guidelines for the office staff could be a matter of life and death in the pediatric office. It is important for the physician to establish the guidelines to ensure the truly sick child gets attention quickly and to screen the other calls effectively. Office staff should be well trained in handling calls and triaging appropriately. In some states triaging can only be done by nurses and is beyond the scope of medical assisting practice. Every medical assistant should be aware of his or her state's regulations.

OFFICE RECEPTION ROOM

The reception room in a pediatric office must be bright, welcoming, and interesting. Toys for various age groups should be available. Easy-to-clean plastic toys without tiny pieces are most practical. The reception room is a place for well children to pass the time before their appointment. Sick children

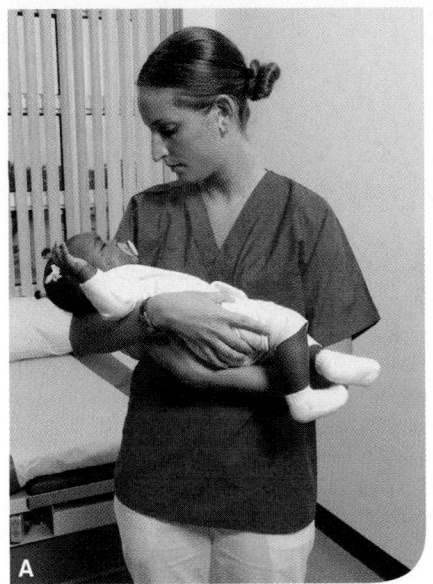
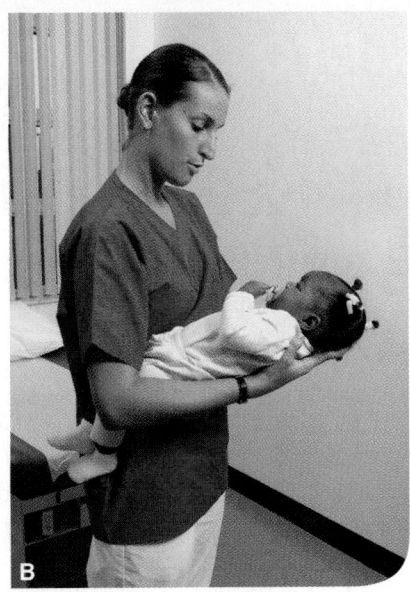
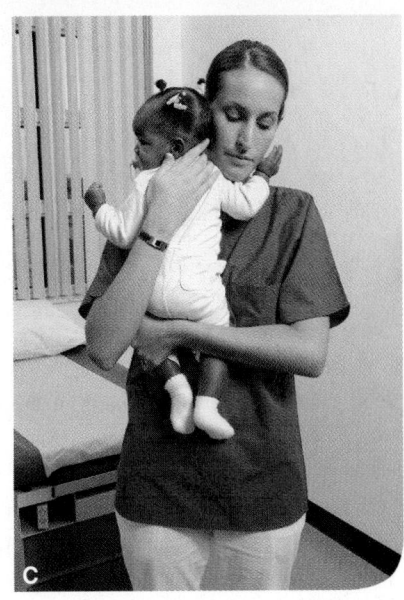

FIGURE 40-1   (A) the cradle hold; (B) the football hold; (C) the shoulder hold.

should be brought directly into an examination room, if possible, to avoid spreading infection. During office hours, toys should be picked up as needed and put away to prevent falls. Sanitizing toys should be done on a regular basis.

PATIENT SAFETY

Once the child enters your office, his or her safety is your prime concern. No child should be left alone on an examining table, scale, toilet, or other place that could pose a danger. Always place your hand on the infant to protect him or her from falling. When carrying an infant, it is helpful to have noticed the way the caregiver holds the child; this position is most likely preferred by the infant. Three positions used for carrying an infant: the cradle hold, the football hold, and the shoulder or upright hold, are shown in Figure 40-1A–C. Support the infant's head when using the upright position. At times, it may be necessary to restrict the movements of the infant or small child to perform a procedure or evaluation. A small sheet or receiving blanket may be used to wrap the child in "papoose fashion," binding the arms to his or her sides (Figure 40-2). To restrain movement of the head, hold your hands on either side of the head and avoid sealing off the ears or touching the fontanel (soft spots) on the baby's head. Procedure 40-1 provides the steps to follow for correctly wrapping an infant.

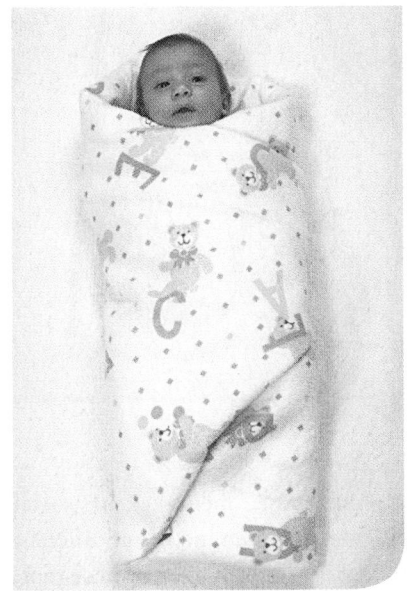

FIGURE 40-2   A baby wrapped for self-containment.

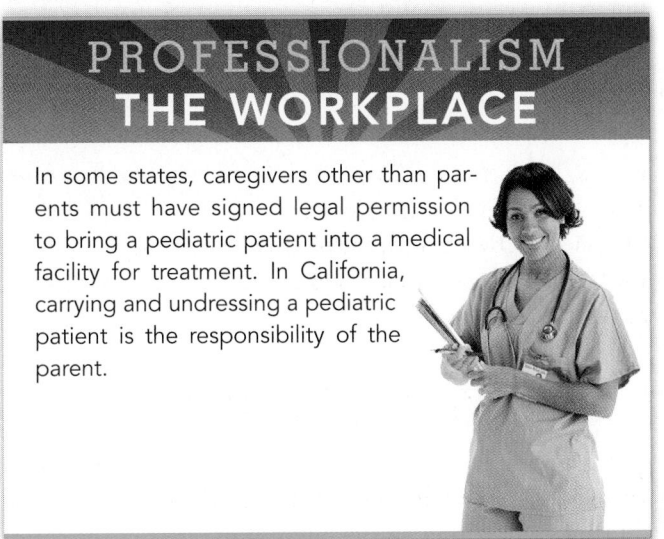

PROFESSIONALISM
THE WORKPLACE

In some states, caregivers other than parents must have signed legal permission to bring a pediatric patient into a medical facility for treatment. In California, carrying and undressing a pediatric patient is the responsibility of the parent.

WRAPPING AN INFANT OR SMALL CHILD

Objective: Wrap an infant or small child securely to restrain movement.

EQUIPMENT AND SUPPLIES

small sheet or receiving blanket; examination table; patient's record; pen

METHOD

1. Introduce yourself to the parent and child
2. Speak to the child in soft soothing tones and explain to the parent or child what you are going to do.
3. Perform hand hygiene.
4. Place the child on the table. Have the parent undress the child or undress as needed.
5. Place a receiving blanket or small sheet on table and fold down the top corner. Fold the bottom corner up.

Note: Size of sheet or blanket depends on age and size of child.

6. Place the child diagonally on the blanket, keeping one hand on the abdomen to ensure safety (Figure 40-3).

7. Wrap the right corner across the torso, covering the right arm, and tuck snugly under the left arm.
8. Wrap the left corner across the torso, covering the left arm, and tuck snugly under the torso.
9. To restrain the head place yourself at the end of the table where the infant's head is located and place one hand on either side of the head. Avoid sealing the ears or touching the fontanels.
10. Speak soothingly to comfort the child and allay fears as much as possible.
11. When the procedure is completed, pick up and comfort the child for a few moments. Then proceed to redress or continue with the examination as directed.
12. Clean the examination room.
13. Perform hand hygiene.

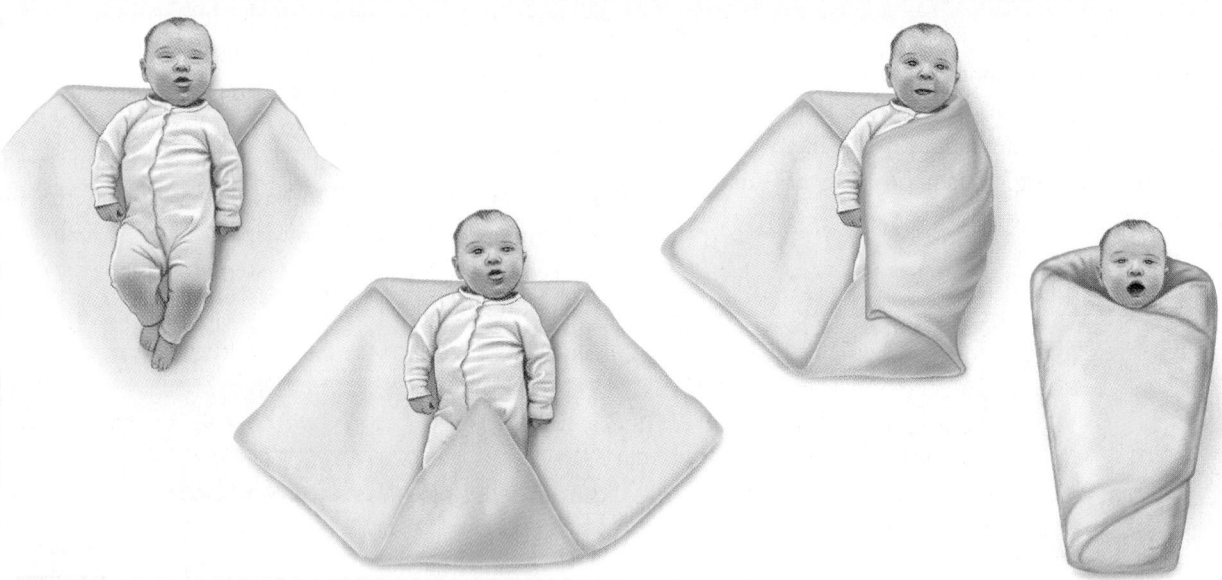

FIGURE 40-3 How to wrap and secure a baby's arms.

The Pediatric Patient

Growth and development refer to changes the child makes as he or she grows and matures. Growth patterns provide valuable information on the physical progress of the child.

Development refers to the motor, mental, and social progress that the child achieves. Children mature at different rates; however, the stages they pass through are consistent, as are the age ranges. The pediatrician looks for markers to detect abnormalities in growth, social, emotional, and

TABLE 40-1 Checklist of Developmental Skills for Young Children from Birth to 5 Years

Age	Developmental Check
Birth to 1 month	Generally helpless, dependent on mother, soothed by rocking motions and soothing sounds.
1–2 months	Raises head from surface when lying on stomach; pays attention to someone's face in his or her line of vision; moves arms and legs in energetic manner; likes to be held.
2–3 months	Smiles and recognizes voices; coos and makes other vocal sounds; rolls partially to the side when lying on back; is startled by loud sounds.
3–4 months	Eyes follow moving object; able to hold head erect; grasps objects in hands; babbles; laughs out loud; rolls from stomach to back; recognizes bottle and familiar faces.
4–5 months	Reaches for and holds objects; stands firmly when held; stretches out arms to be picked up; likes to play peek-a-boo; turns toward sound of a voice; tracks moving objects easily.
5–6 months	Turns from back to stomach; turns toward sounds; sits with a little support; reaches for objects out of reach; listens to own voice; crows and squeals; reaches for and grasps objects and brings them to mouth; holds, sucks, bites cookies and begins chewing.
6–7 months	Transfers an object from one hand to the other; sits for a few minutes alone; pats and smiles at image in mirror; creeps, pulling body with arms and leg kicks; shy at first with strangers; distinguishes emotions by voice tones.
7–8 months	Sits steadily for five minutes; crawls on hands and knees; grasps things with thumb and first two fingers; likes to be near parent; fears strangers.
8–9 months	Says mama or dada; responds to own name; can stand for a short time holding on to support; eats with fingers; can pick up small objects; responds to no.
10–12 months	Pulls self up at side of crib or playpen; drinks from a cup when it is held; walks around holding on to furniture; waves bye bye; repeats a few words; eats solid foods; eats with fingers.
12–15 months	Walks by self; pulls toys while walking; shows wants by pointing and gesturing; scribbles on paper after shown; begins to use a spoon; cooperates with dressing; dumps out toys from container and replaces them.
15–18 months	Builds a tower with blocks; likes to climb and take things apart; can say 6 words; tries to put on own shoes; drinks from a cup held in both hands; follows one-step directions; throws a ball; points to objects or pictures when they are named.
18 months to 2 years	Runs, walks up and down stairs using alternate feet; says at least 50 to 200 words; sometimes uses 2 word sentences; points to objects in a book; undresses with help; capable of bowel control.
2–3 years	Can repeat 2 numbers in a row; knows his or her sex; dresses self except for buttoning; can copy a circle; can follow commands of on, under, or behind (stand on the rug); knows most parts of the body; jumps, lifting both feet off the ground; can build tower of 9 blocks; can name a color; stays dry during the day and night.
4–5 years	Can repeat a simple 6-word sentence; can wash hands and face without help; can copy a cross; can stand on one foot; can catch a tossed ball; can skip; follows three commands.

Note: If a child is late doing several activities in a time period, seek further evaluation. A child born prematurely will be delayed by the number of months he/she was born early.

intellectual development. The earlier a problem is detected, the better the outcome for the child. Information from each office visit is compared to national standards and charts. It is important for you to understand the stages of growth and development in your role as health care provider. Table 40-1 is a checklist of the various physical, mental, and social developmental skills children achieve during their first 5 years.

APGAR SCORING

Immediately after birth the newborn is assessed using the Apgar scoring system. This is a method of evaluating a newborn's condition at 1 and 5 minutes after birth. If a newborn scores less than 7 at 5 minutes after birth, the child must be evaluated every 5 minutes for 20 more minutes. Physicians may intubate an infant if two or more scores are not 7 or higher. Table 40-2 illustrates Apgar scoring.

TABLE 40-2 Apgar Scoring

Sign	0	1	2
Heart rate	Absent	Slow (less than 110)	Over 100
Respiratory Effort	Absent	Slow, irregular	Good crying
Muscle Tone	Flaccid	Some flexion of extremities	Active motion
Reflex irritability	No response	Cry	Vigorous cry
Color	Blue, pale	Body pink, extremities blue	Completely pink

- Newborns scoring 7–10 are considered out of immediate danger.

- Newborns scoring 4–6 are considered moderately depressed.

- Newborns scoring 0–3 are severely depressed.

Pediatric Office Visits and Procedures

Pediatric office visits are divided into well-child visits and sick-child visits. During well-child visits, growth and development are measured, immunizations are given, and health information is provided. Well-baby visits are scheduled routinely after birth: 1 month, 2 months, 4 months, 6 months, 9 months, 12 months, 15 months, 18 months, 24 months, and then on a yearly basis. Immunization schedules for pediatric patients are discussed in Chapter 53.

During a sick-child visit, the ill child is brought in for examination to diagnose and recommend treatment for an illness. Most pediatric offices allow time in the daily schedule for sick-child visits.

Newborns through adolescents come in for both well-child and sick-child visits. Allowing for their differences and providing age-relevant care is vital. Adolescents especially may be embarrassed to be examined by the physician in front of parents and other staff members. Offer them as much privacy as possible, and provide adequate gowns and draping to support their sense of modesty.

GROWTH

The average infant weighs about 7 pounds at birth. By 6 months, that weight has doubled, and at a year the child's length has doubled and the weight tripled. The child will not experience a similar growth spurt until he or she reaches puberty. By 3 years old, the child reaches half his or her adult height. From ages 5 to 10, the child grows 2 to 3 inches and gains 3 to 5 pounds yearly. Infants and small children grow from the top down, with the head growing considerably in the first 4 months. Adult proportions will not be reached until about age 12 years. See Figure 40-4A–E for examples of developmental stages in children.

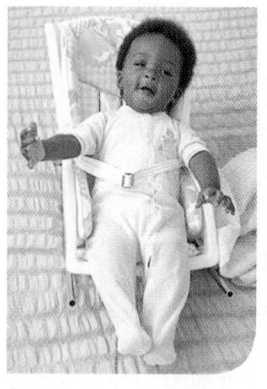 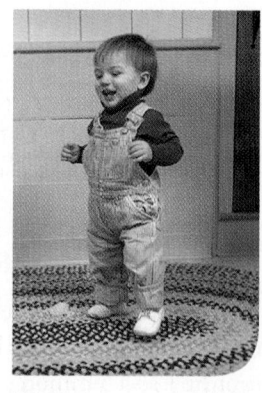 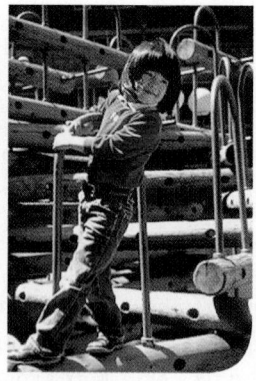 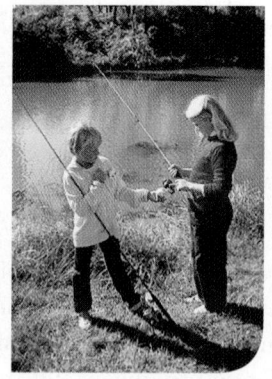 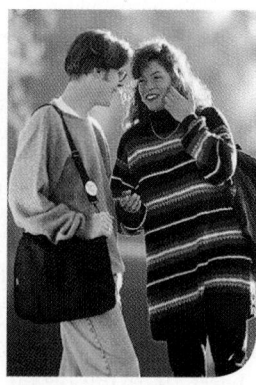

A   B   C   D   E

FIGURE 40-4 (A) Infant: 4 weeks to 1 year; (B) toddler: 1 to 3 years; (C) preschool: 3 to 6 years; (D) school-age (late childhood): 6 to 12 years, or puberty; (E) adolescence: 12 years or puberty to the beginning of adult stage.
Source: Michael Heron Photography.

Failure to Thrive

Gaining insufficient weight according to the standardized baby growth charts is called **failure to thrive (FTT)**. Children have irregular growth patterns; however, if an infant is considerably under the goal for his or her age, normal development could be affected. Babies whose weight is under the third percentile on the growth chart are in the failure-to-thrive syndrome category. The most frequent cause of FTT is inadequate nutrition. For example, colicky babies, new mothers with feeding problems, and mothers who used alcohol or had inadequate nutrition during pregnancy may result in a child with FTT. Other causes could be cleft palate, which affects the ability to suck well, and malabsorption disease, which prevents food from being absorbed normally. In addition, insufficient stimulation and lack of nurturing can cause failure to thrive. Social problems such as abuse, poverty, and drug or alcohol dependence can affect the parent's ability to care for and nourish the child.

MEASUREMENTS

When the child arrives for a well-child visit, the physical examination follows a similar pattern as an adult examination. The physician will examine the patient from head to toe.

Vital Signs

As a medical assistant, it will be your role to obtain temperature, pulse, respirations, and blood pressure measurements. Most pediatricians do not require a blood pressure measurement unless the child has cardiovascular or kidney disorders. Some physicians require blood pressure readings on every patient regardless of age, and others monitor blood pressure once a year after age 3 years. Procedure 40-2 describes steps for measuring pediatric vital signs, including temperature (rectal, aural, and axillary methods), apical pulse, respiration, and blood pressure using a pediatric cuff. Although all the procedures are similar to performing vital signs on an adult, a blood pressure cuff measuring no wider than two-thirds of the child's upper arm must be used. In addition, a pediatric stethoscope has a smaller bell that makes it easier to place over the brachial artery. The blood pressure reading in children is lower than in adults.

In children under age 5 years, temperature should be measured with tympanic or temporal artery thermometers or measuring axillary temperature. The procedures for measuring body temperature in young children are the same as they are in adults. Keeping the child still and calm is the major difference. To measure an infant's body temperature rectally,

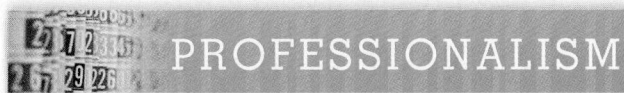

PROFESSIONALISM

THE LAW

Child abuse in the United States affects 1 in 20 children each year. Child abuse is defined by the American Medical Association as "emotional, physical, or sexual mistreatment, or neglect of a child." Children are very dependent on the adults who surround them; therefore, they are very vulnerable. Caregivers, close family members, or friends are usually the abusers, and abuse crosses all socioeconomic, racial, religious, and ethnic backgrounds. Physical and psychological abuse can impact brain development and intellectual growth, delay normal growth and social development, and have long-term health consequences. Moreover, the psychological effects of abuse last although the abuse is over. Abused children are at increased risk of suffering from low self-esteem, depression, and emotional highs and lows. As adults, they often are substance abusers and have eating disorders. Sexual abuse is anything of a sexual nature that the child is asked to witness or participate in without consent and yet does not completely understand.

The pediatrician's office is the first step in suspicion of abuse. The physician is asked to evaluate the child's condition and provide treatment. Physicians are required by the federal Child Abuse Prevention and Treatment Act to report any suspicions of abuse. You, in turn, are required to report your suspicions immediately to the physician. Your role is to be alert to any suspicious bruises, burns, excessive fractures, changes in behavior, and changes in hygiene, any of which may indicate abuse. The effects of abuse cannot be washed away in a short time. In some case, it may takes of years of therapy to resolve the problems caused by child abuse. Victims of any type of abuse will require counseling and assistance from a broad spectrum of social service agencies.

place the infant in the supine position and place your nondominant hand securely under the baby's bent knees. With the other hand, insert the thermometer and hold it securely in place to avoid breakage or the child expelling it. If the child is older, place the child in the prone position, insert the thermometer, and hold it securely in place.

In children under age 2 years, measure the apical pulse by placing the stethoscope on the left side of the chest to the right of the nipple and counting for 1 full minute. Respirations are easy to count due to the visible rise and fall of the chest in a small child. The younger the child, the higher the respiratory rate will be.

MEASURING PEDIATRIC VITAL SIGNS

Objective: Perform all steps of the procedures and provide readings with accuracy according to the instructor's guidelines.

EQUIPMENT AND SUPPLIES

gloves; tympanic thermometer; glass thermometer; electronic thermometer; watch with second hand; pediatric stethoscope; pediatric blood pressure cuff

METHOD

1. Gather the appropriate equipment.
2. Identify the patient, introduce yourself, and explain the procedures to the parent.
3. Speak reassuringly to the child to win his or her trust.
4. Perform hand hygiene.
5. Explain to the parent how he or she can assist you in holding the infant.

OBTAIN TEMPERATURE WITH TYMPANIC THERMOMETER AS FOLLOWS

1. Remove the thermometer from the base and note that it reads "Ready."
2. Attach the disposable probe cover to the earpiece.
3. Gently pull in a downward direction on the outer ear to straighten the child's ear canal.
4. Insert the probe into the ear canal.
5. Press the scan button (Figure 40-5).

6. Observe the temperature reading.
7. Gently withdraw the thermometer and eject the probe cover into a biohazard waste container.
8. Record the temperature reading using "T" to denote the tympanic reading.
9. Return the thermometer to the base.

OBTAIN TEMPERATURE READING USING AXILLARY METHOD AS FOLLOWS

1. Take nonmercury thermometer out of the container and rinse with cool water; inspect for defects.
2. Shake down the thermometer to 95°F/ 35°C.
3. Place the thermometer in the infant's armpit, and hold the infant's arm across the chest for the required 10 minutes.
4. Read the thermometer, then record by designating the reading with "AX" to indicate the method used.
5. Clean and disinfect the thermometer when finished with the patient.

OBTAIN TEMPERATURE READING RECTALLY BY USING A DIGITAL THERMOMETER WITH RED PROBE (RECTAL USE)

1. Put on gloves.
2. Attach the disposable tip to the top of the probe.
3. Lubricate the thermometer to provide easy insertion.
4. Place the child on the bed in a supine or prone position.

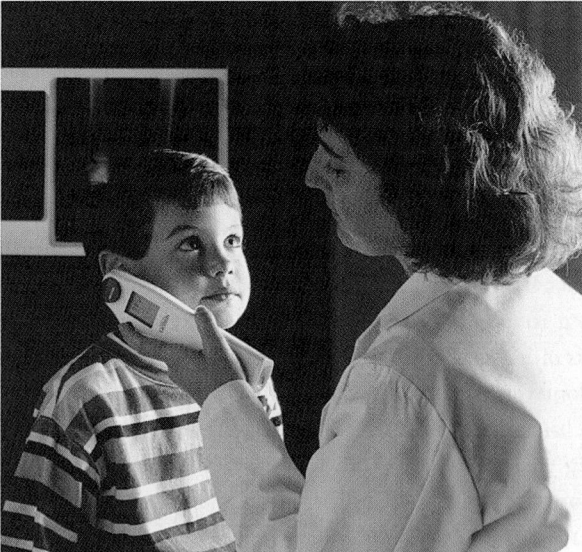

FIGURE 40-5 Tympanic thermometers are particularly helpful for measuring the temperature of a child.

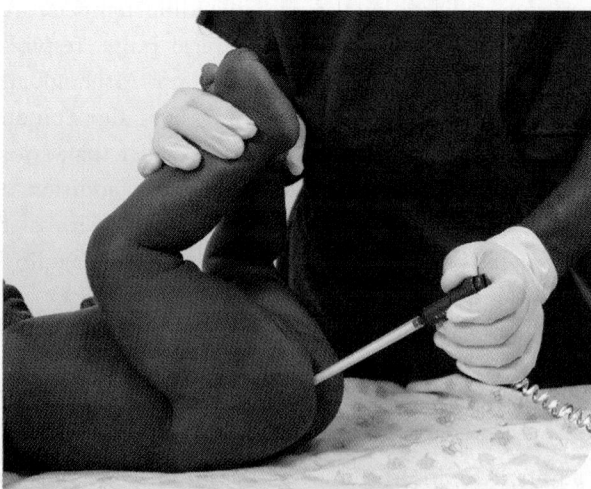

FIGURE 40-6 Obtaining a temperature reading rectally.

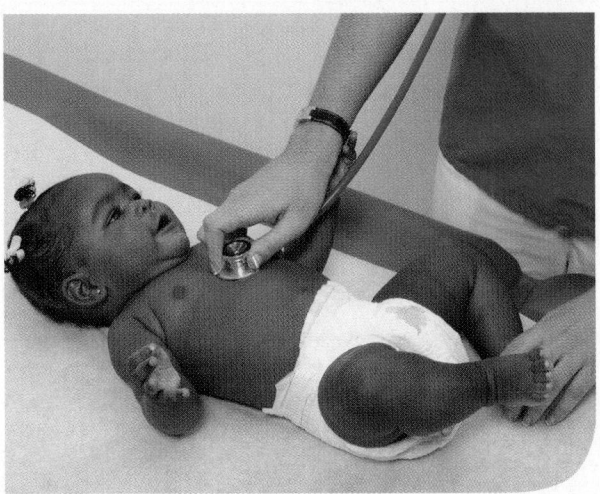

FIGURE 40-7   Measuring the apical pulse of an infant.

5. Insert the thermometer $\frac{1}{2}$ inch into the rectum and hold in place with hand to prevent expelling (Figure 40-6).
6. Hold the child securely to restrict movement.
7. Leave the thermometer in for the required time until it beeps.
8. Remove thermometer, wipe off lubricant, and take the reading.
9. Record the reading using R to indicate method used.

MEASURE HEART RATE/PULSE BY APICAL MEASUREMENT AS FOLLOWS

1. Place the stethoscope on the child's chest at the midpoint between the sternum and the left nipple (Figure 40-7). Distract the child if necessary to obtain the apical pulse.
2. Listen for the apical beat.
3. Count the apical beat for 1 full minute.
4. Record the apical pulse using "Ap" before the pulse to indicate the apical reading.

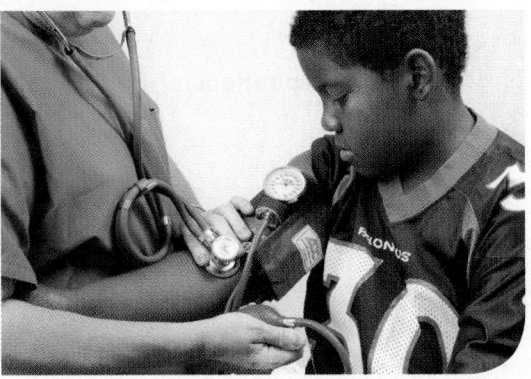

FIGURE 40-8   Taking the child's blood pressure.

MEASURE INFANT RESPIRATIONS FOR 1 FULL MINUTE AS FOLLOWS

1. Place your hand on the child's chest and count the rise and fall of the chest as 1 respiration.
2. Record the results.

MEASURE THE INFANT'S BLOOD PRESSURE USING A PEDIATRIC CUFF AND STETHOSCOPE AS FOLLOWS

1. Wrap the cuff securely around the upper arm (Figure 40-8).
2. Feel for the brachial pulse.
3. Place the stethoscope earpieces in the ears and place the diaphragm near the pulse.
4. Pump up the cuff until the pulse is no longer heard.
5. Release the valve slowly, listening for systolic and diastolic sounds.
6. Record the results.

CHARTING EXAMPLE
4/10/XX T 99°F (T), AP 90, R 20, BP 136/78 · · · · · · · · · · · · · · · · ·
· M. King, CMA (AAMA)

Table 40-3 provides the normal pulse, respiration, and blood pressure values for children from birth to adolescence. Normal body temperature is dependent on the method used. The values are as follows:

- Oral 98.6°F/37°C
- Aural 98.6°F/37°C
- Axillary 97.6°F/36.4°C
- Rectal 99.6°F/37.6°C

Weight, Height, Head, and Chest Circumference

Weight and height measurements covered in Chapter 35 should be reviewed if needed. Infants and children are weighed and measured at each office visit. Infants should be weighed without a diaper to ensure that the most accurate weight is obtained. The length of an infant is measured on the examining table until the child can stand reasonably still on the adult scale. Weight and height are measured without shoes. Procedure 40-3 lists the steps for measuring the infant's weight and height.

Measurement of the circumference of the head is part of each well-baby office visit until age 6 years. Procedure 40-4 provides the steps to measure the circumference of a baby's head. Rapid growth of the head may indicate **hydrocephalus**, which is excessive fluid around the brain that may lead to brain damage. Head growth that falls below the normal percentile

TABLE 40-3 Baseline Pulse, Respiration, and Blood Pressure Values from Birth to Adolescence

Age	Respirations	Pulse	Systolic BP MmHg	Diastolic BP MmHg
Infants	30–60	120–160	74–100	50–70
Toddlers	24–40	90–140	80–112	50–80
Preschoolers	22–34	80–110	82–110	50–78
School Age	18–30	75–100	84–120	54–80
Adolescents	12–16	60–90	107–118	62–67

Note: Pulse and respirations are taken for 1 full minute. The apical pulse is used with a child under age 2 years.

procedure 40-3

MEASURING THE WEIGHT AND HEIGHT OF AN INFANT

Objective: Obtain the weight and height of an infant.

EQUIPMENT AND SUPPLIES

baby scale; patient record; pen; small towel or protector for scale; tape measure

METHOD

1. Introduce yourself and identify the infant by stating the infant's name to the parent. Have the infant remain with the parent or caregiver while you prepare the equipment. Explain the procedure.
2. Perform hand hygiene.
3. Place a towel or paper protector on the baby scale.
4. Balance the scale by placing all the weights to the far left side. Turn the bolt at the right edge of the scale until the balance bar pointer is at the middle of the balance bar.

5. Undress the infant (or ask parent to undress the infant). A clean diaper may be kept in place. Gently lay the infant on the scale. Always keep one hand on the infant until the weights are adjusted. Do not leave the infant unattended at any time.
6. Keeping one hand over the infant's body as a safety precaution, move the large pound weight into the groove closest to the weight estimated for the baby. Move the smaller ounce weight by tapping it gently until it reaches a point in which the pointer floats in the center of the frame. See Figure 40-9A–B for examples of balance and electronic baby scales.

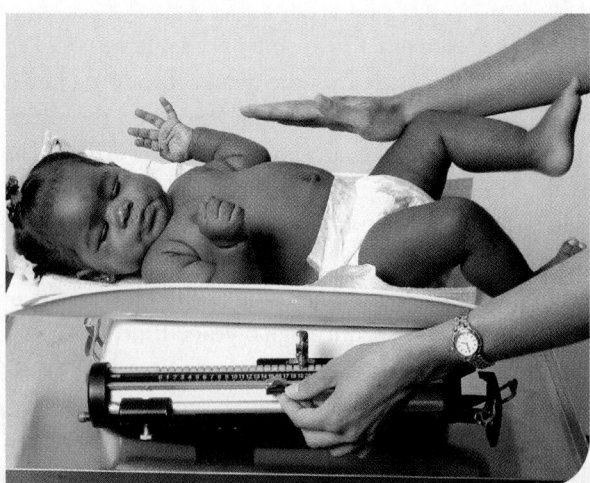 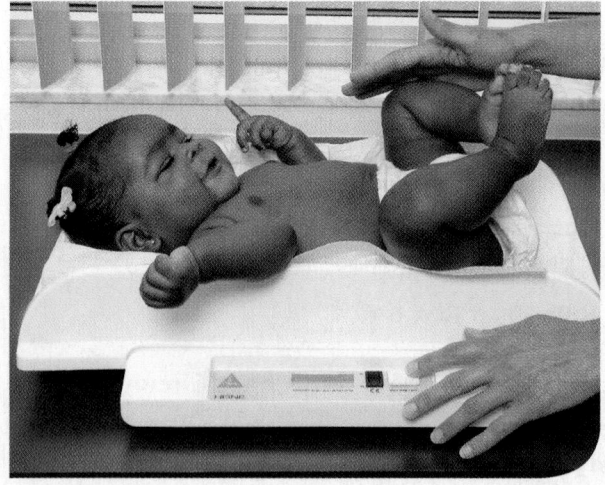

FIGURE 40-9 (A) Balance baby scale; (B) electronic baby scale.

7. Keep the weights in place while the infant is moved to the examination table for height measurement under the caregiver's care while you record the weight.

CONTINUE WITH HEIGHT

8. Holding the tape measure with one hand, place the tape at the top of the side of the infant's head. Stretch the infant out full length as you pull the tape measure down to the bottom of the feet (Figure 40-10). If you are using a table with a measure bar, place the infant's head at one end of the table with the soles of his or her feet touching the footboard so that the toes are pointing toward the ceiling.

Note: It is best, and preferred, to have two people measure the length of an infant. The parent can assist by holding the infant's head still. To measure an active child, make pencil marks on the examination table paper at the top of the child's head and at the bottom of the feet at the heels. When the child is removed, measure the area between the marks.

9. Note the height in inches and fractions of an inch, and write it on the paper covering the exam table.
10. Ask the parent or caregiver to hold the infant while the height and weight are charted in the infant's record.

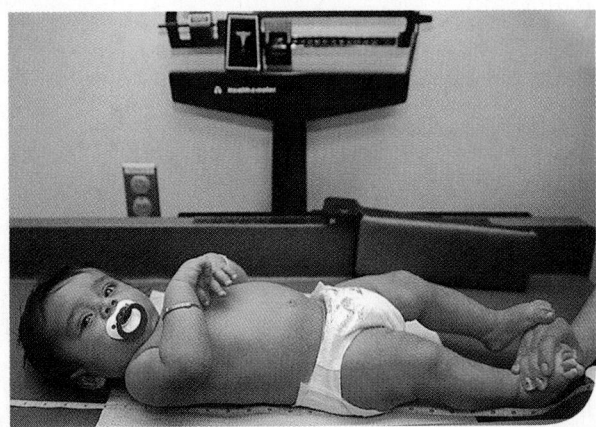

FIGURE 40-10 Measuring the length of an infant from the top of the head to the base of the heels.

11. Tell the measurements to the parent.
12. Discard the paper towel.
13. Perform hand hygiene.

CHARTING EXAMPLE

2/14/XX weight 16 lb. 3 oz., length 30 inches · · · · · · · · · · · · ·
· M. King, CMA (AAMA)

procedure 40-4

MEASURING THE HEAD CIRCUMFERENCE OF AN INFANT OR SMALL CHILD

Objective: Obtain an accurate measurement of the head circumference of an infant or small child head circumference.

EQUIPMENT AND SUPPLIES

flexible tape measure (no elasticity); growth chart

METHOD

1. Identify the patient.
2. Talk to the infant to gain trust.
3. Explain the procedure to the parent or caregiver.
4. Perform hand hygiene.
5. Position the infant on the examination table or have the caregiver hold the infant.
6. Hold the end of tape (0 inches) on the forehead over the patient's eyebrows.
7. Bring the tape around the head and over the ears to meet in front (Figure 40-11).

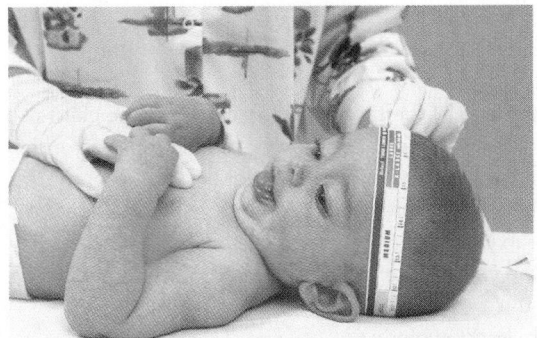

FIGURE 40-11 Measuring the head circumference of an infant.

8. Take the measurement with accuracy to the fraction of an inch or centimeter.
9. Repeat the procedure if in any doubt about the measurements.
10. Document the results, and record them on the growth chart.
11. Perform hand hygiene.

may indicate **microencephaly**. This condition may be caused by a premature closing of the fontanel, constricting brain growth and leading to mental retardation. Normal head circumference at birth should be between 12.5 to 14.5 inches or 31.75 to 36.83 cm. Generally, the head and chest circumferences are equal sometime between ages one and two.

Chest circumference measurement is not normally performed at each visit. It may be performed if the physician suspects over- or underdevelopment of the heart or lungs or that calcification of the rib cage would constrict the growth of organs. To measure the chest circumference, wrap a measuring tape around the chest at nipple level and read the measurement during the resting phase between respirations as described in Procedure 40-5.

Growth Charts

A child is measured during each well-child visit, and the measurements are plotted on a growth chart. Some physicians

procedure 40-5

MEASURING THE CHEST CIRCUMFERENCE OF A CHILD
Objective: To accurately measure the circumference of a child's chest.

EQUIPMENT AND SUPPLIES
disposable tape measure; examination table; patient's record; pen

STEPS
1. Introduce yourself, identify the patient, and explain the procedure to the parent or caregiver.
2. Talk to the patient soothingly to gain trust.
3. Perform hand hygiene
4. Position the child on the table in a supine position. If the child is over age 2 years, he or she may sit on the table for this procedure.
5. Place the end of the tape (0) in the center of the child's chest in line with the child's nipples and slip the tape under the child's body and bring it to meet the other end of the tape. Take a measurement in centimeters to the nearest 0.01 or in inches to the nearest $\frac{1}{2}$ inch (Figure 40-12).
6. Place the child in the caregiver's care before recording the results.
7. Perform hand hygiene.

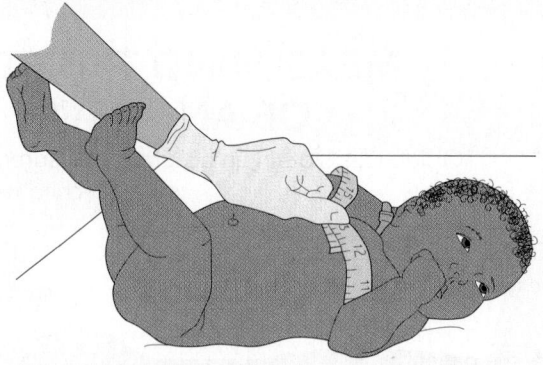

FIGURE 40-12 Measuring the chest circumference of an infant.

require infants to be weighed every time they are seen in the office. A copy of the National Center for Health Statistics growth chart is part of every child's permanent medical record. Individual growth graphs are available for boys and girls aged birth to 36 months and 2 to 20 years. Pediatricians usually provide a growth booklet for each child so caregivers have a copy of the child's measurements. After the measurements are taken, the medical assistant charts the information in both areas. Once the measurements are obtained, the values are plotted according to the child's age and sex and a percentile is obtained. The percentile is used to identify children with growth or nutritional abnormalities. In Figure 40-13 a growth chart for girls 2 to 20 years is

shown. Procedure 40-6 lists the steps necessary to calculate the growth percentiles.

Charts also exist for body mass index (BMI) and head circumference. Once measurements are obtained, it is necessary to record them on the patient's chart and in the growth booklet given to the caregiver.

Hearing and Vision Evaluations

Hearing tests are done in many hospitals at birth as part of special state and federal programs to detect hearing difficulties at an early age. Early detection is important because speech development depends on a child's ability to mimic sounds, word selection, and use of words. If the child tests below normal during the first test, it is repeated at about 6 weeks. Newborns respond to light, and older infants are able to follow light. At the yearly examination, visual acuity is measured on children age 3 years and over using a Snellen eye chart. Procedure 40-7 lists steps for performing a Snellen visual acuity test on a young child.

SICK-CHILD VISITS

When a caregiver brings an ill child into the office, the ill child should be put immediately in an examination room to reduce the possibility of spreading infection among the vulnerable population in the office reception room. Some offices have separate reception areas for sick children. Based on the patient symptoms, the physician may request a urine sample. If the child is toilet trained and over 2 to 3 years old, ask the parents to collect the specimen after providing instruction on cleansing the genital area. The instructions are the same as those for cleansing prior to attaching a urine collection device, which is explained later in this chapter. If the child is too ill or too young, a pediatric urine collection device should be applied as soon as possible to increase the possibility of collecting a sample. When collecting a urine sample, ask the parent or caregiver specific questions to uncover other urinary tract–related problems, such as the following:

- Have there been any changes in the amount of urine produced recently?
- Does the child complain of burning, itching, or pain during urination? (urinary tract infection [UTI])

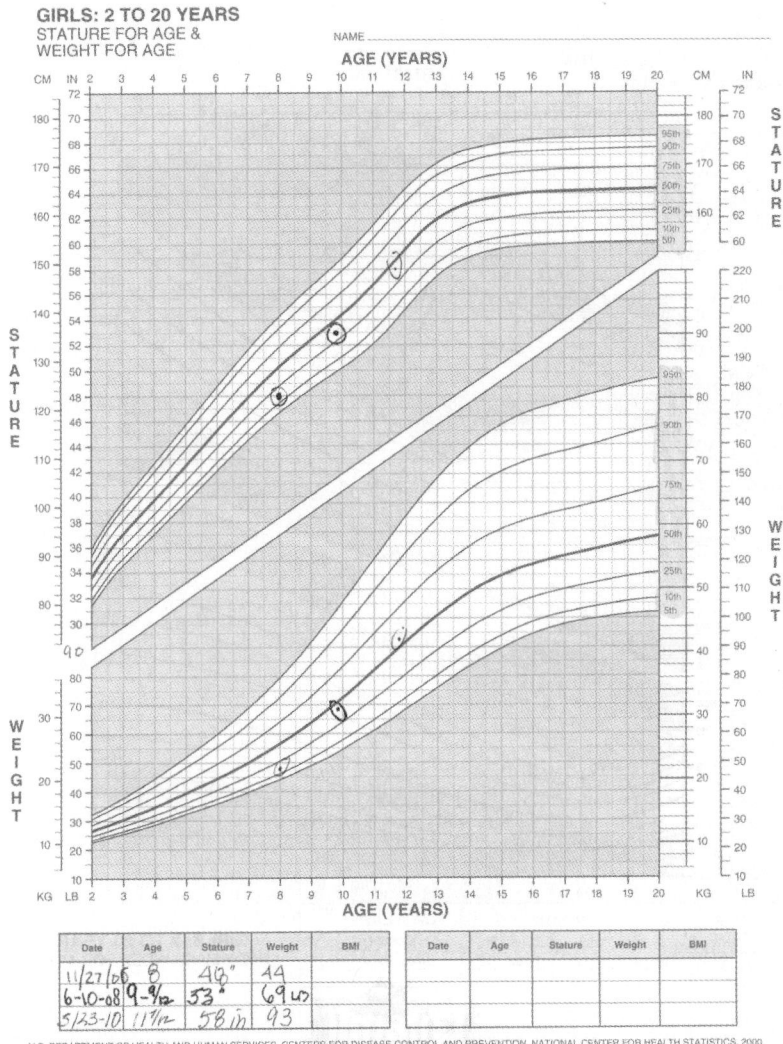

FIGURE 40-13 This pediatric growth chart tracks height and weight for girls ages 2 to 20 years and assigns percentiles. On the initial visit to her pediatrician, this 8-year-old child was in about the 15th percentile and was diagnosed with malnutrition. After 3 years of good nutrition, her most recent visit at age 11 years, 7 months, shows that she is now in the 40th percentile for height and the 55th percentile for weight.

CALCULATING GROWTH PERCENTILES

Objective: To plot the age, weight, and height of a patient and obtain correct percentiles.

EQUIPMENT AND SUPPLIES

patient's record with weight and height values; pen; growth chart

METHOD

1. Select the proper growth chart for the patient. See Figure 40-14 for an example.

2. Locate the child's age in the horizontal axis at the bottom of the chart. Draw an imaginary vertical line on the chart.

3. Locate the proper growth value (in this case weight and height), then draw an imaginary horizontal line on the chart.

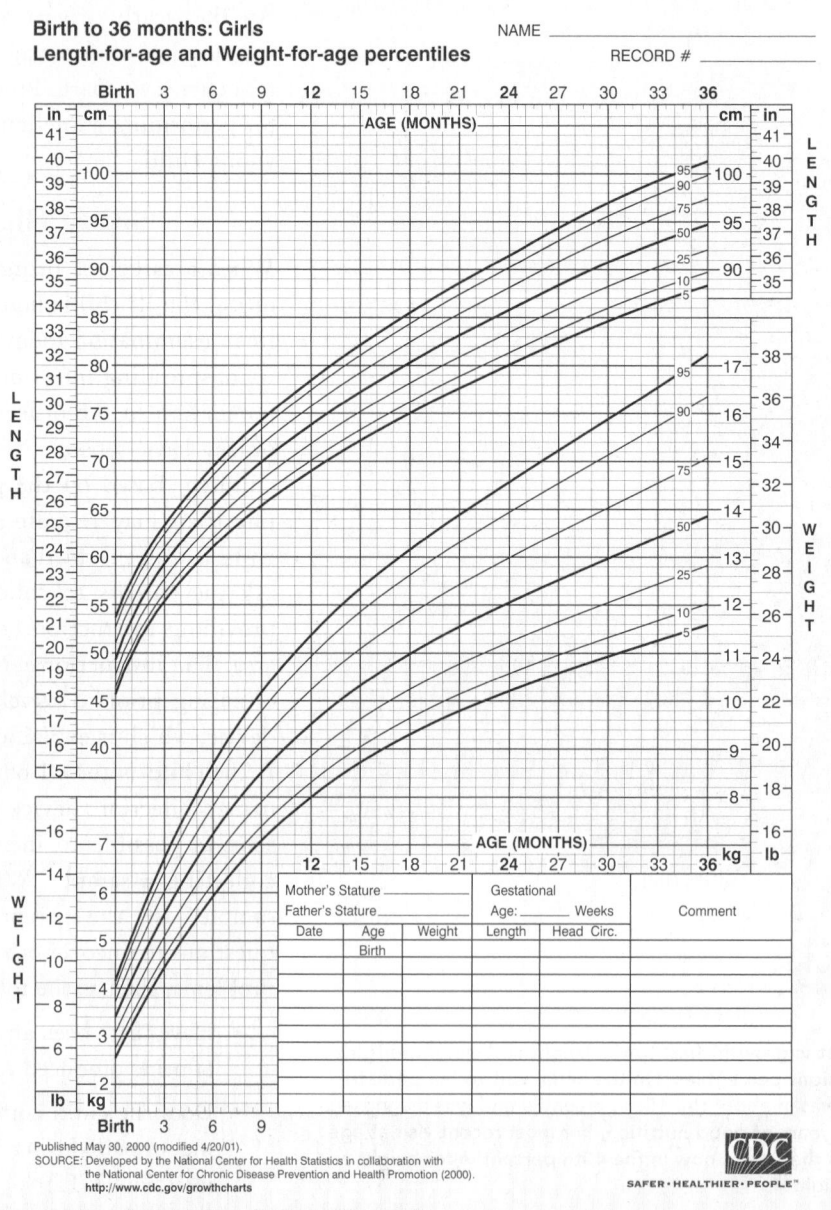

FIGURE 40-14 Pediatric growth chart for girls from birth to 36 months.

4. Find the point at which the two imaginary lines intersect on the graph, then place a dot there.
5. Follow the curved line closest to the dot upward, then read the percentile located on the right side of the chart.
6. If the dot you placed falls between two curved lines, interpolate or estimate the percentile that falls between the two closest percentile lines.
   - For example, if the dot you placed based on the correct age and weight was halfway between the 10 and 25 percentile lines, the difference between 25 and 10 is 15, and half of 15 is 7.5. Therefore, the percentile would be 17.5. The child would weigh more than 17.5 percent of the children his or her age, which is below normal.
7. Record the results in the patient's chart.

CHARTING EXAMPLE
05/25/XX Length 34¾ inches—95th percentile, Wt. 31 lbs—95th percentile.· A. McGrath, CMA (AAMA)

procedure

PERFORM A SNELLEN EYE EXAM ON A CHILD

Objective: Perform a Snellen eye exam for distance acuity on the child.

EQUIPMENT AND SUPPLIES
Snellen E eye chart and occluder; pencil and paper; mark on floor at a distance of 20 feet from the chart

METHOD
1. Assemble the equipment.
2. Introduce yourself and identify the patient.
3. Explain the procedure to the patient and parent or caregiver.
4. Perform hand hygiene.
5. Ask the child to indicate which way the legs on the E are pointing to make sure the child understands the directions.
6. If the child understands, position him or her in front of the Snellen E chart at a distance of 20 feet.
7. Make sure the child is comfortable.
8. Ask the child to hold the occluder over his or her first eye and remind the child to keep both eyes open (Figure 40-15).
9. Point to the Es on the chart. Make sure the child is pointing his or her fingers in the same direction as the E on the chart. Proceed until you have the results from the first eye.
10. Repeat the procedure with the other eye.
11. Document the procedure and record the results using written words (*not* OS, OD, OU).
12. Compliment the child and caregiver on how well the child performed.

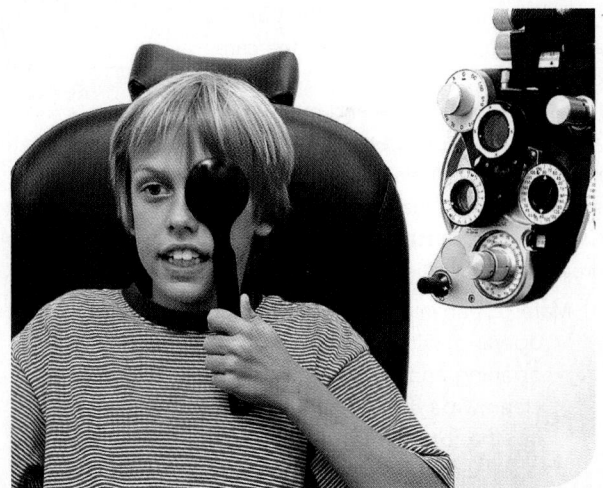

FIGURE 40-15   Testing distance visual acuity using the Snellen eye chart.

13. Perform hand hygiene.
14. Sanitize and replace equipment.

CHARTING EXAMPLE
4/1/10/XX Visual acuity using Snellen E chart Right eye 20/20; left eye both eyes 20/30; OU 20/20 · · · M. King, CMA (AAMA)

- Does the child have persistent diaper rash? (diarrhea, change in urine composition)

- Has the child reverted to bed wetting or loss of bladder control? (stress, UTI)

- Is the child in diapers? If so, how many diapers does the child wet each day? (dehydration)

A positive response to any of the preceding questions could be indicative of urinary tract problems. After obtaining the patient's temperature, pulse, respiration, height, and weight measurements, a urine collection device should be applied. Procedure 40-8 lists the steps necessary to apply a urine collection device on a child who is unable or unwilling to urinate into a container. In some cases, a child may be

procedure
40-8

APPLYING A PEDIATRIC URINE COLLECTION DEVICE
Objective: Properly apply a urinary collection device.

EQUIPMENT AND SUPPLIES
pediatric urine collection bag; laboratory specimen container with label; antiseptic wipes; gloves; biohazard waste container

METHOD
1. Assemble all equipment.
2. Introduce yourself, identify the patient, and explain the procedure to the caregiver.
3. Perform hand hygiene and put on gloves.
4. Ask the parent or caregiver to place the infant on the examination table in a supine position, then remove the diaper.
5. Cleanse the **genitalia** (reproductive organ) area with antiseptic wipes.

   Male: Cleanse the urinary **meatus** (urinary tract opening) with a circular motion, starting at the opening and progressing outward. Repeat with a clean wipe if the infant is uncircumcised, retracting the foreskin to clean the meatus. When finished cleaning, replace the foreskin to the normal position.

   Female: Hold the labia open with your nondominant hand, cleanse the labia from superior to inferior (front to back), wiping in one directional motion. Discard the wipe, and repeat with a new wipe.

6. Make sure the area is dry. Unfold the collection device and remove the upper portion of paper protecting the adhesive surface. Apply to the mons pubis and press to secure. Continue removing paper and applying to perineum, securing the device and making sure it does not stick to the infant's leg (Figure 40-16).

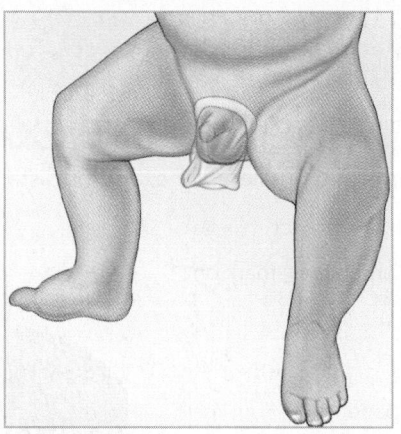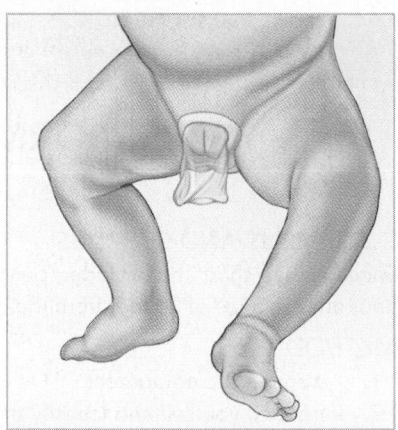

FIGURE 40-16 Applying a urine collection device on a male and on a female infant.

7. Offer water or suggest that the parent try to get the infant to drink to increase the likelihood he or she will produce a urine specimen.
8. When a sufficient urine sample is collected, remove the bag, wipe down the area to which the bag was attached, and rediaper the infant.
9. Pour the sample into a labeled laboratory container and handle according to routine in your facility.
10. Dispose of all used equipment in a biohazard waste container.
11. Remove gloves and perform hand hygiene.
12. Chart the procedure.

CHARTING EXAMPLE
1/10/XX 9:00 A.M. Pedi urine bag attached
    9:25 A.M. No spec obtained
    10:00 A.M. Pt offered H₂O. Recheck at 11:00 A.M. · · · ·
· M. King, CMA (AAMA)

catheterized to obtain a specimen. Urine samples reflect the health status of many systems in the body and are an important diagnostic tool. After these procedures are complete, your duty is to remain ready to assist in the examination in whatever manner necessary. Once the visit is completed, be sure to review the physician's instructions with the caregiver and take a few moments to bond with the child. Remember to document any results.

Pediatric Diseases and Disorders

Children experience frequent colds, gastrointestinal upsets, and other fairly routine conditions, which are seen in a pediatric practice. Additional diseases and disorders for which immunizations are recommended will be discussed in Chapter 54.

UPPER RESPIRATORY DISEASES

The common cold is caused by more than two hundred varieties of **rhinovirus**. It is highly contagious and usually self-limiting after about a week. In infants and children, low-grade fever, nasal congestion, and coughing may be present. During their first 2 years, children may have six to ten colds a year. It may be necessary to instruct the caregiver on the use of a nasal bulb syringe to remove excess secretions and facilitate nursing or bottle-feeding. Treatment of colds is usually with over-the-counter medications to reduce fever. Many physicians no longer recommend the use of decongestants and cough medications since recent studies demonstrate that they have little or no effect in children. Secondary infection such as strep throat or otitis media may result from colds and may require treatment with antibiotics.

Most upper respiratory infections are spread easily by droplets from the nose, throat, or contaminated items handled by the infected person. Children should be reminded to cover their nose and mouth when sneezing, as well as the importance of hand washing. Hand washing is the best defense to ward off upper respiratory infections.

Strep Throat

Strep throat is caused by group A beta hemolytic *Streptococcus pyogenes.* These highly infectious bacteria may lead to other problems, such as scarlet fever and rheumatic fever, which can damage heart valves. The physician may order a throat culture to confirm that strep is the causative agent. Many pediatric offices perform these tests on site with the use of rapid strep testing. Strep throat is treated with antibiotics.

Caregivers should be reminded that children must finish the entire antibiotic prescription to prevent relapse. A child who has recurring strep throat infections may be a candidate for a **tonsillectomy** (surgical removal of the tonsils).

Otitis Media

Otitis media is an infection of the middle ear due to cold, allergies, or other respiratory infections. Fluid builds up and applies pressure to the eardrum, which can cause pain, irritability, and sometimes fever. Treatment of otitis media consists of decongestants, analgesics, and sometimes antibiotics. Repeated infections can lead to damage to the eardrum and loss of hearing. Children with chronic ear infections may require a **myringotomy**, which consists of an incision into the eardrum and a tube inserted through the eardrum to permit drainage of fluid.

Croup

Croup is an inflammation of the larynx and trachea, which leads to a distinctive barking cough and hoarseness. Both types of croup begin with a cold. Spasmodic croup begins suddenly at night with the distinct "seal" type of cough, and viral croup develops more slowly, with swelling, mucous secretions, and **stridor**. Stridor is a high-pitched sound heard during respiration caused by obstruction of the airway. Antibiotics are not effective against viral illness. Croup is treated at home unless breathing is extremely labored and emergency medical help is needed. Sitting in a steamy bathroom, with the door closed for 15 to 20 minutes can help restore normal breathing. Afterward, a cool steam vaporizer or humidifier in the child's room adds moisture to the air and may help breathing. Exposing the child to cool moist night air is also frequently effective.

Bronchiolitis

Bronchiolitis is an inflammation of the bronchioles and is more common in children under 2 years old. Children who have upper respiratory infections, such as colds, may develop bronchiolitis. Children with asthma and those exposed to secondhand smoke are at higher risk. Symptoms include coldlike symptoms such as nasal and chest congestion and low-grade fever. Treatments are the same as those used to treat colds. If excessive coughing is present, using a cool steam vaporizer or humidifier may help add moisture to the air and reduce coughing.

Respiratory Syncytial Virus. Respiratory syncytial virus (RSV), is a common, highly contagious virus that affects the upper and lower respiratory tract. It normally occurs in winter and early spring and is the most common

Box 40-1 Signs of Dehydration in INFANTS

- Decrease in urine output—dry diapers
- Weakness and lethargy
- Dry, pale skin with loss of elasticity
- Decrease in tear production
- Sunken eyes
- Increased thirst
- Confusion

cause of bronchiolitis. RSV can spread by contact with upper respiratory secretions. Hand washing before physical contact with children will help prevent the spread of RSV. By age 3 years most children have had a bout of RSV. When very young or at-risk children are affected, they may need hospitalization for intravenous fluids, bronchodilators, and oxygen therapy. Confirmation of RSV is the presence of viral antibodies obtained from a throat swab or sputum culture.

Asthma

Asthma is the most common chronic disease in children, affecting one out of seven children usually before age 4 years. Inflammation and spasms of the bronchi, mucous secretions, and narrowing of the airways make it difficult to exhale and inhale. Symptoms include wheezing, shortness of breath, and tightness in the chest, difficulty speaking, and anxiety. The cause for asthma is unknown. However, triggers such as allergies, exposure to pollutants, cigarette smoke, cold viruses, and strenuous exercise may bring on an asthma attack.

Children who experience two or more asthma attacks per week should be seen by a specialist. Inhalers or nebulizers may be necessary during attacks. If attacks occur more frequently than twice a week, then daily anti-inflammatory medications will most likely be the treatment. In both cases, an asthma plan should be developed so that the caregiver understands what to do in each stage of an attack, culminating in emergency treatment at a hospital if necessary. Bronchodilators are administered either by inhaler or nebulizers. A peak flow meter may be used to measure the capacity of the child's ability to exhale forcefully. If specific allergens are identified, then removing the offending allergens from the child's environment is helpful.

GASTROINTESTINAL DISORDERS

Diarrhea, nausea, and vomiting are common conditions affecting children. Diarrhea is defined as two or more watery stools within 24 hours.

Diarrhea

Diarrhea may be caused by bacterial, viral, and parasitic infections; food allergies; and medications. Infants and children may have diarrhea with no apparent cause. If diarrhea persists for more than two days, the child may need to be seen in the office.

Diarrhea in infants and small children can rapidly lead to dehydration. Dehydration can trigger an imbalance of electrolytes causing the child to be lethargic and possibly to hyperventilate. Acidosis and death can occur. The signs of dehydration are vital for you and the caregiver to recognize. They are listed in Box 40-1. In addition to dehydration, diarrhea may cause **excoriation**, or painful chafing or rawness of the skin in the diaper area. Other symptoms include cramping, weakness, fever, and irritability. Pediatricians often recommend the **BRAT diet**, consisting of bananas, rice and cereal, applesauce, and toast. Avoiding dairy products is also advised until diarrhea subsides. Foods and dairy products may be reintroduced gradually.

Colic

Colic is severe gastrointestinal pain in infants occurring in both breast-fed and formula-fed babies. The cause of colic is unknown, although some suspect immaturity of the digestive system. Colic is harmless and usually disappears by age 4 months. Symptoms include intense crying, irritability, fussiness, distended abdomen, and gas. Parents and caregivers feel frustrated, angry, at fault, and exhausted. Acting in an empathetic manner can help to ease parental frustration. There is no specific treatment for colic. The trial-and-error approach to feedings and how to hold the baby and soothing remedies like rocking and patting the baby's back serve as the usual treatment. Some babies find relief being held in the football position: lying on their bellies along the parent's arm or leg.

Obesity

Obesity is defined as being 20 percent above the patient's ideal weight with a body mass index over 30. Body mass index (BMI) is a measurement of body weight relative to height and is associated with the amount of body fat. BMI is calculated using the following formula:

$$BMI = weight\ (lb)/[height\ (in)]^2 \times 703$$

See Chapter 35 for more information on how to calculate BMI.

A BMI of 25 to 27 means a child is overweight. Genetic tendencies, family patterns of overeating, poor food choices, and lack of exercise cause children to be obese. Very few children are obese due to endocrine disorders. Fifty percent of the United States population is considered obese. It is estimated that 30 percent of children over age 5 years are obese. According to the Surgeon General's 2007 report *Call to Action to Prevent and Decrease Overweight and Obesity,* overweight adolescents have a 70 percent chance of becoming overweight adults and the rate of type 2 diabetes in children has increased dramatically during the last 20 years. Obesity carries serious consequences to health in the short and long terms and may cause damage to a child's self-esteem. A medical assistant can provide support, encouragement, and educational materials, and serve as a link to community resources for the family dealing with an obese child.

OTHER DISORDERS

Specific conditions and diseases related to genetic or inherited disease are discussed in Chapter 21. Other conditions and disorders that do not fit in any specific category are discussed in the following sections.

Autism

Autism is a nervous system disorder or group of disorders beginning in childhood and affecting the child's ability to relate to others. Autism is four times more frequent in males and is noticeable by age 3 years. Autism affects 1 in 150 children according to the National Autism Association. The cause is unknown; however, recent research indicates that as many as 5 to 20 genes may be involved. Other factors implicated as possible causes are exposure to toxic chemicals during pregnancy, pesticides, flame-retardant chemicals, prenatal or postnatal viruses and exposure to heavy metals such as mercury. There is no link between autism and immunizations according to the latest Centers for Disease Control and Prevention (CDC) research. Symptoms of autism are varied and may include the following:

- Failure to make eye contact
- Engaging in repetitive behavior
- Delayed language skills

- Preference for solitary activities
- Upset by changes in routine
- Indifference to people

No cure has yet been found for autism, but research indicates that early intervention by specialists can be beneficial. The earlier autism is diagnosed and interventions designed to the child's needs are started, the better the prognosis.

Sudden Infant Death Syndrome

Sudden infant death syndrome (SIDS) is the death with no known cause of an apparently healthy infant, usually before age 1 year. SIDS usually occurs during sleep and is a leading cause of death in children in the first year of life. The highest number of deaths occurs between 1 and 4 months of age. SIDS happens more frequently in winter and is more prevalent in boys. Among the probable causes proposed are immature waking centers in the brain leading to **sleep apnea**, abnormal regulation of breathing, heart rates, and lack of airway control. Sleep apnea involves periods of absence of breathing during sleep. Factors that increase the risk of SIDS are low birth weight, premature birth, family history of SIDS, putting the child to sleep on his or her stomach, births from very young mothers, and exposure to alcohol, drugs, or smoking before birth. Possible prevention techniques include having the infant sleep in a back or side position for at least the first 6 months, using apnea monitors, and knowledge of infant CPR by the parents. The loss of a child to SIDS is particularly difficult because parents often feel that they were at fault. Support groups and therapy may help devastated parents. Numerous SIDS associations have local and national chapters that can provide valuable information and help.

Febrile Seizures

Febrile seizures are suffered by some children with high fevers following a rapid spike in body temperature. Seizures can involve jerking arms and legs, loss of consciousness, and stiffening of the child's body. After a seizure, the child may be sleepy and have a headache. Watching a child have a febrile seizure is alarming for parents; however, there is no lasting effect on the child and these seizures are not associated with epilepsy. There is no treatment necessary except to reduce the fever. During the seizure, the child should be placed on his or her side in an area free of sharp objects. Do not put anything in the child's mouth nor restrain the child.

Meningitis

Meningitis or inflammation of membranes surrounding the brain and spinal cord can be caused by viral or bacterial infection. Viral meningitis is more common and is not life threatening, although bacterial meningitis is life threatening and requires immediate medical attention. Usually meningitis results from an infection originating elsewhere in the body and migrating to the brain and spinal cord through the bloodstream. Viral meningitis more often affects those under age 30 years and occurs more frequently in winter. Bacterial meningitis can be caused by several different types of bacteria including *Streptococcus, Staphylococcus, Haemophilus influenzae,* and meningococcus. Bacterial meningitis can affect all ages, but occurs more frequently in children. Symptoms of the bacterial form of the disease include rapid onset of fever, headache, stiff neck, nausea, and vomiting. Some behavioral changes may occur, such as confusion and sleepiness. Evidence of any previous set of symptoms requires immediate medical attention, preferably in a hospital. A lumbar puncture is needed to confirm diagnosis, and large amounts of antibiotics administered intravenously provide the treatment of choice. Complications from the illness include deafness, brain damage, and blindness.

Immunization with *Haemophilus influenzae* type B (HIB) vaccine has greatly reduced the number of meningitis cases in the United States. The Advisory Committee on Immunization Practices (ACIP) recommends that children age 11 to 12 years, teens entering high school, and college freshmen receive the newly licensed (January 2004) meningococcal vaccine. According to CDC statistics, about 2,000 people in the United States develop meningococcal disease annually, 10 to 14 percent of those die, and 11 to 19 percent have permanent disabilities. It is recommended that 11- to 12-year-olds who receive their tetanus–diphtheria booster receive this new vaccine at the same time.

Fifth Disease

Fifth disease, or erythema infectiosum, is a mildly contagious viral disease that occurs during spring in children over 2 years old. It is caused by parvovirus B19. Symptoms, which last about a week, include reddened cheeks, fever, and a lacy rash on the chest, abdomen, arms, and legs. If Fifth disease is contracted during pregnancy, the fetus may suffer damage or die in utero.

Roseola

Roseola is a common early childhood viral infection characterized by a sudden high fever, which can last about 4 days, followed by a rash of tiny pink spots on the head and trunk. Treatment includes bringing down the child's fever with acetaminophen and sponging the body with lukewarm water.

Hand, Foot, and Mouth Disease

Hand, foot, and mouth disease is another mild viral infection and causes blisters to appear in the mouth, on hands, and on feet. It commonly occurs in summer and early fall and affects children up to age 4 years in day care or nursery schools. It is usually caused by the Coxsackie virus and is spread by the fecal–oral route, saliva, or direct contact with blisters. In addition to blistering, symptoms include fever and loss of appetite. Treatments include acetaminophen, rinsing the mouth with warm salty water, and drinking fluids. Hand washing, especially after diaper changes, washing toys, and touching surfaces possibly contaminated by infected children, helps prevent reinfection.

Child Safety Recommendations

The number-one cause of death in children is injury. Injuries cause more deaths than all diseases combined. To reduce risk for children under age 5 years, the following suggestions should be followed:

- Smoke and carbon monoxide detectors should be located on every floor of a home.

- Batteries on smoke and carbon monoxide detectors should be changed every 6 months. Some families choose to change the batteries during the fall and spring when seasonal time changes take affect.

- Protective covers should be placed over electrical outlets.

- Small children should never be left alone in a bathtub or pool, even for a few seconds.

- Side rails should be left up on cribs.

- Night light should be used in halls and bathrooms.

- Dangerous products should be stored out of reach of children.
- Chemicals, cleaning products, and medications should be locked in cabinets.
- The poison control phone number should be posted by the telephone.
- All children should be taught how to dial 911.
- Toys with small parts that could obstruct airways should be kept out of the home.

Adolescence and Puberty

Adolescence is the transition period between puberty and adulthood. It is divided into stages:

- Early adolescence—ages 12 to 14 years
- Middle adolescence—ages 15 to 17 years

Adolescence is a time of dramatic physical, emotional, and social changes. These changes bring with them choices that for the first time teens may make on their own.

EARLY ADOLESCENCE

Puberty marks the beginning of the development of secondary sexual characteristics: body hair, breasts, menstrual cycles, beard, voice changes, and muscle development. Adolescents begin to make their own choices regarding courses of study, sports, and friends. Peer pressure to use drugs, have sex, and drink alcohol increases. In urban areas the threat of violence may be endured on a daily basis. Loosening of parental ties creates sources of conflict for both parents and teens. Eating disorders, depression, and family crises may be prevalent in this age group.

Emotional Changes

Socially, the early adolescent becomes very concerned with body image, clothes, and how friends see them. They are more self-centered, moody, less affectionate toward parents, and more influenced by peer groups. Teens vacillate between having great expectations for themselves and experiencing total lack of confidence in their abilities. Risk taking is common among this group of teens. The CDC notes that the leading cause of death in 12- to 14-year-olds is motor vehicle crashes.

MIDDLE ADOLESCENCE

Developmentally, girls are physically mature at this point. Boys may still be maturing. Body image is important to

PROFESSIONALISM THE LIFE SPAN

Suicide is the third leading cause of death in teenagers and young adults after accidents and homicides. Educating yourself, parents, and caregivers about the warning signs of suicide could save a life. No one knows exactly what causes someone to commit suicide; many factors are implicated. However, others with the same risk factors do not commit suicide. A CDC survey found that 28 percent of high school students had suicidal thoughts, and 8.3 percent had attempted suicide. Girls attempt suicide three times more often than boys. Boys, however, are four times more likely to die in the suicide attempt.

Many people talk about suicide well before they actually make an attempt. This provides a window of opportunity for family, friends, and health care professionals to be alert to their threats and take action to prevent the attempt. Risk factors for teenagers are similar to those of adults, including death of a family member, end of a dating relationship, move from familiar school or house, failure at school, substance abuse, and trouble with the law. Most commonly, depression and substance abuse are implicated in suicides. In teenagers, behavior imitation is sometimes a factor. After a publicized suicide of an idol, for instance, teenage suicide attempts sometimes increase. As health care professionals, you are in a position to identify those who exhibit any of the following behaviors:

- Decline in hygiene
- Access to firearms and prescription drugs
- Preoccupation with morbid thoughts
- Substance abuse
- Family history of suicide
- Dramatic changes in grades, mood, or contact with friends
- Decrease in appetite
- Change in sleep patterns
- Previous suicide attempt

Experts say that any suicide attempt must be taken seriously, even if it is only a couple of scratches on the wrist or a couple of pills. All suicide attempts should be evaluated in a hospital emergency room for treatment or hospitalization. Crisis hotlines are helpful, especially for worried parents and friends. Having information about suicide allows you to be prepared to alert caregivers to suicide risks and to inform them to look for certain behavior.

Box 40-2 Parenting Tips for Teen YEARS

- Be honest and answer questions directly.
- Take an interest in your children's friends and school activities.
- Have family meal times as often as possible.
- Respect the opinions of adolescents.
- Encourage a healthy lifestyle, including proper nutrition and exercise.

- Set clear-cut rules—and stick to them.
- Know where your son or daughter is at all times, and be sure a parent is present.
- Talk about sex and drugs, and really listen.

these teens. Eating disorders may continue to develop among females and some males. Middle teens may be developing more individual opinions and a definite personality. A more clear sense of identity develops, thus they may not be as strongly influenced by peers. Teens may start to assert independence and find employment.

Emotional Changes

During the middle teen years, conflicts with parents may decrease; these adolescents exhibit greater independence and a greater interest in the opposite sex. Middle teens spend more time with peers and less with parents and develop a greater capacity to develop more caring relationships. They have a greater sense of right and wrong, more concern for the future, and better work habits. Some teens experience depression which can lead to problems in all areas of their lives. See Box 40-2 for tips on parenting adolescents.

Eating Disorders

Eating disorders are categorized into three main types: anorexia nervosa, bulimia nervosa, and eating disorders not otherwise specified (EDNOS). Eating disorders are marked by extreme problems with eating behavior. The urge to eat smaller or, in some cases, larger amounts of food spins out of control. Frequently, eating disorders appear in adolescence or in young adulthood.

Although females suffer more frequently than males, eating disorders in males are present in 5 to 15 percent of all patients with eating disorders. The National Institute of Mental Health (NIMH) reports that binge eating affects males and females equally. Some medical and psychological treatments, including family counseling, are effective for some eating disorders; however, no specific treatment is available for chronic cases.

ANOREXIA NERVOSA

Anorexia nervosa is associated with a distorted sense of body image and the persistent quest for thinness, at times to the point of emaciation. Some anorexic patients lose weight by stringent dieting, or **purging** (by vomiting or taking laxatives, enemas, or diuretics). These patients often have coexisting psychiatric or physical illnesses. Patients with anorexia nervosa are ten times more likely to die than those without the illness. Signs of anorexia nervosa include the following:

- Extreme weight loss
- Excessively dry skin and brittle hair
- **Amenorrhea** (absence of menses)
- Low vital signs
- Fatigue
- Osteopenia or osteoporosis
- Electrolyte imbalance

Some patients recover after one episode, others have relapses, and still others have a severe chronic form that leads to health deterioration and, in some cases, death. Treatment includes psychotherapy, including family therapy or intensive inpatient or outpatient therapy, and the use of antidepressant or antianxiety medications. Anorexia nervosa remains a difficult condition to treat.

BULIMIA NERVOSA

Bulimia nervosa patients binge eat and then either use self-induced vomiting, laxatives, diuretics, or all three to rid themselves of the large amounts of calories consumed. These patients appear to be in the normal weight range for their age. Bulimic patients are secretive about their condition and deny any problem with food. Binging and purging may occur several times a week. These patients have coexisting conditions such as depression, anxiety, and substance abuse problems. Bulimic patients exhibit some of the following symptoms:

- Chronic sore throat from vomiting stomach acids
- Worn enamel on teeth from stomach acids
- Dehydration
- Gastrointestinal reflux disorder (GERD)
- Intestinal irritation from laxative use
- Swollen neck glands

Treatment for bulimic patients includes nutritional and psychological counseling, treatment with fluoxetine (Prozac) and appetite suppressants, and behavioral modification.

EATING DISORDERS NOT OTHERWISE SPECIFIED

Eating Disorders Not Otherwise Specified (EDNOS), as the name implies, is an eating disorder that does not fit into the category of anorexia or bulimia. EDNOS is characterized by binge eating episodes that are recurring and lead to obesity. The disorder is often associated with feelings of shame, guilt, depression, and other coexisting psychological disorders. Treatment is much the same as treatment for bulimia, including the possible use of appetite suppressants.

SUMMARY

The medical assistant should be prepared to function competently with pediatric patients of all ages. Medical assistants need an understanding of childhood growth and development and of both the common and uncommon childhood diseases and disorders. As a medical assistant, you must be able to accurately perform such procedures as obtaining vital signs on children, measuring children's height and weight, and assisting with all phases of the sick- and well-child examinations. Sensitive issues of child abuse, suicide, eating disorders, and developmental problems should be handled with understanding, empathy, and safeguarding of the patient's rights. Having contact information readily available to assist parents is a vital part of the medical assistant's responsibility.

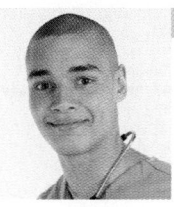

40 CHAPTER REVIEW

COMPETENCY REVIEW

1. Define and spell the terms to learn in this chapter.

2. The pediatrician has asked you to develop a teaching plan for obese children under age 8 years. What is your plan?

3. A new mother comes into the office and is overly concerned about the possibility of her child dying of SIDS. What would you do?

PREPARING FOR THE CERTIFICATION EXAM

1. The average infant doubles his/her weight
   a. at 3 months
   b. at 3 years
   c. at 1 year
   d. at 6 months
   e. at 2 years

2. The Apgar scale is
   a. used to evaluate newborns
   b. used to evaluate preteens
   c. used to measure weight
   d. a component of measuring body mass index
   e. used to evaluate brain function

3. Conditions such as microencephaly or hydrocephalus are evaluated by
   a. diameter of the infant's chest
   b. the length of the infant
   c. the weight of the infant
   d. the size of the infant's limbs
   e. the circumference of the infant's head

4. A normal 1-year-old
   a. prefers to play alone
   b. can wave bye-bye and can walk with assistance
   c. cannot sit up
   d. cannot say any words
   e. prefers to lie in the crib

5. To reduce spread of infection in a pediatric waiting room
   a. only see well patients on specific days
   b. make ill patients wait in a hallway
   c. place ill patients in an examination room at once
   d. spray room with air freshener
   e. raise heat to reduce germs

6. Symptoms of dehydration in infants
   a. are unimportant
   b. include dry skin and loss of elasticity of skin
   c. include increased urine output
   d. include being energetic and alert
   e. include overproduction of tears

7. The respiratory rate of an infant
   a. is lower than that of an adult
   b. is the same as that of an adult
   c. does not need to measured until puberty
   d. is higher than that of an adult
   e. is measured by the parent

8. Bulimia nervosa is an eating disorder that
   a. affects only males
   b. is characterized by bingeing and purging
   c. is curable with antibiotic medication
   d. is characterized by extreme weight loss in all patients
   e. is not important

9. Pediatric blood pressure is measured
   a. at the discretion of the parent
   b. only in newborns
   c. only during yearly exams in teens
   d. yearly after 3 years, or at the discretion of the physician
   e. at every office visit

10. An infant who scores under the third percentile on growth charts
    a. may be suffering from failure to thrive (FTT)
    b. may be normal
    c. must be reported to authorities
    d. will reach normal weight at a year
    e. may suffer from Fifth disease

CRITICAL THINKING

1. What is failure to thrive, and what problems could it cause the child?

2. What are some common causes of FTT in newborns and infants?

3. At age 18 months, what developmental stages should Keyla have mastered?

ON THE JOB

Sara, a 14-year-old, has come to the office for her school physical. She is very remote, moody, and unwilling to answer any questions you ask her as part of her physical exam. She seems to have changed a great deal in the past year, is thinner, more unkempt, and lethargic. You notice also that her mother is constantly badgering her and rolling her eyes in exasperation at her lack of cooperation. What could you do to facilitate the examination? What possible problems could Sara be experiencing?

INTERNET ACTIVITY

Research a childhood disease or disorder that interests you.

MEDMEDIA

Additional interactive resources and activities for this chapter can be found:

On your student DVD: View applicable procedure videos on the DVD-ROM found in the back of this book.

MyHealthProfessionsKit.com: Test your knowledge of this chapter with games and activities. MyHealthProfessionsKit also includes resources, helpful links, and a Spanish audio glossary.

Medical Assisting Interactive: Practice your procedures as a medical assistant in this simulated doctor's office. This can be accessed through MyHealthProfessionsKit.com.

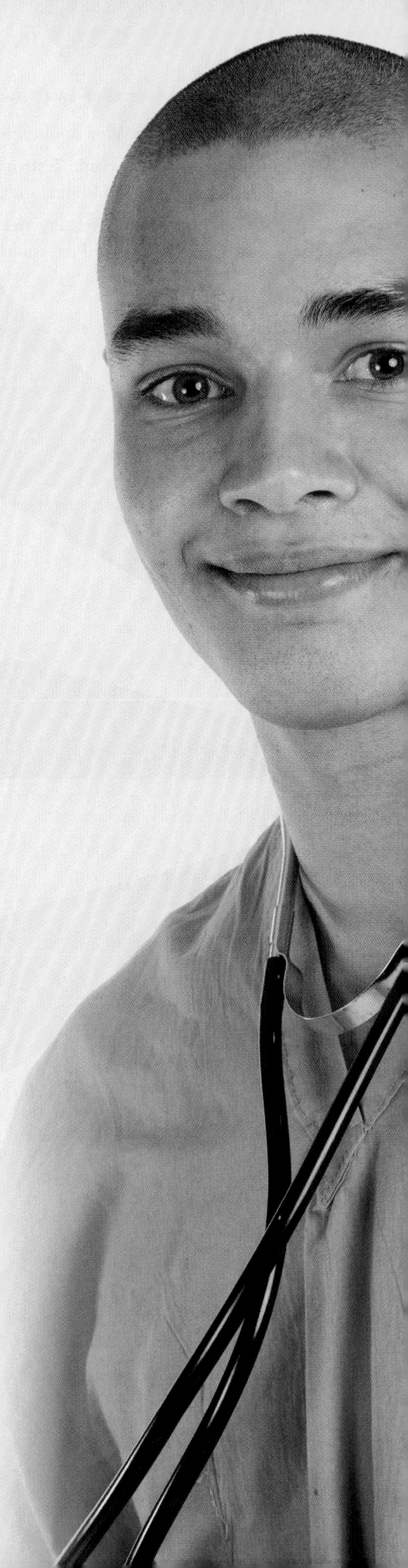

41

Assisting with Life Span Specialties: Geriatrics

LEARNING OBJECTIVES

After completing this chapter, you should be able to:

- Define and spell the terms to learn in the chapter.

- Explain the impact of an aging population on health care in the United States.

- Describe the aging process and its effects on each system of the body.

- Compare and contrast confusion, depression, and dementia in the elderly.

- Summarize guidelines for effective communication with the elderly.

- Identify legal issues of aging patients.

- Identify six safety measures to recommend to caregivers of aging patients.

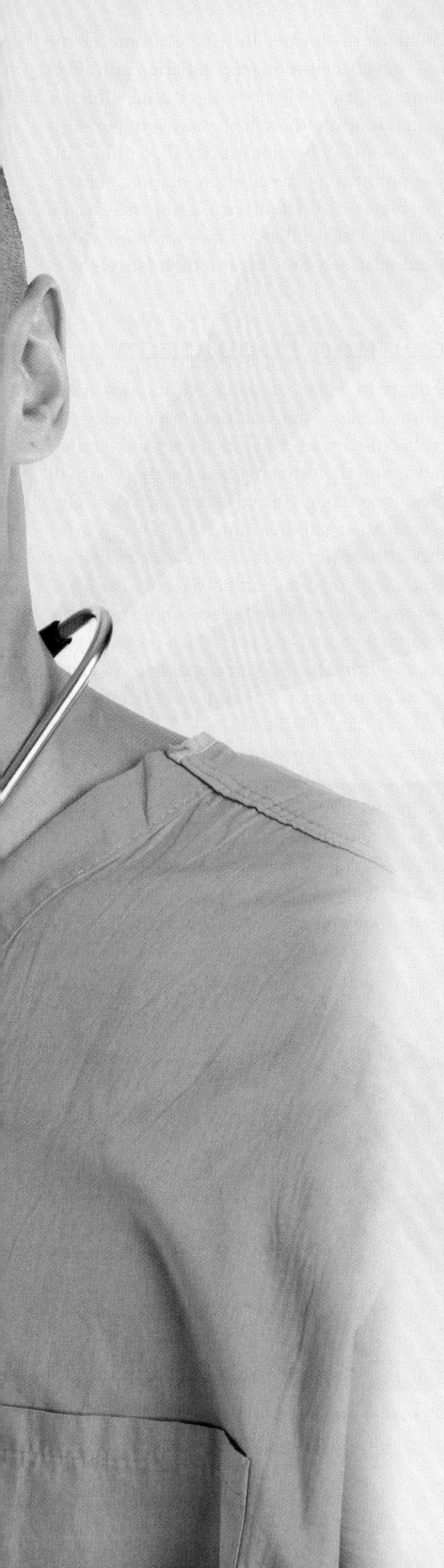

CHAPTER OUTLINE

CASE STUDY

Shandra, an RMA with Pearson Physicians Group, is assigned to work with Dr. Penningworth today. The doctor's next patient is Sylvia Jordan, age 76, who is in the office for her yearly physical. As you escort her to the examination room, Ms. Jordan confides that her husband of 54 years passed away 7 months ago.

ageism

assisted-living facilities

cognitive ability

extended-care facilities

geriatrician

geriatrics

gerontology

Medicare

Medigap insurance

respite care

CERTIFICATION LINK

CMA (AAMA)
Psychology
   Developmental
   stages of the
   life cycle
Communication
   Adapting commu-
   nication according
   to an individual's
   needs
Nutrition
   Special needs

RMA
General medical
assisting knowledge
   Human relations
   Patient education

CMAS (AMT)
Professionalism
   Employ human
   relations skills
   appropriate to the
   health care setting

The field of medicine specializing in the treatment of elderly patients, **geriatrics**, began as early as the early 1900s. In 1914, Dr. Ignatz L. Nascher wrote the first geriatrics textbook, in which the term *geriatrics* was first used. This term is derived from the Greek word *geras,* which means "old age," and from the word *iatrikos,* which means "physician."

Currently the average life expectancy in the United States is 77.8 years, according to the Centers for Disease Control and Prevention (CDC) report published in 2009, a new record high. As a medical assistant you may work in a specialty office that provides services specifically to the elderly population or a general practice that treats patients in every position within the lifespan. This chapter covers the specific differences you may encounter while providing care to the elderly population. **Gerontology**, which is gaining in popularity due to the baby boomer generation, is the study of the process of aging and the effects of aging on people. A **geriatrician** is a physician who diagnoses and treats diseases and conditions that mainly affect older patients, such as osteoarthritis, congestive heart failure, arthritis, emphysema, cerebrovascular accident (CVA), and Alzheimer's disease. In general, some of the same conditions that affect a younger population also affect elders. Surprisingly, the elderly have fewer acute illnesses than younger age groups, although the recovery period is typically longer when they become acutely ill. Chronic illness is the major problem for the older population. Some of the physical problems associated with aging may cause patients to lose their independence; however, many elders remain active and relatively healthy into their late eighties (Figure 41-1).

The Aging Population

Every culture treats its elders according to its own traditions. In the United States, our traditions have undergone change, in part, because we are a mobile society and families are often spread across the country. In the early twentieth century, the older generation had no choice, economically, except to live with their children until they died. Fortunately much has changed in the lives of elders since that time. One of the most important improvements in elders' lives was due to the passage of the Federal Old Age Insurance Law in 1935 under Social Security, which provided elders some financial security. In 1965, in response to an aging population, the Administration on Aging and Older Americans Act, Medicaid, and **Medicare**, a U.S. government insurance program for which persons aged 65 and over and others with special conditions, were all enacted. Several private companies, geared specifically toward the aging population, such as the American Association of Retired Persons (AARP), also offer **Medigap insurance** as a supplement to Medicare. As the numbers of older adults continues to increase, more attention is given to the needs of the elderly

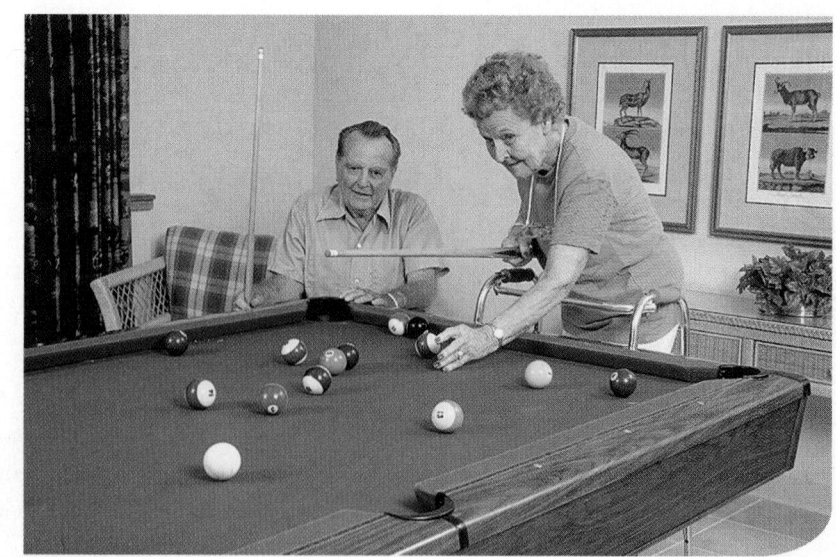

FIGURE 41-1 Older adults can live active lives into their eighties and beyond.

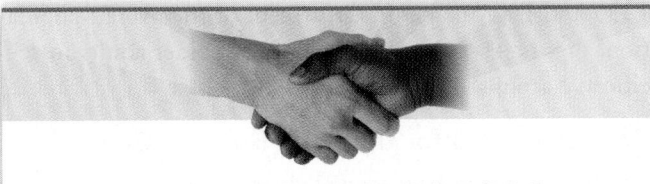

ROFESSIONALISM

CULTURAL CONSIDERATIONS

Native Americans have close family bonds and respect and view elders as teachers and leaders. They believe that each person has a right to make his or her own health care decisions and may find inappropriate the probing questions that health care providers ask.

Many Latino Americans view their health status as God's will. Some consider good health as a reward for living correctly and taking care of your body, whereas being ill is a punishment for not living appropriately. Wearing or having medals and crosses in their rooms is an important part of prayer and healing. Older relatives are held in high regard, and old age is viewed in a positive light.

The traditions of other ethnic or cultural groups are not odd or weird; they are just different. As health care providers, we should seek to honor the traditions of others and not change them. Patients should never be made to feel that their religious beliefs are undervalued or not respected.

in the areas of health care, living conditions, and living a fulfilling life.

In U.S. culture today, many older Americans are still working into their seventies and are enjoying an active social life throughout their eighties and even nineties. These individuals and others do not want to leave their friends by moving across the country or even to another state just so they can live with their children. Box 41-1 lists some famous people who were successful in later years. The elderly are no longer lumped into one group of people over age 65. Sociologists place the elderly into four distinct age groups:

- **Young old:** 65–75 years old
- **Old:** 75–85 years old
- **Old-old:** 85–100 years old
- **Elite old:** 100+ years old

FACTS ABOUT THE ELDERLY

Currently in the United States people over 65 years of age make up 12 percent of the total population. This figure is rising, and it is estimated that in 2050 the elderly will make up 20 percent of the population. Life expectancy is increasing (Box 41-2) due to better living conditions, medical advances, better nutrition, and new medications. Thanks in part to these advances, the elderly are living healthier, happier, and longer lives. Among the elderly population, 40 percent is over age 85. Currently 23 percent of senior citizens report Social Security as their primary source of income. With more people requiring Social Security for longer periods of time, the long-term demands on this beneficial program are obvious. The elderly will be using more health care resources in the coming years. Although **assisted-living facilities** designed for residents who cannot live independently but do not require 24-hour care, and **extended-care facilities**, which provide specialized care, are still viable choices for seniors in need, the number of long-term residents has declined as the option of in-home care services has expanded. Only 5 percent of the older population is in long-term care at any given time; however, one in four elders will spend some time in a nursing home during his or her last years.

THE BABY BOOMER GENERATION

Baby boomers are individuals born between 1946 and 1964. The oldest of this group reaches senior citizen status in 2011. As of 2007, 28 percent of the U.S. population is between 44 and 62 years old. A study by Duke University sociologists Angela M. O'Rand and Mary Elizabeth Hughes has shown that the baby boomers are a diverse generation. The Hispanic and Asian-American groups increased dramatically during the boomer era. A 2000 census study found the early boomers born in foreign countries between 1946 and 1955 make up 12 percent of the overall population. The later boomers born in foreign countries between

Box 41-1 Facts That Counteract Aging ASSUMPTIONS

- Eleanor Roosevelt, wife of Franklin D. Roosevelt, chaired the United Nations Commission on Human Rights from the age of 62 to 67, and she wrote her autobiography at age 74.
- Frank Lloyd Wright designed the Guggenheim Museum in New York City at age 91.
- Nelson Mandela was inaugurated as president of South Africa at age 75 after 27 years in prison and winning the country's first multiracial election.
- Grandma Moses, the famous American painter, started her career in art during her seventies.

Box 41-2 Life Expectancy at Birth for Men and WOMEN

Birth Year	Life Expectancy (in years)
1900	47.3
1940	62.9
1950	68.2
1960	69.7
1970	70.8
1980	73.7
1990	75.4
1995	75.8
2000	76.8
2005	77.4
2006	77.7

Source: Centers for Disease Control and Prevention, National Center for Health Statistics, U.S. Census Bureau, National Vital Statistics Reports, 2009, 57(14), Table 8.

1955 and 1964 make up 15 percent of the overall population. Figure 41-2 shows the number of older adults in specific age groups.

Considerations for the Baby Boomer Generation

The baby boomers have several characteristics that will have an impact on health care and your role as a provider of health care. They have fewer children than previous generational groups or have waited later than previous generations to start a family. Those without the financial safety net of older children will mean that they will be receiving less assistance from family as they age. Baby boomers may also be referred to as the "sandwich generation." Many are facing the reality of caring for an ailing parent and a young child at the same time and are, in a sense, sandwiched between them. This difficult situation makes time and financial management difficult.

The boomer generation has been considered the best-educated generational group. The United States G.I. Bill, also known as the Servicemembers' Readjustment Act of 1944, allowed returning soldiers to obtain a postsecondary education, sometimes becoming the first family member to do so. This increase in education allowed for greater economic freedom and career choices.

Unfortunately, studies show a large inequality in education and financial stability across the boomer generation.

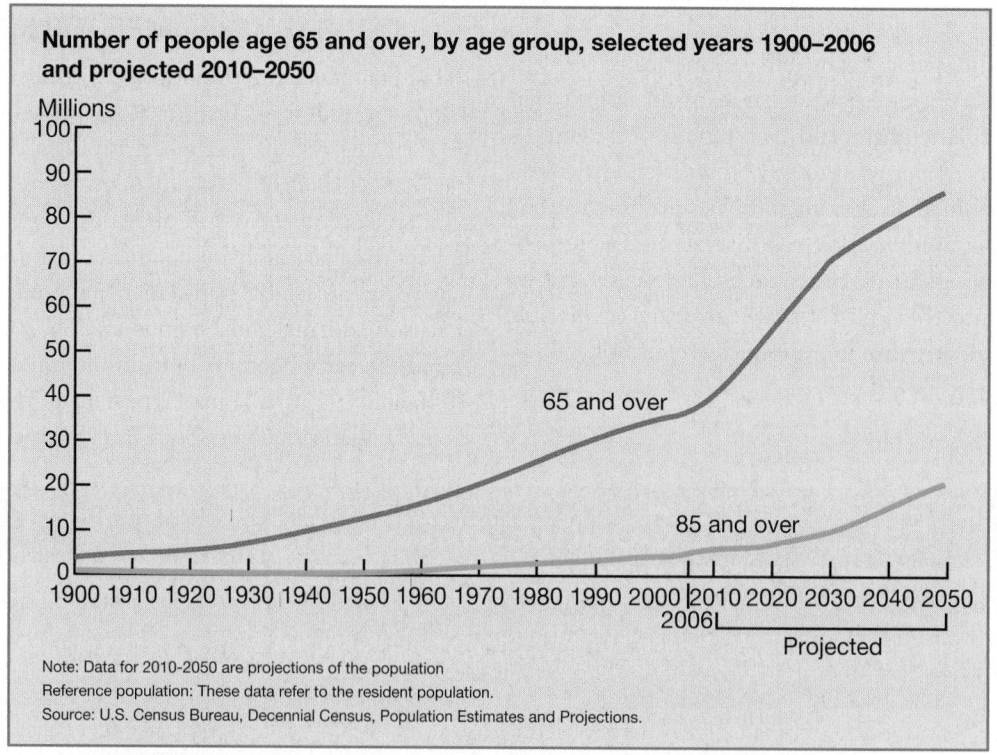

FIGURE 41-2 **Number of older adults in specific age groups.**
Source: U.S. Census Bureau, Decennial Census, Population Estimates and Projections.

The economic hardship, combined with advancing age and deterioration of health, will mean an increased strain on government resources for health care and prescription drug assistance over time.

The Aging Process

The aging process begins at birth and continues until death. This process is a not an illness but a normal part of life that progresses at different rates in each person. There are many theories about the causes of aging. We can identify some factors that impact how we age, such as genetics, lifestyle choices, occupational hazards, poor nutrition, lack of health care, and physical and social environment.

Ageism is defined as a prejudice against and incorrect assumptions about an individual or individuals because of their age. Aging is not easy. Much of our society tends to stereotype the elderly and have many misconceptions. Our goal, as professional care providers, should be to view the aging adult as an individual and provide the best possible health care to him or her.

Understanding the effects that the aging process has on the human body as a whole and on individual body systems will help foster a better awareness of elders' needs. This awareness will help increase the respect and empathy the elderly patient receives from the health care provider.

PHYSICAL CHANGES

Review in Table 41-1 the physical changes of aging on each system of the body and important points that are relevant to each system. If during your time with the patient, you notice new problems in the older patient, chart them accordingly and report them to the physician for immediate evaluation. Table 41-2 lists some diseases that usually affect older people.

Integumentary System

Integumentary system changes within the elderly are often obvious. Observe the patient as he or she prepares for the examination. Pay particular attention to bruises and signs of infection. Since pain receptors are diminished with age, an elderly person may not be aware of an injury. Make sure the examining room is at the proper temperature and that sufficient coverings are available to make the patient comfortable. Since adhesive bandages may damage the skin and cause excoriation or sloughing off during removal, select a type of covering that will cause the least discomfort.

TABLE 41-1 Physical Changes of Aging

Body System	Physical Changes
Integumentary	Hair loses color and becomes thinner; skin dries, becomes less elastic, and wrinkles develop; skin tears easily; skin bruises easily (senile purpura); fingernails and toenails thicken; reduced amount of sweat; increased sensitivity to cold; age spots more common.
Nervous	Problems with balance; temperature regulation off; sensation of pain decreases; deep sleep shortened; more awakening during the night; brain cells lost, but intelligence intact unless pathologic condition present; decreased sensitivity of nerve receptors for heat, cold, pain, and pressure.
Sensory	More difficult to see close objects; night vision may decrease; cataracts (clouding of the lens) more common; peripheral vision and depth perception diminish; hearing diminishes; smell and taste receptors less sensitive.
Musculoskeletal	Less muscle strength; less flexibility; slower movements; arthritis and osteoporosis more common; body is more stooped.
Respiratory	Breathing capacity lessens.
Urinary	Kidneys decrease in size; urine production less efficient; emptying bladder completely more difficult; stress incontinence may develop.
Digestive	Primary taste sensations of salty, sweet, and sour decrease; constipation increases; flatulence increases; movement of food through the digestive tract slows.
Cardiovascular	Blood vessels less elastic and more narrowed; heart may not pump as efficiently; decrease in cardiac output and circulation.
Endocrine	Decrease in estrogen and progesterone; hot flashes, nervous feelings; higher levels of parathormone and thyroid stimulating hormone; weight gain; insulin production less efficient; diabetes mellitus more likely.
Reproductive	*Females:* ovulation and menstruation cease; vaginal walls thinner and drier. *Males:* scrotum less firm; prostate gland may enlarge.

TABLE 41-2 Diseases That Mainly Affect the Elderly

Disease/Condition	Explanation
Alzheimer's disease and other dementias	Brain disorders that lead to progressive loss of memory and other intellectual functions.
Aortic aneurysm	Dilation of the wall of the aorta that can rupture and lead to death if left untreated.
Atrophic urethritis and vaginitis	Thinning of the tissue of the urethra and vagina that can lead to burning on urination and painful intercourse.
Benign prostatic hyperplasia	Enlargement of the prostate gland, which blocks the flow of urine.
Cataracts	Clouding in the lens of the eye, which impacts vision.
Chronic lymphocytic leukemia	A type of leukemia that usually has a long phase with little growth or progression (indolent phase) but has many other characteristic features of cancer.
Decubitus ulcers (bedsores)	Breakdown of skin from prolonged pressure.
Diabetes mellitus type 2	A type of diabetes that may not require insulin treatment, usually begins in middle age.
Glaucoma	Elevation of the pressure in one of the chambers of the eye that can decrease vision and lead to blindness, usually begins in middle age.
Hypothyroidism	Thyroid gland is underactive and produces too little thyroid hormone, can eventually result in anemia, low body temperature, mental confusion, and heart failure.
Osteoarthritis	Degeneration of the cartilage that lines the joints, usually begins in middle age.
Osteoporosis	Loss of calcium from the bones, makes them fragile and leads to fractures.
Parkinson's disease	Slowly progressive degenerative brain disease that leads to tremor, muscle rigidity, difficulty moving, and instability.
Prostate cancer	Cancer of the prostate gland.
Shingles (herpes zoster)	A reawakening of the dormant chickenpox virus that causes skin rash and can lead to prolonged pain.
Stroke	A blockage or bleeding of a blood vessel in the brain that leads to weakness, loss of sensation, difficulty talking, or other neurological problems.
Urinary incontinence	Inability to control urine flow.

Diabetes mellitus is a problem for many elderly and impacts the ability to heal. Examine fingernails and toenails because the patient may not be able to keep them properly trimmed and may cut them too deeply, leading to infection. The patient may need to see a podiatrist or have a visiting nurse trim toenails to reduce chance of infection.

NERVOUS SYSTEM

With age, the nervous system begins to slow down and reaction times are delayed. (Cognitive ability and dementia are discussed later in this chapter.) Allow extra time for older patients to follow directions and respond to questions. Do not finish sentences for older patients or ignore a patient while talking about the patient to his or her family members or caregivers. Slower responses to changes in balance can make the elderly patient more prone to falls and injuries. Offer your arm to patients when walking, and assist them on and off the examination table. Make sure the step stool is secure as patients get on and off the examination table. If you use a beam scale in your office, assist patients onto and off of the platform and provide wall-mount handgrips for additional support. The platform on this type of scale moves in multiple directions and can make patients lose their balance.

Sleep cycles are affected by the aging process in the brain. Ask patients how they are sleeping, how many hours, and if they feel rested. Sometimes the elderly take frequent naps during the day, which can affect their ability to sleep restfully at night.

SENSORY CHANGES

Sensory changes in the eyes, ears, nose, and mouth affect elders' ability to react to the world. Presbycusis (impairment of hearing associated with aging) and presbyopia (inability to focus on objects at close range) reduce elders' ability to interact with the environment around them. As elderly patients prepare for their examination, inquire about hearing and sight abilities. If applicable, ask if their hearing aid is functioning well, whether eyeglasses are helping them to see well enough, if they still drive, and how they react to the glare of lights at night. Speak clearly and slowly enough so patients can understand your message, without being condescending. Sensory information from the nose and mouth declines until about age 80, when approximately half the sense of smell is lost. Taste depends mostly on smell. The elderly may not have much interest in food and therefore may not be taking enough nourishment. Elders often are "tea and toasters." Instead of eating a nutritious meal, they will have tea and toast or crackers periodically during the day. As a result, they feel full; however, they are not consuming the protein, vitamins, and minerals needed to keep them healthy. They may also over-salt or over-season their food due to the reduction in taste. Poor oral hygiene and side effects of medications also can affect eating. Engage elder patients in a discussion of favorite foods and what they normally eat each day. Observe their teeth and oral hygiene, ask if they wear dentures, and check that the dentures fit properly.

Musculoskeletal System

Musculoskeletal system aging is characterized by a decrease in muscle strength and a loss of flexibility. Both of these conditions increase older people's risk of falling and sustaining fractures. Perhaps you can promote regular exercise at the local senior center (Figure 41-3) and provide information about exercises to increase upper body strength that the

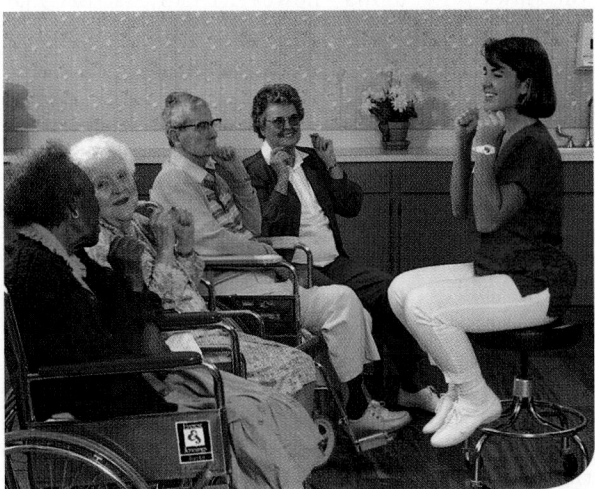

FIGURE 41-3 **Exercise is beneficial and provides socialization.**

elderly can perform at home while seated. Encourage eating proper amounts of dairy products to supply needed calcium. Discuss safety issues at home that can put the elderly patient at risk. Speak to them about how they bathe: Do they have grab rails and chairs in the tub area? Encourage them to use the assistive devices that they may need: cane, walker, and bedside commode (portable toilet). If these assistive devices have not been obtained, check with your office policy regarding the physician prescribing assistive devices for patients. Review safety concerns with caregivers and family members.

Respiratory System

Respiratory system aging is characterized by loss of elasticity in the alveoli and lungs, leading to a reduction in exchange of gases. In addition, as the respiratory muscles become weaker, it becomes more difficult to move air into and out of the lungs. Stridor, or breathing with a high-pitched sound, also can be observed. Inactivity in the elderly, combined with reduced pulmonary function, make them more prone to pneumonia. Breathing exercises can be taught through videos or written materials to help the elderly increase the depth of breathing and exercise respiratory muscles. Any activity that will increase endurance will be beneficial in protecting the elderly from respiratory infections and improving the oxygen supply to all body systems.

Urinary System

Urinary system changes that can occur with aging result in a reduced ability to concentrate urine and slower waste removal by the kidneys. Slower waste removal combined with the number of daily medications taken by most elderly people places older patients more at risk for toxic medication overload that can have significant impact on their quality of life. Decrease in bladder storage capacity and the inability to empty the bladder provide opportunity for infection. Increased frequency of urination, nocturia, and urgency may all become problems for many elderly. Disruption of sleep may make some patients tired and irritable. Urgency makes them feel reluctant to leave home for fear they may embarrass themselves by not making it to the bathroom quickly enough to avoid soiling themselves. Some patients may feel that reducing fluid intake is the way to cope with these problems; however, this can lead to dehydration, electrolyte imbalance, and increased risk of urinary tract infection. Being able to speak to the patient about the consequences of reducing fluids enables the patient to be better informed and possibly to make better choices to get through the day. The proper amount of water and other fluids is critical to maintain homeostasis in the body.

Digestive System

Digestive system aging is characterized by slower passage of food leading to less absorption of food, minerals, and vitamins, along with increased constipation and flatulence. Stressing the importance of proper nutrition that includes all the food groups is helpful. Provide a brochure with a diagram of appropriate food portion sizes as well as lists of foods in each food group, which the patient may take home. Supplying examples will be helpful for the overweight patient as will making sure they are aware of their current body mass index (BMI) and what their goal number should be. If it is obvious that an elderly patient is struggling with nutrition issues, a consultation with a registered dietician may be in order. Since the liver slows down with age, it takes longer for drugs and alcohol to be absorbed, which can cause an increase in the risk of adverse drug interactions.

Cardiovascular System

Cardiovascular changes are age related and are frequently the cause of disease and disorders in elders. However, lifestyle habits such as smoking, high-fat diets, and lack of exercise also take a toll on the cardiovascular system. Hypertension and a decrease in the strength of cardiac contractions decreases cardiac output and reduces the oxygen supply needed by the organs of the body. Orthostatic hypotension occurs in some elderly patients. Orthostatic hypotension is a 20 to 30 mmHg drop in blood pressure that is associated with dizziness and fainting when changing position from lying down or sitting to a standing position. Dizziness can increase elders' risk of injury. The medical assistant should help the patient understand why this may happen and suggest that rising more slowly and holding onto something steady may prevent the dizziness.

Endocrine System

Endocrine system aging is characterized by decreasing levels of estrogen, thyroid hypofunction, and insulin resistance. The decrease of estrogen in females ends menstrual cycles, decreases vaginal secretions, and may lead to hot flashes, night sweats, and sleep disturbances. Thyroid hypofunction can lead to patients being overweight, fatigued, and confused, which can be mistaken for dementia. Many elderly develop diabetes mellitus and will need guidance in menu selections and obtaining and testing blood samples. Encourage elders to have blood work done regularly to screen for endocrine system dysfunctions.

Reproductive System

Since elders are aging more gracefully and are in better health than ever before, it follows that the desire for sex is present in many. Psychologists say that patterns of sexual interest later in life mirror lifelong patterns. Older patients may find it difficult to discuss anything related to sexual matters. If the opportunity presents itself, you must be ready to discuss these issues comfortably and nonjudgmentally. Again, written materials for the patient to read at home are important educational tools. (Other reproductive system changes are discussed in Chapter 31).

MENTAL CHANGES

Mental deterioration is not a normal part of aging. As people age, the risk for mental deterioration increases, as does the risk of age-related disorders. Mental health is the capacity to cope effectively with life changes, manage life's stresses, and achieve a state of emotional balance. Brain function slows with aging; however, many factors may have an impact on a patient's mental status. To maintain good mental health, individuals must participate in activities they find interesting and engage in regular social interactions. For optimal mental health, the elderly should have a sense of self-worth and feel they are of value to society.

Cognitive Ability

Cognitive ability, the ability to think clearly, reason, and perceive, is affected by many factors. Normal aging does not reduce cognitive ability. The psychological status of the mind is altered by health status, genetics, social factors, educational accomplishment, and physical activity. Normally an individual's personality does not change with age unless there is a pathologic problem.

Memory

The three types of memory are short-term memory (things that can be recalled for about 30 seconds or so but, if not repeated multiple times, will fade from memory, such as the name of a one-time acquaintance at a party); long-term memory (memories that have been activated multiple times and committed to the brain); and sensory memory (information gained through the senses and lasting a few seconds). Aging does not mean that a loss of memory or cognitive ability in the elderly is a certainty. With age, the ability to retrieve information from long-term memory may be slower. Basic intelligence is unchanged throughout the life span, as are the abilities for verbal comprehension, arithmetic operations, and problem solving. Learning is not altered by aging. Working memory (the ability to retain information while using other information) slows with age. The expression "Use it or lose it" could apply to the brain as well as other muscles. Keeping the brain active with games, puzzles, and other types of stimulation help maintain memory retrieval. Sleep is equally important. Studies have shown that memories and information are consolidated during sleep and that insufficient physical rest delays the brain's response time. Activities such as knitting and crocheting stimulate the brain. In addition, physical exercise increases oxygen flow and helps maintain blood supply to the brain, improving memory function. Some may find that the first stages of learning something new may take longer, but once learning has taken place, elders as a group are able to keep up with others.

It is important to assist the individual with true memory loss to remain as active and self-sufficient as long as possible. Tips to help with memory loss include placing notes in specific spots to trigger memory, such as a note by the door prompting individuals to remember their keys. Several safety precautions can also be taken, with devices that chime if a window is left open or an automatic stove burner shut-off.

Although there are many types of memory loss, people with memory loss often struggle in four common areas: (1) recalling the distant past, (2) processing new information, (3) remembering people's names, and (4) separating fact from fiction. The following are suggestions that may aid the patient dealing with memory loss:

- **Recalling distant memories**—Caregivers can review with patients souvenirs, pictures, and movies. Looking at pictures and memorabilia will often help jog a distant memory.

- **Problems retaining new information**—Keep new information short and repeat it frequently. If the information has more than three steps, break those steps into smaller segments so they can be learned individually.

- **Remembering peoples' names**—Consistently reintroduce yourself and your intentions (e.g., when you leave the examination room and come back, when the caregiver at home steps away, or any time a lapse in visual contact occurs).

- **Separating fact from fiction**—It is important to correct the patient in a nonthreatening manner.

Effect of Medications on Mental Abilities

Medications taken for other problems may impair mental abilities, especially if said medication is taken in the wrong amount, at the wrong time, or is skipped altogether. Older patients take an average of four to five different medications and one to two over-the-counter medications daily. Providing the patient with a pill organizer, a printed list of the medications he or she is taking, and a record of why he or she is taking them may help decrease incorrect medicating. Caregivers should be provided with these aids if the patient is not competent. Warn the patient in writing and verbally about possible food or drug interactions. When taking a patient history, specifically ask about over-the-counter preparations, vitamins, and herbal supplements since the patient may not view these products as "medications."

Confusion

Confusion is a term used by physicians and health care providers to indicate that the person cannot follow a conversation, answer questions appropriately, understand where he or she is, remember important facts, or make appropriate safety judgments. Confusion is not a normal consequence of aging. Confusion is a broad term that can mean an acute or chronic condition. Acute confusion is a form of confusion with symptoms lasting less than 3 months. Chronic confusion is characterized by symptoms persisting longer than 3 months. Furthermore, confusion can be narrowed down into three categories:

- **Systemic confusion**—occurs when normal brain functions or the metabolic process of the brain are interrupted by factors that are reversible, such as blood sugar spikes or sudden drops.

- **Mechanical confusion**—occurs when a sudden physiologic change in the brain's functioning takes place, such as a blood clot (stroke) or traumatic injury.

- **Psychosocial/environmental confusion**—occurs with the sudden change of the environment, the loss of a life partner, or a move to a different residential setting.

If confusion is demonstrated by a patient, the cause must be determined. Pinpointing the exact cause may be difficult and may have to be determined by the process of elimination of other possible causes.

The most common cause of acute confusion onset in the elderly is a urinary tract infection (UTI). The confusion will resolve with no permanent damage as soon as the infection has cleared. Often family members of the confused individual will be relieved at the quick diagnosis and recovery but also confused by the onset of symptoms. The elderly do not present with the standard UTI symptoms of urinary frequency, burning, and difficulty emptying their bladder. Often acute mental confusion is the first and only symptom.

Sundowner Syndrome. Sundowner syndrome is a type of confusion occurring in patients with Alzheimer's, or other forms of dementia, after sundown or at night. It tends to be more present in those with cognitive impairments. Factors that may increase the incidence of sundowner syndrome include disruption of routine, such as a hospital admission, unfamiliar surroundings, a disturbance in sleep patterns, use of restraints, or excessive sensory stimulation, such as leaving lights on all night or excessive noise. In the morning, symptoms subside. Surrounding the patient with familiar objects, establishing a routine, and controlling room lighting, temperature, and noise level may relieve the problem.

Depression

Depression is defined by the American Medical Association as "an abnormal and persistent mood characterized by sadness, melancholy, slowed mental processes, and changes in eating and sleeping habits." Medical depression is confirmed if these five symptoms have been present daily for at least 2 weeks. Life changes may overwhelm the aging person, causing depression that can worsen with some medication interactions. Depression is often overlooked in the elderly or misdiagnosed as part of another problem, such as dementia.

Maintaining good rapport with elderly patients so they feel comfortable enough to speak to you is beneficial. You can detect changes in their mental state, making you a better member of the health care team. Many medical providers will use the geriatric depression scale form (Box 41-3) to aid in the diagnosis of depression.

Box 41-3 Geriatric Depression (Mood Assessment) SCALE

1. Are you basically satisfied with your life?
2. Have you dropped many of your activities and interests?
3. Do you feel that your life is empty?
4. Do you often get bored?
5. Are you hopeful about the future?
6. Are you bothered by thoughts you can't get out of your head?
7. Are you in good spirits most of the time?
8. Are you afraid that something bad is going to happen to you?
9. Do you feel happy most of the time?
10. Do you often feel helpless?
11. Do you often get restless and fidgety?
12. Do you prefer to stay at home, rather than going out and doing new things?
13. Do you frequently worry about the future?
14. Do you feel you have more problems with memory than most?
15. Do you think it is wonderful to be alive now?
16. Do you often feel downhearted and blue?
17. Do you feel pretty worthless the way you are now?
18. Do you worry a lot about the past?
19. Do you find life very exciting?
20. Is it hard for you to get started on new projects?
21. Do you feel full of energy?
22. Do you feel that your situation is hopeless?
23. Do you think that most people are better off than you are?
24. Do you frequently get upset over little things?
25. Do you frequently feel like crying?
26. Do you have trouble concentrating?
27. Do you enjoy getting up in the morning?
28. Do you prefer to avoid social gatherings?
29. Is it easy for you to make decisions?
30. Is your mind as clear as it used to be?

This is the original scoring for the scale: One point for each of these answers. Cutoff: normal-0–9; mild depressives-10–19; severe depressives-20–30.

1. no 6. yes 11. yes 16. yes 21. no 26. yes
2. yes 7. no 12. yes 17. yes 22. yes 27. no
3. yes 8. yes 13. yes 18. yes 23. yes 28. yes
4. yes 9. no 14. yes 19. no 24. yes 29. no

http://www.stanford.edu/~yesavage/GDS.english.long.html

Dementia

Dementia is a syndrome marked by progressive loss of memory and other intellectual functions. It can occur at any age, but more frequently it is found in the elderly. Over 70 different types of dementia currently are defined. Dementia affects about 7 percent of people over age 65. The onset is usually slow, and because changes in behavior are subtle at first, it may be difficult to detect. Dementia is not a normal consequence of aging (half of those over age 100 have no signs of dementia), and it is irreversible unless caused by a treatable condition such as electrolyte imbalance or thyroid dysfunction. Dementia is different from normal age-related forgetfulness. An older person may misplace keys or fail to remember a person's name, whereas a dementia patient forgets that he or she has a car and fails to recognize the individual at all. Approximately half of dementia patients suffer from Alzheimer's disease. The following may be other causes of dementia:

- Stroke
- Parkinson's disease
- Brain tumor
- AIDS
- Drug and alcohol abuse

Signs and Symptoms.   In patients with dementia, symptoms gradually worsen at different rates over a 2- to 10-year period. The first sign of dementia is usually forgetfulness regarding recent events or places. The individual has difficulty learning new information and may ask repetitive questions. The patient may forget what he or she is doing while in the middle of a task. He or she may forget the correct word for everyday objects, have difficulty with time orientation, and misplace items or put them in an inappropriate place. Often the patient will show a lack of emotion, have mood swings, and demonstrate lack of initiative or disinterest in something he or she previously loved to do. As dementia progresses, patients become unable to follow conversations, unable to perform activities of daily living, and eventually bedridden as the brain shuts down, leading to death.

Alzheimer's Disease

Alzheimer's disease (AD) is a progressive disorder of the central nervous system that eventually destroys mental capacities. It occurs more frequently in the elderly. At this time, there is no known cause or cure for this disease. Genetic factors do play a role. Scientists have pinpointed several gene abnormalities linked to the type of AD that tends to run in families.

AD can have a devastating effect on family members as well as on the patient. One of the first signs of AD is loss of memory. Although there is a normal loss of some memory as people age (forgetting dates, names, and telephone numbers), the memory loss with AD is profound. The patient may not remember where he or she lives or who family members are.

Signs and Symptoms.   In the United States, AD affects about 12% percent of the people over 65 years of age, and 50 percent of those over 85. It costs billions of dollars each year to care for these patients, and the costs will rise as the elderly population increases. Recognizing the symptoms of this and other forms of dementia is necessary for medical assistants so they may be proactive in providing assistance to the patients and caregivers. Box 41-4 illustrates some of the common warning signs of AD.

Diagnoses of dementia and AD are conducted by eliminating other potential factors. A patient who is suspected of having dementia should have a complete physical examination, a blood profile, a thorough medical and family history, an MRI, and a PET scan. After ruling out possible causes, such as thyroid and medication imbalance, the patient should be given the Mini Mental Status Exam, a frequently used mental status examination. This test requires 5 to 10 minutes and consists of a series of tasks to evaluate recall, writing, and math skills. If the patient scores lower than expected for his or her age, more extensive testing should be ordered. A significant portion of the AD/dementia diagnosis depends on symptoms revealed by the patient and family members or caregivers. The ultimate diagnosis of AD may only be confirmed by an autopsy with the detection of plaque (dense protein deposits around the brain's nerve cells) and tangles (twisted protein fibers inside nerve cells).

Initially, dementia patients may try to cover up errors or inabilities and may be unwilling to accept that they are having difficulties. Other symptoms include agitation, restlessness, irritability, an inability to care for oneself, incontinence, and the inability to communicate. AD progresses through various stages over a 2- to 10-year period.

Treatment.   There is no treatment to recover any of the mental functions that have been lost and no way to prevent the loss of more functions in Alzheimer patients. During early stages of dementia, medications, such as Aricept, are purported to slow the progression of the disease. Patients should not drink alcohol, which can worsen the symptoms of AD. Some depressed AD patients may benefit by taking antidepressants in the early stages. Creating a soothing home environment, avoiding criticism, and avoiding constantly

Box 41-4 Alzheimer's Warning SIGNS

1. **Memory loss.** Forgetting recently learned information is one of the most common early signs of dementia. A person begins to forget more often and is unable to recall the information later.

   What's normal? Forgetting names or appointments occasionally.

2. **Difficulty performing familiar tasks.** People with dementia often find it hard to plan or complete everyday tasks. Individuals may lose track of the steps involved in preparing a meal, placing a telephone call, or playing a game.

   What's normal? Occasionally forgetting why you came into a room or what you planned to say.

3. **Problems with language.** People with Alzheimer's disease often forget simple words or substitute unusual words, making their speech or writing hard to understand. They may be unable to find the toothbrush, for example, and instead ask for "that thing for my mouth."

   What's normal? Sometimes having trouble finding the right word.

4. **Disorientation to time and place.** People with Alzheimer's disease can become lost in their own neighborhood, forget where they are and how they got there, and not know how to get back home.

   What's normal? Forgetting the day of the week or where you were going.

5. **Poor or decreased judgment.** Those with Alzheimer's may dress inappropriately, wearing several layers on a warm day or little clothing in the cold. They may show poor judgment, like giving away large sums of money to telemarketers.

   What's normal? Making a questionable or debatable decision from time to time.

6. **Problems with abstract thinking.** Someone with Alzheimer's disease may have unusual difficulty performing complex mental tasks, like forgetting what numbers are for and how they should be used.

   What's normal? Finding it challenging to balance a checkbook.

7. **Misplacing things.** A person with Alzheimer's disease may put things in unusual places: an iron in the freezer or a wristwatch in the sugar bowl.

   What's normal? Misplacing keys or a wallet temporarily.

8. **Changes in mood or behavior.** Someone with Alzheimer's disease may show rapid mood swings—from calm to tears to anger—for no apparent reason.

   What's normal? Occasionally feeling sad or moody.

9. **Changes in personality.** The personalities of people with dementia can change dramatically. They may become extremely confused, suspicious, fearful, or dependent on a family member.

   What's normal? People's personalities do change somewhat with age.

10. **Loss of initiative.** A person with Alzheimer's disease may become very passive, sitting in front of the TV for hours, sleeping more than usual, or not wanting to do usual activities.

    What's normal? Sometimes feeling weary of work or social obligations.

Someone with Alzheimer's Disease Symptoms	Someone with Normal Age-Related Memory Changes
Forgets entire experiences	Forgets part of an experience
Rarely remembers later	Often remembers later
Is gradually unable to follow written/spoken directions	Is usually able to follow written/spoken directions
Is gradually unable to use notes as reminders	Is usually able to use notes as reminders
Is gradually unable to care for self	Is usually able to care for self

Source: © 2009 Alzheimer's Association. All rights reserved. *This is an official publication of the Alzheimer's Association but may be distributed by unaffiliated organizations and individuals. Such distribution does not constitute an endorsement of these parties or their activities by the Alzheimer's Association.*

correcting errors, help reduce the stress for AD patients (Figure 41-4).

By using community resources, patients and caregivers can get help dealing with the complex circumstances caused by this condition. Support groups can help the caregivers establish contact with others in the same situation. Often support groups provide ideas for coping strategies that have worked for others. Helping caregivers locate respite care, which is a temporary interlude of care for the patient to allow the caregiver time for relaxation, can be of great assistance. Many caregivers provide 24-hour care with no outside help for extended periods. This often leads to caregiver burnout and, in some cases, results in elder abuse. **Respite care** (short-term care for the chronically ill) will help caregivers

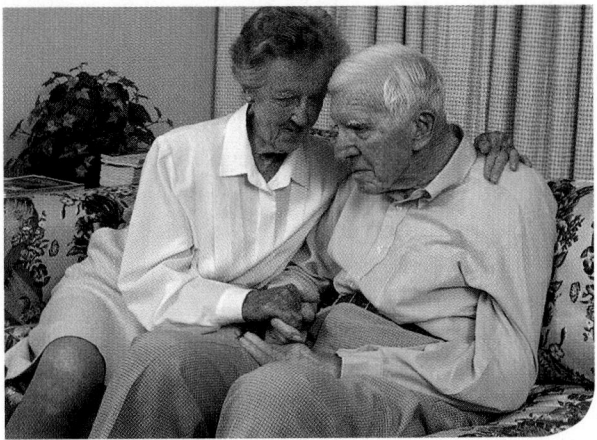

FIGURE 41-4 Familiar objects and a stable environment can reduce behavioral problems in some dementia patients.

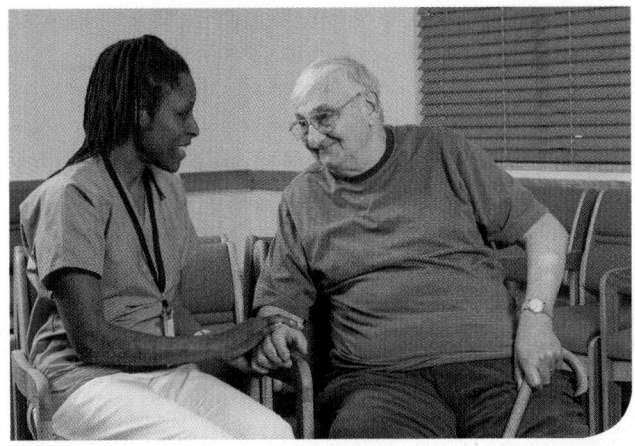

FIGURE 41-5 Effective communication skills are vital to the medical assistant's career.

relieve the extraordinary demands of this disease. Please refer to Box 41-5 for a list of elder care resource phone numbers.

The Dementia Patient in the Office. Dealing with a dementia patient in the office can be challenging. The patient with AD must be kept in safe surroundings with someone observing his or her movements. The patient cannot be left alone in a reception or examination room. Having routines and structure in the AD patient's daily life seems to reduce his or her anx-

iety and stress. Following a simple routine within the office may be helpful. Always tell patients what you are going to do and what to expect next, although they may not comprehend your information (Figure 41-5). Speak to the patient in slow, simple terms and be ready to repeat instructions without exasperation. Make eye contact with the patient, and use appropriate body language. A warm smile is often reassuring, and a simple touch on the arm to guide the patient may encourage him or her to follow your instructions. Sometimes using tactics of diversion

Box 41-5 Elder Care Resource Phone NUMBERS

Emergency (Paramedics, Fire, Police): 911

AARP: 213-380-1800

AMC Cancer Information Center: 800-525-3777

AT&T TDD Hearing Impaired: 800-735-2929

Adult Protective Services: 213-351-5401

Amyotrophic Lateral Sclerosis (ALS) Association: 800-782-4747

Alzheimer's Association 24-Hour Help Line: 800-262-3900

Alzheimer's Disease and Related Disorders Center: 800-621-0379

American Cancer Society: 310-670-2650

American Council of the Blind: 800-424-8666

American Diabetes Association: 800-232-3472

American Dietetic Association Consumer Nutrition Hotline: 800-366-1655

American Heart Association: 800-242-8721

American Kidney Fund: 800-638-8299

American Liver Foundation: 800-223-0179

American Paralysis Association: 800-225-0292

American Parkinson's Disease Association: 800-223-2732

American Mental Health Foundation: 800-443-5959

American Speech and Hearing Association: 800-638-8255

Arthritis Foundation: 800-283-7800 or 213-954-5750

Asthma and Allergy Foundation of America 800-727-8462

Cancer Information Service 800-422-6237

Captioned Films for the deaf (Voice/TDD): 800-237-6213

Elder Abuse Hotline: 800-992-1660

Eldercare Information and Referral: 800-662-1998

Medicare Hotline: 800-638-6833

MedicAlert Foundation International: 800-825-3785

Medicare/Medicaid Fraud Hotline: 800-368-5779

National Alliance for the Mentally Ill: 800-950-6264

National Hearing Aid Society Hotline: 800-521-5247

Random House Audiobooks: 800-733-3000

Recorded Books: 800-638-1304

Recordings for the Blind: 800-499-5525

Simon Foundation for Continence: 800-237-4666

Social Security Administration: 800-772-1213

Social Services/In-Home Services: 800-555-5555

Suicide Prevention Center 24-Hour Hotline: 213-381-5111

and distraction, such as directing attention to something else, works to relieve tension. Keep in mind that the dementia patient cannot control his or her impulses. Allow the patient to maintain dignity, knowing that no one really knows what is going on in his or her mind. On the other hand, the patient may be uncooperative, in which case the physician must decide if the circumstances warrant taking a firm stand with the patient or more extraordinary measures. Procedure 41-1 presents steps for communicating effectively with the elderly. Procedure 41-2 explains how to assist patients according to their needs.

Legal and Medical Decisions

Families of elders who are progressively declining will ultimately face difficult decisions, such as when to take away car keys for safety reasons, when to speak about advance directives, what to do with a living will once it is written, when to take over decision making, and ultimately if and when to place the patient in a long-term-care facility. It is the professional responsibility of physicians and lawyers to provide guidance to caregivers when making these difficult decisions. However, having an understanding of these difficult decisions, an awareness of where to locate materials to help the caregivers, and acting as a go-between to the family and the physician may make things easier for the caregivers.

INFORMED CONSENT

Informed consent must be obtained from the patient and a written document to that effect placed in the patient's chart for any procedure other than basic care. In the case of a

procedure
41-1

COMMUNICATING EFFECTIVELY WITH THE ELDERLY

Objective: Communicate effectively with a new elderly patient preparing for a physical examination.

EQUIPMENT AND SUPPLIES

pen and paper; patient history form; examination table; gown and drapes; other physical examination equipment as needed

METHOD

1. Welcome the patient in the front office warmly with a smile.
2. Face the patient and speak clearly and directly to him or her.
3. Introduce yourself. Be sincere and polite.
4. Address the patient by "Mr.," "Mrs.," or "Ms." unless otherwise instructed by the patient.
5. Observe the patient for cues to indicate comprehension of your remarks.
6. If it appears that the patient does not comprehend, paraphrase using other words and simple gestures.
7. Escort the patient to the examination room. If the patient is using a walker or a cane, walk closely to the patient and offer assistance if needed (see Figure 41-6).
8. Allow sufficient time for the patient to process information.
9. Observe the patient's overall physical ability to comply with your request.
10. Offer assistance if it appears the patient needs it. Allow the patient to do as much for him- or herself as possible.
11. Ask the patient to be seated while you begin to gather information for the patient history.
12. Speak respectfully, and convey a feeling of warmth and empathy. If the patient's replies to questions become too lengthy, gently interrupt and bring the patient back to the subject.

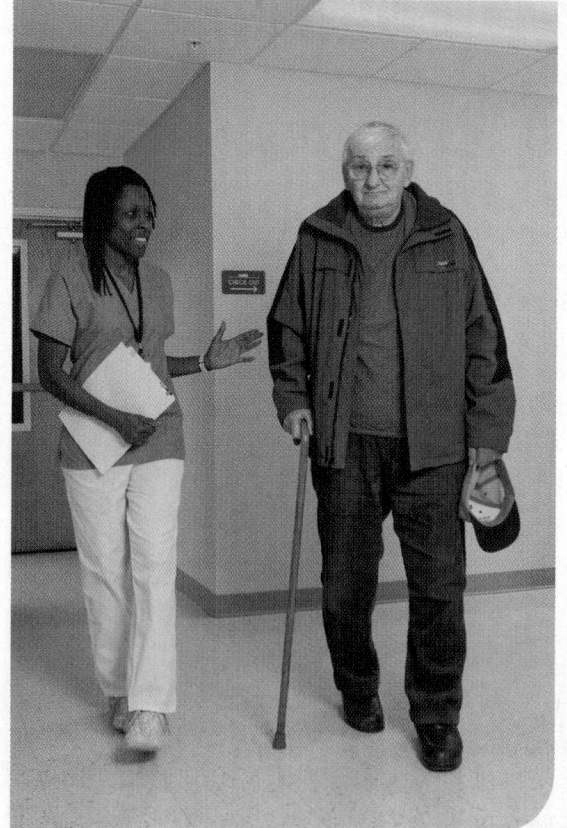

FIGURE 41-6 The medical assistant should provide assistance while promoting independence in patients.

13. Never assume the patient is incapable of understanding you because he or she is old.
14. If answers to some of your questions seem inappropriate, do not correct the patient. Gently distract the ptaient with another topic and proceed with your examination preparations.
15. Set aside questions that received inappropriate answers and ask it of the caregiver or a family member at a later time.
16. Do not leave the patient unattended if he or she is confused.
17. Do not argue with the patient's view of reality. Remember that relaxed body language, facial expressions, and a caring touch are most important in caring for confused patients.
18. Chart all your findings and impressions.

CHARTING EXAMPLE
03/18/XX 11:00 A.M. Pt appeared confused. Unable to follow directions or to undress w/o help. Attitude cheerful. · · ·
· M. King, CMA (AAMA)

procedure

41-2

INSTRUCTING STROKE PATIENTS ACCORDING TO THEIR NEEDS

Objective: Provide patient instruction on the lifestyle changes required after the patient has suffered a stroke. Some stroke victims will suffer irreversible loss of function on one side of their body (hemiplegia).

EQUIPMENT AND SUPPLIES
pen and paper; patient history form

METHOD
1. Welcome the patient in the front office warmly with a smile.
2. Face the patient and speak clearly and directly to him or her.
3. Introduce yourself. Be sincere and polite.
4. Address the patient by "Mr.," "Mrs.," or "Ms." unless otherwise instructed by the patient.
5. Observe the patient for cues to indicate comprehension of your remarks.
6. Ask the patient to follow you to the examination room.
7. Observe the patient's overall physical ability to comply with your request.
8. Offer assistance if you think it appears the patient needs it. Allow the patient to do as much for him or herself as possible.
9. Ask the patient to be seated while you begin to gather information for the patient visit.
10. Follow the physician's recommendation for the patient regarding regular blood pressure screenings. May the patient take the readings at a supermarket's automatic blood pressure machine? Would the physician prefer the patient to come into the office for blood pressure readings?
11. How closely will other medical conditions be monitored now? Conditions such as heart disease, atrial fibrillation, high cholesterol, and diabetes may need closer monitoring. How are the current conditions being controlled? Has medication been prescribed? Will it need adjustments?
12. The stroke may cause stress and depression due to physical limitations, potential loss of income, and financial concerns. The patient should be made aware of depression warning sign and given coping strategies for stress.
13. The patient should be made aware of the factors that he or she cannot change about a recurring stroke risk, such as family history (you are more at risk if someone in your family has had a stroke); age (arteries harden and become furred up with age, which means older people are more likely to have strokes); gender (in people under the age of 75, men have more strokes than women); race (people of Asian, African and African-Caribbean origin are more at risk); medical conditions such as heart disease and diabetes.
14. Once the patient is aware of the risk factors that cannot be changed, provide instruction on how to become proactive toward the factors that can be changed, including smoking, drinking, diet modification, and regular exercise.
15. Once you have given your patient all relevant information, chart all your findings and impressions.

CHARTING EXAMPLE
01/26/XX 2:35 P.M. Pt and spouse were given information regarding instruction on the lifestyle changes that will be required following Pt's recent stroke. Patient understands verbal directions and has taken brochure for review. · · · · · · · ·
· M. King, CMA (AAMA)

patient who is too ill, confused, or suffering from dementia, the family may consent to the procedure. Family members may need to be encouraged to obtain the appointment of a guardian to grant consent for the incompetent individual. It is the responsibility of the court to grant guardianship. You may provide the family with information about how to proceed with obtaining it and identify a state agency that is able to assist. Guardianship invalidates a power of attorney (POA) because POA implies competency of the patient. A person (the principal or grantor) is legally requesting another person (the agent) to make legal and business actions on their behalf. A POA may be limited to a specific time frame, limited to a specific circumstance, or written in general terms. For example, a POA can be contracted for financial obligations only, giving the agent access and authority over the principal's monetary funds and expenses but not their health care decisions.

ADVANCE DIRECTIVES

Issues related to death and dying are very personal and sensitive in nature, and understanding advance directives and do-not-resuscitate (DNR) orders allows the medical assistant to function more professionally to help patients and caregivers. An advance directive or living will provides guidelines or directives formulated by the patient that expresses his or her desires about terminal care. In an advance directive, the individual may state whether or not he or she wants to be resuscitated. Patients and family members should be aware that they need to spell out what other directives they wish to choose if the patient degrades into a persistent vegetative state. These other directives may indicate if the patient wants medicine withheld, except for pain relief, and whether the patient wants feeding and hydration withheld. Patients and families often are under the assumption that when they have a DNR order written it covers all life-sustaining treatments. Providing families and patients with information pertaining to this topic is very helpful. In most states, unless the physician writes a specific order restating what the patient has expressed in the advance directive, a directive is not binding on the staff and facility. Refer to Box 41-6 for a sample advance directive. The U.S. Living Will Registry website is a comprehensive resource that patients and their advocates can use to create advance directives

Box 41-6 Sample Advance DIRECTIVE

Sample Advance Directive Form

This form is a combined durable power of attorney for health care and a living will (in some jurisdictions). With this form, you can name someone to make medical decisions for you if in the future you are unable to make those decisions yourself. You can also say what medical treatments you want and what medical treatments you do not want if in the future you are unable to make your wishes known.

Instructions

Read each section carefully. Before you fill out the form talk to the person you want to name, to make sure that he or she understands your wishes and is willing to take the responsibility. Write your initials in the blank spaces before the choices you want to make. Write your initials only beside the choices you want under Parts 1, 2, and 3 of this form. Your advance directive should be valid for whatever part(s) you fill in, as long as it is properly signed.

Add any special instructions in the blank spaces provided. You can write additional comments on a separate sheet of paper, but you should write on this form that there are additional pages to your advance directive. Sign the form and have it witnessed. Give copies to your doctor, your nurse, the person you name to make your medical decisions for you, people in your family, and anyone else who might be involved in your care. Discuss your advance directive with them.

Understand that you may change or cancel this document at any time.

Definitions to Know

Advance directive—A written document (form) that tells what a person wants or does not want if he or she in the future cannot make his or her wishes known about medical treatment.

Artificial nutrition and hydration—When food and water are fed to a person through a tube.

Autopsy—An examination done on a dead body to determine the cause of death.

Comfort care—Care that helps to keep a person comfortable but does not make him or her get well. Bathing, turning, and keeping a person's lips moist are types of comfort care.

CPR (cardiopulmonary resuscitation)—Treatment to try to restart a person's breathing or heartbeat. CPR may be done by pushing on the chest, by putting a tube down the throat, or by other treatment.

Durable power of attorney for health care—An advance directive that names someone to make medical decisions for a person if in the future he or she cannot make his or her own medical decisions.

Life-sustaining treatment—Any medical treatment that is used to keep a person from dying. A breathing machine, CPR, and artificial nutrition and hydration are examples of life-sustaining treatments.

Living will—An advance directive that tells what medical treatment a person does or does not want if he or she is not able to make his or her wishes known.

Organ and tissue donation—When a person permits his or her organs (such as the eyes or kidneys) and other parts of the body (such as the skin) to be removed after death to be transplanted for use by another person or to be used for experimental purposes.

Persistent vegetative state—When a person is unconscious with no hope of regaining consciousness even with medical treatment. The body may move and the eyes may be open, but as far as anyone can tell, the person cannot think or respond.

Terminal condition—An ongoing condition caused by injury or illness that has no cure and from which doctors expect the person to die even with medical treatment. Life-sustaining treatments will only prolong the dying process if the person is suffering from a terminal condition.

_____

Complete this portion of the advance directive form

I, _____,

write this document as a directive regarding my medical care.

In the following sections, put the initials of your name in the blank spaces by the choices you want.

PART 1. My Durable Power of Attorney for Health Care

_____ I appoint this person to make decisions about my medical care if there ever comes a time when I cannot make those decisions myself. I want the person I have appointed, my doctors, my family, and others to be guided by the decisions I have made in the parts of the form that follow.

Name: _____

Home telephone: _____

Work telephone: _____

Address: _____

If the person cited above cannot or will not make decisions for me, I appoint this person:

Name: _____

Home telephone: _____

Work telephone: _____

Address: _____

_____ I have not appointed anyone to make health care decisions for me in this or any other document.

PART 2. My Living Will

These are my wishes for my future medical care if there ever comes a time when I cannot make these decisions for myself.

A. These are my wishes if I have a terminal condition.

Life-Sustaining Treatments

_____ I do not want life-sustaining treatment (including CPR) started. If life-sustaining treatments are started, I want them stopped.

_____ I want the life-sustaining treatments that my doctors think are best for me.

_____ Other wishes

_____

Artificial Nutrition and Hydration

_____ I do not want artificial nutrition and hydration started if they would be the main treatments keeping me alive. If artificial nutrition and hydration are started, I want them stopped.

_____ I want artificial nutrition and hydration even if they are the main treatments keeping me alive.

_____ Other wishes

_____

Comfort Care

_____ I want to be kept as comfortable and free of pain as possible, even if such care prolongs my dying or shortens my life.

_____ Other wishes

_____

B. These are my wishes if I am ever in a persistent vegetative state.

Life-Sustaining Treatments

_____ I do not want life-sustaining treatment (including CPR) started. If life-sustaining treatments are started, I want them stopped.

_____ I want the life-sustaining treatments that my doctors think are best for me.

_____ Other wishes

_____

(continued)

Box 41-6 *(continued)*

Artificial Nutrition and Hydration

_____ I do not want artificial nutrition and hydration started if they would be the main treatments keeping me alive. If artificial nutrition and hydration are started, I want them stopped.

_____ I want artificial nutrition and hydration even if they are the main treatments keeping me alive.

_____ Other wishes

_____

Comfort Care

_____ I want to be kept as comfortable and free of pain as possible, even if such care prolongs my dying or shortens my life.

_____ Other wishes

_____

C. Other directives

You have the right to be involved in all decisions about your medical care, even those not dealing with terminal conditions or persistent vegetative states. If you have wishes not covered in other parts of this document, please indicate them below.

_____

_____

_____

_____

_____

_____

PART 3. Other Wishes

A. Organ donation

_____ I do not wish to donate any of my organs or tissues.

_____ I want to donate all of my organs and tissues.

_____ I only want to donate these organs and tissues:

_____

_____ Other wishes

_____

B. Autopsy

_____ I do not want an autopsy.

_____ I agree to an autopsy if my doctors wish it.

_____ Other wishes

_____

C. Other statements about your medical care

If you wish to say more about any of the choices you have made or if you have any other statements to make about your medical care, you may do so on a separate piece of paper. If you do so, put here the number of pages you are adding: _____

PART 4. Signatures

You and two witnesses must sign this document before it will be legal.

A. Your signature

By my signature below, I show that I understand the purpose and the effect of this document.

Signature:_____Date:_____

Address:_____

B. Your witnesses' signatures

I believe the person who has signed this advance directive to be of sound mind, that he or she signed or acknowledged this advance directive in my presence, and that he or she appears not to be acting under pressure, duress, fraud, or undue influence. I am not related to the person making this advance directive by blood, marriage, or adoption nor, to the best of my knowledge, am I named in his or her will. I am not the person appointed in this advance directive. I am not a health care provider or an employee of a health care provider who is now, or has been in the past, responsible for the care of the person making this advance directive.

Witness #1

Signature:_____Date:_____

Address:_____

Witness #2

Signature:_____Date:_____

Address:_____

Adapted with permission from the District of Columbia Hospital Association, 1250 Eye St., N.W., Suite 700, Washington, DC 20005.

by following the provided links for their state of residency's Department of Health website.

Elder Abuse

Elder abuse from family members or caregivers may occur at home and in institutions. Elder abuse has many forms, including stealing a patient's belongings; inflicting injury and pain; mishandling funds; withholding care such as food, drink, or medication; sexual abuse; threatening a patient; and confining a patient. As a medical assistant, you must be alert to all signs of abuse. All cases of suspected or known abuse must be reported. Organizations such as the National Center of Elder Abuse, American Association of Retired Persons, and state agencies on aging provide information on abuse.

Safety Guidelines for the Elderly Population

Some of the elderly have to rely on others for care and living accommodations, which makes safety issues a prime concern. Patients and caregivers should be aware of safety risks and interventions to eliminate or reduce those risks.

The elderly may be faced with increased risk of injury and may have a reduced capacity to protect themselves. The U.S. Department of Commerce states that the rate of injury per 1,000 in the population is 100.6 for those under age 12 years, 148.3 for those ages 12 to 21, 98.9 for those 22 to 44, 109.3 for those 45 to 64, and 142.5 for those over 65. The normal aging processes and declining health place the elderly at risk for falling, sustaining fractures, and other injuries. Early identification and correction of health problems help reduce safety risks. Confusion, disorientation, decreased memory, and poor judgment decrease the ability of the elderly to reduce hazards to their health and safety. Environmental risks in the following areas should be identified and corrected:

- **Bathroom**—A small light in the bathroom that is on all the time is helpful. The elderly use the bathroom frequently and can avoid reaching for a switch inside the room. Tub and showers should have nonstick surfaces and grab bars and chairs for support in bathing. Toilets should have grab bars. If the toilet is low, a raised seat attachment may be needed.

- **Electrical cords**—Electrical cords should not be present in traffic flow areas. Overloaded electrical outlets may cause fire.

- **Emergency numbers**—Emergency numbers (including police and fire departments, close relatives, or friends) should be near each phone. The numbers should be posted in a font large enough for individuals with vision problems to read.

- **Floor wax**—Highly polished floors increase the risk of falling.

- **Furniture**—Furniture for the elderly should be sturdy with good armrests lending support for standing. Rooms stuffed with furniture and bric-a-brac increase a patient's risk of falling.

- **Lighting**—Provide adequate lighting and reduce glare. Several smaller areas of light are better in a room than one overhead light that produces glare. The eyes of the elderly are sensitive to glare.

- **Rugs**—All area rugs should be removed.

PROFESSIONALISM

Professional development hinges on becoming a lifelong learner. Keeping current in your field of medical assisting is crucial to maintaining your certification and becoming a better health care provider. To become a lifelong learner, you must seek out groups or facilities that will provide CEU credits for attending seminars. Possibilities include hospitals; local, state, and national medical assisting associations; state medical societies; nursing associations; and community colleges. Because it is not always possible to attend seminars, you will have to find other ways of keeping up to date. Subscribing to professional journals and health magazines provides current information on a regular basis. Learning how to search the Internet and discovering sites, such as the Centers for Disease Control and Prevention or the National Institutes of Health, will provide valid information on a vast array of medical topics.

SUMMARY

The medical assistant should be prepared to function competently with geriatric patients. Medical assistants need to have an understanding of common elderly disorders, uncommon diseases, and genetic disorders. As a medical assistant, you must be able to accurately perform procedures such as obtaining vital signs, measuring height and weight, and assisting with all phases of adult examinations.

The geriatric patient may have many chronic problems that will require medical attention. As a medical assistant, comprehending the aging process and how it affects those over age 65 is vital to providing good health care. Comprehending facts about the aging U.S. population and the impact it will have on health care is also important. The number of dementia, and specifically Alzheimer's, patients will be increasing. You must understand the devastating effects of these conditions and be prepared to provide intelligent assistance to the patient and caregivers. After completing this chapter, you can be an understanding, compassionate, competent caregiver to both categories of patients.

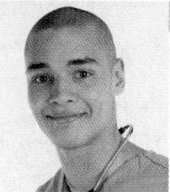

41 CHAPTER REVIEW

COMPETENCY REVIEW

1. Define and spell the terms to learn in this chapter.

2. The physician has asked you to develop a teaching plan for obese patients. What is your plan?

3. Your office has several patients suffering from dementia. Each is in a different stage. Prepare a summary of the different stages and related behaviors for the next staff meeting to help coworkers better understand these patients.

PREPARING FOR THE CERTIFICATION EXAM

1. The slowly progressive degenerative brain disease that leads to tremor, muscle rigidity, difficulty moving and instability is:
   a. Parkinson's disease
   b. Alzheimer's disease
   c. stroke
   d. glaucoma
   e. the normal aging process

2. How many different types of dementia are currently known?
   a. 1
   b. several
   c. at least 70
   d. 7
   e. 17

3. _____ of the people over the age of 100 have no signs of dementia.
   a. One hundred
   b. One-quarter
   c. Three-quarters
   d. Half
   e. One-tenth

4. The Federal Old Age Insurance Law was passed in
   a. 1953
   b. 1935
   c. 1965
   d. 1956
   e. 1955

5. Older patients take an average of _____ to _____ different medications and one to two over-the-counter medications daily.

   a. 1, 2
   b. 2, 3
   c. 3, 4
   d. 4, 5
   e. 3, 5

6. The elderly have _____ acute illnesses than younger age groups.
   a. many more
   b. the same number of
   c. fewer
   d. a few more
   e. many fewer

7. Chronic illness is _____ for the older population.
   a. not a problem
   b. the major problem
   c. a minor problem
   d. the same for the younger population as it is
   e. is less for the younger population than it is

8. When dealing with memory-loss patients it is important to
   a. correct them each and every time they make a mistake so they know fact from fiction
   b. correct them if you need to but weigh the risk for embarrassment and alienation and determine if the correction is truly needed
   c. ask the primary care provider to correct them each and every time
   d. pretend not to notice, ignoring the entire situation
   e. completely ignore the behavior

9. As of 2007, _____ of the United States population is between 44 and 62 years old.
   a. 28 percent
   b. 18 percent

c. 8 percent
d. 12 percent
e. 16 percent

c. sundowner syndrome
d. depression
e. dementia

10. The type of confusion occurring in some older patients after sundown or at night is referred to as
a. cognitive effect
b. confusion

CRITICAL THINKING

1. As Shandra obtains Sylvia's weight, she notes that Sylvia has lost 15 pounds since her last physical examination over a year ago and now only weighs 113 pounds. She appears very frail in her 5'3" frame. What should Shandra do, and what might be the issues surrounding Mrs. Jordan's weight loss?

2. The physician would like Mrs. Jordan to return to the office for nutritional education. She requested that her son, Lewis, accompany her to the visit. What type of patient education materials might Shandra want to prepare prior to the office visit with Sylvia and her son?

ON THE JOB

Olive Johnson is a 62-year-old practicing lawyer and a patient of Dr. O'Brien. She is coming in today for an annual physical examination. On arrival, she seems cheerful, talkative, and cooperative as usual. After placing her in the examination room and giving her instructions about obtaining a urine sample and where to have the gown opening, she seems confused and frustrated. She is unable to open the gown properly and mistakes the door to the hallway for the bathroom door. After directing her to the bathroom, you can hear her crying from the other side of the door.

1. How should you handle the situation?
2. What possible conditions could be causing her confusion?
3. How and when should you inform Dr. O'Brien about Olive's behavior?
4. What tests do you think the doctor should order?

INTERNET ACTIVITY

Select your own ethnic group or one in which you are interested (Greek, Irish, Chinese, etc.) and do an Internet search for issues related to aging in that group using the search term _____-*elderly*.

MEDMEDIA

Additional interactive resources and activities for this chapter can be found:

On your student DVD: View applicable procedure videos on the DVD-ROM found in the back of this book.

MyHealthProfessionsKit.com: Test your knowledge of this chapter with games and activities. MyHealthProfessionsKit also includes resources, helpful links, and a Spanish audio glossary.

Medical Assisting Interactive: Practice your procedures as a medical assistant in this simulated doctor's office. This can be accessed through MyHealthProfessionsKit.com.

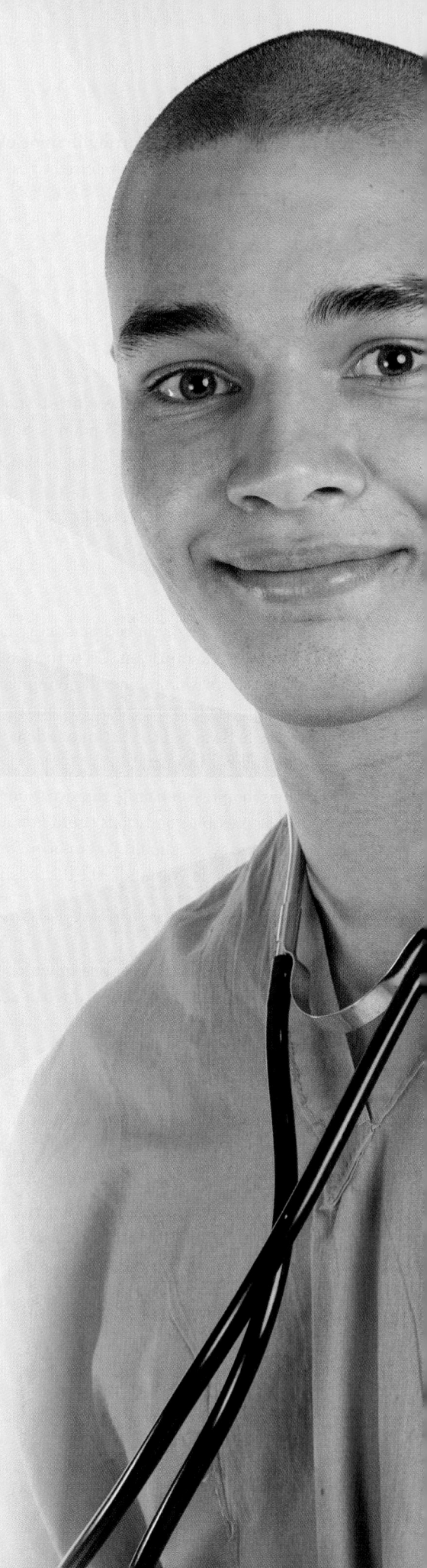

42
Assisting with Minor Surgery

LEARNING OBJECTIVES

After completing this chapter, you should be able to:

- Define and spell the terms to learn for this chapter.

- List and differentiate between the types of ambulatory surgery.

- Discuss all guidelines for surgical aseptic technique.

- Describe the differences between medical asepsis and surgical asepsis.

- List and describe instruments for cutting, dissecting, grasping, clamping, probing, and dilating.

- Give five examples of suture materials, including gauge ranges, with examples of when they may be used.

- Explain the guidelines for handling instruments.

- Describe the preparation of the patient for minor surgery.

- Define informed consent. Discuss the medical assistant's role in the process.

- List equipment and supplies used for preparing the patient's skin for surgery.

- Explain the four types of wounds.

- Describe the stages of healing.

- Describe at least five surgical procedures that can be performed in the physician's office, and indicate the responsibility of the medical assistant for each procedure.

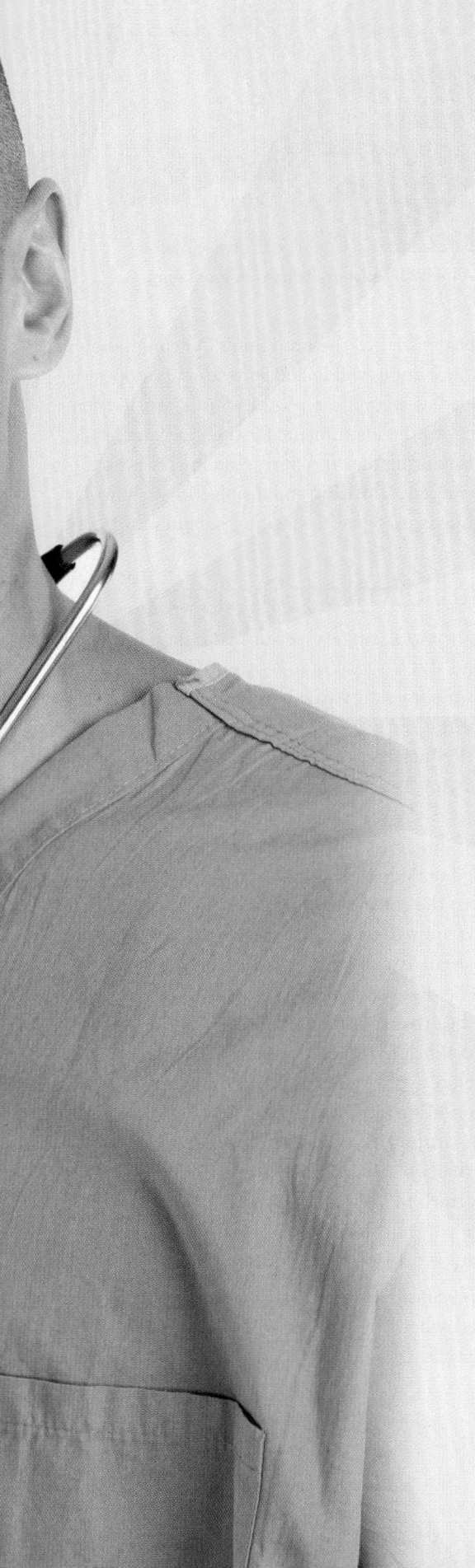

CHAPTER OUTLINE

CASE STUDY

Today, Shandra Wilkinson, RMA, is working with Dr. Penningworth at Pearson Physicians Group. Dr. Penningworth has instructed Shandra to prepare examination room 4 for an I & D of a sebaceous cyst. He will be performing the I & D on Carmen DiStefano, a 32-year-old male who presented to the office with pain and discomfort surrounding the cyst.

CERTIFICATION LINK

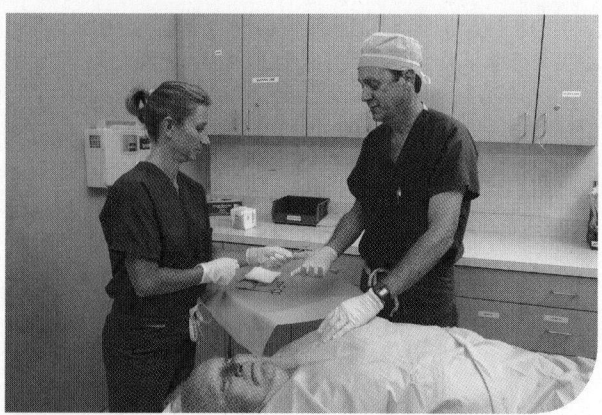

FIGURE 42-1 A medical assistant helps with a dressing change.

This chapter discusses surgical aseptic technique, also known as sterile technique. Procedures requiring sterile technique, such as minor surgical procedures, suture insertion and removal, breast **biopsy** (microscopic examination of tissue to detect cancerous cells), incision and drainage, removal of growths, and wound treatment, are included. Strict adherence to aseptic technique is necessary when assisting with these procedures. It is important to always remember that an item is either sterile or nonsterile. If there is any doubt about sterility, assume it is nonsterile.

Medical assistants perform many duties related to minor surgery (Figure 42-1). Prior to surgery you will perform administrative duties, such as completing insurance forms, obtaining consent forms, and meeting with the patient to answer questions related to the procedure. On completion of the procedure, your duties will include providing postoperative instructions, such as wound care. Other duties will be comprised of setting up the instruments for the procedure, assisting the physician during the procedure, cleaning the procedure room after the surgery, sanitizing and disinfecting or autoclaving the instruments used, and restocking supplies as needed.

Ambulatory Surgery

Ambulatory surgery is surgery performed on a person who is admitted and discharged from a surgical facility on the same day. This includes outpatient surgery in a hospital setting, a surgicenter, or a medical office. Since ambulatory surgery is on the increase, the medical assistant may spend more time assisting the physician with surgical procedures in the office.

Ambulatory surgery, with its option for surgical procedures performed outside the hospital setting, has resulted in a cost savings to the consumer and to the insurer. Hospitalization is not required unless an unexpected complication occurs. The patient is able to return home after a brief recovery time. The disadvantage to this type of surgery is the short time the health care team has for assessing the patient's postoperative condition. It is important for each ambulatory facility to develop a consistent follow-up procedure to track the patient's condition after leaving.

Outpatient surgery is generally limited to procedures requiring less than 60 minutes to perform. Today, many surgeries are performed in free-standing surgicenters or surgical centers that are part of a hospital complex.

Surgeries can be categorized as follows:

- **Elective**—considered medically necessary but can be performed when the patient wishes (e.g., removal of benign growths).

- **Emergency**—required immediately to save a life (e.g., hemorrhage) or prevent further injury or infection.

- **Optional**—may not be medically necessary, but the patient wishes to have it performed (e.g., cosmetic surgery and vasectomy).

- **Outpatient**—does not require an overnight stay in a hospital.

- **Urgent**—to be performed as soon as possible but is not an immediate or acute emergency (e.g., cancer surgery).

Principles of Surgical Asepsis

Surgical asepsis, or sterile technique, is used when sterility of supplies and the immediate environment are required, as in surgical procedures. Sterile technique results in the killing of all microorganisms and spores. It is necessary during any **invasive procedure** (a procedure in which the body is entered), such as when administering an injection, making a surgical incision, or working with an open wound.

Open tissues provide an excellent reservoir (host) for infection. Infections can delay the healing process, cause permanent harm or death to a patient, and result in additional medical costs. Sterile technique prevents microorganisms from being introduced into the body, thereby decreasing the risk of infection.

Both medical asepsis and surgical asepsis are similar in their overall purpose of decreasing the risk of infection. Medical asepsis is a reduction in the number of microorganisms, such as when you wipe a countertop with disinfectant. Medical asepsis results in a "clean" approach in which materials can be handled with clean hands or nonsterile gloves. Surgical asepsis means a complete absence of microorganisms and spores. Surgical asepsis requires a sterile

hand washing or scrub, sterile gloves, and sterile technique when handling materials. A way to remember the difference is to recall "Clean for clean" and "Sterile for sterile." For example, use clean hands when applying a clean bandage to unbroken skin. Use sterile procedure when handling sterile materials, such as using sterile gloves when touching sterile instruments. See Table 42-1 for a comparison of medical and surgical asepsis.

GUIDELINES FOR SURGICAL ASEPSIS

When practicing surgical asepsis, follow the guidelines presented here or those used in your office. Guidelines 42-1 provides some rules for surgical asepsis. Refer to this list of key points often as you read through this chapter. They are the ground rules for establishing a sterile field.

The purpose of personal protective equipment (PPE) is to protect the patient and health care worker from exposure to pathogenic organisms. See Chapter 34 for more information about PPE. Remember that nonsterile scrub suits should not be worn home. All personnel should change to street clothes before leaving a medical facility.

SURGICAL SCRUBS AND STERILE GLOVING

In Chapter 34, medical asepsis and hand hygiene were introduced. Performing hand hygiene is the number-one way to prevent spreading infection. In this chapter, you will learn the procedure for surgical asepsis or a **surgical scrub**. A surgical scrub removes microorganisms more effectively than regular hand washing. It is necessary that the hands be as free from microorganisms as possible in the event that sterile gloves are punctured during a procedure. Procedure 42-1 and Figure 42-2 demonstrate the steps and rationale involved in performing surgical hand

TABLE 42-1 Surgical Asepsis and Medical Asepsis

Surgical Asepsis	Medical Asepsis
Sterile technique used	Clean technique used
Absence of microorganisms	Controls microorganisms
Surgical scrub performed	Basic hand hygiene procedure used
Sterile equipment and supplies required	Clean equipment and supplies
Sterile field	Clean field

SURGICAL ASEPSIS

A sterile item can only touch another sterile item.

- If a sterile item touches a nonsterile item, it is contaminated.
- If a clean item touches a sterile item, it is contaminated.
- A sterile packet that is torn, wet, or punctured is contaminated.
- A sterile packet is contaminated after the date on the packet.
- If unsure of sterility, consider the item contaminated.
- Skin is always considered contaminated. It cannot be sterilized, only disinfected.

A sterile item on a sterile field must be within your field of vision and above your waist.

- If you cannot see an item, it is contaminated.
- If items or your hands are below your waist, they are contaminated.
- If you turn your back on a sterile field, it is contaminated.
- If you leave a sterile field unattended, it is contaminated.

Airborne microorganisms contaminate sterile fields.

- Do not place sterile fields in a draft.
- Avoid extra movements near the sterile field.
- Do not talk, cough, sneeze, or laugh over a sterile field.
- Wear a mask if you need to talk during a procedure.

- Do not reach over a sterile field.
- Avoid spills on a sterile field. A wet field is contaminated.

The edges of a sterile field are contaminated.

- If an item touches any part of the 1-inch border around the sterile field, it is contaminated.

Sterile gloves must only touch sterile items.

- Do not touch the outside of sterile gloves with bare hands.
- Sterile gloves are contaminated if punctured. Remove and dispose of the item and gloves, rescrub, and reglove.

Sterile packets may be touched on the outside with bare hands.

- Outer wrappings are considered contaminated.
- Open sterile packets away from you to avoid contaminating the packet by touching your clothing.
- Never rewrap an unused sterile packet. The unused items must be resanitized, rewrapped, and reautoclaved.

Be honest if you make an error or suspect you have made an error.

- Remove the contaminated item and correct the error.
- Report contamination to your superior.

procedure 42-1

SURGICAL HAND HYGIENE/STERILE SCRUB

Objective: Perform a surgical scrub on hands and arms using the correct procedure for the appropriate length of time.

EQUIPMENT AND SUPPLIES

nail file; germicidal dispenser soap (not bar soap); sterile scrub brush; sterile towel pack (with 2 to 3 sterile paper or cloth towels); sterile gloves (prepackaged); running water (foot pedal preferable)

METHOD

1. Remove all jewelry. With a nail file, remove any gross dirt from beneath fingernails before scrubbing.

   Rationale: Microorganisms can accumulate in crevices of rings or watches and under fingernails.

2. Assemble equipment.
3. Stand at the sink without allowing your body to touch it.

4. Remove your lab coat. Roll up your sleeves above the elbows. Keep your hands and arms above waist level at all times.
5. Regulate running water temperature to warm, not hot.
6. Place hands under running water with hands pointed upward. Allow water to run from fingertips to elbows.
7. Apply a circle of soap from the dispenser and lather well.
8. Vigorously scrub your hands and wrists with a scrub brush (Figure 42-2A). Wash thoroughly between fingers. Scrub under fingernails. Scrub toward the elbows using 5 minutes on each hand (Figure 42-2B–C).
9. Raise hands, bending at the elbow, and place them under running water to rinse off soap (Figure 42-2D).

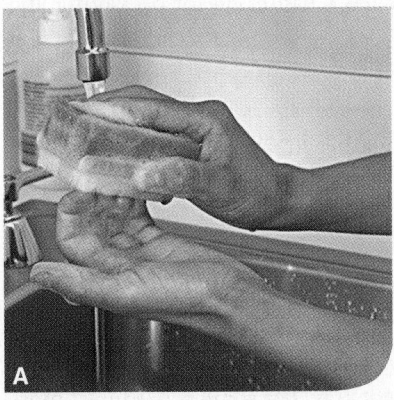

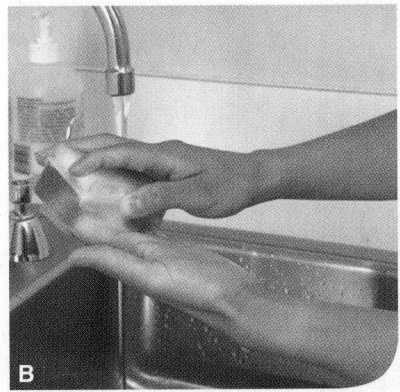

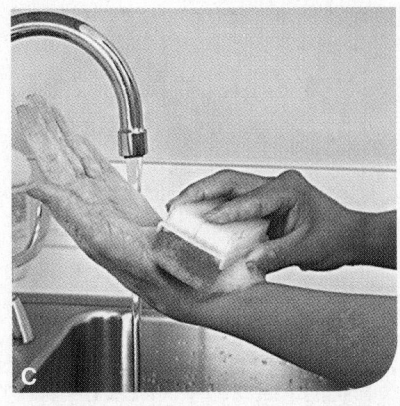

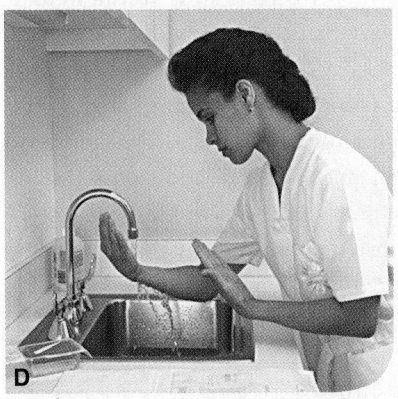

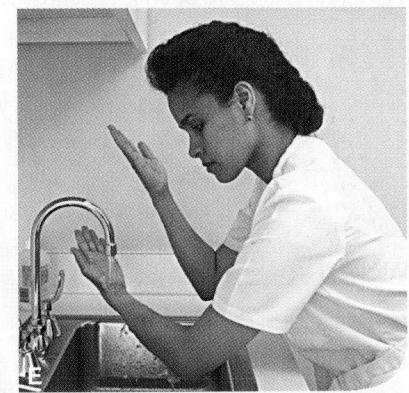

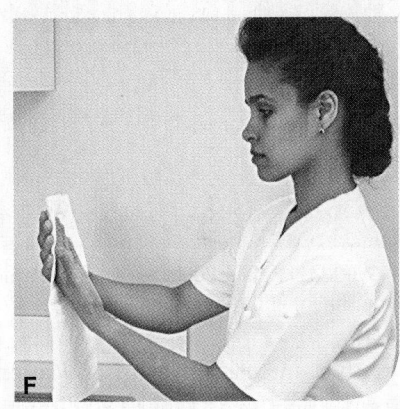

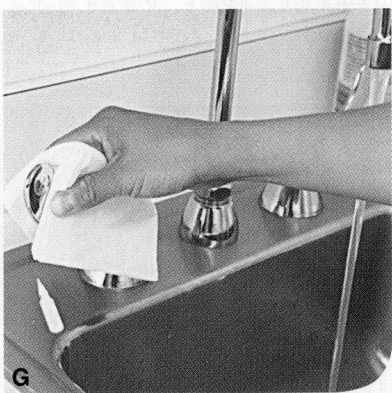

FIGURE 42-2 (A–G) Sterile scrub hand hygiene.

Allow water to flow from fingertips to elbows (Figure 42-2E).

10. If performing a second lather and scrub is the policy in your facility, use 3 minutes for each hand.

11. Using a sterile towel (if possible), pat hands dry moving from fingertips to wrists, and then to elbows. Hands should still be held above the elbows (Figure 42-2F).

12. Turn off the faucet with a fresh towel if foot lever is not available (Figure 42-2G).

13. Glove immediately. Keep hands above waist and folded together until the procedure begins.

hygiene. Figure 42-3 shows a medical assistant in PPE, including face shield, gown, and gloves, preparing to assist with a surgical procedure. PPE provides a barrier between infectious or hazardous material and the wearer. Remember if a sterile glove is punctured or if you touch the outside of the glove with your hand it is considered nonsterile and must be replaced after you perform another surgical scrub.

Procedure 42-2 lists the steps for surgical gloving and glove removal.

STERILE PACKAGING

Sterile packages (packets) are prepared for use in surgery. Each one may contain either a single instrument or piece of equipment or several items packed together. These packets

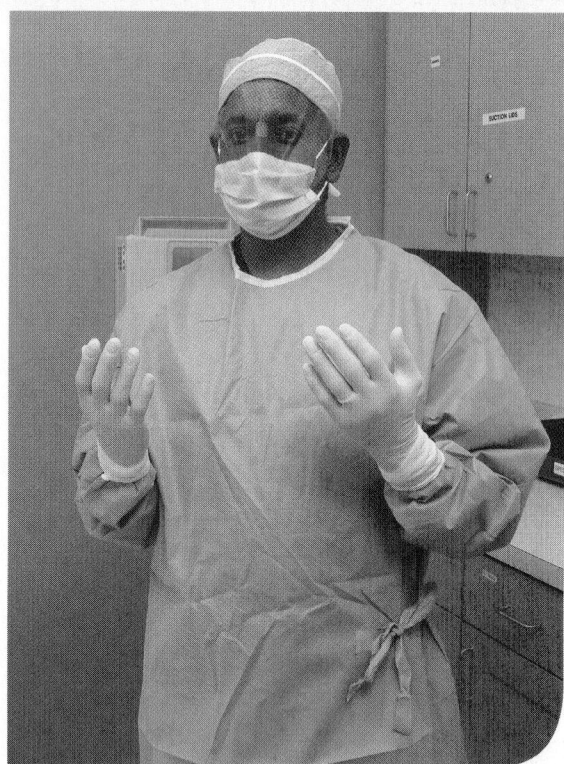

FIGURE 42-3 A medical assistant wearing PPE—gown, face shield, and gloves.

of instruments routinely used in minor surgery (discussed later in this chapter). Review Chapter 34 for packaging and autoclaving procedures.

Sterile packets are used for various procedures. For example, all the instruments needed for a procedure, such as a biopsy, are packaged together in a tray and autoclaved. Procedure 42-3 and Figure 42-5A–F explain the steps for opening a sterile packet.

When assisting the physician or surgeon with the procedure, the medical assistant will set up the specific tray or instruments before the procedure begins. The packets are set up on a **Mayo stand**, a small portable table with enough room to hold an instrument tray. For some procedures, more than one Mayo stand is used. After the sterile packet is opened, the inside of its wrapper becomes the **sterile field** (a specific area free of all microorganisms that will be the work area for a surgical procedure). The outer, 1-inch border all around the open wrapper is considered contaminated. If the field becomes wet, it is contaminated and a new packet must be opened. The physician may want an additional instrument while performing a procedure; you would open a sterile packet and drop the instrument carefully onto the field. Procedure 42-4 and Figure 42-6 show the steps and rationale for dropping a sterile packet onto a sterile field.

Sterile Transfer

In order to place instruments and supplies onto a sterile field or to move them around on the sterile field, you

are then autoclaved with sterilization indicators and dated. Sterile packs may be purchased from a medical supply company or packaged by the medical assistant in the office. To prepare sterile packets, you must know the names and uses

procedure

42-2

SURGICAL GLOVING

Objective: Apply sterile gloves without a break in sterile technique.

Note: This procedure follows a surgical hand scrub.

EQUIPMENT AND SUPPLIES

double-wrapped sterile glove pack

METHOD

1. Assemble equipment and check the tape or seal for expiration date and condition of pack.
2. Place the pack on a flat surface at waist height with the cuffed end of the gloves toward you.
3. Open the outside wrapper by touching only the outside of the pack. Leave the opened wrapper in place to provide a sterile work field.
4. Open the inner wrapper without reaching over the pack or touching the inside of the wrapper. Pull inner wrapper edges to each side without touching the inside of the pack (Figure 42-4A).
5. Using the thumb and fingers of your left hand (if you are right-handed) pick up the glove on the right side of the pack by grasping the folded inside edge of the cuff (Figure 42-4B). The glove can be dangled slightly off the sterile packing material for easier insertion.

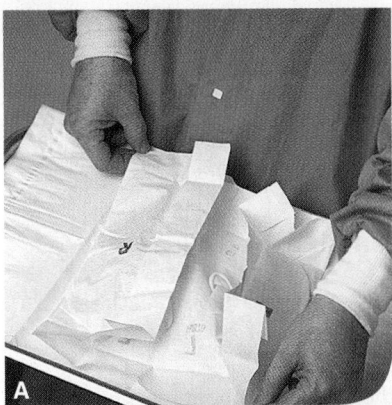

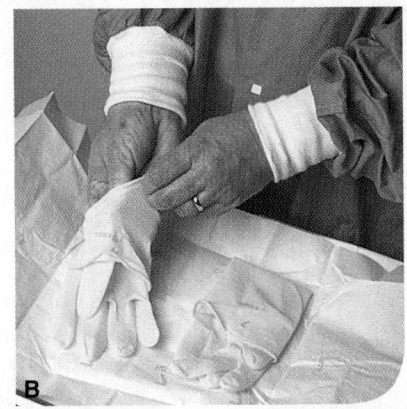

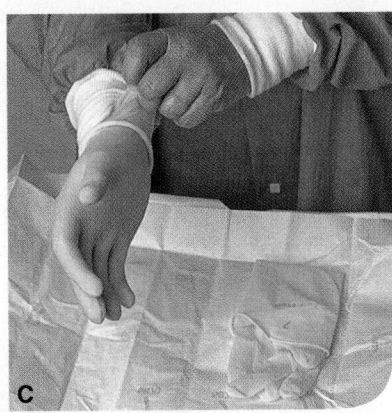

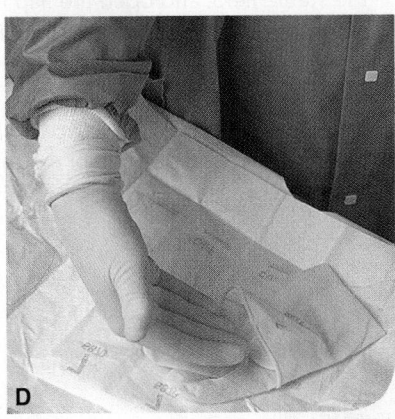

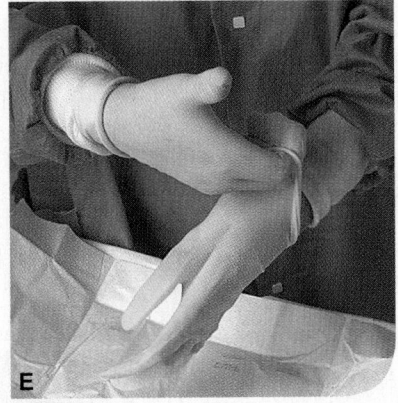

6. Pull the glove onto the right hand using only the thumb and fingers of the left hand (Figure 42-4C). Do not allow fingers to touch the rest of the glove.

7. Place the fingers of the right-gloved hand under the cuff of the left glove and pull onto the left hand and up over the left wrist (Figure 42-4D).

8. With the gloved right hand, place your fingers under the cuff of the left glove and pull up over the left wrist (Figure 42-4E). The thumb should not touch the cuff.

9. After the gloves are in place, the fingers can be adjusted, if necessary, by using the gloved hands.

10. Removing gloves (Figures 42-4F–H): Remove the first glove by grasping the edge of that glove (with fingers of the other gloved hand) and pull the first glove over the hand inside out. Discard the first glove into the proper biohazard waste container. Remove the other glove by grasping the edge of the cuff with your fingers (from the ungloved hand) and pull the second glove down over the hand, inside out. Discard the gloves appropriately.

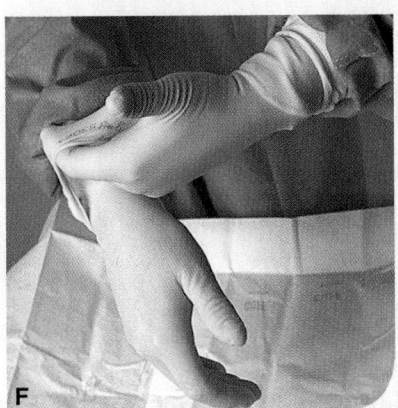

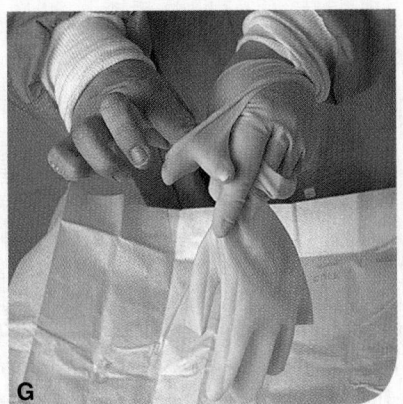

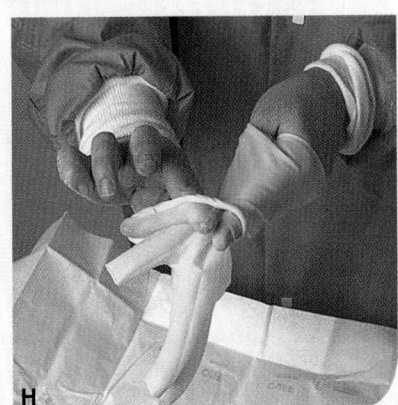

FIGURE 42-4 (A–H) Sterile gloving and glove removal technique.

OPENING A STERILE PACKET

Objective: Open a sterile packet (pack) and use it to set up a sterile field without a break in the sterile technique.

EQUIPMENT AND SUPPLIES

sterile packet; Mayo stand; waste container; sterile forceps

METHOD

1. Perform hand hygiene.
2. Assemble equipment. Adjust the Mayo stand to correct height.
3. Place packet on the Mayo stand with the folded edge on top. Position the packet on the stand so that the top flap will fold away from you.
4. Remove the tape or fastener and check the sterilization indicator and date. Discard in a waste container.
5. Pull the corner of the pack that is tucked under and lay this flap away from you. It will hang down over the edge of the Mayo stand (Figures 42-5A–B).

6. With both hands, pull the next two flaps to each side (Figures 42-5C–D). The packet will still be covered with the last layer of the outer wrapper.
7. Grasp the corner of the last flap, without reaching over the sterile field, and open the flap toward your body without touching it (Figures 42-5E–F).
8. The inside of this outer wrapper is now your sterile field. If you need to arrange items within this field, use sterile forceps. If an inner packet must be opened with an instrument setup, then someone wearing sterile gloves must open it.

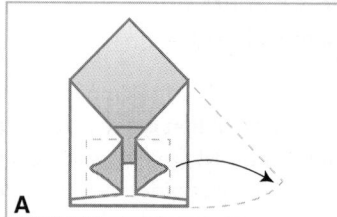
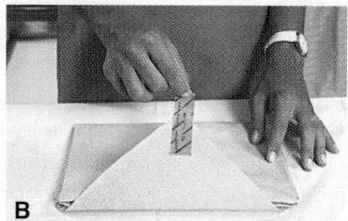
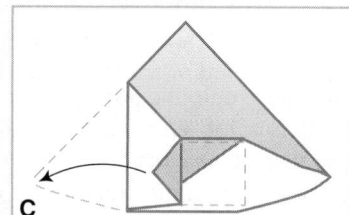
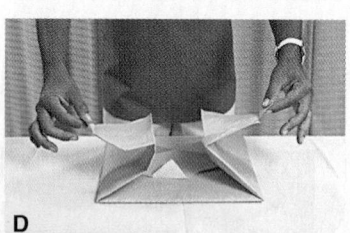
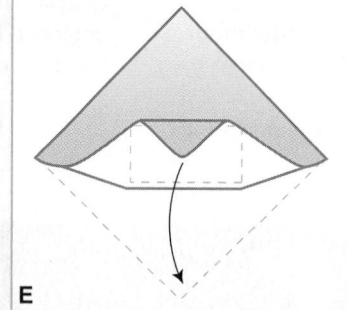
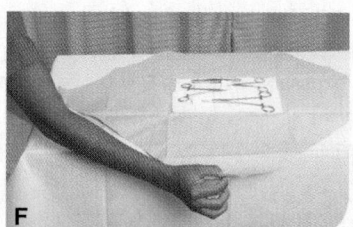

FIGURE 42-5 Opening a sterile packet.

would need to put on sterile gloves or use transfer forceps. Procedure 42-5 and Figure 42-7 illustrate the steps and rationale for transferring sterile objects using transfer forceps. Remember not to reach across the sterile field or turn your back on the field unless it is covered with a sterile towel.

Surgical Instruments

Surgical instruments have been developed over centuries to meet a specific need during an operation such as cutting, suturing, or grasping. In some cases, an instrument developed by a surgeon bears the name of the surgeon—for example,

DROPPING A STERILE PACKET ONTO A STERILE FIELD

Objective: Place (drop) a sterile item onto a sterile field or into a gloved hand without contaminating the packet or the field.

EQUIPMENT AND SUPPLIES

sterile pack (containing, for example, prepackaged items such as a specimen container or needle and syringe in a pull-apart packet)

METHOD

1. Assemble equipment; check expiration date and sealed condition of packet.
2. Locate the edge on the prepackaged item and pull apart by using the thumb and forefinger of each hand. Do not let your fingers touch the inside of the packet. Rationale: The inside of the packet is sterile and the outside is considered contaminated.
3. Pull the packet apart by securely placing the remaining three fingers of each hand against the outside of the packet on each side. The wrapper edges will be pulled back and away from the sterile item.
4. Holding the item securely about eight to ten inches from the sterile field, gently drop the packet contents inside the sterile field (Figure 42-6). Instead of having you drop the item, the physician may wish to remove the item directly from the packet by grasping it firmly with his or

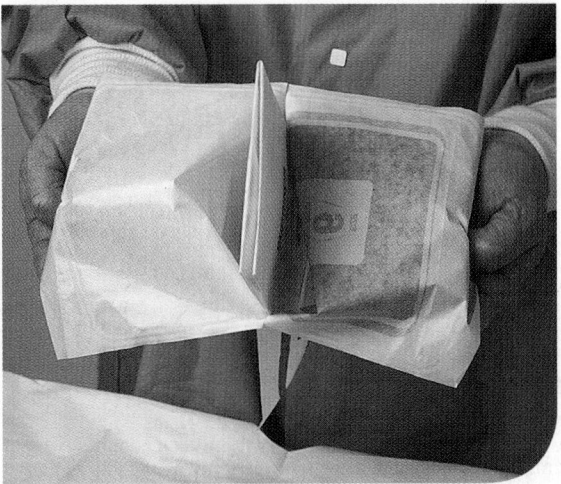

FIGURE 42-6 Dropping a sterile supply onto a sterile field.

her gloved hand. Rationale: Nonsterile hands and arms should not be placed over the sterile field.
5. Discard the paper wrapper in a waste container.

TRANSFERRING STERILE OBJECTS USING TRANSFER FORCEPS

Objective: Move sterile objects, such as instruments and supplies, within or onto a sterile field or into a gloved hand.

EQUIPMENT AND SUPPLIES

sterile transfer forceps in a forceps container with a sterilant solution, such as Cidex; Mayo stand with sterile field setup; sterile 4 × 4 gauze package (opened)

METHOD

1. Grasp forceps handles firmly without separating the tips and remove vertically from the container. Remove vertically to avoid dripping solution onto exposed contaminated portion of forceps.

2. Holding forceps vertically with tips down, gently tap tips together to drop excess solution onto dry sterile 4 × 4 gauze or touch the sterile 4 × 4 gauze to dry the tips.
3. Pick up the sterile item to be transferred by holding transfer forceps vertically with tips down. Do not touch the sterile field. Grasp the article to be transferred firmly at its midsection.
4. Place sterile item within the sterile field (Figure 42-7).
5. Place forceps back into container without touching the sides of the container.
6. Clean and sterilize the forceps and container in the autoclave. Change the solution.

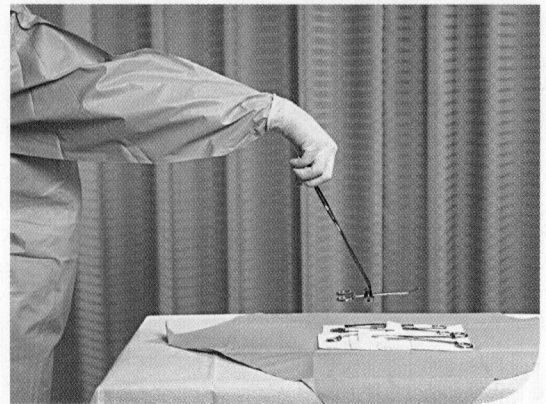

FIGURE 42-7 **Proper technique to handle sterile equipment with transfer forceps in a sterile field.**

Kelly forceps, Halstead mosquito clamp, and Bozeman uterine forceps.

INSTRUMENTS USED IN MINOR SURGERY IN AN OFFICE

The general classification of instruments is based on their use: cutting, dissecting, grasping, clamping, dilating, probing, visualizing, or suturing. Specific instruments are related to individual specialties, such as gynecology; urology; orthopedics; ear, nose, and throat; proctology; obstetrics; and neurology. A minor surgical setup will include a standard group of instruments, such as scalpel, blades, scissors, hemostat, and suture materials. Instruments are usually made of steel and treated to be rust and heat resistant, stainproof, and durable.

It is important to be able to identify common instruments used in your facility. Some physicians will use the full name of the instrument—for example, Pederson vaginal speculum—and others will just refer to it simply as a vaginal speculum. The following tips will help you identify instruments.

- Categorize the instrument by its use: to cut, probe, grasp, clamp, retract, dilate, and so on.
- Examine the types of parts of the instrument, and ask yourself the following questions:
  – What type of handles does it have (e.g., ring, serrated)?
  – What type of tip does it have (e.g., pointed, blunt, teeth, no teeth, serrated)?
  – What type of closure does it have (e.g., spring, boxlock with a screw, ratchet)?
  – What type of edges does it have?
  – How long is it (may indicate for which body part it is used)?
  – Whose name does it bear?

Each time you encounter an instrument you are unfamiliar with, answer the preceding questions to determine its characteristics and remember the name.

Cutting Instruments

Scalpels or knives are used to make **incisions**, which are surgical cuts into tissue. They are small curved instruments

PROFESSIONALISM THE LIFE SPAN

Your role as a medical assistant participating in minor surgery procedures includes not only assisting with the actual procedure but also providing follow-up care, such as changing dressings and educating the patient on wound care at home. The goal in treating any wound is to encourage healing without infection and avoid scarring and loss of function.

Patients will present a variety of health conditions, range of ages, detrimental life habits, and preexisting conditions, all of which impact wound healing. Wound healing may be hindered by poor circulation in patients such as the elderly. A diabetic patient's wound healing is impeded by poor circulation and decreased resistance to infection. HIV patients or those who have been on immunosuppressant medication are slower to heal. Other factors that impact the rate of healing are poor nutrition, obesity, smoking, alcoholism, recreational drug use, excessive stress, and excessive fatigue. Taking a holistic view of your patients will help you to discover factors that may impact wound healing.

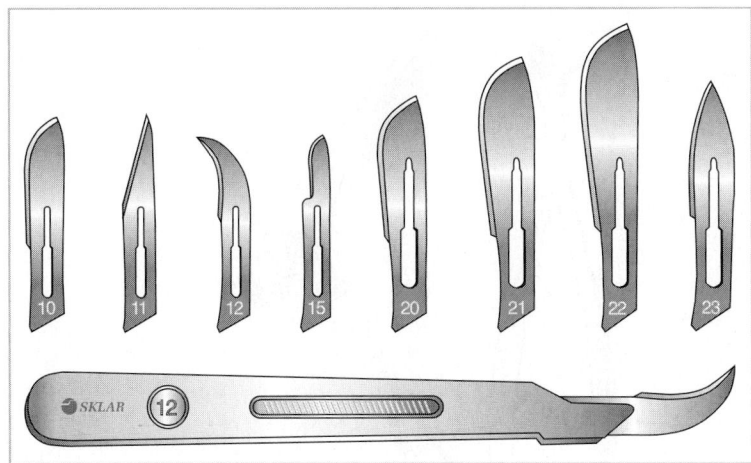

FIGURE 42-8   A variety of scalpels and blades.

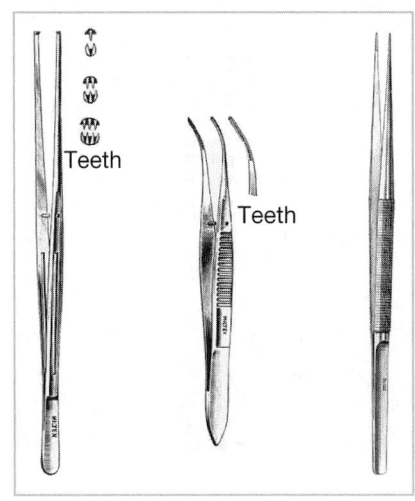

FIGURE 42-10   Types of forceps.

that are made to fit easily into the surgeon's hand. Figure 42-8 illustrates a variety of scalpels and blades. A scalpel blade must be inserted into the scalpel handle. Blades come in various sizes depending on the type of incision and tissue.

Dissecting Instruments

The most common tool for dissecting or cutting tissue is scissors. For example, scissors are used for **debridement** (removal of dead tissue around wound edges using sterile technique) or to cut sutures (thread). Scissors have two blades with sharp edges that come together when the handles are drawn together.

The tips of scissors vary greatly to perform a variety of functions. Some scissors have blunt tips that can slide under bandages and dressings to cut without damaging the skin. Metzenbaum scissors are short, curved, and blunt and intended for use on and to prevent piercing of delicate tissue. Operating scissors or suture scissors are used to cut suture material during surgery; they have a hook on one edge that fits under the suture for ease in suture removal. Dissecting

scissors are also called straight or Mayo scissors. Operating scissors are straight or curved with a combination of blades, such as sharp/sharp (s/s), blunt/blunt (b/b), and sharp/blunt (s/b). Bandage scissors have a blunt tip and a blunt flat edge to allow it to fit easily under a bandage for cutting. Figure 42-9 illustrates a variety of scissors.

Grasping and Clamping Instruments

Forceps are used to grasp tissue or objects (Figure 42-10). One type of forceps is a two-pronged instrument, which has a spring-type handle used to clamp together tightly to prevent slipping. Another type of closure mechanism is a ratchet closure or clasp. The ratchet clasp allows the forceps to close with differing degrees of tightness. Forceps often have serrations or teethlike edges that prevent tissue slipping out of the forceps.

Types of Forceps.   The following are several different types of widely used forceps:

- Tissue forceps have teeth and are used to grasp tissue.
    - Thumb forceps are two-pronged with serrated tips to hold tissue.
    - Splinter forceps are used to grasp foreign bodies.
    - Needle holder forceps are used to grasp needles during suturing.
    - Hemostats are applied to blood vessels to hold vessels until they can be sutured (Figure 42-11).
    - Sponge forceps are used for holding sponges during surgery.
    - Towel clamps are used to hold together the edges of sterile drapes.

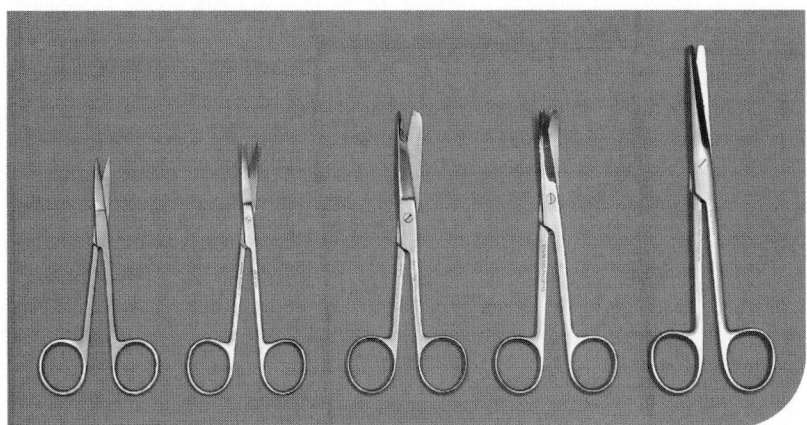

FIGURE 42-9   A variety of types of scissors.

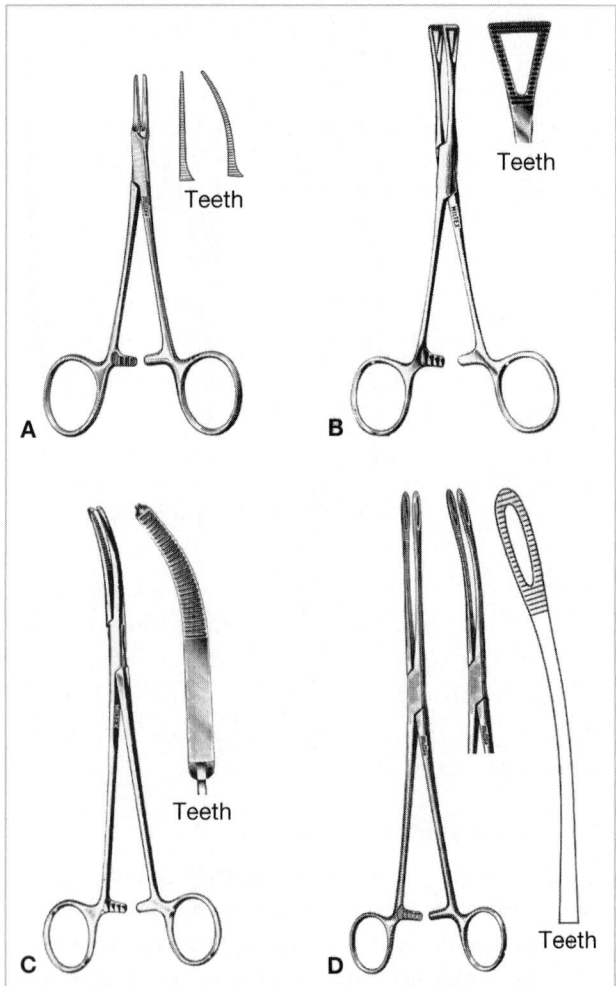

FIGURE 42-11 Hemostats: (A) mosquito forceps; (B) Pennington hemostatic forceps; (C) curved forceps; (D) sponge forceps.

Probing and Dilating Instruments

Instruments used to enter body cavities for probing or dilating purposes include the following:

- **Scope**—usually lighted, it is inserted into a body cavity or vessel to visualize the internal structures. Figure 42-12

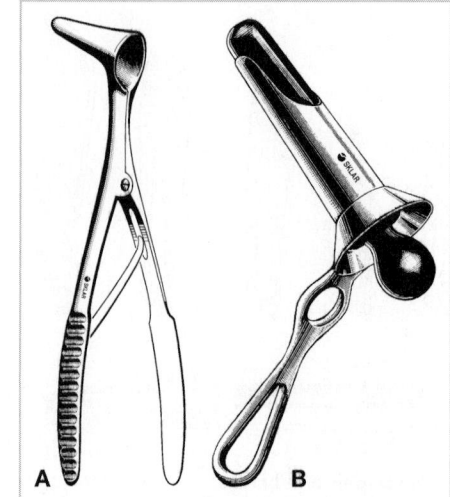

FIGURE 42-13 Specula: (A) Vienna nasal speculum; (B) Ives-Fanster rectal speculum.

shows different sizes of laryngoscopes that are used to look at a patient's voice box or larynx. An obturator is placed inside a scope to guide it into a cavity or canal and then removed during visualization of the surgical site. Some obturators have a point used to puncture tissue.

- **Speculum**—unlighted instrument with movable parts that when inserted into a cavity, such as the nasal cavity or rectum, can be spread apart for ease of visualization and tissue sample removal (Figure 42-13).
- **Probe**—used to explore wounds and cavities usually with a curved, blunt point to facilitate insertion (Figure 42-14).
- **Trocar**—used to withdraw fluids from cavities. It consists of a cannula (outer tube) and a sharp stylet that is withdrawn after the trocar is inserted (Figure 42-15).
- **Punch**—used to remove tissue for examination and biopsy.

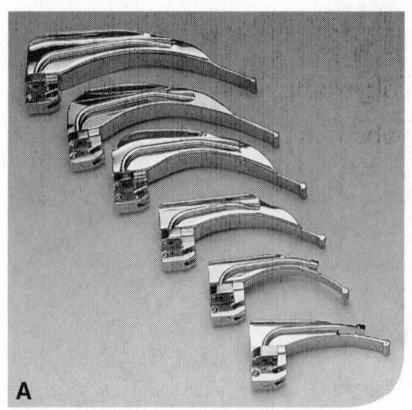

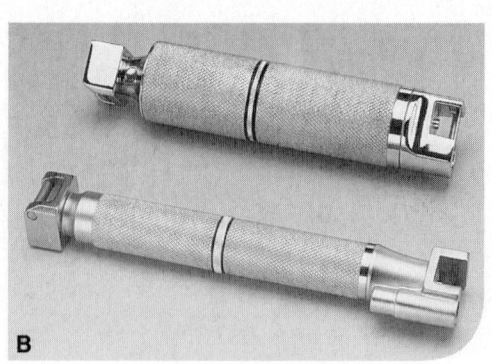

FIGURE 42-12 Laryngoscopes: (A) scopes; (B) handles.

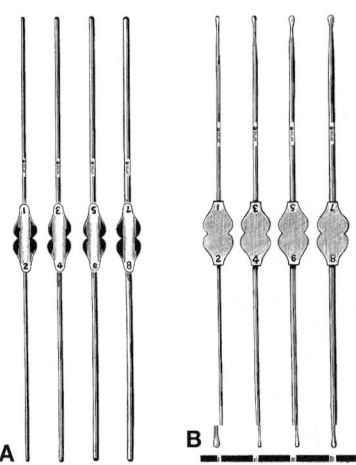

FIGURE 42-14 Lachrymal probes: (A) Bowman; (B) Williams.

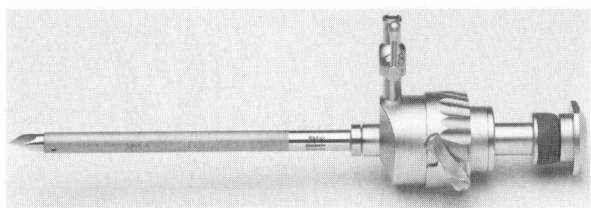

FIGURE 42-15 Trocar.

Specialized instruments are used for disciplines, such as gynecology and obstetrics (Figure 42-16), urology (Figure 42-17), and orthopedics (Figure 42-18).

Suture Materials and Needles

Suture (thread) materials are used to bring together or approximate a surgical incision or wound until healing takes place. Suture materials are added to the surgical tray setup when they are needed for a procedure. Sutures come either with or without an attached needle. The package label will indicate type, size, and length of the suture material. Suture types include absorbable and nonabsorbable.

Absorbable Sutures. Absorbable sutures are digested by tissue enzymes and absorbed by the body tissues. They do not have to be removed. Absorption usually occurs 5 to 20 days after insertion. This type of suture, such as surgical catgut (made from sheep's intestinal lining), or Vicryl, a synthetic material, is used for internal organs such as the bladder and intestines, subcutaneous tissue, and ligating or tying off blood vessels. They include plain catgut, surgical catgut, and chromic catgut. Plain catgut is used in areas

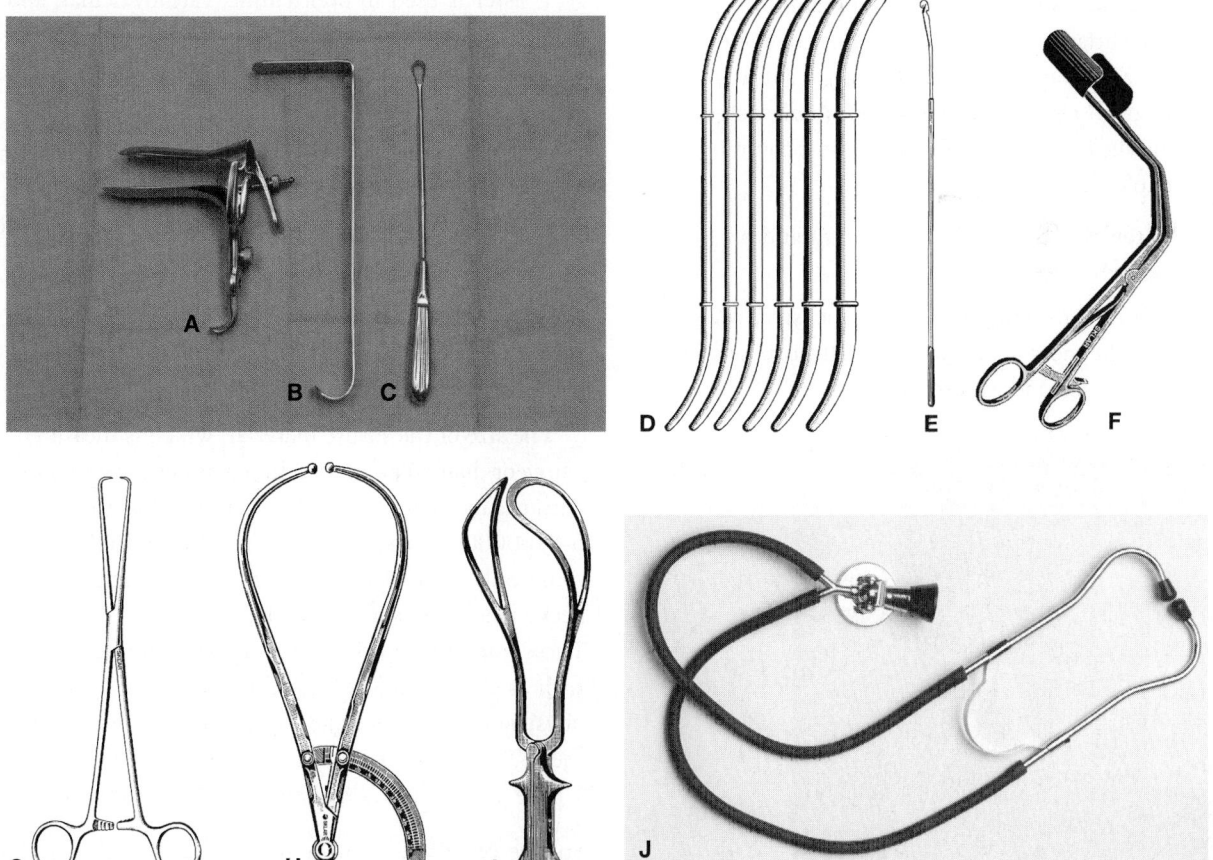

FIGURE 42-16 Gynecological instruments: (A) vaginal speculum; (B) retractor; (C) uterine curette; (D) uterine dilators; (E) IUD extractor forceps; (F) lateral vaginal retractor; (G) Schroeder uterine tenaculum forceps; (H) Martin pelvimeter; (I) De Lee OB forceps; (J) Bowles obstetrical stethoscope.

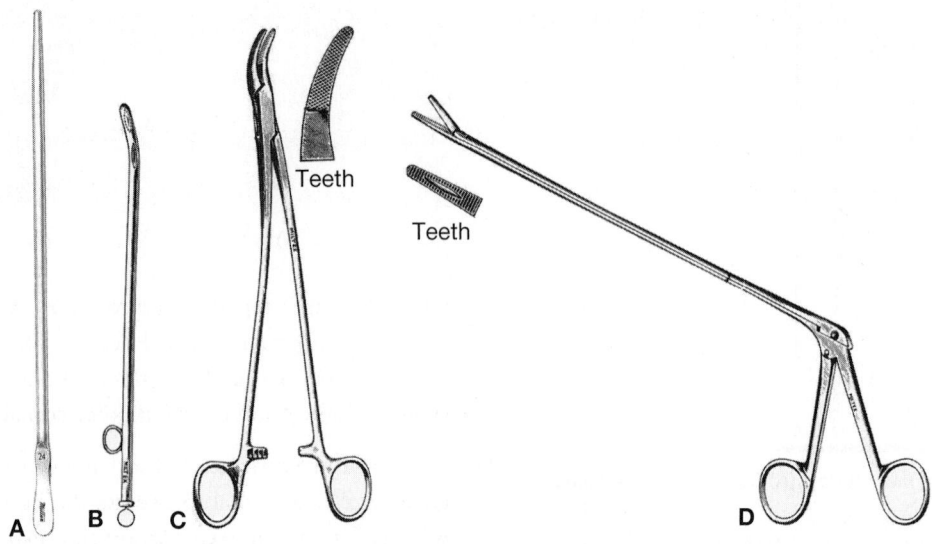

FIGURE 42-17 Urological instruments: (A) sound; (B) female catheter; (C) needle holder; (D) urethral forceps.

where rapid healing takes place, such as highly vascular areas of the lips and tongue. Surgical catgut is used on tissues that are fast healing, such as the vaginal area. Chromic catgut has a slower absorption rate and can be used to hold tissue together longer, such as for muscle repair.

Nonabsorbable Sutures. Nonabsorbable sutures are used on skin surfaces where they can easily be removed after incisional healing takes place. This type of suture material, such as nylon, cotton, silk, Dacron, and stainless steel, is not absorbed by the body. Black silk is the most commonly used nonabsorbable suture.

Suture Material. Suture materials vary and are selected based on how they are used.

- Silk suture, although the most expensive, is also considered the most dependable. An all-purpose suture, it is widely used and easy to tie.

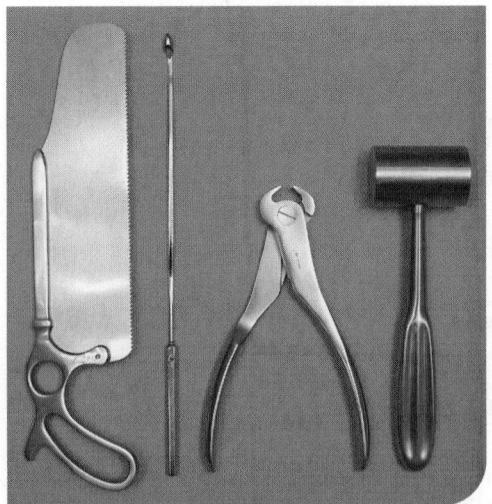

FIGURE 42-18 Orthopedic instruments.

- Nylon suture has elasticity and strength that make it ideal for use in joints and for skin closure. The disadvantage is the difficulty in forming a tight knot.

- Polyester suture is the second strongest of all the standard suture material, and steel is the strongest. Polyester is used in ophthalmic, cardiovascular, and facial surgery, which all require a strong, unbreakable suture since a broken suture could result in permanent damage to the patient.

- Steel is used in staples, as well as nonabsorbable suture wire that is composed of 316L stainless steel, and is the most widely used suture material in major surgery. It is the strongest of all suture material.

- Cotton suture, with less strength than other suture materials, is no longer widely used.

- Linen suture is created from natural flax fiber.

The size of the suture material, which is measured by the gauge or diameter, is stated in terms of 0s, decreasing in size with the number of zeros. For example, 0 is the thickest and 6-0 (000000) is the smallest. Sizes 2-0 through 6-0 are most commonly used. Delicate tissue, on areas such as the face and neck, would be sutured with 5-0 to 6-0 suture material. These fine sutures would leave less scarring. Heavier sutures, such as 2-0, would be used for the chest or abdomen. The physician determines the type and gauge of sutures to be used. Table 42-2 summarizes suture uses, sizes, and types. Figure 42-19 illustrates different suture material.

Suture Needles. Suture needles are available in differing shapes depending on where they are used (Figure 42-20). Needles have either a sharp cutting point used for tissues that provide some resistance, such as skin, or a round non-

TABLE 42-2 Suture Use, Size, and Type of Material

Use	Gauge	Type of Material
Blood vessels	3-0 to 0 3-0 3-0 to 0	chromic gut cotton silk
Eyelid	6-0 to 4-0 6-0 to 5-0	silk polyester
Fascial	2-0 to 0 2-0 to 0 2-0 to 0	chromic gut silk cotton
Muscle	3-0 to 0 3-0 to 0 3-0 to 0	plain gut chromic gut silk
Skin	6-0 to 2-0 5-0 to 3-0 5-0 to 2-0	nylon polyethylene stainless steel

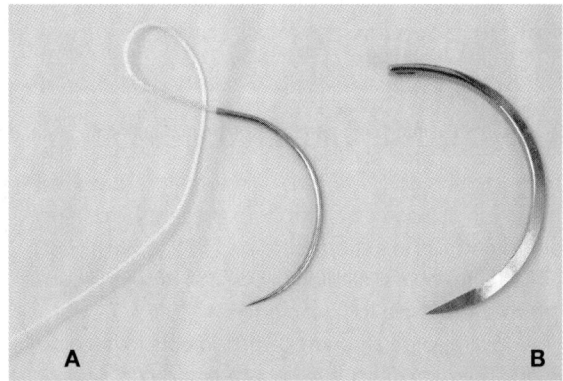

FIGURE 42-20 Surgical needle shapes: (A) taper point; (B) cutting point.

cutting point used for more flexible tissue such as peritoneum. They are available in three shapes: straight, curved, or swaged.

The straight needle is used when the needle is pushed and pulled through the tissue without the use of a needle holder. This type of needle will have an eye that is threaded with the suture material. The suture material thickness will be double when threaded through the needle since it will enter the eye from one side and come out the other.

Curved needles allow the surgeon to go in and out of a tissue when there is not enough room to maneuver a straight needle. This type of needle requires a needle holder.

A swaged needle and suture materials are combined in one length. This offers the advantage of the suture material not slipping off the needle since it is attached. A swaged needle pack will contain a label indicating the gauge, type of needle point (cutting or noncutting), and type and length of the suture material.

Other Wound Closure Materials. Other materials used for wound closure include sterile tapes, such as Steri-Strips (Figure 42-21), staples, and skin adhesives, such as Dermabond. Sterile tapes are nonallergenic and available in a variety of widths. They are used instead of sutures when not much tension will be applied to a wound, such as on a small facial cut. Skin adhesives are composed of cyanoacrylate adhesives that react with water to create an instant, strong, flexible bond. The composition of skin adhesives is similar to Superglue and can be used to close lacerations or small surgical incisions. Staples are made of stainless steel and applied with a surgical stapler.

GUIDELINES FOR HANDLING INSTRUMENTS

Surgical instruments are expensive and may be delicate. They require special care and attention. In some instances, there might not be a duplicate of an instrument. Even slight damage to an instrument can result in malfunction at a

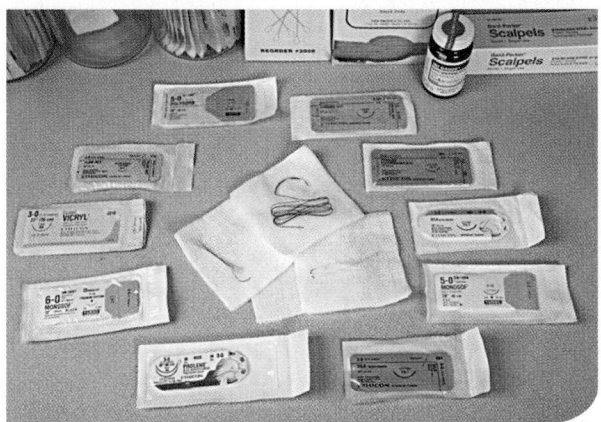

FIGURE 42-19 Types of suture material.

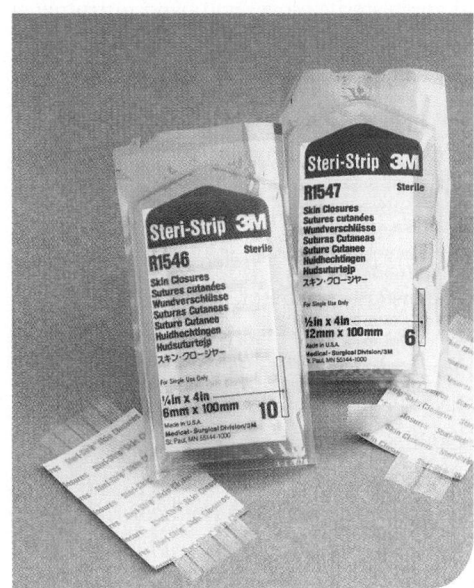

FIGURE 42-21 Steri-Strips from 3M.

critical time during surgery. Guidelines 42-2 provides guidelines for handling instruments.

Surgical Assisting

The medical assistant's role in surgical assisting varies depending on the type of practice and the needs of the physician. For example, an eye surgeon who performs a large number of outpatient cataract operations may employ a full-time **scrub assistant**, scrub technician (scrub tech), or operating technician (OR tech) who will apply sterile gloves and hand instruments to the surgeon. In this case, the medical assistant might act as the nonsterile assistant, who positions the patient, uses transfer forceps to bring additional supplies as needed, holds the vial of local anesthetic while the surgeon draws up the correct dosage into a syringe, and applies dressings. Anyone not in sterile attire and assisting with a procedure can be described as a nonsterile assistant. He or she may also be referred to as a floating assistant, circulating assistant, circulator, or floater.

In many practices, the medical assistant will scrub, apply sterile gloves, and act as the only assistant for the surgeon. A good assistant can help the procedure flow smoothly. The exact surgical tray setup and sequence of passing instruments will vary depending on the procedure and the surgeon's preferences.

A good assistant will anticipate the needs of the physician, use care in handing instruments efficiently, use care that injury does not occur, and account for all materials and instruments used during the procedure. The assistant must maintain an accurate count of absorbent sponges used for cleaning out the wound site during surgery to ensure that all sponges are removed before the patient's wound is closed.

SCRUB ASSISTANT

The scrub assistant performs all procedures in sterile protective clothing using sterile technique. His or her responsibilities include arranging the surgical tray to meet the operating physician's preferences, handing instruments, swabbing (sponging) bodily fluids away from the operative site, retracting the incision area, and cutting suture materials. See Guidelines 42-3 for guidelines on sterile technique for scrub assistants. To become competent as a scrub assistant, practice reaching for an instrument with your eyes closed. This is similar to the conditions under which the physician works since he or she does not look up from the operative site when reaching for instruments.

Instruments should be passed to the physician firmly and by the handle first. An instrument should remain in your grasp until you feel confident that the physician has a firm grip on it. Figure 42-22 illustrates a medical assistant using proper technique when passing instruments to the physician. Procedure 42-6 and Figure 42-23 show the steps for transferring sterile solutions onto a sterile field. All of the preceding procedures are vital for you to master in order to properly assist the physician with minor surgery, as described in Procedure 42-7.

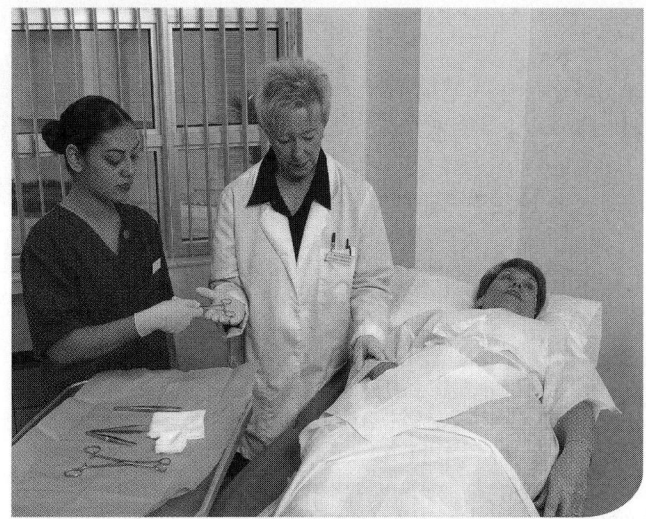

FIGURE 42-22 **A medical assistant using the proper technique when passing instruments to the physician.**

Floating Assistant. The floating assistant performs non-sterile duties during a surgical procedure and thus "floats" between the operating table, supplies, and equipment.

procedure 42-6

TRANSFERRING STERILE SOLUTIONS ONTO A STERILE FIELD

Objective: Pour sterile fluid into a sterile basin on a sterile field without spilling the solution or contaminating the field.

EQUIPMENT AND SUPPLIES
sterile saline or other solution as ordered; sterile basin; Mayo stand or side tray; waste container

METHOD
1. Perform hand hygiene.
2. Assemble all equipment. Check expiration dates on the solution and sterile basin pack.
3. Set up sterile basin on the Mayo tray using inside of wrapper to create a sterile field.
4. Remove cap of the solution and place it on a clean surface with the outer edge down (inside facing up). Avoid touching the inner surface of the cap, which is considered sterile.
5. Check the label on the bottle before pouring the solution.
6. Pour a small amount of the liquid into a waste container for discarding. This will dislodge any bacteria that may have collected on the edge of the bottle after opening it.
7. Pour the bottle with the label held against the palm (Figure 42-23). This protects the label from drips that can destroy the name of the solution.

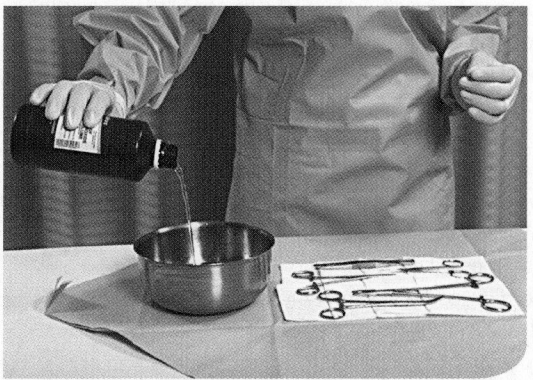

FIGURE 42-23 **Pouring sterile solution into a sterile container.**

8. Hold the bottle about 6 inches above the basin and pour slowly to avoid splashing.
9. Replace the lid immediately after using.

ASSISTING WITH MINOR SURGERY

Objective: Prepare all materials and equipment for immediate use in a surgical procedure using sterile technique.

EQUIPMENT AND SUPPLIES

Mayo stand; side stand; transfer forceps and container; sharps container; waste container/plastic bag; biohazard waste container; anesthetic; alcohol swab; sterile specimen container, depending on type of surgery; sterile pack (2 pairs sterile gloves, towel pack, 4 × 4 sponge pack, patient drape, needle pack, and suture materials); instrument pack(s), including towel clamp pack; syringe pack; 2 sterile basin packs

METHOD

1. Perform hand hygiene.
2. Open sterile tray packs on Mayo stand and side stand. Use sterile wrapper to create a sterile field. The wrapper will hang over the edges of the tray.
3. Use sterile transfer forceps to move instruments on tray or to place equipment from packets. Materials in peel-away packets should be flipped onto the tray.
4. Open the sterile needle and syringe unit and drop gently onto the sterile field. Use care not to reach over the sterile field.
5. Open the sterile drape packs and towel clamp packs.
6. Open a set of sterile gloves for the physician.
7. After the tray is ready with all equipment open and arranged, pull the edge of the sterile towel across the tray, using sterile transfer forceps. The sterile towel will provide a protective covering for the sterile tray until the procedure begins. The medical assistant should not leave the room once the tray is set up (Figure 42-24).
8. When the physician has donned the sterile gloves, remove the sterile towel covering the tray of instruments.
9. Remove the towel by standing to one side and grasping the two distal corners, then lifting the towel toward you so that you do not reach over the unprotected sterile field.
10. Cleanse the vial of anesthetic with a sterile alcohol swab and hold it upside down in the palm of your hand with the label facing toward the physician. Hold it steady while the physician draws up the anesthetic.
11. Stand to one side of the patient and assist the physician as requested. Provide additional supplies as needed. If you assist by handing instruments directly to the physician, you must perform a surgical scrub and wear a sterile gown and gloves.
12. Hold all containers for specimens, drainage, or contaminated 4 × 4s. Wear nonsterile gloves to protect yourself from contact with drainage.

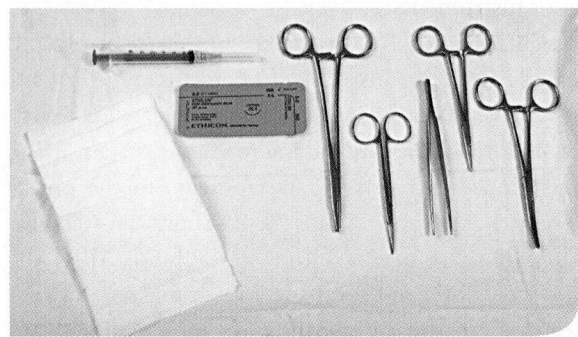

FIGURE 42-24   Sterile instrument setup.

13. Collect and place all soiled instruments in a basin out of the patient's view.
14. Place all soiled gauze sponges (4 × 4s) and dressings in a plastic bag. Do not allow wet items to remain on a sterile field.
15. Immediately label all specimens as they are obtained. Close all specimen containers tightly.
16. Periodically reassure the patient by quietly asking how he or she is doing. Do not touch the patient with soiled gloves.
17. When the procedure is complete, wash your hands before assisting the patient. The patient will often be moved to a recovery area so the surgical area can be cleaned.
   To dispose of soiled dressings, use the following steps:
   a. Remove gloves.
   b. Place one hand into the empty plastic bag.
   c. Using the hand covered with the plastic bag, pick up all the soiled materials. With the other hand, pull the outside of the bag over the soiled dressings.
   d. Dispose of bag in a biohazard waste container.
   e. Perform hand hygiene and document the procedure.
18. Allow the patient to rest and recover from the anesthetic. Periodically, check the patient's vital signs according to your office policy.
19. Provide clear oral and written postoperative instructions for the patient. Make sure the patient is stable before he or she leaves the office.
20. Send the specimen(s) to the laboratory with a requisition slip.
21. Clean, sanitize, and sterilize the instruments. Clean and sanitize the room in preparation for the next patient.
22. Perform hand hygiene.

CHARTING EXAMPLE

11/8/20XX 9:00 A.M. The physician will chart the details of the surgical procedure. · J. Wall, RMA

One of the major roles of the float assistant is to monitor the patient by taking vital signs every 5 to 10 minutes. Other duties include providing additional sterile equipment, opening sterile packets, adding sterile equipment to the field, and performing the necessary counts of supplies utilized, such as gauze squares. Other guidelines for proper floating technique during surgery are listed in Guidelines 42-4.

Either category of assistant may be responsible for setting up the sterile field following appropriate guidelines prior to surgery. A surgical setup for a typical minor surgical procedure would include the following:

- Local anesthetic materials
- 3 cc syringe with needle(s)
- Alcohol sponges to cleanse vial top
- Sterile gloves for surgeon
- 4 × 4 and 2 × 2 gauze sponges
- No. 3 scalpel blades and handle, extra scalpel blades (Nos. 10, 11, and 15)
- Curved iris scissors
- Tissue forceps
- Straight and curved mosquito forceps
- Straight and curved Kelly forceps
- Towel forceps
- Sterile drape towels
- Needle holder with mounted needle and suture materials
- Sterile specimen container with preservative solution

Additional Surgical Supplies

Other surgical supplies may be needed during a procedure. Wound drains such as a rubber Penrose drain may be inserted at the end of a procedure to remove excess fluid. Other packing materials, such as sterile petroleum jelly, saturated gauze squares, or sterilized Iodoform gauze strips of varying lengths, may also be used to pack wounds. Additional sterile syringes may be necessary to irrigate the wound or extra sterile gauze squares may be needed to absorb blood from a surgical area. In preparation for minor surgery and before the procedure begins, check the supply inventory thoroughly.

Preparing the Patient for Minor Surgery

The medical assistant is often responsible for providing instructions before and after minor surgery. Preoperative and postoperative instructions can be presented in a variety of formats, including one-on-one discussion, videotapes, brochures, pamphlets, and models. These instructions must be reinforced through a telephone reminder. It is especially important to provide postoperative instructions in a variety of formats since the patient may not be fully alert right after surgery. Family members should be included in these explanations whenever practical.

Box 42-1 Preoperative and Postoperative Patient INSTRUCTIONS

Preoperative Instructions

- Explain the procedure verbally and provide printed materials.
- Be honest about the level of discomfort expected.
- Advise the patient on the length of the procedure.
- Explain what type of clothing to wear for the procedure.
- Schedule preoperative diagnostic tests—blood, X-ray, etc.
- Describe what at-home preparations the patient will need, such as fasting, and for how long.
- Explain that someone must accompany the patient.
- Inform the patient how long he or she will be out of work.

- Confirm the informed consent form has been signed.
- Answer any questions.
- Measure vital signs.

Postoperative Instructions

- Provide verbal and written instructions for follow-up care.
- Explain when the patient should notify the physician of possible postoperative problems, such as fever, bleeding, swelling, or other symptoms.
- Schedule a follow-up visit, if required.

PATIENT INSTRUCTIONS

Box 42-1 provides guidelines for preoperative and postoperative instructions. For purposes of efficiency, some preoperative patient preparation can take place before the patient arrives for the procedure. For example, patient education with an explanation of the procedure, preoperative and postoperative instructions, and laboratory testing can take place up to a week before the actual procedure. Preoperative instructions might include an explanation of what laboratory testing is needed and when it is to be done, food and fluid restrictions, directions for special bathing/skin cleansing preparations or cleansing enemas, and restrictions on bedtime sedative use. Postoperatively, patients should have a clear understanding of what to expect during recovery and how to care for the surgical incision at home.

INFORMED CONSENT

The patient must be provided by the physician with an honest, thorough explanation of the surgical procedure, including the benefits and risks. (Informed consent is explained in more detail in Chapter 3.) Any invasive procedure with a scalpel, scissors, or other device requires written permission (consent) from the patient. Procedures in which a body cavity is entered for the purposes of visualization, though no incision is made, such as a bronchoscopy, cystoscopy, and colonoscopy, also require written consent. The procedure, with all the risks involved, must be explained by the physician. Every attempt must be made to determine if the patient actually understands the explanation given by the physician. The medical assistant can witness the patient's signing the consent form.

POSITIONING AND DRAPING

Before the surgical procedure, ask the patient to remove all clothing and put on a patient gown with the ties at the back, unless otherwise instructed. Have the patient void before

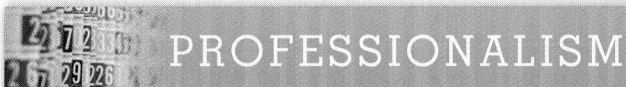

PROFESSIONALISM

THE LAW

All patients must sign an informed consent form before any surgical procedure. It is not enough to just tell the patient what procedure he or she will undergo. The surgeon must also explain the risks, what might occur if nothing is done, and what other options are available. The medical assistant reinforces what the physician has explained and makes sure that there is a patient signature on the consent form before the procedure begins. If there is any doubt about the patient's ability to understand the instructions, the medical assistant must bring this to the physician's attention. Preoperative and postoperative instructions should be read to the patient and clarified, if necessary.

Sterility during a surgical procedure cannot be compromised. The medical assistant has an ethical duty to provide the safest surgical environment possible for the patient.

Confidentiality regarding any surgical procedure a patient undergoes must be maintained. It is the physician's role to give the patient results of surgical procedures, biopsies, and tests.

Insurance information must be accurately documented. It is considered fraudulent to knowingly provide inaccurate information to an insurance company.

assisting him or her onto the operating table, and place him or her in the proper position for the procedure. Every attempt should be made to ensure the patient's comfort since the patient may have to remain in one position for an extended period of time. General guidelines for positioning and draping are discussed in Chapter 36.

ANESTHESIA

Anesthesia, medication that causes the partial or complete loss of sensation, is used to block the pain of surgery. Anesthesia can also relax muscles, produce amnesia, calm anxiety, and cause sleep. Medical assistants do not administer anesthetics, but they should be familiar with them and their effects.

The two types of anesthetics are general or local (conduction).

General Anesthesia

A general anesthetic depresses the central nervous system (CNS) to cause unconsciousness. It is usually administered through inhalation or intravenous (IV) injection. Inhaled anesthetics are generally in the form of gases or volatile liquids. In many cases, these are administered after a patient has received a sedative or narcotic to relieve pain or a tranquilizer to relieve anxiety. Sedatives and narcotics are usually administered intramuscularly before surgery. In some cases, they are administered by IV immediately before the general anesthetic is given.

Anesthetics are hypnotic sedatives that produce anesthesia, or sleep, when given in large doses, such as sodium pentothal. Precautions to be taken when administering a general anesthetic include the following:

- Administering the anesthetic only to a patient on an empty stomach to prevent vomiting and possible aspiration of vomitus into lungs resulting in pneumonia.

- Cautioning patients not to drive or engage in other activity that could result in harm from impaired consciousness. General anesthetics can interfere with the patient's alertness for 12 to 24 hours after the surgery.

- Advising patients to avoid alcohol and depressant drugs for 2 to 3 days before the surgery and 1 day after the surgery.

Local Anesthesia

Local anesthetics provide a loss of sensation in a particular area of the body without overall loss of consciousness. A local anesthetic is also referred to as a conduction anesthetic. The conduction of pain transmission by way of the nervous system is blocked. The following are examples of this type of anesthetic:

- **Topical and local infiltration**—acts on nerve endings

- **Nerve block**—affects pain transmission along a single nerve

- **Regional, spinal, epidural, or saddle block**—affect a group of nerves

A local infiltration anesthetic is injected directly into the tissue that will be operated upon. Examples of a local are lidocaine hydrochloride (Xylocaine) and procaine hydrochloride (Novocaine). This type of anesthetic is used for such procedures as removal of skin growths, skin suturing, and dental surgery. Local anesthesia takes from 5 to 15 minutes to become effective and lasts from 1 to 3 hours. During longer procedures additional injections of anesthetic may have to be administered when the first dosage has worn off.

Epinephrine, a vasoconstrictor that causes superficial blood vessels to narrow, is often added to the local anesthetic when the physician is operating on the face and head. The addition of epinephrine allows for better visualization of the surgical site because it diminishes bleeding. Epinephrine causes local anesthetics to be absorbed by the body more slowly and gives them a longer-lasting effect. Clearly mark anesthetics that have been prepared with the addition of epinephrine. Patients with heart problems could have a reaction to epinephrine that causes tachycardia or other irregularities.

Nerve blocks are administered by injection into a nerve adjacent to the operative site. This type of anesthetic is used for surgery on hands, fingers, and toes.

Topical anesthetics are local pain control medications that are applied to the skin and produce a numbing effect. These can be applied by drop, spray, or swab. They are commonly used in eye procedures. An example of a spray anesthetic is ethyl chloride, which produces a freezing effect on the skin. Benzocaine (Solarcaine) is another example of a topical anesthetic.

Administering Anesthesia

Only physicians or anesthesiologists can administer an anesthetic, and only they must chart the administration. Either the medical assistant or the physician will draw up the local anesthetic. (Using the correct procedure for drawing up medication is discussed in Chapter 54.) The medication vial must be correctly identified and then wiped with an alcohol sponge. If the medical assistant draws up the medication, then he or she must present both the syringe and the vial to the physician so that the physician can read the label. The anesthetic will be injected into the patient's prepared skin by the physician before the physician has donned gloves. This syringe is not placed onto the sterile field because it has been contaminated by the medical assistant's ungloved hands.

If the physician prefers to draw up the anesthetic, it can be done using a sterile syringe after he or she has applied gloves. The medical assistant will hold the vial securely while the physician withdraws the anesthetic without contaminating the needle. The outside of the vial cannot be touched by the physician's sterile gloved hand. This syringe can then be placed onto the sterile field.

Some physicians prefer to change the needle after drawing up the local anesthetic. For example, they may draw up the drug using a 21-gauge needle and then administer the solution using a 23-gauge or 25-gauge needle.

PREPARATION OF THE PATIENT'S SKIN

Although skin cannot be sterilized, it can be cleaned using medical aseptic technique. Careful cleansing of the skin before performing a surgical procedure will reduce the number of microorganisms on the skin. This will decrease the chance of carrying infection-producing microorganisms through the skin during the invasive procedure (incision into skin or entrance of a probe).

In some situations, the physician may order the surgical site to be shaved since bacteria can reside in hair. See Procedure 42-8 and Figure 42-25 for skin preparation and shaving instructions. Care must be taken to avoid scraping or cutting the skin during the shaving process. The physician will order either a wet shave (moistening the skin with soap and water) or dry shave (Figure 42-26). Some physicians feel that shaving the skin presents more risk of skin injury and prefer only to have the patient's skin cleansed carefully.

procedure 42-8

PREPARING THE PATIENT'S SKIN FOR SURGICAL PROCEDURES

Objective: Prepare the patient's skin for surgical procedure using sterile scrub and shave.

EQUIPMENT AND SUPPLIES

antiseptic germicidal soap; sterile saline; antiseptic such as Betadine; 8 sterile applicators; Mayo tray; waste receptacle (may be included in sterile pack); biohazard waste container; plastic bag for soiled dressings; sterile pack (sterile gloves, 3 to 4 towel packs, sterile basin pack with 3 basins, patient drape, 4 × 4 gauze sponge pack with 12 to 24 sponges, shave preparation kit)

METHOD

1. Perform hand hygiene.
2. Assemble equipment by placing packs on Mayo stand or side tray and opening outer wraps from all packs.
3. Identify the patient and explain the procedure.
4. Have the patient remove appropriate clothing and put on gowning. Ask the patient to void, if necessary.
5. Position and drape the patient to provide exposure of the operative site.
6. Unwrap the basin pack. Pour germicidal soap solution into one basin, sterile saline into the second basin, and antiseptic into the third.
7. Wash hands using sterile scrub, and apply sterile gloves.
8. Drape the skin with two towels placed 3 to 5 inches above and below the surgical site.
9. With a sterile gauze or sponge, apply soapy solution to patient's skin. Use a circular motion starting at the site of

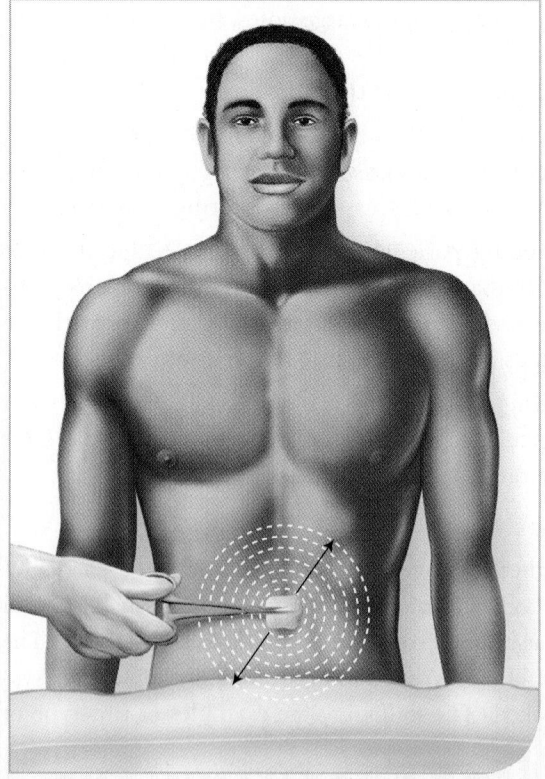

FIGURE 42-25   Preparing the patient's skin at the surgical site.

the proposed incision and move outward (Figure 42-25). Pass over each skin area only once. Place each used sponge into a waste receptacle immediately.

INSTRUCTIONS FOR A DRY SHAVE

Some physicians prefer the patient receive a dry shave. To remove hair, electric clippers are preferred to razor blades because they lessen the likelihood of accidental nicks in the skin.

    a. Clip the hair as short as possible with scissors.

    b. Apply firm traction to the skin with the nondominant hand.

    c. Remove hair in the direction of hair growth. Never shave against the grain as this will cause unnecessary irritation to the skin and increase the likelihood of nicks.

10. Take a fresh sterile gauze or sponge for each cleansing wipe. Repeat this process until the area is completely washed. The last area cleansed will be the outer edges.

11. Rinse using sterile saline on a clean gauze or sponge. Pat dry with a dry gauze only on the area that has been washed. Avoid touching any other skin area.

If shaving is ordered, then proceed with the following steps.

1. Apply soap solution to the site area. Remove razor from shave preparation pack. Pull the skin taut and shave the surgical site in the same direction as the hair is growing. Rinse with a saline solution using the single-pass, circular motion as before and pat it dry.

2. Reapply soap solution to the area and repeat the preceding process according to your office policy (around 5 minutes).

3. Pat the entire area dry with the third sterile towel.

4. Apply the antiseptic solution using two cotton applicators together in the same single-pass, circular motion.

5. Cover the prepared surgical site with the remaining sterile towel.

6. Properly dispose of gloves and soiled materials in a biohazard waste container.

CHARTING EXAMPLE

3/12/XX 11:00 A.M. Pt arrived for removal and biopsy of growth on outer aspect of left forearm. Surgical site prepared using Betadine. No cuts or lesions noted. · · · · · · · · · · · J. Wall, RMA

Postoperative Patient Care

Postoperative care includes monitoring the patient during recovery from anesthesia, wound care, applying dressings, and communicating patient instructions. Patient education addresses more about instructing patients on home care of wounds.

RECOVERY FROM ANESTHESIA

Topical and other local anesthetics take effect either immediately or within a few minutes. Their effects wear off quickly. The use of large amounts of local anesthetic, beyond normal dosages, is not recommended and may result in an

adverse reaction in patients. Some patients are allergic to anesthetics and may slip into anaphylactic shock, which requires emergency treatment (see Chapter 43). An emergency tray or cart stocked with drugs used to counteract shock should always be available in the office. Many facilities require employees to have current CPR certification.

To prevent choking on food or burning the mouth, the patient treated in his or her mouth or throat with a local anesthetic should be advised not to eat until the effects of the anesthetic wear off. Table 42-3 contains examples of local anesthetics. Patients must be observed carefully after surgery for signs of adverse reaction to the anesthetic, bleeding, and circulatory problems. The patient's vital signs (blood pressure, temperature, pulse, and respiration) should

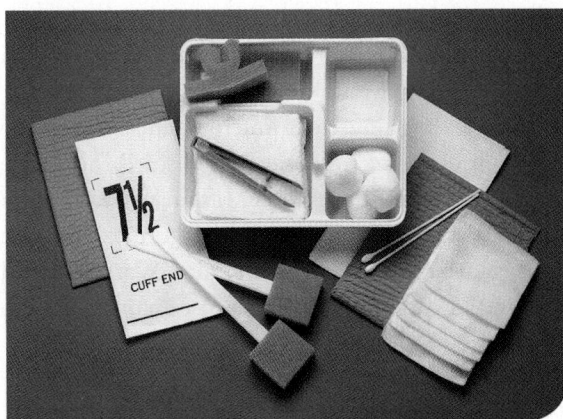

FIGURE 42-26 Dry skin prep tray.

TABLE 42-3 Local Anesthetics

Anesthetic Agent	Use
Benzocaine	Topical use only
Chloroprocaine	Nerve block, epidural
Lidocaine (Xylocaine)	Infiltration or topical
Mepivacaine	Infiltration nerve block
Procaine (Novacaine)	Infiltration; seldom used now
Tetracaine	Infiltration, topical nerve block, spinal

be monitored immediately after surgery and then every 15 minutes for the first hour. Never give fluids to a patient who is not fully alert. This can result in choking. Oral medications for pain, nausea, and vomiting have to be withheld until the patient is fully recovered from anesthesia. Medications may be given by injection until recovery occurs.

Excessive disorientation and inability to revive within a normal recovery time should be reported immediately to the physician. The patient should be observed for nausea and vomiting. Medications may be ordered by the physician to counteract nausea and vomiting.

TYPES OF WOUNDS

The skin acts as a protective barrier and is the body's first line of defense. Any break in the skin, whether from injury or a surgical incision, is referred to as a wound. A surgical procedure requiring an incision through the skin is considered an invasive procedure because a wound is created when the skin is entered. Wounds cause blood vessels to rupture and blood to seep into tissues, which results in skin color changes. Typically, skin coloration will change from erythema in a fresh wound to a greenish yellow color during the healing process, which involves oxidation of blood pigments. There are four types of wound classification:

- **Abrasion**—outer layers of skin are rubbed away due to scraping; will generally heal without scarring.
- **Incision**—smooth cut resulting from a surgical scalpel or sharp material, such as razor or glass; may result in excessive bleeding and scarring if deep.
- **Laceration**—edges are torn in an irregular shape; can cause profuse bleeding and scarring.
- **Puncture**—made by a sharp, pointed instrument such as a bullet, needle, nail, or splinter; external bleeding is usually minimal, but infection may occur due to penetration with a contaminated object, and there may be scarring.

THE HEALING PROCESS

Wounds pass through various stages of healing, including inflammation, as the body starts to fight off potential infection. Inflammation is the body's protective response to trauma and invasion by microorganisms; it is generally localized around the site of trauma or infection. Signs of inflammation are redness or erythema, swelling, warmth, and pain. Wounds go through three phases before healing or restoration of structure and function take place:

- **Inflammatory phase (3 days)**—blood clot forms to stop bleeding and plug the opening of a wound; **eschar** or scab forms to keep out microorganisms.

- **Proliferating phase (3 to 21 days)**—fibrin threads extend across opening of wound and pull edges together; cells multiply to repair the wound.
- **Maturation phase (21 days to 2 years)**—tissue cells strengthen and tighten the wound closure, form a scar; scar eventually fades and thins.

Wound Complications

Wound complications include infection—signs of inflammation, purulent or puslike drainage, fever; hemorrhage or bleeding; **dehiscence**, separation of wound edges; and **evisceration**, separation of wound edges and protrusion of abdominal organs. Uneven or ragged-edged wounds and large wounds take more time to heal. Without proper wound care infection will set in. Infection is the result of wound contamination during or after the injury or surgical procedure. Drainage occurs as fluid and cells escape from the tissues during the inflammatory phase of wound healing. The amount and type of drainage observed on a dressing should be charted. The following are types of wound drainage:

- **Serous drainage**—clear, watery drainage, such as the fluid in a blister.
- **Sanguineous drainage**—bloody (bright red is fresh blood, dark red is older blood); the amount and color of sanguineous drainage is important.
- **Serosanguineous drainage**—thin watery drainage tinged with blood.
- **Purulent drainage**—thick puslike drainage that is green, yellow, or brown.

CLEANSING A WOUND

A wound must be cleaned before a sterile dressing can be applied. The physician will indicate which of the many products available for wound cleansing he prefers. Warm water and soap are used to remove surface dirt from around the wound area.

To clean a wound using sterile gauze or swab, work from the clean area near the wound outward to less clean areas. This will prevent dragging more microorganisms into the wound. Wipe in one direction and then discard the sterile swab or gauze. Cleanse a linear wound from top to bottom with one stroke per sterile gauze or swab (Figure 42-27). Use a new sterile gauze or swab for each stroke. Work outward from the wound in parallel lines. To cleanse an open wound, such as a pressure ulcer, work in circles, half or full, beginning in the center and working outward (Figure 42-28).

Always clean at least 1 inch beyond the edge of the dressing to be applied. If no dressing is to be applied, clean

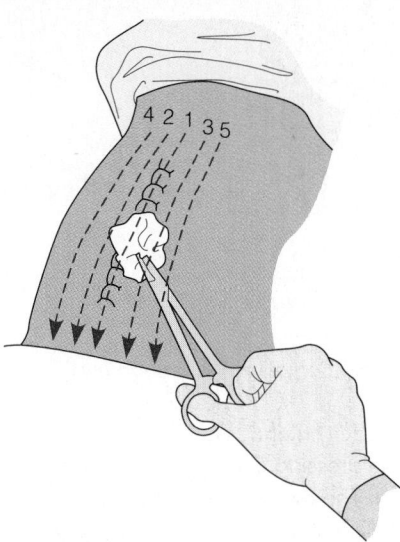

FIGURE 42-27 Cleanse a linear wound by using a new sterile gauze pad for each stroke, beginning next to the wound and working from the top to the bottom of the wound area.

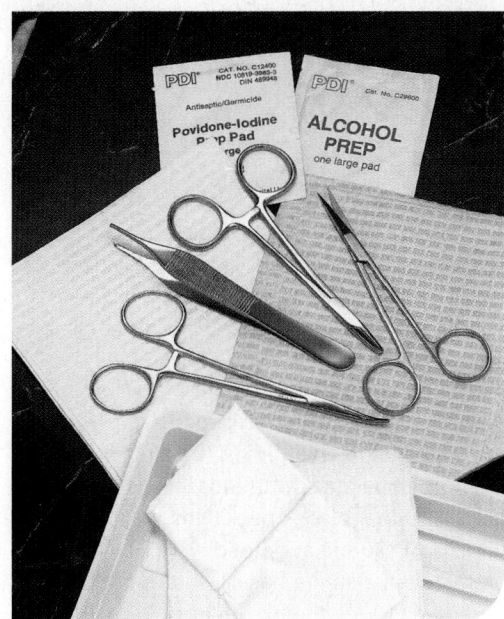

FIGURE 42-29 Wound closure kit.

2 inches beyond the edges of the wound. Use a new gauze pad for each circle.

The size and shape of the dressing needed will depend on the size, location, and amount of drainage from the wound. Sterile 4 × 4 gauze pads ("four by fours") are used for most dressings. If drainage is expected from the wound, a prepared dressing, such as Telfa, may be used to prevent the dressing from sticking to the wound. See Figure 42-29 for an example of a wound closure kit.

Each patient should be asked how long it has been since he or she received a tetanus shot. In the event that the shot was not received within the last 10 years, the physician should be informed.

SUTURES

A suture is a thread used to sew together body tissues. Sutures used to attach tissues beneath the skin are often made

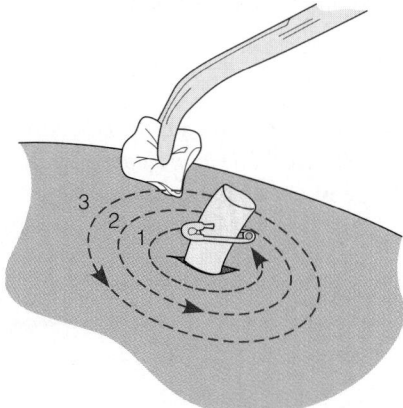

FIGURE 42-28 To cleanse an open wound, begin close to the wound and work outward in full or half circles.

of an absorbable material that disappears in several days. Skin sutures, by contrast, are made of nonabsorbable materials such as silk, cotton, linen, wire, nylon, and Dacron (polyester fiber). Silver wire clips or staples are also available. Sutures or staples are inserted by the surgeon at the end of a procedure to hold tissues in alignment during the healing process. The steps necessary to assist with suturing are given in Procedure 42-9. Sutures generally remain in place 5 or 6 days and then have to be removed if they are nonabsorbable. If sutures remain in the body too long, they can cause skin irritation and infection. The suture acts as a wick to carry bacteria through the skin and into the subcutaneous tissues. Suture removal times differ depending on the site:

- Facial sutures may be removed after only 24 to 48 hours to prevent scarring.

- Head and neck sutures remain in place for 3 to 5 days.

- Abdominal sutures remain in place for 5 to 7 days.

- Sutures over weight-bearing joints and large bones may remain 7 to 10 days.

The medical assistant prepares the patient for suture or staple removal by taking off the dressing, if one is present. Each edge of the dressing is removed by pulling toward the suture line. If the dressing is adhering to the suture line, then a small amount of sterile saline or hydrogen peroxide can be used to moisten the dressing to ease removal.

In some office practices and in some states, medical assistants are permitted to remove sutures. The procedure should be explained to the patient, reminding them that they may feel a pulling sensation. The skin is then thoroughly cleansed

procedure
42-9

ASSISTING WITH SUTURING
Objective: Assist with suture repair of an incision or laceration using sterile technique.

EQUIPMENT AND SUPPLIES
Mayo stand; side stand; anesthetic; sterile transfer forceps; sterile saline; waste container/plastic bag; biohazard waste container; sharps container; sterile gloves (2 pairs); sterile pack(s) (patient drape, towel pack with four towels, 4 × 4 gauze sponge pack); scalpel blades pack (Nos. 10 and 15); needle and syringe pack; suture and needle pack (according to physician's preference); 2 sterile basins; suture pack (scalpel handle, needle holder, thumb forceps; 2 scissors; 3 hemostats)

METHOD
1. Use a sterile scrub and gloving procedure.
2. Stand across from the physician.
3. Place two sponges ready for the physician near the wound site.
4. Assist by using additional sponges to keep the wound dry.
5. Pass instruments, such as scissors, to the physician using a firm snap of the handle into his or her hand without letting go until the physician hasa firm grasp.
6. The blade is placed into the scalpel using a hemostat.
7. Hand the scalpel to the physician with blade edge down to avoid cutting the physician.
8. Continue to use sponges to keep the wound free of drainage.
9. Pass all instruments to the physician as requested. Try to anticipate the next instruments that the physician may need, such as another hemostat or scissors for cutting a suture.
10. Pass the toothed forceps to the physician if laceration edges need to be grasped.
11. Mount the needle into the needle holder and pass as one unit to the physician, using care to keep the suture within the sterile field. Pass the needle holder with the needle pointing outward. Hold the suture with the other hand, and do not let go of it until the physician sees it.
12. Using the suture scissors, prepare to cut the suture as directed by the physician (usually $\frac{1}{8}$ to $\frac{1}{4}$ inch from the knot).

13. Sponge the closed wound once with a sponge and discard.
14. Repeat this step with each suture.
15. Apply a layer of sterile dressing over the wound, such as a sterile gauze pad. The medical assistant may use forceps if preferred. The sterile dressing should extend a minimum of 2 inches past all edges of the wound.
16. Apply a second layer of gauze over the wound site.
17. Add a final third layer of wound dressing, such as a SurgiPad.
18. Secure the edges of the dressing with paper tape or similar product. Some physicians will prefer the wound be covered with a clear, waterproof membrane such as Telfa. Paper tape is often used because it contains a less intense adhesive, lowering the risk for adverse skin reactions.
19. After they are used, place all soiled instruments on the sterile field if they will be used again; discard others in the instrument basin.
20. When the procedure is complete, remove your gloves and perform hand hygiene before assisting the patient.
21. Allow the patient to rest and recover from the anesthetic. Periodically check the patient's vital signs according to your office policy.
22. Provide clear oral and written postoperative instructions for the patient. Make sure the patient is stable before he or she leaves the office.
23. Clean, sanitize, and sterilize the instruments. Clean and sanitize the room in preparation for the next patient.
24. Perform hand hygiene.

CHARTING EXAMPLE
2/14/XX 1:00 P.M. Cleansed wound with antiseptic. Assisted physician with suturing Pt. Instructed on wound care, signs and symptoms of infection, and given follow-up appointment. · M. King, CMA (AAMA)

The physician will chart the details of the surgical procedure.

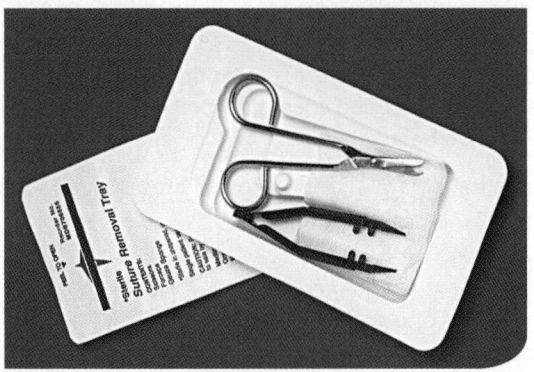

FIGURE 42-30 Disposable suture removal set.

with an antiseptic such as alcohol or Betadine solution. After opening the sterile suture packet (Figure 42-30) and creating a sterile field with the wrapper, the knot of the suture is gently picked up using a thumb forceps. The suture is then cut with suture scissors below the knot as close to the skin as possible. The suture is removed by pulling the long remaining suture out. Suture material that is outside of the skin should not be pulled through the skin due to the danger of pulling infection-causing microorganisms along with it. Very little of the suture is actually pulled through the skin. (Procedure 42-10 and Figure 42-31 illustrate the steps to remove sutures.)

procedure 42-10

REMOVING SUTURES

Objective: Remove sutures using proper sterile technique, following the physician's order.

EQUIPMENT AND SUPPLIES

suture removal pack (suture scissors; sterile gauze squares; thumb forceps; skin antiseptic; sterile gloves; bandages; biohazard waste container)

METHOD

Removal of Sutures

1. Perform hand hygiene.
2. Assemble equipment and check expiration date on pack.
3. Identify the patient.
4. Explain the procedure to the patient, and assist him or her into a comfortable position.
5. Perform hand hygiene.
6. Remove old dressing using proper technique.
7. Perform hand hygiene.
8. Open suture or staple removal pack using proper technique.
9. Apply sterile gloves using proper technique.
10. Cleanse the wound as needed.
11. Place a gauze square next to the wound for placement of sutures or staples as they are removed.
12. Grasp the knot of the suture with thumb forceps and lift gently (Figure 42-31).

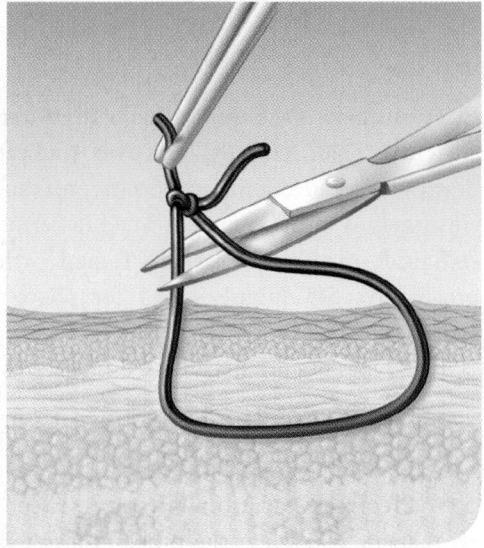
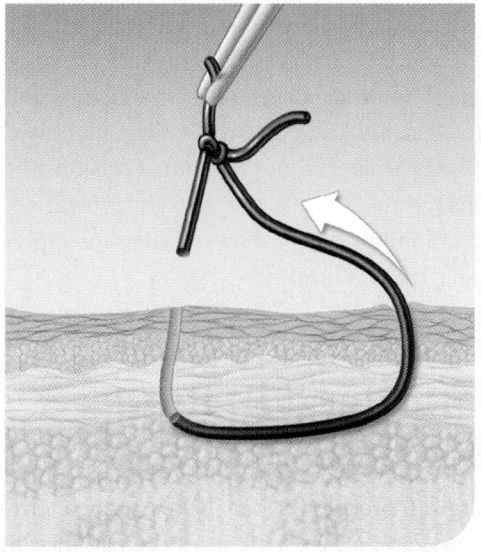

FIGURE 42-31 Removal of sutures.

13. Insert the suture scissors and cut suture at skin level. Pull out the suture.
14. Place the cut suture on the gauze.
15. Repeat these steps until all sutures are removed.
16. Count sutures to make sure that all have been removed.

Removal of Staples

1–10. Perform steps 1 through 10 above.
11. Place the lower tips of a sterile staple remover under the staple.
12. Squeeze the handles together until they are completely closed. (Pressing the handles together causes the staple to bend in the middle and pulls the edges of the staple out of the skin.) Do not lift the staple remover when squeezing the handles.
13. When both ends of the staple are visible, gently move the staple away from the incision site.
14. Hold the staple remover over a disposable container, release the staple remover handles, and release the staple.

15. Place the staple on the gauze, repeat these steps until all staples are removed, and count the number of staples to ensure all have been removed.

Closing Steps for Removal of Sutures or Staples

16. Clean the wound with antiseptic and allow it to dry.
17. Dress wound as ordered.
18. Properly dispose of equipment and supplies.
19. Remove gloves and perform hand hygiene.
20. Instruct the patient on wound care.
21. Document the procedure, including condition of wound, number of sutures or staples removed, and patient instructions on wound care.

CHARTING EXAMPLE

2/14/XX 11:00 A.M. Removed sutures and cleansed wound with antiseptic. Wound healing well. Pt. instructed on wound care. · M. King, CMA (AAMA)

STERILE DRESSING

A dressing is the application of a sterile covering over a surgical site or wound using surgical asepsis. A patient who has sustained an injury or undergone a surgical procedure may need to schedule an appointment to remove the old dressing and apply a new sterile dressing. Procedure 42-11 and Figure 42-32A–C demonstrate the steps for changing a sterile dressing.

BANDAGING THE WOUND

After the wound is dressed, the physician may instruct you to apply a bandage to hold the dressing in place. Bandages may be gauze, fabric, or elasticized and need not be sterile (Figure 42-33). Bandages are available in various sizes, lengths, and shapes. Some bandages are self-adhering and easier to apply to awkward areas. Elastic bandages are used to support an injured part and reduce swelling. Care must be taken not to bandage too tightly and restrict circulation. Procedure 42-12 and Figure 42-34 show the steps for applying a bandage to a patient's forearm.

Surgical Procedures Performed in the Medical Office

Many minor surgical procedures can be performed efficiently in the physician's office. This saves the patient the time and expense of having to go into an ambulatory surgical facility or a hospital. The basic surgical setup is the standard setup with the addition of specific instruments for each procedure. Some minor procedures performed in the medical office include biopsy, cautery, colposcopy, cryosurgery, laser surgery, endocervical curettage, endoscopic procedures, suture removal, removal of foreign bodies, incision and drainage, vasectomy, and removal of growths and tumors.

The medical assistant does not administer these procedures but must understand them and their effects so that he or she can assist the physician and the patient. A brief description of some procedures follows.

ELECTROSURGERY

Electrosurgery is the application of high-frequency electrical currents. These currents are used to heat tissue to cut, destroy, or remove it in very specific areas and patterns. Electrosurgery is most often performed in dermatological, gynecological, cardiac, ocular, ENT, and orthopedic surgical procedures. See Figure 42-35 for photo of a disposable cautery unit.

Five types of currents are used in electrosurgery:

- **Electrocoagulation**—destroys tissues and controls bleeding by coagulation.

- **Electrodessication**—destroys tissue by creating a spark gap when the probe is inserted into unwanted tissue.

CHANGING A STERILE DRESSING

Objective: Change a wound dressing using proper sterile technique.

EQUIPMENT AND SUPPLIES

disposable gloves; antiseptic solution; solution container; prepackaged dressing pack; thumb forceps; sterile cotton balls; sterile gloves; sterile dressing; adhesive tape; scissors, if necessary for tape; waste container/plastic bag; biohazard waste container; Mayo stand or side tray

METHOD

1. Perform hand hygiene.
2. Assemble equipment using the Mayo stand.
3. Prepare the sterile field, utilizing aseptic technique and prepackaged dressing packet. Employ sterile transfer forceps to place additional sterile items on the sterile field.
4. Explain the procedure to the patient.
5. Assist the patient into a comfortable position with the area to be dressed resting on a support, such as an examination table.
6. Apply nonsterile gloves.
7. Remove dressing from the wound by loosening the tape with gloved hands or forceps and pulling it from both sides toward the wound (Figure 42-32A). Without passing the soiled dressing over the sterile field, place it into the soiled waste bag. Do not allow the dressing to touch the outside or edges of the bag (Figure 42-32B).
8. Inspect the wound for signs of infection and inflammation. Note any discharge by its type, amount, and odor (Figure 42-32C).
9. Discard gloves and contaminated forceps properly. Place disposable gloves and forceps in a biohazardous waste container. Reusable forceps are placed in the basin for later cleaning.
10. Drop the antiseptic onto several cotton balls until they are moist but not saturated.
11. Open sterile gloves and apply properly.
12. Cleanse the wound by using sterile forceps to hold the cotton while moving from top to bottom of the wound once. Use a new cotton ball with antiseptic for each wipe. Move from the inside of the wound to the outside edges.
13. Pick up the sterile dressing with gloved hands and place over the wound.
14. Discard gloves and forceps.
15. Apply adhesive tape to hold the dressing in place. Do not apply too tightly as to restrict circulation. The strips of tape should be long enough to hold the dressing in place. Do not wrap the tape entirely around an extremity or completely cover the dressing.
16. Instruct the patient on dressing care, and to schedule a follow-up appointment to see the physician.
17. Chart the procedure, including the date, time, location, and condition of the wound and the instructions given to the patient.

CHARTING EXAMPLE

2/14/XX 11:00 A.M. Dressing change on right anterior forearm. Moderate amount of serous drainage with slight erythema surrounding wound. Incision healing well with edges aligned. Cleansed with Betadine. Sterile dressing applied. Pt. instructed on wound care. · · · · · · · · · · · · · · · · · · · M. King, CMA (AAMA)

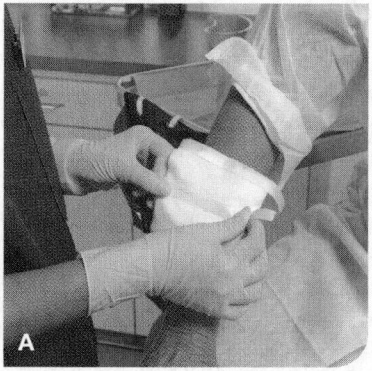 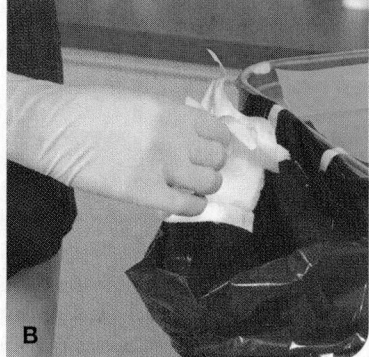 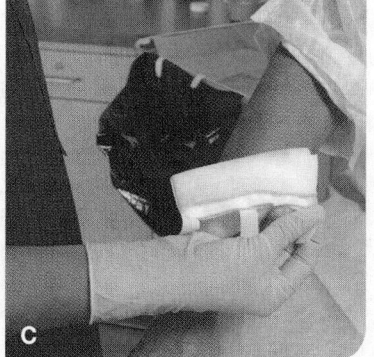

FIGURE 42-32 Wound dressing (A) removal; (B) disposal, and; (C) inspection.

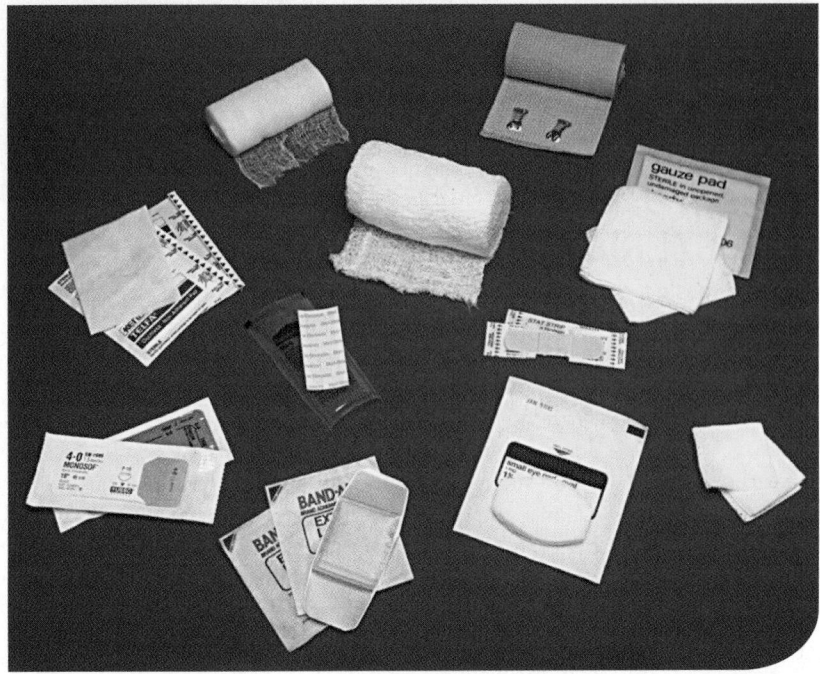

FIGURE 42-33   Various types of bandages.

- **Electrofulguration**—destroys tissue with a spark emitted from the tip of a probe positioned a short distance away from the unwanted tissue.
- **Electrosection**—uses electric current to incise and excise the tissue.
- **Electrocautery (or cautery)**—uses high-frequency, alternating electric current to destroy, cut, or remove tissue. Electrocautery is also used to coagulate small blood vessels, thereby reducing bleeding and cell loss. Some physicians have a **hyfrecator**, which is a miniature electrocautery unit (Figure 42-36).

In some offices, either the electrosurgical unit (ESU) or the ultrasonic surgical unit (USU) is taking the place of electrocautery. The ESU is able to provide a more controlled,

procedure
42-12

APPLYING A BANDAGE OVER A STERILE DRESSING
Objective: Apply a bandage to the forearm.

EQUIPMENT AND SUPPLIES
nonsterile gloves; bandage material prescribed by physician or office procedures; bandage scissors; tape

METHOD
1. Identify the patient.
2. Perform hand hygiene.
3. Apply nonsterile gloves.
4. Explain the procedure.
5. Hold bandage against the skin with nondominant hand 1 inch below the dressing.
6. Wrap bandage around the wrist two to three times to secure (Figure 42-34A).

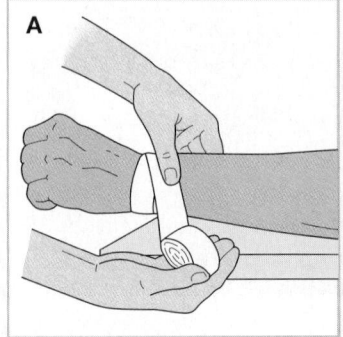
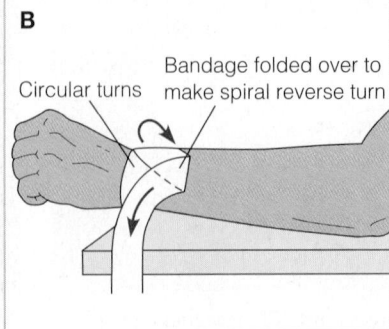
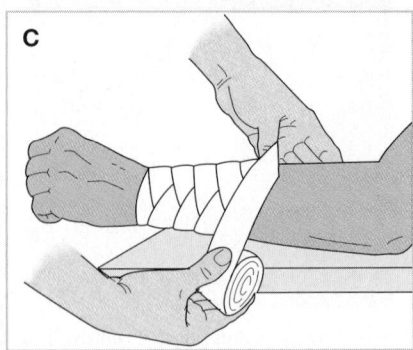

Circular turns

Bandage folded over to make spiral reverse turn

FIGURE 42-34   (A–C) Bandaging a forearm.

7. Wrap forearm from distal (part farthest away from the body) to proximal (closest to the body) with overlapping spiral turns (Figure 42-34B).
8. Check that the bandage is not restricting blood flow.
9. Continue wrapping to at least 1 inch above the dressing (Figure 42-34C).
10. Wrap two more times to secure the bandage, then cut.
11. Tape the cut end to the bandage; do not tape the end to the patient's skin.
12. Check again for any blood flow restriction.
13. Remove gloves.
14. Perform hand hygiene.
15. Explain home care to the patient.
16. Document the procedure accurately.

CHARTING EXAMPLE

1/18/XX 9:30 A.M. Applied bandage to sterile dressing. Pt instructed on home care for dressing. · · · M. King, CMA (AAMA)

---

less damaging form of electric current through the use of a variety of attachments. For example, an incision can be made using ESU with a small electrode blade. The blade cauterizes as it cuts, thus minimizing bleeding. Other attachments can be used to coagulate and suction. The USU uses high-frequency sound waves to break apart calcified or sclerosed tissue that can be removed in small segments. Some models have the ability to suction as they break apart and dissolve body calcifications.

In some forms of electrosurgery, a local anesthetic may be administered.

LASER SURGERY

The term *laser is* an acronym for **L**ight **A**mplification by **S**timulated **E**mission of **R**adiation. A laser emits an intense beam of light and originally was used to treat diseases of the retina. Today laser surgery is used to treat a wide variety of diseases and conditions, including vascular, neurological, orthopedic, and dermatologic problems. Laser surgery has the advantage of promoting quick healing and not destroying surrounding tissue. A medical assistant may need extra training to assist with laser surgery. When a room is to be used for laser surgery, it is important to shut out any stray light rays, post OSHA's laser warning sign, and make sure everyone, including the patient, is wearing safety goggles. After surgery is complete, the wound should be cleaned with antiseptic and dressed with a sterile dressing.

COLPOSCOPY

Colposcopy is an examination of the vagina and cervix performed using a colposcope, a lighted instrument, with the patient in the lithotomy position. The colposcope allows the physician to observe the tissues of this area in great detail through light and magnification. Abnormal areas of tissue or cells can then be removed for biopsy to detect cancer. In some cases, cryosurgery using freezing temperatures to destroy cells is then applied.

Colposcopy is performed in the following cases:

- When an abnormal tissue development is observed by the physician during a routine pelvic examination

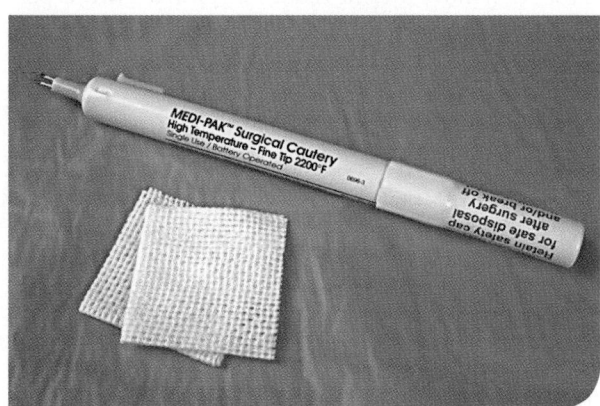

FIGURE 42-35 A disposable cautery unit.

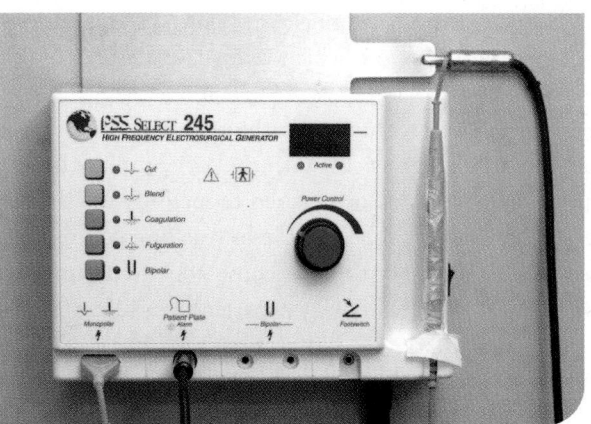

FIGURE 42-36 A hyfrecator, an electrocautery unit.

- When a Papanicolaou (Pap) smear result is in the abnormal range

- For magnified visualization

- To obtain a biopsy specimen

If the physician is unable to visualize the entire cervical canal during the colposcopy, he or she may perform an endocervical curettage (ECC) to scrape endocervical cells from inside the cervical canal. These cells are then sent for further testing to determine any abnormality. Abnormal cell growth can be a sign of a precancerous condition that, if untreated, could lead to the development of cancer.

The patient may experience slight bleeding after a colposcopy if a biopsy is taken. In such cases, provide a perineal pad for the patient with instructions for home care. The patient should receive instructions to call the physician if abnormal pain or bleeding is experienced after this procedure.

ENDOSCOPY

An endoscope is an instrument used to look into a hollow organ or body cavity. An endoscope is used to examine the larynx, bladder, colon, sigmoid colon, stomach, abdomen, and some joints. Some attachments are utilized with some endoscopes, such as a light source, suction, a monitor, and a video recorder. Great care must be taken with these sensitive instruments. In most instances, the patient will need preparation prior to the examination—for example, fasting, taking a laxative, or administering an enema.

Figure 42-37 is an example of a flexible colonoscope with monitor and video recorder.

CRYOSURGERY

Cryosurgery is the use of subfreezing temperatures to destroy tissue. This procedure is also known as cryocautery, rooted in the term *cautery,* which refers to a destruction of tissue.

One example of cryosurgery is the treatment of cervical erosion and chronic cervicitis. With the patient in the lithotomy position, the colposcope is used to magnify the surface of the cervix. Then a probe capable of reaching subfreezing temperatures is placed within the colposcope to destroy abnormal cells. The patient may experience mild cramping and a watery discharge after the procedure. The physician may advise her to take a mild analgesic, such as acetaminophen (Tylenol). The patient should be advised against using

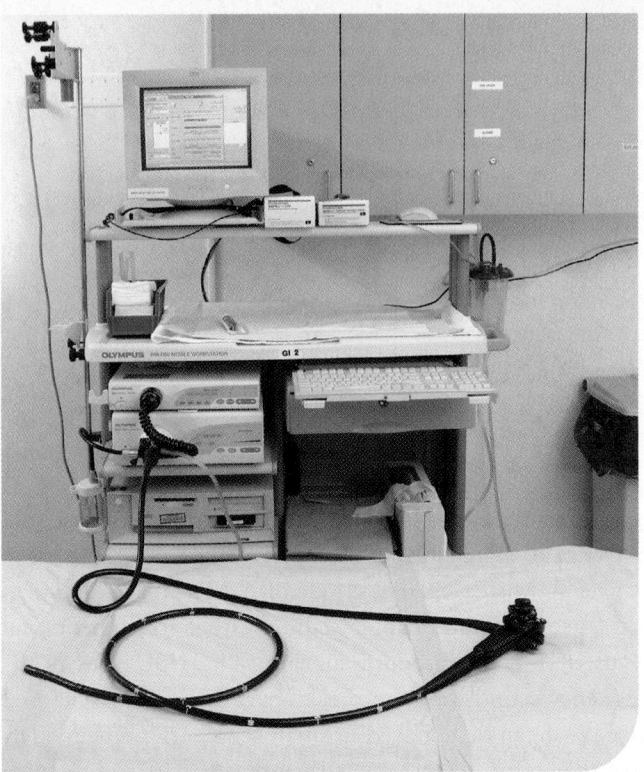

FIGURE 42-37 A flexible colonoscope with monitor and video recorder.

a tampon for at least a month since it could irritate sensitive tissues. Additional instruction should include details on reporting any unusual pain or foul discharge, abstaining from sexual intercourse for 1 month, douching, and when to return for a follow-up visit.

The probe used in cryosurgery must be sterilized according to manufacturer's instructions immediately after use.

ENDOMETRIAL BIOPSY (EMB)

An endometrial biopsy (EMB) consists of using a curette or suction tool to remove uterine tissue for testing. EMB is performed for a variety of reasons:

- To detect precancerous and cancerous conditions of the endometrial lining of the uterus

- To detect inflammatory conditions

- To determine if polyps are present

- To assess abnormal uterine bleeding

- To assess the effects of hormonal therapy

- To screen for early detection of endometrial cancer (particularly if risk factors are present)

An EMB is performed with the patient in the lithotomy position. The physician performs a bimanual examination of the uterus and administers a local anesthetic. A uterine curette is sounded into the uterus, indicating depth and direction, after the anesthetic has taken effect. The specimen is taken by means of a curette or with a suction device to aspirate a specimen. The specimen is sent to the laboratory in a container containing a 10 percent formalin preservative solution.

Provide a perineal pad for the patient with instructions for home care. The patient should receive instructions to call the physician if abnormal pain or bleeding occurs after this procedure. The patient may experience mild cramping for which the physician may advise her to take a mild analgesic. She should be advised against using a tampon, douching, or having sexual intercourse for at least 72 hours.

INCISION AND DRAINAGE

The incision and drainage (I & D) procedure is performed to relieve the buildup of purulent (pus) material as a result of infection. The purulent discharge may be cultured to determine what microorganism is causing the infection and, thus, what antibiotic would be effective. The procedure is performed using sterile surgical technique, keeping in mind that the purulent material may be highly infectious. All soiled dressings and 4 × 4s immediately should be placed in a plastic waste container and then disposed of properly using OSHA guidelines.

A tray setup for an I & D would include the following:

- Scalpel handle and blades (No. 11)

- Curved iris scissors

- Tissue forceps

- Kelly hemostat

- Retractor

- Thumb dressing forceps

- 4 × 4 gauze squares

REMOVAL OF FOREIGN BODIES AND GROWTHS

A foreign body can include a variety of materials from a small splinter or fishhook to a large object, such as an arrow that is embedded in tissue. Splinter forceps are needed on an instrument tray for foreign body removal.

Growths include tumors, warts, moles, and cysts. The most frequent growth removal procedure in the medical office is for cysts, which are enclosed fluid-filled sacs. Some growths will be sent to the laboratory for biopsy testing depending on the physician's instructions. The removal of a foreign body or neoplasm (new growth) requires a surgical setup that includes the following:

- Thumb dressing forceps

- Retractor

- Scalpel handle and blades (Nos. 10 and 15)

- Curved tissue scissors

- Tissue forceps

- Hemostats

- Blunt probe

- Splinter forceps

- Needle holder

- Suture materials and needles

- Sterile 4 × 4 gauze

Figure 42-38 shows a surgical tray for biopsy removal. Figure 42-39 shows a medical assistant holding a specimen container so the physician can place the biopsy specimen into it without touching the rim or outside of the container and the contaminating tissue.

VASECTOMY

The vasectomy procedure, tying and cutting of the vas deferens, on the male patient is a surgical procedure that is now commonly performed in the urologist's office. A vasectomy provides a permanent form of birth control for the male. As with any surgical procedure, a consent form must be signed and placed in the patient's record before beginning this procedure. The patient should be instructed to have someone available to drive him home after the procedure. The patient will be uncomfortable for a short period of time (2 to 3 days). He should be given detailed instructions on home care including activity level and sexual intercourse. The instructions may vary somewhat from one urologist to another. A typical vasectomy tray will include the following:

- Scalpel handle and blade (No. 15)

- Dressing forceps

- Towel clamp

- Straight and curved mosquito forceps

- Curved tissue scissors

- Tissue forceps

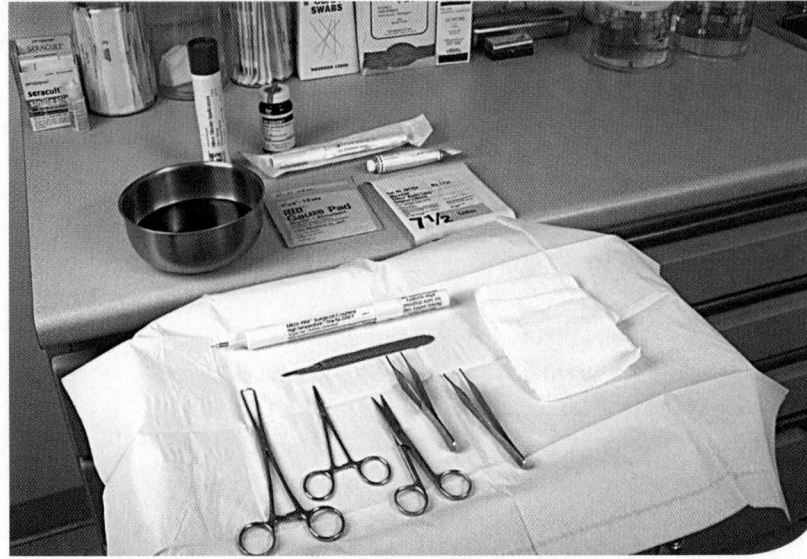

FIGURE 42-38 **Surgical tray set up for a biopsy procedure.**

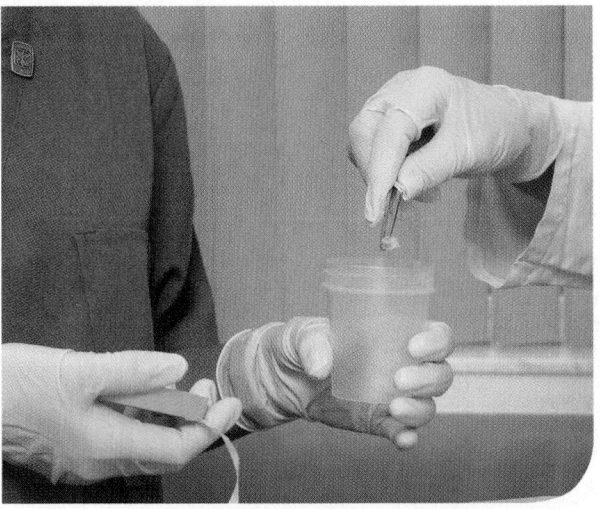

FIGURE 42-39 **A medical assistant holds a specimen container to receive a biopsy sample.**

- Retractor

- Needle holder and suture material

- Suture scissors

SUMMARY

Assisting with surgery includes maintaining aseptic technique, a thorough knowledge of gowning, gloving, surgical hand hygiene, setting up sterile instrument trays, passing equipment to the physician, packaging and surgical setup, and preparing the patient for the procedure. Assisting with surgical procedures carries with it a grave responsibility to maintain absolute sterile technique. The medical assistant incorporates a variety of clinical skills when assisting with a surgical procedure.

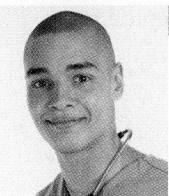

42 CHAPTER REVIEW

COMPETENCY REVIEW

1. Define and spell the terms to learn for this chapter.

2. Perform hand hygiene using medical aseptic technique; do the same using surgical aseptic technique.

3. Identify by name the pieces of equipment needed for
   a. suture removal
   b. incision and drainage
   c. suture of a laceration
   d. cervical biopsy
   e. removal of a foreign body
   f. dressing change with a wound culture
   g. endometrial biopsy

4. You have an open sore on your hand. What procedure should you follow when preparing to assist the surgeon?

PREPARING FOR THE CERTIFICATION EXAM

1. Which of the following is NEVER considered an outpatient surgery?
   a. elective
   b. urgent
   c. optional
   d. organ transplant
   e. tonsillectomy

2. To open a sterile packet you may do all EXCEPT
   a. touch the outside with bare hands
   b. open the sterile packet away from you
   c. rewrap any unused packets
   d. touch the outside with sterile gloves only
   e. open the package on a Mayo stand

3. Which of the following is not used to categorize instruments?
   a. cutting
   b. probing
   c. grasping
   d. closing
   e. suctioning

4. _____ are used to grasp foreign bodies.
   a. splinter forceps
   b. tissue forceps
   c. thumb forceps
   d. sponge forceps
   e. addison forceps

5. _____ is used to remove tissue for examination and biopsy to detect cancerous cells.
   a. speculum
   b. trocar
   c. punch
   d. probe
   e. hemostat

6. The most expensive suture material is
   a. nylon
   b. silk
   c. polyester
   d. cotton
   e. linen

7. If you were to assist in suturing an eyelid, which gauge of silk would you choose?
   a. 3-0
   b. 5-0
   c. 2-0
   d. 7-0
   e. 8-0

8. _____ anesthesia is specifically injected into a nerve adjacent to the operative site. This type of anesthetic is used for surgery on hands, fingers and toes.
   a. local
   b. general
   c. nerve block
   d. topical
   e. spinal

9. This type of local anesthetic is used as a topical nerve block:
   a. benzocaine
   b. procaine (Novacaine)
   c. tetracaine
   d. chloroprocaine
   e. epinephrine

10. This type of wound has edges that are torn in an irregular shape and can cause profuse bleeding and scarring.
   a. puncture
   b. laceration
   c. incision
   d. abrasion
   e. contusion

CRITICAL THINKING

1. What is an I & D, and why is it usually performed?

2. What supplies would Shandra need to gather in order to have the examination room ready for the I & D to be performed by Dr. Penningworth?

3. Dr. Penningworth informs Shandra that the patient has had the cyst for a significant amount of time and would like to send a sample, which will be collected during the procedure, to the laboratory. What type of sample will likely be collected, and why would the physician want to send it to the laboratory for testing?

ON THE JOB

Victor Krenz is assisting Dr. Connors with the fifth cataract surgery for the day. The patient is Kathy Wall, a diabetic patient, whose condition has been stable enough for her to undergo a surgical procedure. Victor has performed a 6-minute surgical scrub on his hands before each of the five procedures. Dr. Connors indicates that he is in a hurry to get back to his office for a heavy afternoon schedule of patients. After both Dr. Connors and Victor are scrubbed, gowned, and ready to begin the operation, Victor feels a slight prick on the tip of his gloved finger as he moves the sterile syringe and needle on the tray. Dr. Connors, who does not notice the accidental needlestick to Victor's glove, states again that he is in a hurry to finish this procedure. Victor knows that it will delay the surgery if he has to change gloves. He also knows that his hands have had a surgical scrub five times that morning and that they are clean.

1. Can Victor justify not changing into new gloves?
2. What could happen to Ms. Wall as a result of Victor's needlestick?
3. How should Victor handle this situation?

INTERNET ACTIVITY

Research the Internet for the newest information about using laser surgery to reduce or remove facial wrinkles. After examining the information, do you think you would elect laser surgery to remove wrinkles? Would you recommend this procedure to others?

Additional interactive resources and activities for this chapter can be found:

On your student DVD: View applicable procedure videos on the DVD-ROM found in the back of this book.

MyHealthProfessionsKit.com: Test your knowledge of the chapter with games and activities. MyHealthProfessionsKit also includes resources, helpful links, and a Spanish audio glossary.

Medical Assisting Interactive: Practice your procedures as a medical assistant in this simulated doctor's office. This can be accessed through MyHealthProfessionsKit.com.

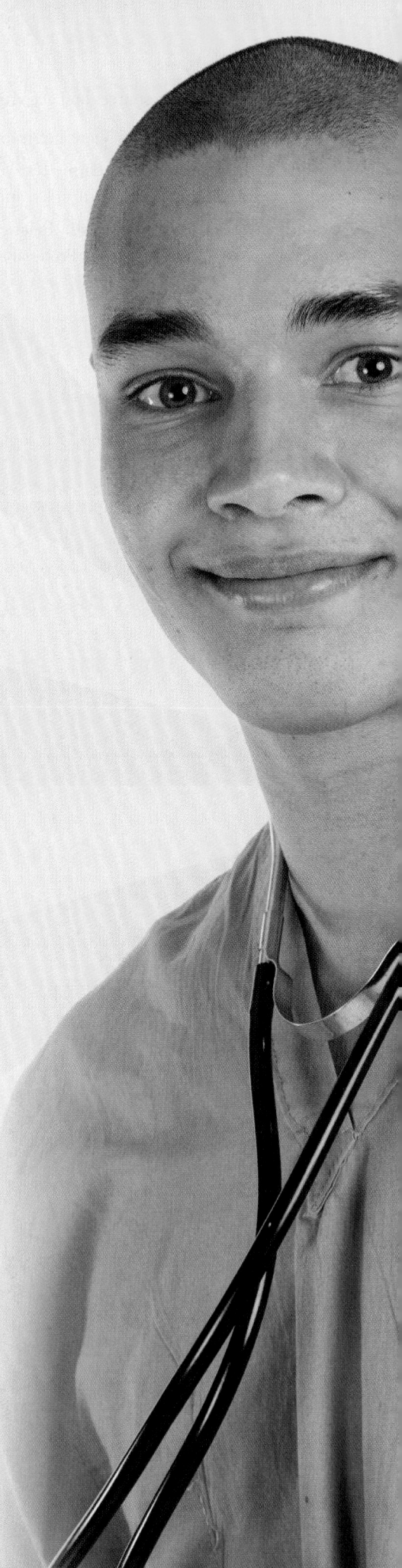

43

Assisting with Medical Emergencies and Emergency Preparedness

LEARNING OBJECTIVES

After completing this chapter, you should be able to:

- Define and spell the terms to learn for this chapter.
- List the steps of a primary assessment.
- Explain ABCD as it applies to CPR and obstructed airways.
- List the signs and symptoms of respiratory distress and chest pain.
- Explain the difference between insulin shock and diabetic coma.
- Identify and describe various types of soft tissue wounds.
- Discuss first-, second-, and third-degree burns as well as the Rule of Nines.
- Identify steps to take for a patient with syncope.
- Explain the concept of and the medical assistant's role in emergency preparedness.

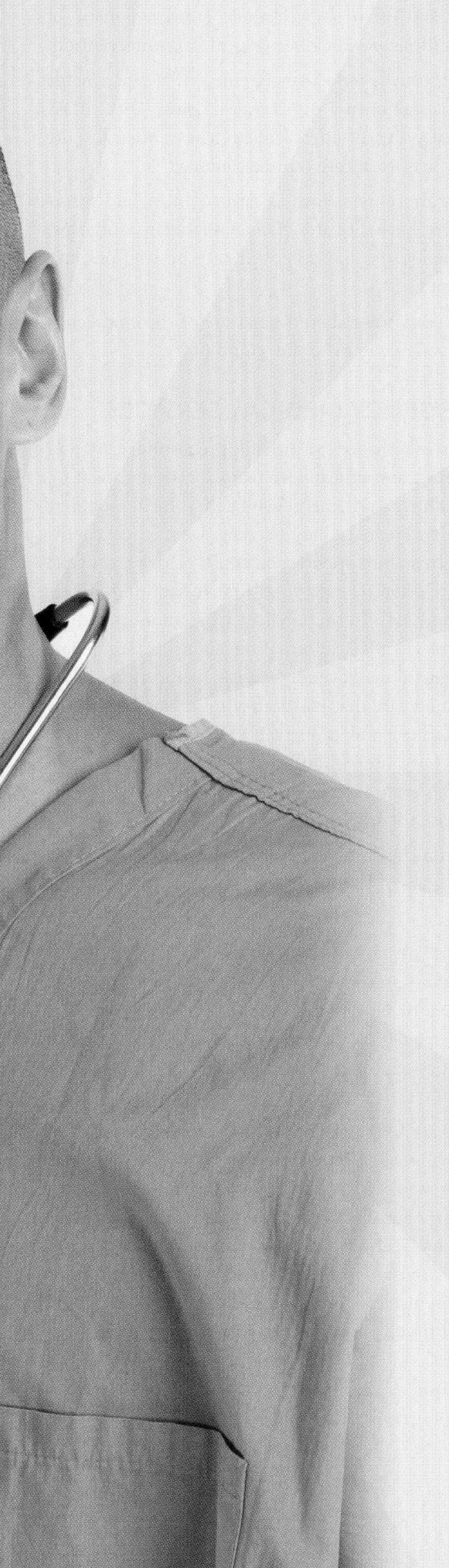

CHAPTER OUTLINE

CASE STUDY

It is a very busy day at Pearson Physicians Group. The examination rooms are full, and three patients are still in the reception area waiting to be seen. Many of the patients have been discussing the odd weather patterns of alternating rain and hail. Lewis Jordan, RMA, is working on medical billing in the front office when he notices that the weather has finally calmed down. Within minutes Lewis hears a fire siren and immediately hears an emergency broadcast on the radio station announcing an immediate tornado warning. All individuals within the listening area are advised to take immediate cover.

CERTIFICATION LINK

CMA (AAMA)
Emergencies
   Prepared action
   Assessment
   and triage
   Emergency
   preparedness
First aid
   Identifying and
   responding to
   various medical
   emergencies

RMA
Clinical medical
assisting
   First aid and
   emergency
   response

CMAS (AMT)
Medical office
emergencies
   Recognize
   and respond
   to medical
   emergencies
   Employ first
   aid and CPR
   appropriately
   Report
   emergencies as
   required by law

A variety of medical emergencies are presented in this chapter. The physician must be notified immediately regarding all medical office emergencies. In some cases you will need to notify the Emergency Medical Services (EMS) system by calling 911. To ensure every patient's safety until additional medical help arrives, medical assistants are cautioned not to perform procedures outside their scope of practice.

Emergency Resources

Those seeking medical care in an emergency have several options:

- During normal office hours, minor emergencies may be handled in a medical office. Some physician group practices may have an emergency clinic where emergency service is provided both during and after office hours.
- Freestanding clinics or urgent care centers provide emergency care during and after hours until late in the evening and often on weekends. However, many of these facilities do not offer critical care intervention.
- Hospitals usually have 24-hour emergency departments (EDs) that are open 7 days a week. These "24-7 EDs" can usually handle most emergencies and transport patients to critical care trauma centers.
- Critical care centers, such as cardiac, burn, and surgical centers, have specialty-trained physicians, surgeons, anesthesiologists, and other critical care staff on duty at all times.

The medical assistant should be aware of the emergency care options available in his or her community.

EMERGENCY MEDICAL SERVICES

The EMS was established to provide prehospital care and safe and prompt transportation from any location, including the medical office, to an emergency facility. EMS providers are individuals who are trained to recognize medical conditions, initiate basic life support, and access other parts of the system, and are often referred to as **first responders**. Firsts responder would look to the medical assistant as a medical professional for detailed information about patient complaints, immediate and overall history, medications taken and allergies, and care that has been administered up to the point of the first responders' arrival.

Guidelines have been established for consistency in care and for ongoing evaluation of the system's services. The following comprise the role of the EMS:

- Provide on-the-scene intervention and treatment.
- Prepare the patient with injuries, trauma, or illness for transport.
- Transport the patient to the emergency facility. Emergency transportation is accomplished by ambulance, helicopter, or fixed-wing aircraft. Once the patient is safely delivered to the receiving facility, the patient's care is passed to medical personnel at that facility (Figure 43-1).

Paramedics are EMS personnel who may **intubate**, which involves inserting a tube into the trachea as an emergency airway, and they may start an intravenous (IV) line in seconds. They carry ample oxygen supplies and an assortment of emergency medications, and they are licensed to perform other invasive procedures. EMS personnel are accustomed to working with health care professionals. One of them will ask the office staff for all the pertinent patient information and make sure that observations become part of the patient chart. In addition, this communicator will operate the radio system that connects your patient to the receiving hospital.

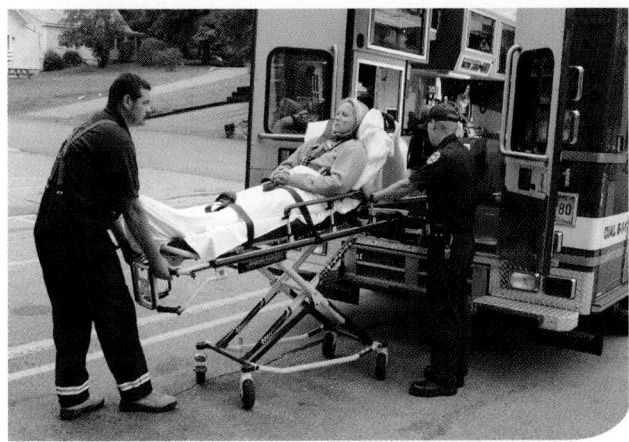

FIGURE 43-1 EMS personnel respond to emergencies and transport patients to the hospital.

SPECIALIZED RESOURCES

Apart from emergency response teams, the medical assistant will occasionally need to consult with specialists in such areas as poison control, pediatrics, trauma, and burns. Some consultations will be under emergency conditions, so make sure the specialists' telephone numbers are displayed prominently near the phones in the office.

GOOD SAMARITAN LAWS

A health care professional who volunteers in an emergency situation is generally protected by various state laws that hold the medical professional not legally liable when rendering first aid.

These laws are often referred to as Good Samaritan laws. A health care professional has a commitment to render care to a patient according to the scope of his or her license, certification, or training. He or she must remain with the patient until relieved by another health care professional with an equal or higher level of training. It is important that every health care professional be aware of the laws in his or her own state and remember that the standard of care must be met within his or her license, certification, or training.

Guidelines for Providing Emergency Care

Medical assistants and other staff members must stay up to date on the emergency plans of the office, facility, and community. These plans should be reviewed on a regularly scheduled basis. For major or catastrophic events, the disaster plan of the American Red Cross (ARC) should be considered. Local law enforcement and emergency management agencies direct rescue, treatment, and transportation efforts after catastrophic events. The standard policy is to treat the least seriously injured ("the walking wounded") as soon as possible in case they can assist in any rescue attempts.

Medical assistants need to be able to handle emergencies in three types of situations. The most common is on the telephone, when a patient or patient's relative calls to ask for advice during an emergency outside the office. Another type occurs when an emergency occurs near the doctor's office and someone brings the patient to the office. The third type occurs when an emergency occurs in the office setting.

In some states, **triage**, or assessing the emergency care needed by patients, is not within the scope of practice of the medical assistant. In these states the medical assistant should not work alone in the medical office.

In an emergency the medical assistant must be able to look at someone or listen to them on the phone and quickly assess whether that person is ill or injured and does or does not require emergency care. The medical assistant may ask the physician for advice anytime he or she is in the office or may make the decision to activate EMS by calling 911.

PROFESSIONALISM

THE LAW

As a medical assistant, you have three primary legal responsibilities in the face of an emergency. The first is obviously a duty to act within your scope of practice. Even though we all feel a little intimidated by the thought of an emergency, you are a medical professional. As such, in case of an emergency you are accountable to yourself, your employer, and the public for actions that measure up to your degree of medical training.

Your second legal responsibility is to document the constant emergency readiness of the office in which you work. You not only need to check your equipment when you come to work every day or as deemed by your employer (an ethical responsibility), but you need to be able to prove that you did so (a legal responsibility). That means documentation, by means of timed, dated, and signed logs as required by your office. When a piece of equipment that you were supposed to check, but did not, fails, the failure is at least partially on your shoulders.

Your third legal responsibility, which you share with others in your workplace, is to do all you can to prevent emergencies, for example, creating environmental exposure preparedness plans. Educating patients and their families about their own safety is also part of emergency prevention.

PRIMARY ASSESSMENT

Every patient contact by a medical professional begins with a few simple questions and a basic patient examination, the **primary assessment**. This assessment is critically important for the medical assistant, whose role it is to organize the process of caring for patients and maintain control of an emergency situation. The steps to obtaining a primary assessment include the following:

1. Determine the patient's name, approximate age, and gender.

    When you ask patients their name, they must quickly go through an extensive neurological process in order to give a simple appropriate answer. They must be able to do the following:

    - Hear you
    - Localize the sound of your voice, using both ears and both eyes
    - Look at you with a symmetrical gaze and focus on you with both eyes
    - Reason that you are a caregiver, and then process the meaning of your words, hopefully in your own language (but maybe not)
    - Remember their name, and formulate a meaningful response
    - Answer in coherent speech and with a symmetrical face

    During that brief period of time, you may learn a lot about a patient's mental function by observing other details, such as facial expressions and body language.

2. Determine the patient's need for intervention.

    A patient who cannot be aroused or who cannot stay awake deserves serious concern. Does the patient seem too weak to stand up? Does the skin color seem very pale or perhaps blue? Is the patient very sweaty for no apparent reason (such as hot weather or recent exercise)? Is the patient bleeding uncontrollably or struggling to breathe? Table 43-1 states various symptoms of conditions based on the necessity of intervention.

3. Obtain the history of the event.

    The immediate history can reveal a lot about the nature of a problem. For instance, a patient who feels "dizzy" on awakening in the morning with a cold is a lot different from a patient who feels the same way after several episodes of dark-colored, foul-smelling diarrhea. Although both of these patients have the same complaint (dizziness), their histories differ. By itself, the first patient's history suggests an ear infection, whereas the second patient's history points to gastrointestinal bleeding. Another example would be a caller who describes where his terrible headache is located and then loses consciousness. The data reported in the patient's history would prompt the initial decisions and actions of an entire team of people who would then care for that patient.

    Past medical history is also important in emergency situations. The best way to gather the past medical history is to use a checklist, whether mental or written. The questions you ask may depend on your employer's standard procedures, but should probably be the same for every patient, regardless of the complaint. Specifically, they might include the following:

    - Heart problems (Heart attack?)
    - Lung problems (Does the patient have both lungs?)

TABLE 43-1 Emergency Intervention

Life-Threatening Condition	Not Life-Threatening: Immediate Intervention	Not-Life Threatening: Intervention as Soon as Possible
- Extreme shortness of breath (airway or breathing problems) - Cardiac arrest - Severe, uncontrolled bleeding - Head injuries - Poisoning - Open chest or abdominal wounds - Shock - Severe burns, including face, hands, feet and genitals - Potential neck injuries	- Decreased levels of consciousness - Chest pain - Seizures - Major or multiple fractures - Neck injuries - Severe eye injuries - Burns not on face, hands, feet, or genitals	- Severe vomiting and diarrhea, especially in the very young and elderly - Minor injuries - Sprains - Strains - Simple fractures

- Asthma or allergies
- Kidney problems (Does the patient have both kidneys?)
- Diabetes (Does the patient take insulin? Has the patient had insulin today and, if so, when?)
- High or low blood pressure (Which?)
- Seizures
- Fainting spells
- Pregnancy, if possible (OB/GYN history? Last menstrual period?)
- Previous similar events (When, treatment, outcome?)

4. Gather medication information.

A medication list can provide information regarding medical history. Also, many medical conditions are caused by interactions among medications or by a patient's reaction to one or more of them. It is important to ask the patient both the name of each drug and the dosage taken.

5. Determine patient's allergies.

Most caregivers underestimate the importance of allergies. People can go into **anaphylactic shock**, a severe allergic reaction that causes respiratory distress due to swelling of the upper airways. This condition must be treated immediately. (Anaphylactic shock is discussed in more detail later in this chapter). Thousands of patients may experience anaphylactic reactions to medications that are dispensed every day. Many wear some kind of identifying jewelry as a reminder, in the form of bracelets, wristbands, or necklaces. Usually they are keenly aware of their allergies, but it happens sometimes during a medical crisis that people will either forget about their allergies or become unable to communicate about them. It is good practice to check for warning tags and jewelry during the patient examination, even if a patient denies having any allergies.

6. Take the vital signs.

With the patient's permission, take his or her vital signs. Take the patient's temperature, then count respirations for about 30 seconds. Then spend 30 seconds checking the pulse, followed by taking the blood pressure. Record these readings on the chart. If the patient has a potentially serious complaint, or if anything in the vitals or the patient's appearance concerns you, terminate the physical examination and notify the physician immediately. If the physician is unavailable, call 911. Have the patient lie down on the examination table, and make him or her comfortable. Oxygen may need to be administered, as ordered by the physician.

PROFESSIONALISM THE LIFE SPAN

It is necessary to consider the age and body structure of a patient who you are treating in a medical emergency. Just as there are specific guidelines for administering CPR to a child, there are factors to take into consideration when performing an emergency intervention on the elderly. As discussed in Chapter 41, the aging body undergoes various systemic changes. For example, as patients enter their seventies and eighties, it is likely that their skeletal structure may be frailer than that of patients who are in their twenties and thirties. Keep this in mind when performing emergency interventions such as abdominal thrusts, chest compressions, and CPR. The amount of force necessary to achieve the desired effect may not be as great in the elderly.

Office Emergency Crash Kit

Every doctor's office has an **emergency kit** or box (sometimes called a **crash cart**) that contains all supplies that may be needed during an emergency and that is instantly accessible to anyone in the office (Figure 43-2). A crash cart

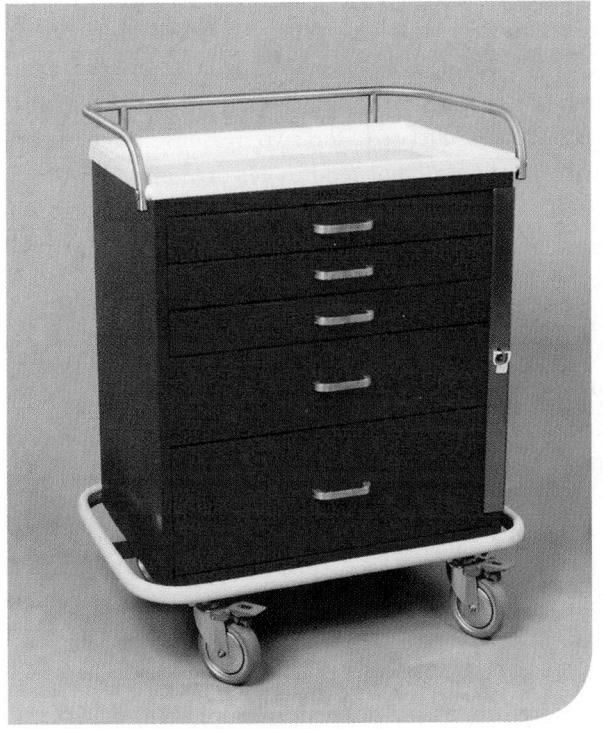

FIGURE 43-2 Emergency crash cart.

TABLE 43-2 Drugs Commonly Stocked in an Emergency Medical Box

• Activated charcoal	• Nitroglycerin
• Atropine	• Normal saline
• Diphenhydramine	• Phenobarbital
• Epinephrine	and diazepam
• Furosemide	• Sodium bicarbonate
• Instant glucose	• Solu-Cortef
• Insulin	• Spirits of ammonia
• Lidocaine	• Syrup of ipecac
• Local anesthetics	• Verapamil

resembles a large roll-around toolbox with drawers that can be used to store emergency medications, intubation equipment, needles and syringes, assorted small instruments, a resuscitator, a heart monitor–defibrillator, an oxygen supply, and airway and suction devices. The emergency medical or drug box is kept on or close to the crash cart. Table 43-2 lists some of the drugs that may be stocked in an emergency medical box.

Each office determines which drugs are appropriate for its practice, as established by emergency algorithms. This cart may contain items that are not within the scope of practice for a medical assistant. However, a physician or nurse may use them. In a small office, a crash kit can be brought to the side of any patient within moments of an emergency, or a "code."

The emergency supplies must be checked routinely. It is suggested that the cart be restocked after every use and maintained at least once a month on a regular basis, with expiration dates checked, for two reasons. First, emergency medications do not tend to get used often, and they expire. The same is true of the batteries that power monitor–defibrillators, laryngoscopes, and suction devices. When these items do get used, someone who is not currently dealing with the aftermath of an emergency must double-check them. Second, being able to use emergency equipment under pressure in an emergency situation requires comfortable, hands-on familiarity with the equipment. When emergencies are infrequent, as in the case of most physicians' offices, familiarity can only come from handling the equipment during frequent maintenance checks. Mock practice sessions can also help medical assistants become more familiar with the equipment and how to respond.

Finally, crash cart supplies must include a checklist that names every drug container and every piece of equipment

the cart contains. (The physician should decide what equipment and supplies should be stocked in the emergency cart.) The checklist should provide space for a daily date and signature, and someone in the office should be accountable for maintaining the cart; however, everyone who is likely to use the cart must check it personally as well, for the sake of their own performance.

Medical Emergencies

The following sections of this chapter present an overview of the descriptions and treatment of medical emergencies that are seen in the medical office.

CARDIOPULMONARY RESUSCITATION, AUTOMATED EXTERNAL DEFIBRILLATION, AND OBSTRUCTED AIRWAYS

Respiratory and cardiac arrest may be caused by an occluded airway, electrocution, shock, drowning, heart attack, trauma, anaphylaxis, drugs, poisoning, or traumatic head or chest injury. Intervention must be immediate if resuscitation is to be successful. For individuals experiencing acute chest pain, loss of consciousness, or respiratory arrest, follow cardiopulmonary resuscitation (CPR) protocol. Guidelines are similar for respiratory arrest, cardiac arrest, and obstructed airways but vary somewhat according to age group. Table 43-3 lists the major differences in the performance of CPR-related skills as defined by the American Heart Association (AHA). Early access to EMS is important. Access for the adult patient is initiated by calling 911 as soon as it has been determined that the patient is unconscious and not breathing.

In general, "Phone first" for an unresponsive adult. With children and infants, EMS access is made after 2 minutes of CPR. In general, perform "CPR first" for unresponsive children and infants. The sequence normally followed is ABCD (Airway, Breathing, Circulation, Defibrillation).

Airway

First, roll the patient onto his or her back, using the logroll technique. Next, assess the unconscious patient for responsiveness. With an adult or child, shake the shoulders and ask, "Are you choking?" With an infant, sharply poke or snap the bottom of the feet. Do not shake the shoulders, as shaking may cause shaken baby syndrome. If the patient does not respond, check the airway. With an adult, child, or infant, place the palm of one hand on the forehead and two or three fingers under the lower jawbone to gently tilt the

TABLE 43-3 Adult, Child, and Infant CPR Skills

CPR Skill	Adult: 8+ years	Child: 1 year to puberty (approximately 12 to 14 years)	Infant: under 1 year
EMS access by calling 911 and giving emergency information	If sudden collapse is witnessed, immediately activate EMS and get AED. If asphyxiation (e.g., drowning, injury, overdose) suspected, first perform 2 minutes of CPR (or 5 cycles), then activate EMS.	If sudden collapse is witnessed, immediately activate EMS and get AED. Otherwise perform 2 minutes of CPR (5 cycles), then activate EMS.	If sudden collapse is witnessed, immediately activate EMS. Otherwise, perform 2 minutes of CPR (5 cycles), then activate EMS.
Assessment of unresponsiveness	Shake the shoulders.	Shake the shoulders.	Sharply poke the feet. Do *not* shake the shoulders.
Rescue breathing and chest compression rate	*Single rescuer:* 30:2 *Two rescuers:* 15:2	*Single rescuer:* 30:2 *Two rescuers:* 15:2	*Single rescuer:* 30:2 *Two rescuers:* 15:2
Obstructed airway foreign body	Abdominal thrusts if patient is conscious Chest compressions if patient is unconscious	Abdominal thrusts if patient is conscious Chest compressions if patient is unconscious	Back slaps and chest thrusts if patient is conscious Chest compressions if patient is unconscious
Pulse check location	Carotid	Carotid	Brachial or femoral
Compression landmarks	Center of chest, between nipples	Center of chest, between nipples	Center of chest, just below the nipple line
Compression technique	One hand placed on top of the second hand with the fingers linked with bottom hand	One hand placed on top of the second hand with the fingers linked with bottom hand	*Single rescuer:* 2 fingertips on sternum *Two rescuers:* 2 thumbs touching on sternum and hand encircling chest and back technique
Compression depth	$1\frac{1}{2}$ to 2 inches	$\frac{1}{2}$ to $\frac{1}{3}$ depth of chest	$\frac{1}{2}$ to $\frac{1}{3}$ depth of chest

head backward (Figure 43-3). If cervical or other spinal injuries are suspected, a jaw-thrust maneuver must be used to open the airway (Figure 43-4). When the airway is opened, the patient may begin spontaneous breathing be-

cause the tongue is lifted from covering the trachea. While keeping close to the patient's mouth, listen for air movement, look for chest movement, and feel for air movement on your cheek. If you do not feel air on your cheek, remove

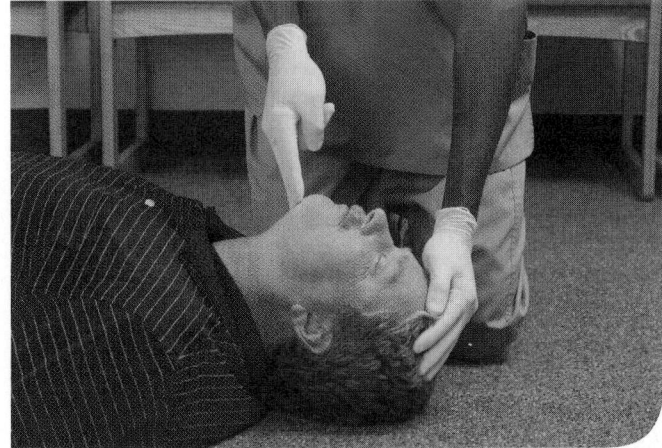

FIGURE 43-3 Head-tilt, chin-lift maneuver.

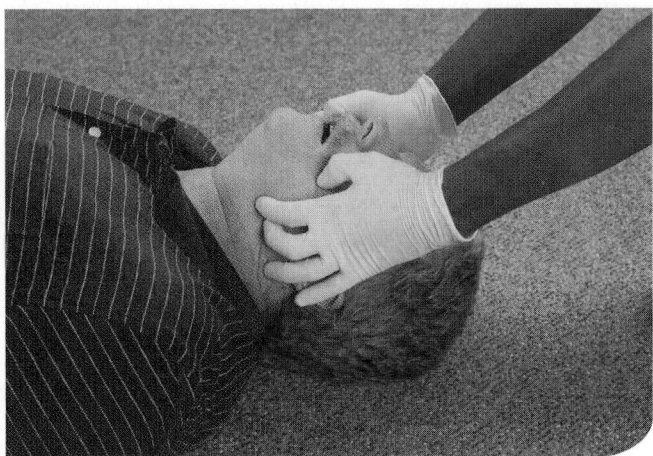

FIGURE 43-4 Jaw-thrust maneuver.

any clothing from the patient's neck. It is possible the patient has a tracheotomy (a surgically created opening for breathing), which may be the reason you do not feel air movement.

Breathing

If you have looked, listened, and felt for breathing and found none, pinch the patient's nose shut, seal your lips tightly around the patient's mouth, and deliver 2 breaths, each lasting 1 second.

You will know the artificial ventilation is effective if the patient's chest rises with each delivered breath. For a patient with a tracheotomy, it may be necessary to close the mouth and nose and administer breaths to the tracheotomy.

Circulation

According to the most recent AHA guidelines for basic life support, the rescuer should check for signs of circulation, defined as pulse, color and warmth of the skin, and patient movement. After you deliver breaths to the patient, check the pulse. In an adult or child, feel the carotid pulse in the neck. In an infant, feel the brachial pulse. Count the pulse for at least 5 to 10 seconds (no more than 10 seconds) because it may be erratic and weak. If the pulse is very weak, erratic, or nonexistent and no signs of circulation are present, begin compressions as appropriate to the patient's age (Figures 43-5, 43-6, and 43-7). If a second rescuer is available, instruct him or her to monitor compression quality by checking the carotid, brachial, or femoral pulse. If your compressions are effective, a pulse will be felt. If the compressions do not generate a palpable pulse, the second rescuer should take over the compressions in two-person CPR or the entire sequence in one-person CPR. The one-person sequence allows the original rescuer to rest or get help. Procedure 43-1 details the proper procedure for adult and one-rescuer sequences, and

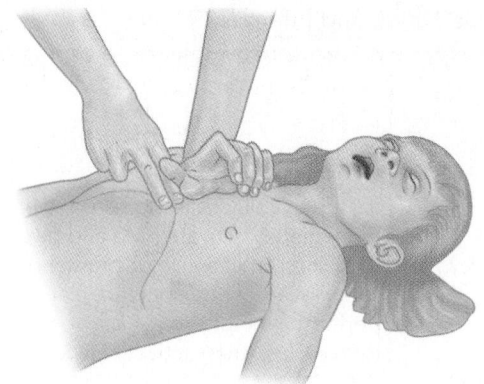

FIGURE 43-6 Compressions for a child.

Procedure 43-2 details the proper procedure for infant/child and one-rescuer sequences.

Defibrillation

Automated external defibrillation (AED) is highly effective when provided immediately after or within minutes of an adult cardiac arrest. Most cardiac arrests in adults are related to fatal electrical arrhythmias of the heart and are correctable with defibrillators. The defibrillator gives verbal directions to the rescuer or rescue team that are easy and safe to follow. AED is not applied to infants. Guidelines have recently been established for the use of AED on children 1 to 8 years old. AED may be used after 1 minute of CPR. It is recommended that child-size defibrillator pads and cables, rather than adultsize, be used. Procedure 43-3 demonstrates the use of an AED.

Heimlich Maneuver

An obstructed airway prevents the movement of air into or out of the respiratory tract. Certain disease conditions, such as anaphylactic shock or epiglottitis, can cause an anatomical blockage, but most obstructions are caused by foreign objects. With small children, the cause is usually food or

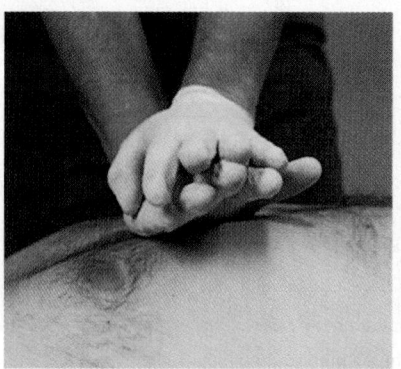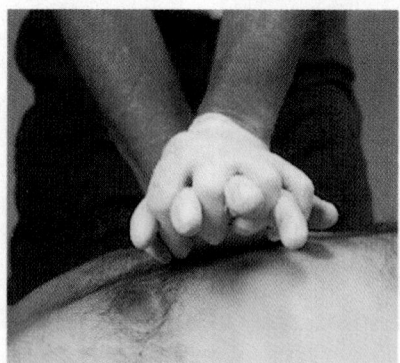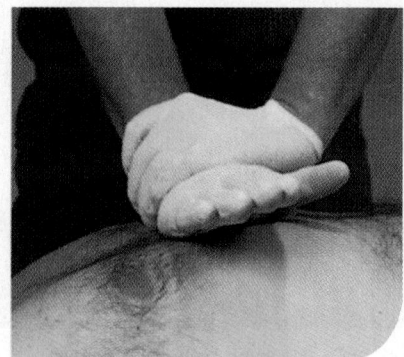

FIGURE 43-5 Location and position of hand during chest compressions on an adult.

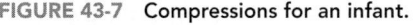

(A) For a very small newborn, encircle chest with fingers and overlap thumbs on the sternum just below an imaginary line connecting the nipples.

(B) For an average-size newborn, encircle chest with fingers and place thumbs side by side on the sternum just below an imaginary line connecting the nipples.

(C) For an infant who is older or too large for you to be able to encircle the chest, place middle and ring fingers on sternum one finger-width below imaginary line connecting nipples. Measure distance by first placing, then raising, index finger.

FIGURE 43-7 Compressions for an infant.

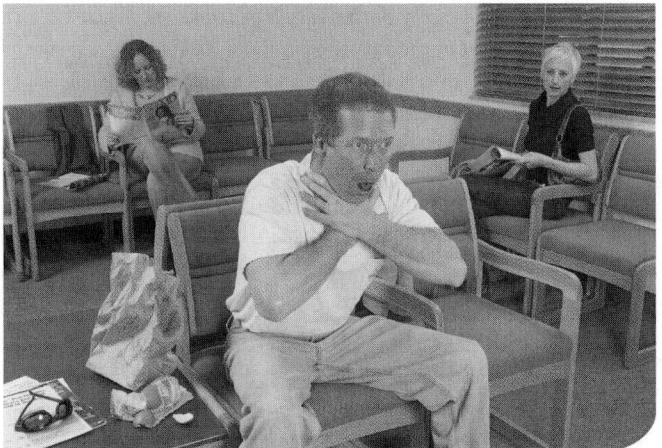

FIGURE 43-8 The universal choking sign.

small toys. With adults, an obstructed airway may be the result of the following:

- Not chewing large pieces of food properly
- Talking too excitedly or laughing too much while eating
- Drinking alcohol before and during eating
- Choking on body or extraneous fluids, such as vomit or blood

The medical assistant should know how to respond to the following choking scenarios:

- **Partial airway obstruction with good air exchange**—The patient is conscious, is capable of speaking, and is making a strong effort to cough.

- **Partial airway obstruction with poor air exchange**—The patient is conscious but is weakening in clinical condition and ability to cough.

- **Total obstructed airway**—The patient is unconscious, and there are no signs of breathing or the patient is unable to vocalize. The conscious choking adult may use the universal choking sign—crossing the hands at the throat—to signal for help (Figure 43-8).

A partial airway obstruction may allow some air into the respiratory tract and is characterized by a high-pitched noise from the patient. The patient may be able to cough and expel the foreign object. If a phone call comes into the medical office and the caller states "My child is not breathing" and you hear the child crying in the background, the airway

procedure 43-1

PERFORM ADULT RESCUE BREATHING AND ONE-RESCUER CPR

Objective: Administer rescue breathing for an adult and one-rescuer CPR for an adult correctly, within the time frame designated.

EQUIPMENT AND SUPPLIES
approved mannequin; gloves; ventilator mask; mouth guard

METHOD
1. Assess the patient and determine if help is needed. Shout "Are you okay?" while gently shaking the patient's shoulders.

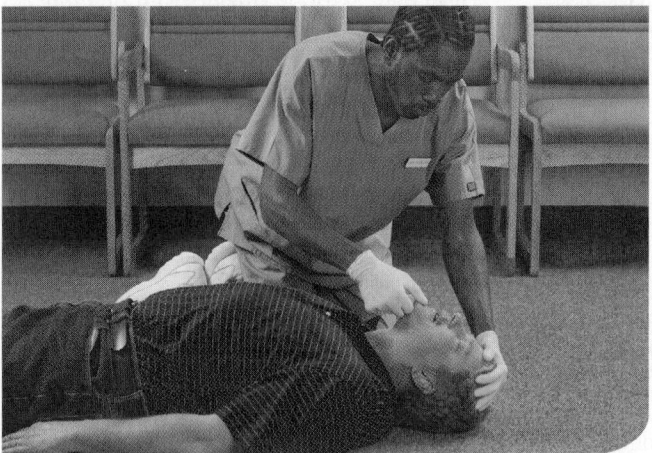

FIGURE 43-9   Establish an open airway.

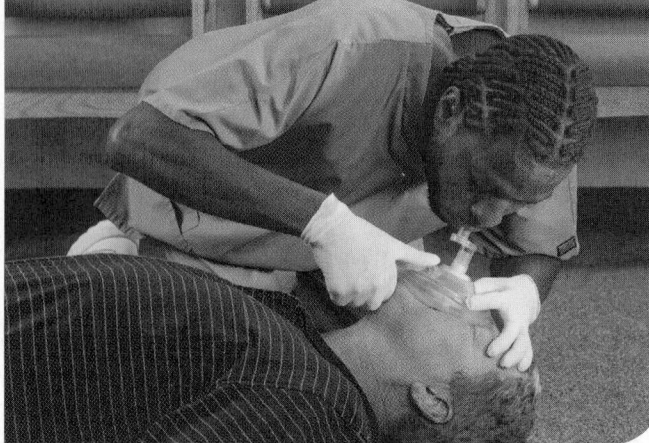

FIGURE 43-11   With mouth guard in place, administer 2 rescue breaths.

2. If the adult patient is determined to be unresponsive, activate EMS immediately by calling 911, then get an AED if available.

3. Assess the ABCs. To check the airway, perform a head-tilt, chin-lift maneuver or, if a neck injury is suspected, a jaw thrust (Figure 43-9). Look and feel for breath and chest movements (Figure 43-10). Attempt to get another person to call 911. If you are alone, begin the rescue sequence for 1 minute, and then attempt to call 911 yourself. If gloves are available, put them on. If you have a ventilator mask, place it on the patient.

4. If breathing is absent, put on a mouth guard and administer 2 rescue breaths (Figure 43-11). If your breaths do not cause the chest to rise, look in the patient's mouth and remove an object if you see one. If you see no onstruction, make a second attempt to administer a rescue breath.

5. If the breaths cause the chest to rise, assess the patient's circulation by feeling for a pulse at the carotid artery (Figure 43-12). If you feel a pulse, begin rescue breathing. Administer 1 breath every 5 seconds, or 10 to 12 breaths every minute. After 1 minute, reassess the patient for breathing and pulse.

6. If you do not feel a pulse, begin chest compressions. Kneel at the patient's side. Place your hand in the center of the chest between the nipples.

7. Place your other hand on top of the first hand, making sure to lift your fingers off the chest, using only the heels of your hands to administer compressions.

8. Keeping your shoulders directly over your hands, compress the chest $1\frac{1}{2}$ to 2 inches, then allow the sternum to relax (see Figure 43-5). Do not lift your hands off the chest.

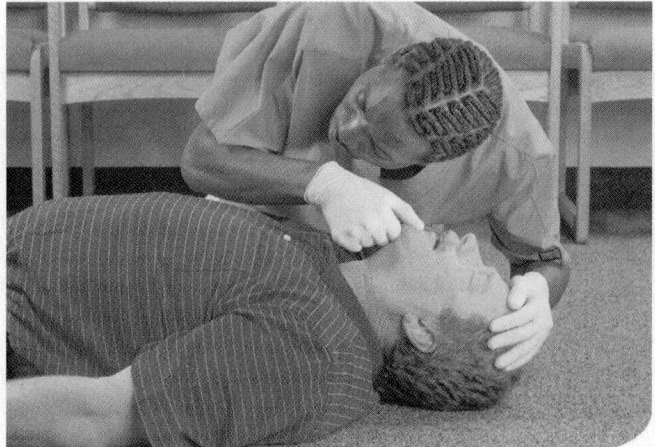

FIGURE 43-10   Look and feel for breath and chest movements.

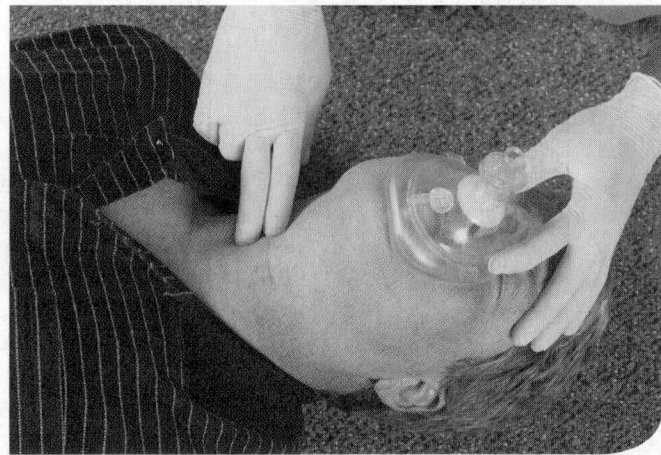

FIGURE 43-12   Assess the patient's circulation by feeling for a pulse at the carotid artery.

9. Continue to compress the chest a total of 30 times, then administer 2 breaths.
10. Repeat this sequence for 4 total cycles. Reassess the patient.
11. If necessary, continue CPR until pulse and breathing return or you are relieved by more advanced medical personnel.
12. Wash your hands and document the incident in the patient's chart.

procedure 43-2

PERFORM INFANT OR YOUNG CHILD RESCUE BREATHING AND ONE-RESCUER CPR

Objective: Administer rescue breathing for a child and one-rescuer CPR for an adult correctly and within the designated time frame.

EQUIPMENT AND SUPPLIES

approved mannequin; gloves; ventilator mask; mouth guard

METHOD

1. Assess the patient and determine if help is needed. Shout the name of the infant or child, and sharply poke at the feet. Never shake an infant.
2. If the infant is determined to be unresponsive, perform CPR for 2 minutes prior to activating EMS immediately by calling 911 and then get an AED, if available.
3. Carefully place the patient on the back, being cautious not to move the head or allow the neck to twist, especially if a spinal cord injury is suspected.
4. Gently, with two fingers, tilt the patient's head and open the airway.
5. Place your ear close to the patient's ear to listen for breathing sounds, watch to see if the chest rises or falls indicating breathing, and feel for any breathing from the patient's nose or mouth.
6. If breathing is absent, secure a mouth guard over the patient's mouth and nose. Administer 2 rescue breaths. If your breaths do not cause the chest to rise, look in the patient's mouth and remove any object seen. If no object is seen, make a second attempt to administer a rescue breath.
7. If the breaths cause the chest to rise, check the patient's pulse at the brachial artery. If you feel a pulse, begin rescue breathing by administering 1 breath every 5 seconds or 10 to 12 breaths every minute.
8. If you do not feel a pulse, begin chest compressions. Place two fingers in the center of the chest just below the nipple line. Compressions should be made one-third to one-half the depth of the chest. Perform 30 quick compressions.
9. Give 2 more rescue breaths followed by 30 more compressions. Continue the 30:2 ratio of compressions and breaths.
10. After 2 minutes, leave the infant and call 911 if you are still alone. Continue compressions and breaths until the infant recovers or EMS arrives.
11. Wash hands and document the incident in the patient's chart.

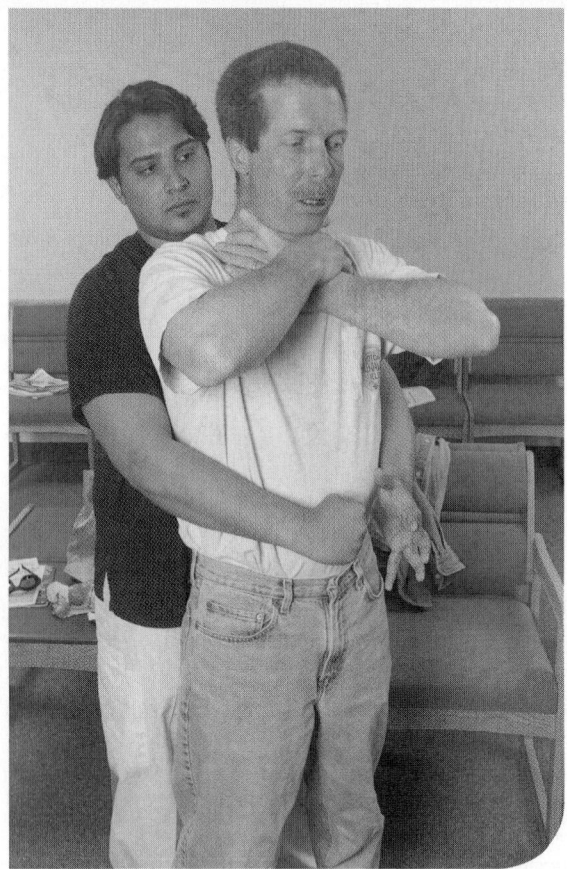

FIGURE 43-13 **Abdominal thrusts are delivered with a firm thrust into the patient's abdomen with an upward movement.**

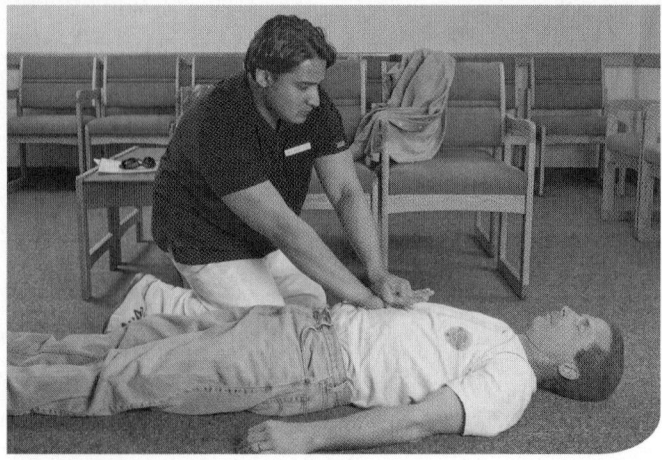

FIGURE 43-14 **Heimlich maneuver.**

is not obstructed. Anytime the patient can speak or cry, air is moving in and out of the airway. As a rescuer, ask the patient "Can you speak?" If the patient responds by shaking the head, the airway is obstructed and immediate intervention is required. Request permission to assist the patient and perform the Heimlich maneuver for the adult or child (or abdominal thrusts for the supine patient (Figures 43-13 and 43-14) and back blows and chest thrusts for the infant (Figure 43-15). You should also use the Heimlich maneuver

if the patient's coughing weakens or if the patient cannot speak.

To perform the Heimlich maneuver, stand behind the patient and put your arms around his or her chest halfway between the xiphoid process of the sternum and the umbilicus. Make a fist with one hand, with the thumb turned into the fist. Wrap your other hand around the fisted hand and pull the fisted hand in and up toward the diaphragm. This force against the diaphragm is usually sufficient to loosen the foreign object and propel it out of the mouth. If the patient becomes unconscious, ease him or her to the floor to prevent any additional injuries, and proceed with the technique described below for unconscious obstructed airway. Procedure 43-4 explains how to respond to an adult with an obstructed airway. For very obese people and visibly pregnant women, the Heimlich is adjusted to chest thrusts that are identical to the chest compressions of CPR. If the patient is unconscious, you will need to add artificial ventilations to the obstructed airway procedure. If the obstruction is loosened during the procedure, it may be possible to get oxygen around the object and into the bloodstream.

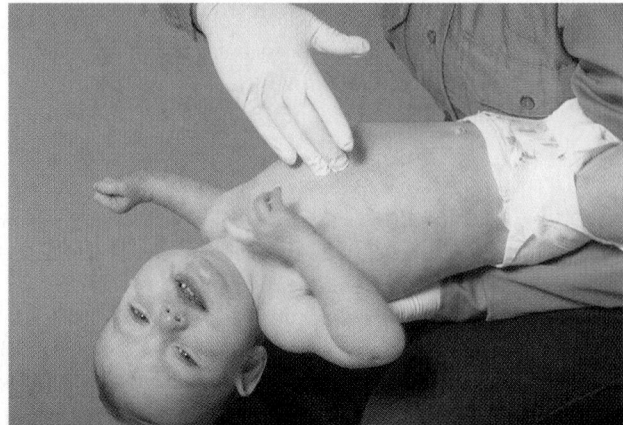

A

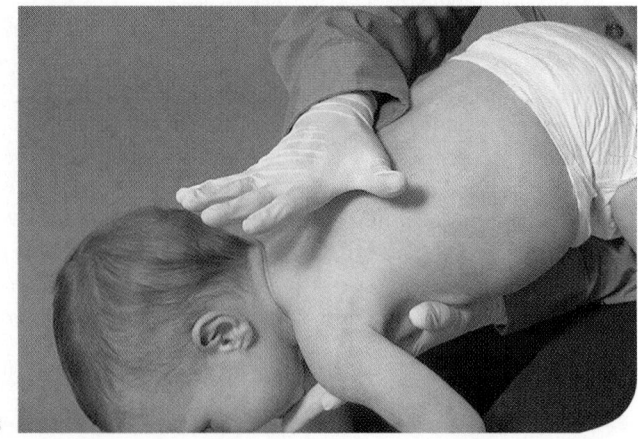

B

FIGURE 43-15 **(A) Use chest thrusts followed by; (B) Back blows.**

procedure

43-3

USE AN AUTOMATED EXTERNAL DEFIBRILLATOR

Objective: Use an automated external defibrillator (AED) correctly within the time frame designated by the instructor.

EQUIPMENT AND SUPPLIES
AED machine; patient chart

METHOD

1. Place the AED (Figure 43-16) next to the patient's left ear. This position allows the rescuers clear access to the chest and airway for continued rescue measures.
2. Turn the AED on and follow the voice prompts.

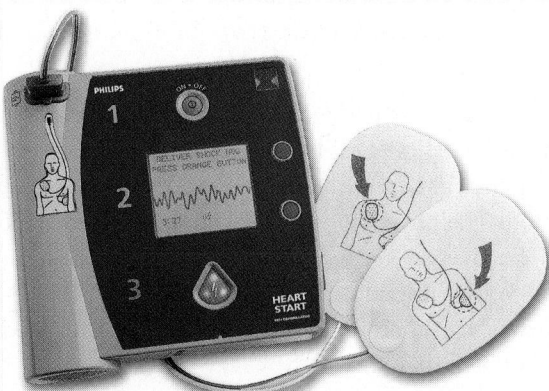

FIGURE 43-16   Automated external defibrillator.

3. You will be prompted to attach the electrode pads to the patient's chest on the sternum and at the apex of the heart, following the diagram for correct placement. Use adult-size electrode pads on patients 8 years of age and older. Child-size electrode pads are used for patients between the ages of 1 and 8 years or under 55 pounds.
4. Next, you will be directed to allow the machine to analyze the heart rhythm to determine if it is a shockable rhythm. CPR should cease while the machine is analyzing.
5. The machine will begin a charging sequence prior to shocking and warn rescuers to stand back. The voice prompt will then tell you to press the SHOCK button to administer the electrical current to the patient.
6. If the machine indicates "No shock is advised," assess the patient for breathing and circulation. Continue CPR as needed until advanced medical personnel arrive.

CHARTING EXAMPLE

11/25/XX 3:30 P.M. Patient found in stairwell, unresponsive, with absence of pulse and respirations. 911 protocol initiated with two-rescuer CPR. Third rescuer initiated AED response, and patient was analyzed for shockable rhythm. CPR and AED shocks administered a total of 8 cycles prior to advanced medical support arriving. Patient released to EMS care and transferred to Sacred Heart Medical Center. · · · · · · · M. Cowan, CMA (AAMA)

procedure

43-4

RESPOND TO AN ADULT WITH AN OBSTRUCTED AIRWAY

Objective: Administer the Heimlich maneuver to an adult correctly, within the time frame designated.

EQUIPMENT AND SUPPLIES
approved mannequin; gloves; ventilation mask with one-way valve for unconscious patient

METHOD

1. Once it has been established that the patient is choking, with no air exchange, direct someone to call 911 and shout "Are you choking?" or "Can you speak?" If

the answer is no—as indicated by a head shake—tell the patient you are going to begin emergency treatment.
2. Stand behind the patient with your feet slightly apart, placing one foot between the patient's feet and one to the outside. This stance will give you greater stability, and if the patient should pass out, you can safely guide him or her to the ground by sliding him or her down your thigh.

3. Place the index finger of one hand at the person's navel or belt buckle to mark that spot. If the patient is a pregnant woman, place your finger above the enlarged uterus.

4. Make a fist with your other hand and place it, thumb side to patient, above your other hand. If the person is very large or far along in pregnancy, you may have to do chest compressions.

5. Place your marking hand over your curled fist and begin to give quick inward and upward thrusts (see Figure 43-13).

6. There is no set number of thrusts to give to an adult who remains conscious. Continue to give thrusts until the object is removed or the patient becomes unconscious.

7. If the patient becomes unconscious, gently lower him or her to the ground.

8. Activate EMS and put on gloves.

9. Immediately begin CPR with 30 chest compressions and 2 rescue breaths.

10. Before administering the rescue breaths, open the airway with the head-tilt, chin-lift maneuver. Look for a foreign body in the patient's mouth and remove any that is visible. Blind finger sweeps are no longer recommended and should not be performed.

11. Continue with cycles of 30 compressions and 2 rescue breaths until the foreign body is expelled or advance medical personal arrive to relieve you.

12. Wash hands and document the event in the patient's chart.

CHARTING EXAMPLE

10/25/XX 11:30 A.M. Jason Jones exhibited signs of choking at lunch. Jason grabbed his throat and was unable to cough or make noise. Tina Muller, RMA, alerted the physician and placed a call to 911. Abdominal thrusts were given until the piece of apple was expelled. EMS arrived and checked Jason for signs of throat irritation and swelling. · · · · · · · · · · · · · · · ·
· J. Walker, CMA (AAMA)

RESPIRATORY DISTRESS

Respiratory distress may be a reaction to a long-term debilitating disease, such as chronic pulmonary obstructive disease (COPD), or to an emergency situation, such as anaphylactic response to medication. It also can be the result of other disease processes, including obstructive conditions, such as asthma, chronic bronchitis, and emphysema, pneumonia, and acute pulmonary edema. Conscious control is usually not a factor in respiratory distress. Being unable to get enough oxygen causes extreme anxiety, and the medical staff should be prepared to give the patient emotional support. Signs and symptoms vary, depending on the cause. One of the most serious conditions is an occluded airway that causes the patient to grasp at the neck and attempt to cough. Unconsciousness soon follows, then cardiac arrest. Other conditions of respiratory distress may cause symptoms such as the following:

- Acute anxiety with gasping breaths
- Bradypnea, abnormally slow breathing (fewer than 8 breaths per minute)
- Cyanosis
- Failure of the chest to rise and fall
- Nasal flaring
- Pursing of the lips
- Noisy breathing (snoring, gurgling, wheezing, rattling, or stridor)
- Tachypnea (abnormally rapid breathing, more than 24 breaths per minute)

If respiratory distress is the result of a known diagnosis, the patient will need medical follow-up with an emergency facility or physician, depending on the severity or change in the condition. The physician may ask the medical assistant to administer oxygen to the patient. This is shown in Procedure 43-5. If respiratory distress is caused by an obstructed airway, the appropriate sequence for an obstructed airway should be initiated.

Shortness of Breath

Any individual experiencing shortness of breath (SOB) needs immediate intervention. A **patent**, or unobstructed, airway is necessary to support life. If the person can speak, air is moving in and out. Ask the patient about the onset for difficult breathing and what activity caused it. This information helps to identify the problem. The patient experiencing SOB may be gasping for air, looking pale or cyanotic, and exhibiting nasal flaring and extreme anxiety (Figure 43-17). Usually the patient sits in an upright position and may be quite weak. If the airway is partially obstructed, the patient may cough in an attempt to clear the passages. It the patient is not in a sitting position, help him or her to a sitting position with support to the back. Call out for assistance.

Hyperventilation

Hyperventilation is quick, shallow breathing or rapid, deep breathing that results in decreasing carbon dioxide in the blood, dilation of blood vessels, and lowered blood pressure.

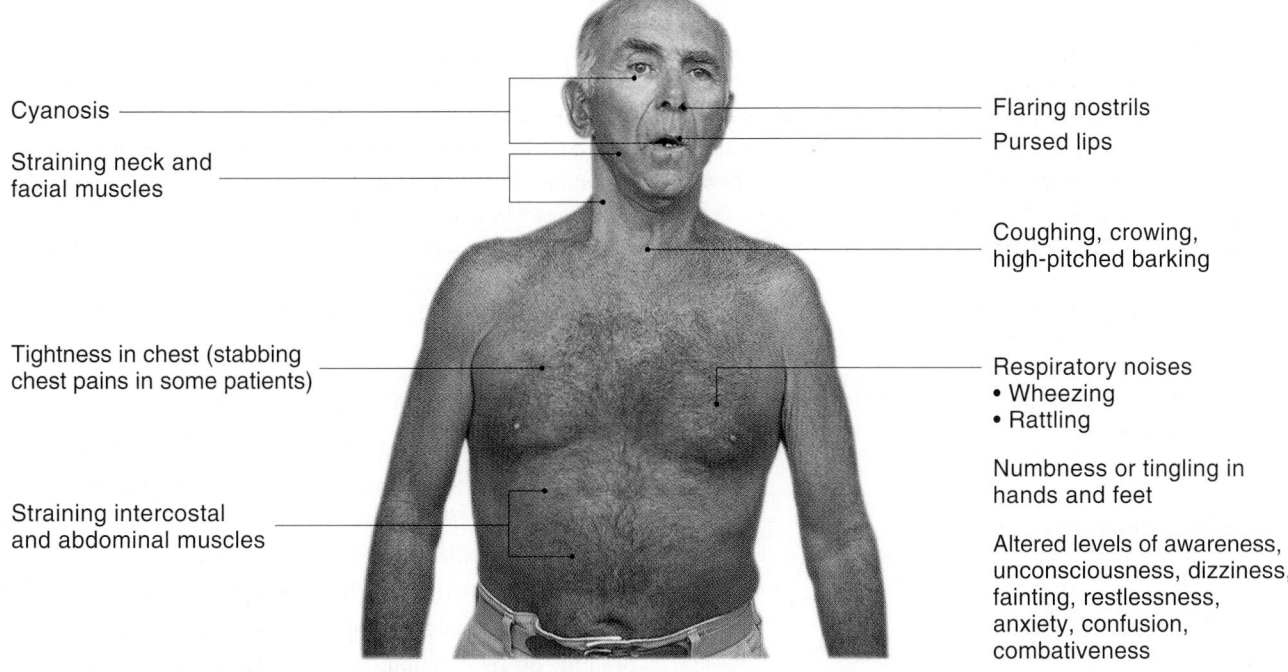

Cyanosis

Straining neck and facial muscles

Flaring nostrils

Pursed lips

Coughing, crowing, high-pitched barking

Tightness in chest (stabbing chest pains in some patients)

Respiratory noises
• Wheezing
• Rattling

Numbness or tingling in hands and feet

Straining intercostal and abdominal muscles

Altered levels of awareness, unconsciousness, dizziness, fainting, restlessness, anxiety, confusion, combativeness

FIGURE 43-17 **Signs and symptoms of breathing difficulty.**

procedure
43-5

ADMINISTER OXYGEN

Objective: Administer oxygen therapy to an adult correctly within the time frame designated by the instructor.

EQUIPMENT AND SUPPLIES

portable oxygen tank; pressure regulator; oxygen flow meter; sterile, prepackaged, disposable nasal cannula with tubing; gloves; oximeter; patient chart

METHOD

1. Gather all needed equipment.
2. Perform hand hygiene.
3. Identify the patient, and confirm the physician's order for oxygen therapy.
4. Check the pressure reading on the oxygen tank to ensure it has enough oxygen in it.
5. Start the flow of oxygen by opening the cylinder.
6. Attach the cannula tubing to the flow meter. Adjust the oxygen flow to the physician's order.
7. Hold the cannula tips over the inside of your wrist, without touching the skin, to determine if the oxygen is flowing.
8. Apply gloves if necessary. You may prefer to wear gloves with patients who demonstrate a chronic cough, have a nasal drip, or exhibit other characteristics of potential exposure.

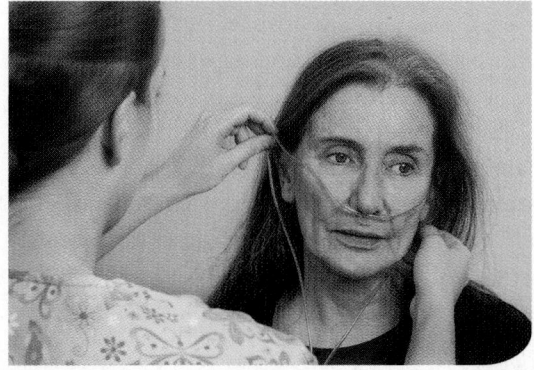

FIGURE 43-18 **Adjust the tubing around the back of the patient's ears.**

9. Place the tips of the nasal cannula into the patient's nostrils. Wrap the tubing behind the patient's ears (Figure 43-18).
10. Instruct the patient to breathe normally through the mouth and nose. Some patients instinctively hold their

11. Check the patient's oxygen level with an oximeter. Place the probe over the index finger and record the reading. If necessary, have the patient take a short walk to verify that the oxygen flow rate is sufficient for activity.

12. Wash hands and document the procedure in the patient's chart.

The patient feels faint or light-headed and may experience any of the following:

- Chest tightness

- Cardiac palpitations

- Rapid pulse

- Deep sighing breaths

- Anxiety

Inform the physician and encourage the patient to breathe slowly. Have the patient breathe into an oxygen mask (not connected to any oxygen), block one nostril, or breathe into a brown paper bag. One of these methods is usually effective. This condition can generally be resolved quickly and without further intervention.

Chronic Obstructive Pulmonary Disease

Asthma, chronic bronchitis, and emphysema are considered COPDs. Air is trapped in the lungs, and the patient is unable to expel all the carbon dioxide from the alveoli. Although each condition has specific signs and symptoms, they share many of the same problems. A person with COPD has SOB and a rapid heart rate and experiences weakness. Asthma may also be characterized by audible wheezes, diaphoresis, and tightness in the chest. Inform the physician in all cases and, if ordered, administer oxygen. Depending on the situation, the physician may order administration of medications, delivery of oxygen, or transport to an emergency facility by EMS.

Pulmonary Edema

Fluid accumulation in the lung tissue and alveoli results in a condition known as pulmonary edema. The patient presents with difficulty breathing, wheezing sounds, cyanosis, rapid heartbeat, distended neck veins, extreme anxiety, and orthopnea. Inform the physician. Place the patient in a sitting position with feet and legs up on a bed or cart. Administer supplemental oxygen if ordered and available. Call EMS for transport to an emergency facility.

CHEST PAIN

Heart attacks are the leading cause of death for both men and women. The patient experiencing chest pain may display various symptoms. The primary complaint will be pain in the middle or left side of the chest, described as sharp, stabbing, crushing, squeezing, or aching. The pain may radiate to the left arm, to the back, or up the neck. Sometimes the pain is brought on by exertion, but other times onset is sudden and unexplained. Other symptoms are nausea, weakness, SOB, apprehension, and the feeling of impending doom. The skin may be clammy, moist, pale, or cyanotic. Denial is common, as the individual tries to explain the pain as heartburn or indigestion.

The first intervention is to have the individual stop what he or she is doing and sit down, with the feet elevated if possible. Immediately request help from a coworker. Ask the coworker to stay with the patient while you inform the physician of the situation. If instructed by the physician, or if a physician is unavailable, call EMS. If oxygen is available, administer it according to office protocol by nasal cannula at 6 to 8 liters per minute (L/min) until the physician or emergency personnel arrive. If the patient has previously been diagnosed with angina and has nitroglycerin tablets, insert one tablet under the tongue (Figure 43-19). Tablets may be administered every 5 minutes up to three doses. If the pain is not relieved, inform

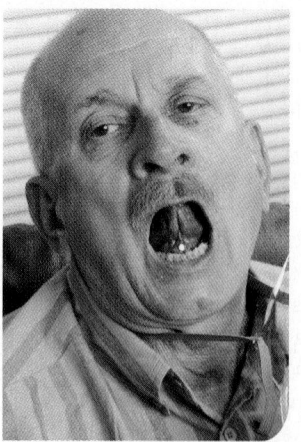

FIGURE 43-19 Nitroglycerin is administered sublingually.

the physician or EMS on the scene. Do the following if a patient calls on the telephone complaining of chest pain:

- Keep the caller on the line while asking for help from another office staff member.
- Write down the caller's name and location. (If someone is calling for the patient, ask the caller for the patient's name and location.)
- Follow office protocol regarding assisting patients with chest pain. Oftentimes offices will want all patients calling with chest pain sent to the emergency department. If this is the case, call EMS for the patient and remain on the phone with the caller until EMS has arrived.

SHOCK

Shock, the collapse of the cardiovascular system, is caused by insufficient cardiac output. Blood supply and nourishment (oxygen and nutrients, including glucose) to the tissue and perfusion to the organs are inadequate. Untreated shock can progress very rapidly to death. Shock may be the result of many insults to the body, including anaphylaxis, cardiac failure, hemorrhage, extreme emotional upset, respiratory distress, neurological collapse, severe metabolic insult, and sepsis. Some of the symptoms that may occur after the initial crisis are listed in Table 43-4.

Anaphylactic Shock

Anaphylactic shock, as mentioned previously in this chapter, is a severe allergic reaction to a foreign substance. Examples of foreign substances include medications, bug bites, and latex gloves. Inform the physician immediately, and call EMS. The physician may order epinephrine with or without an antihistamine. An IV may also be started. Prevention is the most important factor in anaphylactic shock. Always ask the patient about allergies to any medication before administering it and record this information on the front of the chart in red. After administering medication, ask the patient to wait 20 minutes before leaving the office, and observe for any potential reactions. In offices where antibiotics and allergy injections are given on a

regular basis, you must be alert to possible reactions and prepared with an emergency drug box for rapid intervention.

ASSISTING PATIENTS IN SHOCK

Patients go into shock for varied reasons, including blood loss, infection, and pain. The most common signs of shock include pale, gray, or bluish skin; moist, cool skin; dilated pupils; a weak, rapid pulse; shallow, rapid respirations; and extreme thirst. Regardless of the cause, immediate, aggressive intervention is required to stop the progression of the condition and the possible death of the patient. When patients exhibit signs of shock, medical assistants should ensure that those patients have an open airway and proper circulation. Assistants should encourage patients to lie down with their legs elevated to return blood to the vital organs. Next, assistants should cover patients with blankets for warmth and keep them calm until emergency personnel arrive. The medical assistant should inform the physician, call EMS for further assessment and transport, monitor the patient's vital signs, and provide emotional support.

Most emergency treatments for shock patients will need to be administered by a physician or emergency personnel. Oxygen may be administered, if ordered and available, by trained personnel. Table 43-5 outlines the cause and treatment of different types of shock.

TABLE 43-5 Treatment for Shock in the Medical Office

Cause	Treatment
Anaphylactic shock	Epinephrine
Cardiogenic shock	IV dopamine, immediate transport to the emergency department
Hemorrhagic shock	Stop bleeding, replace volume, immediate transport to the emergency department
Hypovolemic shock	Replace volume
Insulin shock	Sugar given to patient by any means tolerated
Neurogenic shock	IV dopamine, immediate transport to the emergency department
Poisoning	Consult the poison control center for treatment specific to the poison
Respiratory shock	Intubation and immediate transport to the emergency department
Sepsis	Fluids, IV dopamine, and immediate transport to the emergency department

TABLE 43-4 Symptoms of Shock Following a Crisis Situation

- Weakness
- Rapid heartbeat
- Thirst
- Nausea
- Dizziness
- Restlessness
- Pallor
- Cool skin
- Clammy skin
- Cyanosis
- Confusion
- Disorientation
- Unresponsiveness
- Shallow breathing

INSULIN SHOCK AND DIABETIC COMA

A patient with diabetes may exhibit signs of either **hypoglycemia** (low blood sugar level) or **hyperglycemia** (high blood sugar level). Both conditions may cause the rapid onset of altered levels of consciousness. The greater risk for a patient is hypoglycemia, which can develop into insulin shock. Hypoglycemia, in which blood sugar falls below 70 mg per deciliter (mg/dL), may be the result of a skipped meal, vomiting after taking diabetic medications, excessive exercise, or an unknown reason. A patient may appear to be intoxicated (slurred speech, balance disturbances, and uncharacteristic behavior), have cold clammy skin, and be anxious or combative.

Intervention must be immediate and consists of some form of glucose administration. If the patient is conscious, ask about the last intake of food and diabetic medication. If the patient is able to swallow, glucose paste may be placed inside the mouth behind the lip and along the cheek, or the patient may drink orange juice with added sugar. If the patient is unconscious, IV glucose is administered.

The person experiencing hypoglycemia is in grave danger when the blood glucose drops below 40 mg/dL. The brain requires glucose to survive, and brain cells begin dying unless glucose is administered promptly. If possible, blood glucose levels should be checked with a blood glucose monitor. Contact EMS if a physician is not available to administer IV glucose. If there is doubt about whether the patient is hypoglycemic or hyperglycemic, glucose may be administered. It will raise the glucose 25 to 50 points, but this rise can be reversed with an insulin injection as soon as an elevated glucose is diagnosed. The hyperglycemic individual may experience acidosis or diabetic coma. With acidosis or diabetic coma, the patient's breath develops a sweet, fruity odor, indicating the presence of ketones.

The patient may progress to an unconscious state, reversible with insulin. The physician orders the amount and administration route of the insulin. Whether the patient is hypoglycemic or hyperglycemic, keep him or her as warm and comfortable as possible on an examination table until the physician arrives.

BLEEDING

Bleeding can be either external or internal. External bleeding occurs when the skin is broken. Internal bleeding occurs with tissue damage and intact skin. Bleeding can originate from any of the three types of blood vessels: arteries, veins, and capillaries.

Arterial bleeding is usually copious, rapid, and bright red. The blood often spurts, echoing the heartbeat. Arterial bleeding must be brought under control as soon as possible. Pressure applied directly over the exit wound may halt the

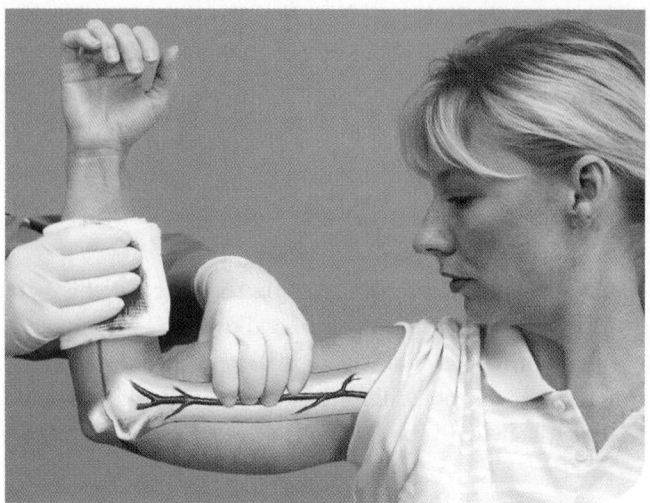

FIGURE 43-20 Apply direct pressure to the patient's wound.

flow of blood. If this is not successful, external pressure on the pressure points may be. Elevating the injured part higher than the heart may also slow the blood flow.

Venous blood flows more slowly, is darker in color, and can usually be controlled by direct pressure. Blood from capillaries oozes rather than flows and can also be halted with direct pressure. Bleeding from the scalp or face is often copious because of the many circulatory vessels in the area. Caution must be exercised if a fracture in the area is suspected. Direct pressure is applied by placing a sterile dressing over the wound and holding it in place (Figure 43-20). A pressure bandage may be wrapped around the injured part to maintain pressure on the site. If blood seeps through, reinforce the bandage by applying more dressings and bandages over it. Do not remove the original dressing.

Pressure Points

Pressure points may be used to help control external bleeding (Figure 43-21). Pressure is applied to the artery where it lies close to the skin and can be compressed against an underlying bone. These arteries include the temporal, carotid, facial, brachial, radial–ulnar, subclavian, femoral, and dorsalis pedis. It is possible to control external bleeding in regions distal to the pressure point.

Open Wounds

Open wounds are seldom life threatening, unless they penetrate the head, chest, throat, or abdomen. These cases are serious emergencies that warrant EMS transport to an ED. Most soft tissue injuries are uncomplicated. They typically require irrigation, debridement (or surgical trimming), sutures, and antibiotics. Wounds that involve important structures such as nerve or muscle tissue, the genitalia, the eyes, and possibly the hands, require specialized care and will probably be referred.

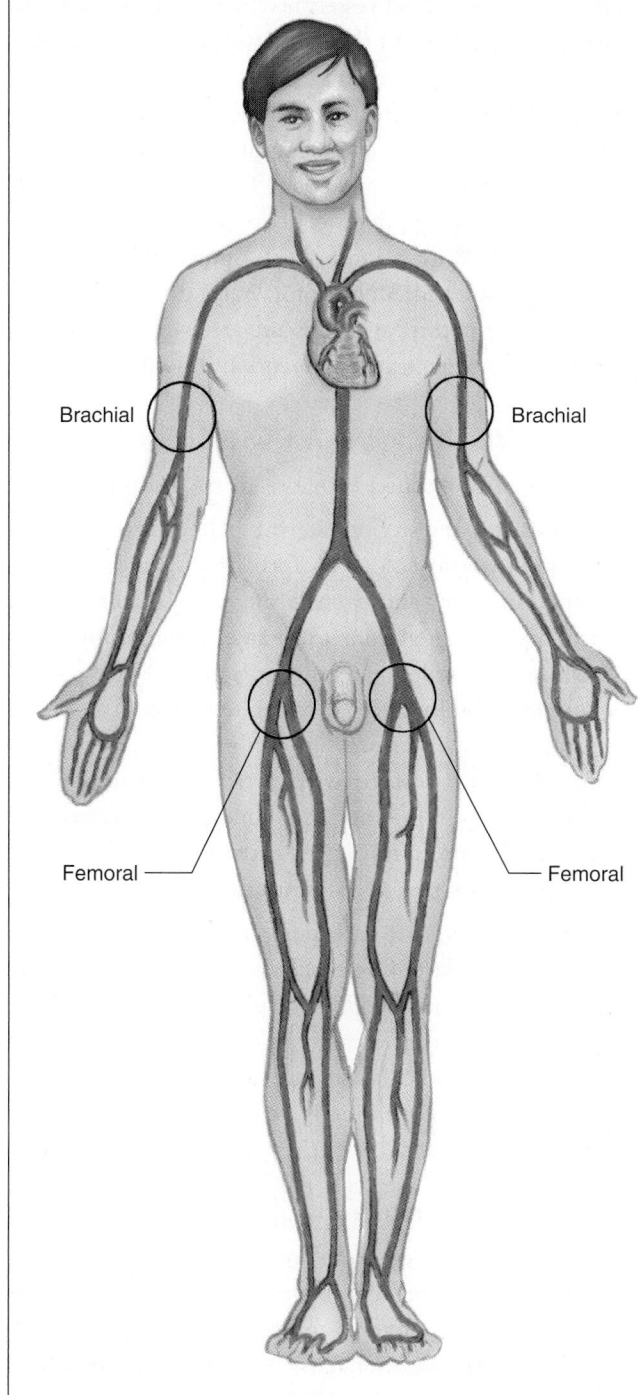

FIGURE 43-21 Brachial and femoral pressure points.

of abrasions include friction burns, rug burns, road rashes, and scrapes. Bleeding is usually in the form of oozing, and the injury is quite painful because nerve endings are exposed or damaged. As with all open wounds, the area is cleansed and any debris removed. Depending on the physician's choice, antibacterial ointment may be applied to the area and covered with a sterile dressing. Large areas of abraded tissue may require burn treatment.

Avulsions and Amputations

An avulsion is the tearing away of skin or tissue. Avulsions usually occur on limbs and appendages, including fingers, toes, hands, arms, feet, legs, nose, and penis. The body part may become entangled in machinery or be injured in a motor vehicle accident or a confrontation with an animal. Cleanse minor avulsion wounds with soap and water and return any skin flap to its normal position. Apply direct pressure, then apply a dressing when bleeding is controlled. If the body part has been amputated and recovered, cleanse the dismembered part with sterile saline. Wrap it with moist, sterile gauze, seal it in a plastic bag, and place the plastic bag in a container on ice. Prompt medical attention and preservation of the body part enhance the chances for successful reattachment. Cover the wound or stump with a sterile dressing until advanced treatment is available.

Lacerations and Incisions

A laceration is an open wound in which the skin and underlying tissue are torn. It usually has jagged edges that may interfere with the healing process. When vessels are torn, bleeding results and must be controlled by direct pressure, pressure on pressure points, or eventual suturing or application of Steri-Strips. Cleanse the laceration with soap and water or an antiseptic solution, removing all debris and foreign matter. If bleeding is severe, a physician should direct the cleansing process. On minor lacerations, after cleansing, the edges are approximated and then held together with a small dressing, such as a Band-Aid, Steri-Strip, or sterile butterfly. Lacerations over a joint may require joint immobilization for a few days while healing progresses. An incision is a cut with smooth edges made with a knife or other sharp object. It is treated in the same manner as any laceration. If the wound is deep or extensive, the physician usually performs a surgical intervention consisting of debridement, hemostasis, and trimming away of the jagged wound edges. If there is damage to underlying tissue, such as a tendon or ligament, further surgical intervention is required.

Puncture Wounds

A puncture wound results from a pointed foreign body penetrating the skin and tissue. Often the wound edges close,

You may see some industrial soft tissue injuries that appear quite dramatic but which will probably heal well after office treatment. The one thing that should matter to you most is something you can almost always control, and that is bleeding.

Abrasions

An abrasion occurs when the outer layer of skin is scraped away, leaving the underlying tissue exposed. Common types

trapping pathogens and debris in the tissue. Depending on the nature of the pointed object, cleansing may consist of simply soaking the area or may require invasive irrigation. After cleansing, a dressing is applied. Bleeding from a puncture wound is usually minimal.

Impaled Objects

A patient who has been impaled by an object such as a large piece of glass or sharp metal requires special treatment. The general rule is to leave the object in place until it can be safely removed by trained personnel. Stabilizing the object is critical to preventing further damage. Control bleeding and stabilize the impaled object with a bulky dressing held in place with tape or other bandages. Splint the area to prevent movement. For a small penetrating object, a small paper cup may be used. Make a hole in the bottom of the cup, place it over the object with the lip of the cup against the skin, and secure it with bandages.

Soft Tissue Injuries

Soft tissue trauma involves both the skin and underlying tissue. Abrasions, incisions, lacerations, and puncture wounds are easily identified as open-wound skin injuries. Avulsions, amputations, and thermal insults are considered soft tissue injuries because tissue as well as skin are involved. Contusions are closed soft tissue wounds in which the skin is not broken. Damage to the underlying tissue may involve blood vessels, nerves, muscles, and subcutaneous tissue. The tearing

of minute to larger blood vessels results in bleeding into the tissue and discoloration of the area. Swelling may exert pressure on nerve endings, creating pain. Crush injuries result when force is applied to the tissue. Depending on the area involved, the crush may be similar to pinching of tissue or so severe as to involve organs and bones. Elevating the body part above the heart and applying cold are often the only intervention needed. With a more severe injury, the body part should be immobilized. Monitoring vital signs and observing skin color, temperature, and moisture are essential to deciding whether more extensive intervention is needed.

WOUND CARE POINTERS

Following is a list of concepts that relate to dressing wounds:

- A **dressing** is a sterile covering placed directly over a wound to absorb blood and other body fluids, prevent contamination, and protect the wound from further trauma. Dressings come in many commercially available forms: sterile and nonsterile gauze (2×2s, 4×4s), compress (bulky sterile dressing to help control bleeding), occlusive (creates an airtight seal), petroleum (sterile gauze covered with petroleum that prevents the wound from sticking), and premedicated and packed dressings (medicated gauze for application over a wound, or strips to pack into the wound).

- A **bandage** is a strip of binding material used to hold a dressing in place. Commonly used dressings are roller gauze (e.g., Kerlix and Kling) and elastic bandages (e.g., Ace and Coban). A dressing or compress prefastened to a bandage is called a bandage compress (e.g., a Band-Aid). A pressure dressing is a compress held in place by an elastic bandage. All of these devices come in various widths. Choose the type and size that fit the wound. Bandage types depend on where the injury is located.

  Circular bandage turns are used to hold and secure a dressing in place. A figure-eight bandage is used for holding a dressing in place, bandaging joints, and providing immobilization of the area. A spiral turn is used to cover cylindrical (round) body parts such as the forehead. A reverse spiral turn is used for covering cone-shaped body parts such as the lower leg and forearm.

Simple direct pressure (as discussed) with a dressing (bulky if needed) will usually stop bleeding from a soft tissue injury. Once the direct pressure is determined to be sufficient, keep the dressing in place with a bandage as ordered by the physician. The priority will be to prevent infection by dressing the wound properly. That always begins with cleansing. Cleanse the wound from the center outward, beginning with vigorous irrigation using a disinfecting solution

PROFESSIONALISM
THE WORKPLACE

An important part of professionalism in the workplace includes time efficiency and preparedness. Many ideas can be implemented when working in a medical office to increase time efficiency, especially in the event of medical emergencies. For instance, you might suggest to the office manager or clinical supervisor the idea of creating wound care kits. These kits would include all necessary materials in the event that a patient with an open wound would present to the medical office. The kit may include alcohol, Betadine, gauze pads or rolls, sterile dressings, suture packs, and anything else determined appropriate by the physician. By having a prepared pack on hand, the medical staff will save time gathering supplies in emergency situations when time is of the essence.

DEMONSTRATE THE APPLICATION OF A PRESSURE BANDAGE

Objective: Correctly demonstrate the application of a pressure dressing.

EQUIPMENT AND SUPPLIES

dressing supplies or makeshift materials; gloves and other available PPE

METHOD

1. Escort the patient immediately to an examination room.
2. Perform hand hygiene.
3. Put on disposable gloves.
4. Under the physician's supervision, apply direct pressure with a dressing placed on the open wound. If possible, elevate the affected part.
5. After assessment, the physician will decide if EMS should be contacted.
6. Apply additional dressings as needed. Do not remove the original dressing.
7. Apply pressure to pressure points as necessary and with the physician's supervision.
8. If bleeding is controlled, anchor the dressing to maintain pressure.
9. If the physician orders, prepare the patient for transport to an emergency care facility.
10. Dispose of waste in a biohazard waste container.
11. Remove and discard gloves.
12. Perform hand hygiene and document the procedure in the patient's chart.

CHARTING EXAMPLE

08/31/XX 8:00 A.M. Pt came to office with 6" laceration to right forearm. Injury occurred from fight with 7-year-old brother when patient fell into glass patio door. Bleeding profusely. Physician called to examination room. B/P 96/60 P 100, regular but weak. R 26. Pt appears very nervous. Pt transported to ED to further control bleeding and take to surgery. Pt is alert and talking to parents. · · · · · · · · · · · · · · · · · S. Porter, CMA (AAMA)

---

prescribed by the physician. Wipe the edges of the wound in all directions away from the wound with sterile gauze, then cover with a sterile dressing and fasten the dressing in place. The use or nonuse of antibacterial ointments or creams should be specified by the physician. Procedure 43-6 describes the application of a pressure bandage, and Procedure 43-7 demonstrates the application of triangular, figure-eight, and tubular bandages.

DEMONSTRATE THE APPLICATION OF TRIANGULAR, FIGURE-EIGHT, AND TUBULAR BANDAGES

Objective: Correctly apply triangular, figure-eight, and tubular bandages.

EQUIPMENT AND SUPPLIES

elastic bandage; roller bandage; Kling bandage; tubular gauze and applicator; triangular bandage; tape; scissors

METHOD

1. Escort the patient immediately to an examination room. You may need to assist the patient, depending on the severity, location, and type of injury.
2. Explain the procedure to the patient.
3. Perform hand hygiene.
4. Gather necessary supplies.
5. Apply the bandage as follows.

TRIANGULAR BANDAGE

- Keep the injured arm as immobile as possible.
- Carefully slide the triangular bandage under the area to be held. The two shorter sides of the triangle should be

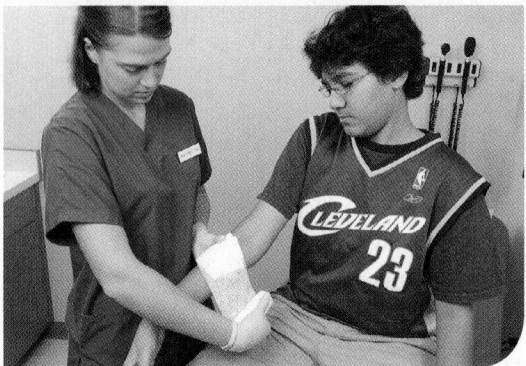

FIGURE 43-22 Complete one circle around the extremity or body part.

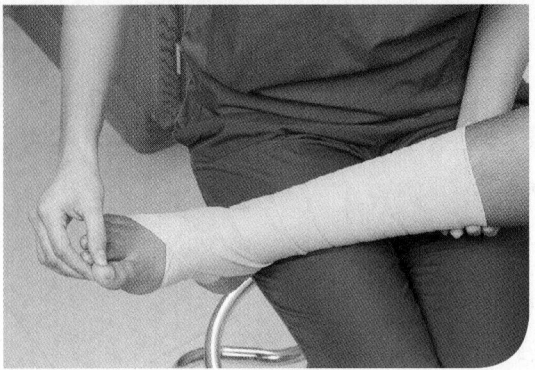

FIGURE 43-24 Bandage the patient's foot with toes exposed for monitoring circulation.

pointing toward the elbow, and the remaining longer edge should be parallel to the opposite body side.

- Bring the lowest side of the triangle up and over the arm.
- Tie the ends of the bandage behind and slightly to the side of the neck. Tuck the peak of the bandage in toward the elbow point of the bandage.
- The triangular bandage may also be wrapped around the head as a turban to anchor dressings onto the head.

FIGURE-EIGHT BANDAGE

- Place the thumb of one hand on one end of the bandage.
- Anchor the bandage with your other hand, then complete one circle around the extremity or body part (Figure 43-22).
- Continue to alternate wrapping above and below the body joint or dressing and circling behind the joint or dressing area until the injured area is covered adequately (Figure 43-23). If applying a bandage to a foot, ensure that toes are exposed to evaluate circulation (Figure 43-24).

TUBULAR BANDAGE

- Choose an applicator that is larger than the extremity to be bandaged.
- Cut an approximate amount of tubular gauze bandage and slide the gathered bandage onto the applicator (Figure 43-25).
- Slide the applicator over the extremity (Figure 43-26).

- Hold the bandage against the proximal end of the extremity and pull the applicator approximately 1 inch past the distal end (Figure 43-27).
- Twist the bandage gauze one complete turn.
- Next, slide the applicator toward the proximal end of the injury (Figure 43-28).
- Hold the proximal end of the tubular bandage gauze in place, and pull the applicator toward the distal end.
- After pulling past the distal end, complete one twist.
- Slide back and forth, and twist the distal end of the dressing until the injured area is adequately covered.

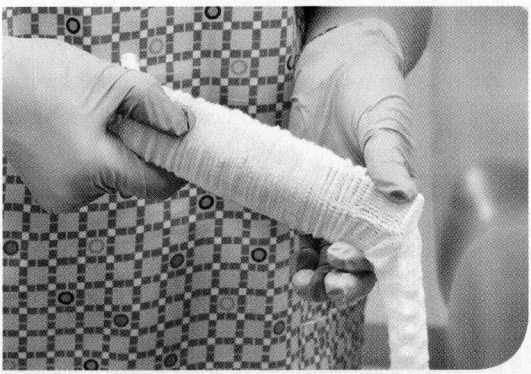

FIGURE 43-25 Gather the gauze bandage onto a tubular gauze applicator.

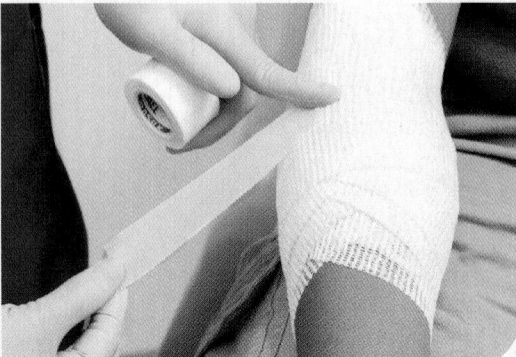

FIGURE 43-23 Wrap above and below the body joint or dressing.

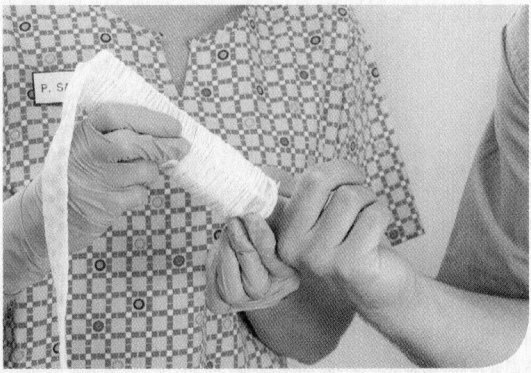

FIGURE 43-26 Slide the applicator on the body part.

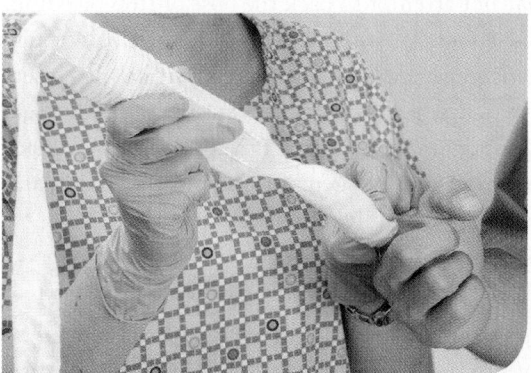

FIGURE 43-27 Position the applicator 1 inch past the distal end.

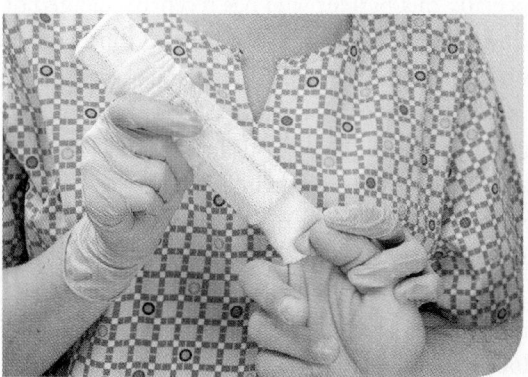

FIGURE 43-28 Slide the applicator toward the proximal end of the injury.

- Cut excess dressing but remember to anchor the bandage at the proximal end.
6. Instruct the patient to watch for signs of circulation impairment.
7. Perform hand hygiene.
8. Document the procedure and patient teaching.

CHARTING EXAMPLE

07/22/XX 9:30 A.M. Figure-eight bandage applied to arm as instructed by physician. Pt stated that arm feels supported and less painful. Pt stated awareness of follow-up appointment and that he will call if pain and swelling become worse. · · · · · · · · ·
· M. Mason, RMA

Figure 43-29 provides a classification of open wounds for injuries. Open soft tissue wounds can be superficial (penetrating only the skin) or deep (penetrating the fascia, or connective layer beneath the skin, and other structures that lie deeper still). Once bleeding is controlled and the wound dressed, obtain a complete set of vital signs and allow patients to remain in the supine position or the position that brings greatest comfort while you take the time to document in the chart. Watch for signs of shock and treat as needed. Next, get patients into a sitting position and make sure they are not dizzy and that they understand their home care instructions. When patient is ready, provide assistance to a standing position, again ensuring stability prior to allowing the patient to leave. If there are signs of shock, notify the physician immediately and do not leave patients alone. If instructed by your physician, contact EMS.

Epistaxis

Nontraumatic epistaxis (nosebleed) may be messy and embarrassing, but it is usually a benign (not life threatening) occurrence. Nosebleeds tend to occur most commonly in dry weather or in dusty conditions and are usually easy to treat.

Bleeding from both nostrils tends to be more serious than bleeding from just one nostril. A nosebleed that occurs after a head injury and does not stop should be considered a serious emergency until proven otherwise. Even if there is no history of trauma, at least three other circumstances should worry

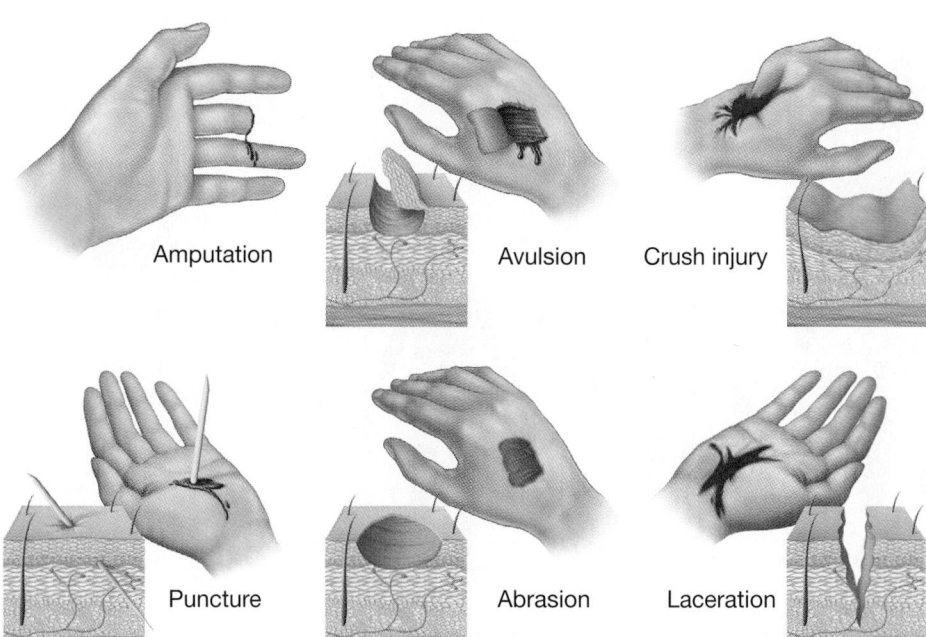

FIGURE 43-29 Classification of open injuries.

a caregiver about persistent nosebleeds. One is high blood pressure, especially in a patient who has recently changed or stopped taking medicines for the condition. Another is a clotting disorder of some kind. The third is a patient history of nosebleeds that have caused shock in the past.

Nosebleeds severe enough to cause changes in a patient's vital signs are rare, but they do occur. If the patient's vital signs are normal in the absence of trauma, the patient should be seated upright. If the vital signs are compromised, the patient should lie on the affected side and may need oxygen.

If the blood emerges from both nostrils, its origin is not in the nose but somewhere above it, and it requires the immediate attention of a physician or **stat** (immediate) transport to an emergency department. A nosebleed that emanates from one nostril is easily treated by a physician. To stop it, the physician will grasp a facial tissue by one corner and twist that corner firmly into a Christmas-tree shape about 4 inches long. The physician inserts the pack deeply into the patient's affected nostril, while continuing to twist it and until the nostril is firmly packed. Then a washcloth is placed over the patient's upper face, and the patient is instructed to hold a chemical cold pack against the washcloth so it fits the bridge of the nose like a saddle.

Bleeding should stop after only a few minutes, at which time the packing can be removed. If bleeding does not stop, electrocautery may be necessary. The physician may be able to perform this treatment in the office, or the patient may require transport to an emergency department.

If trauma is a possible factor in the medical office, the physician may not attempt to pack the nose or stop bleeding. In this case, contact 911 immediately and anticipate transport to the emergency department. The physician may insert an oral airway if the patient is unresponsive. (Do not use a nasal airway in a patient with this type of condition.) Place the patient on high-flow oxygen by nonrebreather mask, and monitor the patient carefully for changes in status.

BURNS

A burn injury occurs when an area of tissue is destroyed by the action of physical heat, chemical activity, high electrical current, or heavy exposure to radiation. The severity of a burn depends on the amount and depth of tissue injury. Survival depends on those factors in addition to the amount of surface area that is destroyed. Destruction of skin surface is an important consideration because of all the skin functions that are lost: insulation, regulation of fluids, sensation, and protection from infection. All of these are crucial to life.

If directed by a physician, the medical assistant may help stop the burning and remove any metal jewelry from the burn patient.

Classification of Burns

Burns are classified in two basic ways: by surface area and by depth. The **Rule of Nines** is a useful tool for estimating body surface area (Figure 43-30). For an adult, each of the following areas represents 9 percent of the body surface: head and

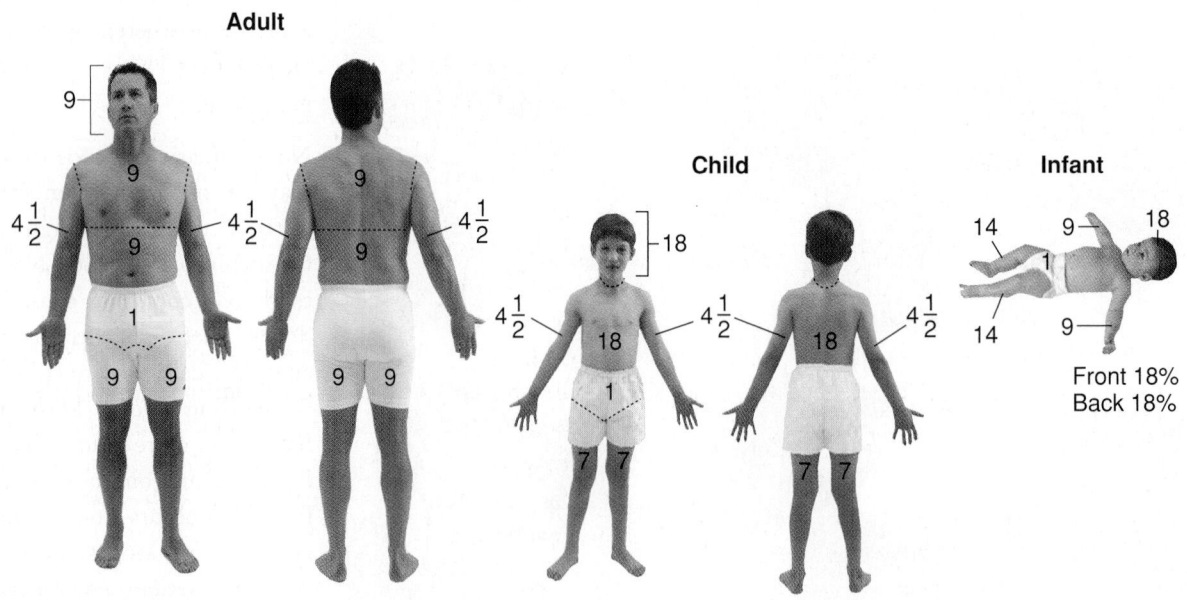

Adult

Child

Infant

Front 18%
Back 18%

Note: Each arm totals 9% (front of arm $4\frac{1}{2}$%, back of arm $4\frac{1}{2}$%)

FIGURE 43-30 Rule of Nine for burns.

TABLE 43-6 Classification of Burns

Degree	Characteristics
First	Reddening, swelling of epidermis (like a mild sunburn)
Second	Reddening, swelling of epidermis and outer dermis; blisters noted
Third	Charring of all layers of skin and at least some deeper structures

neck, each upper extremity, chest, abdomen, upper back, lower back and buttocks, the front of each lower extremity, and the back of each lower extremity. These make up 99 percent of the body's surface. The remaining 1 percent is assigned to the genital region.

In the Rule of Nines, the percentages are modified for infants and young children, whose heads are much larger in relationship to the rest of the body. In addition, Table 43-6 will give you a basic idea of burn severity by depth.

First- and second-degree burns are extremely painful, even those involving very small areas. Third-degree burns tend not to be painful immediately because, along with the entire dermis, this kind of burn destroys sensory nerve endings. However, it also disrupts all the normal functions of skin, including its self-regenerative properties and its ability to resist infection. Third-degree burns are profound injuries, even if they only involve a small amount of surface area.

Certain special considerations can also help determine the seriousness of a burn:

- The mortality of serious burns is higher for elderly patients and for very young patients.

- The mortality is higher if the patient was burned in a closed area (partly due to the possibility of carbon monoxide poisoning and partly due to the possibility of airway burns).

- Burns of the genitalia are always considered serious, regardless of depth.

- Always consider the possibility of other injuries besides burns, especially in a patient who was burned in an auto or industrial accident.

- Patients with chemical burns should have the area irrigated immediately with large amounts of water. If the burns resulted from an alkali substance, irrigation should be continued for a minimum of 20 minutes. Contact EMS as soon as you encounter such a patient to be sure that you have access to the proper resources

as early as possible if you are dealing with a hazardous substance that cannot be rendered harmless.

- Electrical burns serious enough to leave marks on the body are considered serious burns because of the probability of internal injuries. (Electrocution by lightning is always considered serious until proven otherwise.)

These factors are all regarded as stand-alone admission criteria by trauma centers in most places. Treatment for first-degree burns involving less than 10 percent of the body surface includes pain relief by means of cool water. That instantly relieves pain, but it is not appropriate for larger surface areas. Damaged skin may not be able to regulate body temperature, so the use of cooling measures over large surface areas can cause hypothermia. Analgesic creams and ointments are appropriate for use on first-degree burns only if ordered by the physician.

Cool water can also be used to soothe second-degree burns for small surface areas, as long as there are no broken blisters. Second-degree burns of any size should not be treated with creams or ointments, due to the risk of breaking blisters and the resulting potential for infection.

Burns of any kind that involve broken skin may need to be debrided (removal of dead or damaged tissue) by a physician. If third-degree burns are present in any amount, the patient warrants treatment at a trauma center. Burns should be dressed with dry sterile dressings, and pain should be managed with injectable analgesics as ordered. If paramedics transport the patient, they will start the IV and administer analgesics via that route if the physician has not already done so.

Upper airway burns constitute a dire emergency and always warrant prompt intubation by the physician or EMS with the largest tube that can be inserted. The epiglottis can swell quickly and make intubation very difficult or impossible at a later time. If the patient sounds even slightly hoarse or complains of difficulty breathing, or if you notice stridor in any burn patient, consider the possibility of airway burns and notify the physician right away. Administer oxygen as ordered by the physician.

Large surface-area burns should be dressed with dry sterile sheets that are wrapped entirely around the patient's body. These patients benefit most from prompt transport to a trauma center. All burn patients should be monitored for signs of shock, especially in the case of large surface-area involvement.

HEAT EXHAUSTION

Heat exhaustion, which is an extreme fatigue due to heat, occurs as the result of sodium and water depletion from the body. Strenuous activity often precedes heat exhaustion, as the individual becomes overheated and perspires profusely. The skin is moist, pale, and cool, and body temperature is normal. The individual may complain of headache, muscle cramps, weakness, dizziness, and nausea. He or she should be moved to a cooler environment and encouraged to lie down. Apply cool compresses and give sips of water if the individual is conscious. Heat exhaustion can usually be prevented by taking salt pills and drinking lots of water before, during, and after strenuous activities in a warm environment.

HYPERTHERMIA

Prolonged exposure to extremely hot temperatures often results in an elevated body temperature, or **hyperthermia**. The loss of water and salt through perspiration leads to a state of mild shock. If the body's cooling mechanisms fail, heat exhaustion can progress into heat stroke. An individual experiencing heat stroke usually fails to perspire and has a body temperature of 105°F or higher. The skin is dry, red, and hot to the touch. Headache, shortness of breath, nausea or vomiting, dizziness, weakness, and dry mouth are common symptoms. At the onset the pulse is rapid, but it gradually slows and becomes weak, and the blood pressure begins to drop. Mental confusion may appear, possibly accompanied by irritability and hysterical behavior. In some cases the patient collapses. If he or she remains exposed to heat, brain cells begin to die and permanent brain damage or even death may eventually result. The patient must be removed from the environment immediately. Loosen the clothing and cool the body down as quickly as possible by pouring cool water over the patient or sponging with a cool, wet cloth. If heat stroke is suspected, after the initial emergency treatment EMS should be contacted to transport the patient to an emergency facility where vital signs and cardiac status can be monitored. The patient should not be left alone and should be assessed by a physician as promptly as possible.

HYPOTHERMIA

The patient with **hypothermia** is also at great risk. Hypothermia results from prolonged exposure to cold or cold water and can cause the core temperature to drop below 95°F. The patient shivers and experiences a numbness and tingling throughout the body. The skin becomes very cool to the touch and is pale with a blue or ashy tinge. Respirations are slow and shallow, and the patient becomes disoriented and eventually unconscious as body functions and organs slow down to the point of complete shutdown.

Treatment involves removing any cold, wet clothing and wrapping the patient in warm blankets. Heat packs may be used but not directly on the skin. Once the patient is conscious, offer sips of warm liquid. When possible, the patient should be transported to a treatment facility for assessment by a physician.

SEIZURES

Convulsions, or seizures, are produced by disorganized electrical activity in the brain and are characterized by involuntary muscle contractions that alternate between the contraction and relaxation of muscles. In some cases the convulsions are generalized, involving the entire body, or localized and limited to a specific area of the body. Convulsions can result from a number of problems or combinations of problems.

By themselves, convulsions are not life threatening, but the muscle spasms that come with full-body seizures can restrict breathing. Seizure patients may also bite their tongues, causing bleeding and swelling, which can obstruct the airway. Finally, seizure patients are sometimes injured when their convulsions cause them to fall.

Once a seizure stops, especially a full-body seizure, it is normal for a patient to remain unconscious for as long as 15 minutes. During that time, most patients cannot control their secretions—for example, urine—the way they would in normal sleep.

A medical assistant can do two important things for a seizing patient. First, prevent injuries. Keep the patient from falling, and prevent the head from striking anything until the seizure stops. Second, pay close attention to what the patient is experiencing so you can describe it later. Observations will eventually be very important to the patient's neurologist. If breathing seems adequate, note the patient's response, apply oxygen as ordered, and place the patient on the left side to allow any secretions to drain. Listen for noise in the airway, and be prepared to assist the patient.

You must immediately notify your physician. If the physician is not available, contact EMS and anticipate transport. Continue to assess the patient until EMS personnel arrive, and communicate your findings to them.

FAINTING

Many serious disorders cause unresponsiveness. Fainting, or syncope, is the sudden loss of consciousness. It seems to be caused by a brief interruption in the body's ability to control the brain's circulation. Fainting often occurs just after a patient has received an emotional shock of some kind. The patient usually collapses and becomes unresponsive but, within a minute, should awaken and return to normal function. Patients seldom become incontinent or have seizures as a result of simple fainting but may be injured in the course of a fall.

There is always a reason for unresponsiveness, and determining the reason is, of course, important. However, early in your contact with any unconscious patient, your first concern should be to take care of the ABCDs. A patient who suddenly becomes unresponsive may be experiencing arrhythmia such as ventricular fibrillation or ventricular tachycardia. If a patient has fainted and there is no response, provide oxygen if the physician orders this. Check the ABCs and call for help. If the patient is breathing well but will not wake up, place him or her on the left side and contact your physician. If your physician is not available, contact EMS. While you await their arrival, try to get a good set of vital signs and if possible obtain a blood sugar reading. Procedure 43-8 illustrates how to assist a patient who has fainted.

MUSCULOSKELETAL INJURIES

Musculoskeletal injuries involve bones, muscles, tendons, and ligaments and include fractures, dislocations, sprains, and strains. Definitive diagnosis is made by X-ray, but these injuries must be considered fractured bones until determined to be otherwise. Therefore, the affected part must be immobilized.

Fractures

In a closed or simple fracture, the bone is broken but does not penetrate the skin (Figure 43-31). In an open or compound fracture, the bone pierces the skin, or the skin is torn open by the bone or by an external force (Figure 43-32). Fractures may also be single or multiple breaks in the bone. Bone breaks can be complete, twisted, or splintered. The affected part is immobilized and examined for impaired circulation to the distal aspect. The location of the fracture and the possible presence of heavy bleeding or bruising are also determined. Knowing the cause of the injury is very helpful in this assessment. A fracture may occur in any bone. Special precautions must be taken for suspected fractures of the spinal column or skull. For any injury caused by sudden acceleration and deceleration, the cervical spine must be immobilized. Other injuries to the spinal column require extreme caution when moving the patient. The best response is to call 911. Allow EMS professionals to immobilize the cervical spine with a cervical collar, then logroll the patient onto a spine board for transport to a facility where X-rays can be taken to determine the extent of the injury. Suspected fractures of the thigh (femur) and pelvis also require

procedure

43-8

RESPOND TO A PATIENT WHO HAS FAINTED

Objective: Correctly care for a patient who has fainted, within the time limit set by the instructor.

EQUIPMENT AND SUPPLIES

blanket; foot stool or box

METHOD

1. If the patient communicates a faint feeling, help the patient sit, bend forward, and place the head on the knees. If the patient collapses with no warning, do not move the patient. The patient may have sustained a neck or back injury.
2. Immediately notify the physician.
3. Loosen any tight clothing, and cover the patient with the blanket for warmth.
4. If the physician directs, use the foot stool to support the patient's legs in a raised position.
5. If the physician directs, call for EMS.
6. Once the emergency passes, obtain a full set of vital signs and document all activities in the patient's medical record.

CHARTING EXAMPLE

6/8/XX 10:45 A.M. Patient in exam room states that she feels faint. Patient was instructed to lower her head to her knees. Instructed to and assisted with loosening of clothing. Physician notified. BP 116/62, P 82 and regular, R 20. Patient remained in position for 3 minutes until symptoms subsided. Patient transferred to exam room and physician notified and evaluated patient. · M. Jimenez, RMA

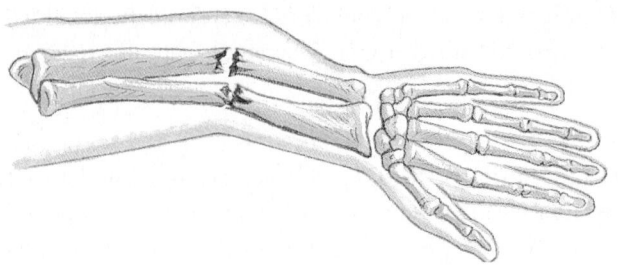

FIGURE 43-31 A closed fracture.

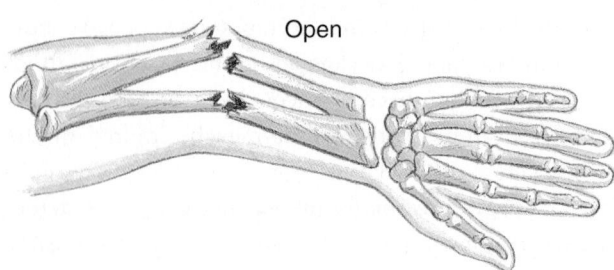

Open

FIGURE 43-32 An open fracture.

immobilization and transport and are best handled by the EMS. In open or compound fractures, the soft tissue injury must be tended. Cover the open wound with a sterile, saline-moistened dressing, then place a sterile occlusive dressing over that. Generally, the tissue must be surgically cleaned and debrided.

Splint Application

Fractures of long bones require immobilization by splinting to prevent joint movement above and below the fracture.

In addition to preventing additional damage to the bone and surrounding soft tissue, the splint helps to relieve pain and allows safe movement of the injured part. Another comfort measure is the application of cold, usually after splinting, to prevent swelling. Procedure 43-9 lists the proper steps for splint application.

Sprains, Strains, and Dislocations

A *sprain* occurs when muscles, tendons, or ligaments are torn. It may be the result of trauma or cumulative overuse of

procedure
43-9

DEMONSTRATE THE APPLICATION OF A SPLINT

Objective: To correctly apply a splint with minimal movement to the affected extremity and without impairment to circulation or neurological status.

EQUIPMENT AND SUPPLIES
makeshift or sterile dressing supplies; stiff or solid materials to immobilize the extremity; bandages or strips of material to secure splint materials

METHOD
1. Identify the patient and introduce yourself.
2. Obtain vital signs.
3. Ask the patient, if conscious, to speak his or her name.
4. Ask about medication allergies and any prescription or over-the-counter medications the patient may be taking. Also inquire about the patient's medical history.
5. Assess the area of suspected fracture for bruising, bleeding, and open areas or protruding bones.
6. Moving the limb as little as possible, and with gentle traction on the distal side, place the splint with padding under the limb or alongside the limb. You may have to ask other clinical staff for help to ensure the least amount of discomfort for the least amount of time.

7. Place sterile dressings or clean makeshift dressings gently over open areas.
8. Secure the splint by wrapping bandages or strips of material around the splint and the limb. The ties must be above and below the joints on both sides of the suspected fracture.
9. Add additional ties as necessary along the length of the splint.
10. If possible, leave an exposed area, such as toes or fingers, so that circulation can be monitored.
11. The splint should be snug enough to immobilize the limb but not tight.

CHARTING EXAMPLE
12/23/XX 8:30 A.M. Pt came to office with splint applied to lower leg and foot. Pt states that brakes failed on bike, he swerved to miss a dog, and was thrown from bike when it ran into a tree. A passerby called his wife, who splinted the lower leg. Pt complains of severe pain and has pliable cold pack applied to area of leg pain. Pt is able to move toes, which are pink and warm.··················· W. Hughley, CMA (AAMA)

the joint. A *strain,* often called a pulled muscle, occurs when a muscle or tendon is overextended by stretching. The patient complains of pain and may be unable to use the joint. In the lower extremities, weight bearing is painful and sometimes impossible. In a *dislocation,* the bone is actually pulled away from the joint, stretching or tearing the ligaments and tendons. A deformity is generally noted. Dislocations must be reduced and the bone reinserted into the joint. The injured body parts should be immobilized to prevent additional damage and reduce pain. Applications of cold also help with the pain and slow edema. The physician assesses the injury and usually orders radiographs to eliminate the possibility of fracture and diagnose sprain, strain, or dislocation.

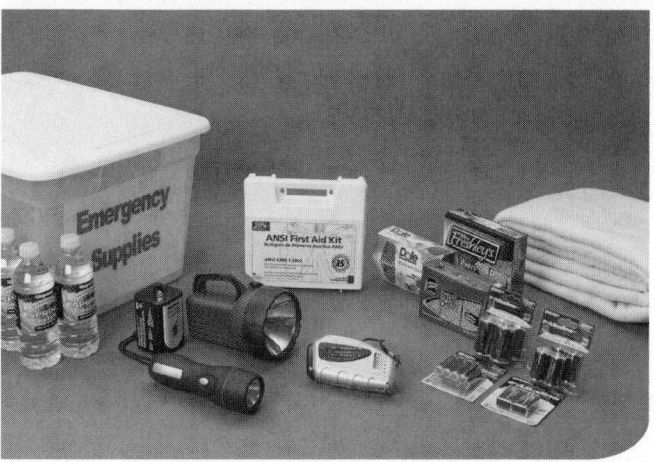

FIGURE 43-33 Every medical office should keep emergency supplies in a waterproof container.

Emergency Preparedness

The medical assistant should be knowledgeable in the area of emergency preparedness. This includes knowing how to respond in the event of a human-caused disaster, such as a terrorist event, and to a natural disaster, such as a hurricane. Remaining calm in the event of an emergency is paramount to the success of handling it. Through proper education, preparedness, and simulation, a medical assistant can play a key role in emergency response.

EARTHQUAKES

Because earthquakes can happen at any time, and without any warning, the medical assistant must know how to respond to this type of emergency. One of the first steps to preventing injury during an earthquake is to prepare before an earthquake happens. Advance preparation may save lives as well as prevent injuries. According to the Federal Emergency Management Agency (FEMA), six steps are involved in planning ahead for an earthquake as well other emergency situations:

1. Check for hazards around the facility.
   - Make sure shelves are fastened securely to walls.
   - Keep large or heavy objects on lower shelves.
   - Store any breakable items in low, closed cabinets equipped with locks.
   - Do not hang heavy items on walls above where patients will sit or lie.
   - Secure overhead light fixtures.
   - Repair any defective electrical wiring or leaky gas connections.
   - Strap water heaters to wall studs and bolt them to the floor.
   - Repair any deep cracks in ceilings or foundations.

   - Store all flammable products on the bottom shelves of closed cabinets with locks.

2. Identify safe places indoors and outdoors.
   - Under sturdy furniture
   - Against an inside wall
   - Away from glass that could shatter
   - Away from bookcases or furniture that could fall over
   - In the open, away from buildings, trees, telephone or electrical lines, overpasses, or elevated expressways

3. Educate yourself and your coworkers.
   - Contact the local EMS office or American Red Cross chapter for information.
   - Teach all staff members how and when to turn off gas, electricity, and water.

4. Have disaster supplies on hand (Figure 43-33).
   - Flashlight and extra batteries
   - Portable battery-operated radio and extra batteries
   - First-aid kit and manual
   - Emergency food and water
   - Extra blankets

5. Develop an emergency communication plan.
   - In case staff members are separated from one another during an earthquake, have a plan in place for reuniting after the disaster.
   - Define the expectations of each staff member: Who will escort patients from the building? Who will check the treatment rooms?

6. Help your community get ready.
   - Provide literature for patients on how to prepare for an earthquake.

procedure
43-10

DEVELOP AN ENVIRONMENTAL EXPOSURE PLAN

Objective: To develop an environmental exposure plan.

EQUIPMENT AND SUPPLIES

pen; paper; computer; copy machine; various emergency supplies; waterproof containers

METHOD

1. Create an emergency kit that can be used by your office in the event of an environmental emergency. Supplies may include flashlights, batteries, bottles of water, nonperishable food, bandages, alcohol and hydrogen peroxide, blankets, vinyl or latex gloves, tweezers, scissors, self-powered radio, and medications (ibuprofen, acetaminophen, antihistamines, antibiotic ointment, tetanus vaccines, etc.).
2. Enclose the kit in a waterproof container.
3. Place the kit in a safe area, such as a medicine closet or storage closet.
4. Create evacuation plans and make sure that every room in the medical office has a detailed exit route posted.
5. Create a delineation chart that outlines responsibilities of office staff members in the event of an emergency.
6. Create a list of safety zones that can be used in the event of an emergency (e.g., a safety zone in the event of a tornado, an outdoor safety zone in the event of a fire, a safety zone in the event of a flood).
7. Make photocopies of the safety zone list, evacuation plan, and delineation chart for everyone in the office. Laminate and hang copies in the employee break room.
8. Train all office staff on the environmental exposure plan within 10 days of hire.

Procedure 43-10 includes the steps to creating an environmental exposure plan.

TORNADOS

According to FEMA, tornados are the most violent storms occurring in nature. Very erratic in nature, tornados can strike with very little or no warning. The warning signs of a tornado include thunderstorms with heavy rain and large hail; dark, almost greenish colored skies; and dark, low-lying clouds. Many people have related the sound of a tornado to that of a freight train.

Often tornado watches and warnings are issued before a tornado touches down. A tornado watch indicates that the weather conditions are right for a tornado and a tornado is possible, whereas a tornado warning indicates that a tornado has been sighted and all persons are to take shelter immediately.

It is important to designate a safe area within the office should a tornado watch occur during working hours. This often will be the basement of a building or the lowest level of a structure. If a basement is not available, it is advisable to seek shelter in a closet or interior hallway. Above all else, stay away from windows, doors, and outside walls. Avoid elevators and use the stairs to reach the lowest level of the facility.

Prior to the occurrence of a tornado (or an earthquake, hurricane, or other natural disaster), it is important to educate yourself, fellow office staff, and the community about safety precautions. The role that a medical assistant will play in the event of a natural disaster is discussed toward the end of this chapter.

FIRES

Because more than 4,000 Americans die and more than 25,000 are injured in fires each year, the medical assistant should be prepared to respond to this type of disaster. Fire spreads quickly, and typically no time is available to gather belongings or make a telephone call. In just 2 minutes, a fire can become life threatening, and in 5 minutes a fire can engulf a building. Heat and smoke from fire are often more dangerous than the flames.

The medical office should be equipped with properly working smoke alarms. These should be placed on every level of the building and in every room, either on the ceiling or high on the walls. Every smoke alarm should be tested and cleaned once per month. The batteries in every alarm should be replaced at least once per year, and every individual alarm should be replaced once every 10 years.

The medical assistant should know the escape routes to use in the event of a fire. Staff members should practice those escape routes. If the office is located above the first level, escape ladders may be used.

Any flammable items must be stored in well-ventilated areas, and care must be taken in placing any items near a heat source or heating vent. Any defective wiring must be repaired to avoid a fire hazard. Fire extinguishers should be located throughout the office, and staff should be trained in their use.

During a fire, the medical assistant should be aware that if a person's clothes are on fire, that person should stop, drop, and roll until the fire is extinguished. Running makes the fire burn faster.

When escaping a fire, the medical assistant should check closed doors for heat before opening. This is done by using the back of the hand to feel the top of the door, the doorknob, and the crack between the door and the door frame before opening the door. If the door is hot, it should not be opened, and another route of escape should be sought. If the door is cool, it should be opened slowly. The medical assistant should crawl low under any smoke on the way to the exit and close doors as they are passed through to delay the spread of fire. Once out of the building, the medical assistant should not attempt to reenter until or unless the fire department declares that action to be safe. (Chapter 6 also deals with basic fire safety within the medical office).

FLOODS

FEMA declares floods to be the most common hazard in the United States. Some floods can develop over days of rainy weather; others may be in the form of flash floods and may come on very quickly. The medical assistant should be aware of the flood dangers that exist in his or her local area. During a flood, the medical assistant should listen to the radio for information. In the event of a flash flood, the medical assistant should move to higher ground. If there is time before evacuating, the medical assistant should disconnect any electrical equipment and shut off utilities at their main valves. When evacuating,

the medical assistant should be careful not to walk through moving water. Only 6 inches of moving water can make a person fall.

HURRICANES

Hurricanes can strike with little warning, although most will allow for some advance warning, giving the medical office staff time to prepare. If the office is in the path of a hurricane, the windows may need to be secured; this can be done using permanent storm shutters or $\frac{5}{8}$-inch plywood cut to fit and ready to install. Trees and shrubs around the office should be well trimmed. Secure rain gutters, and clean clogged ones. If the medical office is to be evacuated before a hurricane, the medical assistant should listen to the radio or television for information and instructions provided by local emergency management personnel. During the hurricane, the medical assistant should listen to the radio or television for additional information.

TERRORISM

In the event of a terrorist attack, the medical assistant should be aware of the steps to take in each of the following types of emergencies.

Explosions

In the event of a bomb threat, the medical assistant should try to obtain as much information from the caller as possible. The following questions should be asked:

1. When is the bomb going to explode?
2. Where is the bomb right now?
3. What does it look like?
4. What kind of bomb is it?
5. What will cause it to explode?

Any information obtained should be immediately provided to the police, and their instructions should be followed. If an explosion has occurred, the medical assistant should respond by following the steps as if an earthquake or fire has occurred.

Biological Threats

There are four methods of delivery of a biological agent:

1. **Aerosols**—Agents are dispersed into the air, forming a mist that may drift for miles.
2. **Animals**—Some diseases are spread by insects or animals.

3. **Food and water contamination**—Some agents are placed in the food or water supply.

4. **Person to person**—Some spread of agents is possible via direct contact among people.

To prepare for a biological attack, the medical facility may have a high efficiency particulate air (HEPA) filter installed. In the event of a biological attack, the medical assistant should be prepared to move away from the contaminant quickly, wash with soap and water, contact authorities, listen to the radio for instructions, and remove and bag clothing if contaminated. (Chapter 34 provides a detailed explanation regarding bacteria, viruses, and other agents that can cause illness and death in humans, animals, or plants).

Nuclear Blast

In the event of a nuclear attack, the medical assistant should take cover as quickly as possible, below ground if the building has a basement. The medical assistant should remain in a safe location, listening to the radio for instructions. The medical assistant should not look at the flash or fireball but should lie flat on the ground with the head covered and seek shelter as quickly as possible.

MOCK ENVIRONMENTAL EXPOSURES

Medical assistants can play a vital role in the event of an environmental emergency. It is helpful to be prepared for such events by understanding how to help patients and provide assistance to other health care providers. Organizations within the community, colleges, and hospitals may offer mock environmental exposure events. These events provide real-life scenarios and situations that may arise during times of disaster. Examples of mock environmental events include a tornado site with injured patients, an exposure to a biological chemical, or treating injured patients of flash floods or hurricanes. The role of the medical assistant will vary in every situation; however, overall, medical assistants may be able to provide assistance in numerous ways:

- Aiding in evacuation plans

- Triaging patients to determine which patients require immediate attention

- Assisting in first-aid response for wounded individuals

- Administering tetanus and other vaccines under the direction of a physician

- Facilitating order and organization in the midst of chaos

- Implementing and following through on an environmental safety plan

SUMMARY

Each team member must know what procedures to follow in a medical emergency. As a medical assistant, you will need advanced training in CPR, AED, and treating specialty office emergencies, such as allergic reactions. Patients may experience fainting, seizures, anaphylactic shock, and other conditions when visiting the medical office for other health reasons. Contacting the physician and EMS, if necessary, is part of office protocol. Good Samaritan laws were established to encourage health care professionals to volunteer in emergencies without fear of financial liability. It is important that health care professionals render emergency care according to the scope of license, certification, or training until relieved by another health professional. EMS may be called for on-the-scene care, stabilization of the patient, and transport to the appropriate emergency department for further assessment and treatment. Equipment is kept for medical emergencies in the medical office. Medical assistants must have an understanding of the various facets of emergency preparedness. Students are encouraged to create an environmental exposure control plan as well as participate in mock environmental exposure scenarios.

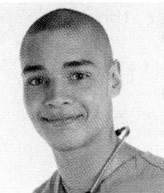

43 CHAPTER REVIEW

COMPETENCY REVIEW

1. Define and spell the terms to learn for this chapter.

2. Elicit a good primary assessment without wasting time.

3. Discuss the signs and symptoms of, as well as treatment for, insulin shock and diabetic coma.

4. Correctly perform CPR on an adult.

5. Identify when it is appropriate to use abdominal thrusts in a patient with an obstructed airway.

6. Correctly demonstrate the application of a splint.

7. Identify supplies that are necessary to create an emergency kit for the medical office.

PREPARING FOR THE CERTIFICATION EXAMINATION

1. Which of the following is not a role of EMS?
   a. provide on-the-scene intervention and treatment
   b. prepare the patient for transport
   c. diagnose patients
   d. administer emergency medications
   e. intubate a patient

2. Who decides the equipment and supplies to have stocked on a crash cart?
   a. medical office manager
   b. certified medical assistant
   c. clinical supervisor
   d. physician
   e. malpractice insurance company

3. When assessing an unconscious infant for responsiveness you should
   a. sharply poke the feet
   b. gently shake the shoulders
   c. locate a pulse
   d. shout the infant's name
   e. immediately begin CPR

4. Another term for an abrasion is
   a. avulsion
   b. amputation
   c. friction burn

   d. puncture
   e. laceration

5. A severe allergic reaction to a substance is known as
   a. metabolic shock
   b. anaphylactic shock
   c. hypoallergenic shock
   d. neurological collapse
   e. sepsis

6. Hypoglycemia is present when a patient's
   a. blood sugar is above 120 mg/dL
   b. blood sugar is between 80–90 mg/dL
   c. blood sugar is below 200 mg/dL
   d. blood sugar is above 300 mg/dL
   e. blood sugar is below 70 mg/dL

7. Arterial bleeding is
   a. slow and bright red
   b. rapid and dark red
   c. slow and dark red
   d. rapid and bright red
   e. pulsating and dark red

8. Hyperthermia occurs when a person's body temperature reaches
   a. 105°F
   b. 95°F

c. 109°F

d. 89°F

e. 103°F

9. Syncope is another term for

  a. vomiting

  b. a blood infection

  c. fainting

  d. dizziness

  e. respiratory distress

10. FEMA declares this disaster to be the most common hazard in the United States:

  a. hurricane

  b. flood

  c. tornado

  d. earthquake

  e. bioterrorism

CRITICAL THINKING

1. What should be Lewis's immediate concern and action on hearing the emergency tornado warning announcement?

2. How can Lewis assist in ensuring the safety of the patients and staff members of the medical office?

3. How could Lewis and the other staff members of Pearson Physicians Group prepare for natural disasters, such as the tornado?

ON THE JOB

Mary Ann, a medical assistant, works in a busy primary care office operated by two physicians, Dr. Johnson and Dr. Laskar. It is Saturday, so the staff consists of just Mary Ann, Dr. Johnson, and another medical assistant named Valerie. On Saturdays, the office is only open until 1:00 P.M., but it is already 11:00 A.M. and the office has been extremely busy. Valerie has not had time to do her morning checks yet, and the reception room is full of crying children.

As Mary Ann is looking over the schedule, she hears a commotion out front, followed by sudden quiet, and then Valerie's call for help. When Mary Ann gets to the reception room, there is a worried-looking man bent over a 35-year-old woman who is supine on the floor. She appears to be awake, but her eyes are closed and she is grimacing. She seems very short of breath. Her face is profusely diaphoretic and pale. "She had some indigestion last night when she went to bed," the man says, "and she did not sleep much last night. This morning when she got up to go to the bathroom, she stated she was very nauseated."

When asked, the lady responds with her name and says she is having some really sharp pain in her right lower abdomen. She points to it with one finger. Dr. Johnson is notified immediately to further evaluate the woman. As instructed, Mary Ann and Valerie help the woman into a wheelchair and wheel her into an examining room. She immediately complains of dizziness and increased pain, and now her breathing becomes extremely labored. She cannot seem to talk at all in response to questions.

What is your response?

1. What is your clinical impression of this woman?

2. In what position should she be placed?

3. What kind of history would you be especially curious about?

4. What kind of initial treatment would you administer?

5. Considering the available resources and this patient's status, what would you like to see happen next?

INTERNET ACTIVITY

Find a website for the poison control center. What types of information does the center have that you might be able to share with your pediatric patients, for educational purposes, to help remind them not to consume unknown substances or items that could poison them.

MEDMEDIA

Additional interactive resources and activities for this chapter can be found:

On your student DVD: View applicable procedure videos on the DVD-ROM found in the back of this book.

MyHealthProfessionsKit.com: Test your knowledge of the chapter with games and activities. MyHealthProfessionsKit also includes resources, helpful links, and a Spanish audio glossary.

Medical Assisting Interactive: Practice your procedures as a medical assistant in this simulated doctor's office. This can be accessed through MyHealthProfessionsKit.com.

44

The Clinical Laboratory

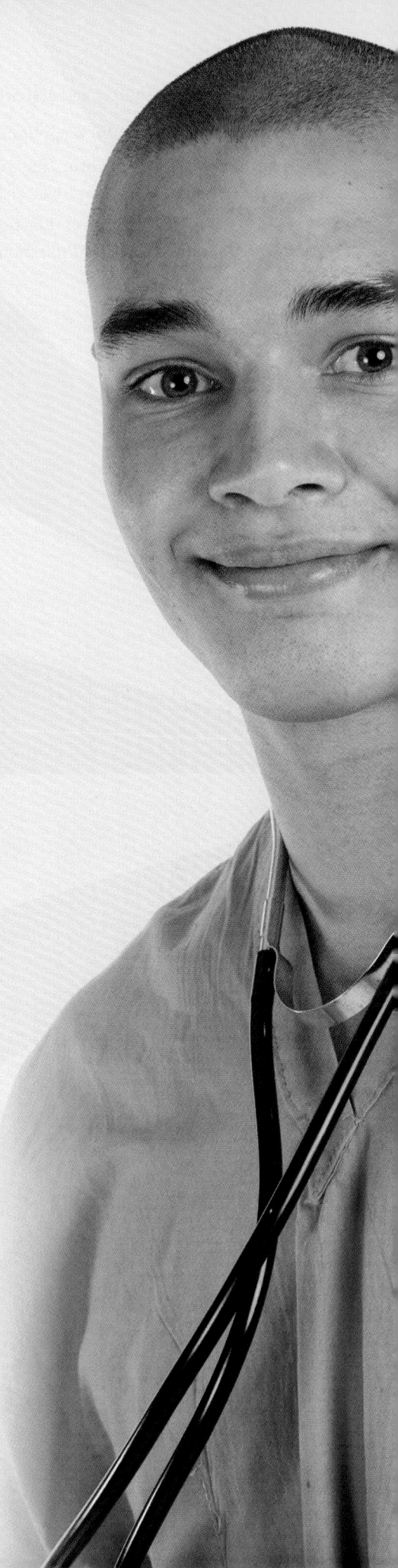

LEARNING OBJECTIVES

After completing this chapter, you should be able to:

- Define and spell the terms to learn for this chapter.

- Explain the role of the clinical laboratory in patient care.

- Identify and explain three types of clinical laboratories and their roles.

- Describe the role of the medical assistant in the physician's office laboratory.

- Summarize Occupational Safety and Health Administration laboratory safety regulations.

- Explain the three Clinical Laboratory Improvement Amendments categories of testing.

- Define quality assurance and list at least five components of a quality assurance program.

- Perform quality control measures.

- Identify several different types of laboratory equipment found in a physician's office laboratory.

- Identify and explain the parts of a microscope.

- Operate and properly care for a microscope.

- Communicate effectively with patients regarding laboratory test preparation and specimen collection.

- List patient information necessary to complete a laboratory request form.

- Monitor and follow up on patient laboratory test results.

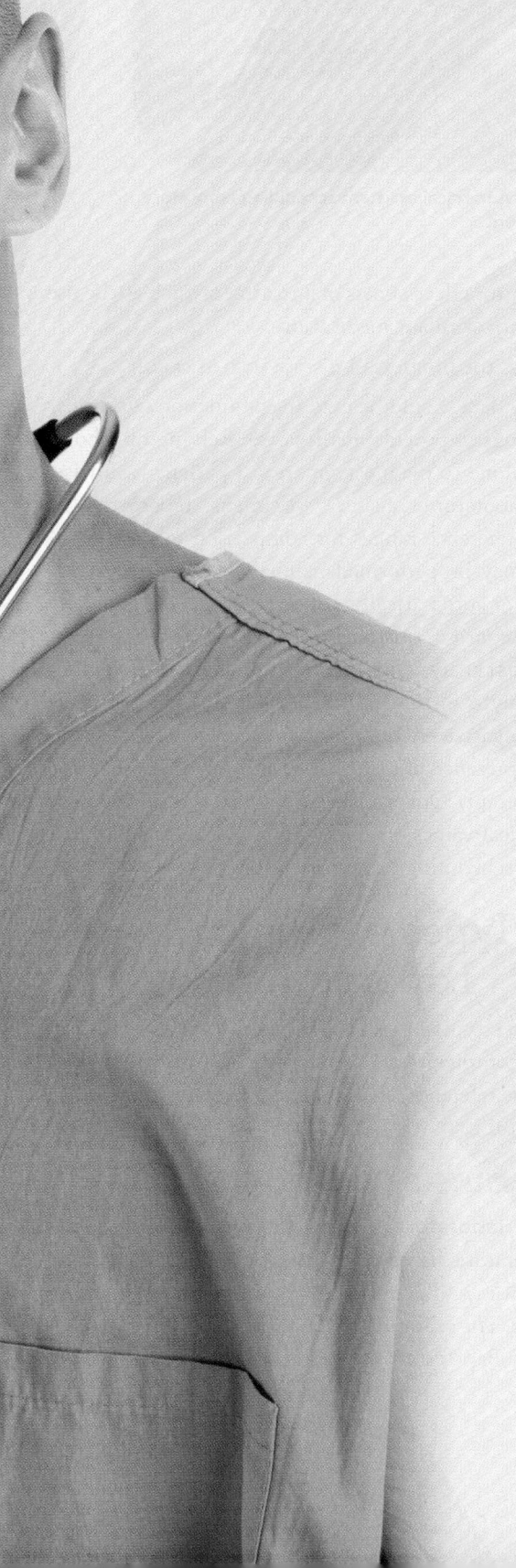

CHAPTER OUTLINE

CASE STUDY

Susan Schultz, CMA (AAMA), is working in the clinical lab of Pearson Physicians Group. Dr. Miller has sent Ravi Patel back to the clinical laboratory with a lab requisition for a urinalysis and blood glucose screening. He also has asked Ravi to schedule an appointment to come back to the office to have a 2-hour postprandial glucose test performed.

975

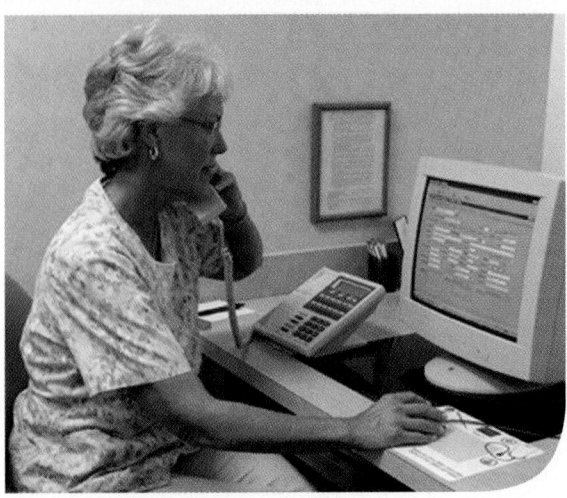

FIGURE 44-1 A medical assistant scheduling laboratory tests for a patient.

- To monitor effectiveness of a treatment such as the use of an anticoagulant medication

- To assess the progress of disease such as cancer

Laboratory data should be used in conjunction with other clinical findings to provide quality care. Relying on laboratory results alone to diagnosis or treat a patient is unwise.

Clinical laboratories analyze specimens, report results, and provide reference ranges for comparison of patient results. Tests may be performed manually, using specialized instruments, or automatically. Laboratory tests fall generally into two categories: qualitative or quantitative tests. A **qualitative test** analyzes for the presence or absence of a substance or **analyte** in the specimen and may be reported as positive or negative. A **quantitative test** analyzes a specimen for the presence of a substance and the amount of the substance present. Quantitative tests are usually reported using numerical values or units. Figure 44-1 shows a medical assistant scheduling laboratory tests.

Types of Clinical Laboratories

There are three types of clinical laboratories in which varying levels of complexity are performed. They are the outside laboratory, the reference laboratory, and the physician's office laboratory (POL).

OUTSIDE LABORATORY

The **outside laboratory**, either a hospital-based or independent laboratory, handles specimens collected from many types of facilities and performs tests ranging from simple to very complex. For example, the local hospital in your town may perform Pap tests collected in gynecologists' offices.

Most of us have had laboratory tests performed at one time or another on samples of blood, urine, or tissue. Clinical laboratory tests provide part of the framework on which physicians base their diagnoses and monitor patients' health.

The Role of the Clinical Laboratory in Patient Care

Clinical laboratory test results are an essential part of patient care and may be helpful in the following ways:

- To screen for disease

- To confirm a condition suspected by the physician

- To rule out a condition such as pregnancy

Box 44-1 Testing Departments of a Large Clinical LABORATORY

Clinical chemistry	Routine and Special Chemistry Testing	Histology	Preparation of tissue samples, slides from biopsies, autopsies
Cytogenetics	Genetic testing	Microbiology	Detection and testing for bacteria, viruses, parasites, and fungus
Cytology	Review Pap tests and other cell detection testing	Specimen collection and processing	Draw blood samples, process for testing, prepare for transportation to outside or reference lab
Hematology and coagulation	Blood counts (CBC) coagulation tests (PT, PTT)		
Immunohematology	Transfusions, blood banking	Urinalysis	Urine analysis (UA), special urine testing
Immunology, serology	Antibody detection testing for many illnesses		

Or your physician may have a contract with a managed care company that requires all specimens to be tested at a specific laboratory named in its contract.

REFERENCE LABORATORY

The **reference laboratory** may be associated with a specific teaching hospital or medical school or be independently owned. This type of laboratory handles more complex tests than an outside laboratory and those tests that are infrequently requested. Tests performed on a regular basis at a reference lab may provide more accurate results than tests performed a few times a year in an outside laboratory.

PHYSICIAN'S OFFICE LABORATORY

A **physician's office laboratory (POL)** is a laboratory in which some of the tests that the physician orders are performed right in the office. In the POL the doctor has the advantage of receiving the results more rapidly than if tests are done outside the office. **Turnaround time** is how long it takes for the test to be performed and the results generated, sent back for physician review, and added to the patient's chart. Disadvantages to the POL are that in-house testing may require more employees and the purchase of expensive equipment.

Clinical Laboratory Departments

Clinical laboratories are divided into various departments that perform specific categories of tests. The typical clinical laboratory may include departments such as specimen processing, chemistry, special chemistry, hematology, blood bank, microbiology, histology, urinalysis, cytology, serology,

parasitology, and toxicology. A physician's office lab performs a narrower range of tests, mainly those related to chemistry, hematology, urinalysis, and microbiology. Box 44-1 lists testing departments of large clinical laboratories.

Clinical Laboratory Personnel

As mentioned in Chapter 2, several different categories of health professionals and paraprofessionals may be employed in the clinical laboratory. The director of a clinical lab is usually a pathologist/MD or a clinical laboratory scientist with a doctorate degree. The clinical laboratory scientist (CLS) or medical technologist (MT) supervises and performs laboratory tests; These professionals have a 4-year degree and additional clinical training and have passed a national examination. A medical laboratory technician (MLT) usually has a 2-year degree, has undergone additional training, and has passed a national examination. The medical laboratory assistant (MLA), clinical laboratory assistant (CLA), certified medical assistant (CMA [AAMA]), and registered medical assistant (RMA) have some specialized training and have passed a certification or registration examination. Other categories of personnel, such as phlebotomists who draw blood samples and specimen processors who process and prepare samples, may be employed in the laboratory.

THE MEDICAL ASSISTANT'S ROLE IN THE CLINICAL LABORATORY

Medical assistants are particularly suited to working in POLs and clinical laboratories because of their cross-training in administrative and clinical areas. All medical assistants are trained in phlebotomy and have basic knowledge of laboratory testing. In addition, their multiskilled abilities help them to perform the many administrative tasks needed in the laboratory field. The patient-oriented training that medical assistants receive helps them be empathetic caregivers.

Laboratory Safety Regulations

Patients are entitled to quality medical care, and health care personnel deserve to work in a safe environment. The safety of both patients and personnel must be the central concern of every clinical laboratory, regardless of size. The accuracy and validity of test results are crucial to the health of the patient. (In the following paragraphs laboratory safety issues and regulations impacting clinical laboratories are discussed).

Several agencies and committees set and review safety guidelines affecting clinical laboratories. They include the Occupational Safety and Health Administration (OSHA); the Centers for Disease Control and Prevention (CDC); the Clinical Laboratory Standards Institute (CLSI), previously known as the National Committee for Clinical Laboratory Standards (NCCLS); the Environmental Protection Agency (EPA); and the College of American Pathologists (CAP). It is important that medical assistants have a working knowledge of the guidelines and regulations of these agencies and keep up to date on changes in order to provide better health care.

OSHA REGULATIONS

In 1970 Congress established OSHA within the U.S. Department of Labor to create safeguards covering nearly every employee in the United States. Two programs of standards under the OSHA umbrella particularly impact the clinical laboratory. They cover exposure to chemical hazards and bloodborne pathogens. Both have been discussed in some detail in Chapter 34, so they are only briefly considered here. OSHA develops and implements specific guidelines governing particular fields and requires adherence. If no specific guidelines exist, then the "general duty clause" must be followed, which means that all employers must provide a safe work environment free of hazards that may cause serious injury or death.

OSHA enforces CDC precautions. In 1996 the CDC developed and published new guidelines for isolation precautions in hospitals, and these were termed standard precautions. Standard precautions combine major features of universal precautions and body substance isolation precautions into one set of recommendations. Copies of these general guidelines can be obtained on the Internet.

CLINICAL LABORATORY IMPROVEMENT AMENDMENTS

In 1988 Congress enacted the **Clinical Laboratory Improvement Amendments (CLIA)** in response to widespread concern over the accuracy of laboratory tests. The government mandates that all laboratories that test human specimens must be regulated to help ensure accurate patient test results. CLIA divides laboratories into the three categories discussed previously and specifies what types of test may be performed in each and who may perform them. States may have their own laboratory safety requirements, but they must be at least as stringent as the federal government regulations. Information regarding state regulations may be obtained from state health departments. In 1992 CLIA was updated to reflect changes in standards, accrediting programs, fees, and enforcement. Tests are classified as Certificate of Waiver tests, Level I tests, and Level II tests.

Certificate of Waiver Tests

Certificate of Waiver Tests (WTs) are the least complex and present the least risk if performed incorrectly. Many of these tests have been approved by the Food and Drug Administration for home use. The early pregnancy detection kit is an example of such a test.

A POL must apply to perform WTs and is then restricted to performing none of the more complex tests from Level I or Level II and is exempt from complying with CLIA 1988 standards. Quality assurance and quality control methods should be observed. The laboratories that perform WTs may be subject to random inspections and investigation if test results are questioned or complaints are made against the laboratory. A Certificate of Waiver is given to laboratories that perform only low-complexity tests. A POL qualified to perform moderate-complexity and waived tests receives a Certificate of Provider-Performed Microscopy (PPM). Box 44-2 lists categories and examples of CLIA tests. A medical assistant employed in a facility with a PPM certificate can perform moderate-complexity tests with further training and under the supervision of a laboratory professional or physician.

Level I Tests. Level I tests are moderately complex and include analysis of specimens in the areas of chemistry, hematology, microbiology, immunohematology, virology, parasitology, and immunology. Any laboratory that wishes to perform Level I testing must be headed by a pathologist/MD or PhD. All personnel must have training past high school. The laboratory must perform proficiency testing and is subject to unannounced inspections. Examples of Level I laboratory tests include a complete blood count (CBC) and cholesterol screenings.

Level II Tests. Level II tests include those that are highly complex; any tests involved in cytology, histopathology, or

Box 44-2 Categories of CLIA TESTS

- **Waived Tests**—Simple procedures approved for home use and POL or POC testing
  - Dipstick urine testing or table testing
  - Fecal occult blood testing
  - Ovulation testing
  - Urine pregnancy testing
  - Erythrocyte sedimentation rate (nonautomated)
  - Hemoglobin testing with CLIA-waived analyzer
  - Spun hematocrit

- Blood glucose using FDA-approved glucose analyzer
- Rapid *Streptococcus* testing
- **Moderate-Complexity Tests/Level I Tests**
  - 75 percent of tests performed daily using automated analyzers for chemistry and hematology
  - Microscopic analysis of urine sediment
- **High-Complexity Tests/Level II Tests**
  - All tests in the field of cytogenetics, cytology, histopathology histocompatibility

---

histocompatibility; and any tests not categorized by the Centers for Medicare and Medicaid Services (CMS), formerly the Health Care Finance Administration (HCFA). The laboratories that perform tests in this category must be subject to unannounced inspections, perform proficiency testing, and be headed by an MD or PhD scientist, and tests may only be performed by qualified personnel as specified in the CLIA 1988 standards.

Laboratory Hazards

The laboratory includes biohazards, chemical hazards, and physical hazards; however, most accidents are preventable. Laboratory safety must be the concern of all who are employed in the laboratory field. Medical assistants must be familiar with the following regulations:

- Hazard Communication Standard
- Universal Precautions and Bloodborne Pathogen Standards
- Hazardous Waste Operations
- Needlestick Safety and Prevention Act

CHEMICAL HAZARDS

Material Safety Data Sheets (MSDS) provide safety information for all in the laboratory environment. MSDS provide product identification, safety information about proper storage and disposal, potential health hazards, handling precautions, and fire and explosion information. All laboratory personnel have the right to know about hazards pertaining to materials they are using and must receive training appropriate to the materials in use. Each hazardous substance must have a hazardous material label attached to the container that provides a shortened version of the MSDS information. Figure 44-2 is an example of an MSDS label.

BLOODBORNE PATHOGENS AND STANDARD PRECAUTIONS

Biohazards have the potential to infect others. As of 1992, OSHA's Occupational Exposure to Bloodborne Pathogen Program must be in place at all working laboratories. In addition the CDC specimen handling precautions known as standard precautions (formerly universal precautions) must be employed when dealing with any infectious materials. All potentially biohazardous material must be labeled with the biohazard label as shown in Figure 44-3. Chapter 34 discusses bloodborne pathogen standards.

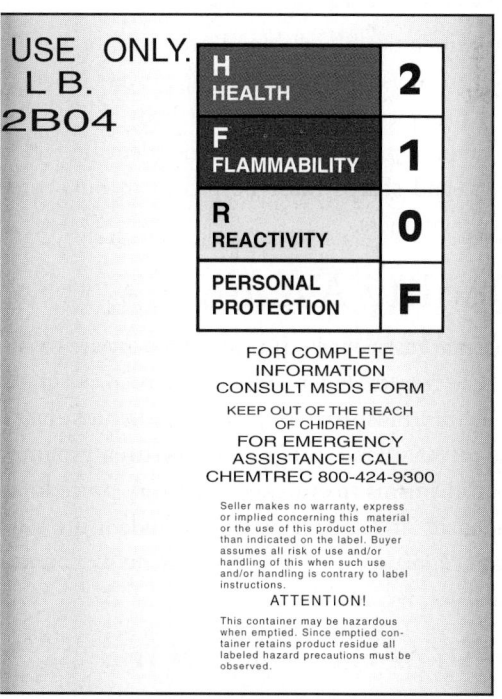

FIGURE 44-2 MSDS labels provide an abridged version of substance hazards information and must be permanently attached to their containers.

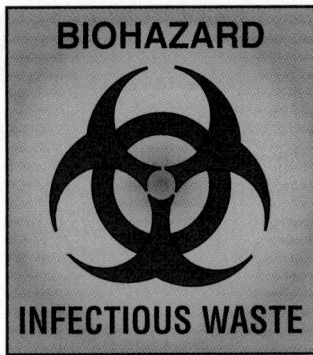

FIGURE 44-3 An orange-red biohazard symbol indicates that bloodborne pathogens may be present, and items should be treated accordingly.

NEEDLESTICK HAZARDS

OSHA revised the bloodborne standards in 2000. Now health care employers must review all new safety devices to lessen the needlestick risks of their employees, and they must ask for safety input from their employees on an annual basis. A detailed report of all contaminated needlestick incidents must be kept.

FIRE AND SAFETY HAZARDS

Staff must take care to reduce the chances of fire and electrical accidents. They also must be familiar with the floor plan, exits, and location of safety devices, such as eyewashes, showers, and safety blankets.

HAZARDOUS WASTE REMOVAL

Hazardous waste includes blood, blood products, body fluids and tissues, cultures, vaccines, sharps, gloves, inoculation loops, and paper contaminated with body fluids. All must be disposed of in proper containers and identified with biohazard labels, and sharps must be placed in puncture-proof, leakproof containers.

Quality Assurance

The most important tasks of the clinical laboratory are to ensure accurate test results and to report them in a timely manner. Each facility must have in place a quality assurance program. A quality assurance program is a written program that includes mechanisms to evaluate laboratory procedures and policies, identify and correct problems, and ensure reliable and prompt reporting of results and testing by competent individuals.

QUALITY ASSURANCE IN THE LABORATORY

The CLIA 1992 standards mandate that written policies and procedures must be in place for a comprehensive quality

assurance program that will "evaluate the ongoing and overall quality of the testing process." To this end, the laboratory is required to do the following:

- Evaluate the effectiveness of its policies and procedures
- Identify and correct problems
- Ensure reliable and prompt test results

- Ensure the competence and adequacy of staff
- Take corrective action if errors are found
- Integrate corrective procedures into future policies and procedures
- Document employee training, and assess competency yearly after the first year
- Maintain the identity and integrity of patient samples during the entire testing process
- Be subject to inspection every 2 years if performing moderate- or high-complexity tests

QUALITY CONTROL

Quality control (QC) programs in clinical laboratories monitor the testing of patient specimens to ensure reliable and consistent results. Patient specimens or samples may be whole blood, serum, plasma, body fluids such as cerebrospinal fluid and urine, feces, tissue, and swabs such as throat, vaginal, or wound.

Control Samples

Control samples are samples similar to the required testing specimen that have been previously tested and have a known value. Controls are usually purchased from a manufacturer, and each batch has an assigned lot number and accompanying value sheet. In addition, information regarding dilution of controls is provided along with information on proper storage.

Reagents

Reagents are substances required for a chemical reaction or used to detect the presence of another substance. For example, when a fingerstick blood glucose test is performed, the reagent is already on the test strip, and it reacts with the patient's blood drop, which is the sample. To determine that the machine and the test strips are working correctly and that the medical assistant is performing the tests correctly, control samples with a known positive and negative result should be performed and the results recorded on QC sheets.

Calibration

Some laboratory tests require the medical assistant to **calibrate** the machine or instrument prior to testing a specimen. To calibrate an instrument, a known standard is used to measure the accuracy of the equipment to be utilized in the test procedure.

Maintenance

All laboratory equipment must be maintained on a regular basis according to manufacturers' instructions. A written record of the maintenance performed must be readily available. In addition, a record of each piece of equipment with model and serial numbers, date of purchase, and manufac-

turers' inserts should be available when repair is necessary or the laboratory is being inspected.

Documentation

Documentation is important for QA. Without a written record of a test result, control result, maintenance performed, or temperature recorded, you have no proof of activity. The end result is the same as if you did not perform the procedure. If it is not written down in the appropriate place, you did not do it.

PROFICIENCY TESTING

Proficiency testing is an external quality control program that monitors the accuracy of test systems by comparing your results to results provided by a survey program of the College of American Pathologists or the American Association of Bioanalysts. Unknown samples are sent to your laboratory periodically throughout the year. Under CLIA 1988 standards, laboratories must participate in proficiency testing three times a year, and if any analyte has an unacceptable rating in two of the three testing surveys, suspension of certification or permission to perform that test occurs. The laboratory may not perform that test for patients until appropriate action is taken and two subsequent proficiency tests are within acceptable limits.

Proficiency tests may be performed on whole blood, serum, plasma, or urine, and the samples will have a range of results similar to any group of patients. Some will be high, some normal, and some low (Box 44-3).

Laboratory Equipment

Clinical laboratories utilize a wide array of equipment. A POL, however, requires less equipment for clinical laboratory testing than does an outside or reference laboratory. An autoclave, centrifuge, photometer, incubator, microscope, and measuring devices are generally found in most POLs.

AUTOCLAVE

The autoclave is discussed in Chapter 34. It is used to sterilize equipment or instruments that are used on patients or in certain test procedures.

CENTRIFUGE

The **centrifuge** is an instrument used to separate specimens into component layers. In the medical office they are used to separate urine so urine sediment can be examined under the microscope (see Chapter 46). A microcentrifuge is used to separate whole blood samples into layers to measure patient hematocrit (see Chapter 47).

Box 44-3 Using Controls to Monitor RESULTS

As a professional in health care, it is important that you comprehend the importance of patient test results and control samples. What would you do if the control sample results were correct according to the manufacturer's value sheet but the patient test results were very abnormal compared to the reference values of your facility? For example, imagine a patient's fasting glucose level is 47 mg/dL when tested. The reference range in your facility is 70 to 100 mg/dL. The control tests were 55 mg/dL and 132 mg/dL, which were in range according to the manufacturer.

- If a result seems incongruous to you, it should not be reported without retesting.
- The test and controls should be repeated.
- The original specimen should be examined to ascertain that the specimen was not **hemolyzed** (red cells burst, causing serum to be a cherry-red color) or **icteric** (bilious yellow-green color). If either problem exists, a new specimen may be required and the test repeated.
- The results from previous tests on this patient should be examined. Is there a pattern among previous test results?
- The patient's results should be flagged and brought to the attention of the supervisor or physician if test and control results were the same as the first test results.
- A protocol should be in place in your POL that establishes the appropriate steps to follow when a result is flagged.
- An **aliquot** (a small portion of the whole) of the original specimen may be sent to an outside laboratory for testing to compare results.

PHOTOMETER

A **photometer** is an instrument that measures light intensity. A glucometer is a type of handheld photometer that is used to test glucose levels in patients.

INCUBATOR

An **incubator** is used to maintain a specific temperature to achieve a specific result. For example, incubators that mimic body temperature are used in POLs to encourage growth of throat and urine cultures. Once the culture has grown sufficiently, identification of the infecting organism can be made (see Chapter 45).

MICROSCOPE

Microscopes are frequently used in the medical office to examine urine sediment, vaginal and bacteriological smears, and differential smears, which categorize types of white cells in a sample. This optical instrument magnifies structures unseen by the naked eye for the purpose of counting, naming, or differentiating. Figure 44-4 shows an example of a **compound microscope** (one that has two sets of lenses, oculars, and objectives). The **resolution** of a microscope refers to the ability to distinguish clearly between two adjacent but distinct objects. Better microscopes have better resolution.

Parts of the Microscope

The following are the components of a microscope:

1. One or multiple eyepieces (monocular or binocular) with magnification imprinted on them
2. Body tube (directional light source)
3. Arm (used in carrying the microscope)
4. Revolving nosepiece (holds objectives and rotates for selection)
5. Objectives (magnification imprinted on each objective: 10, low-power setting; 40, high dry setting; and 100, oil immersion setting (settings are described in the next section)
6. Stage
7. Mechanical stage (movable device that holds slide)

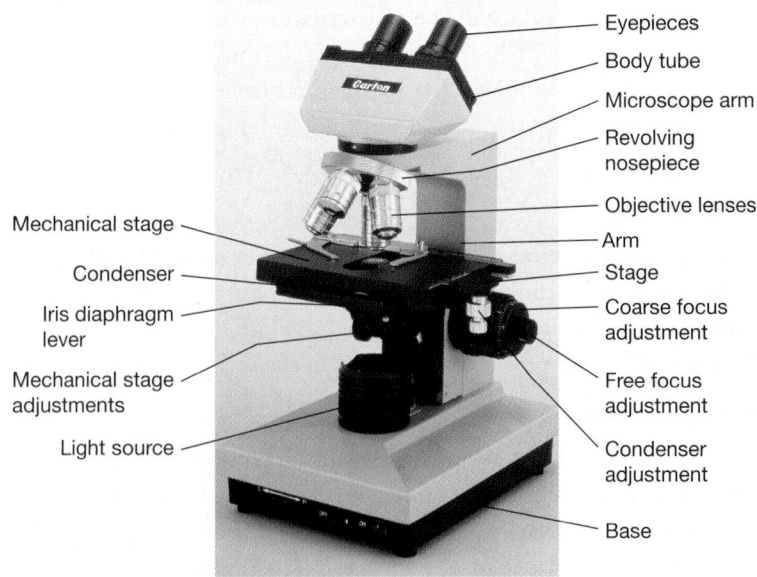

FIGURE 44-4 Binocular microscope with parts labeled.

8. Mechanical stage adjustments (two knobs that control vertical/horizontal movement of slide)

9. Coarse and fine adjustment knobs (small knob atop larger knob that adjusts stage up and down for focusing)

10. Condenser (lens system used to increase light for sharper focus)

11. Condenser adjustment knob

12. Light source (illuminator set in base)

13. Iris diaphragm lever

14. Base (holds illuminator, rheostat, and microscope upright and is used while carrying microscope)

Using the Microscope

The magnification of an object is calculated by multiplying the objective magnification by the eyepiece magnification. On low power, magnification would be 10 (the objective) times 10 (the eyepiece) equaling magnification of 100 times the size of the sample. Procedure 44-1 lists the methods for properly using, cleaning, and storing a microscope.

procedure
44-1

USING AND CLEANING THE MICROSCOPE

Objective: Observe a slide under 10×, 40×, and oil immersion properly, and clean and store microscope correctly.

EQUIPMENT AND SUPPLIES
binocular compound microscope; specimen slide; lens paper; lens cleaner; dust cover for microscope

METHOD
1. Always carry the microscope with one hand on the arm and one hand under the base.
2. Make sure the stage is in the down position before starting.
3. Clean objectives with lens paper starting with 10× and ending with oil immersion (Figure 44-5A).
4. Turn on the light and rotate the nosepiece until 10× objective is directly over the slide (Figure 44-5B). Place the prepared slide on the stage (Figure 44-5C).

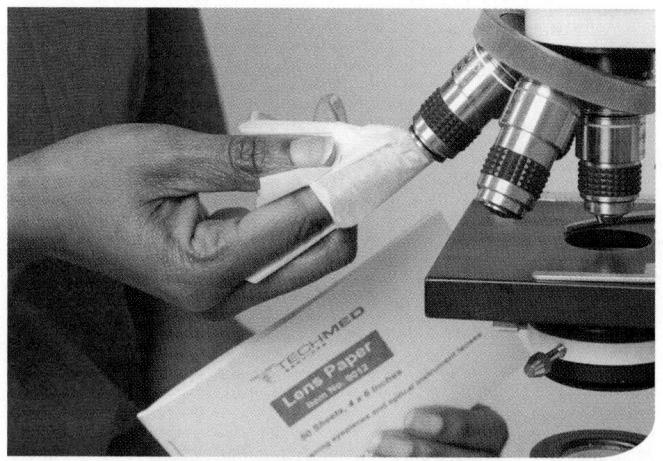

A

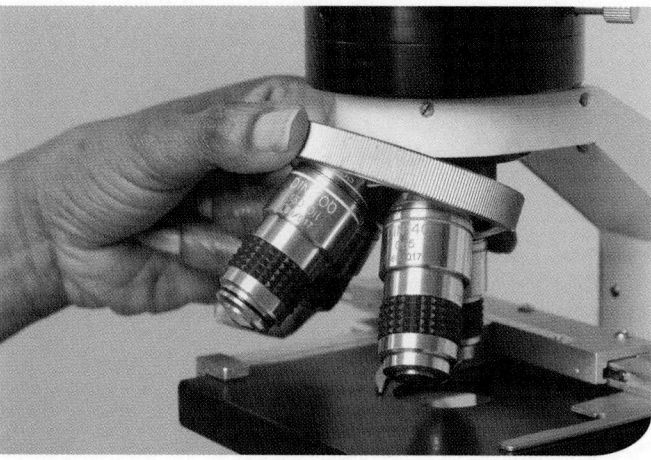

B

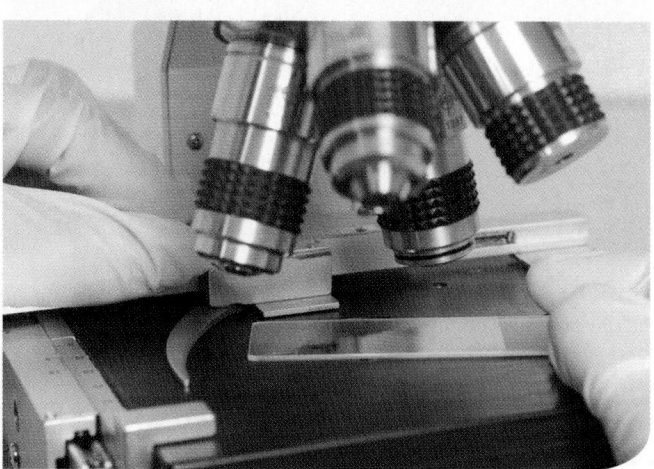

C

FIGURE 44-5   (A) Clean the objective with lens paper; (B) rotate the nosepiece; (C) place the slide on the stage.

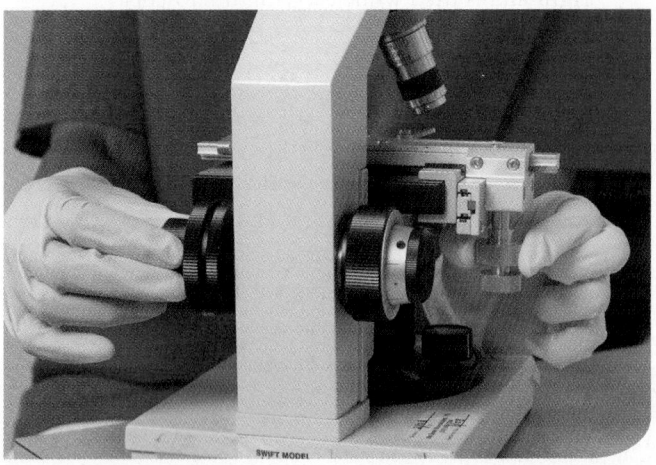

D

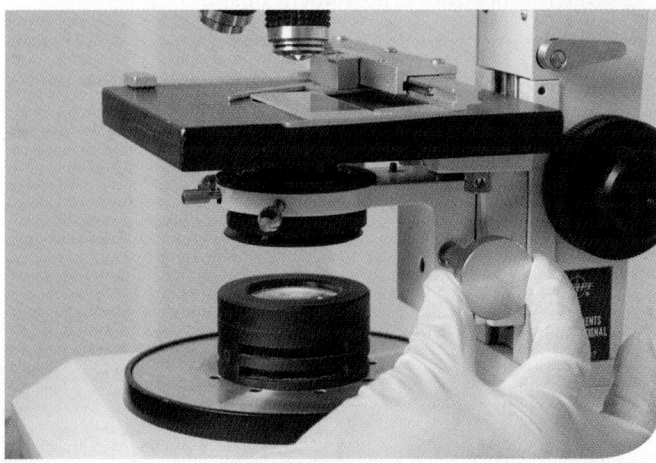

E

5. Use the coarse adjustment knob to raise the stage until the objective is close to the slide on the stage.
6. Look through the eyepiece and adjust the coarse focus knob until the microscope field is seen (a round circle of bright light).
7. Use the fine adjustment knob for a clearer image (Figure 44-5D).
8. Open the diaphragm and, if necessary, adjust the rheostat to focus.
9. Raise or lower the condenser to alter light refraction. The condenser is usually lowered when using 10× power (Figure 44-5E).
10. Observe the slide.

11. Change the objective to 40× and readjust as needed (Figure 44-5F). Move the objective and place a drop of oil on the slide before completing the turn to oil immersion lens.
12. When focusing and examination are complete, lower the stage before removing the slide.
13. Turn off the light.
14. Clean the eyepieces and objectives with lens paper. Clean the oil immersion lens with lens cleaner.
15. Unplug the electrical cord and wrap it around the base.
16. Cover the microscope with a dust cover (Figure 44-5G).
17. Clean the slide and store.

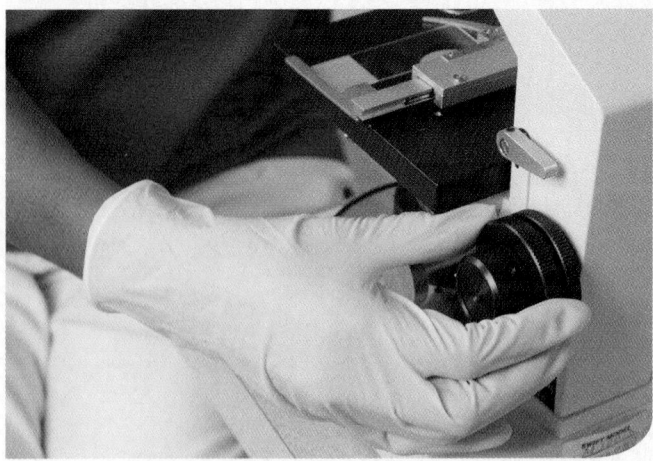

F

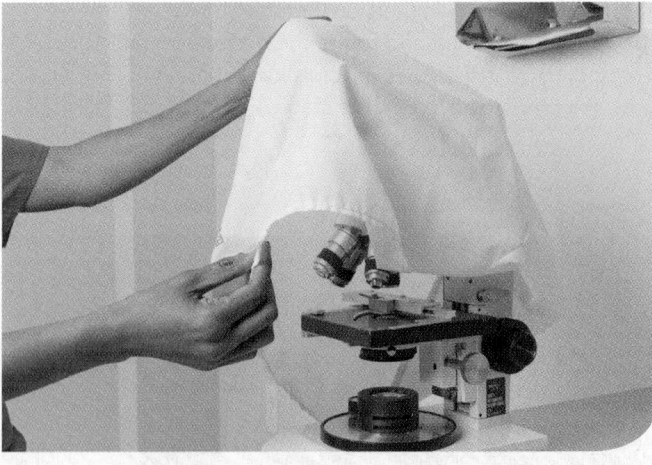

G

FIGURE 44-5 (D) Fine focus with the adjustment knob while moving the slide slightly with the mechanical slide controls; (E) the condenser height control is on the left, and the diaphragm control is on the right; (F) the mechanical stage control moves the slide up and down and back and forth; (G) after cleaning always store the microscope with its protective cover.

CARE AND MAINTENANCE OF A MICROSCOPE

1. Follow cleaning requirements during mandatory daily maintenance.
2. Always use two hands to carry a microscope: one hand to hold the arm of the microscope and one to support the base.
3. Clean oculars, objectives, and stage using only lens paper and lens cleaner.
4. Keep extra light bulbs on hand.
5. Document inspections and repairs in logbook.
6. Store with electrical cord wrapped loosely around base.
7. Cover the microscope with a dust cover when it is not in use.

It is important to use the correct lens for the type of microscopic work to be done. For example, the low-power objective, 10×, is used to view epithelial cells, such as skin scrapings; the high dry setting, 40×, is used for urine RBCs (red blood cells), WBCs (white blood cells), or blood RBCs; the oil immersion setting, 100×, is for differential blood smears (stained with Wright's stain) or bacteria slides (stained with Gram stain). Microscopic work on the high dry setting is done with a cover glass on the specimen.

Care of the Microscope

Microscopes are delicate instruments that will last for many years if maintained properly. Guidelines 44-1 lists the rules for the proper care and maintenance of a microscope.

Laboratory Measurements and Equipment

The validity of laboratory test results depends on accurate measurements and correct calculations using laboratory equipment. Thermometers are used to measure the temperature of various pieces of laboratory equipment, such as refrigerators, freezers, incubators, and water baths, which must be maintained within specific ranges. Each piece of equipment must have its own log of temperature readings with date, time, and the initials of the indi-

vidual who performed the reading. In addition, medical assistants must be aware of the laboratory units of measurement that are used to report results. A laboratory result must never be reported without a unit of measurement after it. Metric system units are used most frequently in the laboratory.

TIME

To ensure accurate test results, all test procedures must be precisely timed. In tests such as the glucose tolerance test (GTT), specimen collection must be timed precisely in order to provide accurate, meaningful test results. Laboratory time is based on the 24-hour clock or military time to avoid confusion that may result from using the A.M. and P.M. designations of Greenwich Time. The 24-hour clock uses four numbers, with noon expressed as 1200 (twelve hundred hours) and midnight as 2400 (twenty-four hundred hours). A time of 4:15 P.M. would be a military time of 1615 (sixteen-fifteen hundred hours), which is calculated by adding 4 hours and 15 minutes to 1200. Some workers are required to use 24-hour time clocks to monitor their work arrival and departure times. Figure 44-6 is an example of a 24-hour or military clock.

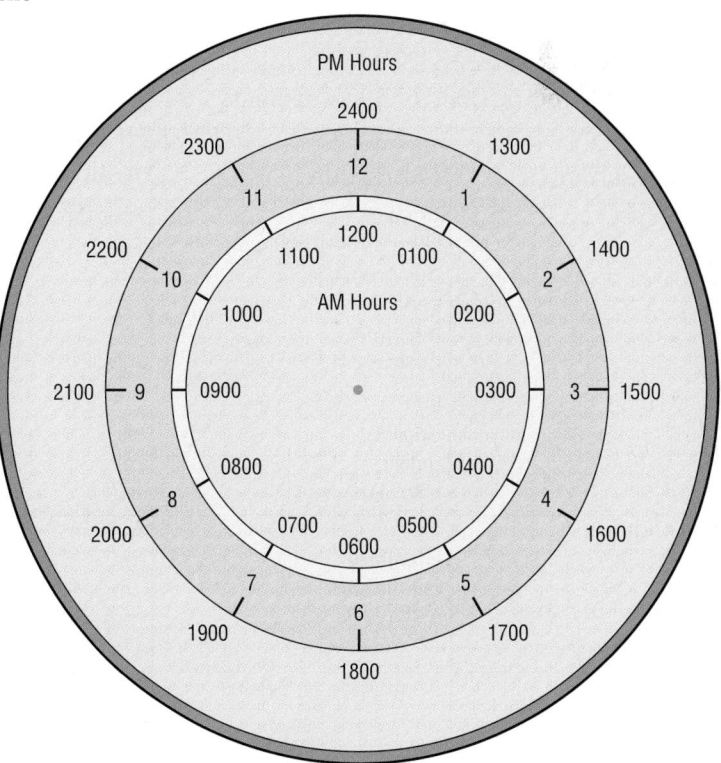

FIGURE 44-6 24-hour clock (military time).

TABLE 44-1 Common Laboratory Temperatures

Laboratory Temperatures	Fahrenheit	Celsius
Autoclave	254	121
Freezer	32	0
Incubator	98.6	37
Refrigerator	41	5
Room	68	20

TEMPERATURE

The two scales used for measuring temperature, as well as the calculations necessary for converting Fahrenheit and Celsius, were discussed in Chapter 35 and are not presented again here. Table 44-1 lists some temperatures routinely associated with the laboratory environment.

LABORATORY UNITS OF MEASUREMENT

The United States uses the English system of measurement in everyday life. The English system uses ounces and pounds for weight; inches, feet, and yards for length; and cups, pints, quarts, and gallons for liquids. In the medical field and throughout most of the world, the metric system is used. The metric system is based on a decimal system combined with various designations—liquid (liter), weight (gram), and length (meter). An apothecary system is also used in pharmacology to measure some medications. These systems and the conversions from one to another will be discussed more fully in Chapters 52 and 53. See Table 44-2 for metric units of measurements.

Most commonly the units used to express laboratory results are the following: millimeter (mm), centimeter (cm), and milligram (mg). The appropriate unit and correct designation must be used when reporting test results. Exact placement of the decimal in a test result is *critical* to the health and safety of the patient. Table 44-3 lists some abbreviations commonly used when reporting patient test results.

MEASURING DEVICES

Various measuring and mixing devices are employed in the laboratory. These include beakers, flasks, cylinders, test tubes, and **pipettes**. They may be made of glass or plastic and be reusable or disposable. Figure 44-7 depicts various types of glassware, and Figure 44-8 depicts pipettes of various types. Beakers and flasks can be used to mix liquids. They are not accurate measuring devices. The graduated cylinder and the volumetric flask are accurate measuring devices.

TABLE 44-2 Metric Units of Measurements

Measurement	Metric Unit	Abbreviation	Comparison to U.S. Units
Weight	gram kilogram = 1000 g decigram centigram milligram microgram	g or gm kg dg cg mg mcg	1 g = approximately 1 raisin 1 kg = 2.2 lbs 1 dg = 1/10 g (0.1 g) 1 cg = 1/100 g (0.01 g) 1 mg = 1/1000 g (0.001 g) 1 mcg = 1/1,000,000 g (one millionth)
Volume	liter deciliter milliliter microliter	L dL mL μL	1 L is slightly more than a quart 1 dL = 1/10 L 1 mL = 1/1000 L; same as cubic centimeter (cc) 1 μL = 1/1,000,000 of a liter
Length	meter kilometer centimeter millimeter	M or m km cm mm	1 M = slightly more than 1 mile 1 km = 1000 M 1 cm = 1/100 M (one hundredth) 1 mm = 1/1000 M (one thousandth) 1 mm = 1/1,000,000 M (one millionth)
Temperature	Centigrade or Celsius	°C	0°C = freezing = 32°F 100°C = boiling = 212°F 37°C = body temperature = 98.6°F

TABLE 44-3 Abbreviations Commonly Used in Reporting Laboratory Results

Unit	Abbreviation
gram	g
milligram	mg
liter	L
milliliter	mL
microliter	μL
microgram	mcg
millimoles per liter	mmol/L
cubic centimeter	cc (mL)
milligrams per deciliter	mg/dL
pint	pt
quart	qt
ounce	oz
quantity not sufficient	QNS

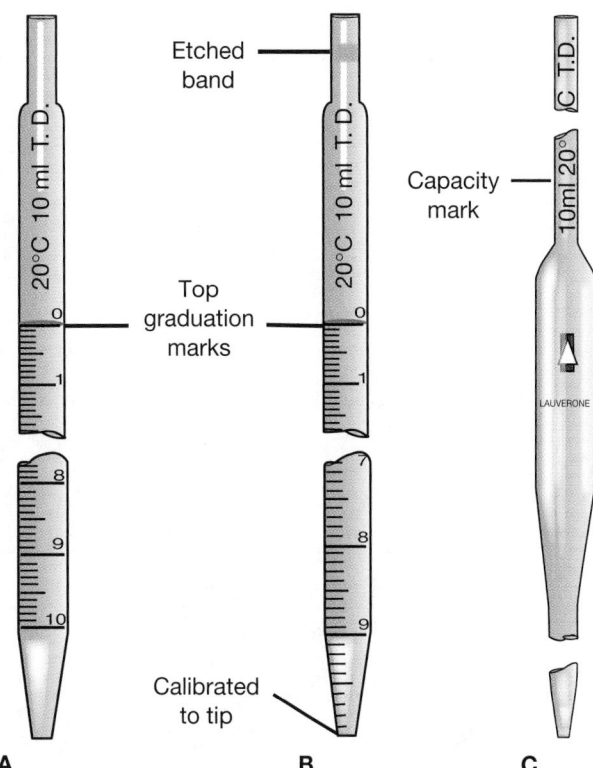

FIGURE 44-8   Types of manual pipettes: (A) graduated; (B) serologic; (C) volumetric.

The graduated pipette is used for measuring, and the volumetric pipette is used for transferring liquid from one vessel to another. The graduated pipette is marked with "TD," which stands for "To Deliver," and it will deliver that spe-

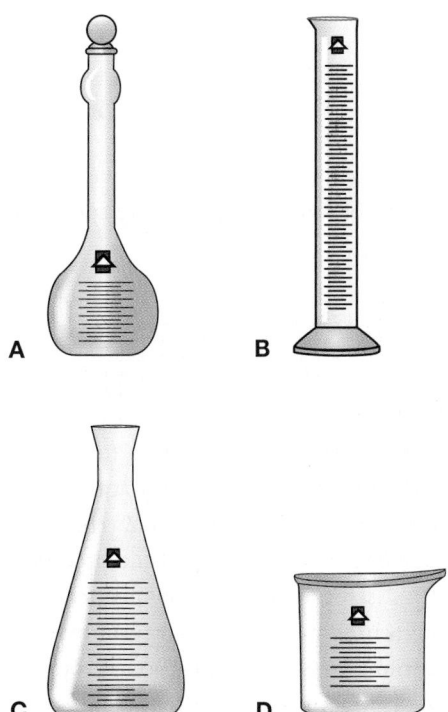

FIGURE 44-7   Laboratory glassware: (A) volumetric flask; (B) graduated cylinder; (C) Erlenmeyer flask; (D) beaker.

cific amount. If it is marked with "TC," "To Contain," it must be emptied completely to deliver the exact amount. A serologic pipette has graduations down to the tip and is used to make serum dilutions in the laboratory. The serologic pipette allows for more rapid flow because of its larger opening but is less accurate and should not be used for making reagent dilutions. Micropipettes are used to deliver very small amounts (microliters) of liquid, and manufacturers' directions must be carefully followed.

Dilutions

For certain types of tests, dilutions of either the reagent or patient sample may be required. The term *dilution* infers that some number of parts is distributed throughout the whole volume of a substance. For example, if a patient's test result is too high to provide an accurate reading, the test directions may say to repeat the test using a 1 in 10 dilution of the patient's serum in a specific diluent (a liquid such as saline or water). A **diluent** is an agent that dilutes a substance or solution to which it is added. The medical assistant would measure out one part of patient's serum and add it to nine parts of diluent. This is a 1:10 dilution of the sample. You could use 1 mL of serum and 9 mL of diluent, or 0.5 mL of serum and 4.5 mL of diluent, and the result would be a 1:10 dilution in either case.

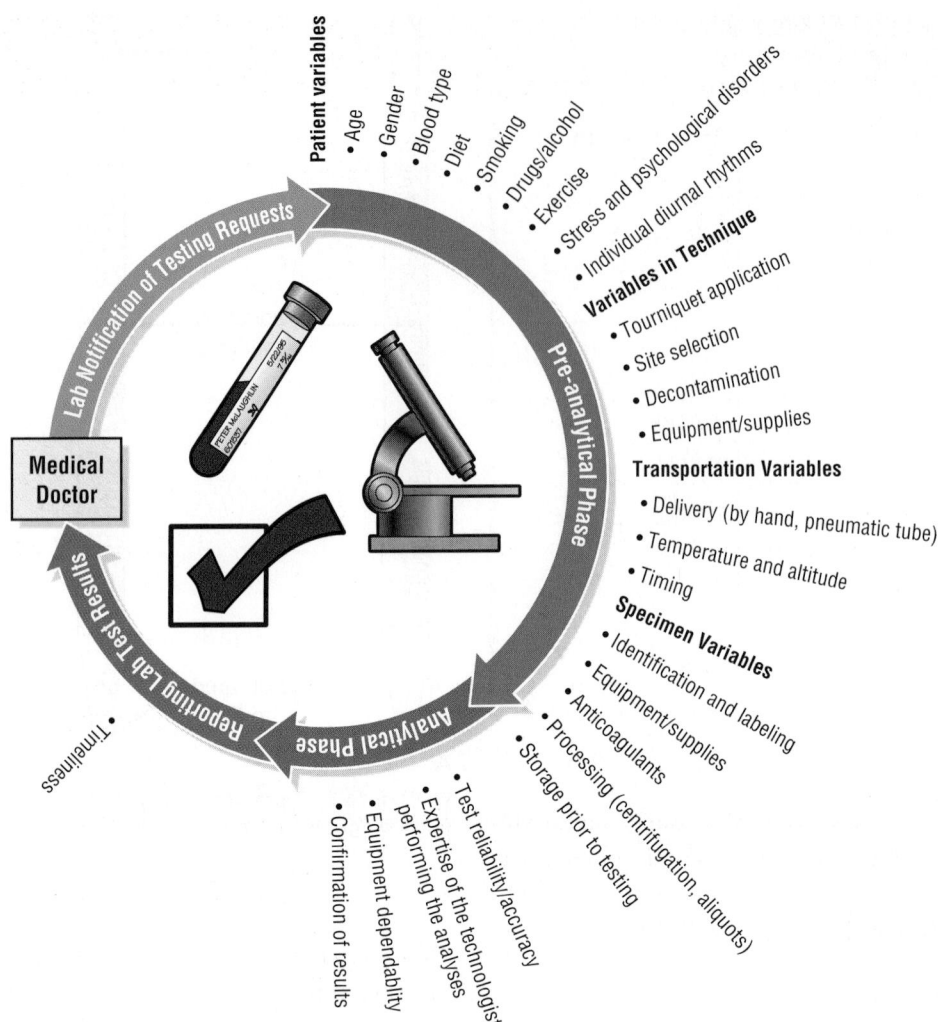

Patient variables
• Age
• Gender
• Blood type
• Diet
• Smoking
• Drugs/alcohol
• Exercise
• Stress and psychological disorders
• Individual diurnal rhythms

Variables in Technique
• Tourniquet application
• Site selection
• Decontamination
• Equipment/supplies

Transportation Variables
• Delivery (by hand, pneumatic tube)
• Temperature and altitude
• Timing

Specimen Variables
• Identification and labeling
• Equipment/supplies
• Anticoagulants
• Processing (centrifugation, aliquots)
• Storage prior to testing

Lab Notification of Testing Requests

Pre-analytical Phase

Analytical Phase

Reporting Lab Test Results

Medical Doctor

• Timeliness

• Confirmation of results
• Equipment dependability
• Expertise of the technologist performing the analyses
• Test reliability/accuracy

FIGURE 44-9 Laboratory testing cycle: preanalytical and analytical.

The Clinical Laboratory and Patient Communication

The laboratory testing cycle is divided into two phases: preanalytical and analytical. The testing cycle begins with the physician's order for specific laboratory tests. The preanalytical phase begins when the laboratory is notified and the specimen is obtained. See Figure 44-9 for an illustration of the laboratory testing cycle. The specimen is transported, processed, and prepared for analysis. The analytical phase includes the actual testing or analysis of the specimen and reporting the results to the physician.

The medical assistant is often responsible for communicating directly with the patient regarding preparation for specimen collection. Test results are only as good as the spec-imen provided for analysis. As a result, the medical assistant must make every effort to obtain the appropriate specimen from the patient.

LABORATORY REQUISITION

The laboratory testing process begins with the physician's request for a test. As a medical assistant you will need to complete a requisition that the patient will bring to the laboratory at the time of the test. If the physician wants the results immediately for a medical intervention, then the requisition must be labeled stat (immediately) and processed accordingly. Box 44-4 lists the information necessary to complete a requisition form. Figure 44-10 is an example of a laboratory test requisition. Be sure to use the appropriate laboratory requisition slip since the office may send specimens to several different testing sites.

Box 44-4 Laboratory Requisition INFORMATION

- Physician's name address, phone number, and account number
- Patient's full name, address, phone number
- Patient's age, sex, date of birth (DOB)
- Patient's complete insurance information
- All relevant diagnostic codes
- Diagnosis, if possible
- Source of specimen
- If fasting or nonfasting specimen
- Date and collection time
- Specific tests requested per physician's orders, including five-digit procedure code
- Patient's present medications
- If request is stat or regular

PATIENT PREPARATION

Various tests require different types of patient preparation. A fasting specimen means that the patient must not consume any food for a prescribed number of hours prior to collecting the specimen. For most tests the fasting period is at least 8 hours. **Postprandial (PP)**, or **post cibum (pc)**, means "after a meal." A **fasting** blood glucose would be drawn after the patient has abstained from eating for at

Lab Services

IMPORTANT
Patient instructions
and map on back

PHYSICIAN ORDERS

Patient ____________ (Last Name) ____________ (First) ____ (M.I.) D.O.B. ________ M ☐ F ☐ Patient SS# ___ — ___ — ___
Address ____________ City ____________ Zip ________ Phone # ________
Physician ____________
ATTACH COPY OF INSURANCE CARD
Diagnosis/ICD-9 Code ____________
(Additional codes on reverse)

Date & Time of Collection: ________ ________
Drawing Facility ________

☐ 789.00 Abdominal Pain
☐ 285.9 Anemia (NOS)
☐ 414.9 Coronary Artery Disease (CAD)
☐ 250.0 DM (diabetes mellitus)
☐ 780.7 Fatigue/Malaise
☐ 272.0 Hypercholesterolemia
☐ 244.9 Hypothyroidism
☐ 272.4 Hyperlipidemia
☐ 401.9 Hypertension
☐ 483.9 URI (upper respiratory infection)

☐ ROUTINE
☐ ASAP
☐ STAT

☐ PHONE RESULTS TO: # ________
☐ FAX RESULTS TO: # ________
☐ COPY TO: ________

HEMATOLOGY

☐ 1021 CBC, Automated Diff (incl, Platelet Ct.)
☐ 1023 Hemoglobin/Hematocrit
☐ 1020 Hemogram
☐ 1025 Platelet Count
☐ 1150 Pro Time Diagnostic
☐ 1151 Pro Time, Therapeutic
☐ 1155 PTT
☐ 1315 Reticulocyte Count
☐ 1310 Sed Rate/ Westergren

URINE

☐ 1059 Urinalysis
☐ 1082 Urinalysis w/Culture if indicated
Urine-24 Hr ______ Spot ______
Ht. ______ Wt. ______
☐ 3033 Creatinine
☐ 3036 Creatinine Clearance (also requires blood)
☐ 3095 Protein
☐ 3096 Sodium/Potassium
☐ Microalbumin 24 Hr______ Spot______

SEROLOGY

☐ 8020 ANA (Antinuclear Antibody)
☐ 8040 Mono Spot
☐ 3494 Rheumatoid Factor
☐ 8010 RPR
☐ 5365 Rubella

CHEMISTRY

☐ 5550 Alpha Fetoprotein, Prenatal
☐ 3000 Amylase
☐ 3153 B12/Folate
☐ 3156 Beta HCG, Quantitative
☐ 3321 Bilirubin, Total
☐ 3324 Bilirubin, Total/Direct
☐ 3009 BUN
☐ 3159 CEA
☐ 3348 Cholesterol
☐ 3030 Creatinine, Serum
☐ 3509 Digoxin (recommend 12 hrs, after dose)
☐ 3515 Dilantin
☐ 3168 Ferritin
☐ 3193 FSH
☐ 3066 ▼ Glucose, Fasting
☐ 3061 Glucose, 1st Post 50 g Glucola
☐ 3075 ▼ Glucose, 2nd Post Glucola
☐ 3060 Glucose, 2nd Post Prandial (meal)
☐ 3049 ▼ Glucose Tolerance Oral GTT
☐ 3047 ▼ Glucose Tolerance Gestational GTT
☐ 3650 Hemoglobin, A1C

CHEMISTRY

☐ 5232 HBsAg
☐ 3175 HIV (Consent required)
☐ 3581 Iron & Iron Binding Capacity
☐ 3195 LH
☐ 3590 Magnesium
☐ 3527 Phenobarbital
☐ 3095 Potassium
☐ 3689 Pregnancy Test Serum (HCG, qual)
☐ 3653 Pregnancy Test, Urine
☐ 3197 Prolactin
☐ 3199 PSA
☐ 3339 SGOT/AST
☐ 3342 SGPT/ALT
☐ 3093 Sodium/Potassium, Serum
☐ 3510 Tegretol
☐ 3551 Theophylline
☐ 3333 Uric Acid

MICROBIOLOGY

Source ________
☐ 7240 Culture, AFB
☐ 7200 Culture, Blood x ________
☐ Draw interval ________
☐ 7280 Culture, Fungus
☐ Culture, Routine
☐ 7005 Culture, Stool
☐ 7010 Culture, Throat
☐ 7000 Culture, Urine
☐ 7300 Gram Stain
☐ 7353 Occult Blood x ________
☐ 7365 Ova & Parasites x ________
☐ 7400 Smear & Suspension (includes Gram Stain/Wet Mount)
☐ 7060 Rapid Strep A Screen (_____)
☐ 7065 Rapid Strep A Screen only
☐ 7030 Beta Strep Culture
☐ 5207 GC by DNA Probe
☐ 5130 Chlamydia by DNA Probe
☐ 5555 Chlamydia/GC by DNA Probe
☐ 7375 Wright Stain, Stool

Additional Tests ________

PANELS & PROFILES

☐ ✗ **3309 CHEM 12** Albumin, Alkaline Phosphatase, BUN, Calcium, Cholesterol, Glucose, LDH, Phosphorus, AST, Total Bilirubin, Total Protein, Uric Acid
☐ ▼ **3315 CHEM 20** Chem 12, Electrolyte Panel, Creatinine, Iron, Gamma GT, ALT, Triglycerides
☐ ▼ **3357 CARDIAC RISK PANEL** Cholesterol, HDL, LDL, Risk Factors, VLDL Triglycerides
☐ ✗ **3042 CRITICAL CARE PANEL** BUN, Chloride, CO2, Glucose, Potassium, Sodium
☐ **3046 ELECTROLYTE PANEL** Chloride, CO2, Potassium, Sodium
☐ ▼ **3399 EXECUTIVE PANEL** Chem 20, Iron, Cardiac Risk Panel CBC, RPR, Thyroid Cascade
☐ **5242 HEPATITIS PANEL, ACUTE** HAVIgMAb, HBsAg, HBsAb, HBcAb, HCVAb
☐ ▼ **3355 LIPID MONITORING PANEL** Cholesterol, Triglycerides, HDL, LDL, VLDL, ALT, AST
☐ **3312 LIVER PANEL** Alkaline,Phosphatase, AST, Total Bilirubin, Gamma GT, Total Protein, Albumin ALT
☐ ✗ **3083 METABOLIC STATUS PANEL** BUN, Osmolality (calculated), Chloride, CO_2 Creatinine, Glucose, Potassium, Sodium, BUN/Creatinine, Ratio, Anion Gap
☐ ✗ **3376 PANEL B** Chem 12, CBC, Electrolyte Panel
☐ ▼ **3382 PANEL D** Chem 20, CBC, Thyroid Cascade
☐ ✗ **3385 PANEL F** Chem 12, CBC, Electrolyte Panel, Thyroid Cascade
☐ ▼ **3391 PANEL G** Chem 20, Cardiac Risk Panel, CBC, Thyroid Cascade
☐ ▼ **3393 PANEL H** Chem 20, CBC, Cardiac Risk Panel, Rheumatoid Factor, Thyroid Cascade
☐ ▼ **3397 PANEL J** Chem 20, Cardiac Risk Panel
☐ **5351 PRENATAL PANEL** Antibody Screen, ABO/Rh, CBC Rubella, HBsAg, RPR
☐ 1059 with Urinalysis Routine
☐ 1062 with Urinalysis w/Culture if indicated
☐ ✗ **3102 RENAL PANEL** Matabolic Status Panel, Calcium, Phosphorus
☐ **3188 THYROID CASCADE** TSH, Reflex Testing

▼ – patient **required** to fast for 12-14 hours
✗ – patient recommended to fast 12-14 hours

LAB USE ONLY
☐ SST ☐ PLASMA
☐ PURPLE ☐ SERUM
☐ YELLOW ☐ SWAB
☐ BLUE ☐ SLIDES
☐ GREEN ☐ DNA PROBE
☐ GREY ☐ B. CULT BTLS
☐ URINE
☐ BLACK
☐ OTHER: ________
RECV. SPECIMEN: ☐ FROZEN
☐ AMBIENT ☐ ON ICE

Special Instructions/Pertinent Clinical Information ________
Physician's Signature ________ **Date** ________
These orders may be FAXed to: 449-5288 LAB 7060-500 (7/96)

FIGURE 44-10 Laboratory requisition slip.

of medication in the patient's system (peak) or the low point (trough) and thus to determine the correct dose to be administered.

SPECIMEN IDENTIFICATION

Any specimen obtained from a patient must be labeled clearly with patient's name, date and time of collection, and specimen processing number if required by the testing laboratory. An improperly labeled specimen should not be tested. The patient or office should be called with a request for a new specimen.

SPECIMEN HANDLING AND PRESERVATION

Once the specimen is obtained and labeled, it must be stored according to the directions provided by the testing laboratory's policies and procedures manual. Prior to obtaining the specimen, the medical assistant should fill out the requisition, check the laboratory manual for type and amount of specimen needed, type of preservative or anticoagulant required, and how the specimen is to be handled after it is obtained. For example, some specimens must be mailed frozen and in dry ice to reference laboratories. Other specimens are to be picked up by a laboratory collection service and must be refrigerated until tested. (Preservatives and anticoagulants are discussed in later chapters.) Chain-of-custody regulations govern the collection of specimens that may have medicolegal implications. Procedure 44-2

least 8 hours. A 2-hour PP or pc glucose means that the patient eats a prescribed amount of food for a meal and that a blood glucose level is drawn exactly 2 hours after completion of the meal. Timing of specimens is important in testing for certain medication levels to assess the highest level

procedure
44-2

COMPLETING A LABORATORY REQUISITION AND PREPARING A SPECIMEN FOR TRANSPORT TO AN OUTSIDE LABORATORY

Objective: Accurately complete a laboratory requisition form for testing as ordered by the physician, obtain the required specimen(s), and prepare specimen(s) for transport to an outside laboratory.

EQUIPMENT AND SUPPLIES
physician's order for laboratory tests; patient's record; pen; laboratory requisition form; gloves; specimen container; laboratory logbook; biohazard waste container; pen

METHOD
1. Check the patient's record for orders for specific lab tests.
2. Verify which lab will be doing the testing and locate their required requisition form (Figure 44-10).

3. Complete the patient demographic section.
4. Complete the section requiring the physician's name, address, phone number, and account number.
5. Complete the patient's insurance and billing information.
6. Mark each box to indicate each test ordered by the physician. If a test is ordered that is not listed on the requisition, write in the name of the test on the lines provided.
7. Indicate the type and source of the specimen to be tested.
8. Enter the patient's diagnosis on the requisition as needed. If no diagnosis has been made, then code the patient's symptoms.
9. Complete the patient authorization to release and assign the benefits as needed.
10. Assemble the equipment and supplies needed to obtain the specimen.
11. Perform hand hygiene and apply gloves.
12. Obtain the specimen required after explaining the procedure to the patient.
13. Label the specimen with the patient's name, date, physician's name, time of collection, and other information required by the facility.

14. Initial the laboratory requisition and complete the date and time the specimen was obtained.
15. Process the specimens, and if they are not to be sent out until later in the day store them according to laboratory policies and procedures manual requirements.
16. Attach the laboratory requisition securely to the specimen before sending.
17. Remove gloves; dispose of them in the biohazard waste container. Perform hand hygiene.
18. Document the patient's record.
19. Record the specimen in the laboratory logbook, indicating date, time of collection, type and source of the specimen, tests ordered, where samples were sent, and the date they were sent.

CHARTING EXAMPLE

08/04/XX 8:00 A.M. Venous blood sample for stat CBC sent to Memorial Lab at 8:40 A.M. Lab will call back with results. · · ·
· R. Patel, CMA (AAMA)

lists the steps to correctly complete a laboratory requisition and prepare a specimen for transportation to an outside laboratory.

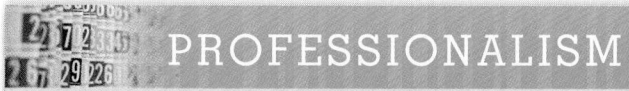

PROFESSIONALISM

THE LAW

Circumstances may arise that require a specimen be obtained from a patient who may have medicolegal implications. Specimen collection in cases of rape; or child, spousal, or elder abuse; or drug or alcohol abuse could have important implications on the outcome of a legal case in a court of law. Proving a chain of custody existed is vital for the specimen to be considered valid. The term *chain of custody* refers to a specific set of procedures used to collect, process, test, and report results on a specimen. A chain-of-custody form must be signed at each step of processing and to prove that the chain of custody was unbroken. Blood alcohol collection kits may be required in certain states for alcohol levels to be considered as evidence in court. Each testing facility should have in place a chain-of-custody procedure for all types of specimens in its policies and procedures manual. Clinical laboratory personnel may be subpoenaed to testify in court about specimens they have collected.

PROFESSIONALISM

In many activities in the medical facility, no one but you knows whether or not you have followed the proper procedure. Whether you wash your hands each and every time you go to a new patient, whether you change gloves as required, whether you perform a test procedure correctly, whether you write down the correct test results, whether you actually perform controls as required are all up to you. Your integrity, honesty, and reliability are on the line every day. Keep in mind the Code of Ethics and the Medical Assistant Creed, which should be followed to uphold the profession and the quality of health care at all times.

MONITORING AND FOLLOWING UP ON LABORATORY TEST RESULTS

Objective: Review incoming laboratory results and follow up with patient per physician's orders.

EQUIPMENT AND SUPPLIES

patient's record; laboratory test results; pen; log of patient's laboratory results

METHOD

Note: Follow the facility policy on contacting patients when results are abnormal. Results are not to be released to the patient unless authorized by the physician.

1. Review incoming lab results and compare with the reference values provided by the analyzing laboratory. Many laboratories highlight or indicate abnormal results on the lab result sheets with H or L.
2. Highlight any abnormal results per facility policy.
3. Obtain the patient's medical record, attach the new laboratory results, and submit the chart to the physician for review. Figure 44-11 shows a medical assistant entering test results electronically. Accuracy when documenting results is critical.
4. Follow the physician's orders regarding scheduling appointments or repeat testing.
5. Document the patient's record accordingly.

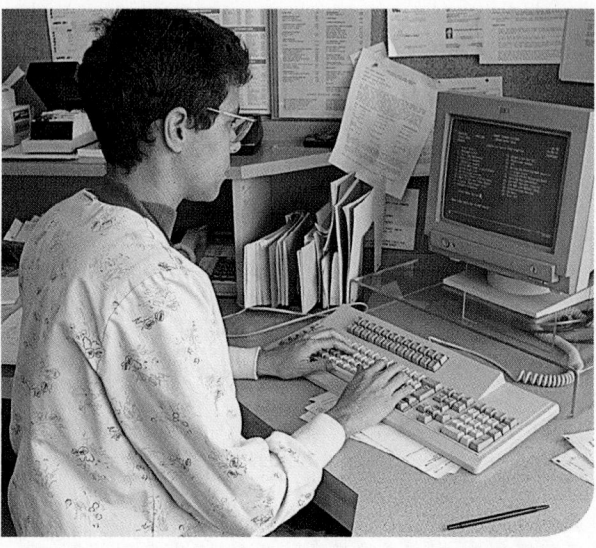

FIGURE 44-11 Correctly documenting laboratory test results in medical records, in writing or electronically, is critical.

CHARTING EXAMPLE

08/04/XX 10:00 A.M. Scheduled repeat lab test and follow up appointment on 08/10/XX per physician's order.· · · · · · · · · · ·
· C. Fisher, CMA (AAMA)

PATIENT RESULTS AND RECORDS

A patient's test results are reviewed by the physician, who will then make them known to the patient (see also "Professionalism"). In some circumstances the physician will allow patient results to be given to the patient by phone. Release of information must comply with HIPAA guidelines to protect patient confidentiality. After the test results are reviewed by the physician, they must be filed according to office policy in the patient's chart. See Procedure 44-3 about monitoring and following up on laboratory test results.

SUMMARY

In this chapter the role of the clinical laboratory in health care has been examined. Different types of laboratories, the types of clinical laboratory departments, and categories of laboratory personnel were discussed. OSHA and CLIA guidelines and laboratory safety issues were considered. The medical assistant has an important role in laboratory testing. It is up to the medical assistant to secure the integrity of the specimen and ensure the proper processing, handling, transporting, and recording of test results. Quality assurance and quality control and their roles in ensuring accurate test results were discussed. The microscope, its parts, and how to utilize it in the POL were covered. Other types of equipment, such as incubator, glassware, centrifuge, photometer, and the microscope, were introduced.

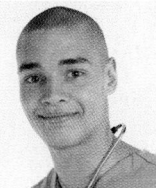

44 CHAPTER REVIEW

COMPETENCY REVIEW

1. Define and spell the terms to learn for this chapter.

2. Define quality assurance and explain its impact on the clinical laboratory.

3. Explain the role of the clinical laboratory in patient care.

4. Explain the three categories of CLIA testing, and give an example of a test that would be performed in each category.

5. Define proficiency testing and how it helps clinical laboratories provide more accurate test results.

PREPARING FOR THE CERTIFICATION EXAM

1. The federal regulations for clinical laboratories specifying guidelines for quality control, qualified personnel and quality assurance is
   a. OSHA
   b. DEA
   c. CDC
   d. NIH
   e. CLIA 1988

2. To change the magnification to a higher objective you would use a
   a. diaphragm
   b. stage
   c. revolving nosepiece
   d. condenser
   e. substage

3. A qualitative test is one that
   a. tests for the presence or absence of a substance
   b. tests for all substances in a sample
   c. tests for the presence and amount of a substance in a sample

   d. is performed only by trained technicians
   e. is only performed at home

4. When using a microscope which of the following is correct?
   a. 10× magnification is used with immersion oil.
   b. Lower the stage after removing the slide.
   c. Only use low with every objective.
   d. Carry the microscope with one hand.
   e. 40× setting is used for high dry power.

5. Which of the following answers is a correct safety rule in the laboratory?
   a. It is unnecessary to supervise new laboratory personnel.
   b. Hands must be thoroughly washed frequently.
   c. Eating and drinking are acceptable in a laboratory
   d. Gloves are unnecessary when working with patients' samples.
   e. Smoking is permitted in the laboratory.

6. The system of scientific measurement used in medical facilities is
   a. the English system
   b. the apothecary system
   c. the metric system
   d. the household system
   e. up to the lab personnel

7. The phlebotomist has the greatest impact on which phase of laboratory testing?
   a. the postanalytical phase
   b. the preanalytical phase
   c. He/she has no impact on lab testing.
   d. analytic phase
   e. result reporting

8. The documentation of all clinical laboratory tests and results is important so
   a. the physician can see the results
   b. any interested party in the facility may see the results
   c. lab directors can monitor the amount of worked performed
   d. quality and coordination of care are monitored
   e. results are available for billing purposes

9. An analyte is
   a. the substance being tested for
   b. a special light in a colorimeter
   c. the same as a sample
   d. the same as a reagent
   e. not important in lab testing

10. A control
    a. is another word for reagent
    b. never needs to be performed when doing lab tests
    c. is similar to the testing specimen with a known value
    d. never needs diluting
    e. is another word for a standard

CRITICAL THINKING

1. What does the clinical laboratory of Pearson Physicians Group need to perform basic laboratory tests (urinalysis, blood glucose screenings, etc.), and how would they go about obtaining what is necessary?

2. Identify the preanalytical phase and analytical phase of the laboratory testing cycle for Mr. Patel's blood glucose screening and urinalysis.

3. Mr. Patel questions why he needs to come back for the 2-hour postprandial blood glucose test. What should Susan tell him?

ON THE JOB

Carmel Lopez has been working in a busy internal medicine office mainly performing clinical procedures. She often performs Certificate of Waiver tests and has helped train new medical assistants to perform them correctly. Carmel observes Rachel not bothering to run the controls that came with a test kit necessary to perform a waived test. Rachel has worked in the office longer than Carmel.

1. Why are controls important when performing a test?
2. What should Carmel do? What should Carmel do if Rachel reacts in a negative way?
3. How would you handle this situation?
4. How might a patient be affected by Rachel's actions?

INTERNET ACTIVITY

Imagine your supervisor asks you to research the Clinical Laboratory Improvement Amendments of 1988 and 1992 and make a short presentation. Do the research and prepare a report.

MEDMEDIA

Additional interactive resources and activities for this chapter can be found:

On your student DVD: View applicable procedure videos on the DVD-ROM found in the back of this book.

MyHealthProfessionsKit.com: Test your knowledge of the chapter with games and activities. MyHealthProfessionsKit also includes resources, helpful links, and a Spanish audio glossary.

Medical Assisting Interactive: Practice your procedures as a medical assistant in this simulated doctor's office. This can be accessed through MyHealthProfessionsKit.com.

45
Microbiology

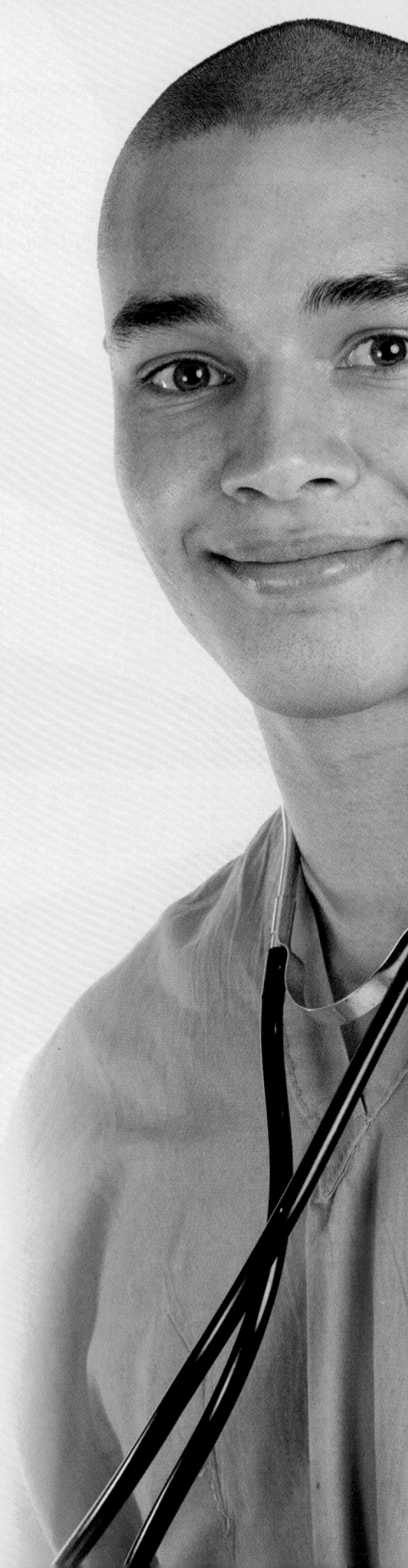

LEARNING OBJECTIVES

After completing this chapter, you should be able to:

- Define and spell the terms to learn for this chapter.

- Define microbiology and its importance in patient care.

- Explain how microorganisms are classified.

- Explain the differences among bacteria, viruses, protozoa, fungi, and parasites.

- Identify three different shapes of bacteria and a disease caused by each.

- Identify a disease caused by each of the five categories of pathogens.

- List general guidelines for obtaining specimens.

- Describe the different growth media needed for culturing microorganisms.

- Explain the purpose of obtaining a specimen.

- Understand how cultures are interpreted.

- Define sensitivity testing and explain how it is done.

- Explain the importance of the Gram stain.

- Describe the basis for serological testing and name three examples performed in a physician's office laboratory.

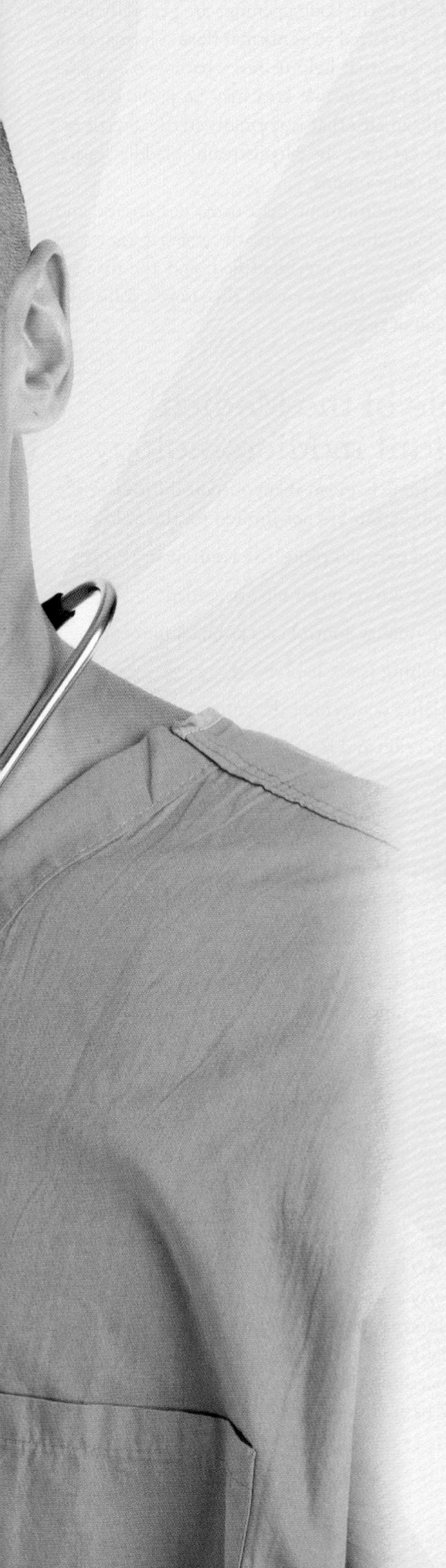

CHAPTER OUTLINE

CASE STUDY

It has been a very busy day at Pearson Physicians Group. David Baker, RMA, has been working with Dr. Penningworth's patients. The next patient that David places in an examination room is 12-year-old Marc Gutierrez. He is accompanied by his mother and is complaining of a very sore throat.

TERMS TO LEARN

acid-fast stain

agar

agglutination

candidiasis

colony

culture media

Culturette

enteritis

eukaryotic

exudates

facultative anaerobes

feces

fixed

inoculated

lawn technique

microbiology

microorganisms

methicillin-resistant
Staphylococcus aureus
(MRSA)

moniliasis

morphology

mycology

necrotizing fasciitis

normal flora

organelles

prokaryotic

sequela

serology

smear

spore

sputum

steatorrhea

subcellular

swabs

viable

wet mount

CERTIFICATION LINK

CMA (AAMA)
Collecting and
processing
specimens; diagnostic
testing
  Methods of
  collection
  Quality control

RMA
Clinical medical
assisting
  Laboratory
  procedures

CMAS (AMT)
Not applicable

The field of **microbiology** is the fascinating study of living organisms too small to be seen with the naked eye (**microorganisms**). Antonie van Leeuwenhoek's invention of the microscope in 1674 allowed humankind to observe for the first time a variety of microbes. Louis Pasteur, the father of microbiology, developed methods for culturing and identifying microbes in the laboratory. Review Chapter 2 for other pertinent facts in the history of medical science.

We are surrounded by microorganisms on our bodies and in the cavities opening to the outside of our bodies as well as in the environment. The microbes that live on the surface of the body and inside the body openings are generally non-pathogenic and are referred to as **normal flora**. Normal flora are beneficial bacteria that help us resist pathogens. A bacterium that is harmless in one area may be pathogenic in another, especially an area that is normally sterile. Sterile areas include body cavities, the bloodstream, bladder, heart, lungs, brain, and other organs.

Bacteria in the environment help us to decompose and recycle waste. This chapter covers the characteristics of microorganisms, how they are identified, and the diseases some pathogens cause. It also covers the proper collection and transportation of specimens.

Role of the Medical Assistant in Microbiology

The medical assistant is given many responsibilities in the office. These include, but are not limited to, the following:

- Proper use of personal protective equipment (PPE)
- Monitoring equipment for repairs needed
- Performing quality control checks on equipment
- Patient teaching (see Chapter 55)
- Confidentiality concerning the patient and test results
- Proper collection and testing of certain specimens

The medical assistant is responsible for instructing patients on the proper collection process for urine, stool, or sputum specimens. It is your responsibility to make the patient as comfortable as possible, particularly when discussing specimens such as stool and urine, which may cause embarrassment.

In some offices, the medical assistant will also test the specimens within CLIA guidelines for waived testing (Chapter 44). If samples are not tested at your facility, you will prepare them for transportation to outside laboratories. No matter what course of action is requested, careful handling of specimens is required for thae safety of the patient and medical assistant and to obtain an uncontaminated sample. Safety guidelines, the infectious process cycle, and infection control are discussed in Chapter 34 and not repeated here.

Observing the Health Information Portability and Accountability Act (HIPAA) regulations concerning privacy must always be one of your chief concerns. Consider the importance of information you will be handling such as test results for sexually transmitted infections (STIs) and HIV. Information concerning the patient should be given only on a need-to-know basis. In other words, the receptionist does

NAMING MICROORGANISMS

Scientists use a binomial system to name all living organisms—animals, plants, bacteria, fungi, and protozoa. Just as we each have two names—a first name and a last name—each organism has two names: the genus (always capitalized) and the species (lowercase). For example, the organism that causes strep throat is known as *Streptococcus pyogenes* (literally, "a chain of round bacteria that produce pus"). The convention is to spell out the entire name at first mention, and then abbreviate with the initial of the genus followed by the species name (e.g., *S. pyogenes*). Although you are not expected to learn all the genus and species names, understanding the system of nomenclature is necessary when you receive laboratory reports over the phone or read a patient's chart.

STRUCTURAL CHARACTERISTICS

The many different types of microorganisms are usually classified by their major structural differences. Differences such as cell structure and the presence or absence of **organelles** (small structures in the cytoplasm of a cell) are used to classify organisms. **Eukaryotic** cells have a nucleus and organelles in the cytoplasm. Protozoa, fungi, and parasites are examples of eukaryotic cells. **Prokaryotic** cells are simpler in structure, without a nucleus or organelles, such as bacteria. **Subcellular** microorganisms, such as viruses, are those comprised of hereditary material (RNA or DNA) with a protein outer coat.

RETENTION OF DYES

Bacteria are also characterized by their reactions to certain stains. A stain is a dye used in coloring microorganisms to allow for visibility under a microscope. The Gram stain, named for Dr. Hans C. J. Gram, a Danish physician, is a commonly used method of staining bacteria. A gram-positive bacterium retains the violet color of the stain used in the staining of the microorganism. Some of the more common gram-positive bacteria are *Staphylococcus aureus* and *Streptococcus pneumoniae*. Figure 45-1 shows gram-positive streptococci.

not need to know the results of the lab test, but the clinical medical assistant does. Certain information should not be shared, even with coworkers in your facility. Although HIPAA regulations affect everyone in the office, those who have most exposure to patients must be informed of methods of enforcement.

Your efficiency can assist the physician in making a proper diagnosis. The physician and the patient are depending on you to complete the test properly and then to accurately document the results.

Classifications of Microorganisms

Although medical assistants are not responsible for identifying and naming specific microorganisms, it is important to understand how they are classified and named. There are many types of microorganisms, and we know already that they are categorized by their ability to cause disease as either pathogens or nonpathogens. Most microbes are nonpathogenic (98 percent to 99 percent); only 1 percent to 2 percent are pathogenic.

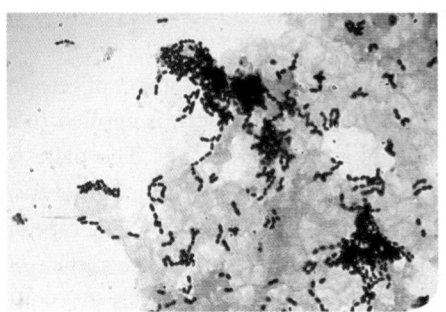

FIGURE 45-1 Gram positive *S. pyogenes* bacteria in chains.

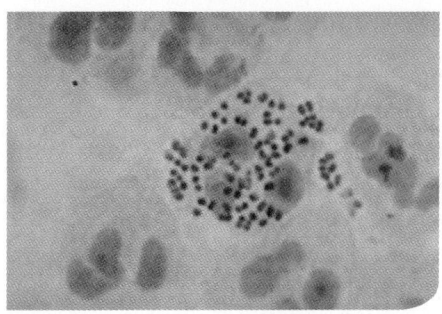

FIGURE 45-2 Gram negative *N. gonorrhoeae.*

A gram-negative bacterium has the pink color of the counterstain used in Gram's method of staining microorganisms. A few of the most common gram-negative bacteria are *Escherichia coli, Neisseria gonorrhoeae,* and *Salmonella typhimurium.* Figure 45-2 shows gram-negative *N. gonorrhoeae.* Some organisms do not stain well with Gram stain and require a special stain, such as the **acid-fast stain** used for the organism that causes tuberculosis.

USE OF OXYGEN

Bacteria also can be categorized by whether they survive in an oxygen-rich environment (aerobes) or die in the presence of oxygen (anaerobes) or are anaerobes that are flexible and can live with some oxygen (**facultative anaerobes**). Successful culturing requires an understanding of the oxygen requirements of bacteria. If the ultimate goal is to grow and identify a sample of the organism that is causing disease in a patient, then we must provide proper oxygen, moisture, nutrition, and temperature in the laboratory setting.

HEMOLYTIC PROPERTIES

Bacteria are also categorized by their ability to hemolyze (burst) red blood cells in the blood agar. When a specimen is collected, it has to be placed on or in a substance called a **culture medium**, to promote growth of microorganisms. **Agar** is a gelatinlike substance made from seaweed that is added to culture media to provide nutrition and a semisolid surface on which microbes can grow. A more detailed discussion of media and cultures follows later in this chapter.

Hemolysis is an important identifying property of certain microbes. A specimen such as a throat swab is applied to a blood agar plate and incubated for 24 hours. The plate is then held up to the light to enhance reading for hemolysis. No change in color around the **colony** (growth of one type of microorganism visible with the naked eye on the surface of culture media) is known as gamma hemolysis or nonhemolytic (the preferred term). A narrow green-colored zone around a colony is known as alpha hemolysis; and a clear zone around the colony is beta hemolysis. Beta hemolysis indicates that the microorganism in that colony has burst the red blood cells, leaving a clear colorless zone around it. The organism that causes strep throat is beta hemolytic.

OTHER IDENTIFYING CHARACTERISTICS

Microbes may be either motile or nonmotile. If they are capable of movement, their means of motility is unique to specific categories of microorganisms. They may possess flagella (long whiplike extensions of the cytoplasm) or cilia (fine hairlike extensions). For example, *Trichomonas vaginalis,* the protozoa that is responsible for one type of vaginitis, has four flagella at one end that produce the characteristic circular whiplike movement seen in wet preparations and microscopic examinations of infected individuals' urine.

Biochemical analysis, often done on semiautomated analyzers, provides the microbiologist with information that assists in identification of certain pathogens, such as enteric organisms.

Types of Microorganisms

Microbes are also divided into groups based on shared special characteristics. Bacteria, viruses, protozoa, fungi, parasites, and other organisms with similar characteristics are discussed next. Table 45-1 provides a list of microorganisms, including descriptions and examples of each.

BACTERIUM/BACTERIA

Bacteria are small, unicellular microorganisms that are capable of rapid reproduction. Their reproductive ability explains how some infections become overwhelming in a short period of time and can be dangerous. For example, one *Escherichia coli* organism, the most common cause of urinary tract infections (UTIs), reproduces in about 30 minutes. By the end of a 24-hour period, this one *Escherichia coli (E. coli)* cell will have produced an enormous number of cells capable of creating an infection if they have been introduced into the bladder.

Bacteria may be named for their **morphology** (shape): cocci (spherical), bacilli (rod shaped), or spirilla (spiral shaped). In the following paragraphs, we consider each group of bacteria classified by their morphology.

Coccus/Cocci

Cocci are round bacteria that are arranged in various configurations. *Staphylococci* are found in grapelike clusters, *Streptococci* in chains, and *Diplococci* in pairs.

Staphylococci. *Staphylococci* are gram-positive, grapelike clusters of cocci, some of which are pathogenic. Nonpatho-

TABLE 45-1 Classes of Microorganisms with Descriptions and Examples

Microorganism	Description	Example
Bacteria	Most numerous of all microorganisms Unicellular Some are pathogenic to humans Identified by shape and appearance	(See cocci, *Bacilli*, and *Spirilla* entries)
• Cocci	Three types of spherical bacteria	
1. *Staphylococci*	Form grapelike clusters of pus-producing organisms	Boils, pimples, acne, osteomyelitis
2. *Streptococci*	Form chains of cells	Rheumatic heart disease, scarlet fever, strep throat
3. *Diplococci*	Form pairs of cells	Pneumonia, gonorrhea, and meningitis
• *Bacilli*	Rod-shaped bacteria	Gram-positive *Bacilli*: tetanus, diphtheria, gas gangrene Gram-negative *Bacilli*: *E. coli* (UTI), *Bordetella pertussis* (whooping cough)
• *Vibrios*		Cholera
• *Spirilla*	Spiral-shaped organisms	Syphilis
• Fungi	Parasitic and some nonparasitic plants and molds Depend on other life forms for their nutrition, such as dead or decaying organic material Reproduction method is budding Yeast is a typical fungus Feed on antibiotics and flourish on antibiotic therapy The Latin word *fungus* means "mushroom"	*Histoplasma capsulatum* (histoplasmosis), *Tinea pedis* (athlete's foot), *Candida albicans* (yeast infection), and *Tinea spp.* (ringworm)
Protozoa	One-celled organism Both parasitic and nonparasitic Can move with cilia or false feet Typically 2–200 mm in size	Trichomoniasis (caused by *Trichomonas vaginalis*), amoebic dysentery, and malaria
Rickettsia	Visible under a standard microscope Susceptible to antibiotics Transmitted by insects (ticks, fleas)	Rocky Mountain spotted fever
Virus	Smallest of microorganisms Can only be seen with electron microscope Can only multiply within a living cell (host) Difficult to kill with chemotherapy since they become resistant to the drug Can be destroyed by heat (autoclave sterilization) but generally not by chemical disinfection More viruses than any other category of microbial agents Feed on antibiotics and flourish on antibiotic therapy	Herpes virus, HIV, ARC, AIDS, common cold, influenza virus, smallpox, hepatitis A, hepatitis B, mumps, shingles

genic *Staphylococci* are found on our skin and in many of our body orifices or openings. *S. aureus* or staph is the major pathogen of this genus and may be found as normal flora in the nose and on the skin. It causes infection especially when resistance is lowered by a break in the skin or in the mucous membranes. *S. aureus* produces infections such as impetigo in children and is associated with infection of wound sites and surgical incisions. It causes pus-producing abscesses

such as boils, carbuncles, and folliculitis. Figure 45-3 shows an example of carbuncles.

S. aureus is a common cause of nosocomial infections and may also cause pneumonia, meningitis, and septicemia in individuals with reduced resistance. Toxic shock syndrome is also caused by this virulent organism. *S. aureus* produces one type of **enteritis** (food poisoning) that occurs within a few hours of eating improperly refrigerated food contaminated

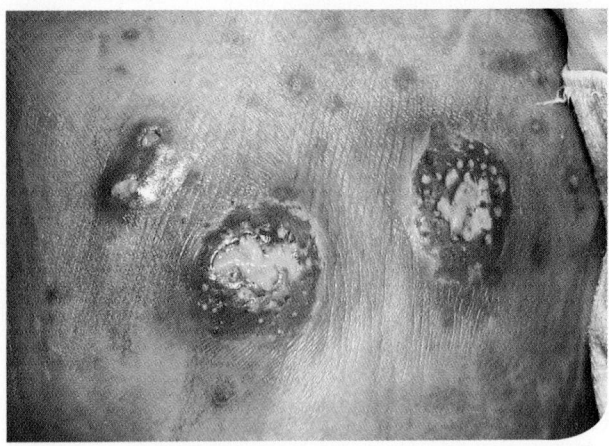

FIGURE 45-3 Carbuncles caused by *S. aureus*.

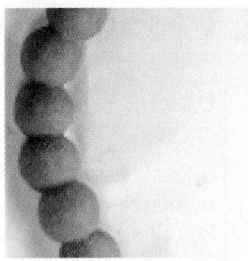

FIGURE 45-4 *Streptococci*: individual bacteria that have a rounded shape and have clumped together to form a chain.

with the toxin produced by the bacteria. This toxin causes nausea vomiting, diarrhea, and abdominal cramping. *S. aureus* is coagulase positive, meaning it produces an enzyme that can be used to help differentiate *S. aureus* from other species of this organism.

Because of increased reliance on treatment with antibiotics to treat low-level infections today, superbugs (various microorganisms that are mutating to produce antibiotic-resistant forms) are becoming common. Of particular interest is **methicillin-resistant *Staphylococcus aureus* (MRSA)**. This form of *S. aureus* produces an enzyme the makes the organism resistant to penicillins and cephalosporins normally used for treatment and renders these antibiotics ineffective. Tests are available to indicate the presence or absence of this enzyme and help determine the most favorable treatment. The problem of antibiotic resistance is a major concern for health care providers and is being experienced worldwide. Additional information on this topic is found later in this chapter.

Streptococci. *Streptococci* are round, gram-positive bacteria arranged in chains, some of which are nonpathogenic, others of which are dangerous to humans. Streptococcal organisms are part of the normal flora of the upper respiratory tract and skin. As previously mentioned, one classification of streptococcal organisms is based on the type of hemolysis the organisms cause on blood agar plates. In addition, *Streptococci* can be classified serologically with antisera specific for antigens in cell walls and specific for each group (A–H and K–V). Identification of the specific group of strep organisms is important in epidemiology, the study of outbreaks of infections.

Group A beta-hemolytic *S. pyogenes* causes a variety of diseases varying from mild such as strep throat to life threatening such as **necrotizing fasciitis** (severe infection due to destruction of subcutaneous tissue and fascia, with a 30 percent mortality rate). This organism also causes other infections, including pneumonia, tonsillitis, scarlet fever, rheumatic fever, acute glomerulonephritis, and bacterial endocarditis, as well as abscesses, wound infections, and bacteremia.

Commercial kits are available for rapid detection of group A beta-hemolytic strep in the office or laboratory setting. Any negative test should be followed up by a culture that includes bacitracin sensitivity. Sensitivity to the antibiotic bacitracin is a useful tool to separate group A beta-hemolytic strep from other strep organisms. The information about rapid strep tests and the procedure for a throat culture with bacitracin are covered later in this chapter. Figure 45-4 shows a model of *Streptococci*.

S. pneumoniae (also called *Pneumococcus* or *Diplococcus pneumoniae*) frequently are found as normal flora in the throat. However, it is the frequent cause of bacterial pneumonia, particularly in the older population, and in middle ear infections in children and meningitis in older children and adults.

Diplococci. *Diplococci* occur in pairs. Some *Diplococci* are gram positive, such as *S. pneumoniae,* which causes bacterial pneumonia. Others such as *N. gonorrhoeae* and *Neisseria meningitidis* are gram negative, the former causing gonorrhea, a sexually transmitted infection, and the latter causing a form of bacterial meningitis and septicemia. Meningococcal meningitis has a high mortality rate and requires immediate treatment. A vaccine for meningococcal meningitis is now available that is recommended for students entering high school or college, those joining the armed services, and other individuals who may be at high risk.

Although these diplococcal organisms are pathogenic, many of the *Diplococci,* both gram negative and gram positive, are normally found in areas such as the upper respiratory tract.

Bacillus/Bacilli

Rod-shaped *Bacilli* may be pathogenic or nonpathogenic. Some *Bacilli* are gram positive, and others are gram negative.

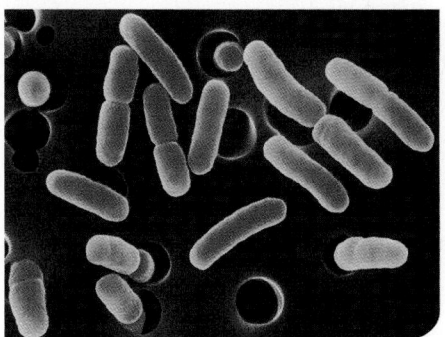

FIGURE 45-5 *Bacilli.*

Figure 45-5 illustrates *Bacilli*. *Bacilli* are responsible for a wide variety of illnesses, including gastroenteritis, UTIs, whooping cough, tetanus, botulism, tuberculosis, and pneumonia.

Gram-Negative *Bacilli*. Enterobacteriaceae are a large family of gram-negative *Bacilli* found mainly in the intestinal tract; however, many of them will cause infections in other body locations. One type, *E. coli*, is most frequently associated with UTIs. Another is the group of *Salmonella* organisms. *Salmonella* organisms are a major cause of foodborne illnesses worldwide. They can be classified serologically to differentiate which among the thousands of members of this pathogenic group are causing the outbreak of disease. Most frequently, outbreaks of food poisoning are caused either by *Salmonella enteritidis* or *S. typhimurium.* Symptoms of enteric food poisoning include rapid onset, abdominal pain, nausea, diarrhea, and in some children even death. Contaminated food such as raw eggs, chicken, or beef is the usual route of transmission.

Typhoid fever is caused by *S. typhimurium* and is frequently found in Third World countries and natural disaster areas where proper sanitation is lacking. Another member of the genus of gram-negative *Bacilli* is a group of *Shigella* organisms that causes bacillary dysentery, characterized by frequent blood-, pus-, or mucous-containing stools. This bacillary dysentery results from inadequate sanitary conditions.

Another gram-negative *Bacillus* not a member of the previously mentioned group is *Helicobacter pylori*, which was discovered in the early 1980s. This organism is found in about half of the human population and causes no symptoms in most individuals. It was discovered that *H. pylori* is the causative agent of peptic ulcers and a risk factor in gastric malignancy in some infected persons. The organism is responsive to a number of antibiotics, including tetracycline. The discovery of *H. pylori* led to major breakthroughs in ulcer treatment. Previously it was believed peptic ulcers were due to nerves or increased acid production, and treatments were generally ineffective.

Gram-Positive *Bacilli*. Gram-positive *Bacilli* may be found in chains or singly and are spore forming or nonspore forming. A **spore** is a thick-walled reproductive cell produced by some organisms that is capable of withstanding unfavorable environmental conditions. Notable in this group are *Clostridium botulinum,* which causes botulism, and *Clostridium tetani,* which causes tetanus. Tetanus immunizations are given to protect from the extremely potent neurotoxin produced by *C. tetani.* Tetanus is a disease resulting from a cut or injury associated with contaminated soil such as a rusty farm implement. Botulism is a severe, possibly fatal form of food poisoning caused by the powerful neurotoxin produced by the anaerobe *C. botulinum;* it is associated with improper canning processes and its potential use as a bioterrorism agent.

Vibrio/Vibrios. *Vibrios* are comma-shaped *Bacilli.* The main pathogen is *Vibrio cholerae,* whose enterotoxin causes cholera. Cholera is characterized by profuse watery stools, vomiting, leg cramps, dehydration, and shock. It is caused by ingesting drinking water or eating shellfish from water contaminated with infected urine, feces, or vomitus. Cholera is common in Asiatic countries, and travelers to these areas can be vaccinated for protection; however, travelers still should boil all drinking water and avoid uncooked foods. Figure 45-6 illustrates a *Vibrio.*

Spirillum/Spirilla

Spirilla, or spirochetes as they are also known, are spiral-shaped or corkscrew-shaped organisms. Technically, they are rods that are twisted in various shapes; however, they are classified as a separate phylum of bacteria. As with other shapes of bacteria, some are nonpathogenic and are found in certain areas of the body and others, such as *Treponema pallidum,* cause the sexually transmitted infection syphilis. *Borrelia burgdorferi* was discovered in the mid-1970s to be the causative agent of Lyme disease. Lyme disease is a deer tick–borne disease named after a town in Connecticut that

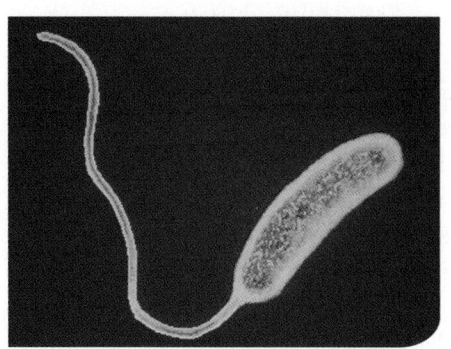

FIGURE 45-6 *Vibrio.*

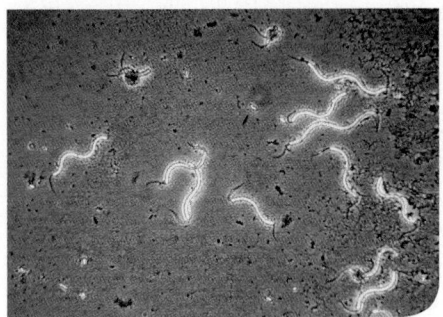

FIGURE 45-7 *Spirilla* bacteria.

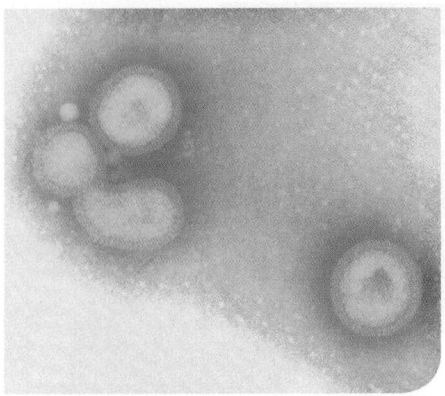

FIGURE 45-8 Influenza virus.

was investigating a cluster of juvenile arthritis cases. Ticks are infected by feeding on deer or rodents, which are natural hosts for the organism. The infected tick then bites a human and transmits the organism. This tick is so tiny that many people are unaware of the bite until the characteristic expanding rash is discovered, followed after a period of time by fever, muscle pain, headache, and fatigue. Immunoassay tests exist to aid in the diagnosis of Lyme disease. Figure 45-7 is an illustration of *Spirilla*.

Special Categories of Bacteria

Some types of bacteria do not fall clearly into any of the previously mentioned groups. These are *Mycobacteria, Rickettsia, Mycoplasma,* and *Chlamydia. Mycobacteria* have a different type of material in the cell wall and can only be stained with an acid-fast stain. Two members of this genus are fairly well known.

Mycobacterium tuberculosis is the causative agent of tuberculosis, and *Mycobacterium leprae* is the cause of leprosy. These organisms do not stain well with a Gram stain. In a positive slide for acid-fast *Bacilli* (AFB), the slender *Bacilli* will appear pink with an acid-fast stain.

Rickettsia, Chlamydia, and *Mycoplasma* are very tiny bacteria in the size range of viruses. *Rickettsia* are bacterial parasites that live in ticks and mites and transmit the disease when they bite humans. Rocky Mountain spotted fever and typhus are both rickettsial diseases. *Chlamydia* is also an obligate parasite, but it does not live in arthropod hosts. *Chlamydia* must invade living cells to reproduce. *Chlamydia trachomatis* is an STI that may be a silent inhabitant of the vagina or cause mild burning sensations and discharge. After repeated infections, this organism may cause scarring in the Fallopian tubes, making conception difficult. *Rickettsia* and *Chlamydia* cannot be grown on artificial media. Tissue cultures or serological testing must be done for identification.

Mycoplasma were thought to be viruses at one time, but they are very tiny bacteria lacking a rigid cell wall. They cause *Mycoplasma* pneumonia and a type of venereal disease.

VIRUS/VIRUSES

Although potent, a virus is the smallest known infectious organism and requires the use of an electron microscope for visualization. A virus, a simpler form of life than a cell, is parasitic, depending on living cells of other organisms for growth. When a virus enters a cell, it may immediately cause a disease, such as influenza, or it may remain dormant for days or even years. Figure 45-8 shows an example of an influenza virus. For instance, herpes zoster may cause an outbreak of chickenpox within 7 to 14 days of exposure. Yet, HIV can lie dormant for a long period of time, sometimes years, before any symptoms are noted.

Viruses cause many common diseases, such as colds, chickenpox, mumps, infectious mononucleosis, and warts. Other illnesses caused by viruses are hepatitis, measles, encephalitis, and herpes. Fortunately, vaccines are available to protect people from diseases such as polio, German measles, measles, hepatitis B, mumps, and chickenpox.

PROTOZOAN/PROTOZOA

Although they are single-celled parasites, protozoa are usually larger than bacteria. Most protozoa live in the soil and receive nourishment from dead or decaying organic material. Lack of proper sanitation can lead to rapid spread of infections. Some protozoa are pathogenic and may cause diseases such as trichomoniasis (a type of STI caused by *T. vaginalis*), or malaria, which is transmitted by the bite of an infected *Anopheles* mosquito. The organism inhabits the red blood cells (RBCs) in the affected individual. Figure 45-9 models malaria protozoa.

FUNGUS/FUNGI

The study of fungi is known as **mycology**. Fungi are present in soil, water, and air. Fungi are unable to make their own food, so they depend on other life forms. Included in this classification are yeasts and molds. In our environment we

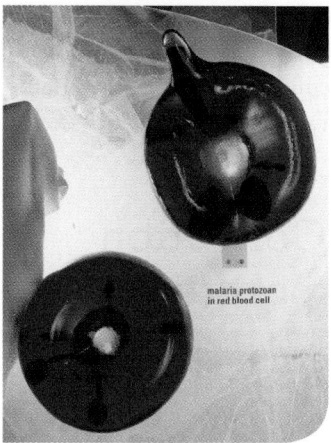

FIGURE 45-9   Model of malaria protozoa in a red blood cell. New parasites are produced and mature in the RBC, then push their way out of the cell.

encounter fungi in the forms of mushrooms and penicillin molds on stale bread. *Penicillium* mold was discovered by Alexander Fleming, and its antibiotic properties changed modern medical treatment. Penicillin is now synthetically produced. Figure 45-10 shows an example of a mold.

Yeasts are single-celled fungi that reproduce by budding. Those fungi that produce spores are molds. Most fungi are not pathogenic and cause few diseases in humans. Of those that do, most will produce only superficial infections, such as athlete's foot (*Tinea pedis*) or ringworm. A few do produce life-threatening illnesses when they invade the internal organs of the body.

Candida albicans is the causative agent of the yeast infection known as **moniliasis**, **candidiasis**, or thrush. Individuals with compromised immune systems or those who have been on long-term antibiotic therapy may develop severe infections. In these cases, the normal flora that protect the openings of the body cavities are killed by the antibiotic therapy and allow fungi a fertile environment in which to reproduce. This type of infection is referred to as a superinfection. As anyone who has endured the unpleasantness of athlete's foot knows, it takes a long time and persistence to get rid of a fungal infection. Fungal infections are resistant to antibiotics and must be treated with antifungal agents.

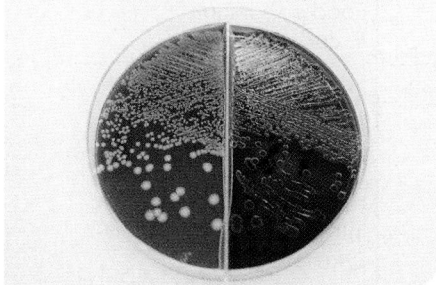

FIGURE 45-10   Mold is growing on red/green agar in a divided Petri dish.

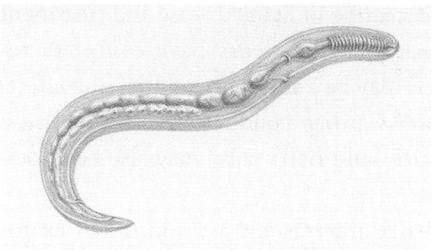

FIGURE 45-11   A female roundworm. Roundworms have long, cylindrical bodies with a tough covering. Eggs laid by the females are excreted in the feces of infected people.

PARASITES

As previously noted, a parasite receives nourishment from another organism. As a result of this activity, the host organism becomes diseased. Parasites may be single celled, such as *Chlamydia,* or multicellular, such as pinworms.

Some examples of parasites include worms and insects:

- **Worms (helminths)**—The person may ingest the egg or an immature form of the worm, or the worm may penetrate the skin. Some of the worms that infect people are flatworms, roundworms, tapeworms, and pinworms. Figure 45-11 shows a female roundworm. Roundworms, flatworms, and tapeworms inhabit the intestines. Tapeworms, for instance, may grow to be many feet in length. The stool or **feces** of the patient can be inspected for the presence of ova and mature forms of the worm. The procedure for collecting stool for ova and parasites (O&P) is covered later in this chapter.

- **Insects**—Insects may bite, burrow under, or attach to the skin of the human. An example of a disease occurring by attachment of an insect is Lyme disease, caused by a tick-transmitted spirochete. Lyme disease has been documented in many parts of North America and has an incubation period of 3 to 32 days. Figure 45-12 shows a tick.

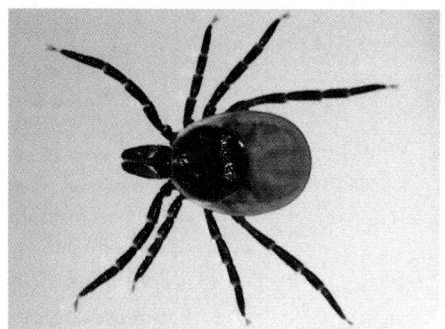

FIGURE 45-12   A deer tick can cause Lyme disease.

With early detection of Lyme disease and treatment with antibiotics, many patients have complete recovery. Arthritis may be a **sequela** (long-lasting effect) of Lyme disease. Cardiac conduction abnormalities, aseptic meningitis, and Bell's palsy may also be associated conditions.

Scabies and lice infestations are additional examples of insect parasites. Both are transmitted by direct contact with bedding or clothing and cause severe itching.

Refer to Table 45-2 for some examples of pathogenic microorganisms, their location in the body, and diseases they produce.

MEDICATION-RESISTANT MICROORGANISMS

Chapter 34 contains a thorough discussion of a variety of medication-resistant microorganisms. Health care costs and the wellness of the population are quite dramatically impacted by these superbugs. Proper and consistent hand and personal hygiene are critically important in decreasing the prevalence of these difficult microorganisms. Bioterrorism and the organisms involved are also discussed in Chapter 34.

Specimen Collection and Transportation

Specimens for microbiology must be collected according to protocols established by the microbiology department of the laboratory performing the testing. One of the first priorities of quality control (QC) is proper specimen collection. No shortcuts may be taken in the collection process. Any incorrect steps could result in a contaminated or altered specimen, delayed diagnosis, and postponed or possibly harmful treatment.

The first step in specimen collection is proper patient education. Many tests require special preparation if accurate

TABLE 45-2 Pathogenic Microorganisms and Resulting Diseases

Body Location	Pathogen	Disease
Respiratory system	Streptococcus pyogenes Corynebacterium diphtheriae Mycobacterium tuberculosis Haemophilus influenzae type B Streptococcus pneumoniae	Strep throat, scarlet fever Diphtheria Tuberculosis Influenza Pneumonia
Central nervous system	Neisseria meningitidis Polioviruses Rabies virus	Meningitis Poliomyelitis Rabies
Genitourinary system	Herpes simplex viruses 1 and 2 Candida albicans (fungus) Chlamydia trachomatis Escherichia coli	Genital herpes Vaginitis Vaginitis Urinary tract infection
Integumentary system	Staphylococcus aureus Varicella zoster virus	Boils, carbuncles Chickenpox Scabies Lice
Gastrointestinal system	Hepatitis A, B, and C viruses Salmonella enteritidis Escherichia coli	Hepatitis A, B, and C Food poisoning E. coli diarrhea
Circulatory system and blood, immune system	Streptococcus pyogenes Staphylococcus aureus Plasmodium falciparum, P. vivax, P. malariae, P. ovale Human immunodeficiency virus Epstein-Barr virus Borrelia burgdorferi	Septicemia, endocarditis Malaria HIV/AIDS Infectious mononucleosis Lyme disease
Tissue	Streptococcus pyogenes	Necrotizing fasciitis

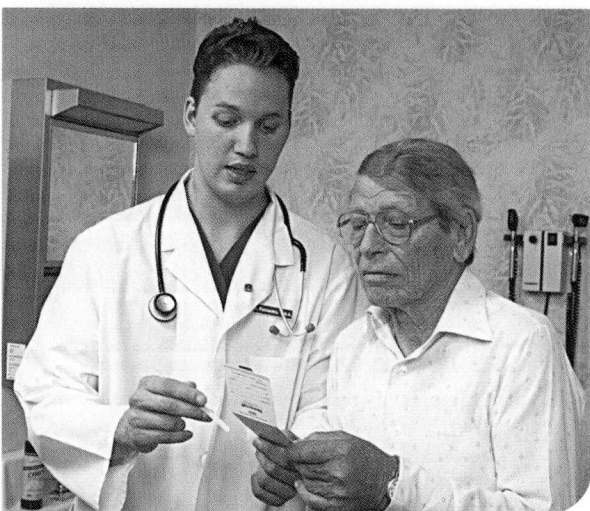

FIGURE 45-13 A medical assistant explains to a patient how to use a specimen collection kit.

results are to be obtained for diagnosis. It is up to the medical assistant to make sure the patient understands and complies with these instructions by doing three things: (1) carefully reading and explaining the instructions, (2) answering any questions the patient might have, and (3) giving written instructions for the patient to follow or refer to at home. (Figure 45-13 shows a medical assistant explaining a laboratory procedure to a patient.) Carefully document any patient teaching and verify that the patient verbalizes understanding of the instructions.

The second important step is to follow the basic guidelines for specimen collection. Guidelines 45-1 provides guidelines for specimen collection. Keep in mind when dealing with microbiological specimens that they are living organisms and must have proper conditions to survive but not to multiply.

LABORATORY REQUEST INFORMATION

In addition to the specimen label information consisting of patient's name, date and time of collection, type and source of specimen, doctor's name, and your initials, the following information should be included on the requisition:

- Patient's address
- Identification number
- Age
- Gender
- Insurance information
- More specific information regarding the type and source of the specimen (e.g., nasal swab, left nostril)
- Test requested

GUIDELINES 45-1

SPECIMEN COLLECTION

The basic rules for specimen collection are:

1. Confirm the identity of the patient by asking the patient to state his or her name and spell it, if necessary.
2. Screen the patient to determine if pretest preparation was followed.
3. Collect specimen prior to beginning antibiotic treatment.
4. Collect sufficient quantity of material for testing.
5. Use only appropriate collection technique by observing proper cleaning and aseptic procedures to control contamination.
6. Use only sterile containers.
7. Select the proper containers for collection that comply with the reference laboratory's or outside laboratory's requirements.
8. Ensure that the collection container is tightly closed and appropriately sealed to avoid leakage and contamination of the specimen and any surface with which the container may come in contact.
9. Label the specimen accurately at the time of collection with the following information:
   a. Patient's full name
   b. Date
   c. Time of collection
   d. Type of specimen
   e. Antibiotic treatment in use, if any
   f. Your initials
10. Fill out the requisition form for the reference lab and double-check that the information matches the label.
11. Deliver specimen promptly to laboratory and document it. Otherwise, maintain proper storage until specimen can be picked up or transported appropriately.

Note: Cerebrospinal fluid always requires immediate delivery.

- Medication patient is currently receiving
- Diagnosis, if available
- Physician's information (name, address, telephone number)
- Special information or orders

A specimen will be rejected by outside laboratories if the information on the label, the requisition, or both is incomplete, or if the specimen is insufficient in quantity or

FIGURE 45-14 Examples of sterile swabs (removed from protective wrappers).

improperly packaged. Tests may have to be repeated and the specimen collected again. This means additional delay and discomfort for the patient.

COLLECTION DEVICES

Sterile **swabs** are frequently used in collection of specimens. The shafts and the tips of swabs vary in terms of the type of material used. They are wrapped in a sterile wrapper or container to preserve sterility. Figure 45-14 shows examples of sterile swabs of various types. Cotton swabs are used less frequently today because certain microbes are inhibited by the natural ingredients in cotton. Polyester and rayon are used for the tips; wood, plastic, or wire are used for the shaft. Swabs also vary in size of tip and flexibility of the shaft to permit collection in difficult-to-reach areas. After a swab is collected, it is placed in a sterile container that may or may not contain culture media.

Swabs, Culture Tubes, and Other Collection Devices

The **Culturette** system is comprised of a disposable, clear plastic tube; a sterile, cotton-tipped applicator swab inside the tube; and a sealed plastic vial of medium (broth containing nourishment for bacteria and a preservative). This system is used to obtain many types of specimens, from sites ranging from the throat, nose, or eyes to wounds and the genital or urethral areas. It is important that these types of specimens, collected in Culturettes, be transported immediately so that microorganisms remain **viable** (capable of living) when they reach the laboratory. Commercially available swab collection and transportation units are used widely. Some of these units contain two sterile swabs, one for culturing and one for preparing the direct smear. A **smear** is a thin layer of microorganisms spread on a glass slide for identification purposes. (Figure 45-15 demonstrates a variety of collection devices, including a swab and Culturette in the lower left of the photograph.) Specimens such as **exudates** (wound drainage material made of serum, white blood cells, and fibrin) may be collected with Culturette units. Collection devices also are available for anaerobic cultures (Fig 45-15). Sterile containers are available for urine, stool, blood, and cerebrospinal fluid. Fluids drained from body cavities may require larger sterile containers.

TRANSPORTING SPECIMENS TO AN OUTSIDE LABORATORY

Specimens may be picked up by courier to deliver to a local laboratory testing site. Or the testing site may be located in a distant location requiring special mailing devices and instructions. In addition to moisture and specific nutrition requirements, specimens must be maintained at appropriate temperatures to ensure viability. Temperatures may differ with the type of specimen. The length of time

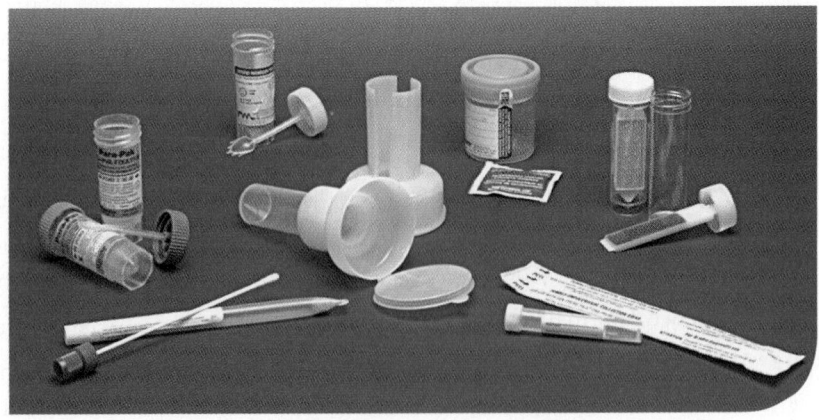

FIGURE 45-15 Examples of specimen collection containers.

between collection and arrival at the testing site can be crucial. Throat cultures and samples for gonorrhea should never be refrigerated. Always consult the office laboratory policies and procedures manual for complete transporting instructions.

Diagnosing Infection

When a patient comes to the office with an apparent infection, exactly what steps are taken to diagnose and begin treatment of the infection? First, the patient is examined and the usual procedures are followed, including gathering information, such as patient identification, vital signs, chief complaint, and present illness. If the infection is one that can be diagnosed on sight by the physician, such as chickenpox, further testing will not be necessary. For an open infected wound, the site should be measured, described, and charted, including information about drainage, odor, and level of patient discomfort.

Next, specimens are collected and labeled and prepared safely for transportation to ensure any organisms remain alive and safety issues are observed. A culture of the specimen may be necessary, in which case a swab of the specimen is streaked on appropriate culture medium in such a way as to allow individual colonies of microorganisms to develop. This permits easier identification. A second culture plate may be heavily **inoculated** (microorganisms placed on or in media) to be tested for antibiotic sensitivity. Certain microorganisms are sensitive to specific antibiotics and resistant to others. The culture plates are incubated at 37°C for 24 hours to allow the organisms to grow.

After 24 hours, a zone of no growth around an antibiotic disk indicates that the organism is sensitive to that drug, and if it is used to treat the patient it should work in the same way. If the patient is allergic to that particular medication, then the antibiotic with the next largest zone of inhibition is chosen for treatment. If direct examination of the specimen is required, then a direct smear is made. This involves placing a thin layer of the specimen material on a slide that is properly labeled, allowed to dry, and then stained. The physician or other qualified personnel will examine it for microorganisms, considering their morphology and stain reactions (gram positive or gram negative). In some cases, a presumptive diagnosis can be made and treatment determined.

Preparation of a **wet mount** may be necessary in cases where the organisms, if present, must be kept alive to observe for motility and morphology. A wet mount is a preparation in a liquid that will preserve motility of the microbe. The ultimate goal of all these steps is to select the most favorable treatment that will restore the patient to a healthy condition. A more detailed discussion of the preceding steps follows.

Microbiology Equipment and Procedures

The equipment and supplies necessary in a microbiology laboratory vary with the size and type of facility. A typical physician's office laboratory (POL) will have a microscope, incubator, autoclave, refrigerator, biohazard waste containers, and a variety of specimen collection devices and containers (all of which are discussed in other chapters). Inoculation equipment, such as loop, needle, and incineration equipment and culture media, are also necessary to process microbiology specimens.

INOCULATING EQUIPMENT

A loop is a long instrument with a small loop on the end designed to pick up fluids and transfer them to culture media. Specifically calibrated loops for urine cultures are available that allow for the transfer of 1 µL (microliter) of urine to a culture plate. This precise amount of urine allows for quantitative evaluation of the number of microorganisms to evaluate whether a UTI is present. Inoculating loops and needles (a needle is a long, straight instrument with a pointed end used to sample individual colonies of microorganisms) may be purchased in sterile, prewrapped packages or may be made of metal for sterilization and reuse. After a prewrapped sterile loop or needle is used, it is discarded in a biohazard waste container. A metal loop or needle requires incineration before and after use to ensure sterility; Bunsen burners requiring a natural gas supply or electric incinerators are used.

CULTURE MEDIA

Once a specimen has been obtained, it must be inoculated onto a medium that will enhance the growth of the microorganism. The most common types of media are broth and agar. A culture is the propagation of microorganisms or living cells in a special media that enhances their growth. Some types of media contain special dyes or ingredients that will enhance the growth of one type of bacteria while retarding growth of others to enable easier identification. The microbiologist observes the culture for a colony and the appearance of the colony, then examines a sample of the specimen under a microscope for morphology and staining properties. Each bit of information about the nature of the microorganism assists in identification and diagnosis.

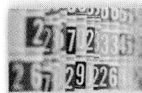

PROFESSIONALISM

THE LAW

Confidentiality regarding any patient testing is paramount. Results of testing are confidential, whether performed in the POL or an outside laboratory. Follow office policy concerning who is or is not allowed to give results to the patient. If you call the patient at home and get an answering machine, do not leave the results of the test as a message. State your name, your facility, and ask the patient to call the office, after assuring the patient that it is not an emergency. If the patient does not return your call within the time limits considered appropriate for your office, call again. Document calls made to your patients.

Careful labeling of specimens will assist in protecting the patient and physician from an incorrect diagnosis. An incorrect diagnosis can lead to delayed treatment.

Because many of the microorganisms present in specimens taken in the office setting are pathogenic, the medical assistant has an ethical responsibility to avoid carrying the microbes outside of the laboratory. This requires strict adherence to policies regarding wearing PPE and hand hygiene.

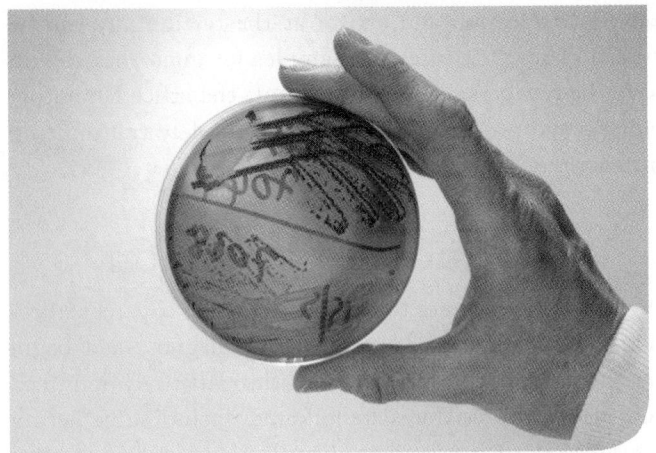

FIGURE 45-16 Petri dish containing fecal bacteria cultures.
Source: Jim Varney.

Commercial units for blood, vaginal, and throat specimens are also available. All media should be inspected for contamination before use to ensure the integrity of the culturing process.

INOCULATING MEDIA

Pathogens are identified by growing cultures (propagating microorganisms) taken from the specimen. Colonies of bacteria can be grown only on certain media. Pathogens are often identified by the manner in which they grow on a particular medium. An example of this would be *Streptococci* bacteria that cause strep throat. Mucus swabbed from a sore throat inoculated on a medium that contains blood will produce pinpoint-size colonies that have a transparent ring around each, which is the result of hemolysis or bursting of red blood cells by the *Streptococci* in the surrounding medium. Table 45-3 lists common culture media and microorganisms that can be isolated on each. Figure 45-17

Media may be solid like a slant (agar in a tube placed in a tilted position to harden), semisolid like agar, or liquid like broth. Media will either inhibit or encourage the growth of certain pathogens and are classified as supportive, selective, differential, or enrichment:

- **Supportive**—used to grow a wide variety of organisms

- **Selective**—encourages growth of some organisms and restricts growth of others (e.g., vaginal and stool cultures.) Figure 45-16 shows an example of a fecal culture growing on selective media.

- **Differential**—includes dyes or chemicals that give organisms a different appearance (e.g., differentiate *Staphylococci*)

- **Enrichment**—contains special organic substances needed to encourage growth of organisms that are fastidious (fussy) (e.g., gonorrhea organisms)

In many POLs, commercial culture units are widely used. For example, units are available for urine that make inoculation easy. A paddle with different media on either side is dipped in a clean-catch or catheterized urine sample and replaced in the vial; it is then incubated for 24 hours.

TABLE 45-3 Culture Media and Isolates

Common Culture Media	Isolates
Blood agar	Most bacteria
Chocolate agar	*Neisseria, Haemophilus*
EMB	Gram-negative bacteria
MacConkey agar	Gram-negative bacteria
Thioglycollate broth	Anaerobic microorganisms
GN broth	Fecal microorganisms

shows a blood agar plate and examples of inoculating needles and loops.

The main goal in growing cultures is to separate pathogenic colonies of organisms from colonies of normal flora. To isolate colonies, the agar must be inoculated properly. The specimen is transferred by rubbing the swab across one small area of the agar near the edge. Next, a wire inoculating loop is sterilized in a Bunsen burner flame or electric incinerator, cooled, and used to streak through the area already inoculated and onto an unmarked area of the agar in a zigzag motion. This procedure is repeated twice more to inoculate the remaining two sections of the agar. This is called quadrant streaking to isolate colonies and is illustrated in Figure 45-18.

After inoculation, the lid or top of the Petri dish is replaced and the agar plate inverted and placed into an incubator (Figure 45-19). The inversion of the agar plate allows moisture to collect on the lid of the Petri dish and not on the culture itself. The culture is allowed to grow in the incubator at 37°C for a 24-, 48-, or 72-hour period. Fungi take longer to grow and may need to grow at slightly lower temperatures.

A secondary culture can be obtained by selecting an isolated colony from the initial agar plate and placing it on another media plate using a sterile loop or needle. This provides a pure culture, a colony containing only one type of organism. Identification of the organism is made by using the pure culture to prepare and stain a slide and by performing various biochemical tests.

Instruments such as Vitek and Autobac use automated technology to facilitate organism identification. The BAC-T Screen Bacteruria-Pyuria Detection Device is an automated

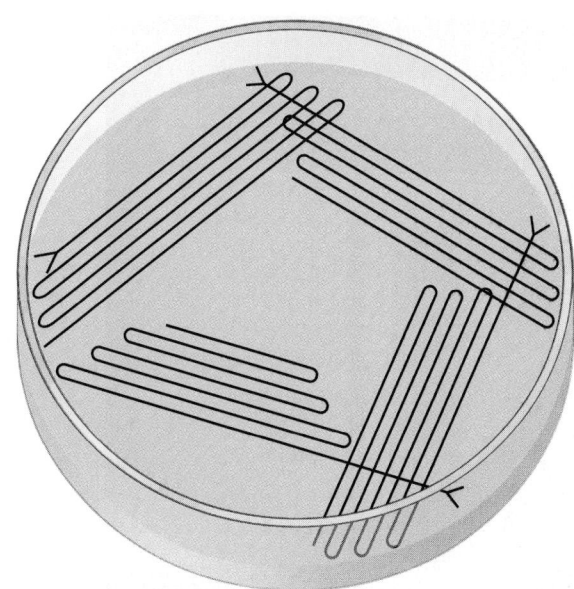

FIGURE 45-18 Quadrant streaking.

system that immediately determines if significant numbers of bacteria are present in a urine specimen, avoiding the 24- to 48-hour wait for complete growth and identification. All the tests mentioned are performed by medical laboratory specialists.

SENSITIVITY TESTING

Once the physician or laboratory specialist identifies the pathogenic organism on the culture, it is necessary to determine which antibiotics will be effective in killing these bacteria. This method of detection is called sensitivity testing. A Petri dish with Mueller-Hinton agar and antibiotic disks are used. The Mueller-Hinton agar is inoculated with the pure culture specimen in overlapping strokes in a technique called the **lawn technique** or colony count (Figure 45-20). The antibiotic disks are placed in a circle on top of the inoculated agar. The lid of the Petri dish is replaced, inverted, and placed in the incubator for 24 hours (Figure 45-21). After 24 hours, the organism will have grown all over except around those disks that inhibit its growth. These zones around the disks are measured to determine the susceptibility of the organism to each particular antibiotic disk. After the most effective antibiotic is identified, the patient is started on drug therapy.

Figure 45-22 is an example of a culture and sensitivity plate after incubation. The more

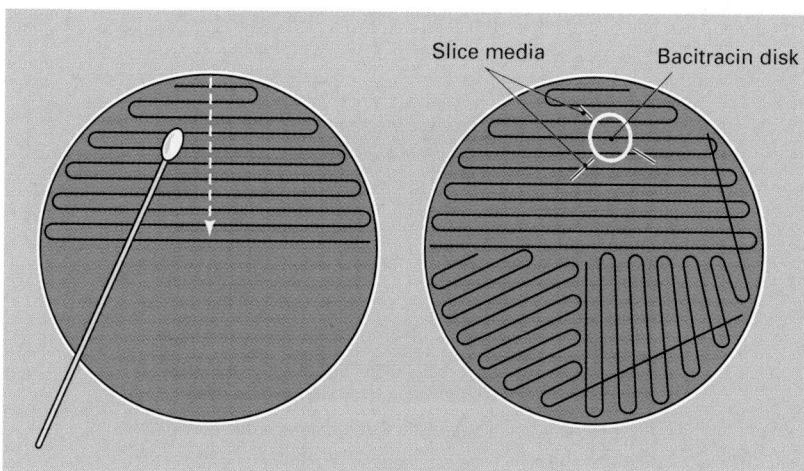

FIGURE 45-17 Swabbing a Petri dish to spread apart colonies. Bacitracin disk is used to prove the presence or absence of *S. pyogenes*.

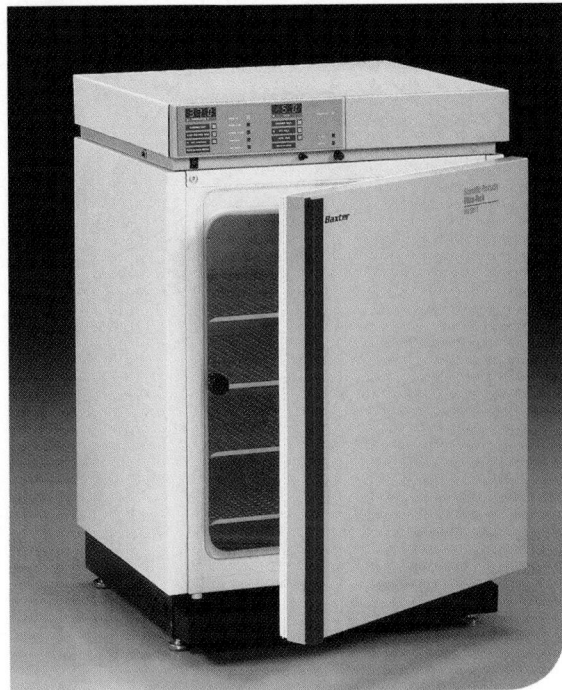

FIGURE 45-19   An incubator for office use.

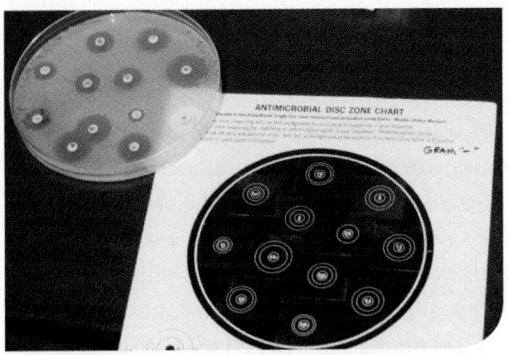

FIGURE 45-21   Paper disks containing various antibiotics are placed on a bacterial culture. If the bacteria are sensitive to that particular antibiotic drug, a large clear zone of inhibition or no growth will appear around that particular disk.

effectively the particular antibiotic killed the organism present, the larger the zone of inhibition or clear zone around a disk. After considering the patient's sensitivity to any antibiotics, the antibiotic with the largest zone of inhibition would be prescribed by the physician.

DIRECT EXAMINATION

Two methods are used to prepare a specimen for direct examination under the microscope: the direct smear and the

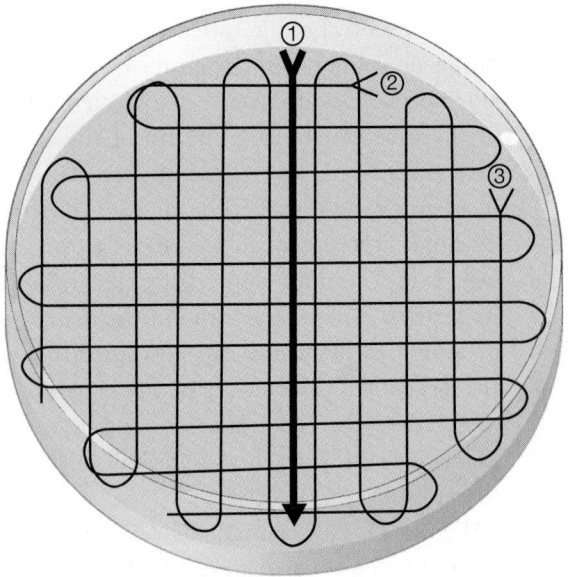

FIGURE 45-20   Lawn spread or colony count streaking.

wet mount preparation. These methods allow the physician to obtain information quickly in the office and thus start treatment immediately.

Direct Smear

A direct smear may be from a swab of the specimen or from a colony on a culture plate (Procedure 45-1). The smear from a specimen is made after the culture is inoculated to prevent contamination of the media since slides are not usually sterile. The swab is rolled carefully across the slide so all areas of the swab touch the slide. The slide is labeled by placing the patient's name and specimen type on the frosted end of the slide. The smear air-dries; do not wave it in the air, which could spread microorganisms. The slide must be **fixed** to ensure that the specimen material remains on the slide during the staining process. It is fixed by passing the clear underneath part of the slide through an open flame three to four times or flooding the slide with methanol and letting it dry. These steps must be done prior to any staining procedure.

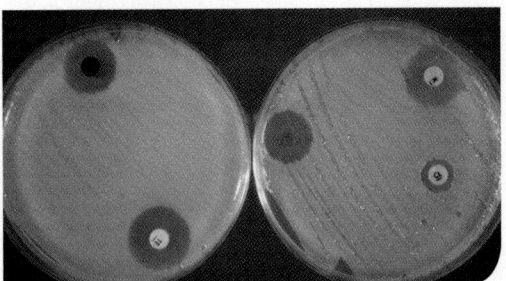

FIGURE 45-22   These two Petri dishes from a urine sample show zones of inhibition around drugs that are effective against *E. coli*, the most common cause of urinary tract infections. The large ring indicates that the bacteria could not grow and that particular drug would be effective in the patient.

procedure 45-1

PREPARING A SMEAR

Objective: Prepare a smear for microscopic examination without error.

EQUIPMENT AND SUPPLIES

frosted slides; specimen from Culturette applicator or inoculating loop; Bunsen burner; inoculating loop (or swab); microscope; oil immersion; gloves; biohazard waste container

Note: Follow standard precautions and safety guidelines when working with body fluid samples. Use care to avoid splashing or spilling body fluids. Wipe up all spills using guidelines established by OSHA.

METHOD

1. Perform hand hygiene and apply gloves.
2. Assemble equipment.
3. Label a clean slide with patient's name, date, and type of specimen.
4. Transfer the specimen to slide to inoculate slide. This is done by rolling a swab over the entire slide (Figure 45-23A–C). Alternatively, place a drop of sterile saline on the slide, and after flaming a needle or loop, pick up the material from one type of colony, place it in saline, and spread it gently over two-thirds of the slide.
5. Allow the slide to air dry for 20 to 30 minutes.
6. Hold the slide with thumb forceps and pass the slide over the Bunsen burner flame. This heat fixes the specimen to the slide in the process known as smear fixation. Let the slide cool. If open flame is unavailable, flood the dry smear with methanol and let it dry to fix the slide.
7. The slide is then ready to be stained.

CHARTING EXAMPLE

11/16/XX Direct smear from abscess RT thigh prepared for staining. · M. King, CMA (AAMA)

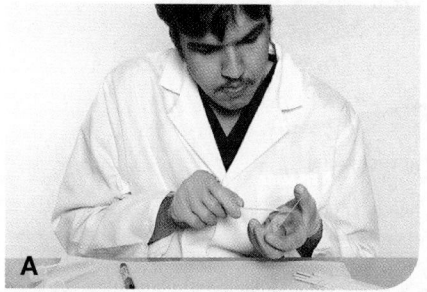 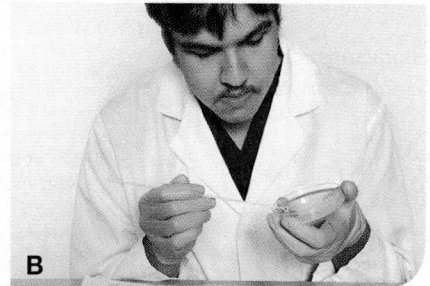 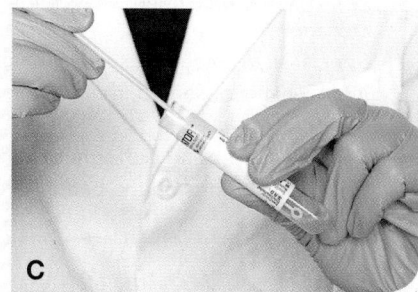

FIGURE 45-23 (A) Roll and turn the swab across the slide; (B) using a loop to pick up a microbial specimen to spread on slide; (C) using a loop to obtain a sample of material from a liquid media.

Wet Mount Preparation

Wet mount preparation involves taking a sample either from a colony or directly from a patient specimen, placing it on a frosted slide, and adding a drop of sterile normal saline and a cover slip. A wet mount preparation such as this allows the physician to observe the motility of the organism and what types of cytoplasmic extensions the organisms have (cilia, flagella). These observations render important identifying information. Refer to Procedure 45-2 for instructions on the preparation of a wet mount slide.

In the POL, a wet mount for fungus often is performed using potassium hydroxide (KOH). Fungus is often difficult to see on direct preparation because keratin from the body, particularly nails, hair, and skin, often obscures the fungal structures. Potassium hydroxide dissolves the keratin, allowing visualization of any fungi present, such as

PREPARING A WET MOUNT SLIDE

Objective: Prepare a wet mount slide for microscopic examination without error.

EQUIPMENT AND SUPPLIES

clean, dry slide, frosted; cover slip; saline; specimen from a Culturette applicator or swab; paper/pen; microscope; gloves

Note: Follow standard precautions and safety guidelines when working with body fluid samples. Use care to avoid splashing or spilling body fluids. Wipe up all spills using guidelines established by OSHA.

METHOD

1. Perform hand hygiene and apply gloves.
2. Label dry slide with the patient's name and date.
3. Inoculate the dry slide by rolling a swab containing the specimen across the surface.
4. Place a drop of saline solution on top of the specimen.
5. Place the cover slip on top of the smeared slide.

Note: The following steps would be performed by a physician or laboratory specialist (Figure 45-24).

6. Observe the wet mount slide immediately under the microscope.
7. Special stains may be used to enhance characteristics.
8. Note what is observed, remove the slide, and dispose of it properly.
9. Remove gloves and perform hand hygiene.
10. Chart the findings on the patient's record.

CHARTING EXAMPLE

11/16/XX Wet mount prepared from vaginal swab for physician to examine. · · · · · · · · · · · · · · · · · · · M. King, CMA (AAMA)

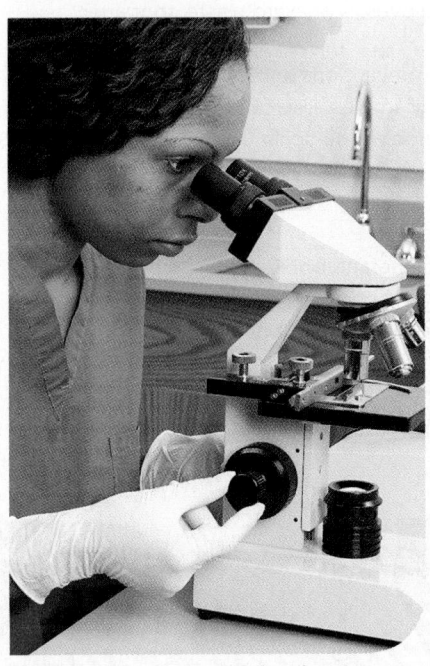

FIGURE 45-24 A medical technician examining a wet mount.
Source: Michal Heron/Pearson Education/PH College

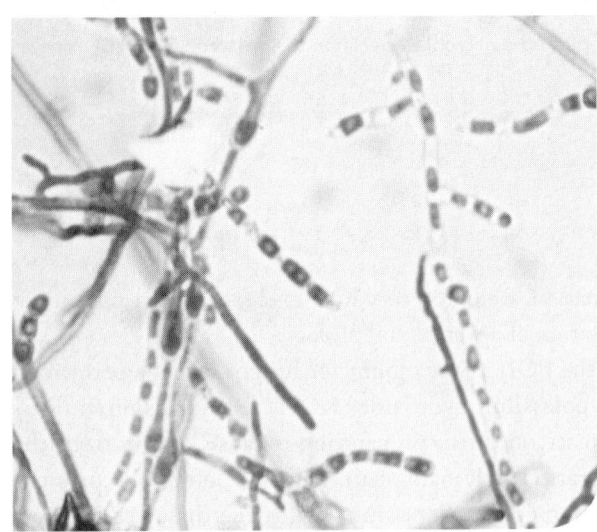

FIGURE 45-25 Example of fungi.

yeast that causes vaginitis (Figure 45-25). To prepare a KOH mount, a specimen is suspended in 1 drop of 10 percent potassium hydroxide and a cover slip is applied. Allow the specimen to sit at room temperature for 30 minutes to dissolve the keratin. The slide will be examined by the physician or laboratory specialist for evidence of fungi in the wet mount.

Staining Specimens

The use of stained smears in microbiology is extensive. The color and shape (morphology) of microorganisms on smears can be observed, for example, in vaginal and nasopharyngeal specimens. The medical assistant should know how to prepare a smear and have a general knowledge of the Gram stain and why it is used. Because several colors are used, the Gram stain will differentiate, or separate, bacteria into two groups: gram positive and gram negative. Different bacteria stain differently, depending on the compounds in their walls. Gram-positive bacteria retain the crystal violet-blue color, and gram-negative bacteria retain only the pink safranine color. Thus, gram-positive (violet) bacteria can be distinguished from gram-negative (pink) bacteria. Precautions must be taken in Gram staining in that temperature, age of specimen, or length of incubation could cause a change in gram-positive bacteria. Gram stains must always be accompanied by culture for microorganism identification.

Procedure 45-3 and Figure 45-26A–F list the steps needed to perform a Gram stain correctly. Particular attention must be paid to the timing of the various steps. Crystal violet is poured on a fixed smear for 1 minute. The stain is washed off with water, and iodine is applied for 1 minute. The iodine is washed off, and the decolorizer is used to wash for 15 seconds. (Care must be taken not to decolorize too long because it will make the slide difficult to evaluate.) Next safranine is applied to the slide for 30 seconds, followed by washing the slide and wiping off the back side of the slide to remove excess stain, then standing it upright to dry.

The staining properties, shape, and size of the organisms can sometimes be used to identify pathogens in specimen samples. As previously noted, *Bacilli* are rod-shaped microorganisms found singly or in groups. *Cocci* are round microorganisms found singly, in pairs (*Diplococci*), in strings (*Streptococci*), or in clusters (*Staphylococci*). *Spirilla,* curved or spiral rods, can be arranged singly or in strands. Some bacteria can produce resistant spores under adverse environmental

procedure 45-3

PERFORMING A GRAM STAIN

Objective: Prepare a slide for a Gram stain to differentiate a gram-positive organism from a gram-negative organism.

EQUIPMENT AND SUPPLIES
Gram-stain kit with decolorizer; culture specimen; slides; Bunsen burner or methanol; staining rack; water wash bottle; water; immersion oil; stopwatch; gloves; slide stand; paper towels; biohazard waste container

Note: Follow standard precautions and safety guidelines when working with body fluid samples. Use care to avoid splashing or spilling body fluids. Wipe up all spills using guidelines established by OSHA.

METHOD
1. Perform hand hygiene and apply gloves.
2. Assemble equipment.
3. Make a smear, label it, air dry the smear, and use heat or methanol to fix.
4. Place slide on staining rack, smear side up.
5. Pour crystal violet solution all over the slide; let it stand 1 minute (Figure 45-26A).
6. Tilt the slide to drain the excess crystal violet stain and rinse with water (Figure 45-26B).
7. Pour Gram's iodine stain all over the slide; let it stand 1 minute (Figure 45-26C).
8. Tilt the slide to drain excess iodine and rinse with water.
9. Gently pour decolorizer with alcohol-acetone all over the slide for 15 seconds or until the color blue stops running (Figure 45-26D).
10. Rinse with water.
11. Pour safranine stain all over the slide, and let it stand for 30 seconds (Figure 45-26E).
12. Tilt the slide to drain the excess safranine and rinse with water. Wipe back of slide (Figure 45-26F).
13. Stand the slide on end on a paper towel or in a slide drying rack, and air-dry.

Note: Examination of a Gram-stained slide is beyond the scope of practice of the medical assistant. It should be performed by a physician or laboratory specialist.

14. Examine under the microscope, using oil immersion lens and oil.

CHARTING EXAMPLE
11/16/XX Gram stain of spec. from abscess of RT thigh prepared for physician to examine.· · · · · · · M. King, CMA (AAMA)

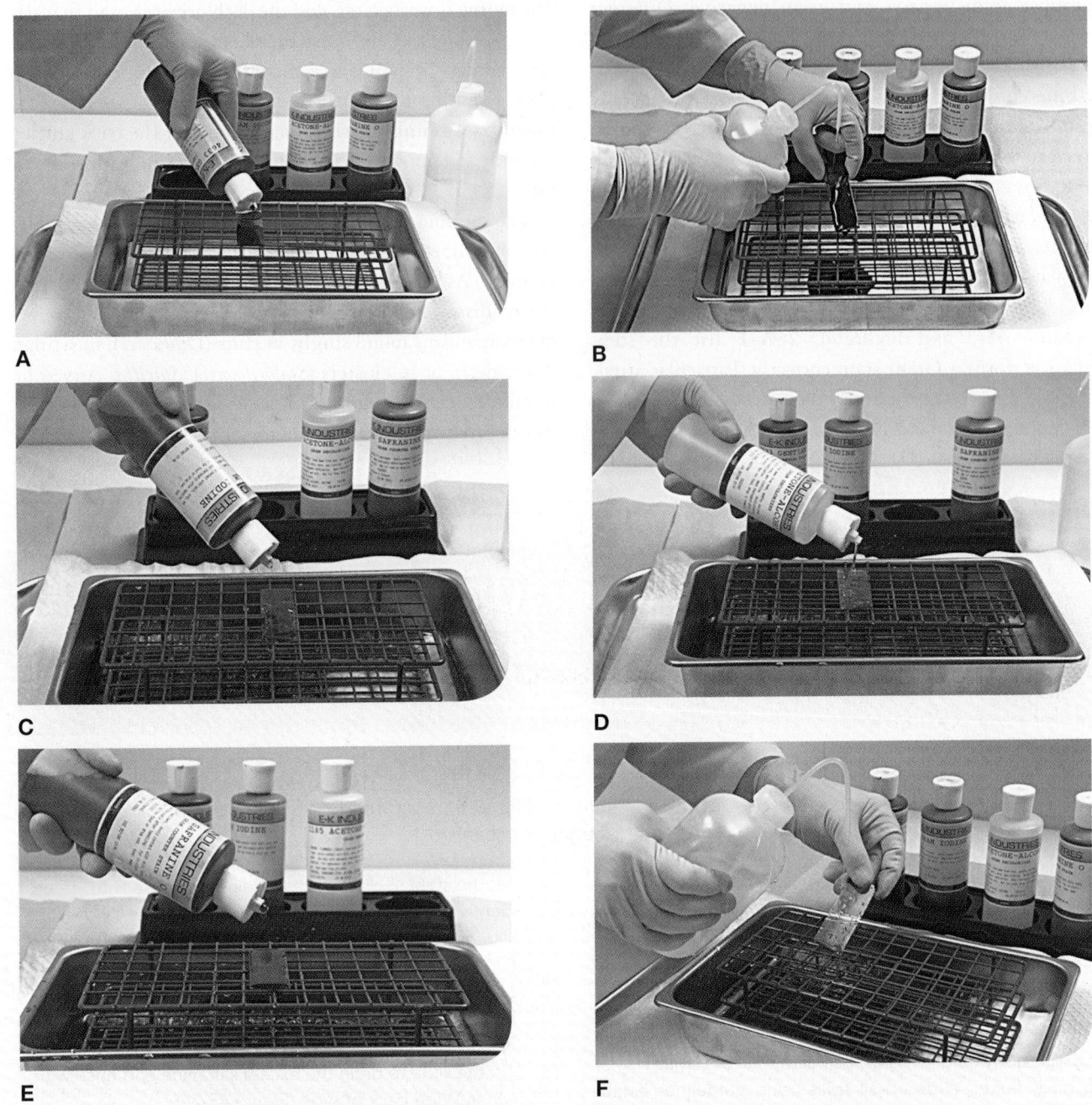

FIGURE 45-26   (A) Pour crystal violet stain over the entire slide and let stand for 1 minute; (B) tilt the slide to drain excess and rinse with water; (C) pour Gram's iodine stain over the entire slide and let stand for 1 minute; (D) gently pour decolorizer with alcohol-acetone all over the slide for 15 seconds or until blue color stops running; (E) pour safraninstain over the entire slide and let stand for 30 seconds; (F) rinse with water and wipe back of the slide.

conditions. Spores can lie dormant for thousands of years and, when conditions are right, can revert back to active form. This trait makes it difficult to destroy these pathogenic bacteria.

Types of Specimens

Pathogens can be observed in specimens of blood, feces, cerebrospinal fluid, mucus, urine, sputum, wounds, tissue, and exudates of other body substances. The following paragraphs discuss these types of specimens and information for obtaining them.

THROAT

One of the most frequently requested specimens in a POL is the throat swab or culture. Based on signs and symptoms the patient presents with, such as upper respiratory infection, sore throat, or sinus infection, the physician will order a throat culture to identify the pathogen involved and begin treatment. Confirmation of *Streptococcus pyogenes* is important because of its virulence and possible complications. When performing a throat culture, it is important not to touch the inside of the mouth or the tongue with the swab to avoid contaminating it. Procedure 45-4 lists the steps for correctly obtaining a throat culture.

If the culture is to be done in house, then it is streaked as mentioned previously. A bacitracin antibiotic disk will be placed on the culture plate in the area with the heaviest inoculation. A zone of no growth around the disk is presumptive evidence that the pathogen is group A beta-hemolytic strep. Other strep organisms are not sensitive to bacitracin. Bacitracin is not used to treat strep throat, only as a differentiating antibiotic. Broad-spectrum antibiotics such as penicillin, ampicillin, and erythromycin are used to treat strep. If strep is suspected, an antigen antibody test for strep may be ordered. These types of tests are discussed later in the chapter.

procedure 45-4

OBTAINING A THROAT CULTURE

Objective: Collect a throat or nasopharyngeal culture without contaminating the specimen.

EQUIPMENT AND SUPPLIES
Culturette system; laboratory requisition; tongue depressor; gloves; biohazard waste container

Note: Follow standard precautions and safety guidelines when working with body fluid samples. Use care to avoid splashing or spilling body fluids. Wipe up all spills using guidelines established by OSHA.

METHOD
1. Assemble equipment and Culturette system.
2. Identify the patient and explain the procedure.
3. Perform hand hygiene and apply gloves.
4. Position the patient facing a light source and have the patient open his or her mouth as wide as possible (Figure 45-27). The gag reflex may be diminished if the patient says "Aaaah."
5. Remove the sterile swab from the Culturette.
6. Depress the tongue, insert the swab, and roll it firmly across the back of the patient's throat or nasopharyngeal area where infected. Be careful not to contaminate the swab on the teeth, lips, tongue, or inside of the cheeks. Avoid touching the uvula to prevent gagging.
7. Insert the swab into a plastic vial. Crush the internal vial of transport medium, making sure that the swab is saturated.

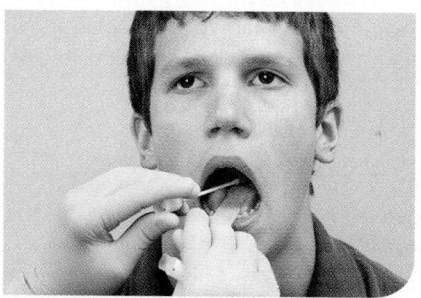

FIGURE 45-27 **Swab the posterior pharynx between the tonsils.**

8. Place the transport medium in labeled mailing or transporting envelope and staple shut if necessary. If being evaluated in the POL, immediately inoculate the culture plate, and apply a bacitracin disk according to office procedure.
9. Remove and dispose of gloves.
10. Perform hand hygiene.
11. Document the procedure in the patient's record.

CHARTING EXAMPLE
2/14/XX 9:00 A.M. Throat culture obtained. Specimen labeled and sent to outside lab. (Specify name of the lab.) ·········
··· M. King, CMA (AAMA)

Nasal swabs are sometimes requested, and care should be taken to label the swabs "Right" and "Left" to identify from which nostril the specimen was taken. Smaller sterile swabs with thinner more flexible shafts are generally used for obtaining nasal specimen.

SPUTUM

To obtain a **sputum** (mucous substance expelled by coughing or clearing the bronchi) specimen, the patient must be carefully instructed to cough deeply and spit up the coughed material into a sterile container. Explain to the patient that this should not be saliva from the mouth. Often it is possible to obtain a good sputum specimen if the patient is reminded to try to collect it on rising in the morning (in a sterile container provided by the POL). The purpose for obtaining a sputum specimen is to isolate and diagnose diseases such as streptococcal pneumonia, influenza, and tuberculosis. Refer to Procedure 45-5 for directions on obtaining a sputum specimen.

procedure
45-5

OBTAINING A SPUTUM SPECIMEN FOR CULTURE

Objective: Collect a sputum specimen without contaminating the specimen.

EQUIPMENT AND SUPPLIES

sterile labeled sputum container with lid; lab requisition form; gloves; biohazard waste container

Note: Follow standard precautions and safety guidelines when working with body fluid samples. Use care to avoid splashing or spilling body fluids. Wipe up all spills using the guidelines established by OSHA.

METHOD

1. Identify the patient.
2. Explain the procedure and give written instructions that the patient can take home, if necessary. Explain that he/she should breathe in or out deeply 2 to 4 times and perform a few low, deep coughs to raise sputum. This avoids getting only saliva. The first morning specimen, collected before eating or drinking, usually provides the best sample.
   a. Cough deeply and expel fluid into center of container and close lid immediately (Figures 45-28A–B).
   b. Make sure no other fluids, such as tears, nasal mucus, or saliva, find their way into the cup.
   c. Fit the lid securely, then write the time and date the specimen was obtained.
   d. Bring the specimen into the physician's office as soon as possible, or place it in a refrigerator for no longer than 2 hours.
3. Perform hand hygiene and apply gloves.
4. Label the transport envelope with information, staple it shut, and transport sample immediately.
5. Remove and dispose of gloves and perform hand hygiene.
6. Document the procedure in the patient's record.

CHARTING EXAMPLE

2/14/XX 10:30 A.M. Sputum specimen collected. Labeled and sent to outside lab. (Specify name of the lab.) · · · · · · · · · · · ·
· M. King, CMA (AAMA)

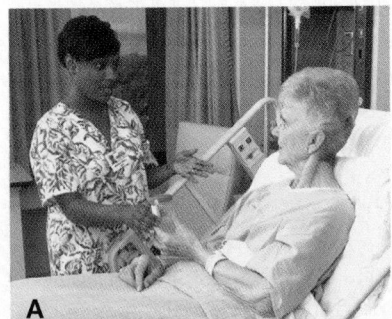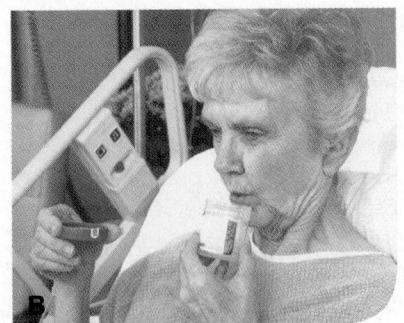

FIGURE 45-28 **(A) Instruct the patient to cough deeply to bring up sputum; (B) instruct the patient to obtain 1 to 2 teaspoons of sputum, then close and seal the container with the lid.**

URINE

Urinalysis is discussed in Chapter 46; however, obtaining a urine culture is an important procedure in this chapter on microbiology. A urine specimen for culture must be either a catheterized specimen or a clean-catch midstream sample (CCMS). Both methods provide sterile samples. Any other type of urine specimen (one for routine analysis for example) would be contaminated by organisms in the container or on the hands or genitals of the patient. See Procedure 46-1 in Chapter 46 for collection of a clean-catch midstream urine specimen from both male and female patients.

Procedure 45-6 provides the steps for performing a urine culture from a CCMS sample of urine. In doctors' offices and smaller facilities, self-contained culture units are purchased and used. Many varieties are available, and each provides specific procedures and charts to facilitate reading the results. Often urine cultures require a means to provide a quantitative result of the number of microorganisms in the sample. By using selective media and an inoculating loop that is specifically calibrated to deliver 1 µL of urine, quantitative results are possible. Each colony growing on the

procedure
45-6

PERFORMING A URINE CULTURE

Objective: Inoculate a urine plate to aid in the identification of a UTI.

EQUIPMENT AND SUPPLIES

lab requisition form; urine specimen (CCMS) collected in a sterile container; incinerator (electric or Bunsen burner); 1.0 µl loop; agar plates (usually blood, MacConkey, and nutrient); gloves; biohazard waste container

Note: Follow standard precautions and safety guidelines when working with body fluid samples. Use care to avoid splashing or spilling body fluids. Wipe up all spills using guidelines established by OSHA.

METHOD

1. Assemble equipment and supplies.
2. Perform hand hygiene
3. Apply gloves and face protection.
4. Verify that the name on the laboratory requisition and the specimen are the same.
5. With the lid on, swirl the urine sample to mix.
6. Sterilize the loop, and remove the lid, replacing it between inoculation of plates.
7. Inoculate each media plate in a pattern to allow for lawn technique, or use the colony count method to isolate colonies (see Figure 45-18).
8. Label the bottom of the plates near the edges with the patient's name, date, and type of specimen.
9. Place media in the incubator with the agar side up for 24 hours.
10. Clean the area, remove and dispose of gloves, and perform hand hygiene.
11. Results will be interpreted (after incubation) by a physician or laboratory specialist.
12. Document the results appropriately.

CHARTING EXAMPLE

2/14/XX 11:00 A.M. Urine culture performed. · · · · · · · · · · · ·
· M. King, CMA (AAMA)

media represents 1,000 colony-forming organisms per milliliter of urine. One hundred colonies represent 100,000 colony-forming units and indicate the presence of a UTI.

STOOL

Stool or feces, (waste product from the bowel) may be tested for bacterial, parasitic, or protozoal infections; for the presence of occult blood; and for excessive amounts of fat (**steatorrhea**). The collection of stool specimens varies with the type of test ordered. Discussing stool sample collection is often embarrassing to both patient and medical assistant; however, correct collection is critical to an accurate result. Fecal specimens must be free of urine, water from the toilet, and toilet tissue.

Stool Culture

To detect bacteria or viruses, a small amount of feces is needed. The collection containers must be sterile, and aseptic technique must be used in the collection process. Once collected, the stool must be sent immediately to the testing facility. Sterile collection devices are available. Sheets of special paper, coverings for the toilet, and bedpans can be used to collect specimens. Sterile tongue depressors or applicator sticks can be used to transfer a small of amount of stool to a sterile container for transport to the laboratory or office. In the office, a sterile bedpan may be used, or a sterile pan may be placed over the bowl of the toilet. Procedure 45-7

procedure 45-7

OBTAINING A STOOL SPECIMEN FOR CULTURE AND SENSITIVITY

Objective: Instruct a patient how to collect a stool sample for culture and sensitivity in a sterile container using correct infection control procedures.

EQUIPMENT AND SUPPLIES

sterile stool collection container; bedpan or container for collection of stool; tongue depressors; sterile applicator sticks; transportation/mailing container; labels; laboratory request form; gloves; biohazard waste container

Note: Follow standard precautions and safety guidelines when working with body fluid samples. Use care to avoid splashing or spilling body fluids. Wipe up all spills using guidelines established by OSHA.

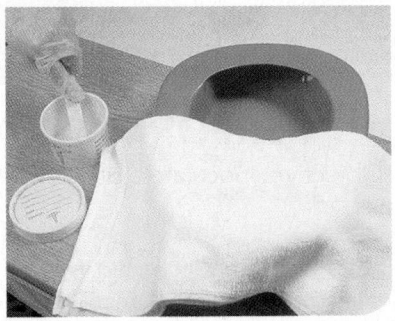

FIGURE 45-29 Equipment for collecting a stool specimen.

METHOD

1. Perform hand hygiene.
2. Assemble equipment.
3. Identify the patient and explain the procedure, giving written instructions as well. Do not overuse medical terminology, which might cause the patient to misunderstand your instructions.
4. Instruct the patient to defecate in a container or bedpan. If the patient is collecting a specimen at home, give the patient a sterile container and written instructions.
5. Using a sterile tongue depressor or applicator stick, take a small amount of stool from different parts of the specimen, and place them in a container, making sure that no other contaminants are included (toilet paper, toilet water, urine, etc.).
6. If the patient provides the stool specimen in a bedpan or other container, proceed using gloves as above (Figure 45-29).
7. Fill out the lab request form and wrap it around the container, securing it with a rubber band.
8. Place the container in a proper mailing container.
9. Deliver or mail the specimen to the outside laboratory facility.

CHARTING EXAMPLE

2/14/XX 9:00 A.M. Stool specimen obtained C&S. Specimen labeled and sent to outside lab. (Specify the name of the lab.)
 · M. King, CMA (AAMA)

lists the steps for collecting a stool sample for culture and sensitivity.

Occult Blood

A stool specimen is required to test for occult or hidden blood that may indicate bleeding in the gastrointestinal tract. Often the patient is given the test units to take home and collect the specimen. Directions are provided on each test unit; however, you should review the instructions each time they are given to a patient. Patients are instructed to write their name, date, and doctor's name on the label of the collection unit. Using one of the wooden spatulas provided, they are to collect a small amount of stool and place it in one of the circles on the back of the booklet, obtain another sample from a different area of the stool, and place this sample on the other circle. Patients should close the unit and take it or mail it to the doctor's office or the laboratory as requested. See Procedure 37-6 in Chapter 37 to review this procedure.

For more accurate results, patients should be instructed to refrain from consuming vitamin C and red meat for 3 days prior to testing because those substances may cause false pos-itives. Also, it is important to check the expiration date of any test kit before giving it to the patient.

Stool for Ova and Parasites

The presence of microbial organisms, such as ova and parasites (O&P), may be determined by testing feces or stool. The presence of ova (eggs) or other forms of a parasite indicate parasitic infestation. Identification of the parasite aids in selecting the correct treatment. Commercial kits are available that provide containers for fresh stool specimens and two additional vials for preserved specimens: one containing formalin and the other containing polyvinyl alcohol. The patient should be instructed to mix portions of stool in each vial and seal. If O&P are suspected, three specimen collections will be requested. The specimen is usually obtained in the early morning. The patient should be instructed to defecate into a stool specimen container or into a bedpan, if available, placed over the toilet. The stool specimen samples should be taken from several different parts of the stool since O&P may be in one portion of the stool and not another. Refer to Procedure 45-8 for collecting a stool specimen for O&P.

procedure
45-8

OBTAINING A STOOL SPECIMEN FOR OVA AND PARASITES

Objective: Instruct a patient to collect a stool sample for ova and parasites using the correct infection control and procedure. Both fresh and preserved specimens are required.

EQUIPMENT AND SUPPLIES

stool collection kit with container for fresh specimen and vials for preserved specimen (formalin and polyvinyl alcohol); bedpan or container for collection of stool; tongue depressors; sterile applicator sticks; mailing container; labels; laboratory request form; gloves; biohazard waste container

Note: Follow standard precautions and safety guidelines when working with body fluid samples. Use care to avoid splashing or spilling body fluids. Wipe up all spills using guidelines established by OSHA.

METHOD

1. Perform hand hygiene.
2. Check orders and assemble equipment and supplies.
3. Identify the patient and explain the procedure, giving written instructions as well. Do not overuse medical terminology, which might cause the patient to misunderstand your instructions. Remind patient not to urinate or put toilet tissue into container.
4. Instruct the patient to defecate in a container or bedpan, if available. If the patient is collecting specimen at home,

give the patient written instructions including diagrams. Figure 45-30 is an example of an ova and parasite collection kit.

5. When the patient returns with the specimen, apply gloves.
6. Using a tongue depressor, take a small amount of stool from different parts of the specimen and place in each vial, using a new depressor or sterile wooden applicator stick for each vial. Make sure that no other contaminants are included (toilet paper, toilet water, or urine).
7. Fill out the lab request form and wrap it around the container, securing it with a rubber band.
8. Place the specimen container in a proper mailing container.
9. Deliver or mail the specimen container to the outside laboratory facility.

CHARTING EXAMPLE
2/14/XX 9:00 A.M. Stool specimen obtained for O&P. Specimen labeled and sent to outside lab. (Specify the name of the lab.) · M. King, CMA (AAMA)

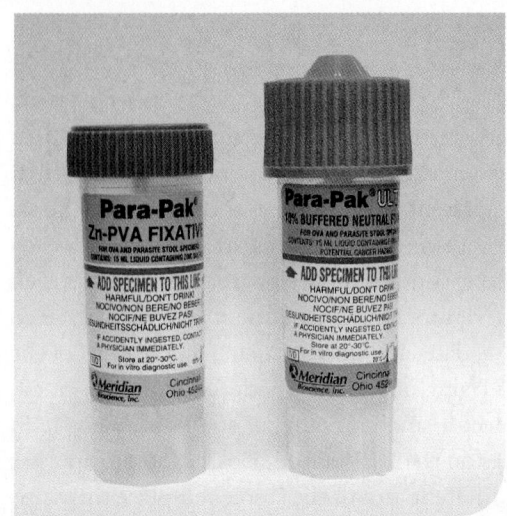

FIGURE 45-30 Ova and parasite collection kit. *Courtesy Meridian Bioscience, Inc.*

Collecting Pinworm Specimens. One examination for ova and parasites may be performed in the office. The pinworm (*Enterobius vermicularis*) is a common parasite that inhabits the lower gastrointestinal tract with mature pinworms migrating out of the anus at night, causing intense itching. Transmission is by the fecal–oral route or by ingesting eggs with hand-to-mouth transmission. Adult worms mate in the colon, and the female migrates out of the anus at night to lay eggs. The eggs stick to the anal area, pajamas, and other items of clothing. Collection of a specimen should be done first thing in the morning before a bowel movement or bathing in order to detect ova or worms. Procedure 45-9

procedure
45-9

OBTAINING A STOOL SPECIMEN FOR EXAMINATION FOR PINWORMS

Objective: Collect a rectal swab using cellulose tape for pinworm examination.

EQUIPMENT AND SUPPLIES
glass slide; tongue depressor; gauze or colon balls; microscope; toluene; lab requisition form

METHOD
1. Gather equipment and supplies.

2. Prepare slide by attaching the sticky side of a piece of cellulose tape to the slide surface and wrapping tape around one end. Leave room to attach a small square of paper for labeling at the other end. Do not use double-sided sticky or Magic Tape (Figure 45-31A).

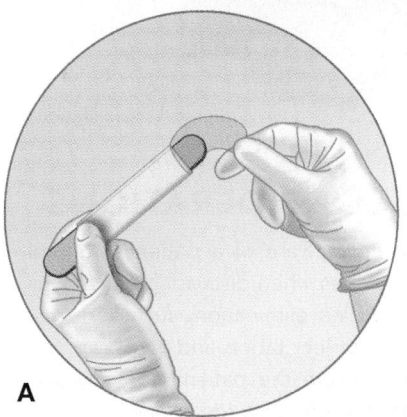
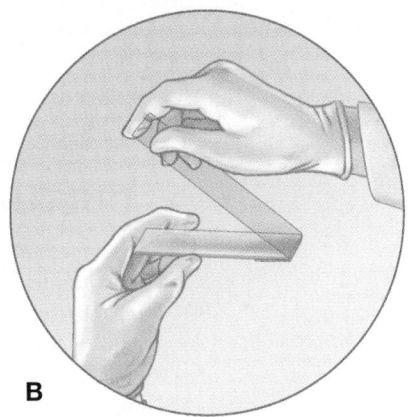
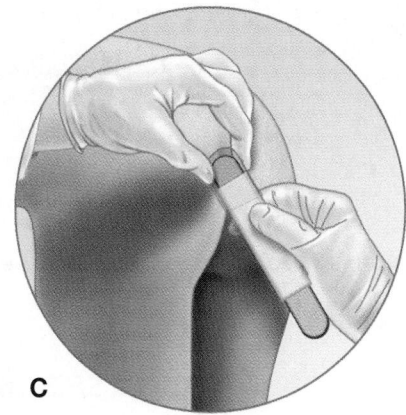

A   B   C

FIGURE 45-31 (A) Attach sticky side of tape to the slide and wrap the tape around one end; (B) peel the tape off the slide and wrap around the tongue depressor with sticky side out. Swab the anal area; (C) replace the tape on slide with sticky side down.

3. Perform hand hygiene and apply gloves.
4. Prepare the patient on examination table or parent's lap with the anal area exposed.
5. Peel the tape off the slide by the labeled end and wrap it around the tongue depressor or swab with the sticky side out (Figure 45-31B).
6. Press the tape to the area around the anus on both sides.
7. Replace the tape on the slide sticky side down, and smooth it with gauze (Figure 45-31C).

8. Label the slide with the patient's name and date. Fill out the lab requisition form.
9. The physician will examine the slide for presence of pinworms or ova (Figure 45-32).
10. Dispose of all waste, perform hand hygiene, and document the procedure appropriately.

CHARTING EXAMPLE
11/16/XX 11:30 A.M. Slide prepared for pinworm examination by physician. · M. King, CMA (AAMA)

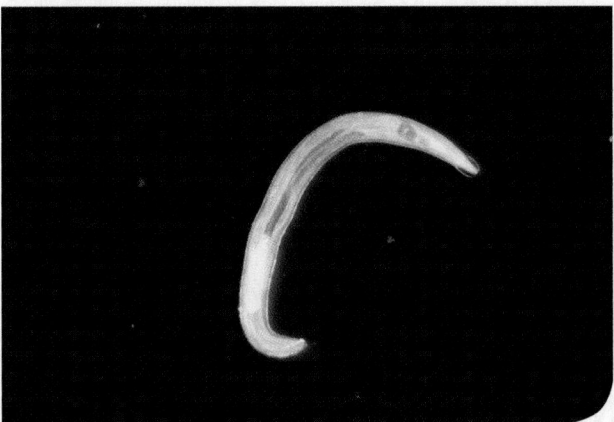

FIGURE 45-32 Microscopic view of a pinworm, *Enterobius vermicularis*.

provides the steps needed either to perform the collection of a pinworm specimen in the office or to instruct a parent to do so at home. Medications are available for treatment, and reexamination is recommended after a cycle of medication has been completed. In addition, parents and other infected individuals must be told to observe strict personal hygiene, including laundering of all bedding and underclothing on a regular basis. It may be necessary to examine other family members and playmates for signs of infection if reinfestation occurs.

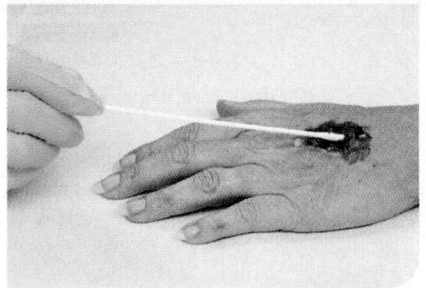

FIGURE 45-33 Swab the inside of the wound.

WOUND SPECIMENS

Sterile swabs are used to obtain a specimen from a wound, abscess, or incision to test for pathogenic microorganisms (Figure 45-33). The procedure is similar to obtaining a throat culture. Several specimens may be necessary from different locations. Be certain to label each appropriately as to the source. Refer to Procedure 37-2 in Chapter 37 on obtaining a wound culture and Procedure 42-11 in Chapter 42 on changing a sterile dressing for additional details on obtaining a wound specimen.

OTHER TYPES OF SPECIMENS

Cerebrospinal fluid (CSF) is always treated as a stat procedure. The procedure to collect CSF is uncomfortable for the patient, and the specimen must be handled with care. Usually three tubes are collected under sterile conditions and sent for testing. The culture and sensitivity test should be performed before chemical and other tests using the second of the three tubes. The first and third tubes are more likely to be contaminated because of the entry and removal processes of collection.

Blood cultures to test for septicemia or bacteremia are covered in Chapter 47. Commercially available containers containing a broth media are widely used. Blood and CSF under normal conditions are free of any type of microorganisms.

Serology Testing

Serology is the study of the antigen and antibody reactions of the body's immune system. The body's ability to recognize a foreign substance (antigen) and produce an antibody against it is the immune response. Antibodies are specific for a particular antigen. For example, polio antibody is specific for polio only.

This antigen–antibody reaction is a frequently used testing tool. It is used to test for pregnancy, rheumatoid

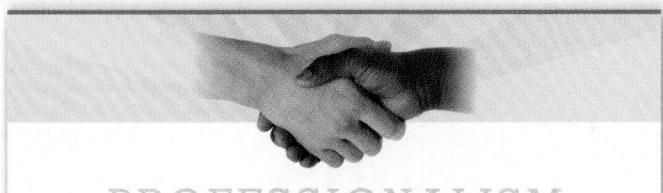

arthritis, mononucleosis, and strep, among other conditions. This testing is serologic since it studies or tests the serum component of the blood. These testing kits contain all the equipment and supplies necessary and assist the medical assistant in ensuring that reagents are fresh and quality control is maintained. The kits standardize testing, thus ensuring accuracy, precision, and quality control. It is absolutely essential to follow exactly the manufacturer's directions.

STREP TEST

The Group A Strep Screen is a test that is done frequently in POLs. It is especially efficient in the pediatric office because it is self-contained and can be done while the patient waits. This screen is an antigen detection test for group A beta-hemolytic *Streptococci* and follows the general procedure for antigen–antibody **agglutination** (clumping together) tests, which produce a clumping of cells. There are many CLIA-waived group A strep kits available that test for the extracted group A beta-hemolytic *Streptococcus* antigen. These self-contained test kits are commercially prepared diagnostic testing kits that include detailed instructions and contain reagents as well as controls and quality control suggestions.

A variety of other serological test kits are available for infectious mononucleosis, rheumatoid arthritis, and HIV, to name a few. The specialty of the physician will determine which tests will be used.

SUMMARY

Microbiology, as practiced by the medical assistant in POLs, is one of the most important aids to diagnosis for the physician. By correct processing and testing of patient specimens, early diagnosis and treatment of disease can take place. The medical assistant plays an important role in the process.

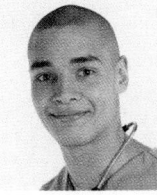

45 CHAPTER REVIEW

COMPETENCY REVIEW

1. Define and spell the terms to learn for this chapter.

2. What does it mean that a microorganism is nonpathogenic?

3. In what ways are bacteria categorized?

4. If a bacterium is aerobic, what does it require to survive?

5. *Tinea pedis* is an example of which type of microorganism?

6. What is the incubation period for a culture?

7. A specimen is sent to an outside laboratory for culture and sensitivity testing. Your office receives a report that the bacterium is resistant to penicillin. What does that mean?

PREPARING FOR THE CERTIFICATION EXAM

1. Invasion of the body by any pathogen is called
   a. contagion
   b. infection
   c. pandemic
   d. epidemic
   e. communicable

2. Material for a CSF specimen is collected from what area?
   a. mouth
   b. throat
   c. lungs and bronchial tubes
   d. pharynx
   e. spinal column

3. *Cocci* occurring in chains are
   a. *Micrococci*
   b. *Diplococci*
   c. *Streptococci*
   d. *Sarcinae*
   e. *Staphylococci*

4. Which of the following is caused by a virus?
   a. candidiasis
   b. malaria
   c. herpes zoster
   d. strep throat
   e. gonorrhea

5. An organism that can live with or without oxygen in its environment is
   a. aerobic
   b. gram positive
   c. gram negative
   d. anaerobic
   e. a facultative anaerobe

6. The test that checks for the susceptibility of an organism to specific antibiotics is the
   a. culture test
   b. sensitivity test
   c. isolation test
   d. screening test
   e. inoculation test

7. After a Gram stain, what color do gram-negative organisms stain?
   a. blue
   b. black
   c. violet
   d. pink
   e. orange

8. *Staphylococcus aureus* is
   a. gram-negative *Bacilli* in chains
   b. gram-positive *Cocci* in chains
   c. a cause of MRSA
   d. gram-negative *Diplococci*
   e. acid-fast *Bacilli*

9. The causative agent of scarlet fever and rheumatic fever is
   a. *Streptococcus pneumoniae*
   b. *Streptococcus pyogenes*
   c. *Neisseria meningitidis*
   d. *Staphylococcus enteritidis*
   e. *Chlamydia trachomatis*

10. The study of ova and parasites is known as
    a. cytology
    b. serology
    c. mycology
    d. parasitology
    e. hematology

CRITICAL THINKING

1. Dr. Penningworth suspects that Marc may have strep throat. He orders a throat swab to be collected and sent to the laboratory. What should David use to obtain the throat specimen, and why?

2. What must David do to ensure that he does not contaminate the throat culture while attempting to obtain the specimen?

3. The laboratory has processed the throat culture and has found that the organism causing the infection is *Streptococcus pyogenes*, confirming Dr. Penningworth's suspicions. What other forms of infection could this microorganism cause?

4. What types of antibiotics are used to treat strep throat?

ON THE JOB

You have been asked to speak to a high school class about the clinical aspects of your job. In particular, the students are interested in microbiology because they have just completed a unit on microorganisms in class.

1. What would you tell them about your functions as a medical assistant?
2. What would you say to those who asked if you looked through the microscope and reported your findings?
3. One student asks what type of training one would need to work solely in microbiology in a laboratory setting. How would you answer her?

INTERNET ACTIVITY

Research a type of bacteria, such as the *Staphylococci,* that can cause gastroenteritis.

Additional interactive resources and activities for this chapter can be found:

On your student DVD: View applicable procedure videos on the DVD-ROM found in the back of this book.

MyHealthProfessionsKit.com: Test your knowledge of this chapter with games and activities. MyHealthProfessionsKit also includes resources, helpful links, and a Spanish audio glossary.

Medical Assisting Interactive: Practice your procedures as a medical assistant in this simulated doctor's office. This can be accessed through MyHealthProfessionsKit.com.

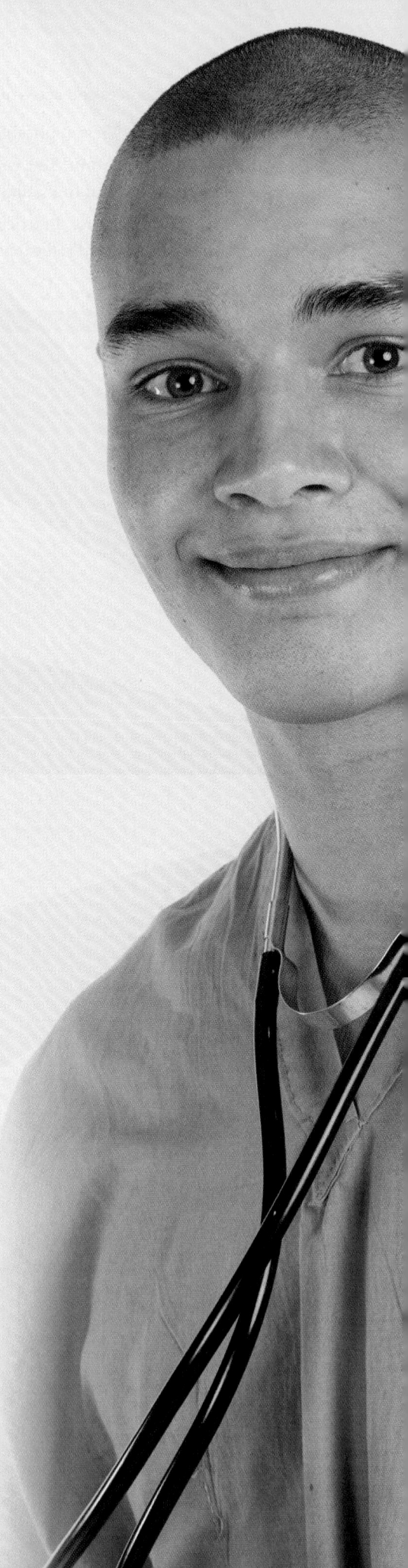

46
Urinalysis

LEARNING OBJECTIVES

After completing this chapter, you should be able to:

- Define and spell the terms to learn for this chapter.

- List nine types of urine specimens that can be collected.

- Understand the purpose of routine urinalysis.

- Describe the steps for collecting a clean-catch urine specimen.

- Describe the physical components of urine.

- Describe the chemical components of urine.

- State normal values for physical and chemical examination of urine.

- Demonstrate the procedure for glucose testing using tablets.

- Demonstrate the procedure for preparing urine for microscopic examination.

- Describe some of the cellular and noncellular elements that might be found during a urine microscopic examination.

- Demonstrate a method for pregnancy testing.

- Discuss quality control as it applies to urinalysis.

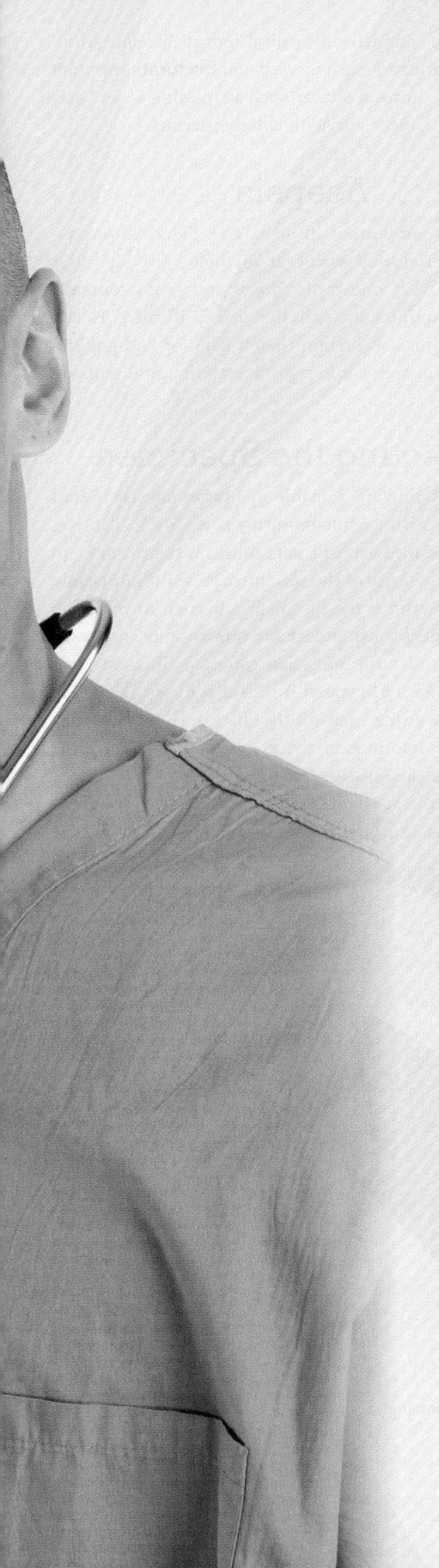

CHAPTER OUTLINE

CASE STUDY

Susan Schultz, CMA (AAMA), has explained the proper collection procedure for a clean-catch midstream urine sample to 65-year-old Shelly Flannery, per Dr. Salpega's orders for completion of a urinalysis. Susan immediately tests the urine using a chemical reagent strip and notices that the urine is dark yellow and cloudy in appearance.

TERMS TO LEARN

amorphous	parasites
anuria	polyuria
bacturia	proteinuria
crystals	renal threshold
glomerulonephritis	sediment
glycosuria	specific gravity
hematuria	spermatozoa
ketones	supernatant
micturate	turbid
occult	urinalysis
oliguria	void

CERTIFICATION LINK

CMA (AAMA)
Collecting and processing specimens; diagnostic testing

RMA
Laboratory procedures

CMAS
Not applicable

Urinalysis refers to the testing of urine for the presence of infection or disease. A routine urine analysis consists of examining the physical, chemical, and microscopic characteristics of urine, and it is one of the most common laboratory tests performed. Urine is readily available, easily collected, and often provides the first clues to illness. Urinalysis provides valuable information about many functions in the body, including kidney functions. The patient must be clearly instructed about methods of collection in easily understood terms. Patients do not necessarily comprehend medical terms; therefore words meaning "to urinate," such as **void** and **micturate**, may not be understood. Instead, phrases such as "passing water" may need to be used, especially with elderly patients.

Asepsis

Asepsis is very important in urinalysis. Standard precautions must be followed whenever any blood or body fluids are handled. Wear nonsterile gloves and avoid contaminating any equipment with the urine. If there is any chance of splashes occurring, then a lab coat and goggles should be worn. See Chapter 34 for a thorough discussion of asepsis.

Collecting the Specimen

Urine samples provide valuable indicators of the overall health of the patient. Although urine is readily available in most instances, medical assistants must do their utmost to maintain the integrity of the specimen. A test result is only as reliable and valid as the specimen collected. Anyone who handles specimens must understand how to store and maintain each type of urine specimen collected. In most cases urine samples are refrigerated if testing will not take place within 2 hours. Always consult the office or laboratory manual for further information about specific storage of urine and addition of preservatives for specific tests.

Generally, at least 10 ml of urine is needed for testing, depending on the test ordered. Figures 46-1A–C show three

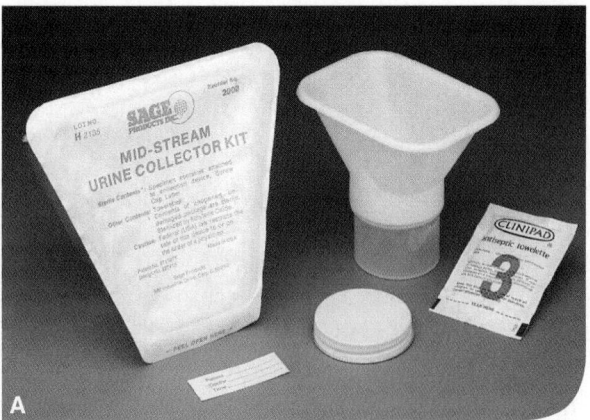
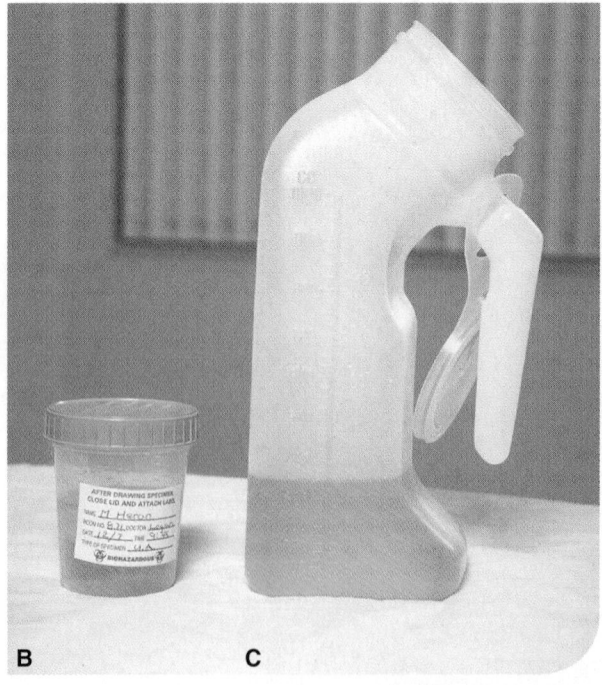

FIGURE 46-1 (A) Midstream collection kit; (B) urine collection cup; (C) 24-hour urine container.

types of urine collection containers. Nine types of urine specimens may be collected:

- Routine (random) sample
- Morning specimen—first voided
- Timed specimen
- 24-hour specimen
- 2-hour postprandial specimen
- Catheterized specimen (sterile specimen)
- Clean-catch midstream (sterile specimen)
- Pediatric specimen
- Suprapubic specimen

ROUTINE (RANDOM) SAMPLE

A random sample of urine is the most commonly collected type of urine specimen. This specimen is collected in a nonsterile container and can be collected in the office during the patient's visit or may be brought in from home. It is preferable to provide the patient with urine specimen containers for any sample to be brought in from home to ensure that containers are clean. Random samples are used only for routine screenings, since the composition of urine changes during the day.

MORNING SPECIMEN: FIRST VOID

A morning specimen (first void) is the most concentrated urine and is collected immediately on arising in the morning. This specimen is used for tests such as pregnancy testing, urine cultures, and microscopic examinations. The patient is given a specimen container and collects the urine when he or she first arises in the morning. The specimen should be brought to the office for testing within 30 minutes to 1 hour. If the examination cannot be performed within 2 hours the sample should be refrigerated, or a preservative added to the container, depending on the test procedure to be completed. See Guidelines 46-1: Collecting Routine Urine Specimens.

TIMED SPECIMEN

Timed specimens are necessary for quantitative analysis of substances such as protein, creatinine, or glucose in urine. Urine specimens must be obtained at specific time intervals. The most common timed specimens are 24-hour and 2-hour postprandial specimens.

24-Hour Specimen

The 24-hour urine test is used to determine the glomerular filtration rate of the kidneys (creatinine clearance), to

GUIDELINES 46-1

COLLECTING A ROUTINE URINE SPECIMEN

1. Provide the patient with a nonsterile container that is labeled with the patient's name and date.
2. Ask the patient to use the bathroom and void into a container. Tell the patient to only fill the container two-thirds of the way to avoid spillage.
3. Explain where you want the patient to leave the container of urine. Place a paper towel in the designated area to avoid contamination of the work area.
4. Wearing nonsterile gloves, take the specimen and test the urine immediately if possible.
5. If you are not able to test the specimen within 30 minutes, place it in the refrigerator. Note, however, that urine should be at room temperature before testing.

check specific hormone levels, and to check for other metabolic abnormalities. It is important to clearly explain to the patient what needs to be done to collect an acceptable 24-hour specimen. Changes occur in urine specimens over time, thus instructions should be given in writing. It should be made clear that when the collection is completed, the specimen should be delivered at once to the laboratory or physician's office. Refrigeration of a specimen slows growth of bacteria and specimen deterioration but does not stop it. Often preservatives are added by the facility before giving the container to the patient. Some of these may be caustic, and containers must be labeled appropriately to prevent injury to the patient and anyone else handling the specimen.

To collect a 24-hour specimen, the patient is given a large, clean, and properly labeled container to take home. Collection begins after the patient voids the first time in the morning. After flushing the first voided urine in the commode, every drop of urine is collected in the container for the next 24 hours, up to and including the first voided specimen on the second morning. Procedure 46-1 includes the method for instructing a patient to collect a 24-hour urine specimen.

2-HOUR POSTPRANDIAL SPECIMEN

A 2-hour postprandial urine specimen is collected 2 hours after a meal has been eaten. This test is used as screening for glucose that may be spilled into the urine once the blood levels exceed the renal threshold. **Renal threshold** is the concentration at which a substance excreted by the kidneys, such as glucose, begins to appear in urine. After the renal threshold is surpassed, the excess glucose is excreted in the urine.

CATHETERIZATION SPECIMEN

Catheterization is used to collect a sterile urine specimen, which results in the ideal urine specimen—one that is

procedure
46-1

COLLECTING A 24-HOUR URINE SPECIMEN

Objective: Instruct a patient how to properly collect a 24-hour urine specimen.

EQUIPMENT AND SUPPLIES

24-hour urine containers (2 may be necessary for some patients); toilet insert for collection; funnel for pouring; label; chemical hazard label as needed; preservatives as required by specific test; graduated cylinder; 10 mL pipette; gloves; written instruction sheet for specific test; requisition slip; patient's record; pen

METHOD

1. Check the patient's record for orders for specific test.
2. Assemble equipment and supplies needed.
3. Consult the laboratory directory for special instructions regarding dietary restrictions and preservative for test ordered.
4. Perform hand hygiene.
5. Label the container with patient's name and dates and times to start and stop collection of specimen.
6. If required, add the exact amount of preservative using a pipette. If preservative is caustic, add a chemical hazard label.

7. Identify the patient and explain thoroughly the directions for collection as follows:
   - Void into the toilet and flush.
   - Note the exact time and date as the beginning of the 24-hour collection.
   - Collect all voided urine after the start time for the next 24-hour period ending exactly 24 hours after the start time on the following day.
   - Note the times and dates on the label.
   - Instruct the patient not to urinate directly into the container or place anything other than urine in the container. Ask the patient to use a toilet or urinal insert for collection of the specimen, then to pour the urine into the 24-hour container. Explain that the specimen may need refrigeration, depending on the test. This means it must be refrigerated for the entire 24-hour period.
   - Patient is to return the container(s) as soon as possible after ending the collection to ensure accurate results.

8. Provide a written copy of instructions to the patient along with the prepared container(s).

9. Record the supplies and instructions given to the patient and the name of the test requested.

10. Verify the collection dates and times with the patient when the specimen is returned to the facility.

11. Check to see if any other additives are to be included before sending the specimen to the testing laboratory.

12. Apply gloves.

13. Mix the urine sample by swirling carefully. Measure the volume of urine collected exactly by pouring into a large graduated cylinder that holds 1 liter.

14. Pour an aliquot of urine into appropriate container for delivery to testing facility. Record the total volume of urine collected and the preservative added. Dispose of the remainder of urine according to laboratory directions (Figure 46-2).

15. Record the date, time, volume of urine, and where the specimen was sent.

16. Clean the cylinder as appropriate. Dispose of the container in a biohazard waste container.

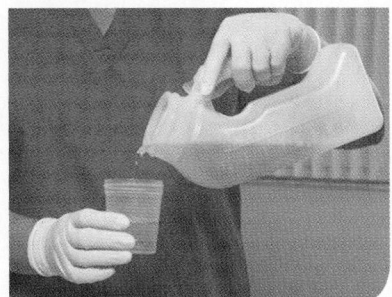

FIGURE 46-2 Mix the urine sample carefully by swirling. Measure the total volume of urine collected; then pour off an aliquot to be sent for testing.

17. Clean the area.

18. Remove gloves and perform hand hygiene.

CHARTING EXAMPLE

08/06/XX 7:00 A.M. Pt given 2 24-hour urine containers for collection of specimen for protein. Timing to begin at 7:00 A.M. 08/07/XX after voiding and discarding first AM specimen. Pt to return containers in 24 hours.·········· C. Cox, RMA

free of contamination. Typically, a nurse will perform this procedure, but the medical assistant may be called to assist. During catheterization, the urethra and its surrounding tissues will be cleaned and thus a sterile field will be created. A small, sterile tube will be inserted through the urethra to the bladder, and the urine will be collected in the sterile container. Figures 46-3A–B show a Foley catheter tray and a Foley catheter, which are used for this procedure.

Catheterization may be performed to test for urine residuals after the patient believes he or she has emptied the bladder, to collect urine from a patient who is unable to void or who is incontinent, to empty the bladder completely before surgery, or to collect sterile urine for diagnostic tests. See Figures 46-4A–B for diagrams of Foley catheters in place in the bladders of a female patient and a male patient.

Intake of fluids and output of urine are often measured in patients with renal disorders, burn patients, and patients

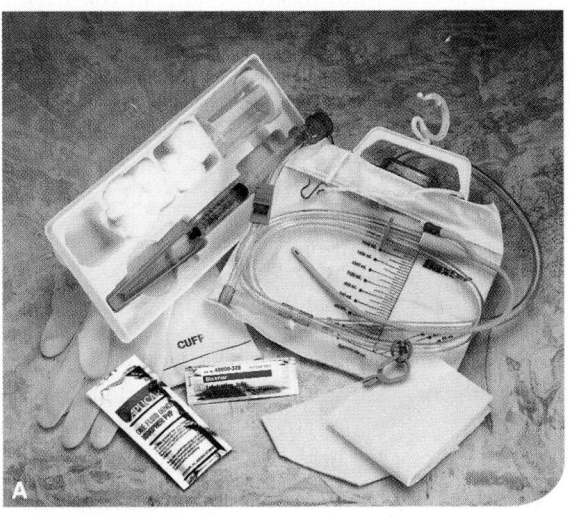

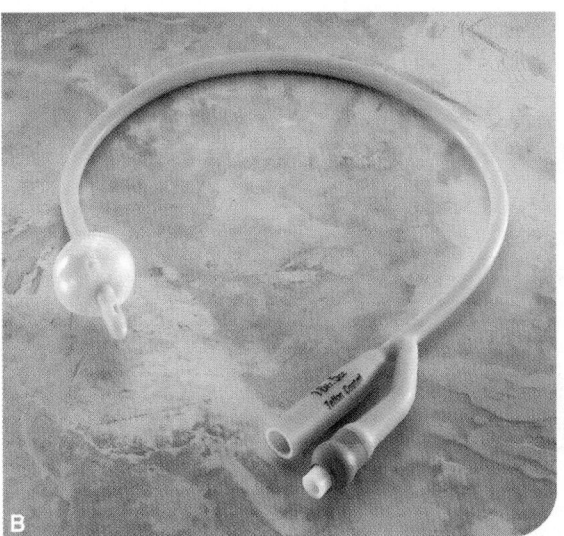

FIGURE 46-3 (A) Foley catheter tray; (B) Foley catheter.

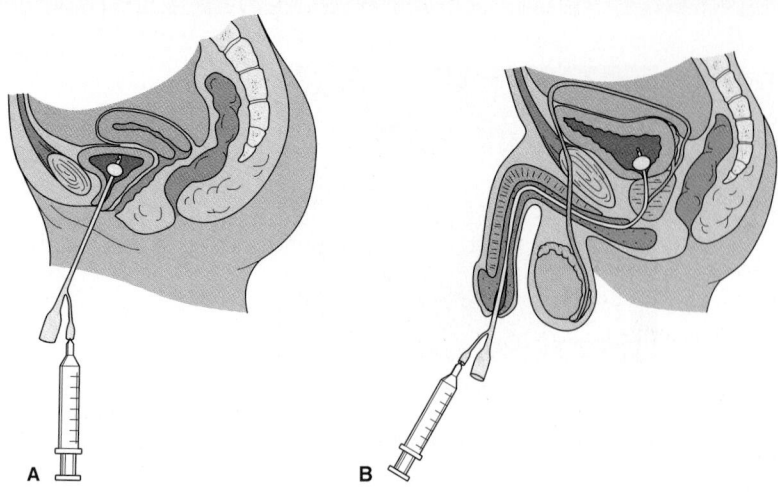

FIGURE 46-4 (A) Foley catheter: The inflated balloon at the tip of the catheter holds the Foley catheter in place in the bladder of a female patient. The catheter drains urine from the bladder continuously as the kidneys produce urine; (B) Foley catheter with balloon in the bladder of a male patient.

with congestive heart failure or dehydration. Figure 46-5 shows a medical assistant measuring urinary output from a patient with an indwelling Foley catheter that drains continuously into a collecting bag.

CLEAN-CATCH MIDSTREAM SPECIMEN

Often it is not practical to collect a catheterized specimen. A clean-catch specimen is a satisfactory alternative. Clean-catch midstream urine samples are used to detect urinary tract infections (UTIs) and other dysfunctions. A clean-catch urine sample may be cultured for microorganisms and tested to determine what antibiotics, if any, will provide effective treatment for the patient. The patient will need clear instructions to obtain a urine specimen that is free of contamination. Procedure 46-2 provides instructions for male

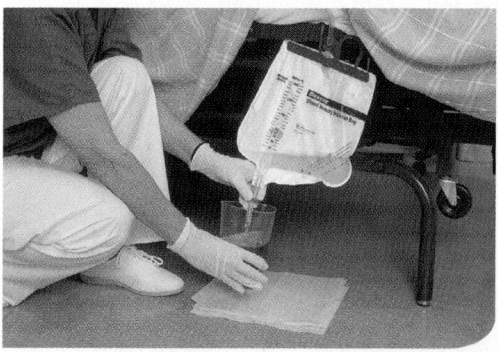

FIGURE 46-5 The medical assistant is measuring the urine output from a patient who has an indwelling Foley catheter that drains into a collecting bag.

and female patients on how to collect sterile midstream clean-catch urine specimens.

PEDIATRIC SPECIMEN

Catheterization or obtaining a midstream clean-catch specimen may not be alternatives for the pediatric patient. Attaching a pediatric urine specimen bag is often the method of choice. This is covered in Chapter 40.

SUPRAPUBIC SPECIMEN

A suprapubic puncture is performed using a sterile needle and syringe so the resulting urine specimen is sterile. This procedure is usually performed by a physician and is used for cytology examinations.

Routine Urinalysis

A routine urinalysis will include a description of the appearance, including color, of the urine. Tests for pH and specific gravity and chemical analyses for glucose, bacteria, protein, and other chemical elements are performed. Lastly, the **sediment**, the solid material settling at the bottom of a test tube after centrifugation, is examined. Table 46-1 is a listing of routine urinalysis categories.

PHYSICAL CHARACTERISTICS

Urinalysis begins with an examination of the physical characteristics of urine: appearance, color, odor, quantity, and specific gravity. Though examining the physical characteristics of urine is not commonly done in and of itself, it is important to understand all the steps and considerations involved. The physical characteristics may be important diagnostic tools for the physician. Evaluating the physical characteristics of urine is covered in Procedure 46-3.

Appearance

When observing a urine specimen, first notice if the specimen is clear or cloudy. If it is cloudy, more specific definitions will include terms such as *slightly cloudy, cloudy with sediment,* or **turbid**, meaning the urine is opaque and does not allow light to pass through. Turbidity (cloudiness) is caused by a number of factors, including bacterial infection; white blood cells, red blood cells, or epithelial cells; or yeast or vaginal contaminants. Always report exactly what is seen in

COLLECTING A CLEAN-CATCH MIDSTREAM URINE SPECIMEN

Objective: Instruct both male and female patients to correctly obtain a contaminant-free, clean-catch midstream urine specimen.

EQUIPMENT AND SUPPLIES

sterile midstream urine container; antiseptic towelettes; written patient instructions

METHOD

1. Perform hand hygiene.
2. Assemble equipment.
3. Identify and greet the patient.

Explain the procedure to a *male* patient as follows:
- Perform hand hygiene.
- Expose the penis. Pull foreskin back if uncircumcised (and hold back until specimen has been collected).
- Cleanse each side of the urethral opening from top to bottom using a separate antiseptic wipe, wiping in one direction only (Figure 46-6A). Cleanse across the top of the urethral opening with a third antiseptic, wiping in one direction only. Be certain to avoid having any body part touch the specimen container.
- Void a small amount of urine into the toilet (Figure 46-6B). Then void into the container, taking care not to touch the insides of the container (Figure 46-6C). Remove the container.
- Continue voiding the remainder of urine into the toilet.
- Recap the container immediately taking care not to contaminate the inside of the lid.
- Deliver the specimen as instructed.

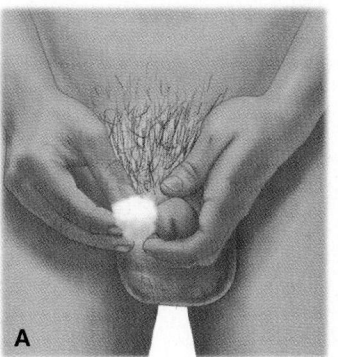

A

Explain the procedure to a *female* patient as follows:
- Perform hand hygiene and remove underwear.
- Expose the urinary meatus by pulling apart the labia and holding the area open with the nondominant hand.
- Use the dominant hand to cleanse around one side of the urinary meatus from front to back with one antiseptic wipe (Figure 46-7A). Use second wipe to cleanse the other side in the same manner. Using a third wipe, cleanse across the opening of the meatus itself. Continue holding the labia apart until the procedure is complete.

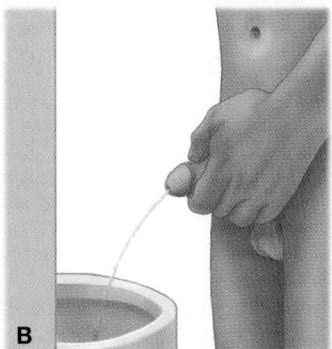

B

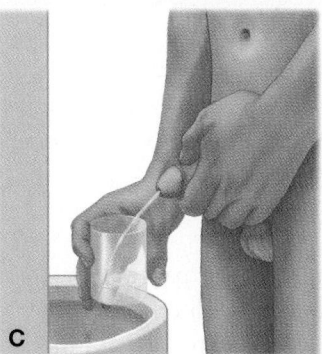

C

FIGURE 46-6 (A) The patient is instructed to cleanse the head of the penis in preparation for a clean-catch midstream urine collection; (B) begin urinating into the toilet; (C) continue urinating into the sterile cup provided for the clean-catch midstream urine specimen.

- Begin voiding into the toilet (Figure 46-7B). Place the container into position and void into the container without touching the inside with fingers (Figure 46-7C.)
- Remove the container and continue voiding into toilet.
- Wipe in the usual manner and cover the container with lid, avoiding contaminating the inside of the lid.
- Deliver the specimen as instructed.
4. Label the specimen container.
5. Perform hand hygiene.
6. Document the chart appropriately.

CHARTING EXAMPLE

4/23/XX Clean-catch midstream urine specimen collected from patient at 11:00 A.M. Sent to lab for C&S. · · · · · · · · · · · · · · · ·
· M. King, CMA (AAMA)

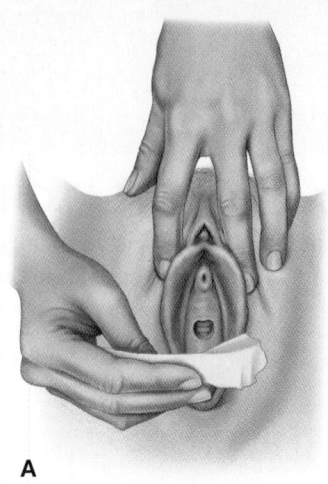

A

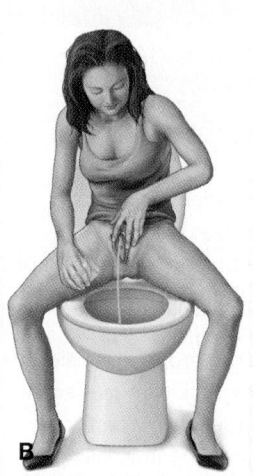

B

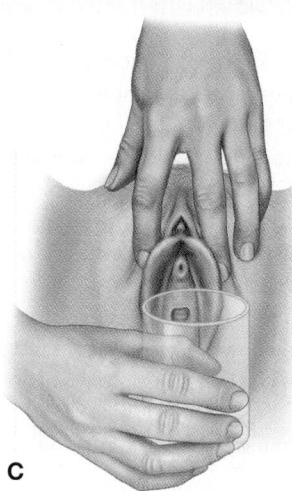

C

FIGURE 46-7 (A) Instruct the patient to spread the labia and expose the urinary meatus, then use towelettes to clean first on side from front to back and then to do the same on the other side; (B) begin urinating into the toilet; (C) urinate into the sterile clean-catch container.

the sample, using appropriate terms. Because crystals can form during the cooling process and change the appearance of the sample, always observe the appearance of the specimen before it begins to cool.

Color

The normal color of urine is straw—a pale yellow color. However, concentrated urine, along with other variables—including medications, vitamins, and some foods—can cause urine colors to range from pale yellow to amber. Occasionally, urine will appear brown or black, indicating a serious illness. Reddish-brown color may indicate bleeding, either in the urinary tract or from menstruation. Orange urine may be a result of Pyridium (a medication used to treat bladder spasms). Large quantities of the B vitamins can cause the urine to appear bright yellow.

Odor

Normally, odor is not recorded, but any abnormal aroma should be documented. Individuals testing positive for ketones (from fat metabolism) may have a "fruity" odor to their urine. This can be indicative of uncontrolled diabetes. Putrid or

TABLE 46-1 Routine Urinalysis Categories

Physical	Chemical	Microscopic
Appearance (clarity/turbidity)	Reaction (pH)	Cells
Color	Protein	Blood (RBCs, WBCs)
Specific gravity	Glucose	Epithelial cells (squamous, transitional, renal)
Odor	Blood	Casts (hyaline, cellular, granular, waxy)
Quantity (24-hour specimen only)	Ketones	Crystals (acid/alkaline)
	Bilirubin	Other: bacteria, spermatozoa, parasites, yeast
	Urobilinogen	Artifacts
	Nitrite	
	Leukocytes	

procedure 46-3

EVALUATING THE PHYSICAL CHARACTERISTICS OF URINE

Objective: Evaluate the physical characteristics of urine, and properly record the results.

EQUIPMENT AND SUPPLIES
urine specimen; centrifuge tube; laboratory slip; personal protective equipment as needed

METHOD
1. Perform hand hygiene and apply gloves.
2. Label the centrifuge tube with the patient's name.
3. Mix the urine by carefully swirling, avoiding spills.
4. Assess the color of the specimen and record observations, using appropriate terms: straw, yellow, dark yellow, amber (other colors if noted). See Figure 46-8 for examples of urines of different colors.
5. Assess and record the clarity using appropriate terms: clear, slightly cloudy, cloudy, and turbid. See Figure 46-9 for examples of urines of different clarity.
6. Clean the area.
7. Remove gloves and perform hand hygiene unless proceeding with complete urinalysis.
8. Document the results.

CHARTING EXAMPLE
4/23/XX Rand urine spec. collected. Clear, pale yellow. · · · · · ·
· M. King, CMA (AAMA)

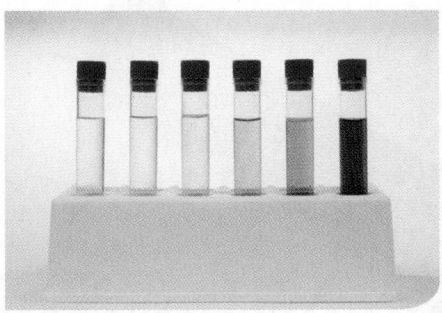

FIGURE 46-8 Colors of urine.

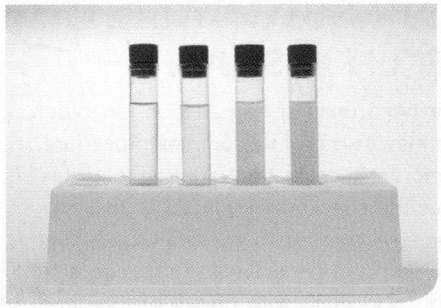

FIGURE 46-9 Appearance of urine (clear to very cloudy).

foul odors might indicate infection. Ammonia odors usually result from urine breaking down over time; they are similar to the odor of old urine on a diaper.

Quantity (Volume)

Quantity is measured when timed urine specimens are collected, but not for routine samples. A 24-hour urine specimen should measure between 700 and 2,000 mL with the average being 1,500 mL (3 pints). This varies depending on the amount of fluid ingested by the patient. **Polyuria** (excessive amounts of urine production) may indicate disorders such as diabetes or kidney disease. **Oliguria** (decreased amounts of urine production) can be indicative of dehydration, bleeding, decreased fluid intake, or kidney disease. If renal failure or an obstruction is present, then **anuria** (the absence of urine) may result. Individuals with these disorders may need to closely monitor their intake and output by recording all fluids ingested and all urine excreted.

Specific Gravity

Specific gravity is the weight of a substance in relation to the weight of the same amount of distilled water. The concentration of urine changes during the day, depending on the amount of fluid intake. Specific gravity is a rough estimate of the amount of substances dissolved in urine. This measurement indicates how well the kidneys can concentrate or dilute urine. Normal specific gravity ranges between 1.010 and 1.030. Readings outside this range may be the first indication that the kidneys may not be working properly. The presence of protein, glucose, or X-ray dyes may increase the specific gravity of urine.

Several methods are used to test urine specific gravity, including the dipstick or reagent strip method, the refractometer method, and (in the past) the urinometer method. This latter method is used infrequently now. Today most facilities perform the dipstick method; however, information and the procedure are offered for the refractometer method of testing in the event that it is being performed in your office.

Dipstick Method. The dipstick method is the most commonly used method of measuring specific gravity. It is performed by dipping a chemically treated piece of plastic (the dipstick) into the sample of urine and then reading the chemical reaction that takes place on the dipstick. The test strip is evaluated by a chemical analyzer or by visual comparison with the results on the side of the test strip bottle.

Refractometer Method. A refractometer may be used to determine specific gravity. A refractometer uses light, a prism, and a calibrated scale to measure the concentration level of the specimen. Figure 46-10 shows a refractometer. Procedure 46-4 provides the steps necessary to accurately measure the specific gravity of urine using a refractometer.

CHEMICAL CHARACTERISTICS

Chemical analyses can provide more detailed information about the patient. The most commonly used method is the dipstick, or reagent strip, method. The dipstick is equipped with small chemically treated pads that react with specific chemicals in the urine to allow for measurement of specific elements. The color changes caused by the chemical reactions are then compared to charts on the outside of the reagent strip container with the normal and abnormal value of each provided or evaluated by chemical urine analyzers. Dipstick tests are available for pH, protein, glucose, ketones, blood, bilirubin, urobilinogen, nitrite, leukocytes, and specific gravity. These tests provide information about the functioning of the kidneys, liver, and other organs. Examples of boxes of reagent strips measuring from two to nine different chemicals in the urine are shown in Figure 46-11. Physicians decide which chemical elements they want to test for, based on the patient's

PROFESSIONALISM
THE LIFE SPAN

Obtaining a urine specimen from an older adult may be a slightly complex procedure, due to the coordination required to ensure that the specimen is placed in the container according to guidelines. Be sure to carefully explain the collection procedure to patients, and provide them with plenty of time and privacy for specimen collection. You may need to be in the lavatory with them to provide help if they are unsteady on their feet or are confused.

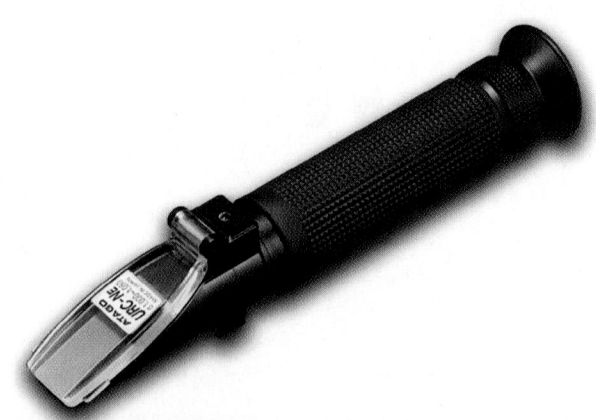

FIGURE 46-10 Portable digital refractometer.

status and possible diagnosis. Obstetricians, for example, usually test for two main elements: glucose and protein. Most physicians test for all nine elements when a patient has an annual physical examination.

Each test has a specific time associated with reading its results, and that information is given on the side of the reagent strip container. The medical assistant must ensure when a strip has been dipped in a specimen that it never touches the outside of the container. This would contaminate the outside of the container. See Procedure 46-5 for the proper steps for evaluating the presence of certain chemicals in the urine using reagent strips.

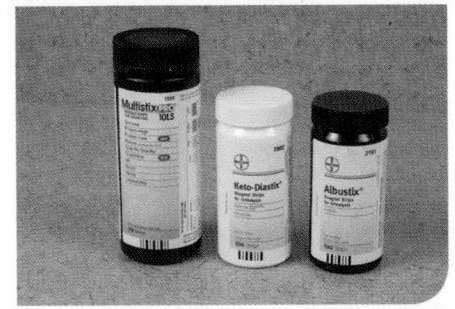

FIGURE 46-11　Variety of chemical reagents strips.

procedure 46-4

MEASURING THE SPECIFIC GRAVITY OF URINE WITH A REFRACTOMETER

Objective: Measure the specific gravity or urine with a refractometer and without error.

EQUIPMENT AND SUPPLIES

antiseptic cleaner; biohazard waste container; blood and body fluid protection: lab coat, protective eyewear, nonsterile gloves; distilled water; medicine dropper/pipette; paper, pen/pencil; paper towels; refractometer; urine specimen

METHOD

1. Perform hand hygiene.
2. Apply gloves and protective clothing.
3. Assemble equipment and materials.
4. Before using the refractometer (Figure 46-12A), perform a quality control check by using a sample of distilled water first. The value with distilled water should be 1.000.
   a. Clean the prism and refractometer cover with distilled water. Wipe dry.

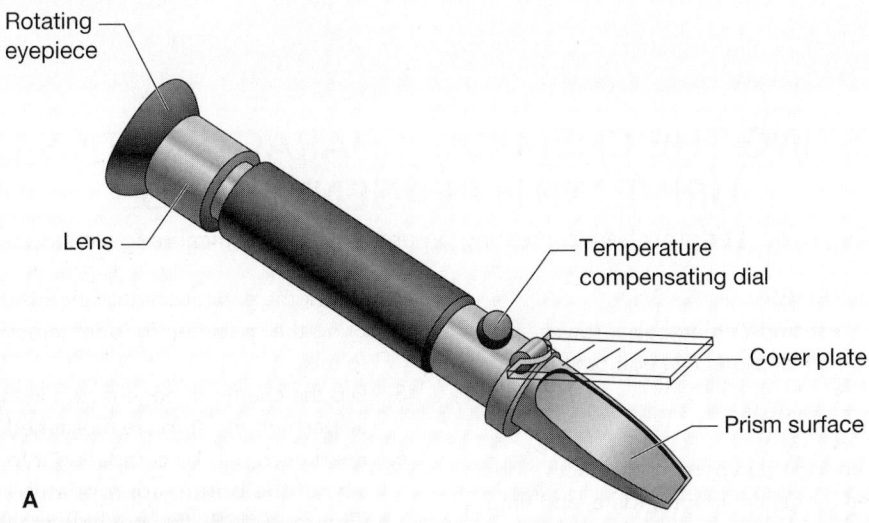

Rotating eyepiece

Lens

Temperature compensating dial

Cover plate

Prism surface

A

FIGURE 46-12　(A) Refractometer with parts labeled.

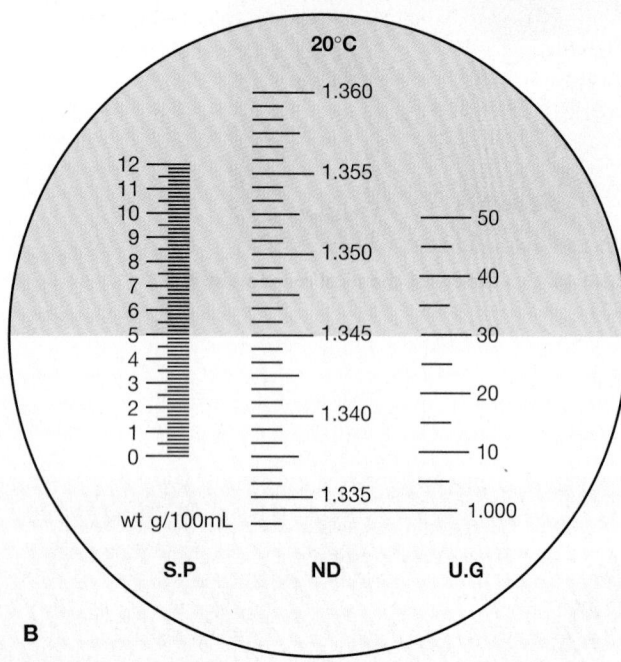

B

FIGURE 46-12 (B) Refractometer scale.

b. Close the cover. Using the medicine dropper or pipette, place a drop of distilled water on the notched area of the cover. If the refractometer does not have an attached cover, place the water directly onto the prism, and then place a cover plate on top of the prism.

c. Tilt the refractometer to allow light to enter. Read the specific gravity by noting the division line between the light and dark area (Figure 46-12B). This reading should be 1.000. If it is not, retest with fresh distilled water.

5. To test the urine sample, swirl the urine specimen gently to avoid splashing. Using the medicine dropper, remove a small sample and place 1 to 2 drops onto the notched area of the cover.

6. Follow the instructions in step 4c to read the specific gravity.

7. Record the reading on a piece of paper.

8. Discard the urine appropriately.

9. Remove gloves and protective clothing, and dispose of them properly.

10. Perform hand hygiene.

11. Document findings in the patient record.

12. Clean the work area and equipment.

CHARTING EXAMPLE
4/23/XX 1:00 P.M. SG 1.012 · · · · · · · · · M. King, CMA (AAMA)

TESTING THE CHEMICAL CHARACTERISTICS OF URINE WITH REAGENT STRIPS

Objective: Perform chemical testing on urine using chemical reagent strips.

EQUIPMENT AND SUPPLIES
urine specimen; reagent test strips; timer; paper towel; laboratory slip; pen/pencil; personal protective equipment as needed

METHOD
1. Perform hand hygiene and don personal protective gear.
2. Check the specimen for patient identity, date, and time of collection.
3. Check the expiration date on the chemical reagent strips.
4. Bring the specimen to room temperature and swirl gently to mix.
5. Dip the chemical reagent strip in the urine, making sure all pads on the strip are moistened (Figure 46-13A).
6. Read each pad by comparing it to the chart on the side of the bottle, appropriately timing each test (Figure 46-13B). (Do not hold the test strip against the

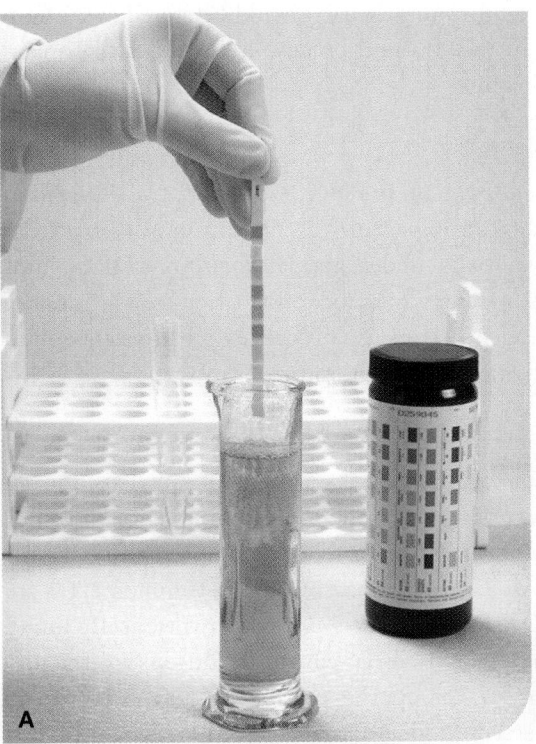

side of the bottle as contamination will result.) Ignore color changes after the prescribed time has elapsed.

7. Record the results on patient's laboratory slip.
8. Clean the work area, remove gloves, and perform hand hygiene.

CHARTING EXAMPLE

Note: Normally a urine test slip would be used to record all results of chemical tests. Then when examination is complete and the physician has reviewed it, the test slip would be placed in the patient's chart.

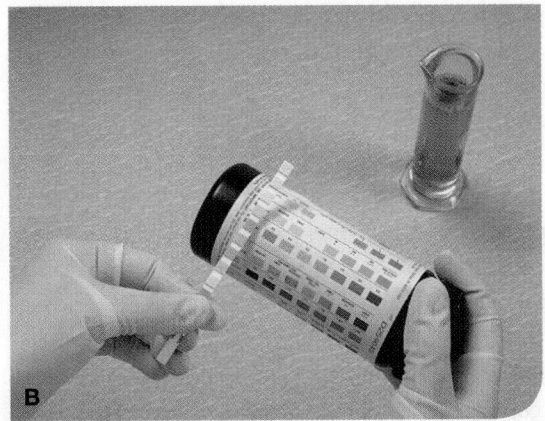

FIGURE 46-13 (A) Dip reagent strip into urine and withdraw; (B) compare color changes on the reagent strip to chart on the side of container without contaminating the container.

Reaction pH

The pH of a solution indicates acidity and alkalinity. The pH is measured on a scale of 0 to 14, with 0 being the most acidic, 14 being the most basic (alkaline), and 7 being neutral (Figure 46-14).

Normally, urine is slightly acidic at about 6.0. The ability of the kidneys to dilute and concentrate urine helps maintain the narrow pH range of blood (7.35 to 7.45) necessary for the body to be in homeostasis. Normal kidneys produce urine with pH ranging from 4.6 to 7.9. In UTIs, the pH is typically more alkaline (higher than 7.0) because some bacteria break down urea to ammonia. Urine samples must be examined when fresh to avoid bacteria multiplying and causing inaccurate results. Higher pH is common in fever, phenylketonuria, and diets high in vitamin C. Some causes of low pH include respiratory acidosis, diets high in fruits or vegetables, and administration of some drugs.

Protein

Protein is normally not found in the urine of healthy individuals. Urine may contain a small quantity of protein after exposure to the cold, after strenuous muscular activity, or after eating large amounts of protein. However, these are considered physiological responses and not symptoms of disease. The presence of protein (**proteinuria**) can indicate renal dysfunction, preeclampsia in pregnancy, congestive

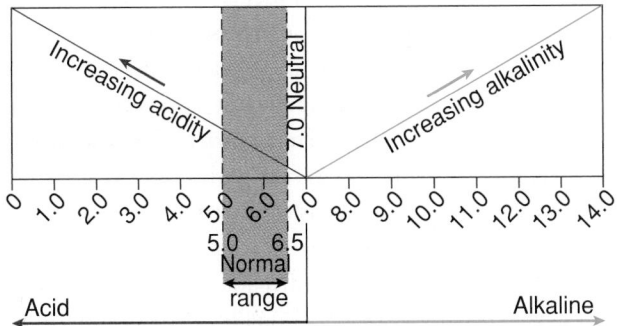

FIGURE 46-14 Urine pH scale.

heart failure, and **glomerulonephritis** (a kidney disease involving inflammation and lesions of the glomeruli).

Glucose

Normal urine should not contain glucose. However, after eating a high-carbohydrate diet, small quantities of sugar may be present in the urine. This, however, is not a normal condition. If urine levels of glucose do not return to normal fairly quickly, it may be indicative of diabetes, gestational diabetes, stress, infection, or Cushing's syndrome, or it may be caused by the use of some medications. **Glycosuria** is the term for the presence of abnormal sugar in the urine. Sugar typically spills into the urine when the blood sugar levels exceed the renal threshold for glucose. The renal threshold for glucose is approximately 160 to 180 mg/dL of glucose in the blood stream.

Blood

Hematuria (blood in the urine) is abnormal unless it is a contamination from menses. The presence of **occult** (hidden) blood in urine may indicate anemia, UTIs, kidney stones, or trauma. It is occasionally caused by some medications. Female patients must be asked if menses is present when collection of a urine sample is required. If a patient is menstruating, it should be noted on the laboratory slip.

Ketones

Ketones are by-products of fat metabolism. Fats normally break down into water and carbon dioxide. If fats are burned as a source of energy instead of glucose, ketones will be found in the urine. If this persists long enough, a condition of acidosis may occur, resulting in coma and death if untreated. Urine normally is negative for ketones. Elevated ketones are typically seen in conditions such as poorly controlled diabetes, dehydration, starvation, ingestion of large quantities of aspirin, and occasionally after general anesthesia. Ketones tend to evaporate at room temperature; therefore, ketone testing must be done immediately or the specimen should be covered and refrigerated.

Bilirubin

Under normal circumstances, bilirubin is not found in the urine. Bilirubin is a product of the breakdown of hemoglobin. Hemoglobin is released from old red blood cells (RBCs) and is converted by the liver into bilirubin and into urobilinogen in the small intestines. The presence of bilirubin in urine may be one of the first signs of liver disease,

obstructive biliary disease, or mononucleosis. Large amounts of bilirubin in the urine will cause the urine to turn yellow-brown to dark orange. If a specimen is found to have large quantities of bilirubin, then it should be stored away from light until further testing, because light causes the breakdown of bilirubin.

Urobilinogen

Urobilinogen is a result of RBC destruction. It is elevated in any condition causing an increase in bilirubin. It is present in small quantities under normal conditions. If no urobilinogen is present, a bile duct obstruction may be present. However, reagents strips usually are not sensitive enough to detect an absence of urobilinogen.

Nitrites

Measurement of nitrites is a method for detection of **bacturia** (bacteria in the urine). Thus the presence of nitrites often indicates a UTI. Nitrites are a by-product of chemical breakdown by certain bacteria. Most common UTIs are caused by *Escherichia coli* (*E. coli*), which is typically found in bowel material. Bacteria, when introduced into the urinary meatus, travel up the urethra to the bladder. The bladder is sterile under normal conditions. An infection may result if enough bacteria are present in the bladder. Females should be reminded after voiding or having a bowel movement to wipe from front to back, away from the urinary meatus, to lessen the chance of developing UTIs.

False positives for the presence of nitrites can happen if the specimen sits at room temperature too long because bacteria can begin to multiply at room temperature. Specimens that cannot be immediately tested should be refrigerated.

Leukocytes

Leukocytes are white blood cells (WBCs), and under normal conditions few leukocytes are found in urine. When leukocytes are present in sufficient quantity, they are usually indicative of a UTI. In the leukocyte esterase test, the reagent strip detects the esterase released by WBCs. The darker the color on the strip, the greater the number of WBCs. When a leukocyte esterase test is positive, always check to see if the results correlate with the rest of the patient's report. If a leukocyte test is positive, then a protein test should be positive, and it is likely that an elevated pH and microscopic bacteria would also be present.

As mentioned, urine samples provide vital information to the physician treating a patient. Usually when an individual has an annual physical, all of the preceding tests are performed on the urine specimen. For example, an abnormal urine glucose result may require a follow-up fasting blood sugar or glucose tolerance test to confirm or rule out diabetes mellitus. An abnormal protein result may indicate bladder infection or infection higher in the urinary tract, or it may indicate hypertension. Follow-up tests such as a 24-hour urine specimen for protein, X-rays of the kidney and a clean-catch midstream urine test, may be ordered for culture and sensitivity. Physicians rely on the initial routine urinalysis to indicate where they may need to follow up with further testing. Never underestimate the importance of the urine test.

REAGENT TABLET TESTING

Some institutions routinely perform tablet testing when a reagent strip test for glucose is positive. It is prudent laboratory practice to repeat any abnormal result before reporting the results using a backup method (other testing method than originally done). In this instance, if the dipstick was positive for glucose, the facility policy should dictate that the medical assistant perform a tablet test or test using another brand or lot number of dipstick before results are reported.

Some facilities use the tablet test in place of the reagent strip. Chemically treated tablets may be used to test urine specimens for substances such as glucose and acetone. Clinitest tablets are chemical tablets that are added to a urine specimen, and the resulting color is compared to a reaction chart to determine the presence of certain sugars. This is no longer used for insulin monitoring because it is specific for lactose and galactose but not glucose. Procedure 46-6 presents the steps necessary to test for glucose using Clinitest tablets.

Acetest tablets are another way of testing for ketones in blood or urine. The reaction is based on the same reaction

procedure
46-6

TESTING FOR GLUCOSE IN URINE USING THE TABLET METHOD
Objective: Perform procedure to test for sugar in the urine without error.

EQUIPMENT AND SUPPLIES
antiseptic cleaner; biohazard waste container; body and body fluid protection—lab coat, goggles, nonsterile gloves; clean glass test tube; Clinitest tablets; distilled water; medicine dropper/pipette; urine specimen

METHOD
1. Perform hand hygiene.
2. Apply gloves and protective clothing.
3. Assemble equipment and materials.
4. Using the medicine dropper or a pipette, place 5 drops of the urine specimen into a clean test tube.
5. Add 10 drops of water. Mix together drops, using the pipette and being careful not to splash the urine.
6. Drop one Clinitest tablet into the urine and water solution. Observe the solution (do not shake) as it reacts in the test tube. Do not touch the bottom of the tube during this chemical process because it becomes very hot (Figure 46-15).

7. At 15 seconds after the reaction (boiling) stops, gently shake the tube to mix the contents.
8. Immediately match the color of the liquid against the color chart on the side of the Clinitest container.

Note: Do not touch the test tube of urine to the Clinitest bottle because this will contaminate the outside of the bottle. Ignore any additional color changes after the 15-second period.

9. Discard the urine according to OSHA guidelines.
10. Remove gloves and protective clothing, and dispose of them properly.
11. Perform hand hygiene.
12. Document findings in patient record.
13. Clean work area and equipment according to OSHA guidelines.

CHARTING EXAMPLE
10/19/XX 4:00 P.M. Clinitest 2+ · · · · · · · M. King, CMA (AAMA)

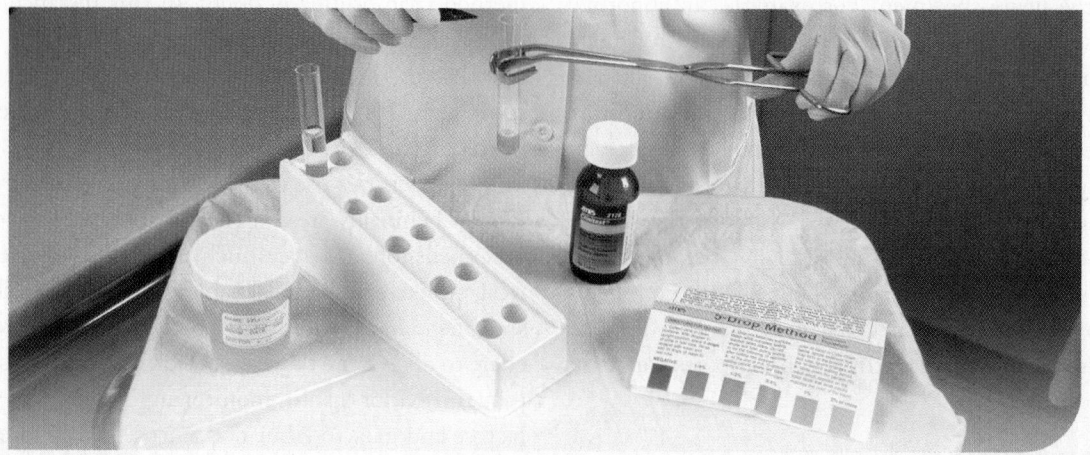

FIGURE 46-15   Do not touch the bottom of the tube when testing with tablets for glucose. The tube is hot from the chemical reaction.

found on the chemical reagent strips. The sulfosalicylic acid turbidity test is used as a confirmatory test for protein in urine; for this test, equal amounts of urine and 3 percent sulfosalicylic acid are combined in a test tube, and cloudiness appears if protein is present. Figure 46-16 shows a variety of tests used to test diabetic urine.

AUTOMATED URINE CHEMICAL ANALYZERS

Automated chemical analyzers for urine are widely used in many types of facilities. These analyzers use light photometry to test the strips, which eliminates the human error associated with color recognition. Some analyzers read the test strips and report the results on a printout sheet. Quality control protocols, including the use of positive and negative controls and proper documentation, must be followed. Figure 46-17 is an example of an automated urine chemical analyzer. Table 46-2 gives normal urine values.

MICROSCOPIC EXAMINATION

Microscopic examination identifies the type and approximate numbers of organisms present in a urine specimen. Microscopic examination helps physicians to determine a disease process. This is not a Clinical Laboratory Improvement Amendments (CLIA) waived test. A certificate of provider-performed microscopy (PPM) procedures is issued

to a physician's office laboratory (POL) that is qualified to perform waived tests, moderate complexity tests, and microscopic procedures. If the PPM certificate is not granted, the specimen may be sent to an outside laboratory. In some states, medical assistants may perform microscopic examinations after further training if the facility has a PPM certificate. Medical assistants must be able to properly prepare a urine specimen for microscopic examination and understand the meaning and importance of the results of a urine microscopic examination.

Preparing a Urine Specimen for Microscopic Examination

After performing the necessary physical and chemical analyses, the urine is placed in a centrifuge tube and then into a centrifuge.

The sediment is the solid material remaining in urine after the **supernatant** (liquid portion) is poured off. The sediment may contain organized material such as RBCs, WBCs, epithelial cells, casts, bacteria, parasites, yeast, fungi, and spermatozoa. The unorganized sediment consists of all chemical materials, including crystals and **amorphous** (without a shape) material. A special stain may be used to provide better contrast to the formed elements present. Specimens that are to be examined under the microscope should be fresh. Ideally, they should be collected by the clean-catch method. Procedure 46-7 presents the steps needed to prepare a urine specimen for microscopic examination.

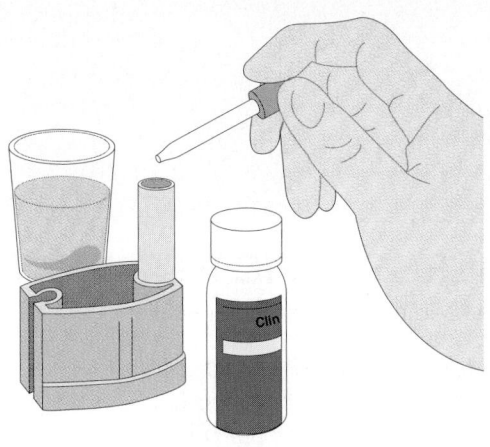

Clinitest

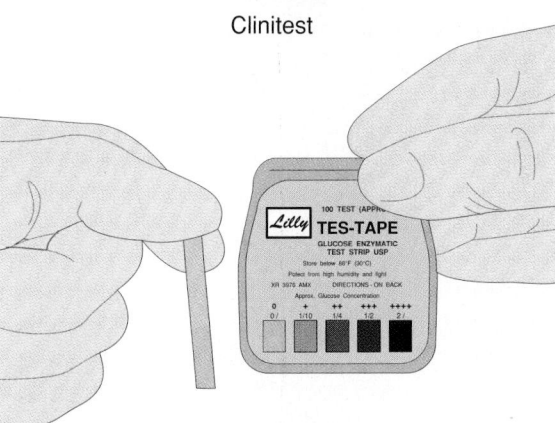

Tes-Tape

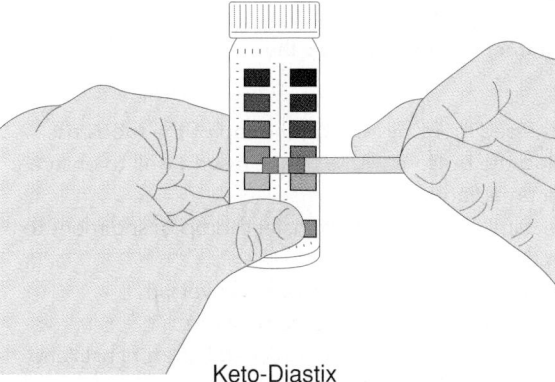

Keto-Diastix

FIGURE 46-16 Three types of urine tests for checking patients' urine for diabetes.

Reporting and Understanding Urine Microscopic Examinations

As mentioned previously, examining urine sediment under the microscope is not a CLIA waived test, and as a medical assistant you should understand CLIA regulations and review your state's regulations regarding these procedures.

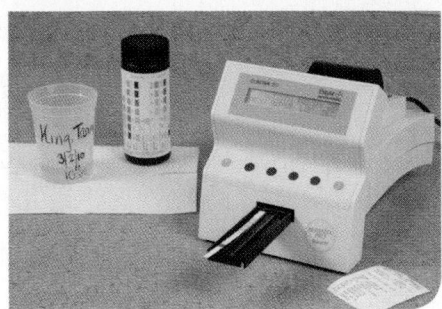

FIGURE 46-17 An example of a urine chemical analyzer.

To better understand the results of a urine microscopic examination, an explanation of the method used to estimate the numbers of formed elements observed is necessary. (The meaning of each individual formed element is discussed in subsequent paragraphs.) Once the slide is made and coverslipped, it is examined first under the low-power field (lpf) setting of the microscope (10×) and low light to locate casts, which if present are found near the edges of the coverslip. Between 10 and 15 fields are scanned, and the number and type of casts or cells are noted. For example, in 10 to 15 fields the examiner sees a range of 0 to 4 hyaline casts. This means that some fields contained no casts and others contained one, two, three, or four casts, thus the report of 0–4 hyaline casts per lpf. Counting and reporting procedures are the same when using 40×, or the high-power

TABLE 46-2 Normal Values for Urinalysis Testing

Element	Normal Values
Color	Straw, pale yellow, yellow, darker yellow, amber
Appearance	Clear, slightly cloudy
Specific gravity	1.010–1.030
Odor	Aromatic
Reaction/pH	4.6–7.9
Protein	Negative to trace
Glucose	Negative
Ketones	Negative
Blood	Negative
Nitrites	Negative
Bilirubin	Negative
Urobilinogen	Less than 2 Ehrlich units/dL
Leukocytes	Negative

PREPARING A URINE SPECIMEN FOR MICROSCOPIC EXAMINATION

Objective: Perform microscopic examination of urine sediment for casts and cells.

EQUIPMENT AND SUPPLIES

biohazard waste container; body and body fluid protection—lab coat, goggles, nonsterile gloves; capillary pipette; centrifuge; centrifuge tube; microscope; microscope slide; paper, pen/pencil; Sedi-stain (optional); urine specimen

Note: Medical assistants are not expected to perform a microscopic examination. They may be requested by the physician to prepare the specimen to step 11.

METHOD

1. Perform hand hygiene.
2. Apply gloves and protective clothing.
3. Assemble equipment and materials.
4. Mix the specimen gently to stir up the sediment that has settled to the bottom.
5. Place 10 mL of urine into the centrifuge tube. Place cap on tube. Place the tube in the centrifuge and balance this with another tube of 10 mL of water on the opposite side of the machine (Figure 46-18).
6. Set centrifuge timer for 5 minutes.
7. After the centrifuge has stopped, remove the tube and pour off the supernatant fluid (the clear liquid left on the top of the specimen after centrifuging), leaving only the sediment (Figure 46-19).

Alternate Method: Some medical assistants prefer using stain (such as Sedi-stain) to help identify sediment more easily. Place one drop of the commercially prepared stain in the test tube.

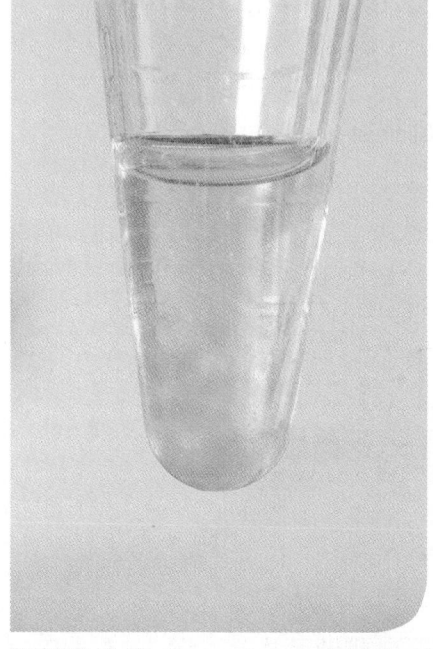

FIGURE 46-19   Pour out most of the liquid supernatant from the tube but keep the sediment.

8. Mix the sediment by holding the top of the tube and tapping the bottom with a finger, mixing well to ensure a correct reading.
9. Use a capillary pipette to transfer 1 drop of sediment to a clean slide (Figure 46-20).
10. Cover the drop of sediment with a coverslip.
11. Place the slide on the microscope stage.
12. Focus under low power and reduced light for casts and epithelial cells.

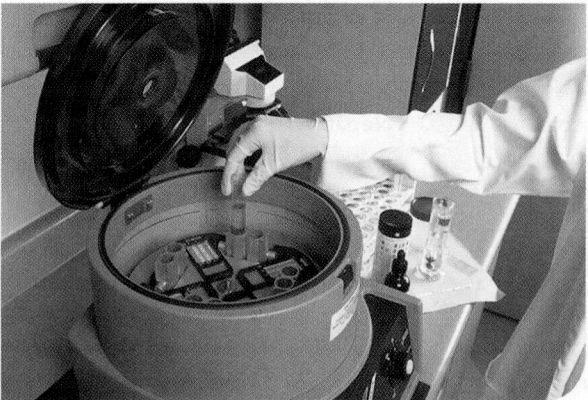

FIGURE 46-18   The centrifuge is used to spin urine specimens in preparation for a microscopic examination.

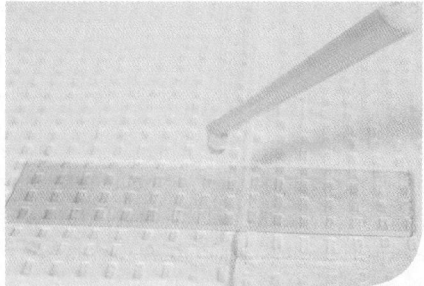

FIGURE 46-20   After mixing the sediment well, use a dropper to place a drop of urine on the slide.

13. Carefully examine for anything abnormal, paying close attention to the edges, which are where casts are seen if present.
14. Examine 10 to 15 fields using low power. Count the number of casts or other abnormalities seen in each field. If there is nothing in one field, then record 0 (zero). Average the count from the 10 to 15 fields for the final result.
15. Use the high-power magnification and adjust for more light, reviewing the 10 to 15 fields. Identify casts if present. Count RBCs, WBCs, round cells, transitional cells, and squamous epithelial cells. Average the count from the 10 to 15 fields for each formed element seen, and record appropriately.

16. Observe for crystals and identify. Observe for bacteria, sperm, yeast, and parasites. Report them as few, moderate, or many.
17. Discard the urine according to OSHA guidelines.
18. Remove gloves and protective clothing, and dispose of them properly.
19. Perform hand hygiene.
20. Document findings in patient record.
21. Clean work area and equipment according to OSHA guidelines.

field (hpf), setting. It is preferable to use a numerical range when reporting formed elements. Other elements may be reported using the following words to estimate the amounts:

- Occasional   0–3
- Few   3–6
- Moderate   6–12
- Many   12 or more
- TNTC   Too numerous to count

Cells

Cells that may be found in urine are epithelial cells, RBCs, and WBCs. The presence of RBCs, an excessive number of white cells, and certain types of epithelial cells indicate urinary tract conditions or disease.

Epithelial Cells.   Epithelial cells are classified as squamous, transitional or bladder, and renal epithelial cells. Squamous epithelial cells line the urinary tract from the external meatus to the bladder. Therefore, a few epithelial cells (0–5 per hpf) are to be expected in a urine sample. They also line the vagina and may be considered vaginal contaminants in urine. Finding bladder or renal epithelial cells is an abnormal finding and may indicate the presence of disease in the bladder or kidneys.

Red Blood Cells.   Anything more than 1 to 2 RBCs per hpf is considered abnormal. The presence of RBCs could represent a bladder infection or kidney disorder such as nephritis. RBCs are pale, round, have no nucleus (core), and are nongranular. They indicate that bleeding may be taking place somewhere in the urinary system. Acidic

urine may cause the RBCs to rupture and be invisible or mistaken for WBCs under microscopic examination. RBCs may be an indication of menstruation in female patients.

White Blood Cells.   WBCs contain a nucleus and a granular surface and are larger than RBCs. A normal count is 0 to 5 WBCs per hpf. Large numbers of WBCs may indicate an infection in the urinary system. Further testing would be needed to pinpoint the infection location.

Casts

Casts result from protein formation in the kidney tubules. Different types of casts are classified according to the substances that form them. Casts are counted under the low power of the microscope but are identified under high-powered magnification. Casts may be identified as hyaline, granular (coarse or finely granular), cellular (WBC, RBC, or epithelial), mixed (containing more than one type of cell), or waxy. Hyaline casts, in large quantities may be indicative of kidney disease. RBC casts are found in diseases such as glomerulonephritis. Waxy casts are rarely seen and are indicative of severe renal disease.

Bacteria

Bacteria are not normally found in fresh urine. A specimen can become contaminated during collection or with vaginal secretions. Large numbers of bacteria in the urine indicate a UTI. A specimen with bacteria and WBCs can be considered a confirmation of a UTI. A urine culture may be done to determine the type of bacteria and the correct antibiotic therapy.

Yeast

Yeast may be present in the urine of a female who has a vaginal yeast infection (moniliasis). It can also be present in both males and females with diabetes mellitus.

Parasites

Parasites are organisms that live within other organisms. They may be present in urine as a result of contamination from vaginal or bowel excretions. *Trichomonas vaginalis* is the most frequently found parasite in urine, and it causes vaginal infection.

Spermatozoa

Spermatozoa, the male reproductive cell, can be seen in both male and female urine after sexual intercourse.

Crystals

Crystals are formed by the precipitation of urinary salts when pH, temperature, or concentration changes occur. Crystals can form in the urine in the kidney, in the bladder, or in a standing specimen. Crystals are found in both acid and alkaline urine. As urine cools, solid crystals will precipitate out. The presence of crystals is not usually clinically significant unless found in large numbers. Crystals are identified by their appearance and the pH of the urine in which they are found. In certain metabolic disorders, abnormal crystals such as leucine or tyrosine or cystine may be found. In addition certain drugs, such as sulfa drugs, may cause the production of crystals.

Contaminants

Many substances can cause contamination of a urine specimen, including clothing fibers, mucous threads, hair, talc, or other body contaminants. A contaminant-free specimen is never completely guaranteed, but patient education can minimize the chances of specimen contamination. Figure 46-21 identifies different structures that may be found in a urine microscopic examination.

Urine Pregnancy Testing

There are two types of pregnancy tests: one tests a urine sample, and the other tests a blood sample. Both tests are based on the detection of human chorionic gonadotropin (hCG), which is produced by the placenta and is present in the urine and blood of pregnant women. Levels of hCG may be detectable as early as 10 days after fertilization has taken place. A first morning specimen is preferred for urine testing because the concentration of the hormone is greatest at that time. There are different types of urine tests for pregnancy, and they can be performed at home or in a clinic or physician's office. One type uses a dipstick, and the other relies on a midstream sample. Blood pregnancy tests must be sent to a laboratory for analysis and generally are more accurate earlier than urine tests.

The technology of the pregnancy test is fairly complex, but the tests themselves are easy to perform. CLIA-waived pregnancy tests performed in POLs fall into two categories: agglutination or enzyme immunoassay. The more frequently used enzyme immunoassay (EIA) tests involve the reaction of antigen and antibody and a second antibody attached to an enzyme. Many CLIA-approved pregnancy tests are available over the counter. They are considered to be 97 percent accurate when directions are followed correctly. Pregnancy tests are produced with built-in controls that are run along with the patient test to provide quality control. Procedure 46-8 lists the steps necessary to perform a urine pregnancy test using the EIA testing method.

Quality Control

Quality control is a system of ensuring that patients' test results are accurate and reported in a timely manner. Each testing product typically is sold with a quality control testing program. Testing should be done on a regular schedule, following the appropriate protocol, and all documentation should be kept in a quality control log. Before any test is used, the expiration date of the product should be checked to be sure the product has not expired. The tests used for urinary pH, protein, blood, glucose, ketones, bilirubin, nitrite, urobilinogen, and specific gravity should be checked periodically by using solutions that contain a known amount of each of these substances. It is important to precisely follow

---

PROFESSIONALISM THE WORKPLACE

One member of the clinic or office team will be designated as an OSHA officer. That individual is responsible for ensuring that all OSHA policies are followed and that all team members are educated appropriately in following OSHA policies. Sharps containers should be provided in any exam room or lab where needles or other sharps are used. Material data safety manuals must be kept up to date, listing all the chemicals used in the facility.

Per OSHA standards, standard precautions must be observed at all times. When a medical assistant is in a situation where exposure to blood and body fluids is a possibility, gloves must be worn. If appropriate, a lab coat and goggles and in some cases a face mask should also be utilized.

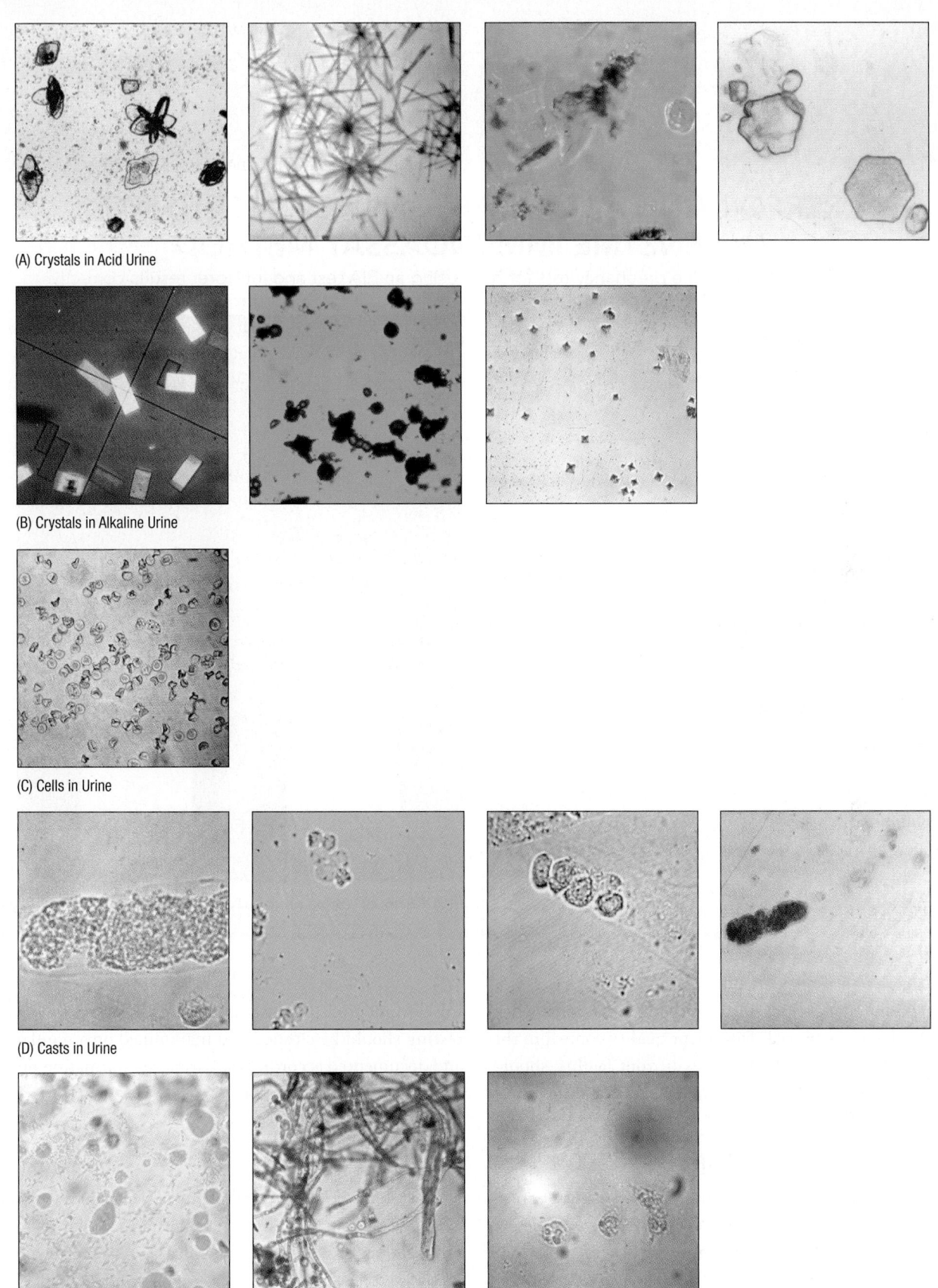

(A) Crystals in Acid Urine

(B) Crystals in Alkaline Urine

(C) Cells in Urine

(D) Casts in Urine

(E) Bacteria, Fungi, Parasites Found in Urine

FIGURE 46-21   Urine sediment chart.

PERFORMING A URINE PREGNANCY TEST USING THE ENZYME IMMUNOASSAY METHOD

Objective: Perform a urine pregnancy test for hCG using an EIA test and interpret results correctly.

EQUIPMENT AND SUPPLIES

patient's first A.M. urine specimen; EIA test kit for hCG; timer; gloves; laboratory report

METHOD

1. Perform hand hygiene and apply gloves.
2. Gather supplies and equipment.
3. Allow the testing materials and specimen to come to room temperature.
4. Label the test with patient name or ID number.
5. Label one area positive and one negative for controls.
6. Place the patient's urine on test chamber following manufacturer's directions.
7. Place positive and negative controls in correct areas (Figure 46-22).
8. Time the test according to the manufacturer's directions.
9. Interpret results correctly.
10. Record results on patient's laboratory slip.
11. Record positive and negative controls in quality control logbook according to office policy.
12. Dispose of equipment and perform hand hygiene.

CHARTING EXAMPLE

10/19/XX 4:00 P.M. Preg test pos. · · · · · M. King, CMA (AAMA)

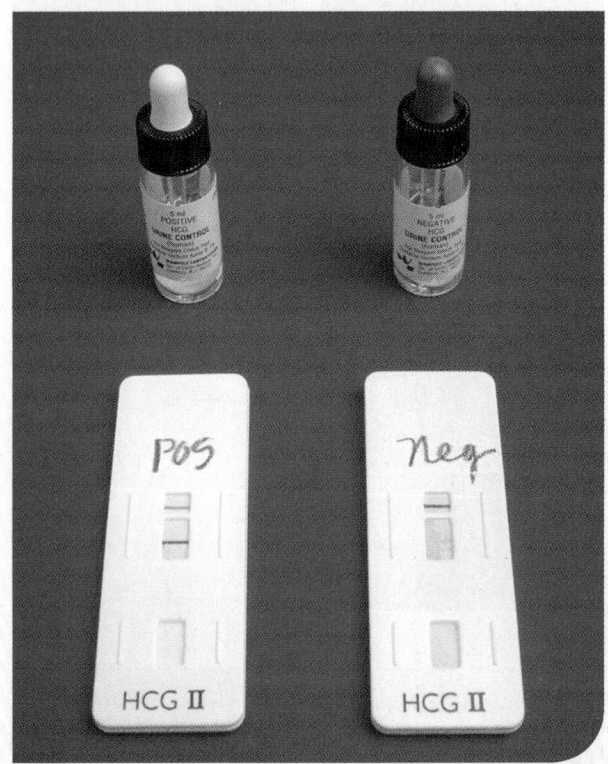

FIGURE 46-22 Urine pregnancy control test—positive and negative.

---

the directions that are supplied by the manufacturer when using this testing material. Document quality control in the quality control log. New employees in your facility should be appropriately trained to perform urine tests and the training documented. All instrumentation associated with urine testing should be cleaned and maintained on a regular basis and documented accordingly. For more information on quality control, see Chapter 44.

SUMMARY

Urinalysis is one of the most common laboratory procedures performed by the medical assistant. Because urine is a body fluid, standard precautions must be observed, including aseptic technique. Many steps are taken to ensure accurate laboratory results, including good patient education, proper specimen labeling, and following laboratory procedures exactly.

The three primary components of a urinalysis include examinations for the physical (appearance, color, odor, volume, and specific gravity), chemical (pH, protein, glucose, blood, ketones, bilirubin, urobilinogen, nitrate, and leukocytes), and microscopic (cells, casts, bacteria, yeast, parasites, spermatozoa, crystals, and contaminants). Quality control is the final component of urinalysis.

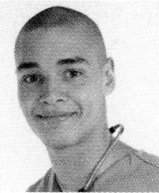

46 CHAPTER REVIEW

COMPETENCY REVIEW

1. Define and spell the terms to learn for this chapter.

2. Explain the procedure for a microscopic examination of urine.

3. Discuss two types of commercial products for chemical analysis of urine specimens.

4. Why do we measure specific gravity?

5. What causes a fruity odor in urine? In what disease condition is it found?

6. What is the purpose of catheterization?

PREPARING FOR THE CERTIFICATION EXAM

1. Pregnancy tests detect pregnancy by the presence in urine or serum of
   a. heterophile antibodies
   b. human chorionic gonadotropin
   c. febrile agglutinations
   d. autoimmune antibodies
   e. anti Rh antibodies

2. To determine the kidney's ability to dilute and concentrate urine, one should measure
   a. glucose
   b. ketones
   c. specific gravity
   d. protein
   e. occult blood

3. In routine urinalysis all of the following are physical properties of urine EXCEPT
   a. color
   b. appearance
   c. specific gravity
   d. odor
   e. glucose

4. Turbid, in regard to urine, would refer to the
   a. odor
   b. color
   c. quantity
   d. cloudiness
   e. specific gravity

5. Normally in a 24-hour period an individual excretes
   a. 70–100 mL of urine
   b. 500–700 mL of urine
   c. 250–2500 mL of urine
   d. 700–2000 mL of urine
   e. 1000–5000 mL of urine

6. Anuria means
   a. no urine production
   b. too much urine produced
   c. scant urine production
   d. kidney stones
   e. bladder infection

7. An indicator of possible urinary tract infection (UTI) is
   a. neutral pH in urine sample
   b. pH greater than 7 in a urine sample
   c. pH much lower than 7 in a urine sample
   d. elevated glucose level in urine sample
   e. elevated amount of hCG in urine sample

8. The presence of which of the following in urine may signal the onset of diabetes mellitus?
   a. leukocytes
   b. erythrocytes
   c. ketones
   d. glucose
   e. nitrates

9. In a normal microscopic urine result there can be
   a. a few epithelial cells, occasional WBC, rare RBC
   b. many epithelial cells, many WBCs, many RBCs
   c. nothing to report
   d. so many cells they cannot be counted
   e. only many RBCs

10. The presence of many red blood cells in a urine microscopic examination is referred to as
   a. polyuria
   b. hematuria
   c. albuminuria
   d. pyuria
   e. leukocytopenia

CRITICAL THINKING

1. After reading the results of the urinalysis, Dr. Salpega diagnoses Shelly with a UTI. What chemical characteristics may have tested positive on the reagent strip that would have led Dr. Salpega to diagnose a UTI?

2. Dr. Salpega informs Susan that he would like the urine sample sent to the lab for a culture. Why might the physician decide to do this?

3. What is a common cause of UTIs in women? What can women do to lessen their chances of developing a UTI?

ON THE JOB

José Menendez is an elderly patient of Dr. Juárez, a board-certified urologist. José has a history of recurrent UTIs dating back more than 10 years. When he becomes symptomatic, he has been instructed to call Dr. Juárez's office and schedule a urinalysis. Dr. Juárez's receptionist has just received a call from Mr. Menendez. He says he knows he is supposed to come in for a urine test but that he just wants a prescription phoned in to his pharmacy instead. The receptionist asks Emilia, Dr. Juárez's medical assistant to take the call from Mr. Menendez.

Emilia listens as Mr. Menendez recounts that he is experiencing dysuria—painful, burning urination. She asks him to come in for a urinalysis, explaining that, as per standing orders, a clean-catch midstream specimen needs to be collected. Mr. Menendez repeats to Emilia that he does not want to come in to the office. "Why can't you call in a prescription for Bactrim? That is what I took last time, and it helped."

What is your response?

1. Should the responsibility for this call have fallen on Emilia, or should the receptionist have either handled the call herself or passed it on to Dr. Juárez?
2. What, if anything, could or should Emilia say to Mr. Menendez to persuade him to come in for the urinalysis?
3. Might the cost of the procedure be a factor in the reason why Mr. Menendez does not want to have a urinalysis, and, if so, what, if anything, can Emilia do or say about the cost?
4. Is it appropriate in this case, given the patient's extensive history, to indeed call in a prescription for Bactrim?
5. If not, how should Emilia handle Mr. Menendez's request for his prescription?
6. If so, what procedure should Emilia follow in order to arrange for a prescription?
7. How should this telephone call be charted?
8. What, if anything, should Dr. Juárez be told about the conversation with Mr. Menendez?

INTERNET ACTIVITY

Use the Internet to research OSHA regulations regarding personal protective equipment.

MEDMEDIA

Additional interactive resources and activities for this chapter can be found:

On your student DVD: View applicable procedure videos on the DVD-ROM found in the back of this book.

MyHealthProfessionsKit.com: Test your knowledge of this chapter with games and activities. MyHealthProfessionsKit also includes resources, helpful links, and a Spanish audio glossary.

Medical Assisting Interactive: Practice your procedures as a medical assistant in this simulated doctor's office. This can be accessed through MyHealthProfessionsKit.com.

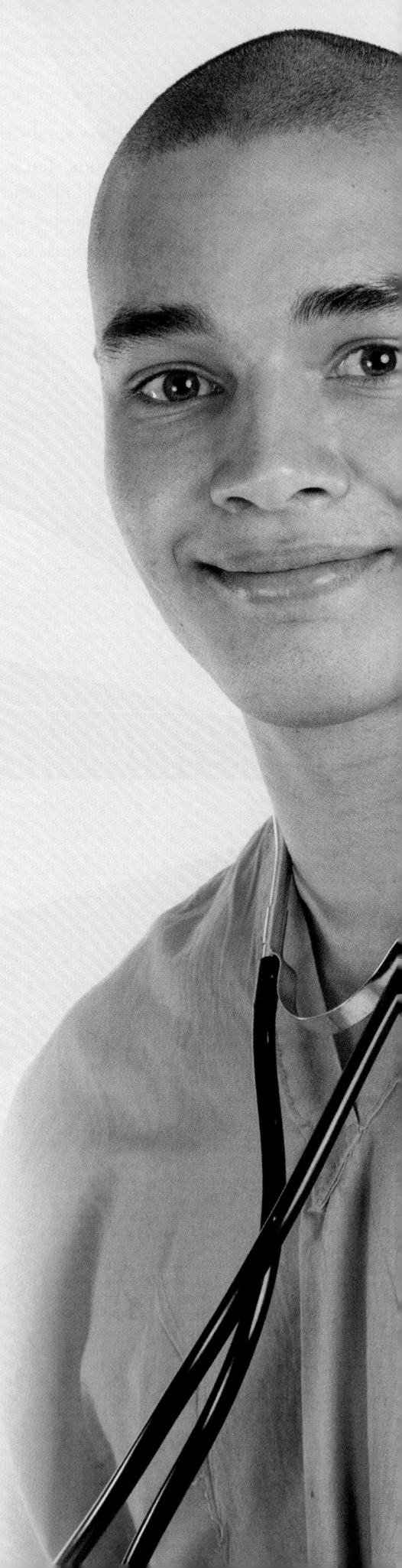

47

Hematology

LEARNING OBJECTIVES

After completing this chapter, you should be able to:

- Define and spell the terms to learn for this chapter.

- List the components of blood, including the liquid and cellular portions and functions of each.

- Describe how to prepare a patient for collection of a blood specimen via venipuncture and capillary puncture methods.

- Discuss how to process a blood specimen for routine testing in a physician's office.

- State the normal values for each of the blood tests discussed.

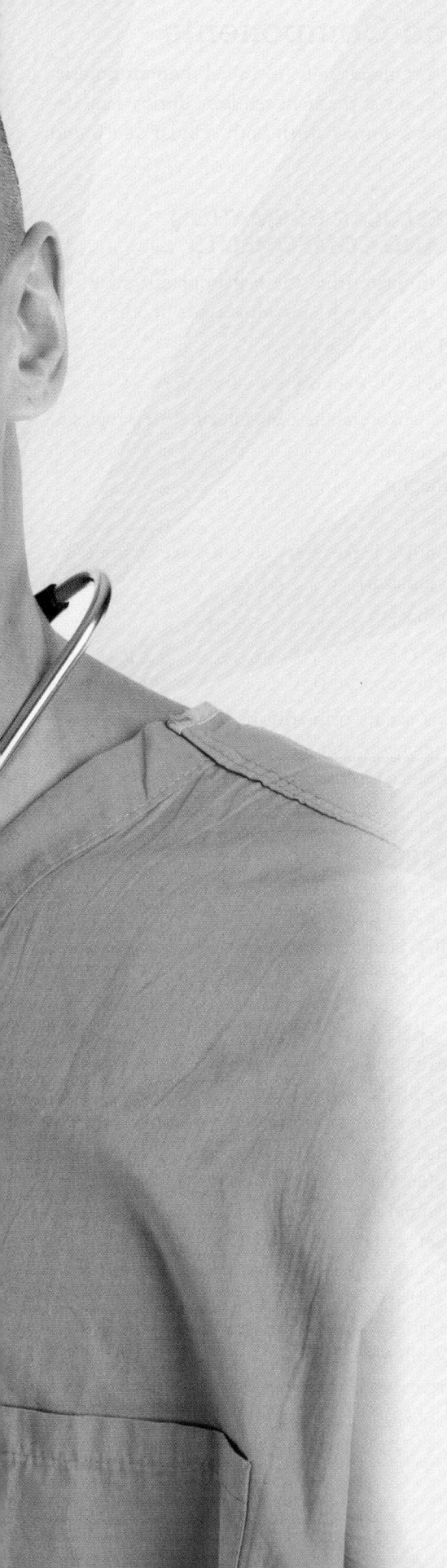

CHAPTER OUTLINE

CASE STUDY

Samra Belkovich, RMA, is working with Dr. Salpega. Dr. Salpega would like Samra to draw blood from Marlene St. Clair in exam room 2. Dr. Salpega has ordered a CBC and a serum chemistry test. He has informed Samra that Ms. St. Clair is a little anxious about having her blood drawn.

CERTIFICATION LINK

CMA (AAMA)	RMA	CMAS (AMT)
Principles of infection control	Clinical medical assisting	Not applicable
Collecting and processing specimens; diagnostic testing	Asepsis	
	Laboratory procedures	
Methods of collection		
Processing specimens		
Performing selected tests		

Hematology is the study of blood and the tissues that produce it. Blood and its components are studied to detect pathological conditions and to determine the appropriate course of treatment. Blood analysis is one of the most common diagnostic tests performed in the doctor's office. As a result, the medical assistant must have a thorough understanding of how to collect, handle, package, and analyze a blood specimen correctly.

The Medical Assistant's Role

When the physician orders a blood test, the role of the medical assistant is to collect the specimen. The actual testing of the blood is not commonly done in the medical office but, rather, is done in an outside laboratory that is contracted with the patient's medical insurance. When a patient's blood is drawn, the medical assistant must ensure that proper specimen labeling has occurred and that the blood is stored correctly until the laboratory courier has arrived for pickup.

Blood Formation and Components

The formation of blood cells is called **hematopoiesis**. Hematopoiesis begins at the stem cell level during fetal development. Blood is formed with both cellular and liquid components.

CELLULAR FORMATION AND COMPONENTS

All blood cells originate from the hematopoietic stem cell but mature into one of seven individual types of cells:

1. Red blood cells (erythrocytes)
2. White blood cells (leukocytes)—five types
   a. Granular leukocytes (have granules in their cytoplasm)
      - Neutrophil
      - Eosinophil
      - Basophil
   b. Nongranular leukocytes (do not have granules in their cytoplasm)
      - Lymphocyte
      - Monocyte
3. Platelets (thrombocytes)

Hematopoiesis occurs primarily in the bone marrow of the adult. Lymphocytes, one of the types of white blood cells, are also produced in the lymph nodes.

Red Blood Cells

Red blood cells (RBCs) are formed in the bone marrow. They are important for the human body because they contain **hemoglobin**, the metalloprotein that aids in oxygen transportation in RBCs. Hemoglobin has two functions. The first is to carry oxygen from the lungs to the cells of the body. The second function is to carry carbon dioxide (a waste product) from throughout the body back to the lungs, where it can be expelled with exhalation. When the hemoglobin is carrying oxygen, it is called **oxyhemoglobin**. When it is carrying carbon dioxide, it is called **carboxyhemoglobin**. Arterial blood has a higher concentration of oxygen, which explains its bright red color. Venous blood is darker in color because of the carboxyhemoglobin.

The formation of RBCs is controlled somewhat by **erythropoietin**, a glycoprotein hormone that controls RBC production and that is secreted by the kidneys in an adult and by the liver in a fetus. When the amount of erythropoietin is decreased, RBCs will not be formed in proper amounts, which may result in certain types of **anemia**, a deficiency of hemoglobin due to a lack of RBCs. For instance, patients who are being treated with chemotherapy may develop anemia that then can be treated with Procrit, an artificial erythropoietin that assists in the reproduction of RBCs. RBCs last for about 4 months and are continuously being reproduced in the body. The normal RBC range for a male adult is 4.5 to 6 million/mm^3. The normal female RBC range is 4 to 5.5 million/mm^3.

White Blood Cells

White blood cells (WBCs), also known as leukocytes, are produced in the bone marrow and are divided into several different types. They originate in the bone marrow from stem cells. WBCs are larger than RBCs, and their principal function is to defend against infection. The five types of WBCs are neutrophils, lymphocytes, monocytes, eosinophils, and basophils. The range of WBCs in an adult is 4.5 to 11 thousand/mm^3.

Neutrophils.   Neutrophils are divided into two categories: segmented neutrophils and nonsegmented neutrophils. Segmented neutrophils have a nucleus that is divided into multiple segments connected by small thin threads. Nonsegmented neutrophils are also called stabs (or bands) and are more immature than segmented neutrophils. The presence of a large number of stabs may indicate the existence of a bacterial infection. Neutrophils are so named because the granules are neutral in color on laboratory-stained slides. The body reproduces neutrophils on an ongoing basis, and they survive only for a few days. Reproduction is increased when bacterial infection is occurring. Neutrophils combat infection by phagocytosis. Phagocytosis is the process in which the neutrophil surrounds, swallows, and digests the bacteria.

Eosinophils.   Eosinophils are assumed also to be produced by the bone marrow. Detection of a large number of eosinophils can indicate a parasitic condition or the presence of certain allergic conditions. Eosinophils have granules that produce a red color on laboratory-stained slides. Eosinophils are so named due to the stain eosin, which is used in the staining of blood smears.

Basophils.   Like other white cells, **basophils** are thought to be produced by the bone marrow, and they produce heparin. **Heparin** is a substance that prevents clotting. When an individual has a condition that is creating inflammation, heparin may be used to assist in diminishing or preventing the occurrence of clotting. Increased amounts of basophils may be found in patients who have had their spleen removed. Patients who have had excessive exposure to radiation also may have increased basophils.

Basophils also contain the vasodilator histamine, and basophils appear in tissues where an allergic reaction is occurring. It is thought that the concentration of basophils may contribute to the severity of allergic reactions.

Lymphocytes.   **Lymphocytes** are produced in the bone marrow and in the lymphoid tissue, such as the spleen and lymph nodes. The function of lymphocytes is primarily to produce antibodies against foreign substances such as bacteria, viruses, and pollens. Lymphocytes are small and large and can proliferate into B and T cells. B cells may convert into plasma cells, which produce antibodies. T cells can produce helper cells, cytotoxic cells, and suppressor cells. To diagnose an individual with HIV, testing is performed to evaluate the type and amount of T cells present. Lymphocytes do not have granules and are nonsegmented.

Monocytes.   **Monocytes** are formed in the bone marrow from stem cells. Monocytes assist in phagocytosis. They ingest foreign particles or bacteria that the neutrophils are unable to digest, and they assist in cleaning up cellular debris that may have been left from the infection. An increase in monocytes is seen in patients who have certain diseases, such as tuberculosis, typhoid, and Rocky Mountain spotted fever.

Platelets

Platelets (also called thrombocytes) are the smallest cells found in the blood and are formed in the bone marrow. The main function of platelets is to assist in the clotting of blood. Platelets increase around an area that is bleeding to assist in the formation of clots. The platelets and the injured tissue release thromboplastin. The thromboplastin combines with other elements in the blood to produce thrombin. The thrombin acts on a protein in the blood called fibrinogen, resulting in the formation of fibrin. Fibrin is tiny threads that create a mesh that catches the RBCs and other cells

PROFESSIONALISM
THE LIFE SPAN

Drawing blood from an older individual can sometimes be challenging due to the condition of their veins. Patients do not want to have any more needlesticks than necessary. To ensure that a successful needlestick occurs requires both experience and patience. If patients will be returning to the office for blood work at a later time, inform the patient to drink a lot of fluids prior to arrival at the office. Being well hydrated is helpful for finding veins. Use of items such as a small ball placed in the patient's hand to squeeze in order to pump up the veins is also helpful. If the hand must be used for the draw site, place a warm cloth over the area to allow for the vein to rise up. All of these techniques can help in making the first try a success.

to form a clot. There are typically between 150,000 and 400,000 platelets/mm^3.

Understanding the process of normal clotting and absence of normal clotting is important because laboratory tests are designed to determine why clotting is not occurring properly, particularly in patients who are receiving anticlotting drugs, such as heparin and Coumadin.

LIQUID BLOOD FORMATION AND COMPONENTS

For the medical assistant to understand how blood is formed requires a thorough comprehension of the cellular and liquid components of blood. The liquid component of blood is called plasma. Plasma is about 55 percent of the composition of blood and carries cellular elements and other substances. Plasma transports substances in the blood to the different parts of the body. Plasma does contain fibrinogen; which converts to fibrin during the clotting process. Plasma without the fibrinogen is called **serum**.

Ninety percent of plasma is water, whereas the other 10 percent is solid substances, called solutes. These solutes may include the plasma proteins (albumin, globulin, fibrinogen, and prothrombin); **electrolytes** also called ionic solutions because they contain free ions (sodium, potassium, and chloride); glucose; amino acids; lipids and carbohydrates; metabolic waste products (urea, lactic acid, uric acid); creatinine; respiratory gases (oxygen and carbon dioxide); and miscellaneous substances (hormones, antibodies, enzymes, vitamins, and mineral salts).

The Function of Blood

The functions of blood are transportation and protection. Blood carries oxygen and nutrients to the body and removes the waste product carbon dioxide. The blood carries the waste products to the liver, kidneys, and skin for elimination.

The heart pumps blood through the body by way of the arteries, veins, and **capillaries**. The capillaries, the smallest of the body's vessels, connect—by way of the arterioles and venules—the arteries and veins that pump the blood to and from the heart. When blood flows away from the heart it flows in arteries, and when it returns back to the heart it flows through veins. Arteries have thick walls that allow them to withstand the pressure sustained when the heart is pumping. The blood carried in the arteries contains oxygen. This blood with its high level of oxygen sustains tissue function. As oxygen is being released from the blood, carbon dioxide is being transported to the lungs to be expelled as a waste product.

The blood regulates body temperature. When the body becomes warm, the capillaries dilate and release heat, which

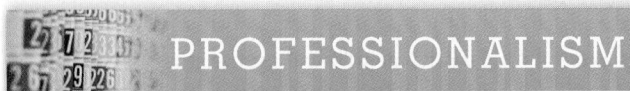

in turn cools the body. When the body is cold, the capillaries constrict, allowing for less blood flow, which increases the body temperature.

Blood Specimen Collection

Laboratory testing of blood and the collection of all blood and body fluids is strictly regulated by OSHA regulations, and the CDC's standard precautions must be followed at all times. CLIA (Clinical Laboratory Improvement Amendments) sets the standards that all laboratories must adhere to, including training of personnel and testing and transport of specimens (see Chapter 44). When performing specimen collection, the medical assistant must follow the regulation guidelines established by these organizations (Procedure 47-1).

The type and amount of specimen to be acquired are dictated by the test to be done. If a very small amount is needed, then the specimen may be obtained by capillary puncture. Larger volumes are collected through venipuncture.

VENIPUNCTURE

Three methods of venipuncture are used: the vacuum tube method, the syringe and needle method, and the butterfly method.

Methods

The most common method of venipuncture is the vacuum container method because multiple samples can be obtained at the same time, requiring fewer sticks for the patient and faster collection for the medical assistant. In using the vacuum container method, it is important to use a large vein because the vacuum can collapse smaller veins. If the patient has no accessible larger veins, then it is appropriate to use a small needle with a syringe to obtain the specimen. See Figures 47-1 and 47-2 and Procedure 47-2 on how to obtain venous blood with a sterile syringe and needle.

QUALITY CONTROL FOR COLLECTING A BLOOD SPECIMEN

Objective: Perform quality control procedure while collecting a blood specimen.

EQUIPMENT AND SUPPLIES

antiseptic cleaner; biohazard waste container; necessary sterile equipment; specimen collection container; disposable alcohol wipe; disposable gloves; appropriate requisition or paperwork required of collection; pen or pencil; patient's chart

METHOD

1. Review request and verify test ordered.
2. Prepare necessary equipment and work area.
3. Perform hand hygiene and apply gloves.
4. Identify the patient and explain the procedure, and make sure he or she understands the procedure.
5. Confirm that the patient has followed any pretest preparation requirements.
6. Collect the specimen properly, using the appropriate equipment and technique.
7. Use the appropriate collection container and the right preservatives.
8. Immediately label the specimen with the patient's name; date and time of collection; test's name; and the name of the person collecting the specimen.
9. Follow correct procedures for disposing of hazardous specimen waste and decontaminating the work area and equipment according to OSHA guidelines.
10. Remove gloves and dispose in appropriate container. Perform hand hygiene. Dispose of all used needles and other equipment in a biohazard waste container.
11. Thank the patient and observe for any signs or symptoms of inappropriate response to the procedure.
12. Document the procedure in the patient's chart.
13. If the specimen is to be transported to an outside laboratory, prepare it for transport in the proper container, with all the appropriate information according to OSHA guidelines.

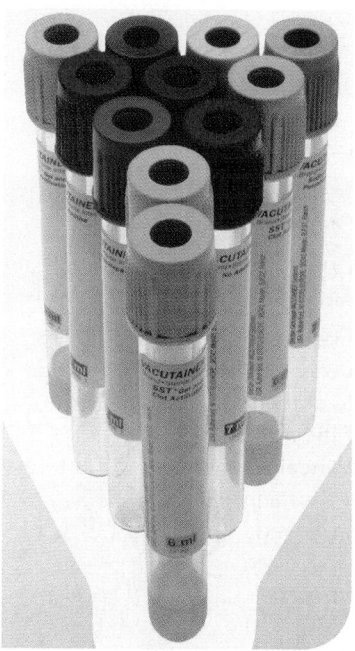

FIGURE 47-1 Vacutainer evacuated specimen tubes with Hemogard closure blood collection tubes. *Courtesy of © Becton Dickinson Company.*

The butterfly method uses a needle that is attached to 6- to 12-inch tubing. The end of the tubing can attach to the syringe or the vacuum container tube holder. The butterfly method is used for small veins that are difficult to draw from with the standard vacuum container method or syringe and needle method. It is called the butterfly method

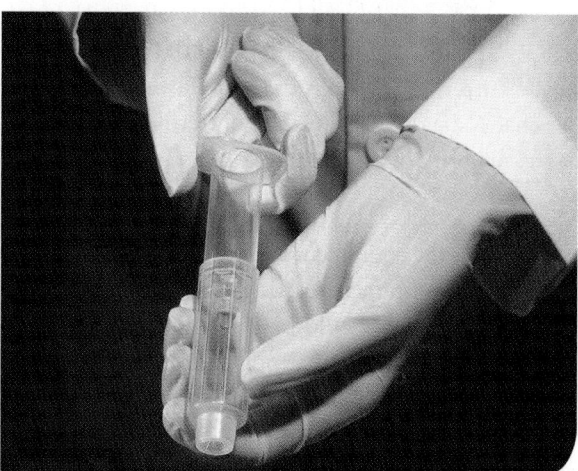

FIGURE 47-2 Vacutainer brand safety lock needle holder.

procedure
47-2

OBTAINING VENOUS BLOOD WITH A STERILE SYRINGE AND NEEDLE

Objective: Perform a venipuncture using the syringe and needle method.

EQUIPMENT AND SUPPLIES

sterile 22-gauge needle and 10- to 20-mL syringe; appropriate vacuum specimen tubes for tests ordered; tourniquet; gloves; alcohol sponge; cotton balls or dry gauze square; adhesive bandage; patient's record; pen; lab coat; biohazard sharps container

Note: Always identify the patient by asking his or her name.

METHOD

1. Perform hand hygiene and assemble necessary equipment and supplies.
2. Apply gloves.
3. Securely attach the sterile needle to the syringe.
4. Apply a tourniquet 3 to 4 inches above the antecubital space.
5. Palpate the vein and clean the venipuncture site with an alcohol sponge, then dry with clean gauze.
6. Have the patient make a fist and hold it shut until told to release it.
7. Make sure there is no air in the syringe and the plunger movies freely.
8. Remove the needle guard and insert the needle into the vein.
9. Slowly pull back the syringe plunger until the proper amount of blood has been obtained.
10. Instruct the patient to open his or her fist.
11. Release the tourniquet and withdraw the needle quickly. Place a piece of cotton or gauze on the puncture site and instruct the patient to hold pressure on the site and raise the arm. This may prevent hematomas from occurring.
12. Fill the appropriate vacuum tubes to the proper level.
13. Discard the used needle and syringe into a biohazard sharps container.
14. Remove the cotton ball to inspect the injection site. Apply a bandage to the puncture site.
15. Remove and discard gloves in the appropriate container.
16. Perform hand hygiene.
17. Record the procedure in the patient's record.
18. Label the tubes and send to the laboratory.

because the needle on the end has a winged portion that keeps the needle from turning and anchors the needle into the small vein. The needle used for the butterfly method is a small 21-, 23-, or 25-gauge needle. The drawback to performing the butterfly method is the cost. The needle is more expensive than a standard needle. The butterfly method is not used for the majority of blood draws due to its expense.

Equipment

Figure 47-3 shows the equipment that a medical assistant will need to perform a venipuncture using the vacuum container method. All equipment should be assembled and the expiration dates checked prior to attempting use. Expired tubes should not be used because they may not have a vacuum. The various types of tubes are distinguished by their color. Each tube has a different chemical additive (anticoagulant) to keep the blood from clotting for different types of tests.

PROFESSIONALISM
THE WORKPLACE

Working in a medical clinic requires efficient skill performance so that the flow of the office is not disrupted. After cleaning the draw site of the patient, it may be difficult to tell if the alcohol has had enough time to dry. A visual reminder that can assist the medical assistant is wiping the back of their gloved hand with the alcohol wipe after they have cleaned the draw site. The alcohol will appear shiny on the glove, and when the alcohol dissipates from the glove surface, the patient's draw site will also be dry.

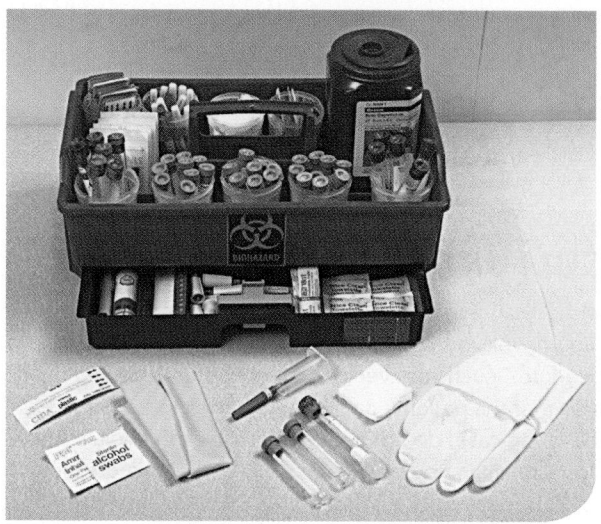

FIGURE 47-3 Venipuncture equipment.

When drawing blood by the vacuum tube method, it is important to fill the tubes in the order of draw recommended by the Clinical Laboratory Standards Institute (CLSI, formerly the NCCLS) in order to prevent contamination of the tubes with skin bacteria or with an additive from another blood tube. The correct order of draw, along with a description of additives and the common laboratory tests run on each individual specimen are listed in Table 47-1.

Some laboratories may use additional tubes. Pink-, tan-, black-, and royal blue–topped tubes are sometimes used for specific laboratory tests. Vacuum blood tubes come in 5-, 7-, 10-, and 15-mL sizes. The amount of blood needed for each test differs, so the tube sizes differ accordingly.

The medical assistant must fill each blood tube completely. Partially filled tubes, especially the light blue tube, can cause erroneous test results, resulting in the patient's blood needing to be redrawn. For each tube being filled, the medical assistant should gently invert the tube 6 to 8 times

TABLE 47-1 Order of Blood Draw

Order of Draw	Vacutainer Color	Additive and Function	Laboratory Use
1.	Yellow	Sodium polyanetholsulfonate (SPS) prevents clotting and stabilizes bacterial growth.	Cultures on blood or body fluid
2.	Light blue	Sodium citrate removes calcium to prevent clotting.	Coagulation tests such as PT/INR and PTT
3.	Red	None	Serum testing, serology, blood bank, blood chemistry
4.	Red marbled	Silica is present to enhance clotting.	Serum testing
5.	Green	Standard heparin (sodium/lithium/ammonium) prevents thrombin formation.	Blood chemistry such as whole blood tests and plasma testing
6.	Light green	Lithium heparin and gel aid in plasma separation.	Plasma determination in chemistry tests
7.	Lavender	Ethylenediaminetetraacetic acid (EDTA) removes calcium to prevent clotting.	Hematology such as CBC or glycosylated hemoglobin
8.	Pink, white, or royal blue	Sodium heparin (may also be referred to as sodium EDTA) prevents thrombin formation and prevents clotting.	Chemistry for trace elements
9.	Gray	Potassium oxalate and sodium fluoride to inhibit glycolysis (the chemical reaction of converting glucose into pyruvate) and removes calcium to prevent clotting.	Glucose tolerance tests and alcohol levels, chemistry tests
10.	Dark blue	Tube contains fibrin degradation product (FDP).	Detects if the patient has had a recent breakdown of clots, which may indicate several conditions such as blood clots in the legs (DVT), hepatic vein obstruction, pulmonary embolus, or stroke

Source: Clinical Laboratory and Standards Institute, January 2004. Retrieved from www.clsi.org. Adapted with permission.

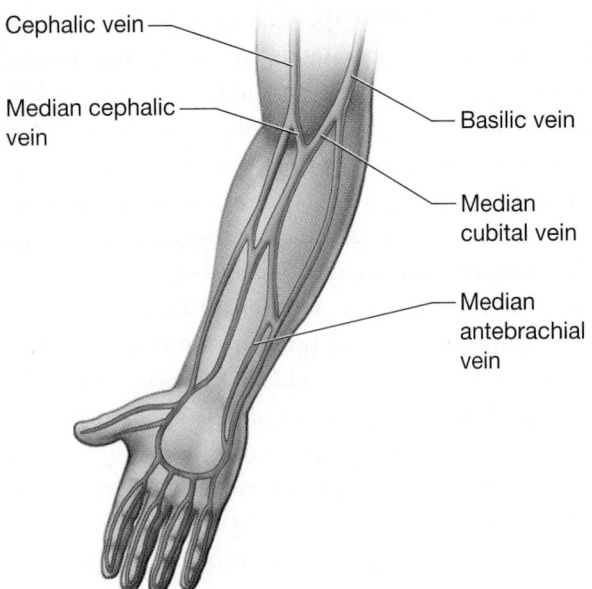

FIGURE 47-4 Anatomy of an arm for venipuncture.

Cephalic vein

Median cephalic vein

Basilic vein

Median cubital vein

Median antebrachial vein

so the anticoagulant and blood have mixed properly. Care should be taken not to shake the tubes, since that action could cause the blood to become hemolyzed. (The process of hemolysis is the releasing of the hemoglobin into the plasma of the cells.)

Sites

The **antecubital space**, the depression in the front of the elbow, is the most commonly used site for venipuncture. This is the space just below the elbow joint. This space has four large veins that are easy to access, making this the site of choice. The most common vein used is the median cephalic vein (Figure 47-4). Depending on the patient's condition, the medical assistant may need to obtain blood using a different site, such as the back of the hand or heel of the foot.

Patient Preparation

The blood tests done in a physician's office typically require little preparation. For some tests, such as a glucose tolerance, cholesterol, or lipids level test, the patient should fast for 12 to 14 hours prior to the test. Few other tests require fasting. If fasting is required, it is important to educate the patient on how many hours to fast prior to the blood draw. If the medical assistant has any question about requirements, such as fasting in preparation for the blood draw, a good resource is the laboratory to which the specimen is being sent. Testing labs typically have a lab assistant available to address these questions.

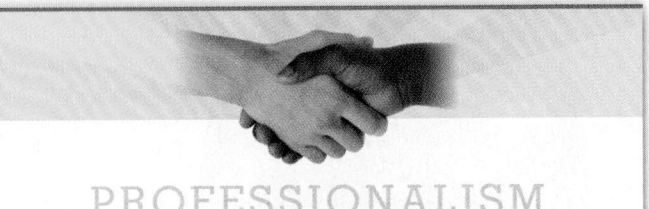

PROFESSIONALISM
CULTURAL CONSIDERATIONS

The medical assistant can help lower a patient's fear and anxiety levels by properly and thoroughly explaining a procedure, such as venipuncture, before beginning. Sometimes the patient's native tongue may not be English. If this is the case, do not assume that you can explain the procedure clearly by speaking slowly and showing examples. You may choose to locate a coworker who speaks the patient's native language or ask a family member who may be present to help translate. It is important to remember that you must request permission from the patient to have his or her family member assist in the explanation and translation, as the patient's confidential medical information may be disclosed. In areas where there are large non–English speaking populations, a medical office may have explanations for various procedures printed in languages common to the area. These can prove to be extremely useful.

At the time of the blood draw, some patients may be anxious. It is important for the medical assistant to communicate clearly what the process involves in order to assist in alleviating the patient's fears. If the patient is a child, the participation of the parent or caregiver may be helpful in calming the patient.

Being prepared at the time of the blood draw can also help in diminishing patient anxieties. A patient is encouraged when sensing that the medical assistant is competent and knowledgeable in performing the blood draw. Competency can be demonstrated by having the appropriate equipment assembled prior to the blood draw and ensuring that the correct blood specimens are drawn correctly. Patients who experience callbacks due to errors such as incorrect specimen handling will lose confidence in the medical assistant and the physician's office.

Unexpected events can happen when performing venipunctures. These include fainting, nausea, excessive anger exhibited by a patient, and uncontrollable bleeding. It is important that the medical assistant remain calm and deal with these situations professionally. When a patient begins to show signs of fainting, it is important to immediately withdraw the needle and request that the patient lower his or her head and arms. The patient may need to lie down to further ensure his or her safety while recovering. Often in treatment rooms, ammonia is available and can be used to help revive a patient. If a patient does not immediately respond, it is important to call another member of the clinical team for assistance.

When a patient becomes nauseous, have him or her breathe deeply through the mouth and provide an emesis basin if necessary. If a patient becomes angry during the procedure, it is important to remain calm and reassuring. If the behavior continues or is disruptive and endangers either the medical assistant or the patient, the procedure should be stopped immediately and the medical assistant should call for assistance in dealing with the situation.

Occasionally, uncontrollable bleeding can occur when the needle is withdrawn. If this occurs it is important to apply pressure to the site. Once pressure has been applied, it is important to call for assistance.

Other complications can make it difficult to perform the procedure or obtain the necessary amount of blood. For example, if a patient has small veins, it is sometimes helpful to apply a hot compress to the area. By doing so, the veins may expand and become easier to access. When veins have a tendency to roll, it is important to place one finger below the area where the needle is to be inserted in order to prevent the vein from moving. An incomplete draw may occur if a patient's vein does not produce enough blood. If this occurs, it will be necessary to obtain blood from a different vein. Some patients present a challenge to the inexperienced phlebotomist. Requesting that a more experienced professional perform the procedure may be necessary.

When drawing blood the medical assistant should wear personal protective equipment such as gloves and a gown or lab coat. Although these items are worn to protect the medical assistant from coming in contact with contaminated items, this attire can also promote a professional image that patients desire in their medical assistant.

See Figure 47-5 for an illustration of the use of venipuncture equipment. To perform a venipuncture utilizing the Vacutainer method, see the procedures as outlined in Procedure 47-3.

CAPILLARY PUNCTURE (MANUAL)

As noted, capillaries are the microscopic blood vessels that connect arterioles and venules. Oxygen and carbon dioxide

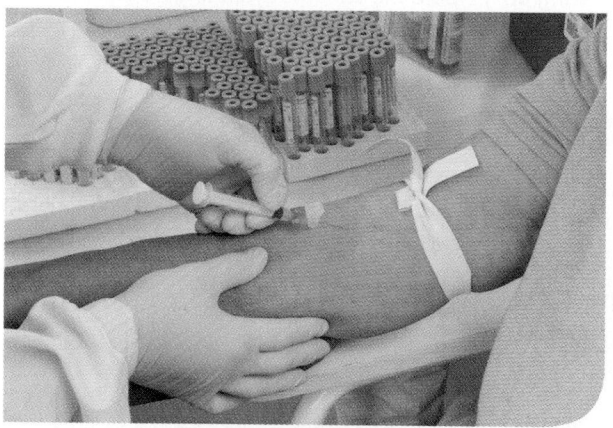
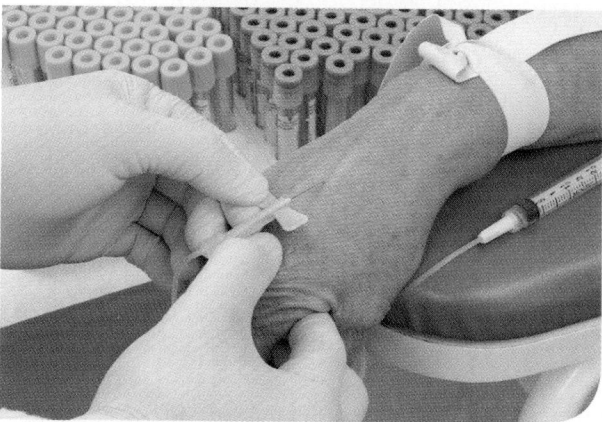
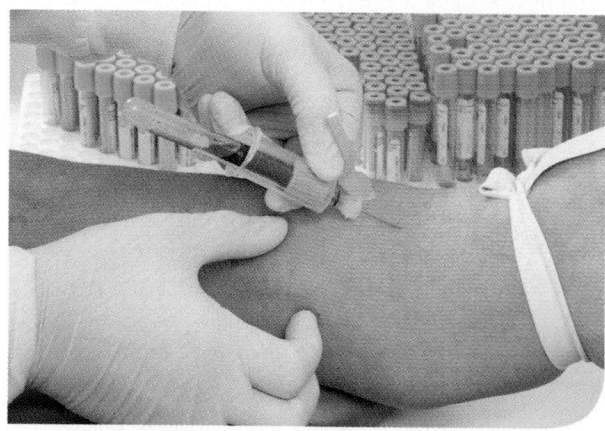
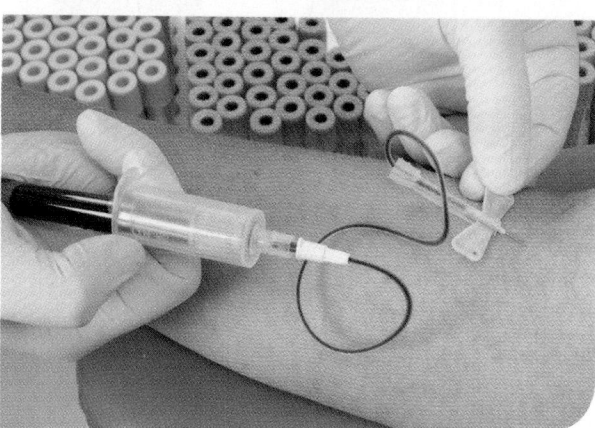

FIGURE 47-5 Demonstrating the use of venipuncture equipment.

PERFORMING VENIPUNCTURE USING THE VACUTAINER METHOD

Objective: Perform venipuncture by correctly assembling, locating, and entering vein and withdrawing blood sample.

EQUIPMENT AND SUPPLIES

biohazard sharps container; Vacutainer tubes; multisample needle; two or three 2-inch gauze squares; alcohol pads; examination gloves; Vacutainer sleeve; tourniquet; bandage; cotton balls; adhesive; ink pen; lab coat; patient record; ammonia ampules

Note: Follow standard precautions and safety guidelines when working with blood samples. Use care to avoid splashing or spilling blood. Wipe up all spills using guidelines established by OSHA.

METHOD

1. Perform hand hygiene.
2. Assemble equipment (Figure 47-6A).
3. Identify the patient and explain the procedure. Have the patient either sit or lie down.
4. Apply gloves.
5. Screw the Vacutainer needle into the plastic sleeve (Figure 47-6B). Insert the tube into the other end of the sleeve. The top of the colored stopper should reach the thin guide line on the sleeve. Do not press tube. If the tube exceeds the line, discard the tube; it may not have a vacuum.
6. Apply the tourniquet about 2 inches above the antecubital space (Figure 47-6C). Place the middle of the tourniquet on the posterior (elbow) side of the arm. Crisscross the ends. While holding one end stable, tuck in the other end. This creates a tie that can be quickly released with one hand. In addition, the tourniquet should apply enough tension to engorge the vein with blood.
7. The arm should be in an extended position with the palm facing up. Palpate the vein with your fingertips (Figure 47-6D). If a vein cannot be felt in one arm, try the other.

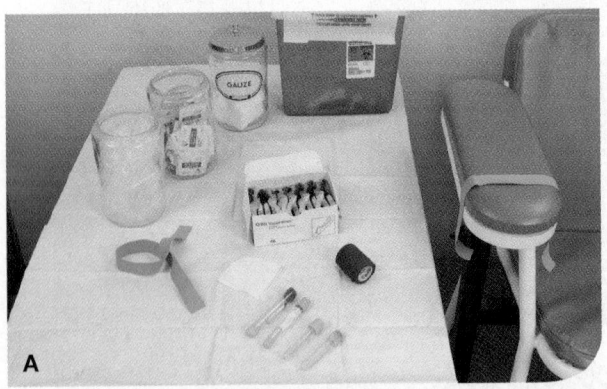

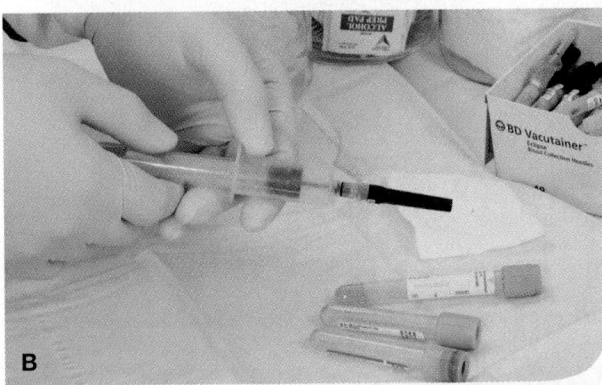

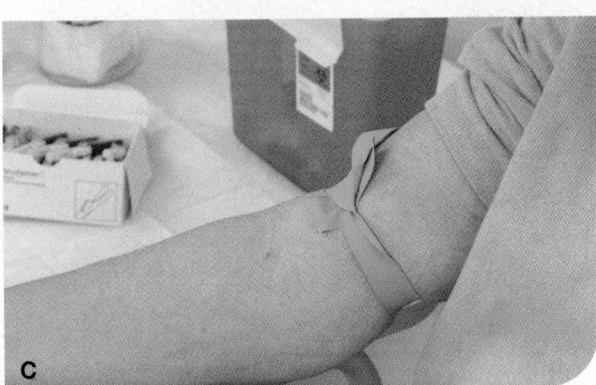

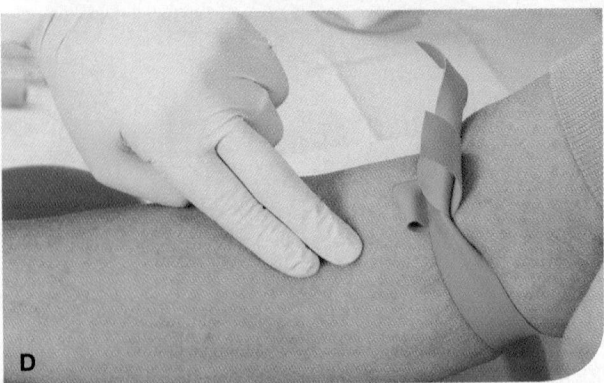

FIGURE 47-6 (A–D) Venipuncture procedure.

8. Wipe the site with an alcohol pad in a circular pattern beginning at the insertion site (Figure 47-6E). Let the alcohol evaporate. Cleanse your gloved finger with alcohol in case you need to repalpate after the site is cleansed.

9. Anchor the vein by placing the thumb of the nondominant hand 2 inches below the insertion site and pulling the skin toward the hand.

10. While holding onto the tube's sleeve with your dominant hand, insert needle smoothly and rapidly at a 15- to 20-degree angle with the bevel up (Figure 47-6F). The needle only needs to be inserted just past the bevel. If inserted too far, it will puncture both vein walls. Also keep the needle in line with the vein. The dominant hand is now considered "fixed," meaning you may not remove it from the tube sleeve until the procedure is over. All other movements must be done with the nondominant hand.

11. While the dominant hand is stabilizing the sleeve, use the nondominant hand to push the tube into the sleeve (Figure 47-6G). Use your thumb to push the tube and hold the sleeve with the index and middle fingers on the flange (Figure 47-6H).

12. Allow the tube to fill. The vacuum will automatically fill the tube to the manufacturer's recommended level for the specific tube used. You should familiarize yourself with the adequate fill level of the individual tubes. Blood collection tubes may contain a weak vacuum due to processing errors, and you will need to redraw those specimens.

13. Remove the tube very carefully without moving the needle and apply a second tube if needed (Figure 47-6I). Gently roll the tube five to six times after removing it from the sleeve to allow the blood to mix with the additive.

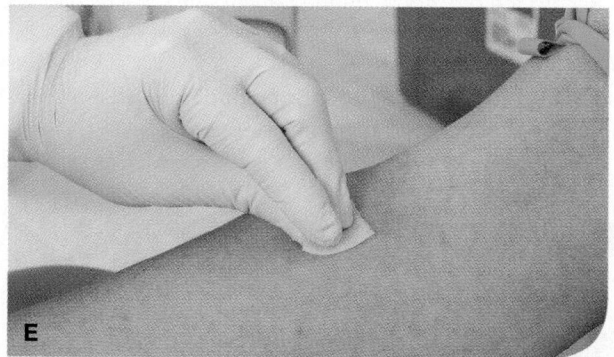

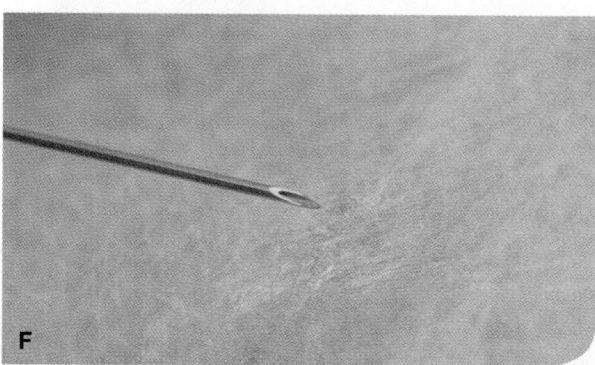

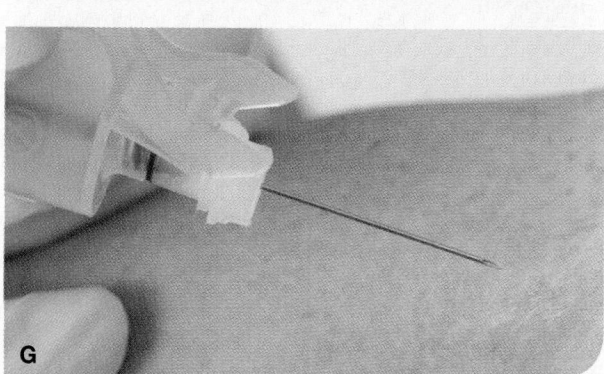

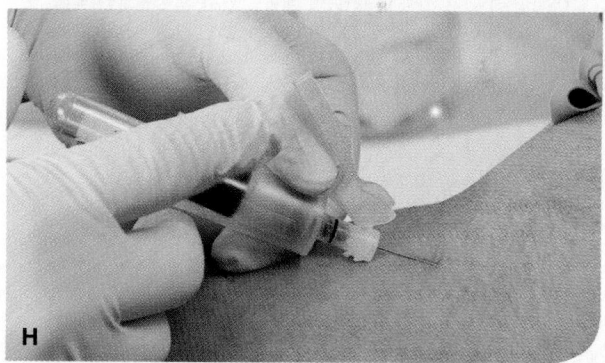

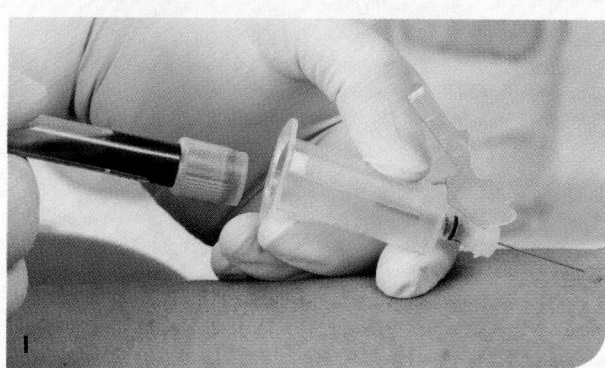

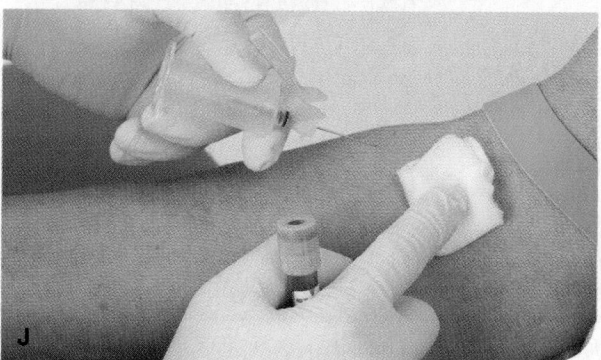

FIGURE 47-6 (E–J) (Continued)

If both a red and purple tube are needed, collect blood in the red tube that contains no additive first.

14. Release the tourniquet once the last tube has been inserted into the adaptor. Fill the last tube, remove it, swiftly remove the needle, and cover the site with a clean gauze pad (Figure 47-6J). Be careful not to push onto the needle when covering the puncture site, since that may cause the needle to scratch the patient's arm. Gently invert the collection tube.

15. Immediately have the patient apply firm, continuous pressure using a cotton ball or gauze square.

16. Properly dispose of needle in biohazard container (Figure 47-6K, 47-6L, and 47-6M).

17. Gently invert all tubes collected eight to ten times in a figure-eight pattern.

18. Assess the patient. Check the venipuncture site for bleeding, then apply some cotton and a strip of adhesive or a bandage (Figure 47-6N). Ask if the patient is dizzy or lightheaded.

19. Label the tubes with the patient's name, date, time, ID number, specimen type, tests to be done, and the phlebotomist's initials. Fill out the laboratory requisition sheet (Figure 47-6O).

20. Remove gloves. Perform hand hygiene.

21. Record the procedure on the patient's medical record.

CHARTING EXAMPLE

2/28/XX 1.00 P.M. Withdrew 10 mL of blood from left arm, no complications. Sent blood to in-office lab for CBC.· · · · · · · · · ·
· M. Garcia, RMA

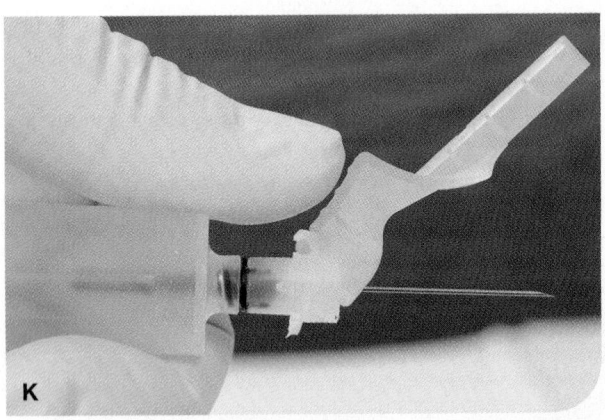

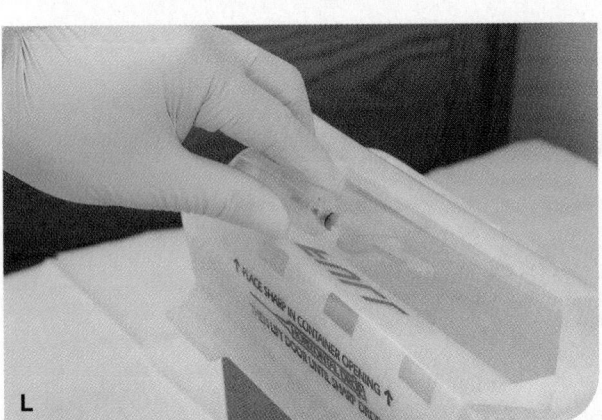

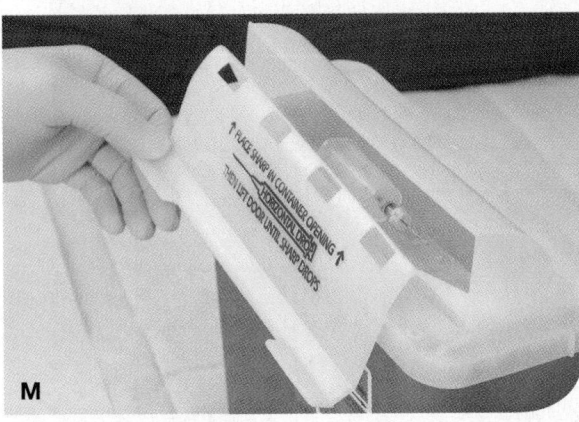

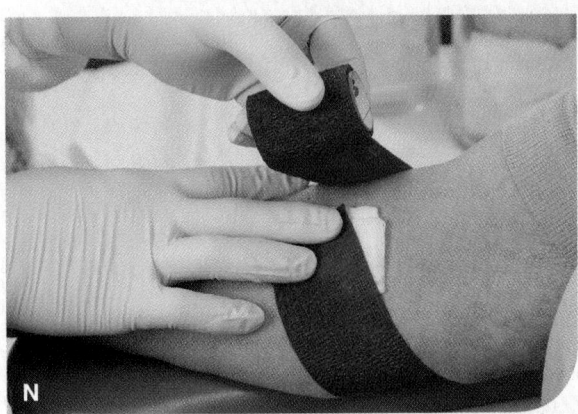

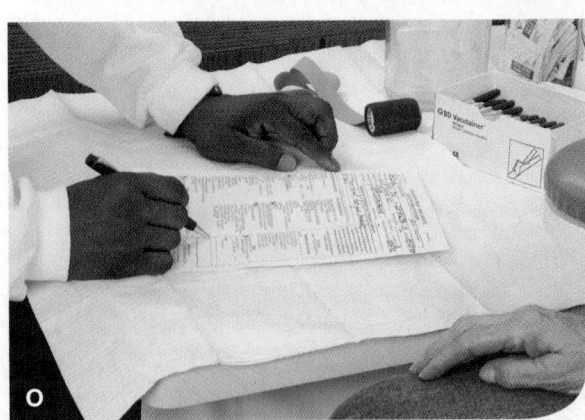

FIGURE 47-6 (K–O) (Continued)

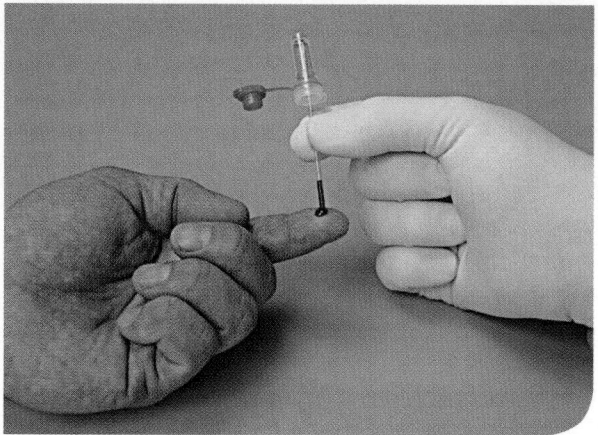

FIGURE 47-7 A finger-stick is useful for obtaining small amounts of blood.

are exchanged at the capillary level. Small amounts of blood can easily be obtained from the capillaries in a capillary puncture or finger-stick (Figure 47-7).

Puncture Sites

Figure 47-8 shows the common capillary puncture sites for adults and infants. When performing capillary punctures, the medical assistant should take precautions to avoid using the thumb because it is often callused. The index finger should also be avoided if possible because it has extra nerve endings that make it more sensitive. The fifth finger is also not a good capillary puncture site because it generally has less tissue. The tissue on the lateral sides of the fingers is less sensitive than that in the middle, but a larger specimen can be obtained from the fleshy area closer to, but not directly in, the middle of the fingers. The puncture should be a minimum of 2 mm away from the fingernail. The medical assistant should take precautions to avoid any area that is callused, burned, cyanotic, red, scarred, or showing signs of injury or infection. Earlobes are also a common puncture site for adults.

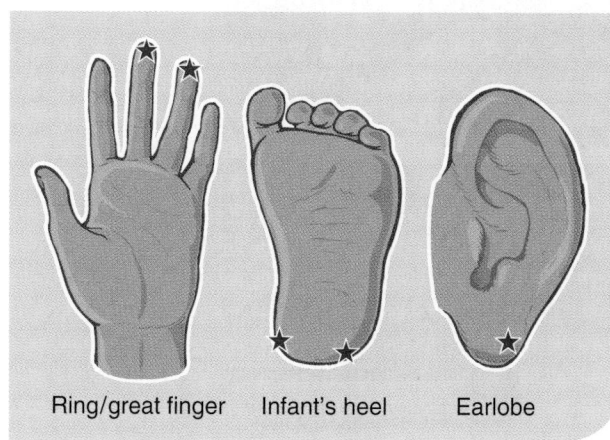

Ring/great finger   Infant's heel   Earlobe

FIGURE 47-8 Capillary puncture sites.

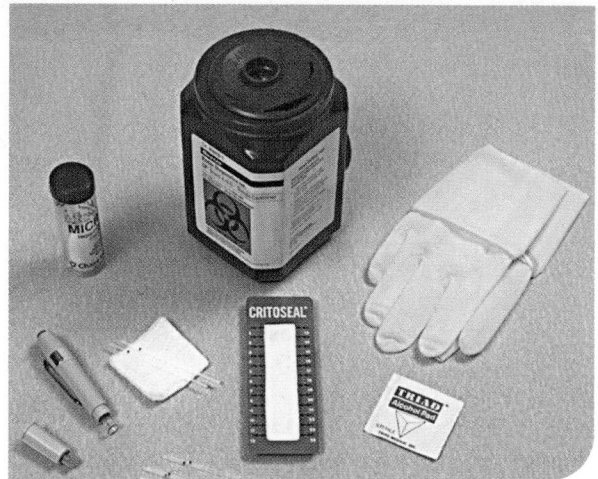

FIGURE 47-9 Capillary puncture equipment.

When doing a capillary puncture on infants, their fingers are not large enough to yield a sufficient sample, so a heel may be a better option. The puncture should occur on the medial and lateral surfaces of the heel. The infant patient can be held by their guardian or another medical assistant with the legs hanging to allow gravity to increase blood flow. The heel should be thoroughly cleaned and warmed prior to the procedure. A warm (never exceeding 42°C, 108°F), moist towel can be applied for 3 to 5 minutes to increase blood flow. The medical assistant should never place an adhesive bandage on patients younger than 2 years. The patient may peel them off and create a choking hazard.

Equipment and Supplies

Figure 47-9 shows the equipment needed for a capillary puncture. Lancets may be either manual or automatic (Figure 47-10). The primary advantage of the automatic lancet is that the depth of the puncture is controlled by a spring-loaded mechanism, causing less pain to the patient. After a lancet is used, it should immediately be placed in a sharps container to prevent needlesticks. Procedure 47-4 outlines the process for a manual capillary puncture.

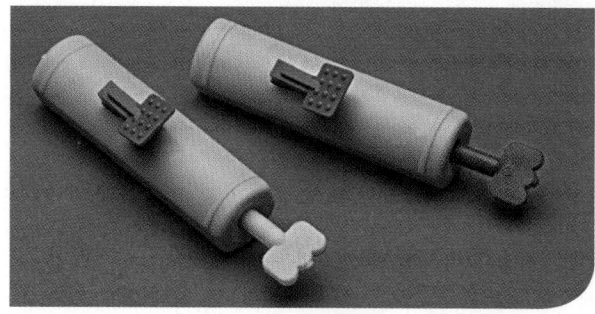

FIGURE 47-10 Spring-activated lancet.

PERFORMING A CAPILLARY PUNCTURE (MANUAL)

Objective: Perform a capillary stick using a lancet or spring-loaded lancet following correct aseptic technique and obtaining an adequate sample.

EQUIPMENT AND SUPPLIES

biohazard sharps container; gloves; alcohol sponge; 2 × 2 gauze square, or cotton balls; lancet or spring-loaded lancet; capillary tubes; sealing clay; ammonia ampules; bandage; lab coat.

Note: Lancets come in a variety of sizes and needle gauges for specific purposes. The majority of capillary punctures performed on adults, requiring only a few drops of blood, can be performed with needle gauges 21G, 25G, or 28G. Pediatrics and micro-collections will require specific lancets and blades.

Note: Follow standard precautions and safety guidelines. Use care to avoid splashing or spilling blood. Wipe up all spills using guidelines established by OSHA.

METHOD

1. Perform hand hygiene.
2. Assemble equipment.
3. Identify the patient and explain the procedure. Have the patient either sitting or lying down.
4. Apply gloves.
5. Select either the ring or great finger on the nondominant hand. Wipe the site with an alcohol sponge. Let alcohol evaporate.
6. Remove plastic protective tip to expose the lancet.
7. Grasp patient's hand and gently squeeze the finger 1 inch below the chosen puncture site.
8. Puncture the site using a quick, jabbing motion across the fingerprints to obtain a full round drop of blood (Figure 47-11A). Do not puncture the direct center of the finger pad since the skin is generally tougher there. Immediately discard the lancet in a sharps container. (A spring-loaded lancet may also be used.)
9. Wipe away the first drop of blood with a gauze square or cotton ball (Figure 47-11B).
10. Obtain the sample using a microhematocrit capillary tube (Figure 47-11C). The finger may be gently massaged to increase blood flow. Seal one end of the capillary tube in a clay sealer (Figure 47-11D).
11. Apply clean gauze over the site and ask patient to apply firm, continuous pressure until the bleeding stops.
12. Assess the patient and the site. Apply a bandage, if needed. Ask the patient if he or she is dizzy or lightheaded.
13. Remove gloves and perform hand hygiene.
14. Record the procedure on the patient's medical record.

CHARTING EXAMPLE

2/28/XX 1:30 P.M. Performed capillary puncture on left ring finger, no complications.· M. Garcia, RMA

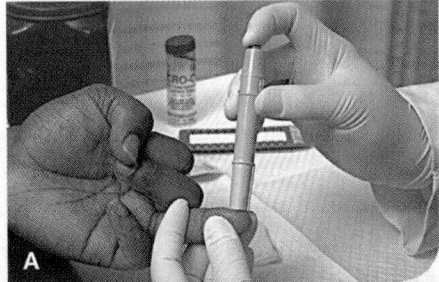
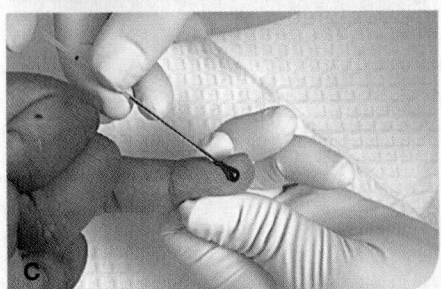
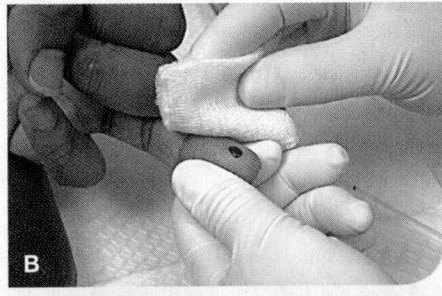
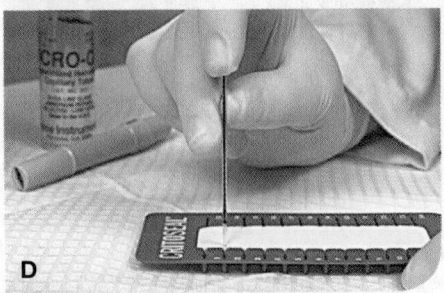

FIGURE 47-11 (A–D) Capillary puncture procedure.

Routine Blood Tests

Blood analysis is one vital and routine tool of medicine. The medical assistant performs routine blood tests and procedures in the physician's office. More complex tests are performed by specially trained individuals, either a medical lab technician (MLT) or medical technologist (MT).

Physicians frequently order a complete blood count (CBC). A CBC typically consists of a microhematocrit, hemoglobin, WBC count, RBC count, platelet count, and differential WBC count (diff).

The medical assistant may be asked to perform a coagulation test. This test is done to determine how well a patient's blood is clotting. It is done on a routine basis with patients who are on blood-thinning medications such as warfarin (Coumadin). This test is called a prothrombin time, more commonly referred to as a protime. Prothrombin is a protein in the blood plasma that is converted to thrombin as part of the clotting process.

Blood tests ordered for patients often are ordered in panels. Common panels include the lipid panel and the liver panel. Included in the lipid panel are such tests as cholesterol, triglycerides, and high-density lipoproteins (HDL). A liver panel includes tests such as SGOT and SGPT, which can be used in the diagnosis of hepatitis. When performing blood tests, it is always essential that the medical assistant utilize the office lab policies and procedures manual to determine how much blood to draw and the specific blood tube required for each test.

Diabetics monitor their blood sugar with a portable machine called a glucometer, such as the OneTouch shown in Figure 47-12A or the Accu-Chek. A patient who is diagnosed with diabetes may be anxious about performing this test. Proper education of patients is helpful if it addresses their concerns. A recheck visit or follow-up call to the patient may be necessary to ensure that the patient's comfort level is achieved. This daily test is very critical to address the patient's diabetic condition. See Procedure 47-5 about how to monitor blood glucose levels in diabetics.

The physician will often order a glycosylated hemoglobin (HbgA1C) to test the long-term control of diabetes. For this test it is critical that the patient be instructed to fast. If the patient fails to fast, the test results will be inaccurate. Concerns expressed by the patient regarding his or her medications should be directed to the physician. The physician will then determine if changes in medication must occur.

Other tests that a physician may order on a diabetic patient could include the glucose tolerance test. Although this test was traditionally done in a physician's office, it is now done more often in the outpatient department at a hospital.

procedure 47-5

MONITORING BLOOD GLUCOSE LEVELS
Objective: Determine blood glucose level using a glucometer.

EQUIPMENT AND SUPPLIES
sterile lancet; testing strips; glucometer; examination gloves; cotton balls; alcohol sponges; gauze squares; pen; lab coat; patient's record

METHOD
1. Identify the patient and make sure the patient is fasting if required.
2. Assemble the equipment and supplies.
3. Perform hand hygiene and apply gloves.
4. Make sure the glucometer has been turned on the required amount of time and has been calibrated for accuracy, according to the manufacturer's instructions.
5. Remove a plastic test strip from the container and place it in the glucometer in the designated slot. Ensure that the "Apply Blood" message appears on the screen (Figure 47-12A).
6. Perform a capillary puncture, preferably on the patient's finger, utilizing a sterile lancet.
7. After wiping away the first drop of blood with a cotton ball, gently touch the test strip to the second drop of blood that has formed on the patient's finger. The glucometer should automatically begin to count down the time that must elapse during the testing. This is usually 30 seconds (Figure 47-12B).

8. At this time provide the patient with a dry cotton ball to hold over the puncture site after wiping the site with an alcohol sponge.

9. The results of the blood glucose test will appear on the screen after the proper amount of time has elapsed. The blood glucose reading will remain on the glucometer until the unit has been turned off. Immediately remove the test strip, and discard all used equipment.

10. Remove gloves and perform hand hygiene.

11. Record in the patient's chart the number of mg (milligrams) of glucose per deciliter (mg/dL) displayed on the glucometer screen (Figure 47-12C).

Note: Several different types of testing instruments may be used to perform this test. It is critical to follow the manufacturer's instructions for the testing equipment provided.

2/28/XX 1:30 P.M. Random blood glucose performed, result 161 mg/dL. · M. Garcia, RMA

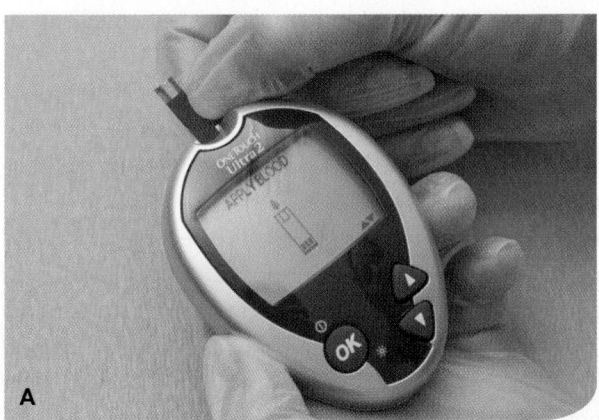

A

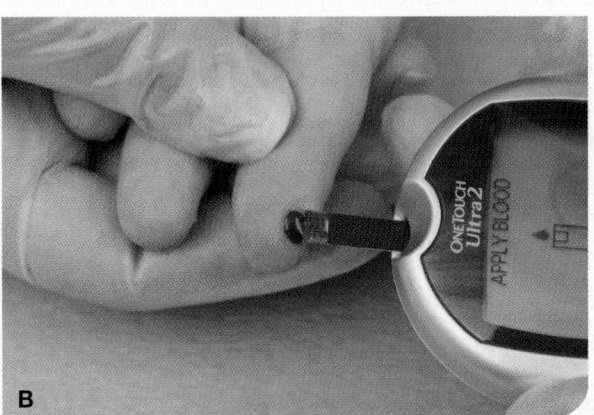

B

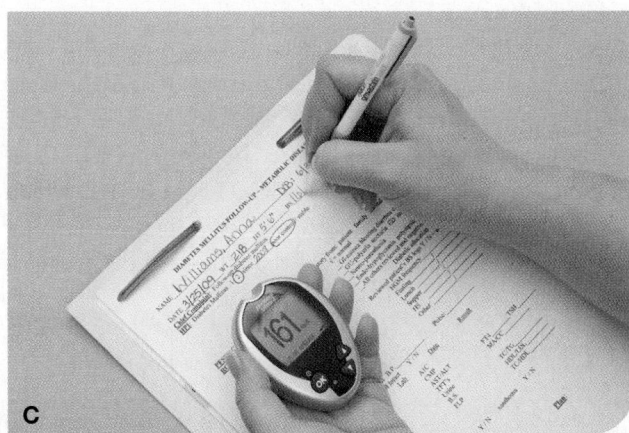

C

FIGURE 47-12 (A) Make sure that the monitor is turned on, and insert a test strip into the glucometer in the designated slot; (B) touch the test strip to the second drop of blood that has formed on the patient's finger; (C) record the blood glucose result in the patient's chart.

The patient should be given clear instructions as to the location of the outpatient hospital department. Often hospitals provide maps that are useful to provide to the patient. The patient should be informed that this test requires several hours. This is due in part to the preparation, which involves drinking a solution and several blood draws.

Laboratory results are reported from the lab to the physician's office in a variety of ways, including phone calls from the laboratory or by copies of the report being faxed or sent by courier. If the medical assistant receives a call from the laboratory with results, it is important to write down the correct results. Often physicians' offices will have standard forms that are used to record laboratory results. Lab slips for common tests such as urinalysis and common blood panels are often provided. This makes the process of recording the phone information easier. If a lab report does come in by phone, it must be followed up with the printed copy containing the results from the lab.

The contents of most lab reports include the patient's name, the written results of the test, and the range values. Table 47-2 provides a list of some commonly performed laboratory tests and the normal range values.

MICROHEMATOCRIT PROCEDURE

The **microhematocrit**, or crit is a hematocrit performed on an extremely small quantity of blood by use of a capil-

TABLE 47-2 Common Laboratory Tests and Their Normal Values

Test	Result
Total cholesterol	130–200 mg/dL
Glucose	70–120 mg/dL
Triglycerides	40–150 mg/dL
Creatinine	0.7–1.4 mg/dL
Uric acid	3.5–7.5 mg/dL
BUN	8–20 mg/dL
Sodium	132–142 mEq/L
Potassium	3.5–5.5 mEq/L
Chloride	98–106 mEq/L
CO_2	25–32 mEq/L
White blood cell count	5,000–10,000/mm^3
Red blood cell count	3.5–5.5×10^6/mm^3
Hemoglobin	12–16 g/dL
Hematocrit	35.5–49 percent
Sedimentation rate	0–10 mm/hr
Platelet count	150,000 and 400,000 per µl^3

lary tube. It provides the physician with information about the patient's RBC volume. A low hematocrit indicates anemia or hemorrhage. An elevated hematocrit indicates dehydration or polycythemia. A normal hematocrit is 40 percent to 50 percent in males and 35 percent to 45 percent in females.

To perform a microhematocrit, the patient's blood must be drawn using capillary tubes. The patient's finger is cleansed with an alcohol swab or sponge and then dried with sterile gauze. The patient's finger is then punctured utilizing an automatic lancet or a manual lancet. The first drop of blood is wiped away with dry sterile gauze. The second and subsequent drops are drawn up using a capillary tube that is either tilted horizontally or slightly downward. When the tip of the tube touches the blood, the tube will automatically draw the blood up by capillary action. The tube should be filled two-thirds to three-quarters of the way full and then sealed on each end. These tubes are then placed in a microhematocrit centrifuge that performs cellular separation. For the complete procedure, see Procedure 47-6.

HEMOGLOBIN DETERMINATION

Hemoglobin (Hgb) provides the physician with information regarding the amount of hemoglobin present in the sample. A low Hgb may indicate iron-deficiency anemia, whereas elevated readings are present in patients with polycythemia and in extreme situations, such as burns. Normal values for adult females are 12 to 16 g/dL and for males 14–18 g/dL.

Hemoglobin can be measured either by an automated blood analyzer or manually by a hemoglobinometer

procedure
47-6

PERFORMING A MICROHEMATOCRIT
Objective: Perform a microhematocrit on a capillary blood sample using proper aseptic technique.

EQUIPMENT AND SUPPLIES
biohazard sharps container; gloves; capillary tubes; sealing clay; microhematocrit centrifuge; whole blood; hematocrit card or other reader

Note: Follow standard precautions and safety guidelines when working with blood samples. Use care to avoid splashing or spilling blood. Wipe up all spills using guidelines established by OSHA.

METHOD
1. Perform hand hygiene and apply gloves.
2. Assemble equipment as shown in Figure 47-13A.
3. Fill two capillary tubes three-quarters full. The blood specimen can be obtained from a vacuum tube of antico-agulated blood using a plain capillary tube or directly from a fingerstick site using a heparinized capillary tube. Seal one end in the sealing clay.

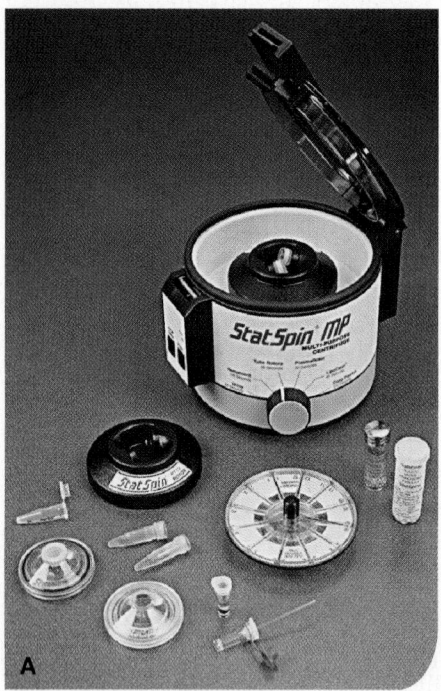

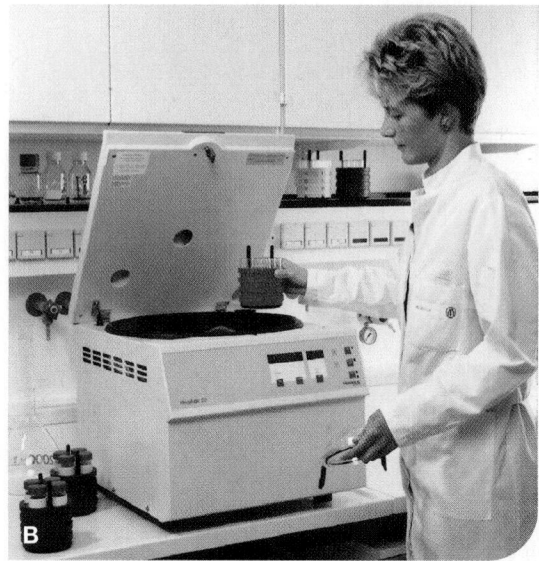

FIGURE 47-13 (A) Centrifuge and supplies; (B) loading a centrifuge.

4. Place capillary tubes in the centrifuge with the sealed ends against the rubber gasket (Figure 47-13B). If more than one patient's blood is being tested, mark down the number of the slot the patient's tube is in. Spin for 3 to 5 minutes at 10,000 rpm. (Always check the manufacturer's recommendations for proper time and speed.) After centrifuging, the sample will be separated into three layers:
   - Top layer is the plasma.
   - Middle layer, or the buffy coat, is made up of WBCs and platelets.
   - Bottom layer is packed RBCs.
5. Remove tubes immediately after centrifuge stops. If tubes are not removed immediately, blood may begin to mix together.

6. Determine the results. Use the Hct card by placing the sealing clay just below the zero line on both tubes. Then on both tubes match the top of the plasma with the 100 line. Read results on both tubes directly below the buffy coat. Then add those results together and divide by 2.
7. Discard the tubes into the sharps container.
8. Remove gloves and perform hand hygiene.
9. Record the value as a percentage on the patient's medical record.

CHARTING EXAMPLE
2/28/XX 1:45 P.M. Hct 47 percent. · · · · · M. King, CMA (AAMA)

(Figures 47-14, 47-15, and 47-16). Typically, the manual method is less accurate and not as reliable as the automated blood analyzer.

Hemoglobin values can be determined utilizing two methods: the specific gravity method or the cyanmethemoglobin method. The specific gravity method is a screening method for blood donors. The cyanmethemoglobin is a more specific and accurate method to give exact hemoglobin levels using hemoglobin analyzers. See Procedure 47-7 for a hemoglobin determination using the hemoglobinometer.

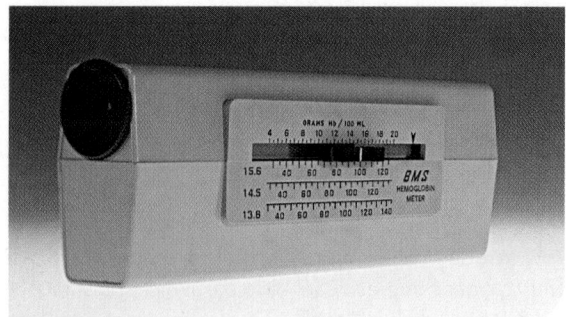

FIGURE 47-14 Hemoglobinometer.

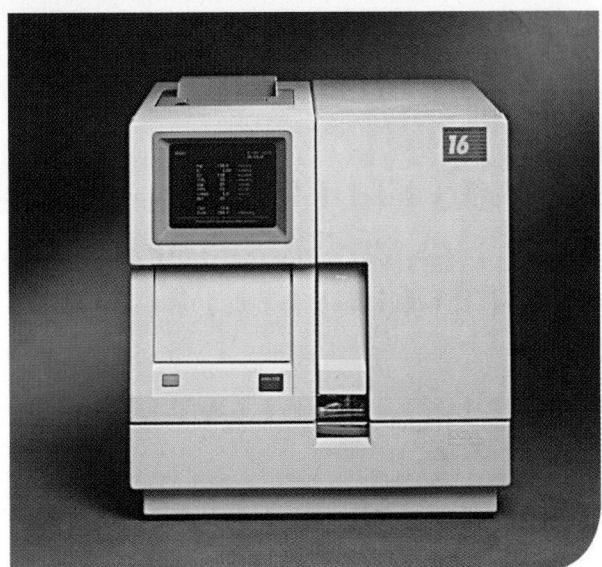

FIGURE 47-15 Nova 16 analyzer.

WHITE BLOOD CELL COUNT

Normal WBC or leukocyte counts in adults range from approximately 4,500 to 11,000 per mm^3. An elevated level usually indicates infection (leukocytosis) or, if grossly elevated, possibly leukemia. A low level usually indicates a viral infection or autoimmune deficiency.

A WBC count can be performed either manually by the medical assistant using a microscope or by an automated blood analyzer. The manual method of obtaining white blood counts is through the use of a hemacytometer. A hemacytometer is a special counting chamber that allows for counting of cells on slides under the microscope. If testing is performed manually, the medical assistant may use an automated tabulator to assist in counting the various

types of cells (Figure 47-17). Always follow the instructions on the automated analyzer exactly to ensure the validity of the results.

RED BLOOD CELL COUNT

Normal RBC volume in an adult female is 4.5 to 5.0 million per mm^3. In the adult male, it is about 5.0 to 6.0 million per mm^3. An increase in the number of circulating RBCs may indicate polycythemia, whereas a decrease may indicate anemia.

A manual RBC count is similar to a manual WBC count. Both require small samples of the specimen to be diluted in a special solution. Then the sample is placed on a hemocytometer, which is placed on a microscope used to count the red and WBCs.

Automated testing for RBCs is more common than manual testing. Always follow the machine's procedure manual exactly. The manual method of counting RBCs is done with the hemacytometer.

DIFFERENTIAL WHITE BLOOD CELL COUNT

A differential WBC count (diff) determines the percentages of each type of WBC, RBC morphology, and platelet estimation. Performing this test manually is a skill that requires practice to achieve proficiency. The testing is done using a microscope with a bright light and 100× magnification with an oil immersion slide. Focus near the edge of the stained slide where the cells are feathered, and where the cells are one layer thick. This test can also be performed by the automated analyzer. See Procedure 47-8 for details about slide preparation.

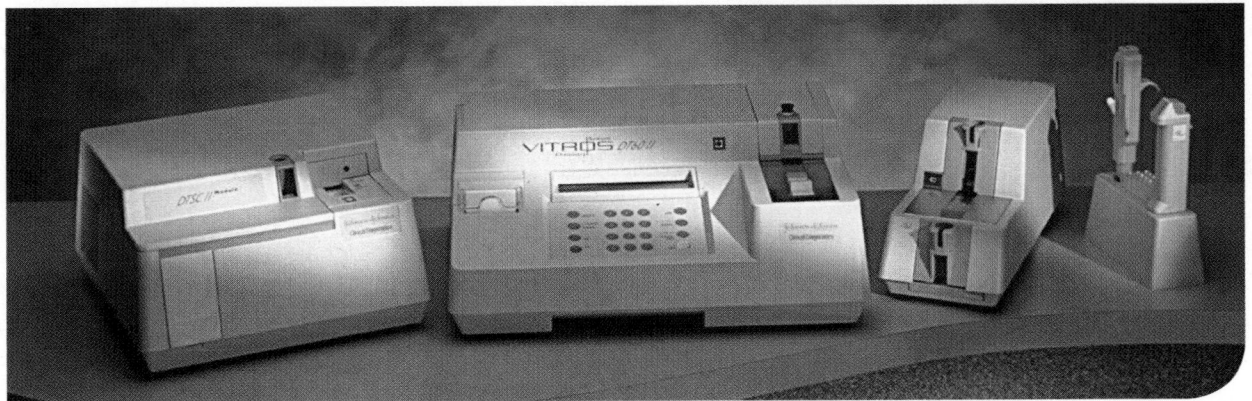

FIGURE 47-16 VITROS DT60II system.

DETERMINING HEMOGLOBIN USING THE HEMOGLOBINOMETER

Objective: Perform a blood test to determine hemoglobin levels using the hemoglobinometer.

EQUIPMENT AND SUPPLIES

hemoglobinometer; glass slide chamber; hemolysis applicator (plastic or wooden); sterile manual or spring-loaded lancet; cotton balls; dry gauze square; alcohol sponges; gloves; patient's record; lab coat; biohazard sharps container

Note: Follow standard precautions and safety guidelines when working with blood samples. Use care to avoid splashing or spilling blood. Wipe up all spills using guidelines established by OSHA.

METHOD

1. Perform hand hygiene and apply gloves.
2. Gather the necessary equipment and supplies.
3. Clean the puncture site with an alcohol sponge.
4. Using a manual or spring-loaded lancet, obtain capillary blood.
5. Pull the glass chamber out of the hemoglobinometer, and position the lower part of the slide so that it is slightly offset.
6. Place a large drop of capillary blood onto the slide.
7. Wipe the patient's puncture site with a cotton ball and provide the patient with a dry gauze square to apply mild pressure to the puncture. This should stop further bleeding.
8. Mix blood with the hemolysis applicator until the blood becomes clear.
9. Push the glass chamber into the clip and place it into the slot on the left side of the hemoglobinometer.
10. Hold the hemoglobinometer in your left hand at eye level while using your left thumb to turn on the light by depressing the bottom button. Look into the instrument to see a split green field.
11. Slide the button on the right side of the meter with your right thumb and index finger while looking into the meter until a matching green field occurs. Leave the sliding scale on the calibrated line where the solid green field appeared.
12. Read the hemoglobin value at the top of the scale. The results are read as grams of hemoglobin per 100 mL of blood (g/dL).
13. Wash the chamber and reusable hemolysis applicator with a detergent solution, rinse, dry, and return to the instrument for the next test.
14. Remove gloves and perform hand hygiene. Discard gloves and nonreusable supplies in appropriate containers.
15. Record the results in the patient's record.

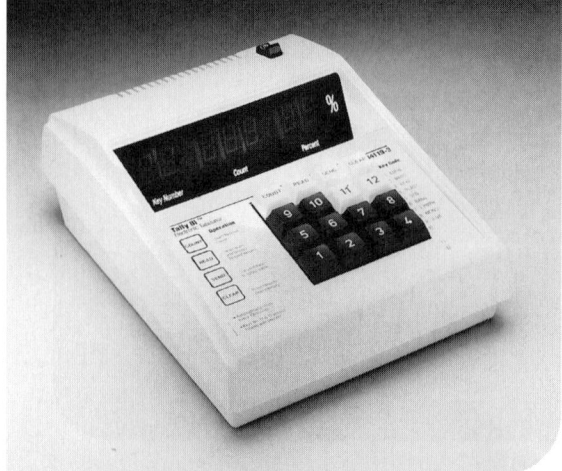

FIGURE 47-17 Electronic tabulator.

Red Blood Cells

RBCs are the most numerous, are salmon colored, and appear oval with a slightly pale center. RBCs have no nucleus or granules. RBCs with a nucleus are called reticulocytes (immature RBCs). Normal-looking RBCs are recorded as "normal RBC morphology."

Platelets

Platelets are the smallest of the formed blood elements. They are about half the size of a RBC. They stain purple and tend to appear in a clump, although they may also exist singly. They have a rough outer edge and contain small granules. There are between 200,000 and 300,000 platelets per mm^3 of blood. There are typically between

PREPARING SLIDES

Objective: Prepare a slide for a differential WBC count using correct aseptic procedure.

EQUIPMENT AND SUPPLIES

clean, glass slides; whole blood (EDTA); gloves; biohazard container; eye dropper; Wright's stain; lab coat; ink pen; patient record

Note: Follow standard precautions and safety guidelines when working with blood samples. Use care to avoid splashing or spilling blood. Wipe up all spills using guidelines established by OSHA.

METHOD

1. Perform hand hygiene and apply gloves.
2. Assemble equipment.
3. Obtain a whole-blood sample using EDTA as the anticoagulant of choice. Blood must be mixed thoroughly before use.
4. Using a dropper, place one drop of room temperature blood on the end of a clean, glass slide (Figure 47-18A).
5. Using the short side of another clean, glass slide, back the slide to the drop of blood. Allow the blood to spread across the short side of the slide (Figure 47-18B). Holding the spreader slide at a 30-degree angle, spread the blood across the length of the slide (Figure 47-18C). Use gentle, continuous pressure, and a smooth gliding motion to create a smear as pictured in (Figure 47-18D. Notice that the smear has a thick side that gradually changes to a thin side. The thin side has a feathered edge, and the blood covers one-half to three-quarters the length of the slide.
6. Allow the slide to air-dry on a rack (Figure 47-19A)
7. Label the patient's name and the date on the frosted edge of the slide.
8. Stain slide using Wright's staining method. Flood slide with stain for exactly 45 seconds or amount of time indicated by manufacturer (Figure 47-19B).
9. Rinse with distilled water (Figure 47-19C). Rinse until water is clear (Figure 47-19D).

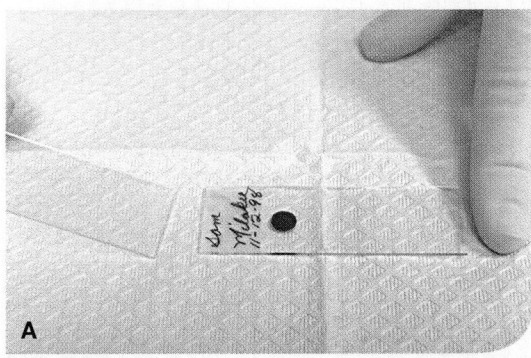

A

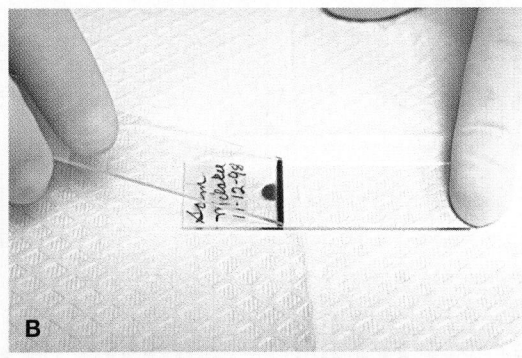

B

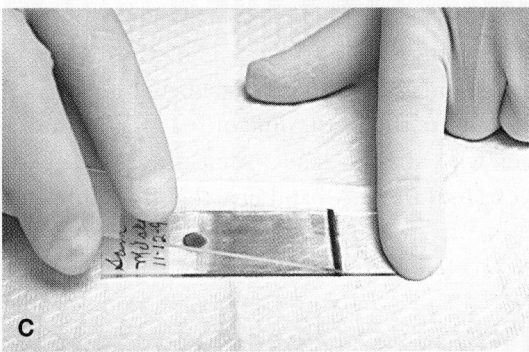

C

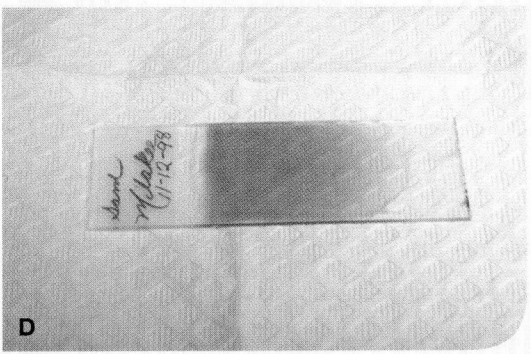

D

FIGURE 47-18 (A–D) Blood smear.

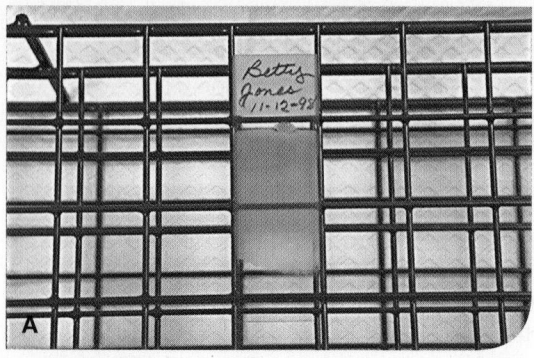

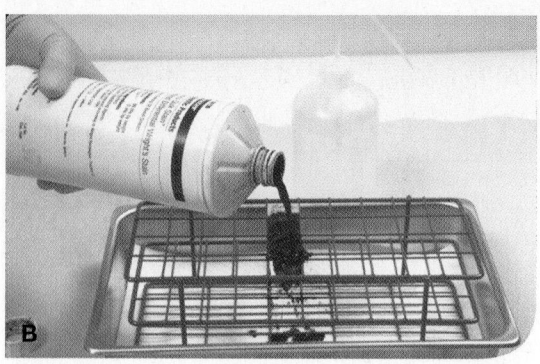

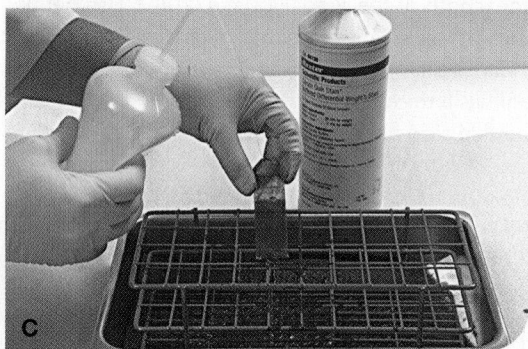

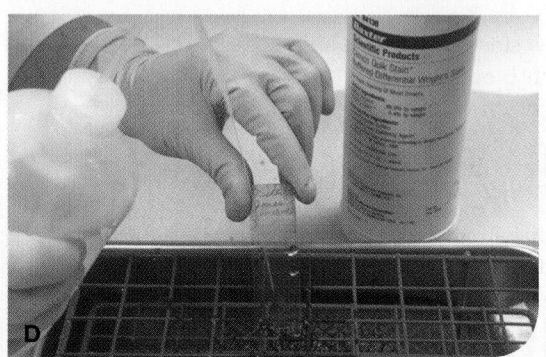

FIGURE 47-19 (A–D) Wright's staining process.

10. Allow slide to air-dry before examining under the microscope.
11. Abnormal findings may need to be referred to a laboratory technician for analysis. Record results on the patient's medical record.

CHARTING EXAMPLE

2/28/XX 2:15 P.M. Differential cell count: neutrophils 62 percent, lymphocyte 28 percent, monocytes 5 percent, eosinophils 5 percent, basophils 0 percent, RBC morphology—normal, adequate platelet estimation. · · · · · · · · · · · · · · · M. Garcia, RMA

5 and 20 platelets in one field of view. If this number is counted, then record the platelet count as "Adequate platelet estimation."

White Blood Cells

There are five types of WBCs, each of which has a distinct identifying characteristic when using the Wright's staining method. Count 100 WBCs, then express each of the cell types as a percentage. Normal values for adults are as follows:

- Neutrophils: 50–70 percent
- Eosinophils: 1–4 percent
- Basophils: 0–1 percent

- Lymphocytes: 20–35 percent
- Monocytes: 3–8 percent

Values may differ between manual and automated analyses.

Granulated White Blood Cells. The neutrophil, or seg, is the most numerous WBC. The neutrophil has small cytoplasmic granules that stain pink or lilac with a multi-lobed nucleus with small strands connecting each of the lobes, which stain purple. A band neutrophil is an immature neutrophil. It appears similar to the neutrophil except that the nucleus is unsegmented and curved with a bandlike structure. Cytoplasmic granules stain blue to pink.

Eosinophils have segmented nuclei and large, reddish staining granules that are found in the cytoplasm. Basophils are rarely seen in a diff count. This WBC has an S-shaped nucleus and large, irregularly shaped purplish-blue granules that almost entirely cover the nucleus.

Angranulocytic White Blood Cells. Lymphocytes have a single round or lightly indented nucleus, which almost completely fills the cell. The cytoplasm is clear and stains a pale blue. Lymphocytes are the smallest WBC.

Monocytes are the largest WBC and have a distinct kidney bean–shaped nucleus. The cytoplasm is abundant and clear, and it stains a grayish blue.

Erythrocyte Sedimentation Rate

The **erythrocyte sedimentation rate (ESR)** (also called the sed rate) is the rate at which RBCs settle at the bottom of a tube. Drawing a patient's ESR can be done utilizing either the Wintrobe or Westergren method. When performing the Wintrobe method, the Wintrobe tube is calibrated in mm/hr. The rate is the height of the RBCs in the bottom of the tube (Procedure 47-9 and Figure 47-20).

Depending on the method used, the normal values may vary. Utilizing the Wintrobe method, the normal ESR in an adult female is 0 to 20 mm/hr and in an adult male 0 to 9 mm/hr. Increased values may mean inflammation. An individual's ESR may also be elevated due to a variety of reasons, including menstruation, pregnancy, and malignant tumors.

An ESR itself is not diagnostic, but it is used in conjunction with other tests for diagnosis. For example, when testing for rheumatoid arthritis or fibromyalgia, an ESR may be done in conjunction with the antinuclear antibody test (ANA).

The sed rate is related to the condition of the RBCs and the amount of fibrinogen in the plasma. When an individual presents with a disease, the surfaces of the membranes of the cells are affected. When a sed rate test is conducted on a patient, the rate at which the RBCs fall indicates the existence of possible conditions.

procedure 47-9

PERFORMING AN ERYTHROCYTE SEDIMENTATION RATE TEST USING THE WINTROBE TUBE METHOD

Objective: Perform an ESR using the Wintrobe tube method and aseptic technique.

EQUIPMENT AND SUPPLIES
gloves; whole blood (EDTA); Wintrobe tube; Wintrobe rack; ink pen; patient's record; lab coat; biohazard sharps container

Note: Follow standard precautions and safety guidelines when working with blood samples. Use care to avoid splashing or spilling blood. Wipe up all spills using guidelines established by OSHA.

METHOD
1. Perform hand hygiene and apply gloves.
2. Assemble equipment.
3. Obtain a whole-blood sample using a purple-top tube. Mix well. EDTA is the anticoagulant of choice.
4. Slowly fill Wintrobe tube with blood. Avoid air bubbles.
5. Adjust the meniscus of the specimen to the zero line at the top of the tube.
6. Maintain the tube in an upright vertical position for 1 hour.
7. After 1 hour, record the number of RBCs that settle. Read the ESR on the same side of the tube as the zero line at the top.
8. Remove gloves and perform hand hygiene.
9. Record the procedure on the patient's medical record.

CHARTING EXAMPLE
2/28/XX 2:00 P.M. ESR (Wintrobe Method) 10 fall of mm/hr. · · · ·
· M. Garcia, RMA

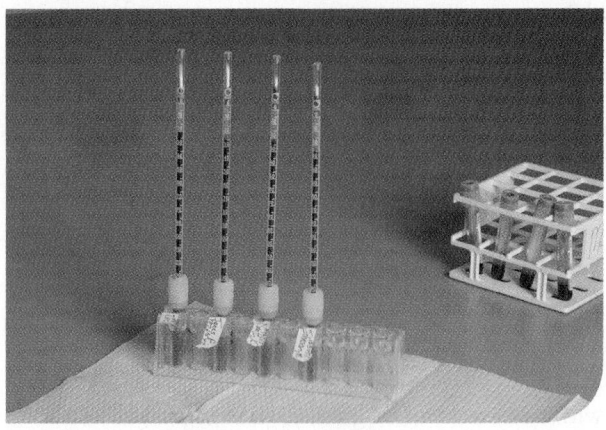

FIGURE 47-20 Wintrobe tube and Westergren tests are used to measure the ESR.

Phenylketonuria

Phenylketonuria (PKU) is a congenital disease caused by a defect in the metabolism of the amino acid phenylalanine. The unmetabolized protein accumulates in the bloodstream and, if undetected and untreated, will result in mental retardation. The PKU test is always performed on newborns to determine the presence of the unmetabolized protein phenylalanine. The test is typically performed in the hospital but may be performed in the office if not done in the hospital. See Procedure 47-10 for steps in performing the PKU test.

Mono Testing

The mono test, which is also known as the mononucleosis spot test, is used to help determine whether a patient has infectious mononucleosis (Procedure 47-11). Infectious **mononucleosis** is also commonly referred to as the "kissing disease" and is a contagious viral infection that frequently is spread through oral contact. It is frequently ordered along with a CBC. A strep test may be ordered with the mono test to determine whether a person's sore throat is due to a streptococcal infection instead of or in addition to mononucleosis.

A mono test is primarily ordered when an adolescent patient has symptoms such as fever, headache, swollen glands, and fatigue that the doctor suspects are due to infectious mononucleosis. The test may be repeated when it is initially negative but suspicion of mono remains high. The physician may order a repeat test in a week or so to see if heterophile antibodies have developed or may order Epstein-Barr

procedure 47-10

PERFORMING A PKU TEST
Objective: Collect blood specimen for PKU testing.

EQUIPMENT AND SUPPLIES
sterile lancet; alcohol sponge; gloves; sterile dry gauze; special filter paper card, typically supplied by the state health department

METHOD
1. Perform hand hygiene and apply gloves.
2. Cleanse the infant's heel with an alcohol sponge.
3. Puncture the lateral portion of the infant's heel with a sterile disposable lancet.
4. Wipe away the first drop of blood with dry sterile gauze.
5. Allow a large blood droplet to form.
6. Touch the blood droplet to the center of the circle on one side of the special filter paper card.
7. Ensure the blood has completely soaked through the paper card by looking at the reverse side.
8. Fill all required five circles on the paper card.
9. Do not squeeze the heel excessively to avoid collecting tissue fluid mixed with blood.
10. Set the card in an appropriate area to air-dry for 2 hours at room temperature.
11. When completely dry, place in the state-provided envelope and mail within 48 hours.

procedure

PERFORMING A MONO TEST

Objective: Perform a mono test.

EQUIPMENT AND SUPPLIES

antiseptic cleaner; biohazard waste container; disposable lancet; gloves; capillary tube; test tube; mono test diluent; mono test stick(s); blood specimen

METHOD

1. Perform hand hygiene.
2. Apply gloves.
3. Assemble equipment and supplies.
4. Perform a capillary puncture on the patient's finger.
5. Fill a capillary tube end to end, dispensing all of the blood into the test tube.
6. Slowly add 1 drop of diluent to the bottom of the test tube.
7. Mix.
8. Remove the test stick(s) from the container. Recap the container immediately.
9. Place the absorbent end of the test stick into the treated sample. Leave the test stick in the test tube.
10. Read result at 5 minutes. Positive results may be read as soon as the red control line appears.
11. Discard used test tubes, lancet, and test sticks in the biohazard waste container.
12. Remove gloves and dispose of them correctly. Perform hand hygiene.
13. Document findings in the patient record:
    Positive: A blue test line and a red control line indicate a positive result.
    Negative: A red control line but no blue test line indicates a negative result.

Note: Although the medical assistant is responsible for reporting abnormal results (or positive results in the case of a mono test) to the physician, "interpreting" such tests as being positive or negative is *not* within the scope of practice for the medical assistant as such and should never be done. The medical assistant is only allowed to report the findings of "positive" or "negative."

14. Clean the work area and equipment according to OSHA guidelines.

---

virus (EBV) antibodies to help confirm or rule out the presence of a current EBV infection.

If a patient has a positive mono test, an increased number of WBCs, reactive lymphocytes, and symptoms of mononucleosis, then the patient will be diagnosed with infectious mononucleosis. If symptoms and reactive lymphocytes are present but the mono test is negative, then it may be too early to detect the heterophile antibodies, or the affected patient may be in the small number of people who do not make heterophile antibodies. Other EBV antibodies and/or a repeat mono test may be performed to help confirm or rule out the mononucleosis diagnosis.

Patients with negative mono tests and few or no reactive lymphocytes may be infected by another microorganism that causes monolike symptoms (such as a cytomegalovirus or toxoplasmosis). If the infection occurs during pregnancy, it is important to determine the cause, because some of the monolike infections (but not EBV infection) have been associated with pregnancy complications and damage to the fetus. It is also important to identify strep throat, whenever present, because it should be treated promptly with antibiotics.

Blood Chemistry Panels

Blood chemistry panels may be ordered by the medical provider as part of the assessment of a particular organ or group of organs. Laboratories have automated blood chemistry analyzers to detect multiple analytes in the patient's blood (see Figures 47-15 and 47-16). Serum is generally needed for most blood chemistry tests. Table 47-3 covers commonly ordered blood chemistry tests.

TABLE 47-3 Common Blood Chemistry Tests

Test	Common Medical Abbreviation	Normal Adult Value	Description	Purpose of Test
Alanine aminotransferase	ALT (SGPT)	<45 units/L	Liver enzyme, may also be found in kidneys	Detection of liver disease or inflammation.
Albumin	No standard abbreviation	3.5–5.0 g/dL	A protein that normally constitutes 60 percent of plasma serum	To detect effectiveness of specific medications such as warfarin because it binds to albumin. High levels may indicate dehydration; low levels may indicate drug toxicity in the liver.
Alkaline phosphate	ALP	20–70 units/L	Enzyme found in all tissues; especially concentrated in the kidneys, bile, liver, bone and placenta	Used to detect several conditions in the bone and liver and blocked bile ducts
Aspartate aminotransferase	AST (SGOT)	<40 units/L	Enzyme found in all tissues; similar to ALT; found in cardiac muscle cells and red blood cells	Used to detect conditions of liver health.
Blood urea nitrogen	BUN	7–18 mg/dL	Metabolic products of protein catabolism	Used to measure the amount of nitrogen in the blood, indicating renal function
Cholesterol	CH, Chol	Total count: <200 mg/dL; LDL <130 mg/dL; HDL >35 mg/dL	Lipids	Annual screening done to determine atherosclerosis and other cardiac related diseases.
Creatinine	Creat	0.2–0.8 mg/dL	The product of creatinine phosphate breakdown in muscle in a fairly constant rate, then filter out through the kidneys	Screening for renal function often used in combination with BUN. Checked prior to contrast studies, such as CT, to assess the kidneys' ability to filter out contrast material.
Glucose Tolerance Test	GTT	70–100 mg/dL	Carbohydrate	To determine how quickly the body is able to filter glucose to help diagnosis diabetes, insulin resistance, and reactive hypoglycemia.
Troponin I and T	No standard abbreviation	<0.4	A specific protein only found in cardiac muscle when it is damaged	Aids in the determination of myocardial infarct.
Thyroid-stimulating hormone	TSH	5–6 units/mL	Peptide hormone produced by thyrotropic cells in the pituitary gland	Assessment of thyroid and pituitary function.

Thyroxine	T4	5–12 mcg/dL	Hormone secreted by the follicular cells of the thyroid gland	Assessment of the body's ability to control the metabolic processes in the body that influence physical development.
Triglycerides	Trig	30–190 mg/dL	Dietary fat	Annual screening done to determine atherosclerosis and other cardiac related diseases.
Uric acid	UA	*Male:* 3.4–7.0 mg/dL *Female:* 2.4–6 mg/dL	Organic compound of carbon, nitrogen, oxygen, and hydrogen	Diagnosis of several conditions, including gout, Lesch-Nyhan syndrome, cardiovascular disease, diabetes, metabolic syndrome, and multiple sclerosis (low levels).

SUMMARY

The proper collection, handling, and processing of blood specimens are vital to reliable test results. In addition, it is critical for a medical assistant to have a thorough understanding of patient preparation and the theory of blood formation, including the cellular and liquid components of blood. Knowledge of and competency in the performance of routine blood tests—CBCs, differentials, hemoglobins, microhematocrits, ESRs—is also essential to proper patient care.

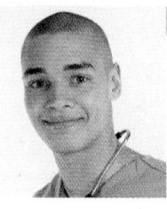

47 CHAPTER REVIEW

COMPETENCY REVIEW

1. Define and spell the terms to learn for this chapter.\

2. List, in order, the steps for performing a venipuncture.

3. Prepare a list of the different types of venipuncture collection tubes. Explain what makes each unique and the order in which they should be used.

4. Make a list of the types of white blood cells and the values of each that are expected in a normal differential.

5. Create a normal list (for male and female, where applicable) for the WBC, RBC, Hct, Hgb, and ESR.

6. List the equipment needed to perform an erythrocyte sedimentation rate test.

PREPARING FOR THE CERTIFICATION EXAM

1. How many types of white blood cells are there?
   a. 5
   b. 1
   c. 4
   d. 3
   e. 2

2. Which of the following is NOT a plasma protein?
   a. albumin
   b. prothrombin
   c. globulin
   d. fibrinogen
   e. urea

3. The most common method of venipuncture is
   a. syringe
   b. butterfly
   c. vacuum container
   d. capillary puncture
   e. heel-stick

4. Which tubes contain heparin and are used for testing whole blood and plasma?
   a. red top
   b. brick top
   c. lavender top
   d. green top
   e. yellow top

5. The most commonly used site for a venipuncture is the
   a. cephalic vein
   b. pulmonary vein
   c. median cephalic vein
   d. antecubital space
   e. basilic vein

6. The normal range for glucose is
   a. 70–120 mg/dL
   b. 40–150 mg/dL
   c. 140–220 mg/dL
   d. 130–200 mg/dL
   e. 132–142 mg/dL

7. The normal RBC volume in an adult female is
   a. 5.0–6.0 million/mm^3
   b. 4.5–5.0 million/mm^3
   c. 6.0–7.0 million/mm^3
   d. 7.0–8.0 million/mm^3
   e. 4.0–5.0 million/mm^3

8. The normal WBC counts range from _____ to _____ thousand in adults:
   a. 4.5, 11
   b. 11, 14
   c. 1.0, 4.5
   d. 6.0, 9.0
   e. 4.5, 5.0

9. The percentage range of basophils in adult blood is
   a. 50–70 percent
   b. 1–4 percent
   c. 0–1 percent
   d. 20–35 percent
   e. 2–3 percent

10. To perform a differential white blood cell count, the microscope must be placed on
   a. 40×
   b. 60×
   c. 80×
   d. 20×
   e. 100×

CRITICAL THINKING

1. Samra will be using Vacutainer tubes to draw blood. Which color of tube top will Samra need for the tests ordered? List the additional supplies that Samra will need to perform the blood draw.

2. What additives, if any, are in the Vacutainers that Samra will be using? What is the correct order of draw, and why is it important to follow a correct order of draw?

3. How can Samra calm Ms. St. Claire's anxiety regarding the procedure?

ON THE JOB

It is Wednesday and Drs. Joseph and Burg are not seeing patients. However, the office is open for blood draws. Angie, a medical assistant, is in the office alone.

Matt, a 17-year-old upcoming college freshman, has just arrived to have his labs drawn so that Dr. Joseph can complete Matt's college physical. He is extremely nervous, although he is trying very hard to exhibit a relaxed manner. Angie tries to reassure Matt, but the more she tries, the more nervous he gets. At Matt's urging to "just get it over with," Angie decides to go ahead and draw his blood. Unfortunately, as soon as the first collection tube begins to fill with blood, Matt notices it and slumps forward. He has fainted.

1. What is the first thing that Angie should do?
2. Was Angie at all negligent in drawing Matt's blood given that he was extremely nervous?
3. Does the fact that Matt is a minor influence how Angie should handle this situation? If so, how?

4. Does Matt have some level of complicity in this incident? If so, describe it.
5. Is this considered a medical emergency?
6. Would the situation have been different or handled differently if Angie had not been alone?
7. Does an incident report of some sort need to be filed? If so, what should be included, and who should receive a copy?

INTERNET ACTIVITY

Go online and research materials to further understand OSHA regulations, the Centers for Disease Control and Prevention (CDC) Standard Precautions, and the laboratory regulations established by CLIA 1988.

MEDMEDIA

Additional interactive resources and activities for this chapter can be found:

On your student DVD: View applicable procedure videos on the DVD-ROM found in the back of this book.

MyHealthProfessionsKit.com: Test your knowledge of the chapter with games and activities. MyHealthProfessionsKit also includes resources, helpful links, and a Spanish audio glossary.

Medical Assisting Interactive: Practice your procedures as a medical assistant in this simulated doctor's office. This can be accessed through MyHealthProfessionsKit.com.

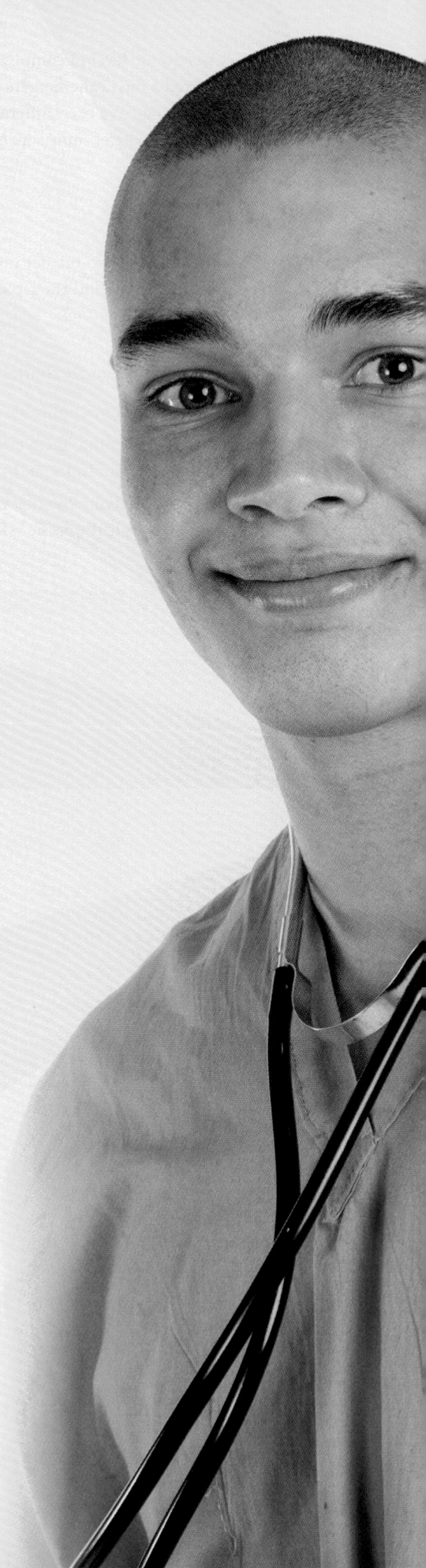

48
Radiology

LEARNING OBJECTIVES

After completing this chapter, you should be able to:

- Define and spell the terms to learn for this chapter.

- List six X-ray procedures that require preparations ahead of time. Describe the preparations.

- List and explain four basic positions used for taking X-rays.

- Describe the process and medical use of fluoroscopy.

- Discuss computed tomography, positron emission tomography, magnetic resonance imaging, and ultrasound.

- Define and discuss the use for radiology, radiation therapy, and nuclear medicine.

- List four side effects of radiation therapy.

- Describe the safety precautions to take for health care workers and patients relating to X-ray procedures.

- Discuss the proper methods for storage of X-ray materials.

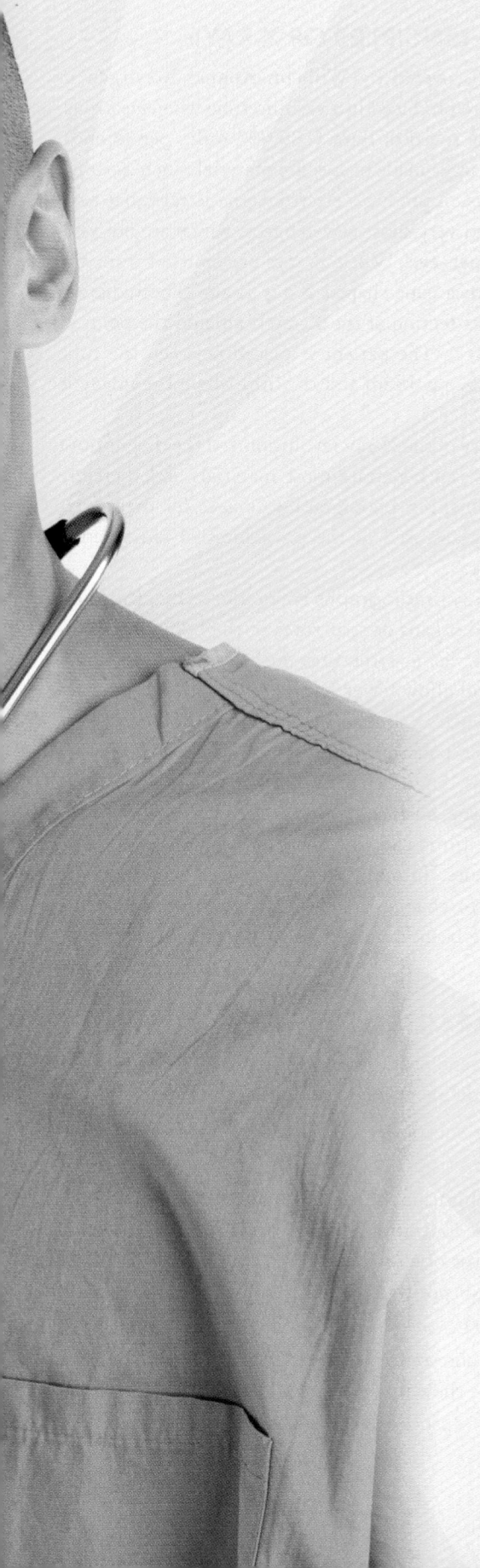

CHAPTER OUTLINE

CASE STUDY

Timothy Adler, a 32-year-old patient, saw Dr. Miller for intense pain in his abdomen, which occurred after eating meals, especially dinner. Dr. Miller suspected that Timothy might have gallstones and ordered an ultrasound of his gallbladder. Unfortunately, the gallbladder ultrasound report came back as inconclusive.

angiography
bucky
claustrophobia
collimeter
cumulative
dosimeter
fluoroscopy
gantry
grid
nuclear medicine
radioactive

radiation
radiographs
radiologist
radiology
radiolucent
radiopaque
rem
retrograde pyelography
transducer
X-rays

CERTIFICATION LINK

CMA (AAMA)	RMA	CMAS (AMT)
Collecting and processing specimens; diagnostic testing Medical imaging	Clinical medical assisting	Not applicable

The study of radiology includes an understanding of the use of X-rays, diagnostic radiology, radiation therapy, and nuclear medicine. A **radiologist** is a physician specializing in radiology. A radiographer or radiologic technologist is involved in making diagnostic radiographs or X-rays. His or her duties include positioning patients for radiographic procedures, determining the proper voltage, current, and exposure time for each X-ray; adjusting radiographic equipment; developing the film; and assisting the radiologist with special procedures. To become a radiologic technologist requires a 2- to 4-year college program. The medical assistant in a radiology department will require additional training in order to assist with radiologic procedures. Safety issues and requirements must also be followed when working in and around X-ray equipment.

Radiology

Radiology is the branch of medicine that uses **radioactive** substances or matter that gives off **radiation** (radiant energy) and various techniques to visualize the internal structures of the body for the diagnosis and treatment of disease. Radiology uses X-rays, radioactive substances, and other forms of radiant energy such as ultraviolet rays.

Radiology can be divided into three specialties: diagnostic radiology, radiation therapy, and nuclear medicine. A discussion of various X-ray, fluoroscopic, and radiologic procedures follows.

PRINCIPLES OF X-RAYS

X-rays were discovered by Wilhelm Konrad Roentgen in 1895. **X-rays** are produced in a vacuum tube when electrons, traveling at the speed of light (186,000 miles per second), collide into a target made of specific materials such as tungsten. This collision produces electromagnetic rays that have high energy and very short wavelengths, which are not visible to the human eye. When X-rays are emitted from the tube, they form a cone-shaped X-ray beam. The radiation field is the cross-section of the X-ray beam and the point of use (Figure 48-1). The patient is placed between the tube producing the X-ray beam and the film where the image is recorded.

The discovery of the X-ray revolutionized the diagnosis of disease. X-rays can penetrate most materials and therefore are useful for making photographic images for diagnostic purposes. They are used in the procedures of radiography and fluoroscopy.

X-ray images or **radiographs** are produced by projecting X-rays through organs or structures of the body onto photographic film. Some structures such as bones are more **radiopaque** and allow fewer X-rays to pass through; other softer tissues, such as skin and lungs, are **radiolucent**, permitting greater penetration of X-rays. Thus radiopaque tissue, such as bone, appears light on the film, and radiolucent tissue, such as the lungs, leave a shadowy, dark image. X-rays films can then be examined for defects in bones and tissues. In addition, X-rays that penetrate the body are able to change the basic structure of body cells. Thus they have been useful in the diagnosis and treatment of tumors.

CHARACTERISTICS OF X-RAYS

X-rays have several characteristics that make them useful in the field of medicine. X-rays can do the following:

- Penetrate substances of different densities to varying degree.
- Cause ionization of the substances through which they pass. Ionization is the process, which causes the gain or loss of electrons from a neutral atom. Loss of electron = positive charge; gain of electron = negative charge.
- Cause fluorescence of certain substances. Internal structures show up dark on a glowing screen as X-rays

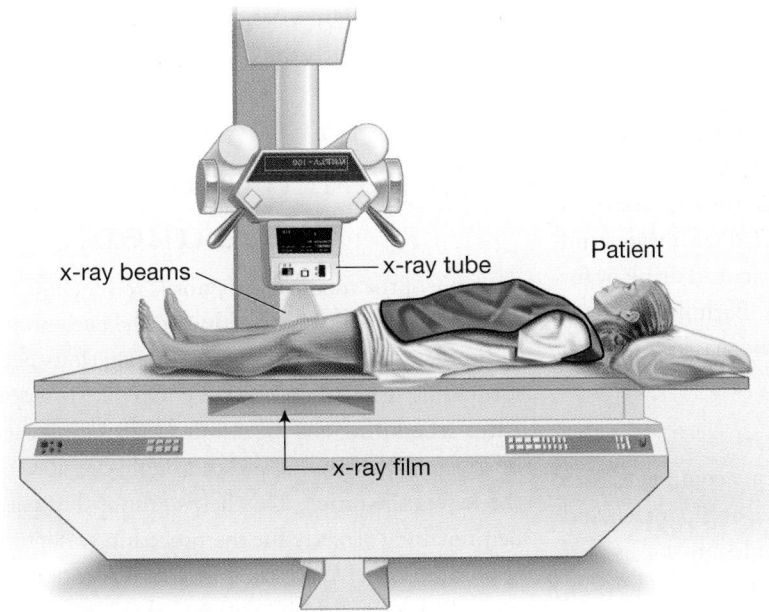

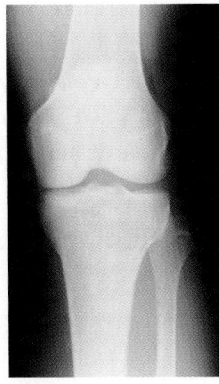

Image Receptor (film)

Knee x-ray

x-ray beams

x-ray tube

Patient

x-ray film

FIGURE 48-1 The patient is placed between the X-ray tube, which emits a cone-shaped X-ray beam, and the film or image receptor. Bones do not allow the X-ray beam to pass through them, resulting in an image of the bones on the film.

pass through, allowing physicians to visualize structures in motion.

- Travel in a straight line so the X-ray beam can be directed at a specific area.

- Destroy body cells and be used to kill cancer cells.

Since X-rays are invisible and produce no sound or smell, precautions must be taken to protect patients and employees from unnecessary exposure. Safety precautions are discussed later in this chapter.

Overview of Diagnostic Imaging

Diagnostic imaging involves the use of X-rays, ultrasound, radiopharmaceuticals, radiopaque media, and computers to produce images of internal structures and processes. Advances in the field of electronics have made possible noninvasive procedures for visualizing organs and processes that previously required surgical procedures.

USE OF A CONTRAST MEDIUM

A contrast medium is a radiopaque substance that does not allow the passage of X-rays but facilitates radiographic imaging of internal structures that are difficult to visualize on a regular X-ray or fluoroscopic screen. The body structure or organ with the contrast medium is seen in contrast to adjacent structures.

Contrast media include liquids (barium), powders, air, and gas. They are administered orally, by injection (parenterally), or by enema. The contrast medium acts to convert an organ or structure into an opaque area. In this way, the actual function of that particular organ or structure can be visualized under fluoroscopy or by film.

PROFESSIONALISM

During your educational program preparing for medical assisting, you have been introduced to the field of radiography. Radiography is a complicated field, and to become a radiologic technologist or radiographer takes advanced schooling and training experience. Radiographers perform imaging procedures ordered by physicians; operate several different types of imaging equipment; and produce images through the use of ultrasound, magnetic resonance imaging, or radionuclide procedures. "Rad techs," as they are known in the health care field, have career opportunities in doctors' offices, private imaging facilities, hospitals, and clinics.

To become a radiologic technologist, a student must graduate from a 2- or 4-year degree program in radiology and pass a national registration examination administered by the American Registry of Radiologic Technologies. Passing this examination earns the candidate the title of Registered Radiologic Technologist (RRT). For more information regarding a career in radiology, contact the American Society of Radiologic Technologists, 15000 Central Avenue SE, Albuquerque, NM 87123-3909, (800) 444-2778.

Barium Sulfate

Barium sulfate and iodine are positive contrast media, which means they have more density and thus can absorb more radiation. Positive contrast media will appear white on X-ray images. This differs from air, a negative contrast medium, which allows more X-rays to pass through. Barium sulfate consists of a chalky compound mixed with water and flavoring to the right consistency for a patient to drink or for a technician to administer as an enema. Barium sulfate is used for fluoroscopic examination of the gastrointestinal tract.

Iodine Contrast Compounds

Iodine compounds used to form radiopaque compounds are employed for thyroid studies, pyelograms, angiograms, and cholecystograms. Iodine compounds should not be used if the patient is allergic to seafood or iodine. In addition, iodine radiopaque compounds interfere with nuclear medicine. Therefore, these two types of studies should not be performed during the same time period.

Negative Contrast

Negative contrast media include air, carbon dioxide, and other gases. These will appear black on X-rays. These media are used to visualize the spinal cord, as in a myelogram, and joints. The introduction of gas and air into the body can result in severe headaches following procedures such as myelograms. Negative contrast studies have largely been replaced with the use of magnetic resonance imaging (MRI).

Preparing and Positioning the Patient

The role of the medical assistant is to schedule the procedure ordered by the physician, educate the patient about the procedure, explain beforehand the preparations needed, and inform the patient how long the entire procedure will take. After scheduling the procedure, written instructions should be given to the patient and thoroughly reviewed before he or she leaves the office. This helps ensure that the patient will be prepared correctly for the procedure when arriving at the appointed time. Once the procedure is concluded, it will be your duty to assist the patient, provide post-procedure instructions, and inform the patient when to expect the test results. For some X-ray procedures, special patient preparation must be performed before the patient can be examined. These procedures are described in Table 48-1.

For many radiology examinations, the patient will be asked to undress and wear a patient gown. Many of the procedures involve positions and interventions that may be embarrassing to the patient. The medical assistant must make every effort to provide an ample size gown and drape the

TABLE 48-1 X-ray Procedures Requiring Special Preparations

Procedure	Preparation
Angiogram	No breakfast if morning examination or lunch if afternoon examination.
Barium enema (lower GI)	Enemas until the bowel return is clear on the evening before the examination, may order rectal suppository in the morning or a cathartic such as 2 oz. of castor oil or citrate of magnesia at 4:00 P.M. the day before the X-ray, clear liquids and gelatin for dinner, nothing by mouth (NPO) after midnight.
Barium meal (upper GI)	NPO after midnight.
Bronchogram	NPO.
Cholecystogram (GB series)	Light supper of non-fatty food such as fruit and vegetables without butter or oil the evening before the X-ray; gallbladder tablets (prescribed by the physician) are taken with water after supper; NPO except for water until X-ray the following day.
Computerized tomography (CT)	NPO for 4 hours before X-ray if a contrast media is used.
Intravenous cholangiogram	NPO.
Intravenous pyelogram (IVP)	Three Dulcolax tablets or 2 oz. castor oil at 4:00 P.M. the day before the X-ray; eat a light supper; NPO after midnight.
Myelogram	NPO.
Retrograde pyelogram	Enemas or laxatives on the evening before X-ray; NPO for 8 hours before the procedure.
Ultrasound	May require a full bladder or laxatives, depending on the type of ultrasound.

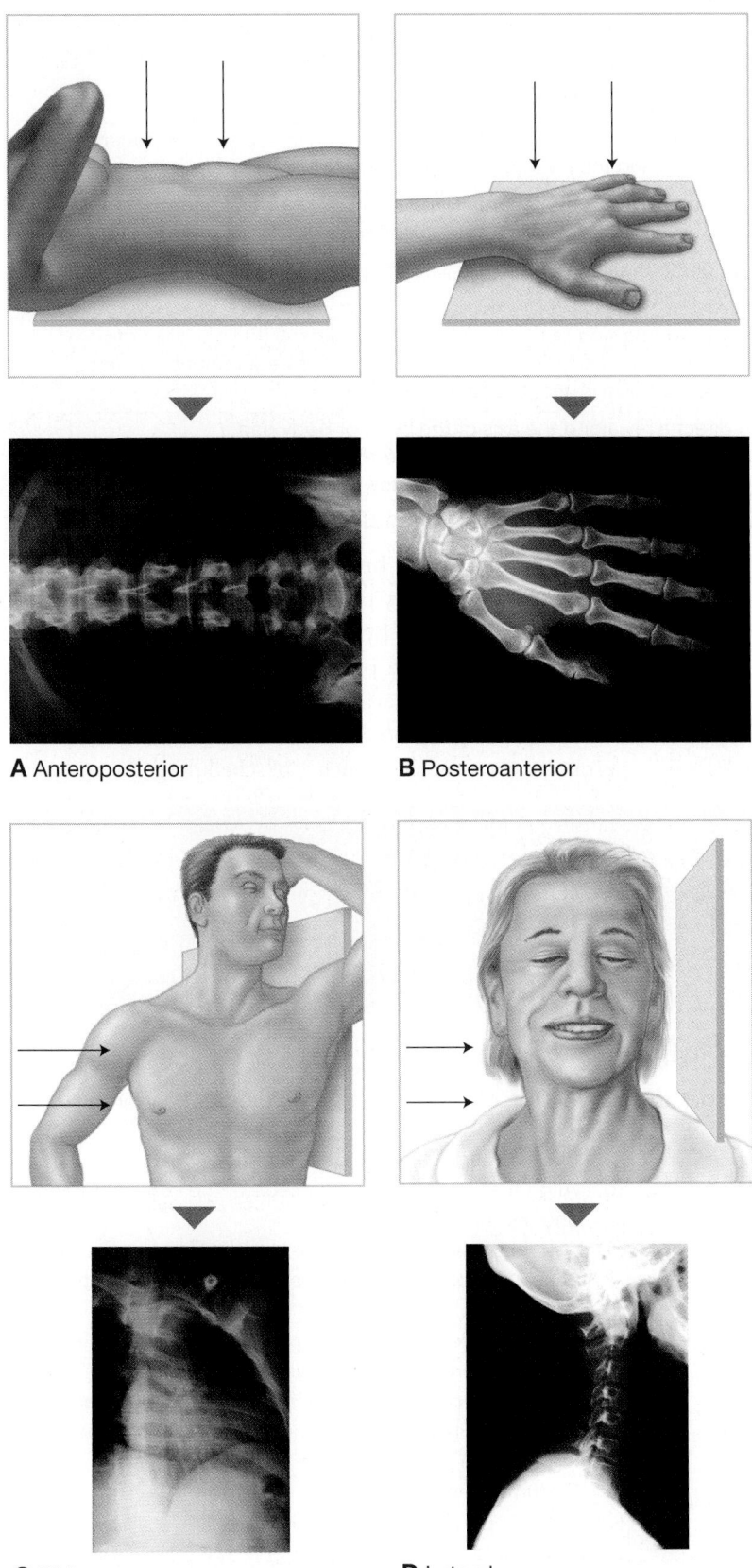

A Anteroposterior

B Posteroanterior

C Oblique

D Lateral

FIGURE 48-2 **(A–D) Examples of the most common X-ray positions and the images they produce.**

patient to preserve his or her privacy. Request that the patient remove all metallic materials such as jewelry, belt buckles, watches, eyeglasses, hairpins, earrings, and hearing aids. In some X-rays of the head, mouth, and neck, the patient may have to remove dentures. Since the patient is not able to wear jewelry during the procedure, a safe container or locker should be provided for personal belongings.

The patient may need assistance getting onto the X-ray table. A footstool should be available if the table is high. X-ray tables do not have side rails. If there is a concern that the patient may become confused, then someone must remain in the room with the patient until the procedure begins. The X-ray technician should be told about the patient's confused state. Children may require special attention and need someone to help them maintain the correct position. Anyone who has to be in the room during an X-ray procedure must follow the strictest safety considerations.

POSITIONING

Although it is unlikely that you will be positioning a patient for a diagnostic imaging procedure, it will be helpful for you to understand that the patient position relative to the source of X-rays determines the images produced. It may be helpful to review anatomical locations on or in the body presented in Chapter 4. Figure 48-2 illustrates X-ray pathways and the image produced when the patient is placed in a specific position. The position of the patient and the position of the X-ray beam must be known ahead of time by the technician. The position of the patient is critical for an accurate X-ray. Table 48-2 lists radiology positions and descriptions of each position. Procedure 48-1 lists the steps for a general X-ray examination.

SCHEDULING GUIDELINES

The medical assistant often has the responsibility of scheduling the patient and providing instruction for radiologic procedures. If the procedure is performed in a facility other than the medical office, you may have to call to make the appointment. When setting an appointment, have the patient's name, type of insurance with pre-certification or approval number, the

TABLE 48-2 Radiology Positions

Position	Description
Anteriorposterior (AP)	The X-ray beam is directed from front to back. Patient may be standing or supine. The patient's front will face the X-ray equipment, and the patient's back will be near the film plate.
Posterioanterior (PA)	The X-ray beam is directed from back to front. Patient will be standing upright. Patient's back will face the X-ray equipment, and his or her front will be near the film plate.
Oblique	The patient is turned at an angle to the film plate so the X-ray beam can be directed at areas that would be hidden on an AP, PA, or lateral X-ray.
Lateral	The X-ray beam is directed toward one side of the body. In the right lateral (RL) position, the patient's right side is near the film plate, and the left side is near the X-ray equipment. In a left lateral (LL) position, the patient's left side is near the film plate.
Axial	The X-ray tube is angled to direct a ray along the axis of the body or body part. *Cephalad angulation:* The X-ray beam is directed at an angle from the feet toward the head. *Caudal angulation:* The X-ray beam is directed from the head toward the feet.

referring physician's name, and type of radiologic procedure to be performed.

Special dietary restrictions in preparation for radiographic procedures often call for an all-liquid diet on the day before the test. All-liquid diets mean that the patient may have any of the following beverages: coffee, tea, carbonated beverages, clear gelatin desserts, strained fruit juices, bouillon, clear broth, and tomato juice. He or she may not have any dairy products. Remind the patient that NPO means "nothing by mouth." It is up to the physician to decide whether the patient should or should not take his or her daily medications.

When multiple procedures are to be scheduled, it is important to consider the sequence of scheduling. Attention to

procedure 48-1

PROCEDURE FOR A GENERAL X-RAY EXAMINATION

Objective: Assist with a radiologic procedure under the supervision of a physician or radiologic technologist.

EQUIPMENT AND SUPPLIES
order for X-ray examination; dosimeter badge; appropriate X-ray equipment—X-ray film; holder; and machine; processing equipment; drape; lead patient shield

METHOD
1. Check X-ray examination order.
2. Check necessary X-ray equipment as needed.
3. Identify the patient.
4. Determine patient compliance with procedure preparation instructions.
5. Explain the procedure to the patient.
6. Instruct the patient to remove all clothing appropriate for the procedure.
7. Ask the patient to remove all jewelry and metals as needed for the procedure.
8. The following steps will most likely be performed by a radiologic technologist.
9. Position and drape the patient correctly.
10. Align the X-ray tube and cassette at the correct distance and set the controls.
11. Ask the patient to hold his or her breath as necessary.
12. Leave the room and stand behind the lead shield to take the X-ray(s).
13. Ask the patient to take a comfortable position while all X-rays are processed and reviewed.
14. Instruct the patient to dress if the X-rays are satisfactory.
15. Label the X-rays and place them in an envelope, according to office procedures.
16. Document appropriately.

CHARTING EXAMPLE
05/05/XX 7:00 A.M. Chest X-ray done. ··· M. King CMA (AAMA)

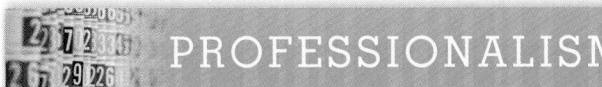

PROFESSIONALISM

THE LAW

To protect the patient and the physician, always have a written order for every procedure. For invasive procedures, a written consent from the patient is necessary before the procedure can be performed.

The procedures discussed in this chapter would not ordinarily be part of the medical assistant's routine work assignment. Assisting with radiologic procedures requires extra training and practice. The medical assistant must refrain from assisting with or performing advanced procedures without adequate training.

In some states, the medical assistant is not allowed to assist with radiologic procedures. If in doubt about the practice and laws within your state, always check with your local medical assistant organization or contact the AAMA office in Chicago, Illinois.

sequencing is important because some procedures, such as those that require the use of contrast medium, may interfere with other tests. In addition, the patient may not be able to tolerate multiple procedures on one day. In general, examinations that do not require the use of contrast medium are performed before examinations with contrast medium. For example, an abdominal X-ray would be taken before a barium enema. Always check with the facility performing the tests to obtain specific instructions for scheduling. Guidelines 48-1 provides guidelines for sequencing multiple diagnostic procedures.

GUIDELINES 48-1

ORDER OF SEQUENCING FOR MULTIPLE RADIOGRAPHIC PROCEDURES

1. All radiographic examinations and tests that do not require contrast media or iodine uptake
2. Radiographic tests of the urinary tract
3. Radiographic tests of the liver and gallbladder
4. CT scans of abdomen and pelvis
5. Procedures requiring barium
6. Lower gastrointestinal series (barium enema)
7. Upper gastrointestinal series

Note: CT procedures that require IV contrast media may be done *after* blood is drawn for an iodine uptake series.

Some procedures require long waiting periods between imaging procedures because it takes time for the contrast medium to move through portions of the body. This should be carefully explained to the patient in order to schedule his or her time appropriately. The patient may have to allow a full morning for a series of X-ray procedures.

Diagnostic Imaging Procedures

Diagnostic imaging procedures can be divided into invasive and noninvasive procedures or divided into categories based on those that use contrast media and those that do not. The latter classification will be used in this chapter. Table 48-3 identifies the most frequently ordered tests and the conditions they are used to diagnose.

RADIOLOGIC IMAGING PROCEDURES REQUIRING CONTRAST MEDIA

Various radiologic procedures involve the use of contrast media. They are as follows: angiography, arthrography, barium enema (lower GI), barium swallow (upper GI), cholangiography, cholecystography, fluoroscopy, intravenous pyelogram (IVP), myelography, nuclear medicine studies, retrograde pyelogram, and sometimes MRI. Contrast media can be administered by mouth, by enema, and by injection through intravenous lines or a catheter.

Fluoroscopy

Fluoroscopy is a technique in radiology for visually examining a portion of the body or the function of an organ using a fluoroscope. This technique allows the radiologist to have immediate images that can be used to assess heart function such as cardiac catheterization. The moving image that is seen on the fluoroscope can then be filmed using a radiograph (X-ray) to obtain a permanent record. Contrast media are often used during fluoroscopic procedures to better visualize organ function and abnormalities. Fluoroscopic procedures include the gastrointestinal series, IVP+, cholecystogram, and myelogram.

Gastrointestinal Series. A gastrointestinal (GI) series is a fluoroscopic study of the digestive tract using contrast media to detect abnormalities such as tumors, ulcers, polyps, and diverticulosis. An upper GI series is an examination of the esophagus, stomach, duodenum, and small intestine. The patient drinks a barium solution, and a fluoroscope outlines the esophagus, stomach, and small intestine as the barium moves through the system. The procedure takes 1 to

Test	Conditions Diagnosed/Treated
Angiography	*Cardiovascular:* Status of blood flow, collateral circulation, aneurysm, hemorrhage, vessel malformation *Cerebral:* Aneurysm, hemorrhage, evidence of CVA, arteriosclerosis *Gastrointestinal (GI):* Upper GI bleeding *Pulmonary:* Pulmonary emboli, evaluation of pulmonary circulation in heart conditions prior to surgery *Renal:* Abnormalities of blood vessels in urinary system
Arthrography	Joint conditions
Barium enema (lower GI)	Obstructions, ulcers, polyps, diverticulosis, tumor, and motility problems of colon or rectum
Barium swallow (upper GI)	Obstruction ulcers, polyps, diverticulosis, tumors, and motility problems of esophagus, stomach, duodenum, and small intestines
Cholangiography and cholecystography	Gallstones, gallbladder, or common bile duct stones or obstructions; ability of gallbladder to concentrate and store bile
Computed tomography (CT)	Aortic and heart aneurysms, disorders of liver and biliary systems, renal and pulmonary tumors, brain abnormalities (tumors, blood clots, CVA, outlines of brain ventricles), GI tract lesions, GI tract disorders (pancreatic cyst, abdominal abscesses, biliary obstruction), breast diseases and disorders, spinal disorders, biopsy guides
Fluoroscopy	Structure, process, and function of organs in motion to detect abnormalities
Intravenous pyelography (IVP), excretory urography, intravenous urography	Urinary system abnormalities, including renal pelvis, ureter, and bladder (kidney stones); abnormal size, shape, or structure of kidneys, ureter, bladder; tumors; cysts; pyelonephrosis; hydronephrosis; trauma to urinary system
KUB (kidneys, ureters, bladder) radiography	Size, shape, and position of urinary organs; urinary system diseases or disorders; kidney stones
Magnetic resonance imaging (MRI)	Cancerous tissue, arthosclerotic tissue, blood clots, tumors, and deformities, particularly of the heart valves, brain, spine, and joints
Mammography	Breast tumors and lesions
Myelography	Irregularities or compression of spinal cord
Nuclear medicine (radionuclide imaging)	Abnormal function, lesions, or disorders of bone, brain, lungs, kidneys, liver, pancreas, thyroid, and spleen
Radiation therapy	Treatment of cancer and some benign tumors or scars
Retrograde pyelogram	Obstruction of ureters, bladder, or urethra
Stereoscopy	Fractures, dense areas that indicate tumor or increased pressure within skull
Thermograph	Breast tumors, breast abscesses, fibrocystic disease
Ultrasound	Abnormalities of gallbladder, liver, spleen, heart, kidneys, gonads, blood vessels, lymph system, fetal conditions: number of fetuses, age, sex, fetal development, position, and deformities
Xeroradiography	Breast cancer, abscesses, lesions, and calcifications

2 hours and produces little discomfort. The barium may cause constipation and white stools for several days following the procedure. The patient should also be advised to drink plenty of liquids to help push the barium through his or her system.

A lower GI series is the administration of a barium enema, which outlines the colon and rectum on a radiographic picture. The lower GI series is done by giving the patient a barium enema and also air to better illuminate the lower part of the digestive tract. Figure 48-3 shows a radiograph of the lower GI tract after a barium enema. Some patients may feel cramping and urgency to move their bowels. They should be encouraged to take deep breaths during the procedure to help relax their abdominal muscles. After the procedure is completed, the patient may defecate, and more X-rays may be taken of the empty colon. The patient should

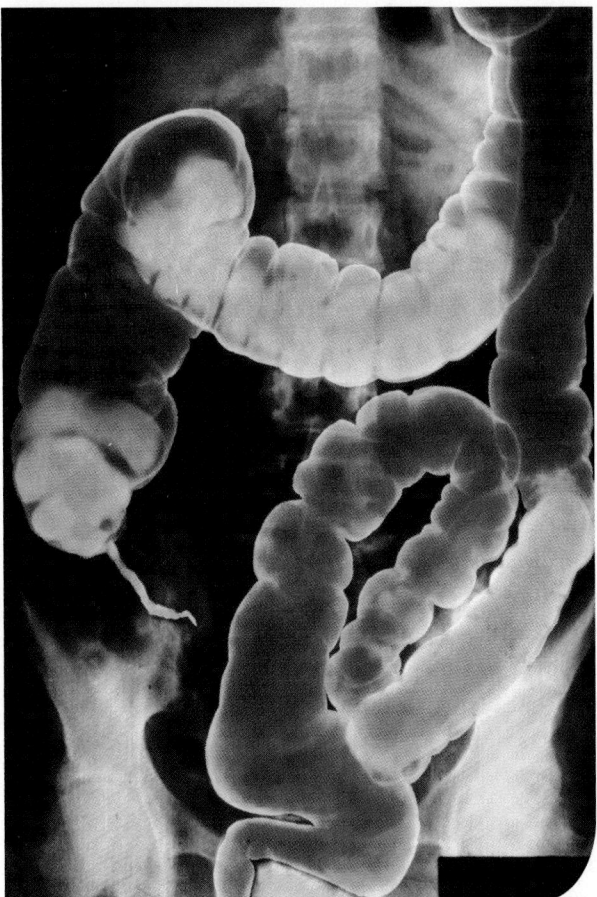

FIGURE 48-3   Radiograph of the colon after a barium enema.

be encouraged to drink water to help move barium out of his or her system and made aware of the possibility of white stools due to the barium.

The patient should receive written instructions prior to these procedures. In addition, the medical assistant should explain the instructions and the procedure. Careful preparation is necessary for good results on these procedures. If the patient's digestive tract is not properly prepared and cleaned, the procedure may have to be repeated. This results in added expense, time, and patient discomfort. Guidelines are provided for the patient who will undergo an upper GI series (Guidelines 48-2) and a lower GI series (Guidelines 48-3).

Intravenous Pyelogram or Excretory Urogram.   The intravenous pyelogram (IVP), also called a pyelogram, intravenous urogram, or excretory urogram, is a radiologic examination of the kidneys, ureters, and bladder. The patient should be screened for iodine sensitivity prior to the procedure. This procedure takes between 60 and 90 minutes. The patient will be instructed to eat a low-residue diet and drink plenty of water the day before the procedure. The patient will be allowed nothing by mouth (NPO) after midnight. A

cathartic, such as castor oil or citrate of magnesia, may be ordered along with an enema to be taken the night before the examination.

The patient will need to undress and wear a patient gown for this procedure. A contrast medium containing iodine is injected into the vein. This substance may cause the patient to have a warm, flushed feeling and a metallic taste in the mouth. The patient should be instructed to notify the radiologist of any unusual symptoms, such as shortness of breath or itching, which could indicate an allergic reaction to the dye.

The patient is tipped into various positions on the X-ray table, which allows the radiologist to view the dye as it flows through the urinary system. The patient may be asked to urinate and then have one final X-ray taken. After the examination, the patient can return to a normal diet. He or she should be encouraged to drink water to flush out the contrast medium through the kidneys.

GUIDELINES 48-3

LOWER GI SERIES

The colon and rectum need to be free of stool for a clear view of the area on X-ray.

Day Before the Examination

- The patient may be instructed to follow a low-residue diet for several days before the test. On the morning before the test, he or she will change to an all-liquid diet (such as water and clear soup) because NO solid foods may be taken until after the procedure.
- A cathartic, such as castor oil or citrate of magnesia, may be ordered to be taken at 4:00 P.M. the day before the procedure. Enemas must be taken until the return fluid is clear.

Day of the Examination

- The patient must undress and wear a patient gown for the procedure. Another cleansing enema may be given before the procedure.
- The patient lies on his or her side on the X-ray table while the technician gives an enema of barium sulfate. The patient is asked to retain or hold the enema within the rectal and colon area.
- The patient is then moved or tipped into different positions on the table while the radiologist observes the flow of barium on the fluoroscope. Radiographs (X-rays) are taken periodically during the procedure.
- The patient is asked to expel the barium into the toilet. Then a final X-ray is taken of the empty bowel.
- The patient may return to a regular diet after this procedure. Whitish stools may be present for 1 or 2 days after the procedure. The patient should be encouraged to drink water to flush out the remaining barium with stool.

Retrograde Pyelography. Retrograde means "against the normal flow,' and **retrograde pyelography** involves inserting a catheter into the urinary tract through the bladder and into the ureters. The dye is sent up the tube into the ureters and kidneys, and X-rays are taken to evaluate the function of the ureters, bladder, and urethra. The post-procedural recommendations are the same as those for the IVP.

Cholecystogram. A cholecystogram is a radiologic examination of the gallbladder using a contrast medium, usually iodine. This procedure is done to detect abnormalities such as the presence of gallstones. Although this procedure has been replaced by ultrasound in many facilities, it is still ordered when ultrasound scanning fails to provide a definitive diagnosis.

It is important for the patient to understand that significant time is involved in preparation the night before and the day of the procedure. The patient is instructed to have a fat-free meal the evening before the procedure and NPO after midnight. The contrast medium, in the form of pills, is taken after dinner. The patient is instructed to take one pill at a time every few minutes with water until the six pills have been ingested. In some facilities, the contrast medium is administered by intravenous (IV) injection. The patient undresses and wears a patient gown for this procedure. An initial X-ray is taken to see if the gallbladder is visible. A study is then conducted using the fluoroscope. Radiographs (X-rays) also are taken. After this portion of the procedure, the patient is asked to eat a fatty meal. This meal stimulates the gallbladder to empty. Another X-ray is taken 1 hour after the meal. The patient can resume a normal diet after the procedure is complete; however, the patient should be told that diarrhea is an expected side effect of the contrast medium used in this procedure. Patients should be encouraged to drink plenty of fluids to replace the fluids lost as a result of diarrhea.

Myelography. Myelography is a fluoroscopic procedure of the spinal cord. A lumbar puncture is done to remove some cerebrospinal fluid (CSF) and instill contrast medium. This procedure produces a myelogram and is used to detect compression of the spinal cord or herniated disks. CT scans and MRIs are more commonly done now; however, a myelogram may be needed if the other procedures do not reveal enough detail. A pneumoencephalograph is performed by injecting air instead of contrast media after some cerebral spinal fluid has been removed. This procedure allows visualization of the cavities of the brain.

Angiography

Angiography is the X-ray visualization of the internal anatomy of blood vessels after a radiopaque material has been injected into the blood vessels. This procedure is used to assist in the diagnosis of many conditions, including myocardial infarction (MI or heart attack), cerebrovascular accident (CVA or stroke), renal artery stenosis as a cause of hypertension, clots, stenosis in arteries in the lower extremities and abdomen, aneurysm of the aorta, and pulmonary emboli or clots.

Since iodine is used as the contrast medium, the patient should be tested for allergy to iodine before the procedure begins. The contrast medium is injected into an artery or vein by way of a catheter and threaded through the vessel until it reaches the correct site, whereupon the radiographic image is recorded. The patient is monitored for a few hours after the procedure for any signs of bleeding from the puncture site.

TABLE 48-4 Radiology Procedures Not Requiring Contrast Material

Type of X-ray	Description and Use
Abdomen	Flat plate or survey of abdomen used for suspected tumors, hematomas, enlarged organs, or abscesses.
Bone	X-ray studies of bones for suspected abnormalities from disease or trauma such as fractures and tumors. Commonly performed spinal X-rays are: Cervical—X-ray of neck area Thoracic—X-ray of the middle back Lumbosacral—X-ray of lower back
Breasts	Mammogram
Chest	Routine chest X-rays are taken to rule out any abnormality and to pick up hidden disease in the lungs and some cardiac abnormalities (cardiomegaly). The patient assumes the posteroanterior erect position and a lateral position.
Kidneys, Ureters, Bladder (KUB)	This abdominal X-ray studies the kidneys, ureters, and bladder, abdominal wall, pelvic bones, and unusual masses.
Paranasal sinuses	X-ray of the sinuses found within the maxillary, frontal, ethmoid, and sphenoid bones for signs of infection, inflammation, and abnormalities.

Angiography may be used to study the blood vessels of the brain—cerebral angiography; the kidneys—renal angiography; and the heart—cardiography. This procedure is usually done in the hospital or a same-day surgical facility and requires the use of local anesthetic. Cardiac catheterization, a form of angiocardiography, is frequently performed to assess the status of the coronary arteries. A catheter is inserted into the femoral artery and fed through the arteries until it reaches the heart. If obstructions are discovered, therapeutic interventions can take place, such as balloon angioplasty or stent insertion or bypass surgery, to relieve blockage of coronary arteries.

Angiographic procedures are costly, carry risks, and are not usually performed unless other procedures have failed to provide enough information. Facilities that specialize in angiography have patient preparation sheets available. It would be helpful for you to have a copy of each preparation in the office as reference material.

Arthrography

Arthrography is a diagnostic procedure used to produce an arthrogram or image inside a joint. It is performed by a radiologist to help diagnose abnormalities of the joints, tendons, ligaments, and cartilage of the knee, hip, or shoulder. The procedure involves injecting a local anesthetic followed by contrast medium or air or both into the joint. A fluoroscope is used to evaluate the function of the joint. The procedure usually takes about 1 hour, and the patient should be advised to expect some slight discomfort and swelling for a day or two. The patient should be advised to rest the joint during that time.

RADIOLOGY PROCEDURES NOT REQUIRING CONTRAST MEDIA

Several diagnostic radiologic examinations do not require the use of a contrast material. Table 48-4 lists several of them. The procedures not requiring contrast media include films of the abdomen, bones, chest, kidneys, ureters, bladder (KUB), and paranasal sinuses.

These examinations or films require that the patient be positioned properly; however, no prior preparation, such as an enema, is required. One of these procedures is the mammogram.

Mammography

Mammography is the radiologic examination of the soft tissue of the breast to provide identification of benign and malignant neoplasms (tumors). Breast masses are often smaller than 1 cm. Women are encouraged to perform monthly breast examinations and check for unknown lumps because finding any mass early increases the cure rate significantly. Contrast medium is not used for this procedure. The patient should be instructed not to use underarm deodorant, talcum powder, body lotion, or perfume prior to the procedure since the clarity of the image could be affected.

The patient stands in front of the X-ray equipment, and the technician positions the patient carefully to have all breast tissue examined under X-ray. The patient should be instructed to follow the technician's direction regarding placement of hands, arms, and body position. Patients of childbearing age are given a lead apron to wear during the procedure.

Each breast is alternately compressed by the mammography equipment to spread the tissue for better viewing. The X-rays are directed at angles into the breast tissue. The procedure takes a few seconds for each view with the entire procedure lasting about 30 minutes. Some patients may feel discomfort during the procedure due to pressure during the breast compression. For most patients, the discomfort is over as soon as the compression is completed (less than a minute). Occasionally patients will complain of discomfort for several days after a mammogram, and the physician may suggest they take an over-the-counter analgesic.

Women over the age of 40 are advised by the American Cancer Society to have a yearly mammogram for early detection of breast cancer. Figure 48-4 shows a woman receiving a mammogram.

Many abnormalities detected on mammograms are benign and present no danger to the patient. Figure 48-5 is an example of a normal mammogram.

If a lump is detected, follow-up with further testing should be commenced immediately without waiting to see if

PROFESSIONALISM
THE WORKPLACE

Mammography aids in the diagnosis of breast tumors—some even too small to be felt—but is a relatively uncomfortable procedure for the patient. The breasts must be compressed to allow less radiation to be used and a clearer picture to be taken. This compression often results in discomfort, swelling, and bruising for the patient. To help reduce the negative effects of the compression, the medical assistant should try to schedule the mammogram as close to, or during, the week following the patient's menstrual cycle. During this time the breast will not be as sensitive. Caffeine can also produce a heightened sensitivity to pain and additional swelling, so patients should be advised to cut back, or completely eliminate, caffeine from their diets at least 1 week prior to the procedure.

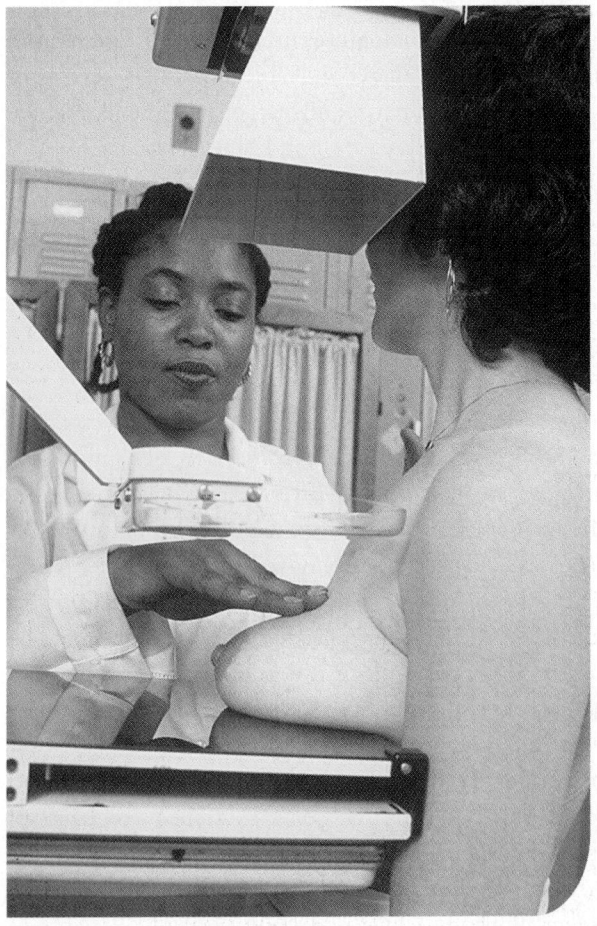

FIGURE 48-4 Compressing the breast between plates provides a better image of breast tissue. Regular mammograms help detect early cancers.

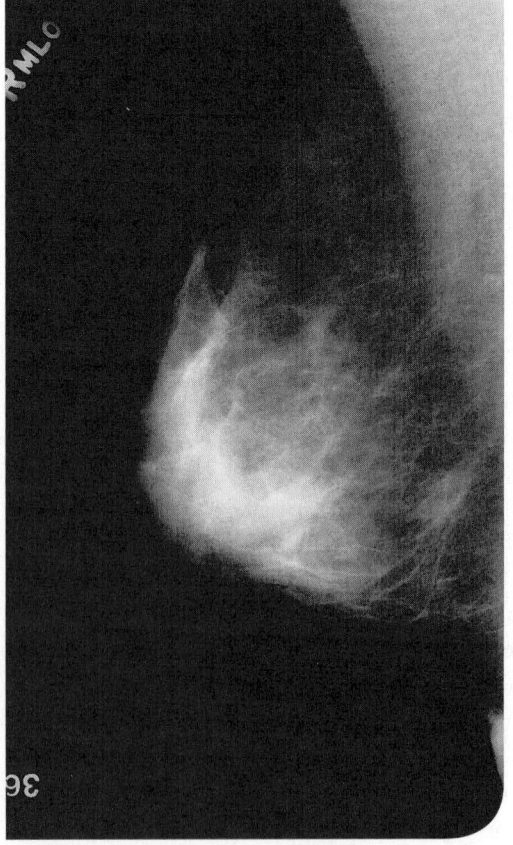

FIGURE 48-5 Normal mammogram.

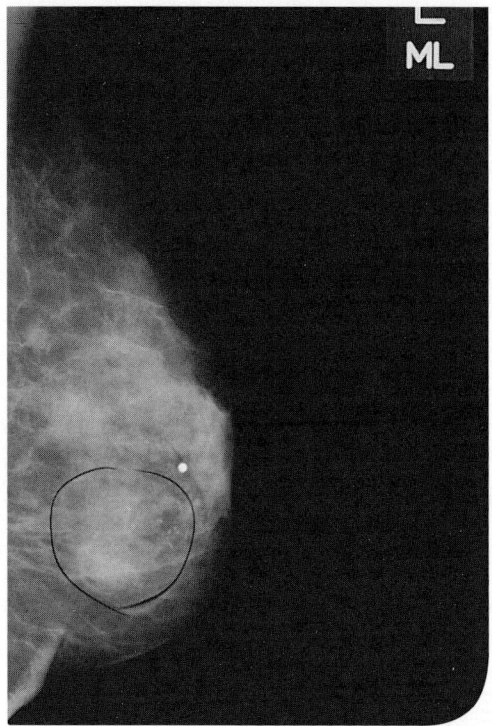

FIGURE 48-6 Mammogram showing microcalcifications.

the lump disappears over time. Once a mammogram reveals suspicious tissue, a breast biopsy should be done to confirm the type of mass detected. A new type of biopsy known as stereotactic breast biopsy is less invasive and less painful than previous types of biopsies. This procedure is done with the patient lying face down with the breast compressed between two paddles with the suspicious mass centered in the window of the paddle. A computer determines the precise positioning of the biopsy needle. A small sample of cells is taken and sent for review by a pathologist. After the examination is complete, the physician informs the patient of the pathologist's findings. Figure 48-6 is an example of an abnormal mammogram showing microcalcifications.

Kidneys, Ureters, and Bladder

A kidneys, ureters, and bladder (KUB) or abdominal flat plate is used to assess the size, shape, and location of the organs of the urinary tract, and to detect kidney stones and diseases of the urinary tract. It is also used to detect the location of an intrauterine device (IUD) or other foreign object.

TOMOGRAPHY

Tomography, or the sectioning of the body using roentgenography, allows the technician to penetrate dense areas of the body that could not otherwise be visualized. When tomography was first introduced it was considered the most significant advancement in diagnostic medicine

since the discovery of the X-ray. Tomography produces tomograms. Tomography has the ability to remove, or blur out, areas that are not within the plane being examined.

Computed Tomography

Computed tomography (CT) combines radiography with computer analysis of tissue density. In CT scans, the X-ray camera rotates completely around the patient, and the computer accumulates cross-sectional slices from each rotation of the camera. The CT scanner consists of a movable table with a remote control; the circular structure, or **gantry**, that houses the X-ray equipment; and an operator console with monitor and computer equipment. Ancillary software and hardware sort, manage, retrieve, and store images. This procedure is painless, noninvasive, and requires no special preparation.

The patient lies on a narrow table that slides into the scanner. A narrow beam of X-ray rotates in a continuous 360-degree motion around the patient to slice the images of the body in cross-sectional angles. The computer then calculates various factors, including tissue absorption, and displays a printout that determines the density of the tissue. In this way, tissue masses, such as tumors, bone displacement, and fluid accumulation are detected. These images are more detailed than those obtained through conventional X-rays.

The CT scan is a valuable diagnostic tool for identifying and discovering tumors such as those found in the brain, liver, gallbladder, and spleen. It is especially valuable in evaluating malignant conditions in the lungs and bones. It can eliminate the need for more invasive procedures. Figure 48-7 is a CT of the skull showing multiple facial fractures.

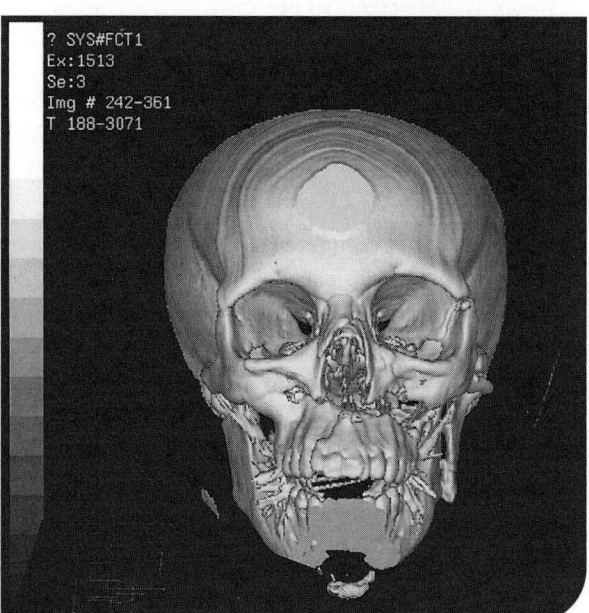

FIGURE 48-7 Three-dimensional CT scan of the skull shows multiple facial fractures.

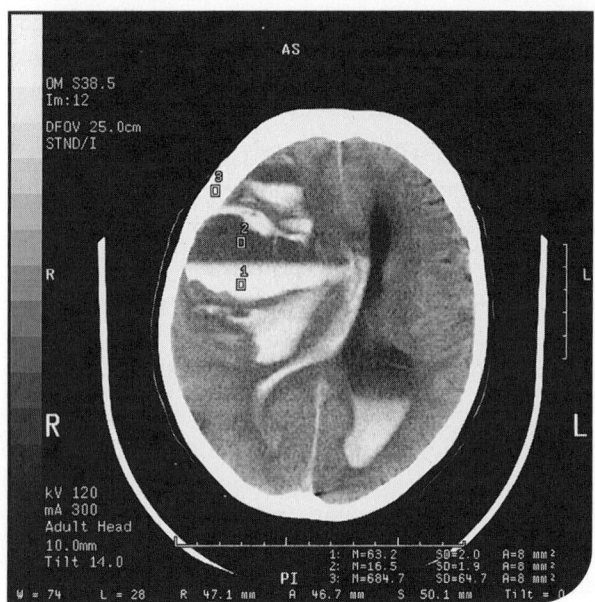

FIGURE 48-8 CT scan of the head shows a massive bleed with a midline shift.

CT scanning and MRI have largely replaced the use of tomography except in areas where these two techniques are not available. CT scans are useful when there is conflicting information about the cause of the patient's condition or when defining exactly where radiation therapy must be directed for tumor masses. Other uses for CT include detecting cerebral abnormalities, such as tumors, hematomas (Figure 48-8), childhood cancers, and abdominal masses, and surveying difficult-to-visualize glands, such as the pituitary gland and tissue. The CT scanner is able to scan the entire body in 15 to 20 minutes, which allows one scanner to scan up to 20 patients in one day.

CT Scan Preparation

In many instances, CT scans involve little prior preparation for the patient. For some CT procedures, a contrast medium is used so the patient may be instructed to have NPO for 4 hours before the procedure.

The imposing size of computed tomography equipment may cause considerable apprehension in a new patient. As with any procedure, a thorough explanation when scheduling the scan helps to relieve patient anxiety. Many patients have never seen a CT scanner, and having a diagram listing the major parts and their basic functions is helpful.

Any metallic objects will interfere with the CT scan, so instruct the patient to remove all metallic objects and inquire whether he or she has a pacemaker or metallic prosthesis.

The table may move continuously in a spiral scanning motion or stop and start, depending on the area being scanned. The patient should be reassured that he or she will not be in a confined space as with an MRI.

POSITRON EMISSION TOMOGRAPHY

Positron emission tomography (PET) is a computerized radiographic method that uses radioactive substances to examine metabolic activity within the body.

For PET scans, the patient is either injected with or inhales a chemical, such as glucose, which carries a radioactive substance. This substance then emits positively charged particles (positrons) that combine with negatively charged electrons found within the body. The rays that are produced are converted into color-coded images that indicate the degree of metabolic activity. PET is used to assist in the treatment of epilepsy, brain tumors, stroke, Alzheimer's disease, blood flow, and metabolism of the heart and blood vessels. This procedure can detect mild early changes in the brain before nerve damage, memory loss, or other symptoms occur. The radioactive elements used in PET are short lived, which results in minimal radiation exposure for patients.

MAGNETIC RESONANCE IMAGING

One of the newest imaging technologies, magnetic resonance imaging (MRI), has changed the field of radiology. The MRI uses a powerful magnetic field to visualize internal tissues, organs, and structures. The images produced with this technique are excellent. All areas of the body can be scanned using the MRI. There is no ionizing radiation used, and the MRI has no known risks. See Figure 48-9 for a color-enhanced MRI image.

The signal or nuclear magnetic resonance produced by the MRI varies with different body tissues. These signals are processed by the computer and form a visual image. An MRI scan can give the viewer a three-dimensional view of tissues or organs of the body in total or as slices. This can be useful for tumor detection.

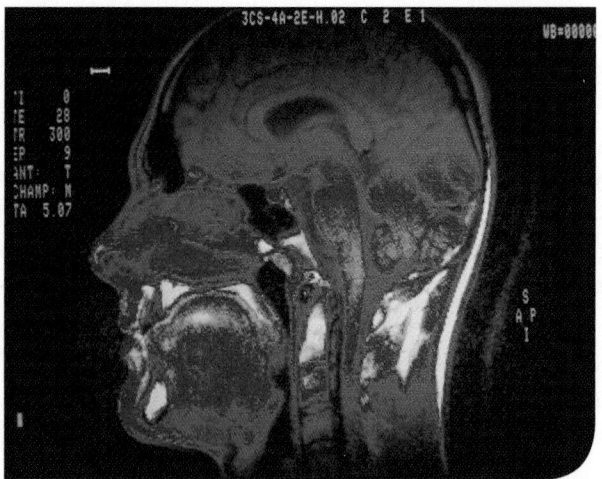

FIGURE 48-9 A color-enhanced MRI image of the skull.

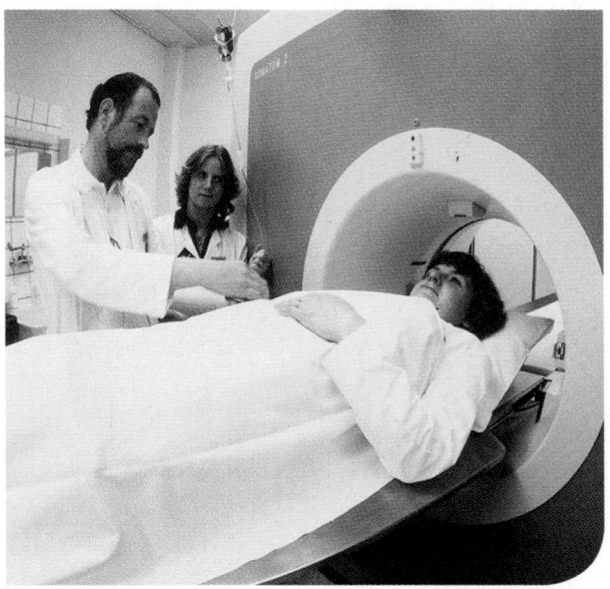

FIGURE 48-10 An open chamber MRI may be more comfortable for the patient, but images may not be as distinct.

Explaining the procedure to the patient should include a description of the type of chamber in which the patient will be placed. One type of chamber consists of a large cylindrical electromagnet. The patient is rolled into it on a pallet. The chamber is sealed, which allows the patient's entire body to come into contact with the electromagnetic field. The procedure, although painless, can be upsetting to patients who have **claustrophobia**, which is a fear of closed-in spaces. The space inside a closed MRI machine is only slightly larger than the average patient. The MRI machine makes loud thumping noises intermittently during the procedure. The patient should be made aware of this noise and be provided with earplugs or earphones to listen to music. In cases of extreme apprehension, the patient may need to be given a medication to promote relaxation. Open MRIs are available for patients who are too large for the enclosed MRI or too apprehensive; however, the images produced may not be as accurate or detailed (Figure 48-10).

Use of the MRI has some limitations. It is not possible to view the hard portion of bone matter. For visualizing fractures and other abnormalities, the CT scan and general X-rays are still used. In addition, the strong magnetic field is not appropriate for patients who have pacemakers or metallic clips on blood vessels. The patient should be instructed to do the following:

- Remove all jewelry, eye shadow, and metallic objects, such as watches, belts, hearing aids, and hairpins.
- Identify which devices, if any, have been inserted within his or her body, such as pacemakers, dental implants, surgical staples, intrauterine devices, joint or

bone pins, prostheses, metallic clips on blood vessels, or metal fragments, such as from a gunshot. These will all be present on the scan and can interfere with magnetic conduction. In addition, metallic clips on blood vessels can become loosened during the procedure.

- Leave credit cards or devices, which contain metallic or magnetic code strips, outside the MRI chamber.
- Use a patient gown if the patient's clothing has zippers or metal snaps.

The technician is not in the chamber with the patient during the procedure. The patient should be told that the technician will be in constant contact with the patient via a microphone and camera. The patient should be instructed to remain still during the procedure. An MRI scan takes from 20 to 60 minutes, depending on the amount of the body to be scanned.

An advancement in MRI technology, the functional MRI, enables physicians to observe the function of organs. Functional MRIs can provide information about nerve activity in the brain and locate areas of the brain activated in memory.

DIGITAL RADIOLOGY

Digital radiology is the use of standard fluoroscopy, which is digitized, stored as computer bits, processed, and then converted into an image on a television or video monitor screen. The image is stored on videotape or digital disc. Digital angiography is used for cardiac and pulmonary arteries and head and neck angiograms.

ULTRASOUND (SONOGRAPHY)

Ultrasound, or sonography, is the use of high-frequency sound waves to image internal structures. Ultrasound imaging consists of projecting a beam of sound waves into the body. The waves at about 20,000 cycles per second bounce back as the beam comes into contact with a structure, such as a fetus, which then produces an outline of the internal structure.

Ultrasound has valuable medical applications, such as fetal monitoring and detecting abnormalities, such as gallstones, tumors, and heart defects. It is used to scan organs such as the liver, heart, kidneys, thyroid, gonads, and blood vessels. Ultrasound is not used to image the lungs, brain, or skeleton since they are made of or surrounded by bone, which sound waves cannot penetrate.

Ultrasound uses no ionizing radiation and is a painless noninvasive procedure. It has been widely accepted as a safe examination of delicate tissues and the fetus. Fetal ultrasound is commonly performed to detect the presence of multiple pregnancies, fetal and placental positioning, and internal organ development. The use of ultrasound is not recommended simply to determine gender of the fetus.

Ultrasound Scanning

To perform an ultrasound procedure, a conduction material such as water, special jelly, or oil is used to conduct the sound waves into the body. An ultrasonic **transducer** (a device that both produces and senses ultrasonic waves) with a conduction head is then placed on or near the skin. As sound waves pass through the skin, they bounce off the body tissues or fetus and remit back to the instrument an echo reflection of the image. These echoes of the body tissue or fetus are then recorded as a series of dots on an oscilloscope (an instrument that displays a visual picture). The record produced is an echogram or a sonogram (Figure 48-11). The patient is often able to view the sonogram on the screen as it occurs. A printout of this visual picture can then be printed for the patient's record and, in some cases, a copy of this printout is given to the patient. Usually, the sonogram will require some interpretation. The medical assistant should not attempt to explain the results to the patient.

Patient preparation for the ultrasound examination is minimal. The patient should wear loose-fitting garments or clothing that is easy to remove since the procedure is performed over bare skin (Figure 48-12). During a fetal ultrasound or pelvic ultrasound, the patient is instructed not to urinate right before the test since a full bladder displaces the intestines and allows for a better view of the uterus. In fact, the patient may be asked to drink a quart or more of water just prior to either of these examinations. For an ultrasound of the gallbladder or liver, the patient may be asked not to eat for several hours before the procedure.

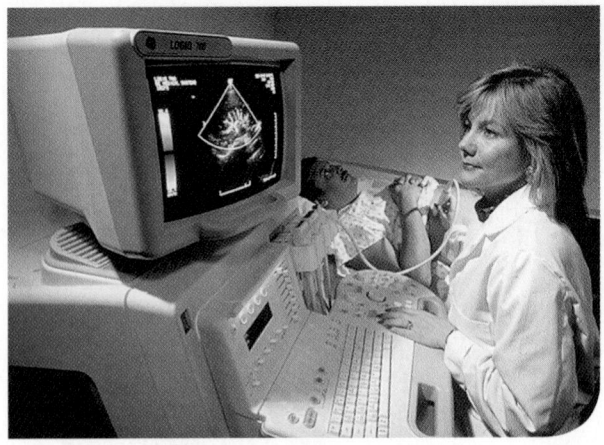

FIGURE 48-12   An ultrasound being performed on a patient.

Ultrasound is also used in physical therapy and is discussed in Chapter 51.

Radiation Therapy

Radiation, as employed in medicine, is the use of a radioactive substance in the diagnosis and treatment of disease. Radiation therapy is the process of administering a particular dosage of radiation to a specific area on the patient's body for the purpose of killing diseased cells, such as cancers. Radiation actually alters the cells so they cannot reproduce and thus eventually die, leaving no new cells to develop. Both diseased and normal cells are altered with radiation. Diseased cells are eventually destroyed; however, normal or healthy cells are able to repair themselves and multiply. Radiation therapy is also known as cobalt treatment, X-ray treatment, or radiotherapy.

RADIATION RAYS

In radiation therapy, the radioactive substances used emit three types of rays: alpha, beta, and gamma. Alpha rays are the least penetrating rays and are positively charged helium particles released by the disintegration of radioactive material. Beta rays are able to penetrate body tissues a few millimeters and are negatively charged electrons released when atoms of radioactive substances disintegrate. Gamma rays have great penetrating power and are electromagnetic waves emitted by atoms of radioactive elements as they undergo disintegration. Gamma rays can penetrate most body tissue but are absorbed by lead. All three ray types are similar to X-rays, but they come from the element's nucleus, while X-rays come from the orbit of the element's atom.

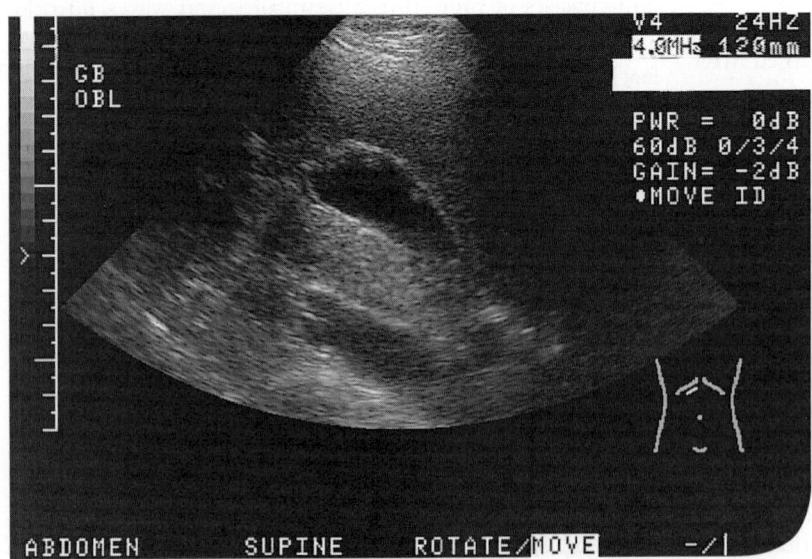

FIGURE 48-11   An ultrasound echogram or sonogram of the abdomen.

USES OF RADIATION THERAPY

Radiation therapy is administered after a tumor is well defined in the patient. Tumors are located through the use of CT scan and ultrasound. The boundary of the tumor can be localized by these radiologic procedures.

There are a few factors to consider when determining whether or not to use radiation therapy to treat a cancer patient: Is the tumor surrounded by normal tissue that can repair itself after radiation treatment? Will the radiation be used to alleviate symptoms if the cancer has metastasized? Is the tumor sensitive to radiation?

Patients receive radiation therapy for a variety of types of cancers including cancer of the ovaries, testes, skin, larynx, and oral cavity. Hodgkin's disease, Wilms' tumor (a type of kidney tumor found in children), and retinoblastoma are also treated with radiation therapy. For some types of malignancies, such as cervical cancer, a combination of radiation and chemotherapy is used. In some cases, when a cure is not probable, radiation may be used to shrink tumors to alleviate pain, relieve pressure, or stop bleeding. In these instances, radiation therapy may improve the patient's quality of life. Certain benign conditions may be treated with radiation, such as keloids (abnormal scars) and malformed blood vessels in the brain, which cannot be accessed any other way.

Radiation Therapy Techniques

There are two methods for administering radiation: external radiation therapy (ERT) and internal radiation therapy (IRT).

External Radiation Therapy. External radiation therapy (ERT) involves administering calculated doses of radiation from a machine positioned at a specific distance from the site (tumor). A marker or tattoo is placed on the patient at the exact site or port of entry. A computer calculates the dosage required to destroy the largest number of malignant cells while causing the least damage to surrounding cells. It may be necessary to schedule a series of ERT treatments over a period of weeks or months.

Internal Radiation Therapy. Internal radiation therapy (IRT) can be administered into the body in two forms: sealed or unsealed radiation therapy. Sealed radiation involves the implantation of sealed containers of radioactive material near the tumor in the body. For example, radium, cesium–137, or cobalt–60 may be sealed in small gold containers or seeds and implanted in or near the tumor site. Unsealed radiation involves introducing a liquid form of radioactive substance into the patient by mouth, bloodstream, or instillation into a body cavity. For instance, radioactive iodine–131, phosphorous–32, and gold–198 may be administered in unsealed forms.

Radiation therapy is not usually disfiguring but may cause side effects in some patients, including hair loss, skin changes, nausea, and diarrhea; irritation of the mucous membranes in the mouth, throat, bladder, and vagina; and chromosome changes. The symptoms vary in intensity and may last 3 to 6 weeks.

Nuclear Medicine

Nuclear medicine is a branch of medicine that uses radioactive isotopes in the diagnosis and treatment of disease. Isotopes are chemical elements that may have several forms but identical properties. Radioactive refers to the ability to give off radiation as the result of the disintegration of the nucleus in an atom. Nuclear medicine is also known as radionuclide imaging.

Radioactive isotopes of iodine, cobalt, and other elements are used in nuclear medicine for the treatment of tumors and for nuclear imaging of certain parts of the body. Radionuclides, which are isotopes whose nuclei (central core) are undergoing decay, are administered to the patient intravenously, orally, or through instillation into body cavities or organs. The radionuclides then travel to a point within the body that attracts them. For example, iodine is attracted to the thyroid and creates an image or outline of that organ or tumor (abnormality). Radionuclides have a short life, which results in very few side effects for the patient. Radionuclide imaging exposes the patient to lower doses of radiation than some other radiologic procedures.

A concentration of radionuclides is referred to as either "hot" or "cold." If the radionuclide is in an area with an abnormality, it is referred to as "hot." If the radionuclide does not concentrate into a tumor but is situated in the surrounding area, it is referred to as "cold." Both hot and cold areas can indicate the presence of abnormalities. Scans of different areas of the body require various preparations and varying lengths of time. The patient must be informed of the expected time. For instance, a bone scan takes about an hour (Figure 48-13); however, the patient is given an injection 2 hours prior to the scan and then must drink a quart of water. Kidney scans last 2 hours. Thyroid uptake may require 2 days; after the patient takes the initial radioactive capsule, he or she must return 24 and 48 hours after the capsule is taken.

Scanning is the process of studying an area with a concentration of a radioactive substance. The technician uses a gamma counter or camera that detects the radiation and converts it into an image or scintigram, which is displayed on a screen. The thyroid, liver, and brain are frequently evaluated using the scanning process.

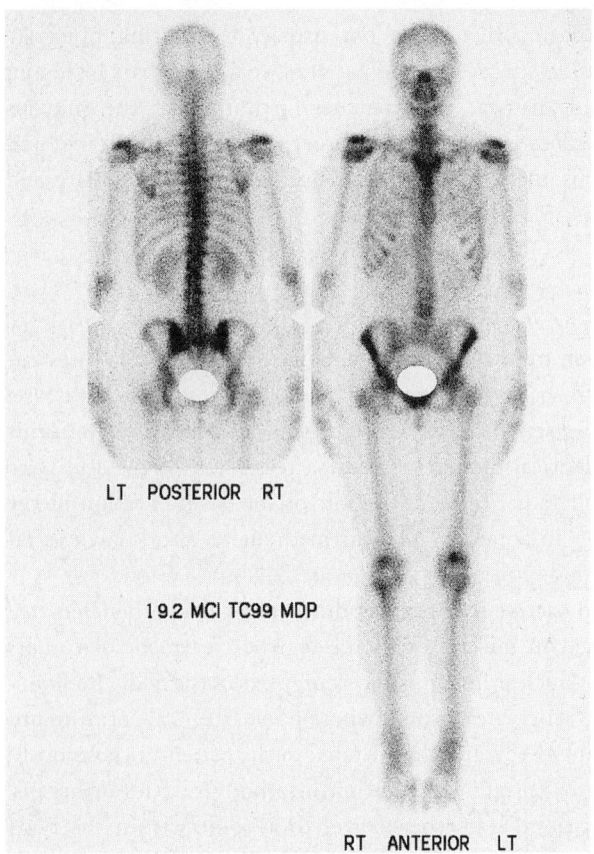

FIGURE 48-13 A nuclear medicine bone scan.

LT POSTERIOR RT

19.2 MCI TC99 MDP

RT ANTERIOR LT

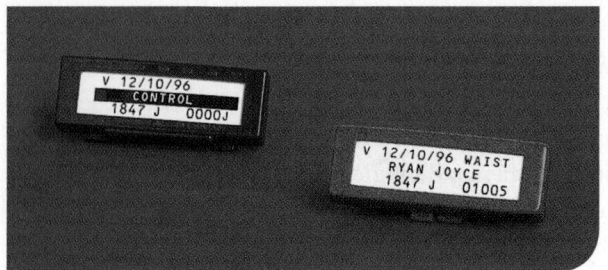

FIGURE 48-14 Dosimeter or personal radiation badge.

If a radioisotope is used in a high dose for treatment, then the patients may have symptoms that are similar to those found with radiation. These include hair loss, nausea, diarrhea, mucous membrane irritation (in the mouth, throat, and bladder), and chromosome changes.

Safety Precautions

Radiation dose is measured in several different units, all of which relate to the amount of energy deposited. The units include the roentgen (R), the gray (Gy), and the sievert (Sv). The sievert and the gray are similar, except that the sievert takes into account the biologic effects of different types of radiation. The biological effect of radiation exposure varies with the type of radiation and its energy. Equal doses of different types of radiation will not always result in the same biological effects. A rad, which stands for radiation absorbed dose, is the unit used to measure the amount of ionizing radiation absorbed during an X-ray procedure. To measure occupational exposure or other exposure that may involve more than one type of radiation, the unit used is the **rem**, which stands for "roentgen equivalent in man." The dosimeter or personal radiation badge containing the occupational exposure dose is reported in rem (Figure 48-14).

RADIATION EXPOSURE

People are constantly exposed to low levels of natural ionizing radiation or background radiation from outer space and radon exposure. In addition, people are exposed to ionizing radiation from human-made sources such as nuclear weapons testing and radiation from medical testing and treatments. On average, diagnostic imaging emits lower doses of ionizing radiation than occur naturally. Advances in diagnostic imaging have reduced the radiation dose a patient is exposed to during a diagnostic procedure. Excessive exposure to radiation causes tissue damage and side effects.

Overexposure to radiation may result in radiation sickness, causing symptoms such as lowered red blood cell and white blood cell counts, bone marrow alteration, burns, damage to ovaries and testes, fetal damage (especially during the first 3 months of pregnancy), and cancer. Radiation sickness from overexposure is usually the result of long-term exposure and is generally delayed. Radiation sickness may result in cancer and premature aging. The severity of radiation sickness depends on the dose of radiation, the type of radiation, duration of exposure, and what areas of body were exposed. Radiation sickness can occur after nuclear reactor accidents.

Cellular Effects of Radiation

At the cellular level, radiation damages the DNA of cells in both malignant and normal cells. Normal cells are better able to repair DNA damage than cancer cells; therefore, treatment with radiation kills the cancer cells, whereas after a period of time damaged normal cells in the area will repair themselves. Sensitivity to radiation of cells increases with their increased rate of cell division. In other words, cells that divide more frequently, such as hair; mucous membranes of nose, mouth, skin, and GI tract; as well as some glands, such as breast and thyroid, are more sensitive. The less specialized a normal cell is, the more affected by radiation it will be. Cells of the bone marrow and germ cells such as sperm and ovum fall into this category. Excessive radiation to embryonic cells causes spontaneous abortion, retardation, genetic abnormalities, and increased risk of leukemia and other cancers. The genetic defects can be passed on to future generations. Some cancers, such as leukemias, lymphomas, and squamous cell carcinomas of the mouth and skin, are more radiation sensitive and are treated using radiation therapy.

PERSONNEL SAFETY PRECAUTIONS

Since X-rays are potentially dangerous to both the patient and the health care personnel, special precautions must be taken.

Radiation is discussed in terms of primary and secondary radiation. Primary radiation strikes the patient for either therapeutic reasons or for an X-ray examination. Once the primary beam strikes the patient, it can then become secondary radiation as it bounces off the patient. Secondary radiation is strongest closest to the patient. Lead has been proven to be an effective barrier to an X-ray beam. Lead aprons, shields, and gloves are provided for personnel coming into close contact with X-ray equipment. X-ray technicians do not normally remain next to the patient during the X-ray process. Rather, they stand behind a lead-shielded divider. X-ray rooms are lined with metal (1 inch thick) as a precaution against X-ray beams escaping from the room. Some facilities have a red light that flashes when X-ray equipment is in use to warn others not to enter.

A film badge or **dosimeter** is worn on the outer clothing of all personnel working with or near radiologic equipment. The badge records the level and intensity of radiation exposure. It is periodically examined to ensure that the health care worker is not exposed to excessive radiation. Radiation exposure is **cumulative**, meaning that each exposure to radiation is added to the effect of all previous exposures. All radiographic equipment should be checked on a regular basis to ensure it is in good working condition and to check for radiation leakage. Radioactive diagnostic materials must be stored in a safe environment and amounts of radioactive material closely monitored. Radioactive materials should be stored in lead containers and handled only with forceps, never with bare hands. Most facilities employ a radiation safety monitor who specifies the requirements for the facility and ensures that OSHA guidelines are observed.

PATIENT SAFETY PRECAUTIONS

The guiding principle in the use of radiation is "as low as reasonably achievable" (ALARA). In other words, the exposure of both patients and workers should always be guided by the idea that it is most prudent to use the lowest amount of exposure to perform the task.

Patient safety requires that a thorough history of the patient be taken. If the patient is female, the 10-day rule about the possibility of pregnancy should apply: an X-ray may be taken only within 10 days of the last menstrual period to avoid taking an X-ray of a female who is unknowingly pregnant. If a patient is unsure about a pregnancy, then a pregnancy test should be performed or the radiographic test postponed until a pregnancy test is completed, unless an emergency situation exists. In cases of emergency, the danger of exposure to the embryo or fetus should be explained to the mother.

Patients should be protected from secondary or scatter radiation by the use of a **grid** during radiographic procedures. Excess scatter may add density to the image and expose the patient unnecessarily. The grid is positioned between the X-ray machine and the patient to absorb radiation scatter before it reaches the film. A Potter–Bucky diaphragm, or a **bucky**, is a type of grid composed of alternating strips of lead and radiolucent material. Not all secondary radiation is absorbed by a grid, so other safety precautions are necessary.

A lead barrier or lead shields should be used by both patients and workers. Patients should be provided with a lead shield for gonads, eyes, breasts, and thyroid whenever appropriate. Employees should use gonad shields, if at the reproductive age (55 years or under), whenever the sex organs are going to be exposed to radiation. For a female patient, the gonad shield should be placed with its lowest margin at the level of the pubic symphysis. In the male, the upper edge of the lead shield should be placed 1 inch below the pubic symphysis.

An implant may present a hazard while the implant is in place in a patient who is undergoing radiation therapy. The length of time the hazard exists depends on the half-life of the material used. The half-life is the time it takes for half of the isotope to decay.

Symptoms caused by radiation therapy will generally not begin for several days after the first treatment. This allows time for the patient and family to thoroughly understand what to expect and what steps to take to make the patient more comfortable. The skin is at most risk, and radiation therapy frequently results in inflammation similar to sunburn. If the burns are deep enough, hair roots are damaged and hair will fall out. Radiation side effects, healing time, and patient interventions are summarized in Table 48-5.

Guidelines 48-4 provides a summary of guidelines for safeguarding the safety of health care workers, and Guidelines 48-5 provides a summary of guidelines for patients.

TABLE 48-5 Radiation Side Effects, Healing Time, and Interventions

Effect On/In Body	Healing Time	Intervention
Alopecia	Hair may grow back in several months.	Shampoo with mild soap, brush, and comb gently; wear scarves or wigs if hair loss is extensive.
Bone marrow and lymphoid tissue	Depends on dosage and degree of damage.	Protect from infection; assess for anemia; watch lymphoid tissue for bleeding and signs of thrombocytopenia; avoid trauma from injections and IVs.
Ear	Depends on dosage and degree of damage.	Assess for blockage of Eustachian tube and bulging eardrum; protect from falls due to dizziness; assess for hearing loss; administer antibiotic for infection.
Eyes	Depends on dosage and degree of damage.	Assess for drying, excessive tearing, conjunctivitis, damage to lens, cataract formation; use artificial tears as needed and antibiotic for infection.
Intestinal mucosa	Several weeks or months, depending on irritation.	Check intake/output levels; assess for diarrhea and vomiting; administer antidiarrheal or antiemetic agents if necessary; encourage intake of potassium-rich food; avoid dairy products; weigh daily.
Nervous system	Necrosis of brain can develop as much as a year after treatment.	Assess for level of cognition, dizziness, slurred speech, weakness, and numbness or tingling in extremities; assess for spinal cord damage, changes in gait, pain; assess for incontinence.
Oral mucosa	Within weeks if irritation not severe.	Increase fluid intake; avoid hot, spicy foods and liquids; restrict smoking; suck ice chips; use lip balm; use artificial saliva if necessary.
Skin: 1st- to 4th-degree burns	7 days to several weeks or months	Assess skin daily; do not use drying substances such as alcohol; avoid lying on area, direct sunlight, and direct heat sources.
Urinary mucosa	Several weeks to months, depending on level of irritation.	Increase fluid intake; measure urinary output; urinalysis; administer antibiotics if infection present.

GUIDELINES 48-4

MAINTAINING PERSONNEL SAFETY

- Wear a film badge on outer clothing at all times when exposed to any form of X-rays. Do not wear a patient gown or lead shield over the badge. These badges are submitted for routine—usually weekly—evaluation of the levels of radiation exposure.
- Health care personnel should stay behind a lead shield in a lead-lined room when the X-ray equipment is in use.
- A sign or lighted display should be visible and the X-ray room door should be closed when X-ray equipment is in use.
- Nonessential personnel should leave the X-ray room.
- All equipment should be inspected on a frequent, routine basis to check for radiation leakage.

- The patient should not be held or supported during radiologic procedures. There are devices that can be used to hold and position the patient.
- If it is necessary to remain in the room with the patient, the attendant should wear a protective lead apron and lead-lined rubber gloves. The attendant should face the patient with the lead apron between the patient and the attendant.
- Periodic blood tests may be required by facilities to determine the presence of blood abnormalities from radiation exposure.

Radiographic Equipment

Medical assistants will not be performing the duties of a radiology technician in most cases. However, you may be employed in a facility where X-rays are taken, thus a basic familiarity with radiographic equipment may be helpful.

The source of the radiation is the X-ray tube, which is located inside a protective covering or housing. The housing protects the X-ray tube and provides places for various attachments that allow the radiographer to move the tube and adjust the size and shape of the X-ray beam. The housing may be attached to the ceiling or mounted on a stand to provide mobility and flexibility of positioning. The X-ray or radiographic table provides support for the patient but also is highly specialized. Figure 48-15 illustrates an X-ray machine with X-ray tube, **collimeter** (device that controls the size and shape of the X-ray field coming from the tube), table, and bucky tray for film and cassette. Some tables have adjustable heights, tilt into various positions, and float to allow ease in positioning the patient. A grid and bucky slide below the table to prevent excess scatter radiation. The bucky holds a cassette tray, which holds the X-ray film. The grid is placed between the tabletop and the film. The bucky moves the grid during exposure so that it is invisible on the X-ray.

The control console is located in the lead-lined booth where the radiographer stands. Here the radiographer determines exposure factors and controls the functions of the procedure.

The cassette provides a rigid structure to hold the film and also holds two intensifying screens, one in front and one behind the film. These screens are coated with phosphors or fluorescent crystals that emit light when exposed to X-rays. Intensifying screens make it possible to use lower doses of radiation on the patient.

Radiographic film is very sensitive to light emitted by the intensifying screens. Routine X-ray film is coated with

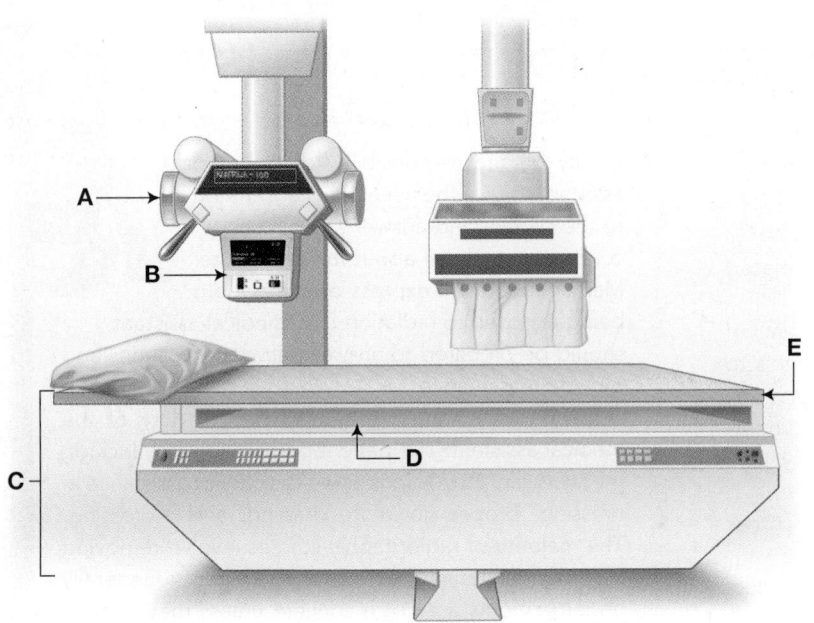

FIGURE 48-15 Generic parts of radiographic equipment: (A) X-ray tube; (B) collimeter; (C) radiographic table; (D) bucky tray for cassette and film; (E) movable table.

an emulsion on both sides so that the film responds to the intensifying screens on both sides. Films and cassettes come in various sizes and are labeled in inches and centimeters.

Processing X-ray Film

Film development takes place in the darkroom of the facility because exposure to light can ruin the film. Red or orange safe lights in the darkroom are dim but provide enough light to see where items are located. The darkroom should always be locked when processing film. Both manual and automated processing methods are used. The automated processing method can meet quality control standards since the equipment can be tested frequently for accuracy. Automated processing may take about 90 seconds or up to 10 minutes, depending on the equipment used. The film is fed into the processor that transports the film through processing chemicals, dries the film, and moves it out of the equipment for the radiologist to view and read.

Storage and Records

X-ray materials for radiologic procedures must be kept in special storage containers that protect the film from damage due to light, heat, chemical fumes, and moisture. For film to remain fresh, it should be kept in a dry, cool place within a sealed package. X-ray film should be stored on end to prevent pressure damage from stacking the film. The expiration dates, which are printed on the top end of the package, can be seen clearly when stored on end. X-ray developer is also

kept in a cool location that is moisture free since damage to this fluid can affect the quality of the film. Film should only be touched with one hand and should be hung vertically to avoid damage. The film packages are only opened in the darkroom of the medical facility because light will destroy the film's imaging ability.

All film records are maintained in a record or logbook that is kept in the X-ray room. Entered in this record are the film identification number, patient's name, date, and type of X-rays taken. Each film taken will have an identification number, which is placed on the film holder or cassette with lead letters or numbers at the time the X-ray film is readied (time of exposure). These ID numbers will identify the physician's name, the date, and the patient's name. These data will then be permanently on the film after it is processed.

Films that have been processed should be stored in custom envelopes and filed in specially designed film cabinets. They are usually filed alphabetically. If a chronological numbering system is used based on the identification number of each film, a master log must be maintained. If a film has to be removed from the file cabinet, an insert explaining where the film was sent is filed in place of the film within the file cabinet.

Ownership of Film

The medical assistant is frequently called on to explain the ownership of film to the patient. Although the patient has paid for the film, it is the property of the medical facility or hospital that performed the X-ray. Written reports prepared by the radiologist are sent to other physicians at the request of the patient, but the film generally remains in the original office or hospital. The reason for this is simple: if the film remains in one location, it can always be accessed for future examination and comparison. Once it leaves the originating facility, it can be misplaced and lost.

Physicians are able to loan their films to referring physicians for further examination. The patient has to sign a release of records form for this to take place, but the film must then be returned to the original facility. Since films are a permanent record of the patient at a particular moment, they must be preserved carefully. It is possible, in some locations, for the patient to obtain a duplicate copy of a film. The patient might have to pay for the copy to be made.

SUMMARY

The use of radiology in medical practice makes it possible to view internal body structures and functions and therefore assist in diagnosis and treatment. These procedures include radiology, radiation therapy, and nuclear medicine.

There are inherent risks to the patients, technicians, and medical assistants in performing these procedures. The use of proper safety precautions can greatly reduce or eliminate these risks altogether.

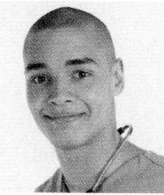

48 CHAPTER REVIEW

COMPETENCY REVIEW

Note: These competencies may only be practiced by a medical assistant if permitted by state law.

1. Define and spell the terms to learn for this chapter.

2. Correctly position the patient for the AP, PA, RL, and LL.

3. Explain radiologic procedures and preparations to patients.

4. Demonstrate safety precautions relevant to radiology procedures.

5. Describe a film badge and its use.

6. Demonstrate how to store X-ray film in the office.

PREPARING FOR THE CERTIFICATION EXAM

1. Some radiographic procedures often call for an all-liquid diet on the day before the test. An all-liquid diet means the patient can eat all of the following EXCEPT
   a. tomato juice
   b. clear gelatin desserts
   c. fat-free milk
   d. bouillon
   e. coffee

2. Iodine contrast compounds used to form radiopaque compounds are employed for
   a. thyroid studies
   b. pyelograms
   c. angiograms
   d. cholecystograms
   e. all of the above

3. Negative media contrast includes all EXCEPT which of the following?
   a. air
   b. carbon dioxide
   c. other gases
   d. barium sulfate
   e. oxygen

4. Which of the following X-ray procedures DOES NOT require the patient to be NPO, unless a contrast media is used?
   a. barium meal (upper GI)
   b. bronchogram
   c. computed tomography (CT)
   d. intravenous cholangiogram
   e. myelogram

5. In which of the following radiology positions is the X-ray beam directed from front to back?
   a. axial
   b. lateral
   c. oblique
   d. posterioanterior (PA)
   e. anterioposterior (AP)

6. In which of the following radiology positions is the X-ray beam directed from back to front?
   a. axial
   b. lateral
   c. oblique
   d. posterioanterior (PA)
   e. anterioposterior (AP)

7. In which of the following radiology positions is the X-ray beam directed toward one side of the body?
   a. axial
   b. lateral
   c. oblique
   d. posterioanterior (PA)
   e. anterioposterior (AP)

8. In which of the following radiology positions is the X-ray tube angled to direct a ray along the axis of the body or body part?
   a. axial
   b. lateral
   c. oblique

   d. posterioanterior (PA)
   e. anterioposterior (AP)

9. In which of the following radiology position is the patient turned at an angle to the film plate so the X-ray beam can be directed at areas that would be hidden on other films?
   a. axial
   b. lateral
   c. oblique
   d. posterioanterior (PA)
   e. anterioposterior (AP)

10. Which diagnostic imaging procedure is used for the treatment of breast tumor, breast abscess, and fibrocystic disease?
   a. thermograph
   b. xeroradiography
   c. mammography
   d. myelography
   e. radiation therapy

CRITICAL THINKING

1. Because Timothy's gallbladder ultrasound did not provide a definitive diagnosis, what radiographic test might Dr. Miller order if he still suspects gallstones?

2. Based on your answer to the preceding question, is a contrast medium used with this test? If so, does it have any side effects the patient should be informed of, and are there any patients who could not use this form of contrast medium?

3. What does the patient need to do to prepare for this test? Be as detailed as possible.

ON THE JOB

Marge Riley, an overweight 50-year-old woman with a history of abdominal pain, has been scheduled for a lower GI series on Monday morning. She states she has board meetings every Monday morning at which breakfast is served and that she will come in for her X-rays after the meeting is over. Marge indicates that she does not understand why she needs these procedures.

1. What, if anything, would you tell the patient regarding her need for these procedures?
2. How would you describe these procedures to the patient?
3. What combination of teaching methods would you use to explain the procedures?
4. You are still concerned, after explaining everything to Marge, that she will not follow the instructions. What do you do?

INTERNET ACTIVITY

Search the Internet for information about the history of radiology. When were X-rays first taken? When did physicians first realize that radiographic waves were dangerous?

MEDMEDIA

Additional interactive resources and activities for this chapter can be found:

On your student DVD: View applicable procedure videos on the DVD-ROM found in the back of this book.

MyHealthProfessionsKit.com: Test your knowledge of the chapter with games and activities. MyHealthProfessionsKit also includes resources, helpful links, and a Spanish audio glossary.

Medical Assisting Interactive: Practice your procedures as a medical assistant in this simulated doctor's office. This can be accessed through MyHealthProfessionsKit.com.

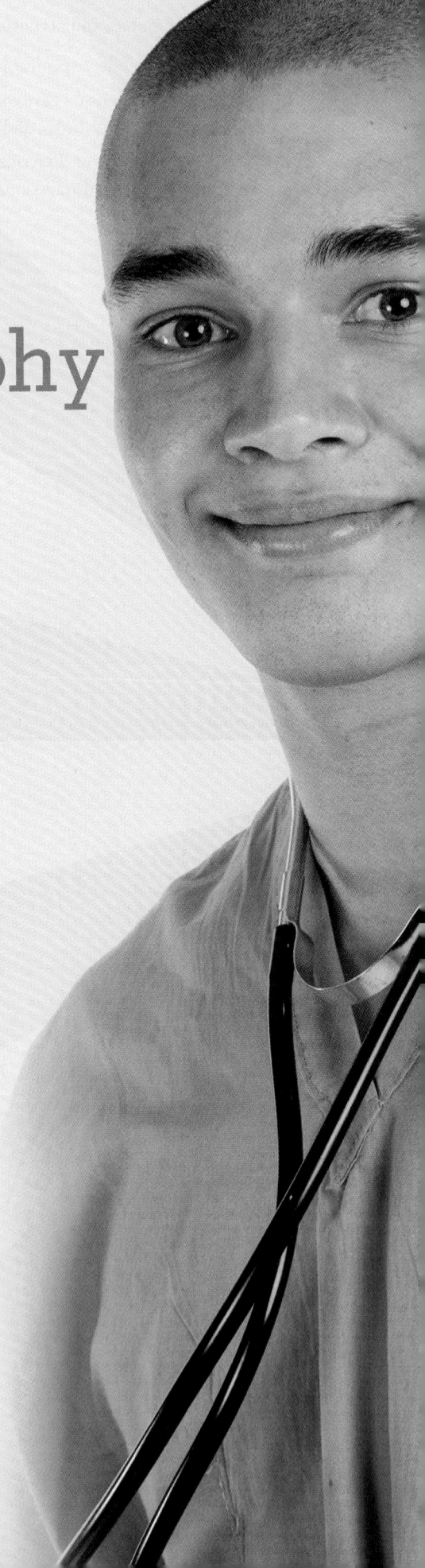

49

Electrocardiography

LEARNING OBJECTIVES

After completing this chapter, you should be able to:

- Define and spell the terms to learn for this chapter.

- Explain the significance of each ECG wave.

- Maintain and operate electrocardiogram equipment.

- Identify by name and function the controls on an electrocardiograph machine.

- Name the standard 12 leads and the locations of their sensors.

- State the cause and correction of artifacts.

- Understand stress testing.

- Comprehend the need for Holter monitoring and how to attach leads.

- Explain telemetry and identify the sites for lead attachment.

- Comprehend the function and placement of pacemakers.

CHAPTER OUTLINE

CASE STUDY

Eliot Masterson, a 41-year-old business owner, was seen by Dr. Salpega for a routine physical. During the office visit, Eliot informed Dr. Salpega that he has had some episodes of chest pain over the past few months that have occurred after exercising. Dr. Salpega decides to have his medical assistant, David, perform an ECG on Mr. Masterson.

1111

artifacts	murmurs
bradycardia	multiple gated acquisition (MUGA) scan
coronary artery disease (CAD)	pacemakers
Einthoven's triangle	perfusion
electrocardiogram (ECG)	rhythm
gallops	stress test
heart rate	submaximal test
Holter monitor	tachycardia
hyperventilating	target heart rate
ischemic	telemetry
leads	thallium
mediastinum	wave

CERTIFICATION LINK

CMA (AAMA)	**RMA**	**CMAS**
Electrocardiography (ECG/EKG)	Electrocardiography	Vital signs and measurements

W ithin the thoracic cavity or chest are the major organs of both respiration and circulation. Because these two systems work together very closely, both are vital for survival, and a problem with one will often lead to a problem with the other. Chapter 50 discusses pulmonary function and the tests associated with lung function. Because many patients suffer with disorders of these two systems, both primary care physicians and specialists monitor and treat these patients. In many clinics, tests associated with these disorders are done by the medical assistant.

All patients visiting a physician should have their heart and lungs assessed, regardless of their chief complaint. A stethoscope is used to evaluate the sounds made as the heart works. These sounds represent the closing of the valves and usually occur closely together followed by a pause, as in "lub-dub . . . lub-dub." Heart sounds are discussed in more detail later in this chapter.

When more specific cardiac information is needed, an electrocardiogram is performed. The **electrocardiogram (ECG)** is a tracing, or recording, of electrical activity as it moves through the heart. The ECG represents only the electrical activity of the heart, not the actual mechanical performance. The physician orders this painless, noninvasive test when the heart sounds are unusual, the rhythm is irregular, or the patient has any heart-related complaints or has a condition that might affect the heart or be due to the heart. A recording will also be made to serve as a reference with which to compare future recordings in evaluating any changes. This may be called a baseline ECG.

Heart Structure and Function

The heart is located in the thoracic cavity between the lungs and behind the sternum in an area called the **mediastinum**. Figure 49-1 shows the mediastinum, lungs, and thoracic cavity. The heart is a hollow triangular organ, about the size of a fist, enclosed within a double-walled sac called the pericardium. The middle layer or myocardium makes up most of the heart wall and is composed of cardiac muscle and fibrous tissue. The endocardium lines the upper chambers, or atria, and lower chamber, or ventricles, of the heart. Figure 49-2 illustrates the layers in the walls of the heart.

The function of the cardiovascular system is to carry oxygen from the lungs to all the tissues of the body. The deoxygenated blood then circulates through the body and discharges carbon dioxide (the waste product of cell metabolism) from the lungs. Figure 49-3 shows the internal anatomy of the heart. For a thorough review of the anatomy and physiology of the circulatory system, see Chapter 27 in this book.

Blood circulates throughout the body and returns from the general circulation by way of the superior and inferior vena cava, to the right atrium, moving in one direction through the heart. When the right atrium is full, the atrium contracts and blood is pumped into the right ventricle through the tricuspid valve. On filling, blood is pumped by contraction of the right ventricle through the semilunar valves into the pulmonary artery going to the lungs. There, blood is oxygenated and returned to the left atrium through the four pulmonary veins. When that chamber is full, it contracts and blood is squeezed into the left ventricle through the mitral (bicuspid) valve. In the left ventricle, blood will enter the aortic semilunar valve and move into all parts of the body except the lungs. Blood travels to all parts of the body via the aorta and then goes into all other arteries. Figure 49-4 illustrates the blood flow pattern through the right and left side of the heart.

The heart muscle receives its supply of oxygen and nutrients through the coronary artery system on the outside of the

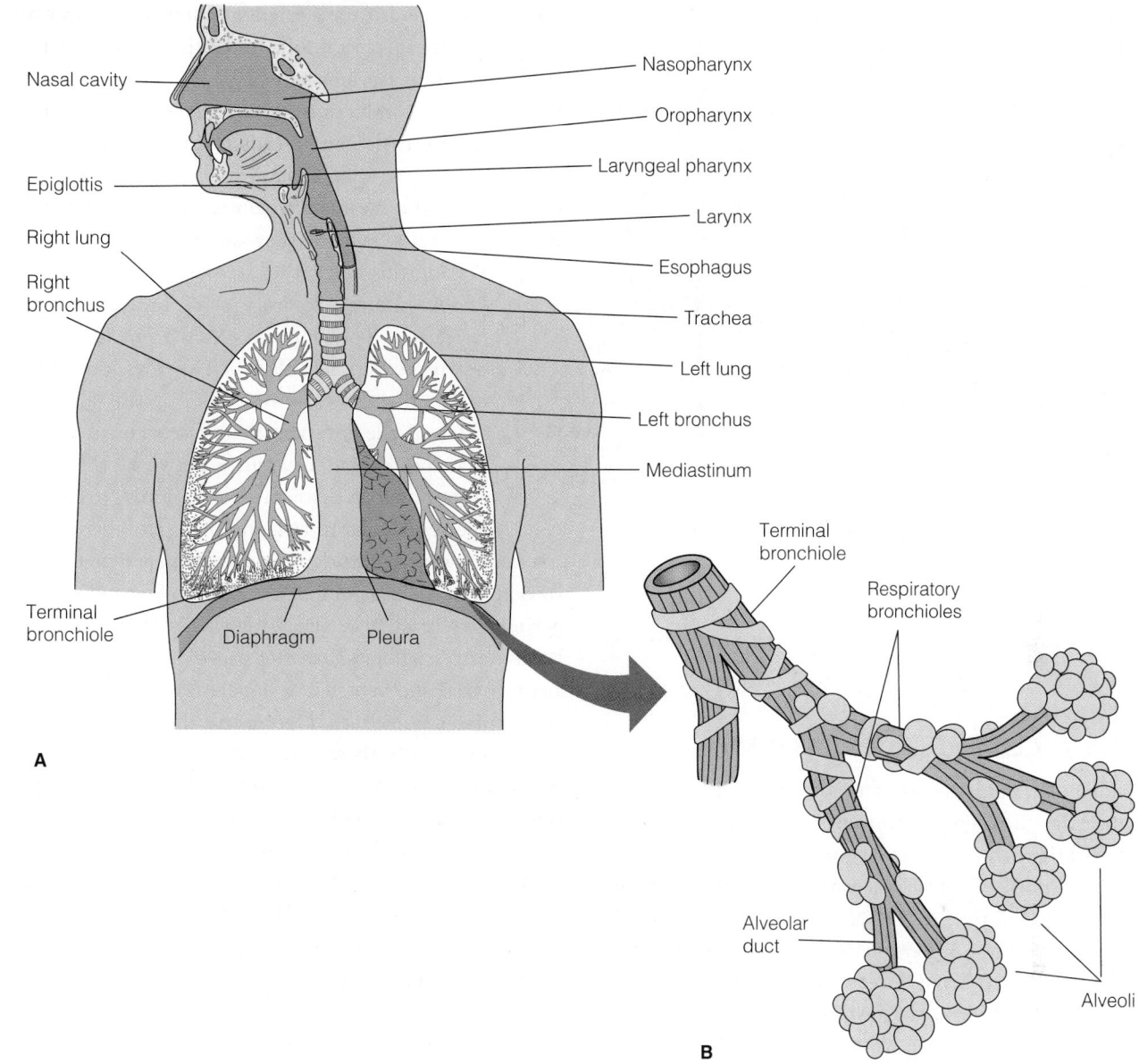

Nasal cavity

Nasopharynx

Oropharynx

Laryngeal pharynx

Larynx

Epiglottis

Esophagus

Right lung

Trachea

Right bronchus

Left lung

Left bronchus

Mediastinum

Terminal bronchiole

Diaphragm   Pleura

A

Terminal bronchiole

Respiratory bronchioles

Alveolar duct

Alveoli

B

FIGURE 49-1   The mediastinum.

heart. The blood that flows through the heart to the body is not used for energy for the heart tissues. As blood leaves the left ventricle rich with oxygen, it enters immediately into the aorta and the coronary arteries to supply the heart muscle. Deoxygenated blood returns to the general circulation through the cardiac veins, which empty into the coronary sinus in the right atrium. See Figure 49-5 for the blood flow in the coronary arteries.

HEART VALVES

Heart valves act as gates to prevent the backward flow of blood. They open and shut in response to the changing pressure brought about by cardiac contraction and relaxation.

The contraction and relaxation of the chambers occur in sequence because electrical impulses move smoothly along the electrical conduction system of the heart.

This conduction system involves the movement of charged particles or ions during different phases. Minerals (sodium, potassium, and calcium) are responsible for smooth contractions and consistent rhythm. At rest, the cells of the heart are polarized—that is, they are charged with energy (negative inside the cell and positive outside). As the cells are stimulated to contract, the mineral particles move like a wave, and the charge within the cells changes to positive inside and negative outside. The cells are depolarized and contraction occurs. The cells then return to a resting state,

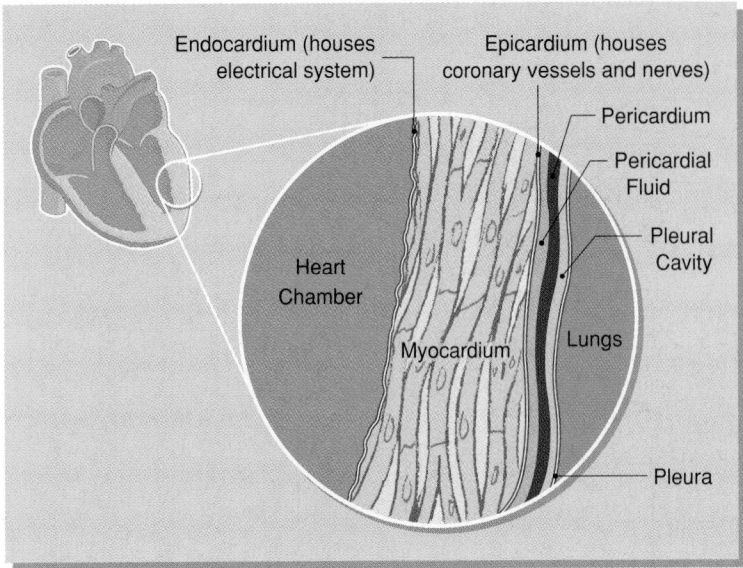

FIGURE 49-2 Layers of the heart wall.

called repolarization, as their electrical charge returns to the original negative inside and positive outside.

CONDUCTION SYSTEM

The four major components of this conduction system are the sinoatrial (SA) node, atrioventricular (AV) node, the bundle of His with right and left bundle branches, and the Purkinje fibers. The heartbeat is controlled by rhythmic impulses that arise in the SA node and move through the conduction system. The SA node, located in the right atrium, is made of modified myocardial cells and acts like a battery. It is known as the pacemaker of the heart because it establishes

the pace. It may accelerate or slow the **heart rate**, or heartbeats per minute, under the influence of the autonomic nervous system.

The conduction system carries the impulse from the SA node and spreads it through the atria. This process is called atria depolarization. The impulses reach the AV node (also made of modified myocardial cells), where they are momentarily delayed. During this delay, the atria rest and recover. This is known as atrial recovery, atrial rest, or atrial repolarization. The impulse passes from the AV node down the bundle of His as it divides into two bundle branches, carrying the impulse along both sides of the interventricular septum. The bundle branches spread to form a network, the Purkinje system, which distributes the impulse to all parts of the ventricular muscle, resulting in ventricular contraction or ventricular depolarization. Ventricular depolarization follows atrial repolarization and is followed by a period of ventricular recovery known as ventricular repolarization or rest. There is a brief pause, and the cycle begins again. Atrial and ventricular depolarization, plus atrial and ventricular repolarization, comprise the cardiac cycle, one pulse and one heartbeat. The term *systole* refers to the contraction phase of the heart, and conversely *diastole* refers to the relaxation phase of the heart. Figure 49-6 illustrates the systolic and diastolic phases of the heart.

A unique property of cardiac muscle is that all conductive tissue has the potential to serve in the role of pacemaker—that is, any area can set the cardiac rate if the SA node fails. Under abnormal circumstances, such as when damage has occurred, other areas may assume the role of the pacemaker. Slower rhythms will be generated by the AV node (40 to 60 beats per minute), by the bundle of His (less than 40 beats per minute), and by the Purkinje system. But normally the SA node generates the controlling impulses at a resting rate of 60 to 80 beats per minute.

Heart sounds are important clues for the physician during an examination. Two types of heart sounds, namely murmurs and gallops, are associated with certain abnormal conditions. **Murmurs** can be caused by damaged valves, regurgitation or backflow of blood through a valve, or high flow rates, all of which cause a kind of turbulence. The timing and intensity and quality of murmurs are described when documenting a patient's record. **Gallops**, or galloping rhythm, is an abnormal rhythm indicated by three distinct sounds in each heartbeat that are similar to the sounds of a galloping horse. The physician documents normal heart sounds, along

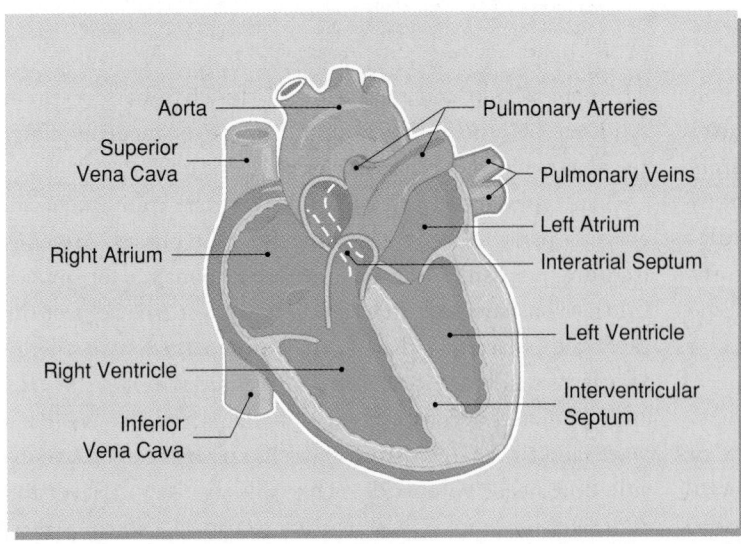

FIGURE 49-3 Internal anatomy of the heart.

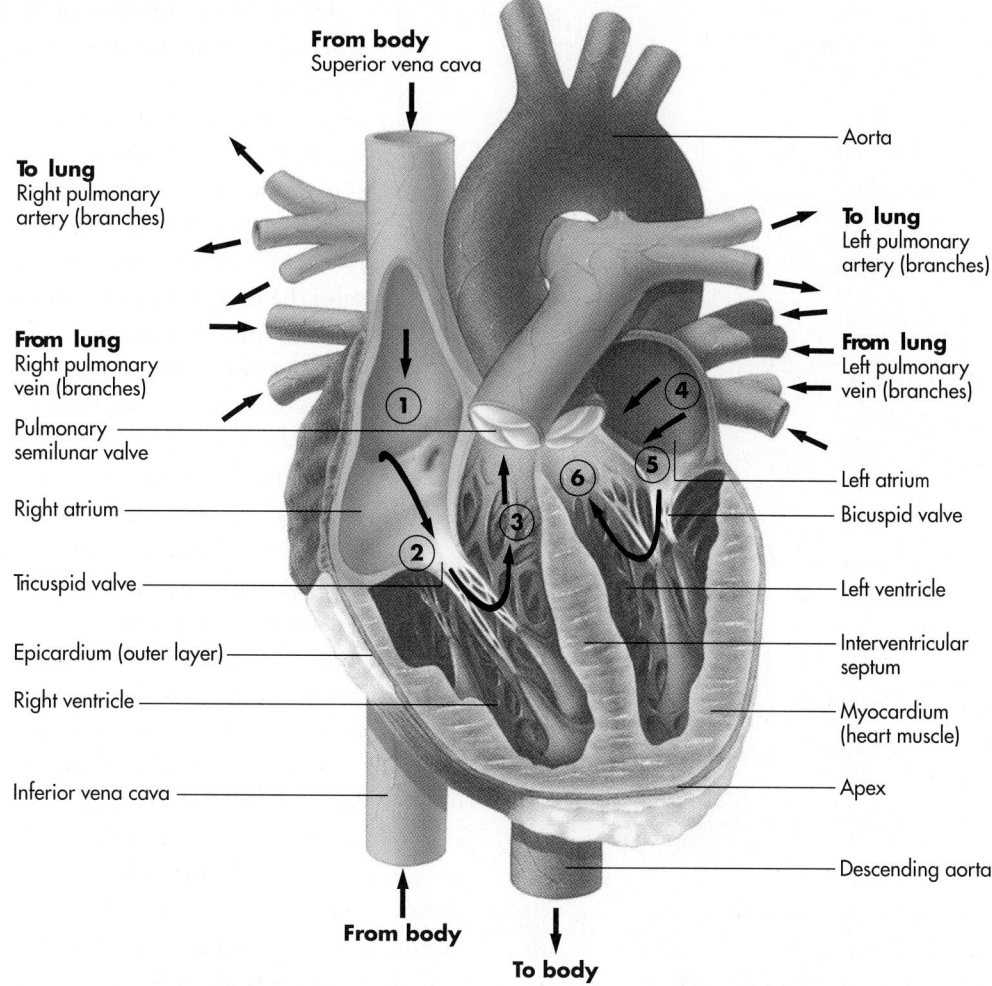

From body
Superior vena cava

To lung
Right pulmonary
artery (branches)

From lung
Right pulmonary
vein (branches)

Pulmonary
semilunar valve

Right atrium

Tricuspid valve

Epicardium (outer layer)

Right ventricle

Inferior vena cava

From body

Aorta

To lung
Left pulmonary
artery (branches)

From lung
Left pulmonary
vein (branches)

Left atrium

Bicuspid valve

Left ventricle

Interventricular
septum

Myocardium
(heart muscle)

Apex

Descending aorta

To body

RIGHT HEART PUMP

1. Deoxygenated blood returns from the upper and lower body to fill the right atrium of the heart creating a pressure against the tricuspid valve.

2. This pressure of the returning blood forces the tricuspid valve open and begins filling the ventricle. The final filling of the ventricle is achieved by the contracting of the right atrium.

3. The right ventricle contracts, increasing the internal pressure. This pressure closes the tricuspid valve and forces open the pulmonary semilunar valve thus sending blood toward the lung via the pulmonary artery. This blood will become oxygenated as it travels through the capillary beds of the lung and then return to the left side of the heart.

LEFT HEART PUMP

4. Oxygenated blood returns from the lung via the pulmonary vein and fills the left atrium creating a pressure against the bicuspid valve.

5. This pressure of returning blood forces the bicuspid valve open and begins filling the left ventricle. The final filling of the left ventricle is achieved by the contracting of the left atrium.

6. The left ventricle contracts, increasing internal pressure. This pressure closes the bicuspid valve and forces open the aortic valve causing oxygenated blood to flow through the aorta to deliver oxygen throughout the body.

FIGURE 49-4 Blood flow pattern through the heart.

with any murmurs, gallops, or other abnormal heart sounds that are present.

The Electrocardiogram

The electrical charges created by the cardiac conduction system can be sensed throughout the body. Electrodes placed in specific areas of the skin can detect those electri-

cal charges and then transmit them to a computer for amplification of the signal and recording on paper for physician assessment. If no energy is sensed, then the equipment records a flat line, or isoelectric line. When the equipment senses an electrical charge, it records it as either an upward or a downward deflection on the readout. Movement away from the baseline is called a deflection or **wave**. The waves

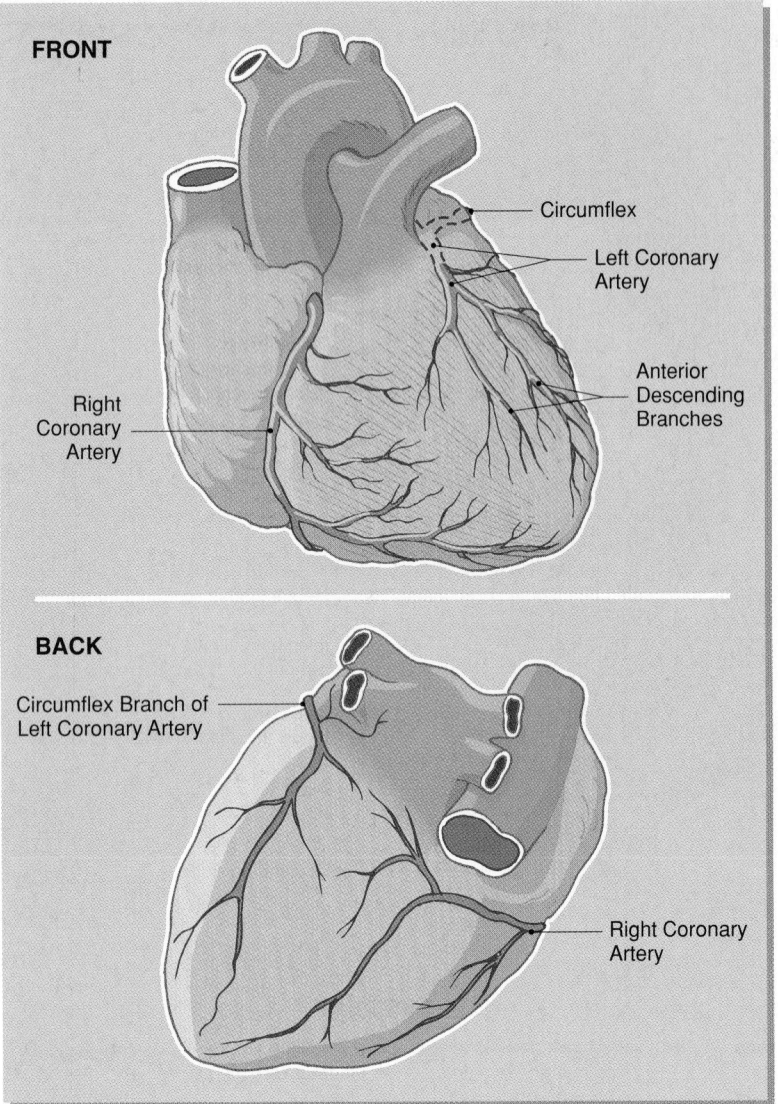

FRONT

Circumflex

Left Coronary Artery

Anterior Descending Branches

Right Coronary Artery

BACK

Circumflex Branch of Left Coronary Artery

Right Coronary Artery

FIGURE 49-5 Coronary circulation showing the coronary arteries.

On an ECG, the horizontal axis (line) represents time; a slower heart rate will have more space between the PQRST complexes. For a patient with a faster heart rate, the cardiac cycles will be closer together. When a heart skips a beat, there is a long flat line between PQRSTs. In addition, the amount of space between the P wave and the QRS complex indicates the time required for the conduction system to carry the impulse from the SA node to the Purkinje fibers.

Recordings are made from a variety of perspectives or angles known as **leads**. Each lead will record from a specific combination of sensors. When completed, the 12-lead ECG produces a three-dimensional record of cardiac impulses. The pattern of deflections will appear quite different on each lead. The pattern of deflections recorded, voltage or amplitude and time, assist the physician in evaluating the status of the patient's heart.

In some instances, it may be necessary to enlarge or shrink the recording. Under ordinary circumstances, a recording is made in sensitivity 1, which represents a 10-mm deflection per 1 millivolt (mV) of electricity. The size is doubled in sensitivity (sensitivity 2) or halved in sensitivity (sensitivity $\frac{1}{2}$).

TIME AND THE CARDIAC CYCLE

The P wave represents the impulse that originated in the SA node and spread through the atria, which is called atrial depolarization. When the P wave is present in normal size and shape, then the stimulus causing the heart to beat originated in the SA node (Figure 49-7).

Normally, the P-R interval (time from the beginning of P to the beginning of QRS) is between 0.12 and 0.20 seconds (three to five small boxes on the ECG graph paper). (See Figure 49-8.) A deviation from these times could represent an abnormality in the electrical system of the heart or in the structure of the heart that impacts the electrical system. This interval represents the time it takes for the impulse to cross the atria and the AV node and reach the ventricles. A P-R interval that is too short means the impulse has reached the ventricles through a shorter-than-normal pathway. If the interval is too long, a conduction delay in the AV node might be assumed.

or deflections may go up (positive) or down (negative) from the baseline and represent amplitude or voltage. The strength or voltage of the electrical impulse will determine the size of the deflection. Large voltages will cause larger deflections, whereas small voltages will create smaller deflections.

The deflections from the heart are labeled P, Q, R, S, and T. (Sometimes a small U wave follows the T wave. This is considered normal and may be due to a potassium deficiency.) A normal cardiac cycle is one series of PQRST waves. The P represents atrial depolarization (change in electrical activity), the QRS complex represents ventricular depolarization, and the T is repolarization (a return to the resting electrical state).

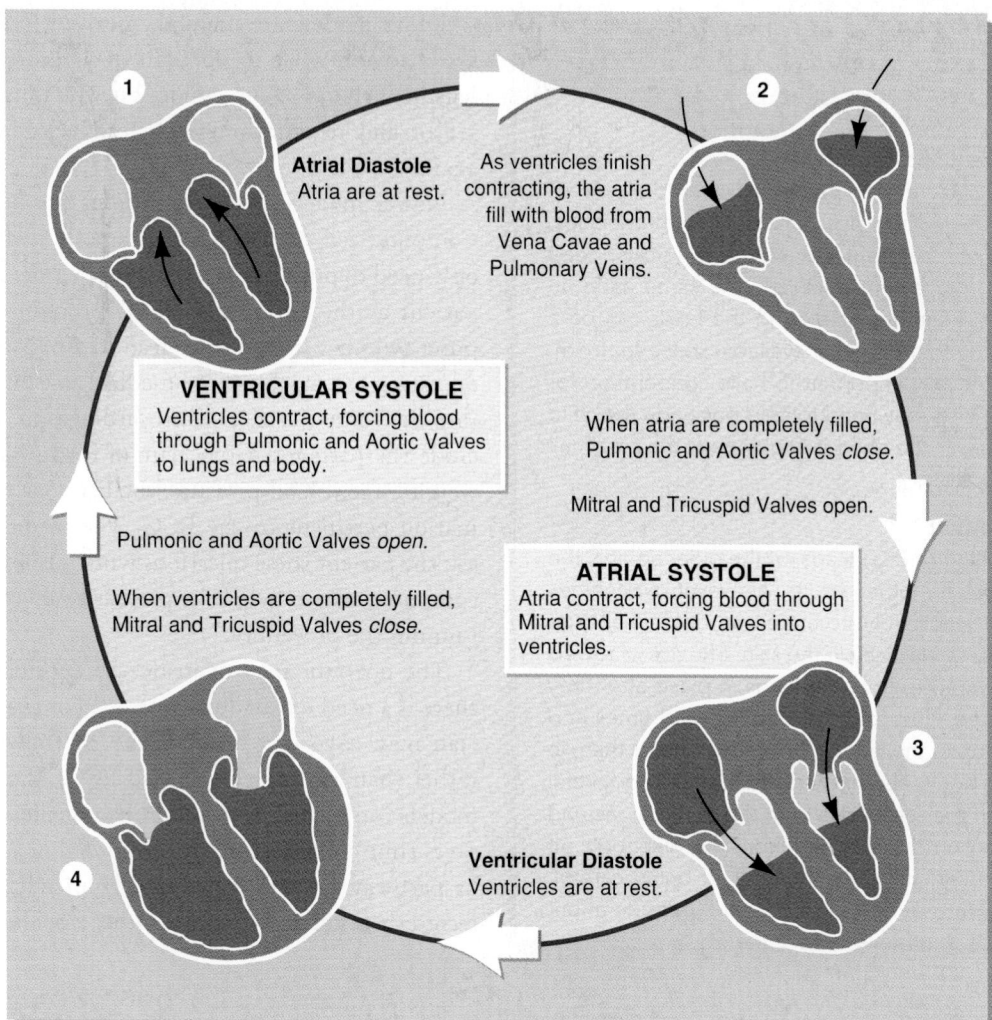

FIGURE 49-6 Cardiac systole and diastole.

In the figure:

1 — Atrial Diastole. Atria are at rest.

As ventricles finish contracting, the atria fill with blood from Vena Cavae and Pulmonary Veins.

VENTRICULAR SYSTOLE
Ventricles contract, forcing blood through Pulmonic and Aortic Valves to lungs and body.

Pulmonic and Aortic Valves *open*.

When ventricles are completely filled, Mitral and Tricuspid Valves *close*.

2 — When atria are completely filled, Pulmonic and Aortic Valves *close*.

Mitral and Tricuspid Valves open.

ATRIAL SYSTOLE
Atria contract, forcing blood through Mitral and Tricuspid Valves into ventricles.

3 — Ventricular Diastole. Ventricles are at rest.

4

The QRS complex represents the time necessary for the impulse to travel through the bundle of His, the bundle branches, and the Purkinje fibers to complete ventricular activation or contraction, which is known as ventricular depolarization. This usually takes less than 0.06 to 0.12 second (three small ECG boxes).

The ST segment and the T wave represent repolarization of the ventricles. The ST segment is normally flat (on the isoelectric line or baseline) or is only slightly elevated. The T wave represents a part of recovery of the ventricles after contraction (Figure 49-9).

The QRS complex and the T wave typically point in the same direction, and T waves that are opposite in direction from the QRS may indicate a problem in the heart or its electrical system. While the medical assistant should not try to interpret the ECG, understanding what is normal in the cardiac cycle is helpful. Figure 49-10 illustrates what is occurring in the heart and how it is represented on ECG tracing.

ECG MACHINES

Many types of ECG machines are in use, but all should be calibrated to align with the international standard. This means that the paper in all machines moves at the same speed of 25 mm/second and, given the same amount of electrical energy, the recording stylus will move the same distance (1 mV of electricity input will cause the stylus to deflect 10 mm), thus giving uniform recordings worldwide. Standardization is a means of verifying that each machine deflects 10 mm in response to 1 mV of electricity in sensitivity.

Older models are manual, meaning someone must tell the machine what to do. You may record from arms and legs in fairly rapid succession, but you must move the chest sensor and record from each lead, then move the sensor again.

Newer models of electrocardiographs are computerized. Computerized models have automatic features so you may only need to push a button. All ten sensors are placed on the patient at the beginning of the procedure, and the computer switches from lead to lead in rapid succession. Before operating the machine, the medical assistant will enter data into the computerized electrocardiograph. Data usually include the patient's name, date of birth, diagnoses, height, weight, age, blood pressure, medications taken, and information pertinent to the ECG. The medical assistant may ask the patient these questions while placing the data in the computer, which helps the patient to relax a bit before beginning the procedure.

The operator may override the automated machines if there is a need for manual controls. For example, the physician may have just ordered one rhythm strip of lead II, rather than a complete 12-lead ECG. Many computerized models can record from more than one lead at once, which saves time and effort. Each is recorded in a separate channel or pathway for the signal and, typically, these machines record three channels at once. Other machines have a built-in

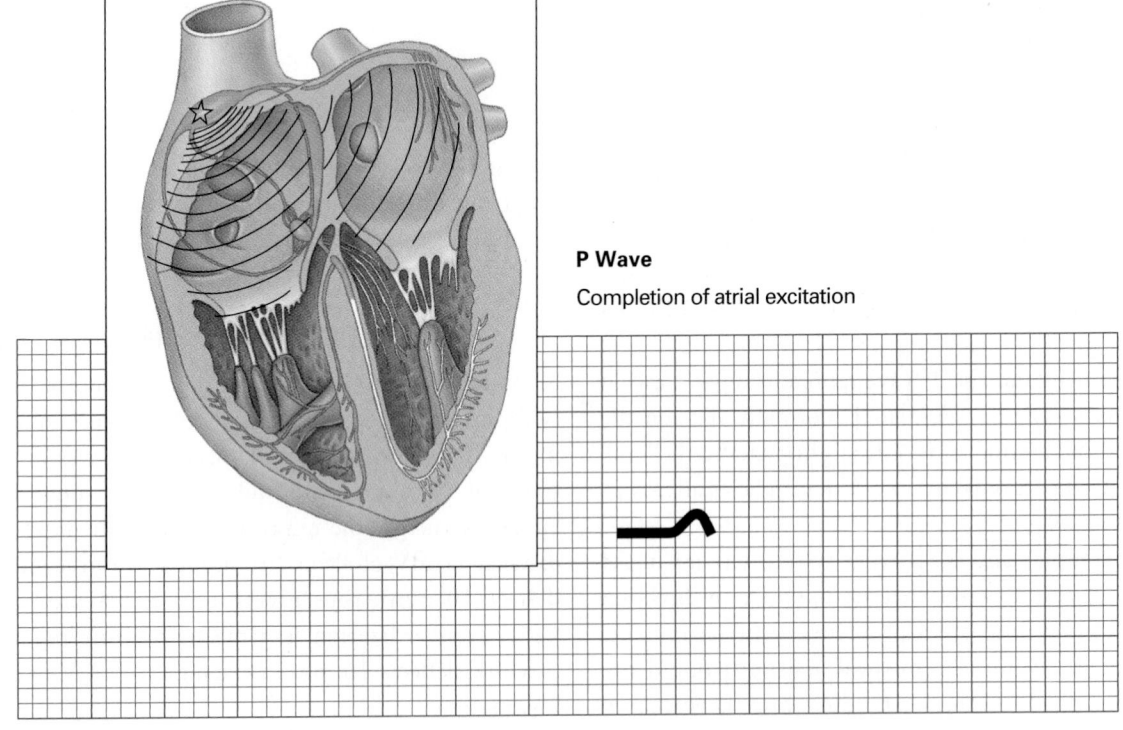

P Wave

Completion of atrial excitation

FIGURE 49-7 P wave (atrial excitation).

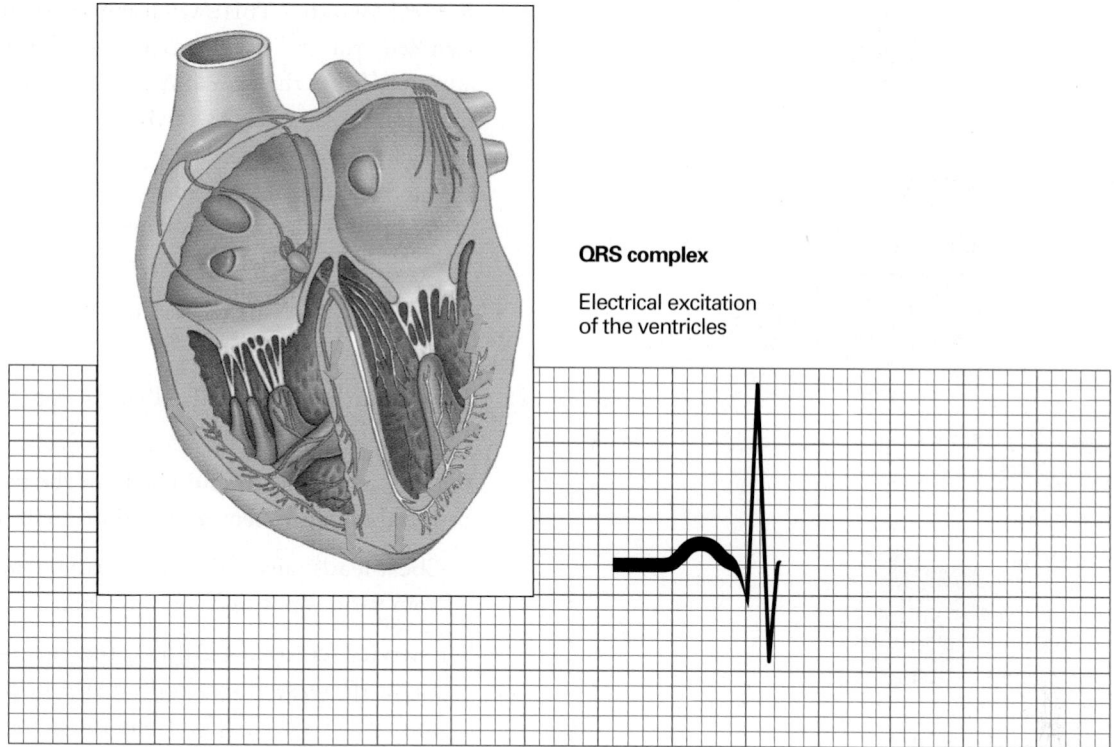

QRS complex

Electrical excitation
of the ventricles

FIGURE 49-8 QRS complex (ventricular excitation).

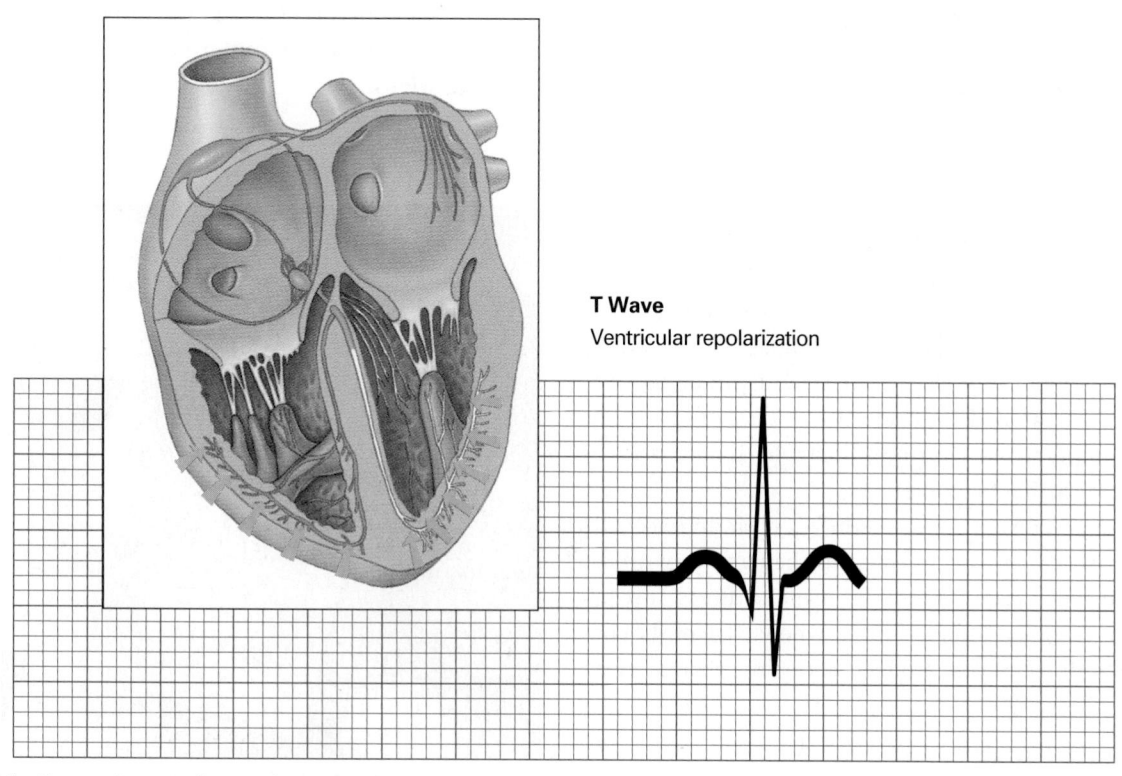

T Wave

Ventricular repolarization

FIGURE 49-9 T wave (ventricular repolarization).

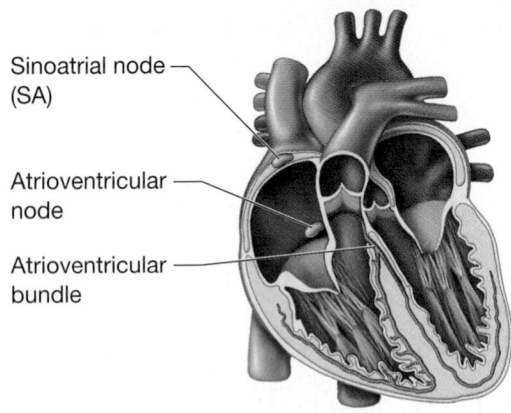

Sinoatrial node (SA)

Atrioventricular node

Atrioventricular bundle

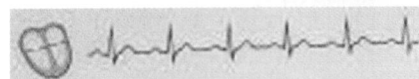

SA Node

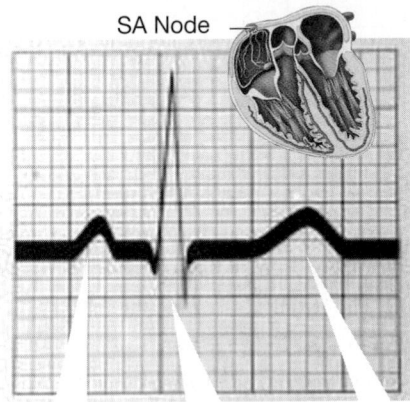

P wave	QRS complex	T wave
corresponds to contraction of the atria	correlates to ventricles contracting	represents preparation for next series of complexes

FIGURE 49-10 The heart and an ECG tracing.

interpretive feature (Figure 49-11) and will print out a statement as to the status of the heart. Others can connect directly via fax with a regional office that will carry out the interpretation function and fax results to your office.

Although computerized electrocardiographs save considerable time in mounting ECGs, care should still be taken to ensure that a clear ECG is made before disconnecting the sensors. Computerized electrocardiographs should still be monitored for **artifacts** (errors).

It is your responsibility to produce a clear and accurate tracing from each patient, so you must be familiar with the machines in your office. Read the manufacturer's instructions for the machine before using it. Knowledge of the control panel will help you produce a tracing that is clear, accurate, and easy to read:

- **Main power switch (off/on)**—Allow for a warm-up time as specified by the manufacture) before using.

- **Record switch**—This switch moves the paper at the standard "run 25" speed (25 mm/sec). ECGs are usually recorded at this speed. Another option is "run 50" (50 mm/sec, or twice as fast). This is used when the heart rate is so rapid that interpretation requires that it be stretched out. This is only used for detailed interpretations because it tends to waste paper and can be more difficult to read.

- **Lead selector**—This determines from which sensors the machine will record:

  - **Standard (limb) leads:** Record from two sensors placed on all extremities.

  - **Augmented leads:** Record from the midpoint between two limb sensors to a third limb sensor.

  - **Chest leads (also called precordial leads):** Record from various positions on the thorax.

- **Sensitivity control**—Allows the operator to increase or decrease the recording size in order to enlarge or shrink the deflections to fit on the paper. When changing from the international standard of sensitivity 1 to sensitivity $\frac{1}{2}$ or sensitivity 2, the operator must include a standard for the interpreter information.

- **Standard button**—Allows verification of calibration to the international standard.

- **Stylus control**—Centers the recording in the middle of the page or the center of each channel by moving the stylus.

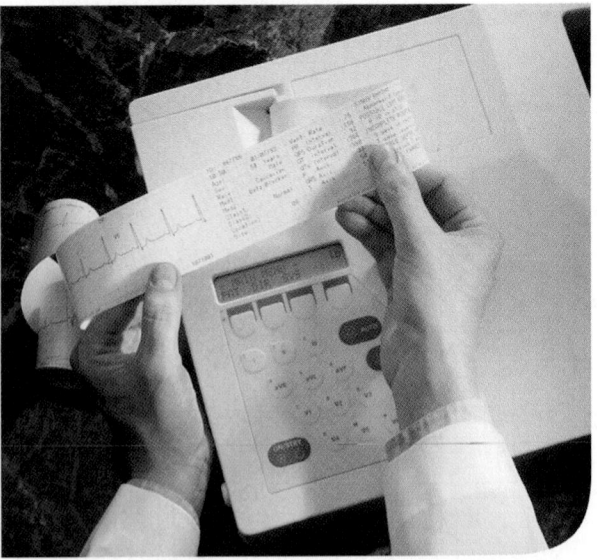

FIGURE 49-11 Single-channel ECG with interpretation of results.

- **Stylus heat control**—Increases or decreases heat and adjusts for the sharpest tracing. New machines use an ink cartridge instead of heat stylus.
- **Marker**—Indicates, by a code, which lead is being recorded.

ELECTROCARDIOGRAM PAPER

Electrocardiogram paper is pressure sensitive and must be handled carefully. If this paper is exposed to light for long periods, the markings will fade with time. Many newer machines use an ink cartridge to supply the stylus and provide a longer-lasting printout. Be sure to read the manufacturer's instructions carefully when changing the ink cartridges in the pens.

"Time" markers, referred to as 3-second markers, are printed on all ECG paper. Look for them at the top of single-channel paper and between channels in multichannel paper. The time markers are small squares with a light line and larger squares with a darker line. The small squares are 1 mm by 1 mm square and represent 0.1 mV of voltage in the height and .04 second time in the width. The larger squares are 5 mm by 5 mm square and represent 0.5 mV of voltage in the height and 0.20 second time in the width. Thus, the paper records both time (horizontally) and voltage (vertically). See Figure 49-12 for ECG paper and markings.

HEART RATE

Heart rate is the same as beats per minute. It is possible to estimate the heart rate from an ECG. Some offices have a

protocol that states you should record some additional cycles if the heart rate is above or below certain numbers. Many cardiologists also expect you to perform an exact calculation of the heart rate before you place the recording in the patient record or on the doctor's desk. Two methods for estimation of the heart rate and one for exact calculation are discussed next.

Note the 3-second markers that are printed by the manufacturer on the paper. To estimate the cardiac rate (beats per minute) from the tracing use the 6-second method. Begin at one 3-second marker and go to the right for two additional markers, for a total of 6 seconds. Count the number of QRS complexes between the first and third markers and add a zero. This is the estimated ventricular rate per minute. A similar atrial estimate can be made by counting the P waves between these markers. This estimate is accurate even if the rhythm is irregular (arrhythmia).

The heart rate can also be estimated by locating a QRS complex close to a 5-mm line, which is the darker line on the paper. Move to the next deflection at the right or the left, counting how many 5-mm lines intersect the tracing before the next QRS complex. Count off at each 5-mm line, beginning at the deflection near the 5-mm line and saying "zero, 300, 150, 100, 75, 60, 50." Stop counting when you reach the next QRS complex. This *count-off method* is an estimate of the ventricular rate. This estimate is accurate only for the complexes where it was done.

To obtain an exact calculation of the heart rate, recall that the paper moves at a standard speed of 25 mm/second, so it will move at 1500 mm/minute (25 mm/second × 60 seconds = 1500 mm/minute). An exact calculation of ventricular heart rate is achieved by counting the millimeter boxes between two QRS complexes and dividing that number into 1500. For instance, if there are 20 mm between

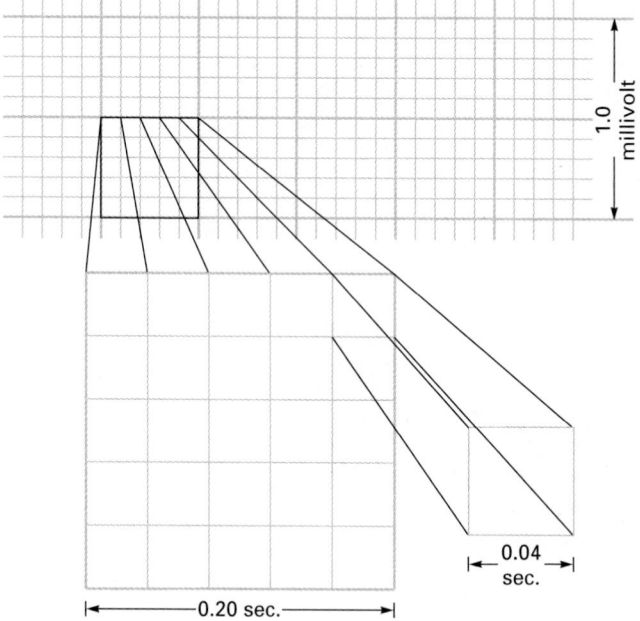

FIGURE 49-12 ECG paper and markings.

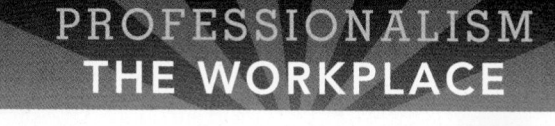

PROFESSIONALISM
THE WORKPLACE

Be aware of the fact that many patients have elevated blood pressure readings just from being in a medical environment. When performing an ECG or monitoring a patient's cardiac rhythms, be alert for signs of instability or life-threatening emergencies such as shortness of breath, chest pain, rapid heart rate, dropping blood pressure, profuse sweating, or changes in mental alertness.

two QRS complexes, 1500 divided by 20 equals 75 beats per minute. An exact calculation of atrial heart rate is achieved by counting the millimeter boxes between two P waves and by dividing that number into 1500. These calculations are accurate only for the complexes where they were done.

Rhythm is the regularity of the occurrence of heartbeats. Ventricular rhythm is determined by measuring the dis-tance between QRS complexes. There should be a fairly consistent space between complexes. Atrial rhythm is de-termined by measuring the distance between P waves. There should be a fairly consistent space between waves. Again, train yourself to look at the rhythm while you are recording. Some offices have protocols about what extra tracings to record in the event the rhythm appears irregu-lar to you.

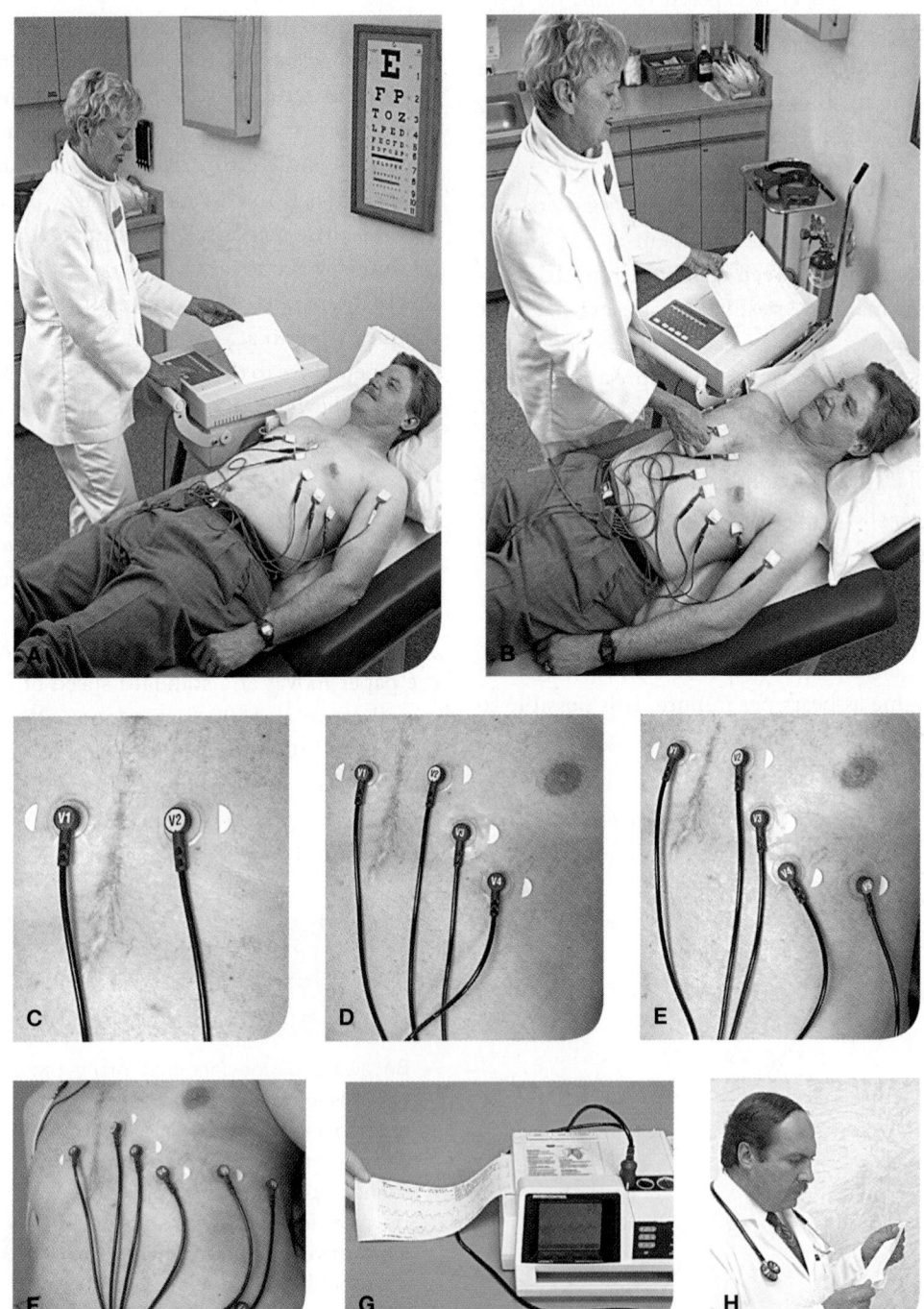

FIGURE 49-13 (A) Performing an ECG; (B) a medical assistant adjusting ECG electrodes; (C) chest or precordial leads V1 and V2; (D) chest leads V1, V2 V3, V4 in place; (E) chest leads V1, V2, V3, V4, V5; (F) the sixth chest lead is added to complete the attachment prior to an ECG; (G) the ECG tracings emerging from the ECG machine during the procedure; (H) the physician is reading the ECG.

TABLE 49-1 Sensor or Lead Placement and Marking Codes

Leads	Placement	Abbreviation	Marking Code
Limb Leads Lead I	Right arm to left arm	RA-LA	•
Lead II	Right arm to left leg	RA-LL	••
Lead III	Left arm to left leg	LA-LL	•••
Augmented Leads AVR	RA-midpoint (LA-LL)	(LA-LL) RA	-
AVL	LA-midpoint (RA-LL)	(RA-LL) LA	--
AVF	LL-midpoint (RA-LA)	(RA-LA) LL	---
Chest Leads V1	4th intercostal space, right sternal border		—•
V2	4th intercostal space, left sternal border		—••
V3	Midway between V2 and V4		—•••
V4	5th intercostal space, midclavicular left		—••••
V5	Left anterior axillary fold, horizontal to V4		—•••••
V6	Left midaxillary, horizontal to V4 and V5		—••••••

SENSOR PLACEMENT

The ECG machine records the cardiac cycle through sensors placed on the patient's bare skin. Sensors are placed over the fleshy part of the inner aspect of both lower legs and either both upper arms or both forearms, avoiding the bony prominences. These locations are abbreviated LA for left arm, RA for right arm, LL for left leg, and RL for right leg. The RL sensor serves as an electrical reference point and is not actually used in the recording. If you have a patient on whom you cannot place one extremity sensor as planned, you must place the sensors on both extremities symmetrically. For example, a patient in a cast up to the knee requires that both sensors be placed above the knee. If a hand and forearm are amputated, both arm sensors must be placed on the upper arm. The chest sensor, abbreviated with V, is used in six locations, with a number following the V, as in V1, V2, and so forth. Placement of chest sensors must be anatomically correct. Figures 49-13A-H show the placement of the leads in a 12-lead ECG.

By recording from different combinations of sensors, the electrical activity of the heart is seen from different angles. A lead selector switch or lead indicator selects the combination of sensors for that lead. One sensor is used for chest (unipolar) leads. A combination may be two sensors, as with standard limb (bipolar) leads, or three sensors, as with augmented limb leads.

With many sensors and many views possible, you must indicate on the tracing from which lead you are recording. An international marking system has been devised using dashes and dots. Some machines automatically mark the code just above the cardiac tracing. Others require manual marking with the international code. Table 49-1 lists limb, augmented, and chest leads and proper placement and marking codes.

It is beneficial to memorize the sensors used in the limb and augmented leads. Then, if you have difficulty getting a clear recording from one lead, you do not have to look at all the sensors, only those involved. Some find it easier to remember all the leads and the sensors being recorded (see Table 49-1) or by picturing **Einthoven's triangle**, which is a pictorial guide to the leads (Figure 49-14).

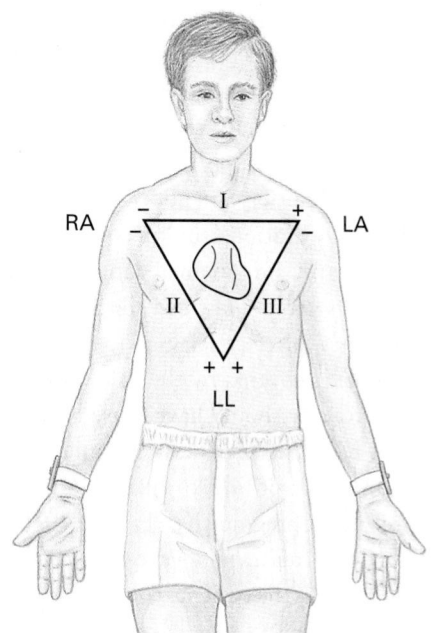

FIGURE 49-14 Einthoven's triangle.

PATIENT PREPARATION

A well-informed patient is more cooperative and less anxious. Explain the equipment and procedure as well as what you will expect the patient to do. The surroundings should be pleasant and the table wide enough for adequate support. Patients must be bare to the waist, so privacy should be provided for disrobing. Offer female patients a gown to be worn with the opening at the front. In addition, you will need access to bare skin on the lower legs. Patients have to remove socks or stockings. Roll long pants legs out of the way. Position the patient comfortably supine with a pillow under the head, and another under the knees if needed to eliminate back strain. If the patient cannot tolerate lying down, use the semi-Fowler's position instead and note that the ECG was done in that position. Jewelry, particularly metal jewelry, must be removed so that it does not interfere with the electrical current of the ECG. Prepare the skin where the sensors will be applied. Any area that has been treated with talcum powder or skin lotion must be rubbed with alcohol to remove the residue to facilitate the adherence of the leads. Some shower gels leave sufficient moisturizer as a residue that can interfere with sensor contact. Such residue must be removed with alcohol before the electrolyte sensors may be applied.

TECHNICAL PREPARATION

If you are to obtain a clear recording of the patient's cardiac cycle, you will need a machine, calibrated and in good working order, with a good supply of paper. You will also need the sensors to place on the skin and a supply of electrolyte or conduction cream, gel, or pads to improve the contact between the skin and electrodes. The sensors may be metal plates that attach with rubber straps, or they may be small suction cups called Welch electrodes. These must be cleaned between patients to prevent the accumulation of electrolyte. Adhesive disposable sensors that contain electrolyte are widely used today.

To begin, assemble the necessary supplies, plug the machine into a properly grounded outlet, and allow it to warm up. Verify that the machine is operational and in compliance with the international standard. Using manual controls, run the machine at the "run 25" setting and push the standard button briefly to release 1 mV of electricity. Stop the machine and count the small boxes covered by the deflection of the stylus. The 1 mV of electricity should have caused a positive deflection of 10 mm. If not, adjust the stylus until the deflection is precisely 10 mm according to manufacturer's directions or call your service representative. Figure 49-15 illustrates correct and incorrect calibration waves.

Identify, interview, and instruct the patient. Following skin preparation, the electrolyte and sensors may be applied. Electrolyte materials come in many forms, including gel, lotion,

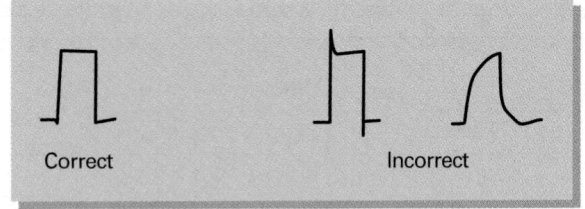

FIGURE 49-15   Correct and incorrect standardization waves.

and paste. Each office selects one that is compatible with the type of sensors they are using and their machines. The most recent development is a disposable, gummy sensor containing electrolyte. It requires that small alligator clamps be added to the sensor wires. These clip onto the edge of the sensor.

The procedure to attach the sensors will vary slightly, depending on the machine you are using. Older machines require sensors to be secured with a rubber strap. One electrolyte-saturated pad is placed on the skin and the sensor plate strapped over it. The limb sensors are attached, and the first six leads are recorded one at a time. Then the one chest sensor is moved from position to position as each lead is recorded.

Newer machines use a small amount of electrolyte lotion and Welch electrodes. Electrolyte and all sensors are placed on the skin at once. All 12 leads are run in rapid succession because the computerized machines can switch from one lead to another quickly.

The placement of chest sensors must be precise. It is possible to complete this task without unnecessary exposure for female patients. The landmarks you will need to palpate or view are the sternum, the fourth intercostal space, both clavicles, and the left axilla. Stand on the left side of the patient and expose the sternum. Locate the right clavicle and the space immediately inferior to it. This is a supracostal space—that is, it is above the first rib and does not count as an intercostal space. Proceed toward the feet at the right edge of the sternum and, using the tips of your fingers, palpate the first rib and first intercostal space, second rib and intercostal space, and so forth until you feel the fourth intercostal space. This space at the right sternal margin is the location of V1. Lead V2 is placed at the same level on the left side of the sternum. Next, you will need to locate V4 to find V3. From the middle of the left clavicle, draw an imaginary line toward the feet, stopping one intercostal space below the level of V2. This is V4 (fifth intercostal space, midclavicular left). Lift a female patient's gown up from the hemline in respect of patient privacy. Lead V4 must be at the base of the breast and, in some patients, under the breast. In males, it should be at about nipple level. Now you can locate V3 midway between V2 and V4. It is on a rib. V5 is at a point where two imaginary lines intersect. Continue to work under the patient's gown. Draw a line from the front of the left axillary fold toward the feet, parallel to the table on which the patient is lying. Draw another line toward the table from V4. Where these lines intersect is V5. Lead V6 is placed at the midaxilla, in line with V4 and V5.

You must practice locating the landmarks and sensor sites on different body sizes and shapes. Remember to keep your female patients covered. You might need to delicately move pendulous breasts to place the sensors beneath them. Review Figure 49-13 for the correct placement of leads. Procedure 49-1 describes the procedure for performing an ECG.

procedure
49-1

RECORDING A 12-LEAD ELECTROCARDIOGRAPH
Objective: Perform an ECG without assistance.

EQUIPMENT AND SUPPLIES
ECG machine with sensors, patient cable, and power cord; ECG paper; electrolyte, if needed; alcohol; screwdriver, for adjustments, if needed; patient gown, if needed

METHOD
1. Perform hand hygiene.
2. Assemble necessary supplies.
3. Attach and plug in the power cord.
4. Verify that the machine is operational and positioned properly.
5. Identify, interview, and instruct the patient on the procedure.
6. Offer female patients gowns to be worn with the opening down the front.
7. Position the patient flat on the table with a pillow under the head and one under the knees if needed.

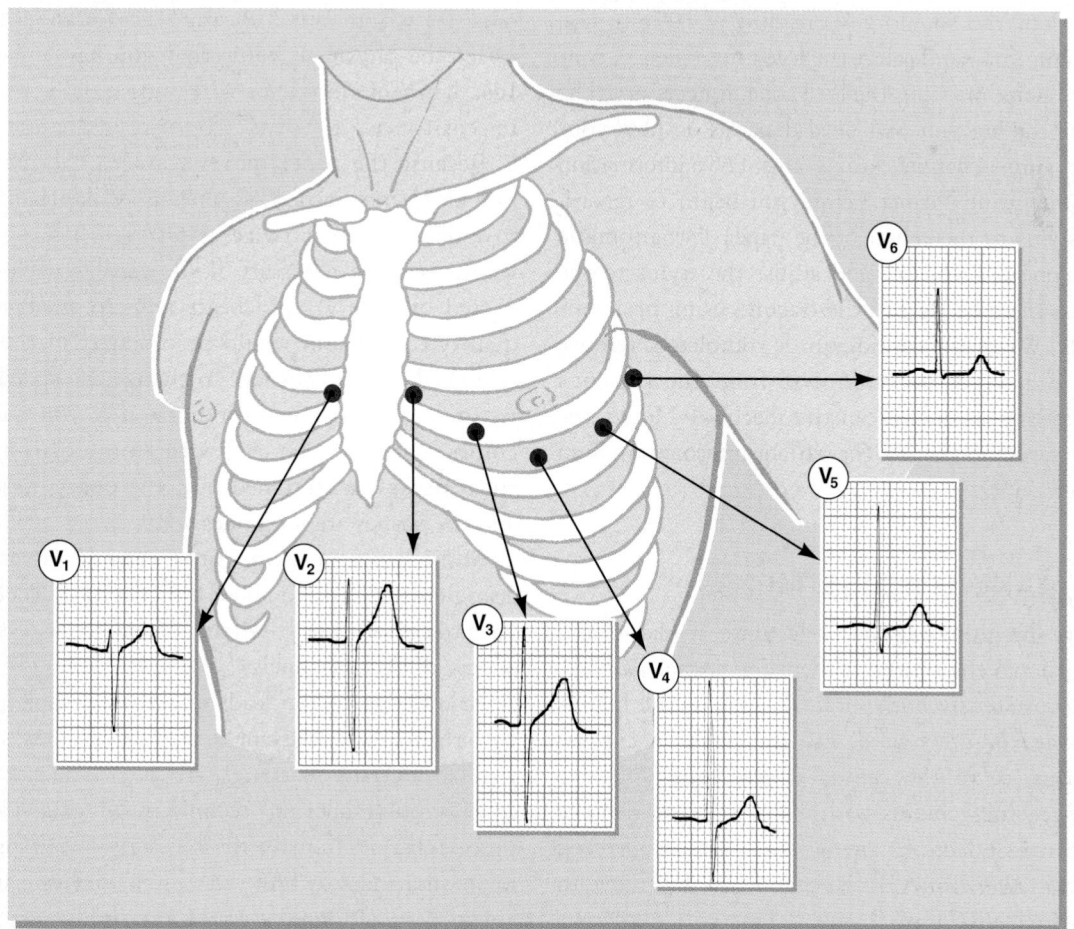

FIGURE 49-16 Electrode placement for chest leads V1–V6.

8. Prepare the electrode sites and attach the electrodes. Limb electrodes should be applied over the fleshy part of the inner aspects of the lower legs and on the upper part of the forearms. Chest leads should be applied as illustrated in Figure 49-16.
9. Connect the patient cable.
10. Instruct the patient to relax, breathe normally, and refrain from speaking.
11. Standardize the machine.
12. Adjust the stylus to the center of the paper or the center of each channel.
13. Record. For automatic machines, depress AUTO-RUN; for manual machines select the leads in sequence and use RUN 25. Use your problem-solving skills if you encounter artifacts.

14. Mark the leads, if necessary.
15. Remove the sensors; wipe electrolyte from the patient's skin, if used.
16. Politely dismiss the patient, aiding the patient in getting up and dressed, if necessary.
17. Perform hand hygiene.
18. Clean the machine, straps, and sensors according to manufacturer's instructions.
19. Mount the ECG if necessary and transfer patient information.
20. Chart the procedure in the patient's record. Sign or initial your work.

CHARTING EXAMPLE

3/11/XX 2:10 P.M. 12-lead ECG performed and given to Dr. Salpega to read. · · · · · · · · · · · · · · · W. Short, CMA (AAMA)

Arrange the patient cable to follow the body contours, avoiding the coils. Connect the patient cable and begin to record by performing a standard (Figure 49-17). For manual machines, select the STD lead, "run 25," and push the standard button. Stop the machine and count the boxes included in the deflection. You should get a reading of 10 mm. Use the lead selector knob and select the leads in sequence, running a 6-inch strip, marking the lead code, if necessary. The length of the tracing you will need depends on how your office mounts single-channel cardiograms. Have information about your mounting format before you begin to record. Adjust the stylus to the center of the paper. For automatic machines, depress "auto-run" and adjust the stylus to the center of each channel. Record the tracing, using problem-solving skills. When the cardiogram is completed, remove the sensors and wipe the electrolyte from the patient's skin. Dismiss the patient. Clean the machine. Mount the ECG, if necessary, and transfer the patient information. Sign or initial your work.

MAKING ADJUSTMENTS

A satisfactory tracing is one that is accurate, readable, and clear; travels down the center of the page; and has a baseline that is consistently horizontal. If the baseline begins to drift upward or downward, use the position control knob to return it to the center of the page. Observe whether the tracing remains within the graph portion of the paper. If the deflections are so large that they exceed the upper and lower limits of the graph, you will have to reduce the sensitivity from 1 to $\frac{1}{2}$. This will make the

tracing half as large, and you will need to include a standard to let the interpreter know what you have done. One mV of electricity will cause a deflection of 5 mm in sensitivity $\frac{1}{2}$. However, if the tracing in sensitivity 1 is so tiny that it is not readable, increase the size by changing the sensitivity from 1 to 2. Again, place a standard on the page to let the physician know that you have made a change. Just 1 mV of electricity will cause a deflection of 20 mm in sensitivity 2.

Because the paper moves through the machine at the rate of 25 mm/second, an option available in recording is to move the paper twice as fast at 50 mm/second. This would only be necessary if the cardiac cycles were compacted by a very rapid heart rate. In this case, a better-quality cardiogram would be produced if the cycles were stretched out. If you have to change the speed or sensitivity, mark the tracing to indicate that you did so. In machines that mark the lead with an international code, the code marks are stretched out; the dots appear as dashes, and the dashes are long ones.

Multichannel machines produce an ECG very quickly on a single sheet of paper about 8 inches by 11 inches. You will have to center three baselines. A sensitivity or speed change affects all three channels.

Knowledge of the leads and their sensor locations will help the medical assistant to trace back to the source any irregular or erratic markings (artifacts). You can also perform other troubleshooting techniques during the recording process. Failure to make the necessary corrections will result in an unsatisfactory or no tracing. The physician will not be able to read and interpret such a recording.

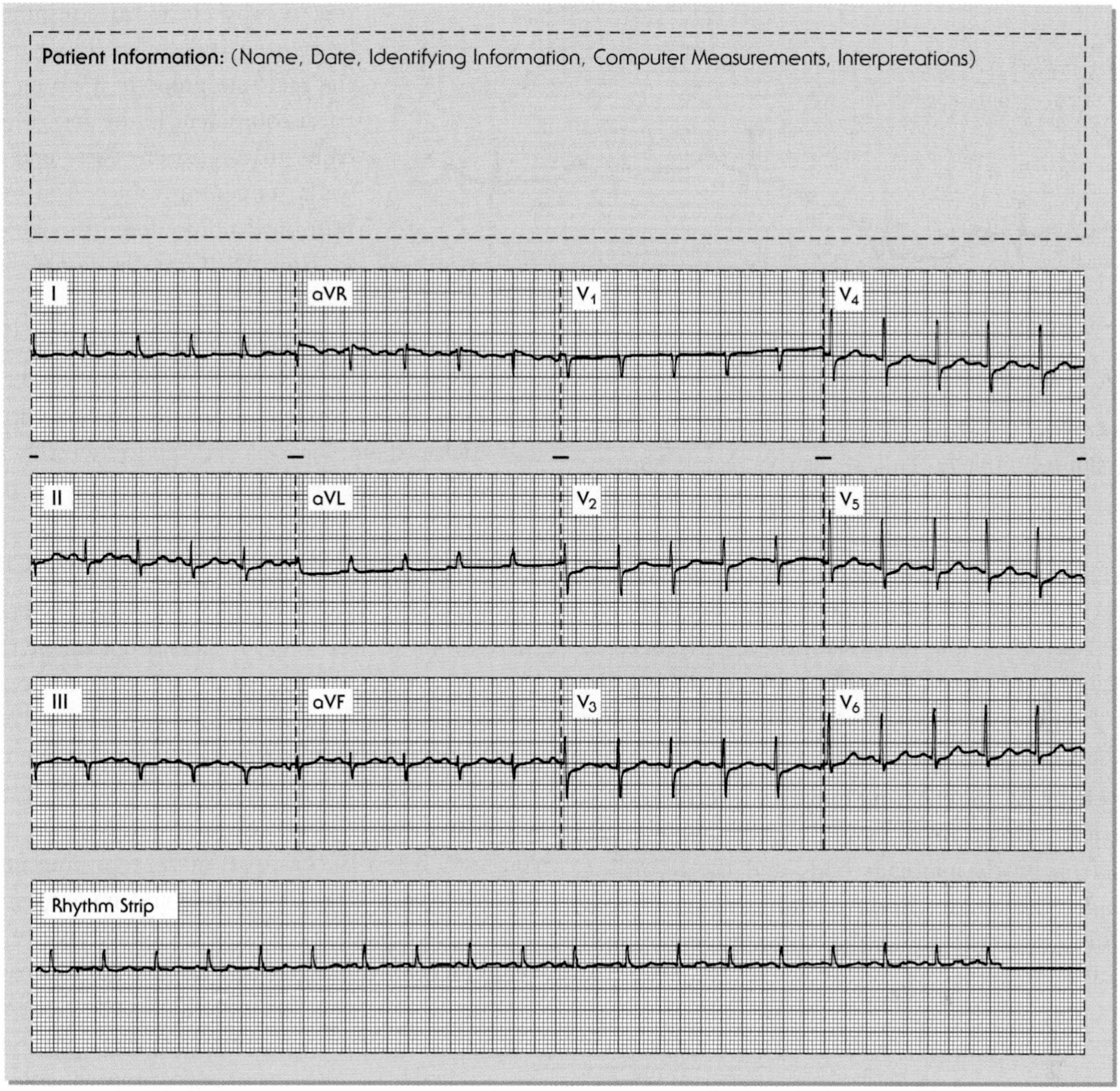

I	aVR	V₁	V₄
II	aVL	V₂	V₅
III	aVF	V₃	V₆

Rhythm Strip

FIGURE 49-17 **Normal 12-lead ECG.**

ARTIFACTS

Occasionally, the sensors will detect electrical activity from a source other than the heart. These deflections or artifacts impair accurate interpretation of the tracing. The medical assistant must find the cause of the artifact and correct it. The different causes of artifacts and how to correct them include the following:

- **Somatic tremor**—A tense muscle or a muscle contraction, even one that you cannot see. It may result from patient discomfort, tension, chills, talking, or moving. Calm and reassure the patient. Suggest that the patient relax, breathe normally, and not talk. If necessary, place

the patient's hands, palm side down, under the hips. This is especially helpful if the patient is not relaxed on the narrow table. This position is also best for patients with a tremor disorder. They will display the smallest number of artifacts in this position. Figure 49-18 illustrates somatic tremors artifacts.

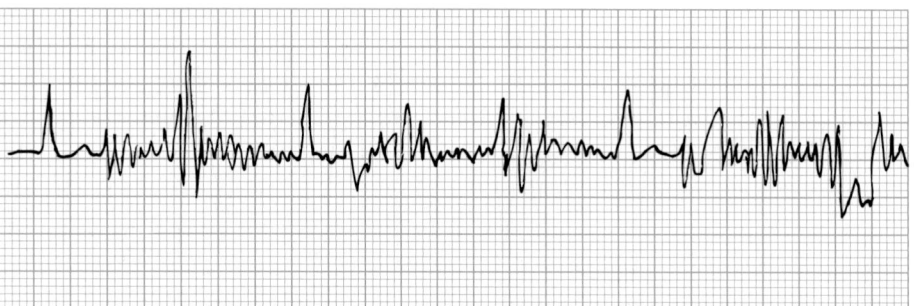

FIGURE 49-18 **Somatic tremors artifact.**

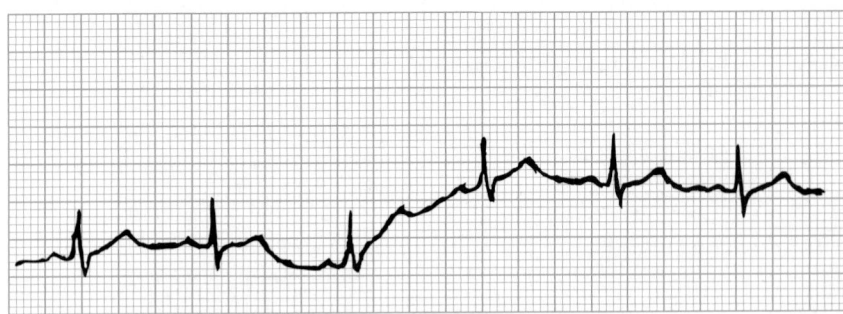

FIGURE 49-19 Baseline sway.

- **Wandering baseline**—Baseline sway and baseline shift (Figure 49-19). This artifact is caused by poor sensor contact with the skin, such as when sensors are dirty or applied too tightly or too loosely, when lotion or talcum prevents good contact with the skin, or when the patient cable slips toward the floor and pulls on the lead wires. You must readjust, reapply, or clean the sensors and place the patient cable securely on the table. You may need to clean the skin with alcohol or cut chest hair.

- **60 cycle or AC (alternating current) interference**—Electrical current in wires and equipment may be picked up by the patient's body and the recording machine. This appears in the recording as small regular spikes or static, and is due to improper ground-ing, nearby electrical equipment in use, or twisted and coiled lead wires. Ground the machine properly. Unplug other electrical equipment in the area. Move the machine to the patient's feet and away from walls containing cables. You may have to wait until a procedure in an adjacent room, such as an X-ray, is completed (Figure 49-20).

- **Erratic stylus**—Loose or broken lead wires cause the stylus to thrash erratically and to go off the page, leading to broken recording. Repair the wires, replace them, or call for service on the equipment (Figure 49-21).

MOUNTING AN ELECTROCARDIOGRAM

Machines that record one lead at a time produce a tracing that is 6 or 12 feet long. To have a document that will fit into the patient record, use a mounting device. Manufacturers make heavy paper folders with pockets or self-stick areas labeled for each of the leads. Many different forms are available. Knowing the form you will use for mounting will help avoid the waste of obtaining a longer tracing than you need. Select the best part of the recording for that lead. It must have a straight baseline and no artifacts. Cut and trim it, and place it in the appropriate area of the folder. Double-check your work to make certain you have read the international code for leads correctly. Repeat the process until all 12 leads have been properly mounted. Employer preference will determine where to place the standardization. Machines that record from three leads at once do not require mounting. The final product fits nicely into a patient record.

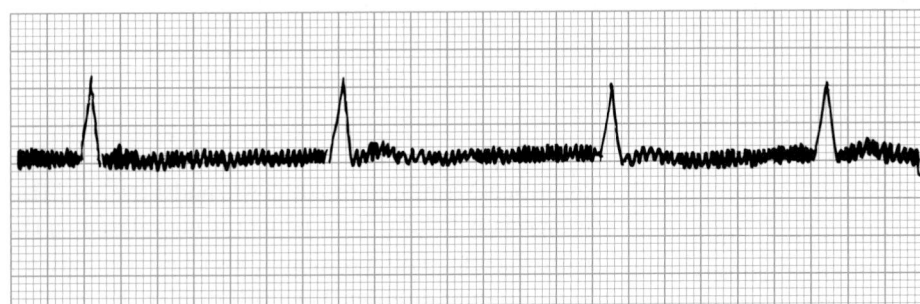

FIGURE 49-20 60-cycle interference.

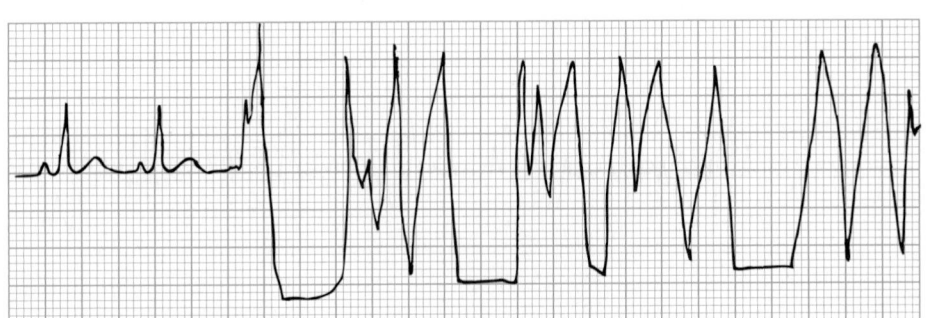

FIGURE 49-21 Broken recording.

WHAT IS NORMAL?

A normal sinus rhythm means that each heartbeat has three distinct waves: a P wave; a T wave; and a QRS complex between the P and T, where the Q is a downward deflection, the R is an upward deflection, and the S is a downward deflection following an R. The beats come at regular intervals, indicating the impulse originates in the SA node. Within the lead being recorded,

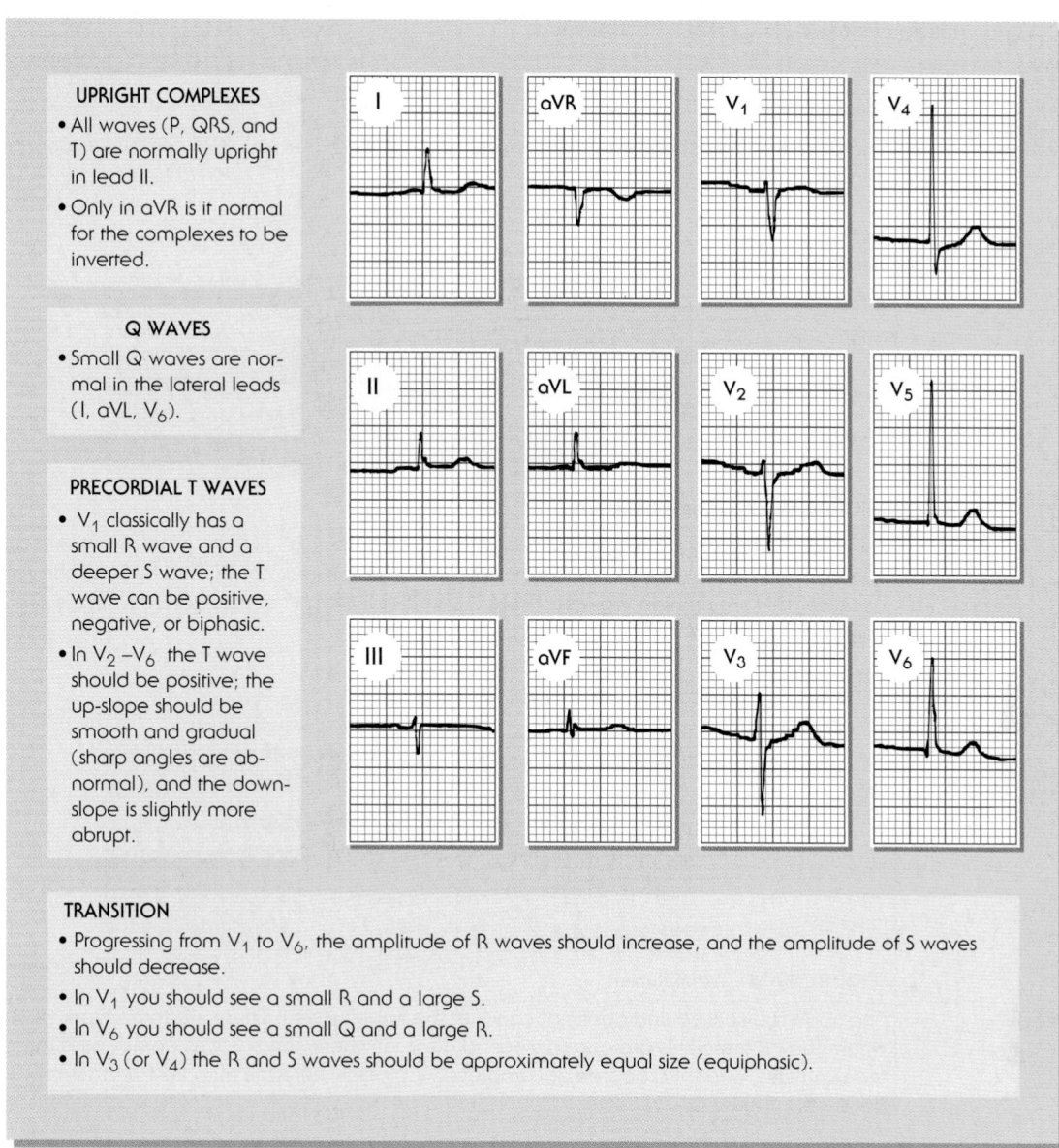

UPRIGHT COMPLEXES
- All waves (P, QRS, and T) are normally upright in lead II.
- Only in aVR is it normal for the complexes to be inverted.

Q WAVES
- Small Q waves are normal in the lateral leads (I, aVL, V$_6$).

PRECORDIAL T WAVES
- V$_1$ classically has a small R wave and a deeper S wave; the T wave can be positive, negative, or biphasic.
- In V$_2$–V$_6$ the T wave should be positive; the up-slope should be smooth and gradual (sharp angles are abnormal), and the down-slope is slightly more abrupt.

TRANSITION
- Progressing from V$_1$ to V$_6$, the amplitude of R waves should increase, and the amplitude of S waves should decrease.
- In V$_1$ you should see a small R and a large S.
- In V$_6$ you should see a small Q and a large R.
- In V$_3$ (or V$_4$) the R and S waves should be approximately equal size (equiphasic).

FIGURE 49-22   Features of a normal 12-lead ECG.

each cardiac cycle appears the same as previous cycles. To recognize abnormalities, you must first be able to recognize what is normal. Figure 49-22 illustrates and identifies features of a normal 12-lead ECG.

ABNORMALITIES

Occasionally a tracing will reveal an abnormality caused by cardiac pathology in the patient. An observant medical assistant will recognize the more common abnormalities and draw them to the attention of the physician or will follow office protocol, which often calls for an additional recording of a particular lead. Table 49-2 lists some cardiac pathology that can be visualized by ECGs, including references to several examples of the abnormalities listed.

PROFESSIONALISM

As health care providers it is important to maintain a healthy lifestyle and set an example for patients. Cardiac risk factors (age, gender, heredity, smoking, obesity, hyperlipidemia, hypertension, stress, and excessive drinking or use of drugs) can affect anyone. Be a living example of a healthy lifestyle by engaging in regular exercise, making healthy food choices, and avoiding use of recreational drugs and excessive alcohol consumption. Encourage patients to do the same.

TABLE 49-2 Abnormalities Caused by Cardiac Pathology

Abnormality	Description
Atrial fibrillation	There are as many as 350 irregular P waves and 130–150 irregular QRS complexes per minute (Figure 49-23).

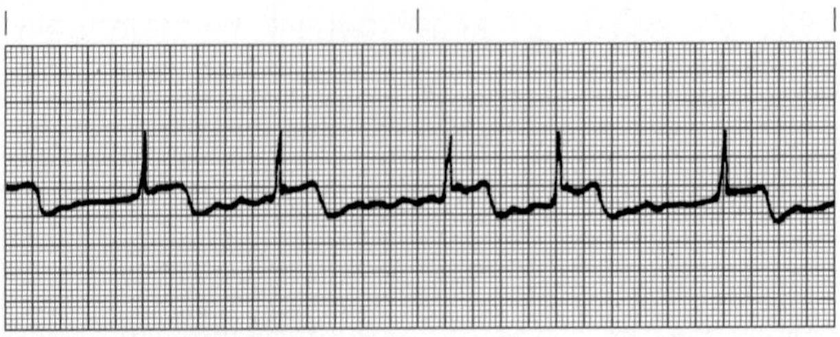

FIGURE 49-23 Atrial fibrillation.

Atrial flutter	This rapid fluttering of the upper chambers looks on the ECG like the pattern of teeth on a saw. The atrial rate is 250–350 per minute. Not all the impulses are conducted through the AV node because they are coming too fast. There is some "blockage" at the AV node. This is one type of heart block (Figure 49-24).

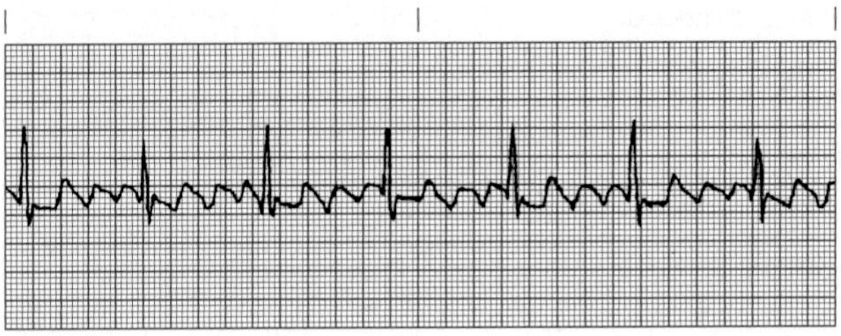

FIGURE 49-24 Atrial flutter.

AV heart block	The node is diseased and does not conduct the impulse well. There are three types: first degree, where the PR interval is prolonged; second degree, where some waves do not pass through to the ventricles; and third degree or complete AV block, where the atria and ventricles beat independently (Figure 49-25).

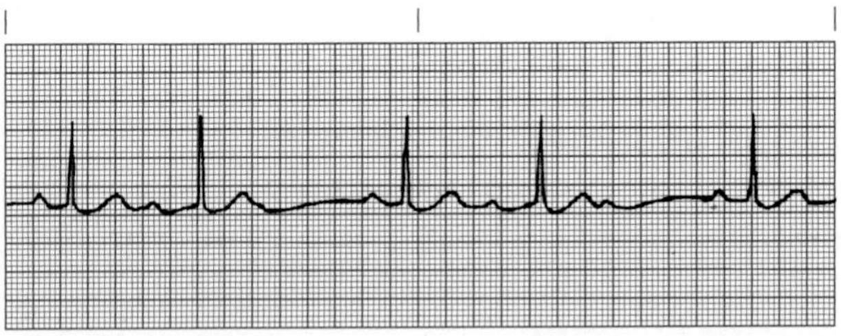

FIGURE 49-25 Third-degree heart block.

Myocardial infarction (MI)	There are broad and deep Q waves. *Old injury:* The ST segment is usually depressed below the baseline. *New injury:* The ST segment is usually elevated above the baseline. Angina pectoris is the name for the syndrome of pain and oppression in the anterior chest due to heart tissue being deprived of oxygen. If this pain lasts 20–30 minutes, suspect a myocardial infarction in which the heart tissue is actually dying.

Paroxysmal atrial tachycardia (PAT)	There is a common arrhythmia, usually seen in young adults with normal hearts. There are no visible P waves because they are hidden by the T wave of the previous cycle. The atrial rate is between 140–250 per minute. In many ways it looks on the ECG like repeated PACs.
Premature atrial contractions (PACs)	A P wave occurs earlier than expected, usually from a source outside the sinus node. Therefore, P waves are distorted.
Premature ventricular contractions (PVCs)	The wide QRS complexes occur without preceding P waves. They may be caused by electrolyte imbalance, stress, smoking, alcohol, or toxic reactions to drugs and in a majority of patients who have had a heart attack (Figure 49-26).

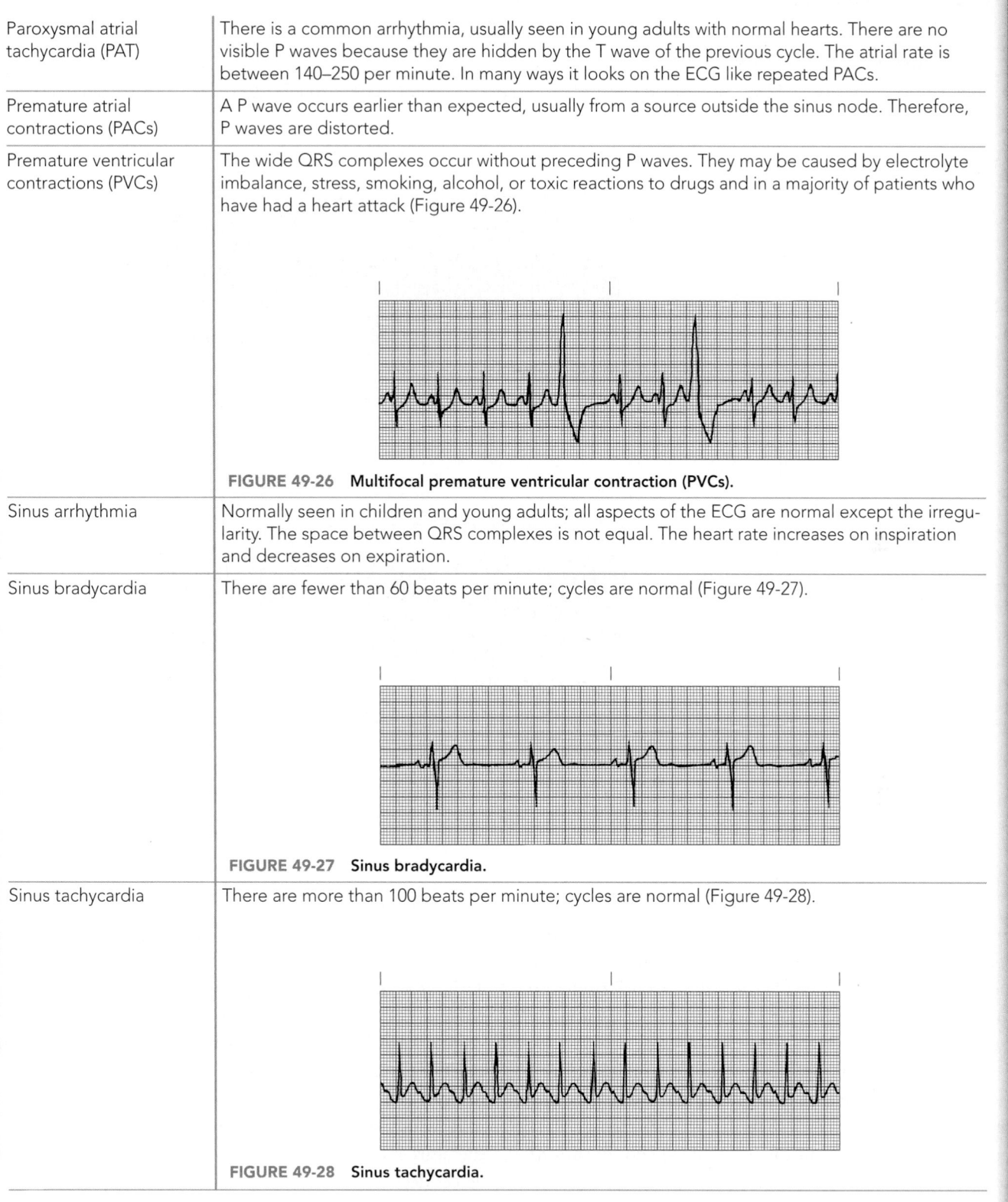

FIGURE 49-26   Multifocal premature ventricular contraction (PVCs).

Sinus arrhythmia	Normally seen in children and young adults; all aspects of the ECG are normal except the irregularity. The space between QRS complexes is not equal. The heart rate increases on inspiration and decreases on expiration.
Sinus bradycardia	There are fewer than 60 beats per minute; cycles are normal (Figure 49-27).

FIGURE 49-27   Sinus bradycardia.

Sinus tachycardia	There are more than 100 beats per minute; cycles are normal (Figure 49-28).

FIGURE 49-28   Sinus tachycardia.

(continued)

TABLE 49-2 (*continued*)

Abnormality	Description
Ventricular fibrillation	The waves are irregular and rounded, the contractions uncoordinated. Death may occur in as little as 4 minutes (Figure 49-29).

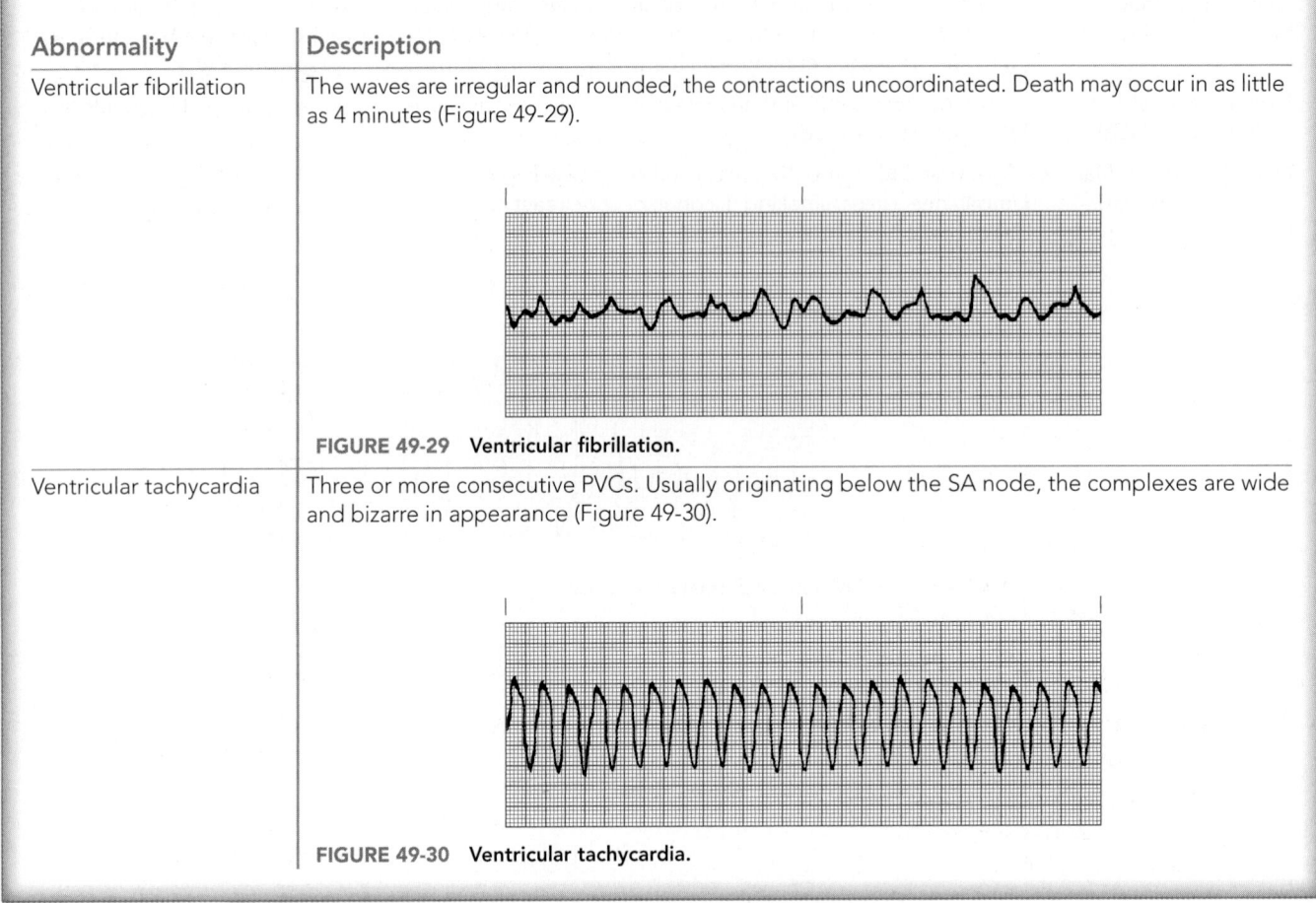

FIGURE 49-29   Ventricular fibrillation.

Abnormality	Description
Ventricular tachycardia	Three or more consecutive PVCs. Usually originating below the SA node, the complexes are wide and bizarre in appearance (Figure 49-30).

FIGURE 49-30   Ventricular tachycardia.

Special Procedures

Some ECG-related diagnostic procedures are performed regularly in the primary care office or in cardiology. The following two procedures involve recording additional lengths of tracings and may be part of written office protocol for cardiograms.

The first one, a rhythm strip, will be run on lead II for 20 seconds at the physician's request or if the medical assistant sees anything that appears abnormal on the tracing. This is not cut and mounted but carefully folded and given to the physician for interpretation.

The second procedure, an inspiration strip, is run on lead II for 10 seconds with the patient holding his or her breath. This is of greatest value when, as the patient breathes, your tracing shows wandering baseline. This will eliminate any respiratory impact on the tracing.

EXERCISE TOLERANCE TESTING

At times patients will have symptoms that are not obvious on a resting ECG. A **stress test** or treadmill test involves an evaluation of the heart's response during moderate exercise while a 12-lead ECG is performed. It is a diagnostic procedure performed to determine the likelihood of **coronary artery disease (CAD)**, blockage of the arteries that supply the heart muscle. The patient is asked to exercise on a bicycle or treadmill, which stresses the heart and requires more oxygen for the heart muscle cells. A faster heart rate makes it easier to detect decreased blood flow.

Stress testing may be used to evaluate patients with a high risk for developing heart disease, known to have early heart disease, or about to begin a strenuous exercise program. This test is also done on patients who have cardiac complaints such as shortness of breath when exercising and as an evaluation of their rehabilitation following cardiac surgery. The treadmill test is noninvasive, and frequent blood pressure measurements are taken while exercise is in progress. The goal of the test is to increase the heart rate to a maximal level and increase the myocardial demand for oxygen. The test continues to a predetermined level or until the patient experiences fatigue or chest pain. The test concludes when the patient's symptoms of chest pain or fatigue or ECG changes indicate significant changes, especially to the ST segment. After the conclusion of the test, the patient rests while the monitoring of blood pressure and heart rate continue until both are within normal range. Complications may occur, and appropriately stocked emergency carts should be on hand.

Patient Preparation

The patient should be given instructions before the scheduled test day to wear comfortable exercise or walking shoes and loose-fitting clothes. Female patients should be instructed to wear a bra to minimize artifacts on the ECG. Instruct all patients not to eat a large meal for at least 4 hours before the test to avoid nausea. Patients should take their normal medications unless instructed otherwise by the physician.

The patient should know that baseline vital signs and a resting ECG are recorded first. Vital signs are measured with the patient in supine position and standing. Another ECG is taken with the patient standing and breathing rapidly (**hyperventilating**). This is done because rapid breathing can produce some changes in the ST segment and the T wave. It is important to know this in advance so the interpretation of the stress test ECG is not compromised. Also, a thorough history is taken emphasizing any symptoms such as shortness of breath or chest pain. Explain to the patient that an ECG will be recorded as he or she walks or bikes at a carefully prescribed pace in the presence of the physician. Increases in rate or incline will be made, but the patient should not feel discomfort or shortness of breath.

The medical assistant prepares the patient, connects the patient to the recording devices (ECG, heart rate, BP), and frequently checks blood pressure during the test. The sensors are all placed on the torso. The precordial sensors (V1–V6) are placed as for the regular ECG, but the arm and leg sensors are put at the midclavicular line on the top of the torso and on the midclavicular line on the abdomen. The electrodes should adhere securely to the skin and may need to be taped in place. If a male patient has a very hairy chest, the hair may be shaved to improve attachment of electrodes. At the conclusion of the test, the physician evaluates the effect of exercise on the heart rate, blood pressure, and ECG. The physician may order the test to be stopped if the patient has trouble breathing or complains of chest pain or significant ECG changes contraindicate continuing the test.

VARIETIES OF STRESS TESTS

The variety of exercise protocols used in treadmill testing involve the speed and incline of the treadmill and how quickly these changes are introduced during the test. The stress test is continued until 85 percent of the maximum target heart rate is achieved or the patient becomes symptomatic. The maximum **target heart rate** is calculated by using the following formula: 220 minus the patient's age = the maximum target heart rate for that person. For a 60-year-old patient, $220 - 60 = 160 \times .85 = 136$, or the maximum target heart rate for this patient. For patients who have had a myocardial infarction (MI), the target heart rate is set lower at 70 percent. This is known as a **submaximal test**.

Thallium (a radioisotope that emits gamma rays and is used in nuclear medicine) is sometimes injected into the patient's vein during a stress test for better understanding of **perfusion** (blood flow to the myocardium). Thallium is injected during the last minute of exercise. The patient lies on a special table, and a gamma camera takes pictures. If the heart muscle is **ischemic** (receiving less than the normal amount of blood flow), poor uptake of the thallium will occur. This is indicated as a "cold spot" on the pictures. Normal perfusion of the myocardium is indicated by "hot spots" on the pictures.

Another type of test, the **multiple gated acquisition (MUGA) scan**, can be done to check blood flow in the myocardium. This involves injection of an isotope and having a nuclear scan performed to detect myocardial perfusion.

procedure 49-2

PREPARING AND MONITORING THE PATIENT DURING A TREADMILL STRESS TEST

Objective: Prepare patient for treadmill test per physician's order, including all preliminary testing of vital signs and ECGs.

EQUIPMENT AND SUPPLIES
treadmill; sensors; blood pressure monitor

METHOD
1. Assemble necessary supplies.
2. Plug in the power cord and turn on the machine.
3. Verify that the treadmill is operational.
4. Identify, interview, and instruct the patient.
5. Measure vital signs and record.
6. Attach the electrode patches securely using tape to hold in place if necessary. Attach limb leads on torso at midclavicular line and on the abdomen of torso at midclavicular line. Attach chest leads as usual.
7. Perform a baseline resting ECG (see Procedure 49-1). If facility protocol requires, perform a standing ECG as well.
8. Disconnect the patient cable from the ECG machine.
9. Attach a sphygmomanometer to the patient's arm.
10. Permit the patient to walk about the room or on the slow-moving treadmill to see what it feels like.
11. Connect the patient to all recording devices.
12. Check with the physician to determine the pace and incline of the treadmill (Figure 49-31).
13. Record BP, ECG, and heart and respiratory rate periodically as you observe the patient's face for redness, difficulty breathing, chest pain, and so forth.

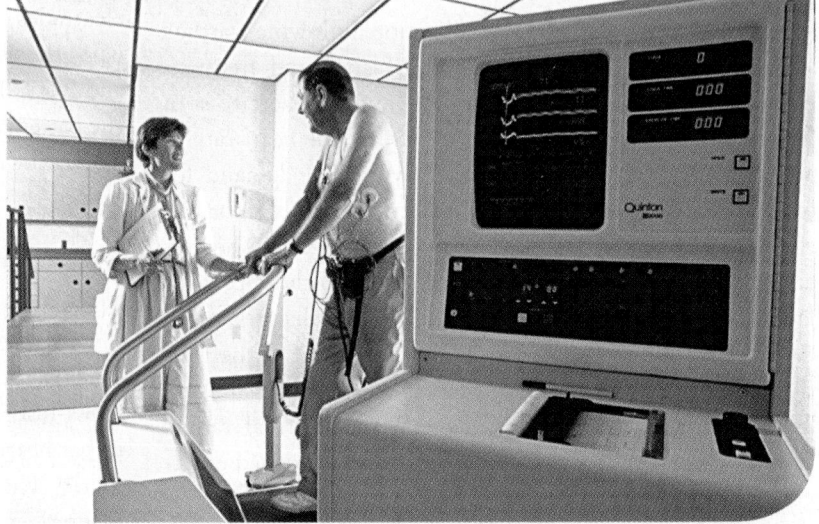

FIGURE 49-31 The patient must be observed closely during a stress test.

14. Allow the patient to rest, and continue monitoring vital signs and ECG as required.
15. When the test is completed, clean the patient's skin and assist with dressing as needed.
16. Organize the documentation into the patient record.

CHARTING EXAMPLE
3/11/XX 3:10 P.M. Stress test performed. Patient observed for 15 minutes after test. Patient tolerated the procedure well. · M. Shapiro, CMA (AAMA)

Pharmacologic stress testing involves no exercise. In this case a medication is given to the patient that causes the heart rate to climb to the target heart rate. Continuous ECGs and vital sign evaluation are performed. This test procedure is useful on patients with physical limitations or the elderly who cannot perform enough exercise to elevate the heart rate.

Because there is always the risk of cardiac arrest, the medical assistant becomes responsible for maintaining emergency equipment that might be needed and having it in the room at the time of the test. Oxygen equipment, a defibrillator, an airway, intravenous solutions, and medications should be periodically checked and replaced, if outdated or not functioning. Figure 49-31 shows the patient being closely observed during a stress test. Always be sure a physician is present when a stress test is done. Procedure 49-2 describes how to perform a stress test.

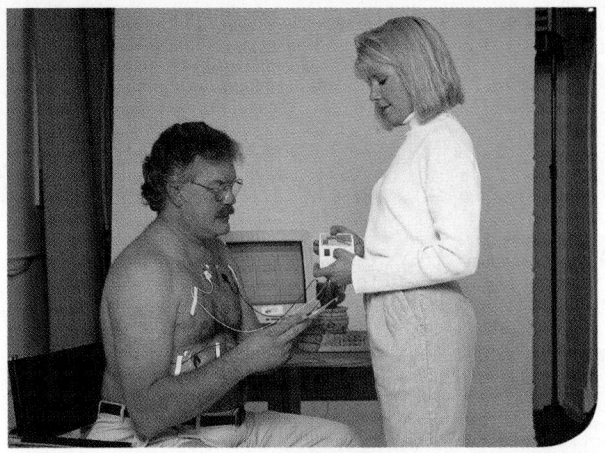

FIGURE 49-32 Discuss the Holter monitor fully with the patient before testing begins.

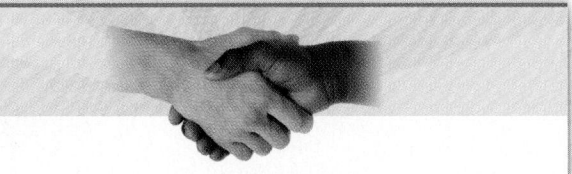

HOLTER MONITOR

The **Holter monitor** records cardiac activity while the patient is ambulatory for at least a 24-hour period. Holter monitoring is performed when the ECG is not conclusive or the cardiac irregularity was not captured on the tracing. A small tape recorder and a patient diary are used to detect heart irregularities that are infrequent and not detected on the standard 12-lead cardiogram (Figure 49-32). It may be set to record continuously and/or to record when the patient presses an "event" button at the onset of symptoms. A medical assistant may instruct the patient and apply the chest sensors.

Patient preparation should stress the importance of the diary. Patients carry out all routine daily activities except showering or bathing. They must also avoid areas of high voltage, as the tape will be affected. Patients use the diary to record their activities during the day. They also indicate in the diary or by depressing an "event button" when they experience any cardiac symptoms, such as chest pain, shortness of breath, or palpitations. Patients should record in the diary such activities as stair climbing, sexual activity, having bowel movements, sleeping, eating, exercising, and so forth. The physician will compare the tape with the activity log to determine which activities were stressing the patient.

The five special disposable chest sensors are attached more securely than in the 12-lead ECG because they must remain in place during all activity. In addition to the usual skin preparation to remove oils, areas for attachment may have to be shaved and an abrasive skin cleaner used. Peel off the cover on the adhesive backing on each sensor and attach one sensor to each of the following locations:

- third intercostal space 2 or 3 inches to the right of the sternum
- third intercostal space 2 or 3 inches to the left of the sternum
- fifth intercostal space at the left sternum margin
- sixth intercostal space at the right anterior axillary line
- sixth intercostal space at the left anterior axillary line

Procedure 49-3 describes the procedure for applying a Holter monitor.

TELEMETRY

Telemetry involves using radio waves to transmit the heart's electrical activity to a central monitoring station. This allows the patient to move around the room or other limited space while the heart is monitored. The patient should be made aware of the range of movement permitted. This type of monitoring is used in inpatient facilities but may be encountered in ambulatory care settings as

procedure 49-3

APPLYING A HOLTER MONITOR

Objective: Apply a Holter monitor, instruct the patient.

EQUIPMENT AND SUPPLIES

Holter monitor with sensors; patient cable; patient activity diary; fresh batteries; blank recording tape; adhesive tape; razor; alcohol

METHOD

1. Assemble necessary supplies.
2. Install new batteries and a blank tape.
3. Verify that the machine is operational.
4. Identify, interview, and instruct the patient.
5. Have the patient remove clothing to the waist (female patients may wear a gown open down the front) and sit on an examination table.
6. Perform hand hygiene.
7. Prepare the electrode sites and attach the electrodes. Remember to attach the sensors in these locations: third intercostal space 2 or 3 inches to the right of the sternum, third intercostal space 2 or 3 inches to the left of the sternum, fifth intercostal space at the left sternum margin, sixth intercostal space at the right anterior axillary line, and sixth intercostal space at the left anterior axillary line (Figure 49-33).
8. Attach the wires so that they point toward the feet, then connect the patient cable.
9. Secure each sensor with adhesive tape.
10. Connect the patient cable.
11. Assist the patient with replacing his or her shirt. Extend the cable between the buttons or under the hem.
12. Place the recorder in the carrying case, and either attach to the patient's belt or to the shoulder strap. Check that there is no tension on the wires.

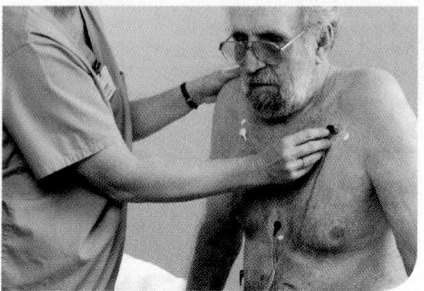

FIGURE 49-33 Medical assistant attaching electrodes for Holter monitoring.

13. Plug the cable into the recorder.
14. Record the starting time in the diary.
15. Ensure that the patient understands what he or she is to do.
16. Confirm the time for the patient to return to the clinic for removal of the Holter monitor.
17. Chart the procedure in the patient's record. Sign or initial your work.

CHARTING EXAMPLE

3/11/XX 4:15 P.M. Holter monitor applied and instruction given. Patient to return in 24 hours with diary and monitor.· · · · · · · · ·
· E. Blodgett, CMA (AAMA)

well. Figure 49-34 illustrates the placement of the electrodes on a patient.

PACEMAKERS

Pacemakers are electronic devices that help the heart maintain normal rhythm. They may be used to increase heart rate in patients with **bradycardia** (slow heart rate) or to override the heart rate in a patient with **tachycardia** (rapid heart rate) or other dysrhythmias. Pacemakers may be temporarily or permanently installed in the patient. Temporary pacemakers are used in acute settings to stabilize and maintain the patient for shorter periods of time. Patients with temporary pacemakers must be hospitalized and continuously monitored. The pulse generator is located outside the body, and leads are either threaded through specific veins (subclavian, femoral, brachial or external jugular) to the

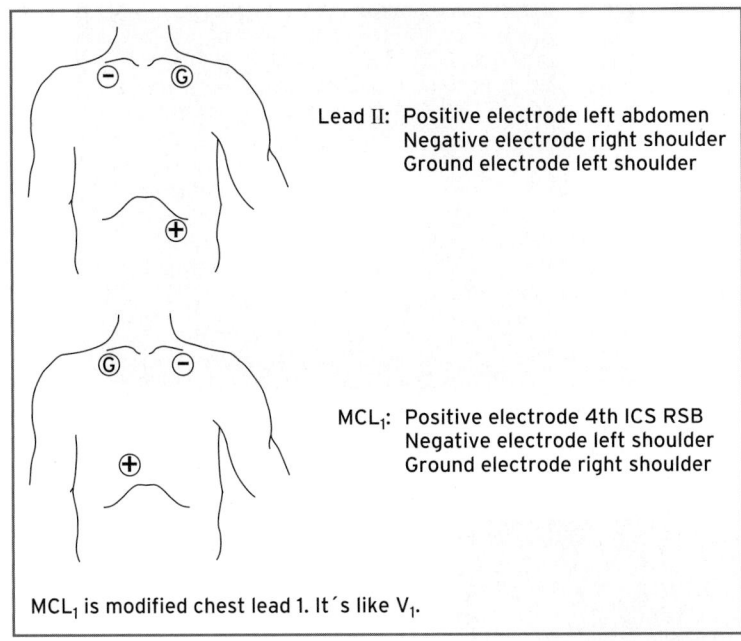

Lead II: Positive electrode left abdomen
Negative electrode right shoulder
Ground electrode left shoulder

MCL₁: Positive electrode 4th ICS RSB
Negative electrode left shoulder
Ground electrode right shoulder

MCL₁ is modified chest lead 1. It´s like V₁.

FIGURE 49-34   Color coded leads are attached as telemetry monitoring.

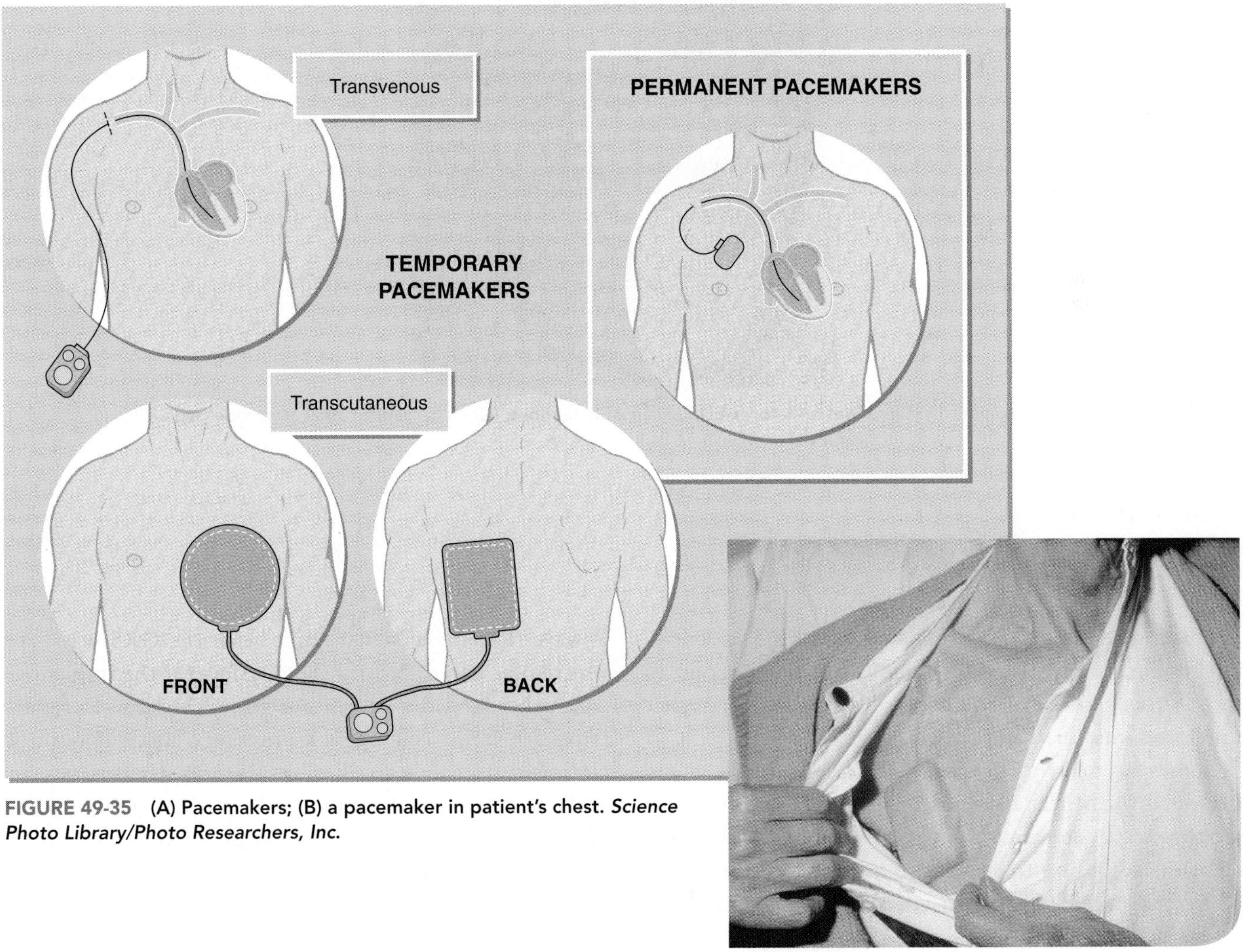

right atrium or the right ventricle. A temporary pacemaker may be attached during surgery to the outer surface of the heart. The wires then exit the chest and are attached to an external pulse generator.

The type of permanent pacemaker implanted depends on the patient's condition and the type of cardiac problem involved. These are long-term devices, and the pulse generator is implanted into the subcutaneous tissue of the upper chest. The leads are inserted into a major vein leading into the heart in the region of the myocardium that is impaired. The opposite ends of the leads are attached to the pulse generator. Figure 49-35A illustrates both temporary and permanent pacemakers.

If the patient has an implanted automatic pacemaker, spikes will appear on the ECG with each cardiac cycle. These spikes should be rhythmically spaced on the ECG if the pacemaker is programmed for a certain rate. In fact, even when a patient is dead,

Transvenous

PERMANENT PACEMAKERS

TEMPORARY PACEMAKERS

Transcutaneous

FRONT

BACK

FIGURE 49-35   (A) Pacemakers; (B) a pacemaker in patient's chest. *Science Photo Library/Photo Researchers, Inc.*

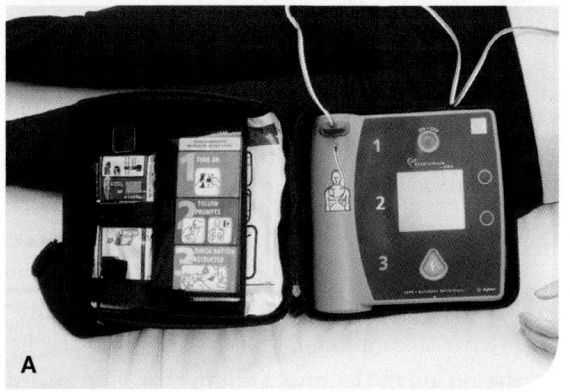

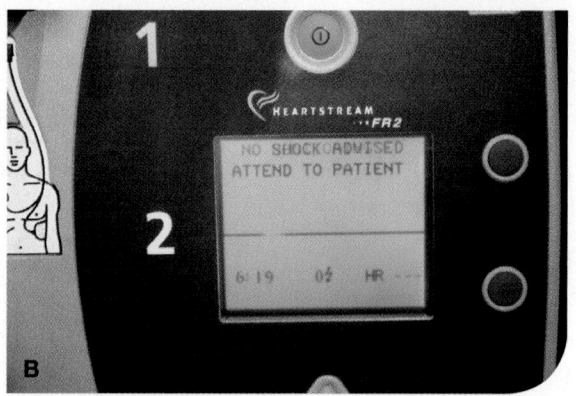

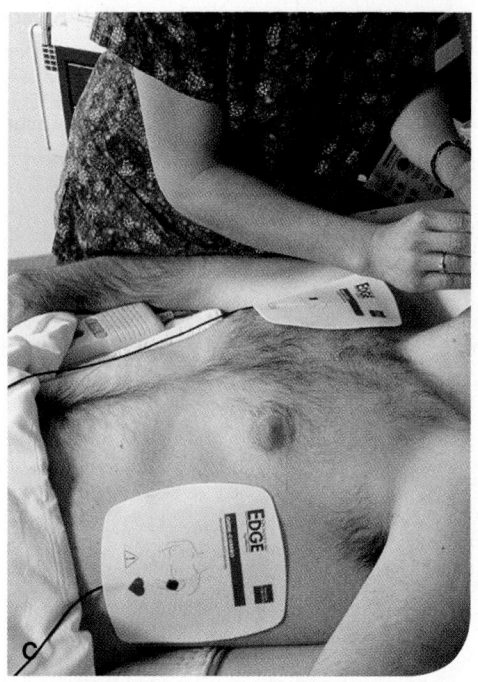

FIGURE 49-36 (A) An automated external defibrillator (AED); (B) an AED readout; (C) placement of AED electrode pads.

the pacemaker spike will be recorded if an ECG is done— but, unfortunately, the heart muscle will not respond to the electrical stimulus. Figure 49-35B shows a pacemaker implanted into a patient's chest.

Some pacemakers are fixed rate or continuous. Some fire only when needed (on demand). Some are rate responsive to physiological changes and respond to the body's demands according to changes in the patient's activities. The atrial-paced pacemaker will show a spike with the P wave. Pacemakers that spike with the QRS wave are ventricular paced. Notify the physician if the implanted pacemaker is visible on the surface of the skin. Defibrillators are used in emergencies to send a small amount of electricity to the heart. Figures 49-36A–C illustrate an AED machine, the readouts, and a patient receiving defibrillation. Figure 49-37 shows an ECG tracing with pacemaker firings.

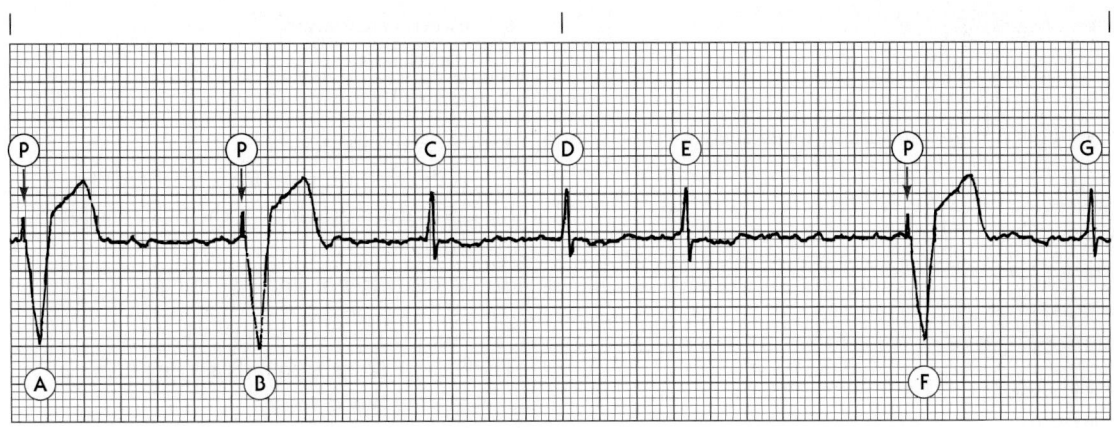

FIGURE 49-37   ECG complexes showing pacemaker spikes (A, B, F).

SUMMARY

The use of electrocardiography for the early diagnosis and treatment of heart disease has contributed to the lengthened life expectancy of many patients and has improved their quality of life. ECGs are usually performed while lying down. Sometimes ECGs are done in combination with stressful exercise to see the effect on the heart. The patient may be monitored for 24 hours with a Holter monitor to see which activities stress the heart. Pacemakers help the patient's heart maintain normal rhythm. Accuracy in carrying out your duties during these tests will provide the physician with the best possible data to make that diagnosis and institute the correct treatment.

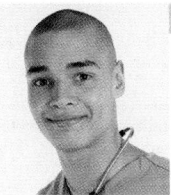

49 CHAPTER REVIEW

COMPETENCY REVIEW

1. Define and spell the terms to learn for this chapter.

2. Describe how to maintain and operate electrocardiograph equipment.

3. Identify by name and location of their sensors the standard 12 leads on an electrocardiograph machine.

4. Name and describe four ECG artifacts.

PREPARING FOR THE CERTIFICATION EXAM

1. In an ECG the electrode used in grounding is
   a. LA
   b. LL
   c. RA
   d. RL
   e. V1

2. When taking an ECG the position of the first chest lead V1 is

   a. third intercostal space, left sternal margin
   b. third intercostal space right sternal margin
   c. fourth intercostal space, left sternal margin
   d. fourth intercostal space right sternal margin
   e. fifth intercostal space mid clavicular line

3. The second wave of the ECG is the
   a. S wave
   b. Q wave

c. P wave

d. T wave

e. R wave

4. When the ECG is running at normal speed the paper is moving at the rate of
   a. 10 mm/sec
   b. 20 mm/sec
   c. 25 mm/sec
   d. 35 mm/sec
   e. 50 mm/sec

5. The sinoatrial node is located in the
   a. right atrium
   b. left atrium
   c. apex
   d. ventricles
   e. septum between the atria

6. The portion of the ECG that relates to atrial depolarization is the
   a. P wave
   b. QRS complex
   c. T wave
   d. U wave
   e. P-R interval

7. A device used to regulate irregular heart rates is
   a. Holter monitor
   b. oscilloscope

c. electrocardiogram

d. pacemaker

e. ventilator

8. A myocardial infarction
   a. is the medical term for a heart attack
   b. indicates a problem in the ECG machine
   c. rarely happens
   d. is an artifact on an ECG tracing
   e. is not important

9. The S1 and S2 heart sounds are caused by
   a. leaking blood vessels
   b. blood clot in the heart
   c. closing of the heart valves
   d. leaky valves
   e. an infectious disease

10. The blood vessels that supply the myocardial tissue with oxygen and nourishment are the
    a. aorta and vena cava
    b. pulmonary arteries
    c. pulmonary veins
    d. carotid arteries
    e. coronary arteries

CRITICAL THINKING

1. Why is it important that David provide Mr. Masterson with a detailed explanation of the procedure? What should David tell him?

2. When Mr. Masterson removes his shirt, David realizes that the patient has a very hairy chest. What should David do, and why?

3. Mr. Masterson informs David that he has trouble lying flat on his back due to a previous injury from a car accident and that he does not think he will be able to lie flat for the ECG. How should David handle this situation?

ON THE JOB

Bonny Glidewell, CMA (AAMA), works in a cardiologist's office. She passes out a questionnaire to all her patients about their lifestyle habits (exercise, eating, smoking, etc.) so she can collect data and then create patient teaching brochures.

1. Which questions should she ask to determine which behaviors are the most prevalent in this practice?
2. What would you expect to be the usual diet of a person with coronary artery disease?
3. What instructions might she give on how to stop smoking?
4. Construct a brochure to give to patients to help them change their diets.
5. Create a patient teaching brochure on the importance of exercise.

INTERNET ACTIVITY

Go to the American Heart Association and the American Lung Association websites, gather information, and create two brochures to teach patients about heart and lung health.

MEDMEDIA

Additional interactive resources and activities for this chapter can be found:

On your student DVD: View applicable procedure videos on the DVD-ROM found in the back of this book.

MyHealthProfessionsKit.com: Test your knowledge of this chapter with games and activities. MyHealthProfessionsKit also includes resources, helpful links, and a Spanish audio glossary.

Medical Assisting Interactive: Practice your procedures as a medical assistant in this simulated doctor's office. This can be accessed through MyHealthProfessionsKit.com.

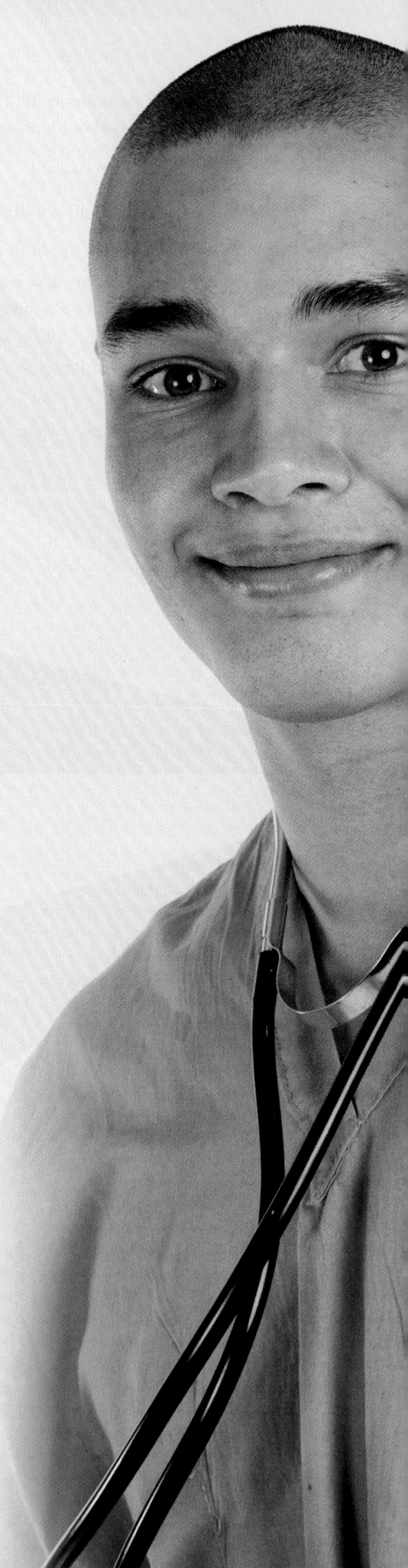

50

Pulmonary Function

LEARNING OBJECTIVES

After completing this chapter, you should be able to:

- Define and spell the terms to learn for this chapter.

- Explain forced vital capacity (FVC), forced expiratory volume in 1 second (FEV1), and maximal midexpiratory flow (MMEF).

- Differentiate between obstructive and restrictive pulmonary disease.

- Operate pulmonary function equipment.

- Identify by name and function the controls on a spirometer.

- Perform spirometry testing.

- Educate a patient to properly perform peak flow testing.

- Operate a pulse oximeter and understand the importance of the results.

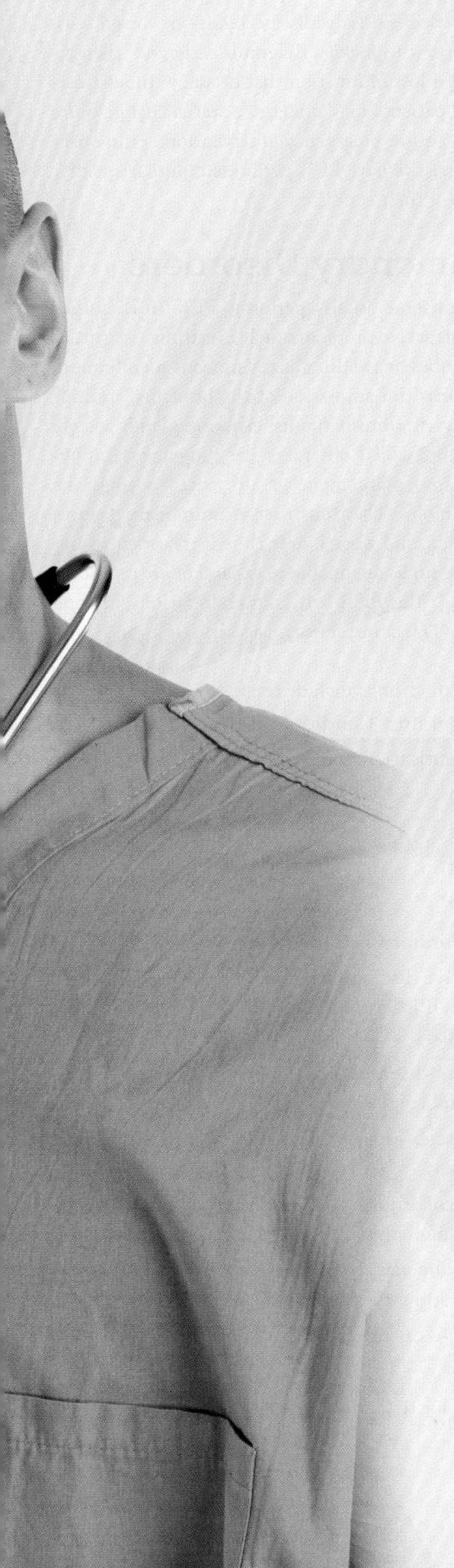

CHAPTER OUTLINE

CASE STUDY

Abigail Lently is a 51-year-old patient who has recently been diagnosed with COPD. She has come in for a follow-up spirometry test since being placed on her maintenance medications. She admits that she has had a very tough time with smoking cessation, and although she has cut back on the number of cigarettes smoked per day, she has not quit altogether.

chronic obstructive
pulmonary disease (COPD)

expiratory reserve volume
(ERV)

forced expiratory volume
(FEV)

forced vital capacity (FVC)

functional residual capacity
(FRC)

inspiratory capacity (IC)

inspiratory reserve volume
(IRV)

maximal midexpiratory
flow (MMEF)

oxygen saturation

peak flow meters

pulmonologist

residual volume (RV)

tidal volume (V$_T$)

total lung capacity (TLC)

vital capacity (VC)

CERTIFICATION LINK

CMA (AAMA)
Principles of
equipment operation

Collecting and
processing specimens;
diagnostic testing

  Respiratory testing

RMA
Laboratory
procedures

Anatomy and
physiology

CMAS (AMT)
Confidentiality

Examination
preparation

Pulmonology is the study and treatment of diseases of the respiratory system. The respiratory system includes the trachea, bronchial tubes, lungs, and alveoli. The primary function of the respiratory system is to transport oxygen to the lungs via the bloodstream to all the cells in the body and to carry waste products (carbon dioxide and water) to the outside of the body for elimination.

Pulmonary Function

Pulmonary function tests (PFTs) are performed to evaluate lung volume and capacity, to assist in the differential diagnosis of patients with suspected obstructive or restrictive pulmonary disease processes, and to assess the effectiveness of drug therapies. These tests may be done by physicians devoted to primary care or allergy care or by a specialist in lung diseases (**pulmonologist**).

Sometimes patients complain of shortness of breath or of difficulty breathing after minimal exertion. Other patients have no symptoms or may have been diagnosed with asthma, chronic bronchitis, emphysema, cystic fibrosis, or a combination of these conditions. An awareness of the long-term effects of smoking and exposure to occupational or environmental toxins has increased the frequency with which PFTs are performed. Because lung disease tends to worsen with age, it is important to make a diagnosis early and, thereby, to slow the rapid loss of function that occurs without treatment. Allergic patients may undergo a status change quite suddenly and require emergency intervention. Pulmonary patients can expect to have PFTs performed quite frequently over the course of their condition.

Pulmonary Disorders

The medical assistant usually performs PFTs in the office for chronic obstructive problems such as asthma (spasms of the bronchial tubes or swelling of the mucous membranes), chronic bronchitis (inflammation of the bronchial mucous membranes), cystic fibrosis (faulty exocrine glands secrete too much mucus, which obstructs the lungs), or emphysema (permanent enlargement of air spaces beyond the terminal bronchioles. These obstructive pulmonary diseases tend to be chronic and worsen over time if treatment is not effective. As the lungs are unable to expand or are restricted from expanding, the PFTs will show alterations in total lung capacity (TLC), inspiratory capacity (IC), and vital capacity (VC).

Respiratory conditions include the following:

Upper Respiratory Conditions

- Acute rhinitis (common cold)
- Sinusitis
- Hay fever
- Pharyngitis
- Laryngitis

Lower Respiratory Conditions

- **Obstructive diseases**—chronic obstructive pulmonary disease (COPD), asthma, acute bronchitis, emphysema (Figure 50-1)
- **Infectious diseases**—pneumonia (Figure 50-2), influenza, tuberculosis, pleuritis, Legionnaires' disease
- **Malignancies**—cancer of the lungs and larynx and other organs
- **Mechanical injuries**—pulmonary emboli, pneumothorax, hemothorax

Patients with pulmonary conditions present with a variety of symptoms, including the following:

- Coughing—dry or productive (sputum)
- Wheezing
- Cyanosis due to lack of oxygen (Figure 50-3)

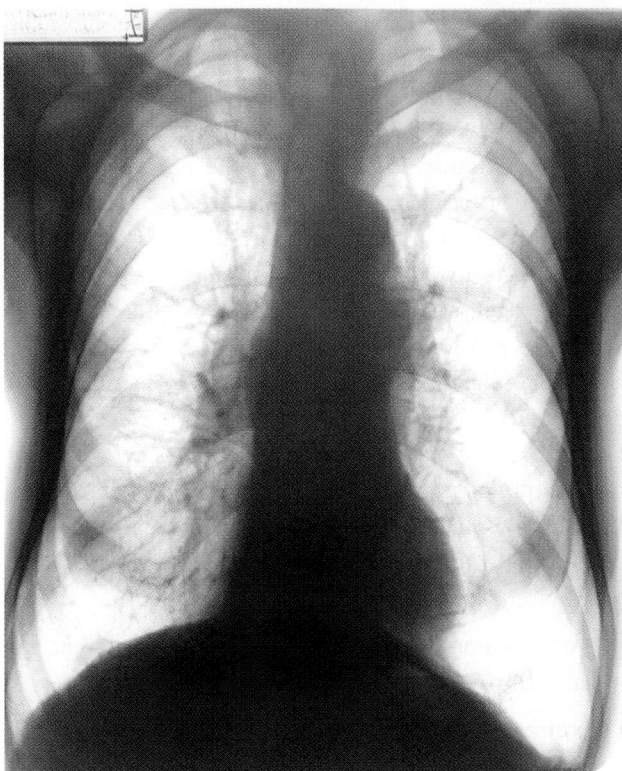

FIGURE 50-1 Chest X-ray of a patient with emphysema.
Source: Scott Comazine, Photo Researchers, Inc.

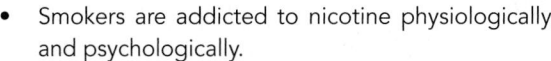
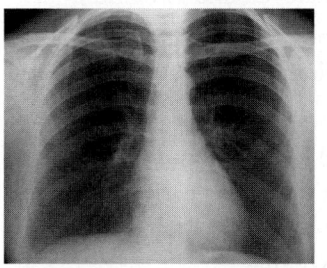 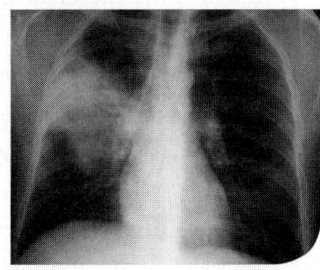

FIGURE 50-2 Chest X-ray of lungs. Normal is shown on the left. The patch gray-white areas on the right show pneumonia.

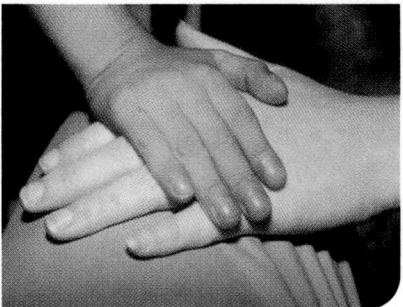

FIGURE 50-3 Cyanosis and clubbing of the fingertips are common symptoms of cystic fibrosis and are caused by low levels of oxygen in the blood.

- Rales—crackles
- Stridor—harsh, high-pitched sounds
- Rhonchus—sounds of wheezing or squeaking heard when listening to chest
- Hemoptysis—blood in sputum

As a medical assistant, you may find yourself doing many PFTs on the same patient to assess whether the drug treatments are effective. (See Chapter 29 for an in-depth discussion of pulmonary disorders and diseases.)

Pulmonary Function Tests

PFTs assess lung function and aid in evaluation and diagnosis of pulmonary disease. The various types of PFTs include spirometry, arterial blood gases, lung volumes, pulse oximetry, diffusion capacity, and cardiopulmonary exercise tests. Spirometry and oximetry are discussed in this chapter.

SPIROMETRY

Spirometry is a noninvasive test that measures the ability of the lungs to exhale. A diagnostic spirometer is employed to evaluate the patient's ability to ventilate during a maximum

The Child

Children need extra time and coaching for pulmonary function tests (PFTs). Take the time to explain to them that they will need to blow "really hard" until you tell them to stop, and then they will need to take a big breath back through the tube. It may take a couple of practice runs the first time this procedure is performed for them to perform the test accurately. If the child cannot perform the procedure correctly it will, of course, change the validity of the results. PFTs are never performed on a child who is unable to cooperate with the testing requirements.

The Older Adult

When doing PFTs, explain the procedure clearly. An older adult may not be able to perform multiple efforts, so each must be a valid try. Watch the patient's technique and offer constructive hints if needed to help improve the validity of each effort. Be very supportive and coach the patient throughout the procedure.

forced exhale. See Figure 50-4 for an example of one type of spirometer. This device measures and records the volume exhaled in a specific length of time (1 second, 3 seconds, etc.). The air movement is recorded on special paper with a vertical mark for each second and a horizontal mark for each liter of oxygen. **Forced vital capacity (FVC)** is the maximum volume of air expelled when the patient exhales as forcibly and quickly as possible following one inhalation. The patient must exhale as much air as possible and continue to exhale it for 6 seconds to be considered a satis-

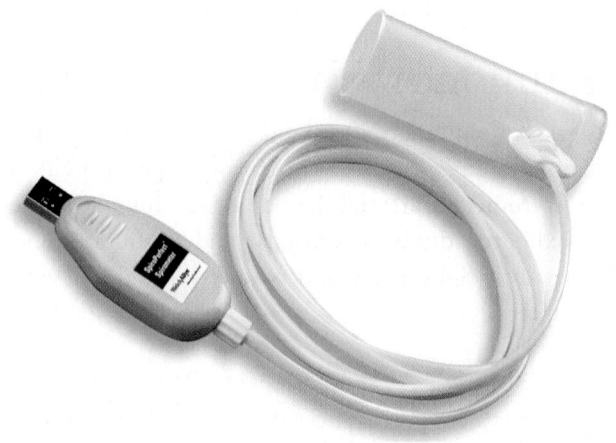

FIGURE 50-4   One type of spirometer.
Source: Courtesy of Welch Allyn.

factory test. At least three efforts at exhaling must be demonstrated. **Forced expiratory volume (FEV)** after 1 second (FEV^1) is the volume of air in liters that is forcefully exhaled in the first second of exhalation. In patients with healthy lungs about, 70 percent to 75 percent of air is exhaled in the first second. The values are often reported as a ratio FEV^1/FVC. Patients with normal lungs may have a ratio of 90 percent. For patients with **chronic obstructive pulmonary disease (COPD)** (a progressive, chronic, usually irreversible condition in which the lungs have diminished capacity for inhalation and exhalation), the ratio may fall below 70 percent.

The first part of the spirometry procedure is performed to discover the amount of air in the lungs when they move normally and how much lung space is available after a normal inhalation and a normal exhalation. These are called pulmonary volume tests, and there are four of them:

- **Tidal volume (V_T)**—the amount of air inhaled or exhaled during normal breathing (about 500 mL).

- **Expiratory reserve volume (ERV)**—the amount of air that can be forcibly exhaled after a normal exhale.

- **Inspiratory reserve volume (IRV)**—the amount of air that can be forcibly inspired after a normal inhale.

- **Residual volume (RV)**—the volume of air left in the lungs at the end of an exhale (around 1200 mL).

From these volume tests, pulmonary capacity can be calculated, based on two or more volumes. Capacities include the following:

- **Total lung capacity (TLC)**—the volume of the lungs at peak inspiration; equal to the sum of the four volumes: tidal volume, expiratory reserve volume, inspiratory reserve volume, residual volume.

- **Vital capacity (VC)**—the amount of air that can be exhaled following forced inspiration and including maximum expiration.

- **Inspiratory capacity (IC)**—the amount of air that can be inhaled after normal expiration.

- **Functional residual capacity (FRC)**—the amount of air remaining in the lungs after a normal expiration.

Total lung capacity and functional residual capacity will increase in COPD because the flow of air out of the lungs is diminished. This results in slow expiratory rate and an increase in residual volume. Patients with asthma have a decreased ability of the lungs to deflate during expiration. In restrictive lung disease, the volumes are decreased because expansion of the lungs is prevented, thereby diminishing total lung capacity, vital capacity, and inspiratory capacity.

These tests are performed by a respiratory care specialist, usually in a hospital setting, as ordered by the pulmonologist. The capacities are included here because, in working with the specialist and pulmonary patients, you will encounter the terms and volumes. Sometimes, however, spirometry testing is done in an occupational medicine office, allergy specialist's office, or pulmonologist's office. It is helpful to know what they describe. To continue monitoring the effects of respiratory disease, an evaluation can be carried out by the medical assistant in an office or clinic.

VOLUME CAPACITY SPIROMETRY

A diagnostic spirometer is employed to evaluate the patient's ability to ventilate during a maximum forced exhale. This device measures and records the volume exhaled and the time required to complete it. This air movement is recorded on special paper with vertical second marks and horizontal liter marks in one of three ways:

- **Forced vital capacity (FVC)**—maximum amount of air exhaled after maximum inspiration during one of the two timed FVCs.

- **Forced expiratory volume (FEV) in 1 second (FEV[1])**—amount of air exhaled during the first second of the FVC maneuver.

- **Maximal midexpiratory flow (MMEF)**—average flow rate during middle half of FVC.

Patient Preparation

The patient must have accurate instructions and reassurance with questions readily answered. Generally, preparation begins when the patient schedules the appointment. Patient preparation for spirometry testing is important and must be thorough. When the procedure is scheduled, a brochure explaining the test should be provided to the patient. Instruct the patient to refrain from smoking and eating a large meal for 4 to 6 hours and not to use bronchodilators or nebulizers for 6 hours prior to the test.

On arrival, again explain the test, review the steps involved, and determine if there are reasons the test should not be performed, such as flu, cold, or allergy. Weigh and measure the patient's height, and measure and record vital signs. The height and weight are necessary for calculations after the test. Demonstrate and explain in simple terms what you would like the patient to do. If the patient is wearing ill-fitting dentures, ask him or her to remove them because lips must be sealed tightly around the mouthpiece. Have the patient loosen any tight clothing, ties, girdles, bras, or belts that could impede the test. The patient should be encouraged to sit because light-headedness may cause

dizziness. The patient's feet should be flat on the floor, legs uncrossed, and head and chin slightly elevated for the entire procedure. This proper upright position must be maintained during a spirometry test. If the patient prefers a standing versus sitting position, it is acceptable because that makes no difference with the results and patient comfort is important.

The test should be repeated three times successfully, and the best two maneuvers should be used to calculate the pulmonary function. Results are considered normal if the patient's best result is 80 percent of pretest calculated values. The effectiveness of bronchodilator medication can be evaluated if the results are abnormal. The patient may be given a bronchodilator and then retested to determine the effectiveness of the medication. Spirometric measurements depend on patient effort, which, in turn, depends on the coaching of the medical assistant. Patients usually need some practice with wrapping their lips around the disposable mouthpiece and forcibly exhaling.

Spirometry Procedure

PFTs to evaluate lung volume and lung capacity are performed mainly in a pulmonary function laboratory. One noninvasive PFT, spirometry, is regularly performed in the office setting. Spirometry assesses lung function by measuring how much air can be held in the lungs and how much and how quickly air can be exhaled. Many types of spirometers are on the market; some are mechanical, others are computerized. All spirometers consist of a mouthpiece and tubing connected to a recording device. The patient is asked to inhale as deeply as possible and then to exhale as forcefully, and as completely, as possible while measurements are being taken. Several different measurements can be made from

PROFESSIONALISM

THE LAW

Many pulmonary patients, especially those who are on oxygen, are apprehensive about having spirometry testing. They worry about being disconnected from their oxygen supply for the duration of the test. You must put them at ease and explain that they will be monitored closely and that the test will be terminated if conditions warrant it. Remember not to promise any outcomes or results in you eagerness to convince patients to be tested. Do not release any results to them either. That is the job of the licensed person in charge: the physician, physician's assistant, or nurse.

TABLE 50-1 Pulmonary Function Tests

Lung Function	Definition
Expiratory reserve volume (ERV)	Maximum volume of air left that can be exhaled after normal expiration
Forced vital capacity (FVC)	Amount of air that can be forcefully exhaled from a maximum inhalation
Functional residual volume (FVR)	Amount of air left in the lungs after normal expiration
Inspiratory capacity (IC)	Maximum amount of air that can be inspired after a normal expiration
Maximal volume ventilation (MVV)	Maximum volume that patient can breathe in and out in 1 minute
Residual volume (RV)	Volume of air left in lungs after forced expiration
Total volume (V_T)	Amount of air inspired and expired in a normal respiration
Vital capacity (VC)	Maximum amount of air that can be expired after a maximum inspiration

a spirometer test. See Table 50-1 for a list of lung capacity tests and definitions.

Spirometry results reflect the elasticity of the lungs, their ability to ventilate, and the strength of the respiratory muscles. These tests are good screening tools for pulmonary function and help the physician determine impaired function due to narrowing or obstruction in conditions such as emphysema, asthma, bronchitis, and diseases that cause muscle weakness such as myasthenia gravis. Spirometry tests can be used to evaluate the effectiveness of a specific dose of medication. To obtain an accurate result, the patient must inhale deeply and then exhale as forcefully as possible for as long as possible. Your role will be to act as cheerleader and coach to induce the patient to give a peak performance. Procedure 50-1 lists the steps necessary to determine a patient's forced vital capacity using a spirometer.

procedure
50-1

PERFORMING A SPIROMETRY TEST TO MEASURE FORCED VITAL CAPACITY

Objective: Perform a forced vital capacity test.

EQUIPMENT AND SUPPLIES
functioning spirometry machine; nose clip; patient mouthpiece; disinfectant; biohazard waste container; paper and pencil; scale for height and weight; sphygmomanometer and blood pressure cuff

METHOD
1. Perform hand hygiene.
2. Assemble all equipment.
3. Calibrate spirometer as necessary, according to manufacturer's instructions.
4. Identify the patient.
5. Question the patient about having prepared for the test by not smoking and not using bronchodilators for the preceding 6 hours.
6. Inquire about general health at present.
7. Explain and demonstrate the procedure to the patient.
8. Weigh the patient and measure the patient's height, and record the results.
9. Measure the patient's vital signs and record them.
10. Explain the proper positioning and, if necessary, assist with loosening any tight clothing.
11. Start the machine and enter the needed data.
12. Review the procedure with the patient. Be sure that the patient knows to breathe forcibly several times into the spirometer.
13. Have the patient place the mouthpiece in his or her mouth and seal his or her lips around the mouthpiece (Figure 50-5A).
14. Apply nose clips (Figure 50-5B).
15. Have the patient inhale deeply.
16. Push the start button at the same time as you give the following instruction to the patient.

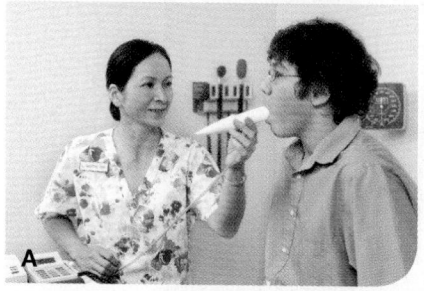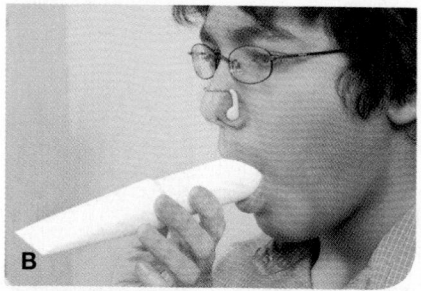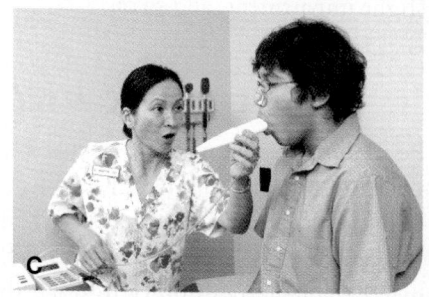

FIGURE 50-5 (A) The patient must close the lips rightly around the mouthpiece; (B) place the nose clip on the patient's nose; (C) direct the patient to blow the air out into the mouthpiece as hard and as fast as possible.

17. Encourage the patient to blast breath out as hard, fast, and long as possible (Figure 50-5C).
18. Make recommendations to improve outcome, if necessary.
19. Obtain the second set of maneuvers.
20. Obtain the third set of maneuvers.
21. Continue until you have three acceptable outcomes. You may facilitate up to eight attempts, if needed, to obtain three good trials. Some computerized machines will select the best attempt and print it.
22. Remove the nose clip and ask the patient to remain until the physician reviews the results.

23. Give the physician the trial information.
24. Record the results in the patient's chart.
25. Clean the tubing and dispose of the mouthpieces using standard precautions and following the manufacturer's directions.

CHARTING EXAMPLE

3/12/XX 8:30 A.M. Spirometry performed with 3 good results submitted to Dr. Penningworth.· · · · · K. Christianson, CMA (AAMA)

Various types of spirometers are available on the market, but they must meet minimum standards for acceptable performance. When using automated computerized machines, the spirometry procedure is complicated by the necessity of dealing with the computer program. You must enter patient data into the computer, such as age, height, weight, vital signs, and medication, depending on the machine and the computer program used. The machine usually makes predictions about what the graphic representation should look like.

Certain changes are anticipated with lung disease. In obstructive lung disease, more time is required for a complete exhale, and in a restrictive pattern, maximum exhale is reached quickly but the volume is small. With the test results, the patient's pulmonary measurement is compared to the predicted values for the patient's height, weight, age, race, and sex by the physician who takes into account the patient's clinical status at the same time. Clinical status refers to the patient's physical condition at the time of the test. A fever, asthma attack, poor night's sleep, scoliosis, or any of a number of other variables could affect the pulmonary function results. A prediction indicator result of 85 to 100 percent

PROFESSIONALISM
THE WORKPLACE

Asthma is hyperactivity of the bronchi and bronchioles (see Figure 50-1) causing bronchospasm (smooth muscle constriction). The patient feels constriction in the chest and difficulty exhaling and inhaling due to the narrowing of the bronchioles. Symptoms include coughing, shortness of breath, mucus production, and wheezing. A prolonged severe attack is known as status asthmatic and is life threatening. Triggers include cigarette smoke, dust, mold, inhaled chemicals, cold air, and emotional stress. Treatment during severe asthmatic attack includes epinephrine (Adrenaline) and oxygen.

It is important for health care professionals to have up-to-date information about chronic life-threatening conditions such as asthma. Asthma occurs more frequently in boys and inner-city poor children. Public health officials feel that cockroach droppings may be a trigger for children who live in the inner city.

would indicate no impairment; 75 to 85 percent would be slight impairment, and so on.

PEAK FLOW METER

Peak flow meters measure the patient's ability to move air into and out of the lungs. Keeping a record of peak flow either daily or when attacks occur helps the physician prepare a treatment plan and establish effective treatments. It may be your responsibility to teach the patient and family members how to use a peak flow meter correctly. Specifically, it measures the fastest rate at which the patient exhales after taking a maximum breath (peak expiratory flow rate, or PEFR). A peak flow meter measures liters per second or liters per minute. See Figure 50-6 for an example of a peak flow meter.

Peak flow meters may be mechanical or computerized. Instruct the patient to put the mouth around the mouthpiece and blow forcibly into the meter, which will measure the peak expiratory flow rate. The patient should keep a diary of the flow rates to see if medication is helping or the disease is getting worse.

A patient may use a flow meter at home to monitor breathing. This information will assist the physician to

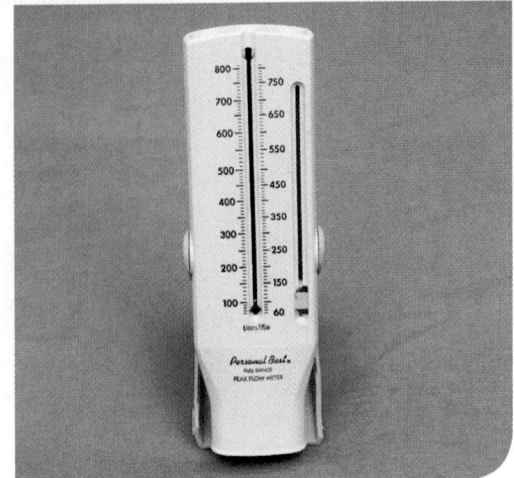

FIGURE 50-6 Peak flow meter with marker for the zero position.

determine the most effective medication regimen. On a "good" day, the patient blows as hard as possible into the device to establish a goal or baseline against which to compare other expiratory attempts. See Procedure 50-2 on how to teach peak flow measurement.

procedure
50-2

TEACHING PEAK FLOW MEASUREMENT
Objective: To instruct patient to correctly monitor peak flow and record results.

EQUIPMENT AND SUPPLIES
peak flow meter; documentation diary/chart; diagram of lungs and breathing processes; pen; patient's record

METHOD
1. Perform hand hygiene.
2. Assemble peak flow meter with disposable mouthpiece or individual peak flow meter for patient use at home.
3. Identify patient and explain the procedure. Include an explanation of breathing processes and importance to overall health. Demonstrate how the mouthpiece fits and explain what the numbers on the side mean. The peak flow meter should always be set on zero to start.
4. Have the patient place the mouthpiece in the mouth and form a tight seal. Explain that better results may be obtained if the patient stands during the test.
5. The patient should be instructed to stand, take as deep a breath as possible, place the mouthpiece in the mouth without biting down on it, and exhale as completely and forcibly as possible (Figures 50-7 and 50-8).
6. Instruct the patient to note the number on the machine where the sliding gauge stopped and to record the results. Reset to zero. Repeat three times. This reading indicates the peak expiratory flow rate (PEFR).

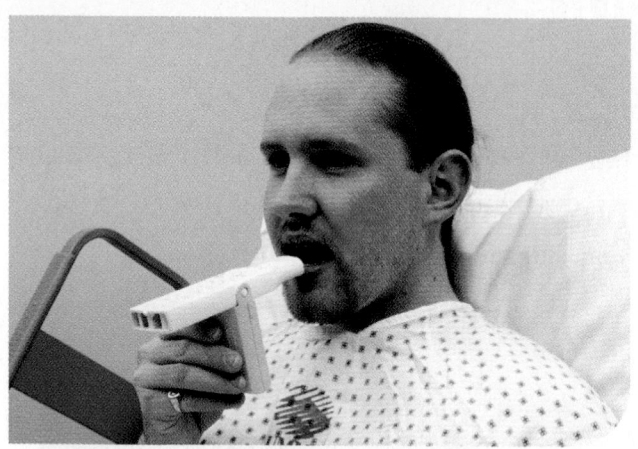

FIGURE 50-7 PEFR measurement.

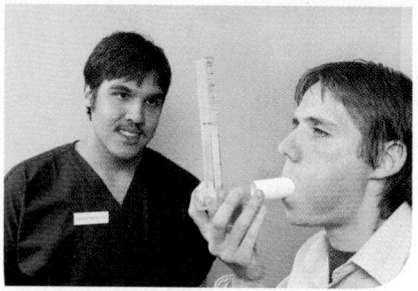

FIGURE 50-8 Ask the patient to exhale as hard and as fast as possible.

7. The patient should follow the physician's orders for when and how often each day to perform this procedure. The "best" result is documented on a chart or in the diary.
8. Demonstrate how to wash the mouthpiece with soap and water without submerging the peak flow meter.

9. Document the instruction.
10. Perform hand hygiene.

CHARTING EXAMPLE
05/16/XX 9:30 A.M. Pt. instructed on use of peak flow meter and recording of results. Returned demonstration easily, verbally confirmed understanding. Peak flow charting form given. Pt. to perform procedure 3× twice/day in A.M. and P.M. Results today: 380 LPM. · · · · · · · · · · · · · · · · · · R. Negri, CMA (AAMA)

OXYGEN SATURATION

For patients suffering from cardiac and pulmonary disorders, it may be necessary to determine the oxygen content of the blood or **oxygen saturation**. An electronic pulse oximeter (a device that can be clipped on the bridge of the nose, forehead, earlobe, or tip of a finger) determines the oxygen concentration in arterial blood. This equipment allows for the measurement of blood oxygenation indirectly at times before clinical signs of hypoxia are present. The measurement is reported as SpO_2 and can help determine whether treatment is needed or not. A pulse oximeter is illustrated in Figure 50-9.

Normal oxygen saturation is 95 to 100 percent, with readings below 70 percent indicating life-threatening situations. Pulse oximeters are selected based on the patient's age, size, and condition. They are available either cordless or with cords. In an adult patient, the fingertip pulse oximeter is generally used. Nail polish should be removed prior to attaching the pulse oximeter. See Procedure 50-3 for the method to measure oxygen saturation.

ARTERIAL BLOOD GASES

Arterial blood gases measure the amount of oxygen, carbon dioxide, and pH of the blood. Blood gas levels are helpful in

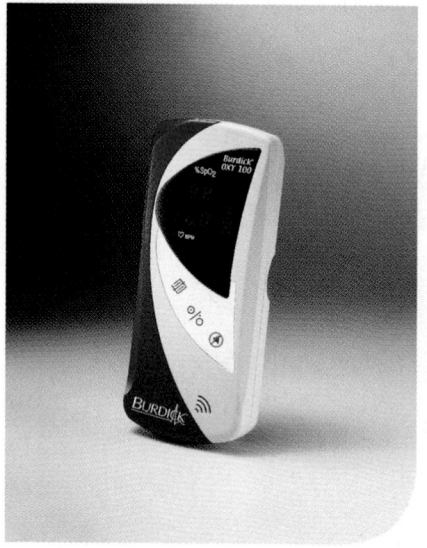

FIGURE 50-9 Burdick pulse oximeter.
Source: Courtesy of Cardiac Science Corp.

MEASURING OXYGEN SATURATION

Objective: Attach and measure oxygen saturation of patient.

EQUIPMENT AND SUPPLIES

pulse oximeter; nail polish remover; alcohol wipe; patient's record; gloves; adhesive tape

METHOD

1. Perform hand hygiene and apply gloves.
2. Assemble equipment based on the patient's size and condition.
3. Identify the patient and explain the procedure.
4. Choose the correct size sensor for the patient. Figure 50-10 is an example of a child-size sensor for measuring oxygen saturation.
5. Determine if the patient is allergic to adhesive tape. If allergic, use a clip-on oximeter.
6. Remove nail polish as needed.
7. Assess the patient's pulse rate.
8. Wipe the site with an alcohol wipe. Attach the sensor following manufacturer's directions. Make sure the sensors are correctly aligned opposite each other.
9. Connect the sensor to the pulse oximeter. Some oximeters are cordless (Figure 50-11).
10. Turn on the machine and set the alarm as directed.
11. Change the position of the oximeter every 4 hours or as directed (Figure 50-12).
12. Compare the pulse previously evaluated with the pulse on the oximeter. If there is a great deal of difference the oximeter may not be functioning correctly and should be checked.

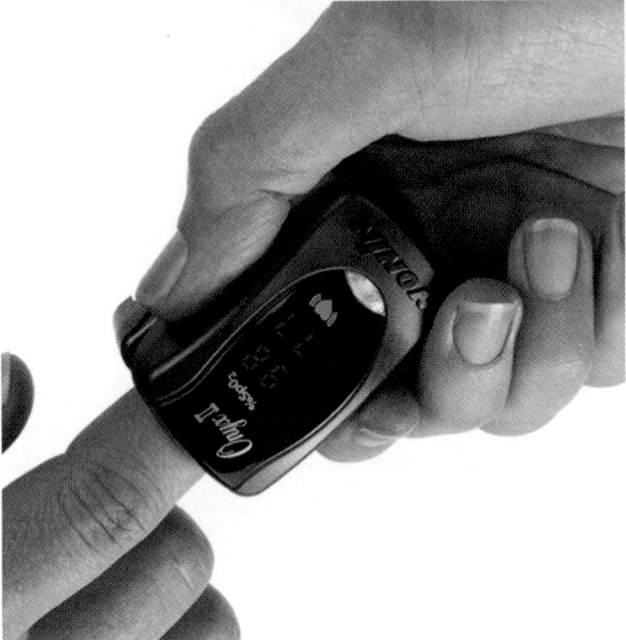

FIGURE 50-11   Cordless fingertip oximeter meter.
Source: Courtesy of Nonin Medical, Inc.

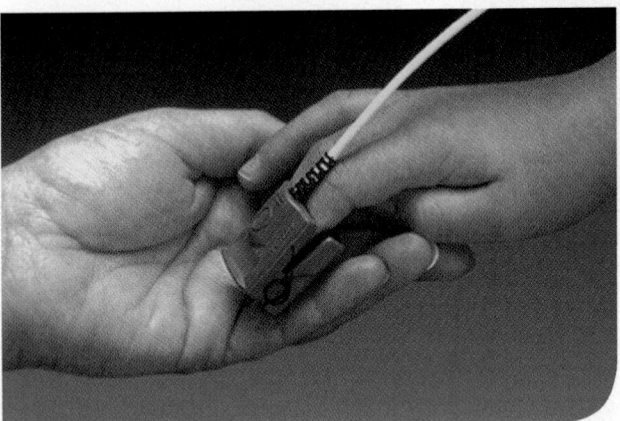

FIGURE 50-10   Fingertip oximeter sensor (child).
Source: Courtesy of Nonin Medical, Inc.

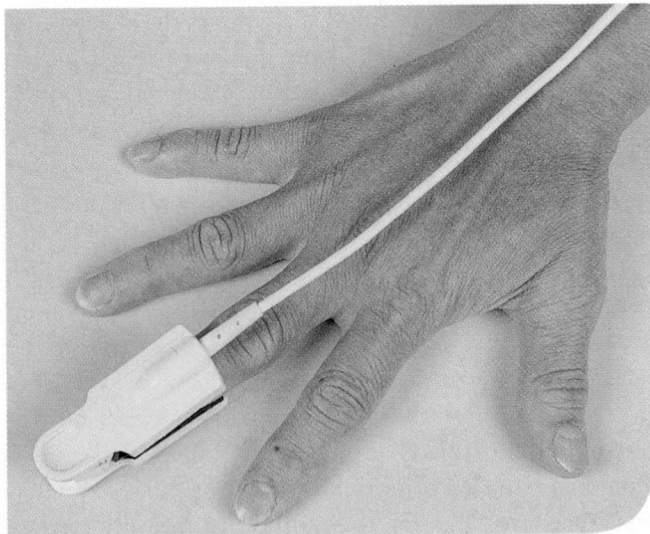

FIGURE 50-12   Fingertip oximeter meter (adult).

13. Record the oxygen saturation level in the patient's record at intervals ordered by the physician.
14. If the oxygen saturation level is abnormal, follow facility protocol for notifying supervisors or the physician.

evaluating breathing conditions such as COPD and pneumonia. They provide information on the effectiveness of oxygen treatment and the pH of the blood. The pH of the blood must be stable between the ranges of 7.35 to 7.45; otherwise, the patient is in a life-threatening situation. The more carbon dioxide increases in the blood, the more acid the blood pH becomes.

Arterial blood gases are usually drawn by respiratory specialists or IV technicians. Arterial blood is drawn from the wrist, groin, or arm after cleansing the site. The specimen must be kept on ice and tested immediately. Direct pressure to the area is applied for 5 to 15 minutes to prevent bleeding.

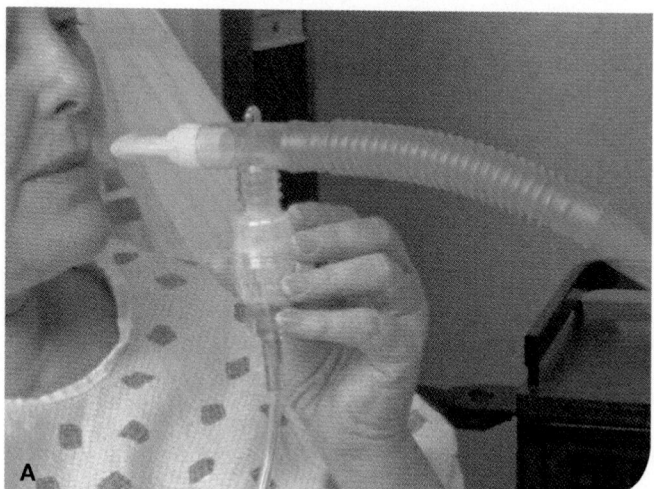

Pulmonary Treatments

Nebulizers and inhalers are used to treat asthma and other respiratory conditions. Nebulizers deliver medication directly to deeper areas in the lungs. Inhalers are used to deliver a measured amount of medication directly into the respiratory tract to dilate the airways.

After a basic spirometry test, some patients are asked to breathe an aerosolized bronchodilator, and the physician evaluates the effectiveness of the drug in improving the lung capacity. The graphic test results become part of the patient's permanent record.

NEBULIZERS

The small-volume nebulizer is sometimes used to treat breathing difficulties. If a handheld nebulizer is used, a small amount of aerosolized liquid medication mixture is placed in a chamber. See Figure 50-13A–B for examples of nebulizers.

Then the patient is asked to put the nebulizer in the mouth and breathe deeply for 8 to 10 minutes. A high-pressure gas stream of either air or oxygen passing through a small opening actually creates the aerosol. The aerosol is then delivered into the patient through either a mouthpiece or a mask. The procedure for a nebulizer is to first note the

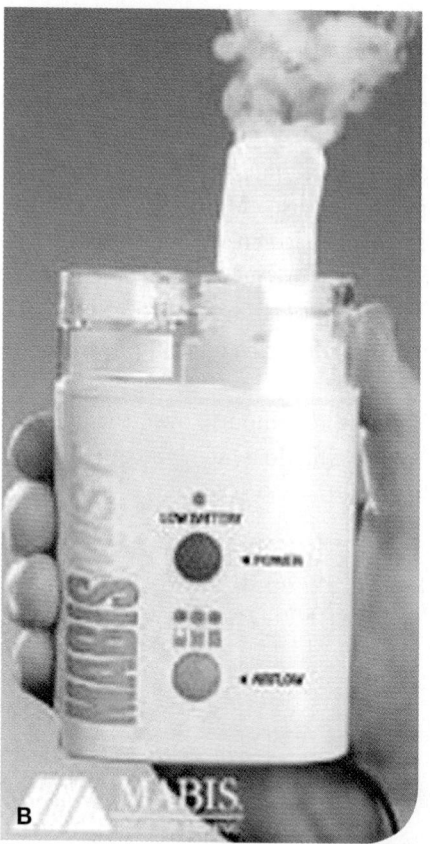

FIGURE 50-13 (A) Nebulizer; (B) ultrasonic nebulizer.

patient's baseline data (auscultation, vital signs, oximeter reading, and peak expiratory flow rate). Then the handheld nebulizer is assembled and a mouthpiece or a mask is selected for delivery. Using a mask can decrease the amount of drug that reaches the lungs by 1 or 2 percent because of deposition on the face. The mask should be used only when the patient is unable to take the treatment with a mouthpiece. The exact method for performing nebulizer treatment is found in Chapter 53: Pharmacology.

Measure the proper dosage of drug and diluent into the nebulizer. Set the gas flow to the nebulizer at 6 to 8 L/min. Position the patient in a semi-Fowler's position. Implement the therapy and encourage the patient to breathe slowly through the mouth. Instruct the patient to deeply inspire periodically and to hold a breath for about 4 to 10 seconds. When no aerosol is flowing, discontinue treatment. Monitor and evaluate the patient's response to the treatment.

Encourage the patient to cough well, quantifying the amount and describing the type of sputum if the cough is productive. Monitor the patient's pulse, breath sounds, peak expiratory flow rates, and blood oxygenation. Disassemble and store the equipment properly. Record the data in the patient's chart.

INHALERS

A metered-dose inhaler (MDI) (one or various types) holds about 200 doses of the prescribed medication in a pressurized container with an attached mouthpiece. Patient teaching is very important because MDIs are frequently misused, resulting in inadequate treatment. As with instructions on how to properly use nebulizers, demonstrate for the patient first and then ask him or her to repeat the demonstration for you. Provide written backup material to the patient as well.

The patient should put the mouth over the mouthpiece of the inhaler and inhale when the medication

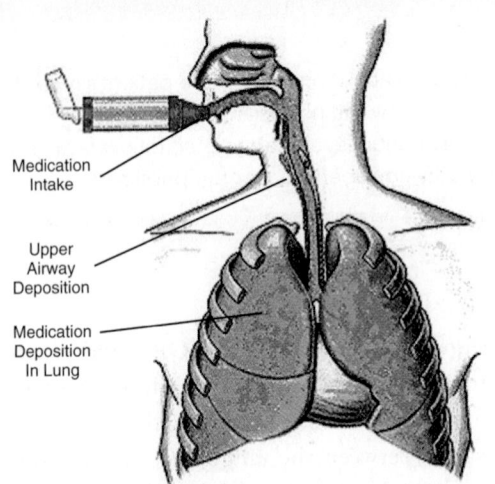

FIGURE 50-15 Delivery of medication to the lungs using a metered-dose inhaler extender.
Source: Courtesy of Trudell Medical International.

container is pressed into the inhaler. Figure 50-14 is an example of a MDI and one with a spacer. An extender is used to improve the delivery and to facilitate absorption of the medication.

The inhaler procedure is also found in Chapter 53 of this text. A puff of medication will be dispensed. After the dose is dispensed, remove the medication and clean the plastic inhaler with soap and water. Figure 50-15 illustrates the delivery of medication to the lungs with a MDI and a spacer.

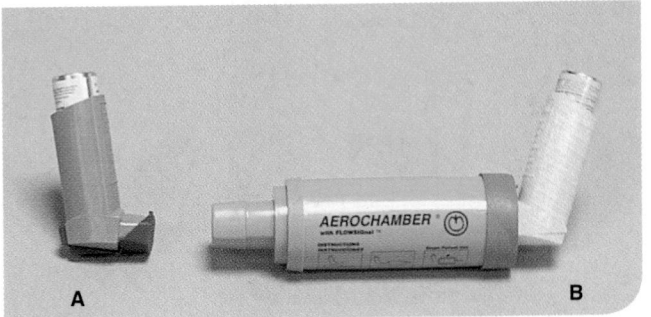

FIGURE 50-14 (A) Metered-dose inhaler; (B) metered-dose inhaler with spacer.

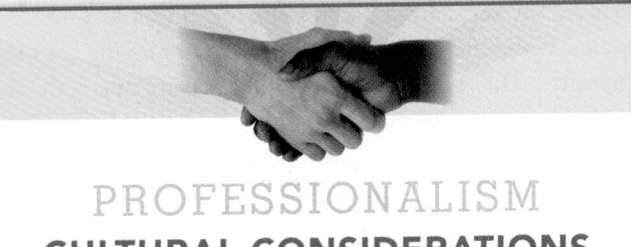

PROFESSIONALISM
CULTURAL CONSIDERATIONS

While working in the medical office, you will find that a person's cultural and spiritual beliefs will play a major role in their health care. Many cultures of eastern and southeast Asia have a very holistic approach to health care. A strong emphasis is placed on hot and cold therapies, yin and yang principles, and harmony with the universe. Some medications, treatments, and tests may be refused by patients from these varying cultural backgrounds. These patients may seek out alternative forms of treatment such as acupuncture and acupressure, massage, and herbal remedies.

SUMMARY

The medical assistant may be asked to perform PFTs (spirometer, oximeter, and peak flow meter) to assess patient breathing function. PFTs are not usually done when the problem is an upper respiratory one. The oximeter can be used to determine arterial blood oxygenation, and spirometers can be used to determine pulmonary response to medications and treatments. Accuracy in carrying out your duties during these tests will provide the physician with the best possible data to make that diagnosis and institute the correct treatment.

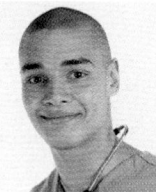

50 CHAPTER REVIEW

COMPETENCY REVIEW

1. Define and spell the terms to learn for this chapter.

2. Describe how to maintain and operate pulmonary function equipment.

3. Explain the differences between obstructive and restrictive pulmonary disease.

4. Explain the purpose of PFTs.

PREPARING FOR THE CERTIFICATION EXAM

1. Which of the following is the amount of air that can be forcibly exhaled after a normal exhalation?
   a. tidal volume
   b. expiratory reserve
   c. inspiratory reserve
   d. total lung capacity
   e. residual volume

2. Pulse oximeter is used to evaluate
   a. vital signs
   b. presence of hypertension
   c. arterial blood oxygen saturation
   d. breathing volumes
   e. nerve function in fingertip

3. To correctly prepare for a spirometry test the patient is told to
   a. follow normal routine
   b. take all medications that day
   c. prepare for test even if ill
   d. not eat a large meal or smoke for 4 to 6 hours prior to test
   e. leave dentures in place

4. Asthma is
   a. a possibly life-threatening, obstructive pulmonary disease
   b. highly contagious
   c. of little consequence to patient
   d. treated with NSAIDS
   e. more prevalent in older women

5. Improper care of a spirometer may result in which of the following?
   a. coronary insufficiency
   b. angina
   c. coronary embolism
   d. cross-contamination/infection
   e. thyroid deficiency

6. When performing a spirometer test on a patient the medical assistant must
   a. leave the patient alone during the test
   b. act as coach to encourage more effort
   c. provide the patient with reading material during test

d. be quiet so patient is not distracted

e. give patient the results right away

7. To measure respiratory function and evaluate medication effectiveness, which of the following tests is performed at home?

a. peak flow meter

b. spirometer

c. oximeter

d. inhaler

e. nebulizer

8. A physician who deals with conditions and diseases of the lungs and respiratory tract is known as a

a. pediatrician

b. podiatrist

c. psychiatrist

d. pulmonologist

e. psychologist

9. Tidal volume is the amount of air inhaled or exhaled during normal breathing. The normal amount is

a. 1000 mL

b. 250 mL

c. 500 mL

d. 900 mL

e. 100 mL

10. A normal oxygen saturation level is

a. 60 percent

b. 50 percent

c. 70 percent

d. 95 percent

e. 40 percent

CRITICAL THINKING

1. Shandra, RMA, is working with Abigail during her appointment today. Abigail says to Shandra, "I don't understand why I am having this test again. I didn't even understand why I had to have it in the first place when I was diagnosed. What does this test do?" How should Shandra respond?

2. What type of data will Shandra need to enter into the computerized spirometry machine that is utilized by Pearson Physicians Group? Why will she need to enter this data?

3. After the spirometry test is complete, Dr. Penningworth looks over the results and examines Abigail. He decides that he would like Abigail to have some medication administered via a nebulizer since she is having some breathing difficulties after the test. Abigail asks Shandra what the difference is between medication being administered via an inhaler versus a nebulizer. What should Shandra tell Abigail?

ON THE JOB

Darla Shulman, CMA (AAMA), works in a pulmonologist's office. Patient Betty Davies is coming in for a volume capacity spirometry test.

1. How can Darla prepare Betty for this procedure?

2. On the day of the appoinment, what would make Darla not want to perform the test?

3. How many times must the test be completed successfully?

INTERNET ACTIVITY

Research any two of the following diseases: cystic fibrosis, bronchiectasis, lung cancer, asthma.

Additional interactive resources and activities for this chapter can be found:

On your student DVD: View applicable procedure videos on the DVD-ROM found in the back of this book.

MyHealthProfessionsKit.com: Test your knowledge of this chapter with games and activities. MyHealthProfessionsKit also includes resources, helpful links, and a Spanish audio glossary.

Medical Assisting Interactive: Practice your procedures as a medical assistant in this simulated doctor's office. This can be accessed through MyHealthProfessionsKit.com.

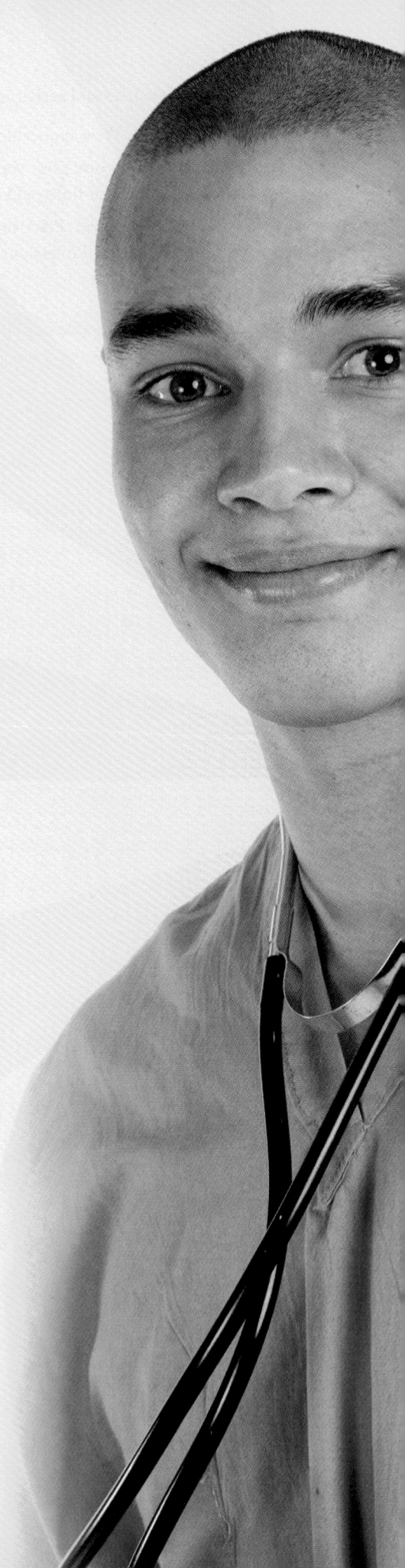

51

Physical Therapy and Rehabilitation

LEARNING OBJECTIVES

After completing this chapter, you should be able to:

- Define and spell the terms to learn for this chapter.
- Differentiate between a physiatrist and a physical therapist.
- Describe ten modalities used in physical therapy.
- Describe AROM, AAROM, and PROM.
- Discuss ten range of motion exercises.
- State the physiologic reactions to the applications of heat and cold. State any contraindications.
- List and discuss three applications of heat and cold therapy and their uses.
- Describe the difference between ultraviolet radiation, diathermy, and ultrasound.
- List and discuss five pieces of adaptive equipment used in rehabilitation.
- Describe the two-point, three-point, and four-point gait in crutch walking.
- Differentiate between electromyography, evoked potential studies, and somatosensory evoked potentials.
- Describe proper body mechanics for transferring a patient from a wheelchair to a chair or examination table.

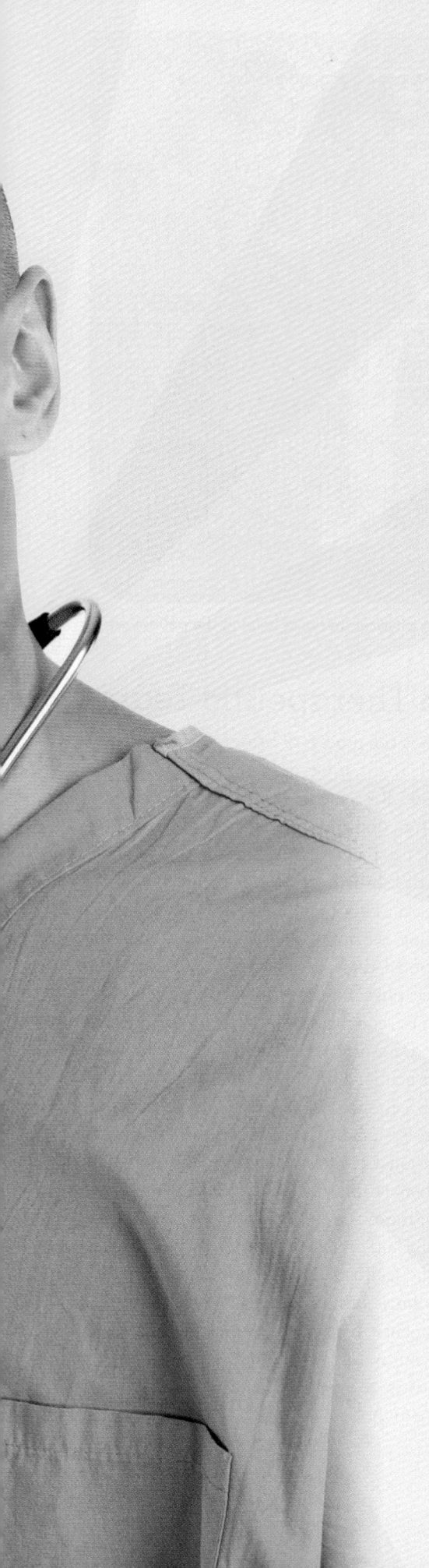

CHAPTER OUTLINE

CASE STUDY

Sylvia Jordan, a 76-year-old patient, arrives to the office with her daughter-in-law, Mary Ellen Jordan. Sylvia is seeing Dr. Miller for a follow-up appointment after being hospitalized for a stroke. Since the stroke, Sylvia has had difficulty walking and uses a wheelchair. Samra, RMA, wheels Sylvia to the examination room to be seen by Dr. Miller.

1159

ambulation

atrophy

contracture

cryotherapy

diathermy

effleurage

erythema

exudate

friction

gait

goniometer

heat hydrotherapy

hemiplegia

holistic

massage

modalities

orthotist

petrissage

physiatrist

physiatry

prosthesis

prosthetist

range of motion (ROM)

rehabilitation

Reiki

suppuration

tapotement

CERTIFICATION LINK

CMA (AAMA)
Patient preparation
and assisting the
physician
  Patient education
Treatment area
  Principles of equip-
  ment operation

RMA
General medical
assisting knowledge
  Patient education
Clinical medical
assisting
  Therapeutic
  modalities

CMAS (AMT)
Not applicable

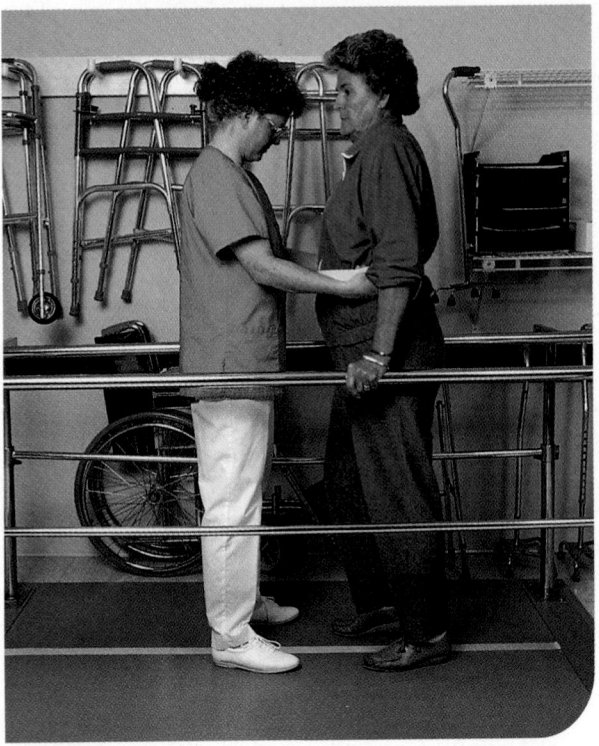

FIGURE 51-1 **A physical therapist helping the patient on parallel bars.**

The Therapeutic Team

Rehabilitation is the process of bringing the patient back as close as possible to his or her normal physical condition after injury or disease. Restorative care is care provided to attain and maintain function and independence.

Patients in need of rehabilitation or physical therapy often require the skilled services of many members of the health care team. This therapeutic team includes the PT, physical therapy assistant (PTA), occupational therapist (OT), occupational therapy assistant (OTA), recreation specialist, exercise physiologist or sports medicine therapist, massage therapist, and prosthetist or orthotist. A **prosthetist** specializes in designing, preparing, and fitting prosthetic devices such as artificial limbs. An **orthotist** designs and fits supportive devices such as braces and splints. Table 51-1 lists several professionals that make up the therapeutic team and the educational requirements for each level of the profession. Members of the therapeutic team may work in hospitals, rehabilitation centers, nursing homes, private physical therapy and occupational therapy practices, schools, sports medicine facilities, and home health agencies. Medical assistants must have a thorough understanding of the different therapeutic team members and their roles in rehabilitation. In your role as a medical assistant, you may schedule appointments for patients and at times assist with patient treatments.

Physical medicine, the branch of medicine called **physiatry**, is the therapeutic use of physical agents for the diagnosis, treatment, management, rehabilitation, and prevention of diseases and debilitating illnesses. A **physiatrist** is a medical doctor or osteopath who must complete 4 years of residency training and obtain licensure in the state where he or she practices.

The treatments that are prescribed by a physiatrist, sports medicine specialist, or a physician usually are carried out by a physical therapist (PT). Physical therapists are licensed professionals who teach patients the correct use of equipment and body mechanics to prevent further injury or disability. Means and methods used in physical therapy consist of rehabilitation, restoration, and the prevention of disabilities. A PT uses a variety of treatments, including heat, cold, massage, exercise, traction, and at times a combination of **modalities** (applications of any therapeutic agent). Figure 51-1 shows a PT assisting a patient on parallel bars.

TABLE 51-1 Careers in Physical Medicine

Career	Education/Experience
Physiatrist (MD or DO)	Medical school graduate, 4-year residency in physical medicine and rehabilitation, state licensure
Physical therapist (PT)	Master's degree, licensure required in all states
Physical therapy assistant (PTA)	2-year accredited program or associate degree plus internship, licensure required in some states
Occupational therapist (OT)	Bachelor's or master's degree and internship, licensure required in all states, certification from American Occupational Therapy Association
Occupational therapy assistant (OTA)	1- to 2-year certificate program or associate's degree and internship, licensure or certification required by most states
Massage therapist	3-month to 1-year accredited massage therapy program; certification, registration, or licensure required in most states
Recreational therapist (TR) or certified therapeutic recreation specialist (CTRS)	Usually a bachelor's degree plus internship; licensure and certification required in a few states, can be certified by National Council for Therapeutic Recreation Certification or registration by Association for Rehabilitation Therapy
Recreational therapy assistants (activity director)	1- to 2-year certificate program or associate degree, can be certified by National Council for Therapeutic Recreation (NCTRC)
Sports medicine (athletic trainer, ATS)	Bachelor's or master's degree, licensure required in some states, can be certified by National Athletic Trainers Association
Prosthetist/orthotist	2 years of college and 2 years of supervised training, national certification available (ABC, BOC)

ROLE OF THE PHYSICAL THERAPIST

A PT receives special training in assisting patients through the use of exercises and equipment to regain body motion and strength (Figure 51-2). The PT is skilled at using special equipment for strengthening muscles and measuring, fitting, and using assistive devices such as crutches, walkers, and canes.

ROLE OF THE OCCUPATIONAL THERAPIST

An occupational therapist (OT) is a vital member of the rehabilitative team. The OT is focused on increasing the patient's ability to function within his or her own environment. The OT assists the patient to relearn and acquire skills for activities of daily living (ADLs) by addressing the following areas:

- **Mobilization**—activities include assisting patients to maintain balance, reach, grasp, move, and turn while sitting.

- **Teaching activities of daily living**—include bathing, dressing, feeding, grooming, household chores, and leisure activities.

- **Coordination, strength, and activity tolerance**—includes teaching the patient techniques for using all physical resources without tiring quickly and while conserving strength.

To illustrate, a patient recovering from a traumatic injury will be treated by physicians and nurses, referred to a physiatrist for therapeutic

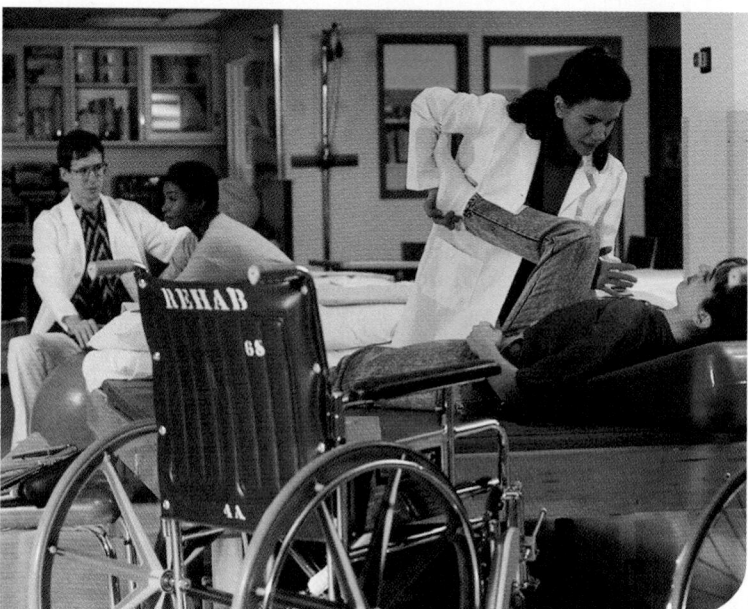

FIGURE 51-2 A physical therapist exercising the patient's leg in a physical therapy department.

rehabilitation, and given a care plan implementing the doctor's prescription by a PT and OT who utilize various modalities to try to bring the patient back to pre-trauma levels of function. Since many recoveries involve long-term treatments, the patient may see a recreational therapist to

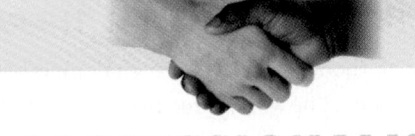

design activities to engage the patient's interest and to boost morale. A PTA or OTA will carry out care plans designed and ordered by the professionals.

ROLE OF MEDICAL ASSISTANT

Although as a medical assistant you would need more training and education to perform many of these duties, carrying out orders for treatments such as heat or cold compresses and exercise may be within your scope of practice. A medical assistant may not recommend a course of treatment to any patient. You may, however, need to instruct and demonstrate to the patient how to appropriately use heat or cold applications at home and assistive devices such as canes and crutches. If in doubt whether or not a specific task is within your scope of practice, obtain information from local, state, or national medical assisting organizations.

Rehabilitation

Rehabilitation is the process of assisting a patient to regain a state of health and the highest level of function possible. Injury, illness, and conditions such as multiple sclerosis cause patients to lose mobility and self-esteem.

The rehabilitation process is a holistic approach to every aspect of the patient's well-being, not just the present disease or injury. **Holistic** medicine focuses on the whole patient and addresses the social, emotional, and spiritual needs of a patient as well as the physical treatment. Goals are set for each patient by professionals on the case and suited to the individual patient's needs. In addition, each patient may have his or her own rehabilitation goal. For some, it may be to return to work, for others to be able to care for themselves and live independently. The patient is assisted to resume activities of daily living, such as feeding, toileting, and providing as much of his or her own care as possible.

Rehabilitation after a long illness or a debilitating disease can cause muscle loss and atrophy, which requires patience from everyone involved: the patient, family members, and caregivers. Special attention should be paid to the psychological problems, such as depression and anger that can occur from a feeling of loss of control over one's life. Rehabilitation programs are useful for the following conditions and diseases:

- Surgery, such as hip and knee replacements

- Trauma, such as broken bones, which can result in long periods of inactivity and muscle weakness

- Catastrophic illness such as stroke

- Disease conditions resulting in muscle atrophy or disuse, such as multiple sclerosis, muscular dystrophy, cerebral palsy

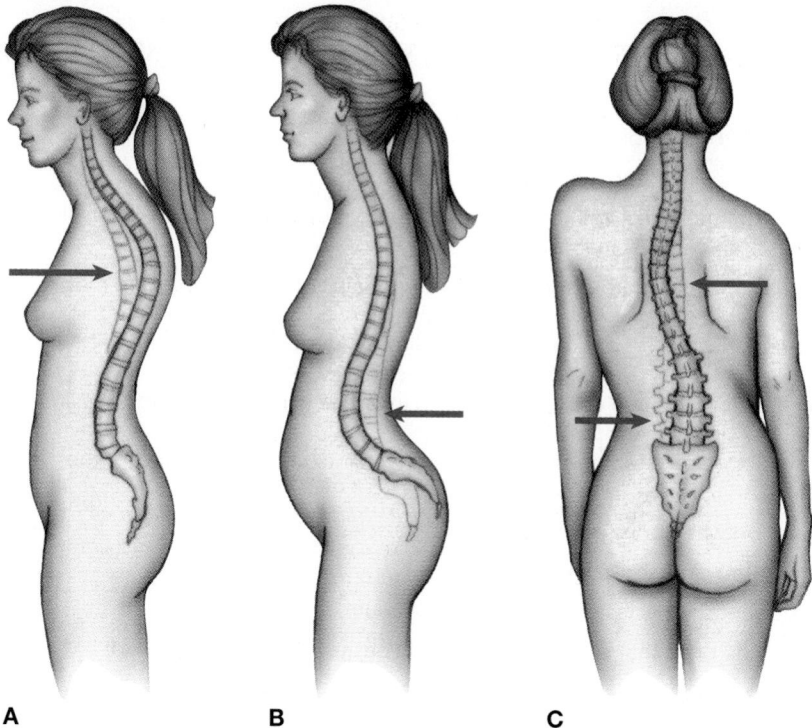

FIGURE 51-3 Three abnormal curvatures of the spine: (A) kyphosis; (B) lordosis; (C) scoliosis.

A formal rehabilitation program begins as soon as the acute phase of an illness or disease has passed. Short-term and long-term goal setting takes place based on the physician's orders and the patient's willingness to cooperate.

A short-term goal would include objectives such as learning crutch walking and range-of-motion exercises. Long-term goals aim at independence and the patient acquiring a feeling of confidence. In this chapter, we focus mainly on the physical aspects of rehabilitation.

Patient Assessment

Prior to actually prescribing rehabilitation treatments, the physician must assess the patient's ability to perform certain functions. The physiatrist will inspect and palpate the patient's limbs and joints to evaluate muscle strength and flexibility. Range of motion, the amount of movement in a particular joint, will be evaluated (see "Range of Motion" later in this chapter). The physiatrist will evaluate the patient's gait (the way a person walks) for clues to specific problems. Posture is also evaluated because the lack of symmetry may indicate scoliosis or curvature of the spine resulting in uneven muscle development. Figure 51-3 illustrates the abnormal types of curvature of the spine. Kyphosis is a thoracic curvature that becomes exaggerated and produces a humpback appearance. Lordosis is an abnormal anterior curvature and is sometimes referred to as swayback. In scoliosis, there is an abnormal lateral curvature of the spine. Scoliosis can occur in individuals sometimes during adolescence or periods of rapid growth. Treatment of any abnormal curvature may include physical therapy exercises, surgery, a body cast, or a brace, depending on the severity.

As a medical assistant, you will assist the physician with these examinations. Once the evaluation is completed, the physician will recommend prescriptions for specific treatments.

Conditions Requiring Physical Therapy

Disease, injury, birth defects, surgery, and amputation all can result in loss of function. Often, the loss of function involves more areas of the body than the specific part affected. For instance, a patient who loses his or her lower leg as a result of diabetes has difficulty with **ambulation** (the act of walking) and other activities of daily living. The loss of the leg forces the patient to use different muscle groups that may become sore when walking with crutches or an artificial limb. Box 51-1 lists common health problems that require rehabilitation.

Box 51-1 Common Health Problems Requiring REHABILITATION

- Alcoholism
- Amputation
- Brain tumor
- Cerebral palsy
- Chronic obstructive pulmonary disease (COPD)
- Traumatic brain injury (TBI)
- Myocardial infarction (MI)
- Spinal cord injury or tumor
- Cerebral vascular accident (stroke)
- Substance abuse
- Mental illness

TABLE 51-2 Conditions Treated by Physical Therapy

Disorder/Pathology	Description
Amputation	Removal of an extremity due to injury or disease
Arthritis	Inflammation of a joint that usually occurs with pain and swelling
Back pain	Pain along and radiating from the spinal column area resulting from back strain, muscular weakness, and disease or pathology of the spinal cord, such as slipped disc
Burn	Damage to the skin from 1st-, 2nd-, or 3rd-degree burns resulting in strictures, decreased mobility, and stiffness *1st-degree:* Damage to superficial layer of skin or outer layer of epidermis with no scarring but resulting in erythema *2nd-degree:* Damage extending through the epidermis and into the dermis causing vesicles and scarring *3rd-degree:* Damage to full thickness (epidermis and dermis) and into underlying layers of the skin with scarring
Bursitis	Inflammation of the bursa between bony prominences and muscles or tendons
Cardiovascular disease	Diseases of the circulatory and cardiac systems
Cerebral palsy	Nonprogressive paralysis due to defects in the brain or birth trauma
Cerebrovascular accident (CVA)	Hemorrhage or clotting in the brain that can result in unconsciousness or paralysis (stroke)
Fracture	Broken bone
Multiple sclerosis	Inflammatory disease of the central nervous system, generally strikes adults between ages of 20–40 and causes progressive weakness and numbness
Muscular dystrophy	Wasting disease of the muscles
Neck trauma	Damage to neck muscles and nerves as the result of trauma or injury (such as whiplash from a car accident)
Osteoporosis	Disease that results in a reduction of bone mass that frequently occurs in postmenopausal women; can result in back pain and fractures
Paraplegia	Paralysis of the lower portion of the body
Parkinson disease	Chronic nerve disease with fine tremors, slow gait, muscular weakness, and rigidity
Poliomyelitis	Acute viral disease that causes an inflammation of the gray matter of the spinal cord, resulting in paralysis in some cases; has been brought under partial control through vaccinations
Quadriplegia	Paralysis of all four extremities of the body
Rheumatoid arthritis	Form of arthritis with inflammation of the joints, swelling, stiffness, and pain
Sprain	Pain and disability caused by trauma to a joint; a ligament may be torn in a severe sprain
Strain	Trauma to a muscle from excessive stretching or pulling

Table 51-2 lists conditions that may necessitate physical therapy and the services of a physical medicine specialist. Patients requiring physical therapy may be inpatients, outpatients, nursing home residents, home health patients, and those in special facilities such as veterans' hospitals.

Physical Therapy Methods

Methods used in physical therapy include massage, exercise, heat and cold applications, electricity, ultraviolet radiation, ultrasonic diathermy, hydrotherapy, and application of hot paraffin. These treatment methods are used to improve circulation, strengthen muscles, relieve pain, and assist the patient in learning to perform all activities of daily living.

MASSAGE

Massage is kneading or applying pressure by the hands to a part of the patient's body to promote muscle relaxation, improve blood circulation, and reduce tension. Massage can consist of the simple act of rubbing an injection site to stimulate absorption and reduce pain. It can incorporate techniques, such as kneading, rolling, stroking, and tapping the skin, that are performed by persons skilled in the art of massage.

Massage is considered a form of passive exercise that is usually applied by someone other than the patient. Terminology related to massage follows:

- **Effleurage**—light stroking movement that may be performed in a circular pattern.
- **Friction**—rubbing or deep stroking that produces an increase in circulation and mild heat within the tissues.
- **Petrissage**—a kneading or rolling method of massage that requires pressing the muscles.
- **Tapotement**—light tapping or percussion to relieve congestion that is performed with the hands, the fingertips, or the hands in a cupping position.

In addition, massage can help restore mobility, decrease swelling, relax muscle spasms, and reduce pain. Physical therapists often incorporate massage in their treatment plans.

Massage therapy is a holistic approach to promoting health that is increasingly valued as a valid form of heath care. Massage therapists require special training and are licensed in many states. They may perform massage in individual private practices and in the hospital setting. Several types or categories of massage are practiced by massage therapists. Traditional or Swedish massage, which is most commonly used in the United States, includes stimulating blood circulation through the soft tissues. Deep tissue massage is used to release chronic patterns of tension or pain by applying massage and pressure at deeper levels. Trigger point massage concentrates finger pressure directly to individual muscles to release trigger points or knots in the muscles. **Reiki** involves channeling the body's energy and spirit through gentle touch and massage.

EXERCISE THERAPY

Being active is an important part of maintaining physical and mental well-being. Inactivity affects every system of the body, and the lack of activity can complicate any physical or mental condition. Any person who has exercised regularly and then suspended the exercise activity for a period knows how quickly muscles lose vigor. **Atrophy**, the decrease or wasting away of muscle tissue, occurs rapidly in an inactive patient. Contractures may result increasing the original disability. A **contracture** is the permanent shortening of the muscle around the joint causing abnormal and sometimes painful positioning of the joint.

Exercise programs are conducted to maintain or regain fitness through planned activity of muscles and joints. Effective exercise programs can help increase or establish lost muscle tone, improve circulation, relieve stress, correct poor posture and body alignment, and increase endurance.

Regular exercise programs, at least three times a week for 20- to 30-minute periods, are recommended for normal adults. Recent research indicates that daily exercise for 30 minutes is actually needed to maintain health. A patient with known medical problems should have a medical consultation with his or her physician to evaluate the medical condition and recommend appropriate exercise.

Types of Exercise

A well-rounded exercise program should involve different types of exercises. In addition to an aerobic exercise program, it is considered beneficial to perform 30 minutes of strength training twice a week to promote healthy bones and improve the ratio of fat to muscle. Various types of exercise are recommended:

- **Aerobics**—strengthens the cardiopulmonary system
- **Isotonic**—maintains uniform (unchanging) tension or tones the muscles on stimulation
- **Isometric**—involves contractions with muscles fixed in place so that the tension occurs without noticeable movement
- **Stretching**—results in muscle elongation

RANGE OF MOTION

Patients who have suffered from a temporary or permanent loss of mobility will need instruction on exercises for range of motion. Range-of-motion exercises can help to maintain muscle tone and flexibility. The medical assistant may need to demonstrate ROM exercises for the patient's family members if the patient is unable to perform the exercises alone.

Range of motion (ROM) is the degree of movement that can be achieved in a specific joint without causing pain; it is measured with a special type of protractor called a **goniometer**. During the patient assessment, the physician lines up the two arms of the goniometer with the bones on either side of the joint being measured. Figure 51-4 is an

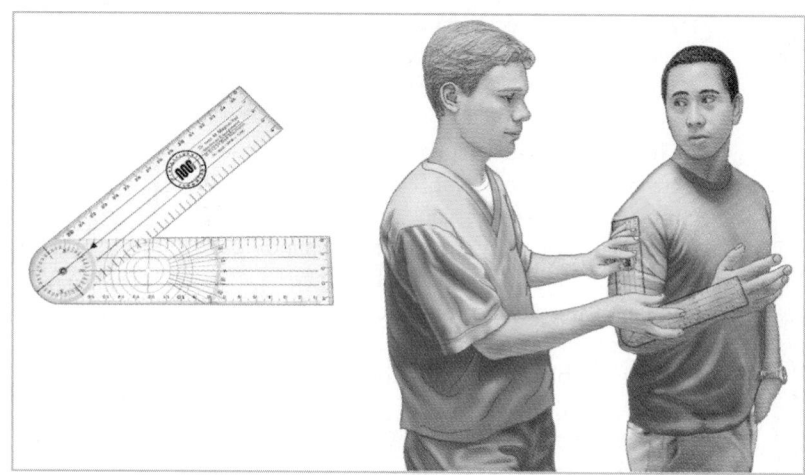

FIGURE 51-4 **A goniometer is used to measure range of motion of the patient's arm.**

example of a goniometer measuring the ROM at the patient's elbow. The degree of movement is read from the scale on the hinged arm of the goniometer. Both active movement and passive movement are measured.

Based on the ability of the patient, the physician may order one of the following types of ROM exercises:

- **Active range of motion (AROM)**—The patient is able to move all limbs through the entire ROM unassisted.

- **Passive range of motion (PROM)**—The patient must have someone else move his or her limbs

GUIDELINES 51-1

PERFORMING RANGE-OF-MOTION (ROM) EXERCISES

- Each exercise should be performed three times unless otherwise ordered by the physician.
- A logical sequence of exercises should be followed so that every muscle and joint receives some movement. In general, ROM exercises begin with the head and move down the body.
- The patient should attempt to do as much as he or she is able to do without assistance.
- Never force any part of the body beyond normal range. Do not exercise to the point of pain.
- Exercise should not be performed if a joint is reddened or swollen.
- Limbs should be supported at the joints when exercising.

through the ROM exercises because he or she is unable to do it.

- **Active assist range of motion (AAROM)**—The patient participates to a limited extent in ROM exercises but requires assistance.

Before beginning ROM exercises, certain guidelines should be explained to the patient (Guidelines 51-1). The patient and the patient's family should be given printed ROM instructions and precautions to take home with them.

Range-of-Motion Exercises

ROM exercises are used to develop and strengthen muscles and joints. Figure 51-5 illustrates the types of body movements used in ROM assessment. Terminology used when discussing movement produced by muscles in ROM exercises is listed in Table 51-3. Most terminology relating to muscle movement is in pairs with opposite meanings. For example, abduction means movement of a body part away from the body, and adduction means movement toward the body. Figure 51-6A–D illustrate ROM exercises performed on a patient's wrist.

APPLICATION OF HEAT AND COLD

Heat and cold are used to treat conditions resulting from trauma and infection. Heat and cold, when used therapeutically, are applied for short periods of time (usually 15 to 30 minutes). Circulation can be impaired if either hot or cold applications remain on a body part for an extended period of time. Tissue damage may result if hot and cold applications are not monitored closely.

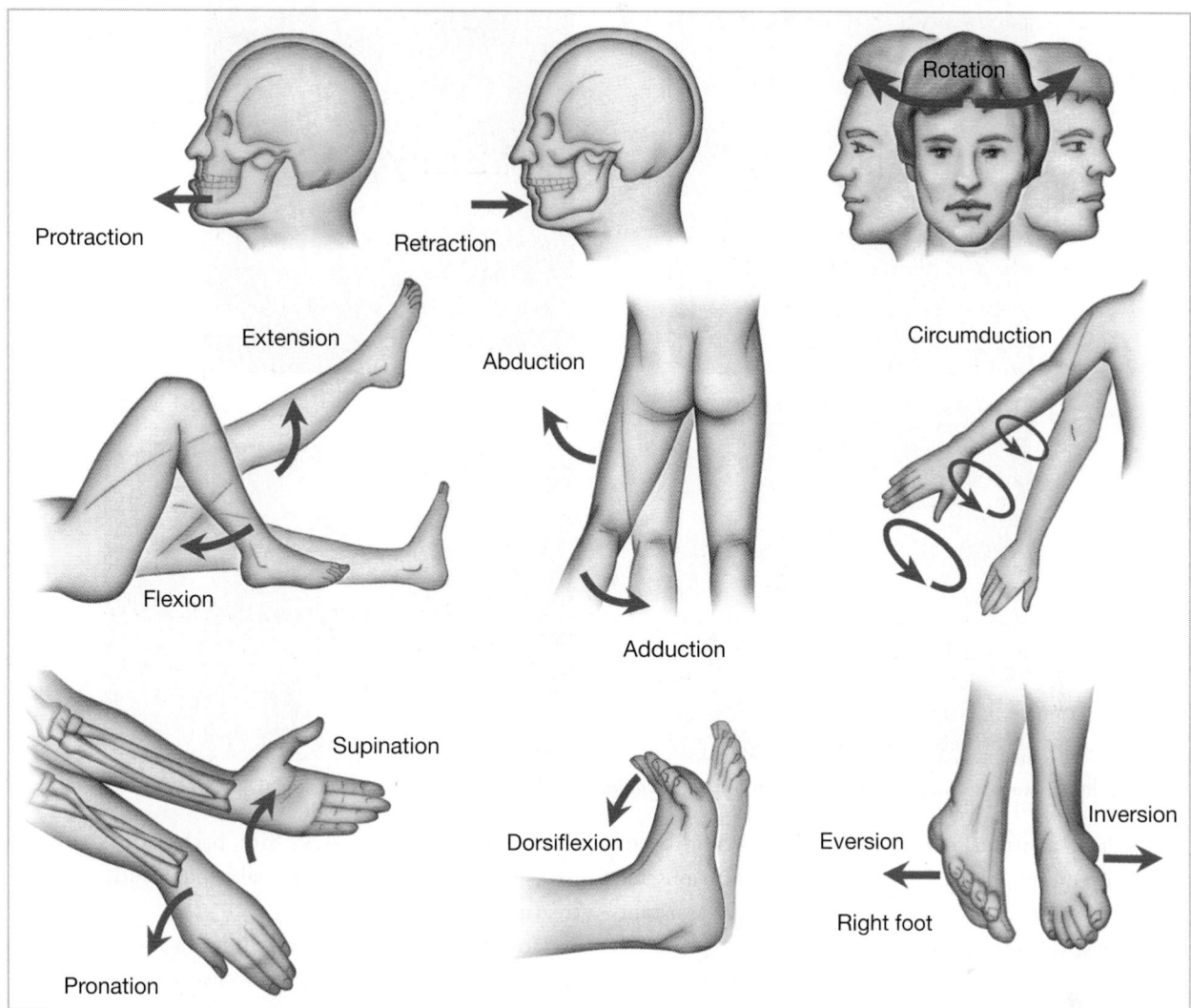

FIGURE 51-5 **Types of body movements used in ROM assessment.**

TABLE 51-3 Terminology for Movement Produced by Muscles

Term	Description
Abduction	Movement away from the midline of the body
Adduction	Movement toward the midline of the body
Circumduction	Movement in a circular direction from a central point
Dorsiflexion	Backward bending (as of a hand or foot)
Eversion	Turning outward
Extension	Movement that brings a limb into or toward a straight condition
Flexion	The act of bending
Hyperextension	Extreme or abnormal extension or stretching
Inversion	Turning inward
Opposition	Ability to move the thumb into contact with other fingers
Plantar flexion	Bending the sole of foot, pointing toes downward
Pronation	Turning downward or backward with the hand or foot; to lie in a prone position (facing downward)
Rotation	The process of turning as if on an axis or a pivot
Supination	Turning of the palm or hand anteriorly, turning of the foot inward and upward, lying in a supine position (face upward)

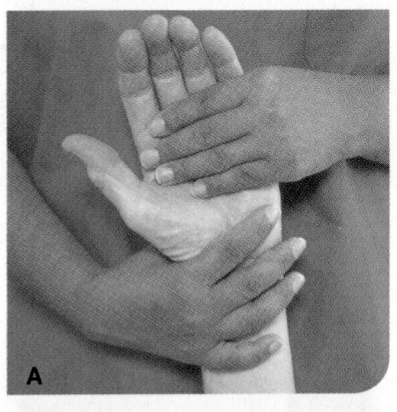
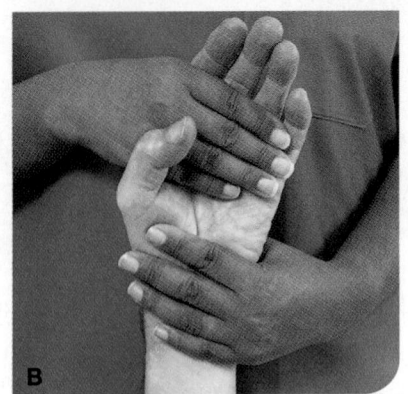
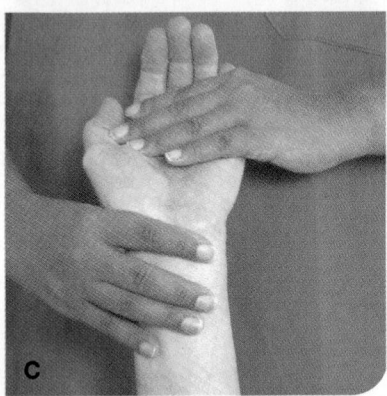
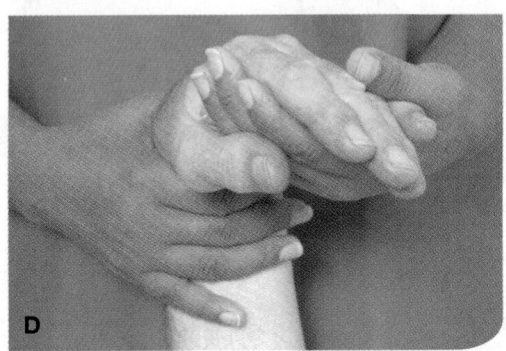

FIGURE 51-6   ROM exercises on a patient's wrist: (A) radial deviation; (B) ulnar deviation; (C) extension; (D) flexion.

The medical assistant may have the responsibility to teach the patient the use of heat and cold applications for therapeutic purposes. In some cases, the medical assistant will apply these devices in the office setting.

Heat Applications

Heat is often used to hasten the healing process. The application of heat to a body part causes dilation of blood vessels and allows more blood to circulate to injured tissues. A condition of **erythema**, or redness of the skin, is caused when the capillaries become congested with blood. This increased circulation assists in providing the body with oxygen and nutrients necessary for repair and healing. Tissue metabolism increases, and healing can occur.

Heat can also assist in relieving pain and muscle spasms. In addition, heat can be used to soften hard crusts of exudate produced by damaged body tissues. **Exudate** is an accumulation of fluid, pus, or serum in tissue that may become hard and crusty. The application of heat, in particular moist heat, can hasten **suppuration**, a process to relieve the internal buildup of pus formation. Heat application can take the form of either moist or dry applications to produce a dilation of blood vessels in the skin.

Moist Heat.   Moist heat application uses heated water that actually touches the skin, such as in a tub or with a wet compress (pad). Examples of moist heat applications include warm to hot compresses, Sitz baths, tub baths, warm soaks, heat hydrotherapy or whirlpool bath, and paraffin treatment.

Hot compresses, often containing a medicated solution, are applied to hasten healing or cleanse open wounds. Any soft, absorbent cloth, such as a washcloth, small towel, disposable woven towels, or gauze squares, can be used as a hot compress. Procedure 51-1 provides the steps for applying a hot compress. The compress may be kept warm by placing a hot water bottle on top of the compress or rewarming the compress. Applying a hot compress to an open wound requires the use of sterile procedures.

Hot soaks involve having the patient put the affected part of the body into a container of water with or without medication for 15 minutes. The water temperature should be no more than 110°F (44°C). Procedure 51-2 provides steps for a hot soak application.

A hot pack is a canvas bag filled with a heat-retaining gel. Hot packs vary in size and are commercially available. They are used to treat larger areas of the body. The packs are placed in hot water and heated, then wrapped in a towel and applied to the affected area. These packs have the advantage of retaining heat longer than hot compresses.

Heat hydrotherapy is the use of warm water as a therapeutic or healing treatment. This can be done in bathtubs, swimming pools, and whirlpools. The whirlpool bath, with

APPLICATION OF A HOT COMPRESS

Objective: Perform a hot compress application and document the procedure.

EQUIPMENT AND SUPPLIES

soaking solution (or water) as ordered by physician; basin; bath thermometer; absorbent cloths such as washcloths or gauze squares; waterproof cover such as plastic wrap

METHOD

1. Perform hand hygiene.
2. Assemble the equipment. If an open wound is present, use sterile equipment and standard precautions.
3. Identify and explain the procedure to the patient.
4. Fill the basin half full of water or medicated solution prepared according to the directions of the physician.
5. Request the patient to remove any necessary clothing because compresses are performed on bare skin. Assist the patient if necessary.
6. Check the temperature of the solution with a bath thermometer. The temperature range for an adult is between 105° and 110°F (41° and 44°C).
7. Position the patient in a comfortable well-supported position.
8. Place the cloths in the basin of hot water or solution. Wring out one cloth until it is wet but not dripping.
9. Gradually place the compress on the patient's body part (Figure 51-7). Ask the patient to tell you how the temperature feels.
10. Frequently test the temperature of the solution. Replace the water as it cools with more warm water.
11. Time the procedure according to the physician's order (15–30 minutes). Check the patient periodically for any signs of change in redness, swelling, or pain.

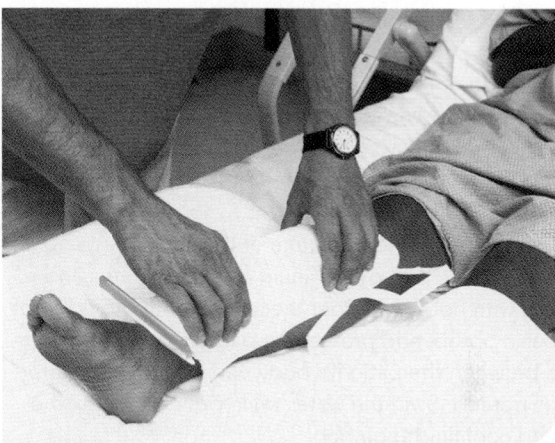

FIGURE 51-7 **Applying a hot compress to the patient's leg.**

12. Gently dry the affected body part.
13. Instruct the patient on any further care such as continued warm compresses at home.
14. Place towels in the laundry. If an open wound is present, then handle the linens according to standard precautions.
15. Clean all of the equipment.
16. Perform hand hygiene and return the equipment.
17. Document the procedure in patient's record.

CHARTING EXAMPLE

6/14/XX 3:00 P.M. Hot compress at 105°F applied to right shin for 20 minutes. Skin with some redness after application. Pt. states there is pain relief. Instructed on application of hot compresses at home. · · · · · · · · · · · · · · · · · M. King, CMA (AAMA)

APPLICATION OF A HOT SOAK

Objective: Perform a hot soak application and document procedure without error.

EQUIPMENT AND SUPPLIES

soaking solution or water as ordered by physician; basin or tub; pitcher; bath thermometer; towels

METHOD

1. Perform hand hygiene.
2. Assemble the equipment. If an open wound is present, use sterile equipment and standard precautions.

3. Identify and explain the procedure to the patient.

4. Fill the basin or tub half full of water or medicated solution prepared according to directions of the physician.

5. Request the patient to remove any obstructing clothing because soaks are applied to the bare skin. Assist the patient if necessary.

6. Check the temperature of the solution with a bath thermometer. The temperature range for an adult is between 105° and 110°F (41° and 44°C).

7. Position the patient in a comfortable well-supported position.

8. Pad the side of the basin or tub with a towel to prevent the patient's body from rubbing on the edge.

9. Gradually place the patient's body part in the solution (Figure 51-8). Ask the patient to tell you how the temperature feels.

10. Frequently test the temperature of the solution. Using a pitcher, remove part of the liquid every 5 minutes and replace it with hot water. Pour the hot water at the edge of the basin or tub, and protect the patient by placing your hand between the patient's body part and the hot water as it is poured. Swirl the water while pouring to mix the hot and cool fluid together.

11. Time the procedure according to the physician's order (15–30 minutes). Check the patient periodically for any signs of change in redness, swelling, or pain.

12. Gently dry the affected body part.

13. Instruct the patient on any aftercare, such as performing warm soaks at home.

14. Place the towels in the laundry. If an open wound is present, then handle the linens according to standard precautions.

15. Clean all the equipment.

16. Perform hand hygiene and return the equipment.

17. Document the procedure in the patient's record.

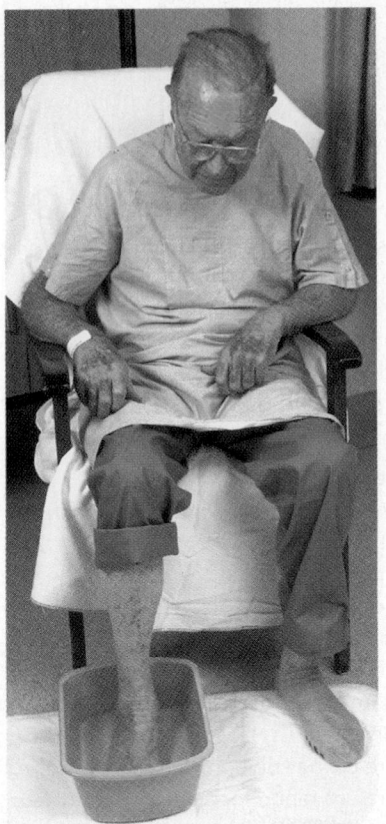

FIGURE 51-8 Place a basin in position for the patient to easily dip his or her foot in water for a hot soak.

CHARTING EXAMPLE

1/15/XX 1:00 P.M. Hot water soak at 105°F applied to right foot for 30 minutes. Skin slightly pink to some redness after application. Pt. states there is pain relief. Instructed on application of hot water soaks at home. · · · · M. King, CMA (AAMA)

continuous jets of hot water reaching the body surfaces, promotes circulation and flexibility of muscles and joints. Arthritis patients are encouraged to participate in exercises in a warm pool to maintain flexibility and reduce pain.

Hot paraffin as a form of heat treatment involves placing the extremities into hot wax to relax the muscles and promote healing. The temperature of the paraffin or wax has to be controlled carefully to prevent burning. Paraffin treatments are usually performed by licensed physical therapists using standard paraffin bath equipment. This therapy is useful for patients with rheumatoid arthritis to relieve the pain and stiffness in joints. The hand or limb is inserted into hot melted paraffin that has been heated to 126°F (54°C). The hand or limb is left in the hot paraffin for about 15 to 30 minutes until there is a thick coating. The relief after this treatment is longer lasting than in some other forms of moist heat treatment.

Note: Burns are a danger if the temperature of the paraffin is not carefully monitored.

Dry Heat. A dry application is a heat application without water, such as with a heating pad. Dry heat, which does not produce moisture, includes infrared radiation (heat lamps), electric heating pads, hot water bottles, chemical hot packs, and aquathermia or aquamatic pads. Figure 51-9 is an example of an aquamatic K-pad, which is an electric, water-filled pad used for dry heat. Another heating pad is a flat electric pad that provides localized heat by regulating a dial.

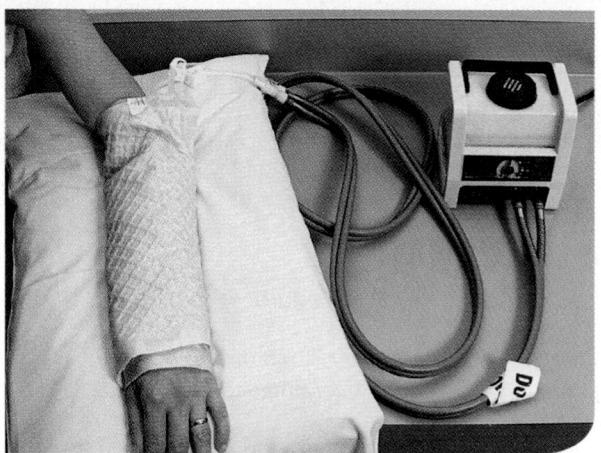

FIGURE 51-9 Aquamatic pad and heating unit provide dry heat treatment to a patient's arm.

The physician should specify the temperature required for the treatment (low, medium, high). Patients should be reminded not to lie on heating pads to avoid burns. Procedure 51-3 lists the application steps for a heating pad.

Heat lamps use infrared bulbs to produce heat. Since the rays from the lamp penetrate the surface of the skin 3 to 5 mm, it is essential that the lamp be placed 2 to 4 feet away from the patient to avoid burning the skin. Treatments usually last about 20 minutes and must be carefully monitored. Ultraviolet lamps are used to treat conditions such as psoriasis or wound infections (see "Ultraviolet Radiation").

A hot water bottle is flat, flexible, and easy to use. The temperature of the water should not exceed 125°F (54°C). For the elderly and children under 2 years old, the temperature should not exceed 115°F (50°C). The water bottle should be filled partially and the remaining air expelled. An overly full bottle is less flexible and harder to conform to the affected body part.

A chemical hot pack is a disposable pack that becomes hot when slapped or kneaded. To use these convenient hot packs, the manufacturer's directions should be followed.

Cold Applications

Cold applications result in constriction of blood vessels, which is the opposite effect of warm applications.

procedure
51-3

APPLICATION OF A HEATING PAD
Objective: Perform a heating pad application and document procedure.

EQUIPMENT AND SUPPLIES

heating pad with protective covering or pillowcase

Note: Perform a preliminary check of the heating pad without bending it to determine that the wires are in good condition.

METHOD

1. Perform hand hygiene.
2. Assemble and test the equipment.
3. Identify and instruct the patient concerning the procedure. The patient should be cautioned against using pins, bending the heating elements within the pad, or lying on the heating pad.
4. Place the heating pad in a protective covering or pillowcase.
5. Connect the heating pad to an electric plug. Set the temperature selector at the setting ordered by the physician (low or medium).
6. Place the heating pad over the patient's affected area. Ask the patient to tell you how it feels. Adjust the temperature as necessary.
7. Instruct the patient regarding the proper temperature setting. Tell him or her not to change the setting.
8. Leave the heating pad in place for the amount of time ordered by the physician (15–20 minutes). Check the patient periodically for any signs of change in redness, swelling, or pain.
9. Remove the heating pad when the procedure is complete. Instruct the patient on any aftercare, such as performing heat treatments at home.
10. Place the protective covering in laundry.
11. Perform hand hygiene and return all the equipment.
12. Document the procedure in the patient's record.

CHARTING EXAMPLE

1/12/XX 9:00 A.M. Heating pad on medium setting applied to left elbow for 20 minutes. Erythema noted over application site. Pt. states there is pain relief and increased mobility in elbow joint. Instructed on application of heating pad at home. · M. King, CMA (AAMA)

APPLICATION OF A COLD COMPRESS

Objective: Perform a cold compress application and document procedure.

EQUIPMENT AND SUPPLIES

water; absorbent cloths or gauze squares; waterproof cover or plastic wrap; basin; ice

METHOD

1. Perform hand hygiene.
2. Assemble the equipment. If an open wound is present, use sterile equipment and standard precautions.
3. Identify and instruct the patient concerning the procedure.
4. Fill the basin half full of cold water. Add ice cubes and compresses.
5. Wring out a compress until wet but not dripping. Wrap the compress in a plastic or waterproof covering to prevent further dripping. Gently place the compress on the patient's affected body part.
6. Check the compress every 3 to 5 minutes, and replace when no longer cool with another cold compress. Add more ice as the water warms.
7. Leave compresses in place for the time specified by the physician (usually 15–20 minutes).
8. Gently dry the affected body part.
9. Place the linens in the proper container. Clean all the equipment.
10. Perform hand hygiene and store the equipment.
11. Document procedure in the patient's record.

CHARTING EXAMPLE

10/23/XX 10:00 A.M. Cold compresses applied to right ankle for 20 minutes. Swelling decreased after treatment. Erythema noted over application site. Instructed on application of cold compress at home. · · · · · · · · · · · · · · · M. King, CMA (AAMA)

Constriction of blood vessels is very useful to prevent or reduce swelling, as in a sprain. Since the blood flow is actually slowed, the amount of body fluids carried into an injured part, such as a leg, is reduced. Additional benefits of cold applications may include the reduction of pain and control of bleeding due to the slowing of blood circulation.

Cryotherapy is using cold for therapeutic purposes. Cold applications can be applied to a body part, such as an ice bag after a tooth extraction. In addition, cold applications can be placed on the entire body to reduce an elevated body temperature. Cold applications consist of cold compresses, soaks, ice packs, and hypothermia blankets. Procedure 51-4 lists the steps for applying a cold compress. Ice in a bag or container (ice pack) is used to treat localized conditions. Procedure 51-5 provides the steps for application of an ice bag. A bag of frozen vegetables, such as peas, makes an effective temporary ice bag.

APPLICATION OF AN ICE BAG

Objective: Perform an ice bag application and document procedure.

EQUIPMENT AND SUPPLIES

ice bag with a protective cover (or small hand towel); ice chips or crushed ice

METHOD

1. Perform hand hygiene.
2. Assemble and test the equipment.
3. Identify and instruct the patient concerning the procedure.
4. Fill the ice bag one-half to two-thirds full of ice. Expel air by squeezing the empty half of ice bag. Replace the cap (Figure 51-10).

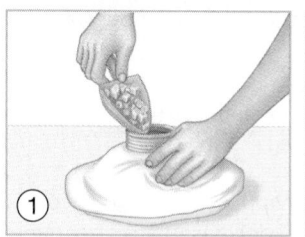 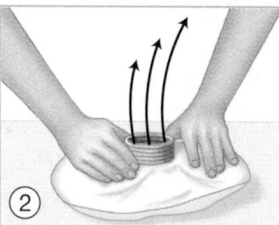 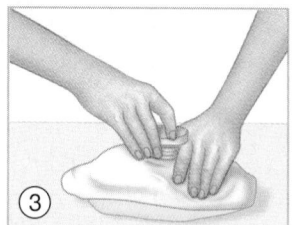 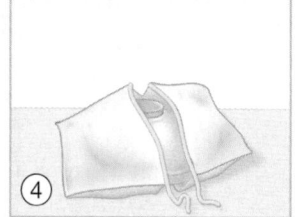

FIGURE 51-10 **Preparing an ice bag.**

5. Dry the bag and place in a protective covering or small hand towel.
6. Place the ice bag over the patient's affected body part. Ask the patient how the ice bag feels.
7. Refill the bag with ice as needed.
8. Leave the ice bag in place for the time specified by the physician (usually 15–20 minutes).
9. Clean the equipment. Allow the bag to air-dry.

10. Perform hand hygiene and store the equipment.
11. Document the procedure in the patient's record.

CHARTING EXAMPLE
2/14/XX 2:00 P.M. Ice bag applied to contusion on right forehead. Swelling reduced after 20 minutes. Erythema noted in treatment area. Instructed on application of ice bag at home. · M. King, CMA (AAMA)

Chemical cold packs are self-contained packets containing a small amount of water in an inner bag that, when released into a chemical contained in the outer bag, causes a chemical reaction that makes the bag cold. This pack can be used as an alternative to an ice pack. Procedure 51-6 lists the steps for applying a cold chemical pack.

Wet cold applications, such as cold compresses, may be used to treat pain and fever. A washcloth or similar cloth is moistened with ice water and applied to an area.

Patient safety and comfort are a concern when using either warm or cold applications.

ULTRAVIOLET RADIATION

Ultraviolet radiation uses rays from natural sources, such as the sun, and artificial sources, such as sun lamps, for healing purposes. Ultraviolet rays stimulate the growth of new epithelial cells and are capable of killing bacteria. These rays are used therapeutically for the treatment of disorders such

procedure
51-6

APPLICATION OF A COLD CHEMICAL PACK

Objective: Perform a cold chemical pack application and document procedure without error.

EQUIPMENT AND SUPPLIES
cold chemical pack; soft cloth

METHOD
1. Perform hand hygiene.
2. Assemble the equipment (Figure 51-11).
3. Identify and instruct the patient concerning the procedure.
4. Shake the bag to allow crystals to fall to the bottom. Squeeze the pack until the inner bag ruptures. Shake the

bag to mix contents. The bag should become cold immediately and remain cold for about 30 minutes.
5. Place the bag inside a soft cloth.
6. Place the cloth-protected bag over the patient's affected body part.
7. Check the patient every 3 to 5 minutes.
8. Leave the cold pack in place for the time specified by the physician (usually 15–20 minutes).

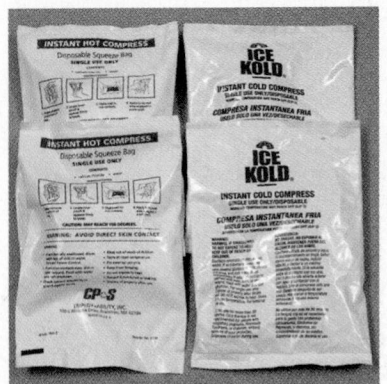

FIGURE 51-11 Examples of disposable hot and cold packs before activation.

9. Discard the ice pack after use in a proper waste container.
10. Perform hand hygiene.
11. Document the procedure in the patient's record.

CHARTING EXAMPLE

7/31/XX 2:00 P.M. Cold pack applied to left cheek over molar area for 20 minutes. Swelling decreased after treatment. Instructed on application of cold chemical pack at home. · · · · ·
· M. King, CMA (AAMA)

as psoriasis. Disorders caused by bacteria, such as acne and pressure sores, are treated effectively with this therapy. The goal of the treatment is to produce a mild redness of the skin to stimulate circulation and kill bacteria.

Ultraviolet-ray lamp treatments must be carefully controlled since the intensity can cause severe first-degree and even second- and third-degree burns. Both the timing of the exposure and the distance of the lamp from the patient must be carefully controlled. A patient can receive a second-degree burn after 1 to 2 minutes of exposure to a lamp set at 30 inches from the patient. Since a patient does not feel this type of burn occurring, he or she cannot warn the operator to stop treatment.

Treatment is ordered by the second, such as a 20-second lamp treatment placed at least 30 inches from the patient and directed only on the area to be treated. Eye protection, in the form of dark goggles, should be worn by both the patient and medical assistant to protect the eyes from ultraviolet ray exposure.

The patient should never be left unattended during this procedure. If you have to leave the room during the treatment, turn off the lamp until you return. The danger of severe burns is great if the timing is not exact.

DIATHERMY

Diathermy is the therapeutic use of a high-frequency current that induces an electrical field within a portion of the body. This electrical field generates heat in various parts of the body and increases blood flow to aid in healing. Diathermy is useful in treating muscular disorders and treatments of tendonitis, arthritis, and bursitis.

The diathermy machine placement must be carefully controlled according to the manufacturer's instructions. Some machines are placed 1 inch from the patient's skin and may have a built-in spacer to assist with exact placement. Others have applicators with pads that require a towel to be placed between the applicator pad and the patient. Due to the danger of burns inherent in diathermy treatment, it has been replaced in many facilities with ultrasound, which is safer.

ULTRASOUND

Ultrasound is sound energy from high-frequency sound waves penetrating deep through tissue layers. It works on the same premise as sonar used in oceanography. Ultrasound waves vibrate at the rate of one million times per second, which cannot be heard by the human ear but produce mechanical and heating effects. The mechanical effect or vibration works on connective tissues, such as ligaments and tendons; the heat effect works on all body tissues. However, ultrasound treatments should be used carefully near bony tissues to avoid causing injury from concentration of waves.

Ultrasound treatments usually are applied for 10 minutes or less, as ordered by the physician. The patient may require several ultrasound treatments to receive the benefit. Ultrasound is used effectively to treat pain, relax muscle spasms, stimulate circulation in patients with vascular disorders, relax tendons and ligaments, and break up calcium deposits and scars. Ultrasound treatments are used in conjunction with other treatments, such as medications, to relieve back spasms.

Ultrasound is administered via a machine with an applicator head attachment that can be placed directly on the skin. The ultrasound applicator head contains quartz crystal that vibrates rapidly when an electric current passes through it. Since these waves do not travel through air, they must be kept in contact with the skin. A conducting medium, such as a special gel or mineral oil, must be placed on the skin to conduct the ultrasound into the body. The ultrasound operator applies the ultrasound head to the patient's skin using a steady up-and-down motion. The operator must keep the ultrasound head in continuous motion over the body part since tissue damage can occur if it is held in one place for a prolonged period of time. Prior to treatment, patients should be asked if they have any implants, such as a hip or joint replacement, since the ultrasound could loosen the implant.

Adaptive Equipment and Devices

Equipment used to assist recovery from physical disorders or disabilities includes adaptive equipment (e.g., wheelchairs, walkers, canes, and crutches) and special furniture (e.g., shower chairs and geriatric chairs). Mobility aids or mobility assistive devices are designed to enable the patient to ambulate. Other devices, including braces, casts, traction, prostheses, splints, and slings, are used by the physical therapist to manipulate the patient's damaged bones and tissues. Adaptive equipment also includes a variety of utensils, such as eating utensils molded to fit the patient's hand and dishes with a wide edge to prevent spilling. Figure 51-12 illustrates adaptive equipment, including a toothbrush, reaching stick, shoe holder, stocking helper, and writing aid.

Special furniture, such as shower chairs made from aluminum or plastic, allows the patient to sit while taking a shower. The geriatric chair, a wheeled chair that reclines with an attached tray for meals, is useful for patients who can feed themselves but may not be able to sit securely in a regular chair.

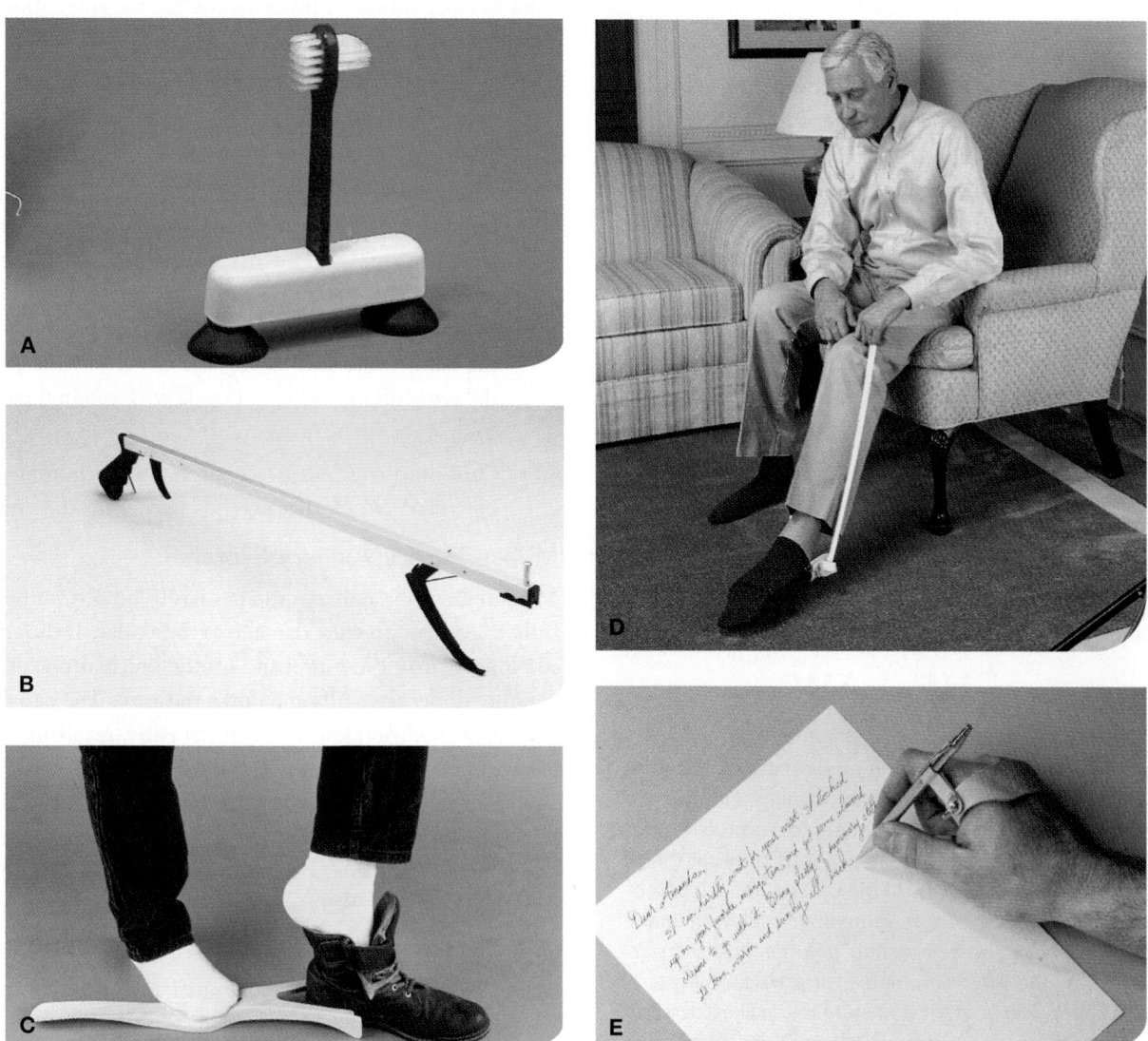

FIGURE 51-12 **There are many types of adaptive devices: (A) a toothbrush; (B) a reaching stick; (C) a shoe holder; (D) a stocking helper; (E) a writing aid.**

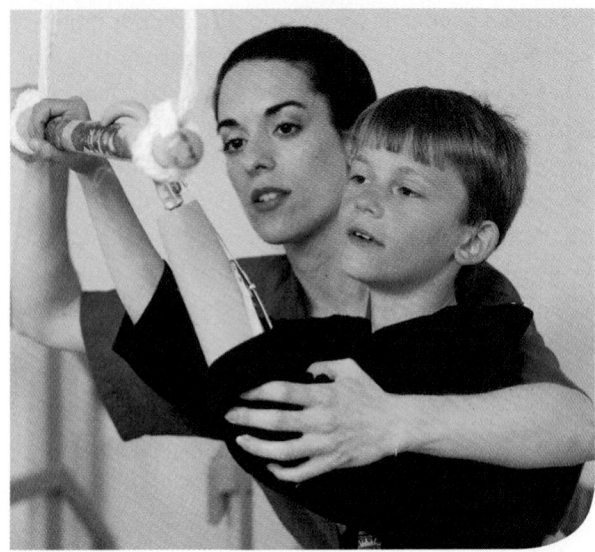

FIGURE 51-13 A therapist assisting an amputee patient to regain mobility and strength after amputation.

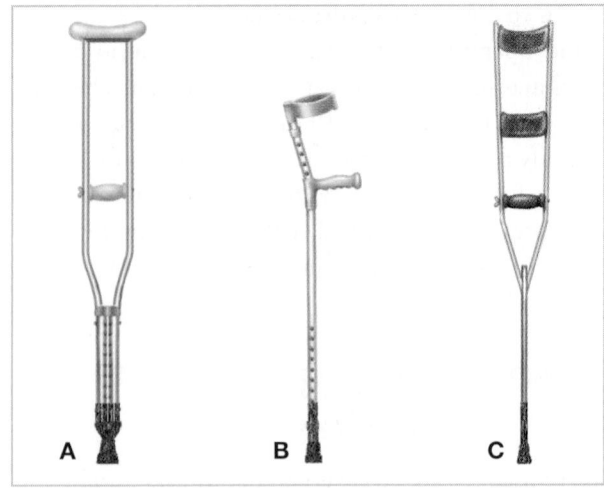

FIGURE 51-14 Three types of crutches: (A) axillary crutch; (B) Lofstrand or forearm crutch; (C) Canadian or elbow crutch.

Adaptive devices are prescribed by the physician; however, the physical therapist may provide the initial instruction on the use of the device. In a general practice setting, the medical assistant will assist the physician with these devices and will provide continuing education and support for the patient when he or she is seen in the physician's office. Figure 51-13 illustrates a physical therapist assisting a patient to regain mobility and strength after an amputation.

CRUTCHES

Crutches allow the patient to walk without placing weight on the healing leg part. Weight is transferred to the arms and hands. Crutches are made from metal or wood and should have a rubber tip at the end to prevent slipping on a smooth floor surface. The following are the three most common types of crutches (Figure 51-14):

- **Axillary crutch**—a tall crutch with shoulder rest and handgrip that reaches from the ground to under the axilla. These crutches are commonly used for a patient who has suffered a fractured leg.
- **Lofstrand (forearm crutch)**—a single aluminum tube with an arm cuff that fits snugly around the patient's forearm and uses a handgrip for weight bearing. This crutch allows the patient to release the handgrip to use the hand while still having the crutch held in place by the arm cuff for support. People with cerebral palsy and paraplegia often choose to use this type of crutch.
- **Canadian or elbow crutch**—a variation of the Lofstrand crutch that extends farther up the arm.

Measuring for Axillary Crutches

Measurement for axillary crutches has to be determined carefully to prevent pressure damage to the axillae. If the crutch is too long it may cause pressure on the brachial plexus (nerve running under the axilla and down the arm). The patient may develop a condition known as crutch palsy, resulting in muscle weakness in the arm, wrist, and hand. Crutches that are too short can result in the patient having to bend forward while walking. Back pain, nerve damage, and injury to the axilla and palms of the hands can occur if the crutches are improperly fitted. The steps for measuring axillary crutches follow:

1. Have the patient wear walking shoes and stand straight.
2. Place the crutch tips 4 to 6 inches to the side and 4 to 6 inches in front of each foot.
3. Adjust the crutch, using the bolts and nuts at the sides of the crutch, so that the axillary crutch bars are three

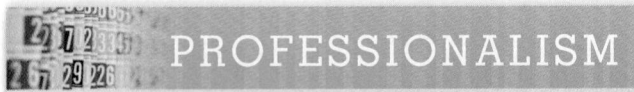

PROFESSIONALISM

THE LAW

Many of the procedures described in this chapter are beyond the scope of practice for a medical assistant beginning his or her first job. Additional training and practice are required before teaching a patient to use crutches, for instance. In some states, only a licensed physical therapist is able to perform many of the procedures discussed. The medical assistant must remember that with many procedures, he or she is "assisting" another licensed person, such as the physician, nurse, or physical therapist. Always check with your local or state medical association regarding the laws in your state. The patient's safety must always be placed first.

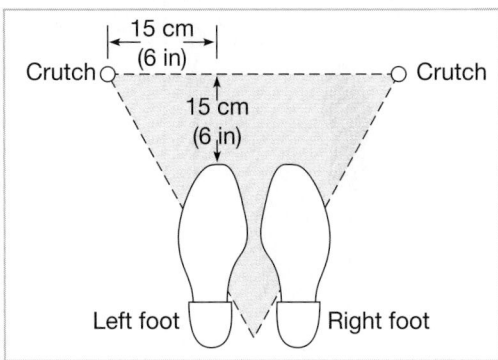

FIGURE 51-15 The correct beginning position for the patient's feet and crutches (tripod position).

finger widths below the axilla. Measure this by inserting your own fingers between the patient's axilla and the crutch bar.

4. Next adjust the handgrips so the patient can flex his or her elbows at a 30-degree angle when the crutch is in place and the patient's hands are on the hand bars.

Instructions both in writing and with an actual demonstration should be provided to the patient who will be using crutches. To teach the patient how to properly use crutches, have him or her start in the tripod position. Figure 51-15 illustrates the correct position of the crutches and the patient's feet. Teaching the patient how to use crutches and proper crutch walking gaits is one of the responsibilities of the medical assistant.

Crutch Walking Gaits

The type of crutch **gait** or walk that the patient will use depends on the amount of weight bearing the patient's leg or legs will support in addition to his or her muscular coordination, age, and overall physical condition. In a crutch walking gait, each foot and crutch is called a point. For example, a two-point gait consists of two points from the total of four points (two legs and two crutches) that are in contact with the ground during each step. The patient should be encouraged to use a slow gait. Common gaits include the four-point, three-point, two-point, swing-to, and swing-through gaits.

The physician determines the type of crutch necessary for the patient and may fit the crutch for the patient in the office. You may be asked to demonstrate the use of crutches and the appropriate gait required by the patient's condition. The patient should be reminded to use a slow pace in crowded areas or when feeling tired. Using crutches requires a great deal of energy and different muscle groups than those the patient is accustomed to using.

Four-Point Gait. The four-point gait is a slow and steady gait and is used when a patient can bear weight on both legs. This is considered the safest of all gaits since the

patient always has three points of support in contact with the ground at all times. This gait is also used by patients who may have muscular weakness and some lack of coordination (Figure 51-16).

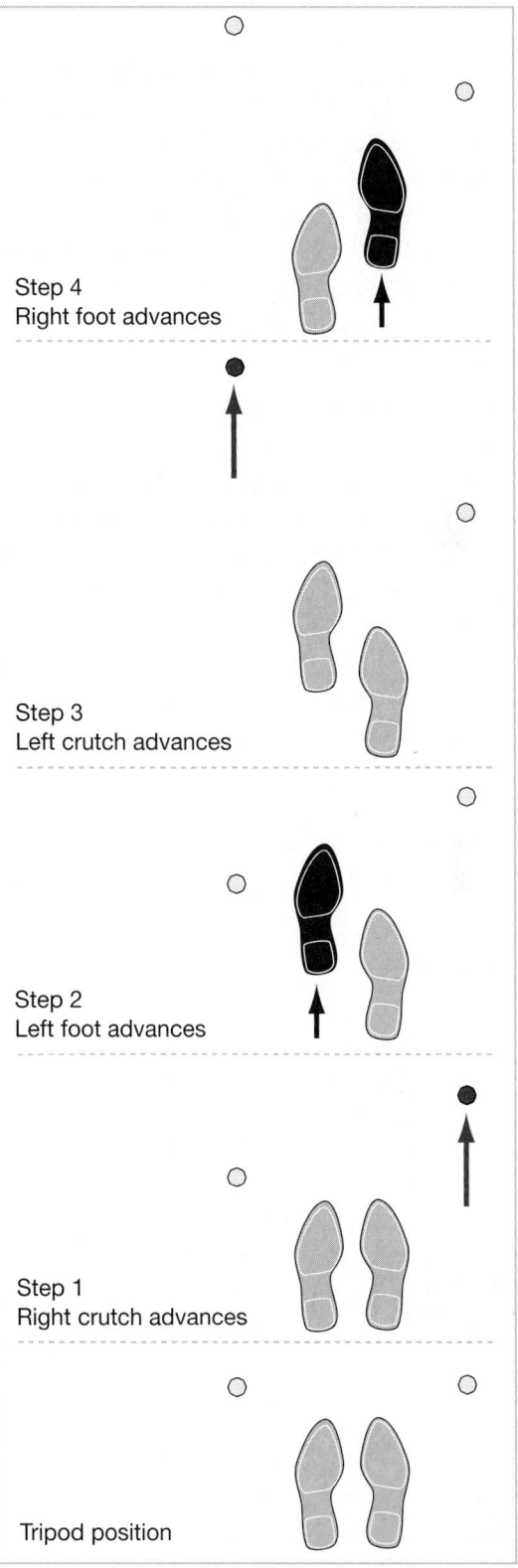

FIGURE 51-16 Four-point gait.

To use this gait, first the right crutch is moved forward, followed by the left foot, then the left crutch, and then the right foot. This is repeated over and over. The patient must be able to move each leg separately to use this gait.

Three-Point Gait. The three-point gait is used when one leg is stronger than the other or when there is no weight bearing on one leg. The patient must have good muscle coordination and arm strength. To use this gait, the patient must be able to support his or her full weight on one leg. Have the patient move both crutches and the affected leg forward and then move the unaffected leg forward while weight is balanced on both crutches (Figure 51-17). This gait requires good coordination and muscle strength. It is used by patients with musculoskeletal disorders (e.g., fractures), recent leg surgery, or amputees without an artificial limb.

Two-Point Gait. The two-point gait is faster moving than the four-point gait and is used by the patient who can bear some weight on both feet and maintain good balance. Two-point gait occurs when a crutch and the opposite foot are moved forward at the same time. For example, the left crutch and the right leg move together (Figure 51-18).

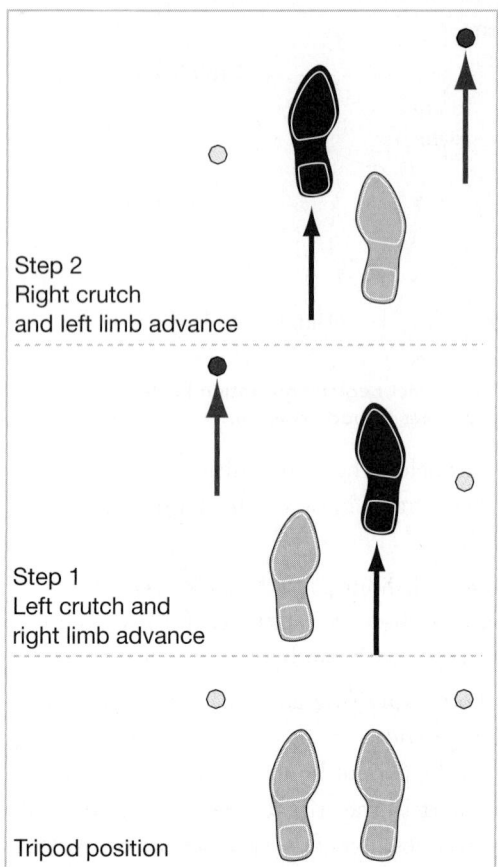

Step 2
Right crutch
and left limb advance

Step 1
Left crutch and
right limb advance

Tripod position

FIGURE 51-18 Two-point gait.

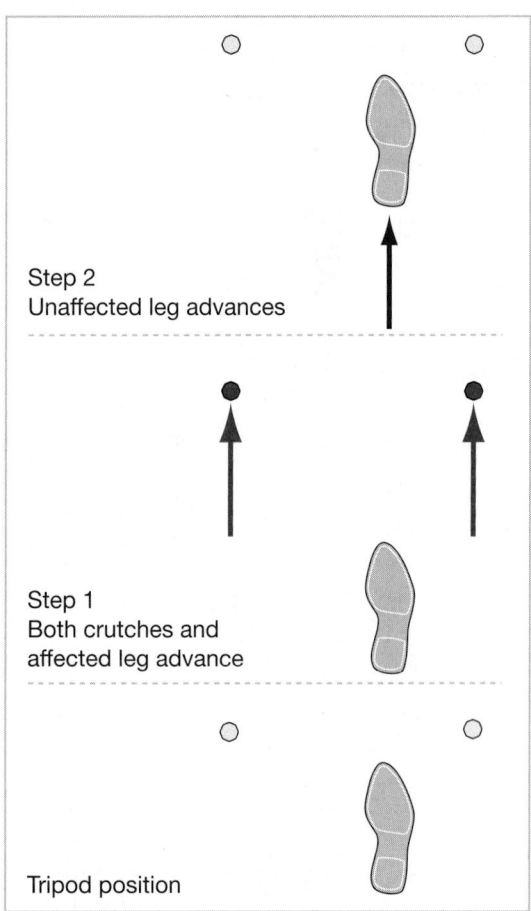

Step 2
Unaffected leg advances

Step 1
Both crutches and
affected leg advance

Tripod position

FIGURE 51-17 Three-point gait.

Swing Gaits. Swing gaits are used by patients with severe leg disabilities, such as deformities or paralysis. They may use either of the two swing gaits: swing-to or swing-through gait.

To use the swing-to gait, the patient moves the crutches forward, lifts his or her body, and then swings the legs up to the same point. Good muscular control is needed for this gait since the patient may lose his or her balance and fall forward with this gait (Figure 51-19A–B).

To use the swing-through gait, the patient moves the crutches forward, as in the swing-to gait, and then swings the legs past the crutches. This provides a good base of support. It is a gait that allows for fast movement. Both the swing-to and swing-through gaits are used by paraplegic patients who are using the forearm type of crutches or by patients with a generalized leg weakness.

Sitting with Crutches

The patient using crutches should be instructed on how to manipulate the crutches and support his or her legs to sit down.

1. The patient should face forward and then back into a straight-back chair with arm rests until the back of his or her legs touch the chair seat.

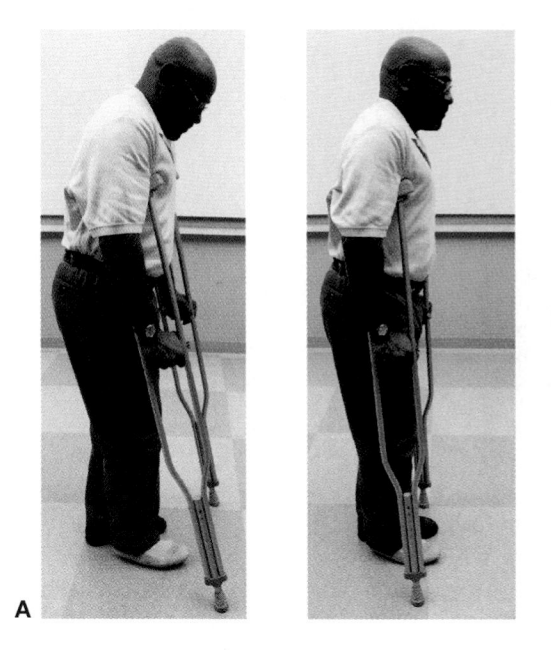

FIGURE 51-19 Swing gaits: (A) swing-to gait; (B) swing-through gait.

2. The crutches should be placed in the hand on the strong side of the body, opposite the weak leg.

3. The patient should grasp the chair arm with the other hand and lower him- or herself gently into the chair.

Standing with Crutches

The patient should be instructed to follow four steps when moving from a sitting to a standing position with the use of crutches.

1. The patient should place the crutches in the hand on the strong side of the body to use as support.

2. The patient should move or slide his or her body forward in the chair.

3. The patient should grasp the chair arm with the free hand on the affected side.

4. The patient should push up to a standing position.

Procedure 51-7 contains the steps for teaching or reinforcing instructions on the correct use of crutches.

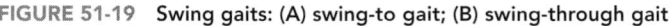

procedure

51-7

INSTRUCTING A PATIENT TO USE CRUTCHES CORRECTLY

Objective: Teach a patient how to use crutches correctly.

EQUIPMENT AND SUPPLIES

crutches; gait belt

METHOD

1. Assemble the equipment requested by the physician's order.
2. Check the crutches to determine that they are in good working condition.
3. Perform hand hygiene.
4. Identify the patient and explain the procedure.
5. Check to see if the patient is wearing sturdy, nonskid shoes.
6. Demonstrate the correct position.
7. Demonstrate the gait requested by the physician.
8. Have the patient stand against a wall or near a chair for support.
9. Adjust crutch length to appropriate height. The distance between the top of the crutch and the axilla should be three finger widths (Figure 51-20).

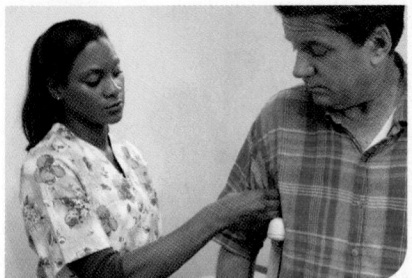

FIGURE 51-20 **The medical assistant measures and adjusts the crutch length for the patient.**

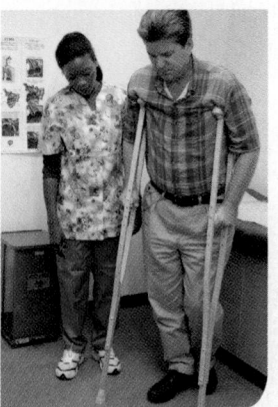

FIGURE 51-21 **The medical assistant instructs the patient how to walk with crutches.**

10. Instruct the patient to keep his or her head up, stand straight with abdomen in, and feet straight with a slight (5 degree) bend at the knee joint. Remind the patient to look ahead and not down while walking with crutches. This will prevent the patient from bending forward.

11. Explain to the patient that the weight should be supported by the hands, not the underarms. The patient should practice standing to maintain balance and place weight on the palms of the hands, and not on the axilla, at the hand bars. Instruct the patient not to rest body weight on the axillary bars for more than 1 or 2 minutes to prevent injury to the brachial plexus.

12. Instruct the patient to assume basic crutch stance or tripod to provide a firm base of support. The basic crutch stance is the tripod to provide a firm base of support. Feet are slightly apart, and the tips of the crutches are 4 to 6 inches in front of and 4 to 6 inches to the side of the toes. An imaginary line drawn from the two crutch points to an area behind the center of the feet will form a triangle (tripod).

13. Instruct the patient to take small steps and swing through when first learning to use crutches. The crutches should only move about 12 inches forward with each step to prevent the crutches from slipping. Have the patient move slowly at first (Figure 51-21).

14. Have the patient practice his or her gait.

15. Remind the patient to report any numbness or tingling in the arms. The crutch shoulders and hand bars can be padded for extra comfort with either sponge rubber or a soft cloth. The patient should then remeasure and adjust the crutches for the correct length.

16. Crutches should always be moved forward and to the side so the feet can swing through.

17. Remind the patient to periodically check the nuts and wing bolts to maintain tightness and to check the rubber tips frequently for cracks. They can easily be replaced.

18. Make corrections on the patient's use of crutches as needed.

19. Chart appropriately.

CHARTING EXAMPLE

9/30/XX 2:00 P.M. Instructed how to use crutches. Adjusted crutches to fit. Pt practiced for 20 minutes. · · · · · · · · · · · · · ·
· M. King, CMA (AAMA)

CANES

Canes are used by patients who have muscle or bone weakness on one side or need assistance with balance. Two common types of canes are the standard cane and the four-point (quad) cane shown in Figure 51-22. Several types of wooden and aluminum canes are available. The aluminum canes use nuts and wing bolts for height adjustments. The wooden canes have to be purchased to size or cut to the correct length. All canes should have a rubber tip on the end to prevent slipping. A standard cane has a curved neck for ease of gripping. It provides support for patients who need only slight assistance. The tripod (three-point) and quad

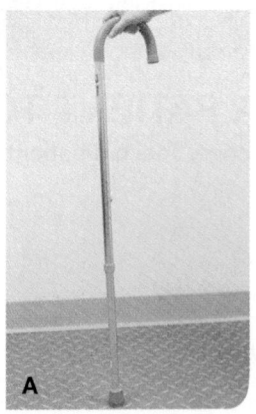
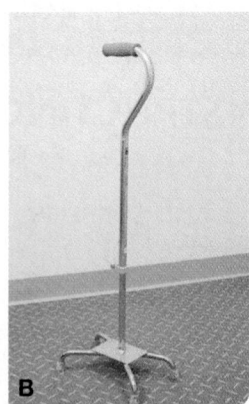

FIGURE 51-22 **(A–B) Two types of canes.**

procedure
51-8

INSTRUCTING A PATIENT TO USE A CANE OR SINGLE CRUTCH CORRECTLY

Objective: Instruct a patient on the correct use of a cane.

EQUIPMENT AND SUPPLIES
cane suited to the patient's needs; gait belt

METHOD
1. Assemble the equipment according to the physician's order.
2. Check the cane height and condition of the cane tip.
3. Identify the patient.
4. Perform hand hygiene and explain the procedure.
5. Check to see if the patient is wearing sturdy, nonskid shoes.
6. Demonstrate the correct position.
7. Demonstrate the gait.
8. Instruct the patient to hold the cane (or single crutch) on the opposite side of the injury or affected limb. As the affected leg moves forward, the cane (or crutch) on the opposite side will move forward to provide support.
9. Place the cane (or single crutch) 6 inches in front of and slightly to one side of the unaffected side. Make sure the cane tip is firmly on the floor and the weight is supported on the strong leg and the cane. The patient's elbow should be slightly flexed during weight bearing.
10. Have the patient look straight ahead, not down at his or her feet.
11. Have the patient move the cane (or single crutch) forward 6 to 12 inches and bring the affected leg forward until it is even with the cane. The weight should be placed on the strong foot and leg.
12. Instruct the patient to move the strong leg forward past the cane and weaker leg. As the unaffected foot moves forward, the weight is shifted to the weak or affected foot and the cane. Thus the cane will provide support for weight bearing on the weaker leg.
13. Have the patient repeat the walking pattern. Evaluate his or her balance and endurance.
14. Document the procedure correctly.

CHARTING EXAMPLE
3/3/XX 1:00 P.M. Instructed on proper use of walking with a cane. Cane height and condition good. Pt balance and gait good. Pt practiced for 10 minutes. · · · · M. King, CMA (AAMA)

(four-point) canes have a wide base with three or four points to provide steadier support; the neck is bent with a T-shaped handle.

A physical therapist determines the most suitable cane for the patient. To determine the correct cane height, the patient should stand tall so that the handgrip of the cane is level with the hip joint and the elbow is flexed at an angle of 25 to 30 degrees. Also, the handle must be suitable for the patient's hand size. Procedure 51-8 lists the steps for teaching a patient the correct use of a cane.

WALKERS

Walkers are assistive devices made of aluminum that provide a base of support for patients who need help with balance and walking. To aid with mobility, many geriatric patients use walkers. The walker should be adjusted to the patient's height and reach just below the patient's waistline (Figure 51-23).

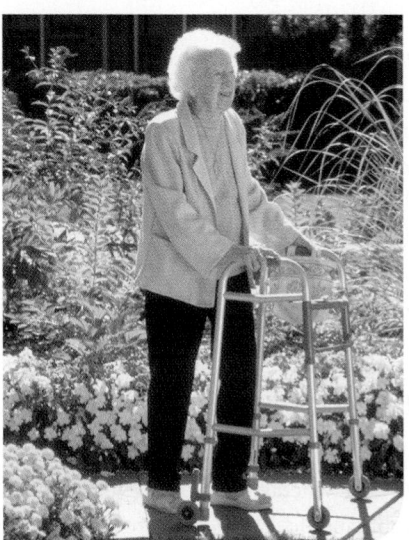

FIGURE 51-23 Walkers help the patient ambulate safely.

TEACHING A PATIENT TO CORRECTLY USE A WALKER

Objective: Teach a patient to correctly use a walker.

EQUIPMENT AND SUPPLIES

walker suited to patient's needs; gait belt

METHOD

1. Assemble the equipment according to the physician's order.
2. Check the condition of the walker.
3. Perform hand hygiene.
4. Identify the patient and explain the procedure.
5. Check to see if the patient is wearing sturdy, nonskid shoes.
6. Demonstrate the correct stance and gait with the walker.
7. Assist the patient into the walker.
8. Evaluate the walker for proper height and fit. (The top of the walker should reach the patient's hipbone and the patient's hands should be on the handgrip with his or her elbow flexed at a 30-degree angle).
9. Instruct the patient to distribute his or her weight evenly between the walker and both legs.
10. Instruct the patient to move the walker 6 to 8 inches ahead with all four legs of the walker hitting the floor at the same time.
11. Instruct the patient to bring his or her weaker foot into the walker.
12. Instruct the patient to bring the stronger foot forward even with the weaker foot.
13. Have the patient continue walking with the walker while you evaluate his or her balance and endurance.
14. Document appropriately.

Note: The walker is not to be used by the patient as a transfer device. Remind the patient to grasp the walker after he or she is in a standing position and not to use the walker to pull up from a sitting position.

CHARTING EXAMPLE

5/31/XX 11:00 A.M. Instructed on proper use of walker. Evaluated walker height to fit. Pt practiced for 15 minutes. · M. King, CMA (AAMA)

A stationary walker must be picked up by the patient, moved forward, and then used as a base of support while the patient walks into it. This requires strong arm muscle development.

A walker with wheels can be used by patients who have good coordination and balance. This type of walker can be dangerous because it might move too quickly, causing the patient to lose his or her balance and fall. Some walkers with wheels have a stop and release bar that the patient presses to unlock the wheels; if the patient lets go of the bar the wheels lock, thus preventing the walker from moving away from the patient. Procedure 51-9 outlines how to teach a patient to use a walker.

WHEELCHAIRS

Wheelchairs are hand manipulated or power driven. Many patients operate their own wheelchairs; however, not all patients are able to (nor should they) operate their own wheelchairs (Figure 51-24). For example, an individual paralyzed on one side or blind or frail may not be able to operate his or her own wheelchair and will need assistance.

Wheelchair Transfer

Always think of moving a patient as the process of transferring him or her from one place to another. In many

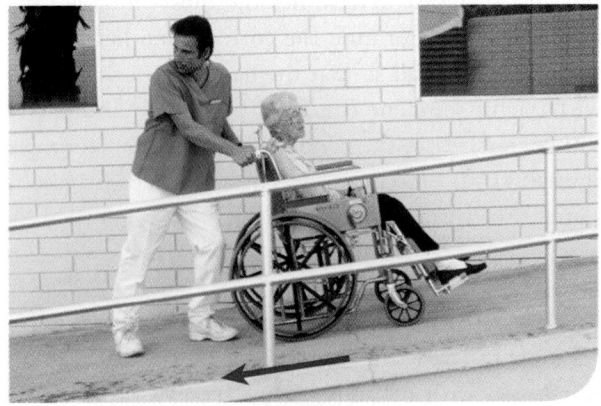

FIGURE 51-24 Wheelchairs are moved down ramps backward.

cases, the patient is familiar with the techniques necessary for the transfer and will be able to assist the medical assistant.

A patient who is paralyzed on one side of the body (**hemiplegia**) or who has a general weakness can be moved from a wheelchair by pivoting the patient so that he or she can use the stronger leg to assist you. Explain to the patient that this transfer technique is used to prevent injury to the patient and to the individual assisting with the transfer. Procedure 51-10 lists the steps to successfully transfer a

procedure
51-10

WHEELCHAIR TRANSFER TO A CHAIR OR EXAMINATION TABLE

Objective: Move the patient from a wheelchair to a chair or examination table without error.

EQUIPMENT AND SUPPLIES
chair or examination table; gait belt, if needed; step stool, if needed

METHOD
1. Perform hand hygiene.
2. Identify the patient and introduce yourself.
3. Explain what you are going to do before you start. Discuss what the patient will do to assist you.
4. Place the wheelchair at a 45-degree angle to the chair or examination table. This provides a shorter distance to pivot the patient from the wheelchair.
5. Put the wheelchair brakes in the lock position on both sides. The patient's legs should be moved off the pedals by supporting the ankle and lower leg. Gently place the patient's feet on the floor and have the patient shift forward in the chair, if possible. Move the foot pedals up and out of the way so the patient has a clear path to move forward.
6. Make sure the examination table or chair is stable before attempting the transfer.
7. Position yourself near the patient's nonparalyzed side so you can provide support and the patient can use his or her stronger limb. You will move the patient toward the stronger side. Do not refer to the patient's "good" or "bad" side.
8. Place one of your feet forward to establish a firm base of support for your body. Move down toward the patient while keeping your back straight.
9. Have the patient place his or her hands on the arm supports of the wheelchair. Then, ask the patient to lean forward and push up as you assist the patient to a standing position, on the count of three (Figure 51-25).

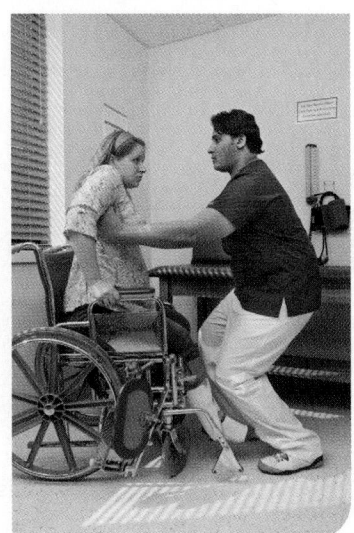

FIGURE 51-25 **A medical assistant helps the patient out of the wheelchair.**

10. Position yourself so that the patient's paralyzed leg is between your knees. Support the paralyzed leg with your knees, if necessary, so the leg will not slip as the patient stands.
11. Place your hands under the patient's armpits and help the patient to stand. Use the muscles in your legs to push your body upward. Do not bend over and use back muscles.
12. Allow the patient to stand for a few moments before attempting to move into the chair or onto the examination table.

13. Assist the patient to pivot (turn) toward the nonparalyzed side by pivoting your own body as you hold the patient under his or her armpits. Do not twist your body. Turn it as a unit.
14. Gently lower the patient into a chair by bending your knees and keeping your back straight.
15. If the patient must move up onto an examination table and can assist you, then support the weak side as the patient places his or her stronger leg onto the step stool. Pivot the patient around so he or she can then sit on the edge of the table. Encourage the patient to move back on the table to eliminate the danger of falling.
16. If the patient is unable to assist you, then ask for another assistant to hold one side of the patient as you support the other side. Count aloud "one," "two," "three," and then lift the patient together. Do not attempt to lift—by yourself—a patient who is unable to help you.
17. When assisting the patient into a supine position, support the paralyzed leg gently onto the table.
18. Never leave a physically challenged (disabled) patient unattended.

patient from a wheelchair to a chair or examination table. Figure 51-26 is an example of moving a patient from a bed to a wheelchair. Figure 51-27 illustrates how to protect a falling patient.

BRACES

A brace is one type of orthotic used to support weakened body parts, correct deformities, and prevent joint movement. Braces may be made out of metal, plastic, or leather and are

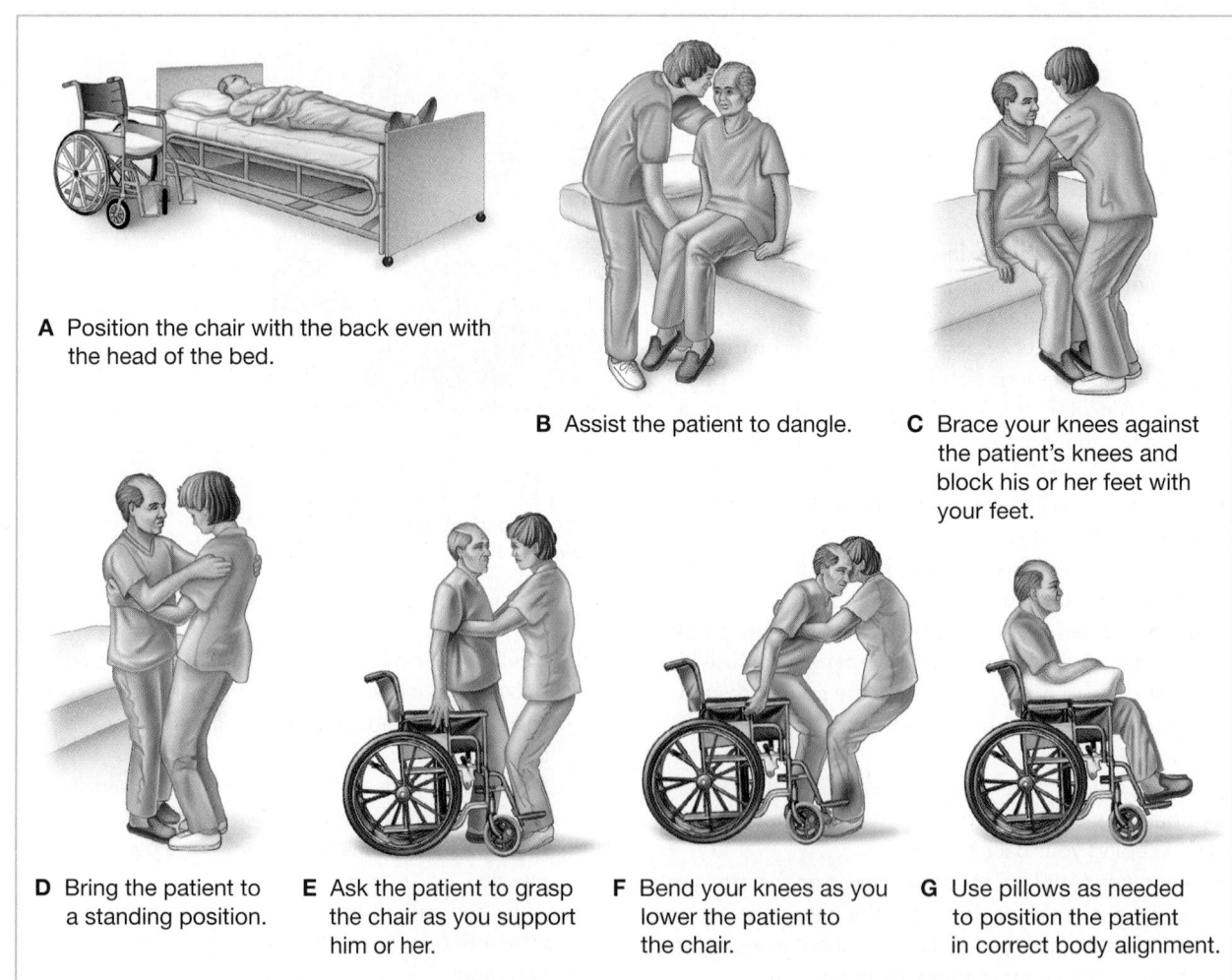

A Position the chair with the back even with the head of the bed.

B Assist the patient to dangle.

C Brace your knees against the patient's knees and block his or her feet with your feet.

D Bring the patient to a standing position.

E Ask the patient to grasp the chair as you support him or her.

F Bend your knees as you lower the patient to the chair.

G Use pillows as needed to position the patient in correct body alignment.

FIGURE 51-26 (A–G) Assisting the patient to transfer from the bed or examining table to a wheelchair.

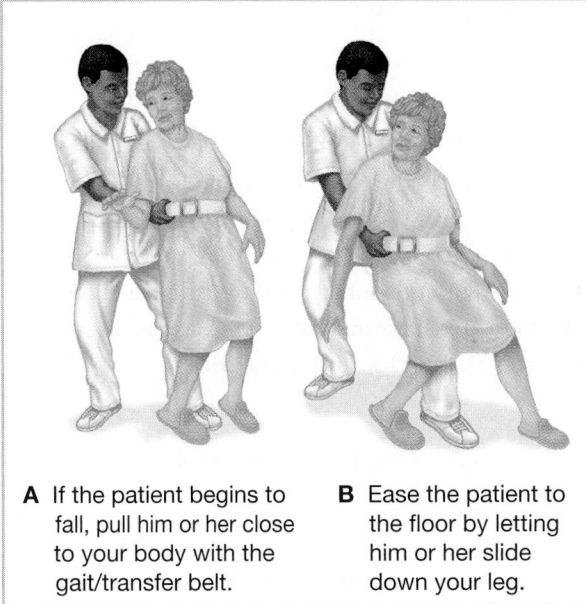

A If the patient begins to fall, pull him or her close to your body with the gait/transfer belt.

B Ease the patient to the floor by letting him or her slide down your leg.

FIGURE 51-27 (A–B) Assisting a falling patient.

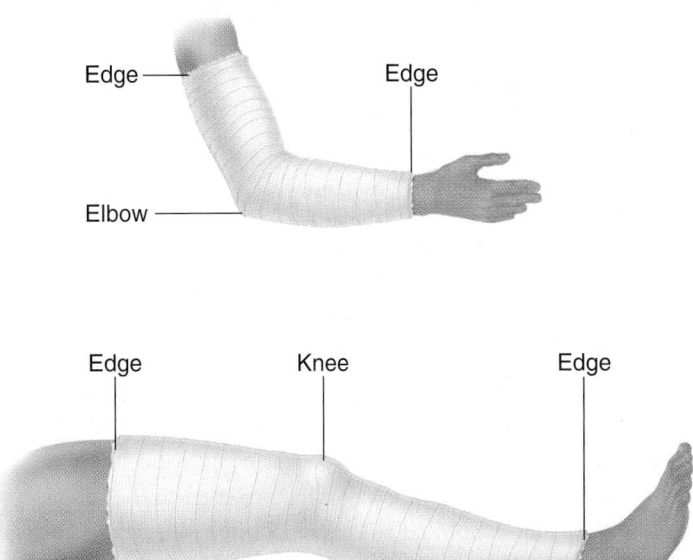

FIGURE 51-28 Check the edges of a cast and report any changes.

customized to the patient's needs and anatomy. To wear this type of assistive leg device, the brace is placed in the patient's shoe, the patient's foot is inserted, and a hook-and-loop strap is used to hold the brace in place. Any orthotic positioned over a bony point must be padded to avoid skin breakdown. Prolonged use of a brace may weaken muscles.

CASTS

Regardless of the type of specialty office that employs you, in your career as a medical assistant, you will encounter patients with casts. Casts are made of plaster, plastic, or fiberglass and are used to hold a bone in place after reduction of a fracture. Casts are applied over a stockinette to protect the skin. Fiberglass and plastic casts dry quickly, while a plaster of Paris cast may take up to 48 hours to dry. Proper cast care and patient assessment are important to avoid further damage to the body part already affected.

Cast Care

Casts are applied for the purpose of immobilizing a broken bone or muscle strain and sprain. A cast may be applied after a surgical procedure on a limb to immobilize the area until healing takes place. Casts are made from a variety of pliable materials that the physician will mold to fit the body part. A cast can be considered to be a form of nonflexible bandage. Casts are generally applied using a wet plaster-type material around a stockinette liner and cotton padding over the limb. As the cast dries, it becomes hard. Newer synthetic fiberglass materials are used to form casts that are lighter in weight than a plaster cast. The medical assistant should use caution when han-

dling fiberglass materials by wearing protective glasses or an eye shield.

The medical assistant may be asked to assist the physician in applying the cast. It may be necessary to hold the limb at the joint areas as the cast is being applied. Remember to handle a damaged limb gently.

After the cast has been applied, it must be left uncovered during the drying process. The limb may need to be supported on a pillow at this time. The patient should be cautioned against moving around until the cast is dry. The cast may become warm or even hot during the drying process. This is normal.

The patient's limb should not become hot or cold once the cast has been applied. Check the edges of the cast and report any changes to the physician (Figure 51-28). The medical assistant should make frequent checks of the patient's circulation. The patient should be instructed to call the physician if any of the following problems are observed:

- Circulation restricted by the cast
- Pain as a result of the cast pinching the skin
- Excessive itching under the cast
- Numbness or tingling of the fingers or toes
- Discolored toes or fingers
- Swelling of the limb around the edge of the cast
- Discoloration soaking through the cast
- Loosely fitting cast
- Foul odor coming from the cast

The physician should advise the patient on the amount of weight and movement that can be safely applied to the cast.

Remind the patient that nothing should be put on the edges of the cast. The cast should not get wet. The patient may be able to tie a strong plastic bag around the cast in order to take a shower.

TRACTION

Traction is a method of pulling or stretching in two directions used to immobilize fractures, correct deformities, and reduce compression of the vertebrae or other musculoskeletal conditions. Skeletal traction, which is performed on inpatients, is applied by the physician to the patient's bone by inserting a pin or wire through the bone. Skin traction is done by the physical therapist by attaching bandages and strips of material to the skin. Weights are then attached to the material, and tension is applied to reduce painful muscle spasm. This type of traction can be set up in a patient's home.

PROSTHESIS

Removal of a limb or part of a limb surgically is known as amputation. Amputations are performed as the result of trauma, bone tumors, severe bone infection, workplace accidents, and disease such as gangrene. Major psychological adjustment is needed to help the patient deal with his or her appearance and limitations on independence. A **prosthesis** is an artificial replacement of a missing body part.

Immediate fitting of a prosthesis involves fitting the patient immediately after the limb is removed, sometimes before leaving the operating room. The benefit of immediate fitting is that the patient is able to begin ambulation the next day. The decision to select a specific type of fitting rests with the physician and must include an assessment of the patient's overall condition, age, and willingness to learn to use the new limb. Many recent improvements in prostheses result in a limb that closely resembles the original and functions efficiently. Prosthetic devices are custom made for the patient, and adjustments may be necessary to ensure a comfortable fit for the patient. In the delayed fitting of a prosthesis, stump conditioning is needed and involves shrinking and shaping the stump before a prosthesis can be fitted. Amputees may feel a phantom pain, which is a normal occurrence for which the cause is unknown. The patient may experience pain in the amputated limb for a short time or, in some cases, for years.

Diagnostic Testing

To determine the presence or full extent of a disabling disease, the physician may order evaluative or diagnostic testing. This may include an examination of the following:

- Muscle strength

- Muscle coordination
- Mobility of joints
- Neuromuscular function
- Circulation and sensory function

Neuromuscular evaluation may include tests, such as electromyography (EMG), nerve conduction studies (NCS), and evoked studies, such as brainstem auditory evoked response (BAER) and somatosensory evoked potentials (SEP), to pick up abnormalities, such as diseases of the peripheral nerves, muscles, and spinal cord.

ELECTROMYOGRAPHY

Electromyography (EMG) consists of using an electromyograph to test the electrical activity of muscles. EMG is most often performed when a patient complains of muscle weakness or numbness. The electromyograph consists of electrodes, an oscilloscope to visually produce the waves of muscle activity, an amplifier, a loudspeaker, an electrical stimulator, and a camera. The patient may receive sedation before this test is conducted since stimulation from the electric current may be painful. The EMG consists of inserting a fine-gauge needle electrode through the skin and into a muscle and then sending a small amount of electric current into the muscle. This procedure permits the physician to examine individual parts of muscles. Abnormal results are found in conditions such as amyotrophic lateral sclerosis (ALS), muscular dystrophy, and peripheral nerve damage.

The electrical activity of the muscle recorded on a graph paper or on film is known as an electromyogram (EMG). This permanent record is then evaluated to determine the adequacy of muscle activity.

A surface electromyogram (SEMG) involves less discomfort for the patient, but the results are less conclusive. In this test, electrodes are attached to the surface of the body to detect electrical activity.

Electrical Stimulation

Electrical stimulation with low-voltage current is helpful to stimulate nerves that supply muscles. An electrical current is applied using disposable gel electrodes. This is a passive means to stimulate muscles when a patient cannot exercise due to injury or disease. This type of stimulation is used to avoid atrophy of muscle tissue.

Transcutaneous electric nerve stimulation (TENS) is another way of using electric stimulation in physical medicine. A TENS unit is attached to the patient in the affected area, and a controlled dose of current is sent to the muscle to help control intractable pain when medication has not been effective. TENS units may be used at home.

EVOKED POTENTIAL STUDIES

Evoked potential studies examine responses within the brain to external stimuli such as light, sound, and touch. These tests are considered noninvasive since no equipment or needle is inserted into the body. Two types of evoked potential studies are these:

- Brainstem auditory evoked response (BAER) is used to assess the auditory nerve pathways. This is useful in diagnosing auditory tumors and lesions.
- Somatosensory evoked peripheral nerves (SEP) are used for diagnosing nerve function defects in peripheral nerves, for example, in the legs.

SUMMARY

Physical therapy involves the use of physical measures, equipment, and body movement to promote mobility and circulation, restore normal function, and relieve pain. The medical assistant, working under the supervision of a physician, is able to teach the patient about proper body mechanics, exercise, and the application of various therapeutic devices such as heat and cold applications. In some cases, the medical assistant will apply these devices.

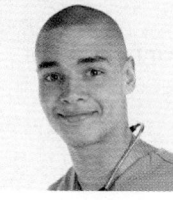

51 CHAPTER REVIEW

COMPETENCY REVIEW

1. Define and spell the terms to learn for this chapter.

2. Instruct a partner on the two-point, three-point, and four-point crutch walking gaits.

3. Create patient education materials for the application of heat and cold applications.

4. Using a partner, demonstrate PROM. Demonstrate AROM yourself.

5. Demonstrate the proper method for wheelchair transfer.

6. Talk to a local physical therapist about a typical day in his or her practice.

7. Describe the following testing methods: electromyography (EMG), nerve conduction studies (NCS), evoked potential studies (EPS), and brainstem auditory evoked response (BAER).

PREPARING FOR THE CERTIFICATION EXAM

1. Which of the following occupations requires a bachelor's or master's degree and internship, licensure in all states, and certification from the AOTA?
   a. speech therapist
   b. occupational therapist
   c. physical therapist
   d. psychologist
   e. respiratory therapist

2. Which of the following is NOT a type of massage?
   a. effleurage
   b. friction
   c. petrissage
   d. tapotement
   e. contracture

3. Which of the following means paralysis of the lower body?
   a. quadriplegia
   b. poliomyelitis
   c. paraplegia
   d. cerebral palsy
   e. muscular dystrophy

4. Which of the following means paralysis of all four extremities of the body?
   a. quadriplegia
   b. poliomyelitis
   c. paraplegia
   d. cerebral palsy
   e. muscular dystrophy

5. Which of the following involves channeling the body's energy and spirit through gentle touch and massage?
   a. effleurage
   b. friction
   c. petrissage
   d. tapotement
   e. Reiki

6. Which of the following can hasten suppuration?
   a. moist heat
   b. moist cold
   c. dry heat
   d. dry cold
   e. ultrasound

7. Which of the following is the bending of the sole of the foot, pointing toes downward?
   a. pronation
   b. rotation
   c. inversion
   d. plantar flexion
   e. dorsiflexion

8. When applying a cold compress, the application should be checked every
   a. 10 to 12 minutes
   b. 12 to 15 minutes
   c. 3 to 5 minutes
   d. 5 to 8 minutes
   e. 8 to 10 minutes

9. Which gait is used by patients who can bear some weight on both feet and have good balance?
   a. four-point gait
   b. three-point gait
   c. two-point gait
   d. swing gait
   e. one-point gait

10. In a hot soak application, the maximum temperature for an adult would be
    a. 41°C
    b. 110°C
    c. 44°C
    d. 54°C
    e. 105°C

CRITICAL THINKING

1. Why is it important that Samra wheel Sylvia to the examination room rather than have Sylvia wheel herself?

2. Sylvia must be transferred from her wheelchair to the examination table before she is seen by Dr. Miller. What are some things that Samra must consider regarding transferring Sylvia, as well as once Sylvia is seated on the table?

3. Dr. Miller is pleased with Sylvia's overall recovery after the stroke; however, he is concerned about her ambulation. He would like Sylvia to be referred to a physical therapist for rehabilitation. What does a physical therapist do and how could this help Sylvia?

ON THE JOB

Jenny Watmore, a medical assistant working in Dr. Cory's orthopedic practice, has been asked to assist Mr. Ivy from the wheelchair onto the examination table. Mr. Ivy, who is 70 years old, is weakened on the left side of his body from a cerebrovascular accident (CVA). He weighs 200 pounds and is reluctant to provide much help to Jenny when she has to transfer him from the wheelchair to the examination table.

1. How can Jenny get Mr. Ivy to help her assist him?
2. Describe the body mechanics that Jenny should use to assist Mr. Ivy.

3. What patient education does Mr. Ivy need?
4. What documentation should Jenny provide on Mr. Ivy's record?

INTERNET ACTIVITY

Select one of the professions listed in Table 51-1. Do an Internet search to discover the duties, the average salary range, where these professionals are usually employed, and the long-term job opportunities of the profession you selected.

MEDMEDIA

Additional interactive resources and activities for this chapter can be found:

On your student DVD: View applicable procedure videos on the DVD-ROM found in the back of this book.

MyHealthProfessionsKit.com: Test your knowledge of this chapter with games and activities. MyHealthProfessionsKit also includes resources, helpful links, and a Spanish audio glossary.

Medical Assisting Interactive: Practice your procedures as a medical assistant in this simulated doctor's office. This can be accessed through MyHealthProfessionsKit.com.

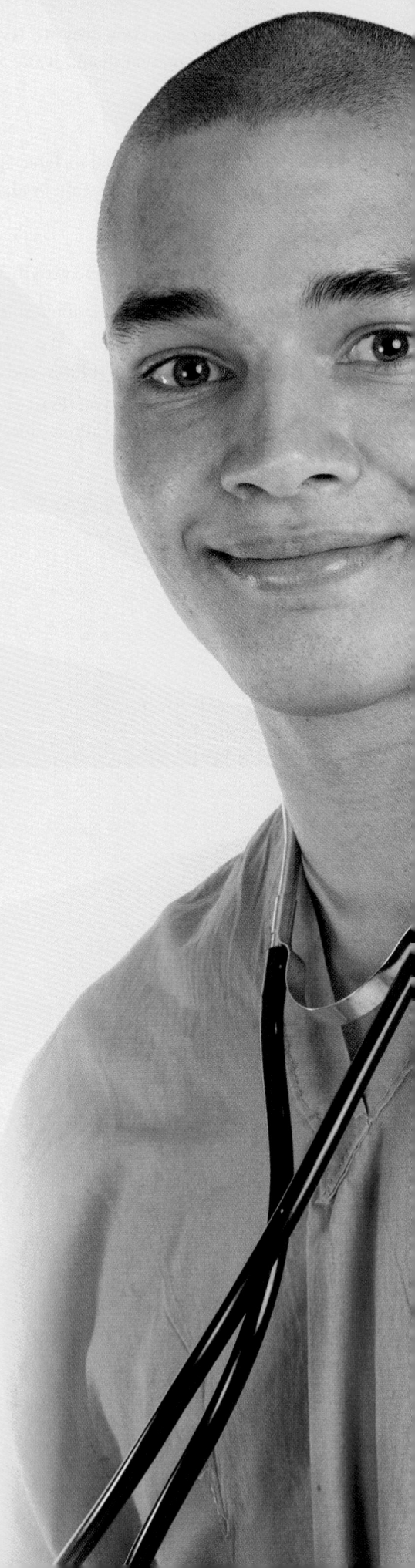

52

Math for Pharmacology

LEARNING OBJECTIVES

After completing this chapter, you should be able to:

- Define and spell the terms to learn for this chapter.

- State the differences between the apothecary and metric systems.

- Identify metric system prefixes and their values.

- Convert dosages between the apothecary and metric systems formula.

- Identify two methods of calculating drug dosages.

- Correctly calculate medication dosages using the mathematical conversions.

- State four rules for calculating pediatric dosages.

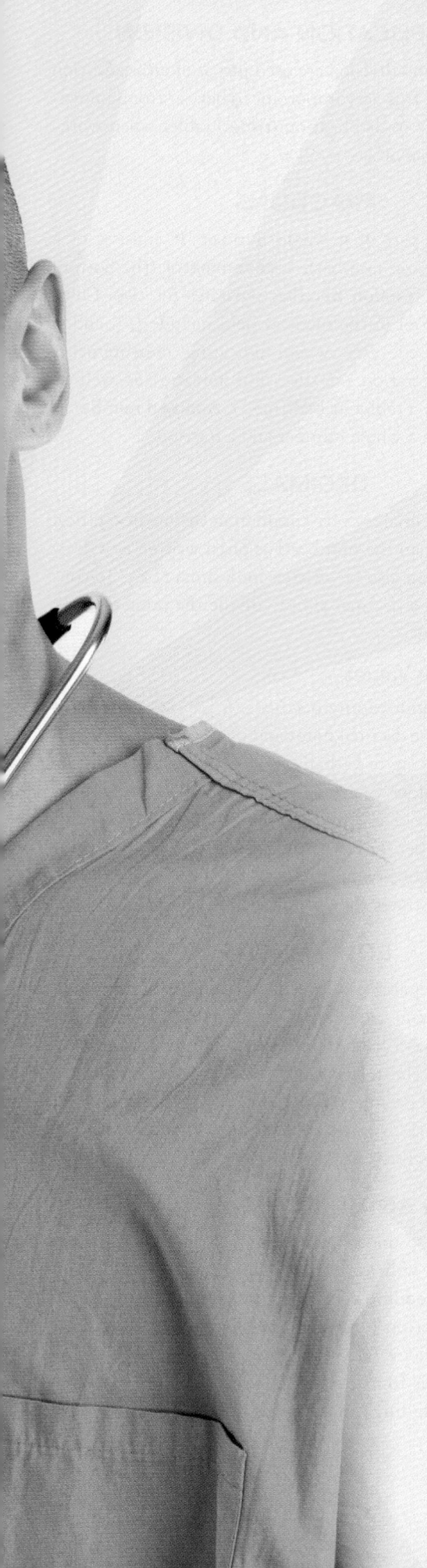

CHAPTER OUTLINE

CASE STUDY

Liu Cheng, a 44-year-old male, is seeing Dr. Salpega because he has had a sore throat and cough that will not go away. He has been sick for the past 2 weeks and says his 4-year-old son Jie is also sick with very similar symptoms. Dr. Salpega diagnoses Mr. Cheng with a severe lower respiratory infection and prescribes 875 milligrams (mg) of Augmentin to be taken twice a day for 10 days. Mr. Cheng asks Dr. Salpega if there is a liquid form of the medication available that he could take because his throat is very sore, and he does not want to swallow pills.

CERTIFICATION LINK

CMA (AAMA)	RMA	CMAS (AMT)
Preparing and administering oral and parenteral medications	Clinical medical assisting	Not applicable
Calculation of dosage	Clinical pharmacology	

It is important to understand correct math calculations and dosing requirements. **Pharmacology** is the study of medications and drugs, including their forms, intentions for use, and effects. A simple error in the calculation of a medication dose can have detrimental effects. An **overdose** (taking too much of a medication) may occur, which could have life-threatening consequences; conversely, an underdose may occur. An **underdose** occurs when not enough medication is given to achieve the desired effect. Over- and underdosing are preventable by proper dosage calculation. General mathematical skills are necessary prior to embarking on dosage calculations.

Mathematics Review

When calculating drug dosages, multiple mathematical calculations are used. These may include addition, subtraction, multiplication, and division. Also, an understanding of fractions, decimals, and ratios is important. Table 52-1 lists reminders and guidelines for many mathematical computations.

ADDITION AND SUBTRACTION

Addition and subtraction are used not only in drug calculation but also in everyday tasks within the medical office. This may include taking inventory as well as collecting payments.

MULTIPLICATION AND DIVISION

Multiplication and division are used just as often as addition and subtraction. It is very important to have a strong knowledge of the basic multiplication (times) tables when working in the medical office.

FRACTIONS

A fraction is a part of a whole number. It consists of a **numerator** (the top number), a **denominator** (the bottom number), and a **fraction bar** that separates the two. Common fractions used in the medical field include $\frac{1}{2}$, $\frac{1}{3}$, and $\frac{1}{4}$. Fractions are used often when indicating measurements (e.g., $\frac{1}{4}$-inch laceration on the right forearm) as well as dosages ("Take $\frac{1}{2}$ a tablet at bedtime."). A **mixed number** is made up of both a whole number and a fraction.

DECIMALS

The usage of decimals is very common in the medical office. Anything less than the number 1 is often written as a decimal. Fractions can also be written in decimal form. To convert fractions to a decimal simply divide the numerator by the denominator.

Decimal Place Values

When writing and reading decimals, it is necessary to correctly identify the decimal point and place value of the number. When speaking or verbalizing decimal values, state the decimal placeholder where the last digit falls. The number 0.9 would be read as "nine-tenths" and not "zero point nine." The number 0.32 would be read as "thirty-two hundredths," and 0.005 would be read as "five thousandths." (Table 52-2 illustrates the decimal point place values.)

EQUIVALENTS

A ratio is a comparison between two numbers. Ratios and their role in dosage calculations are discussed later in this chapter. Table 52-3 lists examples of mathematical equivalents to review the relationship between fractions, ratios, percentages, and decimals. For example, $\frac{1}{2}$ is the same as 0.5 and the ratio of 1:2. A ratio and a decimal are different ways of expressing the fraction $\frac{1}{2}$.

LEADING AND TRAILING ZERO RULES

It is important to understand the placement of a zero in a decimal. When writing decimal number less than 1, you must apply the **leading zero rule**: for example, if you were to write a prescription for a medication that calls for a half teaspoon of medicine you would write 0.5 tsp (*not* .5 tsp). As important as it is to utilize the leading zero rule, you must also follow the trailing zero rule. The **trailing zero rule** states

TABLE 52-1 Mathematical Rules and Guidelines

Function	Rules	Example
Adding and subtracting fractions	• When adding and subtracting fractions, you must have a common denominator. • Remember to multiply the entire fraction by the correct multiplier necessary to obtain the common denominator. • Add the numerators, while the denominator remains the same. • Reduce the final answer to its simplest terms.	$1/8 + 1/3 =$ Common denominator = 24 **Steps:** 1. $\dfrac{1}{8} \times \dfrac{3}{3} + \dfrac{1}{3} \times \dfrac{8}{8} =$ 2. $\dfrac{3}{24} + \dfrac{8}{24} =$ 3. $\dfrac{11}{24}$ $3/5 - 1/15 =$ Common denominator = 15 **Steps:** 1. $\dfrac{3}{5} \times \dfrac{3}{3} - \dfrac{1}{15} =$ 2. $\dfrac{9}{15} - \dfrac{1}{15} =$ 3. $\dfrac{8}{15}$
Multiplying fractions	• If a numerator and a denominator have a common divisor, you may cancel out those terms. • Multiply all numerators across. • Multiply all denominators across. • Reduce the final answer to its simplest terms.	$3/5 \times 10/18 =$ **Steps:** 1. $\dfrac{^{(1)}3}{^{(1)}5} \times \dfrac{10^{(2)}}{18_{(6)}} =$ 2. $\dfrac{1}{1} \times \dfrac{2}{6} =$ 3. $\dfrac{2}{6}$ 4. $\dfrac{1}{3}$
Dividing fractions	• Invert the second fraction of the equation, finding its reciprocal. • Multiply the numerators of the first fraction and the reciprocal. • Multiply the denominators of the first fraction and the reciprocal. • Reduce the final answer to its simplest terms.	$2/3 \div 1/5 =$ **Steps:** 1. $\dfrac{2}{3} \times \dfrac{5}{1} =$ 2. $\dfrac{10}{3}$ $3\overline{)10}$ with quotient $3\frac{1}{3}$, $\dfrac{9}{1}$ 3. $3\frac{1}{3}$
Convert an improper fraction to a mixed number	• An improper fraction is any fraction with a numerator larger than a denominator. • Divide the numerator by the denominator. This becomes the whole number. • The remainder (if any) is then placed over the denominator to form the fractional component of the mixed number. • Reduce the fractional component to its simplest form.	$14/6 =$ **Steps:** 1. $\dfrac{14}{6}$ 2. $6\overline{)14}$ with quotient $2\frac{2}{6}$, $\dfrac{12}{2}$ 3. $2\frac{2}{6}$ 4. $2\frac{1}{3}$

(continued)

TABLE 52-1 (*continued*)

Function	Rules	Example
Convert a fraction to a decimal	• Divide the numerator by the denominator	2/3 = **Steps:** 2 ÷ 3 = 0.67

Adding and subtracting decimals	• Always line up the decimals of every number.
	 • Add zero (0) placeholders to help keep numbers aligned.
		1.9 + 0.33 + 12.344 =
		 Steps:
		    1.900
		    0.330
		 + 12.344
		   14.574

Multiplying decimals	• Multiply the numbers as normal.
	 • Place zero (0) placeholders as needed.
	 • Count the total number of decimal spaces to the right of the decimal point for both numbers.
	 • Place your decimal point with this many numbers to the right of the decimal.
		12.14 × 8.2 =
		 Steps:
		 1. 12.14
		   × 8.2
		    2428
		   97120
		   99548
		 2. 99.548 (Decimal point is placed three spaces in from the right, because there are three decimal placeholders in the original equation.)

Dividing decimals	• If it is not a whole number, move the decimal point of the divisor the necessary number of spaces to make the divisor a whole number. • If the dividend has a decimal, move it to the right the same number of places as you moved the divisor's decimal point. • Add zero (0) placeholders as necessary. • Divide as usual, and then move the decimal directly up in the quotient.	32.4 ÷ 8.5 = **Steps:**
Convert a decimal to a fraction	• Simply place the entire number over the value of the decimal placeholder of the last digit of the number. • Remember to reduce the final answer to its simplest terms.	Convert 0.75 to a fraction. **Steps:** 75/100 • Note that the 5 is located in the hundredths placeholder, thus 75 is placed over 100.

TABLE 52-2 Decimal Point Place Values

Ones	Decimal Point	Tenths	Hundredths	Thousandths	Hundred Thousandths
1	.	0.1	0.01	0.001	0.0001

TABLE 52-3 Examples of Mathematical Equivalents

Fraction	Ratio	Percentage	Decimal
1/4	1:4	25 percent	0.25
1/2	1:2	50 percent	0.50
2/3	2:3	66 percent	0.66
3/4	3:4	75 percent	0.75
7/8	7:8	88 percent	0.88
1/100	1:100	1 percent	0.01
1/200	1:200	0.5 percent	0.005
1/1000	1:100	0.1 percent	0.001

that it is never appropriate to include a zero after a whole number: for example, if a patient were to take 5 milligrams of a medication, you would write 5 mg (*not* 5.0 mg).

These rules have been devised and utilized to reduce the amount of errors in medicine. Too often, a number has been misread because of the placement or lack of a zero. Always remembering and following these rules can help reduce the number of medical errors—and possibly save the lives of patients.

Weights and Measures

Two separate sets of weights and measures are used to calculate medication doses: the apothecary system and the metric system. Generally, most physicians and facilities have moved to the metric system, but the medical assistant must be familiar with both systems because occasionally medications do appear in the apothecary system. Another aspect to remember is that common household measurements, such as teaspoon and tablespoon, do appear, although they are not formal medication measurement units. Most commonly, the household measurements are used in patient education.

APOTHECARY SYSTEM

The **apothecary system** is considered to be the oldest system of measurement. The dry weight measurement was based on the grain (gr). One grain was equal to the weight of 1 grain of wheat. In addition to the grain (gr), the other basic units of dry weight measurement within the apothecary system include the dram (dr, ʒ), the ounce (oz, ℥), and the pound (lb). Fluid measurements include the minims (m), fluid dram (fl dr, flʒ), fluid ounce (fl oz flℨ), pint (pt), quart (qt), and gallon (gal). Such common household measurements as the ounce, pint, quart, and gallon are based on the apothecary system.

Roman numerals are used when numbering in the apothecary system. For example, 3 grains would be gr iii.

Fractions are also used. Three-fourths of a grain would be gr $\frac{3}{4}$. It is important to note that the unit of measure in the apothecary system is placed before the actual number.

To accurately write an apothecary notation the following rules should be applied:

1. The unit or abbreviation comes before the amount.

    Example: qt iii, rather than iii qt

2. Use lowercase Roman numerals to express whole numbers 1 through 10, 15, 20, and 30.

3. Use Arabic numbers for other quantities.

    Example: qt i (1 quart), gr 12 (12 grains), and gr xx (20 grains)

4. Use fractions to designate amounts less than 1.

    Example: gr $\frac{1}{2}$, not 0.50 gr

5. The symbol *ss* is used to designate the fraction $\frac{1}{2}$.

    Example: pt iiiss ($3\frac{1}{2}$ pints)

When interpreting a drug order or reading a drug label, it is helpful to know the common Roman numerals and their Arabic equivalents (Table 52-4).

METRIC SYSTEM

The **metric system** is the most commonly used conversion system for dosage calculations. The following list includes the metric system prefixes and their values:

- kilo = 1000 of a unit
- hecto = 100 of a unit
- deka = 10 of a unit
- base unit of 1

TABLE 52-4 Arabic Numbers, Roman Numerals, and Apothecary Notations

Arabic Number	Roman Numeral	Apothecary Notation	Arabic Number	Roman Numeral	Apothecary Notation
1	I	i, $\bar{\text{i}}$	8	VIII	viii, $\overline{\text{viii}}$
2	II	ii, $\bar{\text{ii}}$	9	IX	ix, $\overline{\text{ix}}$
3	III	iii, $\overline{\text{iii}}$	10	X	x, $\bar{\text{x}}$
4	IV	iv, $\overline{\text{iv}}$	15	XV	xv, $\overline{\text{xv}}$
5	V	v, $\bar{\text{v}}$	20	XX	xx, $\overline{\text{xx}}$
6	VI	vi, $\overline{\text{vi}}$	25	XXV	xxv, $\overline{\text{xxv}}$
7	VII	vii, $\overline{\text{vii}}$	30	XXX	xxx, $\overline{\text{xxx}}$

- deci = 0.1 of a unit
- centi = 0.01 of a unit
- milli = 0.001 of a unit
- micro = 0.00001 of a unit

Metric conversions are simply accomplished by multiplying or dividing by 1000. Multiplying by 1000 would be the same as moving the decimal point three places to the right. Dividing by 1000 would mean that the decimal point moves three places to the left. For further explanation, review the following example:

Convert: 3.5 g to mg

Equivalent: 1 g = 1000 mg. Conversion factor is 1000.

Multiply by 1000: 3.5 g = 3.5 × 1000 = 3500 mg

Or move the decimal point three places to the right: 3.5 g = 3.500 = 3500 mg

Another method is to move the decimal point along the place value chart, either to the right or to the left, depending on the conversion factor. Refer to Figure 52-1 for further review and examples.

Kilo-	Hecto-	Deka-	Numeral w/ base unit (g, l, or m)	Deci-	Centi-	Milli-	Micro-

Example:

Convert 45.2 grams (g) to milligrams (mg).

1. Place 45.2 under the numeral/base unit

Kilo-	Hecto-	Deka-	Numeral w/ base unit (g, l, or m)	Deci-	Centi-	Milli-	Micro-
			45.2				

2. Move the decimal point to the right three times so that the base unit ends in the milli- box:

Kilo-	Hecto-	Deka-	Numeral w/ base unit (g, l, or m)	Deci-	Centi-	Milli-	Micro-
			45.2	452.0	4520.0	45200.0	

3. 45.2g = 45,200 mg

FIGURE 52-1 Metric conversion using the place value chart.

TABLE 52-5 Common Abbreviations for Weights and Measures

Apothecary System		Metric System	Apothecary System		Metric System
Symbol/Abbreviations		**Meaning**	**Symbol/Abbreviations Weights**		**Meaning**
gtt	drop	drop	kg		kilogram
ℳ	min	minim	gm		gram
	dr, ʒ	dram	mg		milligram
	fl dr, flʒ	fluid dram	mcg		microgram
	oz, ℥	ounce	**Symbol/Abbreviations Volume**		**Meaning**
	fl oz, fl℥	fluid ounce	L		liter
O	pt	pint	mL		milliliter
C	gal	gallon	cc		cubic centimeter
	gr	grain			

The common units of measure are the liter (volume), the gram (weight), and the meter (length). Table 52-5 lists common abbreviations for weights and measures. (See Guildelines 52-1 for conversion within the metric system).

Metric System Dosages

In the metric system, the dosage is written as a decimal number first, with the unit of measurement following (2.5 mg). Equivalents are demonstrated in Table 52-6. Common

---

TABLE 52-6 Commonly Used Equivalents for the Apothecary and Metric Systems

Measure Apothecary	Equivalent Metric
1 gr	65 mg or 0.065 g
5 gr	325 mg or 0.33 g
10 gr	650 mg or 0.67 g
15 or 16 gr	1 g
15 or 16 m	1 mL or cc
1 dram	4 mL
1 oz	30 cc, 30 mL, 8 tsp, 8 drams, 2 tbsp
1 lb	450 g
1 lb	0.4536 kg
1 minim (ℳ)	0.06 mL
4 m	0.25 mL
Liquid Measure	
1 fl dr	4 mL
2 fl dr	8 mL
2.5 fl dr	10 mL
4 fl dr	15 mL
1 fl oz	30 mL
3.5 fl oz	100 mL
7 fl oz	200 mL
1 pt	500 mL
1 qt	1000 mL
60 gtts	4 mL

GUIDELINES 52-1

CONVERSION WITHIN THE METRIC SYSTEM

1. No change is required to change milliliters into cubic centimeters because they are equal to each other.
2. To change grams to milligrams, multiply grams by 1000 or move the decimal point three places to the RIGHT.
3. To change milligrams to grams, divide milligrams by 1000 or move the decimal point three places to the LEFT.
4. To convert liters to milliliters, multiply liters by 1000 or move the decimal point three places to the RIGHT.
5. To convert milliliters to liters, divide milliliters by 1000 or move the decimal point three places to the LEFT.

TABLE 52-7 Common Household Measures

Measure	Equivalent
60 gtts (drops)	1 teaspoon (tsp)
3 tsp	1 tablespoon (T)
2 T	1 oz
4 oz	1 small juice glass
8 oz	1 cup or glass
16 T or 8 oz	1 cup
2 cups	1 pint (pt)
2 pints	1 quart (qt)
4 quarts	1 gallon

household measures are presented in Table 52-7, and the comparisons of the three systems for liquid measurements are in Table 52-8.

Drug Calculations

Stock medications are frequently kept in offices for use in the office. However, the stock medications may be a different dosage than the physician's order. Therefore, it is important to understand basic drug calculations to ensure that the correct dose of medication is given. Sometimes, a conversion chart is given, but it is important to double-check and ensure that the dose is correct.

Many factors are involved in calculating the correct dose of a drug, including the patient's age, weight, and current state of health. Another important factor to note is the other medications that the patient is currently taking because they may strengthen or weaken the effects of the new drug.

The first step in the drug calculation is to ensure that the system of weights and measures in the prescription is the

TABLE 52-8 Comparison of Household, Apothecary, and Metric Liquid Measurements

Household	Apothecary	Metric
1 drop	1 minim (♍)	0.06 mL
1 tsp	1 fl dr (fl ʒ)	4–5 mL
1 T	4 fl dr (fl ʒ)	15–16 mL
2 T	1 fl oz (fl ℥)	30–32 mL
1 cup or glass	8 fl oz (fl ℥)	250 mL
2 cups or glasses	16 fl oz, 1 pt	500 mL
4 cups or glasses	1 qt	1000 mL = approximately 1 liter

same as in the container of stock medication. If they are different, the first step will be to covert them to the same system (use Table 52-5 and Table 52-6).

Two methods of drug calculations are explained in this chapter: the ratio method and the formula method. It is important to understand both and then apply the method that seems easiest for you.

RATIO METHOD

Ratios are one method of calculating drug dosages. A **ratio** establishes a relationship between two quantities. The medical assistant would compare the amount of drug ordered to the amount on hand. When there are two ratios to compare, then it is a **proportion**. A proportion resulting from the fraction $\frac{1}{2}$ or ratio could be $10/20 = \frac{1}{2}$ or 10:20::1:2. The proportion is read as 10 divided by 20 equals 1 divided by 2, or 10 is to 20 as 1 is to 2. Even though the numbers are bigger (10 instead of 1), the proportion is exactly the same—the first number is half the size of the second. If you know three of the four numbers for the two ratios, you can solve for the fourth by using mathematical principles. The symbol x is used for the unknown quantity: for example, $10/20 = 1/x$.

To find the unknown quantity, cross-multiply. This means to multiply the top number on the left side of the $=$ sign by the bottom number on the right side, and the bottom number on the left is multiplied by the top number on the right. Then, divide both sides by the number with the x: for example, $10x \div 10 = 1x$ or x and $20 \div 10 = 2$.

This means that $x = 2$.

$$\frac{10}{20} = \frac{1}{x} = 10 \times x = 20 \times 1$$
$$10x = 20$$
$$\frac{10x}{10} = \frac{20}{10}$$
$$1x = 2$$
$$x = 2$$

Another method is to convert $10/20 = 1/x$ into the ratio we saw earlier of $10:20::1:x$. Then, multiply the extremes (the two outer numbers—the 10 and the x) by each other and the means (the two inner numbers—20 and 1) to solve for x, the unknown.

$$10:20::1:x$$
$$10 \times x = 20 \times 1$$
$$10x = 20$$
$$x = 20 \div 10$$
$$x = 2$$

To prove this answer is correct, multiply the extremes and multiply the means. If the answer is correct, they will be equal.

$$\text{So} \ldots 10:20::1:2$$
$$10 \times 2 = 20 \times 1$$
$$20 = 20 \text{— so the answer is correct}$$

Problem: There is a physician order to give 80 mg of Lasix (furosemide). The supply on hand states that there are 40 mg/mL.

There are 40 mg in 1 mL of Lasix. (This is the strength of the medicine.) The problem requires figuring how many mL of Lasix are required to get 80 mg.

$$80\,\text{mg}:x\,\text{mL}::40\,\text{mg}:1\,\text{mL}$$
$$80 \times 1 = 40 \times x$$
$$80 = 40x$$
$$x = 2\,\text{mL}$$

So, 2 mL of Lasix are required to get 80 mg.

Problem: A physician has ordered 60 mg of Prilosec. The supply on hand states 40 mg/capsule.

$$60\,\text{mg}: x\,\text{capsules} :: 40\,\text{mg}: 1\,\text{capsule}$$
$$60 \times 1 = 40 \times x$$
$$60 = 40x$$
$$\frac{60}{40} = \frac{40x}{40}$$
$$1.5 = x$$

So, $1\frac{1}{2}$ capsules are required for the 60 mg dose.

FORMULA METHOD

It is possible to calculate dosages easily using a formula. To determine the amount of the drug needed, set up the following formula:

Calculation formula:

$$\frac{\text{Available strength}}{\text{Ordered strength}} = \frac{\text{available amount}}{\text{amount to give}}$$

Available strength is the strength of the drug in stock. The available amount is the amount of drug in the container. The ordered strength is the physician's order, and the amount to give is the unknown quantity (the x).

For example, the physician order is to give 500 mg of a drug, and an available vial contains 1000 mg/mL.

Calculation formula:

$$\frac{\text{Available strength}}{\text{Ordered strength}} = \frac{\text{available amount}}{\text{amount to give}}$$
$$\text{Strength of the drug in the vial} = 1000\,\text{mg/mL}$$
$$\text{Available amount} = 1\,\text{mL}$$
$$\text{Ordered strength} = 500\,\text{mg}$$
$$\text{Amount to give} = x$$
$$\frac{1000\,\text{mg}}{500\,\text{mg}} = \frac{1\,\text{mL}}{x}$$
$$1000 \times x = 500 \times 1$$
$$1000x = 500$$
$$\frac{1000x}{1000} = \frac{500}{1000}$$
$$1x = 5/10 = \tfrac{1}{2}\,\text{mL} = 0.5\,\text{mL}$$

You would fill the syringe with 0.5 mL of liquid to give you the physician's order of 500 mg of medication.

To solve a problem using other forms of medications, such as tablets, use the same formula:

Physician's order: Give 10 grains of medication.

Available: Tablets containing 2.5 grains each

Calculation formula:

$$\frac{\text{Available strength}}{\text{Ordered strength}} = \frac{\text{available amount}}{\text{amount to give}}$$
$$2.5\,\text{gr} = 1\,\text{tablet}$$

$$10 \, gr \, x \, (\text{number of tablets})$$

$$2.5 \times x = 10 \times 1$$

$$2.5x = 10$$

$$\frac{2.5x}{2.5} = \frac{10}{2.5}$$

$$1x = 4 \, \text{tablets}$$

Problem: Physician's order: Give 60 mg of furosemide.

Available: Tablets containing 40 mg each

Calculation formula:

$$\frac{40}{60} = \frac{1}{x}$$

$$40 \times x = 60 \times 1$$

$$40x = 60$$

$$\frac{40x}{40} = \frac{60}{40}$$

$$1x = 1.5 \, \text{tablets}$$

Another formula that is frequently used is $D/H \times Q$, where

D = desired or ordered dose

H = supply on hand or available supply

Q = quantity available

Problem: The physician ordered penicillin 250 mg. The bottle from the supply cabinet is labeled "Penicillin 500 mg per mL."

Solution: Set up the formula.

$$\frac{\text{Desired}}{\text{Hand}} \times \text{Quantity}$$

The physician's order is placed in the Desired (D) space and the supply you have on hand is placed in the Hand (H) space. The quantity per mL is placed in the Quantity (Q) space:

$$\frac{D}{H} \times Q = \frac{250}{500} \times 1$$

$$\text{Divide 250 by } 500 \times \frac{1}{1} = 0.5 \, \text{mL}$$

The answer is 0.5 mL.

Problem: The physician orders Atorvastatin 70 mcg. The bottle from the supply cabinet is labeled "Atorvastatin 20 mg tablets."

Solution: Set up the formula

$$\frac{\text{Desired}}{\text{Hand}} \times \text{Quantity}$$

The physician's order is placed in the Desired (D) space, and the supply you have on hand is placed in the Hand (H)

space. The quantity per mL is placed in the Quantity (Q) space:

$$\frac{D}{H} \times Q = \frac{70}{20} \times 1$$

$$\text{Divide 70 by } 20 \times 1 = 3.5 \text{ or } 3\tfrac{1}{2} \, \text{tablets}$$

Rules for Conversion

When converting from one system to another, it is important to remember that the equivalents may be only approximate, especially when using conversion tables such as the one in Table 52-9. This table, however, should be learned because the equivalents are very helpful when converting from one measuring system to another. See Guidelines 52-2 for tips on converting from one system to another.

TABLE 52-9 Conversion List

Apothecary	Metric
15 or 16 minims (m)	1 mL or 1 cc
1 fluid dr	4 mL or cc
1 fluid oz	30 mL or cc
1 quart	1000 mL or cc
1/60 grain	1 milligram (mg)
1 grain	0.065 gram
15 grains	1 gram
2.2 pounds	1 kilogram

CONVERSION TIPS

1. To change grains to grams, divide by 15.
2. To change ounces to cubic centimeters (cc) or milliliters (mL), multiply by 30.
3. To change grains to milligrams (mg), multiply by 60. (Use this rule only when you have less than 1 grain.)
4. To change kilograms to pounds, multiply by 2.2.
5. To change cubic centimeters (cc) or milliliters (mL) to ounces, divide by 30.
6. To change drams to milliliters (mL), multiply by 4.
7. To change cubic centimeters (cc) or milliliters (mL) to minims, multiply by 15 or 16.
8. To change minims to cubic centimeters (cc) or milliliters (mL), divide by 15 or 16.
9. To convert drams to grams, multiply by 4.

Calculating Pediatric Dosages

Pediatric medications and their dosages are different from those for adults. Sometimes, those medications used for adults must be calculated for use in children. It is imperative that the calculations be exact when administering medications to a child. Oftentimes, the physician takes the responsibility for this task, but the medical assistant may be asked to assist or to double-check the dosage.

There are several rules or "laws" for the calculations of medications for pediatrics, including Clark's rule, Fried's law, Young's law, West's nomogram, and the body by weight method. Each of these approaches is named for the individual who developed the rule.

CLARK'S RULE

Clark's rule is based on the weight of the child. This is the most common law used in the calculation of drug dosage for children, especially since the weight of different children at the same age can vary significantly. The formula for Clark's rule is

$$\text{Pediatric dose} = \frac{\text{child's weight in pounds}}{150 \text{ pounds}} \times \text{adult dose}$$

This rule is followed by dividing the child's weight by 150 pounds and then multiplying that number by the adult dose.

Problem: Penicillin is ordered for a 3-year-old child weighing 35 pounds. The average dose for an adult is 360 mg. How many mg will the child receive?

$$35/150 \times 360 \text{ mg} = 83.9 \text{ mg}$$

FRIED'S LAW

Fried's law is applied to children under the age of 1 year. Fried's assumption is that a $12\frac{1}{2}$-year-old child could take an adult dose, and a fraction of that is taken to figure dosages on a young child. This is the formula:

$$\text{Pediatric dose} = \frac{\text{child's age in months}}{150 \text{ months}} \times \text{adult dose}$$

This formula uses 150 months in the denominator as the equivalent for $12\frac{1}{2}$ years.

Problem: Augmentin is ordered for an 8-month-old child. The average dose for an adult is 500 mg. How many mg will the child receive?

$$8/150 \times 500 = 26.7 \text{ mg}$$

YOUNG'S RULE

Young's rule is used for children who are over 1 year of age. The formula used for Young's rule is this:

$$\text{Pediatric dose} = \frac{\text{child's age in years}}{\text{child's age in years} + 12} \times \text{adult dose}$$

To use this formula, divide the child's age in years by the same number plus 12. Multiply this number by the adult dose to determine the correct pediatric dosage.

Problem: Benadryl is ordered for a 6-year-old child. The average dose for an adult is 50 mg. How many mg will the child receive?

$$6/18 \times 50 = 16.7 \text{ mg}$$

PROFESSIONALISM
THE LIFE SPAN

The dosing of medication for the elderly requires careful calculations. Older adults have reduced kidney and liver function, in addition to the additional complication of polypharmacy—the use of many prescribed medications for many purposes. These factors can cause an increase in adverse effects of the drugs. It is especially important to ensure that individuals on multiple medications have their medications regularly reviewed by the primary care physician and specialists, with emphasis on any complaints that the patient may have. The medical assistant should instruct patients to bring their medications in their original containers to every visit so that the medications can be properly reviewed.

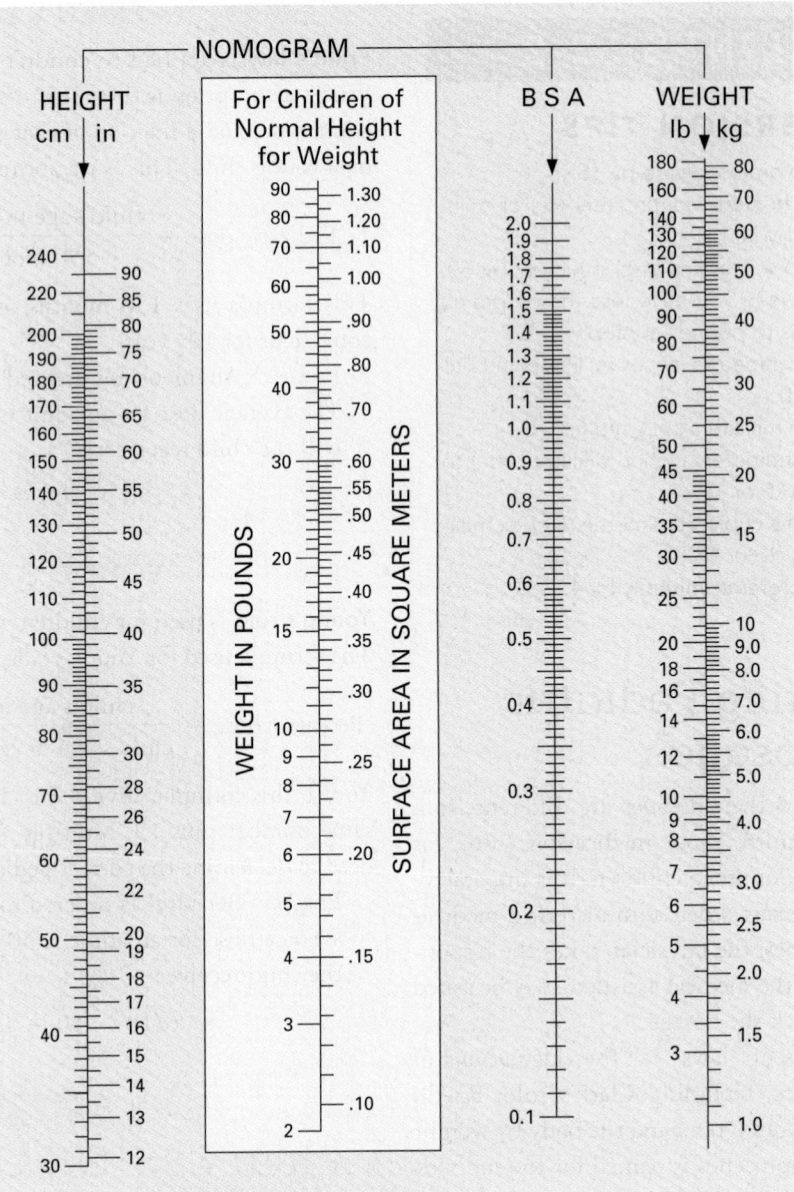

NOMOGRAM

| HEIGHT | For Children of | B S A | WEIGHT |
| cm \| in | Normal Height for Weight | | lb \| kg |

FIGURE 52-2 Nomogram chart.

WEST'S NOMOGRAM

The two methods most commonly used for calculating pediatric dosages are body surface area (BSA) which utilizes West's nomogram, and body weight, which determines the amount of medication to be administered based on the child's weight. **West's nomogram** is the preferred method, particularly for oncology and critical care patients and underweight children. It can be used for both infants and children. The chart is frequently found in pediatric offices, medical textbooks, and dictionaries. It is preferable to other forms of pediatric dosage calculations because it takes into consideration the child's **body surface area (BSA)**, which is based on a calculation of the child's height and weight, and is expressed as m² (meters squared). The chart has three columns (Figure 52-2). To calculate the child's BSA, a straight line is drawn from the patient's height in inches or centimeters across the columns to the patient's weight in kilograms or pounds. The straight line will intersect on the BSA column. This point will give the BSA average. Once a BSA average is calculated, it is applied to the following formula:

$$\text{Pediatric dose} = \frac{\text{BSA of child}}{1.73 \text{ square meters}} \times \text{adult dose}$$

1.73 meters is the standard adult BSA.

BODY WEIGHT METHOD

The body weight method is the other method that is commonly seen in pediatric situations. Medication dosages are often ordered by the body weight method. The body weight method uses calculations based on the patient's weight in kilograms. This requires converting the patient's weight into kilograms. The following provides an example of how this is achieved.

Example: Convert 77 lb to kg.

Approximate equivalent: 1 kg = 2.2 lb

Conversion factor is 2.2

77 lb = 77 divided by 2.2 = 35 kg

Once the child's weight has been converted into kilograms, the correct dosage can be calculated. This is done by calculating the safe drug dosage in mg/kg (as recommended by a reputable drug reference) and then multiplying that amount by the child's weight in kg.

SUMMARY

The medical assistant must be able to calculate dosages correctly since any error has the potential to be fatal to the patient. A general knowledge of mathematical skills is vital for dosage calculations. Always double-check all dosages and, if possible, have someone else double-check your calculations.

Have a copy of the conversion factors in an accessible location to make conversions quickly and accurately. Frequent calculations will keep the medical assistant proficient at medication calculations.

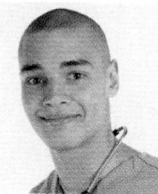

52 CHAPTER REVIEW

COMPETENCY REVIEW

1. Define and spell the terms to learn for this chapter.

2. What are the four rules for pediatric dosage calculations?

3. What is the metric system?

4. What is the apothecary system?

5. What are the calculation formulas for calculating dosages?

PREPARING FOR THE CERTIFICATION EXAM

1. In liquid measures, 1 fluid ounce is equal to
   a. 1 mL
   b. 10 mL
   c. 30 mL
   d. 100 cc
   e. 30 cc

2. With regard to medication, available strength refers to
   a. what actually contains the medication
   b. the potency of the medication in stock
   c. the potency the physician has ordered
   d. the amount of medication that should be administered
   e. the calculated strength

3. According to the rules for converting from one system of measurement to another, to change
   a. grains to milligrams, multiply by 60
   b. grains to grams, multiply by 15
   c. cc to ounces, divide by 50
   d. cc to mL, divide by 15
   e. drams to grams, multiply by 2

4. What is the preferred method of most physicians for calculating pediatric dosages?
   a. Young's rule
   b. Fried's rule
   c. West's nomogram
   d. Clark's rule
   e. body weight

5. Tablets and capsules are measured in metric units of
   a. milligrams
   b. millimeters
   c. cubic centimeters
   d. ounces
   e. grains

6. Sometimes the available dosage of a medication on hand is not the same as that which the physician has ordered. The medical assistant must determine how much of the medication should be used. In the equation used for this calculation, the needed dosage is indicated by
   a. the numerator
   b. the denominator
   c. a whole number
   d. both the numerator and the denominator
   e. numbers less than 10

7. Which of the following choices is NOT a formula used to calculate a dosage of a medication?
   a. West's nomogram
   b. Clark's rule
   c. Young's rule
   d. Fried's law
   e. Blalock-Taussig Law

8. Which of the two following measurements are equal to each other?
   a. milligrams to grams
   b. liters to milliliters
   c. milliliters to grams
   d. milliliters to cubic centimeters
   e. milliliters to liters

9. When converting a larger unit to a smaller unit, you
   a. divide
   b. multiply
   c. subtract
   d. add
   e. measure

10. Which of the following formulas is used to calculate a pediatric dose based on the child's weight in pounds?
   a. Young's rule
   b. Clark's rule
   c. Fried's law
   d. West's nomogram
   e. body weight

CRITICAL THINKING

1. Dr. Salpega informs Mr. Cheng that a liquid form of Augmentin is available. Augmentin is available in an oral suspension (liquid medication) of 250 mg/5 mL. How many mL will Mr. Cheng have to take each time he takes his medication?

2. How many ounces of liquid would this be? (Refer to tables and guidelines in the chapter for conversion amounts.)

3. Using Clark's rule, calculate the Augmentin dosage Dr. Salpega may prescribe for Mr. Cheng's 42-pound son, Jie. Keep in mind that the average adult dose of Augmentin is 500 mg.

ON THE JOB

In the past Mrs. Kennedy has been prescribed Protonix 20 mg a day. Cindy, the medical assistant at Dr. Jones's office, has just spoken to the patient. Mrs. Kennedy tells Cindy that her abdominal pain has increased. After Cindy speaks with the physician on call, the physician increases the dosage to 40 mg once a day. The physician indicates that the patient should take the medication for 2 weeks to see if any further relief can be achieved. Mrs. Kennedy will be stopping by the office to pick up some samples this afternoon. How will Cindy instruct Mrs. Kennedy and document in the patient chart the change in dose?

INTERNET ACTIVITY

Conduct an Internet search for medical assistant pharmacology.

MEDMEDIA

Additional interactive resources and activities for this chapter can be found:

On your student DVD: View applicable procedure videos on the DVD-ROM found in the back of this book.

MyHealthProfessionsKit.com: Test your knowledge of this chapter with games and activities. MyHealthProfessionsKit also includes resources, helpful links, and a Spanish audio glossary.

Medical Assisting Interactive: Practice your procedures as a medical assistant in this simulated doctor's office. This can be accessed through MyHealthProfessionsKit.com.

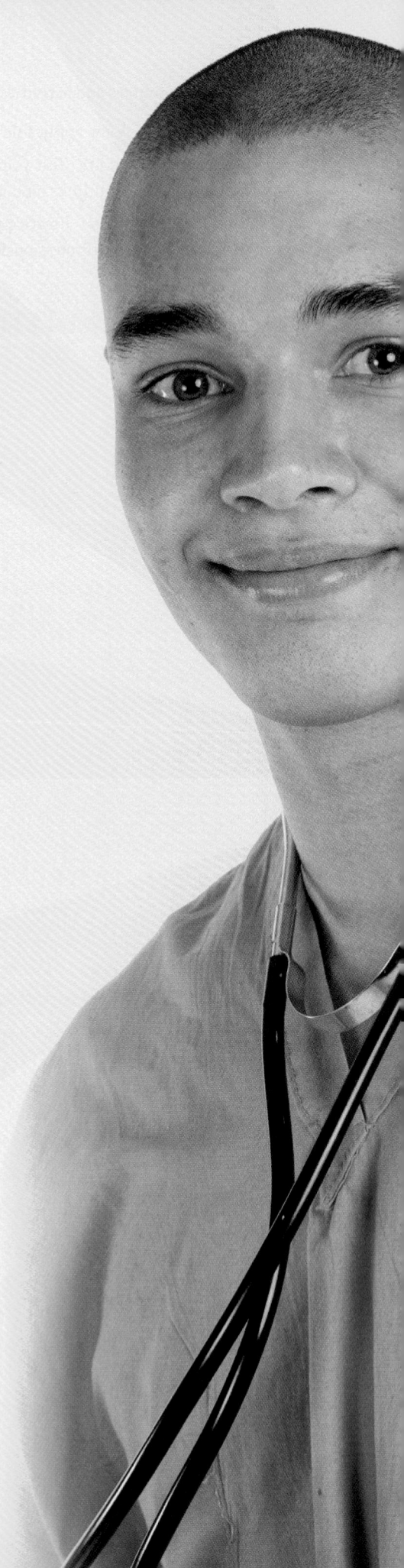

53

Pharmacology

LEARNING OBJECTIVES

After completing this chapter, you should be able to:

- Define and spell the terms to learn for this chapter.

- Differentiate between the legal (generic) and commercial (trade) and chemical names for a drug.

- Describe the drug reference resources that should be accessible in all physician offices.

- List the five schedules of the Controlled Substances Act.

- Differentiate between the routes of drug administration.

- List the "ten rights" to medicine administration.

- Describe the precautions to be observed when administering drugs.

- List and describe drug interactions.

- Identify the parts of a prescription.

CHAPTER OUTLINE

CASE STUDY

Susan Schults, CMA (AAMA), is working the medication refill line for Pearson Physicians Group. She has received a refill request from Adam Lehmke for his diazepam. When she pulls Mr. Lemke's chart, she notices that Dr. Penningworth wrote a prescription for diazepam 3 months ago with two refills and realizes, based on the date, that Mr. Lehmke should still have 2 weeks of medicine.

CERTIFICATION LINK

CMA (AAMA)
Preparing and administering medications
Pharmacology
Prescriptions

RMA
Clinical medical assisting
Clinical pharmacology

CMAS (AMT)
Basic clinical medical office assisting
Pharmacology

Pharmacology is the study of medications and drugs including their forms, intentions for use, and effects. Drugs come from many different sources, including plants, animals, minerals, whereas others are synthetically created. Some drugs, such as vitamins, are found naturally in the foods we eat. Medications, such as penicillin and other antibiotics, come from molds, which are a form of plant life. The vast majority of drugs used in medicine today are **synthetic**, created in a laboratory by artificial means.

Drugs, such as antibiotics or antihypertensives, are given to either help improve or eradicate a condition that a patient already has. If drugs are given **prophylactically**, they are being used to prevent the onset of a condition. For example, birth control pills are taken prophylactically to prevent pregnancy.

The role of the medical assistant is to assist the physician in the treatment of patients. The physician is responsible for prescribing medication for patients. The medical assistant is often required to administer the medication and keep accurate medication records. This requires the medical assistant to develop skills in reading medication orders, properly administering medications, and other aspects of pharmacology.

Drug Names

Any given drug has three types of names. The three names used to describe drugs include the generic name (equivalent to what is sometimes called the "official" or "nonproprietary" name of a drug), the brand name, and the chemical name. The **generic name**, is the single identifying name, is typically noted in lowercase letters, and is considered the legal name for the drug. Generic drugs are required by Food and Drug Administration (FDA) law to have the same effectiveness, safety, active ingredients, quality, strength, purity, and stability as brand name drugs.

The **brand name**, which is typically distinguished by capitalizing the first letter in the drug, is the name given to a drug by a specific manufacturer. This is also called the **proprietary name**. This name is often the most familiar name for a specific drug. The company that holds the patent for the drug can manufacture and produce that drug, under that brand name, for 20 years from the date of the patent. Other companies may manufacture the same drug, but must use their own brand name.

Generic drugs are typically priced lower than drugs with the brand names, and generally are **bioequivalent**, having the same strength and action. It is the active ingredients in generic drugs that are required to be bioequivalent. However, generic drugs are not as closely monitored as the brand name drugs, so their effectiveness may or may not actually be equal. If a physician believes that a specific drug is more effective than a generic version, then the named brand is more likely to be ordered.

The chemical name is the chemical formula typically used by manufacturers and pharmacists. **Pharmacists** are specially trained and licensed professionals who specialize in the preparation and dispensation of drugs. The generic name of a drug is generally somehow related to its chemical name. Table 53-1 shows the three drug names for the drugs Tylenol and Motrin.

TABLE 53-1 The Three Names Given to a Drug

Generic Name	Brand Name	Chemical Name
acetaminophen	Tylenol	N-(4-hydroxyphenyl) acetamide
ibuprofen	Motrin	iso-butyl-propanoic-phenolic acid

Regulations and Standards

The Food and Drug Administration (FDA) is the specific department within the U.S. Department of Health and Human Services responsible for ensuring that human drugs are safe and effective and that these products are honestly, accurately and informatively represented to the public. The Federal Food, Drug, and Cosmetic Act of 1938 stipulates the actual control of drugs. This law was enacted to ensure the safety of food, drugs, and cosmetics that are sold within U.S. borders. The **Drug Enforcement Administration (DEA)** is the agency of the federal government responsible for enforcing drug control. All physicians are required to register with the DEA in order to prescribe, dispense, or administer controlled substances.

References

Many references are available for pharmaceutical products. When administering a medication per a physician's order, the medical assistant must understand the drug that is being administered. The *Physicians' Desk Reference,* the *Hospital Formulary,* and the *United States Pharmacopeia–National Formulary (USP–NF)* are commonly used drug reference books. The *Hospital Formulary* contains up-to-date information about drugs and their usage. It is published by the American Hospital Formulary Service and is used extensively by pharmacists. The USP–NF lists all medicines, dosage forms, drug substances, and dietary supplements authorized for use in the United States; information found in this reference book is enforceable by the FDA.

PHYSICIANS' DESK REFERENCE

The most common drug resource available is the *Physicians' Desk Reference,* also known as the *PDR* (Figures 53-1A–B).

This text is reprinted annually and is a relatively easy-to-read reference published by a private company and purchased by medical offices and hospitals. The *PDR* is divided into six sections that are utilized based on the user's need for information. The six sections include the following:

- The first white section contains current information regarding pharmaceutical manufacturers, including their addresses, phone numbers, and emergency contacts.

- The pink section in the *PDR* is an alphabetical listing of the generic and brand names of each product.

- The blue section in the *PDR* contains an alphabetical listing by category or classification of generic and brand names.

- The gray section provides product identification and color photos of tablets and capsules listed alphabetically by the manufacturer.

- The second white section is devoted to product information. Here you will find information on each drug, including its brand and generic names, description, clinical pharmacology, indications and usage, contraindications, warnings, precautions, adverse reactions, dosage and administration, and how it is supplied.

- The green section provides diagnostic product information. Additional information pertaining to controlled substances, drug pregnancy ratings, poison control, and discontinued products are also listed here.

Updated versions of the *PDR* are published annually. Medical assistants should review and become familiar with each new addition as it will help you to become familiar and comfortable with its use.

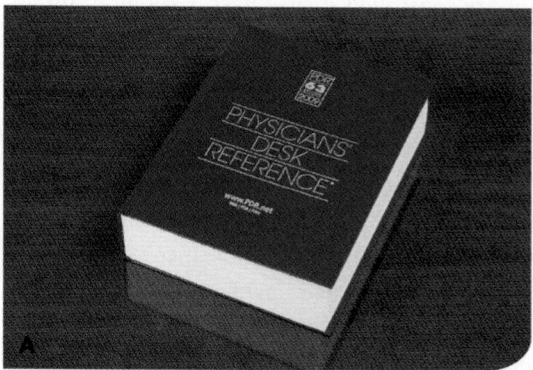
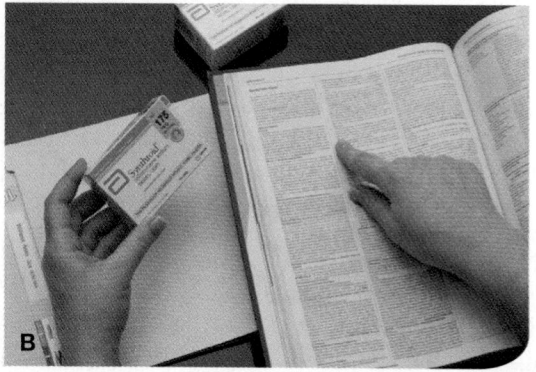

FIGURE 53-1 (A) The *Physician's Desk Reference;* (B) the medical assistant reviews the PDR for information related to a drug.

ONLINE RESOURCES

Many online references are available, including Web MD and Medline, but the medical assistant must be sure to use recognized, reliable resources when searching the Internet for medical information. Because it is impossible for anyone to remember all of the available medications, it is important for the medical assistant to practice using the available medical references and not rely on memory to ensure that patients receive the correct drug. Many names sound alike, and accuracy in prescribing the correct drug for the correct condition is imperative.

Legal Classifications of Drugs

Drugs are classified based on the need for a prescription as well as their addictive potential. It is important that the medical assistant be able to distinguish between prescription and nonprescription drugs and also to stay current on the status of drugs because some drugs change status from prescription to nonprescription.

PRESCRIPTION DRUGS

Physicians are responsible for prescribing medications; however, specially licensed professionals such as physician's assis-

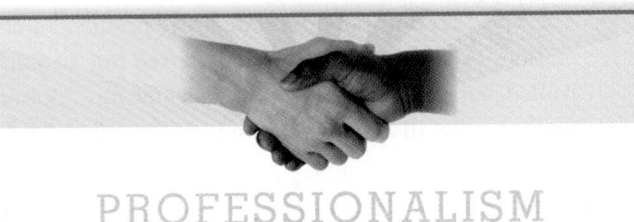

PROFESSIONALISM
CULTURAL CONSIDERATIONS

It is important for patients to understand the instructions when taking medications. If a patient has a difficult time understanding the English language, it is important to overcome this communication barrier. Solutions might include a patient inviting a family member into the treatment room who has a better grasp of the English language. The instructions can then be told to the family member who can then repeat the instructions to the patient in his or her native language. Another solution may be to go online and use an interpretive language program to print out the medication instructions in the patient's language. Use of a trained interpreter would also be an appropriate solution to overcoming this type of communication issue.

tants and advanced practice nurses (such as nurse practitioners and clinical nurse specialists) can also write prescriptions. A prescription is a written explanation to a pharmacist specifying the name of the medication, the dose, the route, and the times of administration. Physicians can also give the prescription verbally to a pharmacist. Examples of prescription drugs include antibiotics, antihypertensives, and pain medications, among others. These drugs must be labeled with the words "Caution: Federal Law prohibits dispensing without prescription."

NONPRESCRIPTION DRUGS

Nonprescription drugs are also known as **over-the-counter (OTC)** drugs. Examples include aspirin, cold medications, and antibiotic ointments such as Neosporin. OTC drugs are found in a variety of stores.

OTC medications are regulated by the FDA. OTC medications are not without dangers, and patients should be educated to read labels and follow the label's directions. If taken incorrectly, some OTC drugs can be unsafe since they may react negatively with a prescription drug the patient is also taking. For example, antacids should not be taken with some antibiotics, and aspirin should not be taken with Coumadin (an anticlotting medication) because of the potential for uncontrolled bleeding. Individuals with stomach ulcers should not take aspirin or ibuprofen because of the risk of bleeding. If the patients have questions about how to take OTC medications, they should ask their pharmacist for guidance. Patients should always let their physician know about all OTC medications they are taking so that there are no complications. Medical assistants should be sure to review and document OTC medications as well as prescription medications that are taken by the patient at every office visit.

CONTROLLED SUBSTANCES

Certain drugs are controlled if they have a potential for addiction or abuse. The DEA enforces the control of these medications. A drug that has the potential for abuse must be placed on the controlled substances list, according to the federal Controlled Substances Act (CSA).

The CSA of 1970 regulates the manufacture and distribution of drugs that can cause dependencies. The CSA has set forth guidelines for controlled substances and divided them into five categories (schedules) based on their potentially addictive level of abuse. See Table 53-2 for examples of these schedules. Controlled substances (also known as

TABLE 53-2 Schedule for Controlled Substances

Level	Description	Comment
Schedule I	Highest potential for addiction and abuse Not accepted for medical use *Examples:* cocaine, heroin, LSD	Not prescribed drugs
Schedule II	High potential for addiction and abuse Accepted for medical use in the United States *Examples:* codeine, morphine, opium, and secobarbital	A DEA-licensed physician must complete the required triplicate prescription forms entirely written in his or her own handwriting. The prescription must be filled within 7 days, and it may not be refilled. In an emergency, the physician may order a limited amount of the drug by telephone. These drugs must be stored under lock and key if they are kept on office premises. The law requires that a dispensing record of these drugs be kept on file for 2 years.
Schedule III	Moderate to low potential for addiction and abuse *Examples:* butabarbital, anabolic steroids, APC with codeine	A DEA number is not required to write a prescription for these drugs, but the physician must handwrite the order. Five refills, which must be indicated on the prescription form, are allowed during a 6-month period. Only the physician can give telephone orders to the pharmacist for these drugs.
Schedule IV	Lower potential for addiction and abuse than Schedule III drugs *Examples:* chloral hydrate, phenobarbital, diazepam	A medical assistant may write the prescription order for the physician, but it must be signed by the physician. Five refills are allowed over a 6-month period of time.
Schedule V	Low potential for addiction and abuse *Examples:* low-strength codeine combined with other drugs to form a cough suppressant	Inventory records must be maintained on these drugs.

narcotics) are generally kept under double lock and key, and strict control must be maintained. A narcotic log must be used to track all narcotics, including the inventory in stock, who administers a narcotic, how much was given, and the date and name of the patient receiving the drug. Most facilities do not allow medical assistants to administer narcotics.

All controlled substances must be labeled according to CSA specifications, showing the drug's assigned schedule. The schedule identification number is written inside a capital letter C, which stands for controlled substance (Figure 53-2). The following are some common controlled substances:

- anabolic steroids
- butabarbital
- chloral hydrate
- codeine
- diazepam
- morphine
- opium
- phenobarbital
- secobarbital
- acetaminophen (Tylenol) with codeine

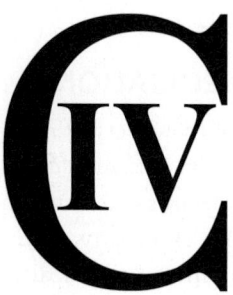

FIGURE 53-2 Label used to indicate a class IV controlled substance.

TABLE 53-3 Injectable Drugs Commonly Stocked in the Medical Office

Name Generic	Trade Name	Route	Usage
amitriptyline HCl	Elavil	IM	Depression
brompheniramine maleate	Dimetane	IM/Subcutaneous	Allergy
chlorpromazine HCl	Thorazine	IM	Psychosis
diazepam	Valium	IM	Anxiety
dimenhydrinate	Dramamine	IM	Nausea/vomiting
diphenhydramine	Benadryl	IM	Allergic reaction
diphtheria, tetanus toxoid	Same name	IM	Immunization active vaccine
furosemide	Lasix	IM	Edema
gentamicin sulfate	Garamycin	IM	Infection
heparin sodium	Same name	Subcutaneous	Prevents clotting
hydromorphone HCl	Dilaudid	Subcutaneous/IM	Severe pain
lidocaine HCl 1 percent, 2 percent	Xylocaine	Subcutaneous	Anesthetic for minor surgery
prochlorperazine	Compazine	IM	Psychosis
promethazine HCl	Phenergan	IM	Nausea/vomiting
sodium chloride with benzyl alcohol 0.9 percent	Bacteriostatic 0.9% Sodium Chloride	—	Diluent for injection
tetanus and diphtheria toxoids	Same name	IM	Immunization (active vaccine)
tetanus antitoxin	Same name	IM	Prevention (passive vaccine)
tetanus immune globulin	Hyper-Tet	IM	Prevention (passive vaccine)
tetanus toxoid	Same name	IM	Immunization (active vaccine)
tuberculin protein derivative	Tine test	ID	Tuberculin testing
water for injection	Same name		Diluent for injection
Emergency Drugs			
bretylium tosylate	Bretylol	IV	Arrhythmia
epinephrine		IV Subcutaneous	Cardiac arrest Allergic reaction
norepinephrine	Levophed	IV	Hypotension
sodium bicarbonate		IV	Acidosis
electrolytes/Ringer's 1000 mL		IV	Dehydration

ID, intradermal; IM, intramuscular; IV, intravenous

Note: Only physicians and nurses may administer IV medications.

INVENTORY OF OFFICE MEDICATIONS

Medical offices maintain an inventory of the variety of medications in stock, including samples from pharmaceutical companies. Commonly stocked injectable drugs are listed in Table 53-3. The medication inventory is usually maintained in a logbook that is the responsibility of the medical assistant. Included in the logbook are the name of each medication, the quantity on hand, and the expiration dates. Typically, a separate section in the logbook is used to indicate when a medication is dispensed to a patient. When distributing a medication to a patient, the patient's name and date of birth are entered into this section of the logbook, along with the quantity, date and time of distribution, and medical assistant's initials. Once a month it is important for the medical assistant to review the inventory to ensure that a sufficient supply of all drugs is available and that no medication has expired.

Physicians are required to register with the DEA in order to prescribe, dispense, or administer controlled substances. A special form, DEA 224, must be completed and submitted to the DEA. Renewal is required every 3 years, using Form 224a.

The expiration dates of all narcotics in stock should be checked regularly, and two staff members should document the destruction of any outdated narcotics. When disposing of expired medications, follow office policy. The signatures of both individuals should be documented on the narcotic log stating that the medications have been destroyed.

Drug Abuse

Although the use of drugs is an important element for treating diseases and conditions, any drug can be abused. Both OTC medications and prescription drugs can be misused. Examples of such drugs include pain medications, sleeping aids, and cold medications. Drug abuse can occur with patients at any age and can lead to dependency or toxicity.

Drug abuse and drug dependency are defined separately. **Drug abuse** is defined as the use of a drug improperly or wrongly. An individual with **drug dependency** is one who relies on the medication or uses the medication for psychological support. Individuals who become physically dependent are those who continuously use a substance to function or to avoid physical pain. For physical dependency to occur, the abused substance produces changes in the nervous system on which the body begins to rely. Once the substance is removed, the individual experiences withdrawal symptoms. Depending on the level of addiction, withdrawal symptoms will be mild to severe.

IDENTIFYING DRUG ABUSE

Medical assistants must be aware of the potential for drug abuse and drug dependency in patients. Table 53-4 lists

TABLE 53-4 Drug Types That Are Commonly Abused

Drug Type	Drug		
Analgesic	Demerol	Vicodin	Percocet
Antianxiety	Valium	Xanax	Librium
Antidepressant	Prozac	Elavil	Tofranil
Sedative	Dalmane	Restoril	Seconal
Illegal drugs	Heroin	Marijuana	Cocaine

drug types that are commonly abused. If the medical assistant suspects a patient to be abusing drugs, the following steps may be taken:

1. Notify the physician. It is not up to the medical assistant to confront the patient.

2. Check local pharmacies to see if the patient is obtaining medications from multiple pharmacies.

3. Tell patients who are frequently calling for refills that another refill will require an office visit.

Items that are important to keep secure in the office include syringes, needles, and prescription pads. Never leave blank prescription pads lying out in examination rooms; prescription pads should always be stored in secure locations. Any dispensing of a controlled substance from the office must be documented in the patient's chart and also in the narcotic log.

General Classes of Drugs

The classification of drugs is based on their action in the body. Table 53-5 presents a comprehensive list of drug classifications with descriptions of the use or function for each classification. Table 53-6 presents a similar list with examples of specific drugs for each classification.

TABLE 53-5 Drug Classification Names and Descriptions of Use

Name	Use
Adrenergic	Increases the rate and strength of the heart muscle. Acts as a vasoconstrictor, dilates bronchi, dilates pupils, and relaxes muscular walls. Used to treat asthma, bronchitis, and allergies.
Adrenergic blocking agent	Increases peripheral circulation, decreases blood pressure and vasodilation. Used to treat hypertension.
Analgesic	Relieves pain without the loss of consciousness. These may be either narcotic or nonnarcotic. Narcotic drugs are derived from the opium poppy and act on the brain to cause pain relief and drowsiness.
Anesthetic	Produces a lack of feeling that may have a local or general effect depending on the type of administration.
Antacid	Neutralizes acid in the stomach.
Antianxiety	Relieves or reduces anxiety and muscle tension. Used to treat panic disorders, anxiety, and insomnia.
Antiarrhythmic	Controls cardiac arrhythmias by altering nerve impulses within the heart.
Antibiotic	Destroys or prohibits the growth of microorganisms. Used to treat bacterial infections. Ineffective in treating viral infections. Must be taken regularly for a specified time period to be effective.
Anticoagulant	Prevents or delays blood clotting. Also referred to as blood thinners. May be administered by intravenous injection, such as with the drug heparin. Oral anticoagulants, such as warfarin, cannot be taken along with aspirin since the interaction between the two medications could cause internal bleeding.
Anticonvulsant	Prevents or relieves convulsions. Anticonvulsants such as phenobarbital reduce excessive stimulation in the brain to control seizures and other symptoms of epilepsy.
Antidepressant	Prevents or relieves the symptoms of depression. Also used in the prevention of migraine headaches.
Antidiabetic	Control diabetes by regulating the level of glucose in the blood and the metabolism of carbohydrates and fat.
Antidiarrheal	Prevents or relieves diarrhea.
Antidote	Counteracts the effects of poisons.
Antiemetic	Controls nausea and vomiting. Generally act on the vomiting center in the brain.
Antifungal	Kills fungus.
Antihelminthic	Kills parasitic worms.
Antihistamine	Counteracts histamine and controls allergic reactions.
Antihypertensive	Prevents or controls high blood pressure. Some antihypertensives block nerve impulses that cause arteries to constrict and thus increase blood pressure. Others slow the heart rate and decrease its force of contraction. Still others may reduce the amount of the hormone aldosterone in the blood that is causing the blood pressure to rise.
Anti-inflammatory	Counteracts inflammation.
Antineoplastic	Kills normal and abnormal cancerous cells by interfering with cell reproduction.
Antipruritic	Relieves itching.
Antipyretic	Reduces fever.
Antiseptic	Prevents the growth of microorganisms.

Antitussive	Controls or relieves coughing. Codeine is an ingredient in many prescription antitussives (cough medicines); it acts on the brain to control coughing.
Astringent	A substance that has a constricting or binding effect by coagulating proteins on a cell's surface. May be used to stop hemorrhage.
Bronchodilator	Dilates or opens the bronchi (airways in the lungs) to improve breathing.
Cardiogenic	Strengthens the heart muscle.
Cathartic	Causes bowel movements to occur. May have a strong purging action and can become habit forming.
Contraceptive	Used to prevent conception.
Decongestant	Reduces nasal congestion and swelling.
Diuretic	Increases the excretion of urine, which promotes the loss of water and salt from the body; since this can assist in lowering blood pressure, diuretics are used to treat hypertension. Potassium in the body may be depleted with continued use of diuretics. Potassium-rich foods, such as bananas, kiwi, and orange juice, along with medications for potassium deficiency, can help correct this deficiency.
Emetic	Induces vomiting.
Expectorant	Assists in the removal of secretions from the bronchopulmonary membranes.
Hemostatic	Controls bleeding.
Hypnotic	Produces sleep or hypnosis.
Hypoglycemic	Lowers blood glucose level.
Immunosuppressant	Suppresses the body's natural immune response to an antigen. Used to control autoimmune diseases such as multiple sclerosis and rheumatoid arthritis.
Laxative	Used to promote normal bowel function.
Miotic	Constricts the pupils of the eye.
Muscle relaxant	Produces the relaxation of skeletal muscle.
Mydriatic	Dilates the pupils of the eye.
Narcotic	Produces sleep or stupor. In moderate doses will depress the central nervous system and relieve pain. In excessive doses will cause stupor, coma, and even death. Can become habit forming (addictive).
Purgative	Stimulates bowel movements.
Psychedelic	Drugs such as lysergic acid diethylamide (LSD) that can produce visual hallucinations.
Sedative	Produces relaxation without causing sleep.
Stimulant	Speeds up the heart and respiratory system. Used to increase alertness.
Tranquilizer	Used to reduce mental anxiety and tensions.
Vaccine	Given to promote resistance (immunity) to infectious diseases.
Vasodilator	Relaxes blood vessels to lower blood pressure.
Vasopressor	Produces muscle contractions that affect capillaries and arteries and elevates the blood pressure.
Vitamin	Organic substances found naturally in foods that are essential for normal metabolism. Most have been produced synthetically to be taken in pill form.

TABLE 53-6 Classification of Drugs by Type or Usage

Type/Usage	Example Brand Name (Generic Name)	Type/Usage	Example Brand Name (Generic Name)
Adrenergic	Isuprel (isoproterenol) Sudafed (pseudoephedrine hydrochloride HCl)	Anticholinergic	Atropine (atropine sulfate) Banthine (methantheline bromide) Donnatal (belladonna)
Adrenergic blocking agent	Aldomet (methyldopa) Inderal (propranolol HCl)	Anticoagulant	Coumadin (warfarin sodium)
Analgesic	Acetylsalicylic acid or aspirin Advil (ibuprofen) Darvon (propoxyphene HCl) Dilaudid (hydromorphone HCl) Demerol (meperidine HCl) Talwin (pentazocine HCl) Tylenol (acetaminophen)	Anticonvulsant	Dilantin (phenytoin sodium) Phenobarbital (phenobarbital)
		Antidepressant	Elavil (amitriptyline HCl)
		Antidiabetic	Insulin and oral medications (Precose and Metformin)
		Antidiarrheal	Kaopectate (kaolin and pectin mixture) Lomotil (diphenoxylate)
Anesthetic	Carbocaine (mepivacaine HCl) Novocaine (procaine HCl) Nupercaine (dibucaine HCl) Xylocaine (lidocaine HCl)	Antiemetics	Atarax (hydroxyzine HCl) Compazine (prochlorperazine) Dramamine (dimenhydrinate) Phenergan (promethazine HCl)
Antacid	Milk of Magnesia (magnesium hydroxide) Mylanta (aluminum hydroxide) Maalox (aluminum hydroxide)	Antifungal	Mycostatin (nystatin)
		Antihelminthics	Vermox (mebendazole)
Antianxiety	Valium (diazepam)	Antihistamine	Adrenalin (epinephrine) Benadryl (diphenhydramine) Chlor-Trimeton (chlorpheniramine maleate) Dimetane (brompheniramine maleate)
Antiarrhythmic	Digoxin (digoxin) Norpace (disopyramide) Pronestyl (procainamide HCl)		
Antibiotics			
• Aminoglycosides	Garamycin (gentamicin sulfate) Kantrex (kanamycin) Mycifradin Sulfate (neomycin sulfate) Nebcin (tobramycin sulfate) Neobiotic (neomycin sulfate)	Antihypertensives	Aldomet (methyldopa) Catapres (clonidine HCl) Lopressor (metoprolol tartrate) Minipress (prazosin HCl)
• Cephalosporins	Ancef (cefazolin sodium) Anspor (cephradine) Ceclor (cefaclor) Duricef (cefadroxil) Keflex (cephalexin)	Anti-inflammatory	Aspirin (acetylsalicylic acid) Indocin (indomethacin) Motrin (ibuprofen) Nalfon (fenoprofen calcium) Aleve (naproxen sodium)
• Penicillins	Amoxil (amoxicillin) Bicillin (penicillin G potassium) Duracillin (penicillin G procaine) Polycillin (ampicillin)	Antineoplastic	Adriamycin (doxorubicin HCl) Cytoxan (cyclophosphamide) Fluorouracil (5FU)
		Antipruritic	Calamine lotion (calamine) Hydrocortone (hydrocortisone sodium phosphate)
• Tetracyclines	Achromycin (tetracycline HCl) Declomycin (demeclocycline) Terramycin (oxytetracycline) Vibramycin (doxycycline hyclate)	Antipyretic	Advil (ibuprofen) Aspirin (acetylsalicylic acid) Tylenol (acetaminophen)
		Antiseptic	Cidex (glutaraldehyde) pHisoHex (hexachlorophene)
		Antitussive	Codeine (codeine phosphate)

Bronchodilator	Alupent (metaproterenol sulfate) Brethine (terbutaline sulfate) Isuprel (isoproterenol HCl) Theolair (theophylline)		Narcotic	Demerol (meperidine HCl) Percodan (oxycodone HCl)
			Psychedelic	LSD (lysergic acid diethyl-amide)
Contraceptive	Ortho-Novum 10/11 (estrogen with progestin)		Sedative and Hypnotic	Amytal (amobarbital) Butisol (butabarbital sodium) Nembutal Sodium (pheno-barbital) Seconal Sodium (secobarbital sodium) Valium (diazepam)
Decongestant	Neo-Synephrine (phenyle-phrine HCl) Sudafed (pseudoephedrine HCl)			
Diuretic	Diuril (chlorothiazide) Hygroton (chlorthalidone) Lasix (furosemide)		Stimulant	Dexedrine (dextroampheta-mine sulfate)
			Tranquilizer	Haldol (haloperidol)
Emetic	Ipecac syrup		Vasodilator	Isordil (isosorbide dinitrate) Nitro-bid (nitroglycerin) Nitrostat (nitroglycerin)
Expectorant	Robitussin (guaifenesin)			
Hormone	Testosterone, Premarin, Estrace			
			Vasopressor	Levophed (norepinephrine)
Hypnotic	Seconal (secobarbital)		Vitamin	Vitamin A Vitamin C Vitamin D Vitamin E Vitamin K
Hypoglycemic	Precose (oral) Metformin (oral)			
Laxative	Dulcolax (bisacodyl)			
Muscle relaxant	Valium (diazepam) Robaxin (methocarbamol)			

Routes and Drug Administration

The route of administration is the method by which the drug is introduced into the body (Figure 53-3). The most common routes of drug administration are as follows:

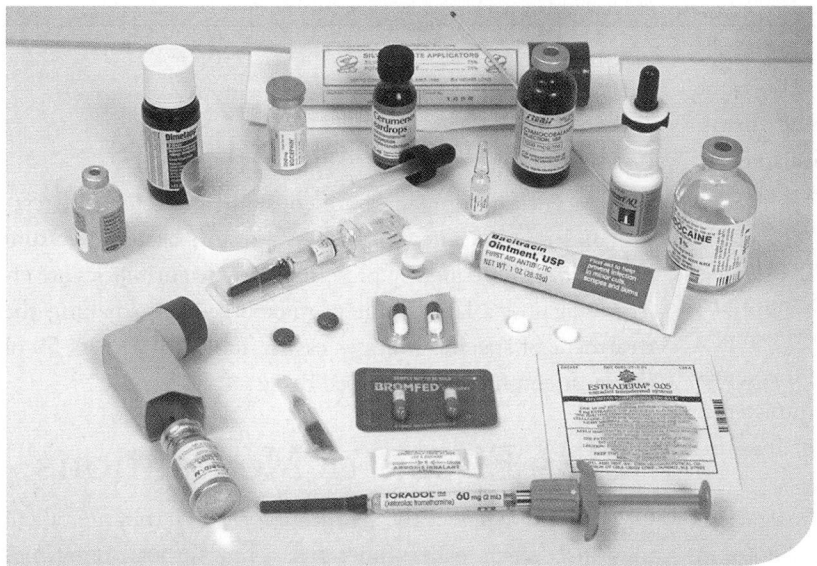

FIGURE 53-3 Different types of medication require different routes of administration.

- **Parenteral**—Parenteral medications are any medications that are given outside of the alimentary canal, such as injections. The parenteral route usually requires the skin to be punctured by a needle with a syringe attached in order to administer the medication. Table 53-7 lists the methods of parenteral administration and describes each method.

  - **Nonparenteral**—Nonparenteral medications include any medications that are given via the alimentary canal. Such medications include oral medications.

  - **Sublingual**—Sublingual drugs are held under the tongue, where they are absorbed through the tissues and into the bloodstream for distribution to the body. Nitroglycerin is commonly administered this way when it is used for treating the heart pains of angina.

Most drugs must be given by specific routes to be effective. It is important to be sure that the patient understands the directions for medication administration because

TABLE 53-7 Methods for Parenteral Administration of Drugs

Method	Description
Intraarticular	Injection into a joint. Corticosteroids are often injected into the joint of the knee or toes.
Intradermal (ID)	A very shallow injection just within the top layer of skin. This is a method commonly used in skin testing for allergies and tuberculosis.
Intramuscular (IM)	An injection directly into the muscle of the buttocks or upper arm (deltoid). This method is used when a large amount of medication is administered or is irritating.
Intrathecal	Injection into the meninges space surrounding the brain and spinal cord.
Intravenous (IV)	An injection into the veins. This route can be set up so that there is a continuous administration of medication, usually after a major surgery or during a major procedure.
Subcutaneous (SC)	An injection under the skin and fat layers. The middle of the upper, outer arm is usually used.

TABLE 53-8 Methods for Nonparenteral Administration of Drugs

Method	Description
Eardrops	Placement directly into the ear canal for the purpose of relieving pain or treating infection.
Eyedrops	Placement into the eye to control eye pressure in glaucoma. Also administered this way during eye examinations to dilate the pupil of the eye for better examination of the interior of the eye. Also used to treat infections.
Inhalation	Inhaled directly into the nose and mouth. Aerosol sprays are administered by this route.
Oral	Taken by mouth and swallowed by the patient.
Rectal	Introduced directly into the rectal cavity in the form of suppositories or solution. Drugs may have to be administered by this route if the patient is unable to take them by mouth due to nausea, vomiting, or surgery of the mouth.
Sublingual or buccal	Placed under the lip or tongue (sublingual) or between the cheek and gum (buccal). Nitroglycerin for anginal pain is administered this way.
Topical	Applied directly to the skin or mucous membranes in ointment, cream, or lotion form. Used to treat skin infections and eruptions. Transdermal patches are also used; examples include Nicotrol, Estraderm, and Nicoderm.
Vaginal	Inserted or spread vaginally to treat vaginal yeast infections and other irritations.

the right route must be followed for the medication to be effective. Drugs are available in many different forms. Table 53-8 lists numerous forms in which medications are prepared and the nonparenteral routes through which they are administered.

Sometimes a drug can be administered in a variety of forms. For example, the female hormone estrogen can be administered orally in the form of a pill or topically in the form of a skin patch. Table 53-9 lists various forms in which medicines are prepared and routes through which they are administered.

Prior to administering a medication to a patient it is important to check the "ten rights."

Guildelines 53-1 discusses medication administration, including the "ten rights," and previews what is discussed in Chapter 54.

Frequently Administered Drugs

Pharmaceutical companies are constantly developing, testing, and releasing new drugs. As a result, **broad-spectrum** antibiotics are frequently prescribed. These antibiotics are effective against a large range of microorganisms, making the treatment of specific illnesses easier. Table 53-10 lists 50 of the most commonly prescribed drugs.

Side Effects of Medications

Drugs not only affect the symptom for which they are taken; they also affect other functions. These other, sometimes undesirable, effects are called **side effects**. Side effects are

TABLE 53-9 Drug Forms and Routes of Administration

Form	Route	Form	Route
Aerosol	Inhalation	Pills	Oral
Caplets	Oral	Powders	Topical
Capsules	Oral	Skin patch	Topical
Elixir	Oral	Spansules	Oral
Liniment	Topical	Spray	Oral, topical
Lotion	Topical	Suppository	Rectal, vaginal
Lozenges	Oral	Syrup	Oral
Ointment	Topical	Tablet	Oral

GUIDELINES 53-1

ADMINISTRATION OF MEDICATION

1. Medications/drugs can only be administered to a patient under the supervision of a licensed physician. To do otherwise is considered "practicing medicine without a license." The medication order must be written and signed on the patient's medical record by the physician.

2. The medical assistant acts as the liaison or intermediary between the physician and the patient. Some of the duties include ordering, storing, rotating, and checking expiration dates on medications.

3. Medications must be checked three times before administration. The "three befores" are these:
   - Before medication is removed from the medication cabinet
   - Before medication is poured, drawn up into a syringe, or placed into a medication cup
   - Before medication is returned to the cabinet

4. Medications cannot be returned to the container once they have been removed. If they are not administered, they must be discarded.

5. Remember the "ten rights" for administering medications (Figure 53-4). The first six rights are:
   - Right patient
   - Right medication
   - Right dosage
   - Right route
   - Right time
   - Right documentation

   It is recommended that you consider four additional rights of medication administration:
   - Right client education
   - Right to refuse

   - Right assessment
   - Right evaluation.

6. Keep a record of all allergies on the patient's medical record. Often these allergies are noted on the front of the medical record as well as within the medical record.

7. The documentation on the patient's medical record must include the following:
   a. Name of medication
   b. Dosage
   c. Route of administration
   d. Site of administration
   e. Signature of the person administering the medication, along with initials designating the person's status (e.g., CMA or RMA)

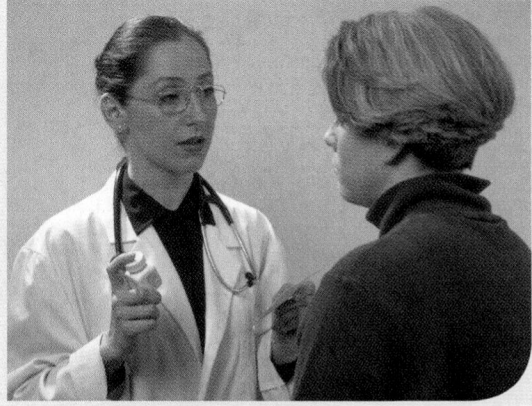

FIGURE 53-4   Remember the "ten rights" when administering medications.

(continued)

8. All narcotics must be documented in a record maintained for that purpose. This is referred to as "logging a narcotic." Every narcotic must be accounted for fully.

9. Be careful that you administer the medication by the correct route. Methods of administration include these:
    a. Oral (by mouth)
    b. Sublingual (under the tongue)
    c. Buccal (in the cheek)
    d. Rectal (inserted into the anal cavity)
    e. Vaginal (inserted into vaginal canal)
    f. Parenteral (by injection)
    g. Topical (applied to the skin)
    h. Inhalation (by breathing the medication)
    Medical assistants do not administer medications by the following routes:

    a. Intrathecal (into the meninges space)
    b. Intracavity (into a body cavity)
    c. Intravenous (IV) (into a vein)

10. Medication labels should be clean and readable. If they become soiled, unreadable, or fall off the container they must be discarded.

11. If you are not familiar with a particular medication, you must look it up in the *PDR*. Never violate this rule.

12. Know the side effects for the medication you are administering.

13. Always advise the patient to take the complete number of doses ordered in the prescription. This is especially important when using antibiotics.

14. Advise the patient to only use medication for the person for whom it was prescribed.

TABLE 53-10 50 Frequently Administered Drugs

Brand Name	Type	Brand Name	Type
1. Amoxil	antibiotic	27. Lasix	diuretic
2. Lanoxin	cardiotonic	28. Voltaren	anti-inflammatory (nonsteroidal)
3. Zantac	antiulcer	29. Darvocet-N	analgesic (narcotic)
4. Xanax	tranquilizer	30. Dilantin	anticonvulsant
5. Premarin	hormone (estrogen)	31. Monistat	antibiotic (antifungal)
6. Cardizem	cardiotonic	32. Augmentin	antibiotic (penicillin)
7. Ceclor	antibiotic	33. Micronase	oral hypoglycemic agent
8. Synthroid	hormone (thyroid)	34. Feldene	anti-inflammatory (nonsteroidal)
9. Seldane	antihistamine	35. Micro-K	potassium supplement
10. Tenormin	beta-blocker	36. Provera	hormone (progestin)
11. Vasotec	antihypertensive	37. Motrin	anti-inflammatory (nonsteroidal)
12. Tagamet	antiulcer	38. Mevacor	cholesterol lowering
13. Naprosyn	anti-inflammatory (nonsteroidal)	39. Triphasil	synthetic hormone
14. Capoten	antihypertensive	40. Prozac	antidepressant
15. Ortho-Novum 7/7/7	synthetic hormone	41. Lo/Ovral	synthetic hormone
16. Dyazide	diuretic	42. Valium	tranquilizer
17. Ortho-Novum	synthetic hormone	43. Retin-A	antiacne
18. Proventil	bronchodilator	44. Cipro	antibiotic
19. Tylenol with codeine	analgesic (narcotic)	45. E-Mycin	antibiotic
20. Procardia	calcium channel blocker	46. Maxzide	diuretic
21. Calan	calcium channel blocker	47. Coumadin	anticoagulant
22. Ventolin	bronchodilator	48. Carafate	antiulcer
23. Inderal	beta-blocker	49. Timoptic	beta-blocker
24. Halcion	sedative	50. Slow-K	potassium supplement
25. Theo-Dur	bronchodilator		
26. Lopressor	beta-blocker		

generally tolerated because the benefit of taking the medication outweighs the unwanted side effects. **Adverse effects** require the patient to discontinue the medication because the negative effects outweigh the benefit of taking the medication. Occasionally, adverse effects can be **lethal**, which means they may cause death. Because of this, it is important that side effects be noted and taken seriously. Sometimes, side effects or adverse effects are specific to the individual (**idiosyncratic**). Food interactions can cause side effects. Other effects can be caused by allergic reactions.

Examples of specific side effects and adverse effects to drugs include the following:

- **Anaphylactic shock**—This is a life-threatening reaction to a drug, food, or insect bite. Symptoms can include respiratory distress, edema (swelling) in the mouth and throat, convulsions, and unconsciousness. If untreated, anaphylactic shock can cause death.

- **Drug tolerance**—This is a decrease in the effectiveness of a drug as the body gets used to having the drug in the system. It will take a larger dose of the drug to achieve the same result. This is common when a patient is repeatedly prescribed the same antibiotic or in patients who require a specific drug, such as a pain control medication, over a long period of time. The dose cannot always be increased, as some drugs can become **toxic** (harmful) with excessive amounts.

- **Habituation**—This is dependence on a drug. Habituation can develop with a variety of drugs, including narcotics and laxatives.

Unexpected side effects can range from rashes to drowsiness, coughing, runny nose, constipation, dizziness, headache, nausea, or vomiting. Patients should be instructed to call the physician if any of these symptoms occur. The physician may adjust the medication dose or completely change the prescription to another drug that may not have the same side effects.

Drug Interactions

Many factors contribute to how a patient reacts to medication. Thus, although a patient may tolerate a medication well, he or she may have a completely different reaction at any time. Factors that contribute to a patient's reaction to a medication include the patient's age, the patient's weight, the method of administration, allergies, and the degree of tolerance and intolerance.

PATIENT'S AGE

Geriatric and pediatric patients specifically are more susceptible to the effects of medications and will usually require lower doses. Due to this fact, when a physician prescribes a

medication for these populations, the medical assistant should review the order to ensure that the correct dosage has been ordered. Some geriatric patients may have special needs that require attention. For instance, medication instructions may need to be typed in a larger font, or medication bottles may need to have easily removable caps (Figure 53-5).

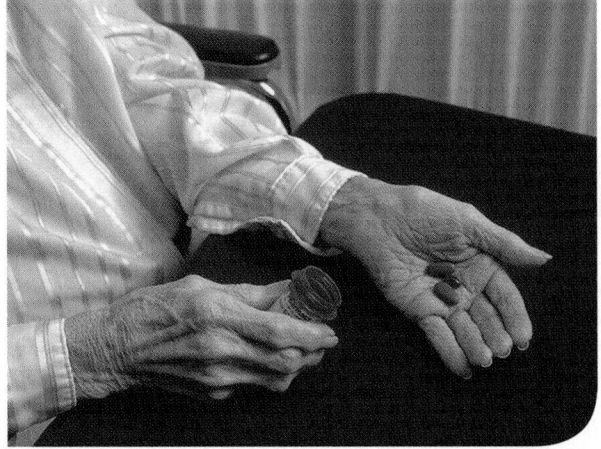

FIGURE 53-5 **Older adults may need special assistance with medications.**

PATIENT'S WEIGHT

A patient's weight is an important factor to consider when calculating the medication dosage. There is a direct correlation between the patient's weight and medication level. The typical medication dosage is based on the weight of a 150-pound adult. A patient's body weight will determine the dosage the physician prescribes. If the medication level is too low for the body weight, the patient will not benefit as much from the medication. At the same time, if the medication level is too high for the patient's body weight, the patient could become ill or even have an overdose reaction.

METHOD OF ADMINISTRATION

The method of administration affects the rate at which the body absorbs the medication. Physicians choose the method of administration depending on the response desired. For instance, for a more immediate response the physician would more than likely order an injectable medication. To offer relief over a sustained period of time, a time-release oral medication may be used.

ALLERGIES

An allergy to a medication can occur at any time. A patient may have an immediate allergic reaction or may develop one over time. An allergic reaction can manifest itself in symptoms such as hives and shortness of breath. This can be moderate to severe. Patients should be educated in what to do if an allergic reaction occurs. Patients who experience an allergic reaction should be told to call the office immediately or, if severe, to go to the nearest emergency room. If a patient has an allergy to any medication, this should be documented in the patient's chart and on an allergy sticker that is placed on the outside of the chart.

TOLERANCE AND INTOLERANCE

Some patients may experience intolerance to a medication. As with allergies, intolerances to medication should also be documented in the patient's chart. Vomiting, diarrhea, or abdominal cramping can be indications of intolerance. If intolerance to a medication is experienced, the patient should alert the physician, who may then adjust the dosage or change the prescription as needed.

After taking a medication for an extended period of time, the patient may develop a tolerance to that medication. If this occurs, the physician may need to change medications or increase the dosage to obtain the desired result.

It is important for the medical assistant to obtain a complete history regarding all medications the patient is taking, including herbal and OTC medications. These medications should be documented in the patient's record. The medical assistant should also review this information with the patient every time he or she is in the office. Any changes to medications should be noted in the patient's medical record. This information is then used by the physician to determine the appropriate treatment for the patient.

Drug Use During Pregnancy

Caution should be used when a pregnant woman decides to take a drug. Very few drugs are considered safe for use during pregnancy. Women who are pregnant should consult with their doctors prior to taking any medication. The FDA regulates and classifies drugs into pregnancy classifications. Every prescription drug should have a pregnancy classification. Pregnancy classifications range from A to X. Class A drugs are the safest for pregnant women, whereas Class X drugs have been shown to cause health risks, deformities, or both to the unborn fetus. Even OTC medications can have harmful effects on a pregnant woman or her fetus. Prior to prescribing a drug for any female, the date of her last menstrual cycle should be ascertained to ensure that she is not pregnant.

DRUG USE AND THE BREAST-FEEDING MOTHER

A lot of medications taken by a breast-feeding mother can appear in breast milk, which would then be swallowed by the nursing infant. A breast-feeding mother can take a few medications, but it is very important that the prescribing physician be aware that the mother is breast-feeding. Several medications, however, are **contraindicated**, which means that the medications are so dangerous for the infant that the mother must stop breast-feeding while she is taking them. These contraindicated medications include the following:

- Tetracyclines
- Chloramphenicol
- Sulfonamides
- Oral anticoagulants
- Iodine-containing drugs
- Antineoplastics

Reading and Writing a Prescription

Reading and writing a prescription are fairly easy tasks when you have some understanding of the symbols used in writing those prescriptions. It is important to be sure that all of the main parts of the prescription, as follows, are filled out completely:

- **Superscription**—Contains the patient's name, address, age, and date on the top line. The symbol (Rx) from the Latin term *recipe,* meaning "take thou," is usually preprinted on the prescription form.

- **Inscription**—Gives the name of the medication, actual ingredients, and dosage.
- **Subscription**—Tells the pharmacist how to mix the drug and how much to provide the patient.
- **Signa (sig.)**—The Latin term for "label." Provides instructions on how the medication should be taken by the patient. This often may be referred to as the signature.
- **Physician's Name, Address, Telephone Number, and DEA Number**—Generally, all but the DEA number are preprinted on the prescription pad.
- **Number of Refills**—Number of times the prescription may be refilled (usually no more than six times).
- **DAW (Dispense As Written)**—This option may be included in the prescription.

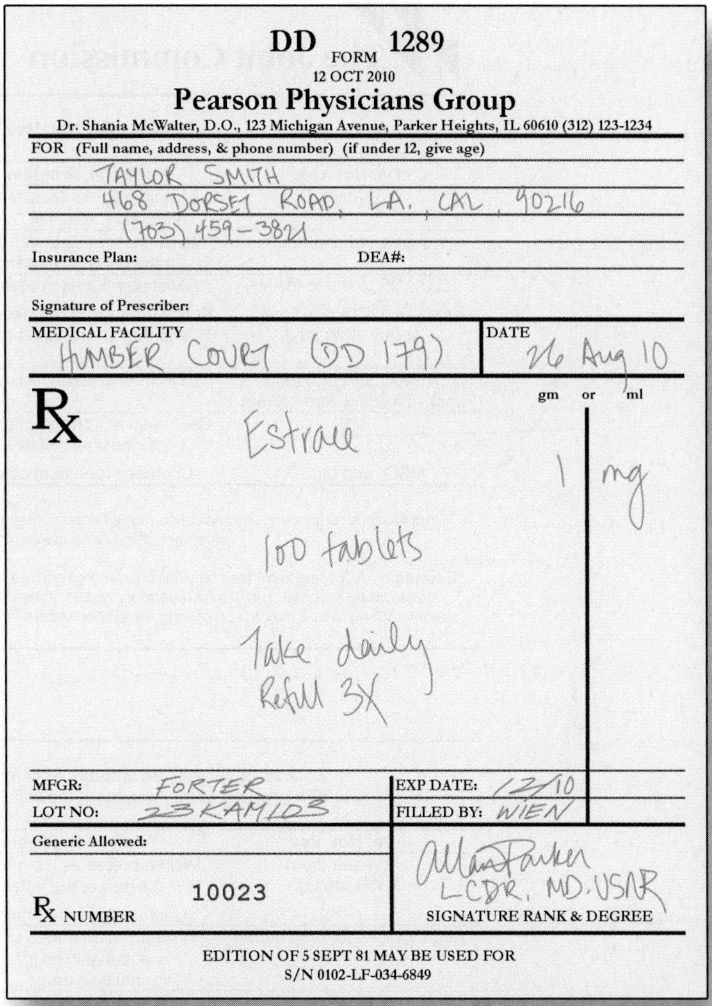
DD FORM 1289
12 OCT 2010
Pearson Physicians Group
Dr. Shania McWalter, D.O., 123 Michigan Avenue, Parker Heights, IL 60610 (312) 123-1234
FOR (Full name, address, & phone number) (if under 12, give age)
TAYLOR SMITH
468 DORSET ROAD, LA., CAL, 90216
(703) 459-3821
Insurance Plan: DEA#:
Signature of Prescriber:
MEDICAL FACILITY: HUMBER COURT (OD 179) DATE: 26 Aug 10
℞ gm or ml
Estrace 1 mg
100 tablets
Take daily
Refill 3X
MFGR: FORTER EXP DATE: 12/10
LOT NO: 23 KAML03 FILLED BY: WIEN
Generic Allowed:
10023
℞ NUMBER
LCDR, MD, USNR
SIGNATURE RANK & DEGREE
EDITION OF 5 SEPT 81 MAY BE USED FOR
S/N 0102-LF-034-6849

FIGURE 53-6 The parts of prescription includes the superscription, inscription, sig., and subscription.

Figure 53-6 shows an example of a prescription and its labeled parts. In this example, the physician has ordered the medication Estrace, which is a form of the hormone estrogen. The prescription tells the pharmacist to give 100 tablets and orders a 1 mg dosage, which is to be taken once a day. The instruction to the pharmacist is to refill the prescription three times and not to substitute with another generic medication. It is important to write out on the prescription the numbers regarding the amount to dispense and the number of refills. This provides a safeguard against tampering with the prescription.

Sometimes a prescription is written for prn refills, meaning that the prescription can be refilled as needed. The physician will fill in the name, address, age of the patient, and date. The physician must also sign his or her name at the bottom of the prescription. A blank prescription form cannot be handed to a patient.

When the pharmacist fills the prescription, the patient instructions will be placed on the label as instructed by the physician, along with special instructions for taking the medication (such as "Take with meals") that can help ensure that the medication is as effective as possible. The pharmacist will also include a package insert with each medication that contains information regarding possible side effects, adverse effects, and contraindications. If the patient experiences any adverse or side effects, the patient should report them to the physician.

Some prescriptions can be filled by telephone. At such times, the patient's record should be pulled for the physician,

PROFESSIONALISM

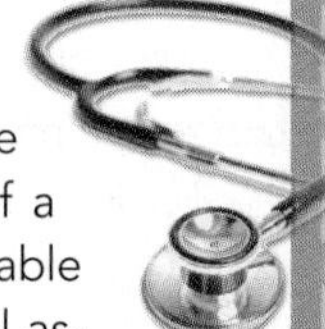

Understanding and being knowledgeable about medication is an important aspect of a medical assistant's job. This includes being able to pronounce medications correctly. Medical assistants will be discussing medications not only with patients but also with physicians and pharmacists when prescriptions are called into pharmacies. If you are unsure of the correct pronunciation of a medication, ask a colleague or a physician about it. Asking such questions will improve your professional image.

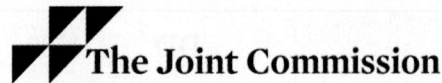
The Joint Commission

FIGURE 53-7   The official "Do Not Use" list as issued by the Joint Commission.
Source: The Joint Commission. Retrieved from http: www.jointcommission.org/PatientSafety/DoNotUseList.

and the refill order or new medications prescribed should be documented. Usually a medication refill form is in the chart. The medical assistant should list what the physician has ordered to be filled: the medication, the name of the medication, and the strength and dosage of the medication. The medical assistant should also document the name of the pharmacy, the name of the pharmacist taking the prescription information, the pharmacy phone number, and the time of the call.

Only physicians are permitted to sign prescriptions. However, the medical assistant in some cases may complete the prescription form, which the physician then checks for accuracy and signs.

It is essential that the medical assistant always safeguard prescription pads. At times, a physician may accidentally leave a prescription pad in an examination room. Medical assistants should always keep a watchful eye for items that are out of place. Maintaining the integrity of the office is, by far, one of the most important elements regarding professionalism.

E-PRESCRIPTIONS

With the focus of emerging technology and Web-based customer service, e-prescriptions are becoming increasingly popular among physicians and patients. E-prescriptions are computer generated and sent via computer through secure and private computer connections. The physician is able to create an e-prescription and send it directly to the pharmacy. Often this is completed before the patient leaves the medical office. Not only do e-prescriptions provide a convenience for the patient, but they also eliminate the error factors involved with the interpretation of a handwritten prescription.

Abbreviations Used in Pharmacology

Medical abbreviations are used in pharmacology, but due to the risk of possible errors taking place in the misreading of information, many physicians choose not to use abbreviations in prescription writing and chart documentation. The Joint Commission, an accrediting body for hospitals and organizations, has recently begun to issue a "Do Not Use" list. This list includes all abbreviations that are not acceptable for use due to the high probability of error. Figure 53-7 lists these unacceptable abbreviations. Table 53-11 lists the most

TABLE 53-11 Commonly Used Pharmacology Abbreviations

Abbreviation	Meaning	Abbreviation	Meaning
@	at	DC, disc	discontinue
ā	before	d/c, disc	discontinue
Aa	of each	dil	dilute
Ac	before meals	disp	dispense
ad lib	as desired	dr	dram
alt dieb	alternate days	dtd#	Give this number
alt hor	alternate hours	dx	diagnosis
alt noc	alternate nights	elix	elixir
am, AM	morning	emul	emulsion
amt	amount	et	and
ante	before	ext	extract/external
aq	aqueous (water)	Fe	iron
ba	barium	fl	fluid
bid	twice a day	G	gauge
C	100	G	gram
c̄	with	gal	gallon
cap(s)	capsule(s)	gr	grain

(continued)

TABLE 53-11 (*continued*)

Abbreviation	Meaning	Abbreviation	Meaning
gt	1 drop	qhs	every night
gtt	2 or more drops	R	right
H	hour/hypodermic	Rx	take
IM	intramuscular	$\overline{s}$	without
Inj	injection	Sig.	Label as follows/directions
IV	intravenous	SL	under the tongue
K	potassium	SOB	shortness of breath
kg	kilogram	Sol	solution
L	liter	ss	one-half
liq	liquid	stat	at once/immediately
M ft	make	SubQ	subcutaneous
mcg	microgram	subling	sublingual
mg	milligram	suppos	suppository
mitt#	Give this number	susp	suspension
mL	milliliter	syr	syrup
mm	millimeter	T, tbsp	tablespoon
noct	night	Tab	tablet
non rep	Do not repeat	tid	3 times a day
NPO	Nothing by mouth	tinc, tr	tincture
NS	normal saline	top	apply topically
$\overline{p}$	after	tsp	teaspoon
PR	per rectum	ung	ointment
prn	as needed	UT	under the tongue
pt	pint	ut dict UD	as directed
pulv	powder	wt	weight
q	every		

commonly used abbreviations. Because it is easy to mistake one abbreviation for another, the medical assistant must be very careful to ensure that the abbreviations used are appropriate, correct, and clear. Always use approved abbreviations—never create your own.

SUMMARY

The medical assistant works directly under the supervision and the license of the physician. No matter what kind of medical practice the medical assistant is working in, it is always important to follow all federal, state, and local regulations regarding the administration, dispensing, and inventorying of all medications. You must remember that you are always ethically and legally responsible for all your actions. Consider all aspects of administering a medication, and follow your checklist. Never administer a medication with which you are unfamiliar, and always get clear instructions from the physician.

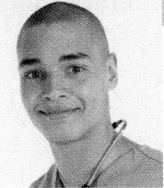

53 CHAPTER REVIEW

COMPETENCY REVIEW

1. Define and spell the terms to learn for this chapter.

2. Name the governmental agency that enforces drug sales and distribution.

3. Name the federal act that controls the use of drugs causing dependency.

4. List the "ten rights" of drug administration.

5. Discuss the "three befores" that must take place before drug administration.

6. Describe what you would do when a patient indicates a drug allergy.

7. Define "logging a narcotic."

8. List the information that must be charted when administering a medication.

9. List the functions of the following medications: diuretic, sedative, anesthetic.

10. A drug may be known by three different names. What are they?

PREPARING FOR THE CERTIFICATION EXAM

1. The generic name for the OTC medication Tylenol is
   a. naproxen sodium
   b. acetaminophen
   c. Naprosyn
   d. Tylenol
   e. Aldomet

2. According to the Drug Enforcement Administration, controlled substances
   a. can be addictive
   b. may have the potential for abuse by a patient
   c. must be kept under lock and key
   d. must be recorded in a narcotics log when dispensed
   e. all of the above

3. An example of a Schedule IV drug is
   a. Xanax
   b. diazepam
   c. vicodin
   d. cocaine
   e. Tylenol with codeine

4. Capoten, which is an ACE inhibitor, is classified as an
   a. antibiotic
   b. anti-inflammatory
   c. antipruritic
   d. antihypertensive
   e. antipyretic

5. Which of the following is a method for the administration of a drug by means of an injection under the skin and fat layers?
   a. intradermal
   b. intramuscular
   c. subcutaneous
   d. intravenous
   e. intrathecal

6. A nonparenteral method of administering drugs would be
   a. inhalation
   b. topical
   c. vaginal
   d. buccal
   e. all of the above

7. The "ten rights" a medical assistant must observe when administering medications include the right medication, the right documentation, and
   a. time
   b. route
   c. dosage
   d. patient
   e. all of the above

8. Which, if any, of the following routes of administration is not used by a medical assistant?
   a. ID
   b. IV
   c. IM
   d. Z-track IM
   e. SC

9. Which part of a prescription precedes the instructions that should be given to the patient?
   a. Sig.
   b. counterscript
   c. superscription
   d. inscription
   e. subscription

10. A common abbreviation, used in pharmacology that means "as needed" is
    a. aa
    b. ac
    c. prn
    d. ante
    e. NS

CRITICAL THINKING

1. Susan knows that there are laws that govern the refilling of diazepam, which is a controlled substance. How do these laws affect Mr. Lehmke?

2. What should Susan do to respond to this medication refill request?

3. After talking with the patient, Dr. Penningworth has approved the request for one refill. What is Susan's next step?

ON THE JOB

Dr. Waring has a solo practice. When she is on vacation, she arranges for Dr. Dumphey to cover her patients. Dr. Dumphey's medical assistant, Theresa, has just received a call from a patient of Dr. Waring. The patient is an elderly woman, with multiple medical problems, who is possibly having a reaction to a medication that Dr. Waring prescribed 2 days ago for bronchitis. Her symptoms include nausea, upset stomach, dizziness, headache, rash on her chest, and extreme exhaustion. Theresa senses that the patient may be exhibiting some disorientation to time and place because it is difficult to elicit consistent responses from her regarding her medications.

The patient reports to Theresa that the newest medication she has been taking is Biaxin. The other medications she takes includes Prinivil, Cardizem CD, Premarin, Prilosec, Robaxin, Zocor, Ambien, Prozac, Fosamax, Seldane, and aspirin. The patient does not know the dosage of any of these medications but is willing to "open up her bag of medicine" and read each prescription label to Theresa. What should Theresa do? What is your response?

1. Does Theresa have an obligation, as Dr. Dumphey's medical assistant, to handle this situation with this patient, or should Dr. Waring simply be notified?
2. Is this an emergency situation or potential emergency situation and, if so, what should Theresa do immediately?
3. Because the patient seems disoriented, should Theresa even trust what the patient is reporting?
4. Should Theresa have the patient read the label of each of her medications?

INTERNET ACTIVITY

To further understand the elements of the *Physicians' Desk Reference,* go online and type "PDR" in the search area.

MEDMEDIA

Additional interactive resources and activities for this chapter can be found:

On your student DVD: View applicable procedure videos on the DVD-ROM found in the back of this book.

MyHealthProfessionsKit.com: Test your knowledge of this chapter with games and activities. MyHealthProfessionsKit also includes resources, helpful links, and a Spanish audio glossary.

Medical Assisting Interactive: Practice your procedures as a medical assistant in this simulated doctor's office. This can be accessed through MyHealthProfessionsKit.com.

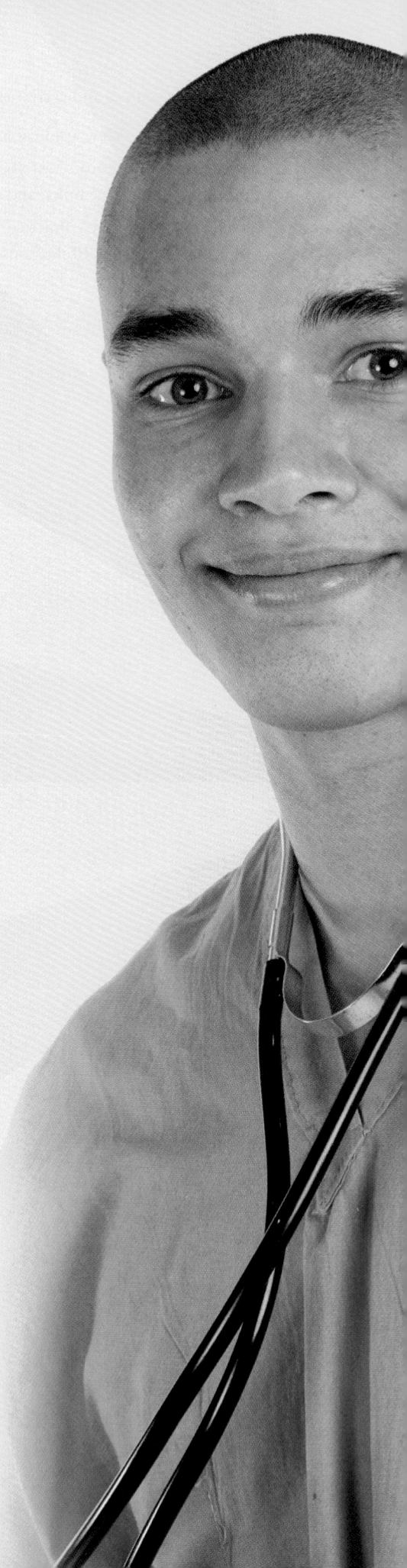

54

Administering Medications

LEARNING OBJECTIVES

After completing this chapter, you should be able to:

- Define and spell the terms to learn for this chapter.
- Correctly describe the procedure for the administration of oral medications.
- Correctly describe the procedure for the administration of parenteral medications.
- List the standard needle lengths and gauges.
- Describe the OSHA standards relating to needlesticks.
- List and define the four sites for intramuscular injections.
- State the rationale for using the Z-track injection method.
- List the precautions used when administering an injection to an infant or small child.

CHAPTER OUTLINE

CASE STUDY

Today, Samra, RMA, is working with Dr. Miller at Pearson Physicians Group. Four-year-old Owen Russiano has been brought by his babysitter for an emergency appointment due to severe nausea and vomiting. Because he is so small, Dr. Miller is concerned that he may be dehydrated. Dr. Miller has ordered medication to be administered stat, via a rectal suppository. Samra is concerned because the boy seems very fearful, and she is worried she will not be able to administer the medication due to the child's behavior.

TERMS TO LEARN

ampules

artificially acquired active immunity

deltoid muscle

diphtheria

dorsogluteal site

hepatitis A

hepatitis B

Hib disease

immunity

immunizations

immunoglobulin

inactivated polio vaccine (IPV)

inhalation medications

Intradermal (ID) injection

intramuscular (IM) injections

liquid medications

measles, mumps, and rubella (MMR) vaccine

oral medication

oral polio vaccine (OPV)

parenteral medication administration

pertussis

pneumococcal vaccine

prefilled cartridge injection systems

subcutaneous injection

tetanus

vaccines

varicella

vastus lateralis muscle

ventrogluteal site

viscosity

Z-track method

CERTIFICATION LINK

CMA (AAMA)

Preparing and administering medications

  Preparing and administering oral and parenteral medications

  Immunizations

RMA

Clinical medical assisting

  Clinical pharmacology

CMAS (AMT)

Not applicable

One of the most important functions of the medical assistant is administering medications. Pharmacology and drug therapy use the skills of physicians, pharmacists, nurses, and medical assistants. The medical assistant's specific role is administering the correct medication to the right patient at the correct dosage, time, and route.

Medication Administration

Medications may be administered orally, topically, vaginally, rectally, by inhalation, and by injection. For all routes of administration, specific procedures must be followed when the medical assistant is ordered to administer a medication. The first step is always to check the order, making sure that you can clearly read the order and that you completely understand what is being ordered. Be sure to review the "three befores" and the "ten rights" discussed in Chapter 53 before proceeding with this chapter. The second step is to ensure that the patient does not have an allergy to the ordered medicine. Third, check the order again, and check the "ten rights." Although this may sound like duplicated effort, this is where mistakes are very often caught, and giving an incorrect medication can be deadly. Medical assistants do not administer medications by intravenous (IV) fluids, nor do they administer chemotherapy drugs or narcotics.

ORAL MEDICATION ADMINISTRATION

Oral medication is swallowed, enters the body through tissues of the gastrointestinal system, and is then rapidly absorbed in the body. These medications can be pills, syrups, or other liquids. The many different types of **liquid medications** include suspensions, emulsions, elixirs, syrups, and solutions. (Medications are also discussed in Chapter 53.) Equipment used for the dispensing of liquid medication includes calibrated cups, spoons,

PROFESSIONALISM

THE LAW

The medical assistant should never give any medication to any patient without a physician order and patient consent. Verbal orders should be written down and read back to the physician, who should sign the order. Always be sure that the "ten rights" and the "three befores" are followed and double-checked.

The medical assistant, and the physician, are liable for all medications that are administered to the patient. Therefore, it is imperative that the medical assistant be familiar with medications prior to administration, and ensure that the calculations for the dosing are correct. NEVER ASSUME ANYTHING relating to medication administration! Do not perform a procedure or give a medication if you are unsure or unfamiliar with it.

It is essential that medication administration be performed strictly by the procedures presented or the facility protocol. This includes good aseptic technique and proper administration. For injections, there is always a potential for infection and inflammation. With any medication, there is a potential for unexpected reactions.

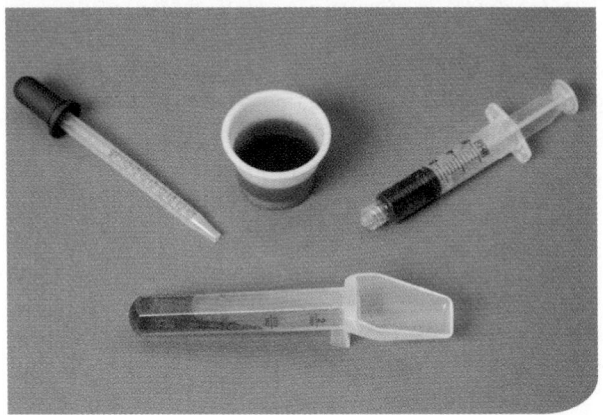

FIGURE 54-1 Calibrated cups, spoons, droppers, and syringes are often used to administer liquid medications.

droppers, and syringes (Figure 54-1). As with any medication, it is important to educate the patient on the proper measurement of these medications. Many liquid medications are prescribed for the pediatric patient due to the ease of administration. Sublingual drugs are held under the tongue, where they are absorbed through the tissues and into the bloodstream for distribution to the body; nitroglycerin is commonly administered this way when it is used for treating the cardiac pain of angina. Buccal medications are placed in the patient's cheek and gum area for distribution through the tissues into the bloodstream. See Procedure 54-1 for administering oral medications. See Procedure 54-2 for administering sublingual or buccal medications.

procedure 54-1

ADMINISTERING ORAL MEDICATIONS
Objective: Administer oral medication.

EQUIPMENT AND SUPPLIES
medication order signed by physician; oral medication; calibrated paper cup or receptacle for medication; water in glass; patient instruction sheet; biohazard waste container; pen

METHOD
1. Assemble equipment.
2. Perform hand hygiene.
3. Select the correct medication using the "three befores." If you are not familiar with the medication, look it up in a reference book, read the package insert, and/or consult the physician.
4. Always double-check the label to make sure the strength is correct since medications are manufactured with different strengths.
5. Correctly calculate the dosage in writing. Double-check your calculations with someone else.
6. Place a medicine cup or container on a flat surface.
7. Gently shake the medication if it is in liquid form.
8. Hold the bottle so that the label is in the palm of your hand to prevent damaging the label with liquid medication.
9. Recheck the label again.
10. Remove the cap from the medicine container and place it upside down on a clean surface. This will keep the

inside of the cap clean, which can then be replaced on the bottle.
11. A. *Liquid medication:* Hold the calibrated medicine cup at eye level and pour the medication into the cup, stopping at the correct dosage line. Pour the medication away from the label side of the bottle. If too much medication is poured into the calibrated cup, do not return it to the bottle. Discard it into a sink.
    B. *Tablet or capsule medication:* Shake out the correct number of tablets or pills into the bottle cap. Then place them in the medicine cup. If you accidentally pour out an extra tablet, do not return it to the medication bottle; discard it.
12. Check the medication again to make sure the dosage is the same as the medication order.
13. Replace the cap on the medication bottle and return the bottle to the storage shelf.
14. Take the prepared medication and a glass of water to the patient.
15. Warmly greet and identify the patient both by stating his or her name and examining any printed identification such as a wrist name band or medical record. Introduce yourself to the patient and ask the patient if he or she has any allergies.
16. Tell the patient the name of the medication and dosage that you are administering per the physician's order. Ask

the patient if he or she has any questions prior to taking the medication.

17. Remain with the patient until the medication has been swallowed.
18. Provide the patient with written follow-up instructions if further medication is to be taken.
19. Chart the medication administration on the correct patient's record, noting the time, medication name,

dosage, route (oral procedure), and your name. After giving the medication to the patient, it is best to have the patient wait in the office for 30 minutes.

CHARTING EXAMPLE

2/14/XX 1:00 P.M. ASA, 500 mg, po, after 30 min. no adverse reactions were noted. · N. Young, RMA

procedure
54-2

ADMINISTERING SUBLINGUAL OR BUCCAL MEDICATION

Objective: Administer a medication to a patient under the tongue or between the cheek and gum.

EQUIPMENT AND SUPPLIES

medication order signed by physician on the patient's medical record; oral medication; paper cup or receptacle for medication; patient instruction sheet; biohazard waste container; pen

METHOD

1. Assemble equipment.
2. Perform hand hygiene.
3. Select the correct medication using the "three befores." If you are not familiar with the medication look it up in a reference book, read the package insert, and/or consult the physician.
4. Always double-check the label to make sure the strength is correct since medications are manufactured with different strengths.
5. Correctly calculate the dosage in writing. Double-check your calculations.
6. Place a medicine cup/container on a flat surface.
7. Shake the tablet ordered into the bottle cap and then into a medication container.
8. Check the dosage again against the medication order.
9. Replace the cap on the medication bottle, and return the bottle to the storage shelf after reading the label again.
10. Introduce yourself and warmly greet and identify the patient, both by stating his or her name and examining any printed identification such as a wrist name band or

medical record. Ask the patient if he or she has any allergies.
11. Tell the patient the name of the medication and dosage that you are administering per the physician's order. Ask the patient if he or she has any questions prior to taking the medication.
12. A. *Sublingual medication:* Have the patient place the tablet under the tongue. Instruct the patient not to swallow until the tablet has dissolved.
    B. *Buccal medication:* Have the patient place the tablet between the cheek and gum area. Instruct the patient not to swallow until the tablet is dissolved.
13. Tell the patient not to take fluids until the tablet is dissolved.
14. Remain with the patient until the medication has dissolved.
15. Provide the patient with written follow-up instructions if further medication is to be taken.
16. Chart the medication administration on the correct patient's record, noting the time, medication name, dosage, route, and your name. After giving the medication to the patient, it is best to have the patient wait in the office for 30 minutes.

CHARTING EXAMPLE

2/14/XX 9:00 A.M. Nitroglycerin tab 1 (gr. 1/100), subling. P = 60. · N. Young, RMA

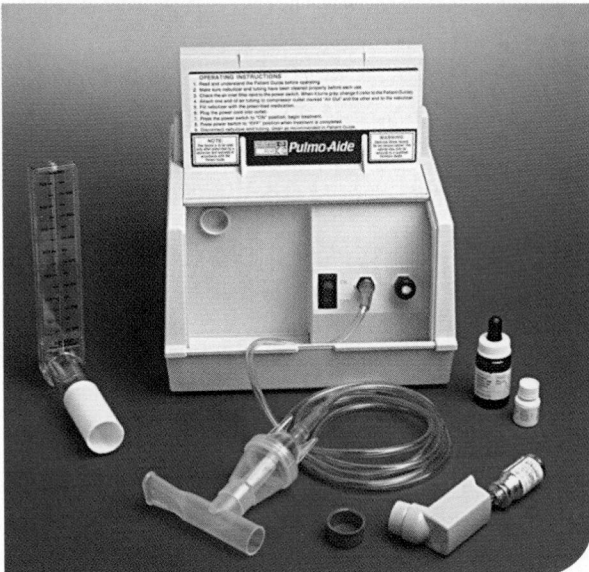

FIGURE 54-2 Equipment used for administering inhalation medications.

INHALATION MEDICATION ADMINISTRATION

Inhalation medications are used for dispensing oral medication into the respiratory tract. The equipment used for this route of administration includes the use of a metered-dose inhaler or a nebulizer (Figure 54-2). When a patient requires this type of medication, the patient may receive the treatment in the office, be sent home with the metered-dose inhaler (MDI), or both. It is the responsibility of the medical assistant to ensure that the patient is trained in the use of the MDI. The patient must clearly understand the use of this equipment prior to taking it home. See Chapter 50 for more information on nebulizers.

TOPICAL MEDICATION ADMINISTRATION

Topical drugs for dermal application and mucosal application come in various forms (Figure 54-3). For skin condi-

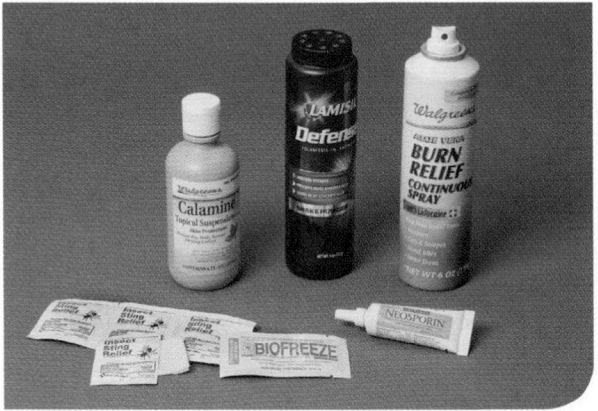

FIGURE 54-3 Topical medications come in a variety of forms.

tions that require treatment, topical drug forms include these:

- Creams and ointments
- Lotions
- Skin patches.

Topical medications that are applied to mucosal membranes include these:

- Eyedrops, eardrops, and nose drops
- Eye ointments
- Vaginal creams
- Rectal and vaginal suppositories
- Sterile douche solutions
- Sublingual or buccal tablets

As with the administration of any form of topical medication, it is important for the medical assistant to wear gloves. When administering ointment to an area, the area should first be cleaned. Once the area has been wiped clean, the ointment should be applied in a thin layer, using either a cotton swab or a tongue depressor. In some instances when a topical drug is applied, the area must then be covered with sterile gauze to keep the area clean. When reapplying ointment to an area, the old remaining ointment should be removed prior to applying a new layer of ointment.

If a patient is to receive a liquid medication such as a lotion or suspension, the bottle should be shaken well and then applied as directed. When administering a liquid medication that is to be sprayed, caution should be taken to ensure that both the patient and the drug administrator do not inhale the spray. See Procedure 54-3 for instruction on administering a rectal or vaginal suppository.

PARENTERAL MEDICATION ADMINISTRATION

Parenteral medication administration means administering a medication through injection. As discussed in Chapter 53, these routes include intramuscular, intravenous, subcutaneous, and intradermal injections. Medication that is given by injection enters the bloodstream more rapidly than medications given by other methods. Parenteral administration allows medication to be targeted to a particular area of the body. For example, a local anesthetic is injected into a specific area on the body. The injection site then becomes numb, allowing the physician to suture the area with no discomfort to the patient.

procedure
54-3

ADMINISTERING A RECTAL OR VAGINAL SUPPOSITORY

Objective: Insert a suppository as ordered by the physician.

EQUIPMENT AND SUPPLIES

medication order signed by physician; lubricant; water; biohazard waste container; patient instructions; vaginal suppository or cream; sterile gloves; sanitary napkin; rectal suppository; nonsterile gloves; 4 × 4 gauze square; pen

METHOD

1. Assemble equipment.
2. Perform hand hygiene.
3. Select the correct medication using the "three befores." If you are not familiar with the medication, look it up in a reference book, read the package insert, consult the physician, or do both.
4. Always double-check the label to validate that the strength is correct since medications are manufactured with different strengths.
5. Correctly calculate the dosage in writing. Double-check your calculations with someone else.
6. Check the dosage again against the medication order.
7. Replace the cap on the medication bottle and return the bottle to the storage shelf or refrigerator after reading the label again.
8. Warmly greet and identify the patient both by stating his or her name and examining any printed identification such as a wrist name band or medical record. Introduce yourself to the patient and ask the patient if he or she has any allergies.
9. Give the patient a gown or sheet. Have the patient remove all clothing from the waist down. Assist the patient as necessary, and provide reassurance as the patient may be uncomfortable with the administration of a suppository.
10. Tell the patient the name of the medication and dosage that you are administering per the physician's order. Ask the patient if he or she has any questions prior to receiving the medication.
11. A. *Rectal suppository:* Have the patient lie on the left side, if possible, with top leg bent. Drape a sheet over the patient. Apply nonsterile gloves. Open the suppository wrapper and place suppository on a gauze square. Moisten the suppository with a small amount of lubricant or water. With one hand separate the buttocks. Pick up the suppository with the other hand. Ask the patient to breathe slowly as you insert the suppository from 1 to $1\frac{1}{2}$ inches through the rectal sphincter. Hold the buttocks together, and instruct the patient not to bear down or push out the suppository. Wipe the anal area with the gauze and discard gauze into a biohazard waste container. Have the patient remain in the side position for about 20 minutes until the suppository melts.

    B. *Vaginal suppository:* Have the patient assume the dorsal recumbent position with legs apart. Drape the patient. Open the sterile glove pack on a flat surface leaving the gloves in place. Use the inside of the glove wrapper as a sterile field. Peel open the suppository container, and drop the suppository on the inside of the glove wrapper. If an applicator is provided, drop it on the sterile surface also. Apply gloves using sterile technique. With one gloved hand, separate the labia minora and hold the folds in place. Using the other hand, insert the suppository one finger length into the vagina. If an applicator is used, place the suppository into the applicator and insert it in a downward direction. Instruct the patient to remain in this position for at least 10 minutes for the suppository to dissolve. Place the applicator into the glove wrapper. Remove one glove by pulling inside out from the cuff. With the remaining gloved hand, roll the contaminated wrapper and contents. Hold these waste items as you remove the remaining glove over them. Dispose of all materials in a biohazard waste container. Give the patient a sanitary napkin.

12. Remain with the patient until the medication has dissolved.
13. Provide the patient with written follow-up instructions if further medication is to be taken.
14. Chart the medication administration on the patient's record noting the time, medication name, dosage, injection site, route, and your name.

CHARTING EXAMPLE

2/26/XX 9:00 A.M. Dulcolax 15 mg. Rectal supp. Patient tolerated medication administration well. · · · M. King, CMA (AAMA)

Equipment Used for Medication Administration

The equipment used for injectable medications includes various types of syringes and needles that are specific to the type of medication and the method of administration. The medical assistant must be familiar with this equipment.

SYRINGES

Understanding the parts of the syringe is necessary so that the device is used correctly. The parts of the syringe include (Figure 54-4) the following:

- **Lumen**—The bore of the hollow needle. The size of the lumen determines the gauge of the needle: the higher the gauge, the smaller the lumen.
- **Shaft**—The actual length of the hollow needle.
- **Hilt**—Connects the shaft to the hub.
- **Hub**—Connects the needle to the syringe.
- **Barrel**—Holds the liquid in the syringe.
- **Flange**—Prevents the needle from rolling on flat surfaces.
- **Plunger**—When pressed, expels medication from the syringe. When pulled, gathers medication into the syringe.

Syringes come in a variety of sizes (Figure 54-5). The smallest syringe is a tuberculin syringe, and the measurements are calibrated in hundredths of a milliliter. Tuberculin syringes are used with 27- or 28-gauge needles to perform tuberculosis (PPD) testing and allergy testing, for which all of the injections are done intradermally (in the skin).

Another type of syringe is the insulin syringe. Units are the measure for insulin administration, which is done with a small needle and injected directly under the skin (subcutaneous). These injections are typically done in the arms, abdomen, or thighs. A 25- or 26-gauge syringe is used for insulin administration.

Larger syringes are calibrated in 2-, 3-, 5-, and 10-mL segments and larger, up to 60 mL. The most commonly used size is the 3-mL syringe, because it is the most accurate with small doses of medication. Most injected doses of medication are less than what the 3-mL syringe can hold. The **viscosity**, or thickness, of the medication being given also determines the gauge of the needle.

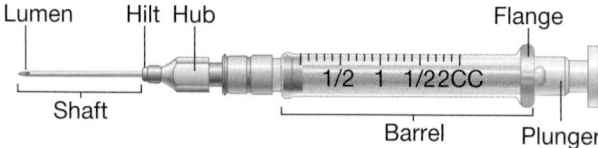

FIGURE 54-4 Parts of a syringe.

NEEDLES

Needles are categorized according to size—both gauge (how large the barrel of the needle is) and length. The larger the size of the needle (lumen), the smaller the gauge. The largest needles available are 14 to 18 gauge and are used only in trauma care. Intravenous (IV) lines are typically placed with 18-, 20- or 22-gauge needles. (IV lines are not a medical assistant responsibility.) Intramuscular injections are usually given with 24- or 25-gauge needles, usually $\frac{5}{8}$ inch to 3 inches long. Subcutaneous injections are given with 25- to 26-gauge needles, whereas intradermal injections are given with 27- to 28-gauge needles. Needle length is very important and varies from $\frac{3}{8}$ inch to 4 inches. The needle length depends on the route used and the area of body to be injected.

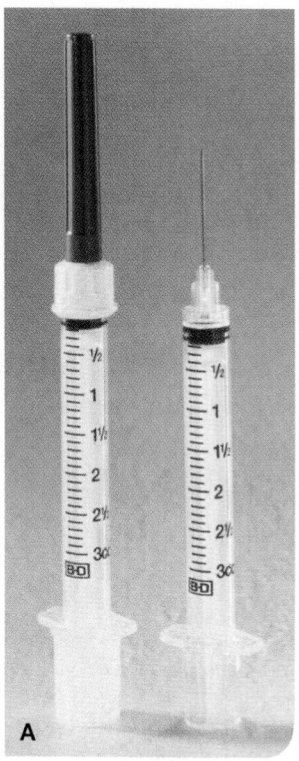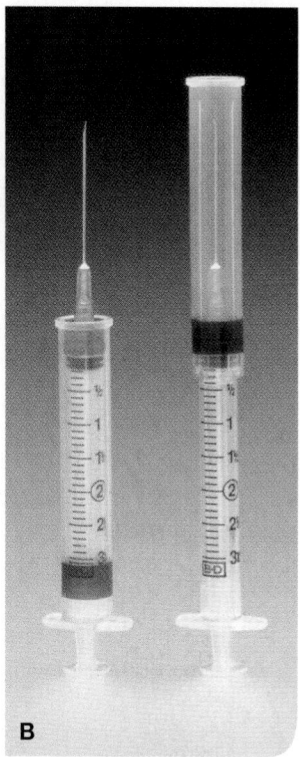

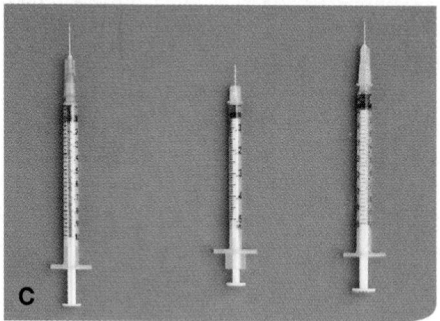

FIGURE 54-5 (A) Med-Saver syringe; (B) Safety-Lok syringe; (C) tuberculin syringes.

Syringes and needles are disposable. There is a puncture-proof sheath or cover on the needle. It is important to check that the sheath is in place any time the medical assistant is changing the needle on a syringe. This prevents needlesticks. *Never handle an unsheathed needle.* Any dirty or used needle should never be handled or recapped (resheathed). After capping the needle, be sure to clean the area with a disinfectant. All needles and syringes should be placed in a red sharps container, needle down as soon as they are used.

As Occupational Safety and Health Administration (OSHA) standards become stricter, more facilities will adapt to using safety needles, where a protective cover can quickly and safely be engaged to protect the user from exposure to a contaminated needle. It is a good idea to practice engaging the safety mechanism on a clean needle to prevent accidents with contaminated ones. Sharps containers are used for disposal of safety needles. No needle should be disposed in any receptacle other than a sharps container.

MEDICATIONS FOR INJECTION

Medications for injection are provided in several forms. The most common forms for injectable medication are single-dose or multiple-dose vials. These are glass vials with rubber stoppers to protect the medications inside. The needle is inserted through the rubber stopper and the correct amount of medication is drawn out. Single-dose vials are meant to be used, as the name implies, one time. Multiple-dose vials are used multiple times, and the stopper is cleaned with rubbing alcohol prior to each use. See Procedure 54-4 and Figure 54-6 for instructions on withdrawing medication from a single-dose or multiple-dose vial.

procedure 54-4

WITHDRAWING MEDICATION FROM SINGLE-DOSE OR MULTIPLE-DOSE VIALS

Objective: Withdraw medication from single-dose and multiple-dose vials.

EQUIPMENT AND SUPPLIES
disposable gloves; biohazard waste container; biohazard sharps container; soap; needle; syringe; alcohol sponge; medication vial; pen

METHOD
1. Check the medication using the "three befores" technique before beginning. Compare the medication vial (bottle) against the physician's order (Figure 54-6A).
2. Select the correct syringe and needle based on the type of medication and location for the injection site.
3. Perform hand hygiene and apply gloves.
4. Roll the medication vial between your hands to mix any medication that has settled on the bottom.
5. Wipe the rubber stopper with an alcohol sponge firmly in a circular motion. Then set the vial on a clean surface while you prepare the syringe (Figure 54-6B).
6. Remove the protective cap from the needle on the syringe. Maintain the sterility of the inner surface of the protective cap since it will be needed to cover the needle again after you have filled the syringe.
7. Withdraw the syringe plunger and allow air to enter the syringe in an amount equal to the amount of medication to be withdrawn. Because the vials are vacuum sealed, this will allow for easier withdrawal of fluid.

8. Turning the vial upside down at eye level and using care not to touch the rubber stopper, insert the needle into the rubber stopper and inject the air into the vial. Be extremely cautious concerning contamination as you enter the multiple-dose bottle.
9. Keeping the upside-down vial at eye level, slowly withdraw the correct amount of fluid medication (Figure 54-6C).
10. While the needle is still in the vial, check to make sure that the dosage is accurate. Any air bubbles in the syringe will give you an inaccurate dose since they take up the space needed for medication. To remove air bubbles, flick your fingers against the side of the syringe until the air bubbles go back into the tip of the syringe (Figure 54-6D).
11. Remove the needle from the vial.
12. If you have accidentally withdrawn too much fluid, discard the excess fluid by shooting it into a sink or waste receptacle. Never return medications to the vial or bottle from which they came.
13. Check the medication vial after you have withdrawn the dosage to make sure you are correct. This is the last step of the "three befores" for checking medications. Also, check to see if the multiple-dose vial should be refrigerated after opening.
14. Remove gloves and perform hand hygiene.

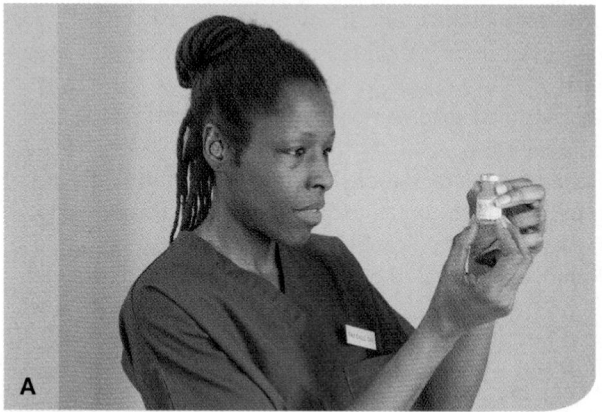
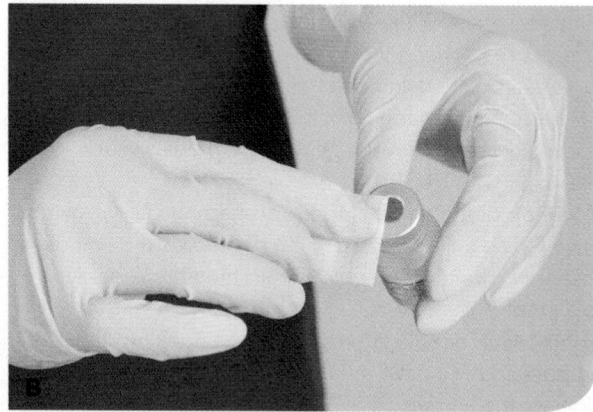
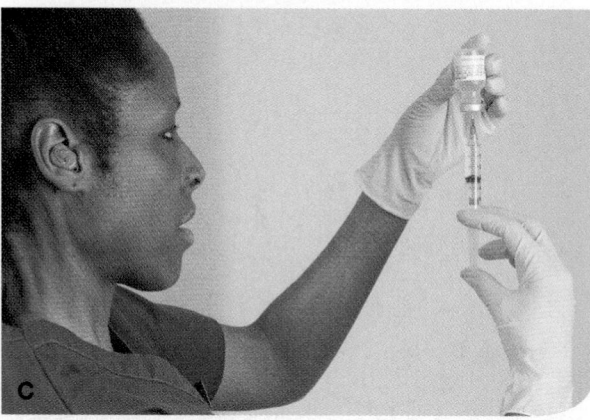
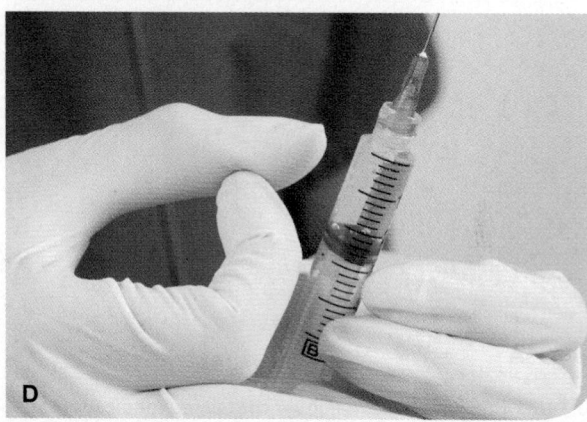

FIGURE 54-6 (A) Read the label on the medication bottle; (B) clean the top of the bottle; (C) with the bottle inverted draw the correct amount of medication into the syringe; (D) remove the needle from the bottle and expel the air or tap out the air bubbles.

Ampules are small, sealed glass bottles containing a single dose of medication. A small indentation in the neck of the ampule designates where to break off the tip to open the container. An alcohol pad or cotton pad must be used to hold the vial to prevent glass cuts when opening ampules (Procedure 54-5 and Figure 54-7).

procedure
54-5

WITHDRAWING MEDICATION FROM AN AMPULE

Objective: Open and withdraw medication from an ampule.

EQUIPMENT AND SUPPLIES

ampule containing medication; soap; alcohol sponge; needle; syringe; disposable gloves; biohazard waste container; pen

METHOD

1. Check the medication against the physician's medication order, following the "three befores."

2. Do not open the ampule until you are ready to withdraw the fluid.

3. Perform hand hygiene and apply gloves.

4. Snap your thumb and middle finger gently against the tip of the ampule to move all the medication away from the neck and into the bottom of the ampule (Figure 54-7A).

5. Clean the neck of the ampule using an alcohol swab.
6. Use gauze between the ampule and thumbs when breaking the ampule. Using one hand to hold the bottom of the vial, and snap the top off with the other hand using a gauze square to prevent a cut when the glass neck breaks (Figure 54-7B).
7. If the top of the ampule does not snap off easily, you may have to use a file to create a cut or "score" the ampule at the neck. The glass ampule should then break easily at this point (Figure 54-7C).
8. Insert a filter needle (attached to a syringe) into the ampule and withdraw the fluid without touching the sides of the ampule.

9. Withdraw all the medication from the ampule. It may be necessary to tip the ampule slightly to withdraw all of the fluid.
10. Discard the broken ampule into a biohazard waste container.
11. Remove the filter needle from the syringe and discard into the sharps container. Place the correct size needle necessary for medication administration.
12. Remove and discard gloves and perform hand hygiene.

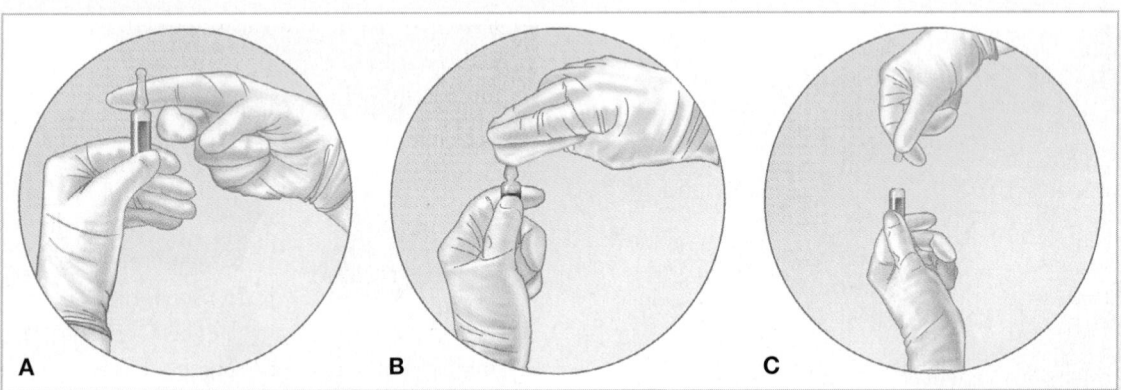

FIGURE 54-7 Breaking a glass ampule containing medication.

Prefilled cartridge injection systems are prefilled, single-dose cartridges that fit into a special cartridge holder. This system is convenient in that medications do not have to be drawn up prior to injections. The cartridge holders are sturdy and long lasting.

Administration Procedures: OSHA Standards

OSHA has established very specific guidelines regarding the disposal of contaminated needles and syringes. The Bloodborne Pathogens Standard has provisions for follow-up procedures for health care workers who are exposed to a needlestick from a contaminated needle.

If a medical assistant is accidentally stuck with a contaminated needle, the physician and medical office manager

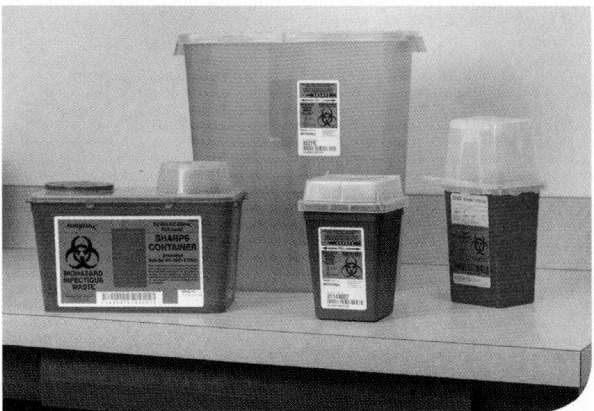

FIGURE 54-8 OSHA regulations require the use of sharps containers to discard used needles.

should be notified immediately. Specific concerns related to a needlestick injury include exposure to human immunodeficiency virus (HIV), which can cause acquired immunodeficiency syndrome (AIDS), and to hepatitis B virus (HBV).

Immediate reporting of needlesticks is important to ensure that testing and prophylactic treatment can be appropriately initiated. The employer is responsible for providing free medical evaluation and treatment for exposure to contaminated sharps or needles while at work. Investigation of the incident is a second reason for early reporting because the employer should begin to seek reasons for the incident. Additional training may be necessary to prevent other injuries in the office.

According to the law, all medical offices must have for the disposal of sharps a puncture-proof, rigid, locked container labeled with an international biohazard sticker (Figure 54-8). Smaller biohazard sharps containers may be placed in all patient examination rooms. When these smaller containers are two-thirds to three-quarters full, they should be closed and placed in a large biohazard container that is in a central location in the office. When the large container is two-thirds to three-quarters full, it should be replaced and disposed of using a waste removal service contracted to incinerate or autoclave the contents. The waste removal service will give the office a document of destruction, which should be kept and filed at the office.

Any time a medical assistant has the potential to come in contact with *any* body fluids—such as saliva, blood, or other substances—standard precautions must be observed and followed. Careful hand hygiene must follow the removal of gloves after such contact. For more on biohazard waste disposal, see Chapter 34.

Charting Medication Administration

Parenteral medications are charted using the same documentation as for oral medications: name of medication, dosage, route, date, site, and signature of person administering the medication. It is a good habit also to chart the manufacturer of a medication, as it is necessary for vaccinations, which will be discussed later in this chapter. Finally, it is also necessary to document that you have provided instructions to the patient regarding follow-up care.

Examples of charting follow:

9/10/XX 9:00 A.M. nitroglycerin, 1 tab, sublingually. Written instructions given to pt. Precautions explained. Told to call office at 1:00 P.M. today to report progress of his condition. · · · · · · · · · · M. Richards, CMA (AAMA)

1/19/XX 11:00 A.M. Monistat-3, 200 mg. Vaginal. Patient tolerated administration. Given written instructions for follow-up care. · · · · · · · · · M. Richards, CMA (AAMA)

10/10/XX 1:00 P.M. Mantoux test, 0.01 mL Tuberculin Purified Protein Derivative, Left forearm, subcutaneous, small wheal noted. Pt. instructed not to rub or cover the area and to return for reading on 10/12/XX. · M. Richards, CMA (AAMA)

Sites for Intramuscular Injections

Intramuscular (IM) injections administer medication directly into muscle tissue and are always given at a 90-degree angle (Figure 54-9). IM injections are given in one of four sites. These sites or muscles are the deltoid, vastus lateralis, dorsogluteal, and ventrogluteal muscles (Figure 54-10).

DELTOID MUSCLE

The **deltoid muscle** is located on the upper outer surface of the upper arm. This site of small muscle mass works well for small-volume injections but not for large ones. Common injections in this site include tetanus boosters in adults. This site should never be used in infants or small children because the size of the muscle is too small.

The deltoid muscle is found by measuring two finger widths below the acromion process of the shoulder. Never give injections in the back of an arm because there are large blood vessels and nerves in this area.

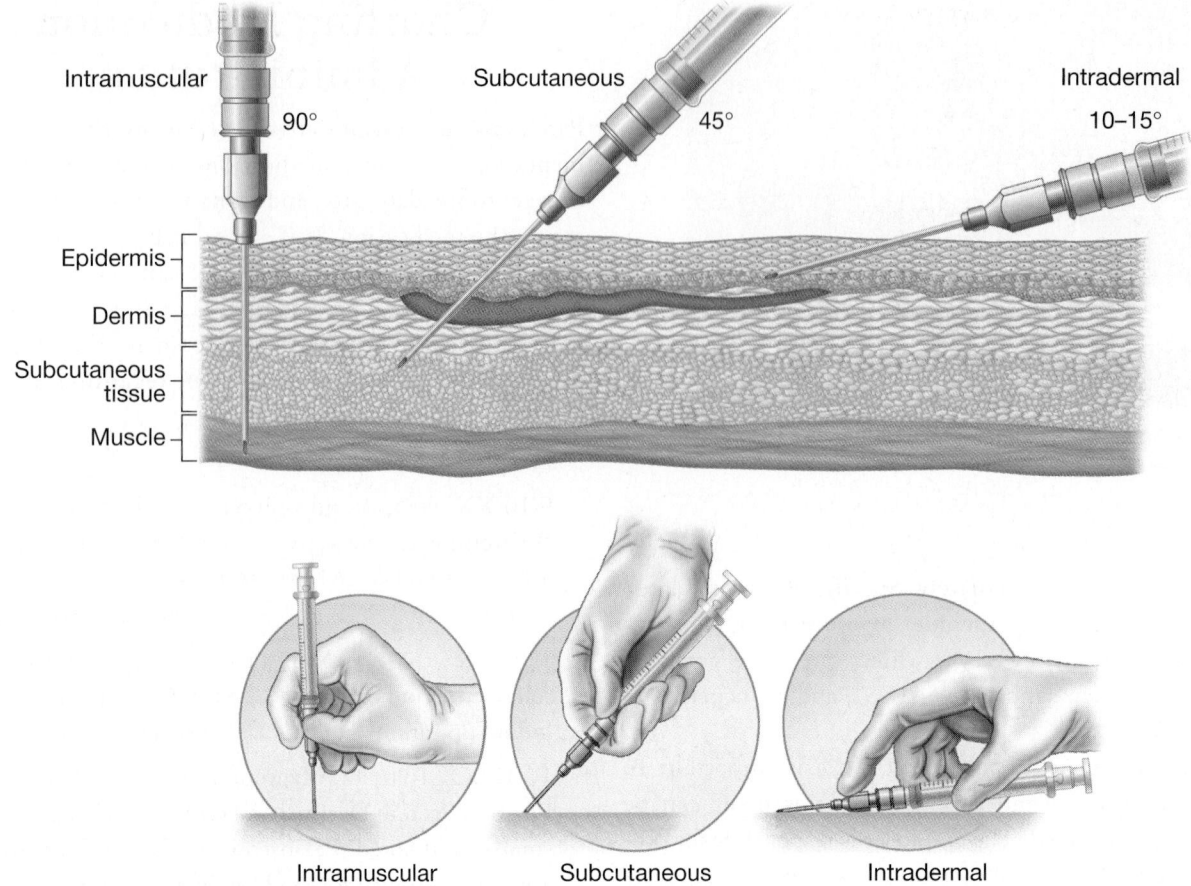

FIGURE 54-9 Angle of insertion for three types of injections.

Use a 23-gauge, 1-inch needle to give injections in the arm. For individuals with small arms, a 25-gauge, $\frac{5}{8}$-inch needle is more appropriate.

VASTUS LATERALIS MUSCLE

The **vastus lateralis muscle** is on the outer portion of the upper thigh and is part of the quadriceps. This site is considered the safest site for IM injections, especially in children or small individuals, because few major blood vessels are in this area. The vastus lateralis muscle lies below the greater trochanter of the femur and within the upper lateral quadrant of the thigh. This muscle is well developed in the infant and recommended by the American Academy of Pediatrics as the preferred injection site for infants and children.

In the adult, the vastus lateralis extends from the middle of the anterior (front) thigh to the middle of the lateral thigh. Typically, it is one handbreadth below the greater trochanter and extends to one handbreadth above the knee. For an injection in this muscle, the patient may be either sitting or lying down (supine).

DORSOGLUTEAL MUSCLE

The **dorsogluteal site** is most commonly used for large-volume, deep IM injections or irritating viscous (thick) medications. It is located on the upper outer quadrant of the buttocks. Antibiotics are often administered with an IM injection. Damage to the sciatic nerve is possible in this area, so this is not the first choice of a site for injections. Landmarks must be carefully observed to ensure proper placement of the injection in this site and to avoid damage to the sciatic nerve.

To give this injection, the patient should be asked to lie prone and point the toes inward. This causes the gluteal muscles to relax. Draw an imaginary line from the greater trochanter of the femur to the posterior superior iliac

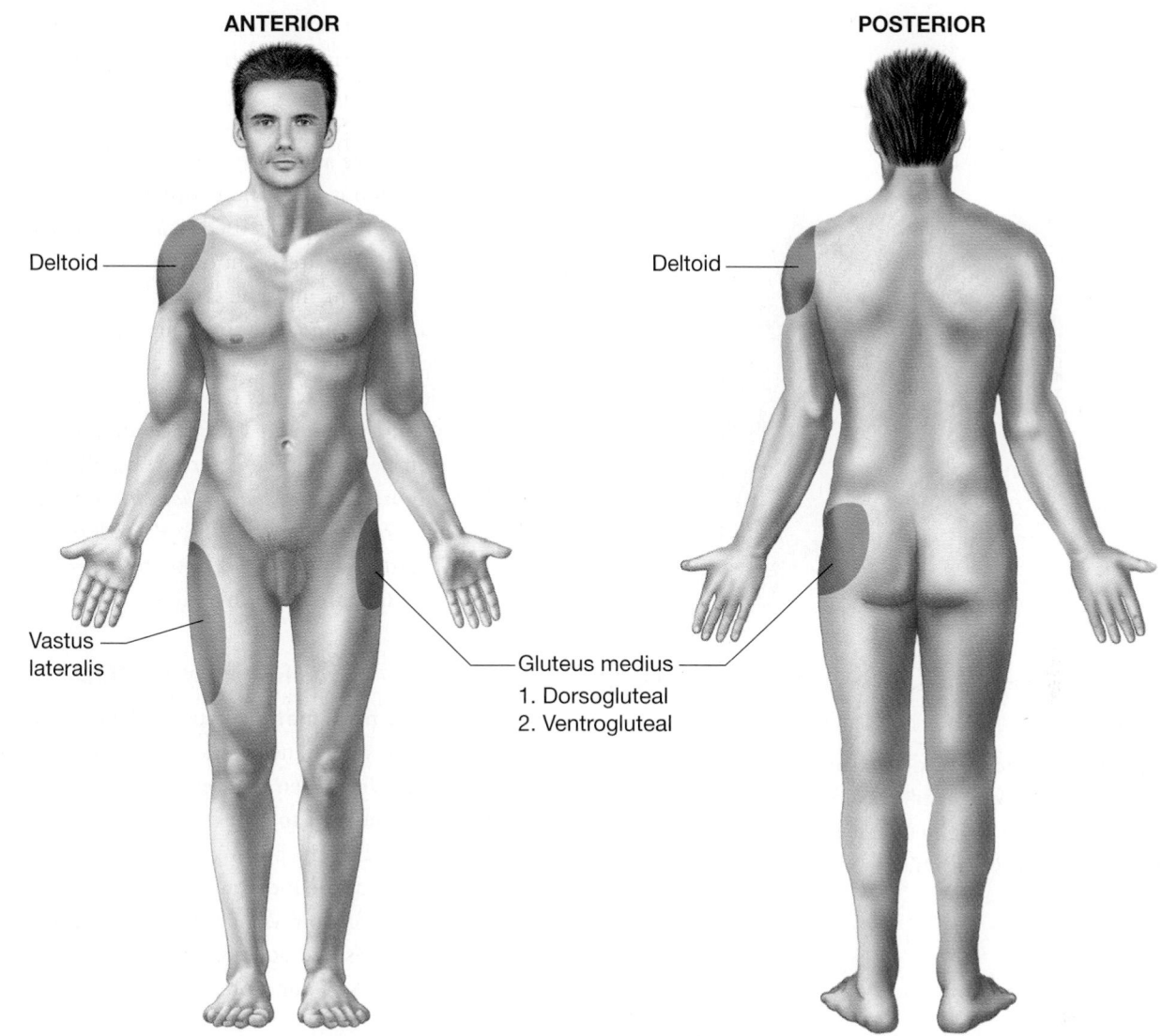

ANTERIOR

Deltoid

Vastus
lateralis

POSTERIOR

Deltoid

Gluteus medius
1. Dorsogluteal
2. Ventrogluteal

FIGURE 54-10 Sites for intramuscular injections.

spine. Give the injection above and lateral to this line. Another method is to divide the buttocks in four equal parts, and give the injection in the upper outer quadrant (Figure 54-11).

VENTROGLUTEAL MUSCLE

The **ventrogluteal site** is considered safer than the dorsogluteal site because there are no major nerves or blood vessels in this muscle. This site is considered safe for infants, children, and adults (Figure 54-12).

To give an IM injection in the patient's left ventrogluteal muscle, place the palm of the right hand on the greater trochanter and the index finger on the superior iliac crest.

Stretch the index finger as far as possible along the iliac crest and then spread the middle finger away from your index finger. The injection is made in the space between the index and middle finger. When using this method to determine the injection location, always use the hand opposite the side of the planned injection on the patient—for example, your left hand and the patient's right gluteus medius.

Subcutaneous Injections

The **subcutaneous injection** is given just under the skin in the fat (adipose) tissue. This method is used for small doses of nonirritating medications such as immunizations,

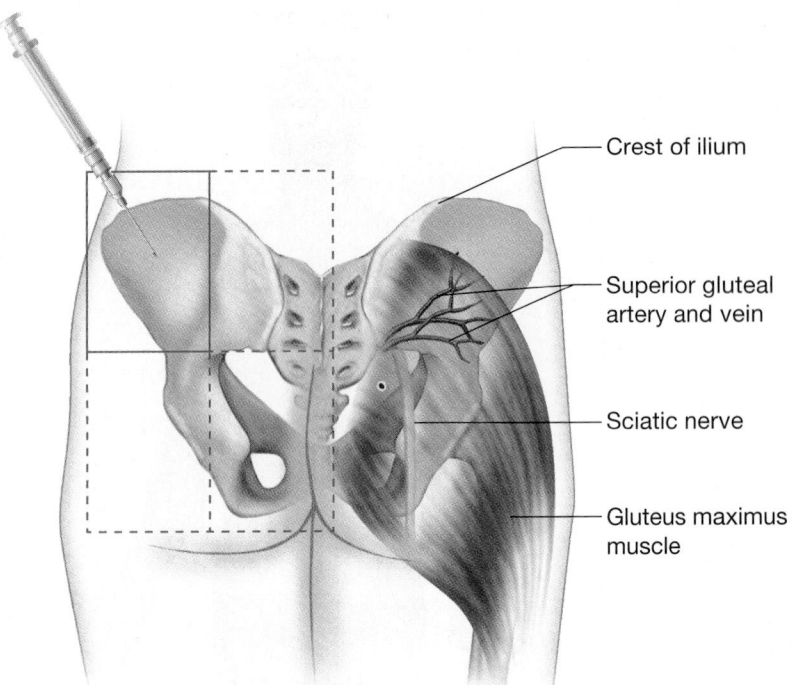

FIGURE 54-11 Injecting the upper outer quadrant of the buttocks.

Crest of ilium

Superior gluteal artery and vein

Sciatic nerve

Gluteus maximus muscle

insulin, and analgesics. The deltoid area is frequently used for these injections, but other areas include the upper back or the abdomen and thighs (when the patient does self-injection, as with insulin). Table 54-1 lists insulin types

Crest of ilium

Injection site

Anterior iliac spine

Head of femur

Greater trochanter of femur

FIGURE 54-12 Injecting the ventrogluteal muscle.

and duration of action. See Figure 54-13 for an illustration of the sites for subcutaneous injections.

The subcutaneous injection is given at a 45-degree angle to the skin surface, unless the injection is heparin or insulin, in which case a 90-degree angle is used. For patients who self-inject, the site of injection must be rotated. The patient must be taught to keep his or her own rotation chart to ensure protection of the skin. (See Figure 54-14 for an example of rotation sites.) Patients receiving allergy injections should remain in the office after their injection per the office protocol, usually 20 or 30 minutes *to ensure that the patient is not having any type of allergic reaction.* See Procedure 54-6 and Figures 54-15 to 54-17 for the steps of administering parenteral injections.

Z-TRACK METHOD

The **Z-track method** is used when a medication is irritating to the subcutaneous tissues or the medication may discolor the skin. When giving a medication using the Z-track method, you need to pull the skin to the side prior to inserting the needle. The pulling of the skin displaces the tissue; then you inject the medication, release the skin, and the medication will not be able to seep back to the skin's surface. See Procedure 54-7 and Figure 54-18 for more on Z-track injections.

Intradermal Injections

The **intradermal (ID) injection** is commonly used for allergy skin testing in which a minute amount of material is injected within the top layer of skin to determine a patient's sensitivity. Common sites to perform an ID injection include the upper chest and upper back, as well as the anterior forearm (Figure 54-19). Because just the top level of skin is entered, a small wheal or bubble that contains the injection fluid appears on the skin. Do not rub the area after giving the injection.

TUBERCULIN SKIN TEST

In addition to allergy skin testing, the tuberculin skin test is also administered intradermally.

TABLE 54-1 Insulin Types and Duration of Action

Insulin Name	Type	Common Name	Action Onset	Action Peak	Action Duration
Crystalline	Rapid action	Regular	1 hour	2–4 hours	6–8 hours
Humulin-N	Intermediate	—	1 hour	4 hours	24 hours
Humulin-R	Rapid	—	15 min	1 hour	6–8 hours
Insulin zinc suspension	Intermediate	Lente	2–4 hours	6–15 hours	24–48 hours
Isophane	Intermediate	NPH	2–4 hours	6–15 hours	24–48 hours
Protamine zinc	Slow action	PZI	3–6 hours	12–20 hours	24–36 hours
Semilentee	Rapid	Regular	1 hour	4–10 hours	12–16 hours
Ultralente	Slow	PZI	8 hours	12–24 hours	36+ hours

A tuberculin skin test is done to see if a patient has ever had tuberculosis. A small amount of TB protein (antigens) is injected under the top layer of skin on the patient's inner forearm. If the person has ever been exposed to the TB bacteria, the skin will react to the antigens by developing a firm red bump at the site within 2 days. The test does not determine if the infection is active or inactive (latent).

The purified protein derivative (PPD) skin test uses a measured amount of TB antigens via an injection that is administered under the top layer of skin on the patient's forearm. A Mantoux test is a good test for a TB infection. It is often used when symptoms, screening, or testing, such as a chest X-ray, show that a person may have TB.

Before administering a tuberculin skin test, the medical assistant should ask the patient the following questions:

1. Have you experienced recent symptoms of TB, such as cough, night sweats, or weight loss for no reason?

2. Have you had a positive tuberculin skin test in the past?

3. Have you had TB in the past?

4. Have you experienced risk factors for TB, such as contact with a person or a health care worker with TB, or have you resided in a country where TB is common?

5. Have you recently been given a TB vaccination?

6. Have you been treated with medicines, such as corticosteroids, that may affect the immune system?

7. Have you been infected with the HIV virus?

8. Do you have a skin rash that may make it hard to read the skin test?

PROFESSIONALISM THE LIFE SPAN

The Child

When giving injections to pediatric patients, it is important to make sure that the patients understand that they are going to be given an injection and that it will hurt for a moment. Never lie to pediatric patients; instead, give them a brief statement such as "I am going to give you some medicine with a shot, and it might hurt for just a minute, but then we will put a bandage on it." Always double-check all pediatric dosage calculations—a slight dosage miscalculation can create significant problems in a pediatric patient.

Never give medications to a pediatric patient without permission from the parent or guardian. Explain why the medication is being given, and be sure that all responsible parties are comfortable with the physician's explanation and have given their signed consent.

The Older Adult

Elderly patients typically take more medications than do younger patients. At every doctor's visit it is important to thoroughly review their medication lists. Include questions about over-the-counter medications. If an elderly patient has difficulty swallowing, be sure that the physician is aware of this so that smaller pills or alternate forms of medication can be prescribed.

Elderly patients often have thinner skin and smaller muscles. So when giving them injections, use a smaller needle and use care not to tear the skin or damage the muscle. Adhesive tape may tear fragile skin, so use gentle pressure on the site, then consider using paper tape if a bandage is needed.

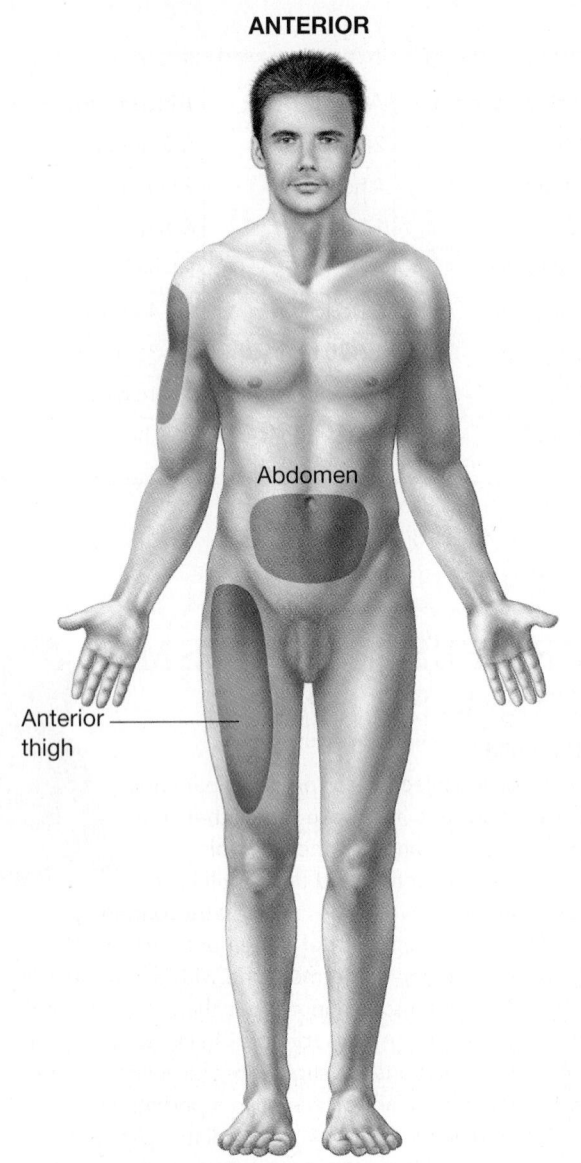

ANTERIOR

Abdomen

Anterior
thigh

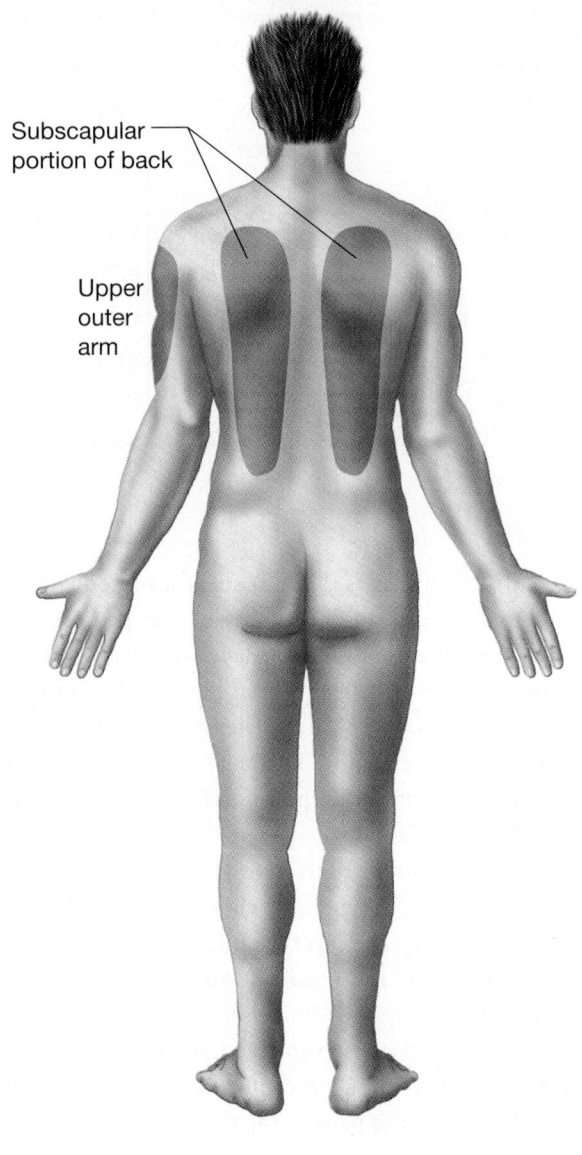

POSTERIOR

Subscapular
portion of back

Upper
outer
arm

FIGURE 54-13 **Sites for subcutaneous injection.**

To perform a tuberculin skin test (Procedure 54-8 and Figure 54-20), ask the patient to sit down and turn up the inner side of his or her forearm. The skin where the test is done should be cleansed and allowed to dry. Using a tuberculin syringe, a small injection of the TB antigen (PPD) is put under the top layer of skin. The fluid makes a wheal under the skin. A circle may be drawn around the test area with a pen. Do not cover the site with a bandage. Tell the patient that some redness at the skin site is expected and that the site may itch but that it is important that it not be scratched because scratching may cause redness or swelling that would make the test difficult to read. Instruct the patient to return to the office within 2 to 3 days after the test to have the skin test checked.

Test Results

Redness alone at the skin test site is a negative reaction. A firm bump is a positive reaction to the skin test. The size of the firm bump (not the red area) should be measured 2 to 3 days after the test to determine the result.

Although the medical assistant is responsible for reporting to the physician abnormal results (or positive results in the case of a TB skin test), interpreting such test results is *not* within the scope of practice for the medical

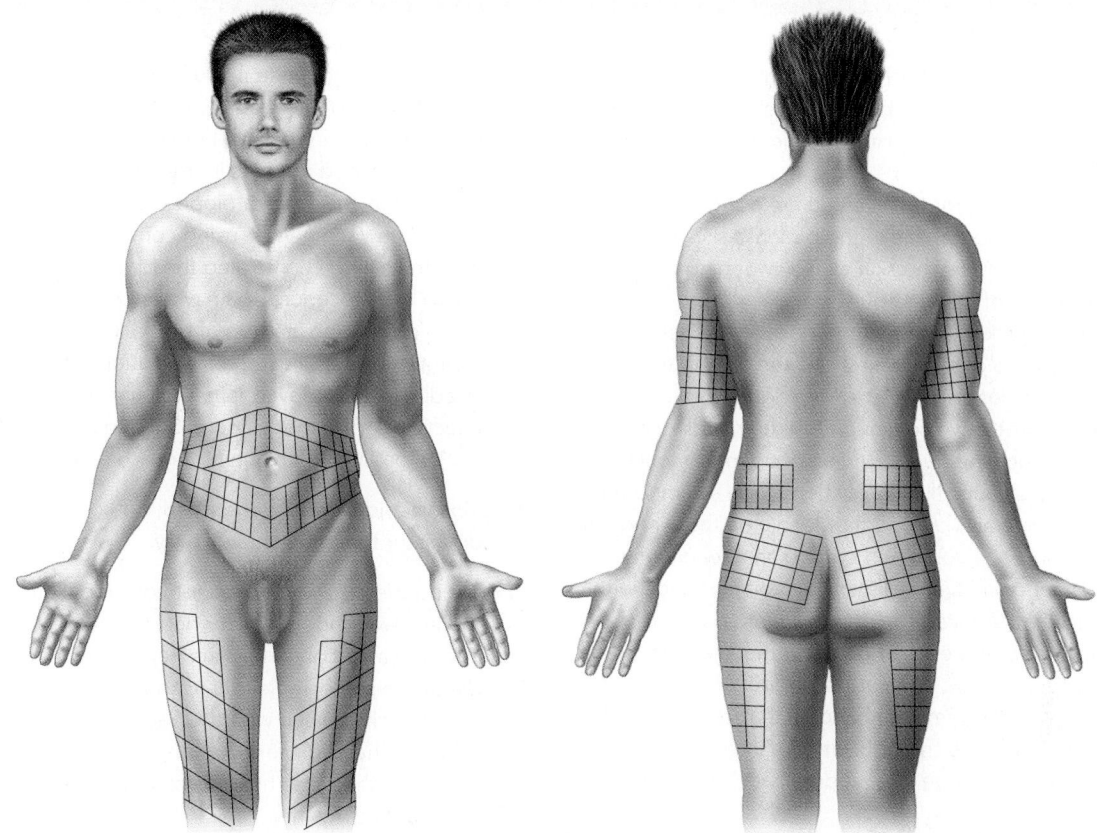

FIGURE 54-14 Rotation sites for administering insulin.

procedure 54-6

ADMINISTERING PARENTERAL SUBCUTANEOUS, OR INTRAMUSCULAR INJECTIONS

Objective: Administer subcutaneous and intramuscular injections.

EQUIPMENT AND SUPPLIES

medication order signed by physician; vial of medication; disposable gloves; alcohol sponges; biohazard sharps container; biohazard waste container

subcutaneous injection: 25-gauge, $\frac{5}{8}$-inch needle for small arm; 23-gauge, 1-inch needle for average arm; disposable 3-mL syringe

intramuscular injection: 22-gauge, $1\frac{1}{2}$-inch needle; disposable 3-mL syringe; pen

METHOD

1. Perform hand hygiene.
2. Apply gloves and follow standard blood and body fluid precautions.
3. Select the correct medication using the "three befores."

Note: Always double-check the label to ensure that the strength is correct since medications are manufactured with different strengths (e.g., 250 mg/mL and 500 mg/mL).

4. Gently roll the medication between your hands to mix any medication that may have settled. Refrigerated medication can be rolled between your hands to warm it slightly.
5. Prepare the syringe using the correct technique. Carefully carry the covered needle and syringe to the patient.
6. Warmly greet and identify the patient both by stating his or her name and examining any printed identification such as a wrist name band or medical record. Introduce yourself to the patient and ask the patient if he or she has any allergies.

7. Tell the patient the name of the medication and dosage that you are administering per the physician's order. Ask the patient if he or she has any questions prior to receiving the medication.

8. Position the patient for the site you are using.

9. Using a circular motion, clean the patient's skin with an alcohol sponge. Wipe the skin with a sweeping motion from the center of the area outward.

10. Once again check the medication dosage against the patient's order to determine if this is the correct time to administer the dose (one of the "ten rights").

11. Remove the protective covering from the needle using care not to touch the needle. If you accidentally touch the needle, excuse yourself to the patient, then return to the preparation area and change the needle on the syringe. If you are using a self-contained syringe and needle unit that does not come apart, discard the entire syringe with the medication and start the process over again.

12. When you are prepared to administer the injection, place a new alcohol sponge or a cotton ball between two fingers of your nondominant hand so that you can easily grasp it when you are through with the injection.

13. Firmly grasp the syringe in your dominant hand like a pencil is held.

14. A. *To administer a subcutaneous injection:* With your nondominant hand, grasp the skin at the injection site and form a small mass of tissue.
B. *To administer an intramuscular injection:* With your nondominant hand, stretch the skin tightly where you will insert the needle.

15. Grasping the syringe in a dartlike fashion, insert the entire needle with one swift movement.

16. A. *For a subcutaneous injection:* Insert into the subcutaneous tissue at a 45-degree angle. (Figure 54-15.)
B. *For an intramuscular injection:* Insert directly into the muscle at a 90-degree angle.

17. Do not move the needle once you have inserted it. If the needle is pushed in farther, contaminants are carried into the skin from the exposed needle.

18. Aspirate to determine if you have entered a blood vessel. To do this, pull back slightly on the plunger with the hand holding the syringe while holding the needle steady in the muscle. If blood appears in the hub area of the syringe, it means that you are in a blood vessel. You will then have to withdraw the needle using correct technique and discard the syringe containing the blood and medication. Begin the procedure again with step 1 and fresh supplies.

19. If you do not see a return of blood in the syringe when you aspirate, slowly inject the medication without moving the needle. Do not move the needle until you have completed injecting all the medication. (See Figures 54-16 and 54-17 for illustrations of intramuscular injections.)

Note: Insert and withdraw the needle quickly to minimize pain but administer the medication slowly.

20. Taking the alcohol sponge (or cotton ball) from between the last two fingers of your nondominant hand, place it over the area containing the needle. Withdraw the needle at the same angle you used for insertion, using care not to stick yourself with the needle.

21. With one hand place the sponge firmly over the injection site. With the other hand discard the needle in a biohazard sharps container.

22. You may gently massage the injection site to assist absorption and ease pain for the patient.

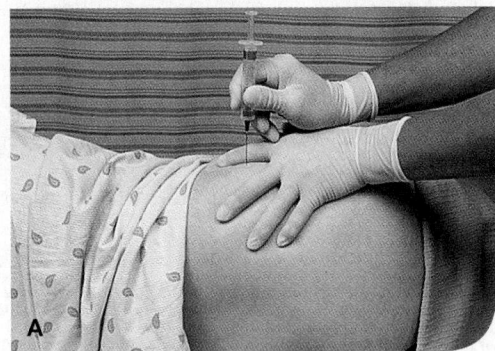

Photographer: Jenny Thomas

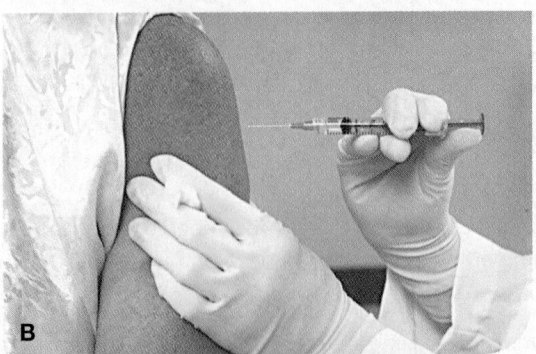

FIGURE 54-15 Subcutaneous injections are administered at a 45-degree angle.

FIGURE 54-16 Intramuscular injection sites: (A) ventrogluteal; (B) deltoid.

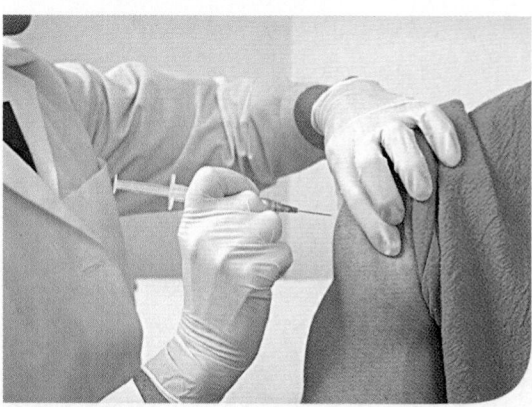

FIGURE 54-17 IM injections are administered at a 90-degree angle.

23. Make sure the patient is safe before leaving him or her unattended. Observe the patient for any untoward effect of the medication for at least 15 minutes.
24. Correctly dispose of all materials.
25. Remove gloves and discard into a biohazard bag. Perform hand hygiene.
26. Chart the medication administration on the patient's record, noting the time, medication name, dosage, injection site, route, lot number on the immunizations, and your name.

CHARTING EXAMPLE
2/14/XX 1:30 P.M. Penicillin G. procaine, 600,000 units IM Right gluteus. Patient tolerated the procedure well. No adverse reactions noted. · · · · · · · · · · · · · · · · · M. King, CMA (AAMA)

procedure
54-7

ADMINISTERING A Z-TRACK INJECTION
Objective: Administer a Z-track injection using proper technique.

EQUIPMENT AND SUPPLIES
alcohol sponges; biohazard sharps container; biohazard waste container; disposable gloves; medication order signed by the physician; pen; sterile needle and syringe; medication vial

METHOD
1–15. Follow steps 1 through 15 of Procedure 54-6 for administration of an intramuscular injection.
16. After withdrawing the medication from the vial, change to a fresh needle. This will eliminate any irritating medication that may be within the needle from coming into contact with the patient's tissue until the needle is placed into the muscle layer (Figure 54-18A).
17. When ready to administer the medication, pull the skin of the buttock to one side and hold it in place with your nondominant hand. You may wish to use a dry gauze sponge if the skin is slippery (Figure 54-18B).
18. With your dominant hand and using a dartlike grip on the syringe, insert the needle up to the hub quickly into the gluteus medius muscle. Do not move the needle once it is in place (Figure 54-18C).

19. While still maintaining a firm hold on the taut skin with your nondominant hand, pull back on the plunger of the syringe to check for blood return with the fingers of the hand holding the syringe. To do this simply move your fingers up the syringe, while keeping the needle steady within the patient's buttocks, until your thumb and index finger reach the top of the plunger. If blood appears in the hub of the syringe, then use the correct technique to withdraw the syringe, discard, and begin with step 1 again.
20. If there is no blood return, then very slowly inject the medication into the muscle.
21. Wait several seconds after injecting the medication before you withdraw the needle. Cover the area with the alcohol sponge, and withdraw the needle at the same angle of insertion. Wait at least 10 seconds before releasing the skin being held by the nondominant hand (Figure 54-18D and 54-18E).
22. Do not massage the area. Observe the patient for at least 15 minutes for any untoward reaction. You may advise the patient to walk around to assist in the absorption process of the medication.
23. Correctly dispose of all materials.

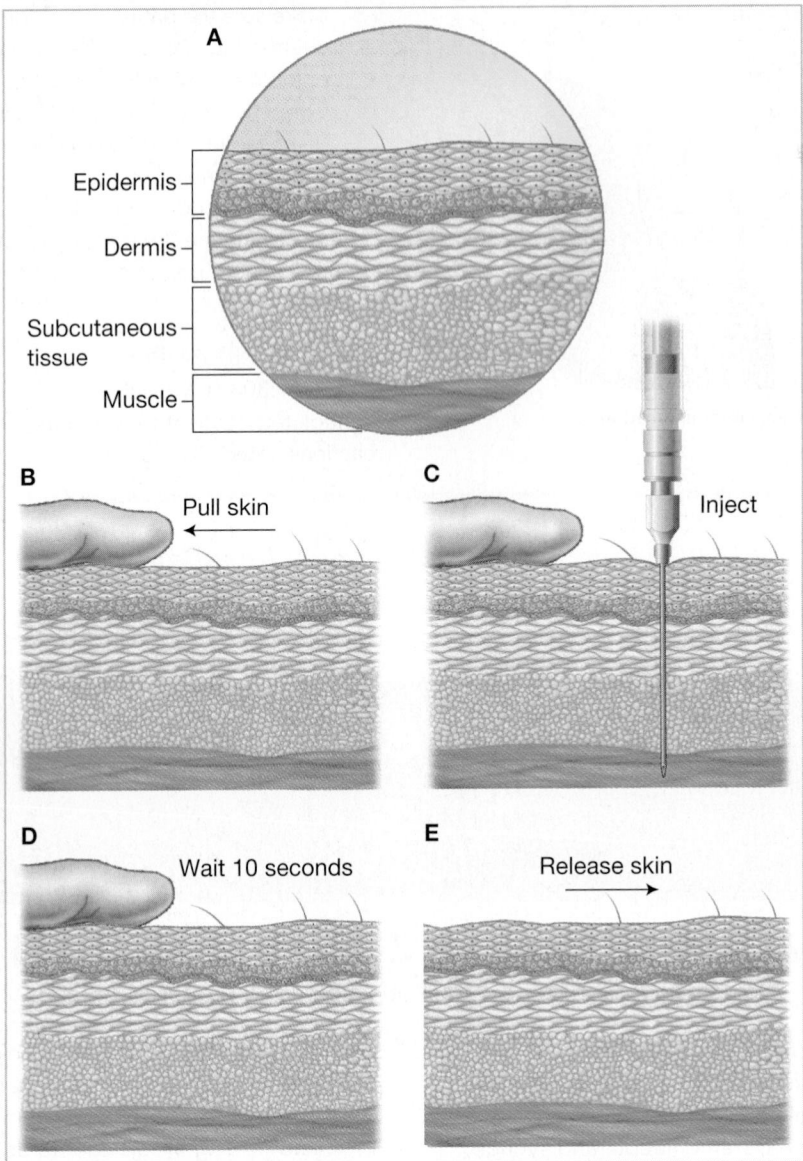

FIGURE 54-18 An example of a Z-track method of injection.

24. Remove and discard gloves and perform hand hygiene.
25. Chart the medication administration on the patient's record noting the time, medication name, dosage, injection site, route, and your name.

CHARTING EXAMPLE

2/14/XX 3:30 P.M. Iron dextran, 50 mg Z-track into left gluteus. No C/O pain and no adverse reactions. · · · · · · · · · N. Young, RMA

---

assistant and, as such, never should be done. The medical assistant is only allowed to report the findings of "positive" or "negative."

Intravenous Therapy

IV therapy utilizes medications or therapeutic solutions that are injected directly into the bloodstream for immediate circulation and use by the body. State practice acts designate which health care professionals can initiate IV fluid therapy and medication administration. Medical assistants must consult their state practices act before attempting any IV procedure. In some states the medical assistant may start IV fluid therapy with advanced training and physician supervision.

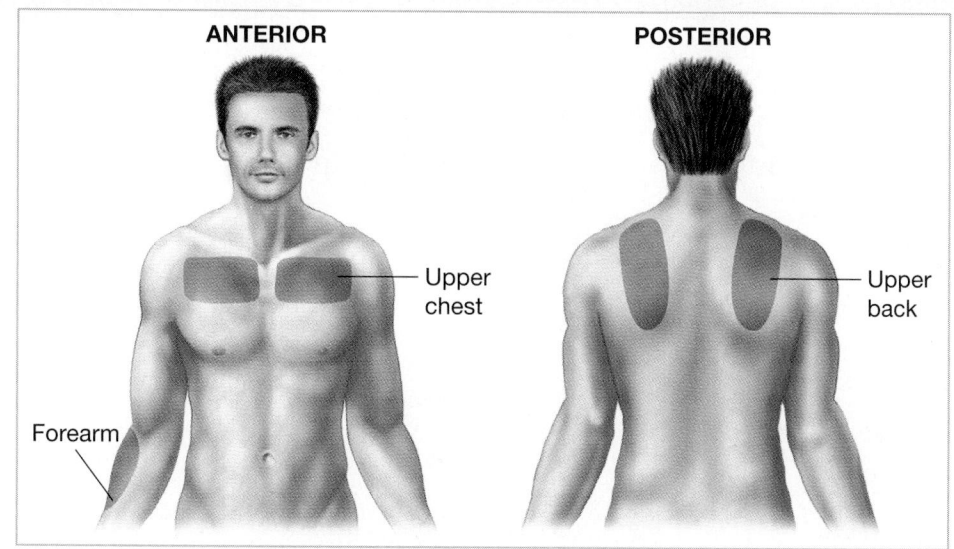

ANTERIOR   POSTERIOR

Upper chest

Forearm

Upper back

FIGURE 54-19   **Intradermal skin injection sites.**

MEDICAL OFFICE SETTINGS AND OUTPATIENT INTRAVENOUS THERAPY

Medical assistants may come into more contact with IV therapy as its use gains more popularity in medical office or outpatient settings. Settings of this nature are only ideal for patients who do not need advanced care and hospital services for close monitoring and treatment of their condition. These settings are becoming more acceptable for a variety of reasons, including the following:

- **Preventing hospital admissions**—Outpatient IV therapy settings allow patients who require IV therapy to receive treatment without being hospitalized. This allows the patient to make scheduled appointments for IV therapy and continue on with their daily regimen without having to be hospitalized for the sole purpose of treatment.

- **Reduction in medical costs**—Utilizing outpatient centers may allow for patients to be discharged earlier from hospitals. This is much more cost effective for both patients without health care insurance as well as insurance companies.

procedure 54-8

ADMINISTERING AN INTRADERMAL INJECTION

Objective: Administer an intradermal injection.

EQUIPMENT AND SUPPLIES

disposable gloves; hazardous waste container; alcohol sponges; sterile needle; sterile syringe; vial of medication; medication order signed by physician; pen

METHOD

I. Preparation

1. Perform hand hygiene.
2. Apply gloves and follow universal blood and body fluid precautions.
3. Select the correct medication using the "three befores." Always double-check the label to make sure the strength is correct because medications are manufactured with different strengths (e.g., 1:10, 1:100, or 1:1000 dilutions).
4. Gently roll the medication between your hands to mix any medication that may have settled. Refrigerated medication can be rolled between your hands to warm it slightly.

5. Prepare the syringe using the correct technique. Carefully carry the covered needle and syringe to the patient.
6. Warmly greet and identify the patient both by stating his or her name and examining any printed identification such as a wrist name band or medical record. Introduce yourself to the patient and ask the patient if he or she has any allergies.
7. Tell the patient the name of the medication and dosage that you are administering per the physician's order. Explain the process of the PPD skin test. Ask the patient if he or she has any questions prior to receiving the medication.
8. Select the proper site (center of forearm, upper chest, or upper back). (See Figure 54-19 for intradermal skin injection sites.)
9. Using a circular motion, clean the patient's skin with an alcohol sponge. Wipe the skin with a sweeping motion from the center of the area outward. This prevents recontamination of the injection site by the alcohol sponge.

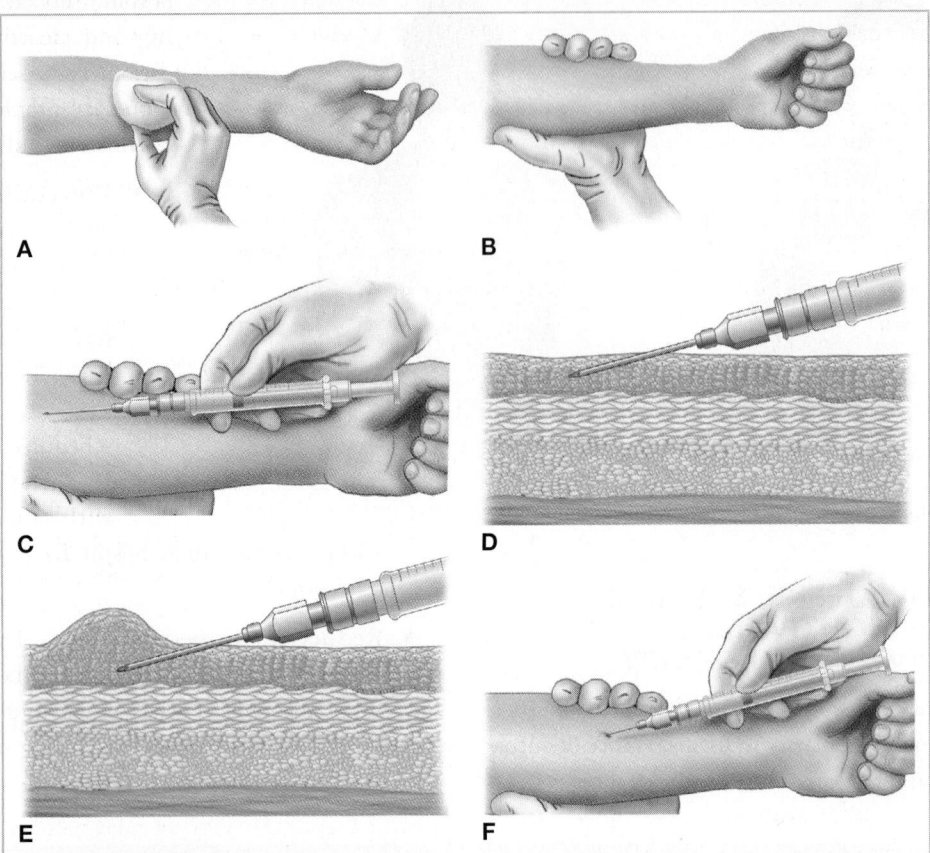

FIGURE 54-20 (A–F) Administering an intradermal skin test.

10. Allow time for the antiseptic on the sponge to dry to reduce the possibility of it reacting with the medication.
11. Check the medication dosage against the patient's order to determine if this is the correct time to administer the dose (one of the "ten rights").
12. Remove the protective covering from the needle using care not to touch the needle. If you accidentally touch the needle, then excuse yourself to the patient. Return to your preparation area and change the needle on the syringe. If you are using a self-contained syringe and needle unit that does not come apart, you will have to discard the entire syringe with the medication and start the process over again.

II. Injection

13. Hold the syringe between the first two fingers and thumb of your dominant hand with the palm down and the bevel of the needle up. Figures 54-20A–F illustrate the steps used to administer an intradermal skin test.
14. Hold the skin taut with the fingers of your nondominant hand. If you are using the center of the forearm, then place the nondominant hand under the patient's arm and pull the skin taut. This will allow the needle to slip into the skin more easily.
15. Using a 15-degree angle, insert the needle through the skin to about $\frac{1}{8}$ inch. The bevel of the needle will be facing upward and covered with skin. The needle will still show through the skin. Do not aspirate.

16. Slowly inject the medication beneath the surface of the skin. A small elevation of skin or wheal will occur where you have injected the medication.
17. Quickly withdraw the needle. With the other hand discard the needle into the biohazard sharps container.

III. Patient Follow-Up

18. Do not massage the area.
19. Make sure the patient is safe before leaving him or her unattended. Observe the patient for any untoward effect, such as an allergic reaction to the medication, for at least 20 to 30 minutes. Tell the patient not to rub the area. Instruct the patient to return to the office within 48 to 72 hours for the reading of the skin test. Make certain that the patient understands the directions and does not have any questions.
20. Correctly dispose of all materials.
21. Remove and discard gloves and perform hand hygiene.
22. Chart the medication administration on the patient's record noting the time, medication name, dosage, injection site, route, appearance of the intradermal site after injection, and your name.

CHARTING EXAMPLE

2/14/XX 10:00 A.M. Mantoux (PPD) tuberculin test, 0.10 mL ID Right anterior forearm. Instructed to return on 2/16 to have test read. · M. King, CMA (AAMA)

- **Patient satisfaction**—Most patients prefer to avoid hospitalization for IV therapy. This allows them more freedom in their schedule and allows them to spend more time with their family. Children who require IV therapy probably would be more comfortable in a non-hospital environment.

INDICATIONS FOR INTRAVENOUS THERAPY

Aside from being a route to administer medication, IV therapy is used for a number of additional indications. Administering blood and blood products, replacing lost fluids and correcting electrolyte imbalances, and aiding in the administration of nutritional supplements are just a few additional reasons that IV therapy is also utilized.

Common Medications Administered via IV Therapy

Some medications that are commonly administered using IV therapy include:

- Chemotherapy medications
- Rheumatoid arthritis medications
- Antibiotics
- Monoclonal antibodies (used to treat inflammatory diseases)
- Analgesics

The IV administration of medications may be *per unit dosage* or may be *continuous*. Examples of unit dosage are bolus, IV push, or scheduled intermittent administration by heparin lock or piggyback medication into an IV port. An example of continuous dosage is an IV drip that may last several hours or around the clock. The flow rate of intravenous lines is regulated by a flow clamp or infusion pump.

Blood Products

Generally, patients who have weakened immune systems require the use of therapeutic blood products, which are administered via IV therapy. These patients are often unable to produce their own antibodies. A common blood product that is utilized is **immunoglobulin**, which contains antibodies.

Patients who have the bleeding disorder hemophilia are lacking clotting factors that are required for proper coagulation. These patients receive clotting factors via intravenous therapy.

KNOWLEDGE RELATING TO INTRAVENOUS THERAPY

IV administration requires extra knowledge and precautions because of the direct access to the bloodstream. Adverse reactions, which can be fatal, may be caused by the specific medication, too many fluids administered too rapidly into the body, violation of any of the medication rights of administration, or certain preexisting medical conditions. Nonfatal reactions include necrosis of tissue (sometimes a reaction to chemotherapy) or swelling or infiltration through the blood vessel into the tissue, obstructing IV flow. Any office in which IV fluid therapy is performed must have emergency equipment, emergency medical access, and established office policies for routine administration, dealing with adverse reactions, and handling emergencies. The patient and the infusion site must be assessed regularly during the infusion for signs of adverse reactions. The following should be reported to the physician immediately: any combination of redness, swelling, heat, bleeding, and loss of feeling at the site of the infusion.

The following information is provided only to acquaint you with the IV therapy process and should not be considered a competency.

Starting an IV requires preparation. Before an IV site is chosen, tubing is selected and connected to the correct solution container, following sterile technique. The tubing is flushed to remove all air. Tape and dressing supplies for the site must also be prepared beforehand. A preparation tray with appropriate IV starter materials and the prepared IV is taken to the patient. The IV solution is hung on an IV pole.

The IV site and the appropriate size and type of catheter are selected. The IV is generally started in the arm, although different medical scenarios may require other sites. The IV catheter includes an outer cannula to thread into the vein and an inner needle to serve as a guide for insertion and then to be removed. A constricting tourniquet is placed above the site. The skin is cleansed, and the catheter is introduced into the vein to obtain an open blood supply. The tourniquet is released and removed. The plastic cannula is advanced into the vein, and the needle is removed. To reduce the patient's anxiety, it is important to mention that the needle has been removed and that only the plastic cannula remains. As soon as the needle is removed and the blood supply has been established, the site is anchored with tape, the IV tubing is connected, and dressing of the site is completed. The IV is regulated with flow clamps or an IV pump as prescribed by the physician. Gloves are worn during the procedure as part of standard precautions. All needles and biohazard materials are disposed according to office policy and OSHA standard precautions.

PREPARING AN INTRAVENOUS TRAY

The most important point about setting up an IV tray is that the medical assistant must have been trained and possess the

procedure
54-9

PREPARING AN INTRAVENOUS TRAY

Objective: Prepare an intravenous (IV) tray.

EQUIPMENT AND SUPPLIES

absorbent disposable sheet; alcohol prep pads; Betadine swabs; disposable tourniquet; IV setup: IV tubing with attached filter; IV catheter; bag of IV fluid labeled with type and patient's name, date, time; paper tape; syringe; port cap; disposable gloves; gauze (2 × 2 or 4 × 4); IV setup tray; IV pole with pump

METHOD

1. Perform hand hygiene.
2. Apply gloves.
3. Prepare IV fluid administration set:
   a. Inspect the fluid bag to make sure it contains desired fluid, that the fluid is clear, and that the bag is free from any leaks and has not expired.
   b. Select the correct administration set (either mini or macro drip) and uncoil the tubing, being careful that the ends of the tubing do not become contaminated.
   c. Close the flow regulator to the fluid bag.
   d. Remove the protective covering from the port of the fluid bag and the protective covering from the spike of the administration set.
   e. Insert the spike of the administration set into the port of the fluid bag with a quick twisting motion, being careful not to puncture yourself.
   f. While holding the fluid bag higher than the drip chamber of the administration set, squeeze the drip chamber once or twice to start the flow of the fluid. Fill the chamber to the marker line. If the chamber is overfilled, quickly lower the bag below the level of the drip chamber and squeeze some of the fluid back into the fluid bag.
   g. Open the flow regulator and allow the fluid to flush all the air from the tubing. A trash can or the wrapper the fluid came in can be used for the overflow of fluid.
   h. Turn off the flow and place the sterile cap back on the end of the administration set (if you had to remove it). Then place this end nearby so it can be easily reached by the person ready to connect it to the IV catheter in the patient's arm.
4. Place the absorbent disposable sheet on the tray.
5. Assemble equipment and supplies on the tray in order of use.
6. If using an IV pole or pump, hang the IV solution (bag) on the pole; do not set it up or calculate drops in the pump; this will be done by the person starting the IV.
7. Notify the appropriate personnel (RN, LVN, physician) that the IV tray setup is ready for administration.
8. Remove and discard gloves and perform hand hygiene.
9. Document the procedure.
10. Clean the work area and equipment according to OSHA guidelines.

---

knowledge necessary to complete such a task (Procedure 54-9). This involves understanding some of the possible side effects that intravenous therapy can cause, such as infections at the site of the needle; phlebitis, which is inflammation of the vein; and the most common side effect, infusion. An infusion occurs when the tip of the IV catheter withdraws from the vein or pokes through the vein into surrounding tissue, or when the vein's wall becomes permeable and leaks fluid. Infusion is frequently encountered with peripheral IVs, and almost always requires replacement of the IV at a different location. Other possible reactions that may occur during IV therapy include blood or drainage from the area of insertion; redness, pain, or swelling in the area; blood backing up into the tubing, and the needle or tube coming loose or being removed by the patient.

Prior to preparing the IV tray, the medical assistant should make sure he or she carefully reads the facility's requirements for this procedure. Instructions for this procedure are frequently located in the office or hospital procedure manual. Once this has been completed, it is important to make sure that you check the doctor's order as to what IV fluid solution is required. When checking the order, remember to check for the following:

- It is the right patient.
- It is the right solution.
- It is the right drug.
- It is the right technique.
- It is the right route.

- The solution is properly labeled with the patient's name, the date and time of administration, and the name of the doctor who ordered it.

Once you have determined that you have the right solution, you will have to prepare the IV administration set. Most facilities have disposable IV administration sets that are ready for use. After you have completed setting up the IV administration set along with your other supplies, they should all be placed on a separate IV or Mayo tray. Make sure you position the items in the order of their usage. Finally, after you have completed the tray setup, notify whoever is going to start the IV that the tray is ready for the patient.

THE MEDICAL ASSISTANT'S ROLE IN INTRAVENOUS THERAPY

Your role as a medical assistant often includes not only setting up the IV tray but also being available to provide the patient with reassurance during the procedure. It also includes making sure that after the procedure has been completed, the patient and the area have been cleaned and that the equipment and supplies have been properly disposed. Most facilities require only that you document the procedure for setting up the tray. Documentation of the actual IV is done only by the person who has started the IV infusion.

Immunizations

Immunizations or **vaccines** are given to humans to decrease the susceptibility to disease. By becoming immunized the human body can resist the invasion of germs that can cause disease to develop. If an individual's immune system is compromised, then the individual is more at risk of becoming sick.

Antibodies are protein substances produced by lymphocytes in the spleen, lymph nodes and tissue, and bone marrow. Antibodies respond offensively to antigens or foreign substances. This process occurs when an individual develops an illness, such as the measles. During the illness, the body begins to develop antibodies to fight off the disease. After the individual has recovered from the measles, the individual is less likely to contract the same strain of measles due to the fact that the body has developed antibodies to fight off the cause of this disease. When this occurs the individual is said to have developed **immunity**, or a resistance, to the disease.

Immunity can be either genetic or acquired. Antibodies are not involved when genetic immunity occurs. Acquired immunity, however, does involve the development of antibodies. This type of immunity may be either natural or artificial and may be acquired either through an active or passive means.

Artificially acquired active immunity develops in response to receiving vaccinations with inactive (dead) or attenuated (weakened) organisms. Through the delivery of immunizations and vaccines, an individual's body can be prepared to fight off a disease. For instance, the flu vaccine is given each year right before the flu season begins. Individuals who are more susceptible to contracting the flu, such as elderly adults, receive the flu vaccine. By receiving the flu vaccine, individuals are establishing immunity to the flu within their bodies and are increasing their chances of being able to fight of the disease. Each year the Centers for Disease Control and Prevention (CDC) recommends that certain individuals receive the influenza vaccination. These individuals usually include the following:

- Children aged 6 months up to their 19th birthday
- Pregnant women
- People 50 years of age and older
- People of any age with certain chronic medical conditions
- People who live in nursing homes and other long-term care facilities
- People who live with or care for those at high risk for complications from flu, including:
  a. Health care workers
  b. Household contacts of persons at high risk for complications from the flu
  c. Household contacts and out-of-home caregivers of children less than 6 months of age (these children are too young to be vaccinated)

Immunizations or vaccines are produced by taking a dead infectious agent of a disease and injecting it into the human body. Typically this creates no harm to the patient. Sometimes, an immunization or vaccine can cause an individual to experience some mild symptoms of the disease or to develop feverlike symptoms at the site of injection. For example, some children after receiving the diphtheria, tetanus, and pertussis vaccine (DTaP) will experience some redness and swelling where the injection was given. A fever may also be a temporary symptom. (To learn more about the immune system refer to Chapter 28.)

CHILDHOOD AND ADOLESCENT IMMUNIZATIONS

An annual recommended childhood and adolescent immunization schedule is issued each year by the American Academy of Pediatrics, the Advisory Committee on Immunization Practices of the CDC, and the American Academy of Family Physicians. The schedule indicates the recommended

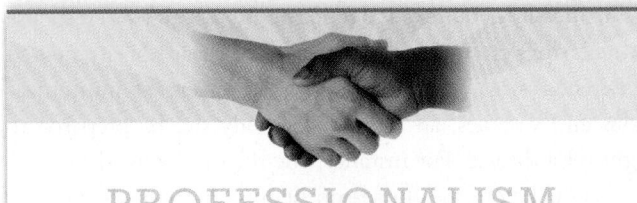
ages for routine administration of childhood vaccines (Figure 54-21). In addition, the CDC provides vaccine information sheets (VIS) that are to be given to parents or guardians prior to the administration of a vaccine to a child. The parent or guardian is generally required to sign a statement acknowledging receipt of the VIS and consenting to the immunization administration. Figure 54-22 provides a sample VIS for the varicella vaccine discussed later in this chapter.

Diphtheria Vaccine

Diphtheria is an acute infectious disease. Transmission of diphtheria is by direct and indirect contact and is diagnosed

by obtaining a throat culture. Individuals with diphtheria typically experience symptoms such as headache, fever, and sore throat. Diphtheria is treatable but can be quite serious. The vaccine for diphtheria is given to children in five separate doses. The fifth dose is given between the age of 4 and 6 years.

Pertussis Vaccine

Pertussis, also known as whooping cough, is a respiratory disease that is most common in children under the age of 4 years. It is known as whooping cough due to one of the symptoms being a violent cough with a whooping sound. Pertussis is caused by bacteria and is transmitted by direct and indirect contact. Once a child is immunized with the pertussis vaccine the child is no longer susceptible to contracting this disease.

Tetanus Vaccine

Tetanus is a disease of the nervous system and is caused by a bacterium that enters the body through a break in the skin. Individuals with tetanus may experience fever, elevated blood pressure, and severe muscle spasms. Tetanus is not contagious and rarely occurs in individuals living in the United States. Occurrence of death with tetanus is low but can occur in people over the age of 60.

DTaP Vaccine. When children receive a vaccine for tetanus, it is usually given in a combination vaccine of diphtheria, tetanus, and pertussis also known as the DTaP vaccine. Five DTaP shots are required to fully protect a child. The last booster is given between the ages of 4 and 6 years. If a child has a reaction to the first dose of DTaP, the child will then, depending on age, be given the tetanus and diphtheria (Td) vaccine or the diphtheria and tetanus toxoids (DT) vaccine. The Td vaccine does not contain pertussis vaccine and contains less diphtheria toxoid than what is contained in the DTaP vaccine. The DT vaccine, which contains diphtheria and tetanus toxoids but no pertussis, may be given to children who have a reaction to their first dose of the DTaP vaccine. The Td vaccine is given to children 7 years and older, and the DT vaccine is given to children under the age of 7.

Haemophilus Influenzae Type B (Hib) Conjugate Vaccine

Although the **Hib disease** is not well known, a recent statistic from the CDC indicated that 1 out of every 200 children in the United States under the age of 5 years contracts Hib. Meningitis, which is a result of Hib, affects about 12,000 children a year. Hib is caused by a bacterium, is spread through the air, and enters the lungs or

Recommended Immunization Schedule for Persons Aged 0 Through 6 Years—United States • 2009

For those who fall behind or start late, see the catch-up schedule

Vaccine ▼ Age ▶	Birth	1 month	2 months	4 months	6 months	12 months	15 months	18 months	19–23 months	2–3 years	4–6 years	
Hepatitis B[1]	HepB	HepB	*see footnote 1*		HepB							Range of recommended ages
Rotavirus[2]			RV	RV	RV[2]							
Diphtheria, Tetanus, Pertussis[3]			DTaP	DTaP	DTaP	*see footnote 3*	DTaP				DTaP	
Haemophilus influenzae type b[4]			Hib	Hib	Hib[4]	Hib						
Pneumococcal[5]			PCV	PCV	PCV	PCV				PPSV		Certain high-risk groups
Inactivated Poliovirus			IPV	IPV		IPV					IPV	
Influenza[6]						Influenza (Yearly)						
Measles, Mumps, Rubella[7]						MMR		*see footnote 7*			MMR	
Varicella[8]						Varicella		*see footnote 8*			Varicella	
Hepatitis A[9]						HepA (2 doses)				HepA Series		
Meningococcal[10]										MCV		

This schedule indicates the recommended ages for routine administration of currently licensed vaccines, as of December 1, 2008, for children aged 0 through 6 years. Any dose not administered at the recommended age should be administered at a subsequent visit, when indicated and feasible. Licensed combination vaccines may be used whenever any component of the combination is indicated and other components are not contraindicated and if approved by the Food and Drug Administration for that dose of the series. Providers should consult the relevant Advisory Committee on Immunization Practices statement for detailed recommendations, including high-risk conditions: http://www.cdc.gov/vaccines/pubs/acip-list.htm. Clinically significant adverse events that follow immunization should be reported to the Vaccine Adverse Event Reporting System (VAERS). Guidance about how to obtain and complete a VAERS form is available at http://www.vaers.hhs.gov or by telephone, 800-822-7967.

1. Hepatitis B vaccine (HepB). *(Minimum age: birth)*

At birth:

- Administer monovalent HepB to all newborns before hospital discharge.
- If mother is hepatitis B surface antigen (HBsAg)-positive, administer HepB and 0.5 mL of hepatitis B immune globulin (HBIG) within 12 hours of birth.
- If mother's HBsAg status is unknown, administer HepB within 12 hours of birth. Determine mother's HBsAg status as soon as possible and, if HBsAg-positive, administer HBIG (no later than age 1 week).

After the birth dose:

- The HepB series should be completed with either monovalent HepB or a combination vaccine containing HepB. The second dose should be administered at age 1 or 2 months. The final dose should be administered no earlier than age 24 weeks.
- Infants born to HBsAg-positive mothers should be tested for HBsAg and antibody to HBsAg (anti-HBs) after completion of at least 3 doses of the HepB series, at age 9 through 18 months (generally at the next well-child visit).

4-month dose:

- Administration of 4 doses of HepB to infants is permissible when combination vaccines containing HepB are administered after the birth dose.

2. Rotavirus vaccine (RV). *(Minimum age: 6 weeks)*

- Administer the first dose at age 6 through 14 weeks (maximum age: 14 weeks 6 days). Vaccination should not be initiated for infants aged 15 weeks or older (i.e., 15 weeks 0 days or older).
- Administer the final dose in the series by age 8 months 0 days.
- If Rotarix® is administered at ages 2 and 4 months, a dose at 6 months is not indicated.

3. Diphtheria and tetanus toxoids and acellular pertussis vaccine (DTaP). *(Minimum age: 6 weeks)*

- The fourth dose may be administered as early as age 12 months, provided at least 6 months have elapsed since the third dose.
- Administer the final dose in the series at age 4 through 6 years.

4. *Haemophilus influenzae* type b conjugate vaccine (Hib). *(Minimum age: 6 weeks)*

- If PRP-OMP (PedvaxHIB® or Comvax® [HepB-Hib]) is administered at ages 2 and 4 months, a dose at age 6 months is not indicated.
- TriHiBit® (DTaP/Hib) should not be used for doses at ages 2, 4, or 6 months but can be used as the final dose in children aged 12 months or older.

5. Pneumococcal vaccine. *(Minimum age: 6 weeks for pneumococcal conjugate vaccine [PCV]; 2 years for pneumococcal polysaccharide vaccine [PPSV])*

- PCV is recommended for all children aged younger than 5 years. Administer 1 dose of PCV to all healthy children aged 24 through 59 months who are not completely vaccinated for their age.

- Administer PPSV to children aged 2 years or older with certain underlying medical conditions (see *MMWR* 2000;49[No. RR-9]), including a cochlear implant.

6. Influenza vaccine. *(Minimum age: 6 months for trivalent inactivated influenza vaccine [TIV]; 2 years for live, attenuated influenza vaccine [LAIV])*

- Administer annually to children aged 6 months through 18 years.
- For healthy nonpregnant persons (i.e., those who do not have underlying medical conditions that predispose them to influenza complications) aged 2 through 49 years, either LAIV or TIV may be used.
- Children receiving TIV should receive 0.25 mL if aged 6 through 35 months or 0.5 mL if aged 3 years or older.
- Administer 2 doses (separated by at least 4 weeks) to children aged younger than 9 years who are receiving influenza vaccine for the first time or who were vaccinated for the first time during the previous influenza season but only received 1 dose.

7. Measles, mumps, and rubella vaccine (MMR). *(Minimum age: 12 months)*

- Administer the second dose at age 4 through 6 years. However, the second dose may be administered before age 4, provided at least 28 days have elapsed since the first dose.

8. Varicella vaccine. *(Minimum age: 12 months)*

- Administer the second dose at age 4 through 6 years. However, the second dose may be administered before age 4, provided at least 3 months have elapsed since the first dose.
- For children aged 12 months through 12 years the minimum interval between doses is 3 months. However, if the second dose was administered at least 28 days after the first dose, it can be accepted as valid.

9. Hepatitis A vaccine (HepA). *(Minimum age: 12 months)*

- Administer to all children aged 1 year (i.e., aged 12 through 23 months). Administer 2 doses at least 6 months apart.
- Children not fully vaccinated by age 2 years can be vaccinated at subsequent visits.
- HepA also is recommended for children older than 1 year who live in areas where vaccination programs target older children or who are at increased risk of infection. See *MMWR* 2006;55(No. RR-7).

10. Meningococcal vaccine. *(Minimum age: 2 years for meningococcal conjugate vaccine [MCV] and for meningococcal polysaccharide vaccine [MPSV])*

- Administer MCV to children aged 2 through 10 years with terminal complement component deficiency, anatomic or functional asplenia, and certain other high-risk groups. See *MMWR* 2005;54(No. RR-7).
- Persons who received MPSV 3 or more years previously and who remain at increased risk for meningococcal disease should be revaccinated with MCV.

The Recommended Immunization Schedules for Persons Aged 0 Through 18 Years are approved by the Advisory Committee on Immunization Practices (www.cdc.gov/vaccines/recs/acip), the American Academy of Pediatrics (http://www.aap.org), and the American Academy of Family Physicians (http://www.aafp.org).

DEPARTMENT OF HEALTH AND HUMAN SERVICES • CENTERS FOR DISEASE CONTROL AND PREVENTION

CS103164

FIGURE 54-21 Recommended childhood and adolescent immunization schedule, 2009.

Source: http://www.cdc.gov/vaccines/recs/schedules/downloads/child/2009/09_0-6yrs_schedule_bw.pdf.

CHICKENPOX VACCINE

WHAT YOU NEED TO KNOW

Many Vaccine Information Statements are available in Spanish and other languages. See www.immunize.org/vis.

1 Why get vaccinated?

Chickenpox (also called varicella) is a common childhood disease. It is usually mild, but it can be serious, especially in young infants and adults.

- It causes a rash, itching, fever, and tiredness.

- It can lead to severe skin infection, scars, pneumonia, brain damage, or death.

- The chickenpox virus can be spread from person to person through the air, or by contact with fluid from chickenpox blisters.

- A person who has had chickenpox can get a painful rash called shingles years later.

- Before the vaccine, about 11,000 people were hospitalized for chickenpox each year in the United States.

- Before the vaccine, about 100 people died each year as a result of chickenpox in the United States.

Chickenpox vaccine can prevent chickenpox.

Most people who get chickenpox vaccine will not get chickenpox. But if someone who has been vaccinated does get chickenpox, it is usually very mild. They will have fewer blisters, are less likely to have a fever, and will recover faster.

2 Who should get chickenpox vaccine and when?

Routine

Children who have never had chickenpox should get 2 doses of chickenpox vaccine at these ages:

  1st Dose: 12-15 months of age

  2nd Dose: 4-6 years of age (may be given earlier, if at least 3 months after the 1st dose)

People 13 years of age and older (who have never had chickenpox or received chickenpox vaccine) should get two doses at least 28 days apart.

Chickenpox	3/13/08

Catch-Up

Anyone who is not fully vaccinated, and never had chickenpox, should receive one or two doses of chickenpox vaccine. The timing of these doses depends on the person's age. Ask your provider.

Chickenpox vaccine may be given at the same time as other vaccines.

Note: A "combination" vaccine called **MMRV**, which contains both chickenpox and MMR vaccines, may be given instead of the two individual vaccines to people 12 years of age and younger.

3 Some people should not get chickenpox vaccine or should wait

- People should not get chickenpox vaccine if they have ever had a life-threatening allergic reaction to a previous dose of chickenpox vaccine or to gelatin or the antibiotic neomycin.

- People who are moderately or severely ill at the time the shot is scheduled should usually wait until they recover before getting chickenpox vaccine.

- Pregnant women should wait to get chickenpox vaccine until after they have given birth. Women should not get pregnant for 1 month after getting chickenpox vaccine.

- Some people should check with their doctor about whether they should get chickenpox vaccine, including anyone who:
  - Has HIV/AIDS or another disease that affects the immune system
  - Is being treated with drugs that affect the immune system, such as steroids, for 2 weeks or longer
  - Has any kind of cancer
  - Is getting cancer treatment with radiation or drugs

- People who recently had a transfusion or were given other blood products should ask their doctor when they may get chickenpox vaccine.

Ask your provider for more information.

FIGURE 54-22 Vaccine Information Sheet (VIS) provided by the CDC for the varicella vaccination.
Source: http://www.cdc.gov/vaccines/pubs/vis/downloads/vis-varicella.pdf.

bloodstream. The Hib vaccine became available in 1985, and since then the cases of Hib disease have decreased dramatically.

Hepatitis A Vaccine

Hepatitis A, which is caused by a virus, is the most common type of hepatitis in the United States. Hepatitis A affects the liver but does not cause long-term effects. It is spread through personal contact or by eating contaminated food or drinking contaminated water. The vaccine is given to children 2 years or older to prevent the risk of contracting hepatitis A. It is recommended that children who live in Alaska, Arizona, and Oregon should receive the vaccine because of high disease incidence. Individuals who travel to other countries are also encouraged to obtain this vaccine.

Hepatitis B Vaccine

Hepatitis B is caused by the hepatitis B virus (HBV) and is transmitted by contaminated serum in blood transfusions or through the use of contaminated needles or instruments. Hepatitis B is a form of viral hepatitis, is highly contagious, and can be fatal. By immunizing children the potential of this disease becoming an epidemic is minimized. It is recommended that soon after birth all infants be given the first dose of hepatitis B. Only infants whose mother's hepatitis B surface antigen (HBsAg) is negative may be given the first dose by age 2 months. A child should receive a total of four doses of the vaccine. The last dose should not be given to the infant before age 24 weeks. When delivering the hepatitis B vaccine, special attention should be paid to the CDC's vaccination requirements for infants born to HBsAg-positive mothers or infants born to mothers whose HBsAg status is unknown.

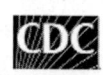
FIGURE 54-22 (Continued)

Measles, Mumps, and Rubella (MMR) Vaccine

The **measles, mumps, and rubella (MMR) vaccine** is given to children to protect them from developing measles, mumps, and rubella. Once a child is given the MMR, the child is protected for life. The MMR is given in two doses. If necessary the vaccines for measles, mumps, and rubella can also be given separately. Due to the MMR vaccine, very few children today contract these diseases.

A virus causes measles, and prior to development of the measles vaccine almost all children came down with the measles. Measles is extremely serious and can result in brain damage, deafness, or death.

Mumps was also a very common childhood disease prior to the development of the vaccine. Mumps is not as serious a disease as the measles but could result in some undesired side effects, including meningitis, encephalitis, and deafness.

Rubella, also known as German measles or 3-day measles, is typically a mild disease that affects an individual for about 24 hours. Rubella is caused by a virus and is spread through close contact. Rubella can strike adults and unborn children. Unborn babies can be infected if the woman gets rubella early in the pregnancy. If a pregnant woman does have rubella, there is a high probability that the infant will be born with birth defects. Since the development of the rubella vaccine, only several hundred cases are reported each year.

Pneumococcal Vaccine

The **pneumococcal vaccine**, until very recently, was not licensed for children under the age of 2 years. Typically, older adults have received this vaccine to protect them from contracting the *Streptococcus* pneumonia bacteria. According to the

CDC, this bacteria kills more people in the United States each year than any other vaccine-preventable disease. By obtaining the vaccine, individuals are protected against the seven strains of the pneumococcal bacterium. The pneumococcal bacteria are spread through the air. Winter and early spring are the most common seasons when pneumococcal infections occur.

Varicella Vaccine

Varicella, or chickenpox, is one of the most common childhood diseases. Chickenpox, thus named due to the blisters that look like chickpeas, is caused by a virus and is spread through the air. Although chickenpox is an uncomfortable illness, it is usually not serious. The varicella vaccine became licensed in the United States in 1995, and since then the number of varicella cases has diminished significantly. Although the vaccine has not eradicated the disease, it has dramatically lowered the percentage of individuals infected by it.

Polio Vaccine

Polio is caused by a virus and is spread through contact with the feces of an infected person. Although paralysis is not a result for all individuals who contract polio, it is an event that does affect some children.

Since 1955 the polio vaccine has been available, resulting in the disappearance of the disease in the United States. However, polio is still common in some parts of the world. A polio epidemic could appear in the United States due to individuals bringing in the disease from another country. Thus, it is important that children even in the United States be immunized.

There are two types of polio vaccines: **inactivated polio vaccine (IPV)** and live **oral polio vaccine (OPV)**. For many years children received the polio vaccine orally (OPV) rather than by injection (IPV). Due to the fact that the oral polio vaccine was found in rare situations to cause polio in children, it is now recommended that all children receive the polio vaccine by injection.

ADULT AND OTHER IMMUNIZATIONS

In addition to the influenza vaccination, adults 65 years of age and older should receive the pneumococcal polysaccharide vaccine (PPV).

Adults and children who travel abroad must also obtain prior to travel the additional vaccines, immunizations, and preventive medications recommended by the CDC. The recommendations are categorized according to the region of travel. For instance, if one were to travel to South Asia, vaccine and medication recommendations would include hepatitis A, hepatitis B, malaria, and typhoid; the recommendations might be different for Africa, and so on.

Reconstituting a Powdered Medication for Administration

Some medications are supplied in a powdered or dry form. Medications supplied in powdered form generally have a longer shelf life. To be injected, these powdered medications must be reconstituted with diluents, usually sterile water. Once the diluent is added to the powder and mixed well, the appropriate dose is drawn up and administered to the patient. To reconstitute a powdered medication, see Procedure 54-10.

procedure 54-10

RECONSTITUTING A POWDERED MEDICATION FOR ADMINISTRATION

Objective: Reconstitute a powdered medication.

EQUIPMENT AND SUPPLIES
alcohol swab; disposable gloves; medication label; medication order signed by physician; pen; sterile needle; biohazard sharps container; vial of medication

METHOD
1. Gather supplies, perform hand hygiene, and apply gloves.
2. Select the correct medication and diluent, perform the "three befores," verify the dosage against the physician's order, and calculate dosage if necessary.

3. Remove the top from the powder medication and the top from the diluent, then wipe the tops of both vials with separate alcohol swabs.
4. Insert a sterile needle through the rubber stopper on the vial of diluent.
5. Withdraw the appropriate amount of diluent and add to the powder medication.

6. Remove the needle from the medication vial and discard in the sharps container.
7. To ensure that the medication is mixed well, roll the vial between the palms of your hand.
8. Label the mixed vial with the strength of the prepared medication, time and date, your initials, and expiration date.

SUMMARY

Administering a medication is one of the medical assistant's most important duties and responsibilities. The medical assistant is expected to be knowledgeable about the medication and its side effects. Medications come in many forms including oral, parenteral, and inhalants. Medications are always given under the supervision of the physician. The physician must be physically present within the facility at the time that the medical assistant dispenses the medication.

When administering medications, the medical assistant must always observe the "three befores" and the "ten rights." Although errors rarely occur, if an error does occur notice must be given immediately to a supervisor so that the situation can be handled quickly for the safety and well-being of the patient.

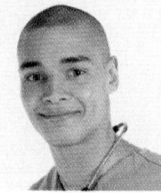

54 CHAPTER REVIEW

COMPETENCY REVIEW

1. Define and spell the terms to learn for this chapter.

2. What are the "ten rights" of drug administration?

3. What would you do if you saw a small amount of blood appear in the plunger of a syringe as you withdrew the plunger?

4. What is the process for giving an oral medication?

PREPARING FOR THE CERTIFICATION EXAM

1. When administering oral or sublingual medication, which of the following is NOT required?
   a. assemble all of the equipment and use aseptic technique
   b. select the correct medication using the "three befores"
   c. double-check the label on the medication
   d. identify the patient by name and date of birth
   e. provide patient with a vaccine information sheet

2. When giving parenteral medication, a smaller gauge needle is used for which type of injection?
   a. intramuscular
   b. Z-track
   c. subcutaneous
   d. intradermal
   e. intravenous

3. Subcutaneous injections are administered at an angle of
   a. 15 degrees
   b. 90 degrees
   c. 45 degrees
   d. 5 to 10 degrees
   e. 25 degrees

4. Which site, because there are fewer major blood vessels, is considered the safest for an intramuscular injection?
   a. vastus lateralis
   b. deltoid
   c. dorsogluteal
   d. ventrogluteal
   e. gluteus medius

5. Which of the following is NOT a common site for intradermal injections?
   a. right forearm
   b. anterior chest
   c. upper back
   d. abdomen
   e. left forearm

6. Which vaccine guards against chickenpox?
   a. DTaP
   b. varicella
   c. CPV
   d. IPV
   e. tetanus

7. Which is the preferred location for intramuscular injections on a toddler?
   a. deltoid
   b. vastus lateralis
   c. gluteus medius
   d. gluteus maximus
   e. biceps

8. What connects the needle to the syringe?
   a. flange
   b. hilt
   c. hub
   d. shaft
   e. barrel

9. A tuberculosis test has to be read within how many hours after being administered?
   a. 12 hours
   b. 24 hours
   c. 48 hours
   d. 36 hours
   e. 16 hours

10. The Hib vaccine helps protect against
   a. human papillomavirus
   b. meningitis
   c. tuberculosis
   d. hepatitis B
   e. tetanus

CRITICAL THINKING

1. How should Samra proceed in order to follow Dr. Miller's instructions?

2. What should Samra do to help her administer the medication to the patient?

3. Since Owen's babysitter has brought him in for the office visit, will Samra need to obtain parental permission before administering the medication?

ON THE JOB

Mrs. Conners comes into Dr. Tyler's office to be seen for a sore throat and fever. The examination reveals that Mrs. Conners has tonsillitis. Dr. Tyler writes an order in the patient's chart for an injection of antibiotic to be given today. The patient is also given a prescription for an oral antibiotic to be taken for the next 10 days.

Joe, the medical assistant, while administering the injection to Mrs. Conners, accidentally punctures his finger with the dirty needle.

What is your response?

1. What should Joe do?
2. Is an incident report necessary?
3. If an incident report is filed, where should it be placed?

INTERNET ACTIVITY

Choose three common drugs, and perform searches to get information about them. Select nationally recognized websites that you know you can access again when seeking information for patients.

MEDMEDIA

Additional interactive resources and activities for this chapter can be found:

On your student DVD: View applicable procedure videos on the DVD-ROM found in the back of this book.

MyHealthProfessionsKit.com: Test your knowledge of this chapter with games and activities. MyHealthProfessionsKit also includes resources, helpful links, and a Spanish audio glossary.

Medical Assisting Interactive: Practice your procedures as a medical assistant in this simulated doctor's office. This can be accessed through MyHealthProfessionsKit.com.

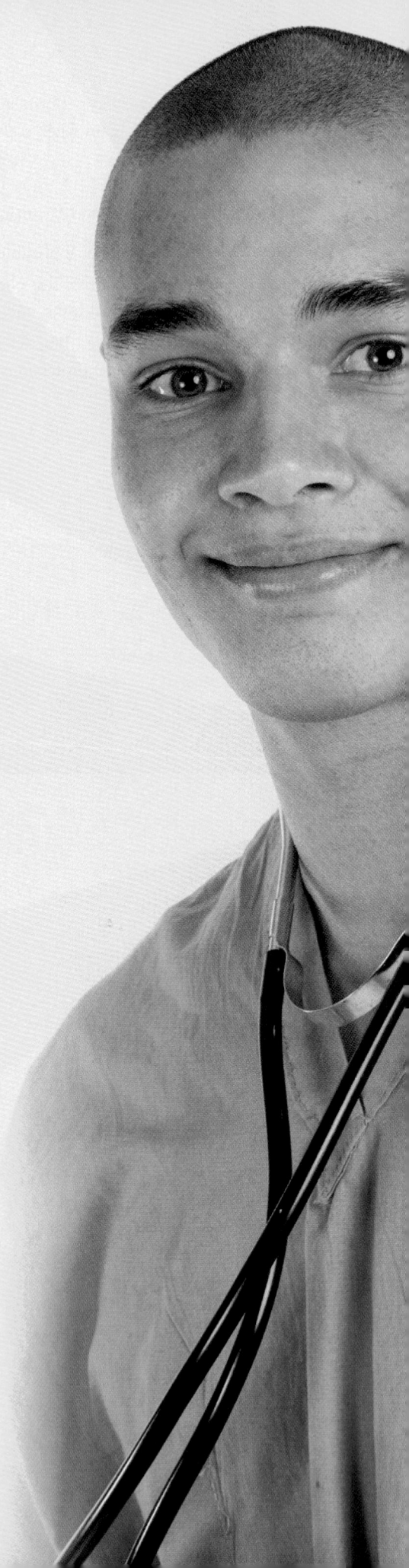

55 Patient Education

LEARNING OBJECTIVES

After completing this chapter, you should be able to:

- Define and spell the terms to learn for this chapter.

- List and describe five methods that help adults learn.

- Create a public relations brochure for the office.

- State 15 teaching methods and strategies to use for patient education.

- Discuss 12 tips for clear writing.

- Discuss how you would adapt education for patients with hearing impairments, patients who do not see well, or those who do not speak English.

- Describe the four changes that take place as people age.

- Describe the process used when developing a teaching plan.

- Describe how you would adapt education for culturally based needs.

- Discuss some of the reasons for noncompliance with patient education.

- Discuss cast application, care, and removal.

CHAPTER OUTLINE

CASE STUDY

Pearson Physicians Group has decided to begin offering group patient-education classes for their patients who struggle with a variety of health-related issues. The office manager, Tania, will organize the classes. Though the physicians require final approval on all decisions, they have given Tania a lot of freedom and responsibility in designing the new patient education programs.

TERMS TO LEARN

acute pain	evaluation
assessment	implementing
chronic pain	learning outcomes
dexterity	noncompliance
document	plan

CERTIFICATION LINK

CMA (AAMA)
Communication
  Adapting communication according to an individual's needs
Resource information and community services
  Patient advocate
Patient preparation and assisting the physician
  Patient education

RMA
General medical assistant knowledge
  Human relations
  Patient education

CMAS (AMT)
Medical assisting foundations
  Professionalism

One of the rights patients have is to receive instruction on how they can manage their own health needs. The medical assistant is often the person of choice to provide patient education. Patients become familiar with the medical assistant who escorts them into the exam room, is often present during the examination process, and will see them when the exam is complete. This familiarity and comfort level of the patient assists in the learning process.

Patient Education

Patient education should not be an afterthought. The medical assistant, knowing the patient's needs, must be prepared to educate the patient on behavior that might improve the patient's health, prepare the patient for a procedure, improve patient compliance on a therapy or medication, or educate the patient about his or her own health behaviors. The education process begins with **assessment**, or evaluation of the patient's needs. For example, the patient may need to lose weight to decrease stress on joints, prevent or reverse obesity, promote fitness, and increase life expectancy. The next step would be to **plan** or determine how to begin the task of teaching. Perhaps the medical assistant could give the patient a pedometer and suggest that she walk for 20 minutes each day. **Implementing** the plan involves actually teaching the patient what to do. For example, the medical assistant could teach the patient how to use the pedometer and record daily walking distance. The medical assistant must then **document** this teaching by charting it in the patient's medical record to ensure continuity of care. The medical assistant would also remind the physician at the next visit to ask the patient how the exercise plan is going; this phase is called **evaluation**. After evaluating the effectiveness of the teaching plan, new teaching plans can be constructed. For example, the physician might then teach the patient how to modify caloric intake to decrease the possibility of obesity.

Most of the patients you will be teaching will be adults. If children need instruction, their parents should be present so they can reinforce the teaching, although communication must be adapted to the learner's level of comprehension. Most patient education concepts apply to both the child and adult learner. Some specific learning concepts, however, relate to the adult based on language skills, previous experience, and motivation.

How Adults Learn

Adult learning is an active process, and adults prefer to participate actively. Therefore, activities and techniques that call for participation, such as role-playing, will achieve more learning faster than those that do not. For example, a lecture is not as useful as role-playing for patient learning. The medical assistant, then, will need to adapt the mode of teaching to the patient. Teaching sessions can begin with explaining how the training will help the patient. For example, role-playing relaxation techniques in a childbirth preparation class may be used before, during, and after childbirth.

Learning must be self directed for adults. Therefore, the clearer and more relevant the statement of desired learning outcomes is, the more the learning that will take place.

Learning outcomes are the goals of patient education. They are what the patient should achieve as a result of the teaching. In health care settings, patients must be taught the advantages of healthy lifestyles and how to achieve their goals. Practical application of learning is desired by most adult learners. Any learning that is applied immediately by the patient is retained longer. For example, a patient in an obstetrician's office might have just been told she is pregnant. She is eager to do what is best for her and her child. This is an excellent time for a medical assistant to refer the patient to community resources such as preparation for childbirth, good nutrition, CPR/first aid, and child care

procedure 55-1

CREATING A COMMUNITY RESOURCE BROCHURE

Objective: Create a brochure that educates patients about available community resources.

EQUIPMENT AND SUPPLIES

computer; computer program that allows the creation of a brochure; printer; pen; phone book; Internet access; newspaper

METHOD

1. Identify community resources that are available to help patients with disease prevention or health promotion, such as smoking cessation or weight loss. Research information found in a phone book, newspaper, or website.

2. Create an attractive brochure for distribution to patients that includes the name, location, phone number, and services offered by the resources.
3. Check your brochure for spelling and grammatical errors prior to printing.
4. Print one copy and perform another spelling and grammar check on the printed document.
5. After the brochure has been polished, obtain approval from the office manager or physician to print and then distribute the brochures in the office waiting room.

---

courses. Sometimes the physician asks the medical assistant to create a list of community resources that the physician can recommend for the patients. Sometimes the new patient requests education about the physician's office itself. Perhaps the new patient would like information about the office,

such as operating hours, other locations where the physician sees patients, and office policies. Creating a brochure is one form of education. For instructions on creating a community resource brochure and a public relations brochure see Procedures 55-1 and 55-2.

procedure 55-2

CREATING A PUBLIC RELATIONS BROCHURE

Objective: Promote the office by creating a brochure for distribution to current and potential patients.

EQUIPMENT AND SUPPLIES

computer; printer; office information; pen

METHOD

1. Gather the necessary data and create a brochure to advertise your office. Be sure to include the following:
   - Office name (e.g., Pearson Physicians Group)
   - Type of practice (e.g., family medicine)
   - Office hours
   - Office address
   - Names and information about physicians
   - Insurance plans accepted

   - Payment expectations (e.g., co-payments are expected before visit begins; all methods of payment are acceptable except cash)
   - Emergency management procedures (e.g., after hours, contact the answering service at 312-321-4321)
2. Check your brochure for spelling and grammatical errors prior to printing.
3. Print one copy and perform another spelling and grammar check on the printed document.
4. After the brochure has been polished, obtain approval from the office manager or physician to print and then distribute the brochures to patients.

The adult often prefers a group learning atmosphere because of the mutual support a group setting offers. For learning to be effective, it must be reinforced. This can be done either through the group or by the teacher. Weight loss centers have used this technique effectively by announcing successful weight loss to others in group meetings.

Learning of new material is facilitated when it is reinforced by material that is already known. For instance, when instructing a new colostomy patient on the necessity for meticulous hand washing before and after handling the colostomy material, it is important to build on the patient's previous knowledge of hand washing.

Motivational incentives for adult learners are better health, improved appearance, pride of accomplishment, self-confidence, and praise from others. In addition to frequent praise, the adult learner learns more rapidly when he or she is made aware of progress. The time an adult spends on learning is related to many factors, including the following:

- Number of years spent in school
- Reading level
- Use of vocabulary
- Satisfaction with previous attempts to learn
- Health status of family member

Teaching Methods and Strategy

A combination of teaching techniques should be used for patient education rather than just one. For example, when instructing a newly diagnosed diabetic patient, a combination of brief lecture, models of anatomical sites for injections, injection procedure demonstration, printed handouts, diagrams of injection site rotation, and videos might all be used at different points in the educational process.

Using language and communication skills that are not suited to the learner creates roadblocks to effective patient learning. Some roadblocks to effective patient learning are these:

- Ordering, commanding, and directing the patient to learn
- Warning or threatening
- Moralizing or preaching ("ought to do," "should do")
- Judging
- Criticizing
- Name calling, stereotyping, labeling
- Sarcasm
- Anxiety
- Culturally inappropriate treatment plans
- Speaking loudly to a blind person
- Age-inappropriate speech

Culture influences learning and can affect readiness, values, feelings of inclusion, what aspect of learning the patients choose, and how they apply it in their own homes. Use of personal space, distances maintained, facial expressions, body movements, gestures, and expressions can be misinterpreted in certain cultures and must be considered when educating a patient. Patient education should be

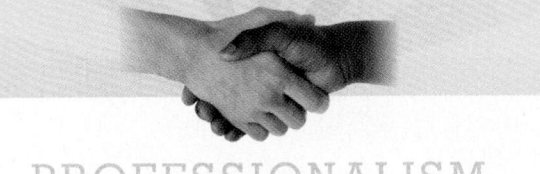

PROFESSIONALISM
CULTURAL CONSIDERATIONS

When creating patient education materials, the medical assistant may need to be sensitive to cultural considerations. Although sketches may be appropriate for a brochure, some cultures do not approve of seeing pictures of actual body parts on patient education information.

In some cultures, patient education includes educating family members. Frequently male family members are expected to assist older women with medical appointments. In some cultures, men should not see women undressed, so they may need to be excluded from the procedure. At the patient's request, family members may be included or excluded from the examination and procedures. An example of this is the varied cultural view of childbirth practices. In the United States, childbirth classes can include male relatives or even friends. In some cultures, only women learn about childbirth and parenting techniques.

PROFESSIONALISM
THE LAW

You must be able to communicate with your patients, especially to get truly informed consent about certain procedures. A responsible office will hire a medical assistant or physician with good foreign language skills or a medical interpreter to ensure patient understanding and compliance.

modified to the appropriate developmental stage to reach each child. A good example is the importance of teaching a child with asthma to use a nebulizer properly. The approach would need significant modification from the approach used to teach an adult.

Attitudes and illness have powerful impacts on learning readiness. Some patients may distrust education due to previous negative experiences. In addition, illness affects individuals in different ways; fatigue and pain can be obstacles to learning. It is important to create a learning environment that encourages patient readiness. Consider rescheduling the session if the patient is not feeling well at the time.

Because of differences in the learning readiness and processing capabilities of older adults and also of special needs patients, such as non-English-speaking patients and those with developmental delays or hearing or visual impairments, the medical assistant must carefully prepare any brochures or materials given to patients.

Table 55-1 describes several teaching methods that can be used effectively for adults and children. As mentioned

TABLE 55-1 Patient Teaching Methods

Method	Description	Advantage	Disadvantage	Usefulness
Lecture	Formal report or instructions delivered to the patient with little interaction between teacher and learner	Efficient No limit to number of learners	No interaction to handle individual learner confusion May be boring for learner	Patients who need general knowledge (new mothers) Large groups (smoking cessation, weight reduction)
Role-play	Short play in which the learner participates in "playing out" the story	Learner sees how others might do something Learner involvement	Time consuming Learner must be willing to "play" the role	Patients with chronic diseases (hypertension, diabetes) Patients learning new interactions (how to direct home health aide) Handling unusual situations that cannot be demonstrated, such as calling 911 in an emergency
Case problems	Applies information to real situations	Believable Concrete rather than abstract	Significant facts may be missing Effectiveness depends on teacher	Patients who must apply new knowledge (patient with angina, new mothers, diabetes)
Demonstration/return demonstration	Showing patients how to do something and then immediately having them do the same procedure	Presents standards for performance both visual and oral Allows learner to know it can be done	May be difficult to see Limited to small group Patients may be nervous	Patients who need to understand cause and effect Patients who must learn new skills (colostomy care, diabetic injections, baby care, CPR)
Contracting	Setting up goals with clear behaviors and responsibilities for the patient	Requires learner involvement Promotes learner's strengths Identifies acceptable goals	Requires learner decision making May be threatening Time consuming	Patients with chronic disease Well patients who wish to change health habits
Use of significant other	Teaching a close relative/friend the same information the patient receives	Provides learner support and reinforcement Learning continues at home	Other person must be willing to help Other person may be a negative influence Other person may foster dependence	Elderly patients and those with disabilities Patients whose compliance is in question

(continued)

TABLE 55-1 (*continued*)

Method	Description	Advantage	Disadvantage	Usefulness
Past experiences	Building learning on what has been learned in the past rather than creating a new set of knowledge	Identifies potential problems Makes the patient more comfortable	Depends on ability to recall Requires insight	Patients who are anxious or overwhelmed Patients who must change behavior (take medication, use proper diet, exercise)
Group teaching	Bringing together patients who have common learning needs	Efficient and economical Participants support each other Participants are actively involved	Group may digress Some cultures discourage open discussion Transportation may be a problem Difficult for all to agree on a time	Patients and families with common learning needs (weight reduction, smoking cessation)
Programmed instruction	Printed instructions that force the learner to understand one concept before going on to the next Every correct response builds toward the next question Can be computer assisted	Active learner participation Individual pacing Encourages independence Provides immediate feedback	May be impersonal and boring Patient must be literate Lack of personal involvement between patient and teacher Patient must be self-motivated	Self-motivated learners Accommodates lower reading level
Simulations (games)	To create a pretend scenario for learning purposes	Involves the patient in the learning process Non-threatening Allows patients to see knowledge previously learned	Some patients dislike competition Some patients do not like games Some patients have difficulty following directions or with abstract ideas	Adults and children with acute problems (cast care), chronic problems (asthma) or health promotion issues (dental care, weight control)
Tests of knowledge	Short questions that relate to the patient's knowledge of the subject	Evaluates patient's knowledge at that moment Gives patient a feeling of accomplishment Raises patient's awareness	May make patients anxious Time consuming May embarrass patients with lack of knowledge	Adults and children who must apply knowledge (diabetic patient, postsurgical patient with a dressing change)
Printed handouts	Brochures or instruction sheets printed for the main purpose of imparting knowledge to the patient	Promotes consistency Gives visual reinforcement	Must be accompanied by verbal teaching Difficult to create since clarity and simplicity are required	Well patients (health maintenance literature) Patients who must remember difficult information (presurgical instructions, medication information)
Diagrams	Picture models of concepts	Offers visual reinforcement Attracts attention of the patient Shows proportions and relationships	Must be accurate May require artistic skill to produce	Preschoolers People with limited reading or vocabulary levels

| Models | A miniature (usually) representation of an object produced in a substance, such as clay or plaster | Encourages patient participation Offers direct application of skill | May be expensive | School-age children Adults practicing a skill (CPR, breast self-exam, bathing a child) |
| Video | A slide presentation or moving picture | Recreates real-life situations Effective for patients with limited reading skills | Too fast for the elderly adult May be expensive Takes time to set up and run | Groups of patients Health maintenance material (nutrition, preventive dentistry) Video player in waiting room |

previously, a combination of methods may prove useful. Box 55-1 provides an extensive list of tips on how to prepare printed material that is easy for patients to read. Guidelines 55-1 describes additional means for improving instruction. Also see Procedure 55-3 about instructing patients according to their health maintenance and promotion needs.

TEACHING CHILDREN

Children have special educational needs and should not be treated as small adults. Depending on their age and rate and stage of development, they should have instruction tailored to them. Coloring books can be used to teach concepts. Stickers can be given to reward children. Children may need to see a treatment or procedure performed on a doll before tolerating it well. Many children like to touch equipment that will be used on them, such as a stethoscope or a blood pressure cuff. Older children may like to see videos about the process of a surgery or other treatment they are expecting to have. As children age, they should be included in discussions and decision making about their health care. Older children also will have numerous questions about their treatments and should receive adequate explanations in response.

TEACHING PATIENTS WITH DISABILITIES AND SPECIAL NEEDS

Patient education should be adapted to the patient. Many patients will have special needs. Patients who have hearing or visual impairments, are developmentally delayed or mentally retarded, or do not speak English pose special challenges.

Patients who have hearing impairments frequently read lips. Face the patient and speak slowly. Be sure you do not stand with your back to the window because such positioning will throw shadows over your mouth. Remove barriers or face masks when speaking to clients with hearing impairments. You may need to hire an interpreter for the deaf. Get a microphone to boost the volume of your voice and give specific written instructions to clients with hearing impairments.

Patients who have visual impairments may not understand written instructions unless the type is very large—and some will not be able to read at all. The medical assistant may need to make audiotaped instructions of information that is usually written. Be sure to clear clutter from the office that might impede the patient and hold the patient's hand to lead him or her to examinations and procedures.

Box 55-1 Tips for Clear WRITING

1. Begin the material with a short introduction to state the purpose and to orient the reader.
2. Use titles and headings that clearly define the topics.
3. Use boldface, italics, or underlining to emphasize important words and ideas.
4. Use a summary paragraph to end a section or recap a point.
5. Use one important idea per paragraph.
6. Start each paragraph with a strong topic sentence.
7. Vary the length of sentences.
8. Use frequent examples to clarify ideas with which the reader may not have had experience.
9. Use active rather than passive voice.
10. Avoid polysyllabic words whenever possible. Use shorter words.
11. Avoid using a specialized vocabulary such as medical terminology.
12. Avoid abbreviations except when commonly understood.

EFFECTIVE HEALTH INSTRUCTION

1. Always address the patient by name. Do not use the patient's first name unless you have asked permission to do so.
2. Be well organized. Have together all materials, models, and brochures so that you will not have to leave the patient during the education process.
3. Have either a verbal or written order from the physician for teaching medical procedures, such as for self-injection.
4. Assume the patient can learn. Do not equate intelligence level with educational level. Avoid talking down to patients.
5. Write or print instructions large enough to be clearly read by the patient.
6. Do not overwhelm the patient with technicalities. The patient does not have to know everything you know.
7. Do not use medical abbreviations when discussing medical procedures or conditions with patients.
8. Define necessary medical terms for patients using simple explanations. Never use "street language" to discuss bodily functions. However, if the patient does not understand you may have to adapt some medical terms to more common terms or expressions (e.g., "passing water" for urination).
9. Correct patient errors in the learning process without harsh judgment. Reemphasize the correct information.
10. Do not teach by performing the procedure over and over for the patient. Give a demonstration of a procedure, such as drawing up insulin for the diabetic patient. Then immediately allow the patient to practice. If the technique is not perfect, reinforce learning by having the patient perform the procedure again.
11. Establish a quiet, unhurried, nonthreatening atmosphere for patient education. It should not be conducted in a waiting room or hallway.
12. Remember that if a patient is facing you as you demonstrate a procedure, such as bathing a baby or giving CPR, the patient's hands will be reversed when performing the procedure. Whenever possible, have the learner stand next to you during a one-on-one demonstration.
13. Avoid criticism. Always stress the positive with comments such as "You're doing fine. Let's try it one more time."

procedure
55-3

INSTRUCTING PATIENTS ACCORDING TO THEIR NEEDS FOR HEALTH MAINTENANCE AND PROMOTION

Objective: Instruct a deaf individual to prepare for outpatient surgery by creating a brochure on steps to minimize infection postoperatively.

EQUIPMENT AND SUPPLIES

computer; printer; pen; stapler

METHOD

1. Create postoperative instructions for the deaf patient, including information about activities, medications, dressing changes, diet, and follow-up care. Create a copy for the client and one for the chart.
2. Face the patient so your lips can be read easily.
3. Greet the patient, using the patient's name.
4. Discuss the contents of the postoperative instructions with the patient.
5. Obtain feedback from the patient to show understanding.
6. Give a copy of the information to the patient.
7. Have the patient sign one copy of the brochure and keep one copy for the patient chart.
8. Document the education.

CHARTING EXAMPLE

Instructed patient on postoperative instructions as highlighted in attached brochure. February 20, 20XX. · · · · · · · · · · · · · ·
· Emily Blodgett, CMA (AAMA)

Patients who have developmental delays or mental retardation may have trouble understanding instructions. The medical assistant may need to instruct the caregiver instead or to give the patient simplified, pictorial directions.

Patients who are illiterate or do not understand English pose special challenges. Ask the patient when an appointment is made if he or she would like an interpreter for patient care. Sometimes the patient prefers to bring a relative who speaks English. Be sure to get patient permission to discuss health information with relatives. Send written instructions home with the patient. If a large percentage of patients in the office speak a certain language other than English, it may help to construct brochures in other languages. Consider culture and diet compliance along with patient likes and dislikes for compliance.

All teaching should have the purpose of patient understanding and retention. With all special needs patients, the medical assistant should ensure understanding of teaching by requesting feedback or demonstration from the patient after teaching. The medical assistant should adjust the teaching to the patient, and may need to cover the same topic several times until understanding is demonstrated.

TEACHING THE OLDER ADULT

Older adult patients' abilities, motivations, and social circumstances differ from those of younger patients. Their intellectual capacity does not diminish; it merely changes. Some changes that take place as a person ages include slower processing of new material, decreased short-term memory, decreased **dexterity** (ability to use their hands effectively), and increased anxiety over new situations.

One type of intellectual ability is based on the intelligence absorbed during life—for example, vocabulary, arithmetic, and the ability to reflect on and evaluate past experience. This type of intelligence can increase with age. Therefore, the older person is able to learn quickly if the learning requires information acquired in the past. When teaching the older adult, it is wise to explore past experiences using concrete examples, such as "Tell me how you calculate the amount of food you eat on your diabetic diet."

Slowed Processing Time

Older patients need more time to think through and absorb new information; therefore, the medical assistant should break down information into small units. When teaching from a list of things, take time to explain each item on the list. For example, when the instructions are "Call your doctor for the following reasons: temperature over 99 degrees, drainage from the incision, inability to take the medication, or pain," each of these reasons should be explained separately.

These explanations should be accompanied by a description of the relationship of each item to the patient's problem. It is also helpful to give written instructions so the patient can process the instructions more slowly later.

Decreased Short-Term Memory

The older adult patient can remember easily things that happened in the past but may have difficulty remembering new information that was acquired yesterday. Learning then becomes very frustrating for them. The medical assistant should work with the patient to devise methods to reinforce instruction or prod the memory. The new information should be linked to a well-known past experience when possible. Always attempt to reinforce old ways of doing things rather than introducing new behavior. For example, when teaching the signs and symptoms of an infection to an older diabetic patient, ask the patient to recall the symptoms experienced in the past with an infected wound or cut.

Decreased Dexterity

Due to arthritis and other physical changes, some elderly patients are not able to do the same things they could when they

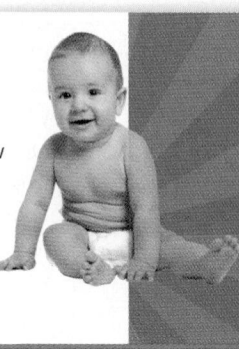

were younger. Advising an overweight elderly patient who uses a cane and is on a reduction diet to get more exercise by walking for 1 hour a day may not be appropriate. Some procedures requiring small muscle dexterity, such as flossing teeth and opening medication bottles, are almost impossible for the elderly person with arthritis. Adaptive equipment may have to be advised for these patients (see Chapter 51).

Increased Anxiety About New Situations

The medical assistant must give the elderly patient a feeling of confidence. This can alleviate some of the anxiety that may surface during a new learning situation. Patients will relax when they see that they are able to manage the situation, and learning will take place.

Teaching methods to use with the older adult range from using handouts with large print to utilizing video and audio displays. Slow-moving slides are preferable to a fast video or movie since the slide can be stopped to reinforce learning. Role-playing can be useful as long as the patient's energy level can be maintained. Family members should be included in the teaching process whenever possible. The elderly person is accustomed to being in control and may not wish to learn anything new if he or she does not see the advantage of doing so.

Developing a Teaching Plan

An effective teaching plan for both the adult and child learner must include desired outcomes. A teaching plan that the medical assistant develops for a condition, such as hypertension (high blood pressure), can be used with some adaptations for all patients with hypertension. Box 55-2 illustrates a sample teaching plan.

Learning Environment

It is important to create a good learning environment when educating patients. Patients may not be honest and open in a busy place where they lack privacy. It is ideal if patient education can take place in a well-lit room with privacy. Sometimes placing patient education materials in racks in examining rooms allows patients to take brochures discreetly. If a medical assistant is teaching a patient how to use equipment, that equipment should be available to show the

---

Box 55-2 Sample Teaching Plan for HYPERTENSION

Content
- I. Basic anatomy and physiology of the heart and blood vessels
- II. What is hypertension?
- III. Symptoms of hypertension
- IV. Risk factors related to hypertension
- V. Situations that might precipitate hypertension
- VI. Home treatment for hypertension
- VII. Handling medications
- VIII. Reasons to contact the physician
- IX. Follow-up
- X. Community resources/support groups

Learning Objectives
- I. The patient describes the anatomy and physiology of the heart muscle and blood vessels in simple terms.
  - a. The heart muscle is a strong hollow organ that acts as a pump. It pumps blood throughout the body and lungs.
  - b. Blood vessels throughout the body carry oxygen to the tissues and cells.
  - c. When the blood vessels become narrowed or do not function properly, the heart may have to work harder. Eventually, pressure within the vessels will rise.
- II. The patient states in simple terms the definition and causes of hypertension.
  - a. Hypertension is an elevation in blood pressure in which the systolic pressure is 140 mmHg or above and the diastolic pressure is 90 mmHg or above.
  - b. An elevated blood pressure reading is a signal that there is a problem that could affect the heart action or even cause a stroke.
  - c. Hypertension (high blood pressure) may be caused by a buildup of fatty substances (cholesterol) on the lining of the blood vessels that feed the heart.
- III. The patient states the most common symptoms of hypertension.
  - a. This is generally a "silent" disease, which means there are few or no symptoms.
  - b. The patient may feel very well.
  - c. The best indicator is an elevated blood pressure reading on several occasions.
  - d. May have headaches or dizziness.
  - e. Patient's symptoms are _____.
- IV. The patient defines risk factors and describes controllable and uncontrollable risk factors.
  - a. Risk factors are habits or characteristics that increase the probability of developing a narrowing of the blood vessels.
  - b. Controllable factors are:
    1. Obesity (20 percent over the average weight for the age, sex, and height)

2. Cigarette smoking
3. Increased amount of fatty substances in the blood
4. Stress
5. Lack of exercise
6. Diet
   c. Uncontrollable factors are:
   1. Family history
   2. Diabetes
   3. Over the age of 50
   d. Patient's risk factors are:
   Controllable _____

   _____

   Uncontrollable _____

   _____

V. Patient states situations that may precipitate hypertension.
   a. Diet heavy in fats and salt
   b. Stress
   c. Smoking
   d. Family history
   e. Age
   f. Lack of exercise
   g. Patient's hypertension may be precipitated by the following:

   _____

   _____

VI. The patient states the home treatment of hypertension.
   a. Monitor blood pressure with home equipment. Record blood pressure readings.

   b. Take medications on a regular basis at the same time every day.
   c. Adjust diet by eliminating salt and fat and reducing calorie intake.
   d. Use stress reduction techniques.
   e. Exercise moderately.
VII. The patient states how to handle medications.
   a. Patient must call physician for a prescription renewal every 3 months.
   b. Patient must have a supply of medication on hand when traveling.
   c. Patient must come in to have blood pressure checked by physician every 2 weeks.
VIII. The patient states reasons to contact the physician or go to the emergency room.
   a. Dizziness or fainting
   b. Blood pressure reading of 160/98 or higher
IX. The patient provides the following:
   Physician #: _____
   Emergency Room #: _____
X. The patient provides a list of community resources/support groups for hypertension.

If the patient and/or significant others are unable to complete some or all of this teaching plan, document evaluation in progress notes on chart.

patient. For example, if a patient with diabetes is learning how to check blood sugar with a glucometer, a glucometer similar to the one to be used should be handy. If the patient asks a question that the medical assistant cannot answer, the assistant should admit not knowing the answer and should get back to the patient about the question.

Teaching Resources

Teaching resources are available for purchase, or the medical assistant can develop handouts for the office. The medical assistant may need to use DVD players, compact disks, videos, or pamphlets. Patients have different learning styles, and the teaching should match the learner's preferred style. See Table 55-2 for reputable websites for patient education.

Patient Issues

Some patient issues, such as skills and abilities, culture, finances, health beliefs, medication errors, and noncompliance, can make educating patients challenging. The medical assistant must remember that each patient is an individual with special needs and learning style.

PATIENT SKILLS AND ABILITIES

Education must be oriented to the skills and abilities of the patient. If a patient is a child or illiterate, the medical assistant may need to use teaching resources that do not involve terminology that the patient cannot understand. Sometimes using pictures rather than words is more appropriate for those who do not speak English well. In some cases, the medical assistant may need to instruct a caregiver how to perform a procedure or give a medication because the patient is unable to assume self-care. Before teaching patients new skills, the medical assistant must be aware of any physical impairments they might have. If an elderly patient cannot easily open medication bottles because of arthritis, the medical assistant may need to teach coping techniques.

CULTURE AND PATIENT EDUCATION

Each patient brings his or her culture to the educational experience. Cultural expectations can interfere with teaching. The best way to find out about a patient's culture is to ask the patient. The medical assistant can ask a patient how he or she would like to be educated. Then the medical assistant

TABLE 55-2 Reputable Websites for Patient Education

Web Site	Information
American Lung Association	Smoking cessation, asthma, hay fever, lung cancer (www.lungusa.org)
American Diabetes Associations	Nutrition and recipes,weight loss and exercise, diabetes prevention (www.diabetes.org)
Hospice	Guides for caregivers of and patients with terminal illnesses, talking to children about death, pain control, advance directives, finding a local hospice, healing after a loss (www.americanhospice.org)
American Heart Association	High blood pressure, controlling cholesterol levels, diet and nutrition (www.americanheart.org)
Alzheimer's Association	Living with Alzheimer's, guides for caregivers (www.alz.org)
American Parkinson Disease Association	Local support groups (www.apdaparkinson.org)
ALS Association	Local support groups, guides for caregivers (www.alsa.org)

can respect those wishes. Sometimes a patient may prefer to be educated by someone who is older or a certain gender. If at all possible, respect those wishes.

Cultural beliefs can impact the patient's health care. Some cultures believe that they have little control over their health. Others assume a great deal of control over balance in health. The family may be a very important part of the treatment team in many cultures. Family members can be key allies in assisting the patient with learning and with reinforcing the medical assistant's teaching.

Religious beliefs also impact health. For example, a Jehovah's Witness may refuse blood products. The medical assistant should ask the patient if special religious beliefs could interfere with the ability to comply with a treatment. For example, the patient may need to fast for religious reasons, in which case it may not be a good time to schedule a procedure requiring swallowing barium.

IMPACT OF FINANCES ON PATIENT EDUCATION

Finances also can have a huge impact on the patient. The patient may want to comply with a treatment or medication but be inhibited in doing so because of lack of money. Creating an environment where the patient is free to share monetary information without shame will help the patient to be more open with the medical assistant. For example, if a patient lacks funds for a special diet, an alternative diet can be created. Patients may not even be able to afford good shoes for an exercise program. The wise medical assistant will create a list of local resources that can help patients who need financial assistance.

PREVENTIVE MEDICINE

Obviously, it is preferable that patients not become sick. Many illnesses are related to lifestyle behaviors—for example, smoking tobacco, overeating, and lack of exercise. Continuously high stress levels can affect the immune system. Drug abuse leads to addiction and toleration of medications. On the other hand, routine immunization and diagnostic tests can prevent diseases. The medical assistant should use the patient visits to educate the patient about preventive medicine. See Table 55-3 for common risk factors for disease.

PREVENTING MEDICATION ERRORS

Medication errors are the fifth leading cause of death in the United States. It is very important that the medical assistant

TABLE 55-3 Common Risk Factors

- Smoking or tobacco product use
- Poor physical fitness
- High alcohol intake
- Poor diet and nutrition
- Disregarding auto safety measures
- High stress level
- Occupational health and environmental hazards
- Drug abuse
- Lack of immunizations
- Poor dental care
- High or very low blood pressure
- Family history of cancer, heart attack, stroke, or diabetes
- Unsafe sex
- High or very low heart rate
- Unhealthy body mass index (BMI)
- Risk-taking behavior

TABLE 55-4 Patient Education Follow-Up Plan

Objective	Performance	Date Needed
Self-administer insulin injections with 100 percent accuracy	1. Understand types of insulin	2/14/XXXX
	2. Practice drawing up insulin × 3	2/14/XXXX
	3. Practice injection on anatomical model × 3	2/16/XXXX
	4. Demonstration on patient by instructor using saline	2/18/XXXX
	5. Return demonstration using saline	2/18/XXXX
	6. Injection of insulin	2/18/XXXX
	7. Follow-up to check technique	3/1/XXXX

ensure not only that patients are given the correct drug but also that they know to speak up whenever they have doubts about receiving the correct drug. For example, the medical assistant can say that the pill is usually a round, blue pill. If the patient does not receive a round, blue pill, the patient should know to ask the pharmacist if the pill is the correct one.

HANDLING NONCOMPLIANCE

Noncompliance—that is, not following a physician's orders—can seriously jeopardize a patient's health and recovery. For instance, a patient with hypertension who fails to take prescribed medication can develop uncontrolled hypertension and have a stroke or heart attack. In addition, health care costs escalate with noncompliance.

Several groups of patients, including those who have had heart bypasses or hemodialysis, have been followed up to determine their compliance level. In both situations, the compliance levels were around 50 percent. Lack of compliance may be indicated by failure to (1) take medication as ordered, (2) return for follow-up appointments, (3) practice dietary changes, and (4) follow an exercise program. On the other hand, patients with cystic fibrosis, a serious disease causing respiratory problems and failure, were found to be more than 80 percent compliant with their medication regimen. This compliance was attributed to the possibility that these patients and their families perceived the very serious consequences of failing to take cystic fibrosis medications.

Noncompliance with instructions is a problem for all age groups, but children have the least problem as long as their parents are compliant and assist them. Patients who have formed a positive relationship with their health care provider, physician, and other staff, such as the medical assistant, have been found to be more compliant. To help form

this positive relationship with the physician, you may choose to create a public relations brochure. See Procedure 55-2 for instructions.

One of the best methods for encouraging patient compliance is to convey to the patients the knowledge they need to make educated decisions about their health care. For instance, the cystic fibrosis patients just mentioned were more compliant after realizing the seriousness of their disease.

In addition to having greater knowledge, the patient must also want to comply. The medical assistant can reinforce learning, and reduce noncompliance, by working out a follow-up plan with regular evaluation of progress. This plan should include an objective stating what the patient should be able to do, along with a date indicating when the objective should be accomplished. Table 55-4 is an example of a patient education follow-up plan.

Health and Wellness

Wellness is the ongoing process of practicing a healthy lifestyle. Balancing physical and psychological stress, and doing what can be done not to overreact to stressors can improve wellness. Patients must choose to practice behaviors that improve wellness and decrease illness. Good teaching from the medical assistant can empower the patient to make positive life changes.

Role modeling healthy behaviors is important. If the medical assistant's uniform smells of cigarette smoke, it is unlikely that the patient will respect the medical assistant's teaching on how to stop smoking. Positive reinforcement when a patient performs can be very powerful. If the medical assistant commends the patient for doing even a little bit of exercise, the patient will be more likely to continue to

TABLE 55-5 Wellness Guidelines

- Keep a positive attitude.
- Cherish your values.
- Exercise your mind, body, and spirit.
- Control your stress.
- Soothe your fears.
- Think happy thoughts.
- Stay active.
- Challenge your mind.
- Forgive and forget.
- Avoid dangerous drugs.
- Watch your sugar intake.
- Walk briskly.
- Enjoy the outdoors.
- Maintain a healthy weight.
- Eat a well-balanced diet.
- Rinse fresh fruits and vegetables before eating.
- Practice cleanliness.
- Take medications as directed.
- Stop smoking.
- Lower your blood pressure and cholesterol.
- Learn to breathe deeply.

exercise. See Table 55-5 for some wellness guidelines that can be taught to patients.

Mind-Body Connection

The mind-body connection refers to the fact that the way a patient thinks and feels affects the body's wellness. Endorphins are released when patients are happy. These proteins have analgesic properties, benefit physical functioning, and boost immunity to disease. On the other hand, negative feelings such as fear, anger, and grieving can cause increased heart rate, tightened muscles, and a fight-or-flight response. The medical assistant must recognize this connection to assist the patient to release or cope with negative emotions to promote healing.

Teaching the Patient

Some of the areas in which patients may require teaching include pain, nutrition, weight loss, exercise, stress reduction, smoking, substance abuse, and cast care.

TEACHING ABOUT PAIN

Pain is an unpleasant sensory and emotional experience. Patients respond differently to pain, depending on tolerance and pain threshold. It is important for the medical assistant not to put subjective value on the patient's pain. Pain is a subjective experience for the patient. Pain is what the patient describes it as. It can be **acute pain**, such as surgical pain. Acute pain will be intense after surgery usually and

will lessen over time. **Chronic pain**, on the other hand, is pain that continues over time. Arthritic pain is chronic pain. The long-term effects of chronic pain include anger, helplessness, sadness, depression, decreased activity, decreased sleep, increased irritability, fatigue, chemical and/or medication dependency, mood swings, lowered self-esteem, and impaired ability to handle stress. Pain can be physical and psychological. Sometimes pain is referred, because it is felt in another area than the actual pain. For example, spleen pain is often felt in the shoulder.

It is important for the medical assistant to assure the patient that pain relief is possible. Before surgery, for example, the medical assistant should reassure the patient that he will be asked to describe his pain in the hospital and that severe pain will be managed. Through this preparatory teaching, the medical assistant can decrease stress on the patient. See Figure 55-1 for a pain rating scale.

TEACHING ABOUT NUTRITION AND WEIGHT LOSS

The medical assistant should be prepared to teach patients how to maintain a healthy weight. The food pyramid that used to be used for teaching encouraged large amount of carbohydrates. That has been shown to be detrimental to health. The new MyPyramid that has been developed by the U.S. Department of Agriculture is individualized and includes activity, moderation in eating, personalization of diet, proportionality, variety, and gradual improvement. For more information about nutrition and healthy weight loss, go to the MyPyramid website. See Chapter 56 for information about good nutrition.

TEACHING ABOUT EXERCISE

Human beings are not meant to maintain a sedentary lifestyle. It is important for patients to get exercise. Before starting any exercise program, a patient should visit the physician's office to ensure that it is safe to exercise. Some patients with heart or respiratory problems may need to have a modified exercise plan. They generally have regular appointments at the physician's office, at which time they can expect the medical assistant to assist in establishing and maintaining an exercise regimen. Patients must be taught how to properly stretch, warm up, and exercise without becoming injured.

TEACHING STRESS REDUCTION

Since stressors abound in life, it is important for the medical assistant to teach the patient how to cope with stress. Some ways to reduce stress are to practice breathing exercises, meditate, use guided imagery, visualize, and exercise. Relaxation, listening to music, and performing yoga can also reduce stress.

 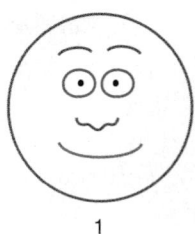 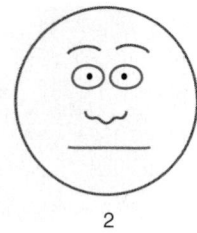 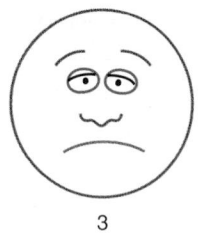 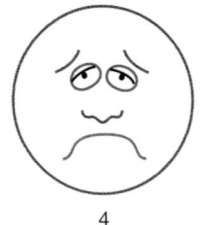 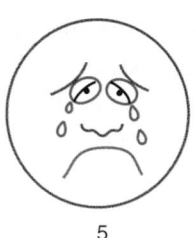

0	1	2	3	4	5

1. Explain to the child that each face is for a person who feels happy because he or she has no pain (hurt, or whatever word the child uses) or feels sad because he or she has some or a lot of pain.

2. Point to the appropriate face and state, "This face..." :
   0—"is very happy because he (or she) doesn't hurt at all."
   1—"hurts just a little bit."
   2—"hurts a little more."
   3—"hurts even more."
   4—"hurts a whole lot."
   5—"hurts as much as you can imagine, although you don't have to be crying to feel this bad."

3. Ask the child to choose the face that best describes how he or she feels. Be specific about which pain (e.g., "shot" or incision) and what time (e.g., Now? Earlier before lunch?)

FIGURE 55-1 The Wong/Baker FACES Rating Scale.
Source: From *Hockenberry MJ, Wilson D, Winkelstein ML: Wong's Essentials of Pediatric Nursing*, ed. 7 St. Louis, 2005 p. 1259. Used with permission. Copyright, Mosby.

TEACHING ABOUT SMOKING AND SUBSTANCE ABUSE

If a patient does not manage stress well, the patient may turn to nicotine or other substances in an abusive manner to cope. These are not healthy coping techniques. The medical assistant should distribute literature that encourages and empowers the patient to select healthy ways to cope with stress. To stop smoking, the American Cancer Society recommends that individuals use nicotine or replacement therapy, utilize various nicotine substitutes, choose the right method to quit, seek telephone support, participate in support groups, and receive information about success rates.

TEACHING ABOUT CAST CARE

The medical assistant may need to educate a patient about cast care. If, for example, a patient has had a cast placed on an injured extremity, the patient must be taught before leaving the office about how to care for the cast. If necessary, the medical assistant must review in advance how to do cast care. To ease the patient's fear, the medical assistant also can discuss each phase of the cast treatment as it is occurring.

Applying a Cast

Casts (a form of inflexible bandage) are applied for the purpose of immobilizing a broken bone or a strain or sprain. A cast may be applied after a surgical procedure on a limb to immobilize the area until healing takes place. The medical assistant can explain the purpose of the cast to the patient.

The medical assistant may be asked to lay out the instruments required for putting on a cast. Equipment includes the cast material (bandage roll or tape), container of warm water, stockinette, Webril (sheer wadding) padding rolls, bandage scissors, rubber gloves, and sponge rubber (for padding). The patient may be curious about each instrument, and the medical assistant can provide information about them. Since none of these items are sterile, the patient could even be allowed to touch the cast material.

Casts are made from a variety of pliable materials that the physician will mold to fit the body part. While encouraging the patient to stay still during application of the cast, the medical assistant can discuss cast materials. The type of casting material is a physician preference and also depends on the body part to which a cast is being applied.

Casts are generally applied using a plaster-type material, which is applied wet around a stockinette liner with cotton padding over the limb. To create this type of cast, the medical assistant will wet a bandage roll impregnated with calcium sulfate and the doctor will mold it to the injured body part. As the cast dries, it becomes hard.

Newer fiberglass materials are being used to form casts since they are lighter in weight than plaster casts. They are formed by using tapes with either a polyester–cotton combination, fiberglass, or plastic resin embedded in the tape. The medical assistant should wear protective glasses or an eye shield when handling fiberglass materials.

Air casts are a type of inflatable immobilizer that uses air to apply firm pressure to the wounded limb. They are used primarily for postcast pressure or sprains. External fixation devices are sometimes used to create appropriate pressure without using casting material. The skin around the fixation pins must be cleaned. The medical assistant should teach, and then have the patient demonstrate before departure, how to clean fixation pins.

The medical assistant may be asked to assist the physician in applying the cast. It may be necessary to hold the limb at the joint areas as the cast is being applied. Remember to handle a damaged limb gently. The time spent holding the limb provides an excellent opportunity for medical assistants to teach about cast care.

After the cast has been applied, it must be left uncovered during the drying process. The limb may need to be supported on a pillow at this time. The patient should be cautioned against moving around until the cast is dry. The cast may feel warm or even hot during the drying process. Reassure the patient that this is normal.

The patient's limb should not become hot or cold once the cast has been applied. Frequent checks of the patient's circulation will alert the medical assistant to any change in the patient's circulation. The patient should be instructed to call the physician if any of the following problems are observed:

- Circulation restricted by the cast
- Pain as a result of the cast pinching the skin
- Excessive itching under the cast
- Numbness or tingling of fingers or toes
- Discolored toes or fingers
- Swelling of the limb around the edge of the cast
- Discoloration soaking through the cast
- Loosely fitting cast
- Foul odor coming from the cast

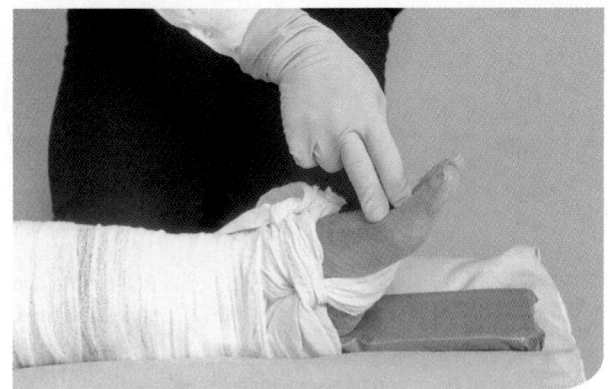

FIGURE 55-2 Checking distal pulses.

The physician should advise the patient on the amount of weight and movement that may be applied to the cast. Remind the patient that nothing should be inserted in the edges of the cast and the cast should not get wet. The patient may be able to tie a strong plastic bag around the cast in order to take a shower.

The patient is an excellent source of information about what is happening under the cast. The injury that caused the fracture leads to swelling, which can create pressure under the cast. Also remember that when the cast dries and hardens, it may constrict blood flow. Always check distal pulses and notify the physician if any abnormality is noted, in which cast the physician may need to remove and replace the cast. Figure 55-2 shows how to check circulation distal to the immobilized area.

The following are some types of casts:

- **Short arm cast (SAC)**—extends from the finger to just below the elbow. Used for a fracture or dislocation of the wrist or forearm.
- **Long arm cast (LAC)**—extends from the fingers to the axilla, with a bend at the elbow. Used for a fracture of the upper arm.
- **Long and short leg casts**—extend from the thigh to the toes (LLC) or from below the knee to the toes (SLC). Usually include an embedded walking heel.

Home Care for a Cast

Before allowing the patient to leave the office, the medical assistant should instruct the patient on how to care for the cast. Educational topics include the following:

- Clean the cast with a damp cloth.
- Do not cut or trim the cast. If the edge seems sharp, apply masking tape to the sharp edge or use a nail file to trim it down.
- Elevate the extremity with the cast on it to reduce swelling and pain.

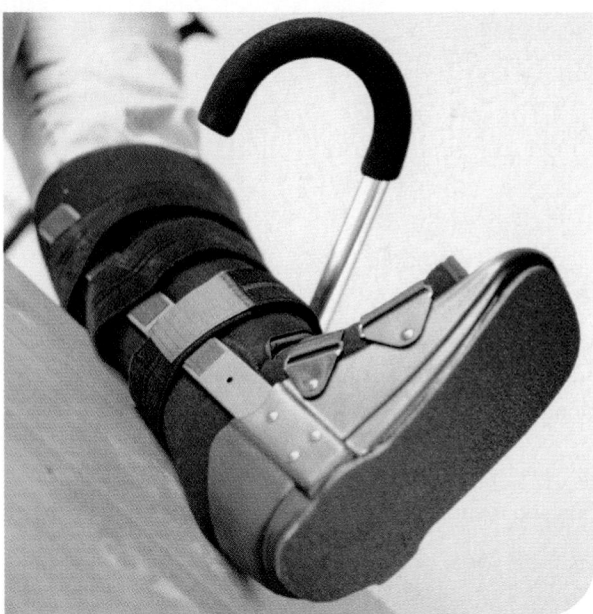

FIGURE 55-3   Cast boot.

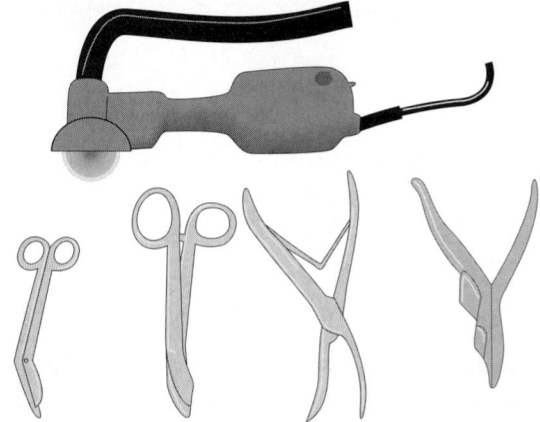

FIGURE 55-4   Cast removal equipment.

Figure 55-3 shows a cast boot given to a patient with a leg cast before leaving the office. After being sure that the patient understands the importance of cast care, the medical assistant must document the teaching in the patient chart.

Removing a Cast

The medical assistant may need to assist the physician with removing a cast. Equipment needed (see Figure 55-4) includes a cast cutter, cast spreader, bandage scissors, bag for disposing of cast materials, and a drape. After washing hands and draping the patient, the medical assistant will explain the process to the patient—for example, the cutter vibrates and does not spin, and the patient may feel some pressure and warmth. The patient may be shocked to see that the skin under the cast has become white and that the muscle tone has decreased. He or she may need some reassurance that physical therapy will improve the function and appearance of the limb.

The medical assistant should stand near the physician and hand the necessary equipment as requested. After the cast is removed, the medical assistant should provide written instructions for postcast care to the patient, clean the equipment, wash hands, and document the procedure in the patient chart.

- Observe the fingers and toes for color changes, temperature changes, pain, tingling, or decreased sensation.

- Allow the cast material to dry by exposing it to the air and keeping it uncovered, even during the night. If you apply pressure to the cast before it is dry, you can damage the tissue underneath.

- Do not try to scratch under the cast by putting objects into the cast. This will result in broken skin that can lead to infection.

- When decorating a cast, use only water-soluble paints or marking pens. Otherwise the cast will not be able to breathe.

- Call the physician's office if you smell a bad odor coming from the cast, lose sensation or blood flow beyond the cast, feel a burning sensation, or notice blood coming from the cast.

SUMMARY

One of the vital tasks of a medical assistant is to provide patient education, as needed and as directed by a physician. Examples of patient education include, but are not limited to, teaching health promotion, describing office policies, and adapting education to special needs. Many diseases can be prevented by patients receiving education from a medical assistant about stopping smoking, losing weight, exercising, using sunscreen, and so on. Good patient education involves effective communication (Chapter 5). For patients with dis-

abilities or special needs, education should be adapted to the patient in terms of both method of presentation and memory aids. Education also must be adapted to the age and developmental stage of the patient. In fact, patients can be educated during procedures, such as casting. In addition, the medical assistant often plays a critical role in handling noncompliant patients (e.g., a diabetic patient who will not adhere to the prescribed diet). Again, patient education is the most effective means of resolving such a situation.

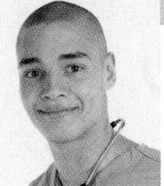

55 CHAPTER REVIEW

COMPETENCY REVIEW

1. Define and spell the terms to learn for this chapter.

2. Create a patient brochure describing a typical medical office. Be sure to include office location, times when patients are seen, contact numbers, physicians, type of practice, and insurance information.

3. Develop a teaching plan for health promotion.

4. Create a community resource brochure (e.g., one containing information about support groups, such as a Lions Club or the Red Cross).

PREPARING FOR THE CERTIFICATION EXAM

1. The most effective combination of teaching methods for the small child is
   a. lecture, printed materials, models
   b. lecture, return demonstration, programmed instruction
   c. role-play, group teaching, return demonstration
   d. video, test of knowledge, group teaching
   e. all of the above

2. When writing instructional booklets to teach diabetics nutritional planning, which of the following statements is FALSE?
   a. Use of pictures is helpful with children.
   b. Sprinkle material with medical abbreviations so the patient will know this is medical education.
   c. Present small amounts of information at a time.
   d. Ask the patient to demonstrate procedures he or she will need to do.
   e. Show diagrams of injection rotation sites.

3. Which of the following is a potential legal dilemma for the CMA (AAMA)?
   a. The patient asks for information regarding an alternative treatment for breast cancer.
   b. The patient asks for a list of the foods that her newborn infant can eat.
   c. The patient is discharged after day surgery for a hernia repair with only an instructional pamphlet.
   d. The patient states that he or she will not follow the instructions, so none are given.
   e. All of the above

4. Which of the following should NOT be included in an office brochure?
   a. where the physician was educated
   b. office location

c. insurance plans accepted
d. physician's home telephone number
e. emergency phone numbers and after-hours plan

5. Which of the following is the most important statement at the end of patient education?
   a. Let me show you a video about your disease.
   b. Please show me how you will do this procedure at home.
   c. This is what you ought to do.
   d. I will show you how to do this.
   e. Take this pop quiz on your disease when you get home.

6. Which of the following is NOT true about teaching the elderly?
   a. slowed processing time
   b. decreased dexterity
   c. decreased short-term memory
   d. should not be asked to demonstrate
   e. increased anxiety about new situations

7. Which of the following would NOT be said by a medical assistant in teaching cast care?
   a. "You can touch the casting materials."
   b. "If you need to scratch, use a ruler."
   c. "You should frequently check the color of your nails beyond the cast."
   d. "Elevate your extremity (arm or leg) when you are at rest."
   e. "When decorating a cast, use only water-soluble paints or marking pens."

8. The best aids for a patient who is hearing impaired would be
   a. a DVD that explains the procedure
   b. a booklet that explains the procedure

c. verbally explaining the procedure

d. showing the materials used in the procedure to the patient

9. The best way to teach a patient with vision impairment would include all of the following EXCEPT

a. verbally explaining the procedure

b. letting the patient touch the materials used in the procedure

c. showing a DVD that explains the procedure

d. providing a booklet in Braille about the procedure

e. a model of the body part involved

10. When teaching children, good ways to teach them include all of the following EXCEPT

a. rewarding them with stickers

b. letting them touch nonsterile instruments and materials

c. showing a 1-hour DVD of the procedure

d. showing the procedure on a doll

e. role-playing the procedure

CRITICAL THINKING

1. To begin her task of creating a patient education program at PPG, Tania is planning to create a list of patient education topics for proposed classes. With the physician's approval she will then begin to formulate the classes. What are some topics that Tania might want to consider for patient education classes?

2. The classes that PPG is going to offer are going to be geared toward its adult patient population. What are some things that Tania should take into consideration when planning education classes for the adult learner?

3. Tania calls Pearson General Hospital to speak with the director of community education for some advice prior to the start of the classes. The woman she speaks with warns her of the roadblocks to patient learning. What would be some of these roadblocks?

ON THE JOB

Bonny, a CMA (AAMA), works in a dialysis clinic. Most of her patients have diabetes mellitus, an endocrine disorder that can destroy the kidneys and leave the patient dependent on dialysis. The patients are usually on the dialysis machine for several hours 3 days per week. This gives Bonny a chance to do a lot of patient teaching.

1. Is it appropriate for the CMA (AAMA) to do patient teaching?

2. What would be the best way for Bonny to teach her patients?

3. If the patient has diabetic retinopathy, what would be the best way to teach this patient?

4. If the patient is old and claims to be "set in my ways," what would be good strategies for teaching the patient about healthy lifestyles?

5. Should family members be involved in the teaching plan? If so, how?

6. Describe a possible teaching plan for diabetic patients.

INTERNET ACTIVITY

Choose a patient education topic that interests you. Do an Internet search to gather information. Then create a patient teaching brochure.

MEDMEDIA

Additional interactive resources and activities for this chapter can be found:

On your student DVD: View applicable procedure videos on the DVD-ROM found in the back of this book.

MyHealthProfessionsKit.com: Test your knowledge of this chapter with games and activities. MyHealthProfessionsKit also includes resources, helpful links, and a Spanish audio glossary.

Medical Assisting Interactive: Practice your procedures as a medical assistant in this simulated doctor's office. This can be accessed through MyHealthProfessionsKit.com.

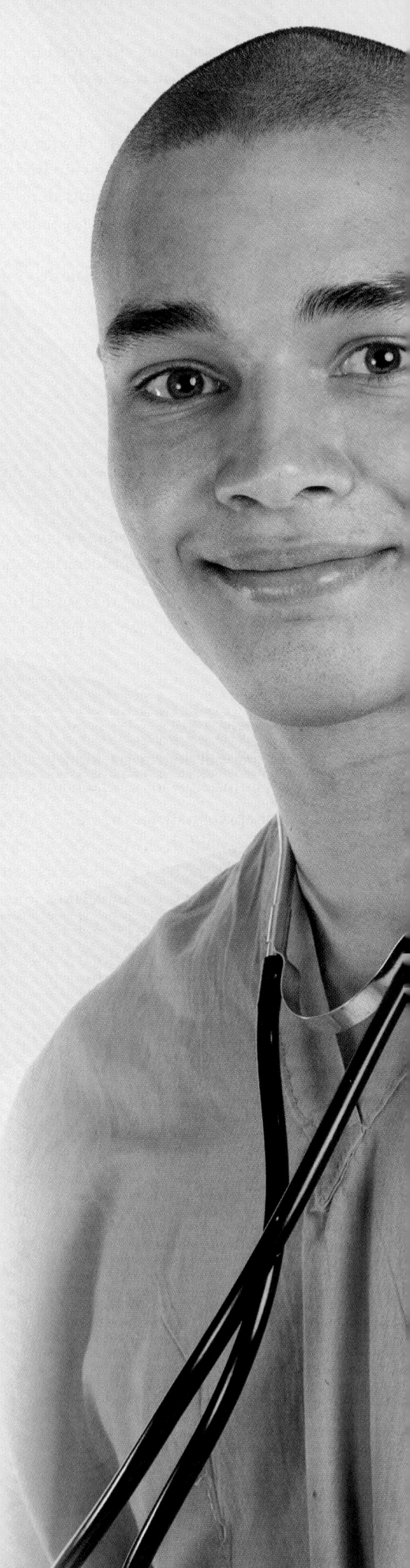

56 Nutrition

LEARNING OBJECTIVES

After completing this chapter, you should be able to:

- Define and spell the terms to learn for this chapter.

- List and describe six types of nutrients.

- Discuss the difference between saturated and unsaturated fats.

- Discuss the difference between LDL and HDL in cholesterol.

- Describe the Food Guide Pyramid and state its importance for patient education.

- Discuss calories as the term relates to proteins, carbohydrates, and fats.

- State the formula for determining the percentage of calories in a food that are supplied by fat.

- List and discuss six important dietary guidelines.

- State 12 diet modifications and why the physician might order them.

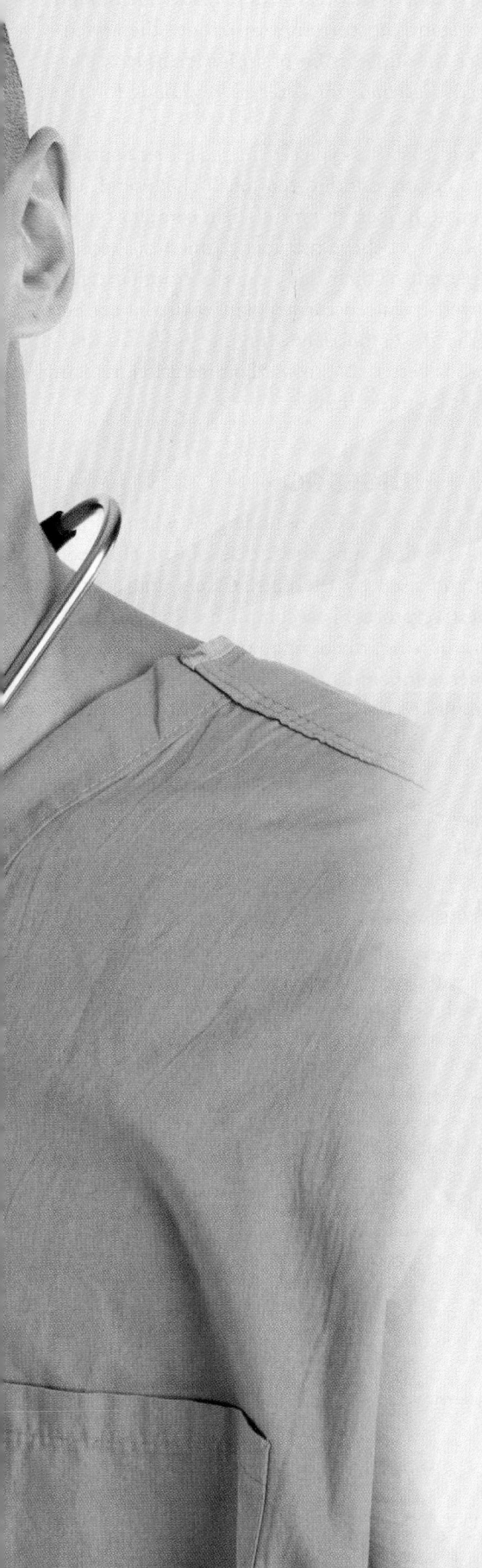

CHAPTER OUTLINE

CASE STUDY

Jaden Henderson is seeing Dr. Salpega for a follow-up to blood work that was completed last week. She tells David, the medical assistant, that she has been extremely fatigued during the past few months. She learns from Dr. Salpega that she has pernicious anemia. In addition, she has broken her right wrist since the time she had her blood drawn last week.

calorie

cholesterol

digestion

hydrogenation

lactating

lactose

lipids

macrominerals

metabolism

minerals

monosaccharides

nutrients

polysaccharides

Recommended Dietary
Allowances (RDAs)

refined sugars

vitamins

CERTIFICATION LINK

CMA (AAMA)
Nutrition
  Basic principles
  Special needs

RMA
General medical
assisting
  Patient education

CMAS (AMT)
Not applicable

N utrition includes all of the processes involved in using foods for growth, repair, and maintenance of the body. The nutrition process includes ingestion, digestion, absorption, and metabolism. Some nutrients are capable of being stored in the body and can be used when the food intake is insufficient. Other nutrients, such as vitamin C, are not stored and must be continually replenished.

Nutrition

Interest in nutrition has been ongoing for a long time. For example, debilitating diseases such as scurvy, rickets, and beriberi were found to be caused by deficiencies in the diet. Scurvy was discovered to be a disease of sailors and others who did not receive fresh fruits and vegetables for long periods of time. When sailors began to take lemons and limes along on their sea voyages, the symptoms of scurvy (hemorrhages, anemia, weakness, sallow complexion) disappeared. A lack of vitamin C was the culprit. Rickets, caused by a deficiency of vitamin D, produced bowed legs in young babies and children until this vitamin was added to milk to fortify it. Beriberi, more commonly found in rice-growing regions, caused neurological and cardiovascular abnormalities until thiamine was added to the diet of patients. The cures for these diseases resulted from research into what people were eating.

Nutritionists and dietitians study and teach about nutrition. Among their other activities, nutritionists provide information on foods and nutrition, and dietitians promote good health through implementation of proper diet and the use of diet in the treatment of disease. Although the medical assistant can certainly distribute dietary information under the supervision of a physician, it is usually a registered dietitian who creates regimens for the patient.

It has been said that the typical American diet contains too much fat, too many calories, too much cholesterol, too much salt, not enough fiber, and insufficient complex carbohydrates. Nutritionists believe that many Americans receive more than 40 percent of their daily calories from fats. The best diet is a well-balanced eating plan with the correct proportion of the major nutrients (Figure 56-1). A well-nourished person is better able to ward off infection, remain alert, and perhaps even live longer.

DIGESTION

Digestion is the process the body undergoes when it converts food into chemical substances that can be absorbed into the blood and used by the body tissues and organs. The actual digestive process is accomplished by physically breaking down, diluting, dissolving, and chemically splitting into simpler compounds the food substances we consume. For example, proteins are broken down into amino

PROFESSIONALISM
THE WORKPLACE

Perhaps the most important patient education the medical assistant can provide is about healthy lifestyles. Poor diet contributes to many diseases, such as diabetes, heart disease, stroke, and gout. The physician should ask about nutritional habits at annual checkups, but if your physician is too pressed for time, you might prepare some brochures to educate patients about a healthy diet. Be sure that you know what comprises a healthy diet before creating the brochures and have your office manager or physician approve them. In this way, teamwork in the office can improve the patient's health and improve outcomes for the medical office.

NUTRIENT CLASS	BODILY FUNCTIONS	FOOD SOURCES
CARBOHYDRATES 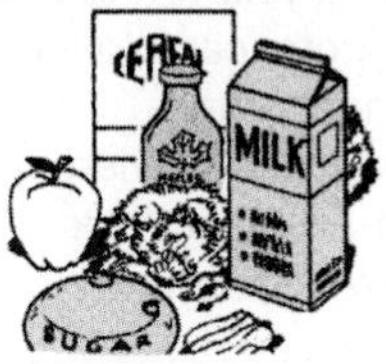	Provides work energy for body activities, and heat energy for maintenance of body temperature.	Cereal grains and their products (bread, breakfast cereals, macaroni products), potatoes, sugar, syrups, fruits, milk, vegetables, nuts.
PROTEINS 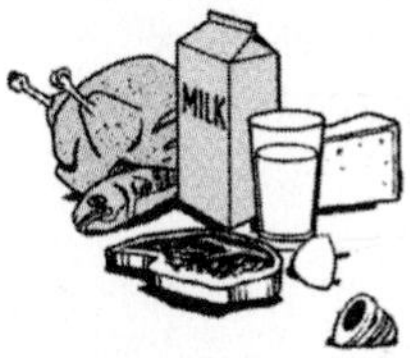	Build and renew body tissues; regulate body functions and supply energy. Complete proteins; maintain life and provide growth. Incomplete proteins; maintain life but do not provide for growth.	Complete proteins: Derived from animal foods—meat, milk, eggs, fish, cheese, poultry. Incomplete proteins: Derived from vegetable foods—soybeans, dry beans, peas, some nuts and whole grain products.
FATS 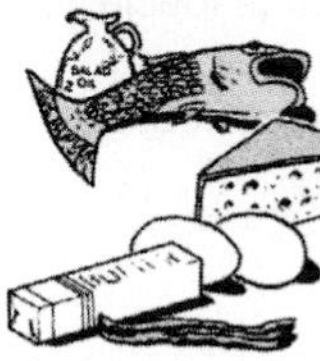	Give work energy for body activities and heat energy for maintenance of body temperature. Carrier of vitamins A and D, provide fatty acids necessary for growth and maintenance of body tissues.	Some foods are chiefly fat, such as lard, vegetable fats and oils, and butter. Many other foods contain smaller proportions of fats—nuts, meats, fish, poultry, cream, whole milk.
MINERALS Calcium 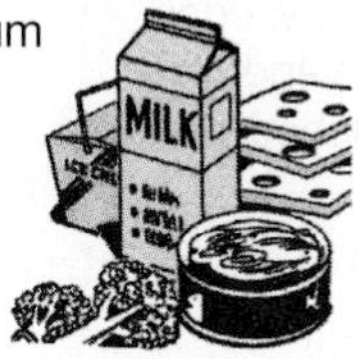	Builds and renews bones, teeth, and other tissues; regulates the activity of the muscles, heart, nerves; and controls the clotting of blood.	Milk and milk products except butter; most dark green vegetables; canned salmon.
PHOSPHORUS 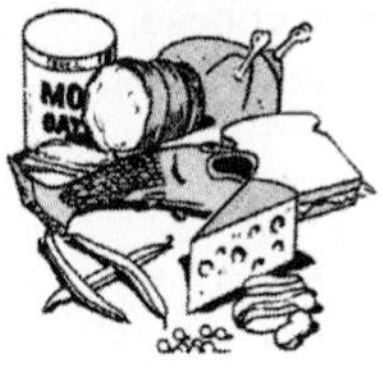	Associated with calcium in some functions needed to build and renew bones and teeth. Influences the oxidation of foods in the body cells; important in nerve tissue.	Widely distributed in foods; especially cheese, oat cereals, whole wheat products, dry beans and peas, meat, fish, poultry, nuts.
MINERALS Iron 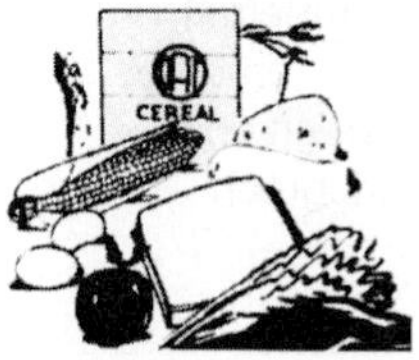	Builds and renews hemoglobin, the red pigment in blood which carries oxygen from the lungs to the cells.	Eggs, meat, especially liver and kidney; deep-yellow and dark green vegetables; potatoes, dried fruits, whole-grain products; enriched flour, bread, breakfast cereals.
Iodine 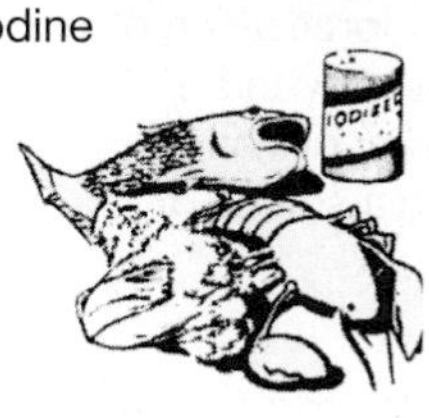	Enables the thyroid gland to perform its function of controlling the rate at which foods are oxidized in the cells.	Fish (obtained from the sea), some plant-foods grown in soils containing iodine; table salt fortified with iodine (iodized).

FIGURE 56-1 A balanced diet begins with eating foods from the basic food groups.

NUTRIENT CLASS	BODILY FUNCTIONS	FOOD SOURCES
VITAMINS A	Necessary for normal functioning of the eyes, prevents night blindness. Ensures a healthy condition of the skin, hair, and mucous membranes. Maintains a state of resistance to infections of the eyes, mouth, and respiratory tract.	One form of vitamin A is yellow and one form is colorless. Apricots, cantaloupe, milk, cheese, eggs, meat organs, (especially liver and kidney), fortified margarine, butter fish-liver oils, dark green and deep yellow vegetables.
B Complex B_1 (Thiamine)	Maintains a healthy condition of the nerves. Fosters a good appetite. Helps the body cells use carbohydrates.	Whole grain and enriched grain products; meats (especially pork, liver and kidney). Dry beans and peas.
B_2 (Riboflavin)	Keeps the skin, mouth, and eyes in a healthy condition. Acts with other nutrients to form enzymes and control oxidation in cells.	Milk, cheese, eggs, meat (especially liver and kidney), whole grain and enriched grain products, dark green vegetables.
VITAMINS Niacin	Influences the oxidation of carbohydrates and proteins in the body cells.	Liver, meat, fish, poultry, eggs, peanuts; dark green vegetables, whole grain and enriched cereal products.
B_{12}	Regulates specific processes in digestion. Helps maintain normal functions of muscles, nerves, heart, blood—general body metabolism.	Liver, other organ meats, cheese, eggs, milk, leafy green vegetables.
C (Ascorbic Acid)	Acts as a cement between body cells, and helps them work together to carry out their special functions. Maintains a sound condition of bones, teeth, and gums. Not stored in the body.	Fresh, raw citrus fruits and vegetables—oranges, grapefruit, cantaloupe, strawberries, tomatoes, raw onions, cabbage, green and sweet red peppers, dark green vegetables.
D	Enables the growing body to use calcium and phosphorus in a normal way to build bones and teeth.	Provided by vitamin D fortification of certain foods, such as milk and margarine. Also fish-liver oils and eggs. Sunshine is also a source of vitamin D.

FIGURE 56-1 (Continued)

NUTRIENT CLASS	BODILY FUNCTIONS	FOOD SOURCES
WATER	Regulates body processes. Aids in regulating body temperature. Carries nutrients to body cells and carries waste products away from them. Helps to lubricate joints. Water has no food value, although most water contains mineral elements. More immediately necessary to life than food—second only to oxygen.	Drinking water, and other beverages; all foods except those made up of a single nutrient, as sugar and some fats. Milk, milk drinks, soups, vegetables, fruit juices. Ice cream, watermelon, strawberries, lettuce, tomatoes, cereals, other dry products.

FIGURE 56-1 (Continued)

acids, carbohydrates are broken down into **monosaccharides** (simple sugars), and fats are absorbed as fatty acids and glycerol (glycerin).

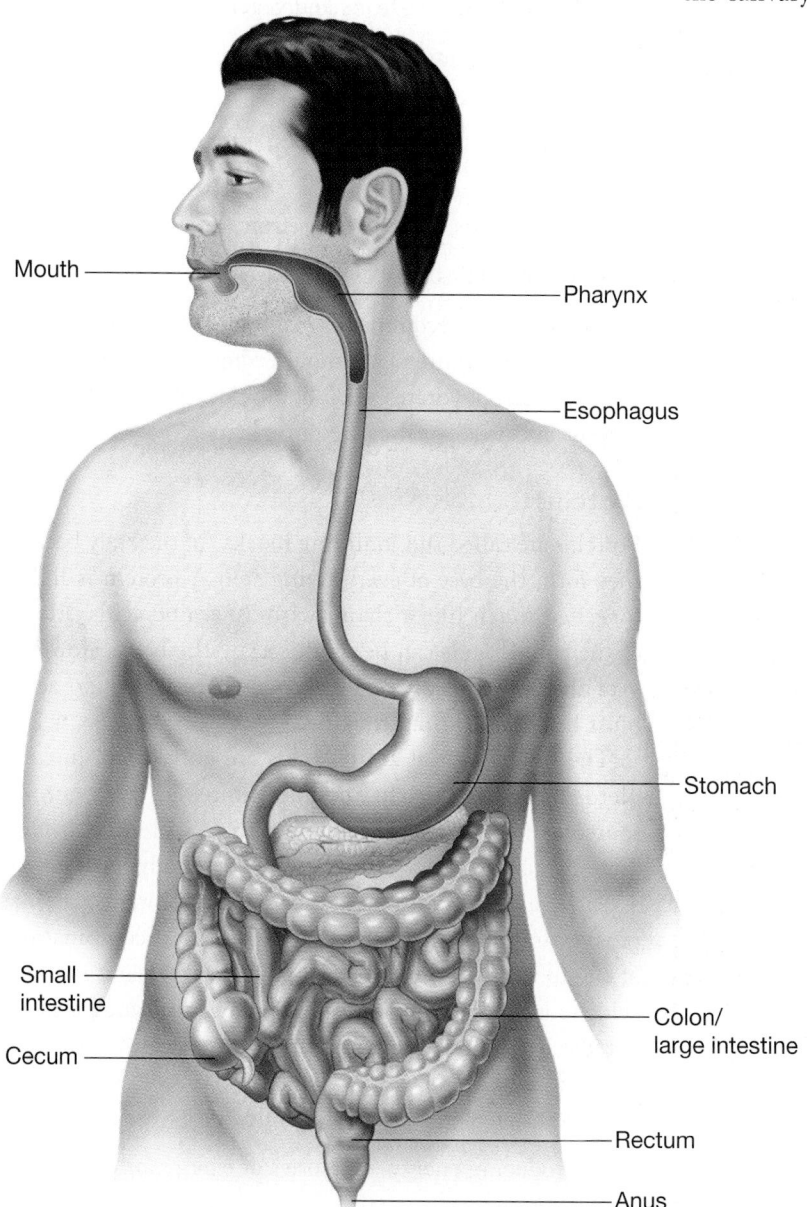

FIGURE 56-2 The digestive system.

Actual digestion takes place in the alimentary canal, also referred to as the digestive system or the gastrointestinal (GI) tract (Figure 56-2). Accessory organs, including the salivary glands, liver, gallbladder, and pancreas, provide essential enzymes for digestion through their secretions. Water, minerals, some vitamins, and some of the carbohydrates in fruit are absorbable as soon as they are ingested.

The average adult stomach holds about $1\frac{1}{2}$ quarts of food and liquid. The stomach will reach a peak in the digestive process 2 hours after a meal and may take 3 to 5 hours to empty into the small intestine. It may take 20 minutes for the brain to register that food has entered the system.

Digestion is influenced by emotions as well as the enzyme and chemical actions of the digestive system. A quiet, calm atmosphere at mealtime can enhance the digestive process.

METABOLISM

Metabolism is the sum of all physical and chemical changes that take place within the human body. It is the process of changing food, air, water, and other materials into substances absorbed into the body through the blood and respiratory system. Specific enzymes that are required to maintain metabolism are amino acids, carbohydrates, vitamins, and essential trace minerals.

Approximately 23 percent of all energy released by nutrients is used by the body to carry on its normal functions, such as respiration, digestion, reproduction, muscular movement, circulation, and cellular regrowth. The remaining 75 percent of the energy becomes heat. Eating and drinking the wrong foods can negatively affect metabolism.

CLASSIFICATION OF NUTRIENTS

Nutrients are the organic and inorganic chemical substances found in foods that supply the body with the elements necessary for metabolism. Certain nutrients (carbohydrates, fats, and proteins) provide energy; other nutrients (water, electrolytes, minerals, and vitamins) are essential to the metabolic process.

There are six main classifications of nutrients, and more than 50 nutrients are required for the human body to function properly. These nutrients must be consumed in the diet on a daily basis. The six classifications of nutrients are as follows:

1. Carbohydrates
2. Proteins
3. Fats
4. Water
5. Vitamins
6. Minerals

Carbohydrates

The main source of energy from foods is carbohydrates. Carbohydrates are the sugars (simple carbohydrates), starches (complex carbohydrates), and fiber (cellulose) that are found mainly in plants. They are stored in the body as glycogen in virtually all tissues but mainly in the liver and muscles. They form an important source of reserved energy in the body.

Sugars include simple sugars (monosaccharides of glucose, galactose, and fructose) and complex sugars (disaccharide or sucrose, lactose or milk sugar, and maltose). Starches are **polysaccharides**, which are reduced to glucose during the digestive process and transported into the blood. Most sugars are produced naturally by plants, especially fruits,

sugar cane, and sugar beets. However, **lactose**, a combination of glucose and galactose, is found in animal milk. Processed or **refined sugars** (e.g., table sugar, molasses, and corn syrup) have been extracted and concentrated from natural resources.

Carbohydrates provide 4 calories of energy for every gram of carbohydrate. Complex carbohydrates are considered ideal foods for a healthy diet since they are generally low in fat, high in fiber, and a good source for vitamins and minerals. Excess carbohydrates are stored in the body as fat.

The following are some sources of simple carbohydrates (simple sugars):

- Refined table sugar, honey, jelly, syrup, candy
- Natural sugar in fruits and vegetables

The following are some sources of complex carbohydrates (starches):

- Vegetables (yams, potatoes, broccoli, carrots, peas, beans)
- Citrus fruits (oranges, grapefruit, lemons, limes)
- Whole grains, cereals, and pastas

Nutritionists recommend that only 10 percent of the body's calorie requirements should come from refined sugar. Complex carbohydrates should provide 50 percent to 60 percent of the daily calorie requirements.

Proteins

Proteins are called the "building blocks" of the body because they form the base of every living cell. A protein is linked together, much like a chain, with 20 amino acids. Eleven of the amino acids can be produced by the body. However, 9 of the amino acids, referred to as essential amino acids, must be obtained from the diet.

The nine essential amino acids are only found in complete proteins, which include proteins from animal sources, such as meat, cheese, eggs, fish, and milk. Incomplete proteins, which cannot supply the body with all the essential amino acids, include vegetable proteins, such as peas, beans, and wheat. Fortunately, various combinations of the incomplete proteins can supply the essential amino acids (e.g., legumes and rice). It is recommended that 12 percent to 15 percent of the daily calories consumed come from proteins.

Proteins are necessary for the following:

- Producing energy (4 calories of energy for every gram of protein consumed)

- Promoting growth and repair of tissues

- Providing the framework for bones, muscles, and blood

Fats

Fats, also called **lipids**, are fatty acids that can be chemically classified as saturated or unsaturated. Fats do not dissolve in water. Some fat is necessary in the diet since the fat-soluble vitamins A, D, E, and K are all carried into the bloodstream by way of fats. Two critical fatty acids, linoleic and linolenic, are "essential" to the diet.

Fat is a major source of energy for the body. Fat can be found in both animal and plant food products. When eaten moderately, fat is important for proper growth, development, and maintenance of good health. Fat provides taste, consistency, and stability and helps you feel full. Parents should be aware that fats are an especially important source of calories and nutrients for infants and toddlers (up to 2 years of age), who have the highest energy needs per unit of body weight of any age group.

Saturated fat is produced by animal sources, such as meat, eggs, lard, and dairy products, and certain oil-producing plants, such as coconuts and palms. Many commercially prepared cakes, cookies, and nondairy creamers contain hidden saturated fat. Saturated fat has many negative effects on the body, including raising the level of blood cholesterol. It is recommended that no more than 10 percent of the daily calorie intake should come from saturated fat. Fat reduction can also reduce the risk of disease (e.g., certain types of cancer, heart disease, and stroke).

Unsaturated fats are of two types: polyunsaturated fat and monounsaturated fat. Polyunsaturated fat is found in vegetable oils and fish oils (omega-3 fatty acids). Unsaturated fat is normally liquid at room temperature but can be converted into a solid fat through the process of **hydrogenation**. Hydrogenation turns liquid unsaturated fat into margarine by adding hydrogen.

Monounsaturated fat is considered to be a more desirable type of unsaturated fat since it has the ability to lower cholesterol levels and low density lipids (LDLs). Monounsaturated fats include canola oil, olive oil, and peanut oil. Fats, in moderation, are beneficial for the body because they provide the following:

- A concentrated source of energy (9 calories of energy for every gram of fat consumed)

- Assistance in the transportation of soluble fat vitamins A, D, E, and K

- A source of energy

- Some taste to foods

- A feeling of satiety

- Lubrication for skin and internal tissues

- Energy stores for future use

Unfortunately, many Americans are eating more fat than they need. Many foods contain hidden fat. Fat content is indicated on the packaging of many foods. However, food labeling can be confusing and misleading. A high-fiber muffin may actually contain polyunsaturated fat, eggs, sugar, and very little fiber. See Table 56-1 for an example of food labeling components mandated by the U.S. Department of Health and Human Services and the U.S. Department of Agriculture.

Trans Fats. Beginning in 2006, all labels must identify the *trans fats* in food. Basically, trans fat is formed when manufacturers add hydrogen to vegetable oil. Hydrogenation increases the shelf life and flavor stability of foods containing these fats.

Trans fat is frequently found in vegetable shortenings, some margarines, snack foods, and other foods made with or fried in partially hydrogenated oils. A small amount of trans fat is found naturally, primarily in dairy products, some meat, and other animal-based foods. Most of it is manufactured.

Whereas unsaturated fats (monounsaturated and polyunsaturated) are beneficial when consumed in moderation, saturated and trans fats are not. Saturated fat and trans fat raise LDL cholesterol levels in the blood. Dietary cholesterol also contributes to heart disease. Therefore, it is advisable to choose foods low in saturated fat, trans fat, and cholesterol as part of a healthful diet.

When comparing foods, look at the Nutrition Facts panel on the label, and choose the food with the lower amounts of saturated fat, trans fat, and cholesterol. Health experts recommend that you keep your intake of saturated fat, trans fat, and cholesterol as low as possible while consuming a nutritionally adequate diet. However, these experts recognize that eliminating these three components entirely from your diet is not practical because they are unavoidable in ordinary diets. For resources on nutrition facts, see Table 56-2.

Water

Water is a vital constituent in the body and is necessary for survival. The human body can survive for several weeks without food but cannot live more than a few days without water. Water is an inorganic nutrient with no

TABLE 56-1 Food Label for Snack Crackers

Nutrition Facts			%DV*
Serving size: 16 crackers (29 g) Servings per container: about 4			
Calories Calories from fat	140 50		
Amount per serving		Total fat 6 g Trans fat 2 g Polyunsaturated fat 0.5 g Monounsaturated fat 2.5 g	9 percent 18 percent
		Cholesterol 0 mg	0 percent
		Sodium 170 mg	7 percent
		Total carbohydrate 19 g	6 percent
		Dietary fiber 2 g	
		Protein 2 g	
		Vitamin A	0 percent
		Vitamin C	0 percent
		Calcium	2 percent
		Iron	4 percent

*%DV = Percent Daily Values, which are based on a 2,000-calorie diet. An individual's daily values may be higher or lower depending on calorie needs.

	Calories	2,000	2,500
Total fat	Less than	65 g	80 g
Sat fat	Less than	20 g	25 g
Cholesterol	Less than	300 mg	300 mg
Sodium	Less than	2,400 mg	2,400 mg
Total carbohydrate		300 mg	375 g
Dietary fiber		25 g	30 g

TABLE 56-2 Resources for Nutrition Facts

Resource	Website
Agricultural Research Service	http://www.ars.usda.gov
Food and Drug Administration	http://www.fda.gov
National Agricultural Library	http://fnic.nal.usda.gov
Nutrient Data Laboratory	http://www.ars.usda.gov/main/site_main.htm?modecode= 12-35-45-00
Office of Dietary Supplements, National Institutes of Health	http://dietary-supplements.info.nih.gov
U.S. Department of Agriculture Food Pyramid	http://mypyramid.gov
U.S. Department of Agriculture Healthy School Meals	http://healthymeals.nal.usda.gov

Box 56-1 The Functions of Water in the BODY

Water is used by the body for the following:

- Carries oxygen and nutrients to cells
- Regulates body temperature
- Prevents dehydration

- Replaces water lost through perspiration, respiration, urination, and defecation
- Removes waste products from cells
- Protects organs and tissues

---

caloric value. Approximately two-thirds of the body is water.

The average human body is composed of between 50 and 60 percent water. The male body contains more water than the female due to the greater muscle mass of the male, which can hold more water. The female body, on the other hand, contains a greater percentage of fat than the male body. Fat does not hold as much water as muscle tissue does.

Water in the body is obtained from a variety of sources. Water is found in most fruits and vegetables, ingested as a liquid beverage, or occurs naturally as a result of metabolism. The function of water in the body is described in Box 56-1.

The recommended amount of water to be ingested daily is six to eight glasses. Because water occurs in many foods, such as fruits, vegetables, meats, crackers, and even desserts, most people ingest enough water on a daily basis. Water intake is kept in balance with fluid output through the skin, lungs, urine, and feces. Individuals vary in their requirements for water depending on the following:

- Age
- Body size
- Climate
- Exercise
- Illness
- Metabolic rate
- Pregnancy

Vitamins

Vitamins are organic substances that are essential for metabolism, growth, and development of the body. They are not sources of energy, but they are required for health. A variety of conditions can increase the need for vitamins above the usual recommended dose. These include pregnancy, lactation, excessive use of alcohol, and some illnesses.

In general, most of the vitamins cannot be formed in the body with the exception of vitamin A, which is formed from carotene. Vitamin D is formed by the action of ultraviolet light on the skin (sunlight); vitamin K is formed by bacteria in the intestines.

Vitamins are generally identified by their alphabetic letter. The two main classifications of vitamins are fat soluble (A, D, E, and K) and water soluble (B and C). These classifications are important in patients who have diseases that interfere with the digestion of fat, such as celiac disease, since they will eventually develop a deficiency in the fat-soluble vitamins. The human body cannot manufacture vitamin C; therefore it must be obtained from foods, including citrus fruits, or nutritional supplements. The liver stores the fat-soluble vitamins A, D, E, and K.

Generally, vitamins are thought to be best consumed in natural foods. However, in modern times many foods have been stripped of their vitamins during processing. For that reason, many foods (e.g., breakfast cereals) are vitamin fortified to increase their vitamin content. Because heavily processed foods lack vitamins, many physicians will prescribe multivitamins for the patient whose diet contains processed food products.

A relatively recent trend toward taking megadoses of fat-soluble vitamins (A, D, E, and K) has led in some cases to vitamin toxicity. Taking megadoses of water-soluble vitamins is unnecessary. Most patients only need the daily requirements found in a multivitamin suitable to the patient's age. Men need less iron, and pregnant women need more folate, for example. A medical assistant should educate the patient on the importance of not taking megadoses of vitamins.

The following are some sources for water-soluble vitamins:

- Vitamin B_1: liver, eggs, pork, wheat germ, yeast-enriched cereals, nuts
- Vitamin B_2: milk, liver, egg whites, yeast, wheat germ, almonds
- Vitamin B_6: wheat bran, molasses, liver, soybeans, bananas, raisins, turkey giblets, yellowfin tuna, chickpeas, beef liver
- Vitamin B_{12}: beef, liver, milk, shellfish, cheese, sardines, beef liver, turkey giblets

- Niacin: liver, poultry, enriched cereals, tuna, peanuts
- Biotin: egg yolks, legumes, meat
- Folacin: legumes, green leafy vegetables, cornmeal, orange juice, lentils, pinto beans
- Pantothenic acid: legumes, grains
- Vitamin C: citrus fruits, raw vegetables, strawberries, peaches, papayas, peppers

Some sources of fat-soluble vitamins are these:

- Vitamin A: green and yellow vegetables, animal foods, egg yolks, cheese
- Vitamin D: milk, butter, margarine, sardines, fish liver oils, sunlight
- Vitamin E: wheat germ, corn oil, soybeans, sunflower seeds, almonds, hazelnuts, spinach
- Vitamin K: green leafy vegetables, liver, cabbage, cauliflower

Vitamins provide essential organic substances, but they can be destroyed in foods through improper storage and prolonged cooking. See Table 56-3 for a further description of individual vitamins.

TABLE 56-3 Vitamins and Minerals

Nutrient/Use	Source	Symptoms of Functional Deficiency	Symptoms of Toxicity	Recommended Dietary Allowances (RDA)
Vitamin A (carotene): necessary for formation and maintenance of skin, mucous membranes, teeth and hair, normal vision	Egg yolk, fish-liver oils, liver, leafy green or yellow vegetables, yellow and orange fruits, dairy products	Night blindness, fatigue, scaly skin	Headache, skin peeling, bone thickening, liver and spleen enlargement	5,000 IU/day
Vitamin B_1 (thiamine): carbohydrate metabolism, nerve cell function, heart muscle function	Dried yeast, whole grains, meat (liver and pork), nuts, enriched cereals, potatoes, legumes	Beriberi, fatigue, mental confusion		1.5 mg/day
Vitamin B_2 (riboflavin): releases energy during protein metabolism	Milk, cheese, eggs, liver, enriched cereals, almonds	Anemia, dermatosis, skin cracks		1.2 mg/day
Vitamin B_6 (group): nitrogen and protein metabolism, assists in building body tissue	Dried yeast, liver, whole grain cereals, fish, legumes, bananas, avocados	Anemia, seborrheic dermatitis, nervous system disorders, convulsions, skin cracks	Nerve damage	2 mg/day
Vitamin B_{12} (cyanocobalamin): nervous system function, fat and protein metabolism	Milk products, seafood, meat, liver, cheese	Pernicious anemia, fatigue, nervousness		6 mcg/day
Niacin (nicotinic acid): carbohydrate, fat, and protein metabolism	Dried yeast, fish, liver, meat, legumes, enriched cereals, eggs, peanuts, and poultry	Pellagra, dermatosis, glossitis, central nervous system (CNS) dysfunction, fatigue		20 mg/day
Vitamin C (ascorbic acid): needed to build bones, muscles, blood vessels, and connective tissue; aids in iron absorption	Citrus fruits, tomatoes, broccoli, potatoes, cabbage, green peppers, strawberries and other berries	Scurvy, loose teeth, hemorrhoids, gingivitis, fatigue	Nausea and diarrhea	60 mg/day

Vitamin D: necessary for calcium and phosphorous absorption, bone and tooth development and maintenance; helps maintain nervous system and heart muscle action	Fortified milk, butter, margarine, eggs, fish-liver oils, liver, sunlight	Rickets, tetany, loss of bone calcium	Diarrhea, weight loss, renal failure	400 IU/day
Vitamin E: protects blood cell membranes, body tissues, and fatty acids from destruction	Vegetable oil, wheat germ, margarine, egg yolks, leafy vegetables, legumes, cereals	Anemia, nerve damage, RBC hemolysis, muscle damage		30 IU/day
Vitamin K: normal blood coagulation, prothrombin formation	Leafy vegetables, liver, pork, vegetable oils, fruit, dairy	Hemorrhage in newborn and in person taking blood thinner		No RDA for Vitamin K
Biotin: metabolism of protein, carbohydrates, and fats	Yeast, liver, kidney, egg yolks, nuts, legumes, cauliflower	Dermatitis, glossitis		0.5 mg/day
Folic acid: RBC production	Dried legumes, leafy green vegetables, organ meats	Anemia, GI disorders, mouth cracks		0.4 mg/day
Pantothenic acid: aids in energy release from carbohydrates and fats	Whole grains, meats, vegetables, fruits, legumes	Muscle cramps, fatigue, vomiting		10 mg/day
Calcium: bone and tooth formation, muscle contractility, blood coagulation, myocardial conduction, neuromuscular function	Milk and milk products, meat, fish, eggs, beans, cereals, fruits, vegetables, tofu, fortified orange juice	Hypocalcemia, tetany, neuromuscular excitability, osteoporosis	Hypercalcemia, kidney stones, renal failure	800 mg/day
Chromium: part of glucose tolerance factor (CTF)	Brewer's yeast; widely distributed in other foods	Impaired glucose tolerance in malnourished children and diabetics		No RDA
Cobalt: part of vitamin B_{12} molecule	Green leafy vegetables	Anemia in children		20 mg/day
Copper: enzyme component	Oysters, organ meats, nuts, dried legumes, whole grain cereals	Anemia in malnourished children		0.3 mg/kg per day
Fluorine: bone and tooth formation	Coffee, tea, fluoridated water	Dental caries	Mottling and pitting of permanent teeth	No RDA
Iodine: thyroxine (T_4) and triiodothyronine (T_3) formation, necessary for energy formation	Seafood, iodized salt, dairy products	Goiter, cretinism	Myxedema	150 mcg/day
Iron: hemoglobin, enzymes	Soybean flour, kidney, beef, liver, beans, peaches	Anemia		30 mg/day

(continued)

TABLE 56-3 (*continued*)

Nutrient/Use	Source	Symptoms of Functional Deficiency	Symptoms of Toxicity	Recommended Dietary Allowances (RDA)
Magnesium: bone and tooth formation, nerve conduction, muscle contractility, enzyme activity	Green leafy vegetables, cereals, nuts, wheat bran, grains, seafood, chocolate	Neuromuscular irritability, weakness	Hypotension, respiratory failure, cardiac disturbances	280 mg/day
Phosphorus: bone and tooth formation, acid–base formation	Milk, cheese, meat, fish, poultry, cereals, nuts, legumes	Irritability, weakness, blood cell disorders		300 mg/day
Potassium: muscle activity, nerve transmission, intracellular acid–base balance, water retention	Milk, bananas, kiwi, raisins, vegetables	Hypokalemia, paralysis, cardiac arrhythmia (irregular heartbeat)	Hyperkalemia, paralysis, cardiac arrhythmia	2,000 mg/day
Sodium: maintain acid–base balance, muscle contractility, nerve transmission	Meat (beef, pork), cheese, sardines, olives, potato chips, table salt	Hyponatremia, muscle cramping	Hypernatremia, coma, confusion, high blood pressure	500 mg/day
Zinc: growth, wound healing component of insulin and enzyme	Vegetables	Growth retardation		30 mg/day

IU, international units; mg, milligrams; mcg, micrograms.

Minerals

Minerals are inorganic elements that are of neither animal nor plant origin. They are found throughout the body but mainly in bones and teeth, and they constitute 5 percent of the body. The two classifications of minerals are macrominerals (major minerals) and microminerals (trace minerals). The **macrominerals** include calcium, magnesium, phosphorus, sodium, potassium, chlorine, and sulfur. Macrominerals are required in greater amounts than the trace minerals iron, iodine, copper, manganese, cobalt, fluorine, zinc, selenium, chromium, nickel, tin, and vanadium. Minerals are found in the following sources:

- Vegetables and fruits (calcium, iron, phosphorus, copper, iodine)
- Milk and leafy vegetables (calcium)
- Balanced diet

Minerals do not supply calories or energy; however, they are necessary for physiological processes such as heart contraction and hormonal action. Minerals used to be readily available in fruits and vegetables because they existed in the soil. Soil may have been depleted by the heavy use of fertilizers, overuse of the soil, and failure to add organic compounds. Unless the patient buys organic or fresh foods, the patient may lack vital minerals. For that reason, the physician may prescribe a multivitamin with mineral supplement. See Table 56-3 for more information on minerals.

Cholesterol

Much controversy surrounds cholesterol. **Cholesterol** is a fat-like material that is normally found in the body. It is essential for the function of body systems, such as the nervous system, formation of cell membranes, and many hormones. Animal sources of cholesterol provide saturated fat, which may contribute to elevated blood cholesterol in humans.

Cholesterol moves into and out of the body cells within compounds called lipoproteins. These lipoproteins are classified into either high-density lipoproteins (HDLs) or low-density lipoproteins (LDLs). HDLs are the "good cholesterol," and LDLs are the "bad cholesterol." LDLs are bad since they carry most (60 to 70 percent) of the cholesterol into the bloodstream. This cholesterol is deposited into blood vessels and can lead to a narrowing of the blood vessels that leads to heart disease and stroke. HDLs are good because they only contain 20 to 30 percent of the blood cholesterol and carry cholesterol away from the arteries. It is believed that the

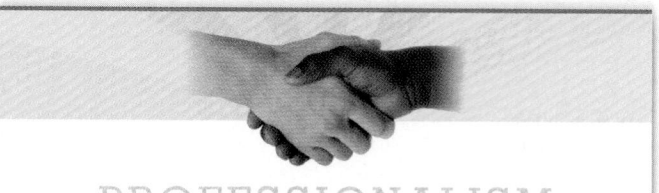
higher the HDL level in the blood, the lower the risk for cardiovascular disease.

An increase in cholesterol level has been tied to an increased risk for heart disease: heart attack and stroke. Evidence indicates that unsaturated fats (olive oil and canola oil) may help to lower the amount of cholesterol in the blood. It is important to examine food labels for the amounts of both cholesterol and saturated fat. Many foods contain no cholesterol but a large amount of saturated fat, which can lead to cholesterol buildup in the body.

BALANCED DIET

The key to a balanced diet is eating a variety of foods in the correct amount. Eating food as recommended in the Food Guide Pyramid published by the U.S. Department of Health and Human Services will be adequate for good health. The size of portions and number of servings will depend on the age, size, and exercise level of the individual. See Figure 56-1 for an illustration of the basic nutrient classifications.

Food Guide Pyramid

A revised Food Guide Pyramid was introduced in 2005 by the U.S. Department of Agriculture to replace the old "basic four" food groups used from 1946 and updated in 1992. Figure 56-3 illustrates the new Food Guide Pyramid. A healthy diet should include a wide variety of foods. Patients can better understand the entire nutritional process if they review the Food Guide Pyramid. Many doctors' offices display a large poster of it on a wall.

The new Food Guide Pyramid customizes a regimen according to age, activity, and gender. If patients want a customized Food Guide Pyramid, they can go to the website to customize an education plan for themselves. The site ad-

dresses appropriate physical activity and describes the six food groups: grains, vegetables, fruits, milk, meat and beans, and fats and oils. The customized pyramid describes an ideal amount for the person to eat daily, with lists of healthy foods in each category. The site promotes fresh, rather than processed, foods. It also suggests the use of healthy oils rather than solid fats. The pyramid suggests the user choose lean or low-fat meat and poultry and foods rich in omega-3 fatty acids. It also describes discretionary calories, such as wine and sweetened cereals, which should be minimized. Sweets, although pleasant to taste, are rarely nutritious.

Recommended Dietary Allowances

The Food and Nutrition Board of the National Academy of Sciences has created standards of recommendations for the amount of protein, vitamins, and minerals that Americans should try to eat and the body weights they should try to maintain for good nutrition. These standards, called **Recommended Dietary Allowances (RDAs)**, periodically change as weight ranges and protein needs are reviewed. The charts can be ordered through the National Academy Press in Washington, D.C.

CALORIES

The intake of food is measured in terms of the energy that it produces. A **calorie** is a measurement of a unit of heat that provides energy. The definition of a calorie is the amount of heat (energy) required to raise the temperature of 1 kg of water 1 degree Celsius ($1°C$).

All food (except water) generates energy in the body. Daily calorie requirements of individuals will vary based on a variety of factors including gender, age, weight, and activity level. Men generally need more calories than women; the young need more calories than older adults; heavier people require more calories to maintain their weight; and active people require more calories because they tend to burn calories faster than individuals who are inactive. Women require more calories during periods of pregnancy and lactation.

When more calories are taken in than are consumed, they are stored as fat. Overall body weight will increase when this happens on a consistent basis. When fewer calories are taken in than are needed, stored calories are used and body weight will decrease.

Calories come from the proteins, carbohydrates, and fats in food. To determine the amount of energy generated by the food eaten, use the following figures:

- Protein: 4 calories of energy per gram
- Carbohydrate: 4 calories of energy per gram
- Fat: 9 calories of energy per gram

Anatomy of MyPyramid

One size doesn't fit all
USDA's new MyPyramid symbolizes a personalized approach to healthy eating and physical activity. The symbol has been designed to be simple. It has been developed to remind consumers to make healthy food choices and to be active every day. The different parts of the symbol are described below.

Activity
Activity is represented by the steps and the person climbing them, as a reminder of the importance of daily physical activity.

Moderation
Moderation is represented by the narrowing of each food group from bottom to top. The wider base stands for foods with little or no solid fats or added sugars. These should be selected more often. The narrower top area stands for foods containing more added sugars and solid fats. The more active you are, the more of these foods can fit into your diet.

Personalization
Personalization is shown by the person on the steps, the slogan, and the URL. Find the kinds and amounts of food to eat each day at MyPyramid.gov.

Proportionality
Proportionality is shown by the different widths of the food group bands. The widths suggest how much food a person should choose from each group. The widths are just a general guide, not exact proportions. Check the Web site for how much is right for you.

Variety
Variety is symbolized by the 6 color bands representing the 5 food groups of the Pyramid and oils. This illustrates that foods from all groups are needed each day for good health.

Gradual Improvement
Gradual improvement is encouraged by the slogan. It suggests that individuals can benefit from taking small steps to improve their diet and lifestyle each day.

MyPyramid.gov
STEPS TO A HEALTHIER YOU

USDA U.S. Department of Agriculture Center for Nutrition Policy and Promotion April 2005 CNPP-16

USDA is an equal opportunity provider and employer.

GRAINS | VEGETABLES | FRUITS | OILS | MILK | MEAT & BEANS

FIGURE 56-3 The 2005 Food Guide Pyramid.

Note: These figures are just for the protein, carbohydrate, and fat content of foods and not the total weight, including fluid, of the food.

Determining the Number of Calories in Food

Using a cookie that contains 1 g of protein, 4 g of carbohydrates, and 4 g of fat, calculate the total number of calories.

$$1 \text{ g protein (4 calories per gram)} = 4 \text{ calories}$$
$$4 \text{ g carbohydrates (4 calories per gram)} = 16 \text{ calories}$$
$$4 \text{ g fat (9 calories per gram)} = 36 \text{ calories}$$
$$\text{Total calories} = 56 \text{ calories per cookie}$$

Determining the Percentage of Calories Supplied by Fat

Use this formula when you want to determine the percentage of calories in a food supplied by fat:

$$\text{Fat calories} = \text{grams of fat} \times 9$$

Place result of calculation over total calories

Using the previous example of a cookie containing 56 calories, determine the percentage of calories supplied from fat:

$$4 \times 9 = 36 \text{ fat calories}$$
$$36/56 = 0.642 = 64.2 \text{ percent}$$

Therefore, 64.2 percent of the calories in this cookie are supplied by fat.

Dietary Guidelines

Under normal disease-free conditions, the average person should observe the following dietary guidelines:

1. Eat a wide variety of foods to acquire the necessary vitamins and minerals.
2. Choose a diet that is low in fat, saturated fat, and cholesterol.
3. Eat a diet that is rich in vegetables, fruits, and whole grains.
4. Limit intake of salt. Try not to add salt to food.
5. Use sugar in moderation.

6. Use alcohol in moderation. Do not use alcohol at all during pregnancy.

DIETARY MODIFICATIONS

The normal (regular) diet can be modified to adjust to specific patient conditions, such as pregnancy, recovery from surgery, gastrointestinal upset, allergies, dental work, and disease conditions such as diabetes mellitus. A modified diet for health reasons is called a therapeutic diet. Diets can be modified based on calorie content, spice and salt content, bulk, nutrients, consistency, and intervals between meals.

Therapeutic diets must be carefully explained to patients. In some cases, the physician will refer the patient to a registered dietitian who can discuss all aspects of a therapeutic diet with the patient.

The medical assistant will often provide dietary education for patients in the medical office. Since lifestyle changes must be made to comply with some of the diets, the patient must be motivated to make the required changes. All the principles of adult education must be considered when teaching patients about dietary changes. For example, when a woman is pregnant, it is more important for her to eat good-quality food (high in folic acid and calcium) than to increase the quantity of food. In fact, a pregnant or **lactating** (producing milk) woman should increase her caloric intake by only 500 calories per day.

Clear Liquid Diet

A clear liquid diet contains no solid food or milk products. A clear liquid diet is frequently required before certain laboratory tests, examinations, or surgery. It may also be prescribed for a patient suffering from gastrointestinal problems. A clear liquid diet is frequently the first diet a patient is placed on after having surgery and a general anesthetic. Patients must not remain on a clear liquid diet for an extended period of time because it has little nutritional value.

Foods included on a clear diet are these:

- Clear soup and broth
- Plain gelatin
- Black coffee
- Tea
- Carbonated beverages

Full Liquid Diet

A full liquid diet is often prescribed for patients who are unable to chew or digest solid food. This may be due to gastrointestinal problems, infections, or oral surgery. This diet is also prescribed as the next diet step for patients who have been on a clear liquid diet.

Foods recommended on a full liquid diet are these:

- All liquids allowed on a clear diet
- Fruit and vegetable juices
- Strained fruit
- Soup (creamed or strained)
- Milk and milkshakes
- Ice cream

As with the clear liquid diet, a full liquid diet is not to be used for extended periods of time.

Mechanical Soft Diet

The mechanical soft diet is recommended for patients who have dental problems, such as a lack of teeth, or who have difficulty swallowing. This diet is often recommended when patients are recovering from surgery.

PROFESSIONALISM
THE LAW

What do you do about patient noncompliance? Perhaps you teach the patient about a healthy diet, but the patient chooses to disregard the teaching and instead eats a diet high in fat and sugar. The patient may develop complications such as diabetes because of this behavior. It is very important for the medical assistant to document teaching. You might choose to place a copy of the diet regimen you recommended to the patient or a copy of the patient brochure in the patient's medical record to show what you taught.

It is important that you perform within the boundaries of medical assisting standards. Do not be tempted to prescribe a diet regimen—that is a physician responsibility. Once the physician orders dietary teaching, you can teach the patient as you have been approved to do.

PROFESSIONALISM
THE LIFE SPAN

Older adults on fixed incomes may have trouble affording fresh fruits and vegetables and meat. Thus, they may select less expensive food choices that have poor nutritional value. Sometimes when elderly adults live alone, they are hesitant to cook for themselves alone. The medical assistant may be able to support the patient by recommending social programs such as Meals on Wheels to bring nutritional food to their homes.

Foods included on this diet are these:

- All soups
- All liquids
- Cooked vegetables
- Canned fruit
- Ground meat and vegetables
- Tender fish and poultry

Bland Diet

A bland diet contains no seasonings or fibers that are irritating. This diet is prescribed for patients who have gastrointestinal problems and allergies. Foods that are gas forming (such as cabbage), contain caffeine or spices, or are high in fiber are eliminated.

Foods included in a bland diet are these:

- Mildly flavored foods
- Low-fiber foods
- Milk products
- Cooked fruit
- Noncitrus juices

BRAT Diet

Children suffering from uncontrolled gastrointestinal upsets can become dehydrated more easily than adults due to the depletion of body fluids. Physicians often recommend foods on the BRAT diet since they are easily digested and do not cause further upsets.

The acronym BRAT stands for the following foods:

Bananas

Rice

Applesauce

Toast

The BRAT combination of foods is prescribed for small children who suffer from vomiting, nausea, and diarrhea. Children should be seen by the physician if symptoms continue.

High-Protein Diet

A high-protein diet is recommended for patients recovering from bone injuries. This diet can aid in healing. Protein foods such as meat, dairy products, and legumes must be eaten along with a variety of fruits and vegetables for a balanced diet. Often a high-protein drink is included for the patient.

Diabetic Diet

A therapeutic diet designed for diabetic patients must consider several factors, including these:

1. Type of insulin therapy the patient receives
2. Severity of the diabetes
3. Activity and exercise level
4. Ability for activity
5. Calories necessary to maintain the patient's weight

A food exchange system is often used for diabetic patients. This allows for variety in the diet since the patient is able to select preferred foods. Foods are grouped into the same six categories discussed in the Food Guide Pyramid: breads, fruits, vegetables, meat, milk, and fat.

Each food plan must be prescribed for the individual patient. All diabetic diets should be given to the patient in writing. The medical assistant will be asked to reinforce the eating plan with the patient.

High-Residue/High-Fiber Diet

The high-fiber diet is used to treat patients with existing problems as well as to provide prevention of heart disease. New research is demonstrating that a diet high in fiber is effective in preventing colon cancer.

Dietary fiber is thought to provide protection against diabetes, breast and colon cancer, gallbladder disease, constipation, irritable bowel syndrome, hemorrhoids, and diverticulosis. Fiber may also reduce the level of cholesterol within the blood, thereby protecting against heart disease.

The recommended daily intake of fiber is between 20 and 30 grams. Dietary fiber is not found in animal products or dairy products.

The following are fiber sources:

- Raw fruits and vegetables
- Whole-grain breads and cereals
- Legumes

Low-Residue/Low-Fiber Diet

A low-residue diet is also called a low-fiber diet. This diet is useful for a variety of patients including those with colitis, diarrhea, indigestion, or a colostomy.

Some low-residue foods are these:

- Cooked vegetables and stewed fruit
- Bananas (the only raw fruit allowed)
- Lean beef, lamb, chicken, and turkey
- Cooked cereal
- Eggs
- Soups, all except creamed soups

Foods not allowed on a low-residue diet are these:

- Fried foods
- Milk or milk products
- Seasonings

Low-Fat/Low-Cholesterol Diet

The average American diet contains between 30 and 50 grams of fat per day. A low-fat diet is aimed at keeping the fat content between 20 and 30 grams of fat per day. This diet is recommended for patients who have an intolerance to fat—for example, patients with gallbladder disease, pancreatic disease, liver disease, or any combination of them. A low-fat diet has been found to reduce the risk of colon, breast, and prostate cancer; heart disease; and obesity.

Foods recommended on a low-fat/low-cholesterol diet are these:

- Fruits and vegetables
- Skim milk
- Whole-grain breads and cereals
- Angel food cake, graham crackers, no-fat wafers

Foods not allowed on a low-fat/low-cholesterol diet are these:

- All fried foods
- Visible fat
- Butter and margarine
- Most desserts

Low-Sodium/Low-Salt Diet

Therapeutic diets vary in the amount of salt restrictions. Restrictions vary from mild to moderate to severe. Diets are restricted in salt (sodium chloride) for patients with hypertension and heart or kidney disease. Salt restriction is also recommended for patients on weight reduction diets since an excess of salt in the diet promotes water retention.

Many foods, especially processed foods, contain salt. A mild sodium-restricted diet (2,000 to 3,000 mg) would result in an allowance of $\frac{1}{2}$ teaspoon of table salt per day and a very limited amount of foods containing salt. A moderate salt-restricted diet allows 1,500 to 2,000 mg of sodium per day. This diet allows $\frac{1}{2}$ teaspoon of table salt, but all processed and canned foods containing salt are prohibited. No salt is allowed in food preparation. This is the most frequently prescribed level of salt restriction.

A severe salt-restricted diet of 500 mg per day would limit all table salt use, cooking salt, and include only salt-free products in the diet. This diet is difficult to maintain using purchased foods. Patients are advised to increase the use of fresh fruits and vegetables and to read labels carefully when on severe salt-restricted diets.

Calorie Content Diet

Weight reduction diets are often prescribed for patients whose health is affected by excess weight. Gaining excess body fat can lead to serious health problems, such as high blood pressure, heart disease, and diabetes.

A 1,200-calorie diet using a balance of the five food groups and low-fat foods will result in weight loss. For a healthy diet, patients are advised to eat at least four choices from the grains group; five meat or bean choices; two vegetable choices; two fruit choices; two milk choices; and not more than three fat choices. These choices add up to 1,200 calories. Examples of these foods are listed in Box 56-2.

Patients are encouraged to keep a food diary of all they eat each day. This helps patients to become more aware of the unhealthy eating they might be doing and to substitute healthy foods for unhealthy ones. Table 56-4 illustrates a sample food diary format.

Healthy Food Choices

Healthy food choices include eating less fat, eating more high-fiber foods, using less salt, and eating less sugar.

Eat Less Fat

- Eat smaller servings of meat. Eat poultry and fish more often. Choose lean cuts of red meat.
- Prepare all meats by roasting, broiling, or baking. Trim off all visible fat. Avoid or limit the use of added sauces or gravy.
- Remove skin from all poultry.
- Avoid all fried foods. Avoid adding fat during cooking.
- Eat fewer high-fat foods such as cold cuts, bacon, sausage, hot dogs, butter, margarine, salad dressing, nuts, lard, and solid shortening.
- Drink skim or low-fat milk.
- Eat less ice cream, cheese, sour cream, whole milk, cream, and other high-fat dairy products.
- Instead of eating foods with trans fats, increase consumption of the omega-3 fatty acids in fish.

Eat More High-Fiber Foods

- Choose dried beans, peas, and lentils more often.
- Eat whole grain breads, cereals, or crackers.
- Eat more vegetables, raw and cooked.
- Eat whole fruit in place of fruit juice.
- Try high-fiber foods such as oat bran, barley, brown rice, bulgur, and wild rice.

Use Less Salt

- Reduce the amount of salt you use in cooking.
- Try not to add salt to already cooked food.
- Eat fewer high-salt foods such as canned soups, ham, hot dogs, pickles, sauerkraut, and foods that taste salty.
- Eat fewer convenience and fast foods.

Box 56-2 Basic Food Group Choices for a 1,200-Calorie Eating PLAN

Grains

Each of the following equals one grain choice (80 calories) and contains 1 gram of fat; for weight reduction, limit to four to six choices a day:

- $\frac{1}{2}$ cup pasta or barley
- $\frac{1}{3}$ cup rice
- 1 slice bread or 1 roll
- 4 to 6 crackers
- $\frac{1}{2}$ English muffin, bagel, hamburger/hot dog bun
- $\frac{1}{2}$ cup cooked cereal
- $\frac{3}{4}$ cup dry, unsweetened cereal
- 3 cups popcorn, unbuttered, not cooked in oil

Vegetables

Each of the following equals one vegetable choice (25 calories); two or more servings are recommended per day:

- $\frac{1}{2}$ cup cooked vegetables
- 1 cup raw vegetables
- $\frac{1}{2}$ cup tomato or vegetable juice

Meat and Beans

Each of the following equals *one* meat choice (75 calories); five to six servings are recommended per day:

- 1 ounce cooked poultry, fish, or meat
- $\frac{1}{4}$ cup salmon or tuna, water packed
- 1 tablespoon peanut butter
- 1 egg (limit to 3 per week)

Each of the following equals *two* meat choices (150 calories). Fat content varies for meat but should be limited to a total of 18 fat grams for meat per day:

- 1 small chicken leg or thigh
- $\frac{1}{2}$ cup cottage cheese or tuna

Each of the following equals *three* meat choices (225 calories):

- 1 small hamburger
- 1 small pork chop

- $\frac{1}{2}$ chicken breast
- 1 medium fish filet

Cooked meat about the size of a deck of cards

Milk

Each of the following equals one milk choice (75 calories); two servings per day are recommended:

- $\frac{1}{4}$ cup cottage cheese
- 1 ounce low-fat cheese, such as mozzarella or ricotta

Fruit

Each of the following equals one fruit choice (60 calories); two servings per day are recommended:

- 1 fresh medium fruit
- 1 cup berries or melon
- $\frac{1}{2}$ cup fruit juice
- $\frac{1}{2}$ cup canned fruit in juice without sugar
- $\frac{1}{4}$ cup dried fruit

Oil

Each of the following equals one fat choice (45 calories and 5 grams of fat each); fat should be limited to three servings per day:

- 1 teaspoon margarine, oil, or mayonnaise
- 2 teaspoons diet margarine or diet mayonnaise
- 1 tablespoon salad dressing
- 2 tablespoons reduced-calorie salad dressing

Do not assume similar products are the same. Be sure to check the Nutrition Facts panel on food labels because even similar foods can vary in calories, ingredients, nutrients, and the size and number of servings in a package. Even if you continue to buy the same brand of a product, check the Nutrition Facts panel frequently because ingredients can change at any time.

Eat Less Sugar

- Avoid adding table sugar, syrup, honey, jam, jelly, candy, sweet rolls, fruit canned in syrup, regular gelatin, desserts, pie, cake with icing, and other sweets.

- Avoid regular soft drinks. One 12-ounce can contains 9 teaspoons of sugar!

- Choose fresh fruit or fruit canned in natural juice or water.

- If desired, use sweeteners that do not have calories, such as saccharin or aspartame, instead of sugar.

- Avoid heavily processed foods.

- Food choices that include hydrogenated fats used to preserve food are not as good as fresh foods.

TABLE 56-4 Food Diary

Calories Each Day: _____		
Meal Time:	Meal Time:	Meal Time:
_____	_____	_____
_____	_____	_____
_____	_____	_____
_____	_____	_____
_____	_____	_____
_____	_____	_____
_____	_____	_____
_____	_____	_____
Snack Time:	Snack Time:	Snack Time:
_____	_____	_____
_____	_____	_____
_____	_____	_____

FOOD SUPPLEMENTS

Physicians prescribe protein–vitamin–mineral food supplements when patients are debilitated due to disease processes, such as AIDS, or they are unable to tolerate a normal diet. In some cases, the liquid supplement may have to be given via a tube feeding until the patient is strong enough to drink the supplement. Supplements to the diet should only be used under the direction of a physician. Megadoses of supplements can be harmful to the body. Be sure to encourage the patient to discuss supplements with the physician before taking them.

EXERCISE

Exercise and physical activity should be included as part of the patient's health plan. Activity helps to metabolize the fat in the diet so that it does not become stored in the body. Almost any patient can exercise, after being cleared by the physician. Exercises in a pool can even be enjoyed by patients with arthritis. Walking is a good exercise and can be done with little extra equipment beyond a good pair of walking shoes. Some patients, however, will exercise more if they have made a monetary commitment to a gym or health club. Patients can lose weight by making simple modifications to their lifestyle, such as taking the stairs instead of an elevator or by parking farther away from the entrance to their workplace.

Even small changes can help with weight loss. It is important to match the exercise with the interests and finances of the patient. If you select an exercise program that is impossible for the patient to comply with, you set up the patient for failure. It is better to keep an exercise program simple and reasonable for the patient.

ALCOHOL

Alcohol is not considered a food product, but it does contain calories and lowers the rate at which calories are burned. Some studies have shown the value of moderate consumption of red wine, but excessive alcohol intake is associated with problems such as alcoholism, auto accidents, and family and work disruptions. Pregnant women are advised to exclude alcohol during pregnancy because of the potential for birth defects such as fetal alcohol syndrome.

SUMMARY

Bodily functions cannot be facilitated without nutrients. Carbohydrates provide energy, whereas proteins build and renew body tissues. Fats provides work energy and help vitamins function. Minerals such as calcium, phosphorus, iron, and iodine facilitate body functions. Vitamins A, B, C, D, E, and K are vital for body regulation. Water is also important for regulating body temperature, carrying nutrients, and lubricating joints.

Good nutritional habits can improve health. One of the vital tasks of a medical assistant is to provide patient dietary education, as needed, and as directed by a physician. An example would be nutritional planning for a diabetic patient. The medical assistant often plays a critical role in handling noncompliant patients, such as a diabetic patient who will not adhere to the prescribed diet. Dietary education should be individualized to the patient and the specific disease or condition the patient has. No one diet works for all, but diet is an important component of health and should be considered with all patients.

Balanced diets are developed according to the age and health of the patients. The Food Guide Pyramid adjusts the diet to individual. Dietary modifications are sometimes necessary for certain diseases and disorders.

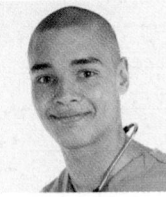

56 CHAPTER REVIEW

COMPETENCY REVIEW

1. Define and spell the terms to learn for this chapter.
2. Design a patient teaching chart based on the Food Guide Pyramid to illustrate the five classifications of nutrients.
3. Develop a sample menu for 3 days based on the Food Guide Pyramid.
4. Determine the number of calories in a piece of pie that has 1 g of protein, 8 g of carbohydrates, and 9 g of fat.
5. Take a food label from a package of cereal and list the number of calories, total fat, cholesterol, sodium, total carbohydrates, dietary fiber, sugars, protein, and vitamins.
6. Write a 1-day food plan for the following therapeutic diets: full liquid, mechanical soft, high fiber, moderate salt restrictive, and 1,200 calorie.
7. Maintain a weekly diary of your intake of food. Analyze each food group intake.
8. List the factors influencing a diabetic patient's diet.
9. List five foods high in iodine.
10. List five food sources for water.

PREPARING FOR THE CERTIFICATION EXAM

1. All of the following are fat-soluble vitamins stored in the liver EXCEPT
   a. vitamin A
   b. vitamin D
   c. vitamin B
   d. vitamin E
   e. vitamin K

2. Which of the following are food sources for carbohydrates?
   a. eggs and fish
   b. milk and salmon
   c. pasta and potatoes
   d. cheese and poultry
   e. butter and fish

3. A BRAT diet has been ordered for David Abilene, who is 2 years old. What foods will be included on that diet?
   a. apple juice
   b. peanut butter sandwich
   c. macaroni and cheese
   d. bananas and rice
   e. pureed vegetables

4. When restricting food on a 1,200-calorie diet that is being adapted for a diabetic patient using food exchange lists, what needs to be remembered?
   a. Alcohol is forbidden for all diabetics.
   b. Exercise increases the need for insulin.
   c. More than 1200 calories may be too much for a diabetic patient.
   d. Water should be restricted with diabetics.
   e. Consider all elements of the Food Guide Pyramid when developing a diet.

5. All of the following are milk products EXCEPT
   a. yogurt
   b. butter
   c. cheese
   d. cereal
   e. ice cream

6. Which of the following statements about cholesterol is TRUE?
   a. All cholesterol is bad.
   b. Good cholesterol is low-density lipoproteins (LDL).

c. There is no evidence that high cholesterol intake is linked to disease.

d. Cholesterol is an essential element normally found in the body.

e. The information "Cholesterol 0 mg" on a food label means that there is no fat present.

7. Which of the following is a good source of iron?
   a. oat cereals
   b. milk
   c. nuts
   d. butter
   e. cantaloupe

8. Milk is NOT a good source for which of the following?
   a. iron
   b. carbohydrates

c. proteins
d. fats
e. calcium

9. Which of the following is NOT a function of water?
   a. removes waste products from cells
   b. carries oxygen and nutrients to cells
   c. regulates body temperature
   d. decreases blood pressure
   e. prevents dehydration

10. Which of the following is NOT allowed on the bland diet?
    a. citrus juices
    b. milk products
    c. mildly flavored foods
    d. cooked fruit
    e. low-fiber foods

CRITICAL THINKING

1. Patients with pernicious anemia, like Jaden, are lacking a particular vitamin. Name this vitamin and list foods that David may suggest Jaden should eat to increase her daily intake to begin to feel better.

2. Jaden tells David that she knows that she also could stand to lose about 45 pounds, which she knows will also help increase her energy level. She was wondering if David had any tips on making healthy food choices. What might David tell Jaden?

3. Jaden expresses an interest in learning more about healthy eating habits that include foods from her ethnic background. She asks David if he has any additional information. What would be a good resource for David to share with Jaden?

ON THE JOB

Gladys Pierce is a 70-year-old patient of Dr. Court Franklin. She is more than a hundred pounds overweight and a newly diagnosed type 2 diabetic. She is concerned that she may lose her eyesight and feeling in her arms and legs if she does not get her diabetes under control. She also may have strokes and even a lethal heart attack. Dr. Franklin asks Dan Tyler, CMA, to create a diet for Ms. Pierce.

1. What general instructions would you give Ms. Pierce?
2. What foods would be good dietary choices?
3. Which foods would be poor choices for her?
4. How should Ms. Pierce prepare foods to decrease fat calories?
5. Would processed foods be a good choice for Ms. Pierce or not?

INTERNET ACTIVITY

Research the Food Guide Pyramid on the Internet and develop an individualized diet for yourself or an imaginary patient.

MEDMEDIA

Additional interactive resources and activities for this chapter can be found:

On your student DVD: View applicable procedure videos on the DVD-ROM found in the back of this book.

MyHealthProfessionsKit.com: Test your knowledge of this chapter with games and activities. MyHealthProfessionsKit also includes resources, helpful links, and a Spanish audio glossary.

Medical Assisting Interactive: Practice your procedures as a medical assistant in this simulated doctor's office. This can be accessed through MyHealthProfessionsKit.com.

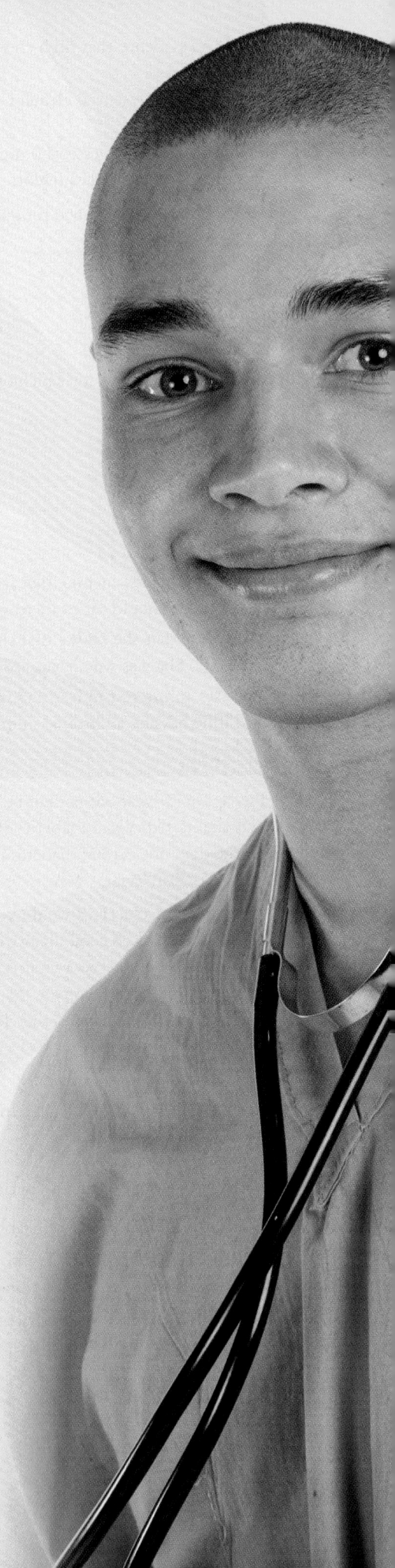

57

Mental Health

LEARNING OBJECTIVES

After reading this chapter, you should be able to:

- Define and spell the terms to learn for this chapter.

- List 13 major diagnostic categories of mental disorders.

- State the difference between behavioral and mental illness.

- Explain psychotherapy, psychopharmacology, and electroconvulsive therapy.

- Discuss heredity and cultural and environmental influences on behavior.

- Discuss interpersonal skills and human behavior.

- Explain how to communicate with a patient who is frightened, angry, or depressed.

- Explain motivation.

- Describe eight ways to cope with stress.

- Describe the five stages of grief.

CHAPTER OUTLINE

CASE STUDY

Sharon, an RMA at Pearson Physicians Group, is preparing Simon Aurora to be seen by Dr. Penningworth. She notes that his blood pressure is 168/92, which is much higher than his blood pressure of 122/76 that was taken last month during a sick visit. He also has lost 7 pounds since that last visit. Today Simon is being seen for a follow-up visit for a bilateral ear infection. While working with Simon, Susan notices that he seems edgy and that his cell phone has already rung three times in the past 10 minutes.

Many patients who come into the physician's office or clinic will have physical or emotional problems that are not the main reason for their appointment. The medical assistant must be able to care for the entire person in a holistic fashion. Although it is easy to focus on the purely physical complaint about which the patient came for help, all patients have psychological and emotional needs as well as needs for physical wholeness.

Psychology

Psychology is the science of behavior and the human thought process. This behavioral science is primarily concerned with human beings acting alone or in groups. A psychologist is one who is trained in the methods of psychological analysis, therapy, and research. A psychologist usually has a PhD (doctorate) in psychology. The psychologist usually administers psychological tests, facilitates psychotherapy, or does research. The psychologist cannot prescribe medication. A **psychiatrist**, however, can prescribe medications. A psychiatrist is a medical doctor who has chosen to specialize in psychiatry. **Psychiatry** is the branch of medicine that deals with the diagnosis, treatment, and prevention of mental disorders. Psychiatrists also can order and perform electroconvulsive therapy (ECT) and facilitates psychotherapy. Other medical doctors also can prescribe psychotropic medications.

Within the study of psychology, a distinction is made between normal and abnormal behavior. All social interactions, such as might occur in the communication process, pose some problems for some people. These problems are not necessarily abnormal. One means of judging if behavior is abnormal is to compare one person's behavior against others in the community. If a person's behavior interferes with the activities of daily living, it is often considered abnormal.

Abnormal psychology is the study of behavior that deviates from the normal. This includes psychoneuroses, psychoses, psychosomatic disorders, personality and sociopathic disorders, and disturbances occurring as a result of intoxication, brain damage, and brain disease.

Psychological Disorders

Psychological disorders can be classified as either mental or behavioral disorders. Mental disorders are caused by organic changes to the brain, such as depression, but exclude substance abuse and other disorders that are primarily behavioral. Behavioral disorders are caused not by brain changes but primarily by the patient's behavior.

Many people will have some type of mental disorder during their life. This is considered normal. A continual state of emotional disorder that disrupts life is considered abnormal. Mental disorders are defined as any behavior or emotional state that causes an individual great suffering or worry, is self-defeating or self-destructive, or disrupts the person's day-to-day relationships.

The guide for terminology and classifications relating to psychiatric disorders is the *Diagnostic and Statistical Manual of Mental Disorders, Fourth Edition, Text Revision (DSM-IV-TR)*, which is published by the American Psychiatric Association. Major diagnostic categories of mental disorders in the *DSM-IV-TR* are described in Table 57-1.

TABLE 57-1 Major Diagnostic Categories of Mental Disorders

Category	Example
Anxiety disorder	Phobias, panic attack, compulsive rituals
Cognitive disorder	Delirium, dementia, amnesia (resulting from brain damage or the effects of toxic substances or drugs), degenerative disorders such as Alzheimer's.
Disorder diagnosed in infancy and childhood	Mental retardation, attention deficit disorders such as hyperactivity or inability to concentrate, and developmental problems.
Disorder with physical symptoms and no organic cause (somatoform)	Paralysis, heart palpitation, dizziness; also referred to as hypochondriasis.
Dissociative disorder	Dissociative amnesia in which important events cannot be remembered after a traumatic event, and dissociative identity disorder (multiple personality disorder) in which two or more personalities or identities are present in one person.
Eating Disorders	Characterized by abnormal eating patterns, distorted body image, fear, guilt, and depression.
Factitious Disorders	Characterized by physical and/or psychological symptoms that are consciously fabricated by the patient, which the patient knows are not real. Patients pretend to be sick (or sicken others) to get attention.
Impulse control disorder	Inability to resist an impulse to perform some act that is harmful to the individual or others such as pathological gambling, stealing (kleptomania), setting fires (pyromania), or having violent rages.
Mood disorder	Major depression, bipolar disorder (manic depression), chronic depressive mood.
Personality disorder	Inflexible behavior patterns that cause distress or the inability to function; these include paranoid, narcissistic, and antisocial disorders.
Schizophrenia and other psychotic disorders	Characterized by delusions, hallucinations, and severe disturbances in thinking and emotion.
Sexual and gender identity disorder	Transsexualism (wanting to be the other gender), sexual performance (lack of orgasm, premature ejaculation, or lack of sexual desire), or unusual or bizarre sexual acts.
Substance-related disorder	Related to either excessive use of or withdrawal from alcohol, amphetamines, caffeine, cocaine, hallucinogens, nicotine, opiates, and other drugs.

ANXIETY DISORDERS

Anxiety disorders are mild emotional disturbances that impair judgment. Patients suffering from anxiety disorders are able to tell the difference between fantasy and reality. Anxiety is a vague feeling of apprehension, worry, uneasiness or dread. A certain amount of anxiety is normal, but when it impairs judgment it is an anxiety disorder. In anxiety disorders, **compulsions**, repetitive acts performed to relieve anxiety, are frequently accompanied by **obsessions** (persistent thoughts). Although a certain amount of anxiety is normal, some patients have abnormal fears (phobias). Anxiety disorders are treated with anxiolytics, which decrease anxiety.

The fear of leaving the home and going out is agoraphobia. Arachnophobia is the fear of spiders. Claustrophobia is the fear of enclosed spaces. See Table 57-2 for more information about common phobias.

COGNITIVE DISORDERS

Cognitive disorders impair the ability of a patient to think clearly. Delirium, particularly if related to substance abuse, can be transient. Delirium is usually treated by easing the person into withdrawal from substances or by treating the underlying cause. However, dementia is a progressive disease that robs the patient of short-term memory, while frequently leaving long-term memory intact. Family members of patients with Alzheimer's disease, a cognitive disorder, also will need support. New medications have been developed to treat dementia, but intervention must be early to be successful. The medical assistant should help

TABLE 57-2 Common Phobias

Phobia	Description	Word Part and Definition
acrophobia	Fear of heights	acrophobia (AK-roh-FOH-bee-ah) acr/o- *extremity; highest point* phob/o- *fear or avoidance* -ia *condition, state, thing*
agoraphobia	Fear of crowds or public places	agoraphobia (AG-or-ah-FOH-bee-ah) agor/a- *open areas or space* phob/o- *fear or avoidance* -ia *condition, state, thing*
arachnophobia	Fear of spiders	arachnophobia (ah-RAK-noh-FOH-bee-ah) arachn/o- *spider, spider web* phob/o- *fear or avoidance* -ia *condition, state, thing*
claustrophobia	Fear of closed-in spaces	claustrophobia (KLAW-stroh-FOH-bee-ah) claustr/o- *enclosed space* phob/o- *fear or avoidance* -ia *condition, state, thing*
microphobia	Fear of germs	microphobia (MY-kroh-FOH-bee-ah) micr/o- *small* phob/o- *fear or avoidance* -ia *condition, state, thing*
ophidiophobia	Fear of snakes	ophidiophobia (oh-FID-ee-oh-FOH-bee-ah) ophidi/o- *snake* phob/o- *fear or avoidance* -ia *condition, state, thing*
social phobia	Fear of being embarrassed or humiliated in front of others or in a public place or fear of being the center of attention	social (SOH-shal) soci/o- *human beings; community* -al *pertaining to*
thanatophobia	Fear of death	thanatophobia (THAN-ah-toh-FOH-bee-ah) thanat/o- *death* phob/o- *fear or avoidance* -ia *condition, state, thing*
xenophobia	Fear of strangers	xenophobia (ZEN-oh-FOH-bee-ah) xen/o- *foreign* phob/o- *fear or avoidance* -ia *condition, state, thing*

family members find local Alzheimer's caregiver support groups.

DEVELOPMENTAL DISORDERS

Sometimes disorders appear before the age of 18 and include developmental delays (such as Down syndrome) and personality disorders (such as antisocial behavior, which is discussed later in this chapter). Developmental delays are usually treated by maximizing the potential of the patient with rehabilitation. *Mental retardation* is a broad term that includes some patients who are profoundly unable to function in the world as well as those who have relatively high intelligence but are slow to learn. Rehabilitation is usually successful at improving the quality of life for the patient with developmental delay but usually will not increase the intelligence quotient. Autism (also known as spectrum disorder) has a range of symptoms. Some patients with Asperger's syndrome (a milder form of autism) may be highly intelligent but may not seek social contact. Other patients may be totally absorbed in their own world, may be hypersensitive to outside stimuli, and may engage in self-soothing behaviors such as rocking back and forth.

DISSOCIATIVE DISORDERS

Dissociative disorders cause a person to withdraw from reality and dissociate at least temporarily from the life issues that give them anxiety. If the person attempts to flee the life he or she is living to assume another identity in another place, it is called dissociative fugue. Amnesia, or forgetting events, is frequently present with dissociative disorders. Dissociative identity disorder (formerly called multiple personality disorder) is a severe dissociative disorder in which the patient assumes multiple personalities. Contrary to frequent depictions of patients with this disorder in the media, these patients have usually been severely victimized and assume multiple personalities as a defense mechanism to protect themselves.

EATING DISORDERS

Anorexia nervosa is a psychiatric disorder in which patients are so starved for affection that they starve themselves while believing that they are overweight. This is a life-threatening disease that can cause permanent heart, dental, and other organ damage. Bulimia nervosa is usually found in slightly overweight individuals who seek to control their lives by overeating, then purging with laxatives or vomiting. Medications to increase appetite can be used, but cognitive behavioral therapy is usually indicated.

Eating disorders are becoming more prevalent, especially among young women. They are also discussed in Chapter 40.

HYPOCHONDRIASIS

Hypochondriasis is a disorder in which the patient is preoccupied with fears of having, or the idea that one has, a serious disease, based on a misinterpretation of one of more bodily signs or symptoms. With this disorder, it is important to rule out physical illness. Therapy would then be directed toward improving the patient's insight and decreasing anxiety.

IMPULSE CONTROL DISORDERS

Some disorders are disorders of impulse control. Attention-deficit/hyperactivity disorder (ADHD), a disorder of impulse control, is thought to be a problem of either the prefrontal cortex or dopamine processing. Although controversial, ADHD is currently treated with stimulants that help the patient to focus better. Other impulse control disorders include excessive gambling, stealing, and setting fires.

MOOD DISORDERS

Mood disorders are disorders of emotional feeling or mood and include a pervasively negative worldview. Depression is a mood disorder characterized by a lack of enjoyment in life's pleasures, such as food, sex, friends, family, and hobbies. It can be life threatening when accompanied by suicidal thoughts. A **bipolar disorder** has two poles: depression and mania (an overactivity of mood). Patients with mania may not stop to eat, rest, relate to others, or sleep. Bipolar disorder is characterized by periods of mood swings from excessive mania to profound depression. Mania is characterized by excessive energy, flight of ideas, weight loss, and cognitive lack of focus. Medication therapy is targeted usually at the manic phase, but antidepressants can sometimes be helpful with the depression phase caused by exhaustion of the manic phase.

Depression is a serious mental illness that affects 20 million people in the United States. One out of four women and one out of ten men will be diagnosed with depression in their lifetime, and unfortunately depression can reoccur throughout the patient's lifetime. Symptoms include sadness, loss of interest or pleasure in activities, change in weight, difficulty sleeping or oversleeping, energy loss, feelings of worthlessness, excessive guilt, and thoughts of death or suicide. Because these symptoms impact the patient's life greatly, depression can be a fatal disease. Depression can be successfully treated with antidepressant medications (including serotonin reuptake inhibitors), and patients can fully recover from this life-threatening disorder. These medications help to stabilize the neurotransmitters in the synapses of nerves, which improves the depressed patient's ability to process information both cognitively and emotionally. Usually treatment for depression includes talk therapy with a psychologist or counselor to process the issues that lead to the depression.

With some mental disorders, particularly severe depression, the patient may become so distraught as to threaten or attempt suicide. Often the suicidal person does not really want to die but just wishes to escape an intolerable situation. A wise medical assistant will always assess for suicidality in patients with mental illness.

PERSONALITY DISORDERS

Personality disorders include narcissistic (self-centered), paranoid (abnormally concerned people will hurt the patient), antisocial (not concerned with laws and other people), histrionic (dramatic), and borderline (impulsive) behavior. Unlike other disorders that may necessitate medication therapy, talk therapy with a psychologist is the treatment of choice for entrenched personality disorders.

Psychopathic personality disorders affect about 1 percent of the population and are characterized by lack of empathy, narcissism, impulsivity, and antisocial reactions such as breaking the law and manipulating others. Cognitive behavioral therapy can be successful with psychopathology, but no medication will help. Patients with this personality disorder tend to be cunning and manipulative. They tend to have problems with following laws.

PSYCHOTIC DISORDERS

Psychotic disorders are severe mental disorders that interfere with patients' perceptions of reality and their ability to cope with the demands of daily living. **Schizophrenia** is a psychotic disorder marked by a variety of symptoms, including **delusions** (fixed false beliefs), **hallucinations** (false sensory perceptions), disorganized and incoherent speech, severe emotional abnormalities, and withdrawal into an inner world. Psychoses must be treated with antipsychotic medications, as delusional individuals cannot respond well to talk therapy.

SOMATOFORM AND FACTITIOUS DISORDERS

Somatoform disorders occur when unresolved mental illness is displaced into body complaints. For example, a woman in a suffocating relationship may complain of having trouble breathing, a man who was just rejected and is heartbroken may complain of chest pain, and a woman who has been raped may complain of urinary problems. Anxiolytics can be used to decrease anxiety and improve the effectiveness of talk therapy.

Factitious disorders are different from somatoform disorders. In factitious disorders, the patient creates illness to seek attention. Sometimes the patient with a factitious disorder might injure another person, such as a spouse or child, in order to get attention too. If the person injures himself, the disorder is Munchausen's disorder. If another person is injured by the patient to get attention, it is known as Munchausen's by proxy. Cognitive behavioral therapy is preferred over medication for this group of disorders.

Substance Abuse Disorders

Addiction is a physiological need for a substance, which in its absence causes withdrawal symptoms. Habituation is the psychological addiction to a substance. Research has shown that some people are particularly drawn to abuse drugs rather than take the ordered amount and to be drawn to self-medicate with drugs that are illegal. The most abused drug in the United States is a legal one: alcohol. Because of this, alcohol sales are controlled in every state, and penalties exist for driving under the influence of alcohol. Because patients are drawn to these substances, they frequently will make poor cognitive choices in order to obtain the substance. A patient may steal, forgo relationships, or abuse others to get the substance. For this reason, treatment usually consists of admitting that the substance is controlling the patient and training the patient to be accountable to a group such as Alcoholics Anonymous or Narcotics Anonymous. A medical assistant may need to give information to a substance abuser about local meetings but also should give information to family members about supportive groups such as Al-Anon/Alateen for family members of patients with a substance abuse problem. When the patient depends on the substance, instead of family and friends, to cope with problems, the patient is dependent on that substance.

Substance abusers may come to the medical office in search of pain medications to which they have become addicted. It is important that the medical assistant document carefully visits to the physician office so that addictive behavior can be traced. Notify the physician if you suspect drug-seeking behavior. Never give a patient unsupervised access to medications in the medical office. Recently prescription drug abuse has become more prevalent, with a surge of parties where patients swap their medications for those of other party members.

Some patients are drawn to illegal substances such as marijuana or cocaine. The patient may not easily admit illegal drug use to the medical assistant. The physician may have to introduce the subject of illegal drug use after the patient has developed a level of trust with the physician.

Some substance abusers use legal drugs but in a nontherapeutic way. Oxycontin is a continuous-release medication that provides appropriate doses of oxycodone to those who need pain relief. However, substance abusers will crush the medication, changing the continuous-release property, and take large doses of it quickly.

A drug that is both habituating and addicting is nicotine. It is found in both chewing tobacco and smoking tobacco. The link between tobacco and cancer is solid. Fortunately, oral medications and transdermal patches are both available and can help the patient wean from this drug. It is important that medical staff not smoke in front of patients, as this reinforces this dangerous habit.

The most abused drug in the United States is alcohol. It is legalized to control it as outlawing it during Prohibition simply led to underground, illegal use of it. Although fairly easy to access even if the patient is young, there is the potential for abuse. Because alcohol is illegal to consume as a young person, younger people tend to drink large amounts and an assortment of types quickly, usually in cars, usually with a group of other young people. All these behaviors can lead to physical and mental health problems. Although some treatments, such as Alcoholics Anonymous, insist that the only cure for alcoholism is abstinence, other treatments include focus on moderate alcohol consumption. Alcoholics Anonymous supports the substance abuser through group support.

In addition to Alcoholics Anonymous, Narcotics Anonymous has similar support groups for narcotics addicts. Narcotics, which reduce pain and induce sleep, are popular coping mechanisms for those who want to escape stress. For that reason, narcotics are highly controlled substances.

The medical assistant should be hypervigilant for the public safety. If a provider in the office is impaired due to substance abuse, the medical assistant should report the behavior immediately to the office manager and perhaps notify the state board of medicine or nursing.

Treatments

Treatments for mental disorders are varied and include psychotherapy, psychopharmacology, and electroconvulsive therapy.

PSYCHOTHERAPY

Psychotherapy is a method for treating mental disorders by mental rather than physical means. This includes psychoanalysis, humanistic therapies, and family and group therapy. Cognitive behavioral therapy helps the patient to change both the way the patient thinks and the way the patient acts. For example, if the patient is afraid of flying, the therapist and patient may discuss the faulty thinking of this fear, and the therapist may challenge the patient to fly in order to process the fears. For some impulse behaviors, the therapist might extract a commitment in contract form from the patient to stop the behavior. The goal of psychotherapy is to help the patent cope with life.

Psychoanalysis is a method of obtaining a detailed account of the past and present emotional and mental experiences from the patient in order to determine the source of the problem and eliminate the effects. It is a system developed by Sigmund Freud that encourages the patient to discuss repressed, painful, or hidden experiences with the hope of eliminating or minimizing the current problem. Because psychotherapy can be lengthy, third-party payers frequently limit the number of visits a patient can have with a psychoanalyst.

Humanistic therapies are also called client-centered or nondirective therapy. The therapist does not delve into the patient's past when using these methods. The patient is helped to feel better by building self-esteem and a feeling that he or she is respected. This therapy was pioneered by Carl Rogers.

Family therapy and group therapy are solution focused. The therapist places minimal emphasis on the patient's past history and places a strong emphasis on having the patient state his or her goals and then finding a way to achieve them. It is usually led by a specialist in this therapy. Figure 57-1 shows a group therapy session.

PSYCHOPHARMACOLOGY

Psychopharmacology relates to the study of the effects of drugs on the mind and brain, particularly the use of drugs in treating mental disorders. The brain is a large soft mass of nerve tissue contained within the cranium. It is the cranial portion of the central nervous system. The mind is the integration of and organization of functions of the brain resulting in the ability to perceive surroundings; to have emotions, imagination, memory, and will; and to process information in an intelligent manner. The quality and quantity of the functions of the mind vary with experience and development. The main classes of drugs for the treatment of

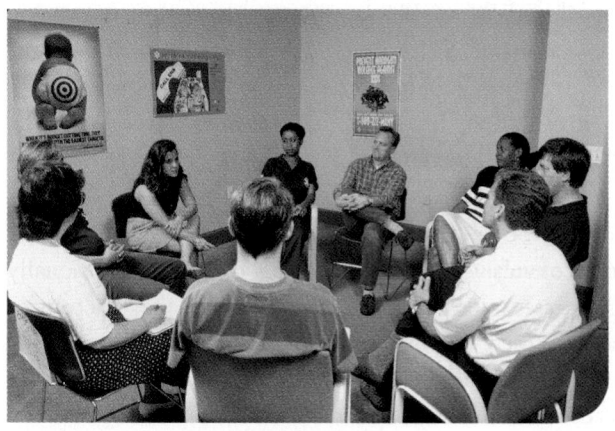

FIGURE 57-1 **A group therapy session.**

mental disorders are antipsychotic drugs, antidepressant drugs, "minor" tranquilizers, and lithium:

- Antipsychotic drugs are the major tranquilizers, which include chlorpromazine (Thorazine), haloperidol (Haldol), clozapine (Clozaril), and risperidone (Risperdal). Drugs have transformed the treatment of patients with psychoses and schizophrenia by reducing the patient's agitation and panic, and shortening the schizophrenic episode. One of the side effects of these drugs is involuntary muscle movements, which develop in approximately one-fourth of all adults who take them.

- Antidepressant drugs alter the patient's mood by affecting levels of neurotransmitters in the brain. An older group of antidepressants, including tricyclic antidepressants, are no longer the first antidepressants prescribed. Serotonin reuptake inhibitors (SSRIs), such as Prozac, Effexor, Paxil, and Zoloft, are more frequently prescribed because they have fewer side effects. Monoamine oxidase inhibitors (MAOIs) require a special diet and therefore are infrequently prescribed. Tricyclic antidepressants are nonaddictive, but they can produce unpleasant side effects such as dry mouth, weight gain, blurred vision, and nausea. Because of these side effects, psychiatrists more frequently prescribe the milder selective SSRIs.

- "Minor" tranquilizers include Valium and Ativan. These are also classified as depressants and are prescribed for anxiety. However, they are the least effective in treating emotional disorders. Patients may develop a problem with **tolerance** (needing larger and larger doses) after taking these drugs for an extended time. In general, antidepressants are preferred to tranquilizers for treating anxiety disorders.

- Lithium, from the salt lithium carbonate, is a special category of drug. It is used successfully to calm patients who suffer from bipolar disorder (depression alternating with manic excitement). The patient on lithium must be carefully monitored because too much of this drug is toxic and too little is ineffective. Blood levels should be regularly drawn to prevent overdose or underdose.

ELECTROCONVULSIVE THERAPY

Electroconvulsive therapy (ECT) is a procedure occasionally used for cases of prolonged major depression. This is a controversial treatment in which an electrode is placed on one or both sides of the patient's head, and brief electric current is turned on, causing a convulsive seizure. A low level of voltage is used in modern ECT, and the patient is administered a muscle

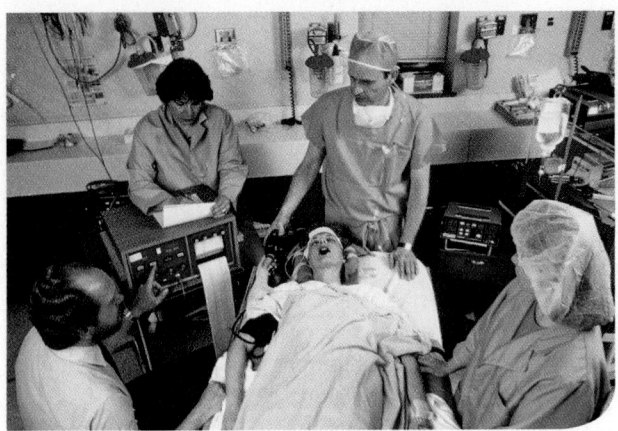

FIGURE 57-2 Electroconvulsive therapy.

relaxant and an anesthesia prior to administration of the current. This helps to prevent violent muscle contractions. Advocates of this treatment state that it is more effective than the use of drugs to treat severe depression. It is not effective with disorders other than depression, such as schizophrenia and alcoholism. It is usually the treatment of last resort. A photo of electroconvulsive therapy is shown in Figure 57-2.

Although the medical assistant will not usually be engaged in psychological treatment with the patient, the assistant may be instrumental in arranging referrals from the medical office to a psychiatrist or psychologist. In some cases, a health psychologist may work in the medical office—providing therapy to the patients in that practice in coordination with the physician. This is a particularly useful model because the psychologist can easily access the patient chart for medical information and give useful feedback to the treatment group.

Developmental Stages of the Life Cycle

When you are caring for patients it will be important for you to understand the developmental stages of life cycles so that you can take better care of your patients. The five main developmental periods are prenatal, infancy, childhood, adolescence, and adulthood. Within each developmental period are subdivisions.

PRENATAL PERIOD

The first period of child development is the **prenatal period**, which covers the process from conception until birth. Throughout this period the structures of the body as well as the organs are formed. At this time development is influenced by the environment and heredity.

INFANCY

The second period of child development is **infancy**. This period of vast changes occurs from childbirth until

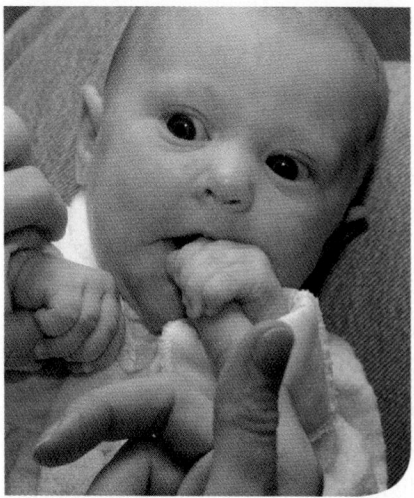

FIGURE 57-3 Infancy.

toddlerhood. During this time an infant gains motor ability and coordination. The infant will also develop language and sensory skills, express basic emotions and feelings, develop trust or mistrust, and become attached to caregivers. Figure 57-3 shows an infant.

CHILDHOOD

Childhood is the last period of child development. Ages 3 to 5 years are considered early childhood. During children's preschool years, their linguistic, physical, and cognitive capabilities will grow rapidly. The concept of self begins to develop, as does socialization. Ages 6 to 11 years are considered middle childhood. During middle childhood, children start to know their world, think logically, and make major advances in reading and writing. Moral and psychosocial development progress rapidly. Achievement is very important to the child during this stage. Childhood is illustrated in Figure 57-4.

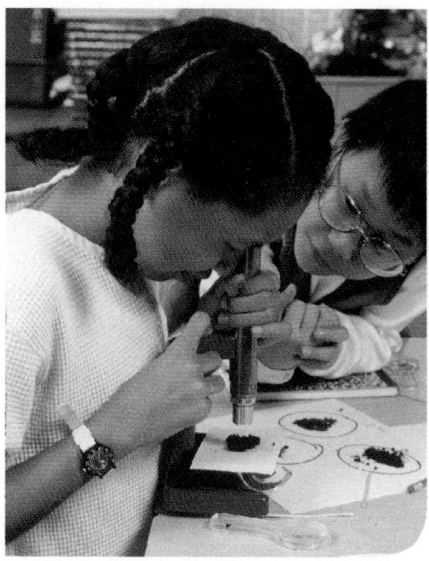

FIGURE 57-4 Childhood.

ADOLESCENCE

Adolescence occurs between childhood and adulthood. Ages 12 to 14 years are considered early adolescence. During this time, the beginning of formal operational thinking and sexual maturation take place. Early adolescents want more independence from their parents, and they start to form companionships with their friends. Late adolescence occurs from ages 15 to 19 years. The psychosocial task of forming positive identity takes place. Late adolescents are completing their high school education, deciding on a career path, and entering the workplace. They are also forming sexual relationships and developing the ability to relate to others.

ADULTHOOD

Adulthood is divided into early, middle, and late. Early adulthood occurs during a person's 20s and 30s. The challenges of career choice, achieving intimacy, and accomplishing vocational success arise during this time. A person in his or her 40s or 50s is considered to be in middle adulthood. Achieving vocational success plus social and personal responsibility occurs during this period. At some point during this period, a person's body and emotional status change. Late adulthood occurs from age 60 until death. During this period many adjustments occur. A person's physical capacities and relationships with others change. New meanings are discovered within family relationships. Life satisfaction and happiness are reported by many during this life stage. Figure 57-5 shows adults engaging in healthy behavior.

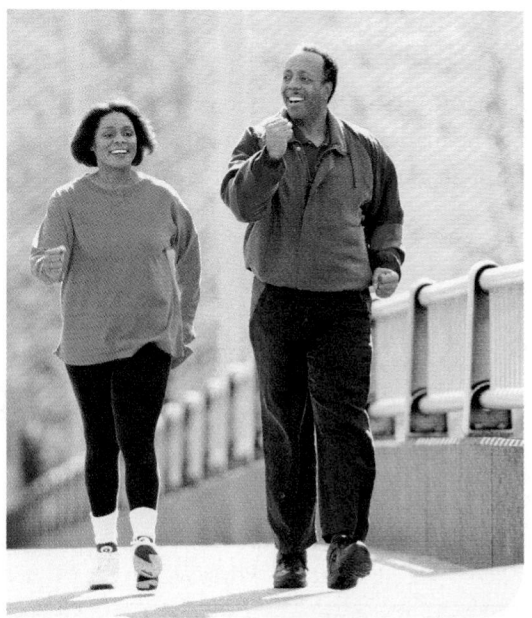

FIGURE 57-5 Adulthood.

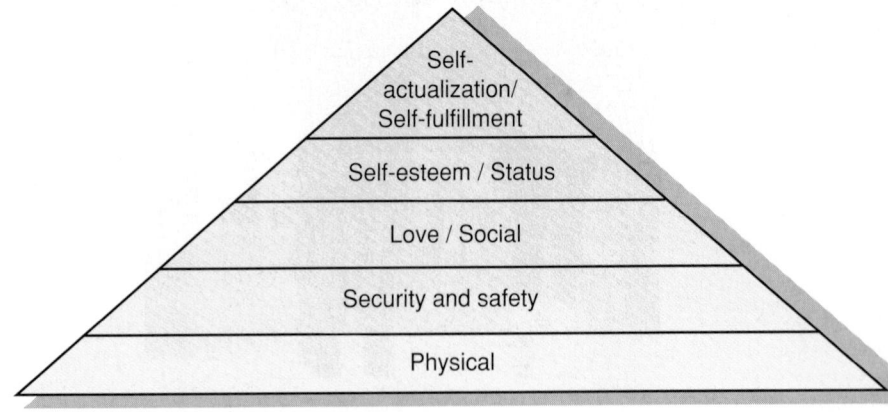

PROFESSIONALISM THE LIFE SPAN

Patients of all age groups have emotional and psychological needs. It is important for the medical assistant to understand life span development and to adapt behavior to the age of the patient. An infant or child may want to be with the parent or caregiver during an examination, but a teenager might not. Also understand that elders want to be respected, included in decision making, and allowed to have more time during physician visits.

Mind–Body Connection

Psychologists have discovered that there is a link between stress and illness. Certain predisposing factors create a tendency or susceptibility to become stressed. These include attitudes and feelings (e.g., emotions such as optimism or pessimism), health habits (e.g., smoking, exercise, drug use, and diet), the individual patient's methods for coping, economic and social resources (e.g., income, kind of job, security), and the state of the patient's immune system.

Many patients with a major illness go through a period of depression. The disease may cause emotional changes. In turn, worry about the disease may cause unhealthy habits such as an increase in smoking or drinking alcohol. Patients who have a physical illness such as heart disease, diabetes, or AIDS may become additionally stressed when confronted with the loss of income or a job.

Maslow's Hierarchy of Needs

Abraham Maslow (1908–1970) developed a **hierarchy of needs** in which he maintained that people had special needs and moved through various levels in achieving satisfaction

in life. The hierarchy of needs is based on five elements or levels:

- **Level I**—physical needs such as food, water, and shelter.
- **Level II**—security and safety needs, which include physical safety as well as security relating to employment.
- **Level III**—love and social needs, which include having a sense of belonging to a group and the need for social interaction.
- **Level IV**—self-esteem/status, which includes having a sense of self-worth and pride.
- **Level V**—self-actualization/self-fulfillment, which occurs when the individual achieves all he or she is capable of achieving and experiences a sense of accomplishment.

Maslow said that he believed a person could not move to a higher level until the basic needs at a lower level were met. For an illustration of Maslow's hierarchy of needs see Figure 57-6. An understanding of Maslow's hierarchy of needs is important for the medical assistant since the patients the medical assistant will encounter daily are at different stages or levels of fulfillment of their needs.

For example, one patient may be at Level I and be concerned about how he or she will pay a medical bill. Another patient, whose Level II and III needs have been met, may wish to see the physician about cosmetic surgery as the patient attempts to have his or her self-esteem needs (Level V) met. Patients who have a life-threatening illness must have their Level II needs for future security met.

Heredity, Environmental, and Cultural Influences on Behavior

Your heredity (nature) plus the environment (nurture) and culture in which you are raised influence your behavior. Some people believe heredity influences behavior more than the environment. Others believe the environment influences behavior more than heredity. Every factor has been determined to be essential for development because all can interact with each other.

Before you can communicate effectively with a patient from another culture you should understand the terms *bias, prejudice,* and *stereotyping.* **Bias** is when a person

Self-actualization/
Self-fulfillment

Self-esteem / Status

Love / Social

Security and safety

Physical

FIGURE 57-6 **Maslow's hierarchy of needs.**

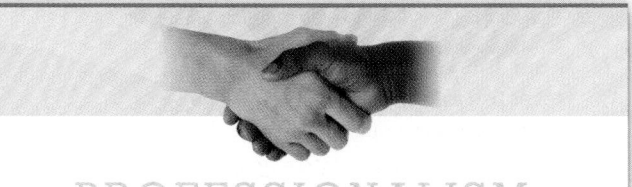

CULTURAL CONSIDERATIONS

Many cultures, particularly some ethnic and some religious groups, have strong opinions regarding mental health disorders. In fact, some Asian cultures view the idea of mental illness as a flaw or weakness in a person's character. Those who follow Scientology often strongly oppose psychology, psychiatry, and medications as a means for treating mental illness or depression. Some religious sects believe that mental illness is a form of demon possession or spiritual attack.

These varying views regarding psychology and mental health will have an impact on the way a patient receives treatment. Above all else, it is the medical assistant's responsibility to be the advocate for the patient and to place the patient's wishes and beliefs above their own.

favors a certain belief or attitude. **Prejudice** is a preformed and unfavorable belief or attitude toward a certain culture or group with little or no information about the culture or group. **Stereotyping** is the formation of negative beliefs or attitudes concerning specific characteristics of a person or group and applying them unfairly to an entire population.

As a medical assistant you will encounter patients from different cultures. Some of these patients will not speak any English, some will speak a little English, and some will be fluent in English. To be an effective communicator with a patient from another culture, you must think about how you would want to be treated if you were a patient in a different culture and could not speak the language of that culture. This will help you relate to how that patient might be feeling, and hopefully it will help you display more patience with the patient. Learning about different cultures, particularly those in your geographic area, will help you be more comfortable around a person from another culture and to communicate more effectively with him or her.

When you are talking to a patient from another country, use simple and common words. Avoid using medical terms if possible. You should never use slang. It is important for you to determine if the patient understands you. Sometimes patients who do not understand English pretend to understand so as not to seem impolite.

It will also be important for you to be aware of your nonverbal communication and that of the patient. As you research the different cultures in your area, you must learn how nonverbal communication varies across the cultures. You must determine if eye contact should be direct or indirect. Not having proper eye placement can interfere with the communication process.

Facial expressions can show a variety of emotions, such as sadness, anger, confusion, and happiness. Facial expressions can also differ from culture to culture. A smile does not always mean kindliness or friendliness; it may also be a sign of fear. It will be important to determine what different facial expressions mean.

Hand gestures also vary across the different cultures. It will be very important for you to understand the appropriate gestures to use for a particular culture. Some hand gestures that are appropriate in U.S. culture are very inappropriate in others (Procedure 57-1).

procedure
57-1

ROLE-PLAYING A SITUATION IN WHICH A PATIENT IS FROM ANOTHER CULTURE

Objective: Learn how to communicate with patients from another culture.

EQUIPMENT AND SUPPLIES
pen or pencil; paper

METHOD
1. Choose a classmate.
2. Select a quiet part of the classroom to conduct the procedure.
3. Determine who will be the medical assistant and who will be the patient.
4. Have the student pretending to be the patient act as if he or she speaks very little English.
5. Be calm, respectful, and considerate (Figure 57-7).
6. Use simple and common words.

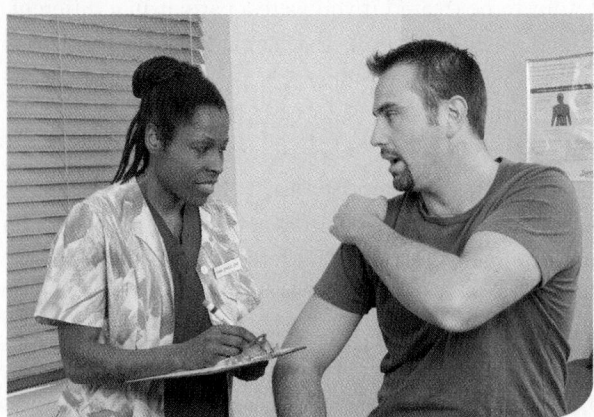

FIGURE 57-7 A medical assistant will work with patients of all cultures.

7. Avoid using medical terms.
8. Never use slang.
9. Pay attention to your eye contact, facial expressions, and hand gestures.
10. Make the patient feel as comfortable as possible.

Note: In a real-life situation, if a staff member who speaks the patient's language is available, have him or her translate the conversation if that would make the patient feel more comfortable.

11. Document the interaction in the patient chart.

CHARTING EXAMPLE

9/30/XX 8:05 A.M. Patient states that he speaks little English. Gave patient handout in Spanish after demonstrating procedure to the patient in the office. · · · · · · · · · C. Glidewell, CMA (AAMA)

Emotions

As a medical assistant you will experience and witness all the different types of emotions, but what are emotions? Most people think of emotions as feelings. Emotions can vary from person to person because of the way we react or because of past experience. Consider this example: Let's say that two medical assistants in the medical office received flowers on the same day. One of the medical assistants smiled and giggled as she received the flowers. The other medical assistant began to cry when she received hers. Both medical assistants received flowers, but each displayed different emotions.

It is normal for everyone to experience emotions, and emotions are an everyday part of life. How boring would it be if we humans did not express emotions? We would be like robots walking around. Emotions are a very important part of communicating with others. Medical assistants can see a person's emotions on the face. Some types of emotions that can be seen on a person's face include anger, sadness, surprise, and confusion.

Communication between people has changed due to the advent of e-mail. Because emotions cannot be seen on an e-mail and showing emotions is an important part of communication for some people, special software programs have been designed that use symbols to express certain emotions because they are so important in communication.

For medical assistants to understand a patient's emotions, they must first understand their own emotions. It is important for medical assistants to understand emotions because being aware of oneself and knowing how to express and react to different emotions will help medical

assistants be more effective with the patients they encounter.

Think of a time when you experienced an emotion. What did your face look like? Were your eyes open or closed? Were you smiling or frowning? Did you laugh or cry? These are important questions to ask yourself so you can become more aware of your emotions.

As a medical assistant working in a medical office, you will encounter patients who are frightened, depressed, and angry. How do you know a patient is experiencing these emotions? How can you help that patient? A scenario follows from which you can learn:

- Holly Sutter, CMA, was given a medication order by Dr. Baldwin for Christine Smith. After preparing the medication she entered the examination room to give Ms. Smith the injection as ordered. Ms. Smith asked, "Am I getting a shot?" Her eyes widened, she began to sweat, and her heart started to beat faster (Figure 57-8).

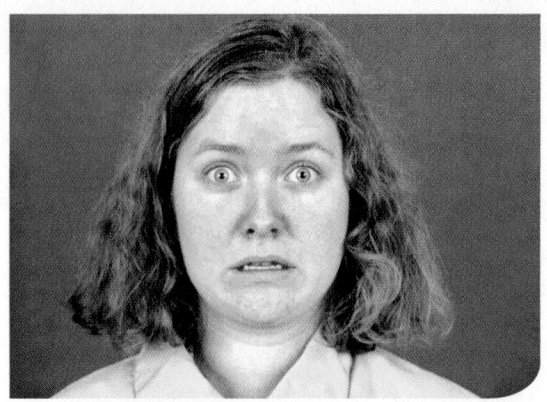

FIGURE 57-8 Emotion: fear.

Holly responded by saying "Yes, I have your injection right here." Ms. Smith stated, "I'm not getting a shot" and walked out of the examination room.

Holly did not recognize that Ms. Smith was displaying the emotion of fear. Holly was only focused on completing the task of giving the injection. Before Holly entered the examination room with the injection, she should have explained to Ms. Smith that she would be receiving the medication Dr. Baldwin ordered by injection. This would have given Ms. Smith the opportunity to express her negative feelings about receiving an injection, and it would have given her the opportunity to maintain control over the situation.

- You are working in the front office when a patient comes to the front reception window and starts screaming, yelling, and cursing at you. How else could you recognize this patient was angry? What should you do?

If a person is angry, he or she may have a reddish color to the face and ears, eyes may be slightly squinted, and fists may be clenched. These are just some of the signs that a person is angry. Once you recognize a person is angry, remain calm. As long as the patient is not being aggressive, allow him or her to communicate the anger. First, let the patient know that you understand he or she is angry. Next, so you can resolve the issue, you should inquire about what is making the patient angry. During the conversation make sure you are empathic so the patient knows you are concerned about his or her issue. Figure 57-9 depicts an angry patient.

- Holly Sutter, CMA, is taking a patient's vital signs when the patient tells her, "I failed all my courses last quarter, and if I fail any more courses I'm going to be kicked out of school." During the conversation the

patient starts crying and tells Holly, "I'm having trouble sleeping, and I am tired of trying so hard in my courses and not succeeding" (Figure 57-10).

During the conversation with the patient, Holly should be empathic and caring. After Holly allows the patient to express his feelings, she should immediately tell the doctor about the conversation as well as the statements the patient made. It is also important for Holly to document the situation

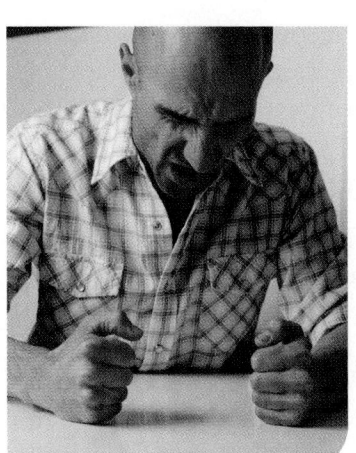

FIGURE 57-9 Emotion: anger.

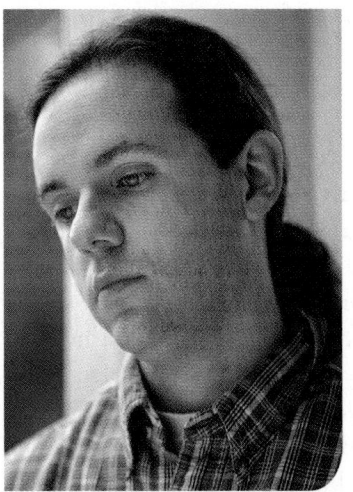

FIGURE 57-10 Emotion: depression.

ROLE-PLAYING A SITUATION IN WHICH A PATIENT IS FRIGHTENED, ANGRY, OR DEPRESSED

Objective: Learn how to deal with a patient who is frightened, angry, or depressed.

EQUIPMENT AND SUPPLIES

pen; medical record

METHOD

1. Choose a classmate.
2. Select a quiet part of the classroom to conduct the procedure.
3. Determine who will be the medical assistant and who will be the patient.
4. Have the student pretending to be the patient express the emotions of being frightened, angry, and depressed.
5. Once you recognize one of these emotions, remain calm.
6. If the patient is not displaying destructive behaviors, allow the patient to express his or her feelings without being interrupted (Figure 57-11).
7. Let the patient know that you understand.
8. Inquire about the issue so you can solve the issue.
9. During the conversation make sure you are empathic so the patient knows you are concerned about his or her issue.
10. Notify the physician of the conversation.
11. Document the conversation in the medical record.

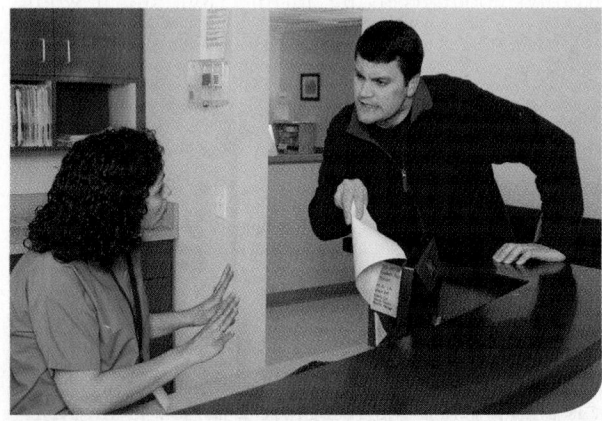

FIGURE 57-11 Medical assistants must calm angry patients.
Source: Michal Heron/Pearson Education/PH College

CHARTING EXAMPLE

3/4/XX 4:00 P.M. Patient expressed concern about not seeing doctor immediately on arrival. Explained physician was delivering baby at hospital and offered patient another appointment later in the day. Patient refused later appointment and agreed to wait in the reception area until physician returned. · M. Tyler, CMA (AAMA)

---

in the patient's medical record. See Procedure 57-2 for a role-play situation in which a patient is frightened, angry, and depressed.

Motivation

When was the last time you were motivated to complete a task or a goal? What was the task or goal you wanted to accomplish? What motivated you to complete that task or goal? **Motivation** is the stimulus that drives us to act. It forms and guides our goal-directed behavior. As a medical assistant there will be many tasks for you to complete every day. Knowing the task or goals you want to accomplish is the first step. Next you need to determine what is motivating you to complete that task or goal. Some people are motivated to complete a task or goal because it challenges

them. People also like the rewards or praise they receive from completing the task or goal.

There are many types of motivators. Medical assistants who are motivated to accomplish tasks or goals on a regular basis will be successful in their careers.

Stress

Stress is the body's reaction to the world around it. Stress can be emotional, intellectual, or physical. It can also be spiritual, economical, or social. Everyone experiences stress at one time or another.

Depending on the level of stress, it can be energizing, motivating, or exhausting. Medical research has shown that a certain amount of stress is not a bad thing. The body's reaction to stress determines if it is good stress or bad stress

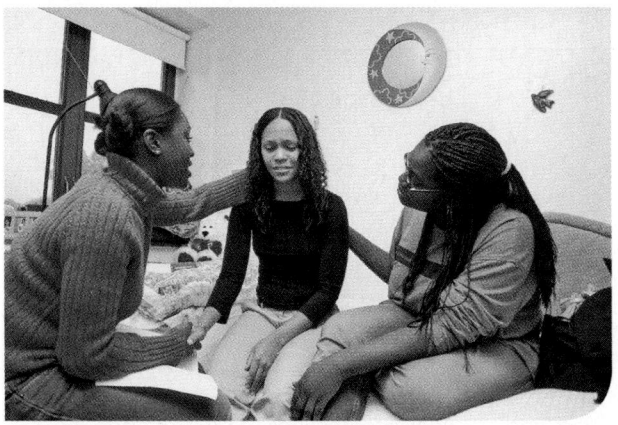

FIGURE 57-12 **Signs of stress.**

(distress). Stress has also been implicated in various illnesses. See Figure 57-12 for an illustration of stress.

A **stressor** is a real or imaginary event that causes stress. Certain major life events such as the death of a loved one, divorce, an unexpected move away from family and friends, unemployment, illness, getting married, delivering a baby, studying for an examination, or purchasing a new car can trigger stress. Each of these life events or others may be positive or negative. For a life event to be stressful, it does not always have to be a negative event.

Symptoms of stress vary from person to person. It is important for you to know what is normal for you and your body. Box 57-1 lists symptoms of stress.

DEFENSE MECHANISMS

Defense mechanisms operate at a subconscious level to manage anxiety by denying, misinterpreting, or distorting reality. They often hinder self-awareness by preventing people from being sensitive to anxiety. Defense mechanisms can be helpful in dealing with anxiety; however, consistent use of certain defenses leads to the development of either good or self-destructive behavior patterns. For example, the basic human need to be loved and cared for by another person can result in a variety of behaviors when the fear of losing love produces anxiety. One person may be driven to constantly look for love and affirmation by engaging in frequent one-night sexual encounters. Another person may seek and develop a warm, intimate relationship. A third person may be so frightened of not finding love and so fearful of rejection that he or she avoids relationships to decrease the anxiety. The management of defense mechanisms may become so time consuming that little energy remains for other aspects of living. Table 57-3 lists examples and uses of defense mechanisms.

POST-TRAUMATIC STRESS DISORDER

Patients who have been exposed to a natural disaster, terrorist attack, physical or sexual assault, military combat, or some combination of them may experience post-traumatic stress disorder (PTSD). In addition to feelings of anxiety, aggression, irritability, tension, and guilt, there can be a numbing of other emotions and a feeling of being detached from others. Memory may be affected, and the patient may experience flashbacks of the event.

COPING WITH STRESS

Before you or a patient can cope with stress, you must be able to recognize it and know how you are being affected by it. You will also need to know what event or events are causing the stress. Recommendations for coping with stress (Figure 57-13) include the following:

- Develop a strong support system including family and friends.
- Find a balance between perfection and fear of failure.
- Eat nutritious meals.
- Avoid harmful habits such as smoking and drinking.

Box 57-1 Symptoms of STRESS

Fatigue	Cramps
Exhaustion	Constipation
Difficulty falling asleep	Diarrhea
Difficulty staying asleep	Flatulence
Restlessness	Sore muscles
Tension	Increased blood pressure
Boredom	Increased heart rate
Lack of interest	Change in eating habits
Inability to concentrate	Increased use of alcohol
Depression	

TABLE 57-3 Defense Mechanisms

Defense Mechanism	Example(s)	Use/Purpose
Compensation Covering up weaknesses by emphasizing a more desirable trait or by overachievement in a more comfortable area.	A high school student too small to play football becomes the star long-distance runner for the track team.	Allows a person to overcome weakness and achieve success.
Denial An attempt to screen or ignore unacceptable realities by refusing to acknowledge them.	A woman, though told her father has metastatic cancer, continues to plan a family reunion 18 months in advance.	Temporarily isolates a person from the full impact of a traumatic situation.
Displacement The transferring or discharging of emotional reactions from one object or person to another object or person.	A husband and wife are fighting, and the husband becomes so angry he hits a door instead of his wife; or a student gets a C on a paper she worked hard on and goes home and yells at her family.	Allows for feelings to be expressed through or to less dangerous objects or people.
Identification An attempt to manage anxiety by imitating the behavior of someone feared or respected.	A student nurse imitates the nurturing behavior she observes one of her instructors using with clients.	Helps a person avoid self-devaluation.
Intellectualization A mechanism by which an emotional response that normally would accompany an uncomfortable or painful incident is evaded by the use of rational explanations that remove from the incident any personal significance and feelings.	The pain over a parent's sudden death is reduced by saying, "He wouldn't have wanted to live disabled."	Protects a person from pain and traumatic events.
Introjection A form of identification that allows for the acceptance of others' norms and values into oneself, even when contrary to one's previous assumptions.	A 7-year-old tells his little sister, "Don't talk to strangers." He has introjected this value from the instructions of parents and teachers.	Helps a person avoid social retaliation and punishment; particularly important for the child's development of superego.
Minimization Not acknowledging the significance of one's behavior.	A person says, "Don't believe everything my wife tells you. I wasn't so drunk I couldn't drive."	Allows a person to decrease responsibility for own behavior.
Projection A process in which blame is attached to others or the environment for unacceptable desires, thoughts, shortcomings, and mistakes.	A mother is told her child must repeat a grade in school, and she blames this on the teacher's poor instruction; or a husband forgets to pay a bill and blames his wife for not giving it to him earlier.	Allows a person to deny the existence of shortcomings and mistakes; protects self-image.
Rationalization Justification of certain behaviors by faulty logic and ascription of motives that are socially acceptable but did not in fact inspire the behavior.	A mother spanks her toddler too hard and says it was all right because he couldn't feel it through the diapers anyway.	Helps a person cope with the inability to meet goals or certain standards.
Reaction formation A mechanism that causes people to act exactly opposite to the way they feel.	An executive resents his bosses for calling in a consulting firm to make recommendations for change in his department but verbalizes complete support of the idea and is exceedingly polite and cooperative.	Aids in reinforcing repression by allowing feelings to be acted out in a more acceptable way.

Regression		
Resorting to an earlier, more comfortable level of functioning that is characteristically less demanding and responsible.	An adult throws a temper tantrum when he does not get his own way; or a critically ill client allows the nurse to bathe and feed him.	Allows a person to return to a point in development when nurturing and dependency were needed and accepted with comfort.
Repression		
An unconscious mechanism by which threatening thoughts, feelings, and desires are kept from becoming conscious; the repressed material is denied entry into consciousness.	A teenager, seeing his best friend killed in a car accident, becomes amnesic about the circumstances surrounding the accident.	Protects a person from a traumatic experience until he or she has the resources to cope.
Sublimation		
Displacement of energy associated with more primitive sexual or aggressive drives into socially acceptable activities.	A person with excessive, primitive sexual drives invests psychic energy into a well-defined religious value system.	Protects a person from behaving in irrational, impulsive ways.
Substitution		
The replacement of a highly valued, unacceptable, or unavailable object by a less valuable, acceptable, or available object.	A woman wants to marry a man exactly like her dead father and settles for someone who looks a little bit like him.	Helps a person achieve goals and minimizes frustration and disappointment.
Undoing		
An action or words designed to cancel some disapproved thoughts, impulses, or acts in which the person relieves guilt by making reparation.	A father spanks his child and the next evening brings home a present for him; or a teacher writes an exam that is far too easy, then constructs a grading curve that makes it difficult to earn a high grade.	Allows a person to appease guilty feelings and atone for mistakes.

- Use physical exercise such as walking, jogging, dancing, biking, and swimming.
- Look outward to develop a social interest by understanding other people's problems and needs.
- Try to see the humor in situations.
- Limit the number of activities to a manageable few.

When you are working as a medical assistant, it will be important for you not to let personal stress affect your job performance. While working in a medical office you will experience stress that is related to work. This type of stress must be left at work when you go home for the night.

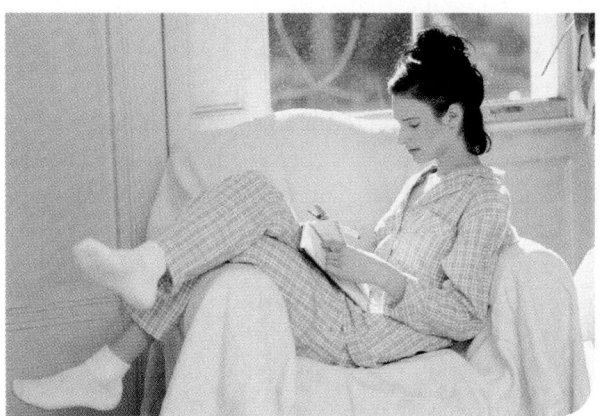

FIGURE 57-13 Coping with stress.

Personal stress and work stress need to be kept separate and should never interfere with one another.

You will experience stress in a medical office each day. You will not be able to predict its onset or eliminate it. While you are working, you can never know what will happen in the next few minutes or hours. Emergencies, being short a staff member, an autoclave that fails to work, or not having certain supplies are just a few situations that could occur and cause stress. If a stressful situation does occur, you must remain calm and focus on the situation. You will be able to handle the situation using the best abilities you possess.

As a medical assistant, you will be taking care of patients who are sick every day. This can be emotionally, mentally, and physically draining. Anytime your stress level is too high and you have trouble coping, you must seek support from a close friend or family member. If a close friend or family member is not able to help you, seek help from a professional.

Encountering a patient who is experiencing stress provides an opportunity for patient teaching. After allowing the patient to discuss the stress and stressors, assess the patient's knowledge of the topic of stress. Doing so will establish a starting point for educating the patient. Next, determine the appropriate reading, language, and education level of the patient so that you can select and prepare materials to use to teach the patient about stress. Some of the educational

DEVELOP A PATIENT TEACHING HANDOUT ABOUT STRESS

Objective: Develop an appropriate teaching tool about stress.

EQUIPMENT AND SUPPLIES

computer; word processor; printer; pen, paper

METHOD

1. Decide what information should be included on the patient teaching handout.
2. Develop an outline of the information you plan to include on the patient teaching handout.
3. Using a word processing program, develop a patient teaching handout.
4. Make sure your patient teaching includes at a minimum the definition, causes, and ways to cope with stress (Figure 57-14).
5. Proofread your patient teaching handout on the computer screen.
6. Make any necessary corrections to the patient teaching handout.
7. Print your patient teaching handout.
8. Proofread the hard copy of your patient teaching handout.
9. Make any necessary corrections to the patient teaching handout.

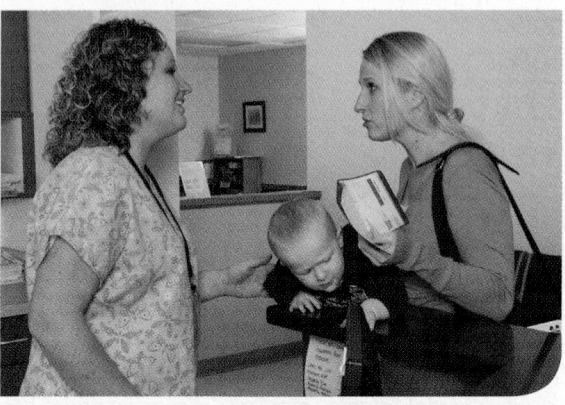

FIGURE 57-14 Medical assistants help patients cope with stress.

10. Turn in the patient teaching handout to your instructor.

CHARTING EXAMPLE

8/27/XX 9:24 A.M. Instructed patient on ways to handle stress and gave patient office handout on stress ················· ································· A. Schuknecht, RMA

---

materials that are used in a medical office include videos, patient teaching handouts (Procedure 57-3), and booklets. After you gather all your equipment and supplies, you will be ready to provide the patient with information about stress. When you have completed the patient teaching, you must document it in the patient's medical record.

Assisting the Patient with a Terminal Illness

The medical assistant will come into contact with patients who have a **terminal illness**. A terminal illness is one that is expected to end in death. This includes many conditions and diseases, including cancer, AIDS, progressive heart disease, amyotrophic lateral sclerosis (Lou Gehrig's disease), cystic fibrosis, and multiple sclerosis.

In cases where the dying process is slow for the patient, the medical assistant may have the opportunity to be with the patient on several occasions during office visits. Although there is always hope of recovery or finding a cure through research for a disease such as AIDS, it is wise to listen to the patient express his or her fears and concerns rather than to offer false hope for recovery.

Death is a natural process that everyone must face. People have various ways of coping with their own death based on a variety of influences, including culture, religion, personal experience, and age.

CULTURE

People learn what their own culture expects of them at a very early age by observing family and friends as they handle life events such as births and deaths. In some cultures death is considered a normal end to the life process and is therefore accepted with peace. In other cultures death may be feared.

The terminally ill patient and family may have already established a very personal approach or method for handling death and dying. The medical assistant may also have a strong cultural attitude toward death.

RELIGION

Religious beliefs play an important role in how patients handle death and dying. Some patients will have a strong belief

TABLE 57-4 Dr. Elizabeth Kübler-Ross's Five Stages of Grief

Denial	A refusal to believe that dying is taking place. In this stage the patient (or family member) may need time to adjust to the reality of approaching death. This stage cannot be hurried.
Anger	At this stage, the patient may be angry at everyone and may express this intense anger at God, family, and even health care professionals. The patient may take this anger out on the person closest to him or her. Usually this is a family member. In reality, the patient is angry about dying.
Bargaining	The third stage of grief involves attempting to gain time by making promises in return. The patient may bargain with God. The patient may also indicate a need to talk at this stage.
Depression	This stage is marked with a deep sadness over the loss of health, independence, and eventually life. There is an additional sadness of leaving loved ones behind. The grieving patient may become withdrawn.
Acceptance	The acceptance stage is characterized by a sense of peace and calm. The patient may make comments such as "I have no regrets. I'm ready to die." It is better to let the patient talk and not make denial statements such as "Don't talk like that. You're not going to die."

in an afterlife. Other patients will follow no particular religious belief. In both cases, the patients' dying process and death can be meaningful and peaceful.

It is considered unacceptable for the medical assistant to attempt to convert the patient to the medical assistant's religious faith. Professionalism mandates that the medical assistant and other staff members recognize and support the patient's right to embrace his or her own religious beliefs.

PERSONAL EXPERIENCE

The past experiences of the patient and the medical assistant will mold how they approach the topic of death. If the patient has been closely involved with the care of someone who has died a painful death, the patient may fear the same kind of death for himself or herself. These patients must be able to discuss their fears. In the same manner, if the medical assistant has had past experiences with the death of friends or relatives, it may be easier to assist the patient. On the other hand, patients who have had little exposure to death may have a more difficult time understanding their feelings or expressing their experience.

AGE

The elderly usually have less fear of death than younger people. In some cases an elderly person may not feel well, and even may have failing eyesight, hearing, and memory, and

may look upon death with relief. If the patient wishes to discuss his or her approaching death, the medical assistant should be ready to listen.

STAGES OF GRIEF

Dr. Elizabeth Kübler-Ross devoted much of her life to the study of the dying process and working with dying patients. She divided the grief process into five stages that she believes all persons go through (Table 57-4). It is helpful to understand these stages when attempting to help the dying patient.

According to Kübler-Ross, all those involved with the dying process may go through the five stages. This would include the patient, family members, and caregivers (such as the medical assistant). The five stages are denial, anger, bargaining, depression, and acceptance. The stages may overlap and may not be experienced by everyone in the stated order, but all are present in the dying person, according to Kübler-Ross.

As the time of death approaches, some of the earlier stages may be repeated. For example, patients who cannot care for themselves may become angry. The critical point to remember when assisting a patient who is dying is that the grieving period is a normal part of the dying process.

Hospice care, which is physical and emotional care provided to the dying person, is a growing movement throughout the United States. The medical assistant should be acquainted with this option of care delivery for the terminally ill.

SUMMARY

Mental and behavioral illness is quite prevalent in today's society. Mental illnesses are caused by changes in brain structure and chemistry. Behavioral disorders are caused by making poor cognitive choices that result in destructive behaviors. The *DSM-IV* is the textbook of classification of

the many psychological disorders. Psychotic patients are out of touch with reality and need to be medicated. Some illnesses require medication. Others, like those with personality disorders, respond more appropriately to talk therapy. Those with substance abuse disorders respond best to group therapy. Electroconvulsive therapy is the therapy of last resort for depression.

According to Maslow, the physical needs of the patient must be met before the psychological ones can be. Mental wellness is greatly influenced by heredity, culture, and the environment. Patients who are frightened, angry, or depressed need special care. Understanding the motivation of the patient enables the medical assistant to aid in the patient's progress.

Poor adaptation to stress influences mental and behavioral health. Kübler-Ross's five stages of grief help the medical assistant to adapt communication to the stage the patient is experiencing at the time.

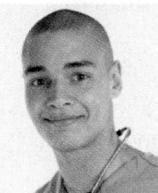

57 CHAPTER REVIEW

COMPETENCY REVIEW

1. Define and spell the terms to learn for this chapter.

2. Describe how you use the eight health habits to cope with stress.

3. Define ten psychological disorders.

4. Discuss the three treatments for mental disorders.

5. Explain how you would communicate with a frightened, angry, and depressed patient.

PREPARING FOR THE CERTIFICATION EXAM

1. Fixed, false beliefs are called
   a. delusions
   b. hallucinations
   c. bipolar
   d. compulsions
   e. obsessions

2. Inflexible behavior patterns that cause inability to functions are
   a. bipolar disorder
   b. depression
   c. schizophrenia
   d. personality disorder
   e. anxiety disorder

3. Phobias are considered
   a. mood disorders
   b. anxiety disorders
   c. personality disorders
   d. bipolar disorders
   e. psychoses

4. Trust and mistrust is the task of which stage of the life cycle?
   a. prenatal period
   b. infancy
   c. childhood
   d. adolescence
   e. adulthood

5. The highest level of Maslow's hierarchy of needs is
   a. love
   b. security
   c. physical
   d. self-esteem
   e. self-actualization

6. The transferring or discharging of emotional reactions from one object or person to another object or person is
   a. identification
   b. denial
   c. intellectualization
   d. displacement
   e. compensation

7. Not acknowledging the significance of one's behavior is called
   a. denial
   b. introjection
   c. minimization
   d. displacement
   e. compensation

8. The stage of grief during which the patient may yell at a family member or physician is
   a. denial
   b. anger
   c. bargaining

d. depression

e. acceptance

9. What is the stimulus that drives us to act?

a. stress

b. defense mechanisms

c. motivation

d. electroconvulsive therapy

e. mania

10. A mother spanks her toddler too hard and says it is all right because he could not feel it through the diaper is an example of

a. regression

b. reaction formation

c. repression

d. rationalization

e. sublimation

CRITICAL THINKING

1. During the examination, Dr. Penningworth asks Simon if any changes have occurred over the past month. Simon sighs and states "What hasn't changed is more like it! My wife has filed for divorce, and my mother was just diagnosed with breast cancer." How might Simon's personal situation be taking a toll on his health?

2. Dr. Penningworth feels that Simon is under a great deal of stress. What are some additional signs and symptoms that Simon may have if he is stressed out?

3. Dr. Penningworth asks Susan to provide Simon with some information regarding stress management as well as a support group for friends and family of people diagnosed with terminal illnesses. When Susan presents this information to Simon he states, "I don't think I will need a support group because I have been doing a lot of extra volunteer work at my church, and I think because of that my mom will begin to feel better." What is Simon displaying, and how should Susan handle this?

ON THE JOB

Amy Freeman is a new medical assistant who has recently graduated and passed the CMA examination. During her education she studied ways to cope with stress. Renee Baker, a full-time student and a young mother of two small children, has an appointment to see Dr. Williams. Ms. Baker tells Amy that she is angry at her husband for not being more supportive and angry at herself for not doing that well in school. Because Ms. Baker has opened up to Amy about her feelings, Amy wants to try to help her. Amy decides to provide Ms. Baker with patient teaching about stress management.

1. What information should Amy give about stress management?
2. How would Amy document the patient teaching she gave Ms. Baker?
3. Does Amy have a responsibility to inform the physician of Ms. Baker's situation?

INTERNET ACTIVITY

Visit the Internet and research one mental illness that interest you. Be able to answer the following questions about this disorder:

1. Define the disorder.
2. Discuss what causes this disorder.
3. What are the symptoms of this disorder?
4. What are the treatments for this disorder?

MEDMEDIA

Additional interactive resources and activities for this chapter can be found:

On your student DVD: View applicable procedure videos on the DVD-ROM found in the back of this book.

MyHealthProfessionsKit.com: Test your knowledge of the chapter with games and activities. MyHealthProfessionsKit also includes resources, helpful links, and a Spanish audio glossary.

Medical Assisting Interactive: Practice your procedures as a medical assistant in this simulated doctor's office. This can be accessed through MyHealthProfessionsKit.com.

Unit One

Unit Two

Unit Three

Unit Four

Unit Five

Career
Assistance

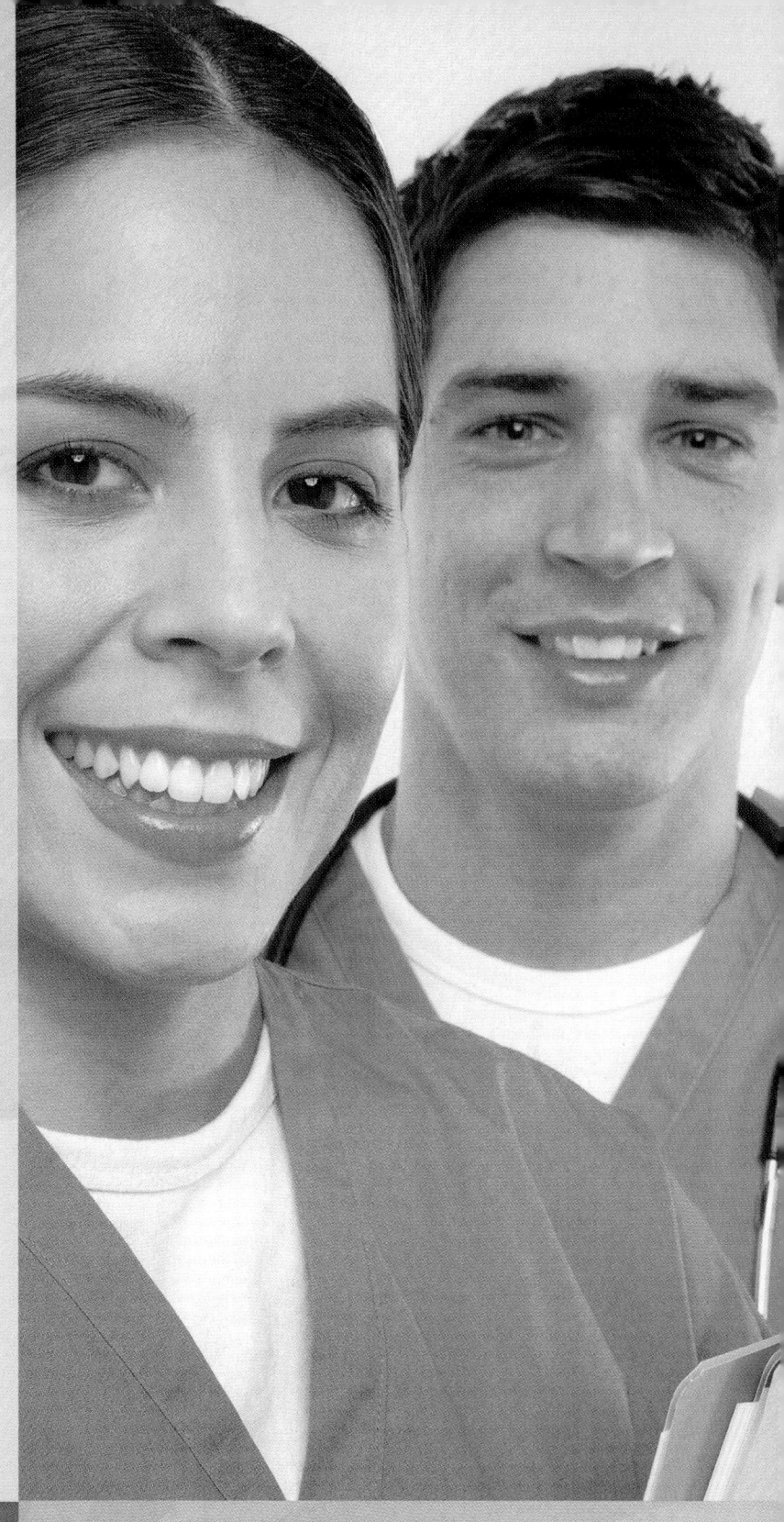

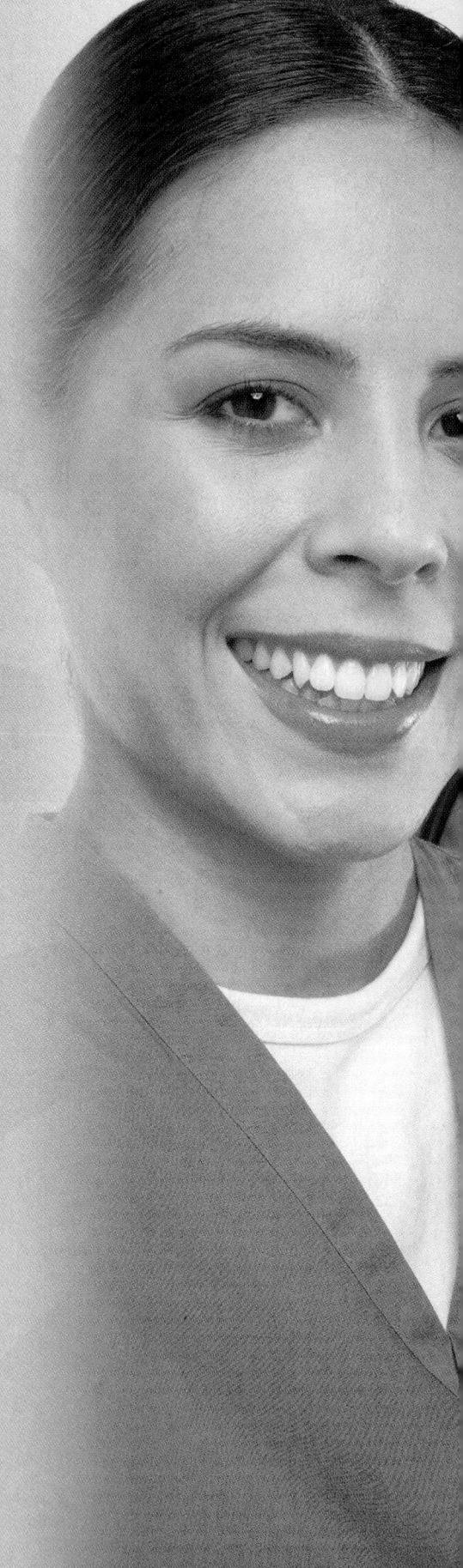

58

Professionalism

LEARNING OBJECTIVES

After completing this chapter, you should be able to:

- Define and spell the terms to learn for this chapter.

- Discuss the importance of professional skills in the workplace.

- Identify the professional skills needed for success in the workplace.

- Explain why professional skills are valued not only by the employer but also by the patient.

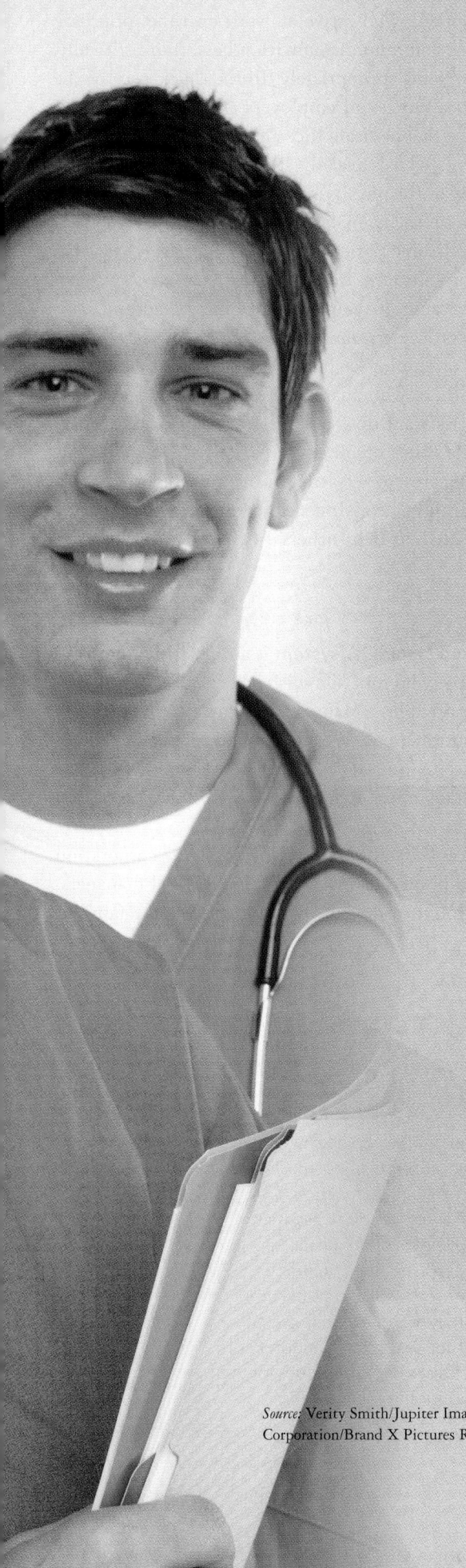

Source: Verity Smith/Jupiter Images/PictureArts Corporation/Brand X Pictures Royalty Free

CHAPTER OUTLINE

CASE STUDY

On a busy morning at Pearson Physicians Group, David, a registered medical assistant, has gotten behind in his work. Susan, a coworker who is also a registered medical assistant, grumbles to Tania that "David never gets his work done." Gossip has begun to circulate that Susan is angry at David and that she thinks he is lazy. David has recently graduated from school, and this is his first job as a medical assistant. He constantly worries that he is not working fast enough and that he will make a mistake.

TERMS TO LEARN

affective	guided imagery
aromatherapy	lifelong learning
biofeedback	persistence
cognitive	psychomotor
diversity	soft skills
encounter note	system

CERTIFICATION LINK

CMA (AAMA)	RMA	CMAS (AMT)
Professionalism	General medical assisting knowledge	Professionalism
Displaying a professional attitude	Human relations	Employ human relations skills appropriate to the health care setting
Working as a team member to achieve goals		Display behaviors of a professional medical administrative specialist
Communication		Participate in appropriate continuing education
Professional communication and behavior		

Health care professionals in the medical office need to have good technical skills, and they also must have soft skills. **Soft skills** are those skills necessary for the smooth functioning of the workplace that are neither **cognitive** (based on knowledge) nor **psychomotor** (coordinating the mind and body) and that display the professionalism of the employee. Although facts and procedural skills are often tested in school, the workplace is the testing arena for professional soft skills. If an employee comes to work not knowing how to perform a procedure but has the professionalism to ask for help, that employee can be trained in that skill. However, if an employee comes to work and does not get along well with others, fails to communicate needs, or handles assignments in a less-than-professional manner, that employee will probably be terminated from the office. **Affective** skills are behaviors that come from feelings and emotions and are truly important in the medical office.

Professional Skills in the Workplace

The physician-employer expects the employee to be competent in performing procedures, understanding anatomy and physiology, and using medical terminology. The physician also needs workers who arrive at work on time, prioritize problems, seek communication with others, think critically, and solve problems appropriately. In the quick pace of the modern medical office, all employees are expected to work for the good of the medical office and its patients.

The patient, who is usually ill, expects competent and courteous help at the physician's office. If a medical assistant cannot prioritize needs, manage time well, display good social skills, and solve patient problems effectively, patients will not return. In fact, frequently patients sue physician offices, not because of poor outcomes but because of poor treatment by office personnel.

The team of employees in the medical office expects to work with others who share similar values and goals. If one medical assistant does not do a fair share of the work, it burdens the other members of the team. Because medical assistants are so versatile, it is expected that even though they might be assigned to one responsibility, they may be expected to help others in the office with other roles.

INTEGRATED SYSTEMS

Every office is a system. A **system** is a regularly interacting group of people who function with an organized set of doctrines and principles. Many times these principles are recorded in a formal policies and procedures manual. Sometimes the system functions a little more informally. The medical assistant must understand how to function within the system.

The medical assistant who works for a large corporation may have had numerous interviews, met several managers, and gone through a long orientation to become familiar

PROFESSIONALISM THE WORKPLACE

Everyone in the workplace would like to work with a supportive team. To ensure that a supportive team functions well in the workplace, every medical assistant must be willing to assume full responsibility as a team member. When teamwork does not occur, the team may need to self-evaluate and construct ways to function more effectively. This is important both for the patients and for the team.

with the office and the hierarchy of people who manage the office. In a smaller office, the medical assistant may have fewer colleagues and managers. This assistant may not have even had a formal orientation but instead just started to work and was expected to ask any questions as they arose. However, the smaller office still will hold the medical assistant accountable for using soft skills at the same level the larger organization does. It is important for the medical assistant to clarify early in the work relationship the expectations in the office. For example, the assistant should know who to contact for what reasons, how to account for time, how and when to expect to be paid, and what to do if time off is needed. Having a clear understanding of managers' expectations makes the system function smoothly.

Truthfulness is very important in the medical office. If a medical assistant does not know how to perform a procedure, an admission must be made to superiors. In that way, the medical assistant can be trained and legal problems may be avoided. Cheating on time cards, lying about previous education, and any lack of truthfulness in general are grounds for dismissal. Every worker in the system must be able to trust each person in the office. Since there are both money and drugs in the office, the medical assistant must be beyond reproach in trustworthiness.

The medical assistant must work well with other allied health professionals. For ideal patient care, the medical assistant should have a network of peer relationships to contact for referrals, support group recommendations, and surgical appointments for patients. Every medical assistant works within a system of health care professionals.

Workplace Communication

Perhaps the most important soft skill to have is effective communication. Communication is important between patient and health care professionals (See Chapter 5), but it is crucially important among members of the health care team to solve many problems. For example, if a physician is out of the office, who is in charge? A medical assistant will communicate with every patient, and the impression of this communication can make a huge difference in how the patient perceives the level of efficiency and empathy of the office. In effect, the medical assistant represents the office with every communication. Therefore, a medical assistant must be aware of how important effective communication is and must incorporate good communication skills with excellent patient care.

Good communication also means knowing when not to communicate. Following Health Insurance Portability and Accountability Act (HIPAA) laws and protecting patient confidentiality are expected of all medical assistants.

ACTIVE LISTENING

Active listening is a key soft skill. If, instead of listening, the medical assistant is thinking of the answer the patient may give to a question or is forming a possible diagnosis while interviewing a patient, the physician may not receive critical information. If the physician is giving an order and the medical assistant is thinking of something else, the results can be disastrous. It is very important that the medical assistant always engage in active listening. Instead of making assumptions about what is being said, the medical assistant with good professional skills will focus on the speaker and will ask for clarification if needed.

SEEKING TO UNDERSTAND

In his book *The Seven Habits of Highly Effective People,* Stephen Covey noted that we should seek to understand before seeking to be understood. A health care professional should enter every conversation, whether with patients or colleagues, seeking to understand the other person. Then communication is facilitated.

SPEAKING TO BE UNDERSTOOD

At the same time the health care professional seeks to understand the person speaking, he or she should speak to be understood. Too often in the busy medical office, personnel use shortened versions of conversation to quickly get work done. A newly hired team member may need to have a fuller explanation of a policy or procedure. Taking the time to explain something well one time will save time in re-explanations later.

When presenting difficult concepts, it is always a good idea to seek feedback from the listener to make sure that he or she understood. When communicating, always take into account the age and culture of the patient. The medical assistant will use a different vocabulary depending on the age and mental capacity of the patient. It is important to address the patient with the title (Mr., Mrs., Ms., Miss) that the patient prefers and with the respect due to age or culture. The wise medical assistant will also address physicians and peers with respect in the medical office.

EFFECTIVE WRITING

The modern age of the Internet and text messaging has led many to assume that short communications are best. In the health care environment, accuracy is more important than brevity. A medical assistant who can write an effective phone message, memo, or letter will be prized by the employer. Although it might take a few minutes to write a longer **encounter note** (documentation of the patient visit to the physician's office), it will be valued in the long run, as it not only provides more information for future reference but also shows the thoroughness of the medical assistant's care for the patient.

Effective instructions given to patients can decrease many potential problems in the office. For example, a patient who is well prepared for a procedure will be less anxious and more compliant because he or she will be less frightened of what will happen.

Critical Thinking

Although cognitive knowledge is important, using facts learned is the goal of learning. In an average day at a medical office, the medical assistant will make numerous crucial decisions. Although some decisions or procedures may be routine, most will involve critical thinking. For proper decision making, the medical assistant must retrieve memorized facts and events, add reflection to the thinking process, and act in the appropriate manner.

Insurance and billing issues often require critical thinking. The medical assistant must advocate for the patient with the patient's insurance company through a maze of complicated rules for reimbursement. Thinking critically can improve reimbursement from the insurance company to the medical practice and greatly relieve a burden on the patient.

A medical assistant should question laboratory results that do not seem consistent with the patient presentation. Although the medical assistant should never diagnose, it is the medical assistant's responsibility to bring abnormal results to the physician's attention. Gathering numerous facts, such as laboratory tests and vital signs, and adding them to how the patient presents and what the patient reports all help to give a true picture of the patient's illness. A critically thinking medical assistant will take in all information before forming a conclusion.

DIFFERENTIATING FACT FROM OPINION

Critical thinking involves differentiating fact from fiction or opinion. A patient may believe that he or she has a particular disease or problem, but a critical thinking medical assistant can discern whether the information (the patient's chief complaints plus the medical assistant's objective notations) actually matches the beliefs of the patient (Figure 58-1). The medical assistant also must critically assess whether he or she has jumped to conclusions during an encounter. If a patient seems angry with the medical assistant for having to wait a long time, perhaps the patient is really angry about the pain he or she is experiencing. There is value in trying to see what the patient needs during an encounter, rather than assuming that the patient has certain emotions toward the medical assistant.

MAKING VALUE JUDGMENTS

A medical assistant must make value judgments on a daily basis. For example, setting the priority for a patient visit should be based on the chief complaint and not on how much the medical assistant values the relationship with the patient. If a physician refuses to give a patient a medication that the patient does not need, the medical assistant may have to reinforce the value of this judgment to

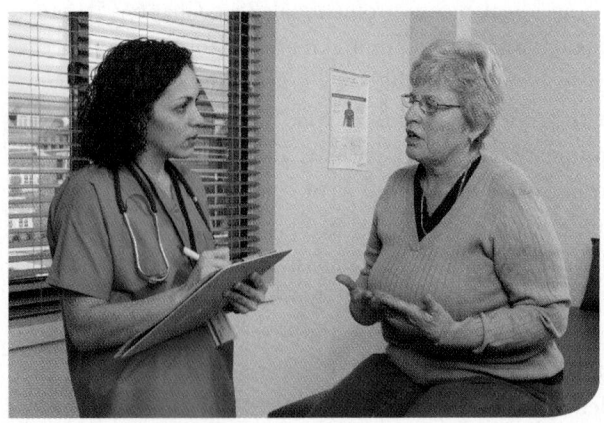

FIGURE 58-1 Medical assistant interviewing a patient.

the patient. Critical thinking should become so habitual that the medical assistant is comfortable with making value judgments.

Teamwork

Teamwork is a critical workplace competency. No matter how small the medical office may be, all the employees must work together. If one employee becomes overwhelmed with responsibilities, the others should be versatile enough in their knowledge to help until the work is caught up. All medical assistants must understand how the team functions and be prepared to share responsibilities. Medical assistants should practice only within the scope of practice; however, within their role delineation, they should maintain competency and a helpful attitude toward working with others (Figure 58-2).

DIVERSITY

In the average medical office, medical assistants and other health care professionals will come from different backgrounds. **Diversity** means "variety." Since the United States is a melting pot of cultures, you can expect to have a variety of both patients and coworkers. It is in everyone's best interest that biases, stereotypes, and prejudices be put aside (see Chapter 5). Holding grudges or rigid beliefs can prevent the

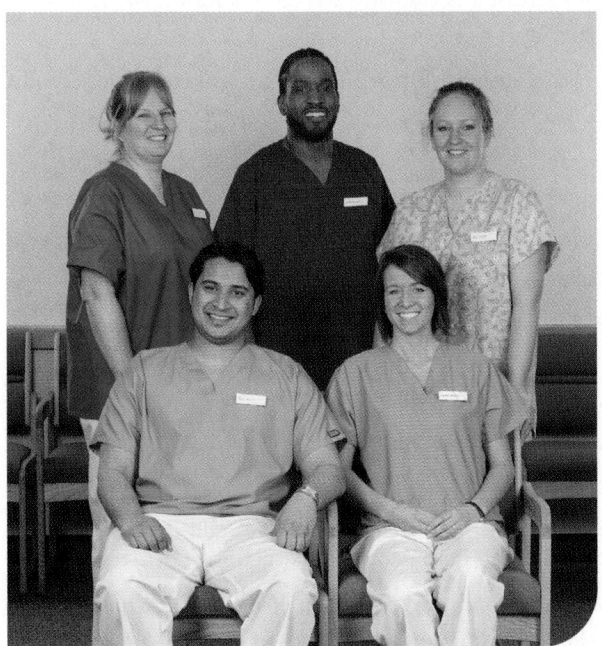

FIGURE 58-2 A diverse team of medical assistants.

team from functioning smoothly, to the detriment of both the patient and the office personnel. Professional medical assistants will work well with a diversity of colleagues and patients.

RESOLVING CONFLICTS

Every medical office will be the scene of some conflict. Conflicts may arise with patients or among team members. They can be as simple as a difference of opinion or as complex as an act of violence. The first step in resolving conflicts is to first seek to understand the situation. Perhaps there is more to the situation than is first noticed. If one person in the conflict is tired, sick, or frustrated, perhaps that is the root of the problem. The medical assistant should also be prepared to look inward. Perhaps something the assistant said or did, intentionally or unintentionally, contributed to the conflict. In that case, an apology can smooth the way to a solution.

It is an important soft skill to not escalate a conflict. If a patient, physician, manager, or peer seems to be getting angry, a wise medical assistant will not escalate the conflict but will seek to understand and solve the problem. Sometimes the solution is as easy as meeting the request of the person—scheduling a new appointment, saying you are sorry, or promising to get a message to the physician. Other times you may need to handle a situation by establishing and defining the problem ("I see you want to have this insurance issue resolved.") and promising to locate someone to help ("That is not something I am authorized to do, but I will get the reimbursement specialist for you.").

If two workers are in conflict, it may be wise to ask a manager to resolve the conflict. The manager should meet with both people separately, then together. It is best not to share the details of the conflict with colleagues, even though that is tempting, because the medical assistant may be perceived as asking colleagues to pick sides in the conflict. When a decision is made in the conflict, it is best to shake hands and agree to work together well in the future. No one wants to work in an office that is seething with hatred, so it is better for both parties to adopt a professional attitude.

Managing Priorities

One of the most challenging soft skills is the ability to manage priorities. Although the medical assistant may plan for the day to go a certain way, patient and workplace priorities may need to be assessed and changed frequently. Patient priorities may be managed by a combination of an efficient schedule and a triage system. However, even the most predictable schedule may need to be adjusted.

Since the medical assistant is very versatile, he or she may be asked to do multiple tasks in a short period of time. Although it is tempting to do several tasks at once, such as filing and talking on the phone, that is not efficient. Focusing on one task at a time will ensure thoroughness.

In the busy medical office, many tasks may have to be deferred to a later time. For example, if a patient calls to speak to the physician about lab results, the return call may have to be deferred until the lab results arrive and the physician is not seeing a patient.

An efficient tickler file system will greatly help the medical assistant. Using outboxes or neat piles to delineate whether a task should be done immediately, done when some other data arrive (such as the lab report), or done at a later time (such as a return call from the physician) can help immensely. Having a tidy workplace and disposing of clutter and trash will facilitate the efficiency of a tickler system.

If a medical assistant is distracted by family issues or other personal problems, it can be distracting and have a negative effect on job performance. For that reason it is wise not to have family and friends call the physician office except in an emergency. That way, the professionals can focus on their work throughout the day. Even text messages on cellular phones can distract the medical professional from the focus of the work. Therefore, those activities should not be done at the office.

When the physician is absent from the office and patients cannot be seen is an excellent time to catch up on lesser priorities that are nonetheless important. Such tasks as inventory or filing may be deferred because of patient care needs, but nonetheless they must be done. The wise medical assistant will efficiently prioritize the tasks needed in the office, so important work is being done even when the patients are not present.

STRESS MANAGEMENT

It is important to decrease stress in the medical office as much as possible. Sick patients can wear down the patience of the staff and leave the medical assistant feeling frustrated. It is important to realize that patients rarely intend to stress the medical assistant—but it is part of the job to deal with people under stress. Therefore, the employees at a medical office may also feel stressed.

One of the best ways to reduce stress in the medical office is to practice stress management. The following are some forms of stress management:

Aromatherapy—Therapy that utilizes pleasant smells such as lavender, have been shown to decrease stress.

Biofeedback—Therapy that utilizes biological information can relieve stress. Wearing biofeedback dots, rings, or patches shows the wearer if stress has constricted blood flow to that area. Knowing when you are stressed is the first step in changing the behaviors that lead to stress.

Deep breathing—Breathing deeply can relax your body, especially the heart and other muscles.

Distraction—Some people find that hobbies or vacations distract them from stress.

Exercise—Mild exercise has been shown to decrease stress in most individuals.

Guided imagery—Taking a few minutes to imagine being in some relaxing place can cause your body to relax in response to that stimulus.

Humor—Laughing at oneself or the bizarre predicaments of life can decrease stress.

Hypnosis—Learning to think more deeply without inhibitions can help people regain control of stress.

Meditation and prayer—Numerous studies have shown that focusing on reflection or prayer can relax the body.

Music—Listening to restful music that you enjoy has been shown to decrease stress.

Relaxation—Even in the office, a few minutes of concentrating on relaxing muscle groups (perhaps in the break room) can be rejuvenating.

Slow breath counting—Taking and counting slow breaths can distract and relax the brain.

Water therapy—Some people find a bath soothing and helps to relieve stress.

Stress can also be caused by pain. If stress results from pain, these techniques are recommended:

Heat—Applying heat to different parts of the body can distract the brain from pain. Many people enjoy a hot bath, for example.

Cold—Applying cold to different parts of the body can distract the brain from pain. Applying a cold pack to the head, for example, can ease a headache.

Pressure—Applying pressure to certain pressure points can reduce pain. Headache pain, for example, can be reduced by massaging the temples.

Usually stress management can only be used for a few minutes at the office, but the medical assistant should plan activities during free time to decrease stress. Sometimes talking to other health professionals about the stress can help the medical assistant to find new ways to reduce stress.

TIME MANAGEMENT

One of the greatest attributes of an effective office manager or medical assistant is the ability to effectively manage time. If the manager is organized, the office is usually organized. Time management requires the ability to prioritize what the important tasks are and to complete them on schedule. This is quite different from doing every task as it comes along. The office manager generally has little control over the tasks presented. The control is in how the tasks are handled and delegated.

One of the main responsibilities of the office manager or medical assistant is to manage all the peripheral office functions so that the physician is free to concentrate on practicing medicine. Tasks such as opening the daily mail, restocking the medical bag, searching for the drug sample to give to a patient, and dealing with pharmaceutical and other sales representatives are handled by the office manager or medical assistant. This can make it possible for the physician to set aside an hour each day to devote to administrative and patient-related tasks that only he or she can do.

Before establishing a time management system, it is important to define the office goals with the physician. Physicians' goals vary from complex to simple and from long term to short term. These goals may include collecting all payments at the time of service delivery, reorganizing or computerizing billing, limiting the practice, adding a partner or new service, writing a textbook, or choosing a benefits package for employees.

After the goals have been established, priorities can be set. The office manager or medical assistant can establish a priority list of the goals. A priority list is a composite of all the tasks that need to be accomplished to actualize each goal. These can be placed on a To Do list as they come to the office manager's attention. Each item is assigned a priority designation of 1, 2, or 3 depending on how critical the item is to completing the task. For example, ordering supplies that are running out is given a number 1, whereas rearranging a linen cupboard or a file drawer might be assigned a 3. Number 1 priority items must be done first and number 3 last. It is often tempting to do the easier tasks first since they take less time and show an immediate accomplishment. Good use of time management would determine that the inventory order should be placed immediately, and the number 3 priority items could be delegated to someone else or completed later, if necessary. It is a good idea to date a To Do list and to cross off items as they are accomplished. Table 58-1 shows an example of a To Do list.

TABLE 58-1 To Do List

Priority	To Do
2	Order paper supplies.
1	Arrange Dr. Christianson's air transportation to medical convention next month.
2	Prepare performance appraisal for Emily Jane Doro.
3	Reorganize storeroom.
1	Type convention speech.
1	Place ad for medical assistant.
3	Ask Ruth to remove old magazines from reception area.
1	Call for Pap test report on Mrs. Glidewell.
2	Block out schedule for next quarter.
3	Ask Belinda to take down Christmas decorations.
1	Prepare agenda for Thursday's staff meeting.

Persistence

One of the most valuable soft skills is persistence. **Persistence** is the quality of being able to stay on task longer than the usual time when necessary, even after others might have given up. Take, for example, the insurance billing process. If a medical assistant sends in an insurance claim and it is denied, persistence in refiling the claim may help the claim to get paid. This effort will be greatly appreciated by the physician and the patient because lack of persistence may cause the patient to have to pay or the physician to have to write the fee off as a loss. When frustrated it may seem easier to give up on a problem than to seek alternative solutions, but the professional medical assistant will creatively think of an alternative approach to the problem and will persist with trying to find a solution.

Professional Image

Although there may have been a relaxed dress code at college, the medical assistant should always project a professional image at work. Sometimes the office policies and procedures manual will be very specific about how the assistant should dress and accessorize, but at other times that will be left to the assistant's discretion. Even though coworkers may dress casually, it is important for the medical assistant to project the best professional image. This means to always wear clean, pressed clothing that does not reveal breasts, waist, tattoos, or underwear. If the medical assistant already has a tattoo, it should be covered when the assistant is at the medical office. Nails should be cut short. Artificial nails can harbor microbes and are inappropriate for most medical assistants. Jewelry also can provide a shelter for microbes and also should be avoided. Hair should be controlled so that it does not fall on the patient or a sterile field. The medical assistant should practice excellent hygiene and avoid perfumes or strong deodorants. Many patients find body piercings, especially those not in the ears, to be offensive. The medical assistant should check on the office policy about piercings and jewelry. Shoes should have closed toes and should be clean. Socks should be worn with shoes. It is also very important that the medical assistant wears a name tag that includes name and title. Name tags inform the patient that the medical assistant is a medical assistant and not a nurse or physician.

Lifelong Learning

Learning is not over upon completing school. Because the field of medicine changes daily, the medical assistant must stay current in professional knowledge. **Lifelong learning** is the process of continuing to learn throughout one's life. The medical assistant may go back to school for a higher degree in medical office management or allied health education, for example. However, even if the assistant does not return to formal schooling, continuing education may be earned through conferences, workshops, training in the office, or online courses.

Even if the medical assistant does not take advantage of these opportunities, the Internet provides a rich library of information. Reading professional journals can also contribute to increasing knowledge. The practice's OSHA officer is usually a good source of information about safety and risk management. Lifelong learning in medicine is a daily event.

SUMMARY

Soft skills, combined with cognitive and psychomotor skills, are vitally important in the medical office. The medical assistant functions within a system, an organized hierarchy of professionals with established policies and procedures. It is important for the medical assistant to communicate well with the patients, physicians, and coworkers. Good communication involves active listening, seeking first to understand, then speaking to be understood, and effective writing. Critical thinking involves discerning fact from opinion and making good value judgments. Teamwork is vitally necessary in the medical office where diverse clients, coworkers, and needs may create conflicts. Medical assistants must prioritize tasks and manage time well.

Stress management for patients, employees, and the medical assistant is also important. Medical careers create stress in the practitioners, so it is important to know how to reduce stress. Time management is critical for the office to operate well. Urgent tasks are not necessarily important tasks. A To Do List can help the medical assistant to list and prioritize tasks.

Persistence also is important in the medical office. The medical assistant may need to focus on a task several times to be thorough. Lifelong learning is the responsibility of the medical assistant, as new breakthroughs and treatments are being developed in medicine perpetually.

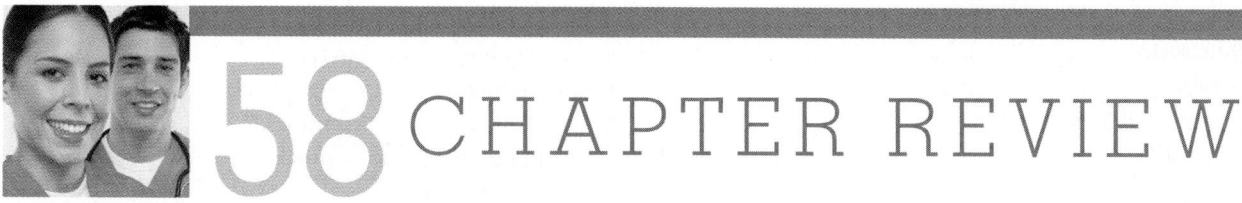

58 CHAPTER REVIEW

COMPETENCY REVIEW

1. Define and spell the terms to learn for this chapter.

2. Describe the system within a medical office.

3. What are the priorities in communication in the medical office?

4. Discuss how a medical assistant can differentiate between what a patient believes and what is measurable.

5. Why are medical offices in the United States composed of a diversity of personnel?

6. How can stereotyping and prejudice affect good patient care?

7. Describe how to resolve conflicts in the medical office.

8. How does a medical assistant determine the daily priorities for the office?

9. Describe a scenario in which persistence is important in the medical office.

10. List five ways for the medical assistant to pursue lifelong learning.

PREPARING FOR THE CERTIFICATION EXAM

1. Taking vital signs is an example of which kind of skill?
   a. critical thinking
   b. cognitive
   c. psychomotor
   d. affective
   e. soft

2. Which of the following is considered a soft skill?
   a. critical thinking
   b. memorizing medical terminology
   c. labeling an anatomical diagram
   d. creating an electrocardiogram
   e. keying patient data into a computer

3. Which of the following is NOT correct about medical assistants?
   a. They should seek first to understand.
   b. They should be able to resolve conflicts.

   c. They should be prejudiced against certain races.
   d. They should communicate effectively.
   e. They should work well with others.

4. A medical assistant continues to submit claims for reimbursement after the claim has been rejected multiple times. What ability does this demonstrate?
   a. cognitive skill
   b. psychomotor skill
   c. persistence
   d. diversity
   e. prioritization

5. If a physician is in surgery, which of the following would be the best priority for the medical assistant?
   a. Treat patients with minor problems in the reception area.
   b. Take inventory of drug samples.

c. Extend the medical assistant's lunch time.

d. Offer to help medical assistants in another office.

e. Return the medical assistant's personal phone calls.

6. Which of the following is NOT appropriate dress for the office?

a. name tag with "Medical Assistant" on it

b. white socks

c. sandals

d. short-sleeved V-neck scrubs

e. short nails

7. Which of the following is considered a source of microbes that could be a significant threat to the patient?

a. wearing the same shoes to work that the assistant wore home

b. having artificial nails

c. wearing a dosimeter badge on the lab coat

d. wearing eyeglasses

e. wearing perfume at work

8. Which of the following would be the first priority of the medical assistant?

a. returning a phone call to a patient wanting lab results

b. a patient calling for help in an examination room

c. a patient completing the registration process

d. obtaining a referral for a patient

e. resubmitting an unpaid insurance bill

9. Lifelong learning for the medical assistant is obtainable at all of the following EXCEPT

a. researching on the Internet

b. attending a professional organization's conference

c. attending local conferences

d. reading professional journals

e. all of the above

10. Which of the following are subjective, not objective?

a. BP 110/60

b. Electrocardiogram shows normal sinus rhythm.

c. Patient states "I feel like I am going to die."

d. Hemoglobin is 15.

e. Height is 44 inches.

CRITICAL THINKING

1. Explain why Susan's attitude toward David's work is detrimental to the office environment.

2. David overhears that Susan has been grumbling about his work performance. What is the best course of action for David to handle this situation?

3. If David is struggling with completing his work during the day, what are some things that could help him manage his time better?

ON THE JOB

Brody is a newly-certified medical assistant in his first job at a family practice office. He notices that the staff rarely wash their hands and sometimes they do not change gloves between patients. When he brings it to the attention of the office manager, she explains that hand hygiene takes so much time, that the office protocol is to wash hands only when patients are infectious. She also explains that using gloves too much will corrode the skin, so Brody should only use them when he is sure that blood is infectious.

1. Should Brody insist on wearing gloves and performing hand hygiene?

2. Where can he go for information on infection control?

3. If he is unable to persuade the office manager to change her protocol, to whom should he report this problem?

INTERNET ACTIVITY

Do an Internet search on professional organizations. Find what professional skills are necessary for the health care professional.

MEDMEDIA

Additional interactive resources and activities for this chapter can be found:

On your student DVD: View applicable procedure videos on the DVD-ROM found in the back of this book.

MyHealthProfessionsKit.com: Test your knowledge of this chapter with games and activities. MyHealthProfessionsKit also includes resources, helpful links, and a Spanish audio glossary.

Medical Assisting Interactive: Practice your procedures as a medical assistant in this simulated doctor's office. This can be accessed through MyHealthProfessionsKit.com.

59

Externship and Career Opportunities

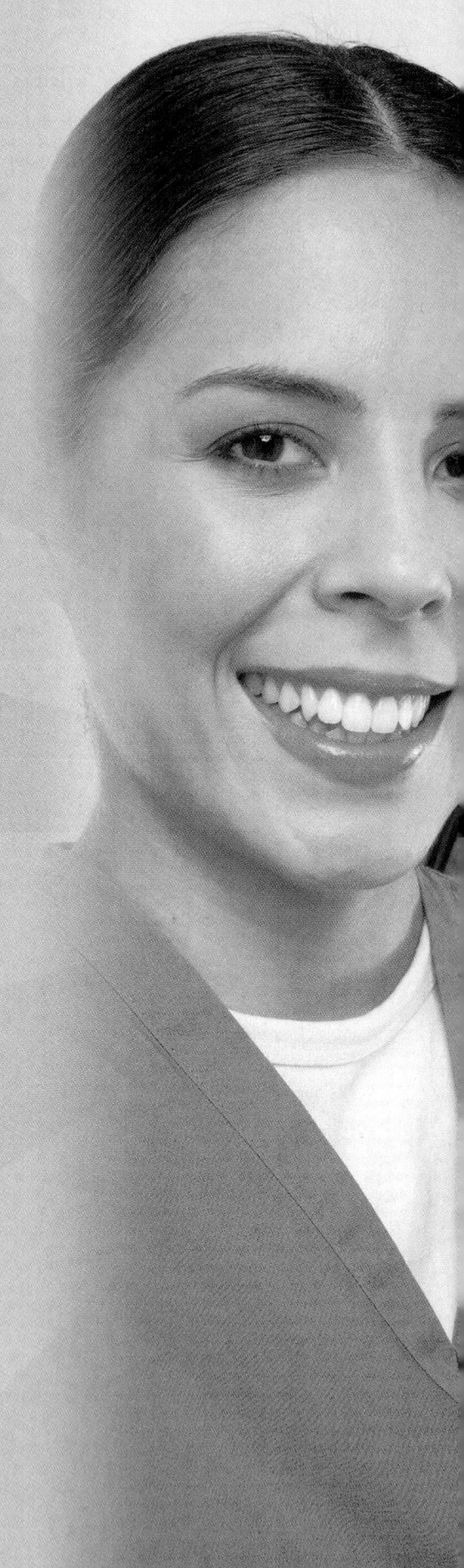

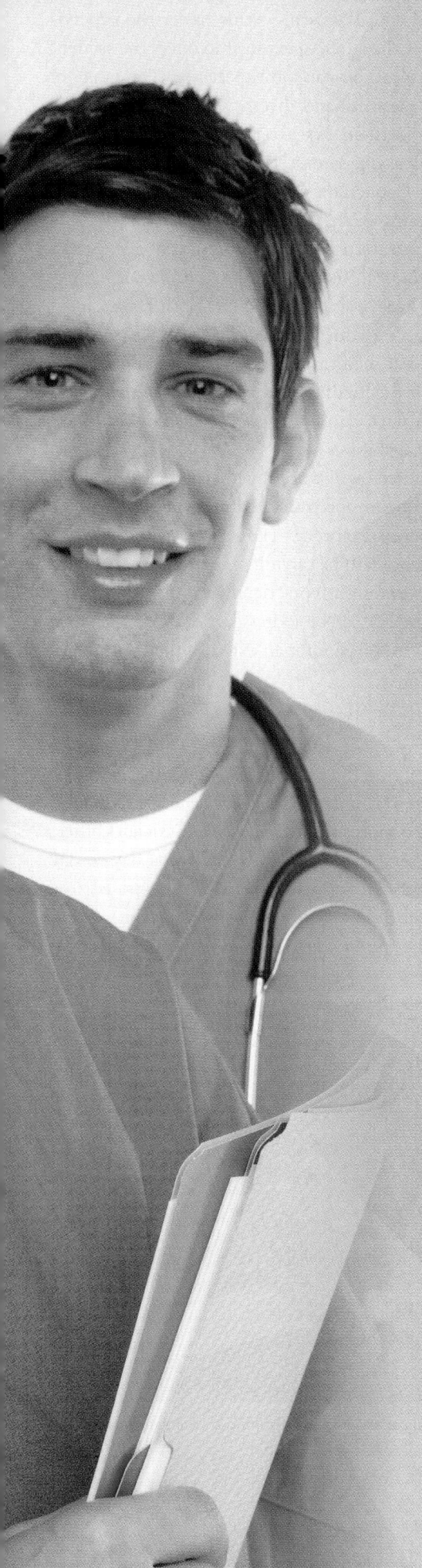

CHAPTER OUTLINE

CASE STUDY

Kenneth Helminski will be graduating from a medical assistant program at a local career school in 2 weeks. He is very eager to be working as a medical assistant and has been sending out many résumés in response to ads that have been posted on the Internet as well as the newspaper. Today, Kenneth has an appointment with Tania, the medical office manager at Pearson Physicians Group.

All indications are that job opportunities for medical assistants are expanding at a rapid rate. The U.S. Department of Labor has projected medical assisting to be one of the fastest-growing occupations. This demand for health personnel means that a well-prepared medical assistant will have a secure future.

One of the best means to facilitate the transition between the classroom and the medical setting is through the externship experience. This experience can be a time of great challenge and learning since the student is able to gain experience while under supervision. To receive the most benefit from the experience, careful preparation must take place. The externship experience is also one of the most exciting components of a medical assisting program.

As the student's formal educational experience in school draws to a close, he or she will prepare for the certification examination offered by the American Association of Medical Assistants (AAMA) or American Medical Technologists (AMT). Most hiring physicians look for this certification. This credential, along with graduation from an accredited program, indicates that entry-level skills have been accomplished.

During this final stage of training, the student will also begin the search for employment. This chapter focuses on skills that are useful to both the externship and job searching.

What Is an Externship or Practicum?

An **externship** refers to a situation in which one leaves the confines of the classroom and works, without payment, in a physician's office, hospital, or other health care setting using newly acquired medical assisting skills under the supervision of someone at the site. An externship offers the student an opportunity to get on-the-job experience. The range of externships is as plentiful and diverse as the medical facilities particpating in them. An externship can be as short as 4 weeks or as long as one semester of school. Schools that are accredited by the Council on Accreditation of Allied Health Education Programs (CAAHEP) in conjunction with the AAMA require an externship of a minimum of 160 hours. The American Medical Technologists require a similar experience that is known as a **practicum**. Both professional organizations expect graduates to have had actual mentoring experiences in a real medical office in order to be certified. The externship or practicum experience should provide the medical assistant with ample experience in both administrative and clinical skills.

Your school and you will work together to select the right externship or practicum for you based on your skills, needs, and place of residency (Figure 59-1). Ideally, the practicum or externship experience will be carefully monitored by the clinical instructor or externship/practicum coordinator so that problems that may arise can be addressed. See Box 59-1 for information on how to prepare for an externship or practicum.

THE EXTERNSHIP/PRACTICUM EXPERIENCE

Students generally find the externship/practicum experience to be the most rewarding part of their school experience. You will have the opportunity to see how a physician's office, ambulatory care setting, or clinic operates on a day-to-day basis (Figure 59-2). In addition, you will be exposed to a variety of different personalities in the work setting. Other advantages of the externship include gaining additional

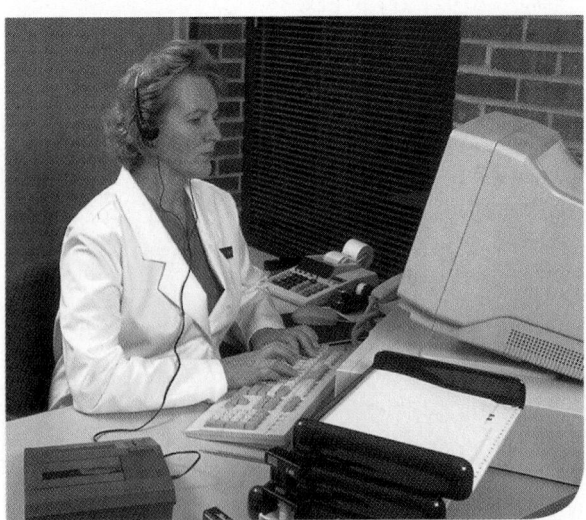

FIGURE 59-1 Medical assistant performing transcription work.

Box 59-1 Preparing for Externship or PRACTICUM

Physicians expect all of their medical assisting externs to have outstanding clinical and administrative skills. However, the physicians and their staff realize that you are inexperienced, and they generally are patient while you are learning. The one area in which physicians and office managers are extremely critical is regarding punctuality. If you are even a minute late for an interview, starting the day, or returning from a break, it will not be overlooked. Because many externships/practicums eventually result in full-time jobs, it is important to establish an unbroken rule that you will NEVER be late. The night before starting at your externship site, you should double-check the setting on your alarm clock. Make sure you get up early enough to eat a good breakfast. The day before your interview, prepare all the paperwork you will need to take with you. Do not forget to make sure that your uniform is pressed.

experience using your skills, such as phlebotomy, taking ECGs and vital signs, conducting urinalysis and hematology testing, using the computer, interviewing patients, performing billing and insurance procedures, and scheduling patients. You will gain experience in budgeting your time and balancing your workday, school day, and home life.

Your performance and behavior will be carefully observed by your supervisor at the externship site. Some of the areas that will be evaluated are these:

- Administrative and clinical skills and techniques
- Caring attitude
- Empathy for patients
- Enthusiasm
- Ethical standards
- Grooming and dress
- Initiative
- Integrity
- Interpersonal skills with patients and coworkers

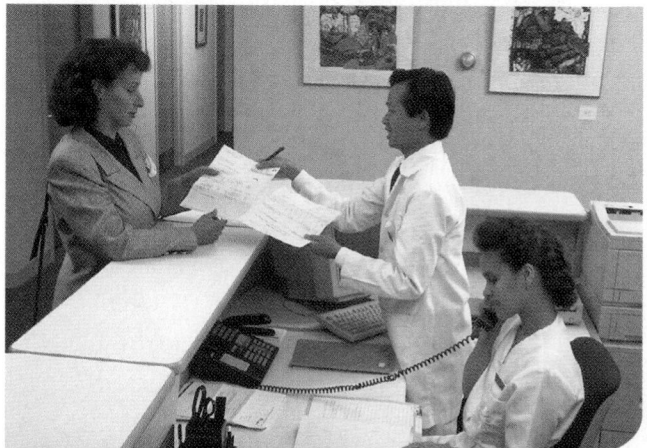

FIGURE 59-2 Medical assistant working in a front office area of a medical office.

- Language skills
- Poise under pressure
- Professionalism
- Punctuality and dependability

Student Responsibilities

The student has an overall responsibility to prepare well in advance of the interview for the externship. This preparation includes a review of skills, updating the résumé, and planning on how to project a professional appearance.

Each externship or practicum site is somewhat unique and may have additional requirements. The externship may require the medical assistant to carry malpractice insurance. Documentation of a recent physical exam and immunizations including hepatitis and tetanus may also be required. A tuberculosis (TB) test is required if you are working near patients. Because some of the immunizations, particularly hepatitis, require several months to complete, it is wise to begin this process 8 to 9 months before your expected practicum or externship. It is the student's responsibility to make sure that necessary physical examinations, paperwork, and immunizations are completed on a timely basis.

You are being given a great responsibility and opportunity by being allowed to gain experience at the externship site. The physician or facility providing an externship or practicum expects candidates to be extremely cautious regarding ethical and legal concerns. Errors can result in malpractice claims against the physician with whom you are working. If an error occurs, it should be reported immediately to the supervisor without alarming the patient. When errors are handled immediately, in many cases they can be corrected. If you cover up an error or mistake, it could result in immediate dismissal. Regular interviews with the office manager provide opportunities for the medical assistant

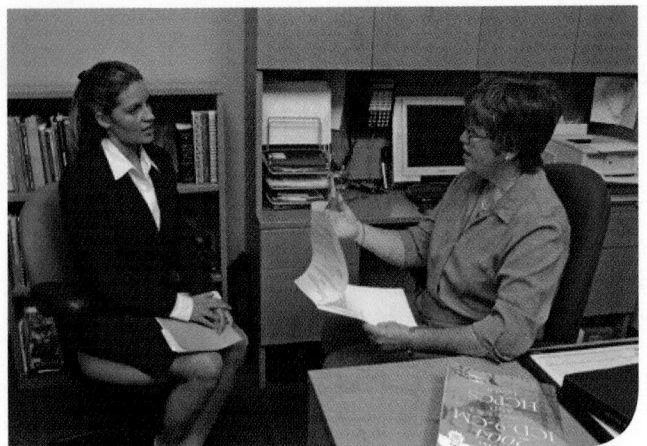

FIGURE 59-3 Medical assistant during an interview with the office manager.

extern to discuss issues that may need clarification (Figure 59-3).

Issues of confidentiality and patient privacy are of great concern to the physician and staff in all facilities. Discussion of information regarding any patient or the physician's practice with anyone outside of a facility is never allowed.

You will receive supervision from your on-the-job supervisor and your practicum or externship coordinator. Be sure to ask questions. The practicum or externship experience is meant to be a learning experience. If you find that you are not receiving the experience you require, bring this to the attention of your clinical supervisor.

Many students are able to take advantage of excellent externship or practicum opportunities simply because of a previous student's good performance in that practicum or externship. Remember, the behavior and work performance of the medical assistant during the practicum or externship is a direct reflection on the school that prepared him or her.

FINDING THE RIGHT SITE

Most schools have an externship coordinator who screens and selects health care sites that are appropriate for training. The screening process requires the coordinator to conduct an interview with the physician or office manager at the site to ensure that the student will benefit from appropriate experiences and receive supervision on site. Often the school has an affiliation agreement with the externship site that is kept on file at the school. Ideally, the externship or practicum site will have a former graduate of your program in their employ who can identify what skills and situations are needed.

Generally, it is not a good idea for students to select practicum or externship sites without the assistance from the school or the externship/practicum coordinator in particular. The school has the responsibility to require that the students are well supervised (Figure 59-4).

THE PRECEPTOR ROLE

The medical assistant at an externship or practicum site always works under the supervision of the physician. However, the physician may designate another member of the health care team as a supervisor for the student. This person performs in the role of a preceptor.

A **preceptor** provides additional instruction and guidance for a student by observing the performance of particular skills. The preceptor will also provide a formal written evaluation for the student, usually at the midpoint and final point. Table 59-1 lists several areas that are included on a typical evaluation form.

The preceptor looks for continual improvement in skills as the student gains confidence. The student should make every attempt to establish a rapport, or comfortable work relationship, with the preceptor.

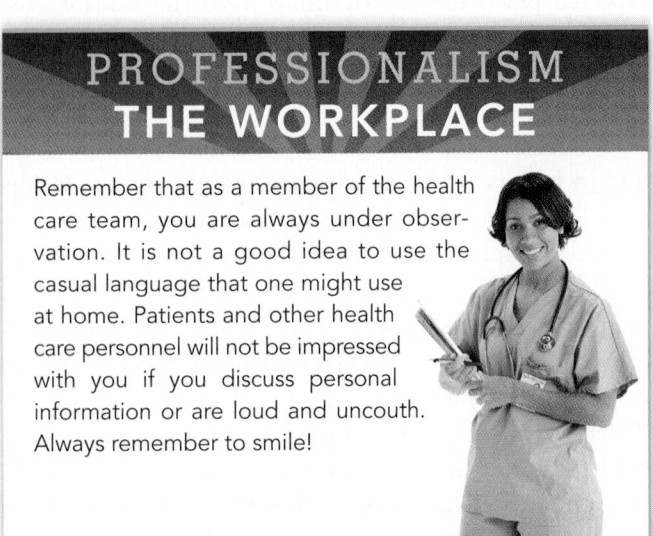

PROFESSIONALISM
THE WORKPLACE

Remember that as a member of the health care team, you are always under observation. It is not a good idea to use the casual language that one might use at home. Patients and other health care personnel will not be impressed with you if you discuss personal information or are loud and uncouth. Always remember to smile!

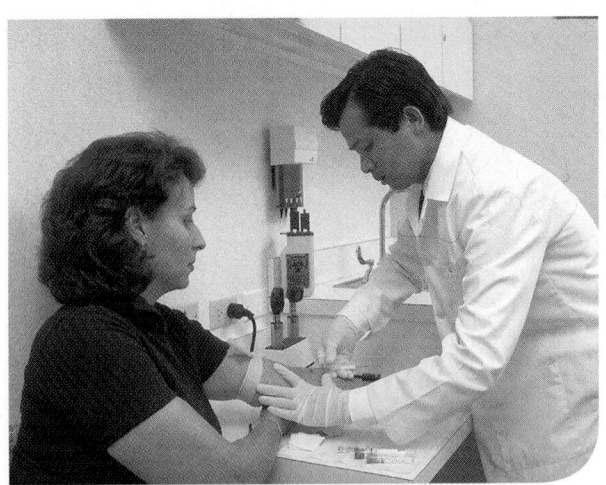

FIGURE 59-4 Drawing blood is one of the procedures the medical assistant may perform in the medical office.

TABLE 59-1 Sample Student Externship Form

Areas Evaluated	Ratings*				
Makes effective use of time	1	2	3	4	N/A
Able to work well with others	1	2	3	4	N/A
Accepts suggestions/criticisms willingly	1	2	3	4	N/A
Expresses concern for patients	1	2	3	4	N/A
Protects confidentiality of physician and patients	1	2	3	4	N/A
Always on time for work	1	2	3	4	N/A
Willingly works until the job is completed	1	2	3	4	N/A
Able to work independently	1	2	3	4	N/A
Demonstrates skill as appropriate	1	2	3	4	N/A
Does not perform skills beyond scope of training, education, and personal capability	1	2	3	4	N/A
Practices principles of aseptic technique	1	2	3	4	N/A
Projects a positive attitude	1	2	3	4	N/A
Recognizes emergencies	1	2	3	4	N/A
Dresses appropriately	1	2	3	4	N/A
Practices good hygiene	1	2	3	4	N/A

*Ratings: 1 = excellent, 2 = good, 3 = average, 4 = needs improvement, N/A = not applicable

EXTERNSHIP/PRACTICUM SITE EVALUATION

At the end of the practicum or externship experience, the student will be asked to provide an evaluation of the site. This evaluation may include the following types of questions:

- Was the overall externship experience positive or negative? Explain.

- Was the supervisor or preceptor approachable and available to answer questions?

- What, in your opinion, could be improved about this externship/practicum site and experience?

- Should this externship/practicum site be offered to other students?

Preparing for the Certification Examination

The **certification examination** to become a certified medical assistant is offered by the AAMA throughout the year. The examination is given at numerous computer centers throughout the United States. It is only available to medical assistants who have completed a CAAHEP-accredited program in medical assisting. The certified medical assistant (CMA [AAMA]) examination is a comprehensive test that includes questions relating to general transdisciplinary knowledge, administrative knowledge, and clinical knowledge. Table 59-2 describes the areas covered under each category.

TABLE 59-2 Major Areas Tested on the CMA (AAMA) Examination

Category	Topics Covered
General	Medical terminology Anatomy and physiology Behavioral science, psychology Medical law and ethics
Administrative	Oral and written communication Records management Insurance and coding Computers and office machines Bookkeeping, collections, credit
Clinical	Examination room techniques Laboratory procedures Pharmacology, medication administration Emergency procedures Specimen collection

The certification examination to become a registered medical assistant (RMA) is given as a computer-based test (CBT) or paper-and-pencil test at various times throughout the year. Eligibility to take this examination is based on completing either 5 years of work experience or a combined training and work program.

Preparation for a certification examination begins as soon as the student begins a training program. All the subject matter taught in a program is interrelated and forms the basis of the student's knowledge. All class notes and information acquired during the training program should be maintained in an organized fashion so that preparation for the examination can be efficient. A variety of examination preparation courses are offered. In addition, several excellent review books provide the student with sample test questions. These review books should be purchased and used well before the actual date of the examination. The study questions are generally related to the three major categories covered on the examination: general, administrative, and clinical. Students should time themselves while answering the sample test questions since the actual examination is timed. See Chapter 1 for a further discussion of the credentialing agencies.

The Job Search

Many offices that offer externship opportunities do not have a full-time position available. Do not think it is a reflection of your work if you are not offered a position at the end of your externship. If your externship experience did not lead to a permanent position, then you must begin the job search in earnest. In some cases, a facility will not want to hire you as a medical assistant until you become credentialed after taking the required examination. However, some facilities will interview you for a permanent position with the understanding that you must pass the certification exam.

Any job search should begin with careful planning. You must prepare a list of information sources for identifying job opportunities, update your résumé, rehearse interviewing, and plan your professional attire for the interview process. Six behaviors are cited as the most common job search mistakes:

1. Having no clear plan
2. Failing to inform others of your job search
3. Spending too much time answering classified ads
4. Looking for the perfect job
5. Limiting yourself to one field
6. Giving up the search too soon

There are several areas to pursue in your search for job opportunities, some of which are listed in Table 59-3.

PERSONAL ASSESSMENT

Before moving ahead with your job search, it is a good idea to perform a **personal assessment** or evaluation of your own strengths and weaknesses. Although it is not a good

TABLE 59-3 Sources for Job Opportunities

Classified ads	Use local and out-of-town newspapers, professional journals, and trade magazines. Use the local public library's access to national newspapers.
Employment agencies	Place your name with the agency and career consultants.
Health care facilities in your area	Contact hospitals, veteran's facilities, extended care facilities, and ambulatory care sites.
Internet	Use various websites such as monster.com, careerbuilder.com, or jobs.com.
Local medical society	Obtain a list of physicians who are looking for help or a list of all the medical practice offices in your area.
Parents, friends	Network with your own friends and relatives. Make sure they know you are looking for employment.
Personal physician	Your own physician may network for you and call his or her colleagues.
Professional organizations	Use both state and local chapters of any professional associations and allied health groups to which you belong.
Publications	American Association of Medical Assistants and other local professional publications.
School placement service	One of the best sources since the staff know your training and skills well. In many cases prospective employers will call schools to identify potential new employees.
State employment office	After completing the required application forms, your name will be on file for available positions.

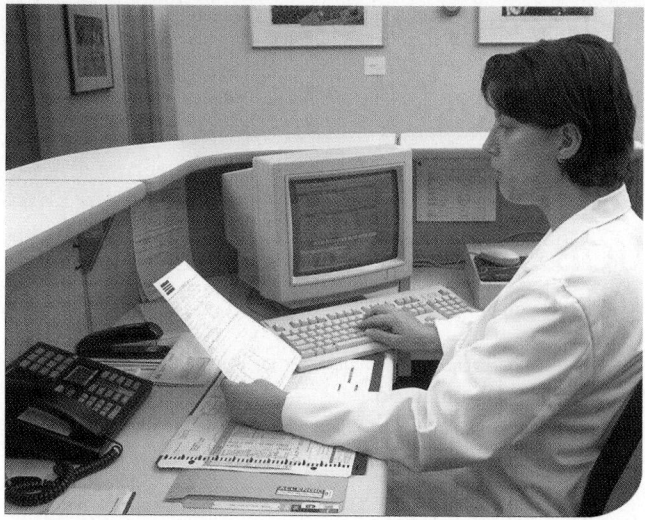

FIGURE 59-5 Medical assistants who perform billing must know and use the proper codes to ensure third-party payments are made correctly by insurance companies.

idea to point out any weaknesses to potential employers, you must be cautious to avoid taking on tasks for which you are not qualified. Employers often ask about weaknesses. State one and indicate what you are doing about it. This shows you are aware of limitations, and it lets the employer know you are serious about improving yourself. By performing a personal assessment, you can determine the fields in which you might enjoy working, which areas require more skill development, and for which positions you are qualified (Figure 59-5).

Ask your instructors for guidance and observations on your appearance, attitude, and skills. You can also ask peers whose opinions you trust and who have been in several classes with you. Although it is never easy to accept criticism, a well-intentioned comment from someone you know about the need to clean your uniforms, eliminate jewelry, change to a more professional hairstyle, or brush up on particular skills may help you obtain the job you are seeking.

You may wish to practice your interview skills with your instructors or in front of a mirror. A good idea is to videotape a practice interview with a friend or instructor and see how you look to others. Use every opportunity to speak up in class to further develop your communication skills. Work on smiling at every opportunity.

CONDUCTING A JOB SEARCH

After planning and performing a self-assessment, it is time to gather the equipment and supplies that will help you to be successful at your job search. At home, at the school you are attending, or at most local libraries you can access a computer and printer to develop and print your cover

letter, résumé, and follow-up letter. If you have computer access to the Internet, you can look on various websites for jobs that have been posted. Searching the Internet has become a very popular way to look for a job. There is no more waiting for a workplace human resource department to open or getting there before it closes. You are able to access the workplace website at your convenience to search for job information.

Many Internet websites can help you with your job search. These websites may focus on résumé writing, job applications, interviewing, job postings, and more. Once you are at one of these websites, you will be able to search for a job by category, keyword, city, state, and zip code. If you want to work for a particular medical office, use any Internet search engine, key in the name of the medical office, the city, and the state to see if the office has a website available. If you already know the website address for the medical office, key it in to the address bar of your Internet browser. Remember, not all medical offices have websites.

Your local or school library can provide classified ads, various publications, and newsletters to use as sources to find a job. If your school has a placement office, it is one of the best places to receive help with your job search. Most school placement offices have a job posting board and will review your résumé, conduct a mock interview, and help as well as encourage you to find a job.

Being organized is a must while searching for a job. A job search organizer or folder is a wonderful place to keep a copy of your cover letters, résumés, follow-up letters, and applications. It can also be used to keep business cards, job advertisements, your contact log, and phone numbers handy. Having all of this information in one place will help you stay organized and keep you focused during your job search. It will also prevent any of these items from getting lost or misplaced.

A contact log is a great reference for information about the offices or people you have contacted about a job search. Keep the names, addresses, telephone numbers,

procedure
59-1

CONDUCTING A JOB SEARCH
Objective: Conduct a job search.

EQUIPMENT AND SUPPLIES
computer; Internet access; newspaper; medical assisting publications; printer; pen; paper; dictionary; thesaurus; telephone; telephone book; job search organizer or folder; calendar; contact log

METHOD
1. Using Table 59-3, determine two sources you will use to conduct a job search.
2. Determine a plan for your job search.
3. Prepare a list of information sources for identifying job opportunities.
4. Update your résumé.
5. Rehearse interviewing with a close family member or friend.
6. Plan your professional attire for the interview process.
7. Perform a self-assessment.
8. Develop a job search organizer or folder.
9. Develop a contact log.
10. Use a calendar to determine what times are available for job searching and interviewing.
11. Select two sources you will use to conduct a job search.
12. Conduct your job searches.
13. Turn in all information gathered during your job search as well as a copy of your résumé and contact log to your instructor.

In your journal, document how you felt about the job search.

CHARTING EXAMPLE
When I went to the Quick Care office for an interview, everyone was very nice to me. I think I would get to use a variety of skills there. I will write a thank-you note tonight and send it to them tomorrow. I sure hope they hire me!

and e-mail addresses of the people you have contacted in your log.

During your job search you also will need access to a dictionary, thesaurus, calendar, and telephone. It is critical that your cover letters, résumés, follow-up letters, and applications be free of errors.

Whether using a wired or wireless phone to call prospective employers, call from a quiet place. If environmental noise is audible in the background when talking to a prospective employer, he or she will think your behavior is unprofessional and rude. It also will make it difficult for you to hear, and you may not be able to give the prospective employer your full attention. If you are unable to give the prospective employer your full attention, you may miss some critical information.

Before calling places that have job openings, you should review your calendar for available dates and times for an interview. This will prevent the prospective employer from waiting while you determine the date and time you can meet for an interview.

Searching for a job is not easy, but if you stay focused and organized, stick to your plan, and perform a self-assessment, you will eventually be successful in finding a job. See Procedure 59-1 for the steps in Conducting a Job Search.

The Résumé

The **résumé** is a summary of your credentials, including your employment history, experience, training, and education. For your first position the résumé is generally one page. Because you will create a first impression with your résumé, it should be carefully written. You may wish to ask your program's career office for guidance when putting together a résumé for the first time. It is also helpful to view examples of résumés on the Internet or in books at your school library or local library.

The most popular résumé format is to present information in chronological order. That is, the events are placed in the order of their occurrence. In this format, your education, work experience, and achievements are listed in reverse chronological order (the most recent events are

```
                         Ralph Taylor
                       222 East Main Street
                       Chicago, IL 60601
                        (312) 555-1212
                         email address
                      taylorr@anywhere.com
```

OBJECTIVE	To obtain a medical assisting position where I am able to utilize my administrative and clinical skills.
EDUCATION	
Associate Degree	Central State College, Hometown, Illinois. Expected date of graduation: June 20XX. Major in Health Science.
Medical Assistant	Central State College, Hometown, Illinois. February 20XX June 20XX. Graduated with honors.
EMPLOYMENT	
Medical Assistant	Dr. Earl Brown, Internal Medicine Externship, 2222 State St., Chicago, IL. Externship duties included: drawing blood, handling medical records, scheduling patients, and patient education. 20XX–20XX.
Nursing Assistant	Jane Young, M.D. Family Practice, 111 Hoyne Ave., Chicago, IL. Duties included taking vital signs. EKGs, assisting with well-baby visits and in treatment room. 20XX – 20XX.
PROFESSIONAL ORGANIZATIONS AND MEMBERSHIP	
	American Association of Medical Assistants Central State College Medical Club
CREDENTIALS	
Medical Assistant	Passed certification examination in January 20XX.
CPR	Certified by American Heart Association, December 20XX.
REFERENCES	Furnished upon request.

FIGURE 59-6 An example of a résumé that uses a chronological format.

listed first). The chronological résumé format is illustrated in Figure 59-6.

Another résumé format is the educational skills résumé. This format is useful if you are just graduating from school and have not had extensive work experience. With this format you concentrate on administrative and clinical skills that have been learned while participating in a medical assisting program.

No matter which type of résumé you use, the medical office manager must be able to understand the information that has been provided. If the reader is unable to understand the information provided on the résumé, he or she will move on to other résumés that are available. Many medical office managers are very busy and only have a short time to glance over résumés. Make sure your résumé is noticed by providing concise information on it.

The résumé should be typed on good-quality $8\frac{1}{2} \times 11$, white or off-white paper. Do not use brightly colored paper. The résumé must be neatly typed and error free. Always use a word processor to prepare your résumé so that you can easily go back and make updates. Always have a backup copy of your résumé stored on a disk, USB drive, or other type of storage device. The spell-checker option on your word processor is not always correct, so also check your spelling using a dictionary.

Proofread your résumé to make sure it is error free in content and typing. Start by reading it on the computer screen. If and when you find errors, correct them and save the document. Next print your résumé and proofread it again. Mark any errors found on the printed copy of your résumé, and then make the changes on the computer and save the document. Now print your résumé again and give it to a close family member or friend to proofread. Correct any errors that are discovered. Once you have determined that your résumé is neat and error free, print at least ten copies of it so that you always have several copies available for distribution.

Spend time working on your résumé. Remember that the purpose of a résumé is to obtain an interview. Keep a personal portfolio in which you gather the names, addresses, and dates of attendance of schools and programs you have attended. Record association memberships and credentialing information, such as certification and registration numbers and expiration dates. This is particularly important if you have earned multiple credentials.

WHAT IS INCLUDED IN A RÉSUMÉ?

Résumés vary somewhat based on the personal preferences of the writers, but several items are standard. These include heading, objective, education, employment, professional organizations and memberships, credentials, and the fact that references are available upon request.

The information you include on your résumé should never be dishonest or misleading. Dishonest or misleading information can be uncovered during the interview or in discussions with personal references. How would you feel if you hired a medical assistant who exaggerated his or her experience on a résumé? Could you still trust this person? Would you still want to work with this person? Clearly it is critical for you to be honest when completing your résumé.

• **Heading**—Your name, address, and telephone number are prepared as a centered heading at the top of the page. If you have a cellular phone number and e-mail address, this information can also be included. When this information is printed in slightly larger type than the rest of the text, it stands out and provides an easy reference for the reader.

- **Objective**—Listing an objective lets the reader know what career goal you would like to achieve. When you write your objective it should be clear and to the point what you want in a career. Your objective may need to be changed depending on where you are sending your résumé.
- **Education**—If you are still a student or a recent graduate with limited work experience, list your education first in reverse chronological order with the most recent school/program listed first. Add any educational experiences you have had, such as workshops, seminars, or courses.
- **Employment**—Your work experience is then listed in the same reverse chronological order. Include externship or practicum experience with a brief description of your duties. Many prospective employers also wish to see part-time employment listed. This is especially necessary and even beneficial if you have other experience in the health care field.
- **Professional organizations and memberships**—Belonging to a professional organization can be a wonderful experience. It helps you to stay current on topics related to your career. Being a member and participating in an organization shows your dedication, commitment, and loyalty to your chosen career field. Many schools have organized a medical assisting club for students to participate in as they are being educated. For a yearly fee, students or graduates can also obtain membership through the AAMA or the American Medical Technologists.
- **Credentials**—Include information about your professional credentials, such as CMA (AAMA) certification or RMA registration. If you do not have any credentials, do not include this section on your résumé.
- **References (upon request)**—The reference section should never include the name, address, and phone number of the references you will be using. You need only to indicate that references are available on request.

When you are developing your résumé, there is some information that prospective employers do not need (or are legally not entitled) to know. Some of this information is very personal to you and does not reflect how you will perform your job duties. The following are some of the items not included on a résumé:

- Age
- General health
- Photograph
- Marital status
- Spouse and children's names

- Salary information
- Names, addresses, and phone numbers of references
- Reasons for leaving previous positions

As you obtain certification, change positions, or perform volunteer work, you will want to update your résumé so that it is always current. You never know when you might need a copy of your résumé to give to a prospective employer. If you continue to update your résumé as it changes, this will prevent you from forgetting information that should be included on it. See Procedure 59-2: Preparing Your Résumé and References.

Professional References

A **professional reference** is the statement of someone who has either worked with you or known you for a period of time. This person will be asked to attest to your skills, personal integrity, or value system. For example, he or she may be asked if you are an honest and sincere person. A prospective employer will call your references before hiring you to ask questions about your work and attendance record.

State at the bottom of your résumé that references will be furnished on request. On a separate piece of paper, prepare a list of at least three references with their addresses and telephone numbers. Names, addresses, and phone numbers of references are generally not included on the actual résumé.

You should obtain permission to use a person's name as a reference. It is wise to include names of professional as well as personal references. Your instructors, dean, and externship supervisor might serve as professional references. A personal reference might include a friend or someone from your place of worship. Parents and spouses do not generally serve as references. Of course, you would not include the name of anyone who may not provide you with an excellent reference.

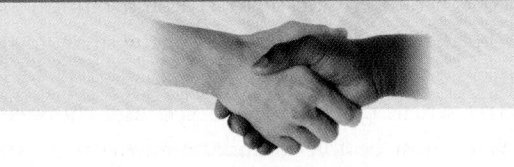

PROFESSIONALISM
CULTURAL CONSIDERATIONS

During your externship experience you will most likely encounter patients with cultural backgrounds different from yours. Most communities are home to residents from various cultures. Learn as much as you can about the cultures in your community. It is very important to include on your résumé any foreign languages that you speak, particularly those that you speak fluently. This is often a tremendous benefit to prospective employers, especially if you are fluent in a foreign language common to your area.

procedure
59-2

PREPARING YOUR RÉSUMÉ AND REFERENCES
Objective: Prepare a résumé and references.

EQUIPMENT AND SUPPLIES
computer; printer; pen; paper; dictionary; thesaurus; telephone book; current and past employment information; current and past educational information

METHOD
1. Gather equipment and supplies.
2. Using Figure 59-6 as an example, prepare your résumé.
3. Using a word processing program, complete the standard parts of a résumé: heading, objective, education, employment, professional organizations and memberships, credentials, and references.
4. Proofread your résumé.
5. Have a close family member or friend proofread your résumé.
6. Make any corrections to errors found on the résumé.
7. Using good-quality white or off-white $8\frac{1}{2} \times 11$ paper, print your résumé.
8. On a separate piece of paper list at least three references with their addresses and phone numbers.
9. Proofread your references.
10. Have a close family member or friend proofread your references.
11. Make any corrections to errors found on your references.
12. Using good-quality white or off-white $8\frac{1}{2} \times 11$ paper, print your references.
13. Save your résumé and list of references on a disk, USB drive, computer hard drive, or other storage device.
14. Update your résumé whenever changes occur.
15. Turn in your résumé and references to your instructor.

The Cover Letter

What is the cover letter? A **cover letter** is intended to introduce you and your résumé to the recipient—the person to whom you send your letter. The cover letter should clearly state the purpose of your correspondence. Because health care institutions may be advertising several positions at the same time, you must state clearly the position that interests you.

The cover letter should be brief. It is not a restatement of everything that is in your résumé. Explain what you can do for the employer and why your qualifications are a good match for the job requirements. Be sure to include an address and telephone number where you can be contacted. Do not add handwritten comments or additional information to your cover letter. Always update or revise information on your résumé and cover letter with a word processor and save the updated file.

Always review the spelling of the employer's name, address, and phone number carefully for accuracy. A potential employer may judge you by your proofreading skills.

If you have word processing capability, you may wish to draft several sample cover letters that you can then access from your computer and add the appropriate heading. For instance, different sample cover letters could be drafted to respond to "blind" ads, classified ads, and unsolicited interview requests at local medical facilities. A **blind ad** does not identify the institution or facility that placed the ad. Unsolicited interview requests are requests for interviews initiated by the candidate or prospective employee, not the institution or facility or individual representing the facility. The following are some of the most common mistakes to avoid when writing a cover letter:

- Not addressing the letter to a specific person in the organization. Be sure to check for name, title, and correct spelling.

- Failing to clearly state the position for which you are applying.

- Sending a cover letter that is too long. One page works best.

- Sending a letter that is poorly worded or has spelling or typing errors. Always send the original cover letter, never a copy.

Ralph Taylor
222 East Main St.
Chicago, IL 60601
(312) 555-1212

May 20, 20XX

James Stark, M.D.
1450 N. Devonshire
Chicago, IL 60611

Dear Dr. Stark:

This letter is in response to your recent advertisement in the May 19, 20XX, <u>Chicago Sun News</u> for a certified medical assistant.

I believe that my qualifications are a good match for your position. During my medical assisting program at Central State College in Hometown, Illinois, I maintained a 3.6 GPA on a 4.0 scale.

My medical assisting program at Central State College was completed in December 20XX. I passed the American Association of Medical Assistants' certification examination January 27, 20XX. Currently I am completing an associate degree program at CSC and plan to graduate in June 20XX.

The enclosed résumé includes my experience as a part-time nursing assistant for Dr. Jane Young in her family practice office.

I look forward to meeting you to discuss your position needs and my qualifications.

Thank you for your consideration.

Sincerely,

Ralph Taylor

Ralph Taylor, CMA (AAMA)

FIGURE 59-7 An example of a cover letter sent in response to a classified ad.

An example of a sample cover letter written in response to a classified ad is illustrated in Figure 59-7. Also see Procedure 59-3: Preparing a Cover Letter.

The Interview

Your library will have reference material on what to expect during the interview process. All interviewers have standard questions, which may include "Tell me why you went into medical assisting?" or "Why do you want to work here?" You should practice responses to these questions before you go to the interview (Figure 59-8).

Another resource for obtaining information about the interview process is the Internet. If you type the word *interviewing* into an Internet search engine, you will find numerous websites that contain information about interviewing topics, such as preparation, questions asked, questions for you to ask, practice interviews, tips, and much more. The information from some of the websites you visit will provide a wealth of knowledge that will help you be successful during the interview process.

Many schools have a placement office or career services office to assist you as you are attending school, after you graduate, or both.

procedure 59-3

PREPARING A COVER LETTER
Objective: Prepare a cover letter.

EQUIPMENT AND SUPPLIES
computer; printer; pen; paper; dictionary; thesaurus; telephone book

METHOD
1. Gather equipment and supplies.
2. Using Figure 59-7 as an example, prepare a cover letter using a word processing program.
3. Proofread your cover letter.
4. Have a close family member or friend proofread your cover letter.
5. Make any corrections to errors found on the cover letter.
6. Using good-quality, white or off-white $8\frac{1}{2} \times 11$ paper, print your cover letter.
7. Turn your cover letter in to your instructor.

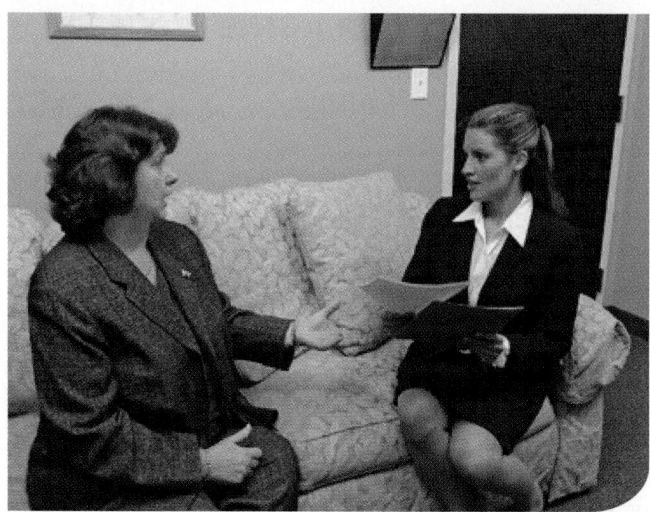

FIGURE 59-8 The job interview.

It is important for you to get to know the staff and to understand the services available. Getting to know the staff will help you become more comfortable when you are seeking assistance from them.

Many placement offices offer these services:

- Help you develop a cover letter, résumé, and follow-up letter

- Review your cover letter, résumé, and follow-up letter

- Conduct a mock interview

- Provide you with current job listings

- Provide career counseling

- Help you with your job search

- Host job fairs for you to attend on campus

- Conduct workshops and seminars about interviewing, cover letters, résumés, and follow-up letters

PREPARING FOR TOUGH INTERVIEW QUESTIONS

In addition to the standard questions, some difficult questions may be asked, such as "We all have our strengths and weaknesses. What is one of your weaknesses?" It is always a good idea to highlight your strengths. Therefore, to answer a tough question, select a strength. For instance, you might make the following response to the question about your weakness: "I am a perfectionist and may sometimes hold myself to a very high standard that is almost unobtainable" or "I care very deeply about people and must work to empathize with them rather than sympathize."

The interviewer may ask you questions regarding any gaps in the chronology on your résumé. Answer all questions honestly, using simple statements such as "I did not work during that year because I was caring for an elderly relative" or "It has been six months since I finished school. I did not seek employment because I was studying for the CMA (AAMA) examination." It is not necessary to provide lengthy explanations for termination from a position. Be especially careful not to criticize the institution or individual who terminated you.

Some of the questions that could be asked during an interview include the following:

- What is one of your strengths?

- What is one of your weaknesses?

- What has been your favorite job? Why?

- What goal or goals do you want to accomplish in the next year?

- What goals do you want to accomplish in the next 5 years?

- Why would you want to work for this medical office?

- Tell me why I should hire you?

- How do you qualify for this position?

- What has been one of your best accomplishments?

- How did you handle a difficult situation at one of your past jobs?

Be prepared to answer the difficult questions with great poise and professionalism. You will have only about 20 minutes to convince your potential employer that you should be the applicant hired. Be absolutely honest about your achievements. However, do not be afraid to talk positively about yourself. There is no one else present at the interview who knows you as well as you know yourself. Guidelines 59-1 lists some guidelines for successful interviewing.

Be prepared with questions to ask the interviewer about the medical office, the position, and the staff. The answers will give you a clearer understanding of the place of employment and will help you decide if you want to be employed there.

The following are some questions you might want to ask the interviewer:

- Why is this position open?

- How many patients are seen in the office per day?

- What are the working hours for this position?

- How long is the probationary period?

- When are evaluations conducted?

GUIDELINES 59-1

SUCCESSFUL INTERVIEWING

1. Learn all you can about the organization. Interviewers are impressed by candidates who indicate knowledge of the facility or organization.
2. Have a specific job in mind when you interview so that you project self-assurance.
3. Know your qualifications for each specific job and task requirement. Rehearse or review possible responses several times before going to the interview. You can role-play with a friend or relative to build your confidence.
4. Prepare responses to the interviewer asking you difficult questions or asking you to describe yourself.
5. Be prepared to discuss where you want to be professionally in 5 years.
6. Carry extra copies of your résumé.
7. Arrive 5 to 10 minutes before your scheduled appointment. You may wish to wait outside the facility if you arrive too early.
8. Dress conservatively to project a well-groomed professional appearance. Generally, a uniform is not required for an interview.
9. Never ask for permission to smoke during an interview. Do not eat anything during an interview unless the interview takes place during a meal. Chewing gum is never acceptable during the interview.
10. Be alert and prompt in giving answers to the interviewer's questions. Do not offer information that is not requested. Keep answers concise.
11. Ask questions about the position and the organization. It is generally not a good idea to inquire about benefits on the first interview.
12. Bring a pen, your Social Security number, driver's license number, extra résumés, and the names of three references with their addresses and telephone numbers.

- How long is the orientation or training period?
- Why do you enjoy working here?

To get a clearer understanding of the medical office, ask for a copy of the job description for the position. If the interviewer has not already given you a tour, ask to meet the rest of the staff and tour the medical office. This will help you decide if you would fit in with the other staff at the medical office.

PROFESSIONALISM AT THE INTERVIEW

The day of the interview you will be judged immediately by your appearance. You should present a conservative, well-groomed professional appearance. Wear little or no jewelry and avoid showy hairstyles, heavy perfume, bright nail polish, and bright clothing. Of course, this is the same appearance that you will want to present on the job.

Women should wear a suit or dress. Men should wear a suit, a plain shirt, and tie. The colors of the attire you wear during the interview should never stand out or be bright. Your attire should be dark blue or black. Your attire should never have any bizarre patterns, designs, or textures. Low-cut shirts and tight-fitting garments are unacceptable and unprofessional for a job interview.

Before you leave for the interview, look at yourself in the mirror. Is the garment you are wearing wrinkled? If so, press it. Never go to an interview with your garment wrinkled. Make sure there is no lint on your garment. Make sure your shoes are clean and polished. Now ask yourself "Would I want to hire that person in the mirror?" If you are still in a medical assisting program, you may wish to wear a clean pressed uniform with your school insignia.

No one should accompany you to an interview. Introduce yourself to the receptionist and wait quietly in the reception room until you are called for the interview. Be very courteous to all office staff. Many physicians will have their entire office team assist in selecting new employees.

Greet the person interviewing you with a firm handshake. Now is an excellent time to give the interviewer a copy of your résumé and reference list. Even if the interviewer already has a copy of your résumé, it is acceptable to give him or her another copy. Interviewers will generally take a few minutes to ask casual questions that will allow you to relax. Be prepared for questions such as "Tell me about yourself." Have good eye contact with the interviewer and answer all questions in a sincere and friendly manner. Never give answers to the interviewer that are misleading or dishonest.

Questions relating to age, ethnicity, place of birth, marital status, and number of children are prohibited by law. Most interviewers are aware of this law and will not ask these questions. You do not have to answer them if they are asked.

Salary and benefits are not generally discussed in the first interview. If you are called back for a second interview or offered a job, the topic of salary and benefits can be discussed at that time. Remember to be pleasant when the interview is

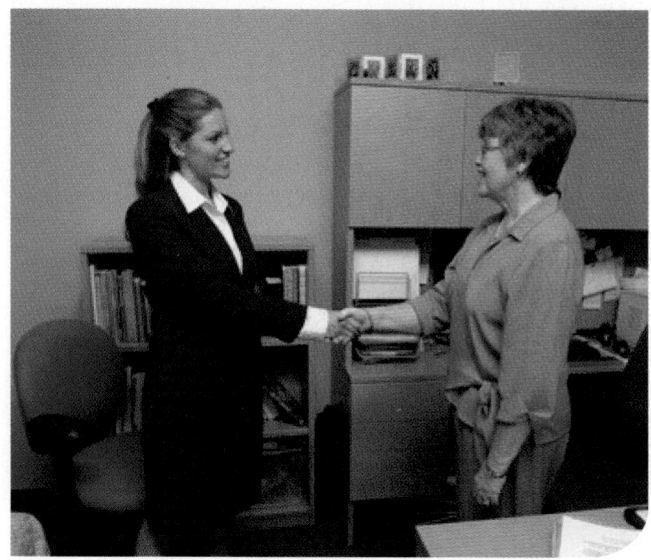

FIGURE 59-9 Medical assistant shaking hands with the interviewer at the close of the interview.

over. The interviewer will usually indicate the end of the interview by standing up and shaking your hand as you leave (Figure 59-9).

Every interview experience is an opportunity for personal growth. If you are not hired on the first or second interview, do not become discouraged. Reassess your interviewing skills. (See Procedure 59-4: Role-Playing an Interview.) Ask your instructor or friend to critique your skills to see how you might improve. Immediately send out more cover letters and résumés until you are hired. According to interviewers, the ten most common mistakes made in interviews are these:

1. Poor eye contact
2. Use of slang or improper grammar
3. Inappropriate dress or poor grooming
4. Lack of enthusiasm
5. Poor posture
6. Smoking or chewing gum
7. Talking too much or projecting an overconfident attitude
8. Arriving late

procedure 59-4

ROLE-PLAYING AN INTERVIEW

Objective: Successfully role-play a job interview.

EQUIPMENT AND SUPPLIES
none

METHOD

1. Determine five questions that may be asked during an interview.
2. Choose a classmate.
3. Select a quiet part of the classroom to conduct the interview.
4. Determine who will be the interviewer and who will be the interviewee.
5. The interviewer will begin the interview process by giving the interviewee a general idea about the medical office and the employees that work there.
6. The interviewer will ask the interviewee the five questions he or she selected in step 1.
7. The interviewer will gather information about the interviewee's past work experience.
8. The interviewer will gather information about the interviewee's educational experience.
9. The interviewee will answer the interviewer questions.
10. The interviewee will ask the interviewer questions about the medical office and the position.
11. The interviewer will answer the interviewee's questions.
12. Repeat the process, with students reversing roles. (Each student should play the part of the interviewer and the interviewee once.)
13. Now the students should discuss the ten most common mistakes made in an interview. Did either student display any of these mistakes?
14. Each student will assess his or her own interviewing skills.
15. Each student will discuss the appropriate attire to wear to an interview.
16. Each student will discuss the successful interviewing guidelines derived from their textbook.

9. Speaking critically of previous employers

10. Inability to ask questions about the organization

THE APPLICATION

If you have had work experience, there should be no gaps on your job **application** or résumé from the time you began to work. An application includes personal information and previous work experience. You may have stopped working temporarily to complete your education. The employer will then expect the dates of employment and schooling to run consecutively. Gaps with no apparent work or schooling indicated should be clarified. If you were unemployed for a period of time, the potential employer will want to know why.

An application is usually completed at the time of the interview. Therefore, bring along a folder containing all of your documentation, such as the following:

- Social Security number

- Updated résumé and an extra copy for the interviewer

- List of three references with their addresses and telephone numbers

- A chronological list of all your work experience

- Driver's license and/or photo ID

The neatness of your handwriting and printing will be demonstrated on your application. Be careful to print if that is requested. Remember that questions relating to age, ethnicity, place of birth, and number of children are prohibited by law. However, some offices and institutions may still have these questions on their application forms. You do not have to answer these questions. Simply leave the questions blank.

Follow-Up After the Interview

Immediately following the interview, on the same day if possible, send a letter thanking the interviewer for his or her time. This is a good opportunity to again express your interest in the position. Be meticulous about proofreading your letter for mistakes. It may be your final professional contact with the interviewer before the decision to hire is made.

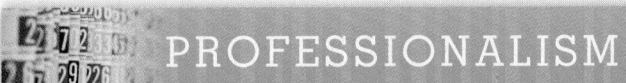

PROFESSIONALISM

THE LAW

You are responsible for providing complete and accurate information on application forms. Be sure all the facts surrounding your education and work experience are absolutely accurate. It is especially important to be honest about your skill level. Do not promise to perform procedures or tasks for which you are not trained. Lying on an application or a résumé is considered cause for termination. In some instances there may even be cause for prosecution.

You may wish to call the office a few days later to ask about the progress made on filling the position. If you are offered a position and decide not to accept it, you would use the same courtesy when turning down an offer as you use when accepting one. See Figure 59-10 for a sample of a follow-up letter and Procedure 59-5: Preparing a Follow-Up Letter.

Ralph Taylor
222 E. Main St.
Chicago, IL 60601
(312) 555-1212

May 30, 20XX

James Stark, M.D.
1450 N. Devonshire
Chicago, IL 60611

Dear Dr. Stark:

Thank you for giving me the opportunity to discuss the medical assisting position that you are seeking to fill in your office. I believe that my skills would be a good match with your needs.

I enjoyed meeting you and your staff today, and I would be very interested in working for you.

Thank you for considering my application. I look forward to hearing from you.

Sincerely,

Ralph Taylor

Ralph Taylor, CMA (AAMA)

FIGURE 59-10 An example of a follow-up letter following an interview.

procedure
59-5

PREPARING A FOLLOW-UP LETTER

Objective: Prepare an interview follow-up letter.

EQUIPMENT AND SUPPLIES

computer; printer; pen; paper; dictionary; thesaurus; telephone book

METHOD

1. Using Figure 59-10 as an example, prepare a follow-up letter.
2. Proofread your follow-up letter.
3. Have a close family member or friend proofread your follow-up letter.
4. Make any corrections to errors found on the follow-up letter.
5. Using good-quality, white or off-white $8\frac{1}{2} \times 11$ paper, print your follow-up letter.
6. Turn in your follow-up letter to your instructor.

If you are offered a position that you wish to accept, send a letter of acceptance no later than 5 days after the offer. Accept the offer graciously, clearly stating the position you are accepting, and express your thanks.

What Does the Employer Want?

Employers are looking for a variety of skills from their employees. To be successful as a medical assistant, you must master six basic skills:

- **Reading**—As a medical assistant you will be reading medical records, orders, instructions, memos, correspondence, resources, references, and much more. You also will read a variety of professional journals to keep your skills current.

- **Listening**—A large amount of your time as a medical assistant will be spent listening to patients. You also will use your listening skills during meetings, telephone conversations, and conversing with other staff members. Good listening skills are critical for every medical assistant.

- **Speaking**—As a medical assistant you will spend a lot of time speaking to patients and other staff members. When you are speaking with others you must speak clearly and use appropriate vocabulary and grammar.

- **Writing**—Documentation in a medical office is a must. It demonstrates that care or treatment has been provided. This could be critical if a physician is called to court for a lawsuit. A medical assistant must make sure all documentation is complete, accurate, and spelled correctly.

- **Problem solving**—Your problem-solving skills will be an asset to the medical office and will allow you to be more efficient in performing your duties. Employers want their employees to be able to take care of changes and think of new ways to improve situations.

- **Teamwork**—A medical office must work as a team for it to run efficiently. As a medical assistant you will share knowledge and responsibilities with other staff members. Good-quality patient care results when all members of the team are working together.

Employers will look for a wide range of values and skills in an employee, although not every employer will seek the same values or skills. Some of the values and skills employers look for are these:

- **Initiative**—When the medical assistant takes on a task without being told to do so, this is initiative. Starting a task on your own will show your employer that you are problem solving and using your critical thinking skills.

- **Enthusiasm**—A medical assistant's enthusiasm can be expressed verbally or nonverbally. When you are enthusiastic, you enjoy what you are doing and are passionate about it. Enthusiasm is a positive quality for all medical assistants to acquire.

- **Honesty**—For the patients, physician, and other staff members to trust you, you must be honest at all times. If you have made a mistake, admit it and learn from it.

- **Dependability**—When a medical assistant is late, leaves early, or misses work, the office must reassign staff and possibly work understaffed for that time. This causes more work for everyone. The physician and other staff members depend on you to be there at the scheduled time.

- **Flexibility**—Most medical offices are very busy, and emergencies do occur. As a medical assistant you must be flexible with the changes that can occur daily or even minute to minute. This also means that you must multitask throughout the workday.

- **Administrative skills**—Part of your job duties may include administrative procedures. Take special care to make sure each one is performed correctly.

- **Clinical skills**—Part of your job duties may include clinical procedures. It is critical for a medical assistant to perform clinical skills with total accuracy.

You will not be perfect at all of these skills, but you can develop each and every one of them with time, practice, and commitment. The more values and skills you have as a medical assistant, the more employable you will be. Just ask yourself, what would you want in an employee? This will help lead you to the values and skills you need to develop.

SUMMARY

One of the most valuable components of a medical assisting program is the externship because it provides an opportunity to practice skills that have been learned in school, under the direct supervision of the externship coordinator. This important stage of the training provides the student an opportunity to gain insight into strengths and weaknesses, allowing students to work on or correct weaknesses before accepting employment.

The job interview process requires the medical assistant to be honest and sincere about capabilities and the desire to work diligently. A fulfilling career demands careful planning, the ability to arrive on time, and the ability to work diligently for an employer while always keeping the patient's needs in mind.

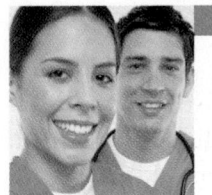

59 CHAPTER REVIEW

COMPETENCY REVIEW

1. Define and spell the terms to learn for this chapter.

2. Describe three areas of student responsibility concerning the externship.

3. List and discuss three externship opportunities in your area that you would like to pursue.

4. List and discuss six areas that your externship supervisor will be evaluating.

5. Write a résumé or update an existing résumé.

6. Select an advertisement for a medical assistant position from your local newspaper's classified section. Write a cover letter in response to that advertisement.

7. Write a follow-up letter after receiving an interview for the position mentioned in question 6.

8. What are three questions you would ask a potential employer during an interview?

9. How would you respond to the question "What is your major strength?"

10. How would you respond to the question. "What is your major weakness?"

PREPARING FOR THE CERTIFICATION EXAM

1. At the end of medical assistant training, working without payment in a health care setting as part of a medical assisting program is called
   a. a clinical rotation
   b. an in-service
   c. an externship
   d. an internship
   e. a preceptor

2. Which of the following is NOT a subject tested on the AAMA (CMA) exam?
   a. medical terminology
   b. pharmacology
   c. bookkeeping
   d. nursing skills
   e. computer skills

3. Which of the following should NOT be brought to an interview?
   a. photo ID
   b. résumé
   c. proof of certification
   d. children
   e. grades received in school

4. Which of the following is NOT a guideline to successful interviewing?
   a. Carry one extra copy of your résumé.
   b. Dress conservatively.
   c. Be alert.
   d. Arrive exactly on time.
   e. Do not chew gum.

5. Which of the following is NOT considered a job hunting mistake?
   a. failing to network with others and tell them that you are looking
   b. knowing your weaknesses
   c. limiting yourself to one field
   d. not having a clear plan
   e. not practicing interviewing skills

6. Which of the following should NOT be included in a résumé?
   a. objective
   b. education
   c. salary expectations
   d. work history
   e. address

7. Which of the following is NOT desired by employers?
   a. honesty
   b. problem-solving ability
   c. negative discussion about previous employers
   d. dependability
   e. clinical skills

8. After an interview, which of the following should be done?
   a. Send a thank-you letter.
   b. Send six copies of your résumé.
   c. Inform the workplace of other job offers you have received.
   d. Send testimonials from your pastor.
   e. Make a thank-you phone call.

9. The name of the type of correspondence that is intended as a courtesy to introduce yourself and summarize your qualifications for the job is called a
   a. cover letter
   b. follow-up letter
   c. résumé
   d. interview letter
   e. calling card

10. Which of the following is NOT considered one of the more common mistakes made in an interview?
    a. making eye contact
    b. being critical of a previous employer
    c. not asking questions about the potential employer's organization
    d. being extremely talkative
    e. using very familiar language such as "yep" instead of "yes"

CRITICAL THINKING

1. Kenneth prepares a list of questions that he would like to ask Tania during the interview. What would be some important questions that Kenneth may ask during the interview?

2. On his way to the interview, Kenneth takes the wrong exit and must turn around to head in the right direction. How should Kenneth handle the situation if he thinks that he may be late for the interview?

3. Tania asks Kenneth about a 6 month gap in his résumé where he did not have a job. Kenneth is embarrassed and flustered while answering the question. What should he tell Tania?

ON THE JOB

Stacy is the lead medical assistant in an ophthalmology practice of ten physicians. The eye clinic sees patients, literally, from all over the world. Several of the physicians are leaders in their specific area of ophthalmology, such as Dr. Keeler, who specializes in retinal diseases.

Today Stacy is going to interview a potential new employee, Sarah Banks. Sarah is currently finishing a CAAHEP-approved medical assisting program at a local college and is searching for full-time employment. She has some on-the-job experience dating back to when she was an after-school receptionist for a general practitioner, but that was more than 10 years ago.

The clinic tends to hire medical assistants who are certified, experienced, and very capable of dealing with patients from different age groups, races, and origins. However, Sarah is being considered for the position because, first of all, her father is a personal friend of Dr. Keeler and, second, medical assistants are difficult to find because of the high demand. What should Stacy do to prepare for the interview with Sarah? What is your response to the situation?

1. Considering that the practice is limited to ophthalmology, would any special requirements be warranted in a medical assistant who was going to work in this area?
2. Considering that the clinic's patient population is mixed by age and race, would any special requirements in a medical assistant be warranted in this case?
3. Is it proper procedure for Sarah to be applying for this position given that she has not yet completed her medical assisting program?
4. Should Stacy, given the circumstances, invest a lot of time in interviewing Sarah? Why or why not?
5. Should the rather dated on-the-job experience be factored into Stacy's decision to hire Sarah or not?
6. If Stacy decides not to hire Sarah, does Stacy need to personally contact the reference and thank him anyway, given that he is a friend of Dr. Keeler?

INTERNET ACTIVITY

Using any Internet search engine, type the phrase *dressing for an interview.* Go to one or more of the resulting websites to answer the following questions:
1. Would a person be ready for an interview if he or she had an eyebrow piercing?
2. Should a person chew gum during an interview?
3. What are appropriate colors for dresses or suits?

MEDMEDIA

Additional interactive resources and activities for this chapter can be found:

On your student DVD: View applicable procedure videos on the DVD-ROM found in the back of this book.

MyHealthProfessionsKit.com: Test your knowledge of this chapter with games and activities. MyHealthProfessionsKit also includes resources, helpful links, and a Spanish audio glossary.

Medical Assisting Interactive: Practice your procedures as a medical assistant in this simulated doctor's office. This can be accessed through MyHealthProfessionsKit.com.

APPENDIX I
General, Clinical, and Administrative Skills* of the CMA (AAMA)

General Skills

Communication
- Recognize and respect cultural diversity
- Adapt communications to individual's understanding
- Employ professional telephone and interpersonal techniques
- Recognize and respond effectively to verbal, nonverbal, and written communications
- Utilize and apply medical terminology appropriately
- Receive, organize, prioritize, store, and maintain transmittable information utilizing electronic technology
- Serve as "communication liaison" between the physician and patient

- Serve as patient advocate professional and health coach in a team approach in health care
- Identify basics of office emergency preparedness

Legal Concepts
- Perform within legal (including federal and state statutes, regulations, opinions, and rulings) and ethical boundaries
- Document patient communication and clinical treatments accurately and appropriately
- Maintain medical records
- Follow employer's established policies dealing with the health care contract
- Comply with established risk management and safety procedures

- Recognize professional credentialing criteria
- Identify and respond to issues of confidentiality

Instruction
- Function as a health care advocate to meet individual's needs
- Educate individuals in office policies and procedures
- Educate the patient within the scope of practice and as directed by supervising physician in health maintenance, disease prevention, and compliance with patient's treatment plan
- Identify community resources for health maintenance and disease prevention to meet individual patient needs

- Maintain current list of community resources, including those for emergency preparedness and other patient care needs
- Collaborate with local community resources for emergency preparedness
- Educate patients in their responsibilities relating to third-party reimbursements

Operational Functions
- Perform inventory of supplies and equipment
- Perform routine maintenance of administrative and clinical equipment
- Apply computer and other electronic equipment techniques to support office operations
- Perform methods of quality control

Clinical Skills

Fundamental Principles
- Identify the roles and responsibilities of the medical assistant in the clinical setting
- Identify the roles and responsibilities of other team members in the medical office
- Apply principles of aseptic technique and infection control
- Practice Standard Precautions, including handwashing and disposal of biohazardous materials
- Perform sterilization techniques
- Comply with quality assurance practices

Diagnostic Procedures
- Collect and process specimens
- Perform CLIA-waived tests

- Perform electrocardiography and respiratory testing
- Perform phlebotomy, including venipuncture and capillary puncture
- Utilize knowledge of principles of radiology

Patient Care
- Perform initial-response screening following protocols approved by supervising physician
- Obtain, evaluate, and record patient history employing critical thinking skills
- Obtain vital signs
- Prepare and maintain examination and treatment areas
- Prepare patient for examinations, procedures and treatments

- Assist with examinations, procedures, and treatments
- Maintain examination/treatment rooms, including inventory of supplies and equipment
- Prepare and administer oral and parenteral (excluding IV) medications and immunizations (as directed by supervising physician and as permitted by state law)
- Utilize knowledge of principles of IV therapy
- Maintain medication and immunization records
- Screen and follow up test results
- Recognize and respond to emergencies

Administrative Skills

Administrative Procedures
- Schedule, coordinate, and monitor appointments
- Schedule inpatient/outpatient admissions and procedures
- Apply third-party and managed care policies, procedures, and guidelines
- Establish, organize, and maintain patient medical record
- File medical records appropriately

Practice Finances
- Perform procedural and diagnostic coding for reimbursement
- Perform billing and collection procedures
- Perform administrative functions, including book-keeping and financial procedures
- Prepare submittable ("clean") insurance forms

*All skills require decision making based on critical thinking concepts.

Reprinted with permission of the American Association of Medical Assistants (AAMA).

A-1

MEDICAL ASSISTING TASK LIST

The various tasks that medical assistants perform include, but are not necessarily limited to, those on the following list. The tasks presented in this inventory are considered by American Medical Technologists to be representative of the medical assisting job role. This document should be considered dynamic, to reflect the medical assistant's evolving role with respect to contemporary healthcare. Therefore, tasks may be added, removed, or modified on an ongoing basis.

Medical assistants that meet AMT's qualifications and pass a certification examination are **certified** as a Registered Medical Assistant (RMA).

I. General Medical Assisting Knowledge

A. Anatomy and Physiology
1. Body systems
2. Disorders and diseases of the body

B. Medical Terminology
1. Word parts
2. Medical terms
3. Common abbreviations and symbols
4. Spelling

C. Medical Law
1. Medical law
2. Licensure, certification, and registration

D. Medical Ethics
1. Principles of medical ethics
2. Ethical conduct
3. Professional development

E. Human Relations
1. Patient relations
2. Interpersonal skills
3. Cultural diversity

F. Patient Education
1. Identify and apply proper communication methods in patient instruction
2. Develop, assemble, and maintain patient resource materials

II. Administrative Medical Assisting

A. Insurance
1. Medical insurance terminology
2. Various insurance plans
3. Claim forms
4. Electronic insurance claims
5. ICD-9/CPT Coding applications
6. HIPAA mandated coding systems
7. Financial applications of medical insurance

B. Financial Bookkeeping
1. Medical finance terminology
2. Patient billing procedures
3. Collection procedures
4. Fundamental medical office accounting procedures
5. Office banking procedures
6. Employee payroll
7. Financial calculations and accounting procedures

C. Medical Secretarial - Receptionist
1. Medical terminology associated with receptionist duties
2. General reception of patients and visitors
3. Appointment scheduling systems
4. Oral and written communications
5. Medical records management
6. Charting guidelines and regulations
7. Protect, store, and retain medical records according to HIPAA regulations
8. Release of protected health information adhering to HIPAA regulations
9. Transcription of dictation
10. Supplies and equipment management
11. Medical office computer applications
12. Compliance with OSHA guidelines and regulations of office safety

III. Clinical Medical Assisting

A. Asepsis
1. Medical terminology
2. State/Federal universal blood borne pathogen/body fluid precautions
3. Medical/Surgical asepsis procedure

B. Sterilization
1. Medical terminology associated with sterilization
2. Sanitization, disinfection, and sterilization procedures
3. Record keeping procedures

C. Instruments
1. Specialty instruments and parts
2. Usage of common instruments
3. Care and handling of disposable and reusable instruments

D. Vital Signs /Mensurations
1. Blood pressure, pulse, respiration measurements
2. Height, weight, circumference measurements
3. Various temperature measurements
4. Recognize normal and abnormal measurement results

E. Physical Examinations
1. Patient history information
2. Proper charting procedures
3. Patient positions for examinations
4. Methods of examinations
5. Specialty examinations
6. Visual acuity/ Ishihara (color blindness) measurements
7. Allergy testing procedures
8. Normal/ abnormal results

F. Clinical Pharmacology
1. Medical terminology associated with pharmacology
2. Commonly used drugs and their categories
3. Various routes of medication administration
4. Parenteral administration of medications (subcutaneous, intramuscular, intradermal, Z-tract)
5. Classes or drug schedules and legal prescriptions requirements for each
6. Drug Enforcement Agency regulations for ordering, dispensing, storage, and documentation of medication use
7. Drug Reference books (*PDR, Pharmacopeia, Facts and Comparisons, Nurses Handbook*)

G. Minor Surgery
1. Surgical supplies and instruments
2. Asepsis in surgical procedures
3. Surgical tray preparation and sterile field respect
4. Prevention of pathogen transmission
5. Patient surgical preparation procedures
6. Assisting physician with minor surgery, including setup
7. Dressing and bandaging techniques
8. Suture and staple removal
9. Biohazard waste disposal procedures
10. Instruct patient in pre- and post-surgical care

H. Therapeutic Modalities
1. Various standard therapeutic modalities
2. Alternative/complementary therapies
3. Instruct patient in assistive devices, body mechanics and home care

I. Laboratory Procedures
1. Medical laboratory terminology
2. OSHA safety guidelines
3. Quality control and assessment regulations
4. Operate and maintain laboratory equipment
5. CLIA-waived laboratory testing procedures
6. Capillary, dermal, and venipuncture procedures
7. Office specimen collection such as: urine, throat, vaginal, wound cultures--stool, sputum, etc.
8. Specimen handling and preparation
9. Laboratory recording according to state and federal guidelines
10. Adhere to the MA Scope of Practice in the laboratory

J. Electrocardiography
1. Standard, 12 lead ECG Testing
2. Mounting techniques for permanent record
3. Rhythm strip ECG monitoring on Lead II

K. First Aid
1. Emergencies and first aid procedures
2. Emergency crash cart supplies
3. Legal responsibilities as a first responder

WHAT KIND OF LEARNER ARE YOU?

To become a successful student, you must evaluate the type of learner you are. Following are the characteristics of the visual, auditory, and tactile learner.

The visual learner

- Tries to envision the word when spelling it out.
- Dislikes listening for long periods of time.
- Becomes distracted by movement when trying to concentrate.
- May not remember names but typically will remember faces.
- Prefers face-to-face meetings.
- Prefers to read descriptions when learning new material.
- Likes to look at pictures when learning new material.

The auditory learner

- Tries to sound out a word when spelling it out.
- Enjoys listening rather than talking.
- Becomes distracted by sounds or noises when trying to concentrate.
- Prefers the telephone to face-to-face meetings.
- Prefers verbal instructions.

The tactile learner

- Writes a word out when learning to spell it.
- Uses gestures and expressive movements when talking.
- Becomes distracted by activity when trying to concentrate.
- Prefers to talk while participating in activities.
- Is not necessarily a good reader—prefers stories that are action oriented.
- Tends to figure things out during the process rather than read directions.

SKILL SETS

Once you've realized the type of learner you are, take steps to use the skills you have in learning new material.

The visual learner might try

- Looking at pictures or diagrams when learning new material.
- Studying in a quiet room with no distractions.
- Asking for descriptions or asking instructors to explain how a topic might apply in the real world (e.g., "Would you demonstrate that skill to the class?").

The auditory learner might try

- Reading aloud or taping his or her voice and playing it back to study new material.
- Taping the instructor's lecture and replaying it later to study.
- Studying in a quiet room with no distractions.
- Working with study groups where students discuss the material they've learned.
- Prefers to hear descriptions when learning new material.

The tactile learner might try

- Writing material down several times in order to memorize it.
- Studying in a quiet area with no distractions.
- Asking the instructor to give examples of how a topic is addressed (e.g., "Would you allow the class to role-play that activity so we can see what it feels like?").
- Practicing activities or skills in order to commit them to memory.

TIME MANAGEMENT

One of the greatest difficulties for new students is time management and organization of priorities. For those students who have trouble in this area, the following steps may help:

- Set aside blocks of time for studying.
- Take periodic breaks when studying—get up and move around, get a drink, close your eyes for a few moments.
- Prioritize your assignments. Many students find it helpful to write down their assignments and place numbers next to each to indicate the order in which they need to be done.
- Study or read while doing other activities. Students can study or read while exercising at the gym or elsewhere.

- Review study material just prior to class on test day.
- Create "to do" lists.
- Use a daily/weekly/monthly calendar. Write down dates of upcoming tests or project due dates, then backtrack to add in dates when certain stages of the project should be completed. For example, if a paper is due 4 weeks from today, add a note to the calendar for 1 week from today that the outline should be completed, a note that 2 weeks from today the rough draft should be completed, and so on.

- Look for study partners for each class. Link up with study partners who are "good" students, not those who are not as dedicated as you are to learning the material. Spend time together each week going over the material from the class and studying or preparing for tests or projects.

Students should always be able to consult the course instructor for clarification of subject matter, or for verification of course progress. Students must keep aware of their progress in any given class and take an active part in ensuring their own success.

AAO	alert, awake, and oriented	ECG	electrocardiogram	NKDA	no known drug allergies
A&O	alert and oriented	EMG	electromyogram	NMR	nuclear magnetic resonance
ABD	abdomen	ENT	ears, nose, and throat	NPO	nothing by mouth
ABG	arterial blood gas			NSAID	nonsteroidal anti-inflammatory
abs	absent	FBS	fasting blood sugar		drugs
AC	before eating	FTT	failure to thrive	NSR	normal sinus rhythm
ACLS	advanced cardiac life support	FU	follow-up		
ADH	anti-diuretic hormone	Fx	fracture	OB	obstetrics
adm	admission			OPV	oral polio vaccine
ad lib	as much as needed	GI	gastrointestinal	OR	operating room
ADR	adverse drug reaction	GSW	gunshot wound		
AFP	alpha-fetoprotein	GTT	glucose tolerance test	PA	posteroanterior
amb	ambulatory			PC	after eating
amt	amount	HA	headache	PDR	Physician's Desk Reference
ant	anterior	H&P	history and physical examination	PE	physical exam
ante	before	HBP	high blood pressure	PKU	phenylketonuria
AOB	alcohol on breath	HCG	human chorionic gonadotropin	PMH	previous medical history
AP	anteroposterior	HCT	hematocrit	PO	by mouth
ASAP	as soon as possible	HDL	high-density lipoprotein	PR	by rectum
		HEENT	head, eyes, ears, nose, throat	PRN	as needed
BCP	birth control pills	Hgb	hemoglobin	Pt	patient
BE	barium enema	HIV	human immunodeficiency virus	PT	prothrombin time, or physical
bid	twice a day	HO	history of		therapy
BM	bowel movement	HR	heart rate	PTT	partial thromboplastin time
BMR	basal metabolic rate	HS	at bedtime	PUD	peptic ulcer disease
BP	blood pressure	HSV	herpes simplex virus		
BPH	benign prostatic hypertrophy	HTN	hypertension	q	every (e.g., q6h = every 6
BPM	beats per minute	Hx	history		hours)
BS	bowel, or breath sounds			qd	every day
BX	biopsy	I&D	incision and drainage	qh	every hour
		ICU	intensive care unit	qid	four times a day
c̄	with	ID	infectious disease		
Ca	calcium	IG	immunoglobulin	R	right
CA	cancer	IM	intramuscular	RA	rheumatoid arthritis
CAD	coronary artery disease	INF	intravenous nutritional fluid	RBC	red blood cell
CAT	computerized axial tomography	IV	intravenous	R/O	rule out
CBC	complete blood count			ROM	range of motion
CC	chief complaint	L	left	ROS	review of systems
CHF	congestive heart failure	LLL	left lower lobe	RTC	return to clinic
CNS	central nervous system	LMP	last menstrual period		
C/O	complaining of	LOC	loss of consciousness, or level of	s̄	without
COPD	chronic obstructive pulmonary		consciousness	SOAP	subjective, objective, assessment,
	disease	LPN	licensed practical nurse		plan
CP	cerebral palsy			SOB	shortness of breath
CPAP	continuous positive airway	MAO	monoamine oxidase	STAT	immediately
	pressure	MBT	maternal blood type	SubQ	subcutaneous
CPR	cardiopulmonary resuscitation	MI	myocardial infarction, or mitral	Sx	symptoms
CT	computerized tomography		insufficiency		
CVA	cerebrovascular accident	mL	milliliter	T&C	type and cross
CXR	chest X-ray	MMR	measles, mumps, rubella	TB	tuberculosis
		MRI	magnetic resonance imaging	tid	three times a day
DC	discontinue, or discharge	MRSA	methicillin resistant staph aureus	TIG	tetanus immune globulin
DNR	do not resuscitate	MS	multiple sclerosis	TMJ	temporomandibular joint
DOA	dead on arrival	MVA	motor vehicle accident	TNTC	too numerous to count
DTR	deep tendon reflexes			TO	telephone order
DVT	deep venous thrombosis	NG	nasogastric	TPN	total parenteral nutrition
DX	diagnosis	NKA	no known allergies	TSH	thyroid stimulating hormone

TT	thrombin time	VO	verbal order	yo	years old
Tx	treatment			YOB	year of birth
		WBC	white blood cell	yr	year
UA	urinalysis	WD	well developed	ytd	year to date
UAO	upper airway obstruction	WF	white female		
UBD	universal blood donor	WM	white male		
URI	upper respiratory infection	WNL	within normal limits		
US	ultrasound	WO	written order		
UTI	urinary tract infection				

APPENDIX V
Glossary of Word Parts

PREFIXES

Prefix	Meaning
a	no, not, without, lack of, apart
ab	away from
ad	toward, near
ambi	both
an	no, not, without, lack of
ana	up
ant	against
ante	before
anti	against
apo	separation
astro	star-shaped
auto	self
bi	two, double
bin	twice
brachy	short
brady	slow
cac	bad
cata	down
centi	a hundred
chromo	color
circum	around
con	with, together
contra	against
de	down, away from
deca	ten
di (a)	through, between
dia	through, between
dif	apart, free from, separate
dipl	double
di (s)	two, apart
dis	apart
dys	bad, difficult, painful
ec	out, outside, outer
ecto	out, outside, outer
em	in
en	within
end	within, inner
endo	within, inner
ep	upon, over, above
epi	upon, over, above
eso	inward
eu	good, normal
ex	out, away from
exo	out, away from
extra	outside, beyond
hemi	half
heter	different
hetero	different
homo	similar, same
homeo	similar, same, likeness, constant
hydr	water
hydro	water
hyp	below, deficient
hyper	above, beyond, excessive
hypo	below, under, deficient
in	in, into, not
infra	below
infer	below
inter	between
intra	within
ir (in)	into
macro	large
mal	bad
mega	large, great
meso	middle
meta	beyond, over, between, change
micro	small
milli	one-thousandth
mon (o)	one
mono	one
multi	many, much
neo	new
nulli	none
olig	little, scanty
oligo	little, scanty
pan	all
par	around, beside
para	beside, alongside, abnormal
per	through
peri	around
poly	many, much, excessive
post	after, behind
pre	before
primi	first
pro	before
proto	first
pseudo	false
pyro	fire
quadri	four
quint	five
re	back
retro	backward
semi	half
sub	below, under, beneath
super	above, beyond
supra	above, beyond
sym	together
syn	together, with
tachy	fast
tetra	four
trans	across
tri	three
ultra	beyond
uni	one

WORD ROOTS/COMBINING FORMS

Root	Meaning
abdomin	abdomen
abort	to miscarry
absorpt	to suck in
acanth	a thorn
acid	acid
acoust	hearing
acr	extremity, point
acr/o	extremity, point
act	acting
actin	ray
aden	gland
aden/o	gland
adhes	stuck to
adip	fat
agglutinat	clumping
agon	agony
agor/a	gathering place
albin	white
albumin	protein
alimentat	nourishment
all	other
alveol	small, hollow air sac
ambul	to walk
ambyl	dull
amni/o	membrane
ampere	ampere
amputat	to cut through
amyl	starch
anastom	opening
andr	man
andr/o	man
ang	vessel
ang/i	vessel
angin	to choke, quinsy
angi/o	vessel
anis/o	unequal
ankyl	stiffening, crooked
an/o	anus
anter/i	toward the front
anthrac	coal
aort	aorta
aort/o	aorta
append	appendix
arachn	spider
arche	beginning

arter	artery	cheil	lip	cutane	skin
arter/i	artery	chem/o	chemical	cyan	dark blue
arteri/o	artery	chlor/o	green	cycl	ciliary body
arthr	joint	chol	gall, bile	cycl/o	ciliary body
arthr/o	joint	chole	gall, bile	cyst	bladder, sac
artific/i	not natural	chol/e	gall, bile	cyst/o	bladder, sac
aspirat	to draw in	choledoch/o	common bile duct	cyt	cell
atel	imperfect	chondr	cartilage	cyth	cell
atel/o	imperfect	chondr/o	cartilage	cyt/o	cell
ather	fatty substance, porridge	chord	cord	dacry	tear
ather/o	fatty substance, porridge	chori/o	chorion	dactyl	finger or toe
atri	atrium	choroid	choroid	dactyl/o	finger or toe
atri/o	atrium	choroid/o	choroid	defecat	to remove dregs
aud/i	to hear	chromat	color	dem	people
audi/o	to hear	chrom/o	color	dendr/o	tree
auditor	hearing	chym	juice	dent	tooth
aur	ear	cine	motion	dent/i	tooth
aur/i	ear	cinemat/o	motion	derm	skin
auscultat	listen to	circulat	circular	derm/a	skin
aut	self	cirrh	orange-yellow	dermat	skin
axill	armpit	cirrh/o	orange-yellow	dermat/o	skin
bacter/i	bacteria	cis	to cut	derm/o	skin
balan	glans penis	claudicat	to limp	dextr/o	to the right
bartholin	Bartholin's glands	clavicul	little key	diast	to expand
bas/o	base	cleid/o	clavicle	didym	testis
bil	bile, gall	coagul	to clot	digit	finger or toe
bil/i	bile, gall	coagulat	to clot	dilat	to widen
bi/o	life	coccyg/e	tailbone	disk	a disk
blast/o	germ cell	coccyg/o	tail bone	dist	away from the point of origin
blephar	eyelid	cochle/o	land snail	diverticul	diverticula
blephar/o	eyelid	coit	a coming together	dors	backward
bol	to cast, throw	col	colon	dors/i	backward
brach/i	arm	coll/a	glue	duct	to lead
bronch	bronchi	collis	neck	duoden	duodenum
bronch/i	bronchi	col/o	colon	dur	dura, hard
bronchiol	bronchiole	colon	colon	dur/o	dura, hard
bronch/o	bronchi	colon/o	colon	dwarf	small
bucc	cheek	colp/o	vagina	dynam	power
burs	a pouch	concuss	shaken violently	ech/o	echo
calc	lime, calcium	condyle	knuckle	ectop	displaced
calcan/e	heel bone	con/i	dust	eg/o	I, self
calc/i	calcium	conjunctiv	to join together	ejaculat	to throw out
cancer	crab	connect	to bind together	electr/o	electricity
capn	smoke	constipat	to press together	embol	to cast, to throw
capsul	a little box	continence	to hold	eme	to vomit
carcin	cancer	cor	pupil	emulsificat	disintergrate
carcin/o	cancer	coriat	corium	encephal	brain
card	heart	corne	cornea	encephal/o	brain
card/i/io	heart	corpor	body	enchyma	to pour
cardi/o	heart	corpor/e	body	enter	intestine
carp	wrist	cortic	cortex	enucleat	to remove the kernel of
carp/o	wrist	cortis	cortex	eosin/o	rose-colored
cartil	gristle	cost	rib	episi/o	vulva, pudenda
castr	to prune	cost/o	rib	equ/i	equal
caud	tail	cox	hip	erget	work
caus	heat	cran/i/o	skull	erg/o	work
cavit	cavity	crani/o	skull	eructat	a breaking out
celi	abdomen, belly	creat	flesh	erysi	red
cellul	little cell	creatin	flesh, creatine	erythr/o	red
centr	center	crine	to secrete	esophag/e	esophagus
centr/i	center	crin/o	to secrete	esophag/o	esophagus
cephal	head	crur	leg	esthesi/o	feeling
cept	receive	cry/o	cold	estr/o	mad desire
cerebell	little brain	crypt	hidden	eti/o	cause
cerebell/o	little brain	cubit	elbow, to lie	eunia	a bed
cerebr/o	cerebrum	culd/o	cul-de-sac	excret	sifted out
cervic	cervix, neck	curie	curie	fasc	a band (fascia)

fasci/o	a band (fascia)	hydr	water	lobul	small lobe
femor	femur	hymen	hymen	locat	to place
fenestrat	window	hypn	sleep	log	study
fibr	fibrous tissue, fiber	hyster	womb, uterus	log/o	word
fibrillat	fibrils (small fibers)	hyster/o	womb, uterus	lopec	fox mange
fibrin/o	fiber	icter	jaundice	lord	bending
fibr/o	fiber	ile	ileum	lucent	to shine
fibul	fibula	ile/o	ileum	lumb	loin
filtrat	to strain through	ili	ilium	lumb/o	loin
fixat	fastened	ili/o	ilium	lump	lump
flex	to bend	illus	foot	lun	moon
fluor/o	fluorescence	immun/o	safe, immunity	lymph	lymph, clear fluid
foc	focus	infarct	infarct (necrosis of an area)	lymph/o	lymph, clear fluid
follicul	little bag	infect	infection	malign	bad kind
format	a shaping	infer/i	below	mamm/o	breast
fungat	mushroom, fungus	inguin	groin	mandibul	lower jawbone
fus	to pour	insul	insulin	man/o	thin
galact/o	milk	insulin/o	insulin	mast	breast
ganglion	knot	integument	covering	masticat	to chew
gastr	stomach	intern	within	mast/o	breast
gastr/o	stomach	ionizat	ion (going)	maxill	jawbone
gen	formation, produce	ion/o	ion	maxilla	jaw
gene	formation, produce	iont/o	ion	maxim	greatest
genet	formation, produce	irid	iris	meat	passage
genital	belonging to birth	irid/o	iris	meat/o	passage
gen/o	kind	isch	to hold back	med	middle
ger	old age	ischi	ischium	medi	toward the middle
gest	to carry	is/o	equal	medull	marrow
gester	to bear	jaund	yellow	medull/o	marrow
gigant	giant	kal	potassium	melan	black
gingiv	gums	kary/o	cell's nucleus	melan/o	black
glandul	little acorn	kel	tumor	men	month
gli	glue	kerat	cornea	mening	membrane (meninges)
gli/o	glue	kerat/o	horn, cornea	mening/i	membrane
glob	globe	keton	ketone	mening/o	membrane
globin	globule	kil/o	a thousand	menise	crescent
globul	globe	kinet	motion	men/o	month
glomerul	glomerulus, little ball	kyph	a hump	ment	mind
glomerul/o	glomerulus, little ball	labi	lip	mes	middle
gloss/o	tongue	labyrinth	maze	mes/o	middle
gluc/o	sweet, sugar	labyrinth/o	maze	mester	month
glyc	sweet, sugar	lacrim	tear	metr	to measure, womb, uterus
glyc/o	glucose, sweet, sugar	lamin	lamina, thin plate	metr/i	womb, uterus
glycos	sweet, sugar	lamp (s)	to shine	micturit	to urinate
gonad	seed	lapar/o	flank, abdomen	miliar	millet (tiny)
goni/o	angle	laryng	larynx	minim	least
gon/o	genitals	laryng/e	larynx	mi/o	less, smaller
granul/o	little grain, granular	laryng/o	larynx	mit	thread
gravida	pregnant	later	side	mitr	mitral valve
gryp	curve	laxat	to loosen	mnes	memory
gynec/o	female	lei/o	smooth	mucos	mucus
halat	breathe	lemma	rind, sheath, husk	mucus	mucus
hallux	great (big) toe	lent	lens	muscul	muscle
hem	blood	lept	seizure	muscul/o	muscle
hemat	blood	letharg	drowsiness	muta	to change
hemat/o	blood	leuk	white	mutat	to change
hem/o	blood	leuk/o	white	my	muscle
hemorrh	vein liable to bleed	levat	lifter	myc	fungus
hepat	liver	libr/i	balance	myc/o	fungus
hepat/o	liver	lingu	tongue	mydriat	dilation, widen
herni/o	hernia	lip	fat	myel	bone marrow, spinal cord
hidr	sweat	lipid	fat	myel/o	marrow
hirsut	hairy	lip/o	fat	my/o	muscle
hist/o	tissue	lith	stone	my/os	muscle
hol/o	whole	lith/o	stone	myring	drum membrane
horizont	horizon	lob	lobe	myring/o	drum membrane
humer	humerus	lob/o	lobe	myx	mucus

narc/o	numbness	path/o	disease	prot/e	first
nas/o	nose	pause	cessation	proxim	near the point of origin
nat	birth	pector	chest	prurit	itching
nat/o	birth	pectorat	breast	psych	mind
necr	death	ped	foot, child	psych/o	mind
necr/o	death	ped/i	foot, child	pudend	external genitals
nephr	kidney	pedicul	a louse	pulm/o	lung
nephr/o	kidney	pelv/i	pelvis	pulmon	lung
neur	nerve	pen	penis	pulmonar	lung
neur/i	nerve	penile	penis	pupill	pupil
neur/o	nerve	pept	to digest	purpur	purple
neutr/o	neither	perine	perineum	py	pus
nid	nest	periton/e	peritoneum	pyel	renal pelvis
noct	night	phac	lens	pyel/o	renal pelvis
nom	law	phac/o	lens	pylor	pylorus, gate keeper
norm	rule	phag	to eat, engulf	py/o	pus
nucl	nucleus	phag/o	to eat, engulf	pyret	fever
nucle	kernel, nucleus	phak	lentil, lens	pyr/o	heat, fire
nyctal	blind	phalang/e	closely knit row	rach	spine
nystagm	to nod	pharyng/o	pharynx	rachi	spine
occlus	to shut up	pharyng	pharynx	rad/i	radiating out from a center
ocul	eye	phas	speech	radi	radius
odont	tooth	phen/o	to show	radiat	radiant
olecran	elbow	phe/o	dusky	radic/o	spinal nerve root
onc/o	tumor	phim	a muzzle	radicul	spinal nerve root
onych	nail	phleb	vein	radi/o	ray
onych/o	nail	phleb/o	vein	rect/o	rectum
o/o	ovum, egg	phon	voice	relaxat	to loosen
oophor	ovary	phone	voice	remiss	remit
ophthalm	eye	phon/o	sound	ren	kidney
ophthalm/o	eye	phor	carrying	ren/o	kidney
opt	eye	phos	light	respirat	breathing
opt/o	eye	phot/o	light	reticul/o	net
or	mouth	phragm	partition	retin	retina
orch	testicle	phragmat/o	partition	retin/o	retina
orchid	testicle	phras	speech	rhabd/o	rod
orchid/o	testicle	physic	nature	rheumat	discharge
organ	organ	physi/o	nature	rheumat/o	discharge
orth	straight	pil/o	hair	rhin/o	nose
orth/o	straight	pine	pine cone	rhonch	snore
oscill	to swing	pineal	pineal body	rhytid/o	wrinkle
oscill/o	to swing	pin/o	to drink	roent	roentgen
oste	bone	pituitar	phlegm	rotat	to turn
oste/o	bone	plak	plate	rrhyth	rhythm
ot	ear	plasma	a thing formed, plasma	rrhythm	rhythm
ot/o	ear	plast	a developing	rube/o	red
ovar	ovary	pleur	pleura	sacr	sacrum
ovul	ovary	pleura	pleura	salping	tube, fallopian tube
ovulat	ovary	pleur/o	pleura	salping/o	tube, fallopian tube
ox	oxygen	plicat	to fold	salpinx	tube, fallopian tube
ox/i	oxygen	pneum/o	lung, air	sarc	flesh
oxy	sour, sharp, acid	pneumon	lung	sarc/o	flesh
pachy	thick	poiet	formation	scapul	shoulder blade
pancreat	pancreas	poli/o	gray	scler	hardening
paque	dark	pollex	thumb	scler/o	hardening, sclera
palat/o	palate	por	a passage	scoli	curvature
palliat	cloaked	porphyr	purple	scoli/o	curvature
pallid/o	globus, pallidus	poster/i	behind, toward the back	scop	to examine
palm	palm	prand/i	meal	seb/o	oil
palpitat	throbbing	presby	old	secund	second
papill	papilla	press	to press	semin	seed
para	to bear	proct	anus, rectum	seminat	seed
paralyt	to disable, paralysis	proct/o	anus, rectum	senile	old
partum	labor	prolif	fruitful	senil	old
parturit	in labor	prophylact	guarding	sept	putrefaction
patell	kneecap, patella	prostat	prostate	septic	putrefying
path	disease	prosth/e	an addition	ser (a)	whey

ser/o	whey, serum	tempor	temples	ungu	nail
sert	to gain	tendin	tendon	ur	urine
sexu	sex	tend/o	tendon	ure	urinate
sial	saliva	ten/o	tendon	urea	urea
sial/o	salivary	tenon	tendon	uret	urine
sider/o	iron	tenos	tendon	ureter	ureter
sigmoid	sigmoid	tens	tension	ureter/o	ureter
sigmoid/o	sigmoid	tentori	tentorium, tent	urethr	urethra
sin/o	a curve	terat	monster	urethr/o	urethra
sinus	a hollow curve	testicul	testicle	urin	urine
situ	place	test/o	testicle	urinat	urine
som	body	thalass	sea	urin/o	urine
somat	body	thel/i	nipple	ur/o	urine
somat/o	body	therm	hot, heat	uter	uterus
somn	sleep	therm/o	hot, heat	uter/o	uterus
son	sound	thorac	chest	uve	uvea
son/o	sound	thorac/o	chest	vagin	vagina
spadias	a rent, an opening	thorax	chest	vag/o	vagus, wandering
spastic	convulsive	thromb	clot	varic/o	twisted vein
sperm	seed (sperm)	thromb/o	clot	vas	vessel
spermat	seed (sperm)	thym	thymus, mind, emotion	vascul	small vessel
spermat/o	seed (sperm)	thyr	thyroid, shield	vas/o	vessel
spermi	seed (sperm)	thyr/o	thyroid, shield	vector	a carrier
sphygm/o	pulse	thyrox	thyroid, shield	ven	vein
spin	spine, a thorn	tibi	tibia	venere	sexual intercourse
spir/o	breath	tinnit	a jingling	ven/i	vein
splen/o	spleen	toc	birth	ven/o	vein
spondyl	vertebra	tom/o	to cut	ventilat	to air
spondyl/o	vertebra	ton	tone, tension	ventr	near or on the belly side of the body
staped	stirrup	ton/o	tone	ventricul	ventricle
steat	fat	tonsill	tonsil, almond	ventricul/o	little belly
sten	narrowing	topic	place	vermi	worm
ster	solid	top/o	place	vers	turning
stern	sternum	tors	twisted	vertebr	vertebra
stern/o	sternum	tort/i	twisted	vertebr/o	vertebra
sterol	solid (fat)	tox	poison	vesic	bladder
steth	chest	toxic	poison	vesicul	vesicle
steth/o	chest	trach/e	trachea	vir	virus (poison)
stigmat	point	trache/o	trachea	viril	masculine
stom	mouth	tract	to draw	viscer	body organs
stomat	mouth	trephinat	a bore	volt	volt
strabism	a squinting	trich	hair	volunt	will
strict	to draw, to bind	trich/o	hair	volvul	to roll
superfic/i	near the surface	trigon	trigone	vuls	to pull
super/i	upper	trism	grating	watt	watt
suppress	suppress	trop	turning	xanth/o	yellow
surrog	substituted	troph	a turning	xen	foreign material
sympath	sympathy	tubercul	a little swelling	xer	dry
synov	joint fluid	tuss	cough	xer/o	dry
syst	contraction	tympan	ear drum	xiph	sword
system	a composite whole	tympan/o	drum	zo/o	animal
systol	contraction	uln	ulna, elbow	zoon	life
tel	end, distant	uln/o	ulna, elbow		
tele	distant	umbilic	navel		

SUFFIXES

-able	capable	-ar	pertaining to	-body	body
-ac	pertaining to	-ary	pertaining to	-cele	hernia, tumor, swelling
-ad	pertaining to	-ase	enzyme	-centesis	surgical puncture
-age	related to	-asthenia	weakness	-ceps	head
-al	pertaining to	-ate	use, action	-cide	to kill
-algesia	pain	-ate (d)	use, action	-clasia	a breaking
-algia	pain	-betes	to go	-clave	a key
-ant	forming	-blast	immature cell, germ cell	-cle	small

Word Part	Meaning	Word Part	Meaning	Word Part	Meaning
-clysis	injection	-ist	one who specializes, agent	-phoresis	to carry
-cope	strike	-itis	inflammation	-phragm	a fence
-crit	to separate	-ity	condition	-phraxis	to obstruct
-culture	cultivation	-ive	nature of, quality of	-phylaxis	protection
-cusis	hearing	-kinesia	motion	-physis	growth
-cuspid	point	-kinesis	motion	-plakia	plate
-cyesis	pregnancy	-lalia	to talk	-plasia	formation, produce
-cyst	bladder	-lemma	a sheath, rind	-plasm	a thing formed, plasma
-cyte	cell	-lepsy	seizure	-plasty	surgical repair
-derma	skin	-lexia	diction	-plegia	stroke, paralysis
-dermis	skin	-liter	liter	-pnea	breathing
-desis	binding	-lith	stone	-poiesis	formation
-dipsia	thirst	-logy	study of	-praxia	action
-drome	a course	-lymph	clear fluid	-ptosis	prolapse, drooping
-dynia	pain	-lysis	destruction, to separate	-ptysis	to spit, spitting
-ectasia	dilatation	-malacia	softening	-puncture	to pierce
-ectasis	dilatation, distention	-mania	madness	-rrhage	to burst forth, bursting forth
-ectasy	dilation	-megaly	enlargement, large	-rrhagia	to burst forth, bursting forth
-ectomy	surgical excision	-meter	instrument to measure	-rrhaphy	suture
-edema	swelling	-metry	measurement	-rrhea	flow, discharge
-emesis	vomiting	-mnesia	memory	-rrhexis	rupture
-emia	blood condition	-morph	form, shape	-scope	instrument
-er	relating to, one who	-noia	mind	-scopy	to view, examine
-ergy	work	-oid	resemble	-sepsis	decay
-esthesia	feeling	-ole	opening	-sis	condition
-form	shape	-oma	tumor	-some	body
-fuge	to flee	-omion	shoulder	-spasm	tension, spasm, contraction
-gen	formation, produce	-on	pertaining to	-stalsis	contraction
-genes	produce	-one	hormone	-stasis	control, stopping
-genesis	formation, produce	-opia	eye, vision	-staxis	dripping, trickling
-genic	formation, produce	-opsia	eye, vision	-sthenia	strength
-glia	glue	-opsy	to view	-stomy	new opening
-globin	protein	-or	one who, a doer	-systole	contraction
-gnosis	knowledge	-ory	like, resemble	-taxia	order
-grade	a step	-orexia	appetite	-therapy	treatment
-graft	pencil, grafting knife	-ose	like	-thermy	heat
-gram	a weight, mark, record	-osis	condition	-tic	pertaining to
-graph	to write, record	-ous	pertaining to	-tome	instrument to cut
-graphy	recording	-paresis	weakness	-tomy	incision
-hexia	condition	-pathy	disease	-tone	tension
-ia	condition	-penia	lack of, deficiency	-tripsy	crushing
-iasis	condition	-pepsia	to digest	-troph (y)	nourishment, development
-ic	pertaining to	-pexy	surgical fixation	-trophy	nourishment, development
-ide	having a particular quality	-phagia	to eat	-type	type
-in	chemical, pertaining to	-phasia	to speak	-um	tissue
-ine	pertaining to	-pheresis	removal	-ure	process
-ing	quality of	-phil	attraction	-uria	urine
-ion	process	-philia	attraction	-us	pertaining to
-ism	condition	-phobia	fear	-y	condition, pertaining to, process

Medisoft Advanced is a medical practice management software program that offers choices of actions through a series of menus. Commands are issued by clicking an option on the menu bar or by clicking a shortcut button on the toolbar. All data, whether a patient's address or a charge for a procedure, is entered into Medisoft through menus on the menu bar or through the buttons on the toolbar. Selecting an option from the menus or toolbar brings up a dialog box. The TAB key is used to move between text boxes within a dialog box.

The menu bar lists the names of the menus in Medisoft: File, Edit, Activities, Lists, Reports, Tools, Window, Services, and Help. Beneath each menu name is a pull-down menu of one or more options.

MENU BAR TITLES

The purpose of each menu is briefly described as follows:

File Menu—The File menu is used to enter information about the medical office practice when first setting up Medisoft. It is also used to back up data, maintain files, and set up program options.

Edit Menu—The Edit menu contains the basic commands needed to move, change, or delete information. These commands are Undo, Cut, Copy, Paste, and Delete.

Activities Menu—Most medical office data collected on a day-to-day basis is entered through options on the Activities menu. This menu is used to enter information about patients' office visits, including diagnoses and procedures performed. Transactions, including charges, payments, and adjustments, are also entered via the Activities menu.

Lists Menu—Information on new patients, such as name, address, and employer, is entered through the Lists menu. The Lists menu also provides access to lists of codes, insurance carriers, and providers.

Reports Menu—The Reports menu is used to print reports about patients' accounts and other reports about the practice.

Tools Menu—The calculator is accessed through the Tools menu. Other options on the Tools menu can be used to view the contents of a file as well as a profile of the computer system.

Window Menu—Using the Window menu, it is possible to switch back and forth between several open windows.

Services Menu—This menu contains links for electronic transmission of insurance claims, electronic prescriptions, and electronic eligibility verification.

Help Menu—The Help menu is used to access Medisoft's Help feature.

BASIC MEDISOFT ACTIONS

In this section we discuss some of the basic tasks that all medical office specialists should be able to perform with the Medisoft software.

Saving Data

Information entered into Medisoft is saved by clicking the Save button that appears in most dialog boxes (those in which data is input).

Deleting Data

The majority of Medisoft dialog boxes have buttons for the purpose of deleting data.

Exiting Medisoft

Medisoft is exited by clicking Exit on the File menu or by clicking the Exit button on the toolbar.

Entering Patient Information into Medisoft

Patient information is entered in the Patient/Guarantor dialog box, accessed by clicking Patient/Guarantors and Cases on the Lists menu. The Patient List dialog box displays a list of established patients. Information on a new patient is entered by clicking the New Patient button at the bottom of the dialog box. The Patient/Guarantor dialog box contains four tabs: the Name, Address tab, Other Information tab, Payment Plan tab, and Custom tab (Figure VI-1).

Name, Address Tab   This tab is completed with information provided by a new patient on the practice's patient information form. Most of the information is demographic: name, address, phone numbers, birth date, gender, and Social Security number. Phone numbers must be entered without parentheses or hyphens. The birth date is entered using

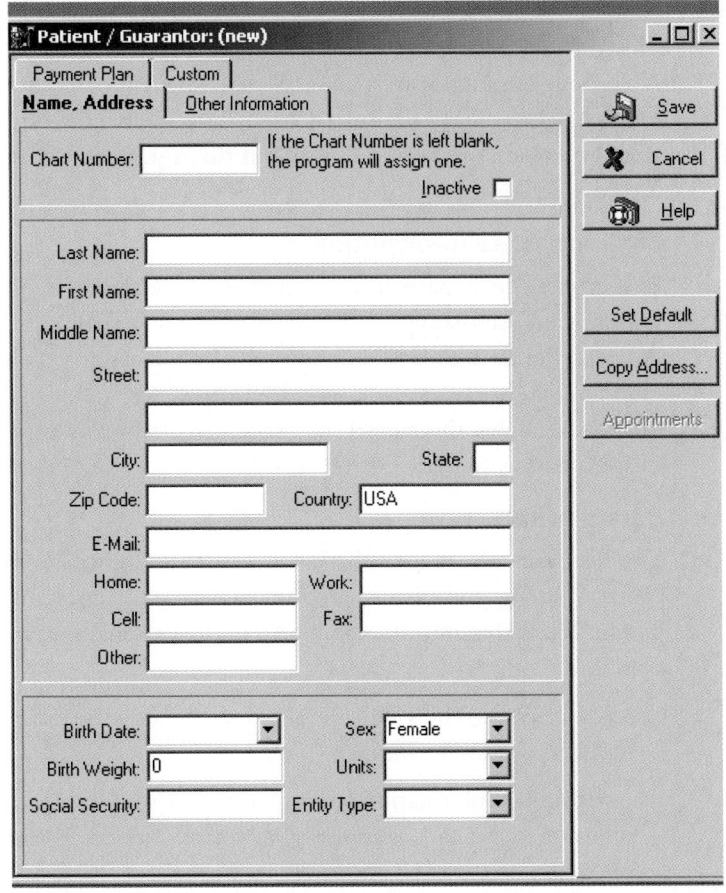

FIGURE VI-1 The Name, Address tab in the Patient/Guarantor window (dialog box).

and other miscellaneous information. The major fields in the Other Information tab are these:

Type—The Type drop-down list designates whether, for billing purposes, an individual is a patient or a guarantor. A guarantor is someone who is responsible for insurance and payment.

Assigned Provider—The code for the specific doctor who provides care to this patient is selected.

Signature on File—A check mark in the Signature on File check box means that the patient's signature is on file for the purpose of submitting insurance claims.

Signature Date—The date keyed in the Signature Date box is the date the patient signed the release of information form.

Emergency Contact—The name the patient/guarantor has written on the patient information form as an emergency contact is keyed in here, along with any phone numbers provided.

Employer—The name of the patient's employer is selected from the drop-down list of employers stored in the database.

the eight-digit MMDDCCYY format. The nine-digit Social Security number should be entered *with* hyphens. Some of the boxes, such as the cell phone number and fax number boxes, are optional.

Chart Number. The chart number is a unique number that identifies each patient. The most common method of assigning a number is to use the first three letters of the last name, the first two letters of the first name, and the digit 0, which represents head of household. If the last name has less than five letters, use more letters of the first name and even of the middle name if necessary. It is not necessary to enter a chart number when entering a new patient. If you choose not to enter one, Medisoft will assign one for you. Once the chart number is set it cannot be changed. To correct an incorrect chart number, the patient and case information would have to be deleted then re-created with the correct chart number.

Other Information Tab The Other Information tab (Figure VI-2) contains facts about a patient's employment

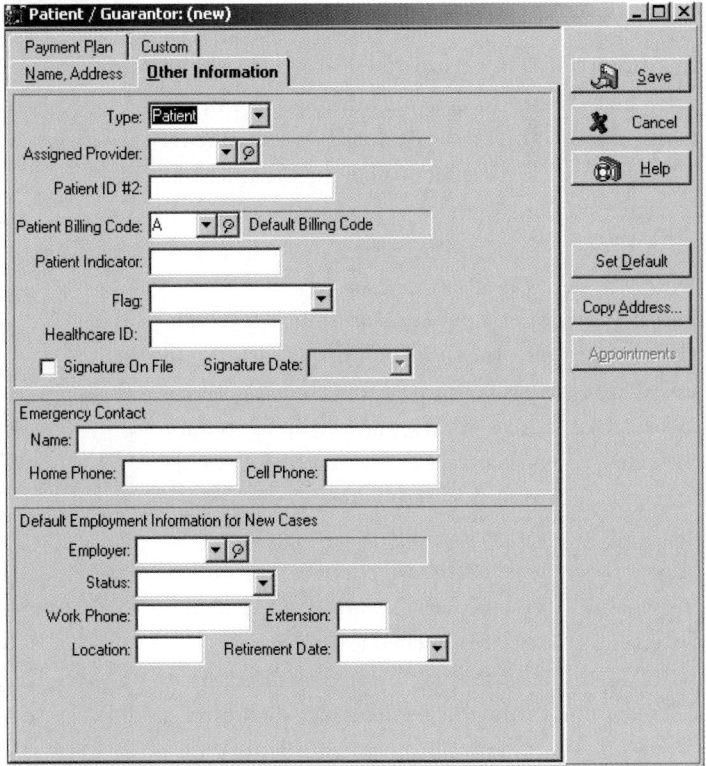

FIGURE VI-2 The Other Information tab in the Patient/Guarantor window.

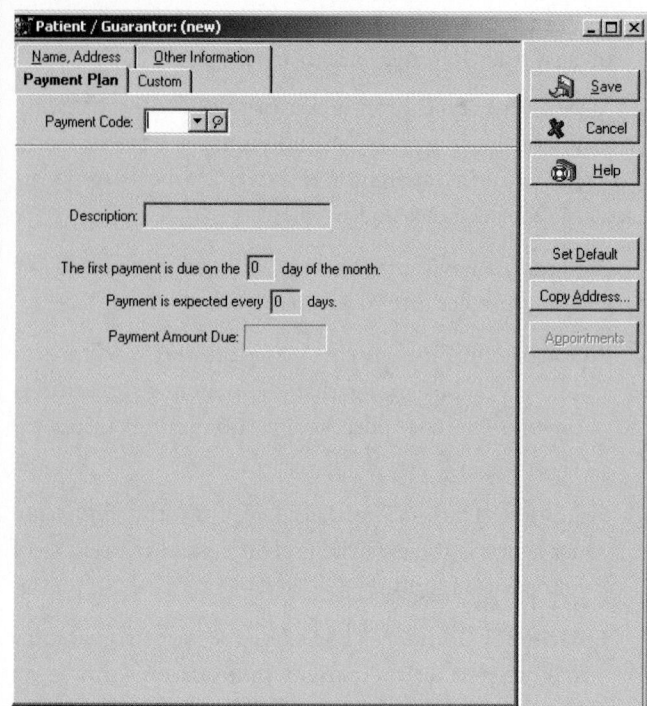

FIGURE VI-3 The Payment Plan tab in the Patient/Guarantor window.

Payment Plan Tab The Payment Plan tab (Figure VI-3) contains data regarding a patient who has signed a financial agreement to pay the facility the balance on the account over a specific period of time.

Custom Tab The Custom tab is designed by the particular facility to contain information important to that facility. In the tutorial data for Medisoft, the Custom tab contains height, weight, and cigarette smoking data.

CASES

Information about a patient's insurance coverage, billing account, diagnosis, and condition are stored in cases. When a patient comes for treatment, a case is created. Cases are set up to contain the transactions that relate to a particular condition. For example, all treatments and procedures for bronchial asthma would be stored in a case called "Bronchial Asthma." Services performed and charges for those services are entered in the system linked to the bronchial asthma case.

In Medisoft cases are created, edited, and deleted from within the Patient List dialog box. When the Case radio button in the Patient List dialog box is clicked, the following buttons appear at the bottom of the Patient List dialog

box: Edit Case, New Case, Delete Case, Copy Case, and Close. These buttons perform their respective functions on cases. For example, to create a new case, the New Case button is clicked. Data recorded in the Case dialog box are stored by clicking the Save button on the right side of the Case dialog box.

Entering Case Information

Information on a patient is entered in 11 different tabs within the Case dialog box: Personal, Account, Diagnosis, Policy 1, Policy 2, Policy 3, Condition, Miscellaneous, Medicaid and Tricare, Comment, and EDI. A twelfth tab, Custom One, allows the facility to create and design its own Custom tabs as well.

Personal Tab

The Personal tab (Figure VI-4) contains basic information about a patient and his or her employment. The most important boxes that must be completed in the Personal tab are as follows:

Case Number—The case number is a unique sequential number *assigned by Medisoft.*

Description—Information entered in the Description box indicates a patient's complaint, or reason for seeing the physician.

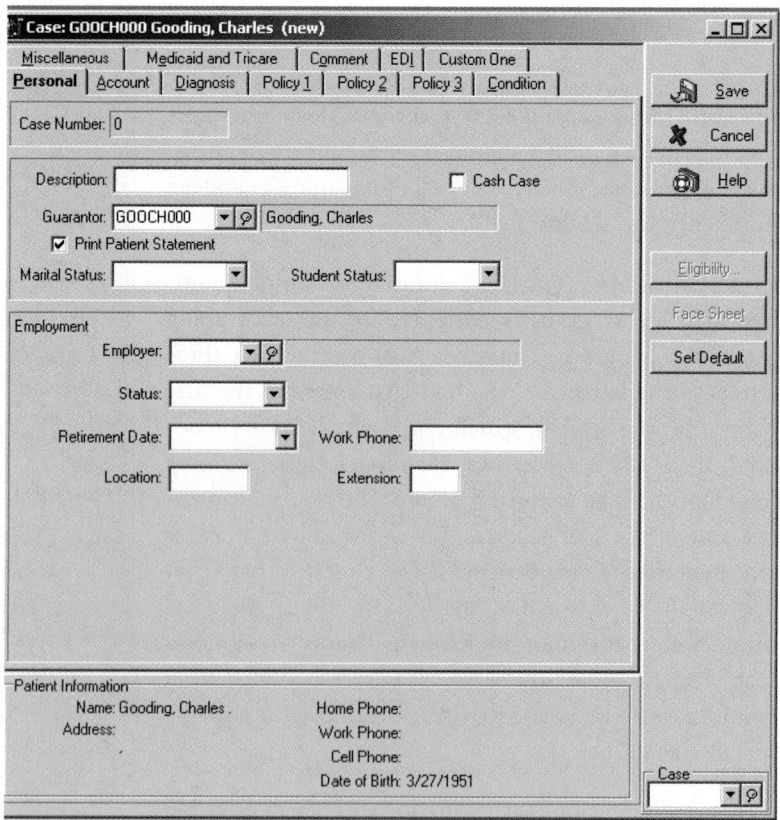

FIGURE VI-4 Case window, Personal tab.

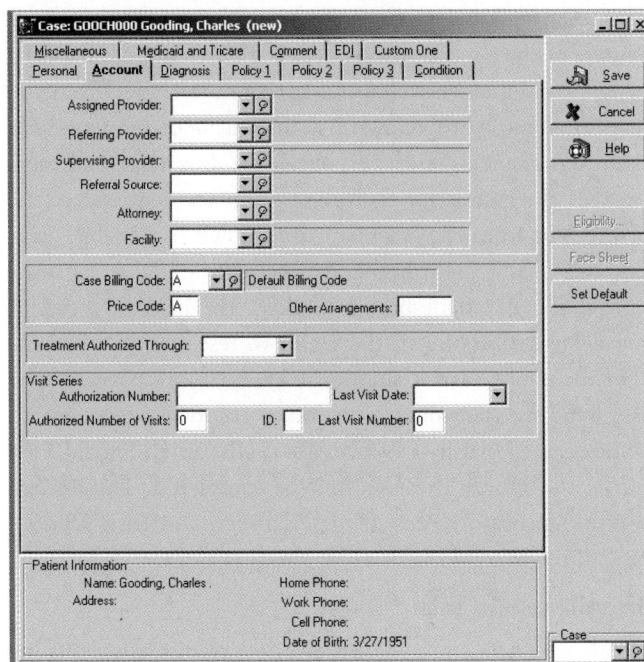

FIGURE VI-5 Case window, Account tab.

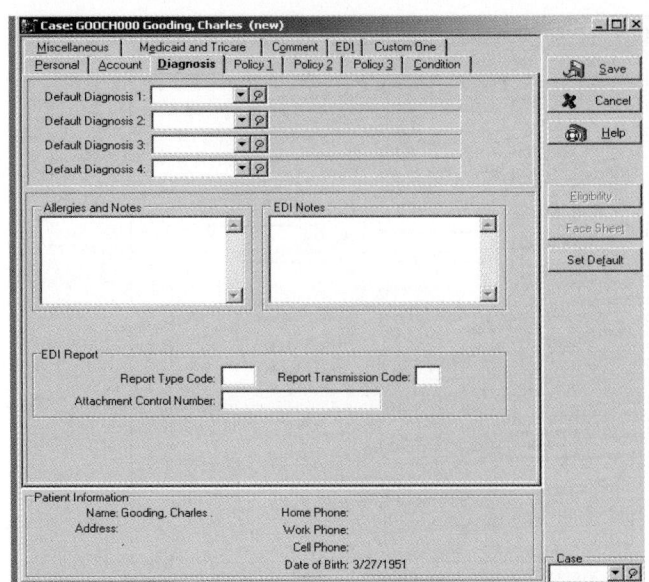

FIGURE VI-6 Case window, Diagnosis tab.

Guarantor—The Guarantor box lists the name of the person responsible for paying the bill.

Account Tab

The Account tab includes information on a patient's assigned provider, referring provider, referral source, as well as other information that may be used in some medical practices but not others (Figure VI-5). The most important boxes that must be completed in the Account tab are as follows:

Assigned Provider—The Assigned Provider box is automatically filled in with the code number and name of the assigned provider listed in the Patient/Guarantor dialog box.

Referring Provider—If the patient was referred to the facility by another provider, choose the referring provider's name from the drop-down list.

Facility—Choose the correct facility name from the drop-down box for the place the services were rendered.

Authorization Number—For patients whose insurance carrier requires a referral/authorization number for services, the number issued should be entered here along with the number of visits authorized and the referral expiration date.

Diagnosis Tab

The Diagnosis tab contains a patient's diagnosis, information about allergies, and electronic medical claim (EMC)

notes (Figure VI-6). The Allergies and Notes box is the most important box that must be completed in the Diagnosis tab.

Allergies and Notes If the patient is allergic to anything it should be entered here. This information is taken from the patient information form. Notes regarding payment arrangements, a forgotten copayment, or anything else are entered in this area as well.

You will not complete the Default Diagnosis 1 through 4 boxes. When you are setting up the case, you will not know the patient's diagnosis. After you have posted the charge transaction, the diagnosis code entered into the charge information will be transferred automatically by Medisoft to the Default Diagnosis boxes in this tab.

Policy 1, 2, and 3 Tabs

The Policy tabs are where information about a patient's insurance carrier and coverage is recorded (Figure VI-7). If a patient has more than one insurance policy, the Policy 2 and 3 tabs are used. The following boxes are the most important ones to be completed in the Policy tabs:

Insurance 1—The Insurance 1 box lists the patient's insurance carrier name, which is chosen from the drop-down list.

Policy Holder 1—This box shows the name of the insured person, which is chosen from the drop-down list. (This may or may not be the patient.) The guarantor must be entered in to the Patient List so that he or she can be chosen from the drop-down list here.

Relationship to Insured—This box indicates the patient's relationship to the individual listed in the Policy Holder 1 box.

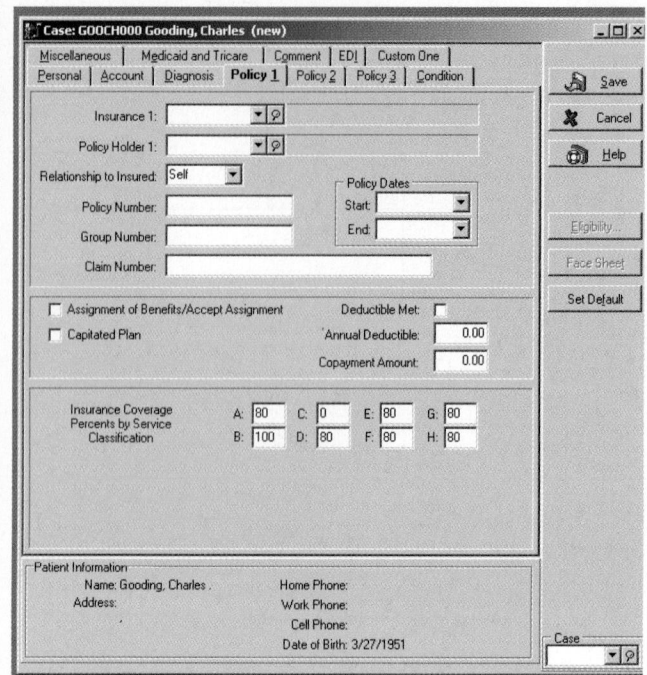

FIGURE VI-7 Case window, Policy 1 tab.

Policy Number—The patient's insurance policy or ID number is entered in the Policy Number box.

Group Number—If there is a group number for a patient's policy, it is entered in the Group Number box.

Assignment of Benefits/Accept Assignment—Check this box if the patient has assigned insurance benefits to the provider.

Insurance Coverage Percents by Service Classification—The percentage of fees that an insurance carrier covers is entered in the Insurance Coverage Percents box. The default entry in this box is 80. The default can be changed by highlighting the default entry and keying the correct percentage over the default. Some insurance policies pay different percentages of charges based on the type of service rendered. For example, a carrier may pay 100 percent for well-man or well-woman exams and 50 percent for lab charges.

Condition Tab

The Condition tab stores data about a patient's illness, accident, disability, and hospitalization. This information is used by insurance carriers to process claims (Figure VI-8).

The top portion of the Condition tab is completed with the date of the illness, injury, or last menstrual period (if the patient is pregnant). Make the appropriate choice from the Illness Indicator drop-down list. If treatment rendered was for an emergency condition, check the box next to Emergency. If the case is for treatment of an accident, select the correct type from the Accident drop-down list. If the "accident" was just a fall at home, it is not considered a true accident. If the Accident box is marked, the insurance carrier may delay processing of the claim to research whether another insurance carrier should be the primary payer. If the case, icluding treatment, is workers' compensation related, the boxes for Unable to Work, Total Disability, Partial Disability, and Hospitalization may be completed. The Return to Work Indicator, Percent of Disability, and Last Worked Date all relate to workers' compensation cases.

Miscellaneous Tab

The Miscellaneous tab records a variety of miscellaneous information about the patient and his or her treatment, including outside lab work, prior authorization numbers, and other information (Figure VI-9). For the authorization number to print out on the CMS-1500 form, it must be entered in the Miscellaneous tab.

Medicaid and Tricare Tab

For patients covered by Medicaid or TRICARE, the Medicaid and Tricare tab is used to enter additional information about the government program (Figure VI-10).

FIGURE VI-8 Case window, Condition tab.

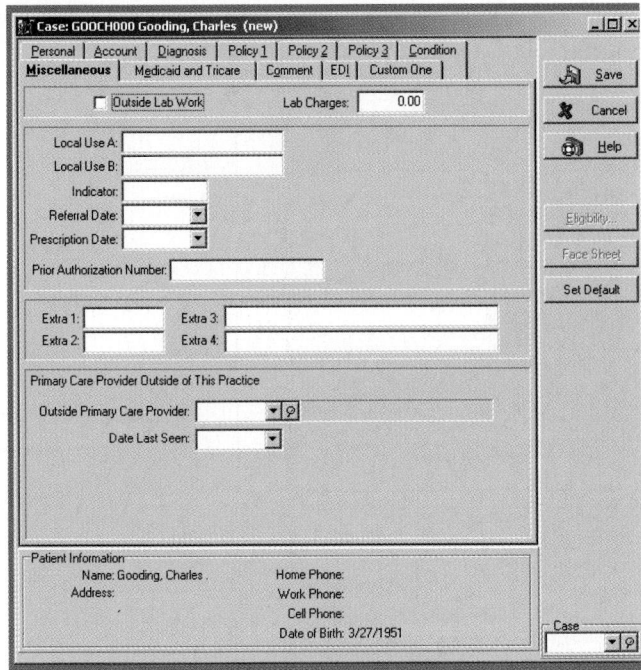

FIGURE VI-9   Case window, Miscellaneous tab.

Comment Tab

Any comments or notes pertinent to this patient's case may be entered into the Comment tab (Figure VI-11).

EDI Tab

Information necessary for the processing or transmission of electronic data interchange (EDI) data is entered in the EDI tab (Figure VI-12).

FIGURE VI-10   Case window, Medicaid and Tricare tab.

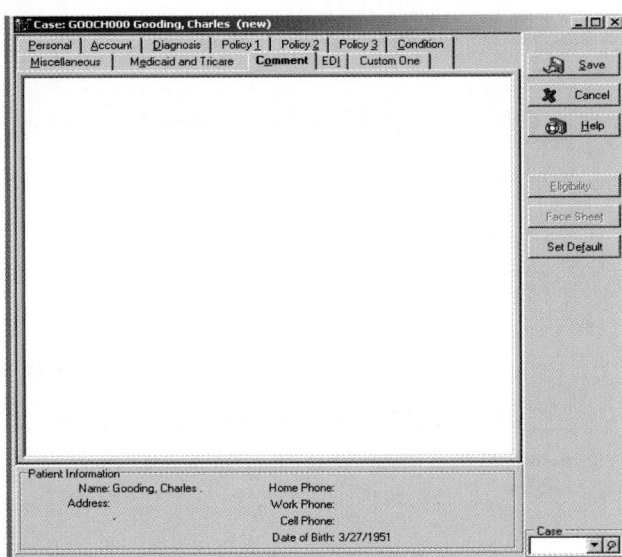

FIGURE VI-11   Case window, Comment tab.

ADDING THE INSURANCE CARRIERS

If, when you are in the patient's Case window and entering the insurance carrier name, you notice the insurance carrier you are looking for is *not* in the drop-down list, you must go to the Insurance Carrier List to add it (Figure VI-13). This can be accessed via a shortcut button or the Lists menu.

Click on the New button to add a new carrier name and address.

In the Address tab of the new Insurance Carrier window, enter the insurance carrier's name, address, telephone

FIGURE VI-12   Case window, EDI tab.

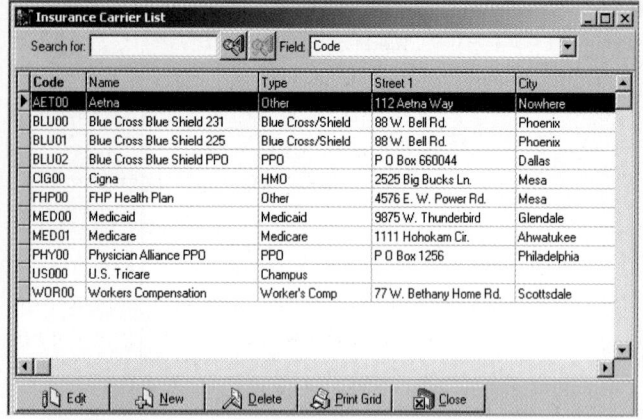

FIGURE VI-13 Adding an insurance carrier in the Insurance Carrier window.

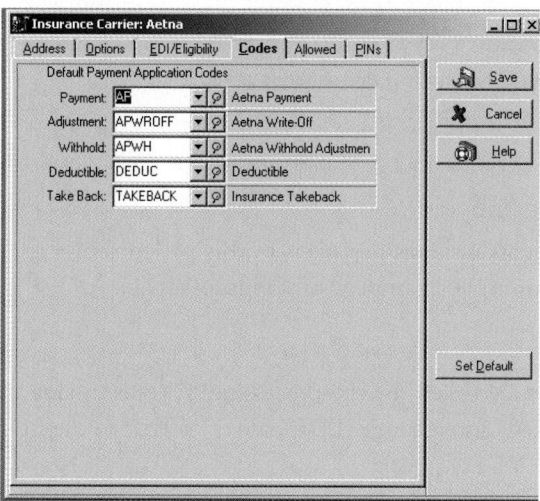

FIGURE VI-15 Insurance Carrier window, EDI/Eligibility tab.

number, fax number, and contact name if you have one (Figure VI-14).

The Options tab in the new Insurance Carrier window is vitally important because it is here that you choose the insurance plan type and indicate whether or not "Signature on File" (SOF) should appear on the claim form. SOF indicates that you have the patient's authorization to release this information and that the patient has assigned benefits directly to the provider (Figure VI-14). (So the payment for the claim will be sent directly to your provider and not the patient.) "Signature on File" should *always* appear on the claim forms you submit.

The EDI/Eligibility tab is used to enter important EDI information for that insurance carrier (Figure VI-15).

The Codes tab is for entering default transactions codes (Figure VI-16).

FIGURE VI-16 Insurance Carrier window, Codes tab.

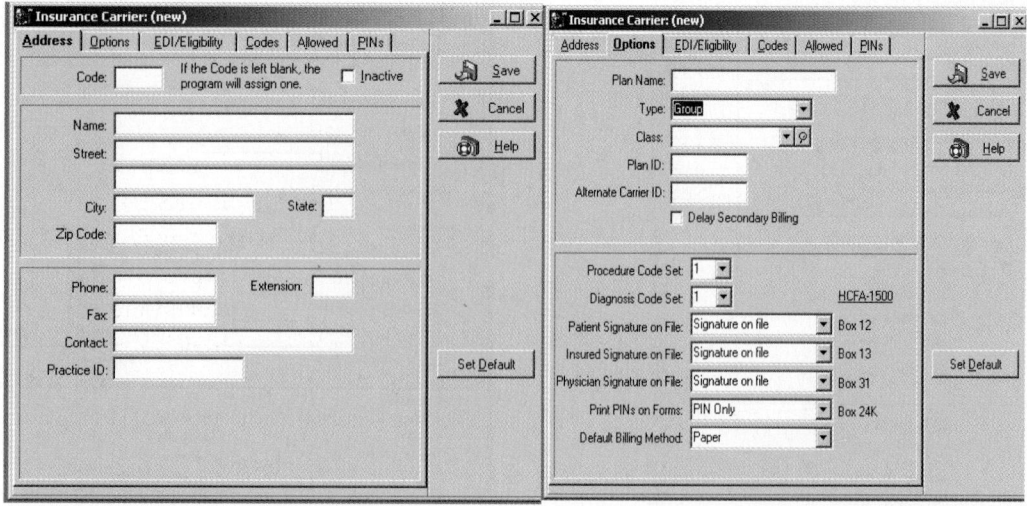

FIGURE VI-14 New Insurance Carrier window, Address tab (left) and Options tab (right).

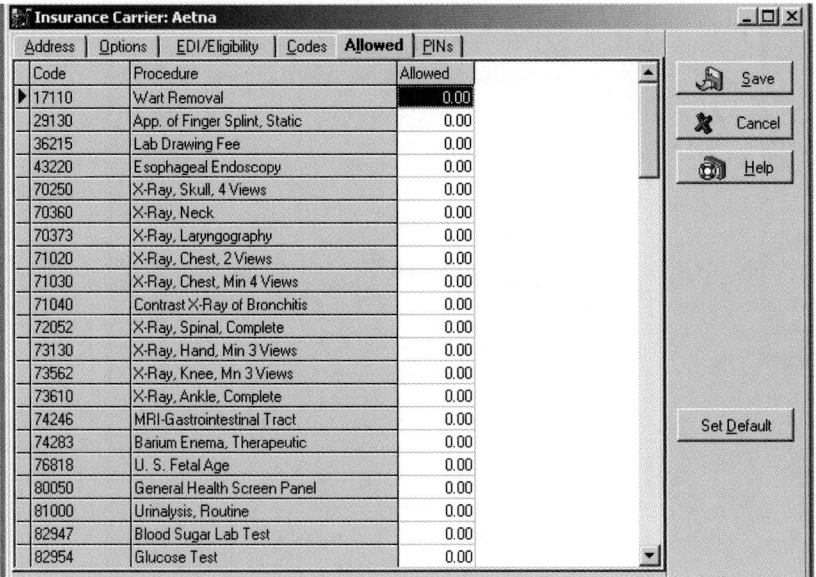

FIGURE VI-17 Insurance Carrier window, Allowed tab.

The Allowed tab may be used to enter the contractual allowed amount per procedure code for that particular insurance carrier (Figure VI-17).

The PINs tab in the Insurance Carrier List is also very important (Figure VI-18). You must first Save your new carrier,

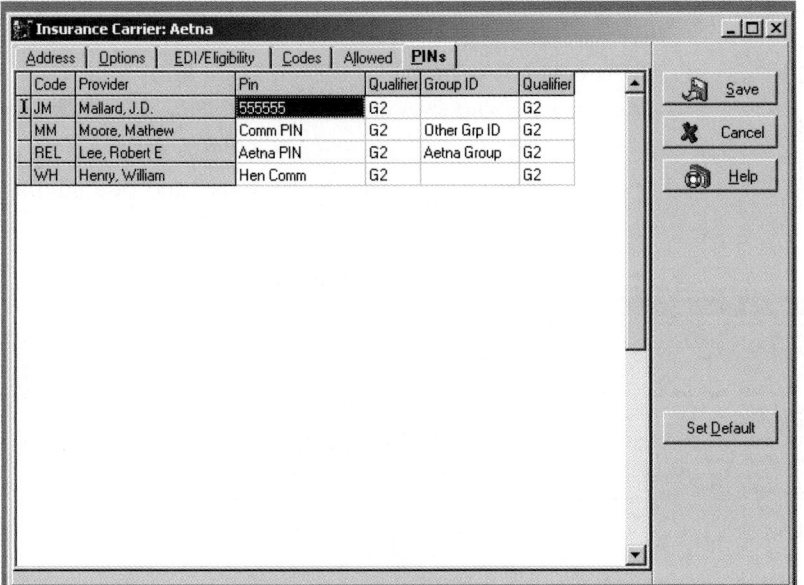

FIGURE VI-18 Insurance Carrier window, PINs tab.

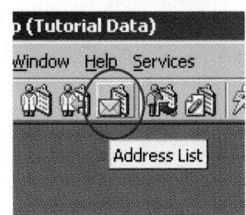

FIGURE VI-19 Address List shortcut button on the taskbar.

then go back in and Edit it to add the provider PINs. PINs are specific to each carrier. Be sure to enter the correct insurance carrier PIN for each participating provider. The appropriate qualifier should also be entered so that it prints on the CMS-1500 claim form.

ENTERING EMPLOYERS

When entering patient and case information, it will be necessary to add the patient's or guarantor's employer name/address into Medisoft. This is accomplished in the Address List, which is accessed from the taskbar using the Address List shortcut button (Figure VI-19).

The Address List contains not only employer addresses but also referral sources (other than physicians), facility addresses, and attorney addresses (Figure VI-20).

Click on the New button to begin (Figure VI-21). Add the employer name, address and telephone number.

If you are entering an employer (and not a referral source, etc.), in the Type field, be sure Employer is shown (Figure VI-22). Click Save when you have finished entering the information.

You can now select the Employer name from the drop-down list in the Patient List or Case windows.

REVIEWING A COMPLETED SUPERBILL

The completed superbill is the primary source of information a medical office specialist needs to record procedure charges. The completed superbill includes the following information: provider's name, patient's name and chart/account number, date services were performed, diagnosis, charge amounts, amount of payment received at time of service, and next appointment time needed.

After a physician completes a patient exam, he or she will place a check mark (or an X or circle) on the superbill next to the procedures performed. As you may recall, the superbill includes only the most common procedures provided by the medical office. If the physician performs a procedure not listed on the superbill, he or she writes the procedure in the "Other Procedures" area or in a blank space on the form.

Insurance carriers will not pay for treatment without a diagnosis code. The diagnosis is the physician's opinion of the patient's condition based on the examination. Therefore,

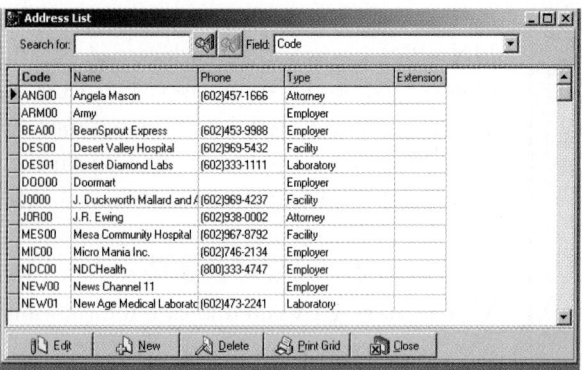

FIGURE VI-20 Address List window.

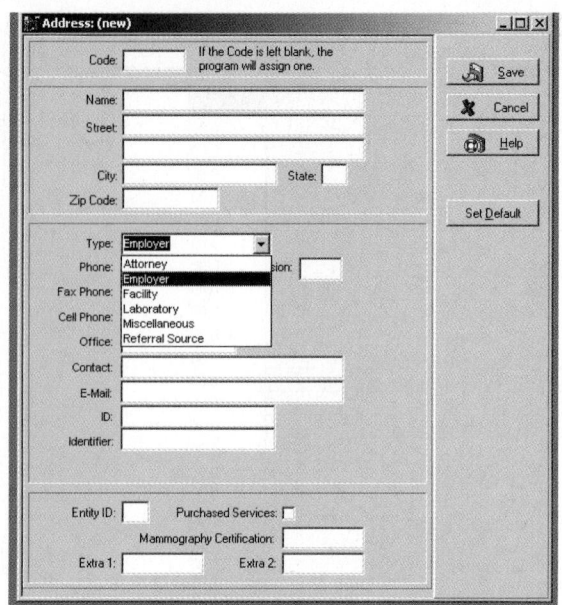

FIGURE VI-22 In the Type field of the new Address window, be sure to choose "Employer" when entering a new employer.

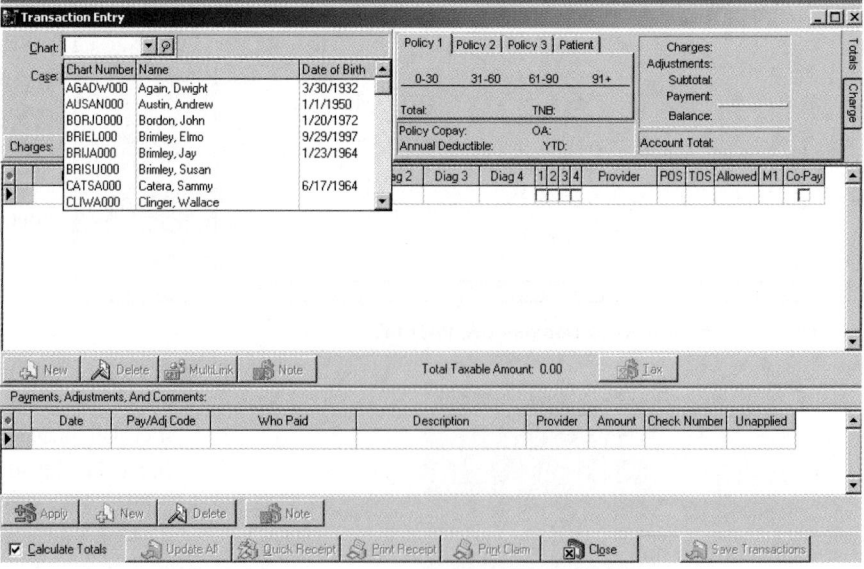

FIGURE VI-21 New Address window.

the physician must record this information on the superbill so that it may be included as part of the procedure charge. If a procedure code or diagnosis is not marked on the superbill, you must ask the physician to mark it. Never demand that the physician do so, and never accuse the physician of forgetting to mark the superbill. Always use respect and tact when addressing members of your medical practice.

ENTERING A PROCEDURE CHARGE

After you review a patient's superbill, you are ready to enter the transaction into Medisoft to record the procedure charge and diagnosis code. You will process all

transactions (charges, payments, and adjustments) in the Transaction Entry window. To access this window, you can use the Activities menu and click on Enter Transactions, click the Transaction Entry shortcut button or click the Accounting menu on the Medisoft side bar and choose Enter Transactions.

After you have opened the Transaction Entry window, *the first thing you must do is choose the correct patient's chart number and case number to which you will post a charge.*

Step 1: Choose a patient chart number and case number (Figure VI-23).

FIGURE VI-23 Begin working in the Transaction Entry window by choosing a patient chart number and case number.

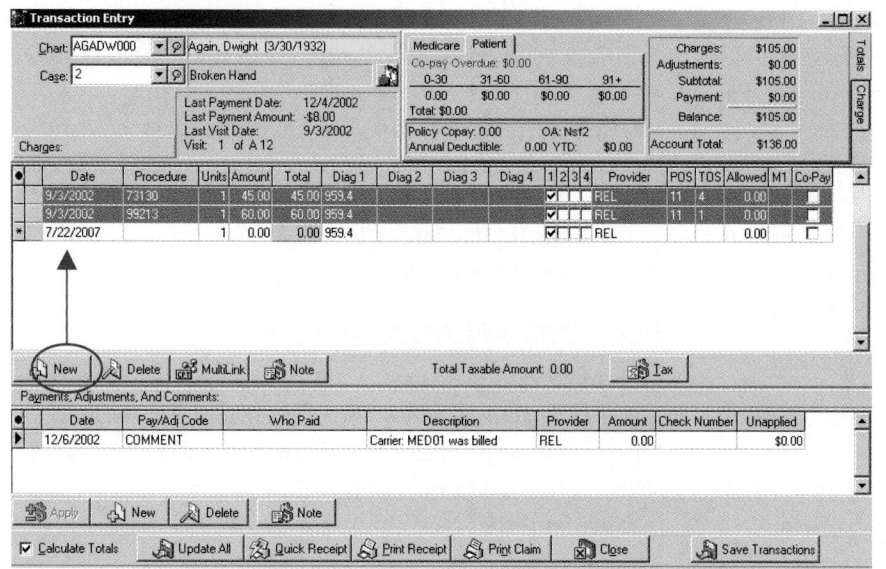

FIGURE VI-24 After choosing the correct patient and case, choose the New button from the middle of the screen.

Step 2: After the correct patient and case have been chosen, click on the New button in the *middle* of the screen (to access the top of the screen) (Figure VI-24).

Medisoft will add today's date by default to the screen. If the date of service is not today's date, type the correct date in the Date field.

Click your mouse inside the Procedure field next to the date. A drop-down menu will be shown. You may either search for the correct procedure code marked on the superbill or type it in.

Once you have entered the CPT code, press Enter or Tab to be taken to the Units field. Most of the time you will not need to change the default units entry.

Press Tab or Enter to move to the Amount field. Medisoft will have already entered a dollar amount associated with that CPT code. If this amount is incorrect, key in the correct amount.

Press Tab or Enter again to be taken to the DIAG1 field. Type in the primary diagnosis code or use the drop-down menu to search for the correct diagnosis. You may enter up to four diagnosis codes per charge transaction.

Tab over to the Provider field to make sure the correct provider is being credited with seeing this patient.

The POS (place of service) and TOS (type of service) fields will automatically be filled in based on the information in the CPT code database.

The Allowed amount field is also completed by default per information in the CPT code and insurance database.

The M1 field is used to enter a two-character CPT modifier if one is marked on the patient superbill.

Complete all these steps again to enter another procedure charge.

When you have finished entering charges, click on the Save Transactions button at the lower right of the screen or the Update All button near the lower left side of the window. When the Update All button is used to save transactions, the Medisoft program checks all fields for missing or invalid information and will display a message if information is needed or invalid.

POSTING A PAYMENT

When the patient (or his or her insurance carrier) makes a payment on the patient's account, you must enter this into the accounting software. Payments are posted in the Transaction Entry window (Figure VI-25). Remember, you cannot enter a transaction without first choosing a patient chart number and case number. It is important to make sure you have chosen the correct case—especially when posting payments from insurance carriers.

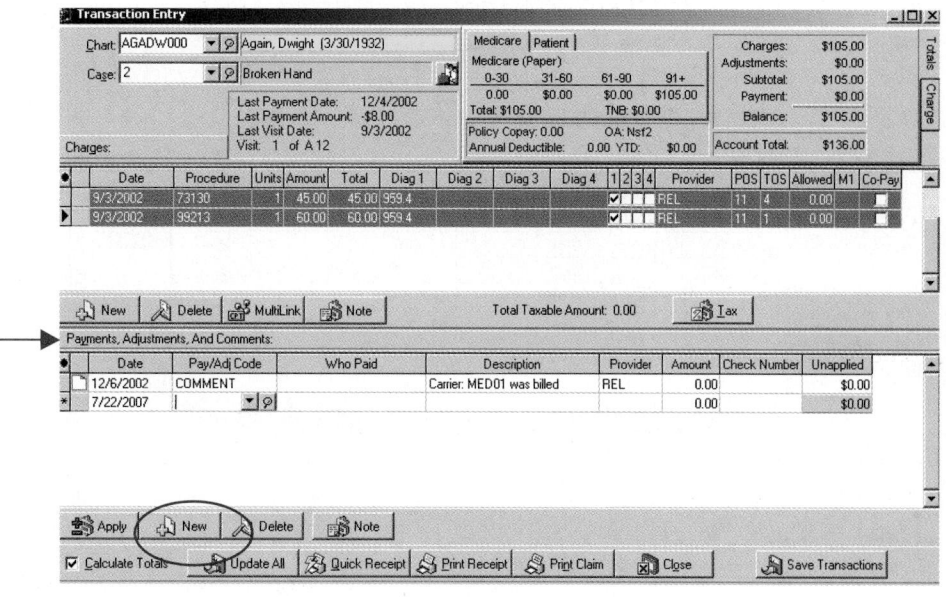

FIGURE VI-25 Posting payments in the Transaction Entry window.

After opening the Transaction Entry window and choosing the appropriate chart and case number, click on the New button toward the *bottom* of the window within the Payments, Adjustments, and Comments section.

Medisoft will start a new entry by adding today's date.

Click in the Pay/Adj Code field and choose the method of payment (personal check, cash, Aetna payment, etc.).

Tab over to the Who Paid field and choose the party that is making the payment.

Enter a description if necessary.

Make sure the correct provider is shown in the Provider field.

Enter the amount of the payment in the Amount field. Enter a check number if appropriate in the next field.

Next, *you must apply the payment to the correct charge(s)*. To do this, click on the Apply button at the bottom left-hand side of the window, to the left of the New button (Figure VI-26).

A new window will open on top of your Transaction Entry window. This is the Apply Payment to Charges window. It is here that you can apply the payment to a specific charge or charges. This is called *line item posting*.

It is most important to post the payment to the correct date of service and the correct procedure code. One payment can be divided among many charges if it is "broken down" that way on the EOB/ERA or the patient has many separate charges and is paying for all of them.

When you have applied the payment to the correct charge(s), click the Close button at the bottom of the Apply Payment to Charges window.

Your Unapplied column in the Payment, Adjustment, and Comments section of the Transaction Entry window should read $0.00 if you applied the entire payment. (A patient's account may have an unapplied balance if he or she is prepaying on surgery, for example.) You must now save the payment transaction.

Click on the Update All or Save Transactions button at the bottom of the window.

POSTING AN ADJUSTMENT

Entering an adjustment into a patient's account is similar to entering a payment and is also performed in the Transaction Entry window. To begin, you must first choose the patient chart number and case number.

Click on the New button toward the *bottom* of the window.

Medisoft will start a new transaction by entering today's date by default.

In the Pay/Adj Code field, select the correct type of adjustment (insurance write-off, charge reversal, courtesy discount, etc.).

Tab over to the Description entry field and type a note about why the adjustment is needed.

Tab over to the Provider field and choose the correct provider, then tab over to the Amount field.

If you are *subtracting* an amount from the patient's account, you must enter a minus (–) sign before typing the amount. If you are adding an amount to a patient's account, you do not need to enter a plus sign before the amount.

Note: Medisoft will assume all adjustments are positive unless you type in a minus (–) sign before the amount.

When you have entered the amount, click on the Apply button at the bottom left of the Transaction Entry window.

When you are applying the adjustment, make sure to choose the correct date(s) of service and CPT code(s). *You must enter a minus sign before the amount in the Apply Adjustment to Charges window.* If you do not, Medisoft *will add* the amount to the patient's account.

When you have entered all the adjustments, click on the Close button to take you back to the Transaction Entry window.

To save all your hard work, be sure to click on Update All or Save Transactions.

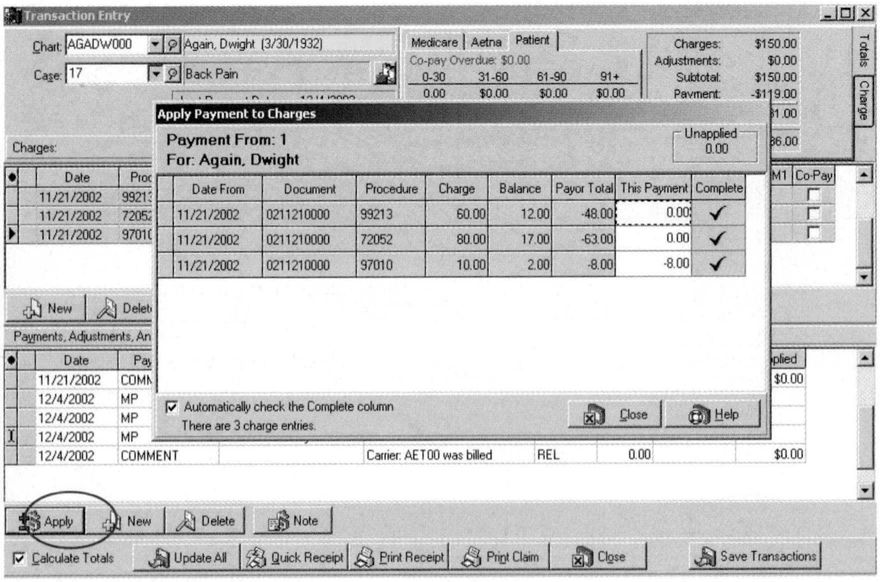

FIGURE VI-26 **Applying a payment to the correct charges.**

USING THE ENTER DEPOSITS AND APPLY PAYMENTS WINDOW

It is easiest to post payments that patients make at the time of service in the Transaction Entry window. However, if you receive a large insurance check that covers claims for many different patients, it is easier to post this in the Enter Deposits and Apply Payments window. This window can be accessed by clicking the Enter Deposits and Apply Payments shortcut button, opening the Activities menu and choosing Apply Deposits/Payments, or by clicking on the Accounting shortcut button on the Medisoft side bar and choosing Enter Deposits/Payments. A Deposit List window will open (Figure VI-27) that contains the following fields:

Deposit Date—The current date is automatically entered. It can be changed by typing a different date in the field.

Show All Deposits—This check box displays all payments entered regardless of date.

Show Unapplied Only—If this box is checked, only the payments that have not been fully applied to charges are shown.

Sort By—This is a drop-down list that allows you to sort deposits by amount, patient chart number, and payer.

Locate and Locate Next—These shortcut buttons allow you to search for a particular deposit.

Detail—This button is used to view a specific deposit in more detail. Highlight the deposit in the window and then click the Detail button.

To enter a new deposit, click on the New button at the bottom of the Deposit List window. After the New Deposit window opens (Figure VI-28), you must choose a Payor Type (patient, insurance carrier, capitation).

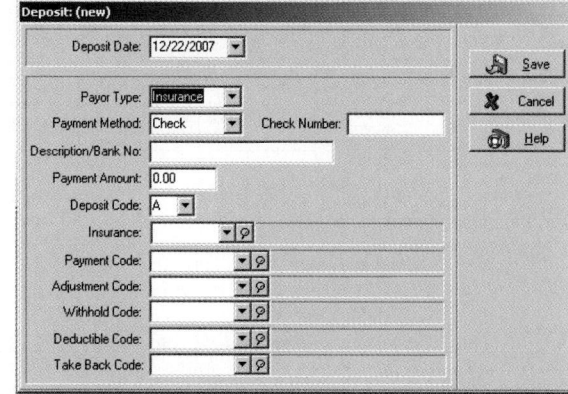

FIGURE VI-28 New Deposit window.

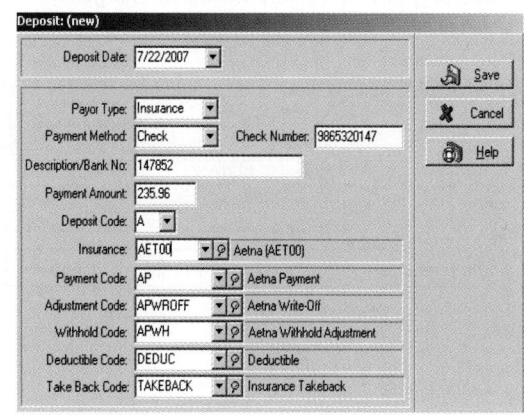

FIGURE VI-29 The various code fields are filled in automatically when the insurance carrier is selected from the Insurance drop-down box.

Choose the Payment Method (check, cash, credit card, electronic) and Enter or Tab over to the Check Number field to enter the check number.

The Description/Bank No. field is used to enter an (optional) description of the check.

Enter the dollar amount of the payment in the Payment Amount field.

The Deposit Code drop-down menu is used by some practices to sort deposits according to practice-defined categories.

Select the insurance carrier making payment from the drop-down menu in the Insurance field.

After you have selected the carrier, the other Code fields are automatically completed (Figure VI-29).

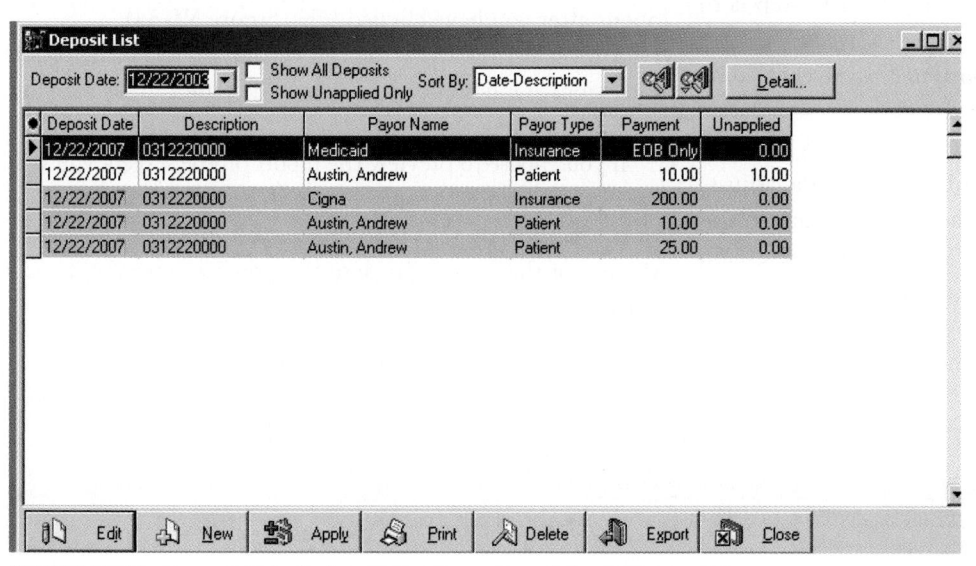

FIGURE VI-27 Deposit List window (Enter Deposits and Apply Payments).

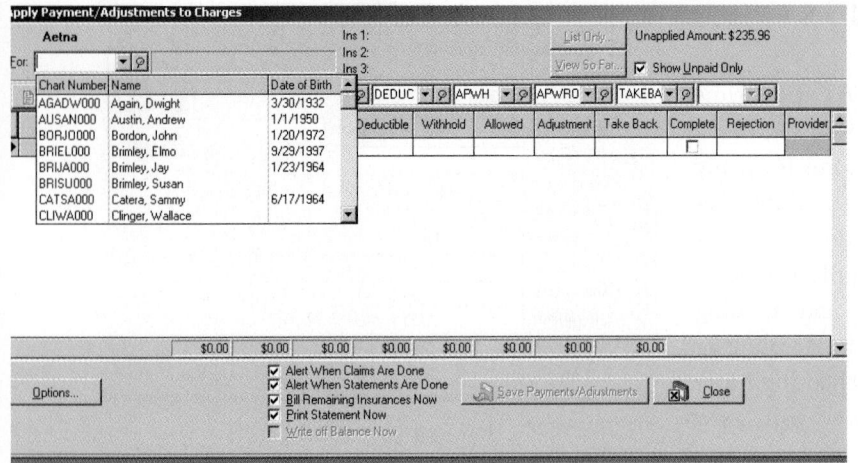

FIGURE VI-30 The Apply Payments/Adjustments to Charges window.

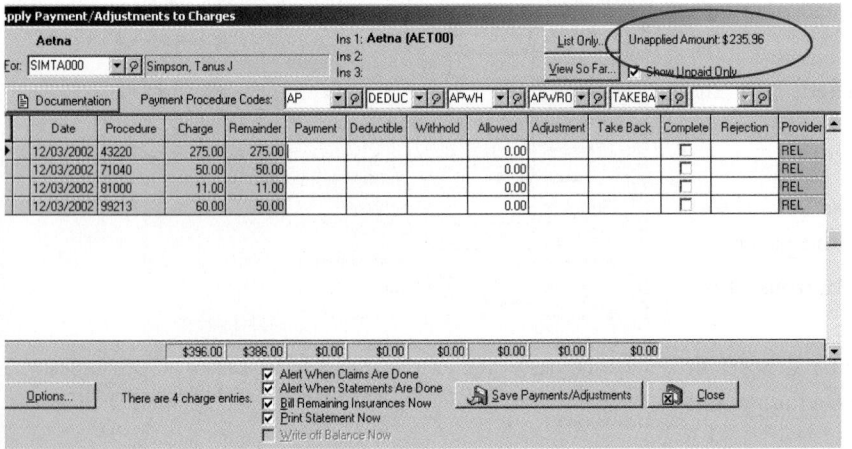

FIGURE VI-31 The Unapplied Amount indicator tells you how much of a deposit remains to be posted.

When finished, click Save.

After entering the check information, the next step is to apply the payment.

Click the Apply button at the bottom of the Deposit List window.

The Apply Payment/Adjustments to Charges window (Figure VI-30) is where you will apply payments and adjustments (if needed) to specific patient accounts. You are able to enter payments and adjustments as well as deductibles and withhold information at virtually the same time.

When you have finished entering payment information on one patient, click the Save Payments/Adjustments button at the bottom right side of the window.

If you have the Print Statements Now box at the bottom of the window checked, after clicking Save, Medisoft

will ask what type of statement you would like to print.

If you have another patient to apply payments to, follow the same steps as before.

The Unapplied Amount indicator in the top right-hand corner of the window will allow you to keep track of how much you have posted and how much you still have to post (Figure VI-31).

WALKOUT RECEIPTS

Throughout the simulation at the end of this appendix, you will be responsible for printing a walkout receipt for each patient who has seen the provider. This task is performed in the Transaction Entry window.

After you have posted the patient's charges and/or payments, click the Quick Receipt button at the bottom of the window to print a receipt for today's visit only (Figure VI-32). A Print Report Where? window will open. After choosing to print to the printer, the receipt will automatically print.

If the patient would like a more comprehensive receipt (one that includes previous visits), click the Print Receipt button instead.

When the Open Report window opens, choose Walkout Receipt (All Transactions), then click the OK button (Figure VI-33). A Print Report Where? window opens after you have clicked OK (Figure VI-34).

After selecting where to print the report, a Data Selection Questions window opens. Choose the date ranges for your receipt and click the OK button.

If you choose to preview the report on the screen, you will see a screen similar to that shown in Figure VI-35. To print from the preview screen, click the picture of the printer at the top of the screen. To close the preview screen, click the Close button.

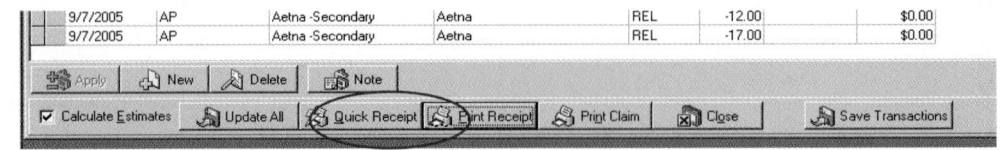

FIGURE VI-32 Quick Receipt button.

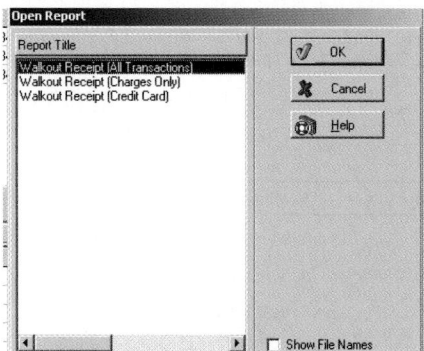

FIGURE VI-33   Open Report window.

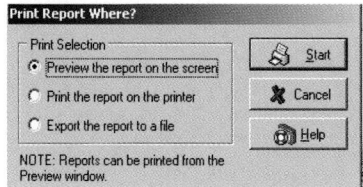

FIGURE VI-34   Print Report Where? window.

PRINTING REPORTS IN MEDISOFT

Let's take a moment to discuss the different reports available in Medisoft.

Patient Day Sheet Report

The Patient Day Sheet report can be accessed in either of two ways: by clicking on the Reports menu or by clicking the Daily Reports menu on the Medisoft side bar.

For the simulation that follows, you will be instructed to stop entering transactions and "batch out." You must compile and run the Patient Day Sheet report. This report, as stated previously, shows all transactions posted in the database for the day. For our purposes, we will use "today's" date.

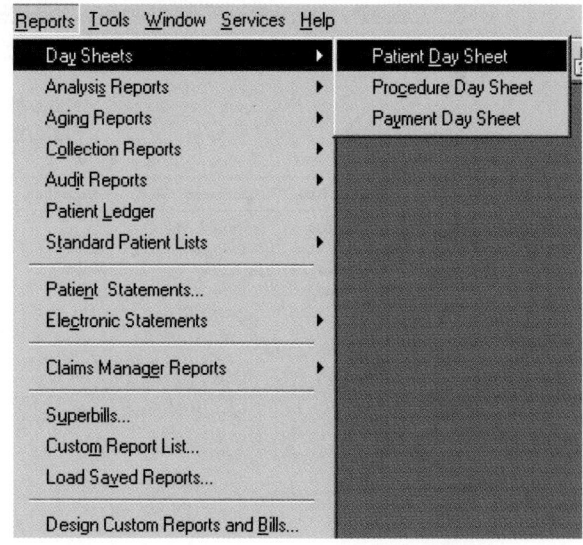

FIGURE VI-36   Selecting the Patient Day Sheet report from the Reports drop-down menu.

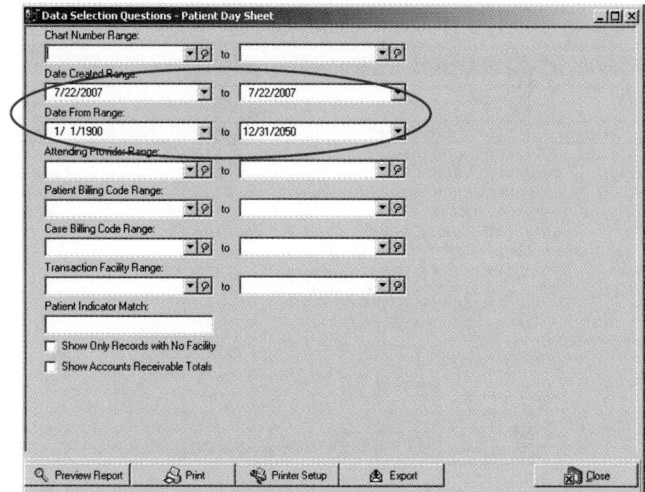

FIGURE VI-37   Data Selection Questions for Patient Day Sheet Reports.

After clicking on Patient Day Sheet in the Reports menu (Figure VI-36), a Print Report Where? window will open. After choosing where to print the report (our example printed it to the screen), another window/dialog box will open: Data Selection Questions: Patient Day Sheet (Figure VI-37).

Click in the Date Created Range field and choose today's date for both the From and To boxes, then click the OK button.

Using the arrows at the top of the screen, go to the last page of the report for your totals. Your totals here should match your

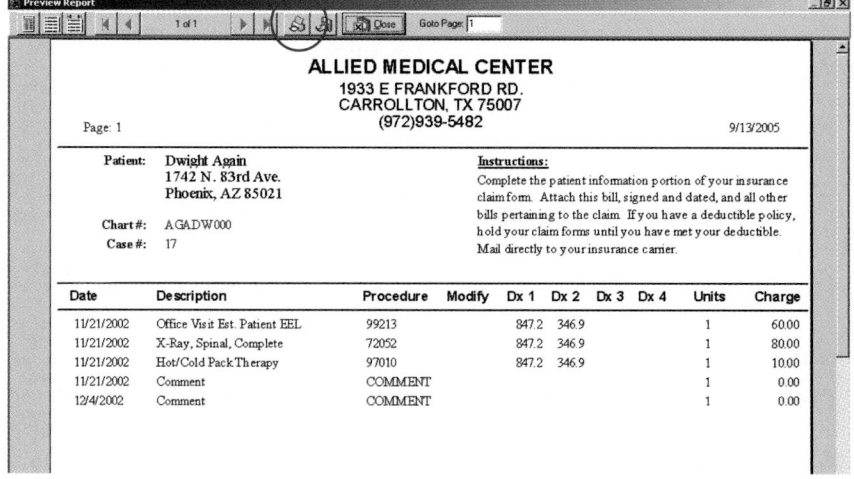

FIGURE VI-35   Sample walkout receipt.

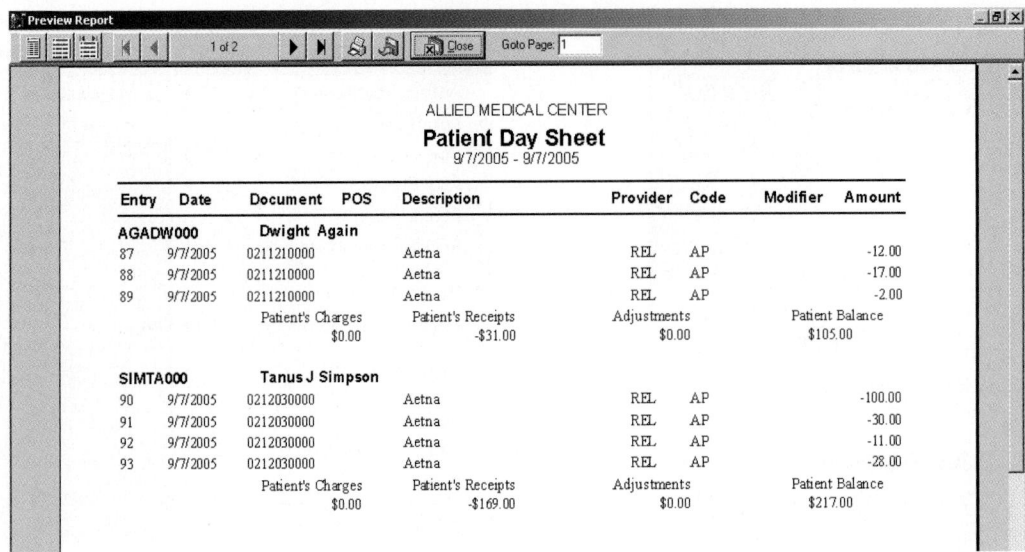

FIGURE VI-38 Sample Patient Day Sheet report.

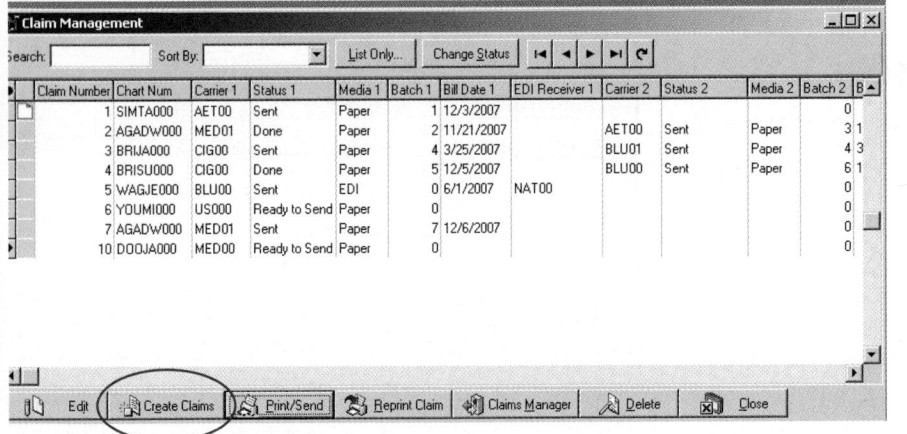

FIGURE VI-39 To process new insurance claims, click the Create Claims button in the Claim Management window.

totals from all the superbills/EOBs you posted throughout the day (Figure VI-38).

CREATING AND PRINTING INSURANCE CLAIMS

During the simulation that follows, you will be responsible for printing paper CMS-1500 claim forms at the end of each day for the patients' accounts to which you posted charges. This task is accomplished in the Claim Management window.

The Claim Management window can be accessed by clicking the Claim Management shortcut button, clicking the Accounting button on the Medisoft side bar, or by opening the Activities menu and clicking Claim Management.

After opening the Claim Management window, the first thing to do is create the insurance claims you want to send. To do this you click the Create Claims button at the bottom of the window (Figure VI-39).

The majority of medical practices print claims several times a week. You will notice, again, that you can sort your claim report many different ways: by transaction dates, chart numbers, primary insurance carrier—you can even create claims for one particular provider name. For the simulation you will be using today's date in the Transaction Dates field (Figure VI-40). After entering the dates, click the Create button on the right side of the window.

As you create a claim, the Claim Management window will be automatically updated. It will show the claims you've just created as "Ready to Send" in the Status 1 column of the Claim Management window (Figure VI-41).

The next step is to look over your claims *before* you print them to make sure they are "clean" claims (meaning no information is missing and all information is correct).

To do this, click on the Print/Send button at the *bottom* of the Claim Management window (Figure VI-42).

A Print/Send Claims window will open and ask you to choose how you wish to send the claims, either on paper or electronically. For our simulation, you will choose the Paper method for claims. Click the OK button on the right side of the window (Figure VI-43).

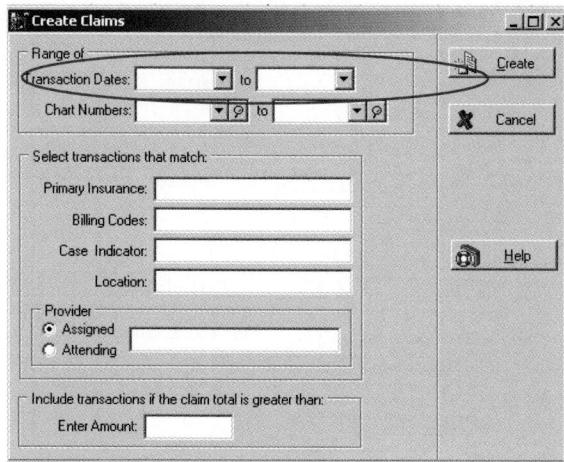

FIGURE VI-40 The Transaction Dates field in the Create Claims window.

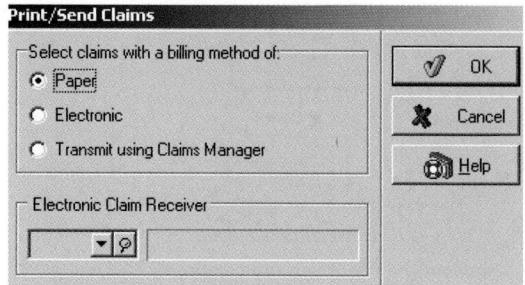

FIGURE VI-43 Print/Send Claims window.

An Open Report window will open next (Figure VI-44). If you are printing Medicare claims, you must choose the CMS-1500 (Primary) Medicare Century report option. If you are printing claims for any other carrier, choose the CMS-1500 (Primary) report option. It is important to choose the correct report type for claims. Medicare prefers a minimum of information on claims, so be sure to choose the correct report/claim format when submitting claims to Medicare. After choosing the report style, click the OK button.

When the Print Report Where? window opens, choose to Preview the report on the screen and click Start (Figure VI-45). You will look over the claims on the screen to be sure they are clean before printing.

A Data Selection Questions dialog box will open for you to choose which claims you want to preview. Use today's date in the Date Created Range fields. You can "filter"

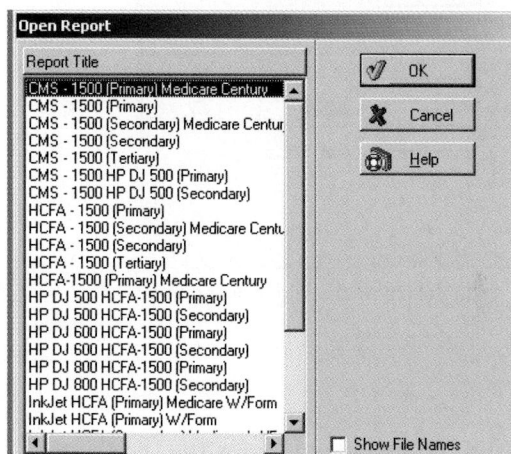

FIGURE VI-44 Open Report window.

those claims you would like to review. Filtering is selecting certain criteria. For example, you may choose to only review claims for a particular insurance carrier (e.g., Medicaid). To do that, you would select the name of the insurance carrier from the drop-down menu from the Insurance Carrier 1 Range boxes. This would filter out all the other

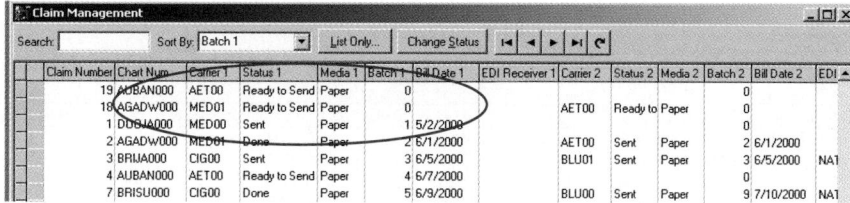

FIGURE VI-41 The Status 1 column indicates which newly created claims are ready to send to insurance carriers.

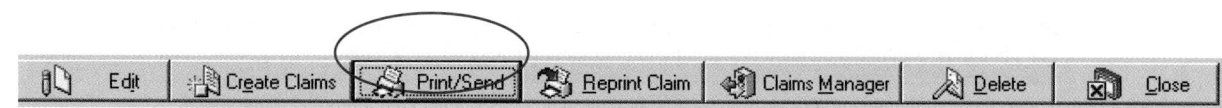

FIGURE VI-42 Print/Send button at the bottom of the Claim Management window.

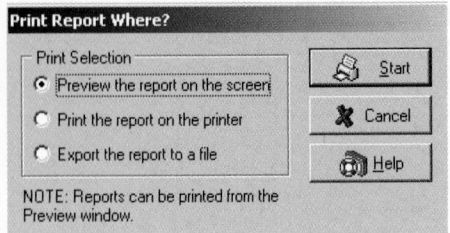

FIGURE VI-45 Preview the report on the screen.

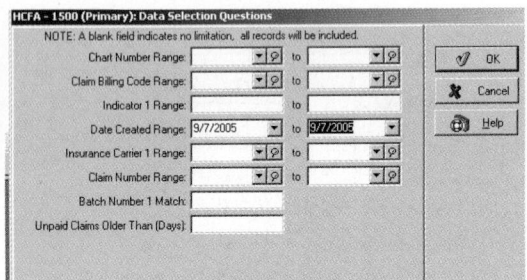

FIGURE VI-46 Data Selection Questions dialog box.

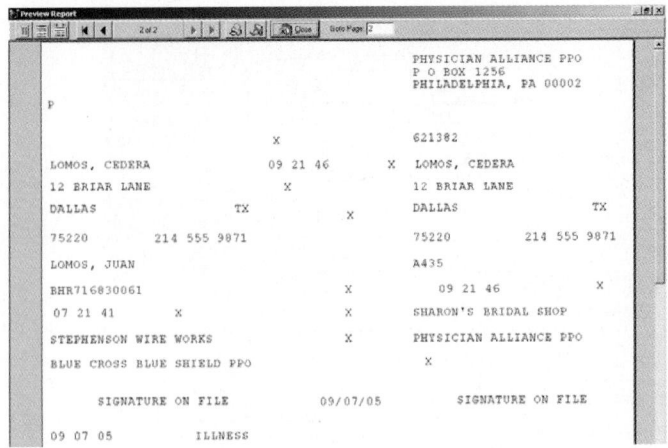

FIGURE VI-47 Sample CMS-1500 Primary claim printed to screen. Note that the locator boxes do not show on screen.

insurance carrier claims and only show you the claims for the carrier you chose from the drop-down menu. You can filter claims by Chart Number Range, Claim Billing Code Range, or Claim Number Range. After choosing your filters, click OK (Figure VI-46). If you want to see all claims created, complete only the Date Created Range boxes.

The claims will be shown on the screen in the format you chose. Note that the CMS-1500 locator boxes will not actually show on the screen because they are instead printed on

the blank claim form originals that you will insert into your printer when you're ready to print claims. However, you may want to refer to a blank printed claim form while checking your claims on screen to see if any information is missing (Figure VI-47).

Once you have checked all your claims and corrected any mistakes if necessary, you are ready to print your claims on CMS-1500 forms that you have loaded into your printer's paper tray.

After you have printed your claims, Medisoft will update your Claim Management window (Status 1 column) to show that the claims have been sent (on paper or electronically) (Figure VI-48).

Table VI-1 shows the relationship between the form locators on the CMS-1500 claim form and the dialog boxes in Medisoft. If, when looking over the claim forms before

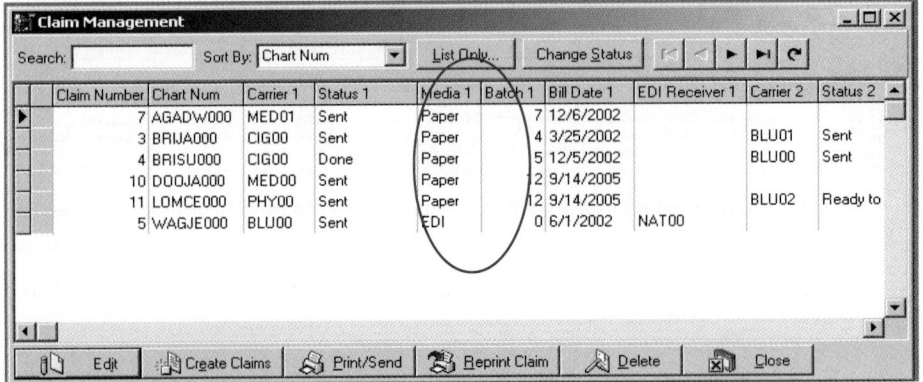

FIGURE VI-48 Medisoft will update your Claim Management window to indicate that the claims have been sent.

Source: CPT is a registered trademark of the American Medical Association.

Patient/Guarantor Information and the CMS-1500 Form

CMS Form Locator	Medisoft		
	Dialog Box	TAB (in Dialog Box)	Field (in Dialog Box)
1	Insurance Carrier	Options	Type
1a	Case	Policy	Policy Number
2	Patient/Guarantor	Name, Address	Last Name, First Name, Middle Initial
3	Patient/Guarantor	Name, Address	Birth Date, Sex
4	Case	Policy	Policy Holder
5	Patient/Guarantor	Name, Address	Street, City, State, Zip Code, Phones
6	Case	Policy	Relationship to Insured
7	Patient/Guarantor	Name, Address	Street, City, State, ZIP Code, Phones
8	Case	Personal	Marital Status
8	Patient/Guarantor	Other Information	Employment Status
9	Patient/Guarantor	Name, Address	Last Name, First Name, Middle Initial
9a	Case	Policy	Policy Number
9b	Patient/Guarantor	Name, Address	Birth Date, Sex
9c	Patient/Guarantor	Other Information	Employer
9d	Insurance Carrier	Options	Plan Name
10a	Case	Condition	Employment Related
10b	Case	Condition	Accident Related To
10c	Case	Condition	Accident Related To
10d	Case	Miscellaneous	Local Use A, Local Use B
11	Case	Policy	Policy Number
11a	Patient/Guarantor	Name, Address	Birth Date, Sex
11b	Patient/Guarantor	Other Information	Employer
11c	Insurance Carrier	Options	Plan Name
11d	Case	Policy 2	Insurance 2
12	Patient/Guarantor	Other Information	Signature on File
13	Patient/Guarantor	Other Information	Signature on File
14	Case	Condition	Injury/Illness/LMP Date
15	Case	Condition	Same/Similar Symptoms and First Consultation Date
16	Case	Condition	Dates Unable to Work
17	Referring Provider	Address	First Name, Middle Initial, Last Name
17a			
17b	Referring Provider	NPI, Qualifiers, PINs, and IDs	Varies with carrier
18	Case	Condition	Hospitalization
19	Case	Miscellaneous	Local Use A, Local Use B
20	Case	Miscellaneous	Outside Lab Work and Lab Charges
21	Case	Diagnosis	Default Diagnosis 1–4
22	Case	Medicaid	Resubmission Number and Original Reference

(continued)

TABLE VI-1 (*continued*)

Patient/Guarantor Information and the CMS-1500 Form

CMS Form Locator	Medisoft		
	Dialog Box	TAB (in Dialog Box)	Field (in Dialog Box)
23	Case	Miscellaneous	Prior Authorization Number
24A	Transaction Entry	Charge	Dates
24B	Procedure Code	General	Place of Service
24C	Emergency	Condition	Emergency check box
24D	Transaction Entry	Charge	Procedure and Modifiers
24E	Transaction Entry	Charge	Default Diagnosis 1–4
24F	Transaction Entry	Charge	Amount
24G	Transaction Entry	Charge	Units
24H-24I	24J Case Provider List/ Insurance Carrier List	Medicaid PINS	EPSDT PINs/National Identifier
25	Provider	PINs and IDs	SSN/Federal Tax ID
26	Patient/Guarantor	Name, Address, or Other Information	Chart Number or Patient ID #2
27	Case	Policy	Accept Assignment or Transaction Default
28	Transaction Entry	Charge	Amount
29	Transaction Entry	Payment	Amount
30	Transaction Entry		Case Balance
31	Provider	Address	Signature on File
32	Case	Account	Facility
33	Provider	PINs and IDs	Last Name, Middle Initial, First Name, Street, City, State, Zip Code, Phone

printing, you notice data missing on the claim, consult this table to discern where to enter it in Medisoft.

MEDISOFT SHORTCUT BUTTONS

The Shortcut Button toolbar is a quick way to navigate to the most commonly used windows/areas within Medisoft. As a helpful reminder, each button is labeled here with a brief description of the use of the window.

Transaction Entry—Use this window to post charges, payments, and adjustments in patient accounts.

Claim Management—Use this window to create, print, and send insurance claims.

Statement Management—Use this window to print and send statements.

Collection List—Use this window to check on open accounts that require collection follow-up and add tickler notes.

Add Collection List Items—Use this window to add multiple collection items at once to the Collection List based on specific criteria chosen from the screen.

Appointment Book—Use this window to set appointments for the practice's providers.

View Eligibility Verification Results—This feature allows the facility to check a patient's insurance coverage online. It is a fee-based service for which the facility must enroll.

Patient/Case (Guarantor) List—Use this window to add or edit patient, guarantor, or case information.

Insurance Carrier List—Use this window to add or edit insurance carriers in the Medisoft database.

Procedure Code List—Use this window to edit or add procedure, payment, or adjustment codes in the Medisoft database.

Diagnosis Code List—Use this window to add or edit diagnostic codes in the Medisoft database.

Provider List—Use this window to add or edit practice providers in the Medisoft database.

Referring Provider List—Use this window to add or edit names of physicians that refer patients to the practice.

Address List—Use this window to add or edit patient/guarantor, employer, attorney, or facility names to the Medisoft database.

Patient Recall List—Use this window to enter appointment recall information.

Custom Report List—Use this window to view every report choice in Medisoft database.

Quick Ledger—Use this window to quickly view any patient's full financial ledger.

Quick Balance—Use this window to view any patient's financial balance.

Enter Deposits and Apply Payments—Use this window as an alternative way to enter patient/guarantor or insurance payments to patients' accounts.

Show/Hide Hints

Medisoft Help Menu

Edit Patient Notes in Final Draft—If notes were entered anywhere in the system, they may be edited here.

Launch Advanced Reporting—Advanced Reporting provides users with enhanced reporting and data viewing capabilities including ad hoc reporting and a set of standard reports that may be customized by users with the report writer.

Launch Work Administrator—The Work Administrator program lets the staff streamline the work process. Use this feature to organize tasks for users and user groups.

Exit Medisoft Program

MEDISOFT MENUS

Each Medisoft menu is shown here as a navigation reminder. Each menu was explained on page A-14.

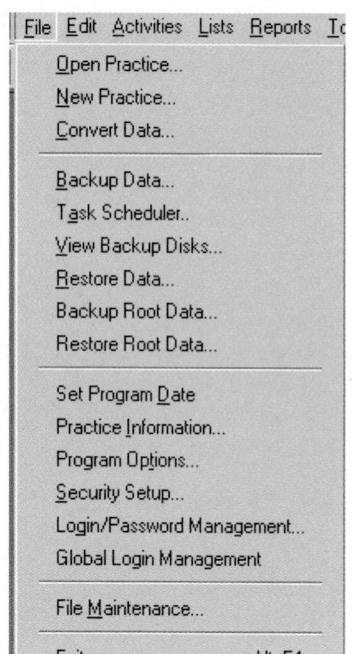

File menu.

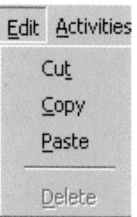

Edit menu.

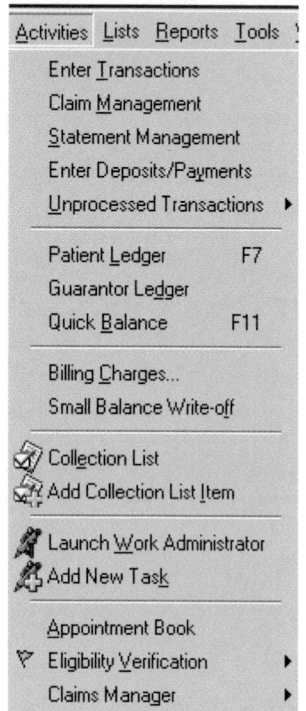

Activities menu.

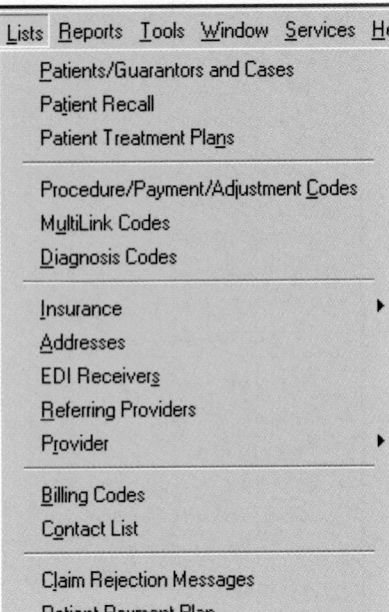

Lists menu.

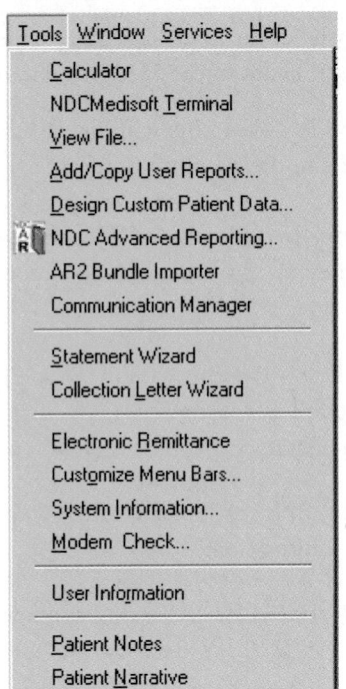

Tools menu.

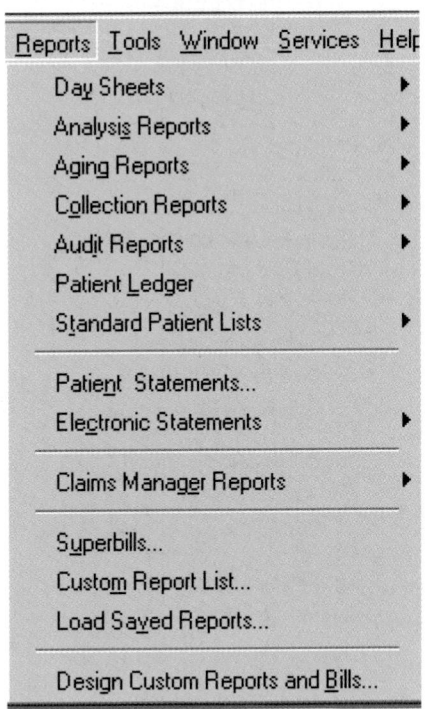

Reports menu.

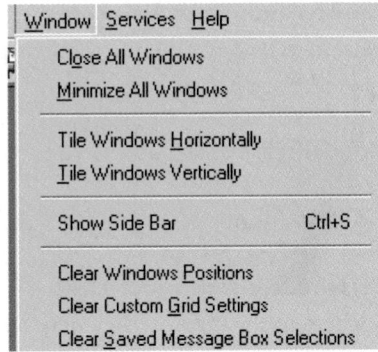

Window menu.

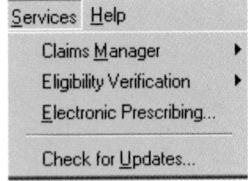

Services menu.

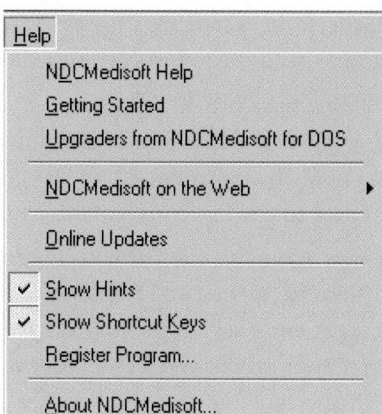

Help menu.

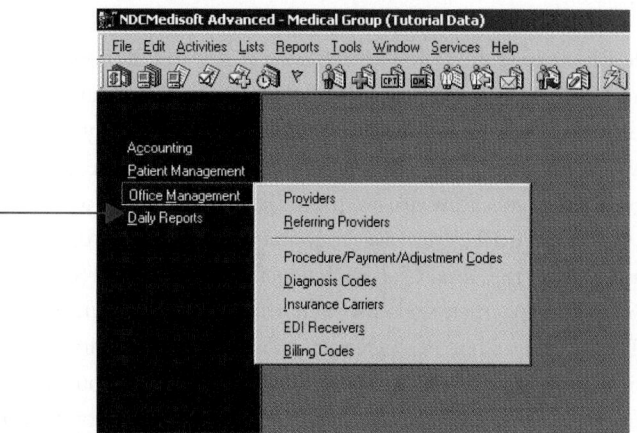

Office Management menu.

MEDISOFT SIDEBAR SHORTCUT MENUS

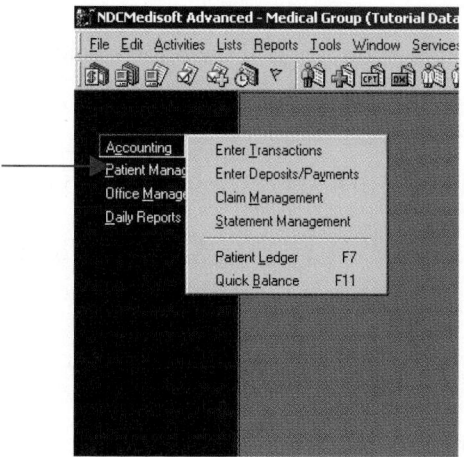

Accounting menu.

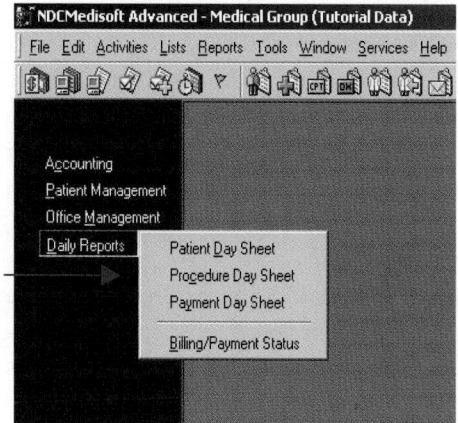

Daily Reports menu.

SIMULATION INSTRUCTIONS

Please use the patient information forms, encounter forms, and Explanation of Benefits forms located at the end of this appendix to complete this simulation exercise.

For this simulation, you are the medical business office specialist for your medical practice. It is your job to enter all patient demographic information, post charges, payments, and adjustments. *It is necessary to enter the ICD-9 and CPT codes and charges exactly as they appear on the superbills.* This may require you to enter them into the Medisoft database (as a new code) as well as into the specific patient's account.

You are responsible for printing a walkout receipt for each patient's account to which you post charges. It is your responsibility to balance your batch at the end of each day and to print insurance claim forms for the patients with insurance.

Some patients may need to come back to the office for follow-up appointments. This will be noted at the bottom of the superbill. If a return appointment is needed, you must schedule the appointment for the patient (in Office Hours).

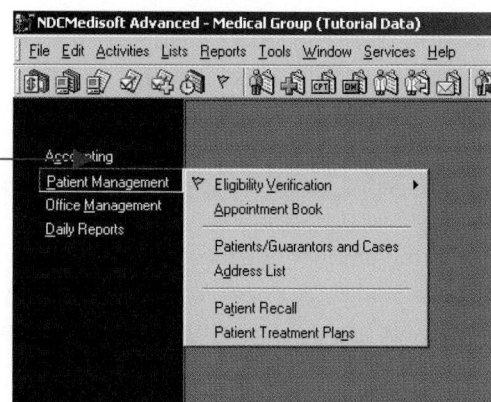

Patient Management menu.

Before class ends each day, you may be instructed to stop posting transactions and "batch out." Access the Reports menu and run the Patient Day Sheet report for today's date. After printing your report, you will use it to make sure you "balance." To do this, you must separately add up all the charges, payments, and adjustments from all the superbills (or EOBs) you posted during the day. Your charges should add up to the amount on the Total Charges line on the Patient Day Sheet report. Your payments should equal the negative amount on the Total Receipts line of the report, and your adjustments should match the Total Adjustments line. If the amounts you totaled from your superbills/EOBs do not match the report totals, you must go over the report patient by patient as you look at each patient superbill/EOB to find the discrepancy.

After you have balanced your totals, your instructor may require you to batch your superbills/EOBs and correct Patient Day Sheet report together and turn them in before you leave each day. If this is the case, it means you will have to remove or copy the superbills/EOBs you posted from your textbook. The Patient Day Sheet report is to be placed on top of your superbills/EOBs, followed by your walkout receipts, and stapled together.

Once your batch is complete, it is time to create insurance claims for the patients for whom you entered transaction information. Medisoft allows you to view your insurance claims on screen prior to printing them or sending them electronically. You must look over the claims on the computer screen to make sure there are no errors. If you find any errors, close the Claims window and go back to the specific patient's account in the computer and correct it. The claim will automatically be updated with the corrected information. Check your electronic claim batch again to make sure all claims are correct. When you are sure there are no errors, print the claims.

Clip your CMS-1500 forms to the bottom of your batch material and turn it in to your instructor.

Tips for Entering Information into Medisoft Advanced

1. First, look over the patient information form. Check the Address List to see if the employer name is already listed in Medisoft. If it is not, add the employer to the Address List.

2. Check the Insurance Carrier List to see if the patient's primary and secondary insurance carriers are already listed in Medisoft. Remember the insurance carrier address must be *exactly the same* as what is written on the patient information form. If the carrier is not listed, add the carrier(s) to the Insurance Carrier List.

3. Check to see if the patient has a Referring Physician (or PCP) listed on the patient information form. If one is listed, check the Referring Provider List to see if the physician is already listed in Medisoft. If the provider is not listed, add the provider.

4. Add the patient to the Patient/Guarantor List if the patient is new. If the patient is not the guarantor, add the guarantor to the Patient/Guarantor List.

5. Make a new Case for the patient. Entering the employer, insurance carrier, and referring provider *prior* to making a patient case allows you to have all the data already entered when you come to the drop-down menus (in the case and the patient/guarantor list) for employer, insurance carrier, etc.). This saves the hassle of closing the patient case, opening the Address Book (or Insurance Carrier List, etc.), adding the data, saving and closing the window, and then opening the patient case again.

Before beginning the simulation, you must enter your physician's information into the Medisoft database. Open the Provider List (accessed either by shortcut button or Lists menu) and click New.

Enter the following information in the Address folder in the window:

Your Name

1933 E. Frankford Rd. #110 Carrollton, TX 12345	office telephone: 972-555-5482 home phone: 214-555-8888 cell phone: 469-555-3657 fax: 972-555-5416
Medicare Participating, Signature on File Specialty: General Practice	License no.: B1740

In the Default PINs folder enter: 75-1234567 for Federal Tax ID Indicator

Medicare PIN: B94765 UPIN: B94765	Medicaid: K89J2 NPI: 1234569860

Be sure to save any data entered. All the patients you enter during the simulation will be seeing you.

There are two more things to do before you begin. Open the File menu in Medisoft and click on Practice Information. Click in the Practice name box. Enter your name as Your Name Medical Clinic.

Click the Save button on the right side of the window.

Go the Address List and enter a new Facility. The facility will be Your Name Medical Clinic, with the address on Frankford Road that you entered for the Practice Name. Click Save and exit the Address List.

You are ready to begin the simulation.

Allied Medical Center
REGISTRATION FORM
(Please Print)

Today's date: _____ PCP: _____

PATIENT INFORMATION

Patient's last name: DUPONT	First: MARGARET	Middle: B	☐ Mr. ☒ Mrs.	☐ Miss ☐ Ms.	Marital status (circle one) Single / (Mar) / Div / Sep / Wid

Is this your legal name? ☒ Yes ☐ No	If not, what is your legal name?	(Former name):	Birth date: 09/21/1946	Age:	Sex: ☐ M ☒ F

Street address: 12 BRIAR LANE		Social Security no.: 717-87-0054	Home phone no.: (214) 555-9871

P.O. box:	City: DALLAS	State: TX	ZIP Code: 12345

Occupation: MANAGER	Employer: SHARON'S BRIDAL SHOPPE	Employer phone no.: (214) 555-8878

Chose clinic because/Referred to clinic by (please check one box): ☐ Dr. ☒ Insurance Plan ☐ Hospital

☐ Family	☐ Friend	☐ Close to home/work	☐ Yellow Pages	Other

Other family members seen here:
LISA DUPONT

REASON FOR THIS VISIT: Persistent cough

INSURANCE INFORMATION
(Please give your insurance card to the receptionist.)

Person responsible for bill: SELF	Birth date: / /	Address (if different):	Home phone no.: ( )

Is this person a patient here? ☒ Yes ☐ No

Occupation:	Employer:	Employer address:	Employer phone no.: ( )

Is this patient covered by insurance? ☒ Yes ☐ No

Please indicate primary insurance:	PHYSICIAN ALLIANCE PPO	Claims Mailing Address:	P O BOX 1256	Philadelphia, PA	12345
		PHONE: 800-555-5522			

Subscriber's name: SELF	Subscriber's S.S. no.:	Birth date: / /	☐ M ☐ F	Group no.: A435	Policy no.: 621382	Co-payment: $10.00

Patient's relationship to subscriber: ☒ Self ☐ Spouse ☐ Child ☐ Other

Name of secondary insurance (if applicable): BLUE CROSS BLUE SHIELD TX PPO	Subscriber's name and DOB: FRANK DUPONT 07/21/1941	☒ M ☐ F	Group no.: 126	Policy no.: BHR716830061

Patient's relationship to subscriber: ☐ Self ☒ Spouse ☐ Child ☐ Other Claims Mailing Address: P O BOX 660044 DALLAS 12345

IN CASE OF EMERGENCY

Name of local friend or relative (not living at same address): SHARON THELANER	Relationship to patient: SISTER	Home phone no.: (469) 555-3259	Work phone no.: (817) 555-8114

The above information is true to the best of my knowledge. I authorize my insurance benefits to be paid directly to the physician. I understand that I am financially responsible for any balance. I also authorize ALLIED MEDICAL CENTER or insurance company to release any information required to process my claims.

Maggie Dupont

_____   _____
Patient/Guardian signature   Date

ENCOUNTER FORM

Patient Information		Payment Method		Visit Information	
Patient ID number		**Primary**	Physician's Alliance	Visit date	
Patient name	Margaret Dupont	Primary ID number	621382	Visit number	
Address	12 Briar Lane	Primary group number	A435	Rendering physician	
City/State	Dallas, TX 12345	**Secondary**	BCBS TX	Referring physician	
Phone number	214-555-9871	Secondary ID number	BHR716830061	Reason for visit	Cough
Date of birth	09/21/1946	Secondary group no.	126		
Age		Cash/credit card			
		Other billing			

E/M Modifiers	Procedure Modifiers	DIAGNOSIS:
21 — Prolonged E&M Service	22 — Unusual, excessive procedure	
24 — Unrelated E/M service during postop.	50 — Bilateral procedure	ACUTE SINUSITIS 461.9
25 — Significant, separately identifiable E/M	51 — Multiple surgical procedures in same day	
32 — Mandated Service	52 — Reduced/incomplete procedure	
57 — Decision for surgery	55 — Postop. management only	
	59 — Distinct multiple procedures	

CATEGORY	CODE	MOD	FEE	CATEGORY	CODE	MOD	FEE
Office Visit — New Patient				**Wound Care**			
Minimal office visit	99201			Debride partial thickness burn	11040		
20 minutes	99202			Debride full thickness burn	11041		
30 minutes	99203			Debride wound, not a burn	11000		
45 minutes	99204	X	135.00	Unna boot application	29580		
60 minutes	99205			Unna boot removal	29700		
Other				Other			
Office Visit — Established				**Supplies**			
Minimal office visit	99211			Ace bandage, 2"	A6448		
10 minutes	99212			Ace bandage, 3"-4"	A6449		
15 minutes	99213			Ace bandage, 6"	A6450		
25 minutes	99214			Cast, fiberglass	A4590		
40 minutes	99215			Coban wrap	A6454		
Other				Foley catheter	A4338		
General Procedures				Immobilizer	L3670		
Anoscopy	46600			Kerlix roll	A6220		
Audiometry	92551			Oxygen mask/cannula	A4620		
Breast aspiration	19000			Sleeve, elbow	E0191		
Cerumen removal	69210			Sling	A4565		
Circumcision	54150			Splint, ready-made	A4570		
DDST	96110			Splint, wrist	S8451		
Flex sigmoidoscopy	45330			Sterile packing	A6407		
Flex sig. w/ biopsy	45331			Surgical tray	A4550		
Foreign body removal—foot	28190			Other			
Nail removal	11730			**OB Care**			
Nail removal/phenol	11750			Routine OB care	59400		
Trigger point injection	20552			Postpartum care only (separate procedure)	59430		
Tympanometry	92567			Ante partum 4–6 visits	59425		
Visual acuity	99173			Ante partum 7 or more visits	59426		
Other				Other			
Other				Other			

Other Visit Information: _____

Lab Work to Order: _____

Referral to: _____

Provider Signature: _____

Next Appointment: _____ RETURN IN A FEW DAYS IF NOT BETTER _____

Fees:

Total Charges: $135.00

Copay Received: $ 10.00

Other Payment: $_____

Total Due: **$125.00**

Allied Medical Center 1933 E.Frankford Rd. Carrollton, TX 12345 **972-555-5482**

Allied Medical Center
REGISTRATION FORM
(Please Print)

Today's date: _____ PCP: _____

PATIENT INFORMATION

Patient's last name: SMYTH	First: SAMANTHA	Middle: M	❑ Mr. ❑ Mrs.	❑ Miss ❑ Ms.	Marital status (circle one) (Single)/ Mar / Div / Sep / Wid

Is this your legal name? ❑ Yes ❑ No	If not, what is your legal name?	(Former name):	Birth date: 03/17/1968	Age:	Sex: ❑ M ☒ F

Street address: 9401 Winding Valley	Social Security no.: 455-94-8204	Home phone no.: (972) 555-9871

P.O. box:	City: PLANO	State: TX	ZIP Code: 12345

Occupation: FOOD SERVER	Employer: WENDY'S HAMBURGERS	Employer phone no.: (972) 555-8936

Chose clinic because/Referred to clinic by (please check one box): ❑ Dr. ❑ Insurance Plan ❑ Hospital

❑ Family ❑ Friend ❑ Close to home/work ❑ Yellow Pages Other

Other family members seen here: _____ **REASON FOR THIS VISIT:** Cholesterol check

INSURANCE INFORMATION

(Please give your insurance card to the receptionist.)

Person responsible for bill: SAMANTHA SMYTH	Birth date: 03/17/1968	Address (if different): Same	Home phone no.: ( )

Is this person a patient here? ❑ Yes ❑ No

Occupation:	Employer:	Employer address:	Employer phone no.: ( )

Is this patient covered by insurance? ❑ Yes ❑ No

Please indicate primary insurance:	NONE	Claims Mailing Address:	
		PHONE:	

Subscriber's name:	Subscriber's S.S. no.:	Birth date: / /	❑ M ❑ F	Group no.:	Policy no.:	Co-payment: $

Patient's relationship to subscriber: ❑ Self ❑ Spouse ❑ Child ❑ Other

Name of secondary insurance (if applicable):	Subscriber's name and DOB:	❑ M ❑ F	Group no.:	Policy no.:

Patient's relationship to subscriber: ❑ Self ❑ Spouse ❑ Child ❑ Other Claims Mailing Address:

IN CASE OF EMERGENCY

Name of local friend or relative (not living at same address): CARRIE TINKHAM	Relationship to patient: FRIEND	Home phone no.: (972) 555-1502	Work phone no.: (972) 555-0074

The above information is true to the best of my knowledge. I authorize my insurance benefits to be paid directly to the physician. I understand that I am financially responsible for any balance. I also authorize ALLIED MEDICAL CENTER or insurance company to release any information required to process my claims.

Samantha Smyth

Patient/Guardian signature   _Date_

ENCOUNTER FORM

Patient Information		Payment Method		Visit Information	
Patient ID number		**Primary**		Visit date	
Patient name	Samantha Smyth	Primary ID number		Visit number	
Address	9401 Winding Valley	Primary group number		Rendering physician	
City/State	Plano, TX 12345	**Secondary**		Referring physician	
Phone number	972-555-9871	Secondary ID number		Reason for visit	Cholesterol Check
Date of birth	03/17/1968	Secondary group no.			
Age		Cash/credit card	CHECK		
		Other billing			

E/M Modifiers	Procedure Modifiers	DIAGNOSIS:
21 — Prolonged E&M Service	22 — Unusual, excessive procedure	Hypercholesteremia 272.00
24 — Unrelated E/M service during postop.	50 — Bilateral procedure	
25 — Significant, separately identifiable E/M	51 — Multiple surgical procedures in same day	
32 — Mandated Service	52 — Reduced/incomplete procedure	
57 — Decision for surgery	55 — Postop. management only	
	59 — Distinct multiple procedures	

CATEGORY	CODE	MOD	FEE	CATEGORY	CODE	MOD	FEE
Office Visit — New Patient				**Wound Care**			
Minimal office visit	99201			Debride partial thickness burn	11040		
20 minutes	99202			Debride full thickness burn	11041		
30 minutes	99203			Debride wound, not a burn	11000		
45 minutes	99204			Unna boot application	29580		
60 minutes	99205			Unna boot removal	29700		
Other				Other			
Office Visit — Established				**Supplies**			
Minimal office visit	99211			Ace bandage, 2"	A6448		
10 minutes	99212	X	35.00	Ace bandage, 3"-4"	A6449		
15 minutes	99213			Ace bandage, 6"	A6450		
25 minutes	99214			Cast, fiberglass	A4590		
40 minutes	99215			Coban wrap	A6454		
Other				Foley catheter	A4338		
General Procedures				Immobilizer	L3670		
Anoscopy	46600			Kerlix roll	A6220		
Audiometry	92551			Oxygen mask/cannula	A4620		
Breast aspiration	19000			Sleeve, elbow	E0191		
Cerumen removal	69210			Sling	A4565		
Circumcision	54150			Splint, ready-made	A4570		
DDST	96110			Splint, wrist	S8451		
Flex sigmoidoscopy	45330			Sterile packing	A6407		
Flex sig. w/ biopsy	45331			Surgical tray	A4550		
Foreign body removal—foot	28190			Other			
Nail removal	11730			OB Care			
Nail removal/phenol	11750			Routine OB care	59400		
Trigger point injection	20552			Postpartum care only (separate procedure)	59430		
Tympanometry	92567			Ante partum 4–6 visits	59425		
Visual acuity	99173			Ante partum 7 or more visits	59426		
Other	82465	X	30.00	Other			
Other				Other			

Other Visit Information:_____

Lab Work to Order:_____

Referral to:_____

Provider Signature:_____

Next Appointment:_____RETURN IN A FEW DAYS IF NOT BETTER_____

Fees:

Total Charges: $65.00

Copay Received: $_____

Other Payment: $65.00 CK #1235

Total Due: $0

Allied Medical Center 1933 E.Frankford Rd. Carrollton, TX 12345 **972-555-5482**

Allied Medical Center
REGISTRATION FORM
(Please Print)

Today's date: _____   PCP: _____

PATIENT INFORMATION

Patient's last name: BAILEY	First: EILEEN	Middle: B	❑ Mr. ❑ Mrs.	❑ Miss ❑ Ms.	Marital status (circle one) Single / Mar / Div / Sep / (Wid)

Is this your legal name? ❑ Yes ❑ No	If not, what is your legal name?	(Former name): EILEEN STANFORD	Birth date: 04/26/1961	Age:	Sex: ❑ M ❑ F

Street address: 2531 BENT TREE COURT		Social Security no.: 555-63-2112	Home phone no.: (972) 555-6058

P.O. box:	City: DALLAS	State: TX	ZIP Code: 12345

Occupation: SUPERVISOR	Employer: DISCOUNT COMPUTER WAREHOUSE	Employer phone no.: (972) 555-6577

Chose clinic because/Referred to clinic by (please check one box):	❑ Dr.	❑ Insurance Plan	❑ Hospital

❑ Family   ❑ Friend   ❑ Close to home/work   ❑ Yellow Pages   Other

Other family members seen here: **REASON FOR THIS VISIT:** Yearly Physical

INSURANCE INFORMATION
(Please give your insurance card to the receptionist.)

Person responsible for bill: EILEEN BAILEY	Birth date: / /	Address (if different): Same	Home phone no.: ( )

Is this person a patient here?   ❑ Yes   ❑ No

Occupation:	Employer:	Employer address:	Employer phone no.: ( )

Is this patient covered by insurance?   ❑ Yes   ❑ No

Please indicate primary insurance:	PHYSICIAN CHOICE EPO	Claims Mailing Address:	P O BOX 9873	Dover, OH	12345
		PHONE: 800-555-8637			

Subscriber's name: EILEEN BAILEY	Subscriber's S.S. no.: 555-63-2112	Birth date: 04/26/1961	❑ M ❑ F	Group no.: K1047	Policy no.: 13056	Co-payment: $

Patient's relationship to subscriber: ❑ Self   ❑ Spouse   ❑ Child   ❑ Other

Name of secondary insurance (if applicable):	Subscriber's name and DOB:	❑ M ❑ F	Group no.:	Policy no.:

Patient's relationship to subscriber: ❑ Self   ❑ Spouse   ❑ Child   ❑ Other Claims Mailing Address:

IN CASE OF EMERGENCY

Name of local friend or relative (not living at same address): MALCOLM JOHNSON	Relationship to patient: FRIEND	Home phone no.: (214) 555-5277	Work phone no.: (214) 555-8788

The above information is true to the best of my knowledge. I authorize my insurance benefits to be paid directly to the physician. I understand that I am financially responsible for any balance. I also authorize ALLIED MEDICAL CENTER or insurance company to release any information required to process my claims.

Eileen Bailey

_____   _____
Patient/Guardian signature   *Date*

ENCOUNTER FORM

Patient Information		Payment Method		Visit Information	
Patient ID number		**Primary**	Physician's Choice EPO	Visit date	
Patient name	Eileen Bailey	Primary ID number	13056	Visit number	
Address	2531 Bent Tree Ct	Primary group number	K1047	Rendering physician	
City/State	Dallas, TX 12345	**Secondary**		Referring physician	
Phone number	972-555-6058	Secondary ID number		Reason for visit	Yearly Physical
Date of birth	04/26/1961	Secondary group no.			
Age		Cash/credit card	CHECK		
		Other billing			

E/M Modifiers	Procedure Modifiers	DIAGNOSIS:
21 — Prolonged E&M Service	22 — Unusual, excessive procedure	Routine Exam V70.0
24 — Unrelated E/M service during postop.	50 — Bilateral procedure	
25 — Significant, separately identifiable E/M	51 — Multiple surgical procedures in same day	
32 — Mandated Service	52 — Reduced/incomplete procedure	
57 — Decision for surgery	55 — Postop. management only	
	59 — Distinct multiple procedures	

CATEGORY	CODE	MOD	FEE	CATEGORY	CODE	MOD	FEE
Office Visit — New Patient				**Wound Care**			
Minimal office visit	99201			Debride partial thickness burn	11040		
20 minutes	99202			Debride full thickness burn	11041		
30 minutes	99203			Debride wound, not a burn	11000		
45 minutes	99204			Unna boot application	29580		
60 minutes	99205	X	160.00	Unna boot removal	29700		
Other				Other			
Office Visit — Established				**Supplies**			
Minimal office visit	99211			Ace bandage, 2"	A6448		
10 minutes	99212			Ace bandage, 3"-4"	A6449		
15 minutes	99213			Ace bandage, 6"	A6450		
25 minutes	99214			Cast, fiberglass	A4590		
40 minutes	99215			Coban wrap	A6454		
Other				Foley catheter	A4338		
General Procedures				Immobilizer	L3670		
Anoscopy	46600			Kerlix roll	A6220		
Audiometry	92551			Oxygen mask/cannula	A4620		
Breast aspiration	19000			Sleeve, elbow	E0191		
Cerumen removal	69210			Sling	A4565		
Circumcision	54150			Splint, ready-made	A4570		
DDST	96110			Splint, wrist	S8451		
Flex sigmoidoscopy	45330			Sterile packing	A6407		
Flex sig. w/ biopsy	45331			Surgical tray	A4550		
Foreign body removal—foot	28190			Other			
Nail removal	11730			OB Care			
Nail removal/phenol	11750			Routine OB care	59400		
Trigger point injection	20552			Postpartum care only (separate procedure)	59430		
Tympanometry	92567			Ante partum 4–6 visits	59425		
Visual acuity	99173			Ante partum 7 or more visits	59426		
Other	82465			Other			
Other				Other			

Other Visit Information:_____

Lab Work to Order:_____

Referral to:_____

Provider Signature:_____

Next Appointment:_____ AS NEEDED _____

Fees:

Total Charges: $160.00

Copay Received: $ 32.00

Other Payment: $_____

Total Due: **$128.00**

Allied Medical Center 1933 E.Frankford Rd. Carrollton, TX 12345 **972-555-5482**

Allied Medical Center
REGISTRATION FORM
(Please Print)

Today's date: _____ PCP: _____

PATIENT INFORMATION

Patient's last name: CATHER	First: JIM	Middle: S	☐ Mr. ☐ Mrs.	☐ Miss ☐ Ms.	Marital status (circle one) Single /(Mar)/ Div / Sep / Wid

Is this your legal name? ☒ Yes ☐ No	If not, what is your legal name? JAMES CATHER	(Former name):	Birth date: 10/01/1953	Age:	Sex: ☐ M ☐ F

Street address: 425 LAVENDER STREET	Social Security no.: 188-38-3833	Home phone no.: (972) 555-3394

P.O. box:	City: GARLAND	State: TX	ZIP Code: 12345

Occupation: SALESPERSON	Employer: MERRY MILER VANS	Employer phone no.: (972) 555-3337

Chose clinic because/Referred to clinic by (please check one box):	☒ Dr. LESLIE MCNEICE	☐ Insurance Plan	☐ Hospital

☐ Family	☐ Friend	☐ Close to home/work	☐ Yellow Pages	Other **AUTH # A569874, 30 DAYS, 3 VISITS**

Other family members seen here: **REASON FOR THIS VISIT:** Hyperglycemia check up

INSURANCE INFORMATION
(Please give your insurance card to the receptionist.)

Person responsible for bill: JIM CATHER	Birth date: / /	Address (if different): SAME	Home phone no.: ( )

Is this person a patient here? ☐ Yes ☐ No

Occupation:	Employer:	Employer address:	Employer phone no.: ( )

Is this patient covered by insurance? ☐ Yes ☐ No

Please indicate primary insurance:	PHYSICIAN ALLIANCE HMO	Claims Mailing Address:	P O BOX 65	TOLEDO, OH	12345

PHONE: 800-555-9865

Subscriber's name: SAME AS PATIENT	Subscriber's S.S. no.: 188-38-3833	Birth date: / /	☐ M ☐ F	Group no.: 145	Policy no.: 188383833	Co-payment: $25.00

Patient's relationship to subscriber:	☐ Self	☐ Spouse	☐ Child	☐ Other

Name of secondary insurance (if applicable):	Subscriber's name and DOB:	☐ M ☐ F	Group no.:	Policy no.:

Patient's relationship to subscriber:	☐ Self	☐ Spouse	☐ Child	☐ Other Claims Mailing Address:

IN CASE OF EMERGENCY

Name of local friend or relative (not living at same address): MARILYN CATHER	Relationship to patient: SIBLING	Home phone no.: (214) 555-3329	Work phone no.: (469) 555-8200

The above information is true to the best of my knowledge. I authorize my insurance benefits to be paid directly to the physician. I understand that I am financially responsible for any balance. I also authorize ALLIED MEDICAL CENTER or insurance company to release any information required to process my claims.

Jim Cather

_____   _____
Patient/Guardian signature   *Date*

ENCOUNTER FORM

Patient Information		Payment Method		Visit Information	
Patient ID number		**Primary**	Physician's Alliance HMO	Visit date	
Patient name	Jim Cather	Primary ID number	188383833	Visit number	
Address	425 Lavender St	Primary group number	145	Rendering physician	
City/State	Garland, TX 12345	**Secondary**		Referring physician	Leslie McNeice
Phone number	972-555-3394	Secondary ID number		Reason for visit	Hyperglyc-emia CK
Date of birth	10/01/1953	Secondary group no.			
Age		Cash/credit card			
		Other billing			

E/M Modifiers	Procedure Modifiers	DIAGNOSIS:
21 — Prolonged E&M Service	22 — Unusual, excessive procedure	Hyperglycemia 790.6
24 — Unrelated E/M service during postop.	50 — Bilateral procedure	
25 — Significant, separately identifiable E/M	51 — Multiple surgical procedures in same day	
32 — Mandated Service	52 — Reduced/incomplete procedure	
57 — Decision for surgery	55 — Postop. management only	
	59 — Distinct multiple procedures	

CATEGORY	CODE	MOD	FEE	CATEGORY	CODE	MOD	FEE
Office Visit — New Patient				**Wound Care**			
Minimal office visit	99201			Debride partial thickness burn	11040		
20 minutes	99202			Debride full thickness burn	11041		
30 minutes	99203			Debride wound, not a burn	11000		
45 minutes	99204			Unna boot application	29580		
60 minutes	99205			Unna boot removal	29700		
Other				Other			
Office Visit — Established				**Supplies**			
Minimal office visit	99211			Ace bandage, 2"	A6448		
10 minutes	99212			Ace bandage, 3"-4"	A6449		
15 minutes	99213			Ace bandage, 6"	A6450		
25 minutes	99214	X	65.00	Cast, fiberglass	A4590		
40 minutes	99215			Coban wrap	A6454		
Other				Foley catheter	A4338		
General Procedures				Immobilizer	L3670		
Anoscopy	46600			Kerlix roll	A6220		
Audiometry	92551			Oxygen mask/cannula	A4620		
Breast aspiration	19000			Sleeve, elbow	E0191		
Cerumen removal	69210			Sling	A4565		
Circumcision	54150			Splint, ready-made	A4570		
DDST	96110			Splint, wrist	S8451		
Flex sigmoidoscopy	45330			Sterile packing	A6407		
Flex sig. w/ biopsy	45331			Surgical tray	A4550		
Foreign body removal—foot	28190			Other			
Nail removal	11730			**OB Care**			
Nail removal/phenol	11750			Routine OB care	59400		
Trigger point injection	20552			Postpartum care only (separate procedure)	59430		
Tympanometry	92567			Ante partum 4–6 visits	59425		
Visual acuity	99173			Ante partum 7 or more visits	59426		
Other	93000	X	45.00	Other			
Other	82954	X	12.00	Other			

Other Visit Information: _____

Lab Work to Order: _____

Referral to: _____

Provider Signature: _____

Next Appointment: _____

Fees:

Total Charges: $122.00

Copay Received: $ 25.00

Other Payment: $_____

Total Due: **$ 97.00**

Allied Medical Center 1933 E.Frankford Rd. Carrollton, TX 12345 **972-555-5482**

Allied Medical Center
REGISTRATION FORM
(Please Print)

Today's date:		PCP:

PATIENT INFORMATION

Patient's last name:	First:	Middle:	☒ Mr. ☐ Mrs.	☐ Miss ☐ Ms.	Marital status (circle one)
BAE	YONG	JOON			Single / (Mar)/ Div / Sep / Wid

Is this your legal name?	If not, what is your legal name?	(Former name):	Birth date:	Age:	Sex:
☒ Yes ☐ No			02/23/1972		☒ M ☐ F

Street address:	Social Security no.:	Home phone no.:
4549 EXPLORER DRIVE #110	661-39-2520	(469) 555-0719

P.O. box:	City:	State:	ZIP Code:
	FRISCO	TX	12345

Occupation:	Employer:	Employer phone no.:
SUPERVISOR	SUGARLAND DAIRY FARM	(903) 555-8663

Chose clinic because/Referred to clinic by (please check one box):	☒ Dr. MALCOLM MAZOW	☐ Insurance Plan	☐ Hospital
☐ Family ☐ Friend ☐ Close to home/work ☐ Yellow Pages	Other **REFERRAL # FOR TODAY–1644401**		

Other family members seen here:	**REASON FOR THIS VISIT:** Shoulder Pain

INSURANCE INFORMATION

(Please give your insurance card to the receptionist.)

Person responsible for bill:	Birth date:	Address (if different):	Home phone no.:
PATIENT	/ /	SAME	( )

Is this person a patient here?	☒ Yes ☐ No

Occupation:	Employer:	Employer address:	Employer phone no.:
			( )

Is this patient covered by insurance?	☒ Yes ☐ No

Please indicate primary insurance:	METLIFE HMO	Claims Mailing Address:	P O BOX 6983	NEWARK, DE	12345
		PHONE: 800-555-6897			

Subscriber's name:	Subscriber's S.S. no.:	Birth date:	☐ M ☐ F	Group no.:	Policy no.:	Co-payment:
SELF	661-39-2520	/ /		62440	661392520-01	$10.00

Patient's relationship to subscriber:	☒ Self ☐ Spouse ☐ Child ☐ Other

Name of secondary insurance (if applicable):	Subscriber's name and DOB:	☐ M ☐ F	Group no.:	Policy no.:

Patient's relationship to subscriber:	☐ Self ☐ Spouse ☐ Child ☐ Other Claims Mailing Address:

IN CASE OF EMERGENCY

Name of local friend or relative (not living at same address):	Relationship to patient:	Home phone no.:	Work phone no.:
YUJIN JEONG	MOTHER	(214) 650-9801	( )

The above information is true to the best of my knowledge. I authorize my insurance benefits to be paid directly to the physician. I understand that I am financially responsible for any balance. I also authorize ALLIED MEDICAL CENTER or insurance company to release any information required to process my claims.

Yong Joon Bae

Patient/Guardian signature	Date

ENCOUNTER FORM

Patient Information		Payment Method		Visit Information	
Patient ID number		**Primary**	MetLife HMO	Visit date	
Patient name	Yong Joon Bae	Primary ID number	661392520-01	Visit number	
Address	4549 Explorer Dr	Primary group number	62440	Rendering physician	
City/State	Frisco, TX 12345	**Secondary**		Referring physician	Malcolm Mazow
Phone number	469-555-0719	Secondary ID number		Reason for visit	Shoulder Pain
Date of birth	02/23/1972	Secondary group no.		**Auth # for today: 1644401**	
Age		Cash/credit card			
		Other billing			

E/M Modifiers	Procedure Modifiers	DIAGNOSIS:
21 — Prolonged E&M Service	22 — Unusual, excessive procedure	Bursitis, Shoulder 726.10
24 — Unrelated E/M service during postop.	50 — Bilateral procedure	
25 — Significant, separately identifiable E/M	51 — Multiple surgical procedures in same day	
32 — Mandated Service	52 — Reduced/incomplete procedure	
57 — Decision for surgery	55 — Postop. management only	
	59 — Distinct multiple procedures	

CATEGORY	CODE	MOD	FEE	CATEGORY	CODE	MOD	FEE
Office Visit — New Patient				**Wound Care**			
Minimal office visit	99201			Debride partial thickness burn	11040		
20 minutes	99202			Debride full thickness burn	11041		
30 minutes	99203			Debride wound, not a burn	11000		
45 minutes	99204			Unna boot application	29580		
60 minutes	99205			Unna boot removal	29700		
Other				Other			
Office Visit — Established				**Supplies**			
Minimal office visit	99211			Ace bandage, 2"	A6448		
10 minutes	99212			Ace bandage, 3"-4"	A6449		
15 minutes	99213	X	45.00	Ace bandage, 6"	A6450		
25 minutes	99214			Cast, fiberglass	A4590		
40 minutes	99215			Coban wrap	A6454		
Other				Foley catheter	A4338		
General Procedures				Immobilizer	L3670		
Anoscopy	46600			Kerlix roll	A6220		
Audiometry	92551			Oxygen mask/cannula	A4620		
Breast aspiration	19000			Sleeve, elbow	E0191		
Cerumen removal	69210			Sling	A4565		
Circumcision	54150			Splint, ready-made	A4570		
DDST	96110			Splint, wrist	S8451		
Flex sigmoidoscopy	45330			Sterile packing	A6407		
Flex sig. w/ biopsy	45331			Surgical tray	A4550		
Foreign body removal—foot	28190			Other			
Nail removal	11730			**OB Care**			
Nail removal/phenol	11750			Routine OB care	59400		
Trigger point injection	20552			Postpartum care only (separate procedure)	59430		
Tympanometry	92567			Ante partum 4–6 visits	59425		
Visual acuity	99173			Ante partum 7 or more visits	59426		
Other				Other			
Other				Other			

Other Visit Information:

Lab Work to Order: _____

Referral to: _____

Provider Signature: _____

Next Appointment: _____

Fees:

Total Charges: $45.00

Copay Received: $10.00

Other Payment: $____

Total Due: $35.00

Allied Medical Center 1933 E.Frankford Rd. Carrollton, TX 12345 **972-555-5482**

Source: Adapted from *Comprehensive Health Insurance: Billing, Coding, and Reimbursement,* by D. Vines, A. Braceland, E. Rollins, and S. Miller, © 2008, Upper Saddle River, NJ: Pearson Education.

Glossary

Number in parentheses ( ) indicates chapter.

abduction—process of moving a body part away from the midline (23)

abortions—fetuses that did not reach the age of viability (38)

accommodation—eye's ability to adjust its optical powers to maintain a clear image of objects at various distances (26)

accounting—system of reporting the financial results of a business (15)

accounts payable (AP)—amounts of money the physician owes to others for supplies, equipment, and services (15, 16)

accounts receivable—money owed to the physician or medical practice (15, 16)

accreditation—process by which an institution voluntarily completes an extensive self-study after which an accrediting association visits the school to verify the self-study statements (1)

Accrediting Bureau of Health Education Schools (ABHES)—accreditation bureau that certifies medical assisting programs; graduates of ABHES accredited programs may take the CMA (AAMA) or RMA examination (1)

acid-fast stain—special stain used to expose the tuberculosis organism (45)

acne vulgaris—common skin condition that occurs when oil and dead skin cells clog the skin's pores; also known as simply *acne* (22)

acquired active immunity—occurs when the person is exposed to a live pathogen, develops the disease, and becomes immune as a result of the primary immune response (28)

acquired immune deficiency syndrome (AIDS)—series of illnesses that occur as a result of infection by the human immuno-deficiency virus (HIV), which causes the immune system to break down (2)

acromegaly—hormonal disorder that results from the overproduction of growth hormone by the pituitary gland, most commonly affecting middle-aged adults (32)

active immunity—introduction of immunity by infection or with a vaccine (28)

active listening—paying attention completely to the speaker, concentrating on the verbal message, watching for nonverbal cues, and offering a response (5)

active records—medical files of patients who are currently being seen by the physician that may cover 1 to 5 years, depending on office policy (13)

active transport—process in cells that requires energy to transport materials to, from, and within the cell (21)

active voice—when the subject of the sentence performs the action (11)

acuity—sharpness (39)

acute conditions—illnesses or injuries that occur suddenly and require treatment but may or may not be life threatening (9)

acute pain—expected pain associated with trauma or surgery that lasts through the recovery of that condition (35); intense pain, usually lessening over time (55)

acute renal failure—condition that occurs when something, such as a blockage, toxins, or a sudden loss of blood flow, causes a change in the filtering function of the kidneys (31)

addendum—addition to the original document (13)

Addison's disease—condition in which the cortex of the adrenal gland is damaged, decreasing the production of adrenocortical hormones, usually resulting from an autoimmune disorder but also caused by infection, cancer, or hemorrhage into the glands (32)

adduction—process of moving a body part toward the midline (23)

adenoids—pharyngeal tonsils (28)

administrative law—laws governing the administration of agency regulations (3)

adolescence—transition period between puberty and adulthood (40, 57)

adrenal glands—endocrine organs that secrete hormones; located on top of each kidney, consisting of the cortex and the medulla (32)

adulthood—age designation from roughly 20 years of age to death (57)

advance booking—when the patient schedules his or her next appointment before leaving the office (9)

advance directive—document that allows patients to request that life-sustaining treatments and nutritional support not be used to prolong their life; includes the durable power of attorney (3)

adverse effects—negative effects that outweigh the benefit of taking a medication and require the patient to discontinue its use (53)

aerobic—requires oxygen to live (34)

afebrile—absence of a fever (35)

affective—behaviors that are based on feelings and emotions (58)

afferent nerves—carry impulses from the sensory receptor to the central nervous system (25)

agar—gelatinlike substance made from seaweed that is added to culture media to provide nutrition and a semisolid surface on which microbes can grow (45)

age analysis—procedure for evaluating accounts receivable by age of the charges incurred (15)

ageism—prejudice against and incorrect assumptions about an individual or individuals because of age (41)

agglutination—clumping together (25, 45)

aggressive—trying to impose one's point of view on others (5)

albinism—inherited disorder that is indicated by the absence of melanin in the skin, hair, and eyes (22)

aliquot—small portion of the whole specimen (44)

allergen—any substance that causes a hypersensitivity reaction (37)

allergy—hypersensitivity to a normally harmless substance (28)

alopecia—baldness or loss of hair (22)

alphabetic filing—filing system based on the letters of the alphabet (13)

alveoli—small air sacs at the end of the bronchioles with a network of capillaries that perform the exchange of gases (29)

Alzheimer's disease—progressive, degenerative disease of the brain characterized by loss of memory and other cognitive functions (25)

amblyopia—a disorder in children caused by the eye muscles being weaker in one eye; also known as *lazy eye* (26)

ambulation—act of walking (51)

ambulatory surgery—surgery performed on a person who is admitted and discharged from a surgical facility on the same day (41)

amenorrhea—absence of menstrual periods (38, 40)

American Association of Medical Assistants (AAMA)—professional association for medical assistants (1)

American Banker's Association (ABA) number—code numbers that identify the bank; found on the right upper corner of a printed check (16)

American Medical Technologists (AMT)—professional association that provides oversight for the registration and testing of medical technologists, medical assistants, and phlebotomists (1)

Americans with Disabilities Act (ADA)—act ensuring that people with disabilities have equal access to structures and options (10)

amorphous—without a shape (46)

amphiarthrotic joint—articulation or joint that permits very slight movement (23)

amplify—to make louder (36)

ampules—small, sealed glass bottles containing a single dose of medication (54)

amyotrophic lateral sclerosis (ALS)—a disease of unknown cause that breaks down the nerves in the nervous system that are responsible for movement; also known as *motor neuron disease* and *Lou Gehrig's disease* (25)

anaerobic—able to live without oxygen (34)

analyte—substance in a specimen being analyzed (44)

anaphylactic shock—severe allergic reaction that causes respiratory distress due to swelling of the upper airways; also known as *anaphylaxis* (37, 43)

anaphylaxis—extreme, often life-threatening response to an antigen or allergen; also known as *anaphylactic shock* (28)

anatomy—body structure; study of the structure of an organism (4, 21)

anemia—condition in which levels of hemoglobin in the red blood cells are insufficient; caused by decreased healthy red cell production by the bone marrow, increased erythrocyte destruction, or blood loss from heavy menstrual periods or internal bleeding (27, 47)

anesthesia—medication that causes the partial or complete loss of sensation (2, 42)

aneurysm—abnormal widening or ballooning of a portion of an artery, related to weakness in the vessel wall (27)

angina—suffocating chest pain (37)

angiography—X-ray visualization of blood vessels after a radiopaque material has been injected into them (48)

angioplasty—surgical vessel repair procedure frequently used to reopen a blocked coronary artery (27)

anorexia nervosa—eating disorder associated with a distorted sense of body image and the persistent quest for thinness, at times to the point of emaciation (40)

answering service—agency that answers phone calls and forwards messages to directed recipients (7)

antagonist—muscle that counteracts, or opposes, the action of another muscle (24)

antecubital space—depression in the front of the elbow that is the most commonly used site for venipuncture (47)

anthrax—deadly infectious disease caused by *Bacillus anthracis* (2)

anthropometry—science of size, proportion, weight, and height (35)

antibodies—specialized proteins that lock onto and have the ability to neutralize specific antigens (28, 34)

antigen—foreign substance that invades the body (28)

antiseptic—agent used for hand hygiene (34)

anuria—absence of urine (46)

aorta—largest artery of the body into which blood enters after it leaves the left ventricle (27)

apical—heart rate that is counted at the apex of the heart (35)

apnea—absence of breathing for more than 19 seconds (29, 35)

aponeurosis—wide, thin, sheetlike tendon, made up of fibrous connective tissue, that typically attaches muscles to other muscles (24)

apothecary system—oldest system of measurement in which dry weight is measured in grains (52)

appendicitis—inflammation of the appendix caused by a blockage of the inside of the appendix (the lumen), which leads to increased pressure, impaired blood flow, and potentially gangrene and rupture (30)

appendicular skeleton—one of the two divisions of the skeletal system, consisting of the 126 bones, including the shoulder and pelvic girdles, as well as the extremities, that are not part of the axial skeleton (23)

appendix—small appendage attached to the cecum, which has no known function in humans (30)

application—form usually completed at the time of the job interview that includes personal information and previous work experience (59)

aqueous humor—watery fluid that fills the anterior cavity of the eyeball (26)

archived—stored for later retrieval (9)

aromatherapy—therapy that utilizes pleasant smells (58)

arrhythmia—irregular heartbeat caused by a disturbance of normal electrical activity of the heart; pulse with an irregular rhythm (27, 35)

arterial blood gases (ABGs)—measurement of oxygen and carbon dioxide in arterial blood (29)

arteriosclerosis—a thickening and loss of elasticity of the arteries; also known as *hardening of the arteries* (27)

arthritis—inflammation of one or more joints caused by various disease processes (23, 37)

articulation—the place where two bones connect, with the positioning of the bones determining the type of movement the joint performs; also known as *joint* (23)

artifacts—errors in an electrocardiograph (49)

artificial active immunity—result of receiving vaccinations with inactive (dead) or attenuated (weakened) organisms (28)

artificially acquired active immunity—immunity that is induced by a vaccine (28, 54)

ascites—fluid in the abdomen (31)

asepsis—state of being free from germs, infection, and any form of microbial life (34)

aseptic—free from germs, infection, and any form of microbial life (34)

asphyxia—suffocation (29)

aspiration—removal by suction of fluid from within a cyst (24)

assertive—to make a point in a positive manner (5)

assessment—evaluation (5, 55)

assignment of benefits—patient's written authorization giving the insurance company the right to pay the physician directly for billed charges (15, 18)

assisted living facility—a resident facility designed to provide assistance and supervision to residents; may include activities of daily living, coordination with health care providers, administration of medication, or personal care by trained staff persons (41)

asthma—chronic inflammatory condition that typically develops when allergens or other irritating substances cause swelling in the lining of the trachea and bronchial tubes, which creates mucus that can cause coughing or difficulty breathing (29)

astigmatism—refractive eye disorder in which irregularities in the curvature of the cornea cause light not to focus on the retina but to spread out over an area and cause overall blurring of vision (26, 39)

asymptomatic—without symptoms (35)

atherosclerosis—narrowing and hardening of the vessel lumen of the arteries due to a buildup of fatty material and plaque (27, 37)

atlas—first cervical vertebra that connects the spine to the occipital bone at the base of the skull (23)

atom—smallest particle of an element that can exist on its own; consists of at least one proton, at least one neutron, and at least one electron (21)

atria—the two upper chambers of the heart (27)

atrioventricular (AV) node—one of the three areas of specialized neuromuscular tissue that initiate the heartbeat; located under the endocardium of the right atrium (27)

atrophy—loss of muscle mass and strength that occurs with the disuse of muscles over time (24, 51)

attitudes—opinions that develop from our value system (5)

audiogram—record of patient responses indicating his or her ability to hear a sound (39)

audiology—study of hearing disorders (26)

audiometer—electronic instrument used to measure hearing ability (39)

audit—reexamination for accuracy (16)

auditory—by ear (5)

auscultation—listening to sounds within the body, such as heart sounds (27, 36)

autoimmune diseases—inflammatory reactions caused when the immune system produces antibodies that stick to the body's own cells, resulting in damage to the body's own cells and in the body attacking itself (28)

automated assistance program—telephone system that directs callers to a recipient based on the caller's answers to questions (7)

autonomic nervous system—part of the peripheral nervous system that is responsible for controlling involuntary bodily functions such as sweating, secretion of glands, arterial blood pressure, and activity of smooth and cardiac muscle (25)

autopsy—examination of the organs and tissues of a deceased body to determine cause of death (2)

axial skeleton—one of the two divisions of the skeletal system, consisting of 80 bones, including the skull, vertebral system, and rib cage (23)

axis—second cervical vertebra that has a pivoting characteristic, allowing the head to turn from side-to-side (23)

bacteremic—pertaining to bacteria in the bloodstream (22)

bacteria—microorganisms that are capable of causing disease (2)

bactericidal—capable of killing bacteria (34)

bacturia—bacteria in the urine (46)

bad debt—amount owed and not collectable (15)

bandage—strip of binding material used to hold a dressing in place (43)

bandwidth—amount of data that can be transmitted in a fixed amount of time (12)

bariatrics—science of obesity (2)

basal cell carcinoma—most common form of skin cancer; most often caused by overexposure to the sun (22)

basal metabolism—rate of metabolism when the body is awake and at rest (35)

baseline—known value with which follow-up values are compared (35)

basophils—granular leukocytes (47)

behavior—the actions others see (5)

Bell's palsy—weakness or paralysis of the muscles that control expression on one side of the face (25)

benefit period—period of time for which payments for insurance are available (17)

benign—noncancerous (37)

benign prostatic hyperplasia (BPH)—an enlargement of the prostate gland, usually occurring in men older than 50 years, which compresses the urethra, restricting the normal flow of urine; also known as *benign prostatic hypertrophy* (33)

bias—unfair preference or dislike of something that prevents an impartial opinion of someone or something; favoring a certain belief or attitude (5, 57)

bicuspid valve—the valve through which the blood leaves the left atrium of the heart; also known as *mitral valve* (27)

bile—digestive juice produced by the liver that emulsifies fats (30)

bimanual—two-handed, deep palpation (36)

bioequivalent—drug that has the same strength and action of another drug (53)

bioethics—ethical decisions pertaining to life issues such as stem cell research, in vitro fertilization, and abortion rights (3)

biofeedback—using biological information to decrease stress (58)

biohazards—biological substances, such as medical waste and samples of a virus or a bacterium, that cause a threat to human beings and are potentially infectious (6)

biopsy—microscopic examination of tissue to detect canserous cells (42)

bipolar disorder—mood disorder characterized by swings of mood between depression and mania (57)

birthday rule—used by insurance claims administrators to determine which parent's benefit plans will pay for the medical bills of a dependent child when the child is covered by the plans of both parents (18)

blepharitis—inflammation of the eyelids (26)

blepharoptosis—drooping of the eyelid (26)

blind ad—advertisement that does not identify the institution or facility that placed the ad (59)

block—style of letter writing in which all lines are flush with the left margin (11)

bloodborne pathogens—microorganisms capable of causing disease in blood (34)

blood pressure—force exerted by the blood on the walls of the arteries (27)

B lymphocytes—cells responsible for production of circulating antibodies (28)

body mechanics—proper coordination of alignment, balance, and movement (6)

body surface area (BSA)—calculation of the child's height and weight, expressed as m^2 (meters squared) (52)

bookkeeping—process of managing the accounts for a business (15)

bounding pulse—full pulse, indicating an increase in blood volume (35)

bradycardia—abnormally slow heart rate of below 60 beats per minute (31, 35, 49)

bradypnea—abnormally slow respiration rate below 12 cycles per minute (35)

brand name—name given to a drug by its manufacturer; with the first letter of the name generally being capitalized; also known as the *proprietary name* (53)

BRAT diet—diet for patients with diarrhea; consists of bananas, rice, cereal, applesauce, and toast (40)

breach of confidentiality—failure to keep patient information confidential; occurs when patient information is released to others without authorization from the patient (18)

breach of contract—failure by either party in a valid contract to comply with terms of the agreement (3)

breast cancer—cancer arising in breast tissue; types include ductal (the most common, which develops in the tiny ducts that run from the milk glands to the nipple), infiltrating lobular (which develops in the lobules), and inflammatory (33)

broad spectrum—refers to antibiotics that are effective against a large range of microorganisms (53)

bronchi—the two main branches of the trachea extending into the lungs that are a passageway for air into the lungs (29)

bronchiolitis—inflammation of the bronchioles or small air vessels commonly seen in children (40)

bronchitis—respiratory system disorder in which the mucous membranes in the bronchial passages become inflamed, resulting in mucus production, coughing, and breathlessness (29)

bronchodilators—medications that open the bronchial passages (29)

bruit—sound made by a heart murmur (27)

bucky—type of grid used in radiography; composed of alternating strips of lead and radiolucent material (48)

buffers—a mechanism within the blood that balances the pH level, thus preventing blood from becoming too acidic or too alkaline (27)

bulbourethral glands—two pea-size glands located inferior to the prostate and on either side of the urethra that secrete a mucous secretion into the seminal fluid before ejaculation; also known as *Cowper's glands* (33)

bulimia nervosa—eating disorder characterized by binge eating and self-induced vomiting and purging (40)

bundle of His—one of the three areas of specialized neuromuscular tissue that initiate the heartbeat; also known as *atrioventricular (AV) bundle* (27)

bursa—sac of fluid that cushions and lubricates an area where joint-related tissues rub against one another (23)

bursitis—inflammation of the bursa (23)

cadavers—dead human bodies used to study human anatomy (2)

caduceus—recognized symbol for medicine; depicts a healing staff with two snakes coiled around it (2)

calibrate—to use a known standard to measure the accuracy of equipment (44)

caller ID—program to identify who is calling the recipient (7)

callus—thickened skin that does not have an identifiable border (22)

calorie—measurement of 1 unit of heat that provides energy (56)

canceled checks—deposited checks that have been processed by the bank (16)

cancellous (spongy) bone—reticular tissue that makes up most of the volume of a long bone; includes red bone marrow, which manufactures most red blood cells (23)

candidiasis—yeast infection; also known as *thrush* (45)

canthus—either of the two corners of the eye where the upper and lower eyelids meet (26)

capillaries—smallest blood vessels; connect the arteries and veins that pump the blood to and from the heart (47)

capital equipment—items that require a large dollar amount to purchase (generally over $500) and have a relatively long life (10)

capitation rate—predetermined amount paid to provider every month regardless of the number of times the patient is seen within the month (17)

carbon dioxide (CO$_2$)—compound of carbon and oxygen, given off in the process of metabolism in the cells and expired from the body through the lungs (29)

carboxyhemoglobin—when hemoglobin is carrying carbon dioxide (47)

carbuncle—a collection of furuncles (22)

carcinoma in situ—cancer in a particular area that has not broken through the basement membrane (38)

cardiac arrest—stoppage of the beating of the heart; also known as *heart attack* (27)

cardiac muscle—type of involuntary muscle found in the heart, roughly quadrangular in shape, cross striated, and having a single central nucleus (24)

cardiac tamponade—congestion of the heart muscle and restriction of heart movement caused by blood or fluid trapped in the pericardial sac (27)

cardiogenic shock—collapse of the cardiovascular system characterized by vasodilation and fluid shifting away from the heart (27)

cardiomegaly—enlargement of the heart (27, 32)

cardiomyopathy—disease of the myocardium, or heart muscle, and the resulting ventricular dysfunction (27)

carditis—inflammation of the heart (27)

carotid artery—artery found on each side of the neck (27)

cash disbursement—payments made to creditors (16)

cashier's check—check guaranteeing payment that is written on a check with the bank as the payer (16)

cataract—clouding over the lens of the eye; prevents light from entering (26)

catch-up time—time built into the morning or afternoon schedule for emergencies (9)

cecum—small pouch that forms the beginning of the large intestine (30)

cell—most basic unit of life; often considered the building block of the human body (21)

cell membrane—the outer covering of the cell (21)

cellulitis—acute, spreading bacterial infection below the surface of the skin, characterized by erythema, warmth, swelling, and pain that can also cause fever, chills, and enlarged lymph nodes (22)

cementum—thin layer of bone that covers the dentin of the root of a tooth; provides protection and anchors the periodontal ligament (30)

central nervous system (CNS)—comprised of the brain and spinal cord (25)

central processing unit (CPU)—the "brain" of the computer, which executes specific sets of instructions (12)

centrifuge—instrument used to separate specimens into component layers (44)

cerebrospinal fluid (CSF)—fluid produced by the choroid plexus in the ventricles of the brain that moves through the spinal canal and the subarachnoid space and surrounds the brain; cushions the brain and spinal cord and nourishes them with oxygen and glucose (25)

cerebrovascular accident (CVA)—sudden death of brain cells that occurs when the blood supply to part of the brain is suddenly interrupted; also known as *stroke* (27)

Certificate of Waiver Tests (WTs)—Clinical Laboratory Improvement Amendments (CLIA) category of least-complex, least-risky laboratory tests if performed incorrectly (44)

certification—issuance by an official body or professional organization of a certificate and credentials to one who has met the education and experience standards of that organization (1, 2)

certification examination—test required for a student to become certified as a medical assistant (59)

certified check—check that is guaranteed because the money has been put aside in the check writer's account (16)

Certified Medical Administrative Specialist (CMAS)—a medical assistant who has met eligibility requirements and who can prove his or her competency to perform entry-level skills through written examination; certification is awarded to candidates who pass the AMT certification examination (1)

Certified Medical Assistant (CMA [AAMA])—multiskilled health care professional who has met the standards of the AAMA by achieving a satisfactory test result and assists providers in an allied health care setting (1)

cerumen—earwax (26, 39)

cervical cancer—rapid uncontrolled growth of severely abnormal cells on the cervix; the two main types are squamous cell (epidermoid) and adenocarcinoma (33)

cervicitis—inflammation of the cervix, usually caused by sexually transmitted infections (STIs) (33)

chancre—syphilitic sore (38)

character—the sum of the values, attitudes, and behaviors a person exhibits (5)

charge slip—record of services for billing and for insurance processing; also known as *superbill* or *encounter form* (15)

chemotherapy—use of chemicals, including drugs, to treat or control infections and diseases such as cancer (2, 28)

chief complaint—reason for the office visit; also known as *presenting problem* (36)

childhood—last period of child development; from ages 3 to 11 years (57)

cholelithiasis—formation of gallstones (30)

cholesterol—fatlike material normally found in the body that is essential for the function of body systems such as the nervous system,

formation of cell membranes, and manufacture of many hormones (56)

chondrocytes—cells that form cartilage (23)

chorionic villus sampling (CVS)—removing a small sample of tissue from the placenta to examine it for chromosomal abnormalities (38)

choroid—membrane that lines the sclera and absorbs extra light entering the eye (26)

chromosomes—microscopic bodies that carry the genes that determine hereditary characteristics (21)

chronic fatigue syndrome (CFS)—immune system disorder of unknown origin that causes depression, sleep disorders, and lack of energy (28)

chronic obstructive pulmonary disease (COPD)—progressive, chronic, usually irreversible respiratory system condition in which the lungs have diminished capacity for inhalation and exhalation (29, 50)

chronic pain—pain that persists longer than 6 months and interferes with functions of life (35, 55)

chronic renal failure—gradual and progressive loss of kidney function (31)

chronological medical record—patient record that follows the patient over a period of time, with each visit consisting of a new entry by date, rather than by symptoms or diagnosis (13)

chyme—semiliquid form of food that is passed from the stomach to the small intestine (30)

cilia—small, hairlike projections that cover the surface of some cells; in the nose they trap dust, pollen, and other foreign matter to prevent them from entering the nasal cavity (21, 29)

ciliary body—part of the middle layer of the surface of the eyeball that holds and moves the lens (26)

circumcision—surgical removal of the foreskin of the penis, performed for religious, cultural, or medical reasons (33)

circumduction—process of moving a body part in a circular motion (23)

cirrhosis—potentially life-threatening condition that occurs when the liver is damaged, usually after years of inflammation, scarring, or fibrosis that replaces healthy tissue and prevents the liver from working normally (30)

civil law—laws governing how people relate to each other and the government (3)

claim—written and documented request for reimbursement of an eligible expense under an insurance plan (17)

clarity—quality or state of being understandable (7)

Clark's rule—most common law used in the calculation of drug dosage for children; based on weight of the child (52)

claustrophobia—fear of enclosed spaces (48)

clean claim—health insurance claim form that has been completed correctly without any errors or omissions (18)

clearinghouse—independent entity that reviews claims, requests clarification from the provider, and "cleans" claims, ensuring accurate information is documented, then submits claims to insurance companies in proper format (18)

clinical diagnosis—preliminary presumptive diagnosis made by physician based on health history and physical examination; also known as *working diagnosis* (35)

Clinical Laboratory Improvement Amendments (CLIA)—enacted by Congress to regulate all laboratories that test human specimens to help ensure accurate patient test results (44)

clock speed—speed at which a computer's central processing unit (CPU) can process instructions (12)

close-ended questions—questions that can be answered with a yes or a no response (5)

closed-panel HMO—facility that is owned by the HMO and in which the providers are employees of the HMO (17)

closed records—medical files of patients who have indicated that they are no longer a patient or who have died, that are kept in storage for legal reasons (13)

CMS-1500—most common health insurance claim form used to file claims for physicians' services (18)

cochlea—bony spiral-shaped structure that forms a portion of the inner ear (26)

cognitive—based on knowledge (58)

cognitive ability—ability to think clearly, reason, and perceive (41)

colic—acute abdominal pain (37)

colitis—inflammation of the large intestine caused by many different disease processes, including infections, primary inflammatory disorders, ulcerative colitis, Crohn's colitis, lymphocytic and collagenous colitis, lack of blood flow, and history of radiation to the large bowel (30)

collating—collecting all records, tests results, and information pertaining to a patient who is scheduled to be seen by the physician (8)

colleagues—fellow members of the profession (20)

collimeter—radiographic device that controls the size and shape of the X-ray field coming from the tube (48)

colon—makes up the bulk of the large intestine and can be divided into the ascending colon, transverse colon, descending colon, and sigmoid colon (30)

colonized—carrying bacteria, such as MRSA, in the nose, throat, armpit, and groin (34)

colony—growth of one type of microorganism visible with the naked eye on the surface of a culture medium (45)

colorectal cancer—collective term for colon and rectal cancer (30)

combining form—word root that has a vowel attached to it in order to add another element (4)

combining vowel—vowel, usually "o," added to a word root before combining (4)

Commission on Accreditation of Allied Health Education Programs (CAAHEP)—body that accredits educational programs that prepare medical assisting students to take the CMA (AAMA) exam (1)

common cold—infection of the upper respiratory tract caused by any one of a number of viruses and differing from other viral infections in its lack of producing high fever or significant fatigue (29)

compact bone—dense, hard layer of bone tissue in a long bone (23)

complement—group of proteins activated by antibodies that assist in destroying bacteria, viruses, and infected cells (28)

complimentary close—courtesy word(s), such as "Sincerely," "Sincerely yours," or "Yours truly," that appear two spaces below the end of the body of a letter (11)

compound microscope—microscope that has two sets of lenses, oculars, and objectives (44)

compulsions—acts performed to relieve anxiety (57)

computer—programmable machine that responds to a specific set of instructions and performs a list of instructions in a programmed language (12)

concussion—injury caused by sharp jarring or a blow to the head that may result in a loss of consciousness (25)

condescending—behavior in which a person adopts a superior attitude and acts as though he or she is better than someone else (5)

conduction hearing loss—result of the obstruction of sound waves (39)

cones—photosensitive cells in the retina that respond to bright light and are used in color vision (26)

conference call—call in which several parties at different locations are on the telephone line simultaneously (7)

confidentiality—the state of safeguarding a patient's confidences, particularly information in the medical record regarding family history, past or current diseases or illnesses, test results, and medications (1)

congenital disorder—genetic disorder that is present at birth (21)

congestive heart failure (CHF)—condition in which the heart cannot pump sufficient blood to the other organs; also known as *heart failure* (27)

conjunctiva—protective mucous membrane lining the underside of the eyelid and the anterior part of the eyeball (26)

conjunctivitis—an inflammation of the conjunctiva frequently caused by a virus, bacteria, sexually transmitted infections (STIs), allergens, and irritants; also known as *pinkeye* (26)

constant information—body of a form letter that is retained in the computer's memory or on an external storage device (11)

constipation—condition in which stools are difficult to pass, involving straining, a feeling of not completely emptying the bowels, and hard or pelletlike stools (30)

contact dermatitis—allergic reaction of the skin caused by irritating substances coming in contact with it, often resulting in red, irritated skin and occasionally in vesicles and rash (22)

continuing education units (CEUs)—credit awarded for additional course work beyond certification; one unit of training or education is granted for each clock hour of workshops, seminars, or conferences (1)

contract law—laws relating to enforceable promises and agreements between two or more persons to do or not to do a particular action (3)

contracture—permanent shortening of the muscle around a joint that causes abnormal and sometimes painful positioning of the joint (24, 51)

contraindicated—when medications have such dangerous effects that their use must be immediately discontinued (53)

contributory negligence—patient's contribution to the injury, which if proven would release the physician as the direct cause (3)

control samples—laboratory samples similar to the required testing specimens that have been previously tested and have a known value (44)

contusion—bruising of the brain (25)

coordination of benefits (COB)—procedures to prevent duplication of payment by more than one insurance carrier (17)

copayments—predetermined amounts of money the patient must pay for medical services at every visit, as determined by the insurance company (8, 15)

corn—thickened area of the skin that has a distinct border with various textures (22)

cornea—clear, transparent covering of the eye; frequently referred to as the "window" of the eye because it allows light to enter (26, 39)

corneal abrasion—lesion or abrasion on the cornea that results from injury or infection (26)

coronary arteries—crown of arteries that supply the heart with freshly oxygenated blood (27)

coronary artery disease (CAD)—blockage of the arteries that supply the heart muscle; also known as *coronary heart disease (CHD)* (27, 49)

cor pulmonale—heart disease that causes the right ventricle to enlarge as a result of primary lung disease; also called *right-sided heart disease* (27)

corpus callosum—largest nerve tract that connects the right and left hemispheres of the brain (25)

cortex—*in the lymph nodes,* portion of node that is mainly populated by lymphocytes; *in the kidney,* outer layer, in which the arteries, veins, convoluted tubules, and glomerular capsules are found (28, 31)

cover letter—letter introducing the applicant to an employer, stating the purpose of the correspondence, the position being sought, and the applicant's match to the stated requirements (59)

crash cart—cart or kit that is instantly accessible to anyone in the medical office and contains all supplies that may be needed during an emergency (43)

credits—funds added to an account (16)

Crohn's disease—a chronic disease of the intestines that primarily causes ulcerations in the lining of the small and large intestines but can affect the digestive system anywhere from the mouth to the anus; also known as *inflammatory bowel disease (IBD)* (30)

crossover claim—patient claim that is eligible for both Medicare and Medicaid; also known as *Medi/Medi* (17)

croup—inflammation of the larynx and trachea characterized by a barking cough (40)

cryosurgery—use of subfreezing temperatures to destroy tissue (42)

cryotherapy—use of cold for therapeutic purposes (51)

crystals—formed by the precipitation of urinary salts when pH, temperature, or concentration occur (46)

culture—values, beliefs, attitudes, views, and customs shared by a group of people and passed on through the generations (5)

culture media—substances that enhance the growth of micoorganisms (45)

culturette—disposable clear plastic tube that contains a sterile cotton-tipped applicator swab and a sealed plastic vial of medium, used to obtain many types of specimens (45)

cumulative—increasing in effect by successive exposures (48)

Current Procedural Terminology **(CPT)**—code book for procedures and services performed by providers (19)

Cushing's disease—rare disorder that develops when too much cortisol is released by the adrenal cortex as a result of stimulation of the pituitary (32)

cyanosis—bluish discoloration of the skin and nail beds due to lack of oxygen in the tissues (27, 29, 35)

cycle time—length of time the average patient spends in the medical office (9, 10)

cystitis—inflammation of the bladder that usually occurs when bacteria infect the lower urinary tract (31)

cytokinesis—division of the nuclei of the cell and distribution of organelles into two daughter cells (21)

cytoplasm—jellylike substance found between the cell membrane and the nuclear membrane (21)

day sheet—used to list or post each day's financial transactions: charges, payments, adjustments, and credits (15)

debits—charges against an account (16)

debridement—removal of dead tissue around wound edges using sterile technique (42)

decibel—intensity of the sound (39)

decubitus ulcer—an area of skin and tissue that breaks down when constant pressure is maintained on it; also known as *pressure sore* or *bedsore* (22)

deductible—amount of eligible charges each patient must pay each calendar year before the insurance plan begins to pay benefits (17)

defamation of character—scandalous statement about someone that can injure the person's reputation (3)

defensive behavior—reaction to a perceived threat that is usually unconscious in nature (5)

dehiscence—separation of wound edges (42)

deltoid muscle—small muscle mass located on the outer surface of the upper arm that is ideal for small dosages of medications (54)

delusions—fixed, false beliefs (57)

demographic—information such as age, gender, ethnic background, education, and Social Security number (8)

denied claim—occurs when procedures or services are not covered by the patient's insurance policy or when the patient has not met his or her deductible (18)

denominator—bottom number of a fraction (52)

dentin—calcified, largely mineral tissue that forms the bulk of teeth (30)

deoxyribonucleic acid (DNA)—provides the cell's blueprint or genetic makeup (21)

deposits—money (cash, checks) placed in a bank account (16)

depreciation—loss in value resulting from normal aging, use, or deterioration (10)

dermis—the middle of the three layers that comprise the skin (22)

desensitizing injections—minute amounts of an allergen injected over an extended period of time to build tolerance for the allergen in the patient's body (37)

dexterity—ability to use one's hands effectively (55)

diabetes mellitus—condition in which the body is unable to produce enough insulin to properly control blood sugar levels by converting sugar and starches into energy (32)

diabetic retinopathy—disease of the retina secondary to diabetes mellitus (26)

diagnosis—determination of the cause and nature of a disease or injury (35)

diagnosis-related groups (DRGs)—Medicare hospital payment system, which classifies each Medicare patient according to his or her illness (2)

dialysis—separation of substances in solution; for renal patients, using a filter other than the kidneys to remove toxins from blood and maintain water balance (31)

diaphoresis—excessive sweating (37)

diaphragm—dome-shaped muscle that separates the chest from the abdomen and helps pump air into, and carbon dioxide out of, the lungs (29)

diaphysis—shaft of a long bone (23)

diarthrotic joint—articulation, or joint, that allows for free movement in multiple directions (23)

diastole—phase 2 of the cardiac cycle in which both atria and ventricles are relaxed, and pressure in the heart chamber is low (27)

diastolic blood pressure—lowest cuff pressure at which the Korotkoff sounds disappear, when the left ventricle of the heart relaxes (27, 35)

diathermy—therapeutic use of a high-frequency current to generate heat within some part of the body (51)

differential diagnosis—determination of which one of multiple possibilities is the cause of a problem (35)

diffusion—moving dissolved particles from an area of greater concentration to an area of lesser concentration (21)

digestion—process by which the body converts food into chemical substances that can be absorbed into the blood and used by the body tissues and organs (56)

dilation—widening of the cervix prior to birth (38)

diluent—agent that dilutes a substance or solution to which it is added (44)

diphtheria—acute infectious disease that has symptoms such as headache, fever, and sore throat (54)

diplopia—double vision (26)

dirty claim—a health insurance claim form that is incorrect because it has missing data or errors (18)

discretion—ability to make decisions responsibly, communicate tactfully with others, be fair, and be familiar with policies and regulations (1)

discriminatory—prejudicial (20)

disinfection—soaking and wiping process used to destroy or inhibit the activity of disease-causing organisms (34)

dislocation—disconnection of the bones that meet at a joint, usually caused by a sudden impact, such that the bones are no longer in their normal positions (23)

diversity—variety (58)

diverticulitis—inflammation or infection of a diverticulum (a small pouch or sac in the wall of the colon) generally caused by stool lodging in diverticula, which can lead to swelling or rupture (30)

diverticulosis—condition of having diverticula (small outpouchings in the large intestine), most typically in the sigmoid colon; increases with age because of the weakening of the colon walls (30)

document—the act of charting a procedure or patient teaching in a patient's medical record (55)

dorsiflexion—the process of bending a body part backward (23)

dorsogluteal site—upper-outer quadrant of the buttocks; ideal location for administration of large-volume intramuscular medications (54)

dosimeter—equipment that measures the level and intensity of radiation exposure (48)

double booking—giving two patients the same time slot without allowing any additional time on the shedule (9)

dressing—sterile covering placed directly over a wound to absorb blood and other body fluids, prevent contamination, and protect the wound from further trauma (43)

drug abuse—use of a drug improperly or wrongly (53)

drug dependency—relying on medication or taking medication for psychological support (53)

Drug Enforcement Administration (DEA)—U.S. government agency responsible for enforcing drug control (53)

drug tolerance—a decrease in the effectiveness of a drug as the body gets used to having the drug in its system (53)

dwarfism—condition characterized by shorter-than-normal skeletal growth (32)

dysmenorrhea—painful abdominal cramps during menstruation (33)

dysplasia—abnormal cells (38)

dysplastic nevus—an abnormal mole (22)

dyspnea—difficulty breathing (27, 29)

dysrhythmia—pulse with an irregular rhythm; also known as *arrythmia* (35)

dysuria—burning or painful urination (31)

eclampsia—condition during pregnancy characterized by severe hypertension, convulsion, possible coma, and death (38)

ectopic pregnancy—growth of a fertilized ovum in the fallopian tube rather than the uterus (38)

ectropion—turning outward of the eyelid (26)

eczema—a chronic skin condition characterized by scaling, itching, and rashes; caused by an allergic-type reaction on the skin; also known as *atopic dermatitis* (22)

effacement—thinning of the cervical walls prior to delivery (38)

efferent nerves—transmit impulse from neural cell body to stimulate target muscle or organ (25)

effleurage—light stroking movement that may be performed in a circular pattern (51)

Einthoven's triangle—pictorial guide to the leads in an electrocardiogram (49)

electrocardiogram (ECG)—tracing or recording of electrical activity as it moves through the heart (49)

electroconvulsive therapy (ECT)—procedure occasionally used for cases of prolonged major depression, in which an electrode is placed on one or both sides of a patient's head and low-voltage current is turned on briefly, causing a convulsive seizure (57)

electrolyte—an ion that is electrically charged and moves to either a negative (cathode) or positive (anode) electrode (21)

electronic health record (EHR)—medical records kept via computer; also known as *electronic medical record* (14)

electronic mail—all written materials that are transmitted electronically; also known as *e-mail* (11)

electronic medical record (EMR)—electronic means of gathering, documenting, and storing information about the patient and the care received in the medical setting; also known as *electronic health record* (13, 14)

electronic signature—electronic version of a person's signature used in electronic medical records (14)

electronystagmograph (ENG)—instrument used to measure involuntary movements of the eyes (39)

embezzlement—unauthorized taking of funds that involves breach of trust (16)

embolus—blood clot that has moved from its place of origin (37)

emergency kit—cart or kit that is instantly accessible to anyone in the medical office and contains all supplies that may be needed during an emergency (43)

empathy—ability to be sensitive to or understand the feelings of another individual and identify with what he or she is experiencing without necessarily experiencing the same thing (1)

emphysema—progressive respiratory system disease in which the tissues necessary to support the physical shape and function of the lung are destroyed, causing shortness of breath and other symptoms (29)

enamel—hardest and most compact part of the tooth, made up almost entirely of mineral; covers the exposed part of the crown (30)

encephalitis—inflammation in the brain, most often caused by a viral infection (25)

enclosure—document included with a letter, such as an X-ray or medical record (11)

encounter form—record of services for billing and for insurance processing; also known as *superbill* or *charge slip* (15)

encounter note—documentation of the patient visit to the physician's office (58)

endocardium—innermost lining of the heart wall (27)

endometriosis—condition in which the endometrium (the tissue lining the uterus) is found outside the uterus, usually in the pelvis or abdominal cavity (33)

endometrium—lining of the uterus (38)

endomysium—connective tissue covering that surrounds an individual muscle cell (24)

endosteum—tough connective tissue membrane lining the medullary canal and containing the bone marrow in a long bone (23)

enteritis—food poisoning (45)

entropion—turning inward of the eyelid (26)

enunciation—clear articulation and pronunciation of words (7)

enuresis—urinary incontinence while sleeping (31)

eosinophil—granular white cell that captures invading microorganisms and antibody-antigen reactions through phagocytosis (37)

epidermis—one of the three layers that compose the skin (22)

epididymitis—inflammation or infection of the epididymis (the long coiled tube attached to the upper part of each testicle), where mature sperm are stored before ejaculation (33)

epiglottis—flap of tissue that covers the trachea during swallowing (29)

epilepsy—disorder associated with misfiring or interference of electrical impulses within the brain, which can lead to seizures (25)

epimysium—thin fascia covering muscles (24)

epiphysis—ends of a developing long bone (23)

episiotomy—incision made in the perineum (the external region between the vulva and the anus) during labor to prevent its tearing during delivery (33)

erectile dysfunction (ED)—inability to achieve or maintain an erection sufficient for sexual intercourse, resulting from insufficient blood supply, from the failure of the smooth muscle to relax, or from the failure of the penis to retain the blood that flows into it (33)

ergonomics—application of scientific information and data regarding human body mechanics to the design of objects and overall environments for human use (6)

erythema—redness of the skin (22, 51))

erythrocytes—biconcave cells produced in the red bone marrow that are small enough to pass through capillaries and carry oxygen to the tissues and organs; also known as *red blood cells (RBCs)* (27)

erythrocyte sedimentation rate (ESR)—rate at which red blood cells settle at the bottom of a tube (47)

erythropoietin—glycoprotein hormone that controls red blood cell production (47)

eschar—scab (42)

esophagus—collapsible tube about 10 inches long along which food is carried from the pharynx to the stomach (30)

established patient—one who has been seen within the past 3 years by any practitioner of the same specialty in the practice (9)

ethnicity—classification of people based on national origin (5)

ethnocentric—belief that one's own cultural background is better than any other (5)

etiology—cause or source of a disease or disorder (23)

eukaryotic—cells that have a nucleus and organelles in the cytoplasm (45)

eupnea—normal breathing (35)

Eustachian tube—auditory tube that extends from the middle ear to the nasopharynx (26)

evaluation—checking to see how the patient is carrying out the teaching plan (55)

Evaluation and Management (E/M)—codes for services such as office visits, consultations, the physician's component for emergency services, and inpatient care (19)

eversion—process of turning outward (23)

evisceration—separation of wound edges and protrusion of abdominal organs (42)

exclusive provider organization (EPO)—combination of PPO and HMO concepts that allows the patient to select from a defined panel of providers (17)

excoriation—painful chafing or rawness of the skin (40)

excreta—waste products (34)

exophthalmos—condition produced by hyperthyroidism in which the eyeballs protrude beyond their normal protective orbit because of swelling in the tissues behind them (26, 32)

expendable supplies—items that are used up in a short period of time and have a relatively inexpensive unit cost (10)

expiration—exhalation (29)

expiratory reserve volume (ERV)—amount of air that can be forcibly exhaled after a normal exhale (50)

extended care facility—assisted living facility that is designed to care for patients with specific care and rehabilitation needs (41)

extended warranty—option of lengthening the time the manufacturer's warranty is in effect once the original warranty expires, usually requiring an additional fee (10)

extension—process of straightening a flexed limb or the spine (23)

external genitalia—external sexual organs (38)

externship—situation, also called a practicum, in which a student works without payment in a physician's office, hospital, or other health care setting for 160 hours over a minimum of 4 weeks during the final stage of his or her training, under the supervision of someone at the site (1, 59)

exudates—wound drainage material made of serum, white blood cells, and fibrin (45, 51)

facsimile (fax)—electronically transmitted document containing print and/or graphic information (8)

facultative anaerobe—able to live with some oxygen (45)

failure to thrive (FTT)—inability to gain sufficient weight in accordance with standardized baby growth charts (40)

Fair Debt Collection Practices Act—law that governs issues regarding debt collection and outlines general rules to follow when attempting to collect overdue accounts (15)

fallopian tubes—structures that extend laterally from either side of the uterus near each ovary and serve as ducts to move ova (egg cells) from the ovary to the uterus and to move sperm from the uterus toward the ovary; also known as *uterine tubes* or *oviducts* (33)

fascia—fibrous sheath that holds together the connective tissue and muscle fibers that make up muscles (24)

fascicles—sections into which a muscle is divided by the perimysium (24)

fasting—refraining from food and drink for a prescribed time period (44)

febrile—having a fever (35)

febrile seizures—convulsions suffered by some children with high fevers following a rapid spike in body temperature (40)

feces—stool (45)

feedback—any response to a communication (5)

fee-for-service—set of fees for services established by a health care provider and paid for by the patient (17)

fee schedule—schedule of the amount paid by a specific insurance company for each procedure or service subject to the managed care contract (17)

fibrocystic breast disease—condition that involves common, benign changes in the tissues of the breast; also known as *mammary dysplasia, benign breast disease,* and *diffuse cystic mastopathy* (33)

fibrillation—quivering or spontaneous contraction of individual muscle fibers (27)

fibromyalgia—musculoskeletal pain and fatigue disorder with no known cause but with evidence pointing to a genetic predisposition to a neuromuscular or neuroendocrine abnormality that disturbs the usual sensory perception, especially of pain signals (24)

filtration—use of mechanical pressure to diffuse dissolved particles through membranes (21)

financial life—a loss in product value resulting from normal aging, use, or deterioration; also known as *depreciation* (10)

first responders—emergency medical service (EMS) providers who are trained to recognize medical conditions, initiate basic life support, and access other parts of the health care system (43)

fissure—a deep groove in the brain (25)

fixed—type of slide preparation that ensures the specimen stays on the slide during the staining process (45)

flagella—tail-like structures that enable a cell to move through a medium (21)

flexion—process of bending (or curving) a flexed limb or the spine (23)

fluoroscopy—visual examination of the body or the function of an organ using a fluoroscope (48)

flutter—trembling of the heart (27)

folliculitis—inflammation or infection of hair follicles that most often appears in areas that become irritated by shaving or the rubbing of clothes, or where follicles and pores are blocked by oils and dirt (22)

forced expiratory volume (FEV)—volume of air that is forcefully exhaled in the first second of exhalation (50)

forced vital capacity (FVC)—maximum volume of air expelled when the patient exhales as forcibly and quickly as possible following one inhalation (50)

formulary—specific to each insurance carrier, a list of medications that will be covered under that insurance plan (17)

fovea centralis retinae—pit in the middle of the macula lutea that contains only cones (26)

fraction bar—bar that separates the numerator and the denominator of a fraction (52)

frenulum lingua—longitudinal fold of mucous membrane under the tongue (35)

frequency—need to void often (31); fluctuations per second of energy in the form of sound waves (39)

friction—rubbing or deep stroking that produces an increase in circulation and mild heat within tissues (51)

Fried's law—pediatric dosage law applied to children under the age of 1 year, based on their age in months (52)

functional residual capacity (FRC)—amount of air that can be inhaled after a normal expiration (50)

fundus—floor of the tympanic cavity (26); top of the uterus (38)

Furuncle—an abscess of a hair follicle and the adjacent subcutaneous tissues; also known as *boil* (22)

gait—one's manner of walking (51)

gallbladder—membranous sac in which bile is stored and concentrated (30)

gallops—abnormal heart rhythm that sounds like a galloping horse (49)

gamete—cell developed through the process of meiosis that contains one-half the chromosomes of its original parent cell (21)

ganglion cyst—benign saclike swelling that typically develops over a joint or tendon (24)

gantry—circular structure that houses X-ray equipment used in computed tomography (48)

gastroesophageal reflux disease (GERD)—condition in which the muscle at the superior portion of the stomach (the cardiac sphincter) does not close tightly or relaxes inappropriately, allowing gastric fluids and stomach contents into the esophagus and the throat (30)

gatekeeper—a primary care provider who refers patients to other providers for services he or she cannot perform (17)

Gender bias—indicating either male or female by the type of language used (11)

generic name—single identifying name, typically noted in lowercase letters, that is considered the legal name for a drug (53)

genetics—study of the makeup of animals or plants (21)

genitalia—reproductive organs (40)

geriatrician—physician who diagnoses and treats diseases and disorders that mainly affect older patients (41)

geriatrics—branch of medicine that specializes in the treatment of the elderly (41)

germinal centers—primary locations where B lymphocytes reproduce and proliferate (28) gerontology—study of the process of aging and the effects of aging on people (41)

gestational diabetes—condition in which the body is unable to produce enough insulin to properly control blood sugar levels by converting sugar and starches into energy, occurring during pregnancy and typically disappearing afterward, but occasionally precipitating ongoing type 2 diabetes (32)

gigantism—condition in which excessive growth hormone is secreted during childhood, before the closure of the bone growth plates, causing overgrowth of the long bones, muscles, and organs; usually caused by a pituitary gland tumor (32)

gingivae—gums of the mouth (30)

glaucoma—condition caused by an increase in the amount of pressure in the eye, leading to an excessive amount of aqueous humor that can lead to damage of the optic nerve and eventually blindness (26)

glomerulonephritis—condition involving inflammation and lesions of the glomeruli that hampers the kidney's ability to remove waste and excess fluids and can lead to kidney failure; also known as *glomerular disease* (31, 46)

glycosuria—presence of abnormal sugar in urine (46)

goiter—an enlarged thyroid gland, most commonly caused by Hashimoto's thyroiditis, an autoimmune inflammation of the thyroid (32)

gonads—sexual organs (38)

goniometer—instrument used to measure the range of motion of a joint (36, 51)

gout—disease caused by the formation of urate crystals in a joint, leading to inflammation (23)

Graves' disease—the most common cause of hyperthyroidism, an autoimmune disorder in which the antibodies produced by the immune system stimulate the thyroid to produce too much thyroxine (32)

gravida—total number of pregnancies (38)

grid—device made of parallel lead strips, used to absorb scattered radiation during radiography before it reaches the film (48)

grievance—complaint (20)

ground fault circuit interrupter (GFCI)—stops electricity from flowing where it can cause harm (6)

gross annual wage—total amount earned in one year before taxes and other debits are deducted (16)

guardian ad litem—adult who will act in the court on behalf of a minor (3)

guided imagery—imagining being in a relaxing place (58)

habituation—dependence on a drug (53)

hallucinations—false sensory perceptions (57)

hallux valgus—an enlargement of the inner portion of the metatarsophalangeal joint at the base of the big toe; also known as *bunion* (23)

hammertoe—a condition in which the toe bends upward like a claw because of the abnormal flexion of the proximal interphalangeal joint (23)

Hashimoto's thyroiditis—autoimmune inflammation of the thyroid that causes hypothyroidism and goiter (32)

hay fever—a seasonal allergy that causes inflammation of the mucous membranes of the nose and eyes; also known as *seasonal allergic rhinitis* or *pollinosis* (29)

Health Information Portability and Accountability Act (HIPAA)—legislative act passed in 1996 and fully enacted in 2003, designed to improve the access and portability of medical information and to decrease waste and the abuse of health insurance (14)

health maintenance organization (HMO)—managed care plan in which a range of health care services provided by a limited group of providers (such as specified physicians or hospitals) are made available to plan members for a predetermined fee (17)

hearing acuity—sharpness of hearing (39)

hearing loss—full or partial decrease in the ability to detect or understand sounds: two most common types are conductive (temporary condition in which sound is not conducted efficiently) and sensorineural (permanent hearing loss caused by damage to cochlea or to nerve pathways from the inner ear to the brain) (26)

heart—four-chambered muscular pump that circulates blood throughout the cardiovascular system (27)

heart murmur—condition in which a damaged or diseased valve allows blood to escape and move backward through the valve (27)

heart rate—number of heartbeats per minute (49)

heat exhaustion—a heat illness resulting in extreme fatigue due to excessive loss of sodium and water contained in sweat (43)

heat hydrotherapy—use of warm water as a therapeutic or healing treatment (51)

hematology—study of blood and the tissues that produce it (47)

hematopoiesis—formation of blood cells (47)

hematuria—blood in the urine (46)

hemiplegia—paralysis of one side of the body, usually caused by stroke (25, 51)

hemoglobin—iron-containing pigment of red blood cells that carries oxygen from the lungs throughout the body (27, 47)

hemolyzed—a condition in which red blood cells burst, releasing hemoglobin and causing serum to be a cherry-red color (44)

hemophilia—hereditary deficiency of clotting factors that predisposes the patient to hemoptysis (coughing up of blood) (29)

hemoptysis—coughing up of blood (29)

hemorrhaging—loss of blood when cut or injured (27)

hemorrhoid—dilated vein in the anus wall and sometimes around the rectum, usually caused by untreated constipation but occasionally associated with chronic diarrhea (30)

hemostasis—stoppage of bleeding as a result of the smooth muscle at the site of a break causing the vessel wall to contract, creating a spasm that reduces the amount of blood loss and initiating the attachment of platelets to the broken area and to each other, which forms a plug (27)

heparin—substance that prevents clotting (47)

hepatitis A—most common type of hepatitis in the United States, a viral disease that affects the liver (54)

hepatitis B—highly contagious form of hepatitis that is transmitted by contaminated serum in blood transfusions or through the use of contaminated needles or instruments (54)

heredity—transmission of genetic makeup from parents to children (21)

hernia—abnormal protrusion of an organ, or part of an organ, through the wall of the body cavity that contains it; the most common types of abdominal hernias are hiatal and inguinal (30)

herpes simplex—viral infection that primarily affects the mouth or the genital areas (22)

herpes zoster—an infection caused by the varicella zoster virus that causes a painful rash; also known as *shingles* (22)

hiatal hernia—condition in which the upper portion of the stomach protrudes into the chest cavity through a weakened or enlarged esophageal hiatus (an opening in the diaphragm normally large enough to accommodate only the esophagus) (30)

Hib disease—lesser known disease caused by a bacterium that is spread through the air and enters the lungs or bloodstream of children (54)

hierarchy of needs—five levels of need identified by Abraham Maslow (57)

hilum—bases of the lungs; the notch in the concave border of each kidney (29, 31)

hirsutism—condition of thick abnormal hair growth that affects men and women (22)

histamine—substance that produces signs and symptoms of allergies (37)

holistic—practice of medicine that focuses on the whole patient; addresses the social, emotional, and spiritual needs of a patient as well as physical treatment (5, 51)

Holter monitor—apparatus used to record cardiac activity while the patient is ambulatory for at least 24 hours (49)

homeostasis—result of an organism's systems working together to maintain balance or equilibrium by adjusting for constant changes (21)

homophones—words that sound alike but have different meanings and spellings (11)

hordeolums—inflamed glands of the eyelid, often caused by a bacterial infection that appears as a pus-filled swelling at the base of the eyelash; also known as *sties* (26)

hospice—facility or company that provides an interdisciplinary program of care and supportive services for terminally ill patients and their families (2)

Human Genome Project—publicly funded international research project (completed in 2001) to sequence and identify human genes and record their positions on chromosomes (2)

human papillomaviruses (HPVs)—group of more than a hundred viruses responsible for the majority of cervical cancer cases and for genital warts (38)

hydrocele—painless buildup of watery fluid around one or both testicles that causes the scrotum or groin area to swell (33)

hydrocephalus—excessive fluid around the brain that may lead to brain damage (40)

hydrogenation—process that turns liquid unsaturated fat into solid fat by adding hydrogen (56)

hyfrecator—miniature electrocautery unit (42)

hyperglycemia—high blood sugar level (43)

hyperopia—farsightedness (26, 39)

hyperpyrexia—markedly elevated body temperature; also known as *hyperthermia* (35)

hypersensitivity—abnormal response to a stimulus (37)

hypertension (HTN)—condition in which blood pressure is consistently higher than 140/90 mmHg; also known as *high blood pressure* (27, 35)

hypertensive retinopathy—retinal disease caused by high blood pressure (26)

hyperthermia—markedly elevated body temperature (35)

hyperthyroidism—condition in which the thyroid produces excess amounts of hormones, potentially leading to exophthalmos, palpitations, atrial fibrillation, enlargement of the heart, and congestive heart failure (32)

hyperventilating—breathing rapidly (49)

hyperventilation—deep, rapid respirations (35)

hypoglycemia—low blood sugar level (43)

hypotension—condition in which blood pressure is consistently lower than 90/60 mmHg; also known as *low blood pressure* (27, 35)

hypothermia—below normal body temperature (35, 43)

hypothyroidism—condition in which the thyroid produces inadequate amounts of hormones, which can lead to an enlarged thyroid gland (goiter) (32)

hypoventilation—shallow respirations (35)

hypoxia—insufficient oxygen supply to the tissues caused by ischemia and infarction (27)

hysterectomy—surgical removal of the uterus (33)

icteric—bilious, yellow-green color (44)

idiosyncratic—side effects or adverse effects that are specific to an individual (53)

immune response—series of immune system attacks on organisms and substances that invade the body systems and cause disease (28)

immune system—tissues, organs, and physiologic processes that identify abnormal cells and foreign substances and defend against those that might be harmful (28)

immunity—resistance to a disease (34, 54)

immunizations—substance that decreases susceptibility to a disease; also known as *vaccines* (54)

immunoglobulin—blood product that contains antibodies (54)

immunology—the study of immunity, the resistance to or protection from disease (2)

immunosuppressants—medications that suppress the immune system (28)

impacted cerumen—earwax that becomes hardened and can impair hearing (26)

impetigo—contagious skin infection, found most commonly in children, caused by bacteria that form round, crusted, oozing spots, typically around the nose and mouth (22)

implementing—teaching the patient what to do (55)

inactivated polio vaccine (IPV)—polio vaccine that is injectable (which is the recommended route of vaccination for children) (54)

inactive records—medical files for patients who have not been seen within the time period established by office policy (generally 1 to 5 years) (13)

incident report—written record of the circumstances of an accident, injury, or unusual occurrence (6)

incisions—surgical cuts into tissue (42)

incontinence—involuntary and unpredictable flow of urine (31)

incubation—period of time between exposure to a pathogen and the appearance of the first symptom (34)

incubator—instrument used to maintain a specific temperature to achieve specific results (44)

incus—bone in the middle ear shaped like an anvil (26)

indecipherable—unreadable (14)

infancy—second period of child development from birth to toddlerhood (57)

infarction—death of heart muscle (27)

infectious mononucleosis—a viral infection caused by the Epstein-Barr virus, part of the herpes family, characterized by an increase in white blood cells that contain a single nucleus, and commonly found in young adults; also known as *mononucleosis, mono* and *kissing disease* (28)

inferior vena cava—large vein that brings blood from below the heart to the atrium (27)

inflection—changes in the pitch and tone of voice (7)

influenza—an illness caused by a viral infection of the respiratory tract; also known as *flu* (29)

informed consent—permission or approval given by a patient who is informed by the physician about the possible consequences of both having and not having certain procedures and treatment (3)

inguinal hernia—condition in which tissue or part of the intestine pushes through a weak spot in the abdominal wall in the groin area, causing a bulge in the groin or scrotum (30)

inhalation medications—route of medication administration that delivers medication directly to the respiratory tract (54)

inoculated—microorganisms placed on or in media (45)

inpatient—services provided to patients who are in a facility overnight or on a long-term basis (2)

input devices—devices, such as keyboards and scanners, that feed data and instructions into a computer (12)

inscription—part of the prescription that gives the name of the medication, actual ingredients, and dosage (53)

insertion—in locations where skeletal muscles attach, the attachment point on the bone that moves (24)

inspection—visual examination of the exterior surface of the body (36)

inspiration—inhalation (29)

inspiratory capacity (IC)—amount of air that can be inhaled after normal expiration (50)

inspiratory reserve volume (IRV)—amount of air that can be forcibly inspired after a normal inhale (50)

instill—to place medication in the eye or the ear (39)

insufflation—introduction of gas, vapor, or powder into a cavity (26)

insulin-dependent diabetes mellitus (IDDM)—condition in which the body is unable to produce enough insulin to properly control blood sugar levels by converting sugar and starches into energy; typically diagnosed in children; also known as *type 1 diabetes* and *juvenile diabetes* (32)

integrated delivery system (IDS)—an arrangement in which provider sites have contracts with an insurance company (17)

integrity—adherence to a code of values, honesty, dependability, and dedication to high standards (1)

intermittent pulse—pulse that occasionally skips a beat (35)

International Classification of Diseases, Ninth Revision Clinical Modification (ICD-9-CM)—code book for diagnosed diseases (19)

International Classification of Diseases, Tenth Revision (ICD-10)—most recent edition of the code book for diagnosed diseases (18)

Internet—communications network enabling the linking of computers worldwide for data interchange (120)

Internet service provider (ISP)—company that sells or gives access to the Internet (12)

interneurons—nerve cells that are located entirely within the central nervous system and work as liaisons between sensory and motor neurons by mediating their impulses (25)

interstitial cystitis (IC)—inflammation of the bladder wall, the cause of which is unknown (31)

intractable pain—pain that is overwhelming, difficult to relieve, and all consuming (35)

intradermal injection—given directly under the first layer of the skin (54)

intramuscular (IM) injections—injections into muscle tissue given at a 90-degree angle (54)

intrauterine device (IUD)—small device placed in the uterus as a form of contraception (38)

intubate—to insert a tube into the trachea as an emergency airway (43)

invalid claim—health insurance claim form that has been completed but contains some type of incorrect information (18)

invasive procedure—procedure in which the body is entered (42)

inventory—supplies and equipment (10)

inversion—process of turning inward (23)

iris—part of the middle layer of the eyeball containing the pigment (color) and a "hole" in the center (pupil), which controls the amount of light entering the eye (26)

irrigate—to rinse the eye or ear (39)

irritable bowel syndrome (IBS)—common intestinal condition characterized by abdominal pain and cramps, diarrhea or constipation or both, gas, bloating, nausea, and other symptoms (30)

ischemia—reduced blood flow to the heart (27, 37)

ischemic—receiving less than the normal amount of blood flow (49)

Ishihara test—test for color blindness (39)

Islets of Langerhans—clusters of cells in the pancreas that secrete glucagons, insulin, and somatostatin (32)

itinerary—travel plan (20)

keloid—skin lesion that results from excessive scarring (22)

ketones—by-products of fat metabolism (46)

kickback—incentive provided by physicians, laboratories, hospitals, or pharmaceutical representatives for using their services (19)

kidneys—paired, bean-shaped organs located at the back of the abdominal cavity and lying on either side of the spinal column in the flank area, against the muscles of the back (31)

kidney stones—deposits of mineral salts in the kidney; also known as *renal calculi* (31)

Kilobyte (K or Kb)—one thousand units of storage, a measure of storage capacity or memory (12)

kinesthetic—involving movement (5)

Korotkoff sounds—sounds heard as the arterial wall distends during the compression of the blood pressure cuff (35)

kyphosis—abnormal curvature of the thoracic spine; also known as *humpback* (23, 37)

labyrinth—located in the inner ear, these bony and membraneous structures contain receptors for hearing and equilibrium (26)

lacrimal apparatus—structures that produce, store, and remove tears (26)

lacrimal canaliculi—ducts at the inner corner of each eye that collect and drain tears into the lacrimal sac (26)

lacrimal gland—gland above the outer corner of the eye that secretes tears onto the surface of the conjunctiva of the upper lid (26)

lacrimal sac—part of the lacrimal duct that collects tears and empties into the nasolacrimal duct (26)

lactating—producing milk (56)

lactose—combination of glucose and galactose found in animal milk (56)

large intestine—tube about 5 feet long extending from the ileocecal valve at the small intestine to the anus; made up of the cecum, appendix, colon, and rectum, which function to complete digestion and absorption (30)

laryngeal mirror—instrument used to visualize the larynx (36)

larynx—muscular, cartilaginous structure lined with mucous membrane at the lower end of the pharynx; also known as *voicebox* (29)

lawn technique—culturing technique that involves inoculating agar with a pure culture specimen in overlapping strokes to test for antibiotic sensitivity (45)

leading zero rule—rule that states you must place a zero before the decimal in a number less than one, such as 0.5 (52)

leads—recordings of heart activity from several angles around the heart (49)

Learning outcomes—goals of education; that is, what the patient should achieve as a result of the teaching (55)

ledger card—record of charges, adjustments, payments, and current balance for each patient (15)

Legionnaires' disease—type of pneumonia or lung infection caused by the *Legionella* bacteria (29)

lens—colorless structure suspended behind the iris that sharpens the focus of light rays onto the retina (26)

lethal—of, relating to, or causing death (53)

letterhead—stationery bearing the name of the physician or practice, address, telephone number, and fax number (11)

leukemia—malignant cancer of the bone marrow and blood, affecting the white blood cells (27)

leukocytes—two types (phagocytes and lymphocytes) of larger blood cells that fight infection and thus contribute to homeostasis also known as *white blood cells* (27, 28)

licensure—granting of a license and authorization to practice one's profession by a government agency (2)

life expectancy—functional life period of the product (2)

lifelong learning—process of continuing to learn throughout one's life (58)

ligament—tough fibrous connective tissue that connects bones or connects cartilage to a joint (24)

lipids—fats or fatty acids classified chemically as unsaturated or saturated (56)

lipolysis—destruction of fats (32)

liquid medications—medications that are taken orally and include suspensions, emulsions, elixirs, syrups, and solutions (54)

lithotripsy—procedure that involves passing shock waves through the body to break down kidney stones (31)

liver—largest glandular organ that plays an essential role in the metabolism of carbohydrates, fats, and proteins (30)

living will—document that allows patients to request that life-sustaining treatments and nutritional support not be used to prolong their lives (3)

lochia—vaginal discharge from the uterus that occurs after childbirth (38)

lordosis—exaggerated inward curvature of the lumbar spine; also known as *swayback* (23, 37)

lung cancer—cancer of the lung tissue (29)

lungs—conical, lobed, spongy, elastic organs in the chest that bring air into contact with the blood and facilitate the exchange of gases in the alveoli and interact with the circulatory system to deliver oxygen and remove carbon dioxide (29)

lunula—crescent-shaped white area at the base of the nail (22)

Lyme disease—caused by the bacterium *Borrelia burgdorferi,* which is transmitted through the bite of an infected tick and results in the telltale round bull's-eye rash (24)

lymph—clear fluid that travels through the body's arteries, circulating through the tissues to cleanse them and keep them firm, and then draining away through the lymphatic system (27)

lymphedema—condition resulting from an interruption of the normal lymphatic flow (28)

lymphocytes—white blood cells created in the bone marrow that allow the body to recognize organisms that have invaded it previously (28, 47)

macrominerals—minerals that are required in larger amounts in the body than trace minerals (56)

macula lutea—yellow spot on the back of the eye (26)

macular degeneration—deterioration of the central portion of the retina (26)

magnetic ink character recognition (MICR)—characters and letters printed on the bottom of the check used as routing information to identify the bank and the number of the individual account (16)

main memory—part of the central processing unit that stores data and program instructions and does not perform any logical operation, such as computation or sorting (12)

malignant—cancerous (37)

malignant melanoma—type of skin cancer, originating in the melanocyte cells of the skin, that develops when the melanocytes do not respond to normal control mechanisms of cellular growth (22)

malleus—bone in the middle ear that is shaped like a hammer (26)

manipulation—passive assessment or movement of the range of motion of a joint (36)

Manometer—part of a sphygmomanometer, a scale that registers the actual pressure reading (35)

massage—kneading or applying pressure with the hands to a part of the patient's body to promote muscle relaxation, improve blood circulation, and reduce tension (51)

mass storage device—equipment that can store much information (e.g., a Zip drive) even when the computer is off (12)

mastication—chewing (30)

Material Safety Data Sheet (MSDS)—printed materials that come with hazardous chemicals and offer basic information needed to ensure the safety and health of the user (6)

matrix—template for scheduling appointments; also known as *nail bed* (9, 22)

maximal midexpiratory flow (MMEF)—average flow rate during the middle half of forced vital capacity (50)

Mayo stand—small portable table with enough room to hold an instrument tray (42)

measles, mumps, and rubella (MMR) vaccine—protects children from developing measles, mumps, and rubella (54)

meatus—urinary tract opening (40)

mediastinum—region of the thoracic cavity between the lungs and the sternum where the heart is located (49)

medical asepsis—destruction of organisms after they leave the body (34)

medical diagnosis—diagnosis arrived at after all examinations, tests, and procedures, are complete (35)

medical emergency—requiring the immediate attention of a physician (8)

medical foundation—a nonprofit integrated delivery system (17)

medical privilege—physician is granted rights to practice medicine in a particular hospital or other health care facility (2)

medical record—source of all documentation relating to the patient; also known as *patient files* or *patient charts* or *patient's record* (14)

Medicare—A U.S. government insurance program for which persons aged 65 and over and others with special conditions are eligible (41)

Medigap insurance—private insurance that is sold to those receiving Medicare to provide additional coverage (41)

medulla—portion of the lymph node that is primarily made up of macrophages attached to reticular fibers; in the kidney, the middle portion, in which the renal pyramids are found (28, 31)

medullary canal—narrow space or cavity throughout the length of the diaphysis in a long bone, which contains yellow bone marrow, made of fat cells (23)

megahertz (MHz)—1 megahertz equals 1 million cycles per second; the higher the MHz, the faster the computer (12)

meiosis—process in which cells reduce their chromosomal number by half in order to form gametes (21)

melanin—pigment that gives the skin its color (22)

melanocytes—cells that produces melanin for pigmentation (22)

memory—storage and retrieval of computerized data (12)

memos—correspondence sent to people within the office or organization; also known as *interoffice memorandums* (11)

menarche—onset of the menstrual cycle (33, 38)

Ménière's disease—condition of the inner ear characterized by vertigo, tinnitus, fluctuating hearing loss, and pressure or pain in the affected ear (26)

meninges—membranes that encompass the brain and spinal cord (25)

meningitis—infection of the meninges that surround and protect the brain and spinal cord, typically caused by a bacterial or viral infection (25)

mensuration—use of special tools to measure the body or specific parts (36)

metabolism—sum of all biochemical and physiological processes that take place in the body (35, 56)

metastasis—process in which cancer cells break away from the original tumor and travel to other areas of the body where they form new tumors (28)

methicillin-resistant *Staphylococcus aureus* (MRSA)—organism that produces an enzyme that makes it highly resistant to antibiotics; two forms: hospital-associated MRSA and community-based MRSA (34)

metric system—most commonly used conversion system for dosage calculations (52)

microbe—one-celled form of life, such as bacteria (45)

microbiology—study of organisms too small to be seen without a microscope (45)

microencephaly—head growth that falls below the normal percentile (40)

microfiche—sheets of microfilm (13)

microfilm—miniaturized photos of records (13)

microhematocrit—hematocrit performed with a capillary tube on an extremely small quantity of blood (47)

microorganisms—living organisms too small to be seen with the naked eye (45)

microprocessor—small chip that processes data in a microcomputer (12)

micturate—urinate (46)

micturition—urination (31)

minerals—inorganic elements that are not of plant or animal origin (56)

mitosis—process during which a cell divides its chromosomes into two identical daughter cells, each having 23 pairs of, or 46, chromosomes (21)

mitral valve—the valve through which blood leaves the left atrium of the heart; also known as *bicuspid valve* (27)

mixed number—number that contains a whole number and a fraction (52)

modalities—applications of any therapeutic agent (51)

modified block—style of letter writing in which the date, complimentary close, and signature line begin at the center of the page, with all other lines at the left margin (11)

modified wave scheduling—modification of scheduling that gives several patients an appointment on the hour, knowing that some will be late (9)

modifier—two-digit code preceded by a hyphen that clarifies the procedure (e.g., a procedure that was done on both arms instead of only one) (19)

molecule—a chemical combination of two or more atoms that forms a specific chemical compound (21)

moniliasis—yeast infection caused by *Candida albicans*; also known as *thrush* (45)

monitor—viewing screen that allows the user to see input and output (12)

monocytes—type of leukocytes that are formed in the bone marrow from stem cells and assist in phagocytosis (47)

monographs—short books published by the American Association of Medical Assistants, each of which contains text and a test, sometimes used to obtain continuing education units for recertification (1)

mononucleosis—a contagious viral infection frequently spread through oral contact; also know as *infectious mononucleosis, mono,* and *kissing disease* (47)

monosaccharides—simple sugars that result from the breaking down of carbohydrates in the digestive tract (56)

morale—employees' feelings about their work and work environment (10)

morbidity rates—rates of disease and illness (2)

morphology—study of the shape of cells (45)

motivation—stimulus that drives someone to act (57)

motor neurons—neurons that control most of the body's movement as they cause muscles to contract, glands to secrete, and organs to function properly (25)

mouse—pointing and selection device for data input (12)

multidrug-resistant organisms (MDROs)—bacteria and other microorganisms that have developed resistance to antimicrobial drugs (34)

multiple gated acquisition (MUGA) scan—nuclear scan to check for blood flow in the myocardium (49)

multiple sclerosis (MS)—chronic, debilitating autoimmune disease in which the body directs the antibodies and white blood cells to attack the myelin sheath surrounding nerves in the brain and spinal cord, which causes inflammation and injury and, eventually, scarring, which results in difficulty with movement, vision, and/or sensation (25)

murmurs—abnormal heart sounds resembling turbulence (49)

muscular dystrophy (MD)—one of a group of genetic diseases characterized by progressive weakness and muscular degeneration (24)

myasthenia gravis (MG)—chronic autoimmune neuromuscular disease characterized by varying degrees of weakness of the skeletal, or voluntary, muscles of the body (24)

mycology—study of fungi (45)

myocardial infarction (MI)—condition that occurs when the blood supply to a part of the myocardium is severely reduced or stopped; also known as *heart attack* (27, 37)

myocardium—middle muscular layer of the heart (27)

myomectomy—surgery that removes uterine fibroids without removing healthy tissue (33)

myopia—nearsightedness (26, 39)

myringa—the eardrum (39)

myringotomy—incision into the myringa or eardrum to drain fluid (40)

myxedema—rare, life-threatening condition that results from long-term untreated hypothyroidism (32)

nares—nostrils (29)

nasolacrimal duct—duct that drains lacrimal fluid into the nasal cavity (26)

National Certified Medical Assistant (NCMA)—credential issued by the National Center for Competency Testing to qualified medical assistants; to continue certification, 14 CEUs must be obtained each year (1)

National Committee for Quality Assurance (NCQA)—national committee that sets standards for and evaluates the quality of health plans (6)

natural immunity—inherited immunity to certain diseases (28)

necrotizing fasciitis—severe infection due to destruction of subcutaneous tissue and fascia with a 30 percent mortality rate commonly caused by group A streptococcal infection (45)

negative feedback—when the body responds to external stimuli by reversing the direction of change (21)

negotiable instrument—actualizes or permits the transfer of money to another person, such as a check (16)

nephrons—functional units of the kidney that remove the waste products of metabolism from the blood plasma (31)

neuralgia—general nerve pain (25)

neurilemma—outer sheath of the nerve composed of Schwann cells (25)

neurology—branch of medicine dealing with the study and treatment of the nervous system (37)

neurons—nerve cells (21, 25)

neutrophils—most common type of phagocyte; primarily attack bacteria (28)

new patient—patient who has never been seen by anyone in the practice, or who has not been seen by any practitioner of the same specialty in the practice for more than 3 years (19)

nocturia—frequent urination at night (38)

noncompliance—not following the physician's orders (55)

non–insulin-dependent diabetes mellitus (NIDDM)—condition in which the body is unable to properly control blood sugar levels, resulting from insulin resistance combined with a relative insulin deficiency; often diagnosed later in life and having a very strong correlation with obesity; also known as *type 2 diabetes* and *adult-onset diabetes* (32)

nonparticipating provider—a physician to whom the patient is expected to pay charges before submitting the claim to the insurance company, which pays the patient directly (18)

nonsteroidal anti-inflammatory drugs (NSAIDs)—medications to decrease inflammation that are not comprised of steroids (37)

nonsufficient funds (NSF)—situation in which the payer's account does not have enough money to cover the amount of the check (16)

nonverbal communication—information conveyed through the language of gesture and actions including body language (5)

normal flora—nonpathogenic microorganisms that live on the surface of the body and inside body openings and organs (34, 45)

no-show—patient who did not show up for a scheduled appointment (8)

nosocomial infections—infection acquired while in a medical facility (34)

nuclear medicine—branch of medicine that uses radioactive isotopes in the diagnosis and treatment of disease (48)

nucleus—control center and part of the cell containing the chromosomes (21)

numerator—top number of a fraction (52)

numeric filing—filing system that assigns an identification number to each person's name (13)

nutrients—organic and inorganic chemical substances in foods that supply the body with the elements necessary for metabolism (56)

nyctalopia—inability to see well in faint light (26)

nystagmus (nystaxis)—involuntary, repetitive, rhythmic movements of the eye (26)

objective symptom—measurable symptom felt by the patient and apparent to observers (36)

obsessions—persistent thoughts (57)

occlusion—blockage (27)

occult—refers to hidden blood in the feces or urine (37, 46)

Occupational Safety and Health Administration (OSHA)—agency of the U.S. Department of Labor that monitors safety on the job and enforces standards for safety (6)

office flow—teamwork, time management, organized and efficient office equipment usage, and patient flow (10)

oliguria—decreased amounts of urine production (46)

oncogenes—genes controlling cell growth and multiplication that are transformed into cancer cells by cancer-causing agents (28)

oncology—branch of medicine dealing with malignant neoplasms or tumors (37)

open-ended questions—questions that require more than yes or no responses (5, 9)

open-panel HMO—HMO in which health care providers are not employees of the HMO and do not belong to a medical group owned or managed by the HMO (17)

ophthalmologist—medical doctor who can perform eye examinations and eye surgery and prescribe medications, eyeglasses, and contact lenses (39)

ophthalmology—branch of medical science that deals with the structure, function, and diseases of the eye (39)

ophthalmoscope—instrument used to examine the interior of the eye, especially the retina (36, 39)

opportunistic infections—infections that take advantage of a suppressed immune system (34)

optical character recognition (OCR)—equipment that scans, reads, and sorts; used by the U.S. Postal Service to sort envelopes (11)

optic disk—area of the retina where the optic nerve enters (26)

optician—technician who specializes in grinding lenses and preparing eyeglasses and contact lenses (39)

optic nerve—nerve that carries information from the eye to the brain (26)

optometrist—a doctor of optometry, not a medical doctor, who can perform eye examinations, prescribe medications, and write prescriptions for eyeglasses and contact lenses (39)

oral cancer—cancer of the mouth, usually starting in the flat squamous cells that line it (30)

oral medication—medication that is swallowed and absorbed through the gastrointestinal system and then rapidly absorbed by the body (54)

oral polio vaccine (OPV)—live, early form of the polio vaccine that was given to children but was shown to cause polio in some cases and is no longer recommended (54) orbit—cavity in the skull that houses each eyeball (26)

organelles—small structures found within the cytoplasm of the cell that have specific functions and purpose to maintain vitality of the cell (21, 45)

organ of Corti—spiral structure in the cochlea that converts the waves of sound that travel through the ear (39)

organs—similarly functioning groups of tissues that serve a common purpose (21)

origin—in locations where skeletal muscles attach, the attachment point on the bone that is more fixed or still (24)

orthopedic physician—physician who specializes in the treatment of diseases and disorders of the musculoskeletal system (23)

orthopedics—branch of medicine dealing with the study and treatment of the musculoskeletal system (37)

orthopnea—condition in which the patient has trouble breathing unless a certain position is maintained, such as with head elevated (29)

orthoses—orthopedic appliances used for support (24)

orthostatic hypertension—severe (20–30 mmHg) drop in blood pressure occurring when standing quickly after lying down or sitting (35)

orthotist—professional who designs and fits supportive devices such as braces and splints (51)

osmosis—form of diffusion whereby water is pulled through a semipermeable membrane, moving from areas of greater to lesser concentration (21)

ossicles—small bones, such as the incus, malleus, and stapes in the ear (26)

osteoarthritis—most common type of arthritis, resulting from years of wear and tear on joints and occurring most frequently in the hips, knees, and finger joints (23)

osteomalacia—adult onset of rickets, literally meaning "softening of the bone" (23)

osteopath—medical professional who places great emphasis on the relationship between the musculoskeletal system and the organs of the body (2)

osteoporosis—progressive loss of bone density and thinning of bone tissue, seen most commonly in older adults, especially postmenopausal women, and in individuals who do not consume enough calcium (23)

otitis media—inflammation of the middle ear caused by viral or bacterial infections (26)

otology—study of hearing (39)

otorhinolaryngologist—specialist in disorders and diseases of the ears, nose, and throat (ENT) (39)

otosclerosis—condition in which the tissue surrounding the bone of the stapes grows abnormally around it, preventing it from transmitting sound vibrations to the inner ear and resulting in profound hearing loss (26)

otoscope—instrument used to examine the eardrum (39)

outpatient—services provided to patients on a walk-in basis where no overnight stay is required (2)

outpatient surgery—surgery that may be done outside of the hospital setting in a surgicenter, a surgical center that is part of a hospital complex, or in a medical office (2, 42)

output devices—components such as a display screen or a printer that allow the user to see what the computer has accomplished (12)

outside laboratory—hospital-based or independent laboratory that handles specimens collected from many types of facilities and performs tests ranging from simple to very complex (44)

ovarian cancer—cancer of the ovaries; the three main types are epithelial cancer, germ cell tumor, and stromal tumor (33)

ovarian cysts—sacs filled with fluid or semisolid material that develop on or within the ovary, typically not disease related and disappearing on their own; formed when the grown follicle fails to rupture and release an egg and, instead of being reabsorbed, forms a cyst (33)

ovaries—two almond-shaped organs on either side of the uterus that produce ova (eggs) and the hormones estrogen and progesterone (33)

overbooking—scheduling more than one patient in the same time slot (8)

overdose—when too much of a medication is administered (52)

over-the-counter (OTC)—nonprescription drugs such as aspirin, cold medications, and antibiotic ointments (53)

ovulation—process of producing an ovum and releasing it into the pelvic cavity and one of the fallopian tubes (33)

ovum—(plural, *ova*) egg or reproductive cell (33)

oxygen debt—inability of the body to absorb enough oxygen to supply the energy required to sustain a high level of activity, resulting in utilization of the anaerobic energy system and in the buildup of lactic acid in the muscles (24)

oxygen saturation—oxygen content of blood (50)

oxyhemoglobin—hemoglobin that is carrying oxygen (47)

oxytocin—hormone that triggers labor (38)

pacemakers—electronic devices that help the heart maintain normal rhythm (49)

palpation—using the hands to feel the skin and accessible underlying organs and other tissues (36)

palpatory method—feeling the radial pulse while the blood pressure cuff is deflating, used to determine systolic pressure (35)

palpebrae—eyelids (26)

palpebral fissure—opening between the eyelids (26)

pancreas—elongated gland behind the stomach that secretes pancreatic juice into the small intestine as well as the hormones insulin and glucagon, which raise and lower blood glucose levels (30)

pancreatic cancer—develops in the exocrine glands with vague symptoms that include pain in the abdomen or back, weight loss, bloating, diarrhea, and jaundice (30)

pandemic—outbreak of a disease that infects many people in different countries at the same time (e.g., bubonic plague) (2)

papilledema—inflammation of the optic nerve (26)

para—number of deliveries after 20 weeks gestation (38)

paraplegia—paralysis from approximately the waist down (25)

parasites—organisms that live within other organisms (46)

parathyroid glands—four glands around the dorsal and lower aspect of the thyroid gland that secrete parathyroid hormone (PTH or parathormone) (32)

parenteral medication administration—medications that are given through injection (54)

Parkinson's disease—progressive disorder caused by degeneration of the nerve cells in the parts of the brain that control movement, resulting in a shortage of the neurotransmitter dopamine, which impairs movement (25)

participating provider—one who has a contractual agreement with an insurance plan to render care to eligible beneficiaries and then bill the insurance carrier directly (18)

parturition—birth (38)

passive immunity—immunity acquired from an outside source, such as breast milk, that lasts for a short time (28)

passive listening—listening to someone without having to reply, such as when listening as a member of an audience (5)

passive transport—process in cells that does not require energy to transport materials to, from, and within the cell (21)

passive voice—the subject of the sentence receives the action (11)

pasteurization—process during which substances, such as milk and cheese, are heated to a certain temperature to eliminate bacteria (2)

patella—the kneecap (36)

patent—unobstructed (43)

pathogens—microorganisms capable of causing disease (34)

pathophysiology—study of diseases or disorders caused by a malfunction or by age, genetic predisposition, or enviornmental influences (21)

payee—person or company named as the receiving party to whom the amount on the check is payable (16)

payer—person signing a check to release money (16)

peak flow meters—devices that measure the ability to move air into and out of lungs (50)

pediatrician—medical doctor who specializes in the treatment of newborns, infants, children, and adolescents (40)

pediculosis—infestation of the head, body, or pubic area with the eggs, larvae, or adults of lice (22)

pelvic inflammatory disease (PID)—inflammation of the vagina, cervix, uterus, and fallopian tubes caused by several sexually transmitted infections (38)

penis—male organ for intercourse or copulation, and the site of the orifice through which urine and semen are eliminated from the body (33)

peptic ulcer disease (PUD)—condition in which a disruption occurs in the lining of the esophagus, stomach, or duodenum (30)

percussion—using the fingertips to tap the body lightly but sharply to gain information about the position and size of underlying body parts (36)

perfusion—blood flow to the myocardium (49)

pericardium—outer lining of the heart wall (24, 27)

perineum—external region between the vulva and the anus, composed of muscle covered with skin (33)

periosteum—membrane that forms the covering of long bones, except at their articular surfaces (23)

peripheral nervous system—made up of nerves that connect the CNS to other parts of the body (25)

peristalsis—involuntary, wavelike, muscular contractions that move the bolus of food through the entire digestive system (30)

permeable—in autoclaving, wrappings capable of allowing the passage of steam through them (34)

persistence—quality of being able to stay on task longer than the usual time when necessary, even after others might have given up (58)

personal assessment—evaluation of one's own strengths and weaknesses (59)

personal digital assistant (PDA)—a lightweight, handheld, usually pen- or stylus-based computer used as a personal organizer (14)

personality disorders—include narcissistic (self-centered), paranoid, (abnormally concerned that people will hurt oneself), antisocial (not concerned with laws and other people), histrionic (dramatic), and borderline (impulsive) behavior (57)

personal protective equipment (PPE)—protective gloves, fluid-resistant lab coats, gowns, safety glasses, surgical masks, shields, and respirators used to protect the health care worker whenever working in an environment where the chance of splash or exposure exists (6, 34)

pertussis—respiratory disease that is most common in children under the age of 4 years; also known as *whooping cough* (29, 54)

petechiae—tiny broken blood vessels on the surface of the skin (27)

petrissage—kneading or rolling method of massage that requires pressing the muscles (51)

phagocytes—several types of white blood cells that attack invading organisms (28)

phagocytosis—process by which leukocytes (white blood cells) actively fight pathogenic microorganisms (34)

phantom pain—sensation felt in a missing body part after it has been removed (35)

pharmacists—specially trained and licensed professionals who specialize in the preparation and dispensation of drugs (53)

pharmacology—the study of medications and drugs, including their forms, intentions for use, and effects (52, 53)

pharynx—musculomembranous tube about 5 inches long that extends from the base of the skull to the cervical spine and connects to the trachea and esophagus that serves as a passageway to the lungs for air and food to reach the stomach (29)

phenylketonuria (PKU)—congenital disease caused by a defect in the metabolism of the amino acid phenylalanine (47)

photometer—instrument that measures the intensity of light (44)

photophobia—sensitivity to light (26)

physiatrist—physician who specializes in the therapeutic use of physical agents (51)

physiatry—therapeutic use of physical agents for the diagnosis, treatment, management, and prevention of diseases and debilitating illnesses (51)

physician's office laboratory (POL)—laboratory that performs some of the tests that the physician orders right in the office (44)

physiology—functions and processes of the body; the study of the function of an organism (21)

pineal gland—gland located in the brain at the posterior end of the corpus callosum; secretes melatonin and serotonin (32)

pipette—narrow glass tube with both ends open; used for measuring and transferring liquids from one vessel to another (44)

pitch—frequency of voice (e.g., high or low) (7)

pituitary gland—organ located near the base of the brain in a small depression of the sphenoid bone; regulates all other endocrine glands; also known as *master gland* (32)

placenta abruptio—tearing away of placenta from uterine wall, resulting in hemorrhage and fetal distress (38)

placenta previa—complication in which the placenta develops in the lower portion of the uterus, blocking the opening in the cervix and causing oxygen deprivation for the fetus and possible maternal hemorrhage during labor (38)

plan—to determine how to begin the task of teaching the patient (55)

plasma—fluid portion of the blood (27)

platelets—smallest cells in blood, formed in the red bone marrow; main function is to assist in the clotting of blood; also known as *thrombocytes* (27, 47)

pleura—thin sheets of epithelium that cover the outer surface of the lungs and the inside of the thoracic cavity (29)

pleurisy—an inflammation of the pleura, the membrane surrounding the lungs, generally stemming from an existing respiratory infection, disease, or injury; also known as *pleuritis* (29)

pneumococcal vaccine—vaccine that is given to guard against contracting the *Streptococcus pneumonia* bacteria (54)

pneumonia—inflammation of the lungs caused by bacteria, viruses, fungi, or chemical irritants, often following influenza in the elderly and debilitated, and most commonly caused in the United States by *Streptococcus pneumoniae* (29)

pneumothorax—air in the chest outside the lungs (29)

point-of-service plan (POS)—insurance plan in which a patient may choose an HMO or a non-HMO provider but must pay a deductible for using a non-HMO provider (17)

polycystic kidney disease (PKD)—disorder in which clusters of cysts, noncancerous sacs of waterlike fluid, develop, primarily within the kidneys (31)

polydipsia—excessive thirst (37)

polysaccharides—starches that are broken down into glucose during the digestive process and transported into the blood (56)

polyuria—production of excessive amounts of urine (37, 46)

portal of entry—entryway for pathogens into the body (34)

portal of exit—opening for the exit of pathogens from the reservoir host (34)

positive feedback—process of encouraging external or internal stimuli to continue, or even accelerate, in order to maintain homeostasis (21)

post cibum (pc)—after a meal (44)

posted—recorded (15)

postprandial (PP)—after a meal (44)

practice of medicine—diagnosing and prescribing treatment or medication (3)

practicum—situation, also called an externship, in which a student works without payment in a physician's office, hospital, or other health care setting for 160 hours over a minimum of 4 weeks, during the final stage of his or her training, under the supervision of someone at the site (1, 59)

preauthorization—requirement to obtain prior approval for surgery and other procedures from the insurance carrier in order to receive reimbursement (17)

preceptor—supervisor who provides additional instruction and guidance for a student in an externship or practicum situation and provides a formal written evaluation of the student (38, 59)

preeclampsia—hypertension that develops during pregnancy (38)

preferred provider organization (PPO)—an insurance arrangement that requires the patient to use a provider under contract to the insurance company, which reimburses the provider at a discounted rate (17)

Prefilled cartridge injection systems—single-dose cartridges that fit into a special cartridge holder which results in medications not having to be drawn up prior to injections (54)

prefix—a word element placed before or affixed to the beginning of a word (4)

prehypertension—in adults over 18 years old, blood pressure ranging from 120/80 to 139/89 mmHg, considered a precursor to hypertension (27)

prejudice—preformed and unfavorable belief or attitude toward a certain culture or group with little or no information about the culture or group (5, 57)

premenstrual syndrome (PMS)—condition affecting certain women with symptoms that may begin 2 weeks before the onset of menstruation; also known as *premenstrual dysphoric disorder* (33)

premium—amount paid for insurance (17)

prenatal period—first period of child development; covers the process from conception until birth (57)

prepaid plan—group of physicians or other health care providers who have a contractual agreement to provide services to subscribers on a negotiated fee-for-service or capitated basis; also known as *managed care plan* (17)

presbycusis—hearing loss from gradual deterioration of the sensory receptors located in the cochlea, associated with aging (26, 39)

presbyopia—the loss of elasticity in the eye's lens, usually as a result of aging that causes an inability to focus on objects at close range (26, 39)

present illness—detailed description of the chief complaint, which must contain symptom(s), including the onset, duration, and intensity of each (36)

primary assessment—asking a few simple questions and doing a simple exam to assess the patient's status (43)

primary care provider (PCP)—gatekeeper provider who refers patients to other providers for services he or she cannot perform (17)

primary insurance—medical insurance coverage provided through the patient's employer (18)

prime mover—muscle that is the primary actor in a given movement—that is, the muscle that produces the movement in muscle contraction (24)

principal diagnosis—diagnosis of a particular condition for which a patient sought care on a particular date, used when performing coding in the hospital setting and when a final diagnosis cannot be determined without further patient follow-up (19)

printer—output device for producing hard copy (12)

privacy screen—apparatus that blocks others from viewing the computer screen, especially when the medical assistant is away from the desk (9)

probationary period—usually the first 3 months (90 days) of employment during which the new employee can be terminated without cause (20)

problem-oriented medical record (POMR)—patient record organized according to diagnoses (13)

procedural coding—process of transferring a narrative description of procedures into numbers (19)

proctologist—physician who treats disorders of the rectum and anus (37)

professional courtesy (PC)—consideration extended by physician not to charge other physicians, staff, family members, or clergy (15)

professional reference—statement from an individual who has worked with or knows someone for a period of time, attesting to the person's skills and personal integrity (59)

proficiency testing—external quality control program that monitors the accuracy of test systems by comparing the facility's results to those of the College of American Pathologists or the American Association of Bioanalysts (44)

prognosis—prediction of the course of a disease and its outcome (35)

prokaryotic—cells without a nucleus or organelles (45)

pronation—process of lying prone, or face downward; also, the process of turning the hand so that the palm points downward (23)

proofread—to review a document for errors in content and typing (11, 59)

prophylactically—drug that is being used to prevent the onset of a condition (53)

proportion—comparison of two ratios (52)

proprietary name—name given to a drug by a specific manufacturer; also known as *brand name* (53)

prostate cancer—malignant tumor that grows in the prostate gland (33)

prostate gland—gland lying behind the urinary bladder that wraps around the first 2.5 cm of the urethra that secretes an alkaline fluid which aids in maintaining the viability of the spermatozoa (33)

prosthesis—artificial replacement of a missing body part (51)

prosthetist—one who specializes in designing, preparing, and fitting prosthetic devices such as artificial limbs (51)

proteinuria—protein in the urine (46)

protraction—process of moving a body part forward (23)

proximate cause—natural continuous sequence of events, without any intervening cause, which produces an injury; in a legal case of negligence, the defendant's acts (or failure to act) that directly cause an injury (3)

psoriasis—common skin condition characterized by frequent episodes of redness, itching, and thick, dry scales that results from a buildup of dead skin cells that, rather than shed off, pile up and form scaly patches (22)

psychiatrist—medical doctor who specializes in psychiatry (57)

psychiatry—branch of medicine that deals with the diagnosis, treatment, and prevention of mental disorders (57)

psychologist—one who is trained in the methods of psychological analysis, therapy, and research (57)

psychology—science of behavior and the human thought process (57)

psychomotor—relating to coordination of the mind and body (58)

psychopathic—personality disorder characterized by lack of empathy, narcissism, impulsivity, and antisocial reactions, such as breaking the law and manipulating others (57)

psychopharmacology—study of the effects of drugs on the mind and brain, particularly the use of drugs in treating mental disorders (57)

psychotherapy—method for treating mental disorders by mental rather than physical means, including psychoanalysis, humanistic therapies, and family and group therapies (57)

psychotic—mental disorder that interferes with patients' perceptions of reality and their ability to cope with the demands of daily living (57)

puerperium—period of 4 to 6 weeks following birth (38)

pulmonary artery—artery that transports blood from the right ventricle to the lungs (27)

pulmonary edema—condition in which fluid accumulates in the lungs, usually caused by failure of the heart's left ventricle but also caused by lung problems such as pneumonia, an excess of intravenous fluids, some types of kidney disease, severe burns, liver disease, nutritional problems, and Hodgkin's disease (29)

pulmonary embolism (PE)—blood clot in the lung, usually originating in smaller vessels in the leg, pelvis, arms, or heart and traveling to the lung, where it ultimately becomes wedged in a vessel too small to allow it to pass, causing that portion of the lung to die from lack of oxygen (29)

pulmonary vein—vein that transports freshly oxygenated blood from the lungs to the left atrium (27)

pulmonologist—medical doctor who specializes in treating the lungs and accessory structures (50)

pulse deficit—difference in readings between the apical and radial pulses (35)

pulse pressure—difference between the systolic and diastolic blood pressures (27, 35)

pupil—"hole" in the center of the iris that controls the amount of light entering the eye (26)

purging—dieting by vomiting, or taking laxatives, enemas, or diuretics (40)

Purkinje fibers—specialized conductive fibers located within the walls of the ventricles, responsible for relaying cardiac impulses to the cells of the ventricles, which then contract (27)

pyelonephritis—infection of the kidney and renal pelvis caused by bacteria, usually *E. coli,* entering the kidneys from the bladder (31)

pyloric stenosis—condition in which a baby's pylorus (the connection between the stomach and the duodenum) gradually swells and thickens, which interferes with food entering the intestine (30)

pyrexia—fever (35)

quadriplegia—paralysis from approximately the shoulders down (25)

qualitative test—laboratory test that analyzes a specimen for the presence or absence of a substance (44)

quality assurance (QA)—the act of gathering and evaluating information about services provided and comparing this information with an accepted standard (6)

quantitative test—laboratory test that analyzes a specimen for the presence of a substance and the amount of the substance present (44)

Queckenstedt sign—compression of the veins in the neck resulting in a rise of pressure of the cerebrospinal fluid (37)

queue—waiting line (7)

quickening—fetal movement (38)

race—classification of people based on their physical or biological characteristics, such as skin color, shape of eyes, hair type, bone structure, or facial features (5)

radiating pain—pain that spreads out from an area (35)

radiation—radiant energy (48)

radiation therapy—use of high-energy waves, such as X-rays, to damage and destroy cancer cells (28)

radioactive—of, caused by, or exhibiting radioactivity (48)

radiographs—X-ray images (48)

radiologist—physician specializing in radiology (48)

radiology—branch of medicine that uses radioactive substances or matter that gives off radiation (radiant energy) and various

techniques to visualize the internal structures of the body for the diagnosis and treatment of disease (48)

radiolucent—penetrable by X-rays (48)

radiopaque—allows minimal penetration by X-rays (48)

random-access memory (RAM)—internal storage area in the computer that can be accessed randomly (12)

range of motion (ROM)—degree of movement that can be achieved in a specific joint without causing pain (51)

rapport—environment of cooperation (5)

ratio—relationship between two quantities (52)

read-only memory (ROM)—internal storage area in the computer where data has been recorded and cannot be removed, only read (12)

reagents—substances required for a chemical reaction or used to detect the presence of another substance (44)

real time—keying in appointments, patient needs, and information within a computer program (9)

reasonable person standard—exercising the ordinary standard of care and the type of care that a "reasonable" person would use in a similar circumstance (3)

receptionist—person, usually a medical assistant, who greets patients as they arrive (8)

Recommended Dietary Allowances (RDAs)—recommended amounts of protein, vitamins, and minerals Americans should eat and the body weights they should try to maintain for good nutrition (56)

reconciliation—process of comparing one's banking records to a bank statement to ensure that both are in agreement (16)

rectum—final portion of the large intestine that stores solid waste until it is expelled from the body through the anus (30)

reduction—procedure used to align and reposition a dislocated joint (23)

Redundant—repeating the same word, expression, or statement (11)

reference initials—letters that indicate the name of who keyed a letter; placed at the lower left margin in lowercase (11)

reference laboratory—laboratory, usually associated with a hospital or medical school, that handles more complex and infrequently requested tests than outside laboratories (44)

referral—the process of sending a patient to or from another physician (7, 17)

referred pain—pain that is felt at a site other than the injured or diseased body part (35)

refined sugars—processed sugars (56)

reflex hammer—instrument used to check reflexes (36)

refraction—process of light rays changing direction when they pass through the eye (26)

Registered Medical Assistant (RMA)—medical assistant who has met eligibility requirements and who can prove his or her

competency to perform entry-level skills through written examination; the RMA is awarded to candidates who pass the American Medical Technologists (AMT) certification examination (1)

registration—health care professional on record as part of an organization or association in a specific health care field who administers examinations, maintains a list of qualified individuals, or both (2)

rehabilitation—process of bringing the patient back as close as possible to his or her normal physical condition after injury or disease with the ability to attain and maintain function and independence (51)

Reiki—a therapy that channels the body's energy and spirit through gentle touch and massage (51)

rem—unit of measurement used for exposure that may involve more than one type of radiation; the Roentgen equivalent in humans (48)

renal calculi—deposits of mineral salts in the kidney; also known as *kidney stones* (31)

renal pelvis—saclike area of the kidney in which urine is collected (31)

renal threshold—concentration at which a substance excreted by the kidneys such as glucose, begins to appear in urine (46)

reservoir host—organism that contains the pathogen that is the beginning of the chain of infection (34)

residual volume (RV)—volume of air left in the lungs at the end of an exhale (around 1200 mL) (50)

res ipsa loquitur—doctrine meaning "the thing speaks for itself"; applies to the law of negligence and refers to the breach (neglect) of duty that is so obvious that it does not need further explanation (3)

resolution—referring to a microscope, the ability to distinguish clearly between adjacent but distinct objects

respiratory cycle—one inhalation and one exhalation (35)

respiratory syncytial virus (RSV)—common viral respiratory infection that affects the upper and lower respiratory tracts (40)

respite care—short-term care for the chronically ill (41)

respondeat superior—Latin term meaning "Let the master answer"; refers to the employer or physician who is liable for the negligent actions of anyone working for him or her; in some states, both physician and employee may be liable (3)

résumé—summary of a person's credentials, including employment history, experience, training, and education (59)

retina—innermost layer of the eye containing rods and cones, which translate light into nerve impulses (26)

retinal detachment—separation of the retina from the underlying choroids layer (26)

retraction—process of moving a body part backward (23)

retrograde pyelography—procedure used to evaluate the function of the ureters, bladder, and urethra in which a dye is sent up a catheter that has been inserted into the urinary tract (48)

review of systems (ROS)—review of each system of the body during physical examination; also known as *head-to-toe exam* (36)

rheumatoid arthritis—autoimmune disorder causing joints to be deformed due to inflammation (23, 28)

rhinovirus—a group of several hundred viruses that cause the common cold (40)

RhoGAM—drug administered to a pregnant woman to inhibit the production of antibodies against the Rh antigen (27)

rhythm—regularity or equal spacing of all the beats of the pulse or heartbeats (35, 49)

ribonucleic acid (RNA)—single chain of chemical bases (21)

rickets—childhood bone disorder that causes bone deformity; caused by lack of vitamin D, calcium, and phosphate (23)

risk management—the planning and implementing of strategies for reducing the physician's risk of a lawsuit in the medical setting (5)

rods—photosensitive cells in the retina that respond to dim light and are used in night vision (26)

Romberg test—patient closes eyes and stands with feet together without swaying (37)

rosacea—chronic disorder, primarily of the facial skin, causing redness on the cheeks, nose, chin, or forehead, often characterized by flare-ups and remissions (22)

rotation—process of moving a body part around a central axis (23)

Rule of Nines—formula for estimating the percentage of body surface area (43)

salivary glands—glands in or near the mouth that produce saliva, which contains amylase, an enzyme that helps in the breakdown of carbohydrates (30)

salpingo-oophorectomy—removal of the fallopian tubes and ovaries (33)

salutation—courteous greeting in a letter, typed at the left margin and spaced two lines below the inside address (11)

sanitization—cleaning process that inhibits or inactivates pathogens by means of careful scrubbing (34)

scabies—contagious disorder of the skin caused by the human or scabies itch mite; causes intense itching and a red rash (22)

scheduling system—process that is followed methodically when giving patients appointments (9)

schizophrenia—psychotic disorder marked by a variety of symptoms, including delusions, hallucinations, disorganized and incoherent speech, severe emotional abnormalities, and withdrawal into an inner world (57)

sciatica—pain along the sciatic nerve that runs from the lower back down the back of each leg, often caused by inflammation due to a pinched nerve (25)

sclera—part of the outer layer of the eyeball; also known as *white of the eye* (26)

scoliosis—abnormal lateral curvature of the spine (23, 37)

screen saver—computer software program that makes the monitor unviewable by others, especially when the medical assistant is away from the desk (9)

scrotum—pouchlike structure behind the penis that contains the two testes (33)

scrub assistant—assistant who has completed sterile asepsis and assists the physician in surgical procedures by handing instruments, swabbing bodily fluids, retracting the incision area, and cutting suture materials, using sterile technique (42)

sebaceous cyst—abscess on the skin caused by infection of the sebaceous glands (22)

sebaceous glands—glands in the skin that produce sebum, an oil that acts to protect and waterproof hair and skin (22)

seborrheic dermatitis—inflammation of sebaceous or oil glands of the skin, caused by an increase in sebum; also known as *cradle cap* (22)

secondary insurance—when the patient has medical insurance through their own employer and the patient's spouse also has medical insurance through their employer, the insurance coverage through the spouse is considered secondary (18)

sediment—solid material settling at the bottom of a test tube after centrifugation (46)

seizure—temporary interference with muscle control, movement, speech, vision, or awareness caused by intense bursts of electrical activity produced within the brain; often associated with epilepsy (25)

self-referral—occurs when a patient chooses to see an out-of-network provider without authorization (17)

semicircular canals—three canals in the inner ear that are part of the labyrinth (26)

seniority—status gained by being the individual who has worked for the physician the longest (20)

sensorineural hearing loss—caused by nerve damage (39)

sensory neurons—attached to the sensory receptors, transmit impulses directly to the central nervous system (25)

septum—wall that separates the left and right sides of the heart (27); cartilaginous wall that separates the internal portion of the nose into the right and left cavities (29)

sequela—long-lasting effect (45)

serology—study of antigen and antibody reactions of the body's immune system (45)

serum—plasma without the fibrinogen (47)

severe acute respiratory syndrome (SARS)—newly identified respiratory illness caused by a previously unknown virus, SARF-CoV, of the coronavirus family, whose members often cause mild to moderate upper respiratory illness, such as the common cold (29)

sexually transmitted infection (STI)—an infection transmitted through exchange of semen, blood, and other body fluids or by direct contact with the affected body areas of another person; also known as *venereal disease* (33)

sheaths—protective membranes that wrap nerve fibers in the peripheral nervous system (25)

side effects—unwanted effects of a medication that are tolerated because the benefit of taking the medication outweighs them (53)

signa—Latin term for *label,* the part of a prescription that gives instructions on how the medication should be taken by the patient; also known as *signature* (53)

signature line—typed four spaces below the complimentary close of a letter; contains the name and title of the writer (11)

sinoatrial (SA) node—one of three areas of specialized neuromuscular tissue that initiate the heartbeat, located in the upper wall of the right atrium; also known as *pacemaker of the heart* (27)

sinuses—cavities (29)

sinusitis—infection or inflammation of the mucous membranes that line the inside of the nose and sinuses, causing them to swell and block the drainage of fluid from the sinuses into the nose and throat (29)

skeletal muscle—voluntary or striated muscle (made up of cylindrical fibers) that allows movement by being attached to bones in the body (24)

sleep apnea—periods of apnea or absence of breathing during sleep (40)

small intestine—tube about 21 feet long extending from the pyloric sphincter of the stomach to the large intestine, made up of the duodenum, jejunum, and ileum, which functions in digestion and absorption of nutrients (30)

smear—thin layer of microorganisms spread on a glass slide for microscopic examination for identification purposes (45)

smooth muscle—type of involuntary muscle found throughout the body, composed of elongated, spindle-shaped cells with the nucleus centrally located and without striations (24)

Snellen chart—tool for assessing distance acuity (39)

soft skills—skills necessary for the smooth functioning of the workplace that are neither cognitive nor psychomotor and that display the professionalism of the employee (58)

software—set or sets of programmed instructions that tell computer hardware what to do in order to complete the required data processing; also known as *program* (12)

solvent—describes a medical practice that is capable of paying bills and salaries (20)

somatic nervous system (SNS)—part of the peripheral nervous system that is made of 12 pairs of cranial nerves and 31 pairs of spinal nerves (25)

source-oriented medical record (SOMR)—patient file organized according to the source of information (13)

specific gravity—weight of a substance in relation ot the weight of the same amount of distilled water (46)

specific time—allotted time period for each patient, depending on the reason for the visit (9, 37)

speculum—instrument for viewing a body cavity (36, 39)

spermatozoa—(singular, *spermatozoon*) male reproductive cell; also known as *sperm* (33)

sphygmomanometer—instrument used to measure blood pressure (27, 35)

spina bifida—most frequently occurring, permanently disabling birth defect, resulting from the failure of the spine to close properly during the first month of pregnancy (25)

spore—thick-walled reproductive cell (45)

sprain—stretching or tearing injury to a ligament (24)

sputum—mucous substance expelled when coughing or clearing the bronchi (45)

squamous cell carcinoma—malignant tumor that affects the middle layer of the skin (22)

stale check—check that has not been presented for payment within the time frame suggested on the check (16)

standard of care—level of knowledge, skill, and care a medical practitioner must provide to all patients for the same care that would commonly be provided by other similar medical care professionals under the same circumstances in the same locality (3)

stapes—stirrup-shaped ear bone (26)

stat—immediately (43)

statute of limitations—maximum time period set by federal and state governments during which certain legal actions, such as a patient filing a lawsuit, can be brought forward (3, 15)

steatorrhea—excessive fat in stool (45)

stem cell—undifferentiated cell that can give rise to other cells of the same type or from which specialized cells can develop (2)

stereotyping—formation of negative beliefs or attitudes concerning specific characteristics of a person or group and applying them unfairly to an entire population (5, 57)

sterile field—specific area free of all microorganisms that will be the work area for a surgical procedure (42)

sterilization—destruction of all living organisms and spores with the use of pressurized steam, chemicals, electron bombardment, extreme temperatures, or radiation (34)

stomach—large, muscular, saclike organ that secretes hydrochloric acid and gastric juices that convert food into chyme (30)

stomach ulcer—condition in which the lining of the stomach or upper part of the small intestine (duodenum) is damaged and the sensitive tissue underneath is exposed to stomach acid; also known as *peptic ulcer* or *gastric ulcer* (30)

stop-payment order—procedure in which the writer of the check instructs the bank (in writing) not to honor the payment of a check (16)

strabismus—a disorder caused by weakness in the external eye muscles, resulting in the eyes looking in different directions; also known as *crossed eyes* (26, 39)

strain—stretching or tearing injury to a muscle or tendon (24)

stress—body's reaction to the world around it, which can be emotional, intellectual, or physical (57)

stressor—real or imagined event that causes stress (57)

stress test—treadmill test that evaluates the heart's response during moderate exercise while an electrocardiogram is performed (49)

striated—having a striped appearance (21, 24)

stridor—high-pitched sound heard during respiration, caused by obstruction of the airway (40, 43)

stroke—the result of a clot or hemorrhage in the brain blocking the blood supply and causing brain cells to die from a lack of oxygen; also known as *cerebrovascular accident (CVA)* (25)

subcellular—microorganisms, such as viruses, comprised of hereditary material (RNA or DNA) with a protein outer coat (45)

subcutaneous injection—injection given just under the skin in the fat (adipose) tissue; used for small doses of nonirritating medications such as immunizations, insulin, and analgesics (54)

subjective, objective, assessment, and plan (SOAP)—Patient chart notes organized according to symptoms, signs, assessment, and plan (13)

subjective symptom—unmeasurable symptom felt by the patient but not apparent to an observer (36)

submaximal test—stress test administered to patients who have had a myocardial infarction in which the maximum target heart rate is set lower (at 70 percent) (49)

subpoena—a legal document that requires the office to present information such as the appointment book to the court (9)

subscriber—person who holds a health benefit plan, contract, or policy that may or may not include other family members (15)

subscription—part of the prescription that tells the pharmacist how to mix the drug and how much to provide the patient (53)

sudden infant death syndrome (SIDS)—the death with no known cause of an apparently healthy infant, usually before age 1 year (40)

sudoriferous glands—glands that occur in nearly all regions of the skin but are most numerous on the palms and soles; also known as *sweat glands* (22)

suffix—word element affixed to the end of a word (4)

sulcus—shallow groove of the brain (25)

superbill—record of services for billing and for insurance processing; also known as *charge slip* or *encounter form* (15)

superior vena cava—large vein that transports blood from the head and upper chest to the heart (27)

supernatant—liquid portion remaining after centrifugation (46)

superscription—part of a prescription that contains the patient's name, address, age, and the date on the top line as well as the symbol *Rx* (53)

supination—process of lying supine, or face upward; also the process of turning the palm or foot upward (23)

suppuration—process to relieve the internal buildup of pus formation (51)

surgery scheduler—person in the surgery department who schedules procedures (9)

surgical asepsis—techniques used to destroy pathogenic organisms before they enter the body (34)

surgical scrub—scrubbing the hands, wrists, and arms in preparation for surgery to remove microorganisms more effectively than regular hand washing (42)

susceptible host—reservoir host that is available and capable of being infected by the pathogen (34)

swabs—sterile devices for collecting specimens (45)

sweat glands—occur in nearly all regions of the skin but are most numerous on the palms and soles; also known as *sudoriferous glands* (22)

symbols—used in the CPT manual to distinguish changes or give instructions for proper coding of certain procedures (19)

sympathy—the feeling of sorrow or pity for a patient (5)

synarthrotic joint—articulation, or joint, that produces no movement (23)

syncope—fainting (35)

synergist—muscle that acts with another muscle to produce movement (24)

synthetic—created in a laboratory by artificial means (53)

syphilis—one type of infectious and contagious sexually transmitted disease (2)

system—group of organs that work together to perform a specific function (21); also, a regularly interacting group of people who function with an organized set of doctrines and principles (58)

systemic lupus erythematosus (SLE)—systemic immune system disorder in which the body produces abnormal antibodies that attack its own tissues rather than foreign organisms (28)

systole—phase 1 of the cardiac cycle in which the atria are contracted and the ventricles are relaxed (27)

systolic blood pressure—upper number of blood pressure measurement indicative of the left ventricle of the heart contracting (27, 35)

tachycardia—abnormally rapid heart rate (27, 35, 49)

tachypnea—abnormally high respiration rate above 40 cycles or 24 breaths per minute (35)

tapotement—light tapping or percussion to relieve congestion that is performed with the sides of the hands, cupped hands, or fingertips to relieve congestion (51)

target heart rate—heart rate for an individual calculated by using the following formula: 220 minus the patient's age = the maximum target heart rate for that person (49)

tax withholding—holding back required taxes from the gross amount due an employee (16)

telemetry—using radio waves to transmit the heart's electrical activity to a central monitoring station (49)

telephone triage—determining which caller's needs are the most urgent and where the call must be directed (7)

tendon—band of connective tissue that attaches muscles to bones (24)

tendonitis—inflammation and irritation of the tendon, caused by microscopic tearing (24)

terminal digit filing—filing system based on the last digits of the ID number that evenly distributes the files within the entire filing system (13)

terminal illness—condition that is expected to end in death (57)

testes—two oval-shaped organs in the scrotum in which sperm and testosterone are produced (33)

tetanus—a disease of the nervous system that is caused by a bacterium that enters the body through a break in the skin, such as a puncture, cut, or open wound; also known as *lockjaw* (24, 54)

thallium—radioisotope that emits gamma rays and is used in nuclear medicine (49)

thesaurus—reference book that lists words alphabetically and gives synonyms for each entry word (11)

third-party check—written as payment of another payee but presented to you (the third payee) as payment (16)

third-party payer—party other than the patient who assumes responsibility for paying the patient's bills (e.g., an insurance company) (15)

thoracentesis—drawing fluid out of the chest; also known as *thoracocentesis* (27)

thready pulse—weak, or barely perceptible force or blood volume (35)

thrombophlebitis—condition that occurs when a blood clot causes inflammation in one or more veins, typically those of the lower extremities (27)

thrombus—blood clot (37)

thymus gland—lymphoid tissue located in the chest, in the anterior mediastinum, that manufactures infection-fighting T cells (28, 32)

thyroid gland—gland in the neck that is responsible for metabolism that secretes thyroxine, tri-iodothyronine, and calcitonin (32)

tickler file—appointment reminder system in which the tickler card (a self-addressed reminder postcard used for annual PAP tests and other types of follow-up appointments) is filed under the date it should be mailed (9)

tidal volume (V$_T$)—amount of air inhaled or exhaled during normal breathing (about 500 mL) (50)

time patterns—scheduling options (9)

tinea capitis—a fungal infection of the skin commonly located on the scalp (22)

tinea corporis—a fungal infection of the skin commonly found on the trunk and extremities; also known as *ringworm* (22)

tinea cruris—fungal infection in the genital area; also known as *jock itch* (22)

tinea pedis—fungal infection of the skin, commonly found on the foot; also known as *athlete's foot* (22)

tinnitus—a ringing in one or both ears that is associated with many forms of hearing loss (26)

tissue—grouping of cells that performs a specialized function (21)

T lymphocytes—cells that circulate through the lymph nodes, bloodstream, and lymphatic ducts to seek out any infection (28)

tolerance—the need for larger and larger doses to achieve the same result after taking a medication for an extended time (57)

tongue depressor—thin, flat disposable wooden blade used to press down the tongue to observe the mouth and throat (36)

tonicity—ability of the body to maintain posture through a continuous partial contraction of skeletal muscles (24)

tonsillectomy—surgical removal of the tonsils (40)

tonsils—lymphoid tissues in the pharynx, consisting of the pharyngeal tonsils (adenoids), palatine tonsils, and lingual tonsils (28, 29)

tort—legal wrong or error resulting in harm (3)

total lung capacity (TLC)—volume of the lungs at peak inspiration equal to the sum of the four volumes: tidal, expiratory reserve, inspiratory reserve, and residual volume (50)

toxic—harmful (53)

trabeculae—inward-pointing structures that subdivide lymph nodes into different compartments (28)

trachea—cartilaginous tube between the larynx and the main bronchi; also known as *windpipe* (29)

tract—group of nerve fibers within the central nervous system (25)

trailing zero rule—rule that states it is unacceptable to place a zero after a decimal point in a whole number (52)

transducer—device that both produces and senses ultrasonic waves (48)

triage—process of sorting patients according to the seriousness of their condition; also, to assess the emergency care needed by patients (9, 43)

tricuspid valve—heart valve from the right atrium to the right ventricle (27)

Truth in Lending form—form that must clearly state the amount financed, the finance charge, and the total of the payments and that protects the consumer from loan-related fraud or deceit (15)

tuberculosis (TB)—highly contagious disease caused by the bacillus *Mycobacterium tuberculosis,* which can grow anywhere in the body but is most commonly found in the lungs, where granular tumors are produced in the infected tissues (29)

tuning fork—instrument used to measure a person's hearing ability (36)

turbid—cloudy (46)

turgor—the resistance of the skin when grasped between the fingers (36)

turnaround time—how long it takes for the test to be performed and the results generated, sent back for physician review, and added to the patient's chart (44)

tympanic membrane—eardrum, which separates the outer and middle ears (26)

tympanic membrane thermometer—calculates the body temperature from the energy generated by the heat waves generated within the ear canal and near the eardrum; also known as *aural thermometer* (35)

tympanum—eardrum (39)

underdose—an amount of medication that is insufficient to achieve the desired effect (52)

universal serial bus (USB) drive—portable computer storage device (12)

upcoding—billing for a service at a higher level than was actually provided (19)

ureters—tubes that carry newly formed urine from each kidney down to the bladder (31)

urethra—musculomembranous tube extending from the bladder to the urinary meatus (31, 33)

urethritis—inflammation of the urethra (33)

urinalysis—testing of urine for the presence of infection or disease (46)

urinary bladder—muscular sac, located in the pelvic cavity, that serves as a reservoir for urine (31)

urinary meatus—the external opening of the urinary system (31)

urticaria—a severe itching due to acute hypersensitivity to medications or environmental stimuli; also known as *hives* (22)

usual, customary, and reasonable (UCR)—refers to the usual fee a physician would charge for services, the customary fee a majority of physicians would charge for the same service, and a reasonable fee that the patient might expect to pay (used to determine medical benefits) (15)

uterine cancer—an adenocarcinoma that usually develops in the glandular tissue of the endometrium; also known as *endometrial cancer* (33)

uterine fibroids—benign tumors made up of muscle cells and other tissues that grow within the wall of the uterus, manifesting as a single growth or a cluster (33)

uterus—hollow, pear-shaped, muscular organ located in the anterior portion of the female pelvic cavity (33)

vaccine—substance that contains the antigen and stimulates a primary response against the antigen without causing symptoms of the disease (28); substance that decreases the susceptibility to disease; also known as *immunization* (54)

vagina—musculomembranous tube extending from the vestibule to the uterus (33)

vaginal speculum—instrument used to hold open the walls of the vagina (36)

vaginitis—inflammation of the vagina usually caused by a change in the normal balance of vaginal bacteria, by an infection, or by reduced estrogen levels after menopause (33)

values—set of standards a person uses to measure the worth or importance of someone or something (5)

vancomycin-resistant enterococci (VRE)—type of bacteria that has developed resistance to antimicrobial drugs (34)

vancomycin-resistant *Staphylococcus aureus* (VRSA)—type of *S. aureus* organism resistant to the antibiotic vancomycin (34)

variables—areas of a form letter that require personalization, such as the date, inside address, and salutation, which can be stored on a separate CD or database from the constant information (11)

varicella—chicken pox (54)

vasectomy—surgery to render the male sterile, involving cutting the vas deferens and tying off the ends to prevent sperm from being transported out of the testes (38)

vastus lateralis muscle—part of the outer portion of the upper thigh that is also part

of the quadriceps and is considered the safest site for IM injections (54)

vendor—supplier (10)

venipuncture—the process of withdrawing blood from a vein for examination; also known as *phlebotomy* (27)

venom—poison (37)

ventricles—two lower pumping chambers of the heart (27)

ventrogluteal site—muscle considered safer than the dorsogluteal muscle for IM injections because it has no major nerves or blood vessels (54)

verbal communication—wide range of words and sounds or tone of voice that a person uses to convey vastly different meanings (5)

vesicles—small blisters (22)

vestibule—middle part of the inner ear; also in the vagina, the space between the lines of attachment of the labia minora (26, 33)

viable—capable of living (45)

viability—able to sustain life independently (38)

visceral pleura—membranes that produce a lubricating fluid that helps the lungs glide smoothly in the chest cavity during inhalation and exhalation (29)

viscosity—thickness of a substance (54)

visual—of, related to, or used in vision (5)

visual acuity—clarity of vision (39)

vital capacity (VC)—amount of air that can be exhaled following forced inspiration and including maximum expiration (50)

vital signs—temperature, pulse, respirations, and blood pressure; pain is considered to be the fifth vital sign (35)

vitamins—organic substances essential for metabolism, growth, and development of the body (56)

vitiligo—pigmentation disorder that causes white patches and large areas of decreased pigmentation to form on the skin (22)

vitreous chamber—posterior cavity of the eyeball located behind the lens (26)

vitreous humor—thick fluid that fills the posterior cavity of the eyeball (26)

voice messaging system—allows voice messages to be left on a recorded device for a specific recipient (7)

void—to urinate (31, 46)

volume—refers to the strength or force of the pulse (35)

vulva—structure in the female reproductive system made up of the mons pubis, labia majora and labia minora, vestibule, and clitoris (33)

warrant—statement issued to indicate that a debt should be paid (16)

warranty—guarantee that a product will work for a fixed period of time (10)

warts—type of infection caused by viruses in the human papillomavirus (HPV) family that can grow on all parts of the body, including on the skin, inside the mouth, on the genitals, and in the rectal area (22)

wave—movement away from the baseline in an electrocardiogram (9, 49)

wave scheduling—scheduling system that is set to begin and end each hour on time, in which each hour is divided into equal segments of time depending on how many patients can be seen in an hour (9)

West's nomogram—chart used to identify body surface area to calculate pediatric dosages (52)

wet mount—preparation in a liquid to preserve the motility of the microbe (45)

wheal—more or less round, temporary elevation of the skin, white in the center with a pale red periphery, accompanied by itching (37)

word root—word or element from which other words are formed (4)

World Health Organization (WHO)—specialized agency of the United Nations that tracks statistical health information throughout the world (19)

World Wide Web (WWW)—communications network enabling the linking of computers worldwide for data interchange; the Internet (12)

write off—to agree to forfeit the amount the insurance company does not authorize (18)

X-rays—electromagnetic rays that have high energy and very short wavelengths and are not visible to the human eye; a photograph obtained by use of X-rays, also known as *radiograph* (48)

Young's rule—pediatric dosage law applied to children over the age of 1 year, based on their age in years (52)

Z-track method—a method of injection that is used when a medication is irritating to the subcutaneous tissues or when the medication may discolor the skin (54)

Index

Cold application
    chemical cold packs, 1173–1174, 1174f
    cold compresses, 1172
    explained, 1166, 1168, 1171–1173
    ice bags, 1172–1173, 1173f
    stress management, 1337
Cold sensation, 434
Colectomy, 777t
Colic, 777, 870
Colitis, 586, 588
Collating records, 163–164
Colleagues, defined, 392
Collect calls, 151
Collection agencies
    billing for services and extending credit, 289
    physician-patient relationship, terminating, 294
    posting a payment from, 298–299
    using, 297–298
Collection devices for laboratory specimens,
        1008, 1008f
Collection letters
    example of, 298f
    explained, 296
    writing, procedure for, 297
Collection List button, A33
Collection practices
    contract law, 49
    laws governing, 49t
    performing, procedure for, 346
Collections
    aging accounts receivable, 295
    bankruptcy, 297
    collection agency, using, 297–299
    collection letters, 296, 297, 298f
    collection techniques, 295
    delinquent accounts, 295
    estates, claims against, 297
    positive collection procedures, 294
    process of, 295
    regulations, 295, 296
    special problems, 296–297
    statute of limitations, 297
    telephone collections, 295–296
College of American Pathologists
    laboratory safety regulations, 978
    proficiency testing for laboratories, 981
Colles' fractures, 465, 465f
Collimeter, 1105, 1106f
Colon
    colorectal cancer, 588
    colostomy, 777t
    described, 581f, 584, 584f
Colonized, defined, 681
Colonoscope, 932, 932f
Colonoscopy, 777t, 782–783
Colony, defined, 1000
Colony count, 1011, 1012f
Color
    file systems, 262–263, 263f, 263t
    urine, 1036, 1037f, 1037t, 1045t
    Vacutainer tubes, and order of blood draw, 1061t
Color laser printers, 202
Color vision
    color deficiency (color blindness), 427
    impairment and testing for, 833–834, 835, 835f
Colorectal cancer, 588
Colorectal surgery specialty, 33t

Colostomy, 777t
Colposcope, 805, 806f
Colposcopy, 809t, 931–932
Combining forms, 72–73, 73f, 77t, A9–A13
Combining vowel, explained, 72, 72f
Comment Tab, A20, A20f
Commercial culture units, 1010
Comminuted fractures, 465, 465f
Commission on Accreditation of Allied Health
        Education Programs (CAAHEP)
    accreditation, providing, 5
    CMA certification examination, 10
    curriculum guidelines, 5–6
    externships, 1344
    medical assisting, history of, 4
    surgical technologist training, 933
Commissurotomy, 771t
Common cold (acute rhinitis), 570, 869, 1001t, 1144
Communicable diseases, reporting requirements
        for, 58t
Communication
    barriers to
        defensive behaviors, 105, 106t
        explained, 104–105, 104f
        medical language, using, 105
        multicultural issues, 105–107, 107t
    CMA skills, A1
    different models of, 105
    elderly people, with, 891, 892, 892f
    examinations, during, 751, 753
    informed consent, 1268
    interviewing patients, 689, 691
    office management, 391
    success as a medical assistant, 139
    workplace, in, 1333–1334
Communication process
    channels of communication, 97–98, 97f, 98t
    units of, 97
Communication techniques
    directive communication techniques,
        101–103, 102t
    feedback, 102–103, 102t
    listening skills, 100–101
Communication: verbal and nonverbal, 94–117
    assertive versus aggressive behavior, 103–104, 104t
    barriers to communication, 104–107, 104f,
        106t, 107t
    case study, 95
    chapter review, 115–116
    chapter summary, 115
    communication process, 97–98, 97f, 98t
    communication techniques, 100–103, 102t
    critical thinking, 116
    Internet activity, 116
    interpersonal dynamics, 96–97
    intraoffice communication, 110–111, 111f
    on the job, 116
    medmedia, 117
    nonverbal communication, 98, 99–100, 99f
    patients' rights, 113–114
    special circumstances
        angry patients, 107–108, 108f
        anxious patients, 108
        hearing-impaired patients, 108–109, 109f, 110
        mentally and emotionally impaired patients, 110
        non-English-speaking patients, 110
        visually impaired patients, 109–110, 109f

    staff arrangements, 111–113, 113t
    verbal communication, 98–99, 100f
Communications clerk, career as, 40–41
Community improvement, responsibility for
    AAMA Code of Ethics, 63
    AMA ethical principle, 62
Community resource brochure, creating, 1267
Community-based MRSA, 681
Compact bone, 455, 456f
Compazine, 1212t, 1216t
Compensation
    defense mechanism, 1322t
    defensive behavior, 106t
Compensatory damages, 48t
Competence, mental, and contracts, 48
Competence, professional
    identifying areas of, 1195
    medical assistants, characteristic of, 9
Complaints about service, responding to, 474
Complement, defined, 553
Complete blood count (CBC) with differential, 754t
Complete decongestive therapy, 557
Complex carbohydrates, 1290
Compliance methods for Exposure Control
        Plan, 125
Compliance plans for medical coding, 384–385
Complimentary close for correspondence, 218
Compound (open) fractures, 465, 965, 966, 966f
Compound microscope, 982, 982f
Compression fractures, 465, 465f
Compulsions, 1309
Computed tomography (CT)
    computer use for medicine, 236f
    conditions diagnosed, 1092t
    described, 1097–1098, 1097f, 1098f
    lymphatic system, 786t
    musculoskeletal system, 789t
    preparation for, 1088t, 1098
Computerized billing, 292, 293f
Computerized bookkeeping systems, 308
Computerized employee payroll records, 327,
        328f, 330
Computers
    capital equipment, 202
    computerized scheduling systems, 181–182, 181f
    defined, 237
    frequently used terms, 243t
Computers in the medical office, 234–247
    case study, 235
    chapter review, 246–247
    chapter summary, 245
    computer components, 237–240, 237f, 238f,
        238t, 240f
    computer system, selecting, 242, 243t
    computer use in medicine, 236, 236f
    computers, types of, 236–237, 237f
    critical thinking, 247
    electronic signatures, 244
    ergonomics, 244–245, 245f
    Internet, 242–244
    Internet activity, 247
    on the job, 247
    Medmedia, 247
    security, 240–241
Concussion, 502
Condescending, defined, 111
Condition Tab, A19, A19f

Infection control (*continued*)
    surgical asepsis, described, 661, 665
        waste disposal, 661, 662–663, 662f, 663f
  pathogens, explained, 654
  personal hygiene, 661
  universal precautions, 658–661, 660f
Infectious medical waste, 123
Infectious mononucleosis. *See also* mononucleosis
  described, 554t, 556
  macrophages in the spleen, 552
  pathogen causing, 1006t
Inferior plane, 82, 83f
Inferior vena cava, 522, 523, 524f
Infertility, 818
Inflammatory bowel syndrome, 587t
Inflammatory phase of wound healing, 924
Inflammatory process, 658, 658t
Inflated phrases in written communication, 214, 214t
Inflection of the voice, 139
Influenza
  described, 571
  influenza virus, 1001t, 1004, 1004f
  lower respiratory condition, 1144
  pathogen causing, 1006t
  vaccination for, 1255
Information
  patient scheduling process, 183
  sharing between physicians, 623
Information services cluster careers, 40–41
Informative power, 396
Informed consent
  battery, 53
  communication skills required for, 1268
  Doctrine of Informed Consent, 52–53
  elderly people, 893–894
  emergency situations, 53
  forms as component of medical record, 256
  minor surgery, preparing patients for, 920
  patient signature, 53f
  role of medical assistants, 60
  sample document, 52f
Infraspinatus muscle, 476
Inguinal area, 745t
Inguinal hernia, 587t, 591–592, 592f
Inhalation, 567, 567f
Inhalation medications, 1218t, 1235, 1235f
Inhalers, 1154, 1154f
I-9 form, 400, 401–402f
Initiative by employees, 1359
Injuries
  aging process, 883
  burns, concurrent, 963
  children, 872
  nervous system, 502
  reporting requirements, 58t
Innate immunity, 553
Inner ear
  anatomy and function, 514, 514f
  common disorders, 516
Inoculated culture plate, 1009
Inoculating loops and needles, 1009
Inpatient care
  career opportunities, 14t
  defined, 33
Input devices for computers, 237
Inscription on prescriptions, 1223
Insects, 1005–1006, 1005f

Insertion of muscles, 475
Inside addresses on business letters, 218
Inspection as examination method, 742, 742f
Inspiration, described, 567, 567f
Inspiration strip on ECGs, 1132
Inspiratory capacity (IC), 568, 1146, 1148t
Inspiratory reserve volume (IRV), 568, 1146
Instant messages, 229
Instill, defined, 830
Institute for Safe Medication Practices, 832
Institute of Medicine, 280
Instruments
  chemical sterilization, procedure for, 676, 676f
  CMA knowledge of, A4
  passing to the physician, 917, 917f
  sanitizing, 670, 670f
  sterilizing in an autoclave, 675–676, 675f, 676f
  wrapping and labeling for autoclaving, 673–674, 673f, 674f
Instruments, surgical
  classification and identification of, 908, 910
  cutting instruments, 910–911, 911f
  dissecting instruments, 911, 911f
  grasping and clamping instruments, 911, 911f, 912f
  guidelines for handling, 915–916
  probing and dilating instruments, 912–913, 912f, 913f, 914f
  suture materials and needles, 913–915, 915f, 915t
  wound closure materials, other, 915, 915f
Insufflation, 515
Insulin
  antidiabetic medication, 1216t
  beta cells of the islets of Langerhans, 616
  diabetes mellitus, 621, 775
  emergency crash kit, 944t
  subcutaneous injections, 1244, 1245t, 1247f
Insulin shock, 955t, 956
Insulin syringes, 1237
Insulin-dependent diabetes mellitus (IDDM), 621.
    See also diabetes mellitus
Insurance. *See* health insurance; medical insurance
Insurance 1 box, A18
Insurance Carrier List, A20–A22, A21f, A22f
Insurance Carrier List button, A33
Insurance claims, creating and printing in Medisoft, A29–A33, A29f, A30f, A31f, A32–A33t
Insurance Coverage Percents by Service Classification box, A19
Insurance fraud
  fraud tips, 384
  fraudulent billing and coding practices, 382, 384
  prevention of, tips for, 382
  reporting, 385
Intal, 568
Integrated delivery system, 341
Integrated provider organization, 341
Integrated systems, 1332–1333
Integrity as characteristic of medical assistants, 8
Integumentary system, 432–450
  accessory structures, 435f, 436–437, 436f
  aging process, 883, 884t
  case study, 433
  chapter review, 449–450
  chapter summary, 448–449
  common disorders (*See also* herpes simplex)
    acne vulgaris, 437f, 439–440, 439f, 767, 1001t

    alopecia, 440, 440f, 1104t
    calluses and corns, 441
    carbuncles, 442, 1006t
    cellulitis, 440, 440f
    contact dermatitis, 440–441, 441f, 765t
    decubitus ulcers, 437f, 441–442, 767, 885t
    eczema, 437f, 442, 765t
    folliculitis, 442–443, 442f
    furuncles, 442
    herpes zoster, 443
    hirsutism, 444, 619t
    impetigo, 444, 444f
    keloids, 444, 444f, 769t
    pediculosis, 444–445, 1006, 1006t
    psoriasis, 437f, 445, 767
    rosacea, 445
    scabies, 446, 446f, 1006, 1006t
    seborrheic dermatitis, 446
    signs of, 437, 437f
    skin cancer, 437–439, 439f, 439t, 678, 769t
    tinea, 446, 446f, 1001t, 1005
    urticaria, 437f, 446–447, 447f, 765t
    vitiligo, 447
    warts, 447
  critical thinking, 450
  explained, 85–86
  functions of, 87f, 425f, 434–435, 435f
  Internet activity, 450
  Medmedia, 450
  pathogens and resulting diseases, 1006t
  premenstrual syndrome, 642f
  size of, 434
  skin care treatments, 447–448
  structure of the skin, 435–436, 435f
  word parts, 88t
Intellectual performance changes with aging, 490
Intellectualization as defense mechanism, 1322t
Intentional torts, 46, 47t
Interjections, 217t
Intermediate care facilities (ICFs), 34–35
Intermittent fever, 696
Intermittent pulse, 706
Internal intercostal muscles, 477
Internal medicine, 32
Internal oblique muscles, 477, 478f
Internal radiation therapy, 1101
Internal Revenue Service (IRS), 191
International Classification of Diseases (ICD)
  data for computerized bookkeeping systems, 308
  history of, 373
International Classification of Diseases, Ninth Revision, Clinical Modification (ICD-9-CM)
  abbreviations and symbols, 375–376
  charge slips, 167
  coding, steps in, 374–375
  formats and conventions, 374
  history of, 373
  overview of, 373–374
  principal diagnosis, 375
  procedure for, 376
  reference material, 224
  shortcomings of, 376, 378
  special codes, 375, 376, 377f
International Classification of Diseases, Tenth Revision (ICD-10), 376, 378
International Headache Society, 498
International health and medical insurance, 345

R